T0399273

The Hippocampus Book

The Hippocampus Book

SECOND EDITION

EDITED BY

Richard Morris, DPhil

Professor of Neuroscience
University of Edinburgh

David Amaral, PhD

Distinguished Professor of Psychiatry and Neuroscience
University of California, Davis

Tim Bliss, PhD

Group Leader Emeritus
Francis Crick Institute, London

Karen Duff, PhD

Centre Director
UK Dementia Research Institute at UCL
Professor in Dementia and Neurodegeneration
UCL Queen Square Institute of Neurology

John O'Keefe, PhD

Professor of Cognitive Neuroscience, Cell and Developmental Biology
Sainsbury Wellcome Center for Neural Circuits and Behavior, University College London

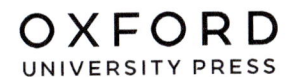

OXFORD
UNIVERSITY PRESS

OXFORD
UNIVERSITY PRESS

Oxford University Press is a department of the University of Oxford. It furthers the University's objective of excellence in research, scholarship, and education by publishing worldwide. Oxford is a registered trade mark of Oxford University Press in the UK and certain other countries.

Published in the United States of America by Oxford University Press
198 Madison Avenue, New York, NY 10016, United States of America.

Library of Congress Cataloging-in-Publication Data
Names: Morris, R. G. M. (Richard G. M.), editor. | Amaral, David, editor. | Bliss, T. V. P. editor. | Duff, Karen (Karen E.), editor. | O'Keefe, John, editor.
Title: The hippocampus book / edited by Richard Morris, David Amaral, Tim Bliss, Karen Duff, and John O'Keefe.
Description: [Second edition] | New York, NY : Oxford University Press, [2024] | Includes bibliographical references and index.
Identifiers: LCCN 2024031955 | ISBN 9780190065324 (hardback) | ISBN 9780190065348 (epub) | ISBN 9780190065331 | ISBN 9780197691212 | ISBN 9780197691229
Classification: LCC QP383.25.H57 2024 | DDC 612.8/25—dc23/eng/20240823
LC record available at https://lccn.loc.gov/2024031955

DOI: 10.1093/med/9780190065324.001.0001

Printed by Integrated Books International, United States of America

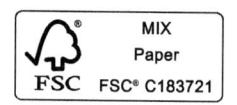

MIX
Paper
FSC   FSC® C183721

Detailed Contents

CHAPTER 4

Development of the Hippocampal Formation 121

Pierre Lavenex, David G. Amaral, Pamela Banta Lavenex, François Guillemot, Ricardo Insausti, and Noelia Urban

CHAPTER 6

Synaptic Function 265

Dimitri M. Kullmann and Kirill E. Volynski

CHAPTER 7

Local Circuits 297

Andres D. Grosmark, Aaron D. Milstein, Attila Losonczy, and Ivan Soltesz

CHAPTER 8

Molecular Mechanisms of Synaptic Function in the Hippocampus 345

Paul G. Donlin-Asp, Anne-Sophie Hafner, and Erin M. Schuman

CHAPTER 9

Adult Neurogenesis 365

Matthew Shtrahman, Sarah L. Parylak, Tomohisa Toda, and Fred H. Gage

CHAPTER 10

Synaptic Plasticity in the Hippocampus 405

Tim Bliss, Graham Collingridge, Sam Cooke, John Georgiou, and Richard Morris

CHAPTER 11

Hippocampal Physiology in the Behaving Animal 501

Julija Krupic and John O'Keefe

CHAPTER 12

The Entorhinal Cortex 565

Benjamin R. Kanter, Edvard I. Moser, and Menno P. Witter

CHAPTER 13

Functions of the Human Hippocampus 605

Daniel N. Barry and Eleanor A. Maguire

CHAPTER 15

Aging and the Hippocampus 723

Sara N. Burke and Carol A. Barnes

CHAPTER 16

Computational Models of Hippocampal Cognitive Function 809

Daniel Bush and Neil Burgess

CHAPTER 17

Stress and the Hippocampus 857

Bruce S. McEwen and Sumantra Chattarji

CHAPTER 18

Mesial Temporal Lobe Epilepsy 895

Matthew C. Walker, Maria Thom, and Umesh Vivekananda

CHAPTER 19

Schizophrenic Psychosis and the Hippocampus: Schizophrenia Mechanisms in the Hippocampus: The Role of Hippocampal Hyperactivity 921

Carol A. Tamminga, Daniel Scott, and Elena I. Ivleva

CHAPTER 20

Alzheimer's Disease 933

Dennis Chan, Tara Spires-Jones, Frank Provenzano, Elizabeth BC Glennon, and Karen Duff

Contributors

David Amaral UC Davis Distinguished Professor Department of Psychiatry and Behavioral Sciences and The MIND Institute University of California, Davis USA

Pamela Banta Lavenex Professor of Psychology Faculty of Psychology, UniDistance Suisse, 3900 Brig, Switzerland

Carol A. Barnes Regents Professor, Departments of Psychology, Neurology and Neuroscience, Director, Evelyn F. McKnight Brain Institute, University of Arizona, Tucson, Arizona

Daniel N. Barry Associate Editor, Nature Communications, Springer Nature, UK

Marlene Bartos Executive Director for the Institute for Physiology I, Albert-Ludwigs-University of Freiburg, Medical Faculty, Freiburg, Germany

Tim Bliss Group leader emeritus, The Francis Crick Institute, London, UK

Neil Burgess UCL Institute of Cognitive Neuroscience and UCL Queen Square Institute of Neurology, London, UK

Sara N. Burke Professor, Department of Neuroscience, McKnight Brain Institute, and Co-Director Center for Cognitive Aging and Memory, University of Florida, Gainesville, FL, USA

Daniel Bush UCL Department of Neuroscience, Physiology, and Pharmacology, London, UK

Dennis Chan Professor, University College London Institute of Cognitive Neuroscience, London, UK

Sumantra Chattarji Director, Center for High Impact Neuroscience and Translational Applications (CHINTA), TCG Centres for Research and Education in Science and Technology, Kolkata, India

Vivien Chevaleyre[†] CNRS Research Director, Sorbonne University, Institute Biologie Paris Seine, Neuroscience Paris Seine, Paris, France

Graham Collingridge Tanz Centre for Research in Neurodegenerative Diseases, Department of Physiology, University of Toronto and Lunenfeld-Tanenbaum Research Institute, Mount Sinai Hospital, Toronto, Canada

Sam Cooke Wolfson Sensory, Pain and Regeneration Centre (SPaRC), Institute of Psychiatry, Psychology and Neuroscience (IoPPN), King's College London (KCL), London, United Kingdom

Paul G. Donlin-Asp Center for Discovery Brain Sciences, University of Edinburgh, Edinburgh, Scotland

Karen Duff, PhD, Centre Director, UK Dementia Research Institute at University College London Professor in Dementia and Neurodegeneration, Institute of Neurology, Faculty of Life Sciences, University College London, London, UK

Mark D. Eyre Institute for Physiology, Albert-Ludwigs-University of Freiburg, Medical Faculty, Freiburg, Germany

Fred H. Gage Laboratory of Genetics, The Salk Institute for Biological Studies, La Jolla, CA, USA

John Georgiou Lunenfeld-Tanenbaum Research Institute, Mount Sinai Hospital, Sinai Health, Toronto, Canada

Elizabeth BC Glennon Senior Researcher, UK Dementia Research Institute, University College London, UK

Francesco Gobbo Centre for Discovery Brain Sciences and UK Dementia Research Institute, The University of Edinburgh, UK

Andres D. Grosmark Assistant Professor, Department of Neuroscience, University of Connecticut Medical School, Farmington, Connecticut, USA

François Guillemot Principal Group Leader, Neural Stem Cell Biology Laboratory, The Francis Crick Institute, London, UK

Anne-Sophie Hafner Professor of Neurochemistry, Donders Institute, Radboud University Nijmegen, Netherlands

Ricardo Insausti Professor of Anatomy, Human Neuroanatomy Laboratory School of Medicine. Biomedical Institute University of Castilla-La Mancha, Spain

Elena I. Ivleva Associate Professor, Department of Psychiatry, UT Southwestern School of Medicine, Dallas, Texas, USA

Benjamin R. Kanter Kavli Institute for Systems Neuroscience and Centre for Algorithms in the Cortex, Norwegian University of Science and Technology; Trondheim, Norway

Julija Krupic Dementia Research Institute at University College London, London, United Kingdom

Dimitri M. Kullmann Professor of Neurology, UCL Queen Square Institute of Neurology, University College London, London, UK

Pierre Lavenex Professor of Neuroscience, Institute of Psychology University of Lausanne, Switzerland

Attila Losonczy Professor, Department of Neuroscience, Columbia University, New York, NY, USA

Sam McKenzie School of Medicine, University of New Mexico, Albuquerque. New Mexico, USA

Eleanor A. Maguire Professor of Cognitive Neuroscience, Department of Imaging Neuroscience, UCL Queen Square Institute of Neurology, University College London, London, UK

Chris J. McBain Scientific Director for NICHD IRP Porter Neuroscience Bldg Eunice Kennedy Shriver National Institute of Child Health and Human Development National Institutes of Health, Bethesda MD, USA

Bruce S. McEwen[†] Laboratory of Neuroendocrinology, Rockefeller University, New York, NY, USA

Aaron D. Milstein Assistant Professor, Department of Neuroscience and Cell Biology, Robert Wood Johnson Medical School, New Brunswick, New Jersey, USA

Richard Morris Professor of Neuroscience, University of Edinburgh, UK

Edvard I. Moser Kavli Institute for Systems Neuroscience and Centre for Algorithms in the Cortex, Norwegian University of Science and Technology, Trondheim, Norway

John O'Keefe PhD, Professor of Cognitive Neuroscience, Cell and Developmental Biology, and Sainsbury Wellcome Centre for Neural Circuits and Behaviour, University College London

Sarah L. Parylak Laboratory of Genetics, The Salk Institute for Biological Studies, La Jolla, CA USA

Rebecca Piskorowski Inserm Research Director, Sorbonne University, Insitute Biologie Paris Seine, Neuroscience Paris Seine, Paris France

Frank Provenzano Assistant Professor of Neurological Sciences, The Taub Institute for Research on Alzheimer's Disease and the Aging Brain, Department of Neurology, Columbia University Irving Medical Center, New York, USA

Erin M. Schuman Director, Max Planck Institute for Brain Research, Frankfurt, Germany

Contributors

Daniel Scott Assistant Professor, Department of Psychiatry, UT Southwestern School of Medicine, Dallas, Texas, USA

Matthew Shtrahman Department of Neurosciences, University of California San Diego, Sanford Consortium for Regenerative Medicine, La Jolla, CA, USA

Ivan Soltesz Professor of Neurosurgery and Neurosciences, Stanford University, Stanford, California, USA

Tara Spires-Jones Professor of Neurodegeneration, UK Dementia Research Institute at the University of Edinburgh, UK
Professor of Neurodegeneration, Director, Centre for Discovery Brain Sciences, University of Edinburgh, Scotland

Nelson Spruston Executive Director and Vice President Janelia Research Campus Howard Hughes Medical Institute, Ashburn, Virginia, USA

Carol A. Tamminga Professor and Chair, Department of Psychiatry, UT Southwestern School of Medicine, Dallas, Texas, USA

Maria Thom Department of Clinical and Experimental Epilepsy, UCL Queen Square Institute of Neurology and National Hospital for Neurology and Neurosurgery, Queen Square, London, UK

Tomohisa Toda Professor of Neural Epigenomics, Friedrich-Alexander Universität Erlangen-Nürnberg, Deutsches Zentrum für Neurodegenerative Erkrankungen e. V. (DZNE), Germany

Noelia Urban Group Leader, Institute of Molecular Biotechnology of the Austrian Academy of Sciences, Vienna BioCenter, Austria

Umesh Vivekananda[†] Department of Clinical and Experimental Epilepsy, UCL Queen Square Institute of Neurology and National Hospital for Neurology and Neurosurgery, Queen Square, London, UK

Kirill E. Volynski Professor of Neuroscience, UCL Queen Square Institute of Neurology, University College of London, London, UK

Matthew C. Walker Department of Clinical and Experimental Epilepsy, UCL Queen Square Institute of Neurology and National Hospital for Neurology and Neurosurgery, Queen Square, London, UK

Menno P. Witter Kavli Institute for Systems Neuroscience and Centre for Algorithms in the Cortex, Norwegian University of Science and Technology; Trondheim, Norway

Abbreviations

5-HT	serotonin
ab	angular bundle
AAC	axo-axonic cell
A/C	associational & commissural input
ACh	acetylcholine
ADP	afterdepolarization
AHP	afterhyperpolarization
AMPA	α-amino-3-hydroxy-5-methyl-4-isoxazolepropionic acid
AMPAR	AMPA-type glutamate receptor
BC	basket cell
BiC	bistratified cell
C/A	commissural/associational
CA	cornu ammonis
CB	endocannabinoid
CCK	cholecystokinin
CR	calretinin
DA	dopamine
DG	dentate gyrus
EC	entorhinal cortex
EPSP	excitatory postsynaptic potential
FB	feedback
FF	feedforward
FFIN	feedforward Inhibition
GABA	gamma-aminobutyric acid
GC	granule cell
GCL	granule cell layer
HICAP	hilar commissural/associational path associated cell
HIPP	hilar perforant path cell
IB	intrinsically bursting neuron
IML	inner molecular layer
IN	interneuron
IPSC	inhibitory postsynaptic current
IPSP	inhibitory postsynaptic potential
ISI	interneuron-specific interneuron
IvyC	ivy cell
LC	locus coeruleus
LEC	lateral entorhinal cortex
LFP	local field potential
LM	stratum lacunosum-moleculare
LRIP	long-range inhibitory projection
LRPI	long-range projecting interneuron
LTD	long-term depression
LTP	long-term potentiation
Luc.	stratum lucidum
mAChR	muscarinic acetylcholine receptor
MC	mossy cell
MEC	medial entorhinal cortex
MF	mossy fiber
MML	medial molecular layer
MOPP	molecular layer perforant path cell
mPFC	medial prefrontal cortex
NA	noradrenaline
nAChR	nicotinic acetylcholine receptor
NGFC	neurogliaform cell
NMDA	N-methyl-D-aspartate
NMDAR	NMDA-type glutamate receptor
NOS	nitric oxide synthase
NPY	neuropeptide Y
O-LM	oriens-lacunosum-moleculare interneuron
OML	outer molecular layer
PC	pyramidal cell
PPA	perforant path associated cell
PV	parvalbumin
RC	radiatum cell
RS	regularly spiking neuron
SC	Schaffer collateral
SCA	Schaffer collateral-associated cell
SLI	spiny lucidum interneuron
SO	stratum oriens
SOM	somatostatin
SP	stratum pyramidale
SR	stratum radiatum
STDP	spike-time dependent plasticity
SWR	sharp wave/ripple events
TL	trilaminar cell
VGCC	voltage-gated calcium channel
VGNa	voltage-gated sodium channel
VIP	vasoactive intestinal polypeptide
VTA	ventral tegmental area

The Hippocampal Formation

The Editors

Buried deep within the medial temporal lobe of the human brain lie 50 million neurons organized into a network quite different from that found anywhere else in the nervous system. This structure, that protrudes into the lateral ventricles of the human brain, has captivated anatomists since the first dissections took place in classical Greece. The hippocampal formation is a group of brain areas consisting of the dentate gyrus, hippocampus, subiculum, presubiculum, parasubiculum, and the entorhinal cortex. The basic layout of cell and fiber layers of the hippocampal formation is much the same in all mammals (Figure 1.1).

There are several reasons why the hippocampus has attracted the interest of scientists in the many different disciplines that now characterize modern neuroscience—the hippocampus truly has something for everyone. Whether you are a psychologist interested in memory, a synaptic physiologist investigating neuronal function or synaptic plasticity, or a computational neuroscientist wanting to build a neural network model, the hippocampus and its associated regions are an attractive set of brain structures on which to work. Quite apart from learning what it does and how it works, lessons learned in such studies have gone on to influence fundamental research in other brain structures—the amygdala, basal ganglia, neocortex, and others. Principles have emerged related to fundamental physiological processes, many of which apply generically elsewhere in the brain despite their differing network architectures. In parallel, clinicians concerned with the basis of neurological conditions such as epilepsy or Alzheimer's disease had their attention drawn to the hippocampal formation because of the associated pathological processes observed to occur there and the opportunities that scientific study of this area of the brain offers for novel therapeutics. The hippocampus has been a neural Rosetta Stone.

The striking discovery, in 1953, that patient H.M. had a relatively pure memory deficit after bilateral surgical excision of the medial temporal lobe for the relief of epilepsy had a profound effect on the study of memory and, through that, on our understanding of the functions of the hippocampus itself. In the last 50 years, the pyramidal shaped cells of the hippocampus have become the most intensively studied neurons in the brain, replacing the ventral horn motoneurons of the spinal cord so beloved of an earlier generation of classical physiologists. As a result, we now know a great deal about the development of hippocampal pyramidal cells, their synaptogenesis, neurotransmitter receptors and ion-channels, cell-biological machinery, and the local circuitry in which they are embedded alongside numerous types of interneurons. No less impressive has been the molecular analysis of neurotransmission in hippocampal cells; what has been learned from its study is an excellent example of the discovery of general properties and principles. We also know something about why and when these cells are activated in the living brain. Recordings from freely moving animals as they navigate around a space with which they have become familiar have shown that individual hippocampal pyramidal cells fire in particular locations. This finding led to the development of new behavioral tools to study the neural mechanisms of memory in animals. Turning to structure, studded along the extensive dendritic arborizations of each pyramidal cell are many thousands of dendritic spines—the sites where the great majority of excitatory synapses are to be found. An important finding is that the efficiency with which these excitatory synapses actually transmit messages can vary as a function of neural activity. The circumstances bringing about this synaptic plasticity are now reasonably well understood, and we are beginning to understand some of the underlying biochemical mechanisms responsible for its induction, expression, and maintenance. Many suspect that synaptic plasticity is a key mechanism of memory, whereas others see it as part of a wider picture of neural activation and neural homeostasis. Another exciting feature of the hippocampal formation is that dentate granule cells are one of the rare types of neurons that continue to reproduce throughout life. Adult neurogenesis is likely to yield important lessons about neuronal growth and survival and could be a phenomenon that contributes to the processing of information entering the hippocampal formation at the level of the dentate gyrus. Adult neurogenesis is also a phenomenon with potential importance for neuronal repair and therapeutic intervention.

These observations have emerged from the widespread exploration of this beautiful structure. As we shall see, several structural characteristics of the hippocampal formation have greatly facilitated its physiological and behavioral analysis and ultimately its contribution to neuroscience.

1.1 Why Study the Hippocampal Formation on Its Own?

Can one profitably focus on one group of brain structures and appear to ignore the rest of the brain? The brain is so heavily

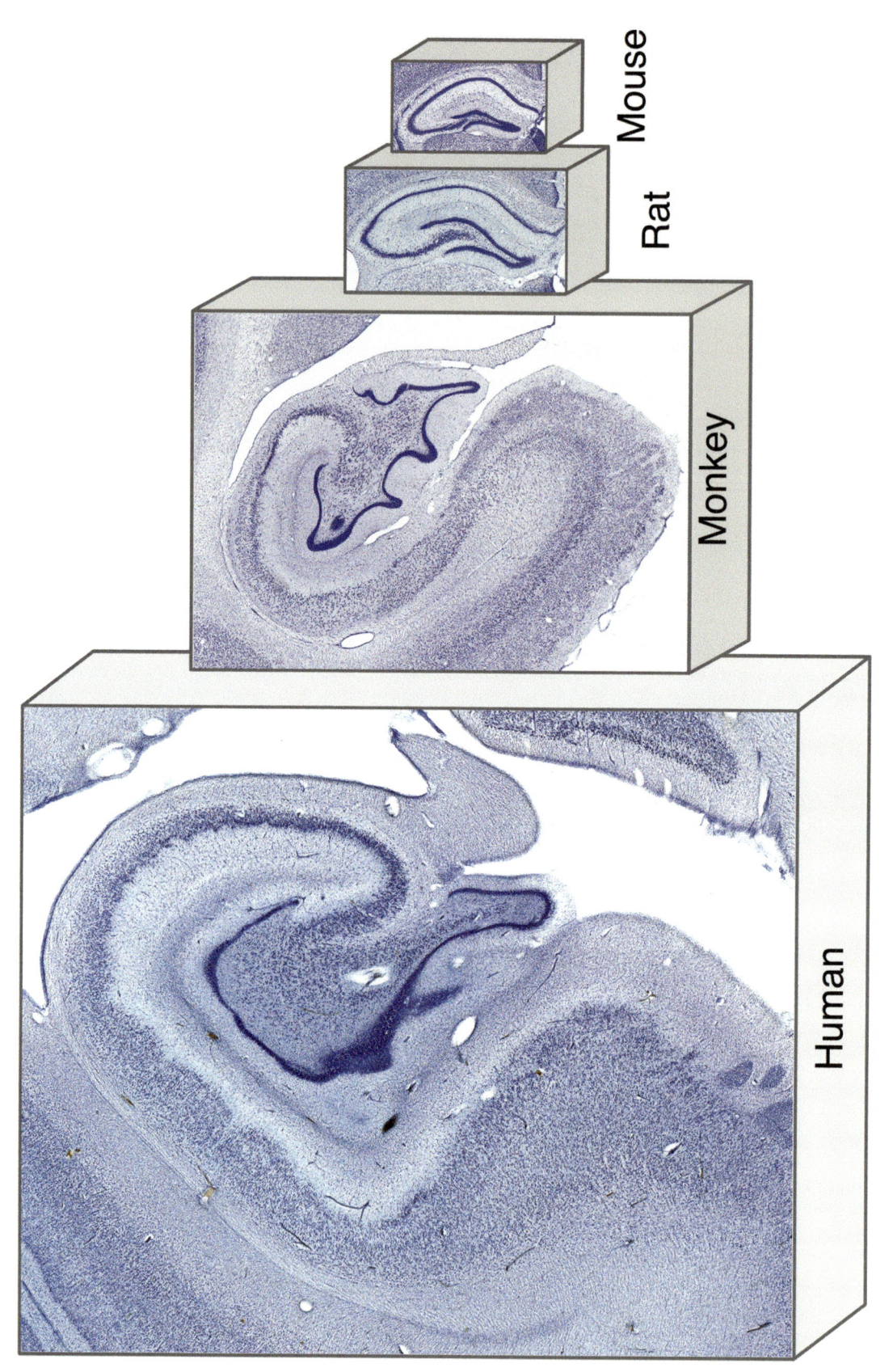

Figure 1.1 Nissl-stained coronal sections through the mouse, rat, monkey, and human hippocampal formation. While there are obvious differences in certain regions, the most striking feature is the general similarity of this brain region across phylogeny.

interconnected that it is potentially misleading to think about the function of one small part of it in isolation. What it does and how it does it might be understood better by routinely comparing it with other brain areas or by thinking about how it works in conjunction with these to realize the seamless fabric of normal brain function. We have sympathy with this view, not least because the general significance of the many exciting discoveries that have been made about the hippocampus will only become clear with a more inclusive approach in which it and other parts of the brain are considered together. Moreover, developments in neuroscience in the contemporary era have repeatedly emphasized network connectivity as a key principle for understanding brain function. We believe, nonetheless, that there is still value in our focused approach.

Specifically, there are three primary reasons for singling out the hippocampal formation as a brain area worthy of a book in its own right, and this second edition of the book touches repeatedly on these themes. These have to do with (1) trying to understand how its unique organization leads to its irreplaceable function(s) within the brain, (2) the way in which work on hippocampal tissue has revealed general principles in neuroscience, and (3) how aging and neurological and psychiatric disorders impact hippocampal function. Considering the first theme, contemporary research points strongly to the hippocampus having a very specific role in memory. There has been a great deal of debate about how that role should be characterized, and after the explosive period of research of the last 50 years, a consensus is beginning to emerge. There is now a general recognition that there are multiple types of memory and that the hippocampus plays a part in only some of these. There is also general agreement that some types of memory are declared, that is, they relate to memories that can be described while other types, such as the process of acquiring actions and then habits, are not. The hippocampus is engaged in remembering information that can be described. That much is clear. Beyond that, there remain many areas of disagreement and debate that continue to fuel imaginative new research in behavioral and cognitive neuroscience. Indeed, the last 15 years have witnessed the emergence of novel ideas about the role(s) that the hippocampus plays in memory, which are discussed in several chapters of the book. Work on the function of the hippocampal formation, arguably more than any other brain area, has led to the development of current concepts about the organization of cognitive systems in the brain.

Some traditionalists still hold that each of the different subjects that make up the biomedical sciences—such as anatomy, biochemistry, and physiology—has a self-contained level of analysis that is logically independent of other levels of analysis. By this view, a physiological problem requires an answer in strictly physiological terms. But a contrasting view emerging at the start of the 21st century is that that each of level of inquiry can profitably inform and guide research at other levels. By way of example, many years of a strictly psychological analysis of learning and memory, beginning with the discovery of Pavlovian conditioning, the ensuing dark phase of behaviorism and the subsequent enlightenment of the cognitive revolution, failed to unravel the existence of multiple memory systems. It was not until a different "brain-systems" approach was taken in the latter part of the 20th century, an approach that emerged in large part from studies of the memory problems faced by patient H.M. and other amnesic patients, that the major breakthroughs in our understanding of the cerebral organization of memory came about. Such thinking led to research which married brain and behavior in single-unit recording

and lesion studies in awake primates and freely moving rodents, to the development of new behavioral tests of learning and memory, and on to pharmacological and molecular-biological analyses. There is a lesson here that we believe is of general applicability to other branches of neuroscience. Specifically, the "brain-systems" approach is one in which there is analytical value in juxtaposing numerous different levels of analysis during the exploration of what bits of the brain do what and how they do it.

The second justification for writing this book is that many general principles of modern neuroscience that were worked out in the hippocampus have now been applied and extended to other brain regions. Fifty years ago, the most widely studied cell in the nervous system was the alpha motoneuron of the ventral horn of the spinal cord. Today it is the pyramidal cell of the hippocampus. One reason for the change of focus has been the unique anatomy of the hippocampus with all principal cells in a compact layer and synaptic inputs confined to well-defined dendritic laminae. This simplified architecture has facilitated recording of both synaptic signals and population discharges. Field potential recording became possible because the well-defined somatic and dendritic laminae allowed identification of current sources and sinks in extracellular recordings made in vivo. It was through these that the basic principle of unidirectional excitatory transmission was first discovered as well as the phenomenon of long-term potentiation. Of particular importance for the study of synaptic function in the context of learning and memory was the fact that field-potential recording of synaptic responses could be made both in the freely moving animal and in the invitro hippocampal slice. In fact, such studies have always been rare, with in vitro brain slices being the preferred technique; the pyramidal cell soon became a popular cell to study because of the analytical potential of brain slice recordings. The first in vitro slices were made from neocortex and pyriform cortex with limited synaptic activation. With its better identification of cells and input fibers, the development of the transverse hippocampal slice revolutionized cortical neurophysiology and neuropharmacology. Of course, many fundamental concepts had been worked out beforehand—in the squid giant axon, the spinal cord, and the cerebellum—but the hippocampal slice made possible the study of cortical cells and identified synapses on an unprecedented scale. Work in the hippocampus has been a major contributor to our understanding of the actions and mechanisms of various types of synapses and of the different classes of receptors for excitatory and inhibitory amino acids, of the many transmitter uptake mechanisms, of activity-dependent synaptic plasticity, and of the deleterious consequences for brain cells of excitotoxicity. It is the laminated architecture of the principal excitatory neurons in the hippocampus, and the strict layering of synapses in the dendritic tree, coupled to its capacity to survive in vitro for long periods of time, that has rendered the design and analysis of electrophysiological and many other types of experiments tractable in a manner that remains difficult in other brain areas and was long thought to be impractical in vivo.

In the last 15 years or so, there has been an exciting revolution in techniques for the study of the nervous system, with the hippocampal formation serving as one test bed in which new techniques could be deployed. In no particular order, these include the development of optogenetics and the opportunity to activate neurons in a cell-specific manner by precisely timed light pulses. Likewise, chemogenetic approaches also enable novel "gain-of-function" studies that had not been possible in a cell-specific manner before with only electrical or pharmacological stimulation. The development and application of multiphoton confocal microscopy, initially in surface structures of the brain such as the neocortex and then in deeper structures such as the hippocampus, is now giving us dynamic images of neuronal activity across tens or even hundreds of pyramidal cells at the same time, and in the different planes of focus of their dendritic arborizations. Electrophysiology is truly moving into the age of light, and this change has created the opportunity for major rethinking in how behavioral studies might be conducted. Confocal work generally requires the animals to be immobilized to secure effective cellular resolution imaging, but the use of head-fixed preparations is now complemented by virtual-reality environments in which animals, although fixed, can nonetheless perceive the world and move on surfaces on air-suspended trackballs. Not every facet of behavior can be studied in this way, but the development of miniature head-mounted endoscopes coupled with viral expression of fluorescent markers of cell activity in a cell-specific manner offers the opportunity to look at real-world navigation, social behavior, and other facets of cognition. Of course, these technologies are being applied in numerous brain regions—but studies in the hippocampal formation have often been pioneering.

Beyond its key role in the development of in vitro techniques and exacting in vivo approaches at cellular resolution, the hippocampal formation has also figured prominently in many types of translational brain research. It is a brain network implicated in disparate neurological disorders, including epilepsy, Alzheimer's disease, schizophrenia, stress, and cerebrovascular disease. Thus, the abnormal electrical activity that is at the root of seizures in epileptic patients is often most easily detected in the hippocampus. Moreover, a hallmark feature of the neuropathology of temporal lobe epilepsy is loss of neurons in several hippocampal fields. In Alzheimer's disease, the characteristic pathological changes are manifest initially within the entorhinal cortex—one of the components of the hippocampal formation—and the disease spreads from there inwardly to the hippocampus proper and outwardly to certain connected regions of the cerebral cortex. Such findings have led to the development of model systems, often based on transgenic mouse preparations, in which pathophysiological events such as these may be studied and, hopefully, ameliorated by treatment. Advancing knowledge of fundamental mechanisms has reached a point where the stage is set for tractable analyses of how hippocampal function changes across the life span and sometimes goes wrong in disease.

These three main reasons for writing the book therefore provide us with intersecting themes that run through many of chapters. One perspective is functional, another generic, and the third translational (Figure 1.2):

- What does the hippocampus do?
- How have general principles derived from the study of the hippocampus informed research on other brain regions and networks?
- Can our developing understanding of the hippocampal formation inform translational studies of neurological and psychiatric disease?

To achieve these three aims, we have broken up our task into chapters that are largely organized along conventional disciplinary lines, but, where appropriate, several strands of thought and levels of analysis are intertwined.

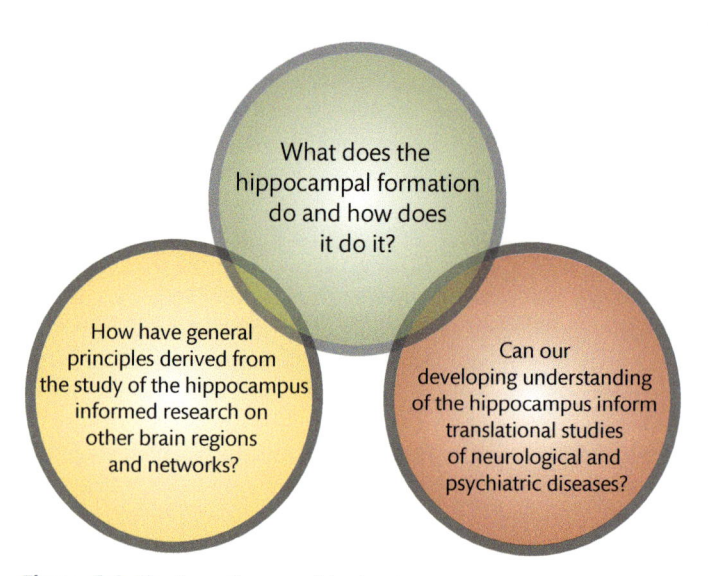

Figure 1.2 The three themes of the book.

1.2 Defining the Contemporary Era

Our starting point in preparing the first edition of this book was to define the contemporary era of research as beginning in the 1960s and to regard discoveries made before that as "modern" and those made afterward as "contemporary." Any division of this kind is arbitrary, but the period of the 1960s and 1970s was a watershed for both functional and mechanistic studies. They saw the first intracellular analysis of synaptic, antidromic, and epileptiform activities of hippocampal neurons; the characterization and interpretation of field potentials signaling excitation and inhibition; and electron micrographs of synapse types and their distribution along the cell bodies and their extensions. It was also at this time that several of the new tract-tracing techniques became available to anatomists, replacing the classical degeneration techniques hitherto used to identify regional connectivity. These made it possible to map the intrinsic and extrinsic connections of the hippocampal formation at a previously unachievable level of sensitivity and detail. In the same decade, hippocampal place cells were discovered, and the phenomenon of long-term potentiation first described in detail. Methodological developments of the 1970s included the hippocampal slice, new tests of recognition memory for primates, and the open-field circular platform (Barnes maze) and the watermaze—behavioral techniques to study learning in rodents that have since been used extensively to analyze the role of the hippocampus in spatial navigation. Mathematicians also started thinking about the hippocampus as a neural network and set in motion a type of theoretical neuroscience that has attracted increasing attention.

As we approached the task of creating a new edition, we have tried to limit the extent to which we are merely repeating those examples of material described at length in the first edition to focus on some of the exciting developments that have unfolded in the last 15 years. This is not always feasible—one example being the need once again to lay out the neuroanatomy of the hippocampal formation in detail as a foundation for material in later chapters of the book. However, certain of the initial discoveries that we highlighted in the first edition are now properly placed in Chapter 2 of the book

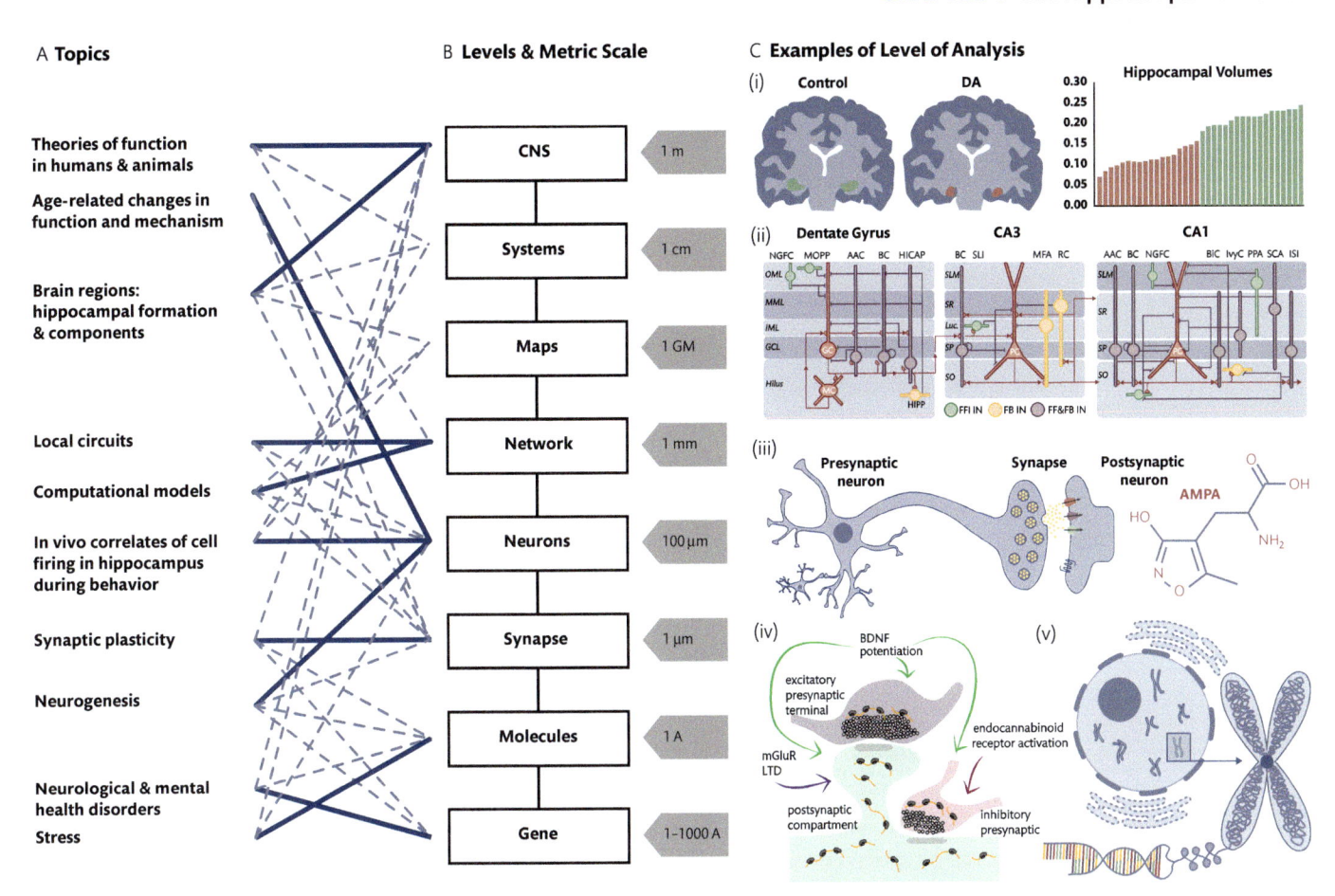

A Topics

Theories of function in humans & animals

Age-related changes in function and mechanism

Brain regions: hippocampal formation & components

Local circuits

Computational models

In vivo correlates of cell firing in hippocampus during behavior

Synaptic plasticity

Neurogenesis

Neurological & mental health disorders

Stress

B Levels & Metric Scale

CNS	1 m
Systems	1 cm
Maps	1 GM
Network	1 mm
Neurons	100 µm
Synapse	1 µm
Molecules	1 A
Gene	1–1000 A

C Examples of Level of Analysis

Figure 1.3 Levels of analysis in the neurobiology of the hippocampal formation. Adaptation of the Sejnowski and Churchland diagram about "levels of analysis" with reference to primary and other levels covered in individual chapters, with exemplar images reflecting new findings of recent years at distinct levels. (A) Examples of chapters and topics. Strong dark blue line indicates the archetypal level of analysis for the particular issue, with gray dotted lines to multiple additional relevant levels. (B) Levels and scales of analysis. (C) Exemplar images of observations: (i) A condition called developmental amnesia is associated with a selective reduction of hippocampal volume and a selective deficit in episodic memory (Chapter 13); (ii) example of complex inhibitory local circuitry in the hippocampus (Chapter 7); (iii) critical role of the synaptic level of analysis for multiple topics; (iv) new structural biology of the NMDA receptor; (iv) protein synthesis in dendrites; (v) gene activation and regulation in hippocampus is increasingly under investigation.

to free up space to discuss the new developments. Decisions on what should stay and what should go are often not clear-cut, since many "classical" discoveries remain directly relevant to currently active domains of research and form the basis for describing more recent findings.

1.3 The Organization and Content of the Book

The organization we have chosen reflects an important facet of contemporary neuroscience—the current perspective that progress in neuroscience comes only from a multifaceted approach to function and dysfunction. First introduced by Churchland and

Sejnowski, we seek to represent these multiple levels of analysis with examples of findings from the study of the hippocampus at all levels and to show how working between levels can be especially instructive (Figure 1.3). Some topics are largely, although not exclusively, focused at one level (e.g., synaptic function) whereas others (e.g., aging) reach to multiple levels.

In coming to a decision about when the contemporary era started, we also recognized the enormous contributions made beforehand and on which so much of modern research rests. Accordingly, we have devoted Chapter 2 to a historical discussion of the key discoveries and concepts of hippocampal neurobiology of the modern era up to about 1970–1990—some 30 to 50 years ago, to which we now turn.

Functions of the Hippocampal Formation, Its Biological Characteristics, and Its Use as a Neurobiological Model

An Historical Overview

Richard Morris, David Amaral, Tim Bliss, Karen Duff, and John O'Keefe

2.1 Introduction

In the first edition of this book, our second chapter provided a selected overview of some historically important proposals concerning the function and neural mechanisms of the hippocampus. Given the importance of the shoulders on which contemporary neuroscientists now stand, we include again some of this historical information, and then go on to identify significant advances in hippocampal neuropsychology and neurobiology in the years leading up to the contemporary era.

As before, we divide the chapter into subsections that emphasize the biological function of the hippocampal formation (sections 2.2 and 2.3 below) and then the nature and possible advantages of the hippocampus as a model system for neurobiological and translational research (sections 2.4 to 2.6). In the 15 years since the first edition, we feel able to move the ravine that divides "history" and the "contemporary era" to a period starting roughly 50 years ago—i.e., around 1970. Clearly this historical divide tends to meander with the defining moments occurring at earlier or later points in time for distinct subdisciplines of hippocampal neurobiology. The most recent advances, notably of the 21st century, are those considered in detail in later chapters; this chapter is primarily an historical overview.

However, before embarking on our historical review, the editors would like to pay tribute here to the late Per Andersen (1930–2020), the driving force behind the first edition of this book (Figure 2.1). His career spanned the latter part of the "historical" era as we are defining it in this chapter through to the contemporary era of neuroscience. Following his early work in Oslo on the interpretation of field potentials in the hippocampus, he joined Sir John Eccles in Canberra in 1961, where the Canberra group's expertise in intracellular recording combined with Andersen's knowledge of hippocampal cellular anatomy led to the first identification of an interneuron in the mammalian brain—the basket cells of the

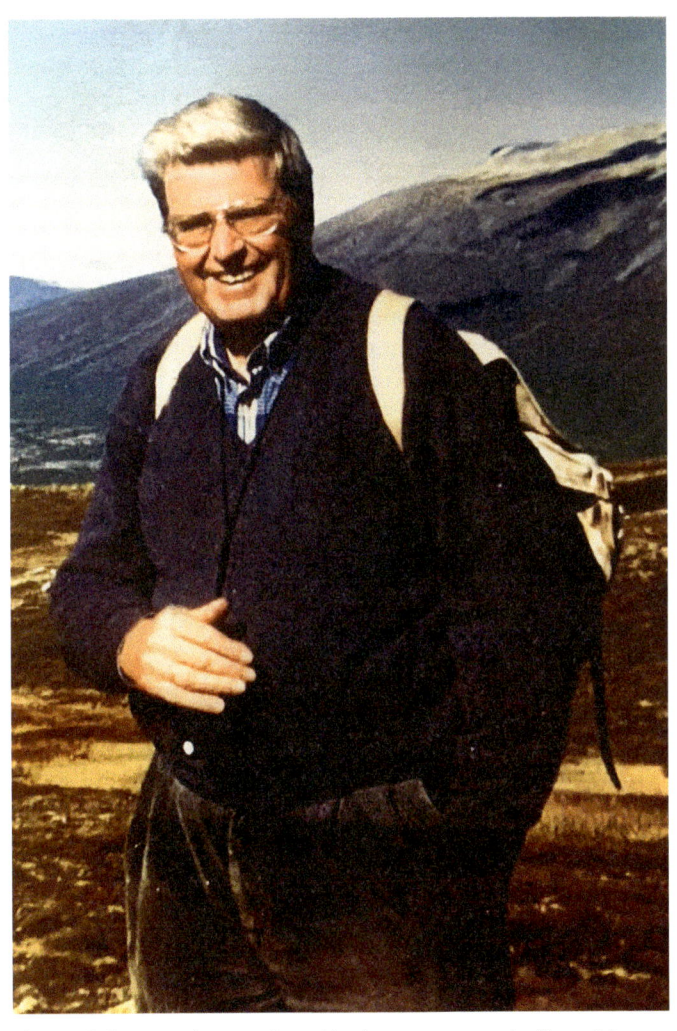

Figure 2.1 Per Andersen, whose idea it was to create the first edition of this book for which he was the driving force. Per was never more at home than amongst his beloved mountains of Norway.

hippocampus. Returning to his native Norway in 1963, he developed in Oslo one of the most influential neurophysiology laboratories in the world. The transverse hippocampal slice, an in vitro preparation still in use in neuroscience labs throughout the world, was developed in Oslo, and the phenomenon of long-term potentiation (LTP) was discovered in his laboratory. Among his last PhD students were Edvard Moser and May-Britt Moser, who went on to discover grid cells in the entorhinal cortex, sharing the 2014 Nobel Prize with John O'Keefe for his discovery of place cells. Per Andersen exerted a profound and enduring influence on physiological studies of the hippocampus.

2.2 The Dawn of Hippocampal Studies

From the very start of investigations into the structure and function of the brain, the hippocampus has been firmly at center stage. No doubt this is due in part to the striking appearance in the human brain of the large, bulging structure impressing itself into the lateral ventricle and clearly visible to the ancient anatomists. Members of the Alexandrian school of medicine were impressed by the elegant, curved structure, which, when seen with its contralateral half, strongly resembles the coiled horns of a ram. Hence, the ancient scholars named the hippocampus "cornu ammonis," Latin for "horn of the ram." This terminology survives in the acronyms for the hippocampal subfields CA1, CA2, and CA3. Over the centuries, this part of the brain has been proposed as the seat of many functions, ranging from olfaction to motor function and even reason, stubbornness, and inventiveness.

The Bolognese anatomist Giulio Cesare Aranzi (circa 1564) was the first to coin the structure "hippocampus," undoubtedly because its shape reminded him of the tropical fish (Figure 2.2). After the advent of microscopy, the hippocampus would have appeared even more impressive, with its characteristic, neatly regimented cellular architecture and interlocking layers of cells. Although the hippocampal formation is organized in a very different way from other cortical areas, it has played an important role in unraveling some of the basic principles of cortical organization.

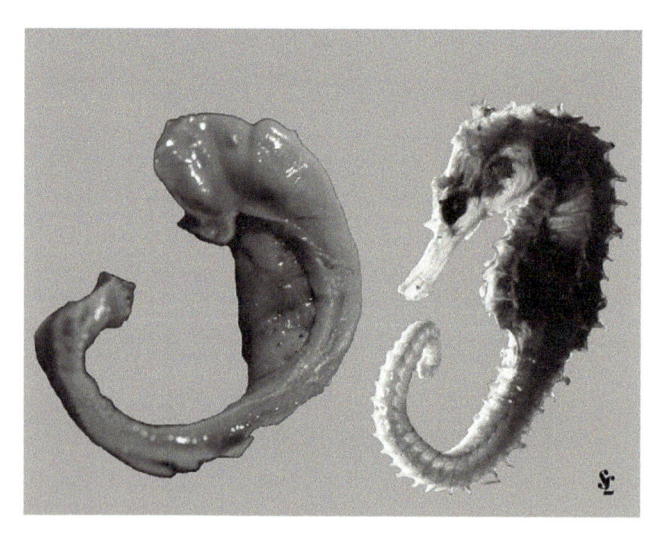

Figure 2.2 Human hippocampus dissected free (*left*) compared with a specimen of the seahorse *Hippocampus leria* (*right*). (Courtesy of Professor Lazlo Seress, University of Pecs.)

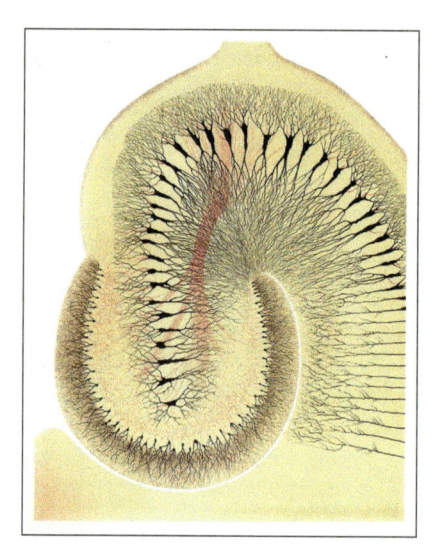

Figure 2.3 Section of a rabbit hippocampus stained with the original Golgi method (1886). Plate 26 from a German edition of Camillo Golgi's *Sulla fina anatomia degli organi centrali del sistema nervoso* (1885). (Golgi et al., 2001.)

The striking organization of the hippocampus, with its cell populations condensed into clearly demarcated layers, has attracted the attention of many investigators of the central nervous system. An early example is Camillo Golgi's illustration from 1885, where he used his revolutionary new technique which stained random individual neurons in full, to illustrate the unique organization of the hippocampus (see Figure 2.3, reproduced from Golgi et al., 2001).

2.2.1 The hippocampal formation and olfactory function

While the hippocampus had been implicated in several functions in the 19th and early 20th centuries, it was considered by many neuroanatomists to be a part of the olfactory system until the 1930s. Perhaps this was because macroscopical investigations left the impression that the hippocampus is especially large in macrosmatic animals like nocturnal insectivores and rodents (with large olfactory mucosa and bulbs). However, in these macrosmatic animals, the absolute sizes of the olfactory parts of the brain are quite small. In fact, it was claimed that the ratio of the volume of the hippocampus to the olfactory bulb is largest in humans (Rose, 1935). Indeed, as observed by Brodal (1947, p. 208), "From a functional point of view, it is worth emphasizing that the development not only of the fornix, but also of the mammillary body, the mammillothalamic tract, the anterior (more particularly the antero-ventral) nucleus of the thalamus and the cingular gyrus, runs roughly parallel with the degree of development of the hippocampus. All these structures reach their peak of development in man."

The idea of an olfactory function for the hippocampus, repeated in numerous textbooks in the first half of the 20th century, possibly arose from some early behavioral and clinical observations. For example, David Ferrier observed "movements of the lip and nostrils on stimulation of the hippocampal lobe in monkeys" (Ferrier, 1876). John Hughlings Jackson and Charles Beevor (1890) reported on a patient who had subjective olfactory sensations during seizures that originate in the periamygdaloid olfactory cortex. Later, Wilder Penfield and Theodore Erickson (1941, p. 56) reported on a patient who had "olfactory sensations as part of his epileptic seizure and where it seems to be the hippocampus which must be the site of the discharge."

In a comprehensive review, the Norwegian neuroanatomist Alf Brodal summarized the evidence that had been put forward for such an olfactory role, but then marshaled a cogent argument against it (Brodal, 1947). He noted that phylogenetic and comparative neuroanatomical studies suggested that the hippocampus develops in parallel with the olfactory portions of the brain and that, indeed, it is prominent in macrosmatic mammals like rodents and insectivores. Moreover, even in the gross brain or in normal histological preparations, fibers from the lateral olfactory tract can easily be traced into brain regions surrounding the hippocampal formation. Even so, Brodal raised a number of arguments against an olfactory role for the hippocampus, suggesting that the association of the hippocampal formation with olfactory function was largely based on circumstantial evidence.

Central to his thesis was the claim that fibers arising in the olfactory bulb did not, in fact, directly innervate any portion of the hippocampus. In particular, while Brodal agreed that some olfactory fibers innervated the anterior portions of the parahippocampal gyrus, these did not extend back into the caudal portion of the gyrus, where the entorhinal cortex resides. He did not entirely dismiss an olfactory role for the hippocampal formation and suggested that the entorhinal cortex "should be considered as concerned mainly with the association and integration of olfactory impulses . . . with other cortical influences" (1947, p. 206). Among other negative evidence, Brodal cited several studies attesting to the fact that the hippocampal formation was present in anosmatic and microsmatic animals such as dolphins and whales (Ries, 1937), and that there was substantial regional differentiation in microsmatic humans. Furthermore, he noted data of William F. Allen in which lesions of the temporal lobe had no effect on the ability of dogs to perform olfactory discrimination tasks (Allen, 1940). Brodal concluded, "No decisive evidence that the hippocampus is concerned in olfaction appears to have been brought forward" (Brodal, 1947, p. 180).

Brodal's review was highly influential in raising doubts about an olfactory role for the hippocampus. However, at least one of the pieces of evidence cited by Brodal—that there are no olfactory projections to the hippocampal formation—has subsequently proven incorrect. More sensitive anatomical techniques have shown that, in the rodent, the entorhinal cortex receives a substantial direct projection from the olfactory bulb as well as secondary olfactory inputs from the piriform and periamygdaloid cortices (Shipley and Adamek, 1984). Even in the monkey, as Ricardo Insausti, David Amaral, and Maxwell Cowan demonstrated in 1987, the anterior portion of the entorhinal cortex is directly innervated by the lateral olfactory tract. The olfactory system retains a privileged position in relation to the entorhinal cortex, as none of the other sensory channels from which it receives information originate in primary or even higher-order unimodal sensory cortices, but rather come from polysensory association cortices. Thus, while Brodal's review was a milestone and is partially responsible for the currently held view that the hippocampal formation is not a major component of the olfactory system, it turns out that olfactory inputs as well as those of other sensory modalities do contribute to functions in which the hippocampus is engaged. Interestingly, olfactory learning and memory tasks are now sometimes used in studies of rodent hippocampal function (see Chapter 14).

2.2.2 The hippocampal formation and emotion

Another influential neuroanatomical hypothesis was proposed by James W. Papez, who suggested that the hippocampus was part of a circuit that provides the anatomical substrate of emotion (Papez, 1937). He was influenced by reports from Walter B. Cannon (1929) and Philip Bard (1934), which indicated that the hypothalamus was essential for evoking the autonomic and visceral aspects of emotional behavior. He accepted the view of Cannon and Bard that emotion has two component processes, emotional behavior and the cognitive appreciation of emotion. In an attempt to explain the anatomical underpinnings of emotion, he proposed a pathway based on circumstantial evidence such as the neuropathology of distemper in animals that interconnected cortical and subcortical structures. In this now famous circuit that bears his name, he viewed the hippocampus as a collector of sensory information which would develop an "emotive state" that could be transferred to the mammillary nuclei. In addition to mediating the appropriate behavioral response to this emotive state, the mammillary nuclei would also relay information to the anterior cingulate cortex via the anterior thalamic nuclei, where conscious appreciation of the emotion would be achieved. As Papez stated:

> The central emotive process of cortical origin may then be conceived as being built up in the hippocampal formation and as being transferred to the mammillary body and thence through the anterior thalamic nuclei to the cortex of the gyrus cinguli. The cortex of the cingular gyrus may be looked on as the receptive region for the experiencing of emotion as the result of impulses coming from the hypothalamic region, in the same way as the area striata is considered the receptive cortex for photic excitations coming from the retina. (Papez, 1937, pp. 725–743)

Again, Brodal provides a robustly skeptical comment. After scrutinizing the anatomical literature, he concluded, "There is no sound biological basis for selecting a few brain regions as being involved in these complex functions (emotions), and today the theory of Papez is of historical interest only" (Brodal, 1981, p. 672). However, it is fair to recognize that the Papez circuit (see Figure 2.4

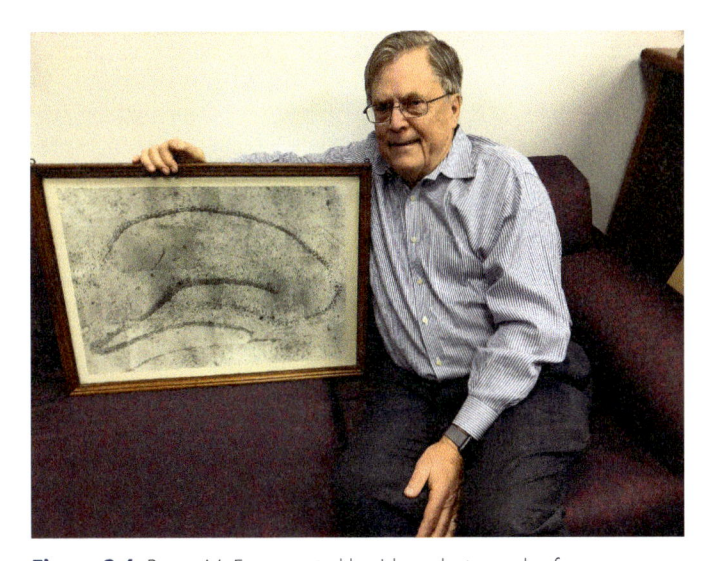

Figure 2.4 Bruce McEwen seated beside a photograph of the distribution of corticosteroid receptors in hippocampus prepared in his laboratory at Rockefeller University. (Courtesy of Sumantra Chattarji.)

of 1st edition) was important historically primarily because it shifted emphasis away from the olfactory functions of the hippocampus. It was one of the early ideas about how the brain might have more autonomy from the environment than suggested by the then-in-vogue "stimulus-response" behaviorism. As we shall see, there is only limited evidence to support the idea that the hippocampus is specifically involved in emotion, an idea that was championed in recent years by Jeffrey Gray (1982), notably in relation to the ventral/anterior regions of the hippocampus. While emotion may no longer be seen as a primary function of the hippocampus, it nonetheless plays a very important role in mediating the impact of stress on cognition. A pioneer in reaching this conclusion was the late Bruce McEwen (Figure 2.4), who before his death in 2020 contributed to the planning of Chapter 17 of this edition. The McEwen laboratory was for several decades at the forefront of the study of estrogen and glucocorticoid actions in the brain, making the important observation that estrogen can increase dendritic spine density in the CA1 subfield of the hippocampus (Woolley et al., 1990). His group also discovered stress-induced dendritic retraction in the CA3 hippocampal subfield. By pioneering the study of the role of both gonadal and adrenal steroid actions in the brain, the McEwen laboratory helped develop the current scientific understanding of stress.

Stepping back some years, Papez's speculations about the role of the hippocampus in emotion appeared to receive support from the experiments of Heinrich Klüver and Paul Bucy that were carried out at around the same time (Klüver and Bucy, 1937). Klüver was a psychologist interested in the neural locus of action of psychotropic drugs such as mescaline. Together with Bucy, a neurologist, he searched for the locus of emotion by removing brain tissue in monkeys and then looking for changes in their behavioral response to drugs. The behavioral changes that followed bilateral temporal lobe removal (which included the hippocampal formation, amygdaloid complex, and temporal neocortex) were interesting enough to warrant extensive description, and the constellation of changes is now known as the "Klüver-Bucy syndrome." This has two important aspects: changes in visually guided behavior and changes in emotional expression. The lesioned monkeys appeared to have a visual agnosia but would nonetheless compulsively follow stimuli brought into their visual field. they continually placed all objects encountered in their mouths, perhaps due to the failure to recognize the objects by sight. In the emotional sphere, they were sexually aberrant and apparently without fear of stimuli that usually frightened them. It was this latter observation which appeared to confirm the role of the hippocampus in emotion predicted by Papez. However, it was subsequently shown that the loss of fear and other behavioral alterations could be attributed to damage to the amygdala and its connections with the visual regions of the inferotemporal cortex (Schreiner and Kling, 1953; Mishkin, 1954; Weiskrantz, 1956; Zola-Morgan et al., 1989; Aggleton, 1993; Hayman et al., 1998). The hippocampus was again a structure in search of a function.

Unbeknownst to Papez, and probably also to Klüver and Bucy, a report appearing nearly a half century earlier by Sanger Brown and Hans Schäfer (1888) described an experiment with a nonhuman primate and, specifically, the results of a large bilateral temporal lobe lesion on a "fine, large, active rhesus" monkey. In addition to describing virtually all of the behavioral and emotional alterations of the Klüver-Bucy syndrome, they also reported disturbances in memory. They commented on the apparent forgetfulness of the monkey in the following way: "And even after having examined an object in this way with the utmost care and deliberation, he will, on again coming across the same object accidentally, even a few minutes afterwards, go through exactly the same process, as if he had entirely forgotten his previous experience" (p. 262). This little-known observation of Brown and Schäfer presaged what has become the most enduring notion of hippocampal function, its essential role in memory.

2.2.3 The hippocampal formation and attention control

Beyond olfaction and then emotion, another prevalent idea was that the hippocampus might be involved in attention. Richard Jung and Alois Kornmüller (1938) had noted that desynchronization of neocortical EEG was temporally linked to a large-amplitude, sinusoidal wave pattern in the rabbit hippocampus, at between 4 and 7 Hz, which they named "theta" activity. Later work suggested that this brain activity was related to enhanced attention (Green and Arduini, 1954). John Green and W. Ross Adey (1956) found that arousal caused an inverse relation between the electrocortical waves of the hippocampus and neocortex. Endre Grastyán et al. (1959), in Hungary, proposed that the theta activity could be coupled to specific learning states (Figure 2.5). Both hippocampal and entorhinal theta waves showed distinct changes during the acquisition of conditioned responses (Holmes and Adey, 1966).

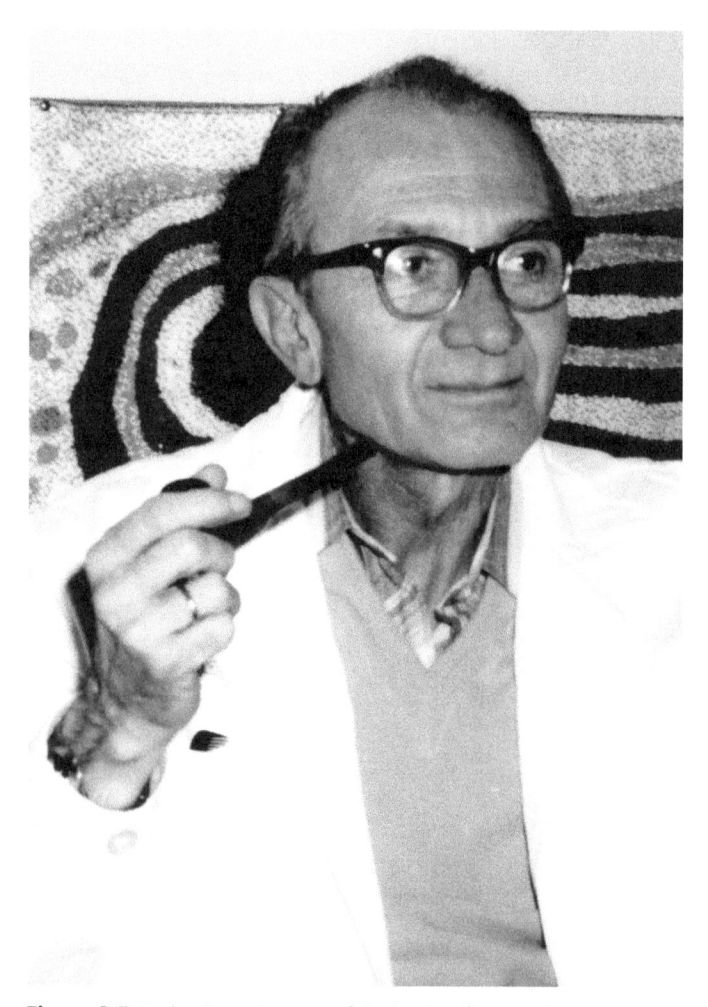

Figure 2.5 Endre Grastyán—one of the leading figures of Hungarian neurophysiology and behavior. (Courtesy of Professor Gyorgy Buzsaki.)

Other signs pointing to a role for the hippocampus in the control of attention came from electrical stimulation of the anterior part of the temporal lobe, including the hippocampus, which led to widespread and long-lasting desynchronization of the EEG in both anesthetized and awake cats (Kaada et al., 1949; Sloan and Jasper, 1950). Such responses were taken as evidence for a general activation of attention. Stimulation of the hippocampus in awake cats produced a peculiar reaction with pupillary dilatation and a slow turning of the head and neck to the contralateral side, as if the animal experienced an unusual sensory stimulus in the contralateral visual field (Kaada et al., 1953). The reaction was associated with enhanced respiration and blood pressure. Similar reactions were elicited from the anterior cingulate gyrus, later to be associated with higher analysis of emotional signals. Modern imaging methods have revealed that this area is deeply engaged in the analysis of emotional aspects of sensory stimuli, suggesting it is a device for estimation of potential conflicts between old and new experiences (Bush et al., 2000; Botvinick et al., 2001; Kerns et al., 2004; Bishop et al., 2004). In summary, this evidence suggests that in animals, and perhaps also in humans, the hippocampus may take part in some form of general attention control together with the anterior cingulate cortex.

2.3 The hippocampal formation and memory

2.3.1 Early ideas about the hippocampus and memory

An early effort to analyze memory functions was made by Théodule-Armand Ribot, a French philosopher and psychologist (Figure 2.6). He proposed that memory loss was a symptom of progressive brain disease. His *Les maladies de la mémoire* (Ribot, 1881) constitutes an influential early attempt to analyze abnormalities of memory in physiological terms. He even proposed that a plausible memory mechanism could be an alteration in the activity of engaged cells in the cortex. This seems to be the first hypothesis suggesting a direct role of nerve cells for memory functions. Strongly influenced by Paul Broca's reports on language localization (Broca, 1861a, 1861b), Ribot's views on localization were further supported by the clinical evidence of John Hughlings Jackson (1865) showing memory loss in human subjects following brain damage and by David Ferrier's 1876

report, mentioned above, on lip and nostril movements following stimulation of the hippocampal lobes in monkeys. Richard Semon, much influenced by Ribot, but working in Berlin, was responsible for coining the term "engram" to signify a memory trace in the form of a physical change in the participating nerve cells (Semon, 1908). This concept has been resurrected in recent chemogenetic and optogenetic studies, notably from the laboratory of Susumu Tonegawa (Figure 2.6), showing that an embedded fear memory could be reactivated, in the absence of the fear-evoking stimulus, simply through stimulation of the engram-encoding nerve cells. Tonegawa switched from immunology (for which he was awarded the 1987 Nobel Prize), to research in neuroscience around 1990. The idea that particular memories can be stored as engrams and reactivated by a physical stimulus has been proposed as a possible way to counter memory loss associated with conditions such as Alzheimer's disease.

Remembering that hippocampal efferent impulses influence many hypothalamic nuclei, most notably the mammillary bodies, the first causal link between memory functions and the hippocampal system was made by three scientists in the 1880s who semi-independently described an affliction causing amnesia. This condition was commonly associated with heavy drinking of alcohol and was later named Wernicke-Korsakov psychosis. Subsequently, this disorder was associated with thiamine deficiency that is often a correlate of inadequate diet in alcoholism. Carl Wernicke (1881) described three patients whose illnesses were characterized by paralysis of eye movements, ataxia, and mental confusion (see image in 1st edition). All three patients, two males with alcoholism and a female with persistent vomiting following sulfuric acid ingestion, lapsed into coma and died. In autopsies of all three patients, Wernicke detected punctate hemorrhages affecting the gray matter around the third and fourth ventricles and near the aqueduct of Sylvius. He considered these to be inflammatory and therefore named the disease polioencephalitis hemorrhagica superioris. Independently, Sergei S. Korsakov (1889, 1890), a Russian psychiatrist, described a similar clinical picture, which he called psychosis polyneuritica, and emphasized that the main symptom was memory deficits. Finally, Johann Bernhard Aloys von Gudden (1896) associated the condition with pathology of the mammillary bodies, the major target for hippocampal efferent pathways via the fornix (see Chapter 3).

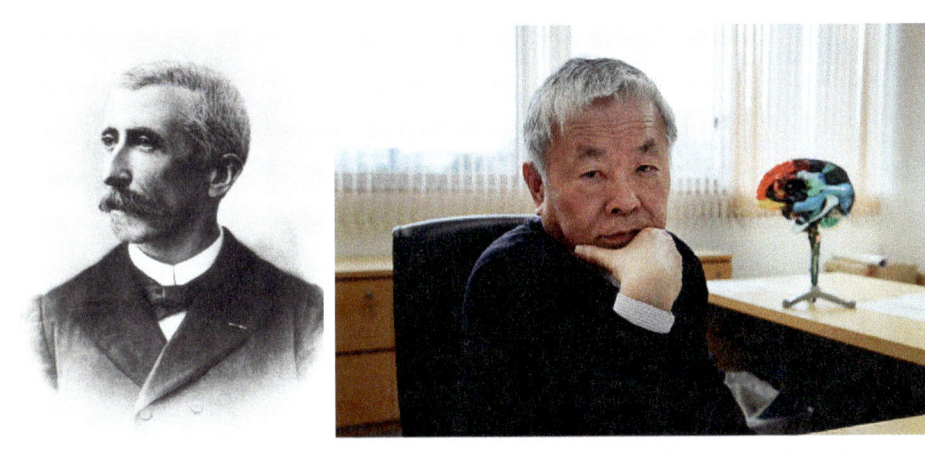

Figure 2.6 Theodule Armand Ribot, who coined the term "engram" as the physical substrate of memory in the 19th century (*left*). The Nobel laureate (for immunology) Susumu Tonegawa (*right*), who has recently brought molecular engineering tools to bear on the neurobiology of memory, has adopted the term "engram," and has introduced techniques to conduct causal studies of how neuronal ensembles may represent information. (Courtesy of Susumu Tonegawa.)

After the first description of the Wernicke-Korsakov syndrome, a similar condition with an emphasis on memory impairment was described by another Russian neurologist, Vladimir Bekhterev (1900), describing two patients with a prominent memory deficit, who were later found on autopsy to have bilateral softening of the hippocampus and neighboring cortical areas. This study appears to be the first hint of a hippocampal localization for memory.

2.3.2 A breakthrough in identifying hippocampal involvement in memory

The major step forward in establishing that the hippocampal formation is intimately associated with memory resulted from observations made on brain-damaged patients by William Scoville and Brenda Milner in 1957. Scoville, a neurosurgeon, removed the medial aspects of the temporal lobes in several patients, in an attempt to relieve a variety of neurological and psychiatric conditions. Drawings based on an MRI scan of the brain of one of these patients 40 years after the operation are shown in Figure 2.7. This patient (H.M.) was a young man whose seizures were resistant to antiepileptic drug treatment. Following surgery, his seizures were reduced, but he was left with a profound global, anterograde amnesia that persisted through to his death in 2008 at the age of 82. H.M. was initially studied by the neuropsychologist Brenda Milner, who, working at McGill University in Montreal, was influenced by the ideas then being developed by Donald Hebb, also at McGill (Figure 2.8).

H.M.—now known to the world as Henry Molaison—had a memory deficit that presented as an inability to remember material or episodes experienced after the operation (an anterograde amnesia) and also included an inability to recall information experienced for some period of time prior to the operation (retrograde amnesia). H.M. could remember items for brief periods, especially if he was allowed to rehearse and was not distracted. Once distracted, however, H.M. rapidly forgot. Thus, he never remembered for any length of time the doctors who tested him, his way around the hospital, nor the contents of any television program or book that he may have been reading. He reported his conscious existence as that of "constantly waking from a dream," and everything looking unfamiliar (see Chapters 13 and 14). The temporal characteristics of H.M.'s retrograde amnesia were controversial. Originally it was thought by Milner to extend up to 2 years prior to the operation, with memories for events earlier than that remaining relatively intact. This was later extended to 11 years (Sagar et al., 1985), with recollection of more distant events preserved. The interpretation of the extent of retrograde amnesia was complicated by the fact that this length of time was approximately equivalent to the period of the preoperative epileptic condition. It is widely accepted that his memory disabilities were due to the removal of a large part of the hippocampal formation and surrounding cortical regions. In addition to the groundbreaking contribution made by Brenda Milner, his memory problems were subject to numerous investigations, including those of the late Suzanne Corkin, whose Clinical Research Center at MIT conducted many tests on H.M. over the years (Figure 2.9) and whose book *Permanent Present Tense* (Corkin, 2013) gives a moving account of her long association with H.M. Four of the editors of the first edition of this book had the privilege of meeting H.M. in Corkin's clinic in 1994, and we experienced his memory problems firsthand. One of Corkin's own research projects included a detailed description of his spared capacity for motor learning, and her wider contributions included enabling access for large numbers of interested scientists to examine and explore the full range of his cognitive and memory abilities.

While Henry Molaison remains the most widely discussed patient with amnesia, there are many other well-known single-case studies, including Kent Cochrane (K.C.) in Canada and Clive

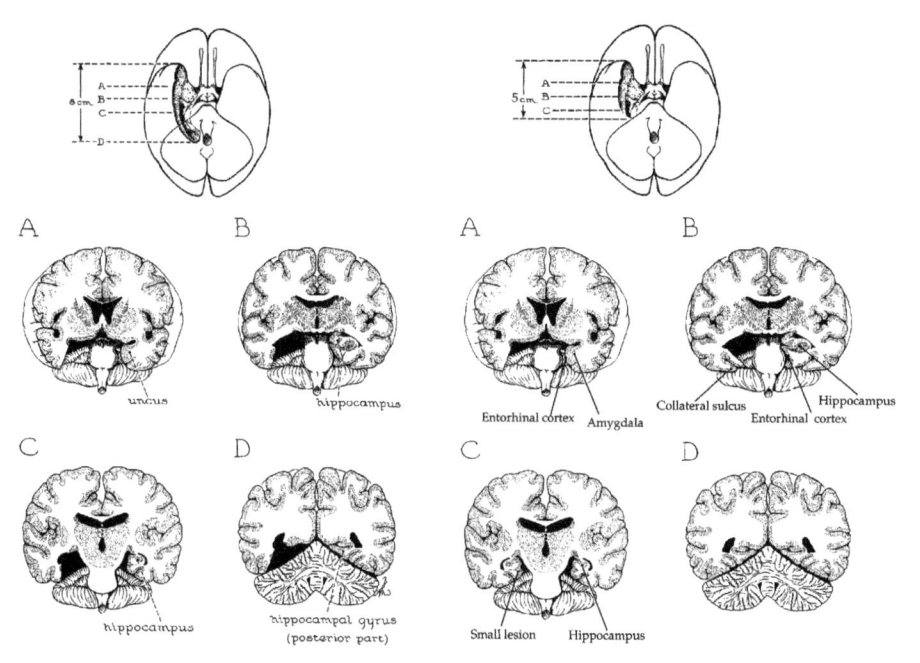

Figure 2.7 Left, Diagram showing the surgeon's estimate of H. M.'s medial temporal lobe resection (adapted from Scoville and Milner, 1957, their Fig. 2, p 13). The inset at the top is a ventral view of the human brain showing the predicted rostrocaudal extent of the ablation. A through D are drawings of coronal sections, arranged from rostral (A) to caudal (D), showing the predicted extent of the lesion. Note that although the lesion was made bilaterally, the right side is shown intact to illustrate structures that were removed. Right, An amended version of the original diagram indicating the extent of the ablation based on the MRI studies reported in Corkin et al. (1997). The rostrocaudal extent of the lesion is 5 cm rather than 8 cm, and the lesion does not extend as far laterally as initially pictured.
This was Figure 2.6 in the first edition.

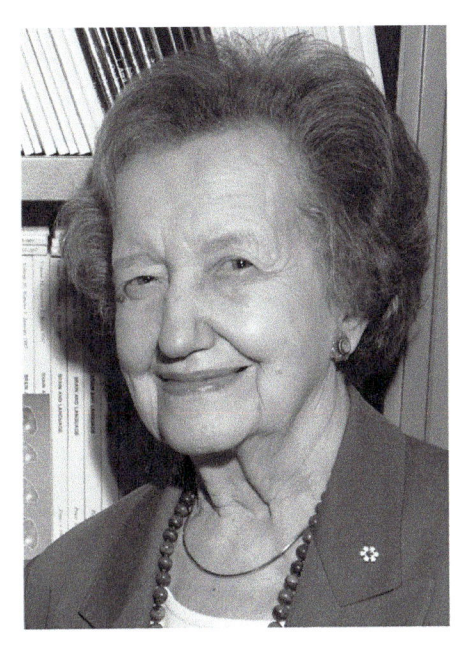 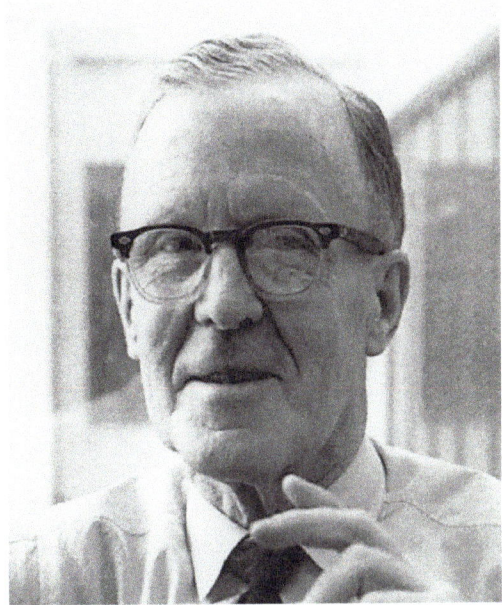

Figure 2.8 Brenda Milner (*left*) pioneered the neuropsychological analysis of the role of the medial temporal lobes in memory. Donald Hebb (*right*) has influenced generations of neuroscientists with his ideas on neural representation and memory mechanisms. (Courtesy of Professor Brenda Milner and www.williamcalvin.com.)

Wearing in the United Kingdom. The existence of several such patients adds confidence to the claim that there are identifiable problems with memory after damage to the medial temporal lobe and associated structures.

However, pointing a precise finger at the hippocampal formation as the critical structure remained controversial in the 1970s and 1980s. This led to a series of animal studies to address this question, as we will describe shortly. A substantial contribution to the issue in humans came from the laboratory of Larry Squire at the University of California, San Diego, and his colleagues. Squire's team carried out careful comparisons of longitudinal neuropsychological data and neuropathological evidence in an extensive series of patients (Figure 2.10). Among other things, Squire demonstrated that the resistance of memory to disruption can develop over long time periods in humans. This finding implied a memory consolidation process that likely reflects a gradual reorganization within

long-term memory itself. Germane to the localization of memory function within the medial temporal lobe, Squire, along with Stuart Zola-Morgan and David Amaral, published a report on patient R.B., who had a memory impairment like H.M.'s, with damage (due to an ischemic episode) confined to the CA1 region of the hippocampus (Zola-Morgan et al., 1986).

The global amnesia reported in H.M. spurred efforts to find an animal model of amnesia. Early studies by Jack Orbach, Brenda Milner, and Theodore Rasmussen (1960) and by R. E. Correll and William Scoville (1967) looked at the effects, in primates, of various temporal lobe lesions on memory tasks such as delayed alternation and delayed response. Deficits were seen with combined lesions of the amygdala and hippocampal formation in the delayed alternation task (where animals are required to alternate their response from one trial to the next), but not in the delayed response task (where animals choose a well-learned response after a delay period). Even

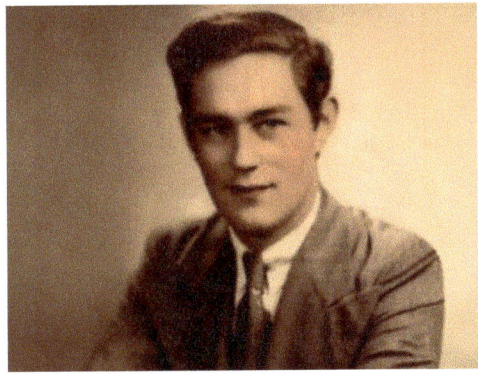 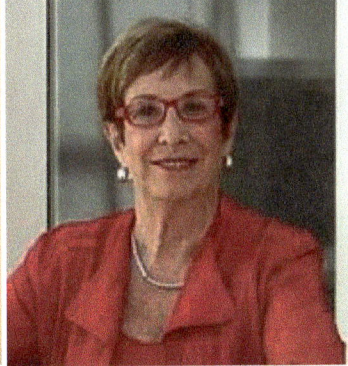

Figure 2.9 Henry Molaison (patient H.M.; *left*) was subject to a bilateral medial temporal lobectomy as a young man by William Scoville to relieve intractable epileptic fits resistant to then-available medications. The operation was discussed extensively with him and his family, but it left him permanently amnesic. Suzanne Corkin (*right*), who took over the neuropsychological testing of H.M. over many years at her clinical research center at MIT, generously allowed many others to conduct tests with him. (Professor Suzanne Corkin.)

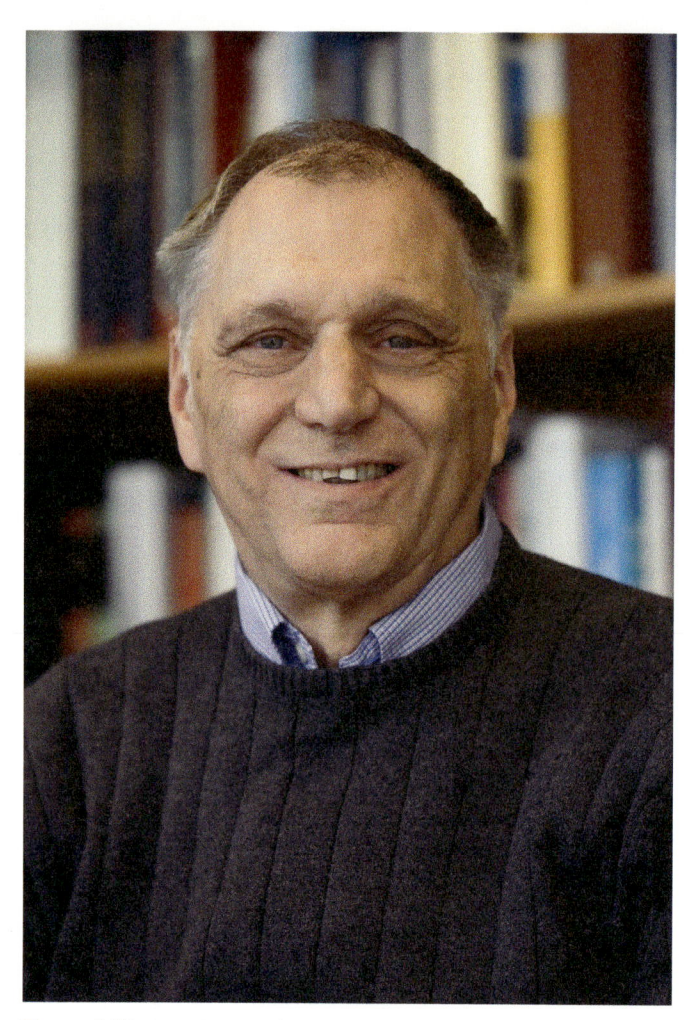

Figure 2.10 Larry Squire, who led a team of neuropsychologists and behavioral neuroscientists whose aim was to understand amnesia and build an animal model of the condition. (Courtesy of Professor Larry Squire.)

lengthening of the delay failed to reveal a deficit in the delayed response task. Thus, these early attempts in the primate were viewed as falling short of developing an animal model of medial temporal lobe amnesia. Work on laboratory rats also failed to find a convincing memory deficit following hippocampal damage. Lesioned rats had no difficulties learning simple sensory discriminations, to press levers in a Skinner box, or to run down alleys to obtain food or avoid punishment. What emerged, however, was a loose constellation of deficits. These included changes in exploration and habituation to novelty. For example, hippocampus-lesioned rats placed in novel environments were hyperactive, i.e., they moved around more than control rats and failed to reduce their activity progressively over time. They also failed to choose alternative arms on two successive runs in a simple T-maze when no rewards were available (spontaneous alternation). Both changes in behavior were attributed to deficits in inhibitory processes and, consequently, a role for the hippocampus in response inhibition or Pavlovian inhibition was postulated by Robert Isaacson and his colleagues Robert Douglas and Daniel Kimble (e.g., Douglas and Isaacson, 1964; Isaacson and Kimble, 1972). Another change was a striking deficit in the ability to withhold a prepotent behavioral response, a finding taken as support for the response inhibition hypothesis.

Hippocampectomized rats learned to run down an alley or press a lever for food as quickly as control animals with intact hippocampi, but were deficient in changing this behavior when the circumstances altered, e.g., when food was withdrawn or when an alternate response was rewarded. Interestingly, they were consistently better at learning one particular type of avoidance task, two-way active avoidance. In this task, the animal must learn to run back and forth between two compartments of a shuttle box to escape punishment. This improved learning seemed anomalous in light of the presumed role of the hippocampus in memory. A third deficit was in complex maze learning. While they had no trouble learning to make a turn in a simple T- or Y-maze, they failed in more complex multichoice configurations (Kaada et al., 1961; Kimble, 1963; Kveim et al., 1964). This confused state of affairs continued until around 1970, when several developments took place that together changed the approach to hippocampal theory. These developments involved alterations in concepts about memory, the introduction of new tests for assessing memory, the application of single cell recording techniques to behaving animals, and the development of field potential recording for assessing changes in synaptic strength in hippocampal circuits in vivo.

A critical step forward took place around this time. It was realized that there might be more than one type of long-term memory, only one of which involved the hippocampus (Gaffan, 1974a; Hirsh, 1974; Nadel and O'Keefe, 1974; Olton et al., 1978). Two related ways of classifying human memory proved particularly influential. The first was Endel Tulving's contrast between memories for episodes set in a spatiotemporal context ("episodic memory") as distinguished from those for semantic items such as facts and other context-independent material ("semantic memory") (Tulving, 1972). The second was the related but different distinction between "declarative" and "procedural" memories, which was originally introduced by Terry Winograd (1975) in the field of artificial intelligence, subsequently applied to studies of amnesia by Cohen and Squire (1980), and extensively promulgated by Larry Squire and his colleagues (Squire et al., 1998, 2004). Declarative memory includes both episodic and semantic memory while the procedural memory refers to skills and other stimulus-response habits. Both memory schemes have influenced research on amnesic patients and animal models of amnesia (Chapters 13 and 14).

The second important development around 1970 flowed from the realization that the behavioral tests for animal memory available at that time were not optimal for testing hippocampal function. David Gaffan (1974b) introduced a trial unique object recognition task. Mortimer Mishkin and Jean Delacour (1975a, 1975b) developed a different version of this task that was to become the standard test for recognition memory in the monkey (see Chapter 14). Following the introduction of these more powerful testing paradigms, efforts to establish memory systems became increasingly fruitful. Mortimer Mishkin's leadership of the Laboratory of Neuropsychology at NIMH was especially influential, building a group that used lesions, single-unit recording, and later magnetic resonance imaging techniques to develop ideas about the dorsal and ventral pathways of vision, the latter projecting information to the perirhinal and parahippocampal cortex to then access the entorhinal cortex and hippocampus (Figure 2.11). A healthy competition between Mishkin's group and that of Squire, Zola-Morgan, and colleagues specifically addressed the question of whether a nonhuman primate model could recapitulate the severe memory disturbances of H.M.

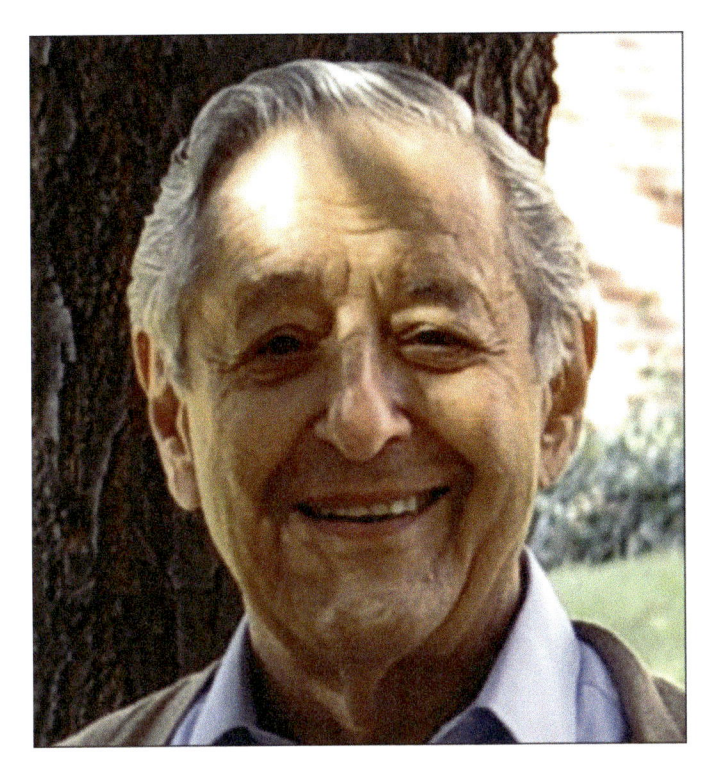

Figure 2.11 Mortimer Mishkin, chief of the Laboratory for Neuropsychology at the National Institutes of Health for many years. Mishkin worked for over 50 years at NIH, where he and many other scientists that he helped to train mapped out the connectivity of the nonhuman primate brain and conducted functional studies. (Courtesy of *The Lancet* and NIH.)

An early assertion by Mishkin (1978) was that only an animal with bilateral lesions of both the amygdala and hippocampus (like the lesion in H.M.) could reproduce the memory impairment. This was challenged by the Squire and Zola-Morgan group, who found that damage to the hippocampus or to the closely related perirhinal and parahippocampal cortices produced a memory impairment in the nonhuman primate but damage to the amygdala without involvement of the hippocampal system did not contribute to the memory loss (see Chapter 14 for a full discussion of this important debate).

We have provided a brief overview of some of the key historical findings concerning the function of the hippocampal formation up to the contemporary era. While there is widespread agreement that the hippocampus is involved in some aspects of memory, surprises may still emerge about other potential functions. An important example, as noted above, is that the hippocampus has been implicated in the modulation of stress responses through inhibitory projections to the hypothalamus (see Chapter 17).

2.4 Development of Methodological Procedures of General Use

Sydney Brenner mischievously noted that, "Progress in science depends on new techniques, new discoveries and new ideas, probably in that order" (Nature, 5 June, 1980). The hippocampal cortex has served as a test bench for the development of a variety of general neuroscientific analyses and experimental techniques. In keeping with the second aim of the book, we discuss some research areas

where hippocampal neurobiology has been instructive for neuroscience in general:

- first use of chronic extracellular microelectrodes for neuronal studies
- development of stereotrodes and tetrodes for multiple single-unit recording from behaving animals
- interpretation of synaptic field potentials and population spikes as extracellular tools for the analysis of synaptic function.
- pioneering use of intracellular recording for central nervous system neurons
- hippocampal slice preparations
- development of histochemical methods for localization of neurotransmitters and receptor types
- studies of morphological plasticity following selective lesions
- neuroplasticity and transplantation studies
- pharmacological studies of central neurons and synapses

2.4.1 The hippocampus as a test bed for microelectrode work

Many of the standard methods used in neurobiology were developed in the peripheral or autonomic nervous systems or in muscle tissue. Recording from single nerve fibers was pioneered by Edgar Adrian and Yngve Zotterman (1926), working on the chorda tympani and lingual nerves. Microelectrodes were developed in studies of cardiac and skeletal muscle by Ralph Gerard's group in Chicago (Ling and Gerard, 1949). In the spinal cord, Chandler McC. Brooks and John Eccles (1947) used microelectrodes to detect what they called a focal potential, a field potential generated by monosynaptic activation of motoneurons by volleys in muscle afferent fibers.

However, the first use of microelectrodes in the brain for extracellular recording of single nerve cell discharges was in the hippocampus (Renshaw et al., 1940). They had greater success in detecting activity of single nerve cells in the hippocampus than in neocortex, possibly because cortex was more depressed at the levels of pentobarbital anesthesia used. In the hippocampus, these authors recorded spontaneous and evoked discharges of what they called "axon-like spikes." In their description they said: "what is evidently the discharge of the same unit—they recur repeatedly with the same waveform" (p. 90). In describing the individual elements with a constant amplitude and predominantly negative polarity they used what later became classic criteria for identification of individual nerve cell discharges. Renshaw et al. (1940) localized such discharges to elements in the pyramidal layer and concluded that the "axon-like spikes" were discharges of individual pyramidal cells. An important development in the analysis of hippocampal function was the use of implanted microelectrodes to monitor single neuronal activity in the hippocampus of the freely moving animal (Hirano et al., 1970; Vinogradova et al., 1970; Ranck 1973; O'Keefe and Dostrovsky, 1971). These experimenters described relationships between cellular activity and a variety of sensory and behavioral parameters, including an account of the "orienting reflex" by the Russian group, who were also the first to note the impact of novelty on hippocampal neural activity (Figure 2.12).

Correlations between the movement of animals and the activity of what he called "theta cells" were made by Ranck (Figure 2.12). Case Vanderwolf (1969), working with rats, discovered that the rhythmic oscillation in the range of 4–10 Hz called "theta" by Jung

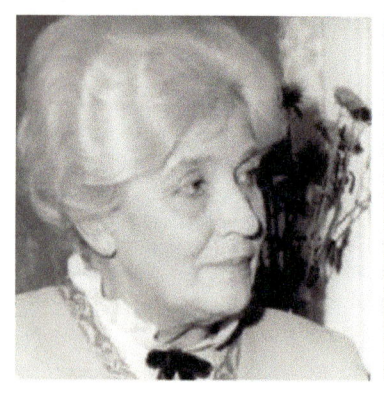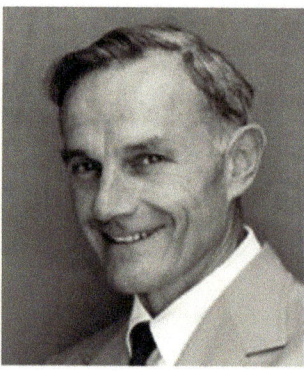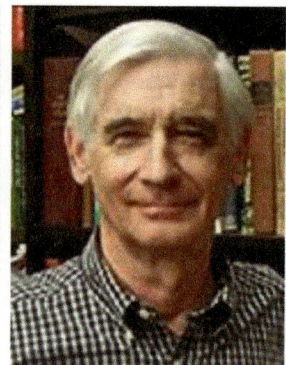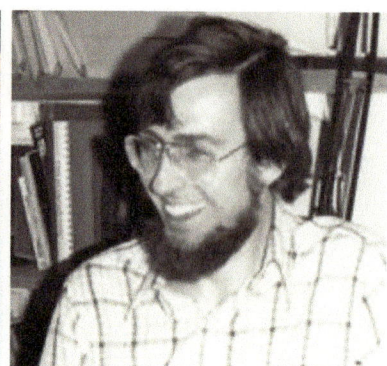

Figure 2.12 Olga Vinogradova, James Olds, Jim Ranck, and John O'Keefe. As described in the text, these neuroscientists were among the pioneers of single-cell recording in the hippocampus in freely behaving animals. (Courtesy of each person.)

and Kornmuller occurred each time the animal initiated a voluntary movement. Whereas Grastyan had linked theta to memory, Vanderwolf adopted a more behavioral description—theta did not occur during movements initiated more automatically or in a reflex-like manner. He also identified two types of theta activity, atropine-sensitive and atropine-insensitive, the former related to attention and the latter to movements (Kramis et al., 1975). Atropine is an alkaloid that blocks muscarinic cholinergic receptors. In elegant analytical studies, Abe Black obtained evidence that the higher-frequency hippocampal theta activity was related to motor activity rather than to learning as such (Black, 1972; Black and Young, 1972; Dalton and Black, 1968; see Chapter 11). Theta activity is also of interest as a means of identifying hippocampal interneurons—the theta cells mentioned above—and relating their activity to behavior (Chapters 8 and 11). In addition, other types of oscillation at different frequencies, including beta and gamma ranges have been studied in hippocampal preparations (Chapter 8).

Another finding that was to become immensely influential was the link between unit activity and an animal's location in an environment. The discovery of place cells by O'Keefe and Dostrovsky (1971; see Figure 2.12) established the link between cell physiology and behavior that gave rise to the cognitive map theory, which has spawned several decades of continuing research into the spatial functions of the hippocampus (O'Keefe and Dostrovsky, 1971; O'Keefe 1976; and Chapters 11 and 14). The theory proposed that the hippocampus in animals is dedicated to spatial memory and mediates navigation in familiar environments. Extension of the theory to humans envisaged the addition of a temporal signal, allowing the hippocampus to act as a spatiotemporal context-dependent (episodic) memory system (O'Keefe and Nadel, 1978). In an early test of the theory, Lynn Nadel, John O'Keefe, and Abe Black (1975) looked carefully at the problems that rats with hippocampal lesions had in avoidance learning. They concluded that deficits were only found when the animals had to learn to avoid places, but not when they were given a clear prominent object or cue to avoid. Subsequently, selective tests for the spatial functions of the hippocampus such as the radial-arm maze and the watermaze were developed (see Chapter 14).

2.4.2 The development of tetrode recording

Following the recording of single cell activity in awake behaving animals (O'Keefe and Dostrovsky, 1971; Ranck, 1973), it became clear that hippocampal cells signaled differently from, for example, visual cortical cells. The latter could be classified as sensitive to contrast

or color and with specific and repeatable patterns to a standardized stimulus delivered to a restricted part of the visual field—the cell's receptive field. In contrast, hippocampal cells showed a much lower rate of discharge, more variability from one trial to the next, and more fuzzy edges of the receptive field (see Chapter 11). Moreover, unlike visual cortical cells, hippocampal place cells could only be identified with distinct types of recording electrodes in freely moving animals. The sharp-tipped electrodes used in acute experiments quickly degenerated when permanently implanted, which limited the period of time for chronic recording. The use of relatively large diameter microwires pioneered by Felix Strumwasser and Jim Olds (Figure 2.12), allowed long-term chronic recordings but made isolation of single units in the densely packed layers of the hippocampus challenging. It also became clear that hippocampal neurons operated in ensembles and that to establish any relation to behavior would require recording from a number of cells at the same time. The solution to both these problems was the use of closely spaced double electrodes called "stereotrodes" (McNaughton et al., 1983) and subsequently, quadruple electrodes called "tetrodes" (O'Keefe and Recce, 1993; Wilson and McNaughton, 1993). Analogous to stereophonic sound recording, which allows the different locations of distinct instruments in an orchestra to be distinguished, such electrode assemblies allow the simultaneous recording of a large number of cells in the freely behaving animal and distinguishes the distinct contributions of different cells. This is achieved, in part, by taking into account the constant shape and form of the discharges on different electrodes of the tetrode of each of the active cells. Furthermore, recordings proved to be stable for several days, facilitating their use during behavioral experiments. An account of the contemporary perspective in this field is offered in Chapter 11. The tetrode technique revolutionized the study of hippocampal neuronal activity and spatial behavior and is now used routinely for chronic recordings in many different brain areas.

2.4.3 Field potential analysis

Field potentials are extracellular responses generated by the synchronous activity of a population of cells. An early study of field potentials was made by Lorente de Nó (1947) studying the signal sequence when a nerve volley traveled antidromically into the hypoglossal motor nucleus. He offered the first theoretical explanation for the generation of such field potentials. In the mid-1950s, several groups started to use field potentials to understand the pattern of activation or inhibition of hippocampal systems.

The stratified histological arrangement of hippocampal neurons and their afferent and efferent axonal projections is highly favorable for field potential studies, allowing both synaptically generated currents and the synchronous action potentials of principal cells to be measured with extracellular electrodes. The dense packing of the cell bodies, with dendrites from a given type of neuron extending into the same region of neuropil, together with the anatomical arrangement whereby excitatory afferents to hippocampal neurons from a given anatomical source project to a restricted section of the dendrites of target cells, are the anatomical features leading to the generation of field potentials. This is most easily seen in the dentate gyrus, where separate projections are restricted to particular regions of the dendrites of target cells—for example, the medial perforant path, containing axons of layer II pyramidal cells in the entorhinal cortex, terminates in en passant synapses on the middle third of the dendrites of granule cells. Weak activation of the medial perforant path elicits a negative extracellular response, which is maximal in the middle third of the molecular layer. With stronger activation a graded spike appears, which reaches a maximum negativity in the granule cell body layer. The practical advantage of field potentials is that an accurate index of synaptic responses can be gained with the simplicity and robustness of extracellular recording (for further details relating to the physics of field potentials see the 1st edition of this book, Box 2.1, pp. 28–29).

If the input is sufficiently strong to discharge the postsynaptic cells, a synchronous extracellular population spike develops; the amplitude of the population spike reflects the number of cells synchronously discharging in response to the afferent volley, and hence the efficacy of the linkage between synaptically evoked depolarization and cell firing. Further information about the location of the synaptic input can be gleaned from the polarity of the evoked field response: the synaptically driven inward current produces maximal negativity in the region of the synaptic input—in the case of the medial perforant path this is in the middle of the molecular layer. The quantitative information about the strength and location of synaptic excitation, coupled to its experimental simplicity, lies at the heart of the popularity of field potential studies.

The final confirmation of the interpretation of field potentials given above came with intracellular recording from dentate granule cells in vivo (Andersen et al., 1966; Lømo, 1971), and later from the comparison of intra- and extracellular responses in hippocampal slices, where intracellularly recorded excitatory postsynaptic potentials (EPSPs) in single CA1 pyramidal cells could be correlated with excitatory field potentials from a population of pyramidal cells in the same area (Schwarzkroin, 1975; Andersen et al., 1980). This now venerable but still widely used extracellular technique has proved particularly useful in the study of hippocampal plasticity, allowing measurement of changes in synaptic efficacy to be followed in the intact animal for many days or weeks, as discussed in Chapter 10.

Brian Cragg and Lionel Hamlyn (1955) were the first to record significant elements of the hippocampal field potentials. However, because they placed their stimulation electrode very close to the recording site, the axonal conduction distance was very short. Consequently, their records of the synaptic component of the field potentials became very brief and difficult to isolate from the rest of the compound signal, or "action potential," in their nomenclature. Nevertheless, they were able to report the first evidence for conduction along apical dendrites and found that the minimal latency was associated with the dendritic position of the activating

synapses. With a commissural input, the shape and conduction of these action potentials were similar to those found with close-range stimulation (Cragg and Hamlyn, 1957).

The large compound action potential following stimulation, later to be called the population spike, was also first noted by Cragg and Hamlyn (1955, 1957), who also gave the first convincing evidence for dendritic conduction in cortical tissue. Although claims to such conduction had been made on the basis of neocortical surface stimulation, the compact and laminated organization of hippocampal circuitry made the interpretation of the records much more compelling. Today, a new and more detailed view of dendritic conduction has emerged, largely due to whole cell patch recordings from dendrites. Again, much of the evidence for dendritic properties has been won from hippocampal preparations (Stuart et al., 1995; Spruston et al., 1995; Johnston et al., 1996; see Chapter 5).

The first to distinguish the synaptically generated component of field potentials from the population spike generated by synchronous action potentials was Per Andersen at the University of Oslo (Figure 2.1). Recording from various dendritic positions, Andersen (1960) described how commissural fibers to CA1 and CA3 gave a local negative field potential in exactly those strata where Theodor Blackstad (1956) had found that the relevant fibers terminated. Such a negative field potential was taken as a sign of excitatory synaptic activity and was called a "field excitatory postsynaptic potential" (fEPSP). Above a given strength, the fEPSP is interrupted by the population spike, which is generated by the synchronous discharge of pyramidal cells. This interpretation was supported by the observation that the great majority of synaptically activated unitary cell discharges fell within the time envelope of the population spike (Andersen et al., 1971a).

When a small bundle of the Schaffer collaterals is electrically stimulated, the amplitude of the synaptic potentials shows a characteristic distribution over the CA1 region. Signals can be detected in the whole transverse extension of CA1. However, within the borders of CA3 and the subiculum, the largest amplitudes are detected along a strip oriented nearly transversely to the longitudinal axis of the hippocampus with responses decreasing on either side, the range spanning nearly half of the length of the hippocampus. With stronger stimulation, the synaptic potentials generate a population spike, the distribution of which displays the same orientation but with more restricted longitudinal distribution (Andersen et al., 1971b). This general arrangement can be found in all four pathways studied: the perforant path, the mossy fibers, the Schaffer collaterals, and the CA1 axons in the alveus projecting to the subiculum. Named the "lamellar organization," this concept was to receive considerable opposition, mostly on anatomical grounds (see Chapter 3), possibly because the name "lamella" suggests an image of thin slices with sharp borders, like the slices of a bread loaf. Instead, the lamella should be seen only as the main orientation of a set of overlapping bell-shaped regions, with axonal density peaking in a direction approximately orthogonal to the septotemporal axis of the hippocampus (Li et al., 1994). The efficiency of the transverse slice, typically cut in widths of around 400 microns, illustrates this organization, although the spread of fiber orientation allows signals to be elicited in slices cut at a less-than-optimal angle.

In summary, extracellular field potentials can be used as a sensitive and quantitative measure of the intensity of both excitatory and inhibitory synaptic drive, and of the efficacy of postsynaptic activation. The final confirmation of the interpretation of field potentials

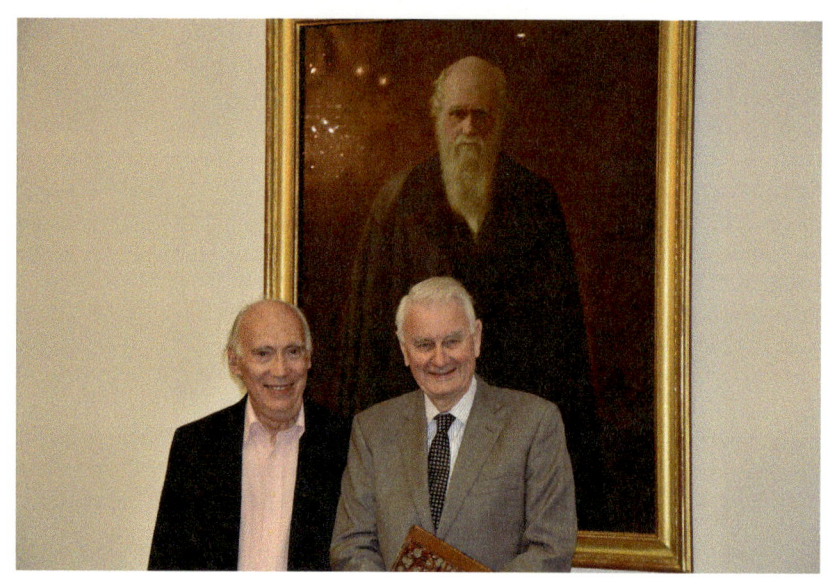

Figure 2.13 Tim Bliss (*left*) and Terje Lømo (*right*) in front of the portrait of Charles Darwin at the Royal Society in London in 2016. They worked together on LTP (long-term potentiation) from 1968 to 1969. (Courtesy of Richard Morris.)

summarized here came with intracellular recording from dentate granule cells (Andersen et al., 1966; Lømo 1971) and from the use of isolated slices, where intracellularly recorded EPSPs in pyramidal cells were correlated with excitatory field potentials in CA1 pyramidal cells (Schwarzkroin, 1975; Andersen et al., 1980). This technique was used by Bliss, Lømo (Figure 2.13), and Gardner-Medwin in their studies of long term potentiation (LTP) in the dentate gyrus of anesthetized (Bliss and Lømo, 1973) and chronically implanted (Bliss and Gardner-Medwin, 1973) rabbits (see Chapter 10).

2.4.4 Pioneers of intracellular recording

The same experimental advantages that facilitated the analysis of field potentials also paved the way for the use of the hippocampus for intracellular recording. The first to succeed in this technically demanding enterprise were Denise Albe-Fessard and Pierre Buser in 1952. They were surprised by the fact that nearly all penetrated cells showed a large and prolonged depolarizing signal. Both its large amplitude and duration rendered interpretation difficult. Initially, they took the response to be an EPSP. Later, it turned out to be an artifactual recording of a large inhibitory postsynaptic potential (IPSP) which, due to chloride diffusion from the recording electrode, resulted in a membrane depolarization. With this approach, however, they did not succeed in recording excitatory synaptic potentials.

The first intracellular records from cortical neurons were made in Oxford by Charles Phillips (1956). He recorded from Betz cells in the precentral gyrus of cats and characterized their responses to both antidromic and orthodromic activation. This too proved a technically difficult task, not least because of the difficulty in finding monosynaptic afferent fibers to stimulate. Fortunately, the situation turned out to be easier in hippocampal preparations. Eric Kandel, W. Alden Spencer, and F. J. Brinley (1961) carried out the first comprehensive intracellular study of hippocampal pyramidal cells. In addition to their analysis of EPSPs and IPSPs (see above), they reported on prepotentials, which were short depolarizing deflections at the very start of the full action potential, interpreted as a sign of dendritically generated action potentials. They also recorded major

features associated with the transition from normal to epileptiform behavior in the form of slow depolarization waves and the occurrence of giant depolarizations with superimposed burst discharges (burst responses) (Kandel and Spencer, 1961a, 1961b) (Figure 2.14). Their discovery was an essential step forward in epilepsy research.

In contrast to the wealth of inhibitory synaptic data, there was a surprising paucity of excitatory synaptic signals. This may be related to the barbiturate anesthesia with its facilitating effect on IPSPs, an effect also noted in hippocampus in a collaboration between Roger Nicoll and John Eccles (Nicoll et al., 1975). As mentioned above in the section on IPSP and EPSP identification, intracellular recording from hippocampal neurons facilitated the identification and localization of inhibitory synapses on the soma and excitatory synapses on dendritic spines.

2.4.5 The hippocampal slice: from seahorse to workhorse

A major technological advance for hippocampal research, and indeed for the field of neurobiology, was the development of the in vitro hippocampal slice preparation. The pioneer in this effort was the neurochemist Henry McIlwain. McIlwain set out to develop a reliable and functional in vitro preparation to investigate how various stimuli and compounds influenced the biochemistry of central nervous tissue (Li and McIlwain, 1957). Despite considerable success using a variety of preparations from the central nervous system, most of the horizontally cut neocortical slices did not allow for a physiologically realistic pattern of afferent impulses. More physiologically relevant data came when he employed slices from the piriform cortex. Here, stimulation of the lateral olfactory tract elicited synaptic and cell activity in neurons of the piriform cortex (Yamamoto and McIlwain, 1966a, 1966b; Richards and McIlwain, 1967; McIlwain and Snyder, 1970). Bliss and Richards (1971) found that field potentials similar to those recorded in the intact animal could be elicited in slices of the dentate gyrus cut parallel the septotemporal axis of the hippocampus. They were nonetheless unable to elicit LTP in these longitudinal dentate slices, it later being shown that addition of a gamma-aminobutyric acid

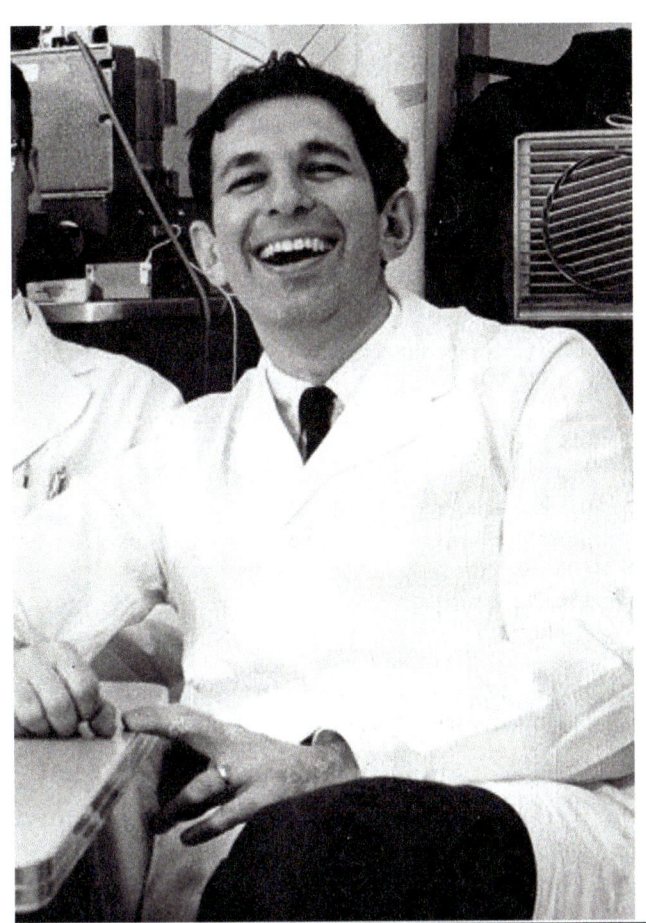

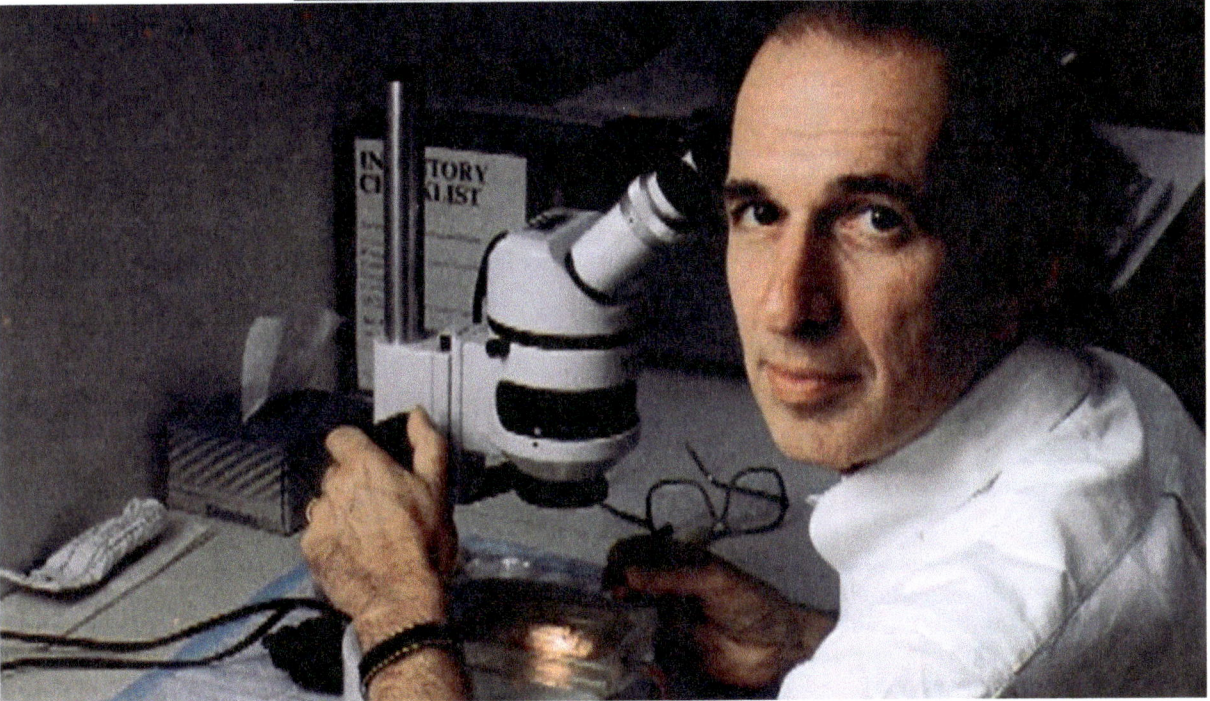

Figure 2.14 Eric Kandel, at Columbia University in 1970, not long after his work with Alden Spencer in which they made the first intracellular recordings in hippocampus. (Courtesy of Professor Tom Carew.)

type A (GABA$_A$) antagonist is required to obtain LTP in the dentate gyrus in vitro. A breakthrough in in vitro studies came with the introduction of the transverse hippocampal slice by Skrede and Westgaard (1971), working in Per Andersen's laboratory. Single cell activity could also be recorded in transvere hippocampal slices from various species (e.g., rat and mouse), and this activity showed similar short-term synaptic plasticity as in intact, anesthetized preparations (Andersen et al., 1972). Distinct advantages included the great stability of the isolated slice preparation, which allowed long-lasting high-quality intracellular recordings to be made from CA1 pyramidal cells (Schwartzkroin, 1975). The first recordings of LTP were made in area CA1 of the transverse slice by Schwartzkroin and Wester (1975) in Andersen's laboratory. Important also was the precision with which electrodes could be placed and lesions performed under visual control, and the possibility of applying and then washing out drugs from the chamber containing the slices. New opportunities arose, since intracellular recording could be combined with iontophoretic delivery of transmitter candidates or blockers from multiple pipettes arranged to hit various parts of the dendritic tree (Schwartzkroin and Andersen, 1975).

2.4.6 Histochemistry was pioneered in the hippocampus

We have become used to the hippocampus being a favored preparation for histological, electrophysiological, or behavioral studies. Less well known is its essential role for the development of neurochemical methodology and for histochemistry. Once again, it was the packing of homogeneous types of cells into compact cell layers and the stratification of afferent fibers and synapses to specific parts of the dendritic tree of principal cells that provided the appeal.

In the middle of the 20th century, virtually all neurochemical analyses were made on homogenized tissue of relatively large samples from various parts of the brain. In an attempt to perform analysis of more discrete CNS elements, Oliver Lowry exploited the synaptic lamination of the hippocampus to perform a detailed neurochemical dissection of cortical tissue. He noted that, "Ammon's horn is a region of the cerebral cortex which is organized in such a manner as to invite quantitative histochemical study." Lowry himself responded to his own invitation by measuring enzyme concentrations and both lipid type and concentration for individual strata of the hippocampal cortex. In a pioneering series of papers (Lowry et al., 1954a, 1954b, 1954c, 1964), Lowry and his colleagues made several fundamental advances. First, they introduced a number of methodological improvements. By dissecting freeze-dried tissue from thin slices of hippocampus under a microscope, they were able to reduce the sample size to 5–10 micrograms of tissue. Second, the accuracy of the enzymatic measurements was greatly improved. The enzymes of interest spanned a large range from acid and alkaline phosphatases through adenosinetriphosphatase, cholinesterases, and aldolase to lactic, malic, and glutamic dehydrogenases. Lowry's group also determined the lipid content and type as related to cortical layers. Third, it was the first instance when a neurochemist explicitly exploited a special histological arrangement for localization of biochemical elements, initially in the hippocampus and then in the cerebellum. His group reported an impressive homogeneity within a single stratum, and often a considerable variation between various strata. In particular, he noted the much higher ATP concentration in the dendritic areas compared with the cell body layer.

Using a similar microdissection method, Storm-Mathisen and Fonnum (1972) were able to give quantitative data for GABA and glutamate concentrations in various hippocampal strata. The amount of GABA was particularly high in the pyramidal layer, in accord with the concentration of inhibitory boutons there. Later

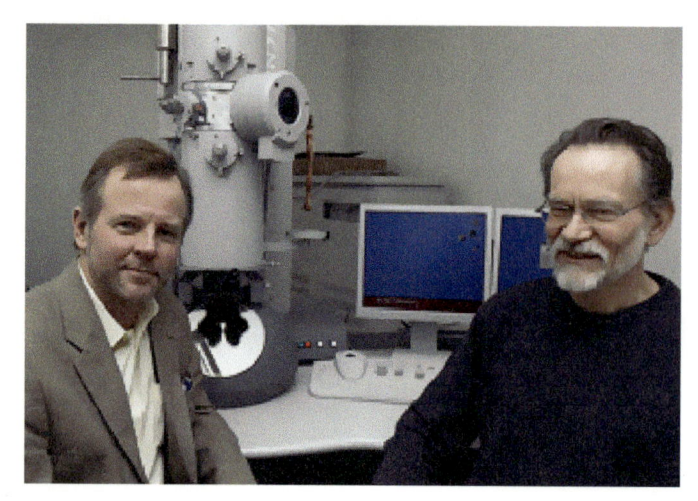

Figure 2.15 Ole Petter Ottersen and Jon Storm-Mathisen, neuroanatomists of the Oslo school, who were the first to visualize glutamate in presynaptic terminals of the hippocampus using electron microscopy. (Courtesy of Ole Petter Ottersen.)

histochemical and immunohistochemical studies largely concentrated on microscopical sections. For this approach, hippocampal tissue has also been a favorite choice. Among these developments, the electron microscopic identification of bouton contents with antibodies raised against an aggregate of amino acids and bovine globulin marked a new and powerful approach (Storm-Mathisen et al., 1972) (Figure 2.15).

After Lowry's pioneering studies, Peter Lewis and Charles Cameron Shute (1967) extended the chemical dissection of brain regions by histochemical analysis of sections from the hippocampus. They showed that the distribution of acetylcholinesterase (AChE) was concentrated in particular laminae, heralding a new approach to chemical analysis of the CNS. This histochemical approach also provided the groundwork for much of the studies on synaptic sprouting that followed in the 1970s (see Chapter 9).

2.4.7 Hippocampal neurons are transplantable with retention of many basic properties

Another remarkable example of neuronal plasticity is the ability of transplanted neuronal cells to emit axonal branches that grow and connect to existing neuronal target cells. The hippocampal formation was the testing ground for analysis of incorporation of embryonic transplants. Following the pioneering work of Geoffrey Raisman on the anatomical plasticity of hippocampal pathways described below (section 2.5.6), Anders Björklund's group (Björklund et al., 1975, 1976) independently investigated the regenerative ability of transplanted monoaminergic tissue to reinnervate normal hippocampal tissue (Figure 2.16). They showed that transplanted tissue containing catecholamine- or acetylcholine-synthesizing neurons could extend axons and reinnervate the hippocampus in a normal fashion. When a graft of noradrenaline-containing neurons, whether from a peripheral source such as the sympathetic superior cervical ganglion or from a central location like the locus coeruleus, was inserted within a noradrenaline-denervated hippocampus, grafted cells were observed to send out axons that entered the hippocampal formation, but only if the endogenous cholinergic septohippocampal fibers were cut (Björklund and Stenevi, 1981, 1984). Lesions of the commissural or perforant path fibers did not

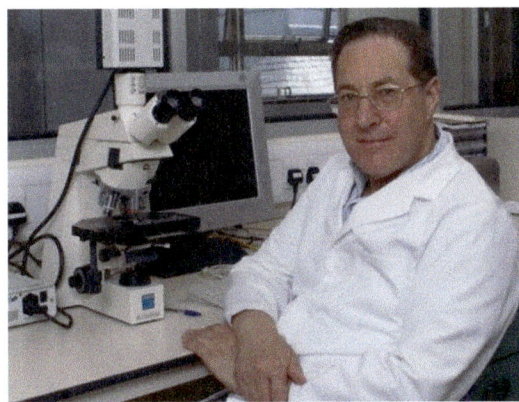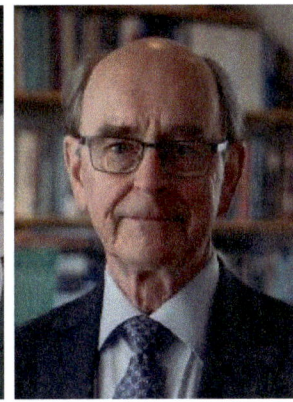

Figure 2.16 Geoffrey Raisman (*left*) and Anders Bjorklund (*right*). Both played major roles in understanding the anatomical plasticity of hippocampal connectivity and pioneered the possible use of neural transplants to correct disorders. (Courtesy of the MRC National Institute for Medical Research, Mill Hill, and Lund University.)

induce such effects. The grafted sympathetic axons respected the lamination borders and formed typical noradrenaline-containing boutons with target neurons.

Similar results were obtained when cholinergically deafferented hippocampi received implants of acetylcholine-containing cells placed in a cavity formed after the original septal region had been removed. Again, regrowth appeared to require vacated synaptic space with which to connect. Both peripherally or centrally located donor neurons were effective and the reinnervation by transplanted cholinergic fibers displayed a homotypic localization. Particularly impressive was the functional recovery of spatial learning ability and the partial restitution of hippocampal place-cell activity (Shapiro et al., 1989) that paralleled the regrowth of cholinergic fibers (Dunnett et al., 1982).

Following these encouraging initial observations, transplantation research in the hippocampal formation flourished. Subsequent efforts were also directed at determining whether cerebellar neurons would survive when transplanted into the hippocampus and, conversely, whether hippocampal tissue might be electrophysiologically active when grafted into the cerebellum. In the latter case, the transplanted hippocampal tissue assumed its original cellular appearance and synaptic lamination and the cells showed electrophysiological properties typical for hippocampus (Hounsgaard and Yarom, 1985). Transplanted material has been proposed as a possible way to repopulate areas of extensive cell loss due to neurodegenerative disease.

2.4.8 Hippocampal cells grow well in culture

The hippocampus also became a favorite source of cells to be grown in various forms of tissue culture. Early successes at defining the parameters for survival and maturation of hippocampal neurons came from the work of Gary Banker in the laboratory of Maxwell Cowan (Banker and Cowan, 1977; Banker and Goslin, 1991). In such cultures both neurons and glial cells are readily identifiable and could be manipulated or recorded as individual elements. A disadvantage that soon emerged, however, was that the original cytoarchitecture disappeared, including such characteristic hippocampal features as laminated inputs with synaptic segregation. This problem led to the development of the organotypic slice by Beat Gähwiler and colleagues (Gähwiler, 1981, 1988; Gähwiler and Brown, 1985). With this technique, thin slices of hippocampal tissue can be grown for several weeks with an impressive capacity

for neuronal growth and differentiation (Zimmer and Gähwiler, 1984). Most neuronal phenomena seen in vivo or in acute slices can be demonstrated in organotypic slices.

2.4.9 Pharmacological analysis of cellular properties

The hippocampus has also been important for the development of ideas on the neuropharmacology of synaptic transmission in the CNS. Following the demonstration of glutamate sensitivity of spinal cord cells by David Curtis and Jeff Watkins (1960), Tim Biscoe and Donald Straughan (1966) found that hippocampal pyramidal cells were sensitive to iontophoretic application of glutamate. Together, these studies suggested what was at the time the radical possibility that glutamate was an excitatory neurotransmitter in the CNS. Exemplar support came from an ingenious study on hippocampal slices in which Nadler et al. (1976) measured Ca^{2+}-dependent release of aspartate and glutamate. Because the release of both compounds was grossly reduced after lesions of commissural or entorhinal fibers, the release is likely to have come from boutons of the two fiber systems, thus supporting the idea that aspartate or glutamate could be excitatory transmitters. Numerous later studies from the University of Bristol group led by Jeff Watkins were instrumental in establishing definitively that glutamate is the major excitatory transmitter of the mammalian brain—a central tenet of contemporary neuroscience.

The postsynaptic inhibition produced by Purkinje cells in the lateral vestibular and deep cerebellar nuclei is mediated by GABA (Obata et al., 1967). As mentioned above, Curtis, Felix, and McLellan (1970) showed that the large and ubiquitous IPSPs in all principal cells of the hippocampus could be blocked by localized application of bicuculline methochloride, establishing that these IPSPs were mediated by $GABA_A$ receptors. The studies of Curtis and his colleagues extended the Obata et al. (1967) results to cortical inhibitory pathways.

2.5 Fundamental research on neurobiological mechanisms of hippocampal function

We now turn to some of the important historical figures who carried out fundamental research on the neurobiological mechanisms underlying hippocampal function. The outcome of some of this research led to general principles of neuroscience (such as the neuron doctrine), whereas other outcomes have established unique features of the hippocampal system (such as the largely unidirectional nature of its intrinsic excitatory connections). In some cases, the motivation for studying the hippocampal formation was to capitalize on some unique aspect of its anatomical and physiological organization that enabled experiments of general interest to neuroscience to be carried out.

2.5.1 Special features of hippocampal anatomy and neurobiology

Several features of the hippocampus have encouraged its use for studies of general neuronal and systems properties relevant to function, some of which have been covered in the previous section on techniques. A short list of additional anatomical and neurobiological features of the hippocampus includes:

- a band of neurons in each subfield, with strictly laminated inputs. This is particularly evident in the rodent hippocampus.
- predominantly, but not exclusively, unidirectional connections between a series of cortical regions.
- extrinsic and intrinsic fibers make en passant contacts with target dendrites, running orthogonal to the main dendritic axis.
- synapses that are morphologically and electrophysiologically highly plastic

Hippocampal studies were important in helping to resolve the 19th-century controversy between the neuron doctrine and the reticular theory. The neuron doctrine proposed that each neuron was an individual cell that contacted, but did not merge with, other target neurons. The reticular theory, on the other hand, posited that nerve cells form a "syncytium," where one cell emits a protrusion or fibril that merges into other cells, thus creating an interconnected network of fibers between large numbers of neurons. This controversy continued for some time because optical microscopes were not able to resolve the spaces (synaptic clefts) that separate pre- and postsynaptic components of connected neurons.

Camillo Golgi, who strongly supported the reticular theory, used observations from the hippocampal formation to bolster his arguments. Employing the "reazione nera" ("black reaction"), as he called his staining technique—later to be called the Golgi method—he repeatedly pointed to the convergence of fine axonal branches from a large number of dentate granule cells to form a dense bundle in the hilus of the dentate gyrus. Here, he believed, filaments from various axons made a large connected feltwork, thus supporting the reticular theory. He also pictured the dendrites of granule cells as being continuous with blood vessels that occupied the hippocampal fissure. Camillo Golgi's most outspoken adversary in the conflict over the neuron doctrine was Ramón y Cajal, whose support of the neuron doctrine came, ironically, from preparations made with Golgi's method. Although he also had many examples from the hippocampal formation, particularly in newborn rodents, Cajal's favorite preparation was the cerebellum. After examining thousands of sections, he became convinced that individual neurons did not form a syncytial network. One particularly important piece of evidence came from observations of individual neurons that were in the process of dying. Adjacent neurons or neurons known to be connected with the dying neurons remained entirely healthy. This

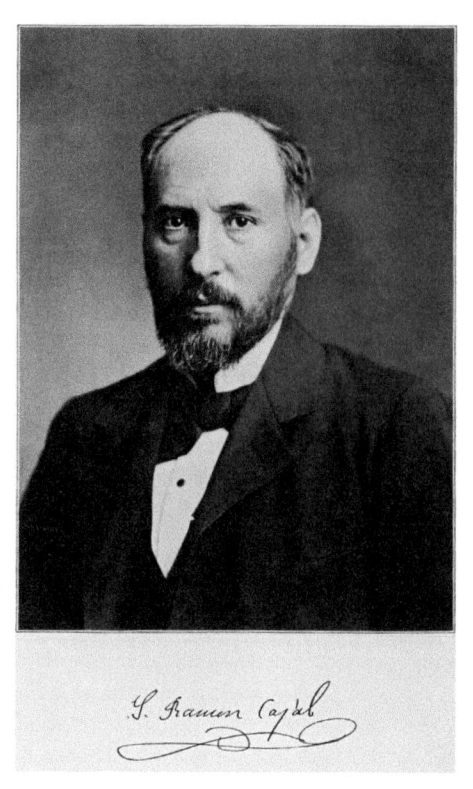

Figure 2.17 Santiago Ramon y Cajal—the pioneering Spanish anatomist—who used Golgi preparations to delineate the cells and connectivity of many brain areas including the hippocampus. (Portrait from the Royal Society London.)

evidence convinced Ramón y Cajal (Figure 2.17) that neurons, like other bodily cells, were individual entities rather than components of interconnected cell groups. The debate lasted for a number of years, involving many participants, and the controversy at times was intense. The final resolution of this classic debate did not occur until the advent of electron microscopy, when Gordon Shepherd's observations conclusively supported the neuron theory by showing neurons as individual entities with narrow gaps (synaptic clefts) between pre- and postsynaptic structures (Shepherd, 1972). Cajal and Golgi shared the Nobel Prize in 1906.

2.5.2 Early neuroanatomical studies of the hippocampus

Hippocampal neuroanatomy benefited from the pioneering investigations of Camillo Golgi and Santiago Ramón y Cajal, but also those of Luigi Sala (1891) and Karl Schaffer (1892). Cajal (1893) described the stratification of the various afferent systems and drew a distinction between cells with long and short axons. This observation made it clear that a hippocampal neuron could influence many different target cells and areas. Even before the formal definition of the synapse by Charles Sherrington in 1897, Ramón y Cajal saw the functional implication of the lamination. He suggested that there was a convergence of afferent inputs onto a single neuron—a notion we take for granted today. His monumental effort, including an analysis of all portions of the hippocampal formation in several animal species, allowed him to propose a now famous functional circuit diagram of this region (Figure 2.18). Following his principle of dynamic polarization—input via the dendrites, and output via the axon and axon collaterals—he placed arrows indicating his view of the direction of impulse flow through the hippocampal formation. Many of these circuit characteristics have stood the test of time. He emphasized the size and variability of the various types of dendritic tree and gave a detailed description of dendritic spines and their distribution.

Contemporaneously with Ramón y Cajal's first studies, the Hungarian anatomist Karl Schaffer, who gave his name to the projection from CA3 cells to target neurons in area CA1, found by meticulous charting of well-impregnated Golgi material not only that axons had short branches but also that some axons could be very long, connecting neurons in neighboring cortical fields (Schaffer, 1892). Nearly 40 years later, Rafael Lorente de Nó (1934), building on the work of his compatriot Ramón y Cajal, greatly extended the analysis of the many hippocampal cell types, and their axonal and dendritic patterns and described many detailed networks of interconnected neurons. Observing the shape of their dendritic trees and their connections, he divided the hippocampal formation into a set of clearly defined divisions and coined the well-known terms CA1 to CA3 after "cornu *ammonis*," the older term for the hippocampus mentioned earlier.

The pioneering neuroanatomists came impressively close to modern-day thinking in their proposed schemata for functional connectivity in the hippocampus. More often than not, the diagrams of Ramón y Cajal (1893, 1911) indicated a correct direction of information flow. Similarly insightful are the detailed drawings of various neurons by Lorente de Nó (1934), in which he used the number of dendritic spines to estimate the relative efficiency of afferents terminating at various positions on the dendrites.

2.5.3 New fiber tracing methods were needed

In parallel with the classical neuroanatomical studies with the Golgi method just described, much work was carried out to trace major afferent and efferent fiber systems in the central nervous system. The early studies exploited the fact that degenerating fibers could be better stained than intact fibers. Temporal gradients in myelinization were also useful. Unfortunately, in the hippocampus, these methods

initially met with limited success. Although the hippocampus contains several fiber systems with moderately thick, myelinated fibers, most of its locally connecting axons, such as the mossy fibers, are much thinner than in other parts of the CNS. These features are probably one reason why the first available methods for experimentally establishing pathways by mapping degenerating fibers did not give satisfactory results. For example, even after appropriate lesions, Vittorio Marchi's original method (Marchi, 1886) stains only a small proportion of degenerating fibers in the alveus and fimbria. In addition, the stained fibers are exclusively among the thicker of those present.

The situation improved greatly when various variants of silver impregnation were applied to lesioned hippocampal pathways. Nauta's method, introduced in 1950, was soon followed by the Nauta and Gygax variant (1954) and Fink and Heimer's method (1967), all of which were remarkably effective in hippocampal tissue. These anatomical techniques revolutionized connectivity studies, a process of innovation that continues to this day. By employing the first variant of Nauta's techniques, Theodor Blackstad (1956, 1958) showed how commissural and ipsilateral afferents to several parts of the hippocampus terminated in layers oriented parallel to the cell layers (Figure 2.19). These data not only verified the general principles established by Ramón y Cajal on stratification of afferent fibers but also showed an astonishing density of presynaptic boutons within the innervated zone. Jens Zimmer continued several of the lines of research initiated by Theodor Blackstad. He and his team were particularly influential in defining aspects of the development and plasticity of the mossy fibers of the dentate gyrus (Zimmer, 1973).

2.5.4 Connectivity between hippocampal subfields is predominantly unidirectional–the dawn of new anatomical tracing techniques

A key aspect of hippocampal connectivity—unidirectionality—was to emerge from these analyses. As the Golgi technique stains a relatively small proportion of the total number of neurons (a feature which allows individual cells to be imaged in their entirety), this picture needed to be complemented by methods giving more quantitative data. Systematic study of each region of the hippocampal

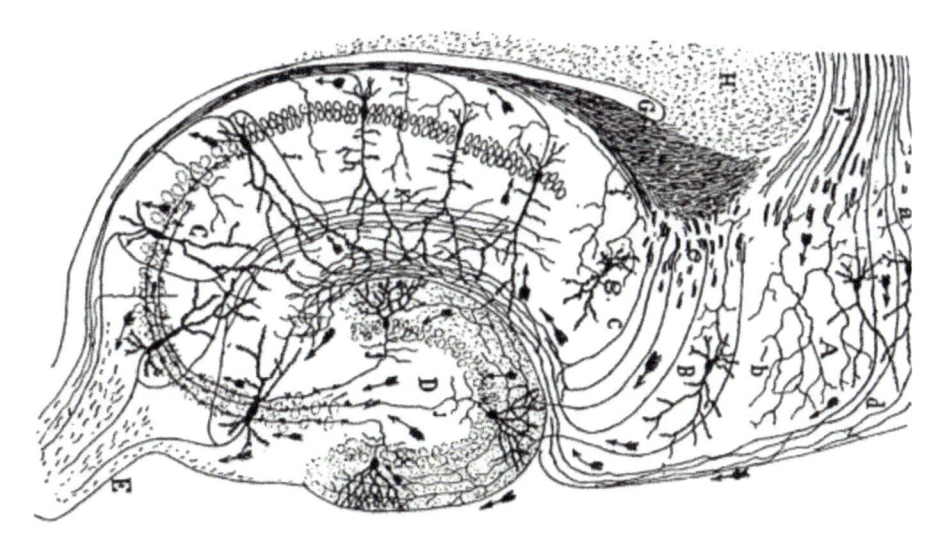

Figure 2.18 Cajal's famous drawing of the hippocampus from his 1911 book *Histologie de systeme nerveux*, published in French in two volumes. The arrows give his interpretation of likely impulse direction. Later functional studies have vindicated his ideas on nearly all points. (Courtesy the Cajal Institute, Madrid.)

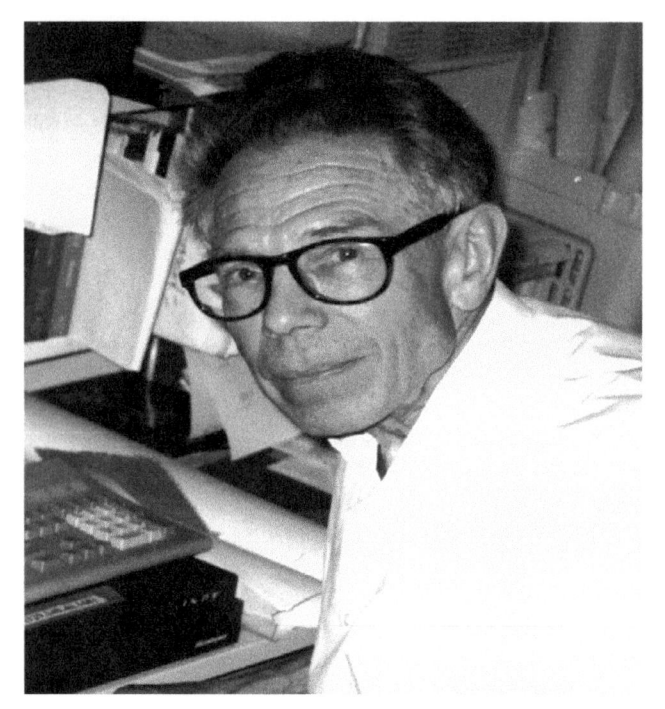

Figure 2.19 Theodor Blackstad, often called the father of modern hippocampal histology because of his groundbreaking studies of external and internal connectivity, made by charting the locations of degenerating fibers through silver staining and electron microscopy. (Courtesy of Jon Storm-Mathisen).

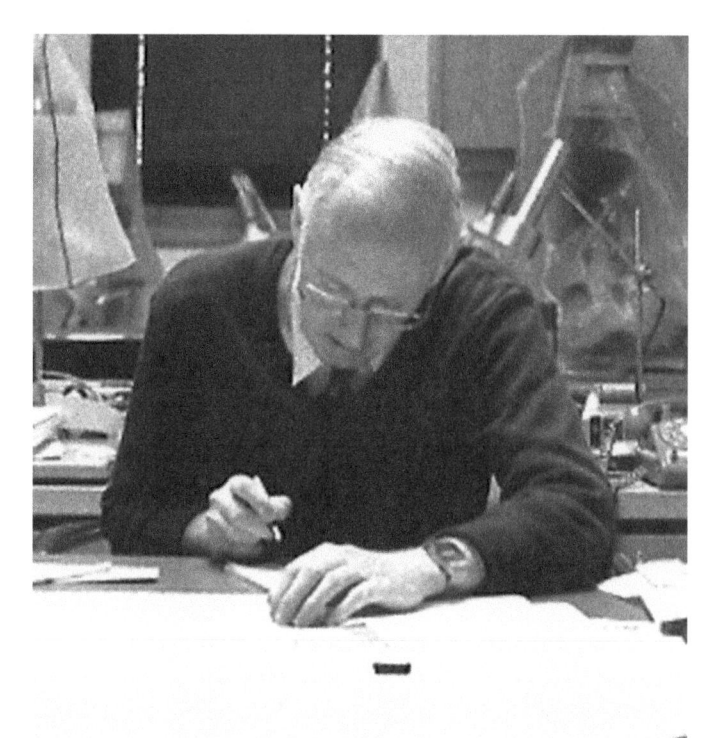

Figure 2.20 W. Maxwell Cowan, the South African–born anatomist, who further developed anatomical studies of the hippocampus and worked with several figures of the contemporary era, including David Amaral, Geoffery Raisman, and Larry Swanson. (Courtesy of David Amaral.)

formation with suitable silver degeneration techniques, later supplemented by electron microscopic and anterograde and retrograde tracing methods, led to the realization that each component of the hippocampal formation projects to its neighboring region but generally does not receive a return pathway from this target (Hjorth-Simonsen, 1973). This was in good accord with previous physiological studies, in which activation of the perforant path led to a sequential activation of CA3, followed by CA1. On the other hand, stimulation within CA1 did not produce synaptic activation in the CA3 region. These findings were the basis for the so-called trisynaptic circuit, comprising the unidirectional excitatory connections from the entorhinal cortex to the dentate gyrus and then sequentially to CA3 and CA1 (Andersen et al., 1966). In this unidirectionality, the hippocampal system differs fundamentally from the reciprocal connectivity of nearly all neocortical areas. This principle of hippocampal neuroanatomy is discussed in detail in Chapter 3, where we also touch on the contemporary idea that predominantly unidirectional connectivity within the hippocampus does not preclude re-entrant circuitry making a major contribution to the dynamics of hippocampal neural activity, most clearly in the extensive re-entrant network between CA3 pyramidal cells. This idea is also developed in Chapters 5 and 12.

As impressive as the degeneration techniques were in advancing our understanding of hippocampal circuitry, they have one major deficit—the fiber of passage problem. When a lesion is produced, it damages not only neuronal cell bodies but also axons that are traveling through the affected area. Thus, new tracing studies using axonal transport of visible markers continued the process of identifying the details of intrinsic hippocampal circuitry. One of the most revolutionary was the use of radioactive amino acids as anterograde tracers—a strategy that was promulgated in the central nervous system by W. Maxwell Cowan and colleagues (Cowan et al., 1972) (Figure 2.20).

Here, they exploited earlier information showing that radioactive proteins could be transported inside axons in both antero- and retrograde directions (Grafstein, 1971; Lasek, 1975). Tritiated amino acids were injected into a location, and resident neurons took them up and produced proteins that were then transported in an anterograde fashion down to the neuron's terminal—also labeling the axons along the way. Since axons do not appreciably take up the injected amino acids, the fiber of passage problem was eliminated.

Cowan, a South African by birth, did his PhD under the mentorship of Thomas Powell at Oxford University. Together, Powell, Cowan, and Geoffrey Raisman were responsible for many of the classical studies of hippocampal and fornix connections (Raisman et al., 1965, 1966). Max Cowan's laboratory in turn spawned a number of hippocampal researchers including Larry Swanson, Brent Stanfield, Clif Saper and David Amaral, who between them have conducted a substantial portion of modern studies on hippocampal connectivity. Led initially by Larry Swanson, the autoradiographic method evolved to using very small and discrete injections placed throughout the hippocampal fields. One important result of this study was the realization that direct hypothalamic projections of the hippocampal formation arose not from the hippocampus proper but from the adjacent subiculum (Swanson and Cowan, 1977).

In addition to the autoradiographic method, new techniques depending on axonal transport of various proteins or plant lectins were also developed (Kristensson and Olsson, 1971; Gerfen and Sawchenko, 1984). The benefit of these techniques was that they allowed a Golgi-like appearance of the cells of origin and the projections of labeled pathways. These techniques have been used extensively in modern studies of intrinsic and extrinsic hippocampal connectivity (e.g., Ishizuka et al., 1990).

2.5.5 The electron microscope brought new opportunities

The first steps toward analysis of the number and types of synapses in the CNS also profited from work on the hippocampus. Following the pioneering work in 1955 of Sanford Palay and George Palade in other brain regions (Palay and Palade, 1955), Lionel Hamlyn (1963) carried out the first electron microscopic analysis of the hippocampus. He provided a comprehensive description of synapses contacting the various portions of the dendritic tree in both CA3 and CA1 pyramidal cells. The introduction of electron microscopy gave an unprecedented view of the detailed structure of the individual cells and synaptic contacts comprising the neural circuitry of the hippocampus and its main target nuclei (Raisman, 1969; see Figure 2.16). In addition, the electron microscope provided a new method for fiber tracing. When a fiber system was lesioned, the resulting degeneration of both fibers and their associated boutons darkened within 1–2 days, a process that could be used for both synapse identification and connectivity studies (Alksne et al., 1966). The early electron microscopic analyses have forged the way for quantitative synaptology studies, prominent among which are those by Kristen Harris and colleagues (reviewed in Harris, 2020).

2.5.6 Neural and synaptic plasticity in response to injury

The term "plasticity" is used to indicate several types of changes. In addition to activity-dependent changes in synaptic efficiency, such as long-term potentiation (see below, and Chapter 10), there are numerous examples of morphological and biochemical changes in the adult brain that occur in response to various stimuli or injury (including changes in cell dimensions and number, in axonal length, branching and connections, and biochemical composition, see Chapter 9).

The hippocampal formation was the first brain region in which axonal sprouting and reactive synaptogenesis were unequivocally demonstrated. Convincing evidence for lesion-induced synaptic reorganization in the hippocampus of the adult rat was described by Geoffrey Raisman (1969). Raisman studied two sets of afferent fibers, one from the hypothalamus and the other from the hippocampus, which converged on cells of the septal nuclei. After long-term lesions

of the fimbria, carrying hippocampal efferents, there was an increase in the number of multiple synapses (boutons in contact with more than one dendritic spine on a target cell), which Raisman interpreted as the result of sprouting from residual axons. Conversely, following removal of hypothalamic afferents, fimbrial fibers were found to contact somata of septal cells, which they rarely do normally. In a further report, Raisman and Field (1973) exploited the fact that fimbria fibers innervate a segment of the lateral septal nucleus on both sides of the midline. A unilateral fimbrial lesion gave rise to a remarkable sprouting from the contralateral fiber system such that the total number of fimbrioseptal synapses remained unchanged. Subsequent work by the same group, using transplantation of embryonic tissue to encourage reinnervation of denervated hippocampal areas (Raisman and Field, 1990), raised interest in the anatomical plasticity of hippocampal afferent and efferent fiber systems. However, the authors also warned that the reorganization was not necessarily adaptive or functionally important.

Nearly simultaneously, lesion-induced sprouting of hippocampal fiber systems was demonstrated with another approach by Gary Lynch, Oswald Steward, Carl Cotman, and their associates (Lynch et al., 1972; Steward et al., 1974; Matthews et al., 1976; Cotman et al., 1977) (Figure 2.21). This group first showed that the AChE-containing septohippocampal fibers innervating the dentate gyrus increased in intensity and distribution if the perforant path fibers to the same region were removed. Electron microscopy confirmed that there was an early postlesion loss of synapses followed by a protracted recovery. After lesions to the perforant path, for example, the maximal reduction of associated boutons in the molecular layer of the dentate gyrus was seen after about 5 days. However, after 2 weeks, there was substantial recovery and after 3 weeks the tissue had regained normal bouton density (Matthews et al., 1976). The remarkably efficient and fast regeneration is an impressive example of the plastic properties of hippocampal neurons and their afferent projections. Later, Christine Gall and Peter Isackson went on to show that the expression of different classes of neurotrophic factor genes are also regulated by physiological activity, by seizures and by neuronal degeneration, reflecting distinct functional demands (Gall and Isaacson, 1989; Isaacson and Gall, 1989). They play critical roles in processes such as activity-dependent neuronal plasticity (including learning) and reactive synaptogenesis following brain

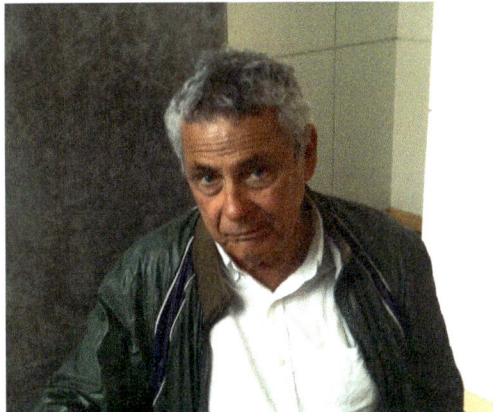 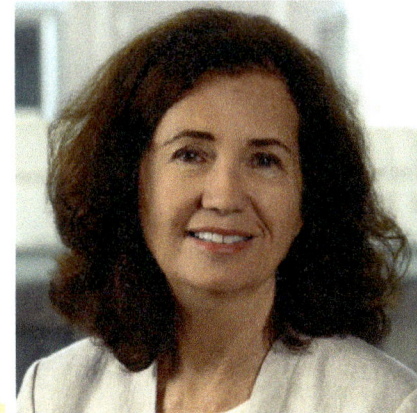 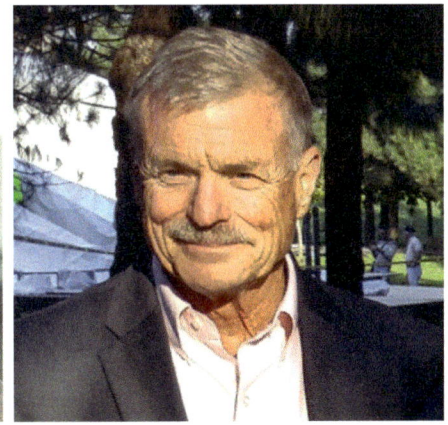

Figure 2.21 Gary Lynch, Christine Gall, and Oswald Steward. figures in the early studies of lesion-induced plasticity in the hippocampus and its underlying mechanisms. Realizing the significance of activity-dependent plasticity, Lynch was an early adopter of brain slice electrophysiology and conducted groundbreaking studies of long-term potentiation and its underlying mechanisms. After observing changes in NGF with activity, Gall was the first to observe altered mRNA expression of BDNF after seizures. Based initially on EM evidence, Steward championed the idea, taken up in Chapter 8, that dendritic protein synthesis may occur. (Courtesy of Professor Gary Lynch.)

damage. Oswald Steward (Figure 2.21) also made major contributions to work concerning how nerve cells create and maintain their connections with each other, and how these synapses are modified after injury, leading to the striking discovery that polyribosomes are localized at the base of dendritic spines (Steward and Levy, 1982; see Chapter 8).

The widely believed view that no neurons are born in the adult brain was challenged by Joseph Altman and Shirley Bayer in the 1960s (Figure 2.22). The original claim for postnatal neurogenesis was based on studies of the granule cells in the dentate gyrus (Altman and Das, 1965) and later extended to the olfactory bulb and cerebellum. It was quantified through progressive and cumulative ^{3}H-thymidine labeling and low-level irradiation (see Bayer, 2016, for details and references). This area of adult neurogenesis is now the subject of extensive research (see Chapter 9).

2.5.7 Ultrastructual identification of excitatory and inhibitory synapses

George Gray (1959) observed that synapses in visual and frontal cortex could be divided into two distinct structural types, which he called type 1 and 2. Type 1 synapses were more heavily stained, and the synaptic specialization was asymmetric in that the presynaptic density was thinner and less intensely stained than the postsynaptic density. Type 1 synapses were usually associated with dendritic spines. Type 2 synapses had pre- and postsynaptic densities with the same moderate staining intensity. These were found mainly in association with dendritic shafts and neuronal somata. As to possible functional consequences of these differences, Gray (1959) was uncertain and concluded, "At present there is no evidence to suggest that type 1 and type 2 synapses are functionally different" (p. 252).

When Gray's colleague Lionel Hamlyn studied hippocampal synapses in the electron microscope, he found the same two synapse types and a similar distribution on dendritic spines and shafts (Hamlyn, 1963). All synapses involving spines were of type 1, while synapses formed on the soma and thicker dendritic trunks or smooth branches were always of type 2. A contemporaneous report by Theodor Blackstad and Per Flood (1963) corroborated these data. What was needed now was a correlation between functional and structural data from the same tissue. Such an opportunity

arose with the advent of intracellular physiological recording from hippocampal neurons, from which key differences in these two types of synapse emerged. It became apparent that inhibitory type 2 synapses are located at the soma of both pyramidal and granule cells in the hippocampus.

Following the initial observations of Kandel and Spencer described above, Per Andersen, John Eccles, and Yngve Løyning (1964a) used a combination of intracellular recording of IPSPs and laminar analysis of the associated field potentials elicited by the same two activation modes. Their results showed that the initial phase of the IPSP in both CA1 and CA3 pyramids and in dentate granule cells was associated with an extracellular positive field potential with a sharp maximum at the cell body layer, indicating synaptic current leaving the somata of many principal neurons. This observation could be explained if basket cells were inhibitory interneurons with synapses terminating on the soma and initial axon. Basket cell synapses were exclusively of Gray's type 2 (Hamlyn, 1963). Andersen, Eccles, and Løyning (1964b) looked for cells that were not antidromically invaded from the alvear fibers and, thus, were not pyramidal cells. They discovered a subset of such neurons that discharged repetitively with a time course corresponding to the rise time of synaptically activated IPSPs in pyramidal and dentate granule cells. The location of such cells corresponded to the basket cells described by Ramón y Cajal (1911) and Lorente de Nó (1934). Hippocampal IPSPs were found to be bicuculline-sensitive by David Curtis, John Felix, and Hugh McLennan (1970), and consequently are mediated by $GABA_A$ receptors.

Thus, basket cells in the dentate gyrus and hippocampus were the first interneurons for which both the functional role and anatomical location of the effective synapses were revealed. Subsequently, the findings from the hippocampal formation served as a template for similar searches in the cerebellum, thalamus, and other parts of the CNS. However, inhibition was far from exclusive to basket cells. Later work, in the cerebellum, hippocampus, and neocortex showed that many more types of inhibitory interneurons and synapses were present (Eccles et al., 1966; Klausberger and Somogyi, 2008; and see Chapters 3 and 7), with Peter Somogyi pioneering the study of single cell connectivity to visualize the differing connection patterns of inhibitory neurons (Figure 2.23). Recent advances

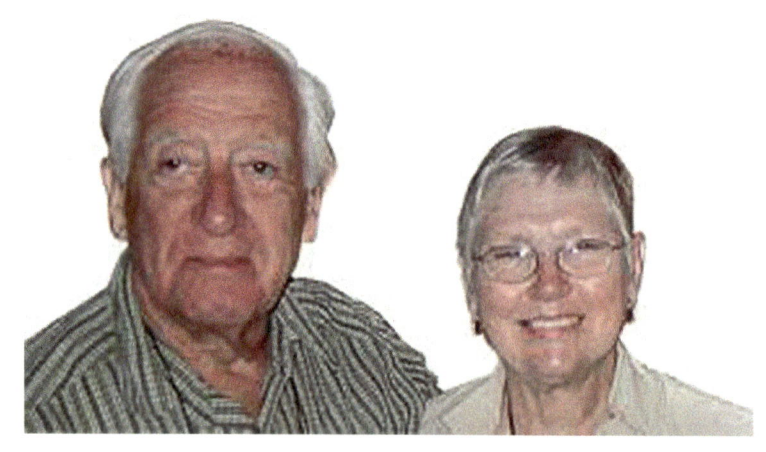

Figure 2.22 Joseph Altman and Shirley Bayer discovered the phenomenon of adult neurogenesis in the dentate gyrus, challenging the then-conventional wisdom that newborn neurons were not to be found in the adult brain. Their work was ignored for many years until it was revisited later with demonstrations also of adult neurogenesis in the olfactory bulb. We devote Chapter 9 to the phenomenon. (Taken from the web.)

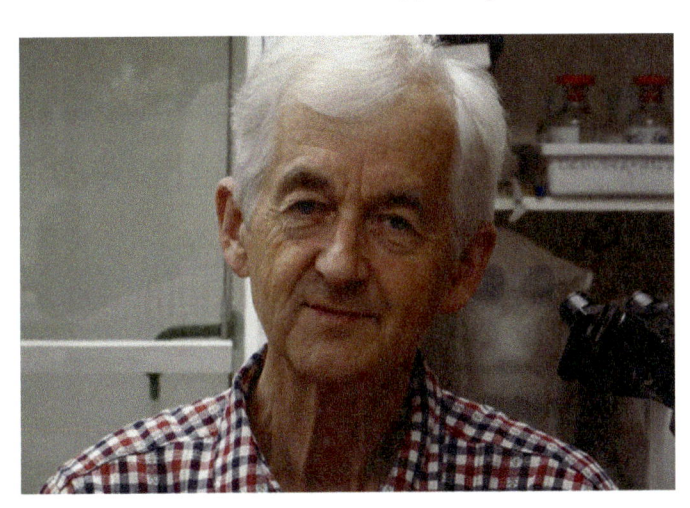

Figure 2.23 Peter Somogyi, the Hungarian neuroanatomist, who used single-cell connectivity and histochemical studies to work out the identity of different classes of inhibitory neurons in the hippocampal formation and their connectivity with excitatory neurons. (Courtesy of Peter Somogyi.)

in transcriptomics-based cell typing techniques continue to reveal the complexity of CA1 inhibitory neuron taxonomy (Harris et al., 2018).

In parallel, it was discovered that excitatory synapses are generally located on dendritic spines and are of Gray type 1. The identification of the morphological and functional characteristics of excitatory synapses was also first carried out in the hippocampus. Kandel et al. (1961) saw examples of EPSPs in cat CA3 and CA2 pyramidal cells in response to stimulation of the subiculum or fimbria but were surprised at how relatively rare such responses were compared with the ubiquitous IPSPs. This relative rarity made them difficult to analyze in detail. In rabbits and rats, field potential recording allowed a better identification of the location of excitatory synaptic activation.

Identification of excitatory synapses and their localization emerged from an analysis of extra- and intracellular responses to various excitatory afferent pathways, along with a new method for marking synapses. In the perforant path projection to granule cells in the dentate gyrus, the first association between an fEPSP and an intracellular EPSP was made by Andersen, Holmqvist, and Voorhoeve (1966), establishing that hippocampal fEPSPs were monosynaptic events and that the synapses in question were excitatory.

Employing a similar approach, several other excitatory synapses were identified. First, activated synapses were identified as excitatory through the use of intracellular recording of monosynaptic EPSPs in rabbits and cats in response to stimulation of four different and independent afferent fiber systems to CA1 and the dentate granule cells. These fiber systems were the perforant path fibers activating dentate granule cells, mossy fibers activating CA3 cells, commissural and local intrinsic fibers in stratum oriens, both types activating CA1 pyramidal cells. In each system, synaptic activation of sufficient intensity gave rise to a localized field EPSP carrying a population spike, proving the excitatory nature of the connection. Following specific surgical lesions to each of these monosynaptic excitatory pathways, the method of Alksne et al. (1966) showed that boutons belonging to all four pathways became electron dense, were closely associated with dendritic spines and were classified as Gray

type 1 (Andersen et al., 1966). Thus, the now widely accepted idea that cortical (and many other) excitatory synapses are of Gray type 1 and are usually located on dendritic spines. originated from these studies in the hippocampal formation.

Thus, within a few years in the 1960s, both inhibitory and excitatory synapses of the hippocampus were identified with respect to location, anatomical type, and function. These findings turned out to be applicable to many other parts of the CNS.

2.5.8 The discovery of place cells and the origin of the theory of the hippocampus as a cognitive map

In 1970, John O'Keefe was recording single units in sensory thalamus, when one of his thalamic electrodes went astray and landed in the hippocampus. He found himself recording hippocampal theta activity and from related theta cells and confirmed the report by Case Vanderwolf (1969) that hippocampal theta had a strong correlation to movements. Intrigued by the existence of clear motor signals in a structure widely believed to be involved in memory following Brenda Milner's description of H.M.'s amnesia, he decided to shift his attention to the hippocampus. He and his student Jonathan Dostrovsky spent several futile months in search of "memory" cells, recording from theta cells and the more prevalent but usually silent pyramidal cells during simple memory tests such as approaching an object or lever pressing for food. They also observed unit activity during simple behaviors such as eating, drinking, exploration, and sleeping. It was during sleep that they first saw sharp wave ripple activity (O'Keefe, 1976) and during exploration that they began to see hints of a spatial correlate for the pyramidal cells.

One day, they saw a clear example of a spatially coded cell that required the animal being in a particular part of the testing box (O'Keefe and Dostrovsky, 1971). In a flash of insight, O'Keefe recognized the possibility that this could be a component of E. C. Tolman's cognitive map, which would provide the neural basis for flexible navigation and could potentially explain many of the effects of hippocampal lesions on running behavior. The hippocampus *was* a memory system, but, at least in the rat, one dedicated to spatial memory. Around this time Lynn Nadel joined the Anatomy Department at UCL, and he and O'Keefe set out to write a small review paper elaborating on this idea, which over several years blossomed into the book *Hippocampus as a Cognitive Map* (O'Keefe and Nadel, 1978). In addition, O'Keefe continued to study the properties of "place" cells including the fact that some of them responded best when the animal found an object in the place or failed to find one that it expected there (misplace cells) (O'Keefe, 1976), and that the cells could be controlled by distal cues that were rotated from one trial to another (O'Keefe and Conway, 1978); see Chapter 11 for further discussion of hippocampal cells in the freely moving animal.

2.5.9 The discovery of long-term potentiation

Prior to the discovery of long-lasting potentiation, many other processes had been studied as potential models for learning. A similar but less persistent phenomenon, posttetanic potentiation (PTP), was a candidate for a number of years. Originally described by Martin Larrabee and Detlev Bronk (1939) in sympathetic ganglia, PTP appeared as a transient enhancement of synaptic responses following a period of high-frequency tetanization of afferent fibers. The main weakness of PTP as a potential mechanism for behavioral learning was its limited duration; in the spinal cord PTP lasted only up to 7 minutes (Lloyd, 1949). This was increased, for up to 30 minutes, by

Alden Spencer (Spencer et al., 1966) using long-lasting tetanization of polysynaptic spinal reflexes.

A limited duration was also the problem in early studies of synaptic plasticity in the hippocampus. Several investigators had noted the remarkable growth of synaptic potentials during a period of high-frequency stimulation (Cragg and Hamlyn, 1955; Kandel and Spencer, 1961b; Gloor et al., 1964). The critical question was: would the enhanced excitability last for a significant period following the cessation of tetanic stimulation? Per Andersen (1960) noted that a period of enhanced synaptic responses to commissural stimulation of CA3 and CA1 cells did indeed follow a short burst of 10–20 Hz stimulation, but the duration was only up to 8 minutes and was initially regarded as a form of PTP.

A few years later, however, it became clear that longer-lasting enhancement could be seen when repeated tetani were given. In 1966, Terje Lømo, a PhD student in Andersen's laboratory, reported a discovery that was to lead to a sea change in the study of the neural basis of learning. In the abstract of a talk that he gave at the annual meeting of the Scandinavian Physiological Society in 1966, (Figure 2.24). Lømo described the long-lasting potentiation of synaptically generated field potentials in the dentate gyrus of the anesthetized rabbit that occurred after repeated episodes of 10–20 Hz stimulation of the perforant path. Thus, unheralded and largely unnoticed, one of the most consequential discoveries of 20th-century neuroscience was ushered into the world. The phenomenon was systematically reinvestigated in the anesthetized rabbit by Lømo and Tim Bliss, working in Andersen's laboratory. Later, in London, Bliss and Tony Gardner-Medwin confirmed that potentiation lasting for weeks could be seen in the awake rabbit. The two sets of results were published together in the *Journal of Physiology* in 1973. An experiment from Bliss and Lømo (1973) is shown in the 1st edition of *The Hippocampus Book* (Figure 10.1). Long-term potentiation (LTP), as the phenomenon came to be known, has spawned a vast literature. Its core features, together with major advances since the first edition, are covered in Chapter 10. Lømo has published his reflections on the discovery of LTP (Lømo, 2018).

2.5.10 Development of computational models of neural networks

In a remarkable set of three papers, published between 1969 and 1971, David Marr developed a theoretical proposal for the mode of operation of three major components of the CNS. Arguably, the triad inaugurated modern computational neuroscience, and the papers incorporate activity-dependent synaptic plasticity as a key mediator of information storage.

Marr started with the cerebellum, for which he proposed the main operation to be a comparison between an initial state of the motor system and the resulting state after an elemental movement had taken place (Marr, 1969). The next paper dealt with the neocortex and how the cortical matrix behaved during perception and

---

XII Scandinavian Congress of Physiology, Turku 1966.
Acta physiol. scand. 1966.68. Suppl. 277.

Lømo, T. (Laboratory of Neurophysiology, Institute of Anatomy, University of Oslo, Norway): FREQUENCY POTENTIATION OF EXCITATORY SYNAPTIC ACTIVITY IN THE DENTATE AREA OF THE HIPPOCAMPAL FORMATION.

Earlier studies on the hippocampus have shown that repetitive stimulation of afferent pathways leads to a marked increase of spike generation. However, the responsible mechanism is largely unknown.

Extracellular responses of dentate granule cells, evoked by repetitive stimulation of the entorhinal area or perforant path fibres, were recorded simultaneously with two microelectrodes, one electrode recording from the layer of perforant path synapses on the granule cell dendrites, the other from the layer of granule cell bodies.

After an initial depression, lasting for a few seconds, repetitive stimulation led to a large potentiated response, compared to the response evoked by a single volley. This effect, frequency potentiation, was seen as an increase of the amplitude and a decrease of the latency of the population spike and as an increase of the rate of rise and amplitude of the extracellular excitatory synaptic potentials. The most effective stimulation frequency was 12 to 15 c/sec. No potentiation was seen with frequencies lower than 6 or higher than 50 c/sec. Presumably, the frequency potentiation is partly due to an increased output of excitatory transmitter. The process may serve as a method for control of nervous activity.

When trains of stimuli (12 c/sec, 10 sec duration) were repeated with intervals of rest of 5—10 min duration, the potentiated responses evoked by the later train were larger, appeared earlier in the train and had shorter spike latencies than the responses evoked by the first train of the series. This represents an example of a plastic change in a neuronal chain, expressing itself as a long-lasting increase of the synaptic efficiency. The effect, which may last for hours, is dependent upon repeated use of the system.

Supported by a US Public Health Service Research Grant NB 04764, from the National Institute for Neurological Diseases and Blindness, which is gratefully acknowledged.

Figure 2.24 The abstract of a talk given by Terje Lømo at a meeting of the Scandinavian Physiological Society in Turku, Finland, in 1966. This contains the first description of long-lasting changes in synaptic function produced by high-frequency stimulation in a monosynaptic cortical pathway. (Reprinted for *Acta Physiologica Scandinavica*.)

attention (Marr, 1970). The third paper contained a description of the mode of operation of the "archicortex" (Marr, 1971), meaning the hippocampal formation. This third paper is probably the best known. Its legacy was assessed in the issue of the *Philosophical Transactions of the Royal Society* celebrating the 350th anniversary of the world's oldest scientific journal (Willshaw et al., 2015). Basing his analysis on its well-known neuronal architecture, Marr proposed that the hippocampus stored a type of simple memory by which the animal could learn from previous experiences to improve important factors for its adapted behavior. Marr was aware of the discovery of LTP and refers to it in a footnote in the 1971 "archicortex" paper. In the process, he described how elemental neurophysiological processes could model certain basic mathematical procedures. For example, inhibition exerted at a dendritic level would cause a relatively small enhancement of the resting membrane potential of the neuron, which could be modeled as a subtraction from the total excitatory drive. In contrast, inhibition at the soma level, produced by basket cells, would trigger a much stronger change of the membrane potential, removing a substantial part of the synaptic drive, that could be described mathematically as a form of division. He also pointed to the recurrent axon collaterals of CA3 as a possible neural basis for attractor networks in which the excitatory interactions between networks of pyramidal cells could form the basis of content-addressable memories and support retrieval of a complete memory from partial information (see Chapter 14, section 14.5). Some electronic memory systems work by retrieving information from a specific address in the computer; a content-addressable system uses the neural representation of one item of an association to retrieve the representation of a separate item with which the first is associated. Such a system is a key element of distributed-associative memory systems. Further description of Marr's work and how it inspired later computational models is found in Chapter 16.

2.6 The hippocampal formation as a test bed for the analysis of several types of neural dysfunction and neuropathology

An era of what funding bodies call "discovery-research" is continuing, but now in parallel with "translational projects" that are intended to take projects from bench to bedside. This trend has unfolded across the entire spectrum of neuroscience, and it is noteworthy that research on the hippocampal formation has played its part in this important development. It is for this reason that this 2nd edition contains four chapters explicitly on translational issues, and frequent reference to applied issues occur throughout the book (Chapters 17–20).

One of the earliest examples is in relation to epilepsy. It is a well-established clinical observation that epileptic patients exhibit a high frequency of temporal lobe foci, often coupled to the neuropathological finding of hippocampal sclerosis (Sommer, 1880; Gastaut, 1956). The hippocampus has thus been a focus of interest in epilepsy research for many years (Schwartzkroin, 1997), being particularly vulnerable to traumatic insults. Spielmeyer (1925) noted that Sommer's sector, which corresponds to the CA1 field of the hippocampus, is a brain structure most vulnerable to ischemic or hypoxic insults. This may be related to a lower level of mitochondrial oxidative enzymes in CA1 pyramidal dendrites than in other

hippocampal subregions (Davolio and Greenamyre, 1995; Kuroiwa et al., 1996).

Hans Berger (1929) gave the first description of the human electroencephalogram (EEG). The EEG has proved invaluable in studies of the electrical activity associated with epilepsy. Richard Jung (1949) reported that electrical polarization (by long-lasting direct current) of the hippocampal formation readily gave rise to electrical after-discharges, similar to those seen during epileptic seizures. He measured the stimulus currents necessary to elicit seizures in various tissues, and concluded that, compared with other cortical areas, the threshold to elicit seizures was considerably less in the hippocampal formation. This observation was in good accord with clinical experience, gained from the electroencephalographic techniques introduced in the mid-1930s, suggesting that many epileptic conditions originated in medial temporal structures.

Progression of an electrographic seizure is often accompanied by a set of depolarizing burst responses, with the extracellular responses characterized by a large local negative wave carrying a number of high-frequency spikes of decreasing amplitude on its back, the so-called burst response (Ajmone-Marsan, 1961). This is associated with epileptiform discharges (Euler et al., 1958; Gloor et al., 1964; Kandel and Spencer, 1961b). After a period with spontaneous high-amplitude burst responses, the electrographic records show diminished activity and all cells cease firing due to a depolarization block. Both in vivo and in vitro hippocampal preparations have been favorite tools in the search for cellular and network properties underlying the generation and spread of epileptiform activity (see Chapter 16). Among these are the epileptiform activity provoked by kainic acid injections in CA3, the GABA blockade by benzyl penicillin, and the effect of ouabain intoxication. An important model for epileptiform activity is kindling, first described by Goddard, McIntyre, and Leech (1969), who elicited seizures by repeated low-strength stimulation of the amygdala. In spite of the ease with which electrographic seizures may be recorded from the hippocampus or the entorhinal area, these areas do not usually develop the kindling phenomenon. While the link between neuropathology of the hippocampus and human epilepsy was forged by Wilhelm Sommer as early as 1880, the precise role of the hippocampus as a generator or victim of epileptic seizures remains unclear. The role of the hippocampal formation in experimental and clinical epilepsy is discussed in Chapter 18.

With respect to the other translationally relevant chapters, we have already touched on the idea that the hippocampus is part of a larger system that reacts to and mediates the impact of stress on facets of cognitive function (Chapter 17). There is also growing interest in the role of the hippocampus in psychiatric disorders such as schizophrenia (Harrison and Weinberger, 2005; see Chapters 10 and 19).

The most prominent example of translational relevance concerns Alzheimer's disease (AD). Early neuropathologists had noted that the hippocampal formation is a major target for pathological changes in patients suffering from dementia caused by AD (Alzheimer, 1907) (Figure 2.25).

The hallmarks of AD are the accumulation of abnormal forms of usually soluble proteins into amyloid plaques composed primarily of amyloid-beta peptides, and neurofibrillary pathology composed of abnormal tau protein in dystrophic neurites surrounding neuritic plaques, neurofibrillary tangles, and neuropil threads. The distribution of neuritic plaques varies widely, but neurofibrillary tangles

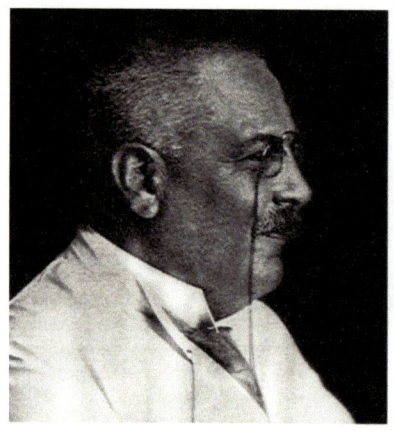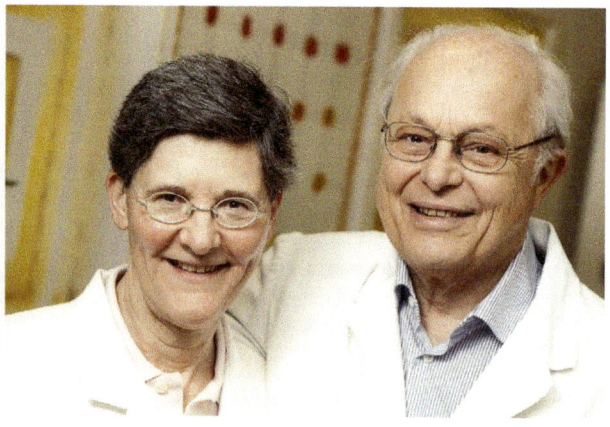

Figure 2.25 Left: Alois Alzheimer, who first identified the disease that bears his name in 1907, and Right: Professors Eva and Heiko Braak who have been pioneers in tracing the pathological progression of the disease. (Courtesy of Heiko Grandel, University of Ulm.)

exhibit a characteristic anatomical distribution pattern, with pathology being first seen in the transentorhinal layer Pre-alpha, then in the medial entorhinal cortex, followed by area CA1 (Braak and Braak, 1991). Later stages are defined by the spread of tau pathology to isocortical association areas. Although pathways associated with the development of amyloid plaque pathology are clearly fundamental for the initiation of the disease, it is the neurofibrillary tau pathology that is most associated with synaptic loss, neuronal degeneration, and cognitive impairment. Despite the great advances made in understanding the causes and consequences of AD, one of the greatest challenges has been to understand the peculiar vulnerability of the hippocampal formation and to identify dysfunction in this region at the earliest stage possible. These advances and challenges are taken up in detail in Chapter 20.

REFERENCES

Adrian ED, Zotterman Y (1926) The impulses produced by sensory nerve-endings: part 2. The response of a single end-organ. *J Physiol (London)* **61**:151–171.

Aggleton JP (1993) The contribution of the amygdala to normal and abnormal emotional states. *Trends Neurosci* **16**:328–333.

Ajmone Marsan C (1961) Electrographic aspects of "epileptic" neuronal aggregates. *Epilepsia* **2**:22–38.

Albe-Fessard D, Buser P (1952) Étude de réponses neuroniques à l'aide de microélectrodes intrasomatiques. *Rev Neurol* **87**:455.

Alksne JF, Blackstad TW, Walberg F, White LEJ (1966) Electron microscopy of axon degeneration: a valuable tool in experimental neuroanatomy. *Ergeb Anat Entwicklungsgesch* **39**:3–32.

Allen WF (1940) Effect of ablating the frontal lobes, hippocampi and occipito-parieto-temporal (excepting pyriform areas) lobes on positive and negative olfactory conditioned reflexes. *Am J Physiol* **132**:81–91.

Altman J, Das GD (1965) Autoradiographic and histological evidence of postnatal hippocampal neurogenesis in rats. *J Comp Neurol* **124**:319–335.

Alzheimer A (1907) Über eine eigenartige Erkrankung der Hirnrinde. *Allg Zeitschr Psychiat Psych-Gerichtl Med, Berlin* **64**:146–148.

Andersen P (1960) Interhippocampal impulses: II. apical dendritic activation of CA1 neurons. *Acta Physiol Scand* **28**:178–208.

Andersen P, Blackstad TW, Lømo T (1966) Location and identification of excitatory synapses on hippocampal pyramidal cells. *Exp Brain Res* **1**:236–248.

Andersen P, Bland BH, Skrede KK, Sveen O, Westgaard RH (1972) Single unit discharges in brain slices maintained in vitro. *Acta Physiol Scand* **84**:1A–2A.

Andersen P, Bliss TVP, Skrede KK (1971a) Unit analysis of hippocampal population spikes. *Exp Brain Res* **13**:208–221.

Andersen P, Bliss TVP, Skrede KK (1971b) Lamellar organization of hippocampal excitatory pathways. *Exp Brain Res* **13**:222–238.

Andersen P, Eccles JC, Løyning Y (1964a) Location of postsynaptic inhibitory synapses on hippocampal pyramids. *J Neurophysiol* **27**:222–238.

Andersen P, Eccles JC, Løyning Y (1964b) Pathway of postsynaptic inhibition in the hippocampus. *J Neurophysiol* **27**:608–619.

Andersen P, Holmqvist B, Voorhoeve PE (1966) Excitatory synapses on hippocampal apical dendrites activated by entorhinal stimulation. *Acta Physiol Scand* **66**:461–472.

Andersen P, Silfvenius H, Sundberg SH, Sveen O (1980) A comparison of distal and proximal dendritic synapses on CA1 pyramids in guinea-pig hippocampal slices in vitro. *J Physiol (London)* **307**:273–299.

Banker GA, Cowan WM (1977) Rat hippocampal neurons in dispersed cell culture. *Brain Res* **126**:397–425.

Banker GA, Goslin K (1991) Primary dissociated cell cultures of neural tissue. In: Culturing Nerve Cells (Banker GA, Goslin K, eds), pp 1–71. Cambridge, MA, MIT Press.

Bard P (1934) On emotional expression after decortication with some remarks on certain theoretical views. *Psychological Review* **4**:Part 1: 309–322; Part 302: 424–449.

Bayer SA (2016) Joseph Altman (1925–2016): a life in neurodevelopment. *J Comp Neurol* **523**:2933–2944.

Bekhterev V (1900) Demonstration eines Gehirns mit Zerstörung der vorderen und inneren Theile der Hirnrinde beider Schlafenlappen. *Neurol Zentralbl* **19**:990–991.

Berger H (1929) Über das Elektroenkephalogramm des Menschen. *Arch Psychiat Nervenkr* **87**:527–570.

Biscoe T, Straughan D (1966) Micro-electrophoretic studies of neurones in the cat hippocampus. *J Physiol (London)* **183**:341–359.

Bishop S, Duncan J, Brett M, Lawrence AD (2004) Prefrontal cortical function and anxiety: controlling attention to threat-related stimuli. *Nature Neurosci* **7**:184–188.

Björklund A, Johansson B, Stenevi U, Svendgaard NA (1975) Re-establishment of functional connections by regenerating central adrenergic and cholinergic axons. *Nature* 253:403–428.

Björklund A, Stenevi U (1981) In vivo evidence for a hippocampal adrenergic neuronotrophic factor specifically released on septal deafferentation. *Brain Res* 229:403–428.

Björklund A, Stenevi U (1984) Intracerebral neural implants: neurological replacement and reconstruction of damaged circuitries. *Ann Rev Neurosci* 7:279–308.

Björklund A, Stenevi U, Svendgaard NA (1976) Growth of transplanted monoaminergic neurones into the adult hippocampus along the perforant path. *Nature* 262:787–790.

Black AH (1972) The operant conditioning of central nervous system electrical activity. In: The Psychology of Learning and Motivation (Bower G, ed), vol 6, pp 47–95. New York: Academic Press.

Black AH, Young GA (1972) Electrical activity of the hippocampus and cortex in dogs operantly trained to move and to hold still. *J Comp Physiol Psychol* 79:128–141.

Blackstad TW (1956) Commissural connections of the hippocampal region in the rat, with special reference to their mode of termination. *J Comp Neurol* 105:417–537.

Blackstad TW (1958) On the termination of some afferents to the hippocampus and fascia dentata. *Acta Anat (Basel)* 35:202–214.

Blackstad TW, Flood PR (1963) Ultrastructure of hippocampal axosomatic synapses. *Nature* 198:542–543.

Bliss TVP, Gardner-Medwin (1973) Long-lasting potentiation of synaptic transmission in the dentate gyrus of the anaesthetized rabbit. *J Physiol (London)* 232:357–374.

Bliss TVP, Lømo T (1973) Long-lasting potentiation of synaptic transmission in the dentate gyrus of the anaesthetized rabbit. *J Physiol (London)* 232:331–356.

Bliss TVP, Richards CD (1971) Some experiments with in vitro hippocampal slices. *J Physiol (London)* 214:7–9P.

Botvinick MM, Braver TS, Barch DM, Carter CS, Cohen JD (2001) Conflict monitoring and cognitive control. *Psychol Rev* 108:624–652.

Braak H, Braak E (1991) Neuropathological stageing of Alzheimer-related changes. *Acta Neuropathol* 82:239–259.

Broca P (1861a) Perte de la parole, ramollissement chronique et destruction partielle du lobe antérieur gauche [Sur le siège de la faculté du langage]. *Bull Soc Anthropol* 2:235–238.

Broca P (1861b) Sur le principe des localisations cérébrales. *Bull Soc Anthropol* 2:190–204.

Brodal A (1947) Hippocampus and the sense of smell. *Brain* 70:179–222.

Brodal A (1981) Neurological Anatomy in Relation to Clinical Medicine. New York: Oxford University Press.

Brooks CM, Eccles JC (1947) Electrical investigations of the monosynaptic pathway through the spinal cord. *J Neurophysiol* 10:251–274.

Brown S, Schäfer EA (1888) An investigation into the function of the occipital and temporal lobes of the monkey's brain. *Philos Trans R Soc B* 179:303–327.

Bush G, Luu P, Posner MI (2000) Cognitive and emotional influences in anterior cingulate cortex. *Trends Cogn Sci* 4:215–222.

Cannon WB (1929) Bodily Changes in Pain, Hunger, Fear and Rage. Appleton-Century-Crofts.

Cohen JD, Squire LR (1980) Preserved learning and retention of pattern-analyzing skill in amnesia: dissociation of knowing how and knowing that *Science* 210:207–210.

Corkin S, Amaral DG, Gonzalez RG, Johnson KA, Hyman BT (1997) H.M.'s medial temporal lobe lesion: findings from magnetic resonance imaging. *J Neurosci* 17:3964–3979.

Corkin S (2013) Permanent Present Tense. Basic Books.

Correll RE, Scoville WB (1967) Significance of delay in the performance of monkeys with medial temporal lobe resections. *Exp Brain Res* 4:85–96.

Cotman C, Gentry C, Steward O (1977) Synaptic replacement in the dentate gyrus after unilateral entorhinal lesion: electron microscopic analysis of the extent of replacement of synapses by the remaining entorhinal cortex. *J Neurocytol* 6:455–464.

Cowan WM, Gottlieb DI, Hendrickson AE, Price JL, Woolsey TA (1972) The autoradiographic demonstration of axonal connections in the central nervous system. *Brain Res* 37:21–51.

Cragg B, Hamlyn LH (1955) Action potentials of the pyramidal neurons of the hippocampus of the rabbit. *J Physiol (London)* 129:608–627.

Cragg B, Hamlyn LH (1957) Some commissural and septal connections of the hippocampus in the rabbit: a combined histological and electrical study. *J Physiol (London)* 135:460–485.

Curtis DR, Felix D, McLellan H (1970) GABA and hippocampal inhibition. *Br J Pharmacol* 40:881–883.

Curtis DR, Watkins JC (1960) The chemical excitation of spinal neurones by certain acidic amino acids. *J Physiol (London)* 150:656–682.

Dalton AJ, Black AH (1968) Hippocampal electrical activity during the operant conditioning of movement and refraining from movement. *Commun Behav Biol* 2:267–273.

Davolio C, Greenamyre JT (1995) Selective vulnerability of the CA1 region of hippocampus to the indirect excitotoxic effects of malonic acid. *Neurosci Lett* 192:29–32.

Douglas RJ, Isaacson RL (1964) Hippocampal lesions and activity. *Psychol Sci* 1:187–188.

Dunnett SB, Low WC, Iversen SD, Stenevi U, Björklund A (1982) Septal transplants restore maze learning in rats with fornix-fimbria lesions. *Brain Res* 251:335–348.

Eccles JC, Llinás R, Sasaki K (1966) The inhibitory interneurons within the cerebellar cortex. *Exp Brain Res* 1:1–16.

Euler C von, Green JD, Ricci G (1958) The role of hippocampal dendrites in evoked responses and after-discharges. *Acta Physiol Scand* 42:87–111.

Ferrier D (1876) The Functions of the Brain. London: Smith, Elder.

Fink RP, Heimer L (1967) Two methods for selective silver impregnation of degenerating axons and their synaptic endings in the central nervous system. *Brain Res* 4:369–374.

Gaffan D (1974a) Loss of recognition memory in rats with lesions of the fornix. *Neuropsychologia* 10:327–341.

Gaffan D (1974b) Recognition impaired and association intact in the memory of monkeys after transaction of the fornix. *J Comp Physiol Psychol* 86:1100–1109.

Gähwiler B (1981) Organotypic monolayer cultures of nervous tissue. *J Neurosci Methods* 4:329–342.

Gähwiler B (1988) Organotypic cultures of neural tissue. *Trends Neurosci* 11:484–489.

Gähwiler BH, Brown DA (1985) Functional innervation of cultured hippocampal neurons by cholinergic afferents from co-cultured septal explants. *Nature* 312:577–579.

Gall C, Isackson PJ (1989) Limbic seizures increase neuronal production of messenger RNA for nerve growth factor. *Science* 245:757–761.

Gastaut H (1956) Étude electroclinique des épisodes psychotiques survenant en dehors des crises clinique chez les épileptiques. *Rev Neurol* 94:587–594.

Gerfen CR, Sawchenko PE (1984) An anterograde neuroanatomical tracing method that shows the detailed morphology of neurons, their axons and terminals: immunohistochemical localization of an axonally transported plant lectin Phaseolus vulgaris-leucoagglutinin. *Brain Res* **290**:219–238.

Gloor P, Vera CL, Sperti L (1964) Electrophysiological studies of hippocampal neurons: 3. Responses of hippocampal neurons to repetitive perforant path volleys. *Electroenceph Clin Neurophysiol* **17**:353–370.

Goddard GV, McIntyre DC, Leech CK (1969) A permanent change in brain function resulting from daily electrical stimulation. *Exp Neurol* **25**:295–330.

Golgi C, Bentivoglio M, Swanson L (2001) On the fine structure of the pes Hippocampi major (with plates XIII–XXIII): 1886. *Brain Res Bull* **54**:461–483.

Grafstein B (1971) Transneuronal transfer of radioactivity in the central nervous system. *Science* **172**:177–179.

Grastyán E, Lissák K, Madarász I, Donhoffer H (1959) Hippocampal electrical activity during the development of conditioned reflexes. *Electroenceph Clin Neurophysiol* **11**:409–430.

Gray EG (1959) Axo-somatic and axo-dendritic synapses of the cerebral cortex: an electron microscope study *J Anat (Lond)* **93**:420–433.

Gray JA (1982) The Neuropsychology of Anxiety: An Enquiry into the Functions of the Septo-Hippocampal System. Oxford University Press, Oxford.

Green JD, Adey WR (1956) Electrophysiological studies of hippocampal connections and excitability. *Electroenceph Clin Neurophysiol* **8**:245–263.

Green JD, Arduini AA (1954) Electrophysiological studies of hippocampal connections and excitability. *Electroenceph Clin Neurophysiol* **17**:533–557.

Gudden JBA, von (1896) Klinische und anatomische Beiträge zur Kenntniss der multiplen Alcoholneuritis nebst Bemerkungen über die Regenerationsvorgänge in periphern Nervensystem *Arch Psychiat Nervenkr* **28**:643–741.

Hamlyn LH (1963) An electron microscope study of pyramidal neurons in the Ammon's Horn of the rabbit. *J Anat (Lond)* **97**:189–201.

Harris KD, Hochgerner H, Skene NG, Magno L, Katona L, Bengtsson Gonzales C, Somogyi P, Kessaris N, Linnarsson S, Hjerling-Leffler J (2018) Classes and continua of hippocampal CA1 inhibitory neurons revealed by single-cell transcriptomics. *PLoS Biol* **16**(6):e2006387.

Harris KM (2020) Structural LTP: from synaptogenesis to regulated synapse enlargement and clustering. *Curr Opin Neurobiol* **63**:189–197.

Harrison PJ, Weinberger DR (2005) Schizophrenia genes, gene expression, and neuropathology: on the matter of their convergence. *Mol Psychiatry* **10**(1):40–68; image 5.

Hayman LA, Rexer JL, Pavol MA, Strite D, Meyers CA (1998) Klüver-Bucy syndrome after selective damage of the amygdala and its cortical connections. *J Neuropsych Clin Neurosci* **10**:354–358.

Hirano T, Best P, Olds J (1970) Units during habituation, discrimination learning, and extinction. *Electroenceph Clin Neurophysiol* **28**:127–135.

Hirsh R (1974) The hippocampus and contextual retrieval of information from memory: a theory. *Behav Biol* **12**:421–444.

Hjorth-Simonsen A (1973) Some intrinsic connections of the hippocampus in the rat: an experimental analysis. *J Comp Neurol* **147**:145–161.

Holmes JE, Adey WR (1960) Electrical activity of the entorhinal cortex during conditioned behavior. *Am J Physiol* **199**:741–744.

Hounsgaard J, Yarom Y (1985) Intrinsic control of electroresponsive properties of transplanted mammalian brain neurons. *Brain Res* **335**:372–376.

Insausti R, Amaral DG, Cowan WM (1987) The entorhinal cortex of the monkey: III. subcortical afferents. *J Comp Neurol* **264**:396–408.

Isaacson RL, Kimble DP (1972) Lesions of the limbic system: their effects upon hypotheses and frustration. *Behav Bull* **7**:767–793.

Ishizuka N, Weber J, Amaral DG (1990) Organization of intrahippocampal projections originating from CA3 pyramidal cells in the rat. *J Comp Neurol* **295**:580–623.

Jackson JH (1865) In: Selected writings of John Hughlings Jackson (2 vols). (Taylor J, ed). **12**:346–357. London: Hodder & Staughton, 1932.

Johnston D, Magee JC, Colbert CM, Christie BR (1996) Active properties of neuronal dendrites. *Ann Rev Neurosci* **19**:165–186.

Jung R (1949) Hirnelektrische Untersuchungen über den Elektrokrampf: die Erregungsabläufe in corticalen Hirnregionen bei Katze und Hund. *Arch Psychiat Nervenkr* **83**:206–244.

Jung R, Kornmüller AE (1938) Eine methodik der Ableitung lokalisierter Potentialschwankungen aus subcorticalen Hirngebieten. *Arch Psychiat Nervenkr* **109**:1–30.

Kaada BR, Jansen JJ, Andersen P (1953) Stimulation of the hippocampus and medial cortical areas in unanesthetized cats. *Neurology* **3**:844–857.

Kaada BR, Pribram KH, Epstein JA (1949) Respiratory and vascular responses in monkeys from temporal pole, insula, orbital surface and cingulate gyrus; a preliminary report. *J Neurophysiol* **12**:347–356.

Kaada BR, Rasmussen EW, Kveim O (1961) Effects of hippocampal lesions on maze learning and retention in rats. *Neurology* **3**:844–857.

Kandel ER, Spencer WA (1961a) Electrophysiology of hippocampal neurons: II. After-potentials and repetitive firing. *J Neurophysiol* **24**:243–259.

Kandel ER, Spencer WA (1961b) Excitation and inhibition of single pyramidal cells during hippocampal seizure. *Exp Neurol* **4**:162–179.

Kandel ER, Spencer WA, Brinley FJ (1961) Electrophysiology of hippocampal neurons: I. Sequential invasion and synaptic organization *J Neurophysiol* **24**:225–242.

Kerns JG, Cohen JD, MacDonald AW, Cho RY, Stenger VA, Carter CS (2004) Anterior cingulate conflict monitoring and adjustments in control. *Science* **303**:1023–1026.

Kimble DP (1963) The effects of bilateral hippocampal lesions in rats. *J Comp Physiol Psychol* **56**:273–283.

Klausberger T, Somogyi P (2008) Neuronal diversity and temporal dynamics: the unity of hippocampal circuit operations. *Science* **321**(5885):53–57.

Klüver H, Bucy PC (1937) Psychic blindness and other symptoms following bilateral temporal lobectomy in rhesus monkeys. *Amer J Physiol* **119**:352–353.

Korsakov SS (1889) Étude médico-psychologique sur une forme des maladies de mémoire. *Rev Philos* **28**:501–530.

Korsakov SS (1890) Eine psychische Störung kombiniert mit multiplen Neuritis. *Allg Z Psychiat* **46**:475–485.

Kramis R, Vanderwolf CH, Bland BH (1975) Two types of hippocampal rhythmical slow activity in both the rabbit and the rat: relations to behavior and effects of atropine, diethyl ether, urethane, and pentobarbital. *Exp Neurol* **49**:58–85.

Kristensson K, Olsson Y (1971) Retrograde axonal transport of protein. *Brain Res* **29**:43–47.

Kuroiwa T, Terakado M, Yamaguchi T, Endo S, Ueki M, Okeda R (1996) The pyramidal layer of sector CA1 shows the lowest hippocampal succinate dehydrogenase activity in normal and postischemic gerbils. *Neurosci Lett* **206**:117–120.

Kveim O, Setekleiv J, Kaada BR (1964) Differential effects of hippocampal lesions on maze and passive avoidance learning in rats. *Exp Neurol* **9**:59–72.

Larrabee MG, Bronk DW (1939) Prolonged facilitation of synaptic excitation in sympathetic ganglia. *J Neurophysiol* **10**:139–154.

Lasek R (1975) Axonal transport and the use of intracellular markers in neuroanatomical investigations. *Fed Proc* **34**:59–72.

Lewis PR, Shute CCD (1967) The cholinergic limbic system: projection to the hippocampal formation, medial cortex, nuclei of the ascending cholinergic reticular system and the subfornical organ and supra-optic crest. *Brain* **90**:521–537.

Li CL, McIlwain H (1957) Maintenance of resting membrane potentials in slices of mammalian cerebral cortex and other tissues in vitro. *J Physiol (London)* **139**:178–190.

Li XG, Somogyi P, Ylinen A, Buzsaki G (1994) The hippocampal CA3 network: an in vivo intracellular labeling study. *J Comp Neurol* **339**:181–208.

Ling G, Gerard RW (1949) The normal membrane potential of frog sartorius fibers. *J Cell Physiol* **34**:383–396.

Lloyd DPC (1949) Post-tetanic potentiation of response in monosynaptic pathways of the spinal cord. *J Gen Physiol* **33**:147–170.

Lømo T (1966) Frequency potentiation of excitatory synaptic activity in the dentate area of the hippocampal formation. *Acta Physiol Scand* **68**(suppl. 277):128.

Lømo T (1971) Patterns of activation in a monosynaptic cortical pathway: the perforant path input to the dentate area of the hippocampal formation. *Exp Brain Res* **12**:18–45.

Lømo T (2018) Discovering long-term potentiation (LTP)—recollections and reflections on what came after. *Acta Physiol* 222.

Lorente de Nó R (1934) Studies on the structure of the cerebral cortex: II. Continuation of the study of the ammonic system. *J Psychol Neurol (Lpz)* **46**:113–177.

Lorente de Nó R (1947) Action potential of the motoneurons of the hypoglossus nucleus. *J Cell Comp Physiol* **29**:207–288.

Lowry OH (1964). Morphological and Biochemical Correlates of Neural Activity. New York: Harper and Row.

Lowry OH, Roberts NR, Leiner KY, Wu M-L, Farr AL (1954) The quantitative histochemistry of brain: I. Chemical methods. *J Biol Chem* **207**:1–17.

Lowry OH, Roberts NR, Leiner KY, Wu M-L, Farr AL, Albers RW (1954c) The quantitative histochemistry of brain: III. Enzyme measurements. *J Biol Chem* **207**:39–49.

Lowry OH, Roberts NR, Wu M-L, Hixon WS, Crawford EJ (1954b) The quantitative histochemistry of brain: II. Enzyme measurements. *J Biol Chem* **207**.

Lynch G, Matthews DA, Mosko S, Parks T, Cotman C (1972) Induced acetylcholinesterase-rich layer in rat dentate gyrus following entorhinal lesions. *Brain Res* **42**:311–318.

Marchi V, Algeri EG (1886) Sulle degenerazioni discendenti consecutive a lesioni in diverse zone della corteccia cerebrale. *Riv Sper Freniatr Med Leg Alien Ment* **14**:1–49.

Marr D (1969) A theory of cerebellar cortex. *J Physiol (London)* **202**:437–470.

Marr D (1970) A theory for cerebral cortex. *Proc Royal Soc Lond B* **176**:161–234.

Marr D (1971) Simple memory: a theory for archicortex. *Philos Trans R Soc B* **262**:23–81.

Matthews DA, Cotman C, Lynch G (1976) An electron microscopic study of lesion-induced synaptogenesis in the dentate gyrus of the adult rat: I. Magnitude and time course of degeneration. *Brain Res* **115**:1–21.

McIlwain H, Snyder SH (1970) Stimulation of piriform- and neocortical tissues in an in vitro flow-system: metabolic properties and release of putative transmitters. *J Neurochem* **17**:521–530.

McNaughton BL, O'Keefe J, Barnes CA (1983) The stereotrode: a new technique for simultaneous isolation of several single units in the central nervous system from multiple unit records. *J Neurosci Methods* **8**:391–397.

Mishkin M (1954) Visual discrimination performance following partial ablations of the temporal lobe: II. Ventral surface vs hippocampus. *J Comp Physiol Psychol* **47**:187–193.

Mishkin M (1978) Memory in monkeys severely impaired by combined but not by separate removal of amygdala and hippocampus. *Nature* **273**:297–298.

Mishkin M, Delacour J (1975a) An analysis of short-term visual memory in the monkey. *J Exp Psychol Anim Behav Process* 326–334.

Mishkin M, Delacour J (1975b) Visual discrimination performance following partial ablations of the temporal lobe: II. Ventral surface vs hippocampus. *J Comp Physiol Psychol* **47**:187–193.

Nadel L, O'Keefe J (1974) The hippocampus in pieces and patches: an essay on modes of explanation in physiological psychology. In: Essays on the Nervous System: A Festschrift for Prof J. Z. Young (Bellairs R, Gray EG, eds), pp 367–390. Oxford: Clarendon Press.

Nadel L, O'Keefe J, Black AH (1975) Slam on the brakes: a critique of Altmann, Brunner and Bayer's response inhibition model of hippocampal function. *Behav Biol* **14**:151–162.

Nadler JV, Vaca KW, White WF, Lynch GS, Cotman CW (1976) Aspartate and glutamate as possible transmitters of excitatory hippocampal afferents. *Nature* **260**:538–540.

Nauta W (1950) Über die sogenannte terminale Degeneration in der Zentralnervensystem und ihre Darstellung durch Silberimprägnation. *Schweiz Arch Neurol Psychiat* **66**:353–376.

Nauta WJH, Gygax PA (1954) Silver impregnation of degenerating axons in the central nervous system: a modified technic. *Stain Technol* **29**:91–93.

Nicoll RA, Eccles JC, Oshima T, Rubia F (1975) Prolongation of hippocampal inhibitory postsynaptic potentials by barbiturates. *Nature* **258**:625–627.

Obata K, Ito M, Ochi R, Sato N (1967) Pharmacological properties of the postsynaptic inhibition of the Purkinje cell axons and the action of γ-aminobutyric acid on Deiters neurons. *Exp Brain Res* **4**:43–57.

O'Keefe J (1976) Place units in the hippocampus of the freely moving rat. *Exp Neurol* **51**:78–109.

O'Keefe J, Conway DH (1978) Hippocampal place units in the freely moving rat: why they fire where they fire. *Exp Brain Res* **31**:573–590.

O'Keefe J, Dostrovsky J (1971) The hippocampus as a spatial map: preliminary evidence from unit activity in the freely-moving rat. *Brain Res* **34**:171–175.

O'Keefe J, Nadel L (1978) The Hippocampus as a Cognitive Map. Oxford: Clarendon Press.

O'Keefe J, Recce ML (1993) Phase relationship between hippocampal place units and the EEG theta rhythm. *Hippocampus* **3**:317–330.

Olton DS, Walker JA, Gage FH (1978) Hippocampal connections and spatial discrimination. *Brain Res* **139**:295–308.

Orbach J, Milner B, Rasmussen T (1960) Learning and retention in monkeys after amygdala-hippocampus resection. *Arch Neurol* **3**:230–235.

Palay SL, Palade GE (1955) The fine structure of neurons. *J Biophys Biochem Cytol* **1**:69–88.

Papez JW (1937) A proposed mechanism of emotion. *Arch Neurol Psychiat* **38**:725–743.

Penfield W, Erickson TC (1941) Epilepsy and Cerebral Localization: A Study of the Mechanism, Treatment, and Prevention of Epileptic Seizures. Springfield, IL: Charles C. Thomas.

Phillips CG (1956) Intracellular records from Betz cells in the cat. *Quart J Exp Physiol* **41**:58–69.

Raisman G (1969) Neuronal plasticity in the septal nuclei of the adult brain. *Brain Res* 14:25–48.

Raisman G, Cowan WM, Powell TPS (1965) The extrinsic, commissural and association fibers of the hippocampus. *Brain* 88:963–998.

Raisman G, Cowan WM, Powell TPS (1966) An experimental analysis of the efferent projection of the hippocampus. *Brain* 89:83–108.

Raisman G, Field PM (1973) A quantitative investigation of the development of collateral reinnervation after partial deafferentation of the septal nuclei. *Brain Res* 50:241–264.

Raisman G, Field PM (1990) Synapse formation in the adult brain after lesions and after transplantation of embryonic tissue. *J Exp Biol* 153:277–287.

Ramón y Cajal S (1893) Estructura del asta de Ammon. *Anal Sociedad español Historia natural* 22. Translated to German by A von Kölliker in *Zeitschr wiss Zool* 56.

Ramón y Cajal S (1911) Histologie du système nerveux de l'homme et des vertébrés. Paris: A. Maloine. Reprinted Instituto Ramón y Cajal, Madrid, 1955.

Ranck JB (1973) Studies on single neurons in dorsal hippocampal formation and septum in unrestrained rats. *Exp Neurol* 41:461–455.

Renshaw B, Forbes A, Morison BR (1940) Activity of isocortex and hippocampus: electrical studies with micro-electrodes. *J Neurophysiol* 3:74–105.

Ribot T (1881) Les maladies de la mémoire. Paris: Ballière.

Richards CD, McIwain H (1967) Electrical responses in brain samples. *Nature* 215:704–707.

Ries FA, Langworthy OR (1937) A study of the surface structure of the brain of the whale (*Balaenoptera physalus* and *Physeter catodon*). *J Comp Neurol* 68:1–47.

Rose M (1935) Cytoarchitektonik und Myeloarchitektonik der Grosshirnrinde. Berlin.

Sagar JH, Cohen NJ, Corkin S, Growdon JH (1985) Dissociations among processes in remote memory. *Ann NY Acad Sci* 444:533–535.

Sala L (1891) Zur Anatomie des grossen Seepferdfusses. *Zeitschr wiss Zool* 52.

Schaffer K (1892) Beitrag zur Histologie der Ammonshorn-formation. *Arch Mikr Anat* 39:611–632.

Schreiner K, Kling A (1953) Rhinencephalon and behavior. *Amer J Physiol* 184:486–490.

Schwartzkroin PA (1975) Characteristics of CA1 neurons recorded intracellularly in the hippocampal in vitro slice preparation. *Brain Res* 85:423–436.

Schwartzkroin PA (1997) Origins of the epileptic state. *Epilepsia* 38:853–858.

Schwartzkroin P, Andersen P (1975) Glutamic acid sensitivity of dendrites in hippocampal slices in vitro. *Adv Neurol* 12:45–51.

Schwartzkroin PA, Wester K (1975) Long-lasting facilitation of a synaptic potential following tetanization in the in vitro hippocampal slice. *Brain Res* 89:107–119.

Scoville W, Milner B (1957) Loss of recent memory after bilateral hippocampal lesions. *J Neurol Neurosurg Psychiat* 20:11–21.

Semon R (1908) The Mneme. London (English translation. First German edition 1904).

Shapiro ML, Simon DK, Olton DS, Gage FH, Nilsson O, Björklund A (1989) Intrahippocampal grafts of fetal basal forebrain tissue alter place fields in the hippocampus of rats with fimbria-fornix lesions. *Neuroscience* 32:1–18.

Shepherd GM (1972) The neuron doctrine: a revision of functional concepts. *Yale J Biol Med* 45:584–599.

Shipley MT, Adamek GD (1984) The connections of the mouse olfactory bulb: a study using orthograde and retrograde transport of wheat germ agglutinin conjugated to horseradish peroxidase. *Brain Res Bull* 12:669–688.

Skrede KK, Westgaard RH (1971) The transverse hippocampal slice: a well-defined cortical structure maintained in vitro. *Brain Res* 35:589–593.

Sloan N, Jasper H (1950) Studies of the regulatory functions of the limbic cortex. *Electroenceph Clin Neurophysiol* 2:317–327.

Sommer W (1880) Erkrankung des Ammonshorns als aetiologisches Moment der Epilepsie. *Arch Psychiatry Nervenkrank* 10:631–675.

Spencer WA, Thompson RF, Neilson DRJ (1966) Response decrement of the flexion reflex in the acute spinal cat and transient restoration by strong stimuli. *J Neurochem* 29:221–239.

Spielmeyer W (1925) Zur Pathogenese örtlich elektiver Gehirnveränderungen. *Zeitschr Ges Neurol Psychiat* 99:756–776.

Spruston N, Jonas P, Sakmann B (1995) Dendritic glutamate receptor channels in rat hippocampal CA3 and CA1 pyramidal neurons. *J Physiol (London)* 482.

Squire LR (1998) Memory systems. *CR Acad Sci III* 321:153–156.

Squire LR (2004) Memory systems of the brain: a brief history and current perspective. *Neurobiol Learn Mem* 82:171–177.

Steward O, Cotman C, Lynch GS (1974) Growth of a new fiber projection in the brain of adult rats: reinnervation of the dentate gyrus by the contralateral entorhinal cortex following ipsilateral entorhinal lesions. *Exp Brain Res* 20:45–66.

Steward O, Levy WB (1982) Preferential localization of polyribosomes under the base of dendritic spines in granule cells of the dentate gyrus. *J Neurosci* 2:284–291.

Storm-Mathisen J, Fonnum F (1972) Localization of transmitter candidates in the hippocampal region. *Progr Brain Res* 36:41–58.

Storm-Mathisen J, Leknes AK, Bore AT, Vaaland JL, Edminson P, Haug FM, Otterson OP (1983) First visualization of glutamate and GABA in neurones by immunocytochemistry. *Nature* 301:517–520.

Stuart G, Spruston N, Sakmann B, Häusser M (1997) Action potential initiation and backpropagation in neurons of the mammalian CNS. *Trends Neurosci* 20:125–131.

Swanson LW, Cowan WM (1977) An autoradiographic study of the organization of the efferent connections of the hippocampal formation in the rat. *J Comp Neurol* 172:49–84.

Tulving (1972) Episodic and semantic memory. In: Organization and Memory (Tulving E, Donaldson W, eds), pp 382–403. San Diego: Academic Press.

Vanderwolf CH (1969) Hippocampal electrical activity and voluntary movement in the rat. *Electroencephal Clin Neurophysiol* 26:407–418.

Vinogradova O, Semyonova TP, Konovalov VP (1970) Trace Phenomena in Single Neurons of Hippocampus and Mammillary Bodies. New York: Academic Press.

Weiskrantz L (1956) Behavioral changes associated with ablation of the amygdaloid complex in monkeys. *J Comp Physiol Psychol* 49:381–391.

Wernicke C (1881) Lehrbuch der Gehirnkrankheiten. Volume 2. Berlin: Theodore Fischer.

Willshaw DJ, Dayan P, Morris RGM (2015) Memory, modelling and Marr: a commentary on Marr (1971) "Simple memory: a theory of archicortex." *Philos Trans R Soc Lond B Biol Sci* 370.

Wilson MA, McNaughton BL (1993) Dynamics of the hippocampal ensemble code for space. *Science* 261:1055–1058.

Winograd T (1975) Frame representations and the declarative/procedural controversy. In: Representation and Understanding (Bobrow DG, Collins A, eds), pp 185–210. New York: Academic Press.

Woolley CS, Gould E, Frankfurt M, McEwen BS (1990) Naturally occurring fluctuation in dendritic spine density on adult hippocampal pyramidal neurons. *J Neurosci* 10(12):4035–4039.

Yamamoto C, McIlwain H (1966a) Electrical activities in thin sections from the mammalian brain maintained in chemically-defined media in vitro. *J Neurochem* 13:1333–1343.

Yamamoto C, McIlwain H (1966b) Potentials evoked in vitro in preparations from the mammalian brain. *Nature* **210**:1055–1056.

Zimmer J (1973) Extended commissural and ipsilateral projections in postnatally deentorhinated hippocampus and fascia dentata demonstrated in rats by silver impregnation. *Brain Res* **66**:293–311.

Zimmer J, Gähwiler BH (1984) Cellular and connective organization of slice cultures of the rat hippocampus and fascia dentata. *J Comp Neurol* **228**:432–446.

Zola-Morgan S, Squire LR, Amaral DG (1986) Human amnesia and the medial temporal region: enduring memory impairment following a bilateral lesion limited to field CA1 of the hippocampus. *J Neurosci* **6**:2950–2967.

Zola-Morgan S, Squire LR, Amaral DG (1989) Lesions of the hippocampal formation but not lesions of the fornix or the mammillary nuclei produce long-lasting memory impairment in monkeys. *J Neurosci* **9**:898–913.

3

Hippocampal Neuroanatomy

David G. Amaral, Pierre Lavenex, and Ricardo Insausti

3.0 Introduction to version 2.0

When approaching the update of this chapter on hippocampal neuroanatomy, we were immediately faced with the question, "What is new with hippocampal neuroanatomy?" Obviously, evolution has not had time to modify the structure and connections of the hippocampal formation, and virtually everything that was presented in the first version of this chapter still stands. Yet, that does not mean that nothing is new. Starting in the early 2000s, new molecular techniques had come to the analysis of hippocampal neuroanatomy led mainly by genetic modifications of the mouse. If you could build a mouse in which a class of neurons fluoresces green, it is obviously an advantage in studying their structure and connectivity. This has led both to a validation of many of the classical concepts of hippocampal neuroanatomy and to a refinement that was not possible with classical techniques. Curiously, there is relatively little cross-referencing between the new molecular neuroanatomical findings and the older classical papers—even when they find the same results! This chapter may be viewed as a bridge between the two eras of neuroanatomical investigation. Much of the text included in the first version is also included here, although we have made every effort to be concise in presenting the classical literature. This is necessary in order to have a framework for understanding the more detailed findings made available by the molecular techniques used mainly in mice.

Clearly, given the rich history of hippocampal neuroanatomy, it would be possible to fill several books with the results that have been obtained. The goal of this chapter is to provide a context for much of the remainder of this book that deals with hippocampal function. To be both thorough and concise, we will highlight a number of excellent reviews that have appeared on various facets of hippocampal neuroanatomy.

3.1 Overview

A key concept in biology is that structure determines function. Thus, how the hippocampus is built will determine, in part, what it can do. In this chapter we aim to describe where in the brain the hippocampus is located and what it looks like. What types of neurons are located here and what connections do they form locally and with other brain regions? What is the difference between the hippocampus and the hippocampal formation? Is the organization of the hippocampus similar in the mouse, rat, monkey, and human brains? What, if anything, is different about the human hippocampal formation? Are the principles of neuroanatomical connectivity similar or different from those found in other brain regions? The beautiful and highly organized neuronal architecture of the hippocampus, and the simplicity and orderliness of its major connections, have been seductive features to neuroscientists for decades. Yet, there are very pragmatic reasons why a working knowledge of its neuroanatomy for the hippocampal neuroscientist is important. First, it is likely that certain peculiarities of the neural organization of the hippocampus, such as its highly associational intrinsic connections, provide important clues to its functions. Second, the design of genetic, electrophysiological, pharmacological, and behavioral studies involving the hippocampus will require an increasingly sophisticated knowledge of its boundaries, cell types, connections, chemical neuroanatomy, and idiosyncratic genetic expression patterns.

3.2 The hippocampus is part of a functional brain system called the hippocampal formation

One of the most captivating features of the hippocampus is its neuroanatomy. The relatively simple organization of its principal cell layers, coupled with the highly organized laminar distribution of many of its inputs, has encouraged its use as a model system for many facets of modern neurobiology. Despite more than a century of neuroanatomical study and literally tens of thousands of research articles on the hippocampus, there is still no consensus concerning certain aspects of its nomenclature. Hippocampal researchers tend to follow one of several implicit "views" concerning what the hippocampus is and what it is not. The view adopted in this book is that the hippocampus, or the hippocampus proper, is one of several related brain regions that together constitute a functional system called the hippocampal formation.

The hippocampus proper has three subdivisions that are labeled, CA3, CA2, and CA1 (CA comes from "cornu ammonis," or "horns of the ram," first used by Lorente de Nó, 1934). The other regions of the hippocampal formation include the dentate gyrus, the subiculum, the presubiculum, the parasubiculum, and the entorhinal cortex. Thus, while the title of this book is *The Hippocampus Book*, a more correct, albeit less melodious title, would be *The Hippocampal Formation Book.* The rationale for grouping these distinct brain regions under the term "hippocampal formation" will be developed throughout this chapter.

3.3 Similarities and differences between the hippocampal formation and other cortical areas

In some ways, such as the occurrence of large, pyramidally shaped projection neurons and smaller interneurons, the neural organization of the hippocampal formation resembles neocortical regions. Yet, in other important ways, such as the largely unidirectional passage of information through intrahippocampal circuits and the highly distributed three-dimensional organization of intrinsic associational connections, the neuroanatomy of the hippocampal formation is unique. Even something as fundamental as the relationship of interneurons to projection neurons appears to be distinct in, for example, the dentate gyrus (Espinoza et al., 2018) compared with other cortical areas. While it has often been touted as a heuristically simple model of neocortical organization, this perspective oversimplifies both the hippocampal formation and the neocortex. It is more reasonable to investigate the distinctive neuroanatomical features of the hippocampal formation as potential clues to its specialized functions and the mechanisms by which they are realized.

The distinctive characteristics of hippocampal neuroanatomy lead to the prediction that whatever processes this group of structures carries out, they are likely to be quite different from those performed in other cortical regions. The hippocampal formation, for example, is one of only a few brain regions that receives highly processed, multimodal sensory information from a variety of neocortical sources (Lavenex and Amaral, 2000; Burwell and Witter, 2002). Moreover, its system of widely distributed intrinsic neuronal networks is ideally suited for further mixing or comparing information (Le Duigou et al., 2014). This ability to integrate information from all sensory modalities may thus be a unique attribute of the hippocampus, conferred by the highly convergent-divergent organization of its connections.

3.4 The hippocampal formation has a unique set of unidirectional (with some exceptions) excitatory pathways

A common organizational feature of connections between different regions of the neocortex is that they are largely reciprocal (Felleman and Van Essen, 1991; Zeki, 2018). If cortical region A projects to cortical region B, then region B usually sends a return projection back to A. As first described by Ramón y Cajal (1893), this is clearly not the case for the main connections that link the various parts of the hippocampal formation (Figure 3.1) although there are several subtle exceptions to the unidirectionality of these pathways that we will explore in further detail below. The entorhinal cortex can, for convenience, be considered the first step in the hippocampal formation circuit. The logic behind this will be developed later in this chapter, but the priority afforded to the entorhinal cortex is based on the fact that much of the neocortical input reaching the hippocampal formation does so through the entorhinal cortex (explained in greater detail later in this chapter and in Chapter 12).

Cells in layer II of the entorhinal cortex give rise to axons that project to the dentate gyrus. The projections from the entorhinal cortex to the dentate gyrus form part of the major hippocampal intrinsic pathway called the perforant path. While the entorhinal cortex provides the major input to the dentate gyrus, the dentate gyrus does not project back to the entorhinal cortex. This pathway is, therefore, nonreciprocated, or unidirectional.

Likewise, the principal cells of the dentate gyrus, the granule cells, give rise to axons called mossy fibers that connect with pyramidal cells of the CA3 field of the hippocampus. The CA3 cells, however, generally do not project back directly to the granule cells (but see Scharfman, 2007). In addition, cells in layer II of the entorhinal cortex also project directly to CA3 and CA2. CA3 and CA2 do not project back to the entorhinal cortex (but see Rowland et al., 2013). The pyramidal cells of CA3 and CA2, in turn, are the major source of input to the CA1 hippocampal field via the Schaffer collateral axons. In addition, cells in layer III of the entorhinal cortex also project directly to CA1 and the subiculum. Following the pattern of its predecessors, CA1 does not project back to CA3. CA1 pyramidal cells then project unidirectionally to the subiculum, providing its major excitatory input. And again, the subiculum generally does not project back to CA1 (but see Xu et al., 2016).

Once one reaches CA1 and the subiculum, the pattern of intrinsic connections becomes somewhat more elaborate. CA1, for example, not only projects to the subiculum but also projects to the deep layers of the entorhinal cortex. And whereas the subiculum does project to the presubiculum and the parasubiculum, its more prominent intrahippocampal projection is directed to the deep layers of the entorhinal cortex. However, as we shall see below, different regions of the subiculum give rise to projections to other, different brain regions (Cembrowski, Philips, et al., 2018; Cembrowski, Wang, et al., 2018). Through these connections, both CA1 and the subiculum close the hippocampal processing loop that begins in the superficial layers of the entorhinal cortex and ends in its deep layers. While this overview of the intrinsic connections of the hippocampal formation leaves out many of the facts that make the system substantially more complex, it does serve to emphasize that the hippocampal formation is organized in a fashion that is distinctly different from most other neocortical areas.

3.5 The hippocampal formation of humans and animals—same or different?

Once one has gained a familiarity with the neuroanatomical appearance of the mouse or rat hippocampal formation, it is not difficult to identify each of the major subdivisions in the monkey or human hippocampal formation (Figure 3.2). Although the volume of the hippocampus is about 10 times larger in macaque monkeys and 100 times larger in humans than in rats (Stephan and Andy, 1970), the basic hippocampal architecture is common to all three species. Yet there are also some striking species differences. The compact pyramidal cell layer in the CA1 region of the mouse or rat, for example, is thicker and more heterogeneous in the monkey and human. Whereas this layer is only about 5 cells thick in the rat, it can be more than 30 cells thick in the human. This may be more than a quantitative distinction. Work carried out in mice indicates that the inputs to CA1 pyramidal cells may be determined by their radial position within the layer (Masurkar et al., 2017) and by their

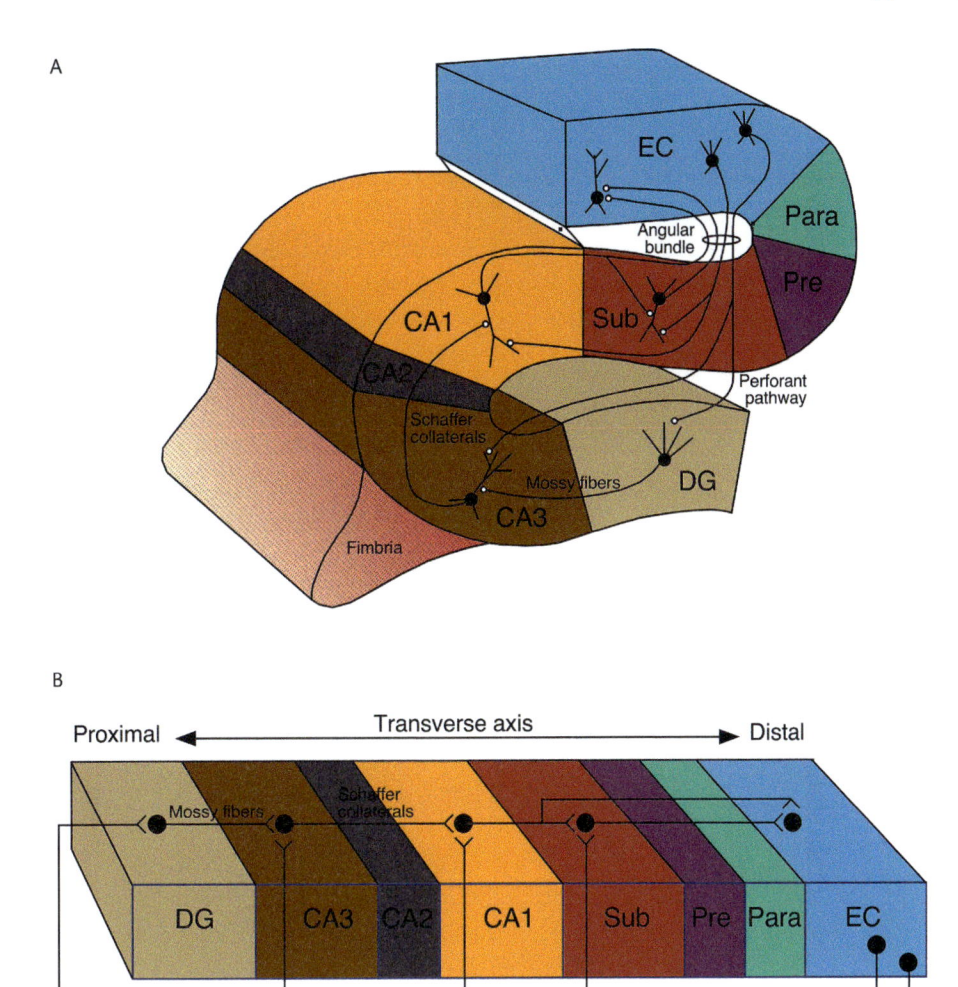

Figure 3.1 Schematic representation of the various cytoarchitectonic fields and major connections that make up the hippocampal formation. (A) Neurons primarily in layer II of the entorhinal cortex project to the dentate gyrus and the CA3 field of the hippocampus via the perforant pathway. Neurons in layer III of the entorhinal cortex project to the CA1 field of the hippocampus and the subiculum via the perforant and alvear pathways (see text for a detailed description). The granule cells of the dentate gyrus project to the CA3 field of the hippocampus via the mossy fiber projection. Pyramidal neurons in the CA3 field of the hippocampus project to CA1 via the so-called Schaffer collaterals. Pyramidal cells in CA1 project to the subiculum. Both CA1 and the subiculum project back to the deep layers of the entorhinal cortex. (B) Block diagram illustrating these projections along the transverse (or cross-sectional) axis of the hippocampal formation; the dentate gyrus is located proximally and the entorhinal cortex distally.

genetic profiles (Dong et al., 2009). If this can be extrapolated to the human hippocampus, one wonders which inputs might target the various strata of the more laminated CA1 pyramidal cell layer. The other region that demonstrates striking species differences is the entorhinal cortex. In the rat, the entorhinal cortex is typically divided into two main, cytoarchitectonically distinct subdivisions, although Insausti et al. (1997) defined as many as six different subdivisions. (For more on the entorhinal cortex see Chapter 12.) In the monkey, seven subdivisions have been identified (Amaral et al., 1987) and in the human brain, recent descriptions (Insausti et al., 1995) recognize eight subdivisions following what is observed in nonhuman primates, although classical cytoarchitectonicists (Rose, 1927) defined as many as 27 subdivisions. Thus, despite the fact that the hippocampal formation is often portrayed as a phylogenetically primitive brain region, it nonetheless demonstrates substantial species evolutionary differences (Barger et al., 2014).

While the patterns of connectivity appear to be generally similar in the rodent and primate brains, there are also striking examples of species differences. The commissural connections of the dentate

gyrus provide one example. In the rat, there is a massive commissural system that provides nearly one-sixth of the excitatory input to the dentate gyrus (Van Groen and Wyss, 1988). In the macaque monkey and presumably in man, however, commissural connections in the dentate gyrus are almost entirely absent (Amaral et al., 1984; Demeter et al., 1985). Another example is the more complex organization of the primate entorhinal cortex, which appears to be associated with stronger interconnections with the associational areas of the neocortex (Munoz and Insausti, 2005). A myriad of other subtle species differences, for example, in the chemical neuroanatomy of the hippocampal formation, have been noted in the literature. And, certain neuroanatomical differences have even been described in different strains of mice that seem too subtle to be worthy of note here, yet could be of enormous practical importance given current interest in the use of genetically modified mice (Lipp et al., 1987; Hausheer-Zarmakupi et al., 1996). An ongoing challenge is to determine how these structural and neurochemical differences affect the functioning of the hippocampal formation, and how detailed information on the functional organization of the hippocampus derived

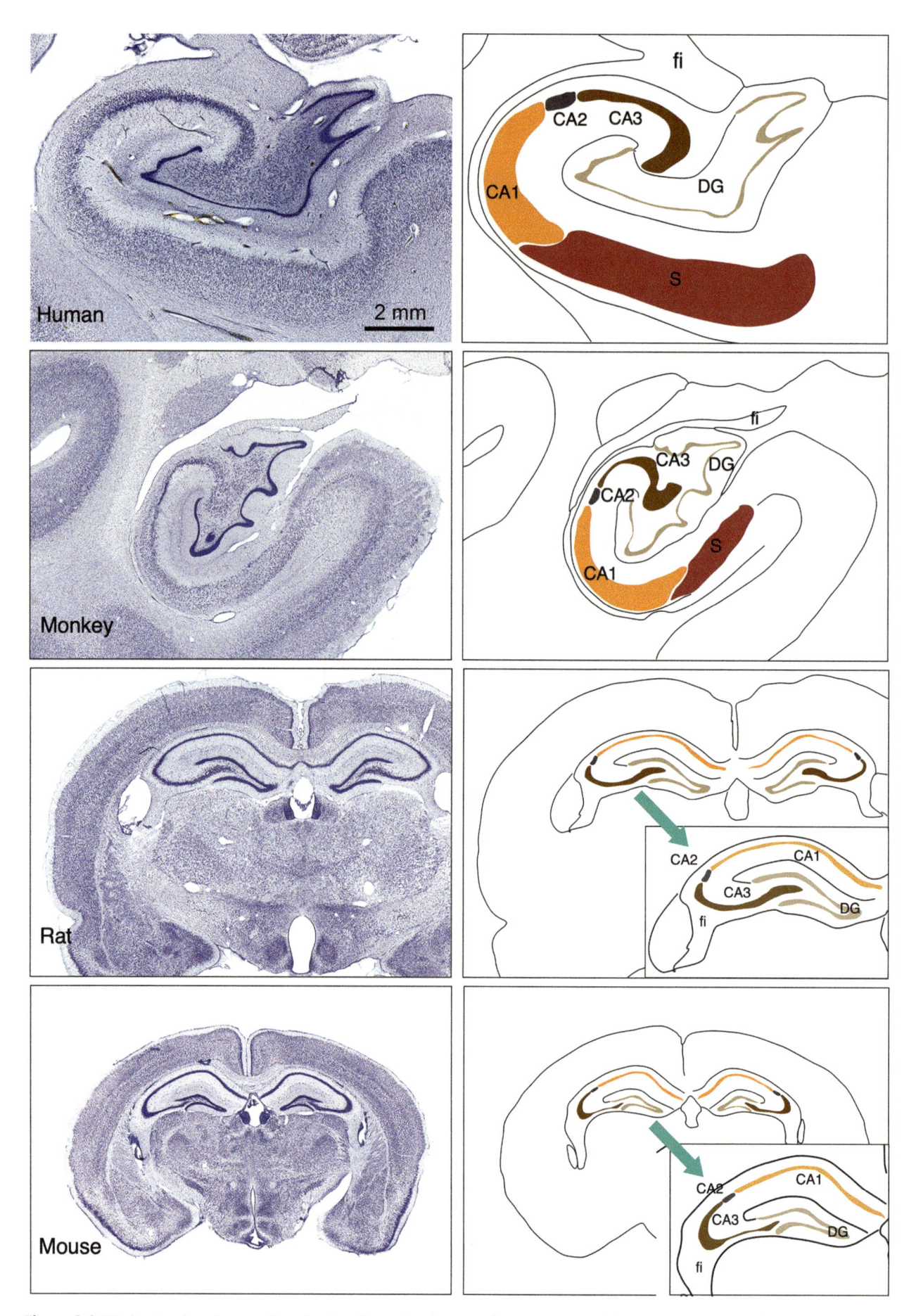

Figure 3.2 Nissl-stained sections and line drawings illustrating the general organization and the similarities of the different subdivisions of the hippocampal formation in the mouse, rat, macaque monkey, and human. These images are all produced at the same magnification. Note the differences in the relative position of the fimbria in the mouse and rat (located lateroventrally) in comparison with the monkey and human (located mediodorsally). Scale bar at top applies to all panels.

from very sophisticated studies carried out in mice can be translated to other species, including humans. Thus, with respect to the question posed in the title of this section, "The hippocampal formation of humans and animals: same or different?," the answer is BOTH.

3.6 Synopsis of the chapter

Our rationale for focusing on the rodent (rat and mouse) hippocampal formation in the first half of this chapter is that much of the available neuroanatomical data have been derived from studies carried out in these animals. While the rat has been used for the vast majority of classical neuroanatomical studies, the mouse has clearly become the choice for molecular biology approaches to understanding the structure and connections of the hippocampal formation. Following a detailed description of regional organization and connectivity of the rodent hippocampal formation, we compare the picture of hippocampal neuroanatomy obtained from studies of the rodent with that of the monkey. In this part of the chapter, we will describe the extensive cortical connections of the entorhinal cortex in the macaque monkey and the prominence of adjacent related brain regions, such as the perirhinal and parahippocampal cortices. We then move on to describe what is known about the structure of the human hippocampal formation.

The chapter concludes with efforts to relate the principles of hippocampal intrinsic circuitry to the flow of information through the hippocampal formation. We also briefly highlight the gaps in our understanding of hippocampal organization in all species and how these may be filled in the future.

3.7 Three-dimensional organization and major fiber systems of the hippocampal formation

The hippocampal formation is positioned quite differently in the rodent and primate brains (Figures 3.3, 3.4, and 3.5). This is due, in part, to the more developed cerebral cortex in primates, which tends to "force" the hippocampal formation into the temporal lobe. While many of the fields of the rodent hippocampal formation are grossly C-shaped and vertically oriented, they tend to be much more linear and horizontally oriented in primates.

3.7.1 The rodent hippocampal formation

The mouse and rat hippocampal formation is an elongated, banana-shaped structure with its long axis extending in a C-shaped manner from the midline of the brain near the septal nuclei (rostrodorsally), over and behind the thalamus into the incipient temporal lobe (caudoventrally) (Figures 3.3, 3.6, 3.7). The long axis of the hippocampal formation is referred to as the septotemporal axis, and the orthogonal axis as the transverse axis. What is not obvious from a surface view of the hippocampal formation is that different regions make up the structure at different septotemporal levels. At extreme septal levels, for example, only the dentate gyrus and the CA3–CA1 fields of the hippocampus are present. About a third of the way back along the septotemporal axis, the subiculum first appears, while the presubiculum and parasubiculum are seen

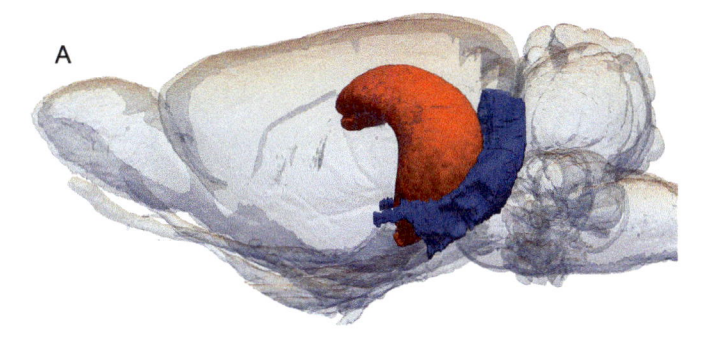

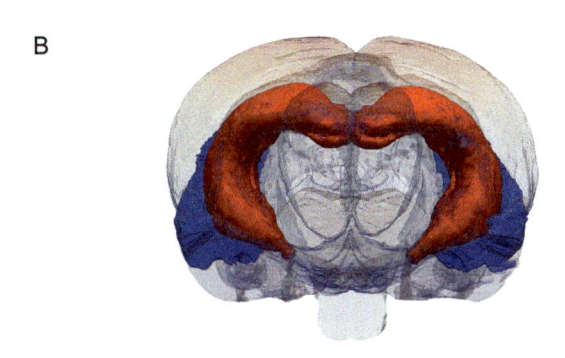

Figure 3.3 Volume-rendered magnetic resonance images of the rat brain illustrating the position of the hippocampus (red) and entorhinal cortex (blue). A illustrates a lateral view of these regions and B illustrates a frontal view. (These images were created by Joshua Lee, PhD, and were based on the high-resolution "Waxholm space atlas of the Sprague Dawley rat brain"; Papp et al., 2014.)

at progressively more temporal levels. The entorhinal cortex is located even further caudally and ventrally. The dorsolateral limit of the entorhinal cortex occurs approximately at the rhinal sulcus, which forms a prominent, rostrocaudally/horizontally oriented indentation on the ventrolateral surface of the rodent brain. This sulcus nominally separates the entorhinal cortex ventrally from the perirhinal and postrhinal cortices dorsally. At rostral levels, however, the perirhinal cortex extends somewhat ventral to the rhinal sulcus and at caudal levels the entorhinal cortex extends just slightly dorsal to the rhinal sulcus.

3.7.2 Major fiber systems of the rodent hippocampal formation

There are several classically defined fiber bundles that either link regions within the hippocampal formation or provide conduits for its inputs and outputs (Figure 3.8). We will describe several of these in this section. We should note that many of the major inputs to the hippocampal formation such as the projections from the perirhinal and parahippocampal cortices to the entorhinal cortex do not have formal names. So, the named fiber systems are in no way the whole story of the hippocampal connectome.

3.7.2.1 Angular bundle

The angular bundle is located between the entorhinal cortex and the presubiculum and parasubiculum. It is the main route taken by fibers originating in the entorhinal cortex as they travel to all septotemporal levels of the other hippocampal fields, particularly the dentate gyrus,

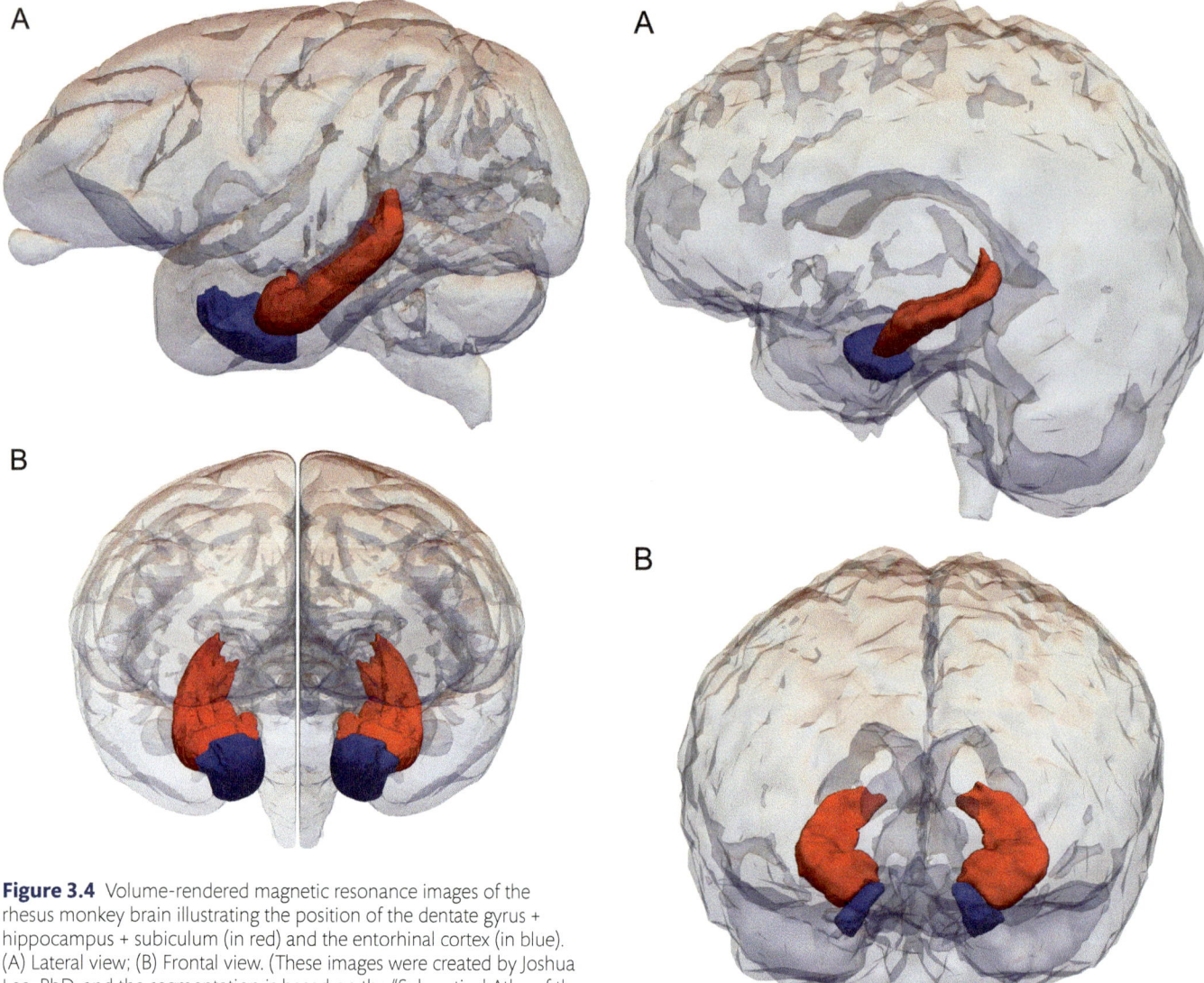

Figure 3.4 Volume-rendered magnetic resonance images of the rhesus monkey brain illustrating the position of the dentate gyrus + hippocampus + subiculum (in red) and the entorhinal cortex (in blue). (A) Lateral view; (B) Frontal view. (These images were created by Joshua Lee, PhD, and the segmentation is based on the "Subcortical Atlas of the Rhesus Macaque (SARM)"; Hartig et al., 2021.)

Figure 3.5 Volume-rendered magnetic resonance images of the human brain illustrating the position of the dentate gyrus + hippocampus + subiculum (in red) and the entorhinal cortex (in blue). (A) Lateral view; (B) Frontal view. (These images were created by Joshua Lee, PhD, from unpublished data from the MIND Institute, UC Davis.)

hippocampus, and subiculum. The angular bundle also contains commissural fibers of entorhinal and presubicular origin, and fibers to and from a variety of cortical and subcortical structures that are interconnected with the entorhinal cortex.

3.7.2.2 Perforant path

The fibers of the perforant path travel within the angular bundle before leaving to *perforate* the subiculum and the hippocampus on their way to the dentate gyrus and hippocampus. This is the main route by which neocortical inputs reach the dentate gyrus and the hippocampus. We will present a more detailed description of the perforant path when describing the inputs to the dentate gyrus and the connectivity of the entorhinal cortex.

3.7.2.3 Temporoammonic alvear pathway

Entorhinal fibers also reach the hippocampus from the alveus via the temporoammonic alvear pathway first described by Ramón y Cajal (1901–1902) and studied in detail by Heinemann and colleagues (Empson and Heinemann, 1995a, 1995b; Gloveli et al., 1997). At temporal levels, most of the entorhinal fibers reach the CA1 field of the hippocampus after perforating the subiculum (via

the classical perforant pathway). At more septal levels, the number of entorhinal fibers that take the alvear pathway is higher (Deller et al., 1996a). In fact, in the septal portion of the hippocampal formation, most of the entorhinal fibers that reach CA1 do so via the alveus (see below). These fibers initially travel parallel to the alveus then make sharp right-angle turns to perforate the pyramidal cell layer, and finally terminate in the stratum lacunosum-moleculare. The alveus is therefore also a major route by which entorhinal fibers reach their targets in CA1.

3.7.2.4 Fimbria-fornix

The fimbria-fornix fiber system provides the major bidirectional conduit for subcortical connections (Daitz and Powell, 1954; Benear et al., 2020). It is perhaps easiest to understand the fimbria-fornix system by analogy with the corticospinal fiber system. The

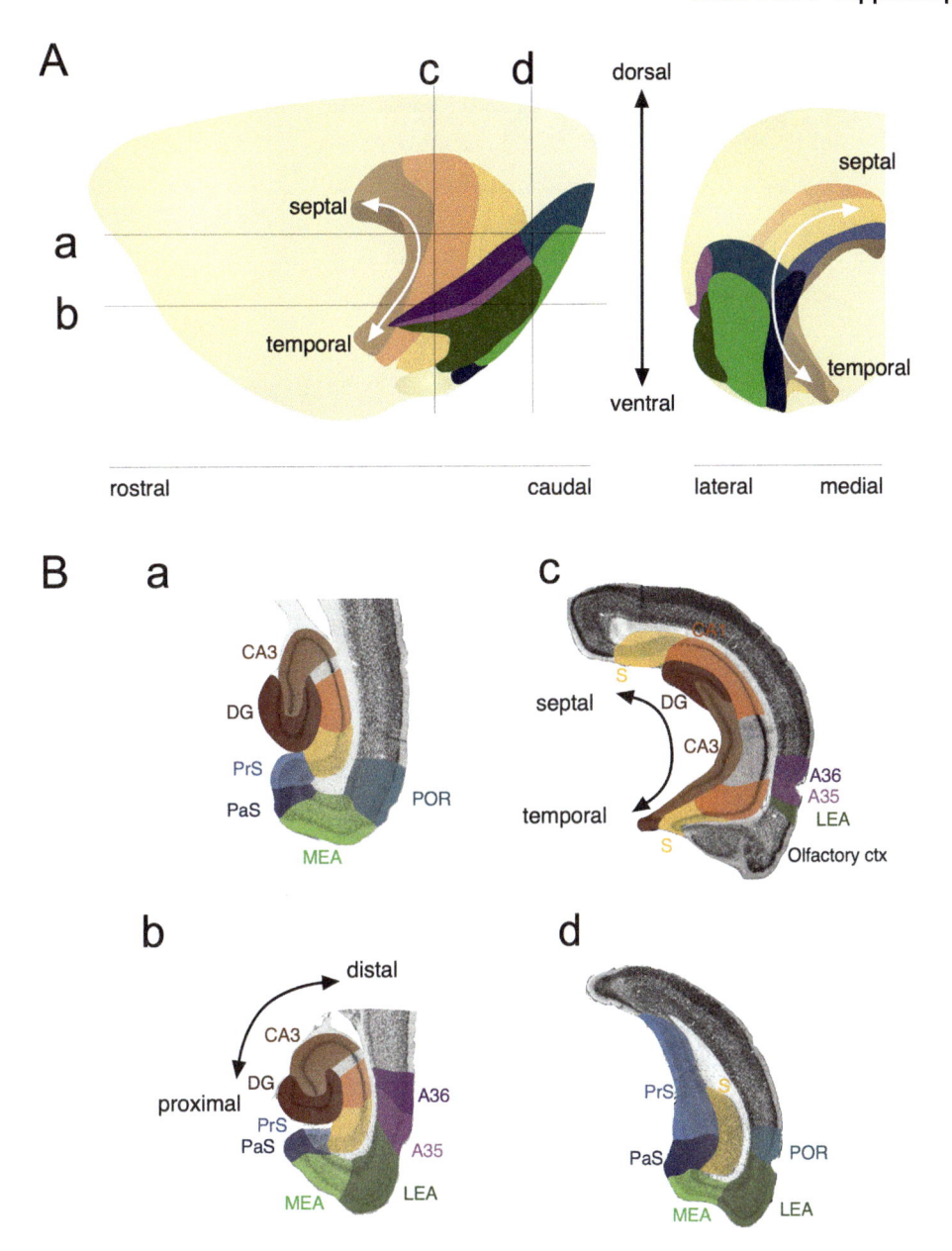

Figure 3.6 Illustrations of the hippocampal formation in the rat brain. (A) Lateral (left panel) and caudal (right panel) views. For orientation in the hippocampal formation—consisting of the dentate gyrus (DG; dark brown), CA3 (medium brown), CA2 (not colored), CA1 (orange), the subiculum (Sub; yellow), presubiculum (PrS; light blue), parasubiculum (PaS; dark blue), and entorhinal cortex (MEA and LEA; shades of green). The perirhinal cortex (area 35 and 36; shades of purple) and postrhinal cortex (POR blue-green) are also shown. The lines in the left panel indicate the levels of two horizontal sections (a, b) and two coronal sections (c, d), which are shown in part B. (Adapted from van Strien et al., 2009, with permission.)

corticospinal fibers are given different names at different points on their journey from motor cortex to the spinal cord. Similarly, the subcortical afferent and efferent fibers of the hippocampal formation are given different names at different points in their trajectory from, or toward, the forebrain and brainstem. Because of this, and because the exact transition between fimbria and fornix is difficult to define, some hippocampal researchers use the term "fimbria-fornix" to emphasize the continuity of fibers in these bundles.

The ventricular or deep surface of the hippocampus is covered by a thin sheet of mainly myelinated fibers called the alveus. These fibers form a white sheet overlying the hippocampus that can be clearly seen when the overlying neocortex is removed. The alveus is a complex fiber system. It contains both connections from other brain regions and fibers forming part of the intrahippocampal network (i.e., the entorhino-CA1 alvear pathway, the CA1-subiculum projection, and the CA1-entorhinal projection). Some alvear fibers originate from the pyramidal cells of the hippocampus and subiculum (Aggleton and Christiansen, 2015) and are en route to subcortical termination sites. At temporal levels of the hippocampal formation, the subcortically directed output fibers extend obliquely in the alveus, from medial to lateral over the surface of the hippocampus and collect in a bundle called the fimbria (from the Latin word for "fringe"). The fimbria gets progressively thicker as it progresses from temporal to septal levels as axons from more septally located pyramidal cells are added to the bundle. The rat fimbria has a flattened appearance, contains approximately 900,000 axons, and is situated

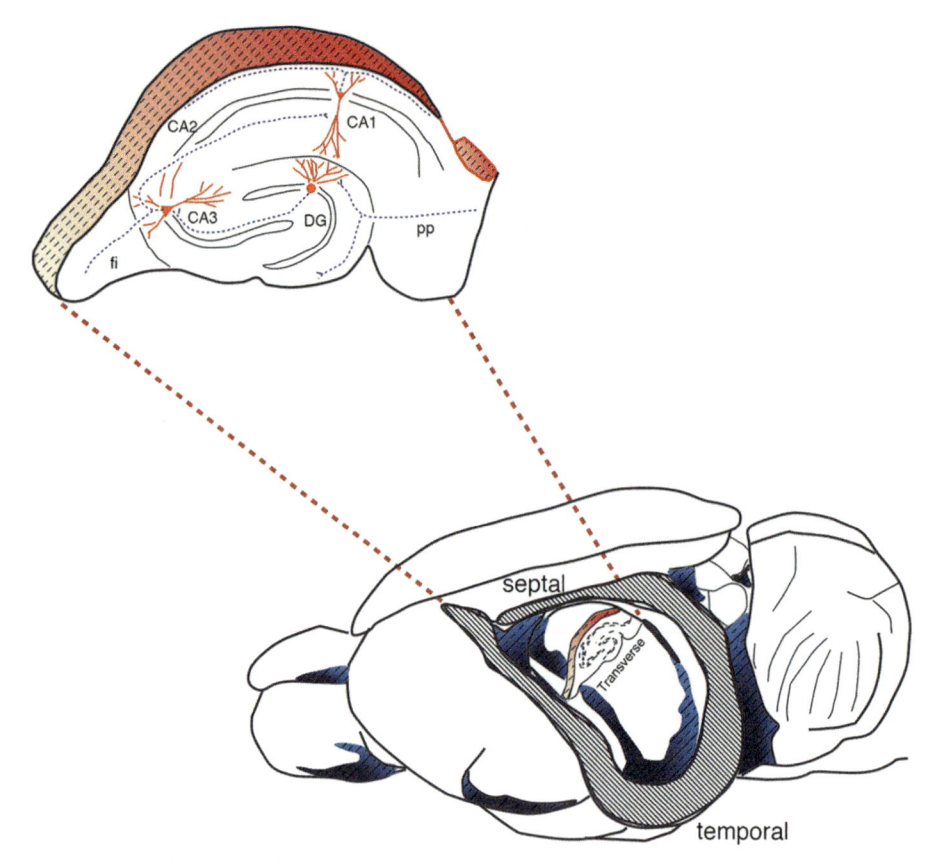

Figure 3.7 Line drawing of the rat brain illustrating the septotemporal and transverse axes of the hippocampal formation. The "slice" that has been removed illustrates several components of the intrinsic circuitry of the hippocampal formation including the perforant path (pp). The fimbria (fi) is also indicated. A dentate granule cell, and CA3 and CA1 pyramidal cells are also illustrated.

along the lateral and rostral aspects of the hippocampus. The fibers of the fimbria are not randomly distributed but are organized in a topographic fashion (Wyss et al., 1980). Axons located medially in the fimbria, i.e., those that are closest to the hippocampus, tend to arise from more septal levels, whereas those located laterally arise from more temporal levels. Fibers from the subiculum are situated deeper (more ventrally) to those from the hippocampus.

The fornix is the continuation of the fimbria and forms a flattened bundle located just below the corpus callosum very close to the midline (fornix is the Latin word for "arch," which is the shape of this tract over the diencephalon). As the fibers of the fimbria descend into the forebrain they are referred to as the columns of the fornix. The fornix splits around the anterior commissure to form a rostrally directed precommissural fornix that communicates with the septal nuclei and nucleus accumbens, and a caudally directed postcommissural fornix that extends toward the diencephalon. As the postcommissural fornix enters the diencephalon (ultimately to reach the mammillary nuclei of the posterior hypothalamus), two smaller bundles split off. One, the medial corticohypothalamic tract, innervates a number of anterior hypothalamic areas. The other, called the subiculothalamic tract, carries fibers to the anterior thalamic nuclei (Canteras and Swanson, 1992; Christiansen et al., 2016).

The fornix and fimbria also carry fibers that are traveling to the hippocampal formation. Many of the subcortical inputs to the hippocampal formation, including those from the septal nuclei,

the locus coeruleus, and the raphe nuclei, enter via the fimbria-fornix. Some subcortical regions have projections that follow other pathways into the hippocampal formation. Fibers from the anterior thalamus, for example, travel through the thalamic radiations and supracallosal stria to innervate the presubiculum. Projections from the amygdala travel to the hippocampal formation via the external capsule.

3.7.2.5 Dorsal and ventral hippocampal commissures

A third major fiber system associated with the hippocampal formation is the commissural system (Blackstad, 1956; Raisman et al., 1965; Laatsch and Cowan, 1967). In the rat, there are both dorsal and ventral hippocampal commissures. Some 350,000 fibers cross the midline in the ventral hippocampal commissure located just caudal to the septal area and dorsal to the anterior commissure. Many of these fibers are true commissural fibers that are directed to the contralateral hippocampal formation. A much smaller number of the fibers are directed into the contralateral descending column of the fornix and ultimately innervate the same structures on the contralateral side of the brain that receive input via the ipsilateral pre- and postcommissural fornix. The dorsal hippocampal commissure crosses the midline just rostral to the splenium (posterior part) of the corpus callosum and carries fibers mainly originating from, or projecting to, the presubiculum and entorhinal cortex. The dorsal hippocampal commissure is the route by which the presubiculum contributes a major projection to the contralateral entorhinal cortex.

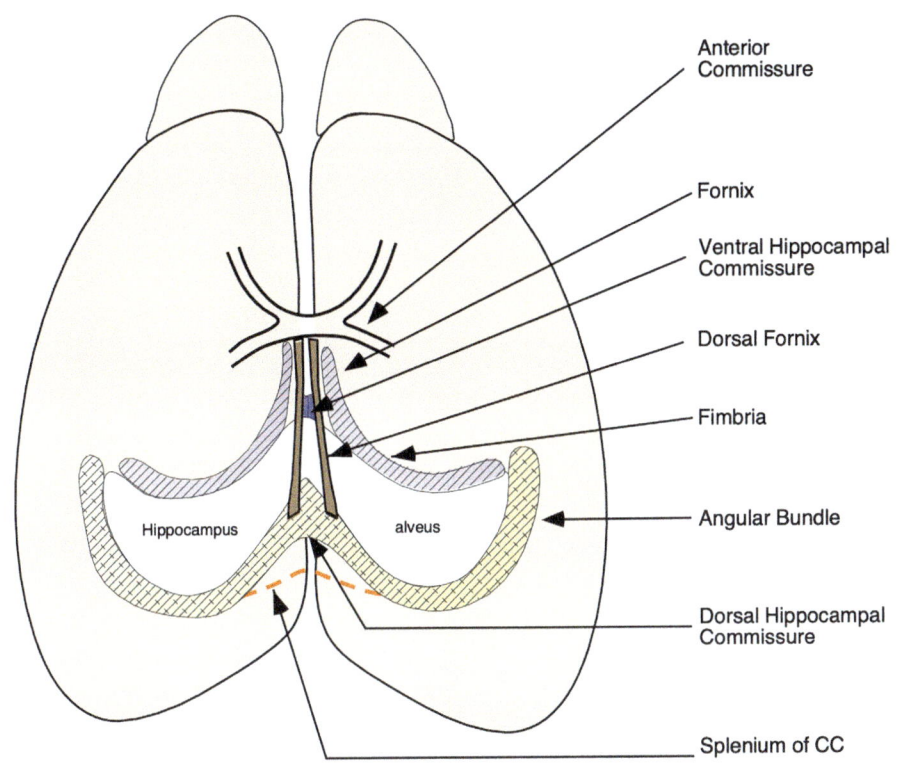

Figure 3.8 Schematic illustration of some of the major fiber systems of the rat hippocampal formation. The brain is seen from above. The surface of the hippocampus is covered by axons of fibers exiting and entering in a thin sheet called the alveus. The fibers of the fibria ultimately converge to form the fornix. The angular bundle is formed by axons from the entorhinal cortex en route to the dentate gyrus and hippocampus. Some of these fibers cross the midline in the dorsal hippocampal commissure. The ventral hippocampal commissure is made up primarily of fibers from the dentate gyrus and hippocampus that are destined for these same structures on the contralateral side of the brain. See text for more details.

3.7.3 The nonhuman primate hippocampal formation

The first question we will address in this section is: How does the appearance and position of the nonhuman primate hippocampal formation differ from that of the rat or mouse? Recently, due to the availability of gene-editing technologies such as CRISPR-Cas9, the potential of carrying out translational models in the nonhuman primate has raised the research profile of the common marmoset (*Callithrix jacchus*), a small nonendangered New World monkey. However, there is relatively little published neuroanatomical information on the marmoset or other New World monkeys. Much of the work on the nonhuman primate hippocampal formation has been carried out in Old World monkeys, primarily macaque monkeys. The description we provide here is for the hippocampal formation of typical research monkeys, such as the cynomolgus and rhesus macaque monkeys (*Macaca fascicularis* and *Macaca mulatta*, respectively). The hippocampal formation in the macaque monkey is not nearly as C-shaped in its long axis as in the rat (compare Figures 3.5 and 3.6). It lies almost horizontally in the temporal lobe and, as in the human, makes up the major portion of the floor of the temporal horn of the lateral ventricle. The major determinant of the change of position of the primate hippocampal formation is the massive development of the associational cortices of the frontal and temporal lobes. As a result of the caudal and ventral transposition of the temporal lobes that takes place developmentally to accommodate the larger cortical surface, the primate hippocampal formation comes to lie almost entirely within the medial temporal lobe. Because of the ventrorostral rotation of the monkey hippocampal formation, the homologue of the

temporal pole of the rat hippocampal formation is located rostrally in the monkey brain, and the equivalent of the septal pole of the rat hippocampal formation is located caudally. Since the term "septotemporal" is not appropriate for the monkey hippocampal formation (since no portion of it approaches the septal area), it is more common to refer to the long axis in the primate as the rostrocaudal axis. The orthogonal axis, however, is still referred to as the transverse axis.

Two additional points should be made about the position of the monkey hippocampal formation. First, at the rostral limit of the lateral ventricle, some fields of the monkey hippocampal formation flex medially and then caudally. This is the monkey homologue of the pes hippocampi that is so prominent in the human brain. At the rostral levels where this flexure occurs, there are actually two representations of the hippocampal formation in standard coronal views of the brain. It is difficult in this flexed region of the monkey hippocampal formation, when viewed in standard coronal Nissl-stained sections, to specify the identity and borders of the subdivisions of the hippocampal formation with certainty. However, genetic profiling, as has been done in the mouse, may ultimately be able to solve this problem. The most medial and caudal portion of the hippocampal formation (i.e., the part that is bent backward) is the actual "rostral" pole of the monkey hippocampal formation, even though it is physically located somewhat caudal to the rostral extreme of the hippocampal formation. In order to make reference to different portions of the monkey hippocampal formation, we call the medial portion of the hippocampal formation the uncal region (because it forms much of the medially situated bulge that in the human would be called the uncus). The flexed, rostrally located portion that runs mediolaterally is called the genu, and the laterally situated, main portion of the hippocampus is the body.

The second point to note is that the monkey entorhinal cortex is physically associated with only the rostral portion of the other hippocampal fields (Figure 3.6). The entorhinal cortex extends caudally just to the level of the lateral geniculate nucleus, whereas the dentate gyrus, hippocampus, and subiculum extend well caudal to this level. The rostral half of the entorhinal cortex extends beyond the rostral limit of the other hippocampal fields and is located ventromedial to the amygdaloid complex. Throughout virtually all of its rostrocaudal extent, the lateral border of the entorhinal cortex is at the rhinal sulcus, just as in the rat.

The fiber bundles of the monkey hippocampal formation are fundamentally similar to those in the rat, though there are a number of minor differences. First, the fimbria is located dorsomedially in the monkey rather than ventrolaterally as in the rat (Figure 3.2). Second, the fimbria leaves the substance of the hippocampal formation at a point near the splenium of the corpus callosum. Thus, the compact bundle of fibers that makes up the body of the fornix travels rostrally as a pendulous, flattened cable hanging beneath the corpus callosum. Upon reaching the level of the anterior commissure, the bundle descends as the columns of the fornix and follows the same trajectories outlined for the rat. Third, the ventral and dorsal hippocampal commissures are relatively less prominent in the monkey than in the rat, reflecting the more restricted commissural connections observed in the monkey brain (Amaral et al., 1984; Demeter, 1985). The more prominent of the two commissures in the monkey is the dorsal hippocampal commissure. It carries fibers from the presubiculum, entorhinal cortex, and parahippocampal cortex to the contralateral side.

3.7.4 The human hippocampal formation

It remains the case to date that there is very little information concerning the organization of the human hippocampal formation. Some of this comes from magnetic resonance imaging (MRI) studies, which we will cover below. There are several human brain atlases that provide a useful description of the human hippocampal formation. The atlas of Mai et al. (2015) portrays the human hippocampal formation through all rostrocaudal levels with boundaries placed between its subfields. Similarly, the atlas originating from the Allen Institute for Brain Science (Ding et al., 2016) also provides a complete account of the longitudinal extent of the human hippocampal formation. A number of review papers on the human hippocampal formation have appeared since the first edition of this book (DeFelipe et al., 2007; Insausti and Amaral, 2012; Schultz and Engelhardt, 2014) and are valuable resources.

The three-dimensional position of the human hippocampal formation is similar to that in the macaque monkey brain (Figures 3.4 and 3.5, respectively). But, due to the larger development of the temporal association cortex, particularly the entorhinal and parahippocampal (temporopolar, perirhinal, and parahippocampal cortices) regions, the structures of the ventromedial surface of the brain, including the gyri, are substantially different in the human and monkey brains. After a brief summary of the gross anatomical attributes of the main or intraventricular portions of the human hippocampal formation, we will review some of the differences of the associated cortical regions.

The classical gross anatomical image of the human hippocampal formation is of a prominent bulge in the floor of the temporal horn of the lateral ventricle (Figure 3.9). As in the monkey, this portion of the hippocampal formation is widest at its rostral extent where the structure expands toward the medial surface of the brain. In this area, 2–5 subtle gyri or digitationes hippocampi form the pes hippocampi (Gertz, 1972). The substance of the pes hippocampi is formed by several of the hippocampal fields, and the constituents differ at different rostrocaudal levels (we will describe this below). Continuing caudally from the pes hippocampi, the main body of the hippocampus gets progressively thinner as it bends dorsally toward the splenium of the corpus callosum.

The fimbria is situated on the medial surface of the human hippocampus, as in the monkey. At rostral levels, the fimbria is thin and flat, but gets progressively thicker caudally as fibers are continually added to it. As the fimbria leaves the caudal end of the hippocampus, it fuses with the ventral surface of the corpus callosum and travels rostrally within the lateral ventricle. The portion of these fimbrial fibers located between the caudal limit of the hippocampal formation and the fusion with the corpus callosum is called the crus of the fornix, whereas the major portion of the rostrally directed fiber bundle is, as in the monkey, called the body of the fornix. At the end of its rostral trajectory, the body of the fornix descends as the columns of the fornix. At about the point where the fimbria fuses with the posterior portion of the corpus callosum, fibers extend across the midline to form the hippocampal commissure. A variety of gross anatomical terms have been applied to this commissure but the term "psalterium" (alluding to a harp-like stringed instrument) is most common. As noted previously, the primate hippocampal commissural connections are much more limited than in the rodent and, as suggested by stereotaxic depth encephalography, there is almost no commissural interaction between the hippocampal formations located on each side of the human brain (Wilson et al., 1987; Gloor et al., 1993; Postans et al., 2020).

The ventral surface of the human temporal lobe is demarcated into mediolateral strips by two prominent rostrocaudally oriented sulci (Figures 3.10, 3.11). The more lateral of the two is the occipitotemporal sulcus, which is often interrupted by small, transverse gyri. The more medial of the sulci, and the one that is more closely associated with the hippocampal formation, is the collateral sulcus. Unlike the situation in the rat and the monkey, the rhinal sulcus is relatively insignificant in the human brain and is associated only with the most rostral portion of the entorhinal cortex (Figure 3.11). It is thus not a useful border for the lateral boundary of the entorhinal cortex in the human. However, the term "rhinal sulcus" has been used to denote the anterior portion of the collateral sulcus (Huntgeburth and Petrides, 2016).

The collateral sulcus forms most of the lateral border of what has classically been termed the "parahippocampal gyrus." The parahippocampal gyrus is a complex region that contains a number of distinct cytoarchitectonic fields and has been defined in different ways by different authors. In recent years, the parahippocampal gyrus has often been broken up into an anterior part that comprises mainly the entorhinal cortex and associated perirhinal cortex, and a posterior part that includes areas TF and TH of Von Economo (1929).

Unlike the situation in the monkey, where the rhinal sulcus forms a reasonably reliable lateral border for the entorhinal cortex, the collateral sulcus does not provide a discrete lateral boundary for the human entorhinal cortex. The lateral boundary of the entorhinal

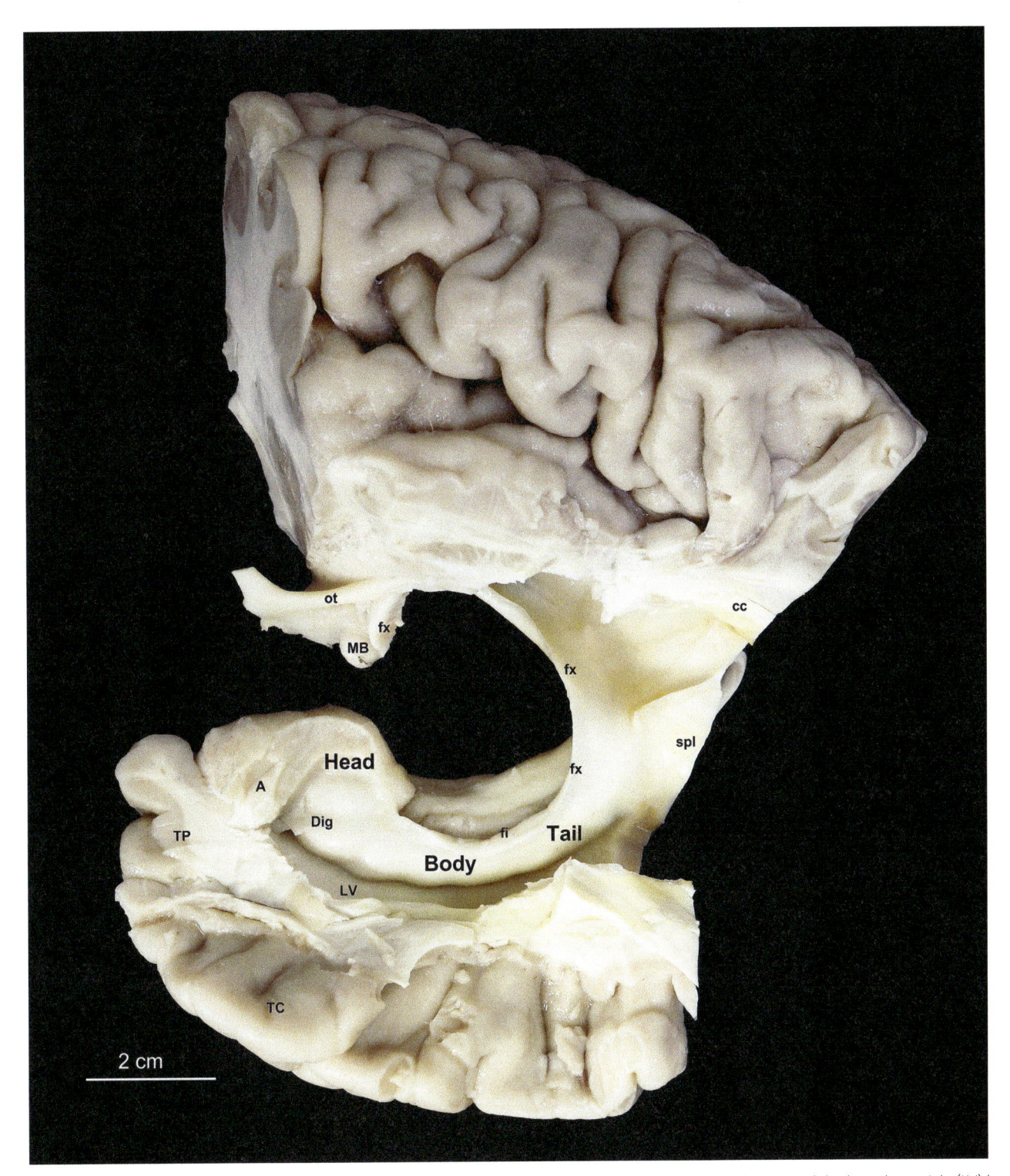

Figure 3.9 Dorsal and lateral view of the human hippocampus after the overlying cortex has been dissected away and the lateral ventricle (LV) has been opened. The gross hippocampus can be divided into a rostral "Head," a mid "Body," and a caudal "Tail," although there are no clear anatomical boundaries between these divisions. The head of the hippocampus is made up of the digitations that represent a bending rostrally and caudally of the fields of the hippocampus as it approaches the rostral extreme of the lateral ventricle. The amygdala (A) is immediately in front and partially overlaps the head of the hippocampus. The thin fimbria (fi) can be seen on the medial surface of the hippocampus as it extends caudally to form the fornix (fx). The fornix extends beneath the corpus callosum as it travels first rostrally and then ventrally to ultimately attain the mammillary body (MB).

cortex may vary along the medial bank to the fundus of the collateral sulcus (Insausti et al., 1998). The two fields of the perirhinal cortex, areas 35 and 36 of Brodmann (1909) form the remainder of the medial bank, fundus, and a portion of the lateral bank of the collateral sulcus, extending into the midportion of the fusiform

gyrus. The perirhinal cortex is massively enlarged in the human brain (Ding and Van Hoesen, 2010) and may account, in part, for the prominence of the collateral sulcus. The border zone between the entorhinal cortex and the perirhinal cortex has been called the "transentorhinal zone" by Braak (1974, 1980). In this region,

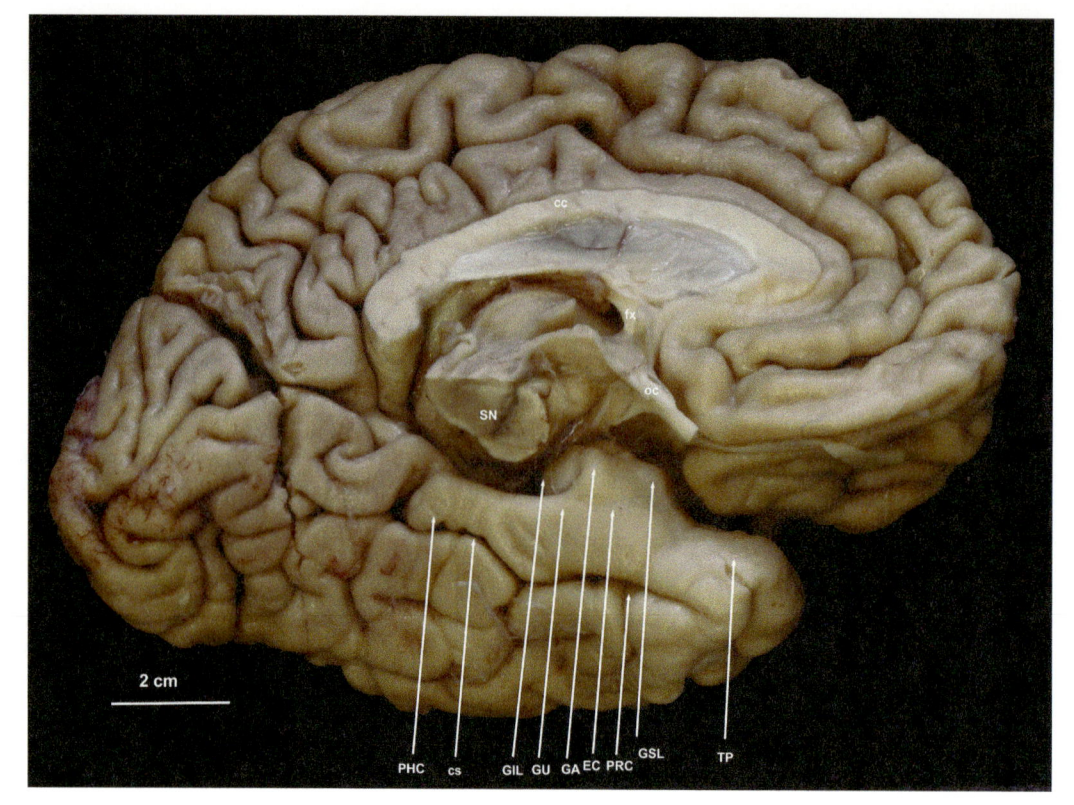

Figure 3.10 Ventromedial view of the left temporal lobe of the human brain. The brainstem and cerebellum have been removed.

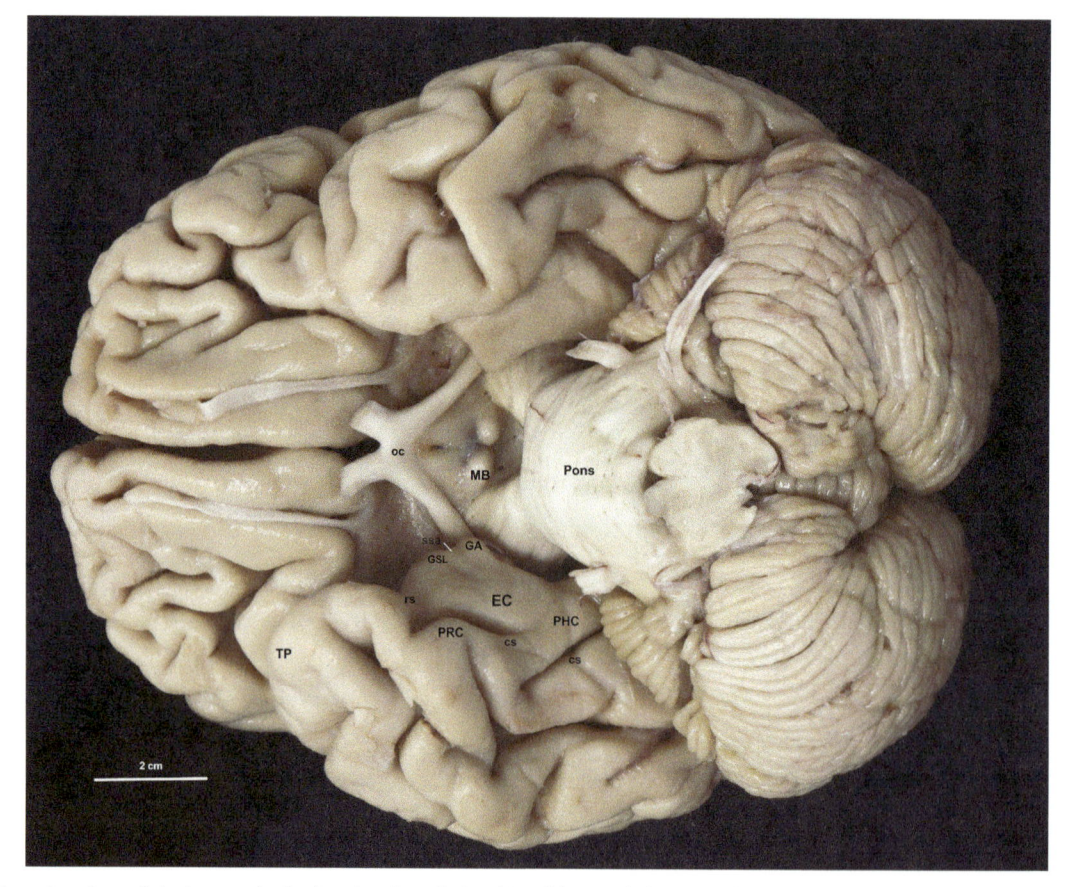

Figure 3.11 Ventral surface of the human brain showing the relationship of the medial temporal lobe to other brain regions.

neuroanatomical markers that label layer II of the entorhinal cortex demonstrate an oblique band of labeled cells, which gives the appearance that layer II is diving down beneath the layers of the perirhinal cortex. Since the perirhinal cortex terminates at a variable point along the lateral bank of the collateral sulcus, it is extremely difficult to define the borders of the entorhinal and perirhinal cortices using imaging modalities such as MRI (Insausti et al., 1998). The only way that it is currently possible to accurately define the border of these fields is through histological analysis, and histological coregistration with MRI scans (Yushkevich et al., 2021). Interestingly, much of the areal extent of the human entorhinal cortex (at least the rostral portions) can be visually identified on the surface of the brain by the conspicuous bumps, named verrucae (Latin for "warts"), which mark its pial surface. These bumps mark the islands of cells that constitute layer II of the entorhinal cortex. Those islands have also been observed in postmortem MRI (Augustinack et al., 2012). The dorsomedial aspect of the entorhinal cortex is marked by a secondary gyrus that forms a conspicuous mound, and is referred to as gyrus ambiens (Brodmann's area 34), but is actually a subfield of the entorhinal cortex (Insausti et al., 2019) (Figure 3.10). The dorsomedial limit of the entorhinal cortex with the amygdaloid complex is marked by the shallow sulcus semiannularis, which is located dorsal and anterior to the gyrus ambiens.

The dorsomedial portion of the entorhinal cortex is continued caudally by a series of prominent bulges on the medial surface of the hemisphere, which is generally labeled the uncus (or hook) in gross anatomical descriptions (Figure 3.10). The most rostral of the uncal bulges is often separately labeled the gyrus uncinatus. Histological sections through the gyrus uncinatus indicate that it is made up of the amygdalohippocampal region (of the amygdaloid complex) and the transition zone between the amygdala and hippocampus, (also known as the amygdalohippocampal transitional area, or HATA). The middle bulge is called the band of Giacomini and is generally composed of the most medial part of the dentate gyrus. The most caudal of the uncal bulges is called the intralimbic gyrus and is composed mainly of a portion of the CA3 field of the hippocampus.

As the parahippocampal gyrus meets the retrosplenial region caudally, a group of small bumps known as the gyri Andreae Retzii are seen on the medial surface of the brain. This irregular region of cortex marks the caudal limit of the hippocampal formation and is composed principally of CA1, with a minor contribution of the subiculum. Two obliquely oriented small gyri located deep to the gyri Andreae Retzii are called the fasciola cinerea (which corresponds to the most caudal part of the dentate gyrus) and the gyrus fasciolaris (which corresponds to the caudal pole of the CA3 field) (Duvernoy, 1988; Insausti and Amaral, 2012). A thin remnant of the hippocampal formation (which is found in all mammalian species) surrounds the splenium of the corpus callosum and is situated dorsal to the corpus callosum to form the induseum griseum (or supracommissural hippocampal formation); this comprises remnants of the subiculum and CA1 field of the hippocampus (Bobic Rasonja et al., 2019).

3.8 Definition of hippocampal areas and terms

3.8.1 Classical definition of hippocampal regions

When a histological section is prepared through the hippocampus and stained for the presence of neuronal cell bodies, it is immediately obvious that a number of cytoarchitectonically distinct structures are encompassed within the region grossly defined as "hippocampus." A number of terminologies have been applied to some of these different regions, and several synonymous terms are still commonly employed. Beyond the problem of different terms being applied to the same region, the borders between several regions of the hippocampal formation are still debated. The terms adopted in this book are based, in part, on converging evidence from cytoarchitectonic, neurochemical, connectional, and functional data and, in part, on personal preference. Most recent data from large-scale gene-expression studies have confirmed the classical definitions of hippocampal regions, but also provided additional means to further subdivide these regions into smaller units based on different patterns of gene expression (Lein et al., 2007; Thompson et al., 2008; Dong et al., 2009; Bienkowski et al., 2021). Early gene expression studies focused on finding individual markers of classical fields, whereas more recent studies aimed at identifying larger groups of genes contributing to broader functional networks associated with distinct connectivity patterns (see section 3.8.2). The main challenge here is to define a common nomenclature that hippocampal researchers working at different levels of investigation can use to communicate. In this context, it is fundamental to not miss the forest for the trees: sequoias will remain the predominant trees of the Redwood National Park in Northern California, even if some other trees are also found in the same ecosystem. Another important aspect to consider is the fact that the vast majority of recent molecular studies are carried out using 3-month-old male wild-type or transgenic mice on a C57BL/6 genetic background. Although the general organization of hippocampal structure is conserved across species (see below), it is not clear that some of the intricate details revealed using very sophisticated techniques in mice will necessarily be confirmed in other animals of different ages and different species, including humans. The question of what level of detail should be considered to define brain regions is not new, however, since Rose (1927) defined as many as 27 subdivisions of the human entorhinal cortex; Insausti et al. (1995) defined eight subdivisions in line with work in rodents and monkeys; and Witter and colleagues (Chapter 12) now argue for the sake of simplicity to subdivide the entorhinal cortex in only two subdivisions, the medial and lateral entorhinal cortex. Hippocampal nomenclature will thus likely continue to evolve, as any language does. Hippocampal researchers may remain, like Americans and Brits, separated by a common language.

The term "hippocampus" has historically been used both as a term for a gross anatomical region of the brain (the bulge or protuberance in the floor of the human lateral ventricle) and for one of the cytoarchitectonically distinct entities that make up the region. As a result, the meaning of the word "hippocampus" is context-dependent and may be ambiguous. We reserve the term "hippocampus" for the region of the hippocampal formation that comprises the CA3, CA2, and CA1 fields identified by the neuroanatomist Rafael Lorente de Nó (1934). The term "hippocampal formation," in contrast, is applied to a group of cytoarchitectonically distinct adjoining regions including the dentate gyrus, the hippocampus, the subiculum, the presubiculum, the parasubiculum, and the entorhinal cortex (Figure 3.1). The adjective "hippocampal" will, by necessity, remain somewhat vague and context-dependent. In general, it is used to refer to the larger area (as in, "hippocampal lesions") rather than to the cytoarchitectonic region. If this seems confusing, the terminological definitions of the next few paragraphs may provide clarification.

The main justification for including the six regions named above under the rubric "hippocampal formation" is that they are linked, one to the next, by unique and largely unidirectional neuronal pathways. The earlier literature on the hippocampal formation emphasized the first three links in the hippocampal circuitry by applying the term "trisynaptic circuit" to the ensemble of the major hippocampal pathways known at the time (Andersen et al., 1971): EC to DG (synapse 1), DG to CA3 (synapse 2), CA3 to CA1 (synapse 3). With the discovery of robust projections from CA1 to the subiculum and entorhinal cortex; direct projections from entorhinal cortex layer II neurons to the dentate gyrus, CA3, and CA2; direct projections from entorhinal cortex layer III neurons to CA1 and the subiculum; and major projections from the deep layers of the entorhinal cortex to the neocortex, it became clear that the trisynaptic circuit was only a portion of the functional circuitry of the hippocampal formation. Given that the subiculum is the main source of subcortical projections and that the entorhinal cortex is the main hub for interactions with the neocortex, the concept of trisynaptic circuit is of historical significance, but is much less influential on current theories of hippocampal function (Chapters 4, 12, 16).

The reader who ventures from the relative safety of this book into the primary literature should be aware that our usage of the term "hippocampal formation" is widely, though not universally accepted. Some authors include only the allocortical (a term applied to cortical regions having three layers) regions as parts of the hippocampal formation (see Chapter 12). Three-layered cortical regions typically have a single neuronal cell layer with fiber-rich plexiform layers above and below the cell layer. In papers employing this usage, the hippocampal formation comprises the dentate gyrus, hippocampus, and subiculum. The remaining fields, the presubiculum, parasubiculum. and entorhinal cortex, are then typically grouped together on the basis of their multilaminate structure either under the term "retrohippocampal" (retro = behind) or "parahippocampal" (para = alongside or near) cortex. In yet other variants, the terms "hippocampus" or "hippocampal complex" are sometimes applied to the combination of the dentate gyrus and hippocampus proper. Because they form a unique functional system, we will scrupulously adhere to the nomenclature in which the hippocampal formation comprises the six structures listed above.

Having outlined the major regions of the hippocampal formation, we now delve more deeply into the subdivisions of each of these regions. Before doing so, however, it is important to note that the terminology we apply to these regions is a hybrid derived from the analyses of classical and modern hippocampal neuroanatomists. The two main contributors to surviving hippocampal terminologies are Santiago Ramón y Cajal and Rafael Lorente de Nó. Some of their subdivisions, based solely on the analysis of Golgi-stained material, have not stood the test of time and the introduction of modern neuroanatomical methods. And many revisions of their nomenclature have been made, as information has become available concerning the connections and the neurochemical and molecular architecture of the hippocampal formation. We considered very carefully the pros and cons of describing more subdivisions, based, for example, on very specific patterns of gene expression. However, we realized that a more detailed description would hinder rather than facilitate communication between hippocampal researchers.

This description should therefore be viewed as a bridge providing fundamental information to facilitate exchanges between different levels of investigation.

3.8.1.1 Subdivisions of hippocampal areas

The dentate gyrus is a trilaminate cortical region that has a characteristic "V" or "U" shape enclosing the proximal portion of the CA3 field of the hippocampus (Figure 3.12). It includes three layers: the molecular layer, the granule cell layer and the polymorphic layer (see section 3.9.1). The portion of the granule cell layer that is located between CA3 and CA1 (separated by the hippocampal fissure) is called the suprapyramidal (above CA3) blade and the portion opposite to this, the infrapyramidal (below CA3) blade. The region bridging the two blades (at the apex of the "V" or "U") is called the crest.

The hippocampus, especially in rodents, can easily be divided into two major regions, a large-celled region that abuts the dentate gyrus and a smaller-celled region that follows from it. Ramón y Cajal called these two regions regio inferior and regio superior, respectively. The terminology of Lorente de Nó has achieved more common usage and is employed here. He divided the hippocampus into three fields: CA3, CA2, and CA1. His CA3 and CA2 fields are equivalent to the large-celled regio inferior of Ramón y Cajal and his CA1 field is equivalent to the regio superior. In addition to the greater size of the pyramidal cells in CA3 and CA2 compared with CA1, the inputs and outputs of these areas are also different. The pyramidal cells of CA3, for example, receive the mossy fiber input from the dentate gyrus via particular branched spines called thorny excrescences, whereas the CA1 pyramidal cells do not.

CA2 was originally defined by Lorente de Nó as a narrow zone of cells interposed between CA3 and CA1. CA2 has large pyramidal cell bodies similar to those in CA3 but, like CA1, CA2 pyramidal cells do not exhibit the typical thorny excrescences of CA3 pyramidal cells. While the existence of CA2 had been questioned, it is now clear that the CA2 field can be distinguished from the other hippocampal fields using a variety of criteria, including connectional and genetic markers (Lein et al., 2005; Bienkowski, 2023). Lorente de Nó also defined a CA4 field, but it is clearly a misnomer. The region that Lorente de Nó called CA4 is actually the polymorphic layer of the dentate gyrus (Blackstad, 1956; Amaral, 1978). In the human, the portion of CA3 that inserts within the blades of the dentate gyrus is often labeled CA4. The term "hilus" of the dentate gyrus can be used synonymously with polymorphic layer.

The subiculum, presubiculum, and parasubiculum are sometimes grouped under the term "subicular complex." Since each of these regions has distinct neuroanatomical features, they are better thought of as independent cortical areas (Insausti et al., 2017). The border between CA1 and the subiculum occurs precisely at the point where the Schaffer collateral projection from CA3 ends. In the rodent, this occurs approximately where the condensed pyramidal cell layer of CA1 begins to broaden into the thicker layer of the subiculum. Some researchers also define a small region between CA1 and the subiculum, called the prosubiculum (Ding, 2013), whereas we and others consider this region as part of the subiculum.

The presubiculum lies adjacent to the subiculum and is typically considered to have more than the three layers that characterize the dentate gyrus, hippocampus, and subiculum. However, the exact delimitation of the deep layers of the presubiculum and

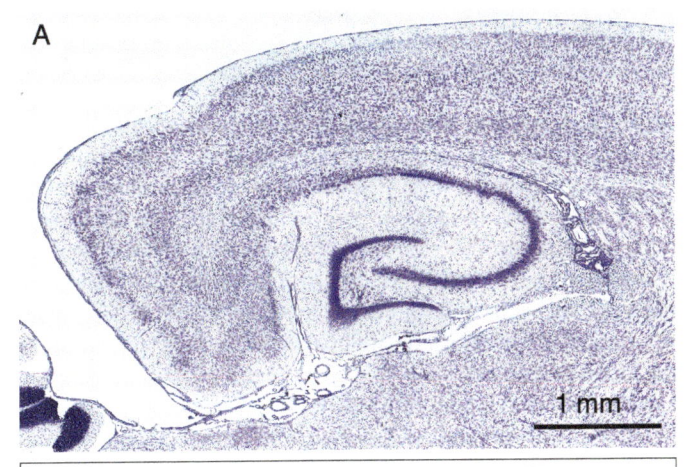

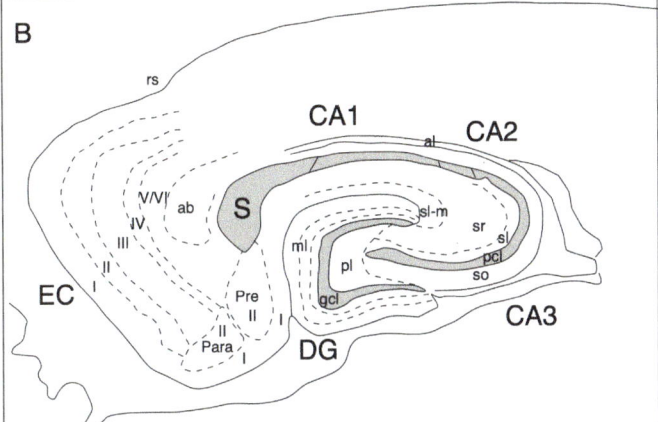

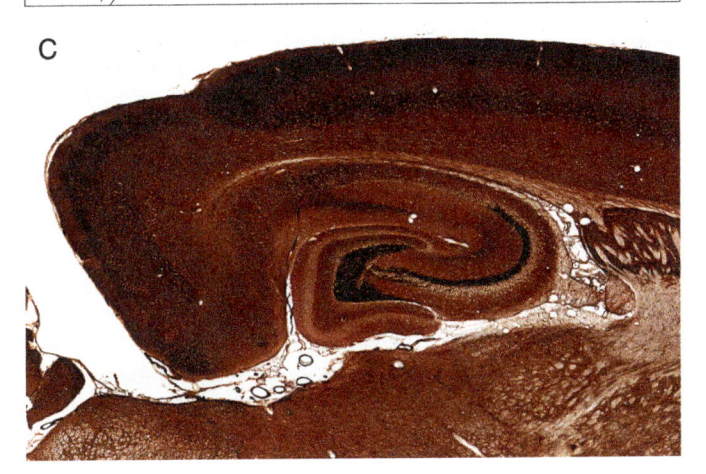

Figure 3.12 Horizontal section through the rat hippocampal formation. (A) Nissl-stained section; (B) line drawing illustrating the different regions, layers, and fiber pathways; (C) Timm's sulfide-silver-stained sections. Note the three bands of the molecular layer of the dentate gyrus in C. The outer band corresponds to the terminal zone of the lateral perforant pathway; the middle unstained region corresponds to the terminal zone of the medial perforant pathway; the inner band corresponds to the zone of termination of the associational and commissural pathways of the dentate gyrus. Scale bar in A applies to all panels.

the differentiation of cells belonging to the presubiculum from those that belong to the deep layers of the entorhinal cortex has never been clearly established. The most distinctive feature of the presubiculum is the densely packed external cellular layer, which

is populated by relatively small and tightly packed pyramidal cells. The parasubiculum is characterized by a wedge-shaped layer II with cells that resemble but are somewhat larger and less compact than those in the presubiculum.

The entorhinal cortex is the only hippocampal region that unambiguously demonstrates a multilaminate appearance. Based on differences in the cytoarchitectonic and neurochemical organization of these layers, as well as patterns of connectivity, the entorhinal cortex has been divided into several subdivisions. We shall return to a description of the subdivisions of the entorhinal cortex later in the chapter (also see Chapter 12).

Before moving on to descriptions of the three-dimensional organization of the hippocampal formation in the rodent, monkey, and human brains, we need to say a few more words concerning nomenclature. We will often want to refer to a specific portion of one of the hippocampal regions. Given the complex shape of the hippocampal formation, no reference system is wholly adequate, and any description inevitably involves arbitrary decisions about where to start or finish, and which direction is up or down, etc. We have adopted a reference system in which the dentate gyrus is considered to be the proximal extreme of the hippocampal formation and the entorhinal cortex is the distal one (Figure 3.1). A portion of any hippocampal field can therefore be defined in relation to this proximodistal axis. For example, the proximal portion of CA3 is located closer to the dentate gyrus and the distal portion is located closer to CA2.

We will also often need to specify subregions within the thickness of a particular hippocampal region. As in most other cortical areas, this radial dimension is usually described along a superficial to deep axis. In six-layer structures, layer I is closest to the pial surface and layer VI is located close to the subcortical white matter. Consistent with this convention, regions closer to the pia or hippocampal fissure are considered superficial and those in the opposite direction (closer to the alveus or ventricle where applicable) are considered deep. The molecular layer of the dentate gyrus, for example, is superficial to the granule cell layer. This superficial-deep nomenclature has the merit of being applicable to all portions of the hippocampal formation and to all of its cytoarchitectonic fields.

3.8.2 Genetic contributions to definition of hippocampal regions

As we have described, the initial demarcation of subregions of the hippocampal formation was based on stains that labeled cell bodies. In time, observations from other types of stains, such as the Timm's stain for heavy metals or histochemical or immunohistochemical stains for neurotransmitter candidates such as acetylcholine or GABA and their related biochemistries, were added to refine regional and laminar descriptions. It is a truism, first poetically stated by Floyd Bloom, that "the gains in brain lie mainly in the stain."

Starting in the early 2000s, spurred by the genetics revolution and the ability to identify expression patterns in tissue of any of the more than 20,000 protein-coding genes found in the mammalian genome, gene expression patterns began to be used for subdividing the hippocampal formation. This effort was enhanced by the publication of the Allen Brain Atlas of gene expression (Lein et al., 2007) that provided a standardized atlas of all expressed genes in the mouse brain. One of the earliest attempts to map gene expression in

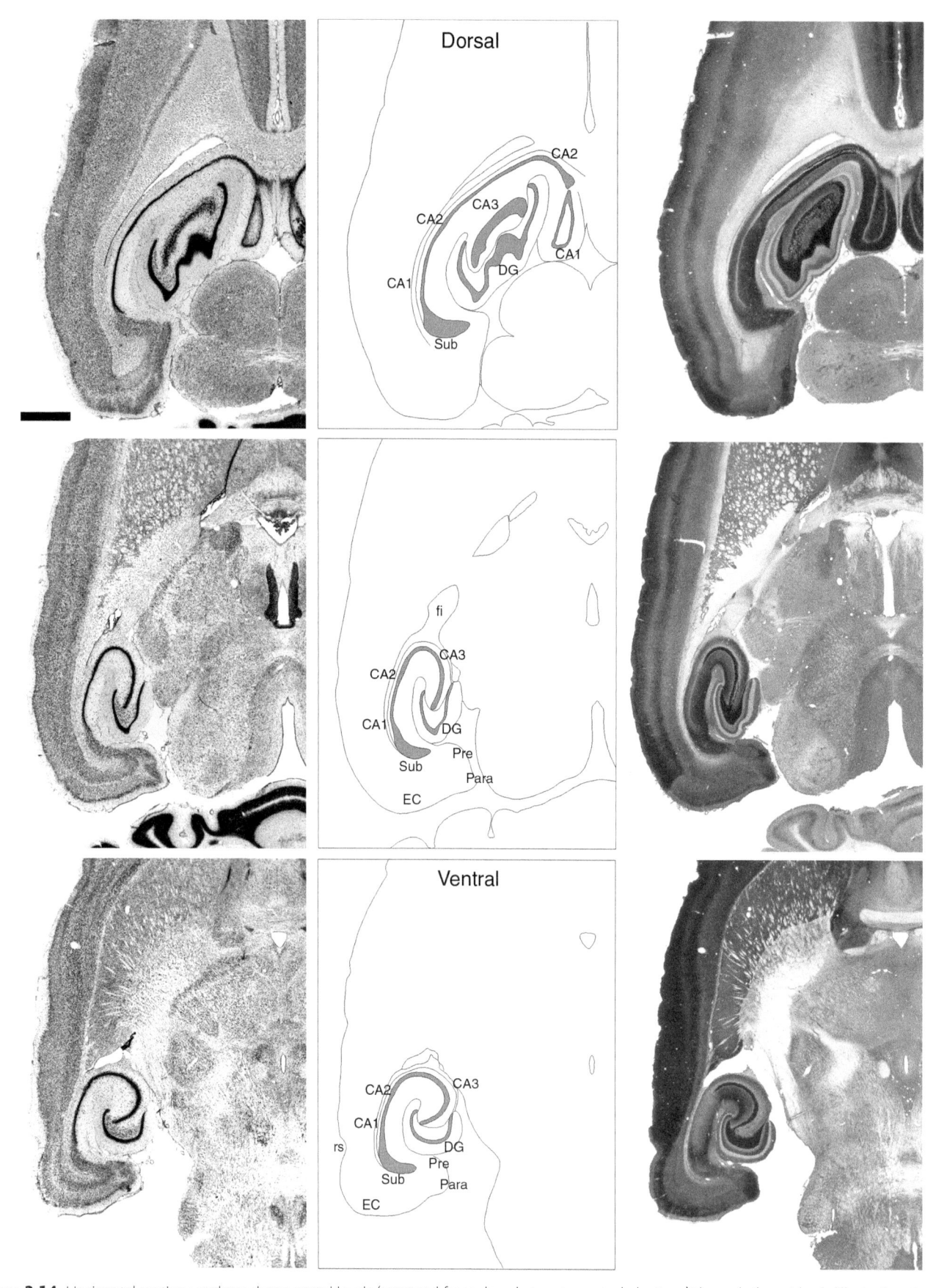

Figure 3.14 Horizontal sections at three dorsoventral levels (arranged from dorsal–top, to ventral–bottom) through the rat brain illustrating the relative position of the hippocampal formation. The three panels on the left are Nissl-stained sections; the three panels on the right are adjacent, Timm's sulfide-silver-stained section; the line drawings (middle column) highlight the different regions of the rat hippocampal formation seen in the stained sections. Scale bar is 1 mm.

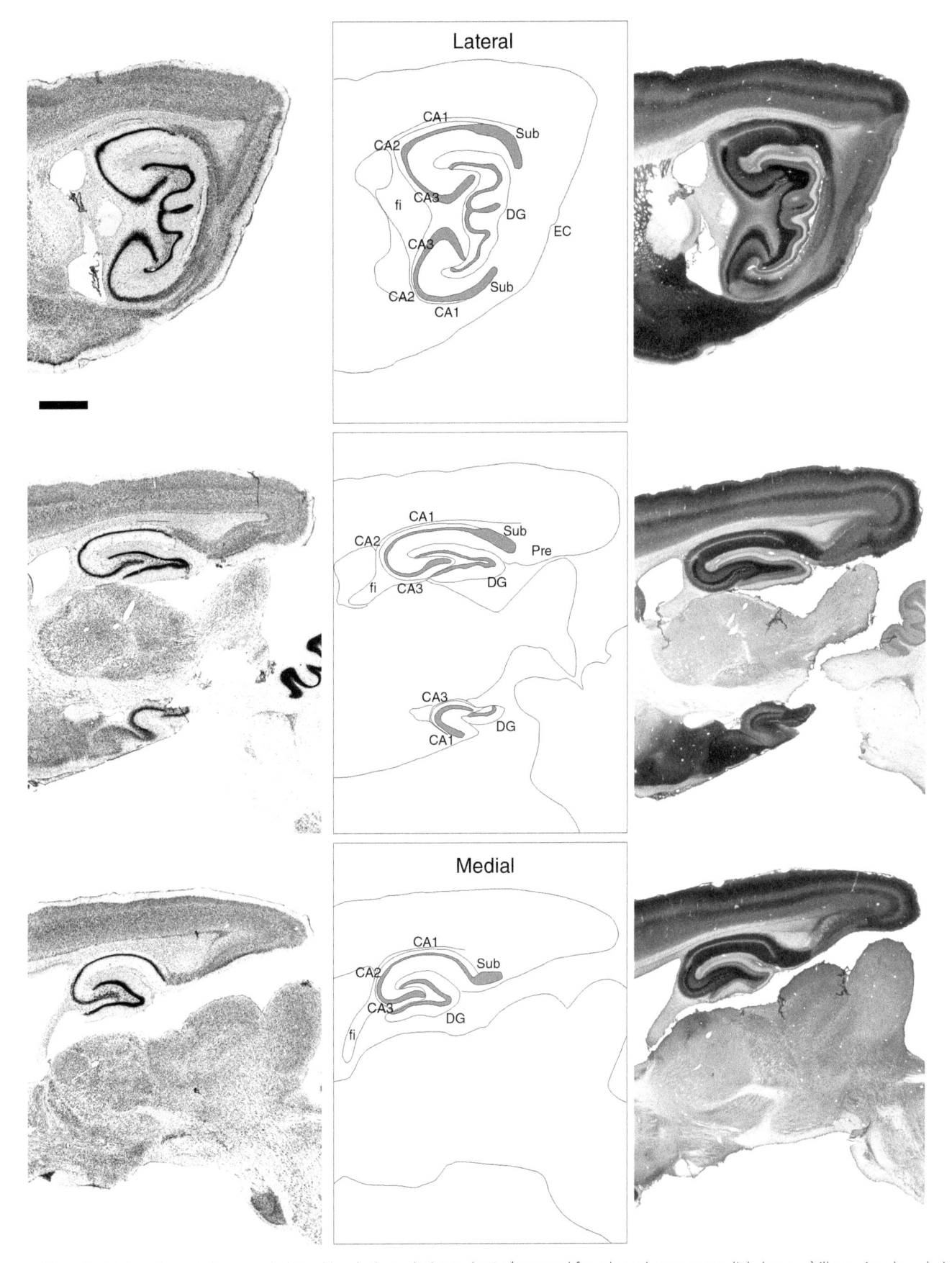

Figure 3.15 Sagittal sections at three mediolateral levels through the rat brain (arranged from lateral–top, to medial–bottom) illustrating the relative position of the hippocampal formation. The three panels on the left are Nissl-stained sections; the three panels on the right are adjacent, Timm's sulfide-silver-stained sections; the line drawings (middle column) highlight the different regions of the rat hippocampal formation seen in the stained sections. Scale bar is 1 mm.

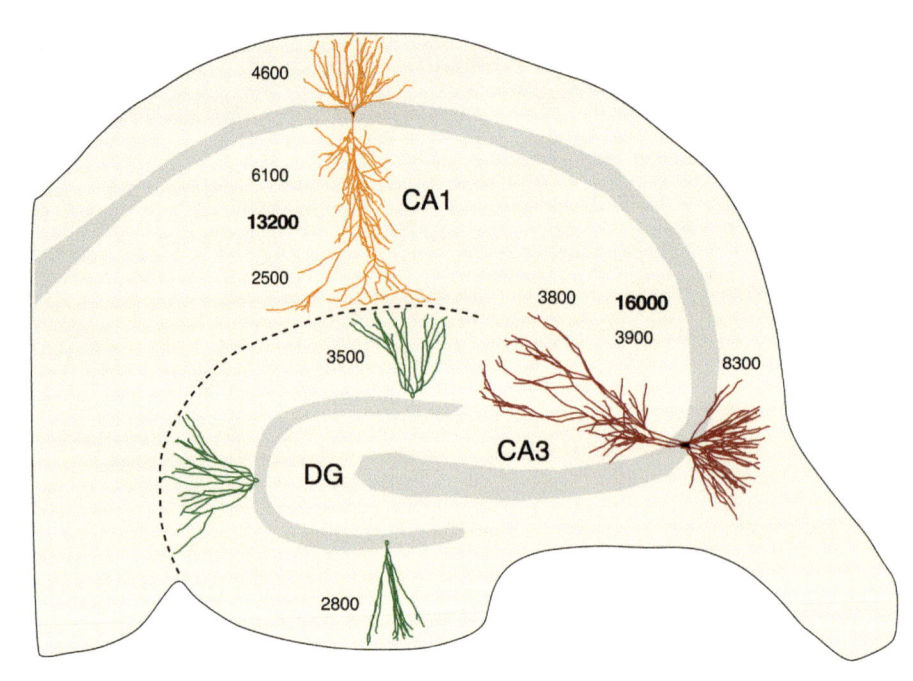

Figure 3.16 Schematic illustration representing the dendritic arborization of the principal cells in the dentate gyrus (granule cells) and hippocampus proper (pyramidal cells) of the rat. Numbers adjacent to the neurons indicate dendritic lengths. Numbers for the granule cells represent total dendritic length. For the CA3 and CA1 pyramidal cells, the total dendritic length in shown in bold. Lengths in the stratum lacunosum-moleculare, stratum radiatum, and stratum oriens are also included.

Table 3.1 Number of principal neurons in distinct regions of the hippocampal formation (in millions)

	Mouse	Rat	Monkey	Human
Dentate gyrus				
Granule cells	0.41–0.48	1.20 20% at birth	7.21 60% at birth	11–18 70% at birth
Hilar cells	0.01–0.02	0.05		
CA3				
Pyramidal cells	0.11–0.21 (+CA2)	0.15–0.25	0.95	2.28–2.83
CA2				
Pyramidal cells	0.02	0.02	0.12	
CA1				
Pyramidal cells	0.16–0.23	0.33–0.38	1.00	6.14–16
Subiculum				
Pyramidal cells	0.11–0.15	0.29	0.47	4.50–5.95
Presubiculum				
Pyramidal cells		0.33	1.45	9.78
Parasubiculum				
Pyramidal cells		0.22	0.21	
Entorhinal cortex				
Layer II		0.10	0.50	0.65–1.10
Layer III		0.25	1.62	3.59–6.09
Layer V(+VI)		0.32	1.41	2.71–6.31
Layer V		–	0.49	1.03–2.06
Layer VI		–	0.92	1.68–4.25
Total		0.68	3.53	6.88–13.50

Mouse studies: (van Dijk, Huang, Slomianka, & Amrein, 2016)

Rat studies: (Merrill, Chiba, & Tuszynski, 2001; Mulders, West, & Slomianka, 1997; Schlessinger, Cowan, & Swanson, 1978; Scorza et al., 2010; West, Slomianka, & Gundersen, 1991)

Monkey studies: (Jabès, Banta Lavenex, Amaral, & Lavenex, 2011; Piguet, Chareyron, Banta Lavenex, Amaral, & Lavenex, 2020)

Human studies: (Gomez-Isla et al., 1996; Harding, Halliday, & Kril, 1998; West & Slomianka, 1998)

Granule cell

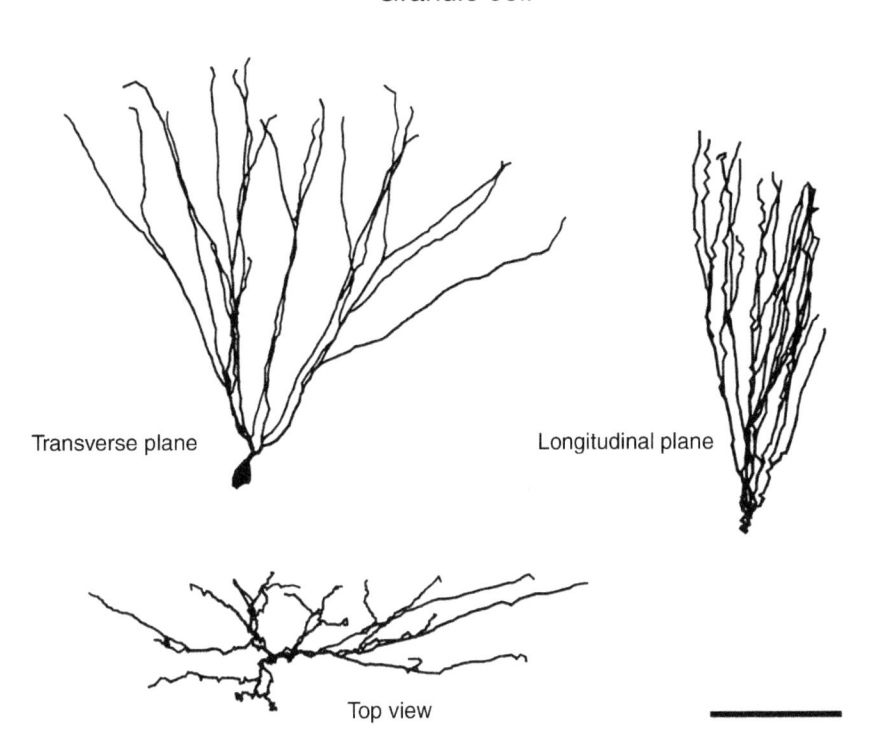

Transverse plane   Longitudinal plane

Top view

Figure 3.17 Dendritic organization of the dentate granule cells. Computer-generated reconstructions of HRP-filled granule cells from the suprapyramidal blade. Scale bar is 100 μm. (Adapted from Claiborne et al., 1990.)

The total number of granule cells in one dentate gyrus of the rat is about 1.2×10^6 (West et al., 1991; Rapp and Gallagher, 1996) (Table 3.1). Although neurogenesis in the dentate gyrus persists in adulthood, and appears to be under environmental control, quantitative stereological studies have shown that the total number of granule cells does not vary in adult animals. Only infant or juvenile mice exposed to running wheels or socially complex, "enriched" environments demonstrate a larger dentate gyrus and a greater number of granule cells that persist in adulthood, as compared with animals raised in standard laboratory cages (Kempermann et al., 1998a). Similar manipulations performed in adult animals can affect cell proliferation and/or survival of newly generated neurons, but they have no significant impact on the volume of the dentate gyrus or the total number of granule cells (Kempermann et al., 1998b). For reviews of adult neurogenesis in the dentate gyrus see (Kempermann et al., 2015; Toni and Schinder, 2015) and Chapter 9.

Before leaving the topic of granule cell number, we should note that the packing density and thickness of the granule cell layers varies somewhat along the septotemporal axis of the dentate gyrus (Gaarskjaer, 1978a). The packing density of granule cells is higher septally than temporally. Since the packing density of CA3 pyramidal cells follows an inverse gradient, the net result is that at septal levels of the hippocampal formation, the ratio of granule cells to CA3 pyramidal cells is something on the order of 12:1, whereas at the temporal pole this drops to 2:3. Since the CA3 pyramidal cells are the major recipients of granule cell innervation, and the number of mossy fiber synapses is roughly the same along the septotemporal axis, contact probability is much lower septally than temporally.

The granule cell is the only "principal" cell of the dentate gyrus, i.e., the only cell type that gives rise to axons that leave the dentate gyrus to innervate another hippocampal field (i.e., CA3). There is one type of neuron, called the mossy cell, whose axon leaves the dentate gyrus of one side of the brain only to innervate the dentate gyrus of the other side. There are numerous other types of neurons, most of which are inhibitory interneurons.

The pyramidal basket cell

The most intensively studied type of interneuron is the pyramidal basket cell (shown schematically in Figure 3.18). These cells are generally located along the deep surface of the granule cell layer. They have pyramidally shaped cell bodies, 25–35 μm in diameter, which are wedged slightly into the granule cell layer. The basket portion of the name refers to the fact that the axon of these cells forms pericellular plexuses that surround and form synapses with the cell bodies of granule cells. Ramón y Cajal first described the pyramidal basket cells as having a single, principal aspiny apical dendrite directed into the molecular layer (where it divides into several aspiny branches), and several principal basal dendrites that ramify and extend into the polymorphic cell layer (Ribak et al., 1978; Ribak and Seress, 1983). These cells contain biochemical markers for the inhibitory transmitter GABA and are thus presumably inhibitory. The number of basket cells is not constant throughout either the transverse or septotemporal extents of the dentate gyrus (Seress and Pokorny, 1981). At septal levels, the ratio of basket cells to granule cells is 1:100 in the suprapyramidal blade and 1:180 in the infrapyramidal blade. At temporal levels, the number is 1:150 for the suprapyramidal blade and 1:300 for the infrapyramidal blade. These data raise a theme that will be repeated throughout this chapter. Namely, despite the apparent cytoarchitectonic homogeneity of the hippocampal fields, there are several differences, especially regarding neurochemical innervation, at different septotemporal

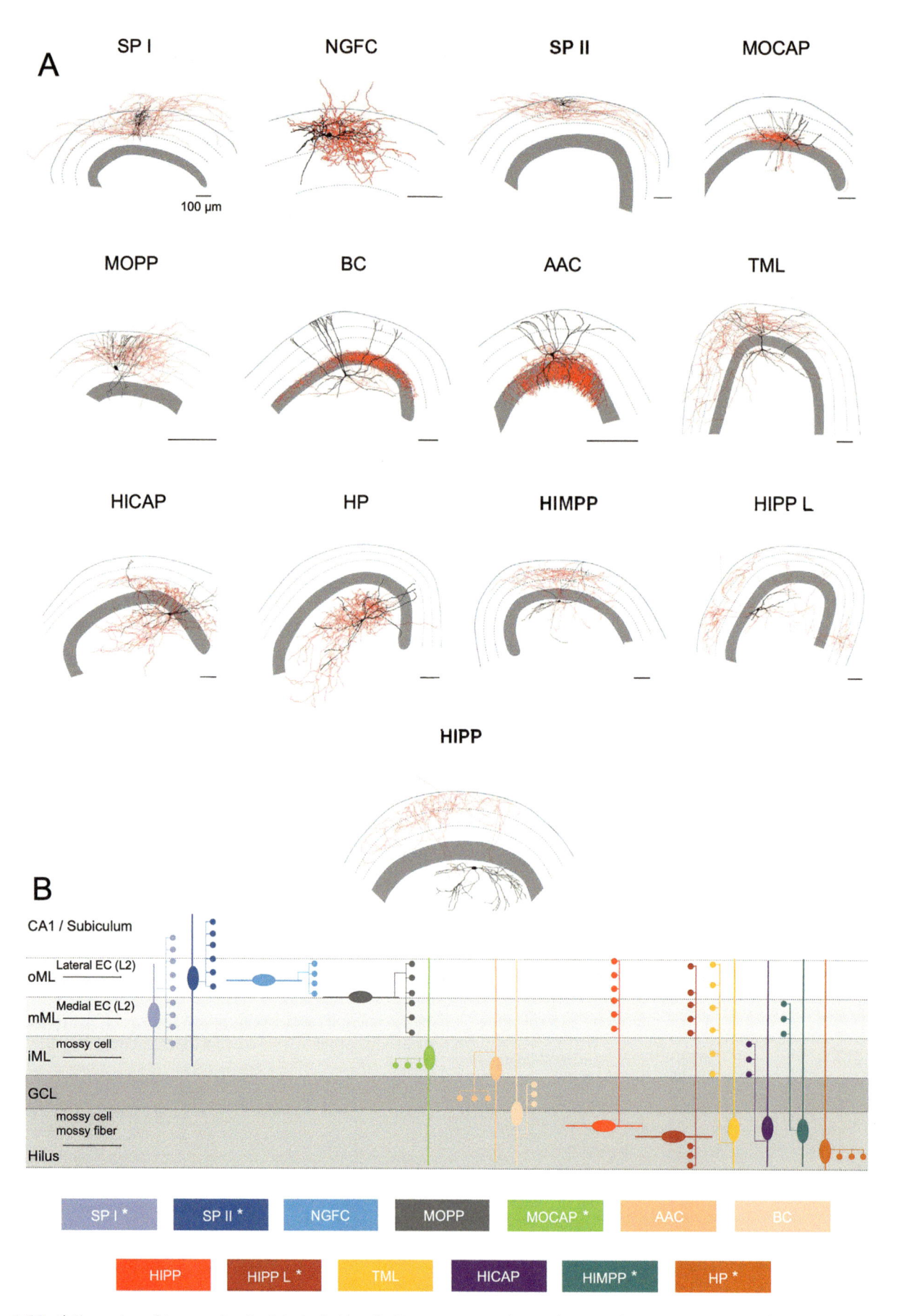

Figure 3.18 A) Illustration of the morphophysiologically identified interneurons in the DG (adapted from Degro et al., 2022). Cell bodies and dendrites are shown in black, and the axon in red. AAC, axo-axonic cell; BC, basket cell; HICAP, hilar commissural–associational pathway associated cell; HIMPP, hilar medial perforant pathway associated cell; HIPP/HIPP L, hilar perforant pathway associated (like) cell; HP, hilar projecting cell; MOCAP, molecular layer commissural–associational pathway associated cell; MOPP, molecular layer perforant pathway associated cell; NGFC, neurogliaform cell; SP I, subiculum projecting cell I; SP II, subiculum projecting cell II; SST, TML, total molecular layer cell. (B) Synopsis of interneuron classes in the dentate gyrus. Schematic overview of dentate gyrus interneuron types superimposed on the layered structure of the dentate gyrus (gray) with afferent pathways indicated by black arrows. Novel interneuron types are marked by an asterisk (*). Somatodendritic distributions are illustrated by oval profiles and thick lines, the axonal distribution is shown as thin lines and circles.

levels of the hippocampal formation. This perspective is elaborated in the recent studies that have identified regional differences in many fields based on transcriptomics (Cembrowski et al., 2016; Cembrowski, Wang, et al., 2018). Elegant patch-clamp recording studies have demonstrated that parvalbumin positive basket cells provide recurrent inhibition (in which the granule cells that excite them are inhibited) 10 times less frequently than lateral inhibition (in which other granule cells are inhibited) (Espinoza et al., 2018). This appears to be a pattern of connectivity that is unique to the dentate gyrus.

Other types of interneurons

There has been an explosion in the number of interneurons identified in the rat hippocampal formation (Freund and Buzsaki, 1996; Booker and Vida, 2018; Degro et al., 2022). Hippocampal interneurons form a heterogeneous population and are designed to carry out different functions. Many of the cell types can be distinguished on the basis of the distribution of their axonal plexus (Figure 3.18). Some have axons that terminate on cell bodies, whereas others have axons that terminate exclusively on the initial segments of other axons. Interneurons have also been distinguished on the basis of

their inputs. Some are preferentially innervated, for example, by the serotonergic fibers originating from the raphe nuclei. Interneurons can also be differentiated from principal cells on the basis of their electrophysiological characteristics. At least some interneurons have high rates of spontaneous activity and fire in relation to the theta rhythm. For this reason, interneurons are often called theta cells (see Chapter 5). A major ongoing research effort is to determine whether different classes of interneurons demonstrate distinct electrophysiological response profiles.

Within the same subgranular region occupied by the cell bodies and dendrites of the pyramidal basket cells are several other cell types with distinctly different somal shapes, as well as different dendritic and axonal configurations (Houser, 2007; Degro et al., 2022) (Figure 3.18). Some of these cells are multipolar with several aspiny dendrites entering the molecular and polymorphic layers, while others tend to be more fusiform-shaped with a similar dendritic distribution. Many of these cells share fine structural characteristics such as infolded nuclei, extensive perikaryal cytoplasm with large Nissl bodies and intranuclear rods. Moreover, it appears that all of these cells give rise to axons that contribute to the basket plexus in the granule cell layer. Many of these neurons

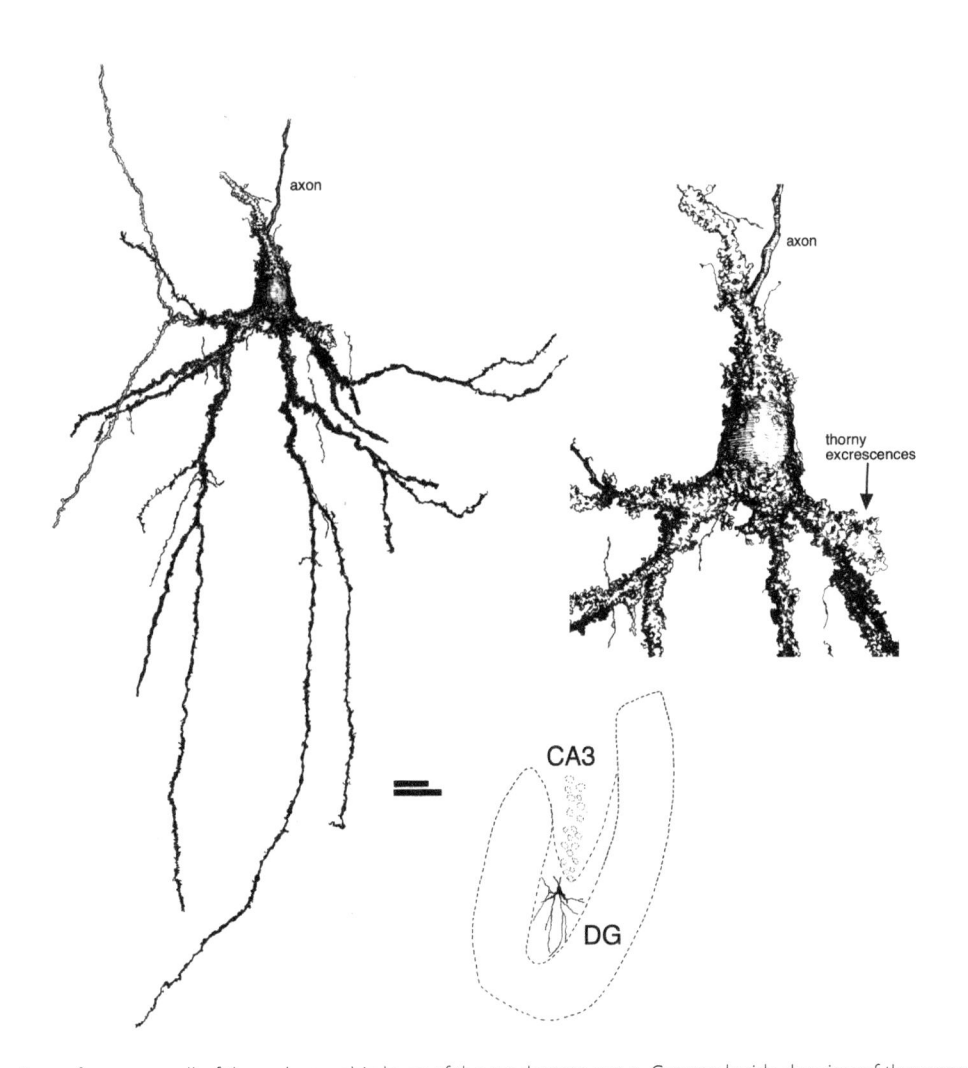

Figure 3.19 Line drawings of a mossy cell of the polymorphic layer of the rat dentate gyrus. Camera lucida drawing of the soma and dendritic arbor (*left*) and the position of the cell is indicated in the line drawing below. Note that the dendrites extend widely within the polymorphic layer but do not penetrate the granule cell layer. The cell body and proximal dendrites are shown at higher magnification on the right. The proximal dendrites are encrusted with many thorny excrescences which are the terminal regions of mossy fiber expansions. Scale bar is 20 μm. (Adapted from Amaral, 1978.)

are immunoreactive for GABA, form symmetrical synaptic contacts with the cell bodies, with proximal dendrites, and occasionally with axon initial segments of granule cells, and therefore function as inhibitory interneurons. These cells are not neurochemically homogeneous, however, since subsets appear to colocalize distinct categories of other neuroactive substances (Booker and Vida, 2018; Degro et al., 2022).

Neurons of the molecular layer

The molecular layer is occupied primarily by dendrites of the granule, basket, and polymorphic cells, as well as axons and terminal axonal arbors from the entorhinal cortex and other sources. At least two neuron types are also present in the molecular layer. The first is located deep in the molecular layer, has a multipolar or triangular cell body, and gives rise to an axon that produces a substantial terminal plexus largely limited to the outer two-thirds of the molecular layer. This neuron has aspiny dendrites that remain mainly within the molecular layer and has been called the MOPP cell (molecular layer perforant path-associated cell). This terminology was proposed by Han et al. (1993) to bring some order to naming interneurons in the hippocampal formation. The lettering system refers to the location of the cell body and to the region where the axon is distributed. There is a second category of interneurons in the outer third of the molecular layer (outer molecular layer cells) that have axons that ramify heavily in the outer two-thirds of the molecular layer but also have collaterals that cross the hippocampal fissure into the subiculum (Booker and Vida, 2018; Degro et al., 2022). A class of small "neurogliaform cells" are located in the outer molecular layer, have few dendrites, and have axons that ramify profusely around the cell body and can cross the hippocampal fissure into the stratum lacunosum-moleculare of CA1.

A second type of neuron in the molecular layer resembles the so-called chandelier or axo-axonic cell originally found in the neocortex (Soriano and Frotscher, 1989). These cells are generally located immediately adjacent or even within the superficial portion of the granule cell layer. The axo-axonic cell is named for the fact that its axon descends from the molecular layer into the granule cell layer, collateralizes profusely and then terminates, with symmetric synaptic contacts, exclusively on the axon initial segments of granule cells. Thus, their shape resembles that of a chandelier. Each axo-axonic cell may innervate the axon initial segments of as many as 1,000 granule cells. Since these cells are immunoreactive for markers of GABAergic neurons and make symmetrical synapses, it is likely that they provide a second means of inhibitory control of granule cell output. The inputs to the axo-axonic cells are currently unknown, though their dendrites remain mainly in the molecular layer, where they are likely to receive perforant-path input from the entorhinal cortex.

Other neurons with cell bodies located in the molecular layer are members of the IS (interneuron specific) class of interneurons that are specialized for termination on other interneurons. These are demonstrated using immunohistochemistry for vasoactive intestinal peptide (VIP), and their axons overlap with the dendrites of the O-LM and HIPP cells (these cell types will be defined shortly).

Neurons of the polymorphic cell layer

The polymorphic layer harbors a variety of neuron types, but little is known about many of them. The most common type, and certainly

the most impressive, is the mossy cell (Amaral, 1978), (Figure 3.19). This cell type is probably what Ramón y Cajal referred to as the "stellate or triangular" cells located in his subzone of fusiform cells and is undoubtedly what Lorente de Nó referred to as "modified pyramids." The cell bodies of the mossy cells are large (25–35 μm) and are often triangular or multipolar in shape. Three or more thick dendrites originate from the cell body and extend for long distances within the polymorphic layer. Each principal dendrite bifurcates once or twice and generally gives rise to a few side branches. While most of the daughter dendritic branches remain within the polymorphic layer, an occasional dendrite pierces the granule cell layer and enters the molecular layer. The mossy cell dendrites virtually never enter the adjacent CA3 field.

The most distinctive feature of the mossy cell is that all of its proximal dendrites are covered by very large and complex spines evocatively called thorny excrescences. These are the distinctive sites of termination of the mossy fiber axons. While thorny excrescences are also observed on the proximal dendrites of pyramidal cells in CA3, they are never as dense as the ones on the mossy cells. The distal dendrites of the mossy cell have typical pedunculate spines that appear to be less densely distributed than those on the distal dendrites of the pyramidal cells in the hippocampus. The mossy cells are immunoreactive for glutamate, presumably excitatory cells, and give rise to axons that project to the inner third of the molecular layer of the ipsilateral and contralateral dentate gyrus, making asymmetric terminations on the dendrites of granule cells. The mossy cells would thus appear to be the major source of the excitatory associational/commissural projection to the dentate gyrus. Interestingly, the distribution of their projections to the molecular layer appears to vary depending on whether they are in the dorsal or ventral dentate gyrus of the rat (Botterill et al., 2021). For this reason, the mossy cell does not fit the classical description of an interneuron. The mossy cells demonstrate a number of interesting species differences. For example, mossy cells in the mouse dentate

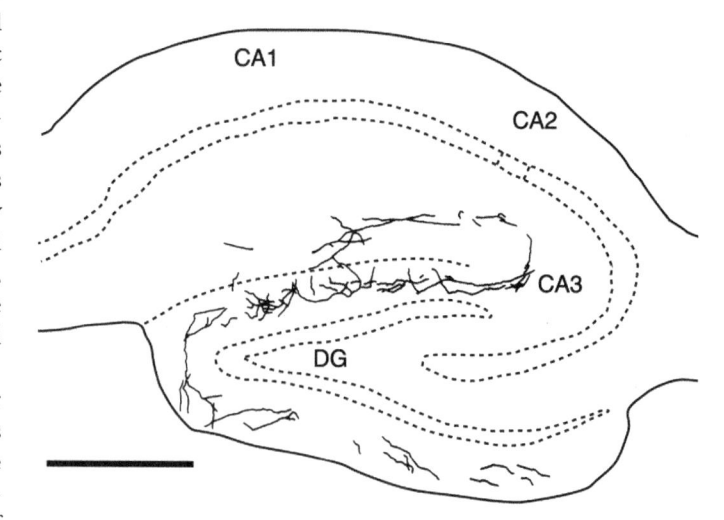

Figure 3.20 Perforant path projections. This illustration shows the distribution of labeled axon branches arising from a single entorhinal cortex layer II spiny stellate neuron. The axon innervates both the molecular layer of the dentate gyrus and the stratum lacunosum-moleculare of the CA2–CA3 fields of the hippocampus. Scale bar is 500 μm. (Adapted with permission of Wiley-Liss, a subsidiary of John Wiley & Sons, from Tamamaki and Nojyo, 1993.)

gyrus, particularly at ventral levels, stain heavily for calretinin but this is not the case in the rat (Houser, 2007). In primates, mossy cells of both New and Old World monkeys demonstrate calretinin staining, but this is far less obvious in the human dentate gyrus (Seress et al., 2008). The mossy cell has undergone intensive research, and many details about this cell type can be found in recent reviews (Scharfman, 2016, 2018). Using single-cell analysis of whole brain connectomes, a subset of mossy cells demonstrates projections outside of the hippocampal formation in the mouse brain (Qiu et al., 2024).

There are also a number of fusiform cells in the polymorphic layer. The main difference between the fusiform cell types is whether they have spines or not. One type, the long-spined multipolar cell has been called the HIPP cell (hilar perforant path-associated cell). This cell type has two or three principal dendrites that originate from the poles of the cell, run mainly parallel to the granule cell layer, and can extend for nearly the entire length of one blade of the granule cell layer. The conspicuous feature of this cell is the distribution of copious, long, and often branched spines over its cell body and dendrites. Intracellular staining techniques demonstrate that these cells have axons that ascend into the outer two-thirds of the molecular layer (i.e., the perforant path zone) and terminate with symmetrical and presumably inhibitory synapses on the dendrites of granule cells. An amazing feature of these neurons is that their axonal plexus can extend for as much as 3.5 mm along the septotemporal axis of the dentate gyrus (the entire length of the dentate gyrus in the rat is only about 10 mm) and may generate as many as 100,000 synaptic terminals. Since inhibitory interneurons typically have aspiny dendrites and relatively local axonal plexuses, this long-spined multipolar/HIPP cell is a very atypical interneuron. At least some of these HIPP cells appear to correspond to the somatostatin/GABA cells that give rise to the somatostatin innervation of the outer portion of the molecular layer.

There are also multipolar or triangular cells in the polymorphic layer with thin, aspiny dendrites that extend within the polymorphic and molecular layers. The axons of these HICAP cells (hilar commissural-associational pathway related cells) extend through the granule cell layer and branch profusely in the inner third of the molecular layer. There are a variety of other neuron types in the polymorphic layer of the dentate gyrus whose axonal plexus have not yet been well described.

Before leaving the typing of interneurons in the dentate gyrus, it is perhaps worth noting that the field has come a long way from believing that interneurons merely damp down neuronal activity. Rather, most current neuroscientists devoted to the study of the hippocampus highlight the heterogeneity of interneurons and see them as integral components of the normal information processing network of the hippocampal formation (see Chapters 5 and 7).

3.9.1.3 Extrinsic connections

Entorhinal cortex projection to the dentate gyrus

The dentate gyrus receives its major input from the entorhinal cortex, via the so-called perforant pathway (Figure 3.20). The projection to the dentate gyrus arises mainly from cells located in layer

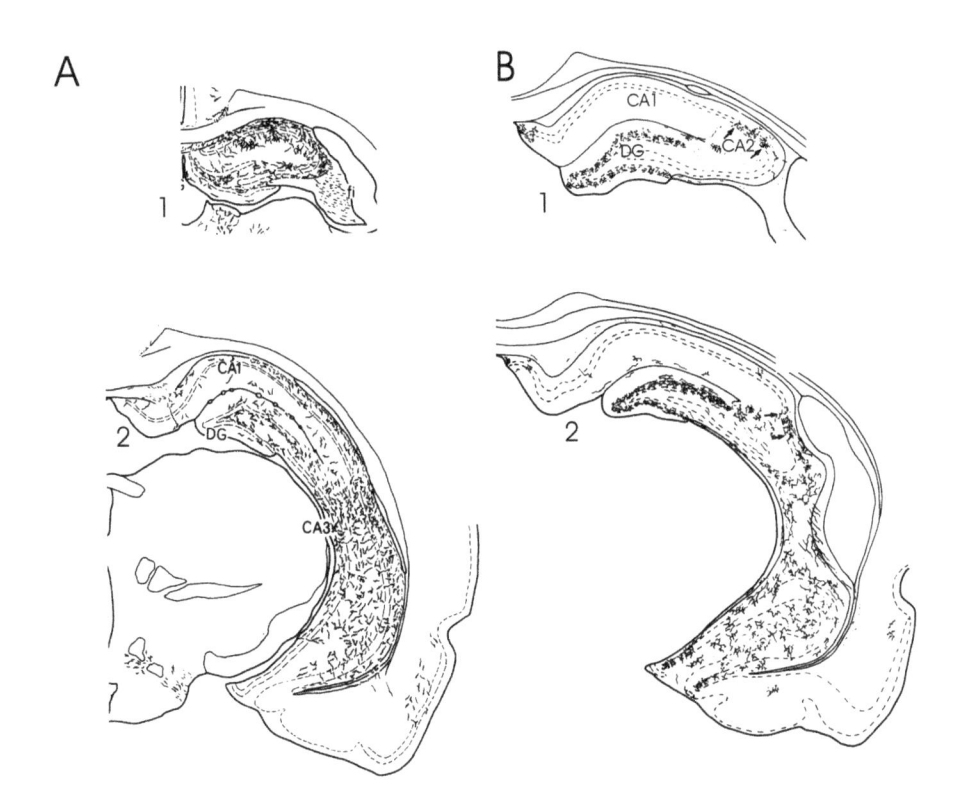

Figure 3.21 Septal and hypothalamic inputs to the rat hippocampal formation. (A) Distribution of labeled fibers in the hippocampal formation resulting from an injection of PHA-L (an anterograde tracer) focused in the medial portion of the medial septal nucleus (adapted with permission from Gaykema et al., 1990). (B) Distribution of PHA-L-labeled fibers resulting from an injection in the supramammillary nucleus. Note the dense plexus of fibers located just superficial to the granule cell layer and in the CA2 region of the hippocampus (between the small arrows) (adapted with permission from Haglund et al., 1984).

II of the entorhinal cortex, although a minor component of the projection also comes from layers V and VI (Steward and Scoville, 1976; Deller et al., 1996a). Layer II of the entorhinal cortex has been subdivided based on the chemical signatures of resident neurons into reelin-expressing neurons and calbindin-expressing neurons and the projection to the dentate gyrus originates mainly from the former (Witter et al., 2017; and Chapter 12). In the molecular layer of the dentate gyrus, the entorhinal terminals are strictly confined to the superficial (outer) two-thirds where they form asymmetric synapses that account for nearly 85% of the total axospinous terminations (Nafstad, 1967; Hjorth-Simonsen and Jeune, 1972). These contacts occur primarily on the dendritic spines of granule cells, although a small number of perforant path fibers also form asymmetric synapses on the shafts of GABA-positive interneurons. The organization of the perforant path projection in the mouse is very similar to that in the rat although there are some detectable species differences such as a more meager commissural connection in the mouse (van Groen et al., 2002; van Groen et al., 2003), which is revealed by a much thinner darkly stained inner band of the molecular layer in Timm's stained material.

The perforant pathway can be divided into two parts based on the region of origin, pattern of termination, and appearance in histochemical and immunohistochemical preparations. In the rat, the two divisions have been called the lateral and medial perforant paths because they originate from the lateral and medial entorhinal areas, respectively. Perforant path fibers originating in the lateral entorhinal area terminate in the most superficial third of the molecular layer, whereas the perforant path fibers originating from the medial entorhinal area terminate in the middle third of the molecular layer. These terminal zones are readily distinguished by the classical Timm's stain method for visualization of heavy metals, which demonstrates dense staining in the outer third of the molecular layer, a near absence of staining in the middle third and a dark staining in the inner third that is associated with the commissural/associational connection (Figure 3.12). Projections from both areas of the entorhinal cortex innervate the entire transverse extent of the molecular layer. The thin axon branches (0.1 μm) in the molecular layer of the dentate gyrus show periodic varicosities with a thickness of 0.5–1.0 μm. The entorhinal layer II spiny stellate cells project up to 2 mm in the septotemporal direction forming a sheet-like axon arbor in the molecular layer (Tamamaki and Nojyo, 1993).

Since the perforant path fibers terminate exclusively in the molecular layer of the dentate gyrus, certain neurons will not be innervated by this input. Cells with dendrites confined to the polymorphic layer do not receive input from entorhinal cortex layer II neurons, although they might receive light input from layer V–VI neurons (Deller et al., 1996a). The mossy cells, for example, are thus likely to receive little or no direct perforant path input, particularly from layer II cells.

In addition to perforant path fibers, the dentate gyrus also receives at least minor projections from the presubiculum and parasubiculum (Kohler, 1985). These fibers enter the molecular layer and ramify in a zone that is interspersed between the lateral and medial perforant path projections. The presubicular axons tend to be thicker than those from the entorhinal cortex and give rise to collaterals that take a radial course in the molecular layer, in contrast to the predominantly transverse orientation of the entorhinal perforant pathway fibers. There has been relatively little recent analysis of the presubiculum projection to the dentate gyrus. Since the presubiculum receives the only direct input from the anterior thalamic nucleus, these fibers provide a potential link by which thalamic information could reach the dentate gyrus.

Basal forebrain inputs: projections from the septal nuclei

The dentate gyrus receives relatively few inputs from subcortical structures. Certainly the most robust and long studied is the projection from the septal nuclei (Mosko et al., 1973; Swanson, 1978; Amaral and Kurz, 1985) (Figure 3.21). The septal projection arises from cells of the medial septal nucleus and the nucleus of the diagonal band of Broca, and travels to the hippocampal formation via four routes: the fimbria, dorsal fornix, supracallosal stria, and a ventral route through and around the amygdaloid complex. Septal fibers heavily innervate cells of the polymorphic layer, including the mossy cell (Sun et al., 2017) particularly in a narrow region just subjacent to the granule cell layer. Septal fibers are lightly distributed throughout the molecular layer (Figure 3.20A).

A major portion of the fibers of the septal projection to the dentate gyrus are cholinergic. Thirty to fifty percent of the cells in the medial septal nucleus and 50–75% of the cells in the nucleus of the diagonal band that project to the hippocampal formation are cholinergic. However, many of the septal cells that project to the dentate gyrus are actually GABAergic. The most interesting facet of this heterogeneous septal projection is that the cholinergic and GABAergic components target different cell types. Fibers of the septal GABAergic projections terminate preferentially on other GABAergic nonpyramidal cells, such as the basket pyramidal cells of the dentate gyrus, and they form symmetrical, presumably inhibitory contacts. The heaviest GABAergic septal termination is on interneurons located in the polymorphic layer. The cholinergic septal projection to the dentate gyrus, in contrast, terminates mainly on granule cells, making asymmetric, presumably excitatory contacts on dendritic spines, chiefly in the inner third of the molecular layer; only 5–10% of the cholinergic synapses are on interneurons.

The septal projection to the dentate gyrus and to the remainder of the hippocampal formation is topographically organized. Cells located medially in the medial septal nucleus tend to project preferentially to septal or dorsal levels of the dentate gyrus, whereas cells located laterally in the medial septal nucleus tend to project to temporal levels. Because the medially situated neurons in the medial septal nucleus tend to be GABAergic rather than cholinergic, septal levels of the dentate gyrus receive most of their cholinergic input from the nucleus of the diagonal band. In contrast, temporal levels of the dentate gyrus receive their cholinergic innervation primarily from the medial septal nucleus.

Supramammillary and other hypothalamic inputs

The major hypothalamic projection to the dentate gyrus arises from a population of large cells, the supramammillary area, which caps and partially surrounds the medial mammillary nuclei (Wyss et al., 1979; Dent et al., 1983; Magloczky et al., 1994; Hashimotodani et al., 2018). The supramammillary projection terminates heavily in a narrow zone of the molecular layer located just superficial to the granule cell layer and only lightly in the polymorphic layer or the remaining portion of the molecular layer (Figure 3.21B). The vast majority of the supramammillary fibers terminate on the proximal dendrites of granule cells. There has been some controversy about

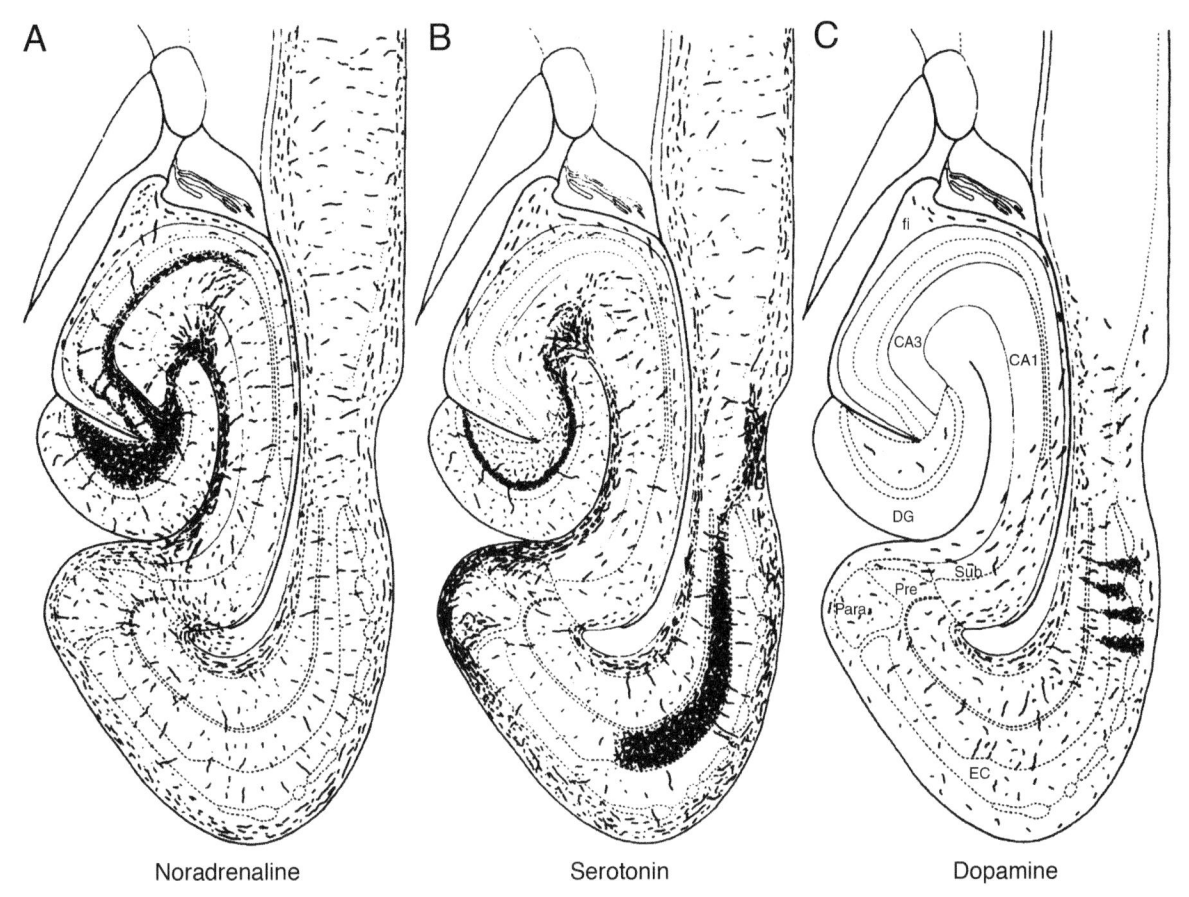

Figure 3.22 Line drawing of horizontal sections through the rat hippocampal formation showing the distribution of noradrenergic (A), serotonergic (B), and dopaminergic (C) fibers and terminals. (Adapted with permission from Swanson et al., 1987.)

the neurotransmitter of the supramammillary projection, but there is substantial evidence that this projection is excitatory and is likely using glutamate as a primary neurotransmitter (Kiss et al., 2000). Most, but not all, of the glutamatergic supramammillary neurons that project to the dentate gyrus also colocalize calretinin; some of these cells also colocalize substance P (Borhegyi and Leranth, 1997). There is additional evidence that supramammillary fibers may release GABA or corelease both glutamate and GABA and can facilitate the firing of granule cells activated by perforant path fibers (Vertes, 2015; Hashimotodani et al., 2018).

In addition to the supramammillary cells, there are additional cells scattered in several hypothalamic nuclei, many of which are in a perifornical position or within the lateral hypothalamic area, that project to the dentate gyrus. While taken together these cells constitute a sizable input to the hippocampal formation, their diffuseness and lack of any distinguishing biochemical marker has made it difficult to study their patterns of termination in the hippocampal formation.

Brainstem inputs

The dentate gyrus receives a particularly prominent noradrenergic input from the pontine nucleus locus coeruleus (Pickel et al., 1974; Swanson and Hartman, 1975; Loughlin et al., 1986). The noradrenergic fibers terminate mainly in the polymorphic layer of the dentate gyrus and extend into the stratum lucidum of CA3, as if preferentially terminating in the zones occupied by mossy fibers (Figure 3.22). The dentate gyrus receives a minor and diffusely

distributed dopaminergic projection that arises mainly from cells located in the ventral tegmental area. The dopaminergic fibers terminate mainly in the polymorphic layer.

The serotonergic projection that originates from median and dorsal divisions of the raphe nuclei also terminates most heavily in the polymorphic layer in an immediately subgranular portion of the layer (Conrad et al., 1974; Moore and Halaris, 1975; Kohler and Steinbusch, 1982; Vertes et al., 1999). A number of GABAergic interneurons appear to be preferentially innervated by the serotonergic fibers. The targets are often the pyramidal basket cells. Fusiform neurons in the region, particularly those that are stained for the calcium-binding protein calbindin, are also very heavily innervated. As with the cholinergic projection from the septum, many of the cells in the raphe nuclei that project to the hippocampal formation appear to be nonserotonergic, but their transmitter is not known.

3.9.1.4 Intrinsic connections

Basket cell and axo-axonic cell innervation of the granule cell layer

As noted previously, there are a variety of basket cells located just below the granule cell layer. These all appear to contribute to a very dense terminal plexus that is confined to the granule cell layer (Struble et al., 1978; Sik et al., 1997; Espinoza et al., 2018). The terminals in this basket plexus are GABAergic and form symmetric, inhibitory contacts, located primarily on the cell bodies and proximal dendritic shafts of apical dendrites of the granule cells. GABAergic neurons in the polymorphic layer are themselves innervated by

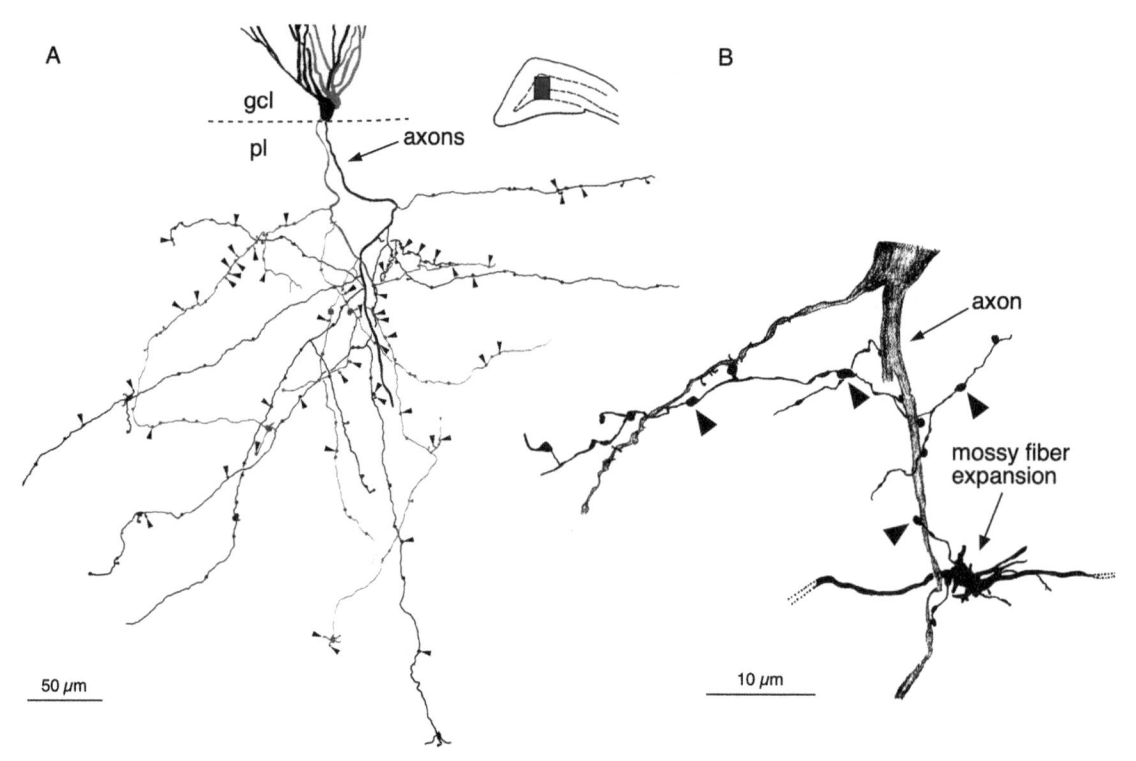

Figure 3.23 Granule cell projections to the polymorphic cell layer. A. Axon arbors of two adjacent granule cells (gray and black) reconstructed from three neighboring 60 μm-thick sections. While the complex mossy fiber expansions terminate on mossy cells in the polymorphic layer or CA3 pyramidal cells, the small varicosities, which are much more numerous, terminate on a variety of neurons including GABAergic neurons. Fifty-two of the 175 small terminals illustrated here innervated GABAergic neurons, whereas large mossy terminals contacted none. Insert shows position of granule cells. (Adapted with permission from Acsady et al., 1998.) B. Line drawing illustrating at higher magnification the varicosities along the length of the mossy fiber axons (arrowheads) make close apposition to the axon and dendrites of a pyramidal basket cell. (Amaral unpublished data.)

other GABAergic terminals, some of which arise from extrinsic sources, such as the GABAergic septal input. This polysynaptic cascade of inhibitory interconnections indicates that the hippocampal circuitry provides for intricate inhibitory and disinhibitory control of cell excitability—an issue discussed in Chapter 7.

Given the small number of basket cells relative to granule cells, the question arises as to how widespread is the influence of a single basket cell. Analysis of Golgi-stained axonal plexuses from single basket cells indicates that they extend for distances greater than 900 μm in the transverse axis and about 1.5 mm in the septotemporal axis. This widely distributed axonal plexus would allow a single basket cell to influence as many as 10,000, or about 1%, of the granule cells. The other inhibitory input to granule cells originates with the chandelier or axo-axonic cells located in the molecular layer. These form symmetric contacts exclusively with the axon initial segment.

Granule cells projection to the polymorphic layer

The granule cells give rise to distinctive unmyelinated axons which Ramón y Cajal called mossy fibers. The mossy fibers have unusually large boutons that form en passant synapses with the mossy cells and with the CA3 pyramidal cells; we shall describe this projection in more detail shortly. What is not generally appreciated is that the mossy fiber axons form a distinctive set of collaterals that also innervate cells within the polymorphic layer of the dentate gyrus (Figure 3.23). Each principal mossy fiber (which is on the order of 0.2–0.5 μm in diameter) gives rise to about 7 thinner

collaterals within the polymorphic layer before entering the CA3 field of the hippocampus. As much as 2,300 μm of collateral axonal plexus is generated by a single mossy fiber in the polymorphic layer (Claiborne et al., 1986). Within the polymorphic layer, the mossy fiber collaterals branch extensively, and the daughter branches bear two types of synaptic varicosities. Numerous small (approximately 2 μm) spherical synaptic varicosities are distributed unevenly along these collaterals. There are about 160–200 of these varicosities distributed throughout the axonal collateral plexus of a single granule cell, and these form contacts on dendrites located in the polymorphic layer. At the end of each of the collateral branches there are also larger (3–5 μm diameter), irregularly shaped varicosities that resemble, although are smaller than, the mossy fiber boutons found in CA3. The mossy fiber terminals in the polymorphic layer establish contacts with the proximal dendrites of the mossy cells (Ribak et al., 1985) and the basal dendrites of the pyramidal basket cells as well as other unidentified cells. The vast majority of granule cell collaterals in the polymorphic cell layer terminate on GABAergic interneurons (Acsady et al., 1998). Since there are 160–200 such varicosities (compared with about 20 of the larger thorny excrescences), mossy fiber axons synapse on a larger number of interneurons than mossy cells or CA3 pyramidal cells. Mossy fiber collaterals may enter the granule cell layer, but they virtually never enter the molecular layer. The collaterals that enter the granule cell layer appear to terminate preferentially on the apical dendritic shafts of pyramidal basket cells. This lack of mossy fiber innervation of the molecular layer is of some importance since in kindling, and in some pathological conditions, such as epilepsy, mossy fibers can be induced to sprout into the molecular layer (see Chapter 18).

Mossy cells projection to the associational/commissural zone

The inner third of the molecular layer receives a projection that originates exclusively from neurons in the polymorphic layer (Laurberg and Sorensen, 1981; Frotscher et al., 1991; Buckmaster et al., 1992; Buckmaster et al., 1996). Since, in the rat, this projection originates both in the ipsilateral and contralateral sides of the hippocampus, it has been called the associational/commissural projection. This projection was initially claimed to arise both from the cells of the polymorphic layer and from the CA3 pyramidal cells located within the confines of the dentate gyrus. It is now clear, however, that the associational/commissural projection arises exclusively from cells in the polymorphic layer, and CA3 cells do not project to the molecular layer of the dentate gyrus. While this statement is generally true, it appears that at least some CA3 neurons in the most temporal extreme of the hippocampal formation might send collaterals into the granule and molecular layers of the dentate gyrus (Scharfman, 2007). This projection appears very minor in relation to other dentate inputs and it is not known why this projection is only observed in the temporal portion of the dentate gyrus. Thus, the principle of unidirectionality, while generally true, may have some exceptions. For all practical purposes, the organization of the commissural projection is similar to that of the ipsilateral associational connection.

The majority of synaptic terminals of the associational/commissural pathway form asymmetric, presumably excitatory synaptic terminals on spines of proximal dendrites of granule cells. Many of the axons contributing to these synaptic terminals originate from the mossy cells of the polymorphic layer, and individual mossy cells contribute a projection to both the ipsilateral associational and commissural projections. The fact that the mossy cells are immunoreactive for glutamate adds credence to the notion that the associational/commissural projection is excitatory. It also appears that the commissural connection is made up, in part, from somatostatin and parvalbumin (presumably GABAergic) neurons, which account for less than 5% of the cells responsible for this connection (Eyre and Bartos, 2019).

There are a number of interesting features of this "feedback" projection from the mossy cells to the granule cells. First, the projection from mossy cells located at any particular septotemporal level of the dentate gyrus is distributed widely along the longitudinal axis, both septally and temporally from the point of origin. Axons from any particular septotemporal point in the dentate gyrus may innervate as much as 75% of the long axis of the dentate gyrus (Amaral and Witter, 1989). Second, the projection to the molecular layer at the septotemporal level of origin is very weak but gets increasingly stronger at levels that are progressively more distant from the cells of origin. Remembering that mossy cells are the recipients of massive innervation from the granule cells at their same level (via the mossy fiber collaterals into the polymorphic layer), it would appear that the mossy cells pass on the collective output of granule cells from one septotemporal level to granule cells located at distant levels of the dentate gyrus. That this is a major role of the mossy cell is supported by the finding that this cell type receives numerically fewer extrinsic inputs except from the septal nuclei (Sun et al., 2017).

The full impact of this longitudinal organization of the associational projection cannot be fully appreciated without one further piece of information. This is that the associational fibers contact not only the spines of the granule cell dendrites but also the dendritic shafts of the GABAergic basket cells that, in turn, innervate the granule cells. Thus, the associational projection may function both as a feedforward excitatory pathway to distant granule cells and as a disynaptic feedforward inhibitory pathway, via the pyramidal basket cell as intermediary.

GABA/somatostatin projection from the polymorphic layer to the outer molecular layer

Antibodies directed against the peptide somatostatin have revealed that neurons scattered throughout the polymorphic layer are immunoreactive for this peptide, and account for approximately 16% of the GABAergic cells in the dentate gyrus (Bakst, 1986; Sik et al., 1997). As noted earlier, the somatostatin immunoreactive cells may correspond, in part, to the HIPP cells. The somatostatin-positive cells all colocalize with GABA and are the source of the somatostatin immunoreactive fibers and terminals in the outer two-thirds of the molecular layer. This system of fibers, which forms contacts on the distal dendrites of the granule cells, provides a third means for inhibitory control of granule cell activity, in addition to the basket cell plexus and the axo-axonic terminals provided by the chandelier cells. Since electron microscopic studies have demonstrated that the somatostatin cells are contacted by mossy fiber terminals, the projection to the outer molecular layer thus constitutes a local feedback inhibitory circuit.

Interestingly, unlike the mossy cell associational projection that terminates more heavily to distant levels of the dentate gyrus, the GABA/somatostatin projection terminates most heavily at the level of the cells of origin, and termination rapidly decreases within approximately 1.5 mm septally and temporally of the cells of origin. Thus, the mossy cell projection and the somatostatin/GABA cell projection have terminal fields that are spatially complementary in both radial and septotemporal axes; the distribution suggests that the two cell types mediate distant excitation and local inhibition, respectively.

3.9.1.5 Dentate gyrus efferent projection—the mossy fibers

The dentate gyrus does not project to any brain region other than the CA3 field of the hippocampus. The axons that project to CA3, the mossy fibers, arise exclusively from the granule cells and terminate in a relatively narrow zone mainly located just above the CA3 pyramidal cell layer (Blackstad et al., 1970; Gaarskjaer, 1978a and 1978b; Swanson et al., 1978; Claiborne et al., 1986). In the proximal portion of CA3, mossy fibers are also located below and within the pyramidal cell layer. The layer of mossy fiber termination located just above the pyramidal cell layer is called stratum lucidum, since the lack of myelin on the mossy fibers gives the layer a relatively clear appearance in fresh tissue (as one might visualize in a hippocampal slice experiment). There is no indication that dentate neurons other than the granule cells project to CA3; in particular, cells in the polymorphic layer do not project to the hippocampus, at least in the rodent. The dentate projection to CA3 has historically been said to stop near the border of CA3 with CA2, and the lack of granule cell input via particular branched spines called thorny excrescences is one of the main features that distinguishes CA3 from CA2 pyramidal cells. The border zone between CA3 and CA2 is not precise, and there are some mossy fibers that seem to enter the region that contain CA2 pyramidal cells. This potential pathway from

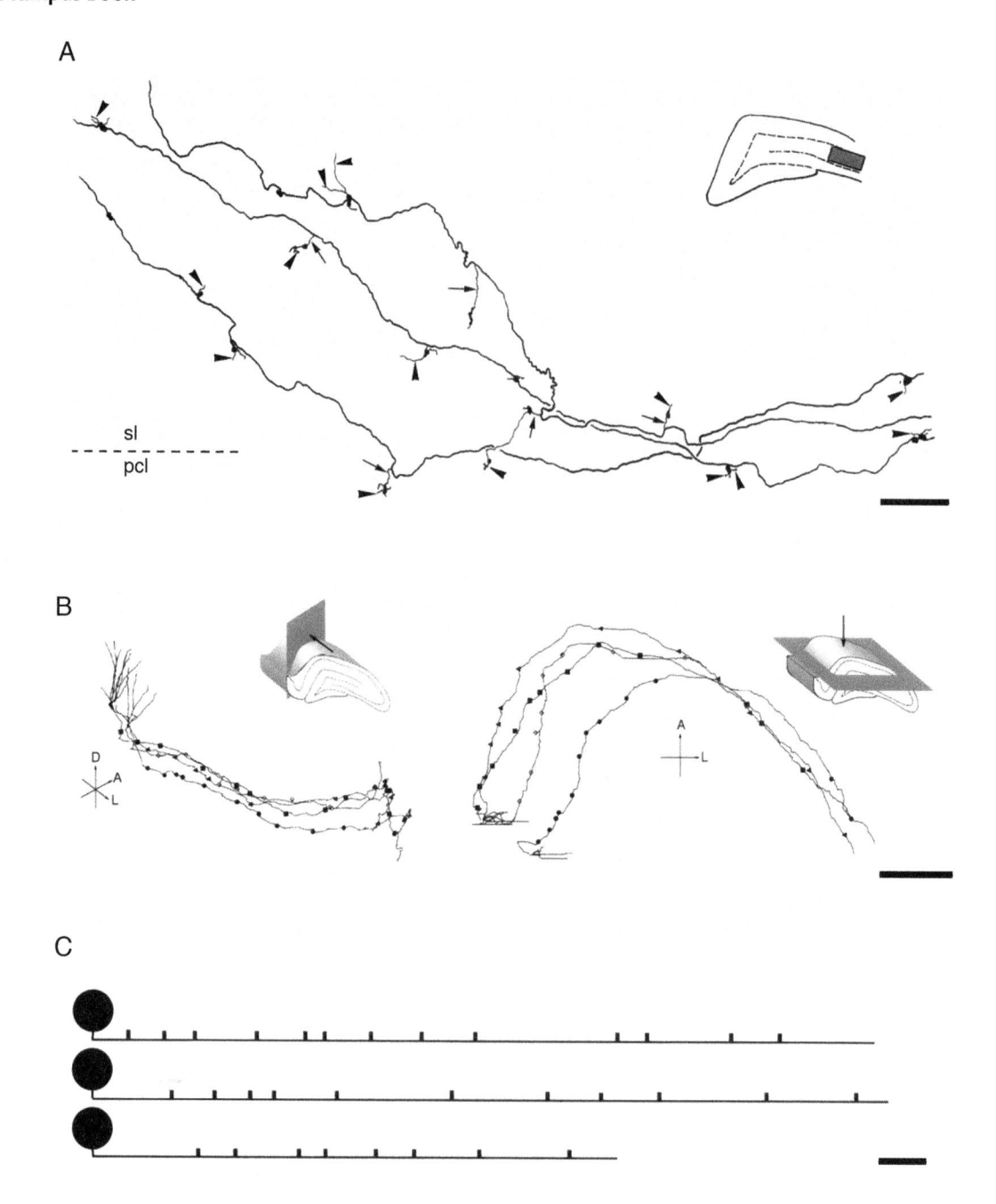

Figure 3.24 Topography of the mossy fibers in the CA3 region. (A) Camera lucida drawing of mossy fibers from three adjacent granule cells (truncated). Note numerous filopodial extensions of the large mossy terminals in A (arrowheads) and thin collaterals of large mossy terminals (arrows). Boxed area in insert in A shows the position of the fibers in CA3. (B) Neurolucida reconstruction of the same three axons shown in A and an additional mossy fiber of a fourth granule cell located posteriorly. The original coronal images are rotated to emphasize the spatial characteristics of the fibers. (C) Wire diagram of the three mossy fibers shown in A, depicting the distribution of mossy terminals. Note that shorter interbouton distance prevails in the proximal portion of CA3. Scale bars: 50 µm in A, 400 µm in B, and 200 µm in C. (Adapted with permission from Acsady et al., 1998.)

the dentate gyrus to CA2 has been emphasized in mouse studies (for example, Kohara et al., 2014), and we shall take this up again when we talk about the fields of the hippocampus.

All dentate granule cells project to CA3, and the axon trajectory is partially correlated with the position of the parent cell body. Before describing features of the mossy fiber projection, it is worth making a few points concerning the organization of the terminal regions within CA3. In the proximal portion of CA3 (close to the dentate gyrus), mossy fibers are distributed below, within, and above the

pyramidal cell layer. The fibers located below the layer, i.e., those that are in the area occupied primarily by basal dendrites, are generally called the infrapyramidal bundle. The fibers located within the pyramidal cell layer are called the intrapyramidal bundle, and those located above the pyramidal cell layer (in the area occupied mainly by proximal apical dendrites) the suprapyramidal bundle; the suprapyramidal bundle occupies the stratum lucidum. At mid and distal portions of CA3, the intra- and infrapyramidal bundles are largely eliminated and virtually all mossy fibers travel in stratum

CA3 pyramidal cell

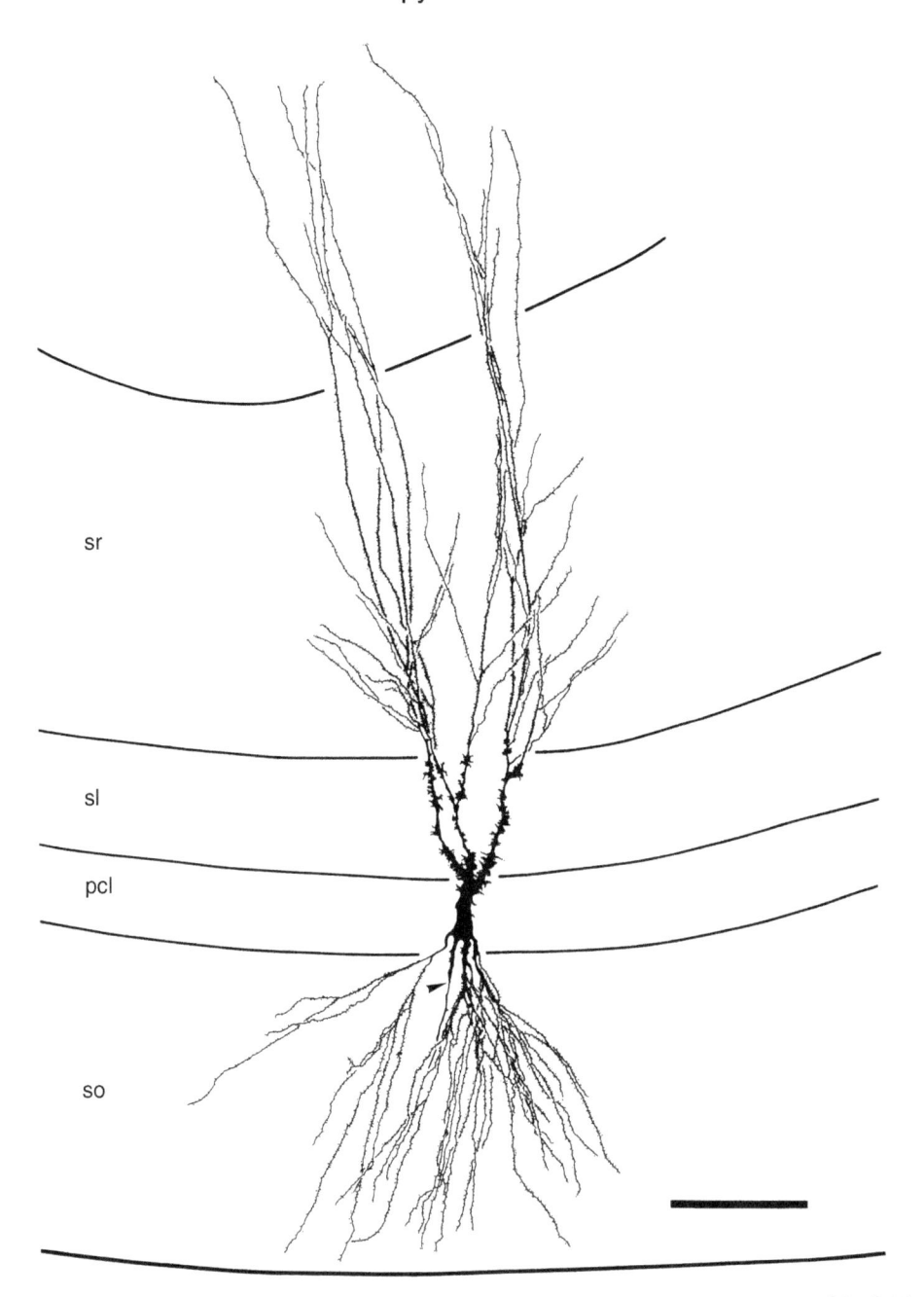

Figure 3.25 Camera lucida drawing of an intracellularly labeled CA3 pyramidal neuron located in the midportion of the field. As this neuron lies outside of the zone of the infrapyramidal mossy fiber bundle, most of the thorny excrescences are located on the proximal apical dendrites. The axon of this neuron is indicated by an arrowhead. Scale bar is 100 μm. (Adapted from Ishizuka et al., 1995.)

lucidum. It is worth noting that variation in the relative size of the intra- and infrapyramidal mossy fibers has been rd across different strains of rats and mice, including mouse strains used widely in transgenic experiments; this variation sometimes correlates with different behavioral profiles (Lipp et al., 1987; Hausheer-Zarmakupi et al., 1996). Granule cells at all transverse positions within the granule cell layer generate mossy fibers that extend for the full proximodistal distance of CA3 (Gaarskjaer, 1981) (Figure 3.24). Cells located in the infrapyramidal blade of the granule cell layer have axons that tend to enter CA3 in the infrapyramidal bundle, but ultimately cross the pyramidal cell layer to enter the deep portion of

stratum lucidum. The axons of granule cells located in the crest of the dentate gyrus tend to enter CA3 in the intrapyramidal bundle and also ultimately ascend into stratum lucidum. Cells located in the suprapyramidal blade of the dentate gyrus give rise to axons that enter CA3 in the stratum lucidum and continue within the most superficial portion of stratum lucidum (Claiborne et al., 1986).

The mossy fibers give rise to unique and complex en passant presynaptic terminals called mossy fiber expansions (Amaral and Dent, 1981). Part of the uniqueness of these presynaptic boutons is their size; they can be as large as 8 μm in diameter but more typically range from 3–5 μm in greatest dimension. Their large size has attracted the attention of physiologists interested in using them for patch-clamp studies of transmitter release (Henze et al., 2000). The mossy fiber expansions form highly irregular, complex, interdigitated attachments with the intricately branched spines called thorny excrescences that are located on the proximal dendrites of the CA3 pyramidal cells. The thorny excrescences are so distinctive that they clearly mark the location of mossy fiber synaptic termination. In the proximal portion of CA3, for example, thorny excrescences are located both on the basal and proximal apical dendrites of pyramidal cells, which are therefore in contact with both the infra- and suprapyramidal mossy fiber bundles. In the mid and distal portions of CA3, however, thorny excrescences are almost entirely restricted to the apical dendritic processes that traverse stratum lucidum (Figure 3.24). The CA2 pyramidal cells are devoid of thorny excrescences (Figure 3.24).

Another distinctive feature of the mossy fiber expansions is the number of active synaptic zones they demonstrate. A single mossy fiber expansion can make as many as 37 synaptic contacts with a single CA3 pyramidal cell dendrite. Three-dimensional analysis of serial sections through these synapses indicates that while a mossy fiber expansion may be in synaptic contact with more than one complex spine originating from the same parent dendrite, it does not typically contact spines on two different dendrites. Thus, one mossy fiber expansion does not typically contact two pyramidal cells. It is now clear that the multiple synaptic contacts of mossy fiber boutons can have nonsynchronized release activity (Rama et al., 2019).

The large mossy fiber expansions occur approximately every 135 μm along the parent axon and each mossy fiber axon forms about 15 of these complex boutons. Thus, each granule cell communicates with only about 15 CA3 pyramidal cells. It is important to point out, however, that these 15 pyramidal cells are distributed throughout the full proximodistal length (transverse axis) of CA3. Since there are approximately 2.5×10^5 CA3 pyramidal cells in the rat and approximately 1.2×10^6 granule cells, each pyramidal cell is expected to receive input from about 72 granule cells. That is, an individual dentate granule cell has the potential to activate about 15 CA3 pyramidal cells, while an individual pyramidal cell receives input from about 72 granule cells. This pattern, not seen elsewhere in the brain, has attracted considerable interest among computational neuroscientists. Since each of the mossy fiber expansions has many release sites, this might ensure highly efficient depolarization of the innervated pyramidal cells.

Early Golgi anatomists indicated that the mossy fiber axons were mainly oriented perpendicular to the long axis of the hippocampus. Mossy fibers do not collateralize once they enter the hippocampus and stay largely within the same septotemporal level as their cells of origin. There is one peculiarity of the mossy fiber projection, however, that has eluded explanation; the mossy fibers actually do change their course and take a longitudinal direction, but not until they reach the distal portion of CA3 (Lorente de Nó, 1934; McLardy and Kilmer, 1970). The extent of this distal longitudinal projection was further clarified using autoradiographic tract tracing (Swanson et al., 1978). Granule cells located at septal levels give rise to mossy fibers that travel throughout most of the transverse extent of CA3 at the same septotemporal level, but, just at the CA3/CA2 border, they abruptly change course and travel toward the temporal pole for nearly 2 mm. The extent of this longitudinal component, however, appears to depend on the septotemporal location of the cells of origin. Granule cells in the mid to temporal portions of the dentate gyrus have mossy fibers that exhibit only a slight temporal inclination at their distal extremity. And mossy fibers that originate at the extreme temporal pole of the dentate gyrus barely extend to the CA3/CA2 border and have little or no longitudinal component. Thus, in the septal half of the hippocampus, there appears to be some overlap of mossy fibers originating from different septotemporal levels, but this occurs only at a restricted distal portion of the CA3 field. On the face of it, this indicates that some CA3 pyramidal cells located very close to the border with CA2 may be contacted by mossy fiber axons from granule cells spread out over a much broader septotemporal extent of the dentate gyrus. They might therefore form a special class of integrator CA3 cells. Not only do mossy fibers travel temporally for 2–3 mm but also they demonstrate typical mossy fiber expansions along this portion of their trajectory (Acsady et al., 1998).

Before leaving this description of the mossy fibers, it should be noted that, in addition to the large mossy fiber expansions, there are also infrequent thin collaterals that emanate from the parent axon or from the mossy fiber expansions. These thin filipodial collaterals, which are much more extensive in neonatal than mature rats, have been found to terminate both on CA3 pyramidal cells and on the GABAergic pyramidal basket cells in the P14 mouse (Martin et al., 2017). It will be important to demonstrate whether this finding is confirmed in mature mice and in other species.

There is substantial evidence indicating that the granule cells use glutamate as their primary transmitter, and the asymmetric contacts made between the mossy fiber expansions and the thorny excrescences would tend to confirm this notion. The mossy fibers are, nonetheless, also immunoreactive for several other neuroactive substances. At least some of the mossy fibers demonstrate immunoreactivity for the opioid peptide dynorphin, and they are also immunoreactive for GABA (Walker et al., 2002). Interestingly, while the granule cells do not normally express mRNA for the synthetic enzymes GAD65 or GAD67, long-duration stimulation of the perforant path can induce GAD messenger expression in rat granule cells. The possible role of GABA or opioid peptides in the synaptic economy of the mossy fibers is discussed in relation to synaptic plasticity at these synapses in Chapter 10.

3.9.2 The hippocampus

3.9.2.1 Cytoarchitectonic organization

An overview of the major fields of the hippocampus was given earlier in this chapter. We will now go into more detail about its laminar organization, which is generally similar for all the fields of the hippocampus. The principal cellular layer is called the pyramidal cell layer. The pyramidal cell layer is tightly packed in CA1 and more loosely packed in CA2 and CA3. The narrow, relatively cell free layer located deep to the pyramidal cell layer is called stratum oriens. This layer contains the basal dendrites of the pyramidal cells and several classes of interneurons. Stratum oriens can be defined as the infrapyramidal region in which some of the CA3-to-CA3 associational connections and the CA3-to-CA1 Schaffer collateral connections are located. Deep to stratum oriens is the thin, fiber-containing alveus. In CA3, but not in CA2 or CA1, a narrow acellular zone, the stratum lucidum, is located just above the pyramidal cell layer and is occupied by the mossy fibers. There is a slight thickening of stratum lucidum at its distal end, where, at least at septal levels, the mossy fibers bend temporally and travel longitudinally. This zone is called the "end bulb" and is more prominent in species such as the guinea pig than in the rat; it marks the CA3/CA2 border. Stratum radiatum is located superficial to stratum lucidum in CA3, and immediately above the pyramidal

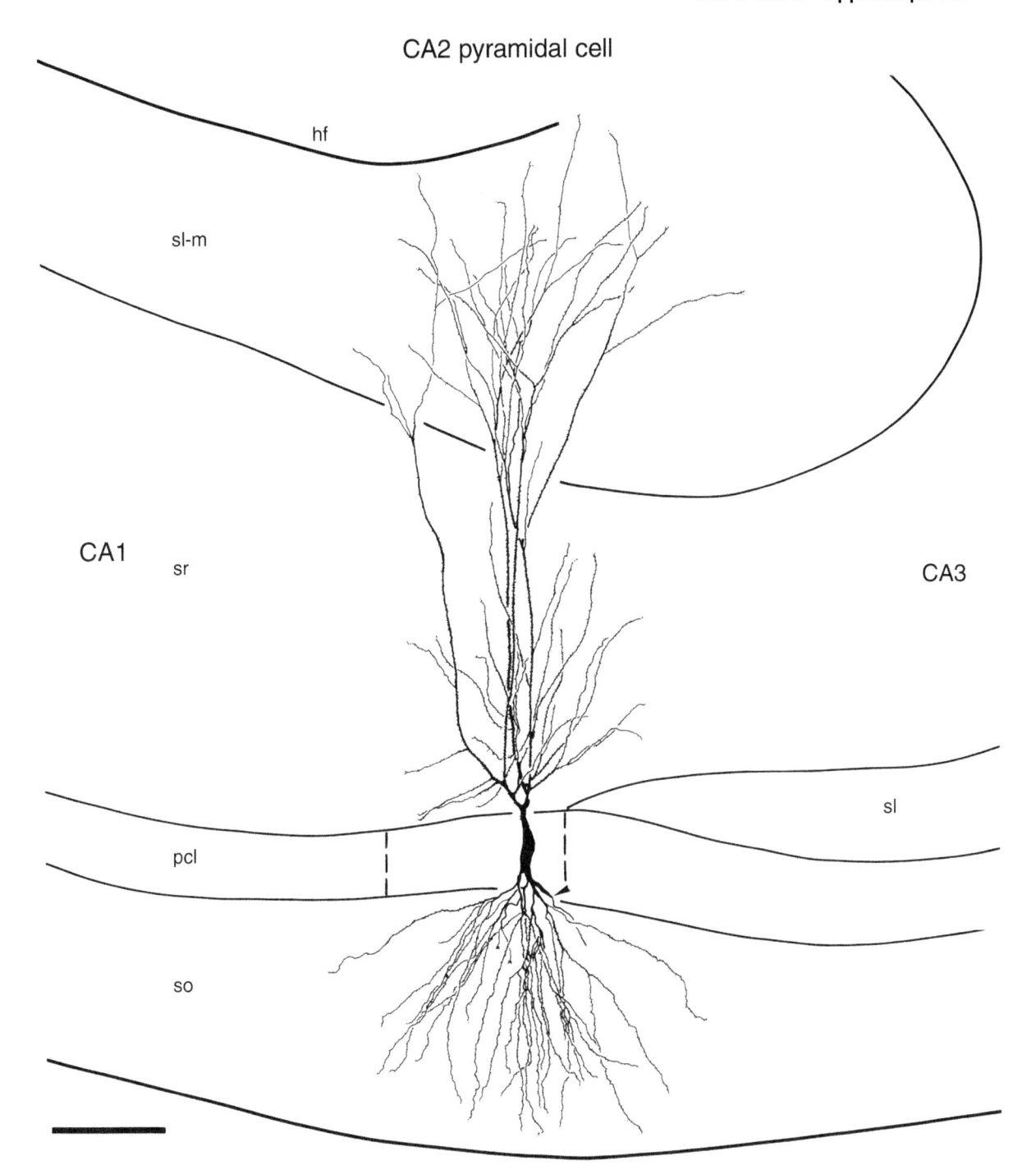

Figure 3.26 Camera lucida drawing of an intracellularly labeled CA2 pyramidal neuron. Note that while the size and general characteristics of this neuron are similar to those in CA3, there are no thorny excrescences on the proximal apical dendrites. Two basal dendrites cut at the surface of the slice are indicated by asterisks. The axon of this neuron is indicated by an arrowhead. Scale bar is 100 μm. (Adapted from Ishizuka et al., 1995.)

cell layer in CA2 and CA1. Stratum radiatum can be defined as the suprapyramidal region in which the CA3-to-CA3 associational connections and the CA3-to-CA1 Schaffer collateral connections are located. The most superficial layer of the hippocampus is called the stratum lacunosum-moleculare. It is in this layer that fibers from the entorhinal cortex terminate. Afferents from other regions such as the nucleus reuniens of the midline thalamus also terminate in stratum lacunosum-moleculare. There are a variety of interneurons in the hippocampus that populate essentially all of the layers.

In the following sections, we will sometimes deal with the organization of the CA3 and CA2 fields of the hippocampus first and then move on to the CA1 field. For other topics, such as the interneurons of the hippocampus, there is not enough known to warrant discussing separately CA3, CA2, and CA1. For these topics, we will discuss data for the entire hippocampus. We should also note that there has been substantially increased interest in the CA2 field as a region particularly involved in social memory (Diethorn and Gould, 2023).

Pyramidal cells of CA3 and CA2

The principal neuronal cell type of the hippocampus is the pyramidal cell, which makes up the vast majority of neurons in the

CA1 pyramidal cell

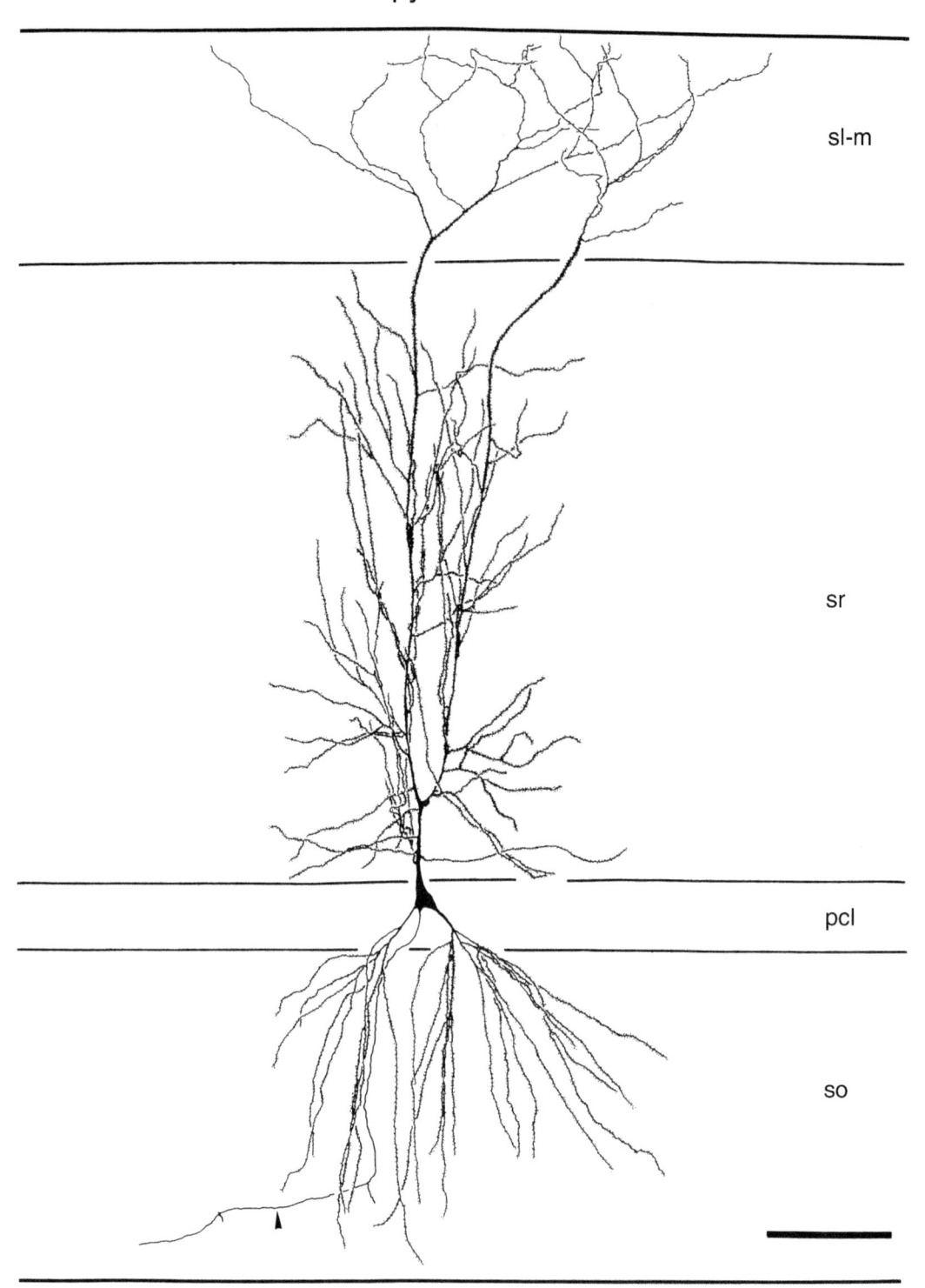

sl-m

sr

pcl

so

Figure 3.27 Camera lucida drawing of an intracellularly labeled CA1 pyramidal neuron from the mid portion of the field. Note that side branches originate from the primary dendrites throughout the full extent of stratum radiatum. Note also the curved and irregular trajectories of dendritic branches in the stratum lacunosum-moleculare. The axon of this neuron is indicated by an arrowhead. Scale bar is 100 μm. (Adapted from Ishizuka et al., 1995.)

pyramidal cell layer. Pyramidal cells have a basal dendritic tree that extends into stratum oriens and an apical dendritic tree that extends into stratum radiatum and stratum lacunosum-moleculare to terminate at the hippocampal fissure.

The dendritic length and organization of CA3 pyramidal cells is quite variable (Ishizuka et al., 1995) (Figures 3.26, 3.28). The smallest cells (with a soma size of about 300 μm² or 20 μm in diameter) are located within the limbs of the dentate gyrus and have a total dendritic length of 8–10 mm. The largest cells (with a soma size of about

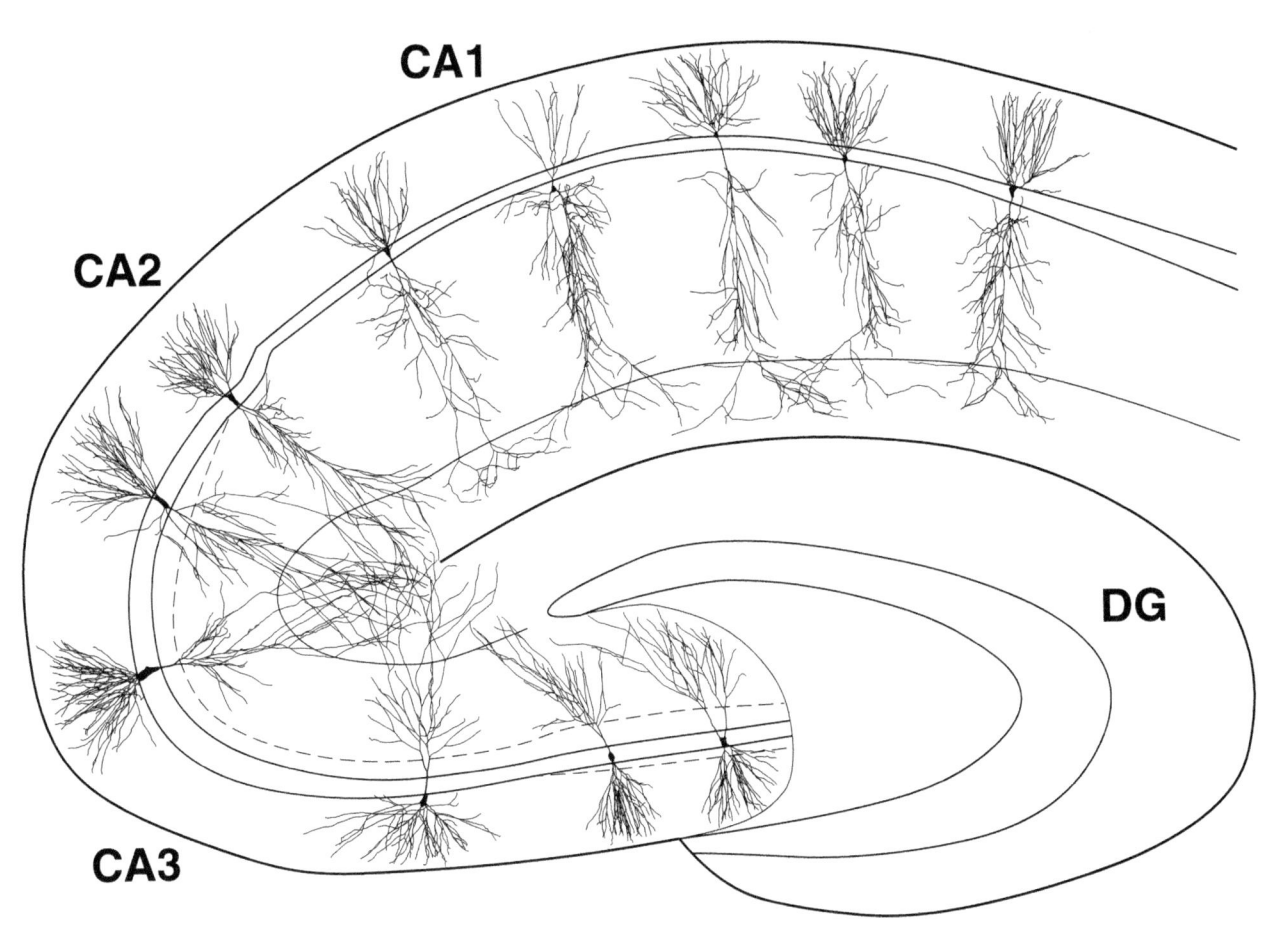

Figure 3.28 Summary illustration of the organization of hippocampal pyramidal cells. Produced as a composite of computer-generated line drawings of neurons from CA3, CA2, and CA1. Dashed line in CA3 marks the region occupied by the infra- and suprapyramidal mossy fibers. While there is substantial variability in the size and dendritic shape of CA3 neurons, the morphology of the dendritic trees of CA1 cells is remarkably homogeneous. (Adapted from Ishizuka et al., 1995.)

700 μm² or 30 μm in diameter) are located distally in the field and have a total dendritic length of 16–18 mm. The distribution of the dendritic trees of CA3 pyramidal cells also varies depending on where the cell body is located. Cells located within the limbs of the dentate gyrus, for example, have little or none of their dendrites extending into the stratum lacunosum-moleculare and thus receive little or no direct input from the entorhinal cortex. These cells, however, receive a larger number of mossy fiber terminals both on their apical and basal dendritic trees, and are thus under greater influence of the granule cells than distally located CA3 cells that only receive an apical mossy fiber input. Recent physiological studies highlight the fact that both the intrinsic membrane properties and functional characteristics of the CA3 pyramidal cells vary along the transverse axis due, in part, to differences in synaptic input (mossy fiber versus entorhinal) (Sun et al., 2017). Cells of the CA2 region are approximately the same size as those in CA3 but typically lack thorny excrescences on their apical dendrites (Figure 3.26).

Pyramidal cells of CA1

In contrast to the substantial heterogeneity of dendritic organization characteristic of CA3 pyramidal cells, the CA1 pyramidal cells show a remarkable homogeneity of their dendritic trees (Pyapali et al., 1998) (Figures 3.27 and 3.28). As well as being more homogeneous, they are also on average smaller than CA3 cells. The total

dendritic length averages approximately 13.5 mm, while the average size of CA1 cell somata is about 193 μm² or 15 μm in diameter. And, regardless of where a pyramidal cell is located within CA1, it has about the same total dendritic length and the same dendritic configuration. Some pyramidal cells have one apical dendrite while others have two. Cells with two apical dendrites tend to have slightly greater total apical dendritic length. Neurons with a single apical dendrite, however, tend to have slightly larger basal dendritic trees and thus, overall, all CA1 neurons have about the same total length of the dendritic tree.

Despite the apparent morphological homogeneity of CA1 pyramidal cells, there is substantial evidence that they demonstrate functional differences. Mizuseki et al. (2011) demonstrated that CA1 pyramidal cells at different depths of the layer demonstrate different properties. Those located more deeply fired at higher rates, were more prone to bursting, and were also more likely to have place fields. Malik et al. (2016) have also demonstrated that there are both gradient-like and segmental changes in the physiological properties of CA1 pyramidal cells along the septotemporal axis of the hippocampus. Cembrowski and Spruston (2019) have summarized a number of other factors contributing to the heterogeneity of CA1 pyramidal cells. They indicated that transcriptional characteristics change in a graded fashion along the septotemporal axis of the hippocampus, and CA1 cells at the extremes of this axis are

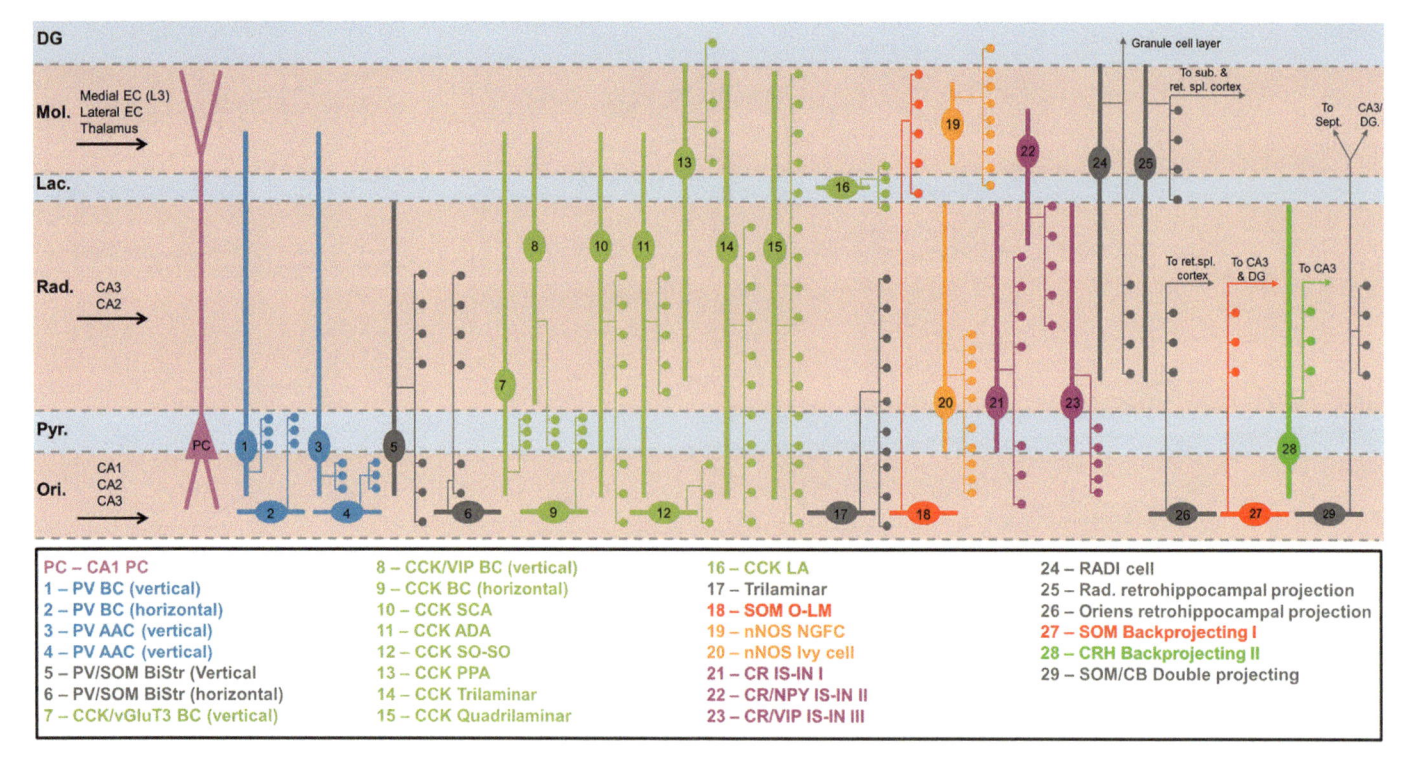

Figure 3.29 Schematic overview of known morphological and neurochemical interneurons in CA1. Somatodendritic domains (thick lines), axonal locations (thin lines) and major terminal fields (circles) are shown with respect to layers of the hippocampus. Afferent inputs are indicated with black arrows. (Adapted with permission from Booker and Vida, 2018.)

quantitatively as different as distinct types of pyramidal cells can be, such as CA3 versus CA1 pyramidal cells at the same septotemporal level. As we will see below, CA1 cells at different laminar and transverse locations also differ in their connections.

Interneurons

Pyramidal neurons are by far the most numerous neurons in the hippocampus. As in the dentate gyrus, however, there is also a fairly heterogeneous group of interneurons that are scattered through all layers. (See Booker and Vida, 2018; Degro et al., 2022 for recent in-depth reviews of hippocampal interneurons.) Most types of interneurons are found in all the hippocampal subfields (Figure 3.29). The two most common types of interneurons are the pyramidal basket cell and the axo-axonic cell. The pyramidal basket cell resides in, or close to, the pyramidal cell layer and its dendrites extend into stratum oriens, stratum radiatum, and stratum lacunosum-moleculare. The dendrites are beaded, aspiny, and receive both asymmetrical and symmetrical synapses. Most of the excitatory inputs are known to arise from hippocampal pyramidal cells. In fact, the dendritic tree of a pyramidal basket cell receives up to 17,000 inputs and the vast majority of these are excitatory inputs (Halasy et al., 1996). Since each pyramidal cell contributes only a single synapse to a particular basket cell, the degree of pyramidal cell convergence on an individual basket cell is enormous. Neurons with basket cell-like axons have a variety of morphologies. There are fusiform-shaped basket cells in stratum oriens and stellate-shaped basket cells in stratum radiatum. In all cases, the axons of these cell types innervate the soma and proximal dendrites of the pyramidal cells. The transverse extent of the basket cell axonal plexus (in a 400 μm in vitro slice preparation) is between 900 and 1,300 μm. Within

this plexus, there are as many as 10,000 synaptic varicosities. And since a basket cell only makes 2–10 synapses on each pyramidal cell, a typical basket cell innervates 1,000 pyramidal cells or more. A single basket cell thus has substantial inhibitory influence over a large population of pyramidal cells.

A second type of hippocampal interneuron is the chandelier or axo-axonic cell. Those found in the hippocampus are very similar to the ones described in the dentate gyrus. Their cell bodies, like those of the basket cells, are located within or adjacent to the pyramidal cell layer and their dendrites span all the hippocampal strata. The axons of the chandelier cells have a transverse spread of approximately 1 mm. They travel just superficial to the pyramidal cell layer and periodically give rise to collaterals that enter the pyramidal cell layer and terminate on the proximal axons of the pyramidal neurons. Each axo-axonic cell terminates on approximately 1,200 pyramidal cell axon initial segments, and each initial segment is innervated by 4–10 axo-axonic cells.

The early Golgi studies of Ramón y Cajal and Lorente de Nó made it abundantly clear that there are a variety of nonpyramidal cell types in stratum oriens, stratum radiatum, and stratum lacunosum-moleculare of the hippocampus. Ribak and colleagues were the first to discover that the vast majority of these neurons are immunoreactive for GABAergic markers, and most are considered to be interneurons (Ribak et al., 1978). Freund and Buzsaki (1996) described the location, dendritic organization, and axonal distribution of these cells based on a classification system dependent on the region of innervation. One class of cells has been called the O-LM cell (oriens lacunosum-moleculare associated cell) and has as its defining feature a dense axonal arbor that is confined to stratum lacunosum-moleculare (a.k.a. cells terminating in conjunction with entorhinal afferents) (Lacaille et al., 1987). The location of the cell body of this class of interneuron varies depending on which hippocampal field it inhabits. The principle seems to be that the cell body and dendritic tree are located in the zones occupied by recurrent pyramidal cell collaterals. In CA3, this includes all strata aside from stratum lacunosum-moleculare, but in CA1 it only includes stratum oriens. The axons of the O-LM cell leave stratum oriens (or whichever layer the cell body is located in) and rise directly to stratum lacunosum-moleculare, ramifying there to form a dense plexus. These axons form symmetrical synapses with the distal apical dendrites of pyramidal neurons. Since most of the excitatory input to the O-LM cells appears to arise from recurrent collaterals of the pyramidal cells, this class of interneuron inhibits activity in the distal dendrites of pyramidal cells in a disynaptic, feedback manner.

Another class of hippocampal interneuron, the bistratified cell, also has its cell body located close to the pyramidal cell layer. The dendritic trees of these neurons are multipolar but do not reach stratum lacunosum-moleculare. The axon of the bistratified cell sends collaterals both into stratum oriens and into the deep portion of stratum radiatum, where a dense terminal plexus is produced. These neurons generate an enormous axonal plexus on the order of 80 mm in total length and up to 16,000 synaptic varicosities. The bistratified cells have axons that terminate both on the dendritic shafts and the dendritic spines of pyramidal cells. While the inputs to these cells have not been thoroughly investigated, their dendrites reside in the zone of associational connections in CA3 and the Schaffer collateral fibers in CA1.

There are other interneurons located in stratum radiatum that have a stellate or multipolar dendritic plexus confined to the layer. The axons of these cells tend to ramify locally in stratum radiatum and terminate primarily on the dendrites of pyramidal cells.

A fairly sizable population of interneurons is located in stratum lacunosum-moleculare or at the border between stratum lacunosum-moleculare and stratum radiatum (Lacaille and Schwartzkroin, 1988). These LM neurons (stratum lacunosum-moleculare interneurons) have dendrites that are oriented horizontally, i.e., within the layer, but occasionally have branches that extend into the pyramidal cell layer. The axon also takes a predominantly horizontal orientation and ramifies mainly in stratum lacunosum-moleculare or in the superficial portion of stratum radiatum. While the connectivity of this class of neurons is not well worked out, their axons do form symmetrical synapses on the distal dendrites of pyramidal cells.

An additional type of interneuron in the hippocampus is the IS neuron (interneuron-selective). Their cell bodies are located in all layers and can be identified by staining with antibodies to the calcium-binding protein calretinin. The IS cells have a number of notable features, including the propensity for their dendrites to form bundles with dendrites of other IS neurons. The major unifying feature, however, is that their axons terminate exclusively on other interneurons. Little is yet known concerning their input/output characteristics. Their dendrites are, however, disposed so that they could be innervated by all major afferent and intrinsic connections of the hippocampus and their axons could potentially innervate all of the interneurons described above.

All of the interneurons that we have described are immunopositive for markers of GABA. As in other cortical regions, the interneurons of the hippocampus colocalize a number of other neuroactive substances. Thus, many of these neurons can be visualized with antibodies to peptides such as somatostatin, vasoactive intestinal peptide (VIP), cholecystokinin (CCK), neuropeptide Y (NPY) or calcium-binding proteins such as parvalbumin, calbindin, and calretinin. It remains something of a mystery what these neuroactive substances are doing in GABAergic neurons. But at the very least, they provide useful markers for establishing subcategories of the large population of GABAergic interneurons.

Currently more than 20 different types of interneurons have been identified in the hippocampal formation (Somogyi, 2010; Degro et al., 2022). However, new interneurons are still being discovered. Francavilla et al. (2018) described in the mouse a VIP-positive interneuron located in the stratum oriens of CA1 that innervates only other interneurons in CA1, but both interneurons and pyramidal cells in the subiculum.

Extrinsic connections

One of the distinguishing features of the connectivity of the hippocampus is that the vast majority of its synaptic input arises from within its own boundaries. CA3 and CA2 pyramidal cells are heavily innervated by collaterals of their own axons (Le Duigou et al., 2014) (i.e., the associational connections) and, in the rodent, from axons of the contralateral CA3 and CA2 (i.e., the commissural connections). CA1, in turn, receives its heaviest input from CA3. A relatively lighter projection arises from the entorhinal cortex, and this terminates on the most distal dendrites of the pyramidal cells in stratum lacunosum-moleculare, as well as on interneurons with dendrites in the same layer. There are relatively few other "extrinsic" inputs to the hippocampus, and these generally account for a relatively small number of synapses.

3.9.2.2 Entorhinal cortex projection to CA3/CA2

While the entorhinal innervation of CA3 is mentioned in most studies of the perforant path projection, the organization of this component of the projection is generally not dealt with in much detail. Indeed, there has been little in-depth research on the entorhinal projections to the hippocampus despite the fact that its prominence suggests it is very important (see Chapter 12 for a more detailed description of this pathway). The perforant path takes its name from the observation that it perforates the subiculum and hippocampal fissure en route to the dentate gyrus, but it is now quite clear that collaterals of fibers that project to the dentate gyrus also project to the hippocampus. In fact, the origin and laminar terminal distribution of the perforant path projection to CA3 are very similar to those to the dentate gyrus (Witter et al., 2017). Entorhinal terminals are distributed throughout the width of stratum lacunosum-moleculare. As with the projection to the molecular layer of the dentate gyrus, projections from the lateral entorhinal area terminate superficially in the stratum lacunosum-moleculare and those from the medial entorhinal area terminate in the deep half of the layer. The laminar origin, types, and numbers of synaptic contacts of this projection are also similar to those to the dentate gyrus. The entorhinal projections to CA3/CA2 originate from cells in layer II, and collaterals of the same layer II cells reach both the dentate gyrus and CA3/CA2, implying that similar information reaches both structures. It is now known that there are two classes of layer II neurons; one is characterized by immunoreactivity for reelin and the other class is calbindin-positive. It is the reelin-positive layer II cells that project to the dentate gyrus and CA3 region. Note that the actual composition

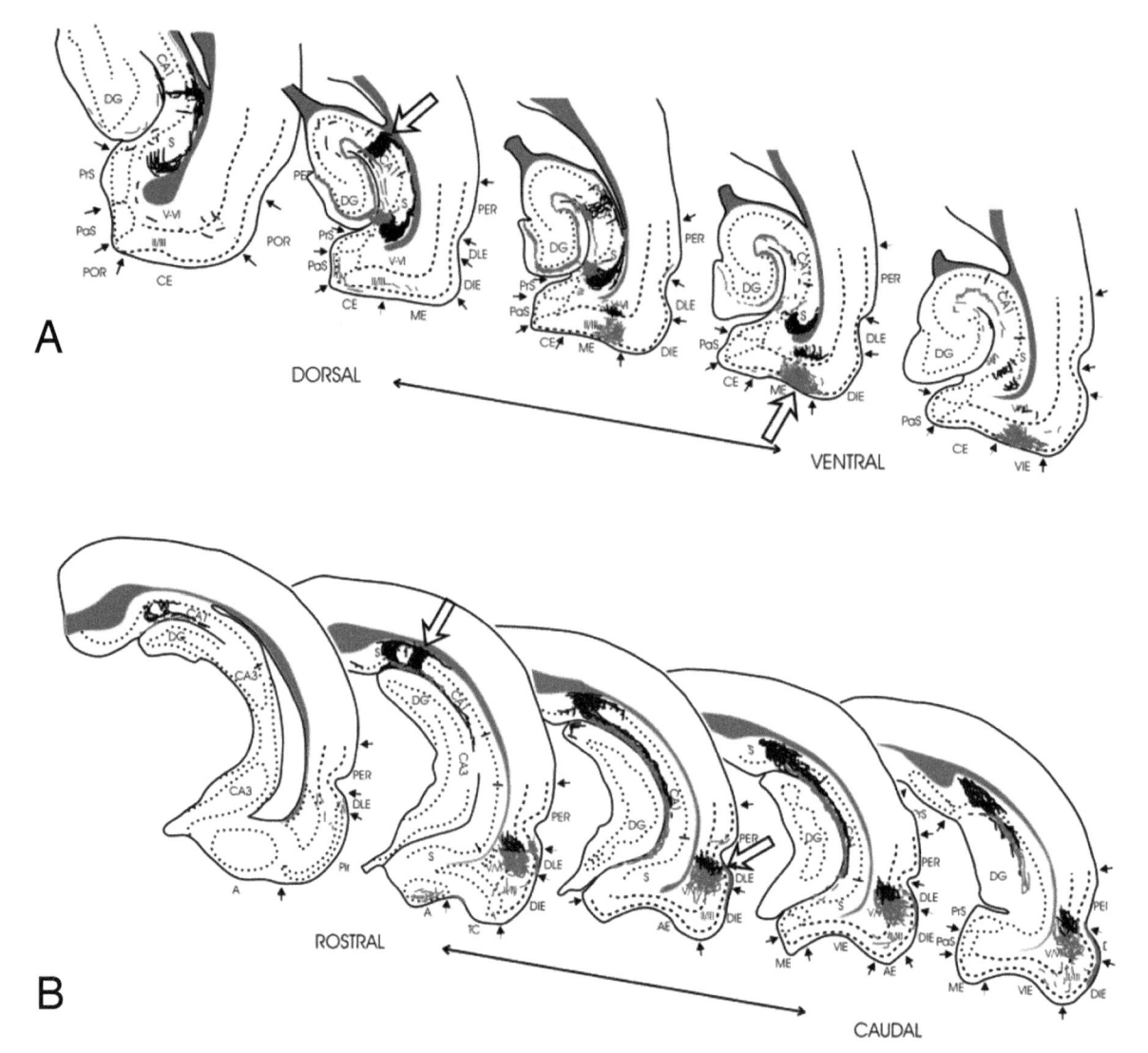

Figure 3.30 Reciprocal entorhinal–hippocampal connections. (A) Distribution of labeled fibers in the hippocampus and entorhinal cortex after combined anterograde tracer injections in the medial part of the entorhinal cortex and the proximal part of the CA1 field of the hippocampus. The terminal fibers originating in the entorhinal cortex overlap with the injection site in CA1, and the terminal fibers originating in CA1 overlap with the injection site in the entorhinal cortex. (B) Distribution of labeled fibers in the hippocampus and entorhinal cortex after combined anterograde tracer injections in the lateral entorhinal cortex and the distal portion of the CA1 field of the hippocampus. The terminal fibers originating in the entorhinal cortex overlap with the injection site in CA1 and the terminal fibers originating in CA1 overlap with the injection site in the entorhinal cortex. The subdivisions of the entorhinal cortex follow the nomenclature of Insausti et al. (1997). Areas CE and ME constitute the medial entorhinal cortex, whereas DLE, DIE, VIE, and AE constitute the lateral entorhinal cortex. (Adapted from Naber et al., 2001.)

of layer II of the entorhinal cortex is more complex than portrayed here (see Chapter 12 for a comprehensive description).

Entorhinal cortex projection to CA1

While the entorhinal cortex also projects to CA1, the organization of this projection is fundamentally different from that of the projection to CA3/CA2. First, the cells of origin are spiny pyramidal cells in layer III rather than in layer II. Second, the pattern of terminal distribution is organized in a topographic fashion rather than in a laminar fashion (Figure 3.30). As in CA3/CA2, the entorhinal fibers terminate throughout the full width of stratum lacunosum-moleculare of CA1. However, fibers originating in the lateral entorhinal cortex terminate in the distal portion of CA1 (closer to the subiculum), whereas fibers originating in the medial entorhinal

cortex terminate in the proximal portion of CA1 (closer to CA2). Thus, depending on where a CA1 pyramidal cell is located in the transverse axis of the hippocampus, it will receive inputs from a different portion of the entorhinal cortex. If this is not complicated enough, Masurkar et al. (2017) have uncovered evidence that the medial entorhinal projections preferentially activate the deep pyramidal cells of proximal CA1, whereas the lateral entorhinal fibers preferentially activate the superficial pyramidal cells of distal CA1.

Hippocampal projections to the entorhinal cortex

Early studies using autoradiographic tract-tracing techniques suggested that all fields of the hippocampus send a return projection to the entorhinal cortex, but it is now clear that only cells located in CA1 give rise to this projection (Naber et al., 2001). The projecting cells appear to send their axons to roughly the same region of the entorhinal cortex from which they receive their input. Thus, proximal CA1 cells project to the medial entorhinal cortex, whereas distal CA1 cells project to the lateral entorhinal area. We will return to a more detailed description of these projections in the section on the entorhinal cortex.

Hippocampal connections with the neocortex and amygdaloid complex

While this book focuses on the hippocampal formation, we shall repeatedly emphasize that no brain structure can be seen in isolation. The hippocampus sends projections to, and receives projections from, numerous other brain regions, and these interconnections are vital to understanding its function. Having said that, and notwithstanding the very important functional relationship between hippocampus and neocortex, it turns out that only selected parts of the hippocampal formation have discrete, monosynaptic connections with the neocortex. The CA3 and CA2 fields of the hippocampus, for example, have no known connections with the neocortex.

Sensitive tracing methods have recently shown that CA3, in particular its temporal parts, receives input from the amygdaloid complex, which was previously thought to send projections only to CA1 and the subiculum (Pikkarainen et al., 1999; Pirker et al., 2000). These inputs originate mainly from the caudomedial portion of the parvicellular division of the basal nucleus and terminate heavily in stratum oriens and stratum radiatum. The best-documented cortical connection, other than with the entorhinal cortex, which we have defined as part of the hippocampal formation, is with the perirhinal (areas 35 and 36) and postrhinal cortices. Cells in the perirhinal cortex give rise to a relatively selective projection to the most distal CA1 pyramidal cells, i.e., those that are located at the border with the subiculum. This projection terminates in the stratum lacunosum-moleculare and overlaps the projection arising from the lateral entorhinal area. The same CA1 cells give rise to a return projection to the perirhinal cortex.

It has been known for some time that CA1 cells in the ventral hippocampus give rise to a projection to the prefrontal cortex (Jay and Witter, 1991). Recent data indicates that this may be constituted by two separate antagonistic pathways that have different physiological roles in the prefrontal cortex (Sanchez-Bellot et al., 2022). CA1 cells located in the septal portion of the hippocampus have also been reported to project to the retrosplenial cortex. One indication that there may yet be undiscovered pathways emanating from CA1 is the finding that a GABAergic neuron with distinct morphology gives rise to long-range projections to the retrosplenial cortex in the mouse (Yamawaki et al., 2019) this finding has not been replicated in other species.

Finally, the temporal two-thirds of the distal portion of CA1 is reciprocally connected with the amygdaloid complex. Projections from the basal nucleus of the amygdala terminate in stratum oriens and stratum radiatum of the CA1/subiculum border region. In addition, the accessory basal and cortical nuclei project to the stratum lacunosum-moleculare. CA1 cells in the same region give rise to a return projection to the basal nucleus of the amygdala.

Basal forebrain connections

The septum provides the major subcortical input to CA3. As with the dentate gyrus, the septal projection originates mainly in the medial septal nucleus and the nucleus of the diagonal band of Broca. The projection terminates most heavily in stratum oriens and to a lesser extent in stratum radiatum (Figure 3.21). CA1 receives a substantially lighter septal projection than CA3, but the fibers are also most densely distributed in stratum oriens.

Until the mid-1970s, it was commonly assumed that the hippocampal fields gave rise to both the precommissural and postcommissural projections to the basal forebrain and diencephalon. Indeed, Ramón y Cajal's classic diagram of the hippocampus shows fibers from CA1 coursing toward the fimbria. Tract-tracing studies employing the autoradiographic method, however, demonstrated that most of these projections actually originate from the subiculum (Swanson and Cowan, 1975). It is now quite clear that the only sizable subcortical projection from CA3 is to the lateral septal nucleus. The CA3 projection to the lateral septal nucleus travels via the fimbria and precommissural fornix and is bilateral; some CA3 fibers cross in the ventral hippocampal commissure to innervate the homologous region of the contralateral lateral septal nucleus. This pathway is topographically organized such that septal portions of CA3 project dorsally in the lateral septal nucleus and progressively more temporal portions of CA3 project more ventrally; proximal CA3 cells tend to project medially in the lateral septal nucleus, and distally situated CA3 cells terminate more laterally. Interestingly, virtually all CA3 cells give rise to projections both to CA1 and to the lateral septal nucleus.

Essentially all CA1 pyramidal cells also project to the lateral septal nucleus. However, the CA1 projection is strictly ipsilateral and some of the fibers travel to the septal nuclei via the dorsal fornix rather than through the larger fimbria/fornix route.

Hypothalamic connections

As we have described previously, the demonstration of differential expression of genes using in situ hybridization has allowed the specification of the borders of hippocampal fields. In a seminal paper by Lein et al. (2005), this strategy identified a region that overlapped with the classically defined CA2 that demonstrated gene expression patterns different from CA3 and CA1. This work has launched a number of studies aimed at defining the connectivity of pathways and functions specific for CA2. It was already known that CA2 receives a particularly prominent innervation from the posterior hypothalamus, in particular from the supramammillary area (Figure 3.21B), and from the tuberomammillary nucleus. These projections terminate mainly in and around the pyramidal cell layer and mainly on principal cells (Magloczky et al., 1994) This projection only goes to CA2 (as well as the dentate gyrus), but not to CA3 or CA1. CA2 projects back to the supramammillary region in the mouse (Cui et al., 2013). Subsequently, CA2 was also shown to receive input from vasopressin containing neurons in the mouse paraventricular nucleus of the hypothalamus (Cui et al., 2013). Vasopressin immunoreactive fibers from the supraoptic and paraventricular hypothalamic nuclei also innervate the rat CA2 region (Zhang and Hernandez, 2013). While beyond the scope of this chapter, a series of studies (reviewed in Piskorowski and Chevaleyre, 2018) have highlighted a particular role for CA2 in social memory. Other reviews of CA2's particular structure and function can be found in Middleton and McHugh (2020) and Robert et al. (2018).

Thalamic connections: nucleus reuniens and other midline nuclei

It has been known for some time that the anterior thalamic complex is intimately interconnected with the presubiculum. However, there are also fairly prominent projections from midline ("nonspecific") regions of thalamus to several fields of the hippocampal formation (Herkenham, 1978; Wouterlood et al., 1990; Dolleman-Van der Weel and Witter, 2000; Cassel et al., 2013). The nucleus reuniens (and to a lesser extent the rhomboid nucleus), located on the midline, gives rise to a prominent projection to stratum lacunosum-moleculare of CA1, where it overlaps with the fibers from the entorhinal cortex. The nucleus reuniens projection travels to CA1 via the internal capsule and cingulum bundle rather than through the fornix and fimbria. This projection innervates all septotemporal levels of CA1, with a preference for the mid temporal levels. The nucleus reuniens fibers terminate with asymmetric synapses on spines and thin dendritic shafts in stratum lacunosum-moleculare on both principal neurons and on GABAergic interneurons.

Brainstem inputs

The hippocampus, like the dentate gyrus, receives noradrenergic and serotonergic inputs from brainstem nuclei (Figure 3.22). Noradrenergic fibers and terminals arising from the locus coeruleus are most densely distributed in the stratum lucidum and in the most superficial portion of stratum lacunosum-moleculare. A much thinner plexus of axons is distributed throughout the other layers of CA3. Serotonergic fibers are more diffusely and sparsely distributed in CA3 than the noradrenergic fibers. Despite the rather low number of fibers, the serotonergic innervation of the hippocampus demonstrates several interesting features. First, there are two calibers of axons, thick and thin, arising from the raphe nuclei that innervate the hippocampus. Most of the serotonergic varicosities, which are located on the thin fibers, do not appear to have standard synaptic junctions and may release serotonin into the extracellular space. The varicosities on the thicker fibers, in contrast, form standard asymmetrical synapses that preferentially terminate on GABAergic inhibitory neurons, specifically on the classes of interneurons that project to the dendrites of hippocampal neurons. Thus, even the relatively few serotonergic fibers that innervate the hippocampus may have a profound action by enhancing the GABAergic inhibitory activity of the hippocampal interneurons. There are few, if any, dopaminergic fibers in CA3. The functional implications of monoaminergic inputs to the hippocampus, in particular in relation to LTP, is considered in more detail in Chapters 6 and 10.

3.9.2.3 Intrinsic connections: CA3 associational connections and Schaffer collaterals

As mentioned earlier, the major source of input to the hippocampus is the hippocampus itself. The CA3-to-CA3 associational connections and the CA3-to-CA1 Schaffer collateral connections are unique in many respects. Perhaps the major distinguishing feature of these projections, however, is their extensive spatial distribution. Through these connections, a particular pyramidal cell in CA3 can, in theory, interact with other hippocampal neurons distributed throughout much of the ipsilateral and contralateral hippocampus. The massive potential for association within the hippocampus is undoubtedly linked to its function. The hippocampal connections, while very widely distributed, are nonetheless systematically organized (Ishizuka et al., 1990; Li et al., 1994).

All CA3 and CA2 pyramidal cells give rise to highly divergent projections to all portions of the hippocampus. CA3 pyramidal

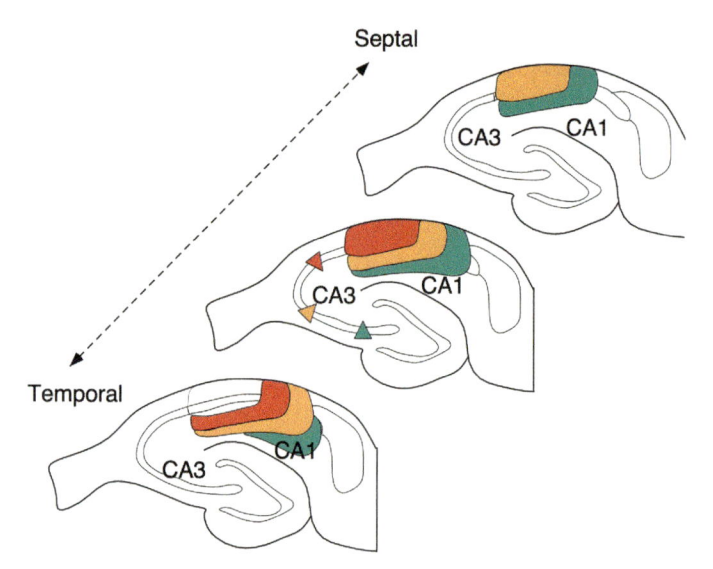

Figure 3.31 Organization of the projections from the CA3 to the CA1 field of the hippocampus (the Schaffer collaterals). The locations of the cells of origin are indicated by small triangles in the middle coronal section. Axonal projections and terminals from these cells are indicated by colors similar to those in the triangles. This illustration highlights the finding that certain CA1 cells are more likely to be contacted by certain CA3 cells and this depends on the transverse location of the CA3 cell and the septotemporal distance of CA1 from the cell of origin (Ishizuka et al., 1990).

cells give rise to highly collateralized axons that distribute fibers both within the ipsilateral hippocampus (to CA3, CA2, and CA1), to the same fields in the contralateral hippocampus (the commissural projections), and subcortically to the lateral septal nucleus. Some CA3 (especially those located proximally) and CA2 cells contribute a small number of collaterals that innervate the polymorphic layer of the dentate gyrus (Scharfman, 2007). While claims of other hippocampal connections are to be found in the literature, it is now quite clear that CA3 does not project to the subiculum, presubiculum, parasubiculum, or entorhinal cortex.

The CA3 projections to CA3 and CA2 are typically called the associational connections, while the CA3 projections to the CA1 field are typically called the Schaffer collaterals. This terminology, however, may be misleading, as one should remember that these two types of projections are true collaterals and, thus, potentially carry the same information to CA3 and CA1. Both the CA3-to-CA3 associational projections and the CA3-to-CA1 Schaffer collaterals demonstrate a systematic gradient-like pattern of projections. While it is somewhat out of sequence to discuss the CA3-to-CA1 projections first, we do so because they have been worked out in somewhat better detail and provide a clear model for the understanding of CA3 projections. Moreover, the organization of the CA3-to-CA1 projection shares many organizational similarities with the CA3-to-CA3 projection.

3.9.2.4 CA3-to-CA1 connections: the Schaffer collaterals

All portions of CA3 and CA2 project to CA1 (Figure 3.31). The pattern of terminal distribution, however, depends on the location of the CA3/CA2 cells of origin. The older notion that a typical CA3 pyramidal cell sends a single axon to CA1 that travels linearly through the field with equal contact probability at all regions within CA1 is clearly incorrect. In fact, each CA3 pyramidal cell gives rise to highly collateralized axons that follow both transverse and oblique orientations through CA1 (Ishizuka et al., 1990). Although Schaffer collaterals are typically illustrated as extending only through stratum radiatum, it should be emphasized that both stratum radiatum and stratum oriens of CA1 are heavily innervated by CA3 axons. Thus, the Schaffer collaterals are as highly associated with the apical dendrites of CA1 cells in stratum radiatum as they are with the basal dendrites in stratum oriens. Moreover, CA3 cells located at any particular septotemporal level distribute some of their collaterals to much of the full septotemporal extent of CA1. This projection is not at random, however, and its topographic organization develops a network in which certain CA3 cells are more likely to contact certain CA1 cells.

The major organizational features of this projection are as follows: CA3 cells located close to the dentate gyrus (proximal CA3), while projecting both septally and temporally, project more heavily to levels of CA1 located septal to their location. CA3 cells located closer to CA1, in contrast, project more heavily to levels of CA1 located temporally (Figure 3.31). At or close to the septotemporal level of the cells of origin, those cells located proximally in CA3 give rise to collaterals that tend to terminate superficially in stratum radiatum. Conversely, cells located more distally in CA3 give rise to projections that terminate deeper in stratum radiatum and in stratum oriens. At or close to the septotemporal level of origin, CA3 pyramidal cells located near the dentate gyrus tend to project somewhat more heavily to distal portions of CA1 (near the subiculum), whereas CA3 projections arising from cells located distally in CA3 terminate more heavily in portions of CA1 located closer to CA2. The truly thick Schaffer collaterals (those that Schaffer originally described) only originate from the proximal CA3 cells. These cells give rise to a thick axon that ascends from stratum oriens into the most superficial portion of stratum radiatum and travels to the distal part of CA1, where it contributes many collaterals. The axons of distal CA3 cells tend to be much thinner and project directly to CA1, either within stratum oriens or through the deep part of stratum radiatum. This is the basic organization close to the cells of origin. However, the position of the terminal field within CA1 varies in a systematic fashion relative to the distance from the cells of origin.

Regardless of the septotemporal or transverse origin of a projection, the highest density of terminal and fiber labeling in CA1 shifts to deeper parts of stratum radiatum and stratum oriens at levels septal to the cells of origin and shifts away from stratum oriens and into superficial parts of stratum radiatum at levels temporal to the cells of origin. Moreover, the highest density of fiber and terminal labeling in CA1 shifts proximally (toward CA3) at levels septal to the origin and distally (toward the subiculum) at levels temporal to the origin. One can think of these projections as a cloud of terminations with a three-dimensional shape that depends on the location of the cells of origin. The shape of the cloud varies in a systematic way as one travels farther from the cells of origin either septally or temporally from the injection site. Interestingly, the projections into different layers of CA1 may have distinctly different synaptic organization. For example, at least half of the synapses in the stratum oriens of CA1 are associated with multisynaptic boutons with one axon terminating on up to seven spines from different neurons (Rigby et al., 2023).

These conclusions are based on the analysis of populations of axons labeled by anterograde tracers injected into CA3. More recent studies using advanced labeling and computational approaches (Druckmann et al., 2014) have demonstrated that there is regional clustering of terminals from CA3 axons within CA1. And, even on a particular CA1 neuron, CA3 axons may terminate preferentially on one dendritic tree. The concept of terminal clustering appears to apply beyond the CA3-CA1 projection since extrinsic axons in stratum lacunosum-moleculare can terminate on adjacent spines of distal but not proximal CA1 pyramidal cell dendrites (Bloss et al., 2018). Bourne and Harris (2008) provide an excellent review of hippocampal connectivity at the ultrastructural level.

The entire axonal plexus of several CA3 pyramidal cells have been labeled by heroic intracellular staining and reconstruction techniques (Li et al., 1994). These studies provide convincing evidence that the axons of individual CA3 pyramidal cells can distribute to as much as two-thirds of the septotemporal extent of the ipsilateral and contralateral CA1 fields. The plexus from a single CA3 neuron comprises as much as 150–300 mm of total axonal length, on which 30,000 to 60,000 synaptic varicosities are formed. While single neurons have not been evaluated at all septotemporal levels, it appears that the extensiveness of CA3 connections is somewhat more restricted at temporal levels. Here, neurons may give rise to axonal plexuses that innervate only the temporal third of CA1.

There are a number of pieces of fundamental information concerning the CA3 projection to CA1 that still remain unknown. For example, it is not clear how many synapses a single CA3 cell makes on a typical CA1 cell. To answer this question using neuroanatomical procedures would be a monumental task (but see "The future of hippocampal neuroanatomy," section 3.13). A number of laboratories have made estimates of the extent of connectivity between CA3 and CA1 cells, and the numbers are always quite low. Work from Harris and colleagues (Harris et al., 1992; Sorra and Harris, 1993) indicates that there are perhaps as few as 2–4 contacts between a single axon in stratum radiatum and a particular dendritic tree, and certainly no more than 10 synapses between typical individual CA3 and CA1 neurons. The surprising state of affairs, however, is that we simply do not know with certainty how many contacts a single CA3 neuron makes with a single CA1 cell. These data are critical for interpreting some of the quantal analysis studies that are described in Chapters 5 and 6.

To summarize, the CA3-to-CA1 projection is the major input to CA1 pyramidal cells. The projection terminates both on the basal dendrites in stratum oriens and on the apical dendrites within stratum radiatum. Individual CA3 axons distribute extensively and may innervate neurons throughout as much as two thirds of the entire septotemporal extent of the hippocampus. The probability that a particular CA1 cell is contacted by a particular CA3 cell is dependent, in part, on the transverse positions of the two cell bodies and their septotemporal distance. At a septotemporal level close to the cell of origin in CA3, a distal CA3 cell is more likely to interact with a proximal CA1 cell, whereas a proximal CA3 cell is more likely to interact with a distal CA1 cell. The proximal CA3 cells are the only ones with classical thick Schaffer collaterals and the thickness of these initial axons is likely to reflect the longer distance that the axon must travel to innervate distal CA1 cells.

3.9.2.5 CA1 to CA3 projections

While it is generally thought that the CA1 field does not provide return projections to CA3, Lin et al. (2021) report projections in the mouse from dorsal CA1 to ventral CA3. These terminate on both excitatory CA3 cells as well as interneurons (Lin et al., 2023). This finding will need to be replicated in other species and even in other mouse strains to determine its significance.

3.9.2.6 CA3-to-CA3 associational connections

The associational projections from CA3-to-CA3 are also organized in a highly systematic fashion (see Le Duigou et al., 2014, for a review). One somewhat idiosyncratic facet of this projection is that cells located proximally in CA3 only communicate with other proximally located CA3 cells. Associational projections arising from mid and distal portions of CA3, however, project throughout much of the transverse extent of CA3 and also project much more extensively along the septotemporal axis. The density of CA3 associational projections also shifts along the septotemporal axis. The radial gradient of termination (superficial to deep in stratum radiatum and stratum oriens) is similar to that described for the CA3-to-CA1 projection. The transverse gradient, however, is the reverse; CA3 projections shift proximally in CA3 at levels located temporal to the cells of origin and shift distally in CA3 at more septal levels.

While initial estimates were that CA3-to-CA3 connections in rat were somewhat sparse (Guzman et al., 2016), more recent studies in mice based on elegant three-dimensional electron microscopy and multiple patch recordings put this number closer to 10% (Sammons et al., 2024). Given the complex topography of CA3 associational connections, it might be expected that the connectivity would vary along gradients and dependent on the somal positions of the pyramidal cells.

3.9.2.7 Commissural connections of the hippocampus

In the rat, the CA3 pyramidal cells give rise to commissural projections to the CA3, CA2, and CA1 fields of the contralateral

hippocampal formation (Blackstad, 1956; Fricke, 1978). In fact, the same CA3 cells give rise to both the ipsilateral and commissural projections. While the commissural projections follow roughly the same topographic organization as the ipsilateral projections, and generally terminate in homologous regions on both sides, there are minor differences in the distribution of terminals. If a projection is heavier to stratum oriens on the ipsilateral side, for example, it may be heavier in stratum radiatum on the contralateral side. The detailed topography of the commissural connections has not been as thoroughly investigated as the ipsilateral connections. As with the commissural projections from the dentate gyrus, CA3 fibers to the contralateral hippocampus form asymmetric synapses on the spines of pyramidal cells in CA3 and CA1, but also terminate on the smooth dendrites of interneurons. Interestingly, Stevens et al. (2024) have studied the CA3 commissural connections to CA1 pyramidal cells that have axons originating either from the cell soma or from a basal dendrite. They find that those with axons originating from a basal dendrite get a substantially stronger input via the commissural fibers which may affect their inclusion in coordinated network activity.

3.9.2.8 CA1 lacks associational connections

Based on bulk labeling of CA1 neurons (Amaral et al., 1991) it appears that pyramidal cells in CA1 give rise to a much more limited associational projection than those in CA3. As the CA1 axons travel in the alveus or in stratum oriens toward the subiculum (see below), occasional collaterals are generated that enter stratum oriens and the pyramidal cell layer, most likely contacting interneurons such as basket cells in stratum oriens, which, in turn, inhibit CA1 pyramidal cells. It is also conceivable that these collaterals might contact the basal dendrites of other CA1 cells. Yang et al. (2014) have used two-photon imaging of intracellularly stained CA1 pyramidal cells and demonstrated that they have a short, longitudinal projection to other levels of CA1. Nonetheless, this projection is numerically modest (though functional) compared with the CA3-CA3 associative network. Similarly, although a weak commissural projection to the contralateral CA1 appears to be present, there is no extensive commissural projection originating in CA1, as is the case in CA3.

3.9.2.9 CA1 projection to the subiculum

CA1 gives rise to two intrahippocampal projections. The first is a topographically organized projection to the adjacent subiculum (Figure 3.32). The second is to the deep layers of the entorhinal cortex. The latter projection will be discussed in the section on the entorhinal cortex.

Axons of CA1 pyramidal cells descend into stratum oriens or the alveus and bend sharply toward the subiculum (Amaral et al., 1991). The fibers re-enter the pyramidal cell layer of the subiculum and ramify profusely in the pyramidal cell layer and in the deep portion of the molecular layer. Unlike the CA3-to-CA1 projection that distributes throughout CA1 in a gradient fashion, the CA1 projection ends in a topographic and columnar fashion in the subiculum. Proximally located CA1 cells project to the distal portion of the subiculum, whereas distally located CA1 cells project just across the border into the proximal portion of the subiculum; the midportion of CA1 projects to the midportion of the subiculum (Figure 3.32). Single CA1 pyramidal cells injected with horseradish peroxidase demonstrate that individual axonal plexuses distribute to about one-third of the transverse extent of the subicular pyramidal cell

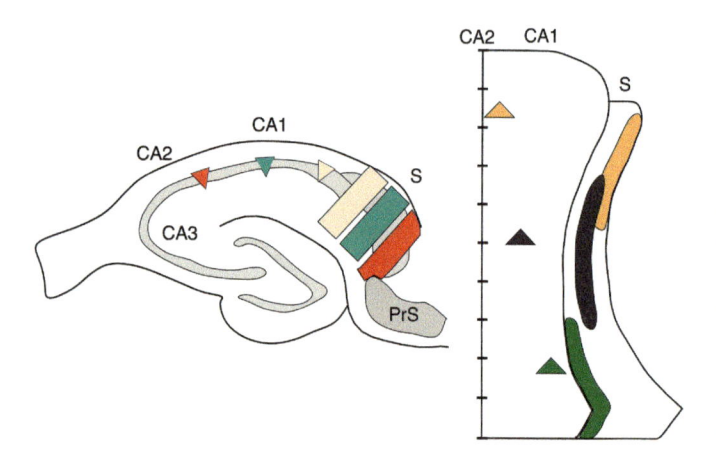

Figure 3.32 Organization of the projections from the CA1 field of the hippocampus to the subiculum. (A) Coronal section illustrating the cells of origin (triangles) and their respective terminal fields indicated by similar colors. (B) Two-dimensional unfolded map of CA1 and the subiculum. The septal portion of these fields is at the top of the figure and the temporal pole is at the bottom; the border between CA2 and CA1 is on the left. The longitudinal extent of the CA1 projection to the subiculum from different septotemporal levels is illustrated. (Adapted from Amaral et al., 1991.)

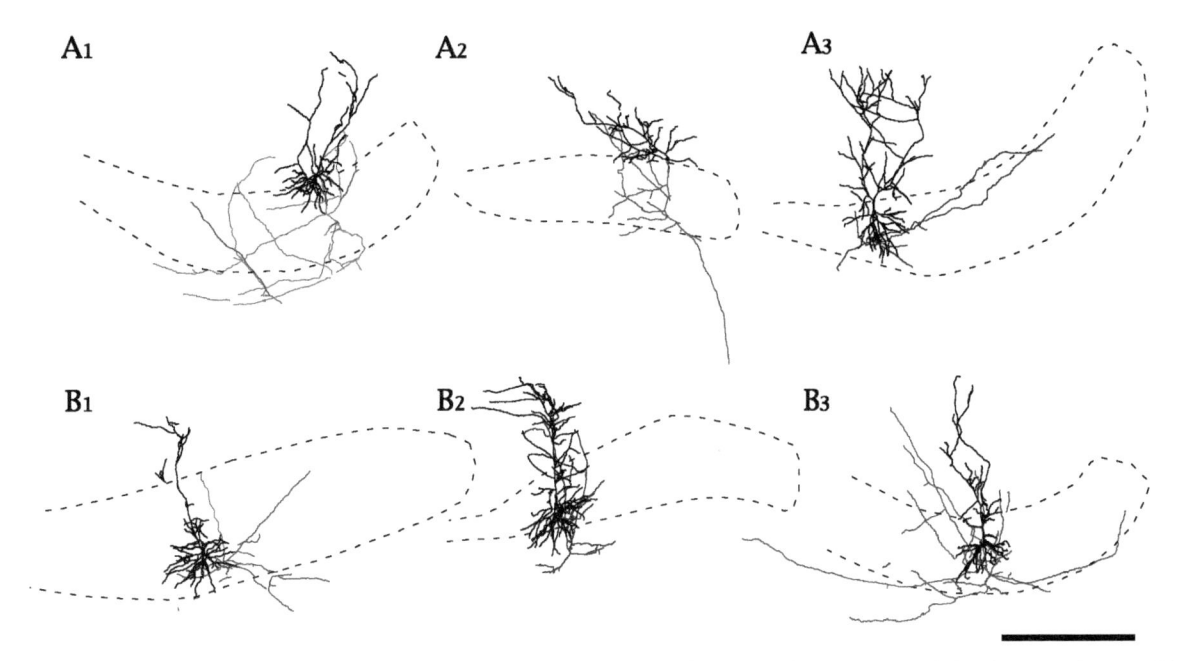

Figure 3.33 Neurolucida reconstructions of pyramidal cells from different regions of the subiculum. Somata and dendrites are shown in black. Axons are shown in gray. Local collaterals tend to be longer in the cell layer for superficially located cells (A1–3); deep cells tend to have axon collaterals that ascend close to the primary dendrite. CA1 is to the left and the presubiculum is to the right. Scale bar is 500 μm. (Adapted with permission from Harris et al., 2001.)

layer and for approximately one-third of the septotemporal length (Tamamaki et al., 1987). The CA1 projection thus segments the subiculum roughly into thirds. This is consistent with recent gene expression studies that indicate that the proximal half of the subiculum is distinctly different from the distal half (Cembrowski, Philips, et al., 2018). The CA1 to subiculum projection, like the CA3-to-CA1 projection, is organized in a divergent fashion, since even a small portion of CA1 projects to about a third of the septotemporal extent of the subiculum.

3.9.3 The subiculum

3.9.3.1 Cytoarchitectonic organization

The CA1 border with the subiculum is marked by an abrupt widening of the pyramidal cell layer and an increased staining intensity with the Timm stain (Figure 3.12). Stratum radiatum of CA1 (as defined as the region that receives CA3 projections) also ends at this border and is replaced with the molecular layer of the subiculum. This layer can be subdivided into a deeper portion that is continuous with the stratum radiatum of CA1, and a superficial portion that is continuous with the stratum lacunosum-moleculare of CA1 and the molecular layer of the presubiculum. The deep portion receives fibers from CA1, whereas the superficial portion receives fibers from the entorhinal cortex. The stratum oriens of CA1 is no longer present in the subiculum. By using gene expression techniques through single-cell RNA-seq, Cembrowski, Philips, et al. (2018) demonstrated that the organization of the subiculum is likely to be much more complicated. They find differential expression patterns that distinguish proximal from distal cells, that distinguish different sublayers of the pyramidal cell layer and differences in pyramidal cells at different septotemporal levels. At least some of these distinctions map onto connectional differences as well.

3.9.3.2 Neuron types

Research on the cytology and connectivity of the subiculum has lagged research on other areas of the hippocampal formation (Wheeler et al., 2015), and with few exceptions (Funahashi and Stewart, 1997; Harris et al., 2001) much of the information on subicular cell types came from the classical Golgi studies of Ramón y Cajal and Lorente de Nó carried out in young mice. The principal cell layer of the subiculum is populated by large pyramidal neurons (Figure 3.33). This layer starts just beneath the distal end of CA1 and continues in a position deep to layer II of the presubiculum. These cells are relatively uniform in shape and size and extend their apical dendrites into the molecular layer and their basal dendrites into deeper portions of the pyramidal cell layer. A subdivision into at least two cell types, however, has been proposed based on their firing characteristics: regular spiking cells and intrinsically bursting cells (Greene and Totterdell, 1997). Although these two cell types do not exhibit distinct morphological characteristics (but see below), they show a differential distribution within the pyramidal cell layer. Bursting cells are more numerous deep in the pyramidal cell layer, whereas regular spiking cells are more common superficially. The two populations can also be distinguished by preferential staining for either NADPH-diaphorase/nitric oxide synthetase (regular spiking neurons) or somatostatin (bursting cells). Both cell types are projection neurons, but they might differ with respect to their connectivity, since there is evidence suggesting that only bursting cells project to the entorhinal cortex. Intermingled among the pyramidal cells are many smaller neurons, presumably representing the interneurons of the subiculum. Little is known, however, about whether the types of interneurons seen in the subiculum are similar to those observed in the hippocampus (Wheeler et al., 2015). Subpopulations of these neurons appear to have characteristics similar to those described for CA1, and among those are GABAergic cells that stain for the calcium binding protein parvalbumin.

Intrinsic connections

The subiculum gives rise to a longitudinal associational projection that extends from the level of the cells of origin to much of the subiculum lying temporally (or ventrally). Interestingly, this projection seems to be largely unidirectional, since few, if any, associational projections course septally or dorsally from their point of origin (Harris et al., 2001). The associational fibers terminate diffusely in all layers of the subiculum. Recent studies have consistently found that the rat subiculum neither gives rise to nor receives commissural connections.

Subicular pyramidal cells provide a strong local input within the pyramidal cell layer and just superficial to it, targeting proximal portions of the apical dendrites. Interestingly, the density of this local intrinsic connection, as estimated by the number of varicosities on locally distributed axon collaterals, is much higher than in CA1. In addition, the two types of subicular pyramidal neurons differ with respect to their local connectivity. Intracellular labeling of electrophysiologically identified bursting cells generally show an axonal distribution that remains within the region circumscribed by their apical dendrites (i.e., a columnar organization), whereas the regular spiking cells generally give rise to an axon that shows more widespread distribution along the transverse axis. It is not known whether differences exist with respect to a possible septotemporal spread. Although much work remains to be done, available data indicate that the organization of the intrinsic connectivity of the subiculum is different from that of CA3 and CA1. There are both crude columnar and laminar organizations, such that the bursting cells form a set of columns and the regular spiking neurons integrate columnar activity along the transverse axis.

Extrinsic connections: the subiculum, a major output structure

The subiculum is a major source of efferent projections from the hippocampal formation. Following the discovery by Swanson and Cowan (1975) that the subiculum, rather than the hippocampus, is the origin of the major subcortical connections to the diencephalon and brainstem (via the postcommissural fornix), evidence has mounted that the subiculum is one of the two primary output structures of the hippocampal formation (Swanson and Cowan, 1975; Swanson et al., 1981; Donovan and Wyss, 1983; Groenewegen et al., 1987; Witter and Groenewegen, 1990; Witter et al., 1990; Canteras and Swanson, 1992; Naber and Witter, 1998; Ishizuka, 2001; Kloosterman et al., 2003; Aggleton and Christiansen, 2015; Christiansen et al., 2016). In broad strokes, the projections of the subiculum are organized both topographically and laminarly. The proximal portion of the subiculum is associated with lateral entorhinal cortex and the perirhinal cortex, the prefrontal cortex, amygdala, and nucleus accumbens. The distal subiculum is more associated with the medial entorhinal cortex and the postrhinal cortex. As initially demonstrated by Ishizuka (2001) cells projecting to the anterior thalamus are located in the deepest part of the subicular pyramidal cell layer, those projecting to the anterior cingulate cortex are located most superficially, and those projecting to the medial mammillary nucleus are located in the middle of the layer.

The subiculum projects to the presubiculum and the parasubiculum

While the subiculum projects to the presubiculum, this projection is not of the magnitude of the other intrinsic hippocampal formation projections. It is probably better to think of the subiculum projection to the presubiculum as one of a series of pathways that distributes information processed in the dentate gyrus, hippocampus and subiculum to a series of cortical and subcortical structures. Subicular fibers terminate mainly in layer I of the presubiculum. The projection to the dorsal part of the presubiculum, however, terminates deep to the prominent layer II, with weaker projections to layers I and II (Kohler, 1985). The projection from the subiculum to the parasubiculum mainly terminates in layer I and the superficial part of layer II. These projections are topographically organized. Septal (or dorsal) portions of the subiculum project to dorsal and caudal aspects of both the presubiculum and the parasubiculum, and temporal (or ventral) portions of the subiculum project to ventral and rostral aspects of the presubiculum and parasubiculum (Witter, 2006; O'Reilly et al., 2013).

The subiculum is reciprocally connected with the entorhinal cortex

Since the perforant path fibers traverse the subiculum on their way to the dentate gyrus and hippocampus, the question of whether some of these might terminate in the subiculum has long been a matter of controversy. Until recently, the collective hunch was that fibers simply passed through the subiculum and probably did not terminate within it. Earlier anterograde tracer studies indicated that perforant path fibers are directed toward the molecular layer of the subiculum, but proof that these fibers formed a terminal plexus among the subicular pyramidal cells was lacking. Witter and colleagues, however, have provided convincing evidence, at both the light and electron microscopic levels, that the subiculum receives a strong projection from the entorhinal cortex (reviewed in Witter, 2006; O'Reilly et al., 2013; and Chapter 12). The topography of the projection is similar to that described for CA1. Fibers are directed toward restricted transverse portions of the subiculum and terminate in the outer two-thirds of the molecular layer. The lateral component of the perforant pathway preferentially projects to the proximal part of the subiculum, i.e., the part of the subiculum that borders CA1, and the medial component distributes to more distal portions of the subiculum, i.e., closer to the presubiculum. The projection originates mainly from layer III, although some of the axons of layer II cells that cross the subiculum on their way to the dentate gyrus and CA3 may also give off collaterals that terminate in the subiculum. Eighty percent of the entorhinal synapses target dendritic spines of presumed principal neurons with asymmetrical synapses, whereas 5%–10% of the asymmetrical synapses terminate on dendritic shafts, most likely belonging to interneurons. Subicular interneurons may also receive a minor inhibitory perforant path input in view of the symmetrical synapses onto dendritic shafts.

The subiculum reciprocates the entorhinal input (Figure 3.34). Projections from the subiculum reach all parts of the entorhinal cortex and terminate in the deep layers; termination is particularly dense in layer V. A minor component of the subicular projection also extends superficially to the lamina dissecans, predominantly

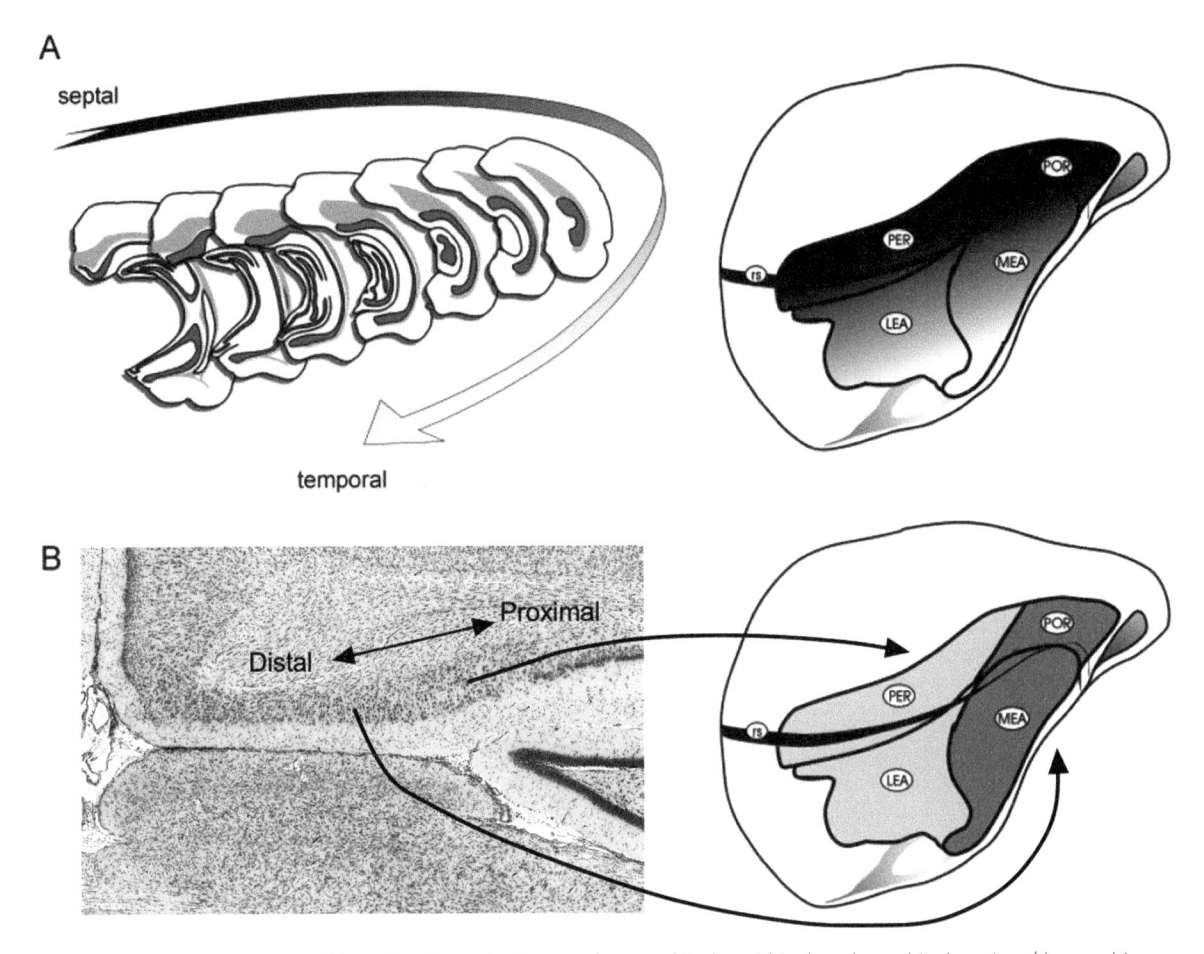

Figure 3.34 Topographical organization of the subicular projections to the entorhinal, perirhinal, and postrhinal cortices (the parahippocampal region). (A) Relationship between the septotemporal origin in the subiculum with a lateral-to-medial termination in the parahippocampal region. The septal portion of the subiculum projects to the perirhinal and postrhinal cortices and the lateral portion of both the lateral and medial entorhinal cortex. The temporal portion of the subiculum projects to medial portions of the lateral and medial entorhinal cortex. (B) Relationship between the proximodistal origin in the subiculum with a rostrocaudal termination in the parahippocampal region. The proximal subiculum projects to the perirhinal and the lateral entorhinal cortex; the distal subiculum projects to the postrhinal and the medial entorhinal cortex. (Adapted from Kloosterman et al., 2003.)

to layer III. Subicular fibers generally form asymmetrical synapses with spines and dendrites located in these layers. A minority of these fibers form symmetrical synapses, suggesting a small inhibitory input from the subiculum to layer V. Therefore, the overall organization of the subiculoentorhinal projection mimics that of the CA1-entorhinal projection. The presence of asymmetrical synapses at the termination of this pathway is consistent with its reported excitatory influences on the entorhinal cortex.

Subicular connections with the neocortex and amygdaloid complex

The subiculum gives rise to prominent projections to the medial and ventral orbitofrontal cortices and to the prelimbic and infralimbic cortices (Verwer et al., 1997; Aggleton and Christiansen). In the orbitofrontal and prelimbic cortices, subicular fibers mainly innervate the deep layers, whereas in the infralimbic cortex, the projection extends into the superficial layers. Subicular projections also reach medial portions of the anterior olfactory nucleus.

The subiculum provides a meager projection to the anterior cingulate cortex, whereas the projection to the retrosplenial cortex is

very substantial (Wyss and Van Groen, 1992; Witter, 2006). The subiculoretrosplenial projection terminates predominantly in layers II and III. The projections to the retrosplenial cortex originate predominantly from the septal two-thirds of the subiculum. The perirhinal cortex receives a strong input from the subiculum, which terminates both in superficial and deep layers.

In the rat, there is a paucity of detailed information regarding direct cortical inputs to the subiculum. Many of the cortical regions that project fairly heavily to the entorhinal cortex (see below) do not project to the subiculum. No inputs, for example, have been reported from the pre- and infralimbic cortices. Similarly, no portion of the retrosplenial cortex projects to the subiculum. Reports of projections from the cingulate cortex have been somewhat contradictory. The perirhinal cortex projects to the subiculum, but this projection terminates only in the proximal third of the field, i.e., at the border region with CA1.

The proximal portion of the subiculum also receives an input from the parvicellular portion of the basal nucleus of the amygdaloid complex, the posterior cortical nucleus and the adjacent amygdalohippocampal area. These amygdaloid inputs terminate mainly at the CA1/subiculum border region, where they preferentially innervate the molecular layer of the subiculum and stratum lacunosum-moleculare of CA1 (Pitkänen et al., 2000).

The temporal one-third of the subiculum gives rise to return projections to the amygdaloid complex. The major component of this projection terminates in the accessory basal nucleus, with more moderate projections reaching several other nuclei but not the lateral nucleus. The ventral subiculum also projects heavily to the bed nucleus of the stria terminalis and moderately to the ventral part of the claustrum or endopiriform nucleus.

Basal forebrain connections—septal nucleus and nucleus accumbens

The most prominent subcortical subicular projections are those to the septal complex, the adjacent nucleus accumbens, and the mammillary nuclei. The projection to the septal area terminates predominantly in the lateral septal nucleus. Closely associated with the septal projection is the equally robust projection to nucleus accumbens and adjacent parts of the olfactory tubercle. Subicular fibers terminate throughout the nucleus accumbens, with the projection to its caudomedial part being most dense. As with other striatal structures, the subicular projection to the nucleus accumbens is unidirectional. Whereas the subicular projections to the lateral septal nucleus are almost entirely confined to the ipsilateral side, those to the nucleus accumbens show a weak contralateral component. The subiculum receives a relatively weak cholinergic projection from the septal complex; fibers originating both from the medial septal nucleus and from the nucleus of the diagonal band terminate in the pyramidal cell and molecular layers.

Hypothalamic connections—mammillary nuclei

The subiculum provides the major input to the mammillary nuclei. The projection is very heavy and is distributed bilaterally in nearly equal density. The subiculomammillary fibers originate mainly from the septal two-thirds of the subiculum. While the temporal one-third of the subiculum also contributes to the mammillary projection, the major hypothalamic target of this portion of the subiculum is the ventromedial nucleus of the hypothalamus. The subicular projections to the mammillary nuclei reach all portions of the medial nucleus but are topographically organized; the lateral mammillary nucleus is only sparsely innervated by the subiculum. Subicular fibers also project to the lateral hypothalamic region located adjacent to the lateral mammillary nucleus.

While the subiculum does not receive a return projection from the medial or lateral mammillary nuclei, the supramammillary region projects heavily to the subiculum, particularly to temporal levels (Vertes, 2015). This portion of the subiculum also receives an input from the premammillary nucleus. It is not clear whether there are any local connections between the medial mammillary nucleus and the supramammillary area or the premammillary nucleus that might complete the subiculohypothalamic loop.

Thalamic connections—nucleus reuniens and other midline nuclei

The thalamic inputs to the subiculum are similar to those to CA1 (Cassel et al., 2013). Thalamic inputs originate mainly in the nucleus reuniens, the paraventricular nucleus, and the parataenial nucleus. The septal and temporal extremes of the subiculum appear to be devoid of an input from nucleus reuniens. The midline thalamic projections terminate mainly in the molecular layer of the subiculum and in stratum lacunosum-moleculare in CA1. Interestingly, the projections to the subiculum and to CA1 originate from different but intermingled populations of neurons in nucleus reuniens. While earlier studies had indicated that the subiculum was interconnected with the anterior nuclear complex, it is now clear that the anterior nucleus projects almost exclusively to the presubiculum and the parasubiculum.

Some of the thalamic regions that project to the subiculum receive a return projection from the subiculum. Subicular fibers terminate bilaterally in the nucleus reuniens, the nucleus interanteromedialis, the paraventricular nucleus, and the nucleus gelatinosus. Although subicular projections to parts of the anterior thalamic complex have been described in the literature, these projections arise from the presubiculum.

Brainstem inputs

Monoaminergic ascending pathways from the noradrenergic locus coeruleus, the dopaminergic ventral tegmental area, and the serotonergic median and dorsal raphe nuclei reach the subiculum, but do not show a preferential innervation of this region. Few details are available concerning the regional localization of these pathways in the subiculum.

Topography of subicular efferent projections

As with the projections from CA3 to CA1 and from CA1 to the subiculum, the subicular efferent projections are topographically organized. In large part, the subicular projections preserve the transverse topography established by the CA1-to-subiculum projection. It is clear that different projections originate from at least the proximal and distal halves of the subiculum. The subiculum also demonstrates a marked septotemporal topography, such that the projections that arise from the septal or dorsal two-thirds of the subiculum are different from those that arise from the temporal or ventral third (Cembrowski, Philips, et al., 2018).

Turning first to the septotemporal topography, it appears that the projections to the entorhinal cortex, the lateral septal complex, the nucleus accumbens, and the medial mammillary nucleus originate from the entire septotemporal extent of the subiculum (Witter and Groenewegen, 1990; Ishizuka, 2001). Different septotemporal levels of the subiculum, however, project to different portions of these fields. In the entorhinal cortex, for example, the septal-to-temporal origin in the subiculum is related to a lateral-to-medial termination within the entorhinal cortex. Septal levels of the subiculum project preferentially to lateral and caudal parts of the entorhinal cortex, i.e., the parts that lie adjacent to the rhinal sulcus. Progressively more temporal levels of the subiculum project to more medially located parts of the entorhinal cortex. Although addressed in more detail below, it is important to point out that this topography is completely in register with the projections from the entorhinal cortex to the subiculum. Thus, cells in the subiculum that receive an input from a subregion in the entorhinal cortex give rise to a return projection to the same region in the entorhinal cortex.

In the nucleus accumbens, the septotemporal axis of origin in the subiculum determines a caudomedial to rostrolateral axis of termination. Dorsomedial portions of the lateral septal complex receive inputs from septal levels of the subiculum, while ventral portions of the lateral septal complex are innervated by fibers originating in more temporal parts of the subiculum.

A similar septotemporal topography has also been described for the subicular projections to the presubiculum and to the medial mammillary nuclei. The latter projection arises mainly from the septal two-thirds of the subiculum, while the ventral one-third gives rise to projections to other hypothalamic regions such as the ventromedial nucleus.

This dichotomy between the septal two-thirds and the temporal one-third of the subiculum is reflected in the organization of other projections. Projections to the amygdala and the bed nucleus of the stria terminalis, for example, originate exclusively from the temporal one-third of the subiculum, whereas projections to the retrosplenial and perirhinal cortices originate predominantly from the septal two-thirds. The subicular projections to the midline thalamus demonstrate even greater septotemporal topography. The most septal part of the subiculum projects preferentially to the anteromedial nucleus, mid-septotemporal levels of the subiculum preferentially project to the nucleus reuniens, and the temporal third of the subiculum projects most heavily to the paraventricular nucleus.

Whereas the septotemporal topography appears to be organized in a gradient or gradual fashion, the transverse organization of subicular efferents is remarkably discrete. Along the transverse axis of the subiculum, two essentially nonoverlapping populations of cells can be differentiated that give rise to projections to specific sets of brain structures. This transverse organization of the outputs of the subiculum is consistently observed along its entire septotemporal axis, although it is clearer septally than temporally. Neurons in the proximal half of the subiculum (closest to CA1) project to the infralimbic and prelimbic cortices, the perirhinal cortex, the nucleus accumbens, the lateral septum, the amygdaloid complex, and the core of the ventromedial nucleus of the hypothalamus. Cells in the distal half of the subiculum project mainly to the retrosplenial cortex and to the presubiculum. Cells projecting to the

midline thalamic nuclei are mainly located in the midportion of the subiculum.

The subicular projections to the entorhinal cortex and to the medial mammillary nucleus do not follow a strict transverse organization, since cells in all proximodistal portions of the subiculum project to these areas. However, the topography of these projections indicates a more subtle transverse organization. Thus, the proximal portions of the subiculum project to rostral medial mammillary nuclei and distal portions of the subiculum project more caudally. A similar situation exists for the subicular projections to the entorhinal cortex. The proximal half of the subiculum projects to the lateral entorhinal area, and the distal half of the subiculum projects to the medial entorhinal area.

Since the proximal third of the subiculum gives rise to projections to at least several cortical and subcortical regions, the question arises as to whether it is the same or different populations of subicular cells that innervate each structure. While the answer initially appeared to be that projections to the septal complex, the entorhinal cortex and the mammillary complex, arise, at least in part, as collaterals from single subicular neurons, it now appears that largely independent populations of intermixed neurons in the subiculum project to each of its terminal regions (Naber and Witter, 1998). Given our earlier assertion that the subiculum is the last staging post of hippocampal processing, this state of affairs would seem to create the possibility that the outputs destined for different target structures can be carrying distinctly different information.

3.9.4 Presubiculum and parasubiculum

3.9.4.1 Cytoarchitectonic organization and neuron types

The presubiculum (Brodmann's area 27), is relatively easily differentiated from the subiculum in standard Nissl-stained material in all species (Ding, 2013). It has a distinct, densely packed external cell layer that consists mainly of darkly stained, small pyramidal cell (Figure 3.35). The most superficial cells are the most densely packed (layer II), while the deeper cells have a somewhat looser arrangement (layer III). The differentiation between layers II and III is more clear-cut at dorsal levels of the presubiculum. The superficial cells are separated by a plexiform layer from more deeply situated cells (layers V and VI) that are continuous with the deep layers of the entorhinal cortex (Witter et al., 1989; van Strien et al., 2009).

The dorsal presubiculum (sometimes called the postsubiculum) has clearly distinguishable superficial and deep cell layers. In the ventral portion of the presubiculum, however, the deep layers are difficult to distinguish from the deep layers of the entorhinal cortex or from the principal cell layer of the subiculum. Deep to the lamina dissecans, one finds one or two layers of large, darkly stained pyramidal cells, and deep to these is a rather heterogeneous collection of pyramidal and polymorphic cells.

The parasubiculum (Brodmann's area 49) lies adjacent to the presubiculum (Tang et al., 2016). Layers II and III of the parasubiculum consist of patches of rather densely packed, lightly stained, large pyramidal cells. This, and other characteristics such as the distinctive staining for heavy metals observable with the Timm's stain method are the major features that differentiate the parasubiculum from the presubiculum (Figure 3.12). There is no clear differentiation between layers II and III. There is little or no association of layers I–III with more deeply situated layers.

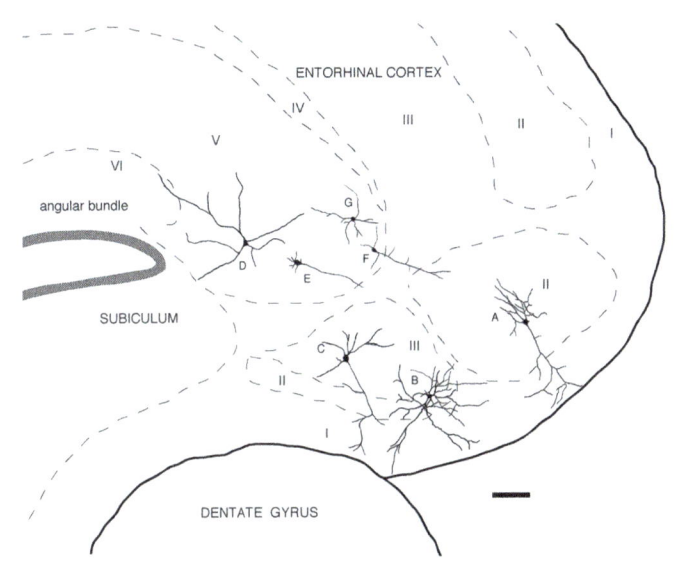

Figure 3.35 Cell types of the presubiculum and parasubiculum. Camera lucida drawings of neurobiotin-filled cells in a horizontal section through the hippocampal formation. (A) pyramidal cell in layer II of the parasubiculum; (B) stellate cell in layer II of the presubiculum; (C) pyramidal cell in layer III of the presubiculum; (D) stellate cell in layer V of the presubiculum; (E) pyramidal cell in layer V of the presubiculum; (F) pyramidal cell in layer V of the parasubiculum; (G) stellate cell in layer V of the parasubiculum. Scale bar is 100 μm. (Adapted with permission from Funahashi and Stewart, 1997.)

3.9.4.2 Intrinsic connections

There are well-developed associational connections in the presubiculum, which interconnect all dorsoventral levels in a highly directional manner. Layer II cells in ventral portions of the presubiculum project to more dorsal levels of the presubiculum. Projections in the opposite direction (dorsal to ventral), however, arise preferentially from cells below layer II.

The parasubiculum also gives rise to associational connections that distribute both dorsally and ventrally from the cells of origin. The dorsally directed projections extend for short distances and are quite weak. The ventrally directed projections are substantially denser and extend for long distances along the long axis of the parasubiculum. The parasubiculum gives rise to a particularly dense projection to the dorsally located area 29e. This small wedge-shaped region was initially described by Blackstad (1956) and later characterized in more detail by Haug (1976). Although the neuroanatomy of area 29e remains sketchy, it might actually be a part of the parasubiculum.

3.9.4.3 Commissural connections

The presubiculum gives rise to strong commissural projections to layers I and III of the homotopic part of the contralateral presubiculum (Van Groen and Wyss, 1990). Commissural projections from the dorsal portion of the presubiculum are relatively sparse. The parasubiculum also gives rise to a commissural projection that terminates most densely in layers I and III.

3.9.4.4 Extrinsic connections

Presubiculum and parasubiculum are reciprocally connected with anterior thalamic nuclei

While the presubiculum and parasubiculum receive a number of subcortical inputs, the one that is unique to these portions of the hippocampal formation is their interconnection with the anterior thalamic nuclear complex, primarily the anteroventral and anterodorsal nuclei and the closely related laterodorsal nucleus (Kaitz and Robertson, 1981; Robertson and Kaitz, 1981; Yoder et al., 2011). Although earlier studies had suggested that the presubiculum also receives inputs from the anteromedial nucleus, the principal projections of this nucleus appear to be directed to the anterior parts of the cingulate cortex rather than to the presubiculum or parasubiculum.

There are topographical differences in the thalamic connections of the ventral and dorsal parts of the presubiculum. The ventral part receives most of its input from the laterodorsal and anteroventral nuclei, whereas the dorsal part receives projections mainly from the laterodorsal and anterodorsal nuclei. The thalamic projections mainly terminate in layers I, III, and IV. The nucleus reuniens also projects to layer I of the presubiculum, but this is a much lighter projection.

Like most other thalamocortical connections, the presubiculum sends a return projection back to the thalamus. The presubiculum projects massively and bilaterally to the anterior nuclear complex. The presubicular projections arise mainly from cells located deep to lamina dissecans (layer VI). The fact that these deep cells are related to the anterior nuclei of the thalamus lends some credibility to the idea that they are, in fact, deep layers of the presubiculum and parasubiculum.

Presubiculum projection to layer III of the entorhinal cortex

The most prominent intrahippocampal projection from the presubiculum is to the entorhinal cortex (Shipley, 1975;

Caballero-Bleda and Witter, 1993; van Strien et al., 2009). This projection has a number of interesting features. First, the presubicular projection is directed only to the medial entorhinal cortex. Second, the projection terminates almost exclusively in layer III and to a much lesser extent in the deep part of layer I. Third, the crossed homotopic projection from the presubiculum to the contralateral entorhinal cortex is every bit as strong as the ipsilateral projection. The projection to the entorhinal cortex is topographically organized. The location of the presubicular terminal field in the entorhinal cortex is determined both by the proximodistal and the dorsoventral location of the presubicular cells of origin.

The parasubiculum selectively innervates layer II of the entorhinal cortex. In contrast to the presubiculum, the parasubiculum projects both to the medial and lateral entorhinal areas, though the projection to the lateral entorhinal area is less robust. While the parasubiculum projects to the contralateral entorhinal cortex, these projections are much weaker than the ipsilateral ones. The topographical organization of the parasubicular projection to the entorhinal cortex is comparable to that of the presubicular-entorhinal projection.

Presubiculum and parasubiculum are connected with some neocortical regions

The presubiculum receives relatively few extrahippocampal cortical inputs. The most prominent one, however, originates in the retrosplenial cortex (Van Groen and Wyss, 1990; Wyss and Van Groen, 1992). Cells located in layer V of the retrosplenial cortex give rise to projections that terminate in layers I and III–V of the presubiculum. A second cortical input originates from layer V of the visual area 18b. This projection mainly distributes to the dorsal half of the presubiculum and terminates in layers I and III. Minor cortical inputs originate in the prelimbic cortex and in a dorsal portion of the medial prefrontal cortex.

Extrahippocampal projections from layer V of the presubiculum reach the granular retrosplenial cortex, where they terminate preferentially in layers I and II. These projections are topographically organized, such that the ventral presubiculum projects mainly to the ventral part of the granular retrosplenial cortex and the dorsal part of the presubiculum projects more dorsally. These projections also exhibit a rostrocaudal organization, such that rostral portions of the presubiculum project to rostral parts of the retrosplenial cortex and caudal portions of the presubiculum project to caudal parts of the retrosplenial cortex. It has been suggested that the dorsal presubiculum projects to the deep layers of the most caudal portion of the perirhinal cortex, though an alternative interpretation is that this projection is directed to the most caudodorsal portion of the medial entorhinal cortex which is difficult to differentiate from caudal perirhinal cortex.

With the exception of the relatively light projections from the retrosplenial cortex and the occipital visual cortex, there are no other known extrahippocampal cortical inputs to the parasubiculum. The laminar distribution of these inputs is similar to that described for the presubiculum.

3.9.4.5 Other intrahippocampal connections

The presubiculum projects to layers I and II of the parasubiculum bilaterally. Anterograde tracing studies have demonstrated that the presubiculum, and perhaps, to a greater extent the parasubiculum, contribute projections, albeit modest ones, to many of the other regions of the hippocampal formation. For example, there is a modest bilateral projection from the presubiculum to the subiculum. There is also a weak projection to all fields of the hippocampus and to the molecular layer of the dentate gyrus. The presubicular fibers to the molecular layer of the dentate gyrus are arranged in a radial manner, which is quite distinct from the predominantly transverse orientation of the entorhinal perforant pathway fibers.

A fact that has not been generally appreciated is that the parasubiculum gives rise to a fairly substantial projection to the molecular layer of the dentate gyrus (Kohler, 1985). Like the lighter projection from the presubiculum, this projection occupies the superficial two-thirds of the molecular layer (with a preference for the midportion of the molecular layer) and fibers have a predominantly radial orientation. Since the parasubiculum receives a projection from the anterior thalamic nuclei, its projection to the molecular layer provides a route by which thalamic input might influence very early stages of hippocampal information processing. The parasubiculum projects weakly to stratum lacunosum-moleculare of the hippocampus and to the molecular layer of the subiculum. The parasubiculum also projects bilaterally above and below layer II of the presubiculum.

Basal forebrain connections

The presubiculum and parasubiculum receive a heavy cholinergic input. The medial septal nucleus and the vertical limb of the diagonal band of Broca mainly innervate layer II of the presubiculum.

Hypothalamic connections—the mammillary nuclei

Cells located deep to layer II of the presubiculum project bilaterally to the medial and lateral mammillary nuclei. The projections to the medial mammillary nuclei are topographically organized in a manner similar to those that originate in the subiculum (Thompson and Robertson, 1987; Allen and Hopkins, 1989; Van Groen and Wyss, 1990).

The presubiculum receives inputs from the area surrounding the mammillary nuclei. Fibers from the supramammillary nucleus terminate preferentially in the deeper cell layers of the presubiculum, although those that are characterized as being alpha-melanocyte-stimulating-hormone positive (an opiate peptide expressed in neurons whose somata are located in the lateral hypothalamic area) terminate in the molecular layer.

Brainstem inputs

The presubiculum receives inputs from various nuclei in the brainstem. A particularly dense innervation arises from the dorsal and ventral raphe nuclei; at least a component of this projection is serotonergic and innervates layer I. The noradrenergic locus coeruleus also innervates layer I.

3.9.5 The entorhinal cortex

The entorhinal cortex (Brodmann's area 28) plays an extraordinarily important role in the flow of information through the hippocampal formation. It not only is the main entry point for much of the sensory information that is processed by the hippocampal formation but also provides the main conduit for processed information to be relayed back to the neocortex. As portrayed in this chapter, the entorhinal cortex is the beginning and the end point of an extensive and complex loop of information processing that takes place within

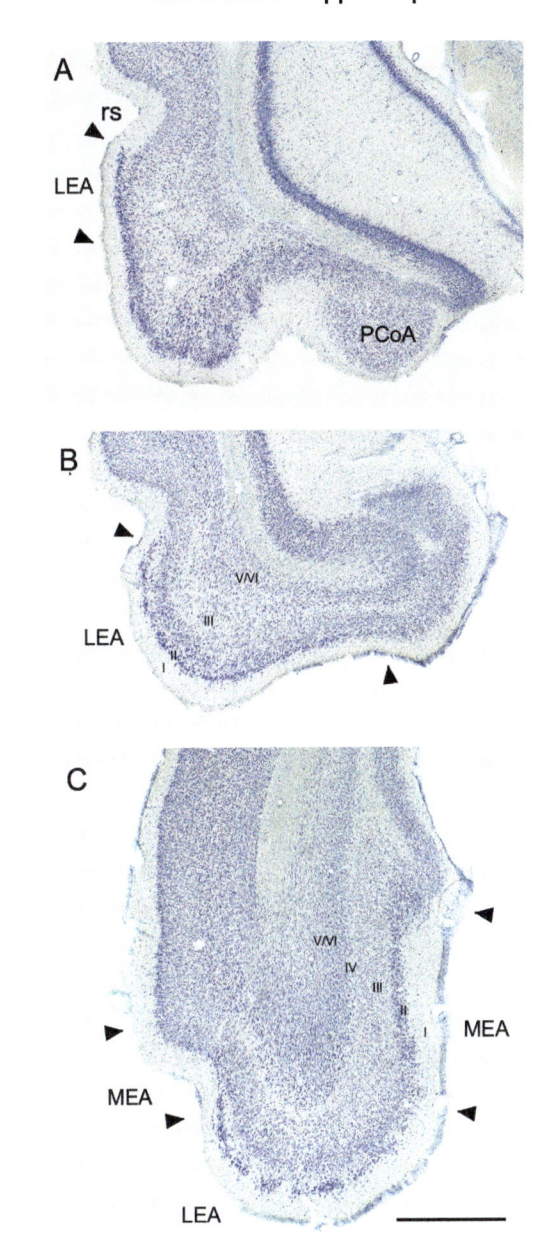

Figure 3.36 Cytoarchitectonic characteristics of the rat entorhinal cortex. (A–C) Photomicrographs of Nissl-stained coronal sections through three selected rostrocaudal levels of the entorhinal cortex, arranged from rostral (A) to caudal (C), showing the lateral (LEA) and medial (MEA) entorhinal area subdivisions. Arrowheads indicate LEA and MEA boundaries. Scale bar is approximately 1 mm.

the various fields of the hippocampal formation. As Ramón y Cajal said (to paraphrase) whatever the rest of the hippocampal formation is doing will depend on what the entorhinal cortex has done. So important is the entorhinal cortex to an understanding of the function of the hippocampal formation, that an independent chapter (Chapter 12) has been dedicated to it. Chapter 12 begins with a comprehensive analysis of the neuroanatomy of the entorhinal cortex. While there are comparative notes in this coverage, the findings are largely based on research carried out in the rodent, mainly the rat, and preponderantly by Menno Witter and colleagues. Witter has produced a series of informative review articles (for example, Witter et al., 2017; Nilssen et al., 2019) in addition to Chapter 12, that the reader is referred to for a detailed view of entorhinal neuroanatomy.

In order to reduce redundancy, we have scaled back the coverage of the rodent entorhinal cortex in this chapter and refer the reader to the first portion of Chapter 12 for that information. We begin our description of the entorhinal cortex with a discussion of some lingering controversies concerning its laminar and regional organization.

3.9.5.1 Cytoarchitectonic organization

Laminar organization

We have adopted the nomenclature for entorhinal layers first suggested by Ramón y Cajal and later modified to more closely resemble the standard six-layer scheme applied to the isocortex (Figure 3.36). According to this scheme, there are four cellular layers (layers II, III, V, and VI) and two acellular or plexiform layers (layers I and IV). The acellular layer IV is also called lamina dissecans. This scheme emphasizes the lack of an internal granular cell layer in the entorhinal cortex. Starting from the pial surface, the layers include: Layer I—the most superficial plexiform or molecular layer, which is cell poor but rich in transversely oriented fibers; Layer II—containing mainly medium- to large-sized stellate cells and a population of small pyramidal cells. These cells tend to be grouped in clusters (cell islands), particularly in the lateral entorhinal area; Layer III—containing cells of various sizes and shapes, but predominantly pyramidal cells; Layer IV (or lamina dissecans)—a cell free layer located between layers III and V. It is most apparent in those portions of the entorhinal cortex that lie close to the rhinal fissure, particularly

at caudal levels of the entorhinal cortex. In the remainder of the entorhinal cortex, groups of cells invade this layer so that it has an incomplete or patchy appearance; Layer V—a cellular layer that can be subdivided into bands. Layer Va forms a band of large, darkly stained pyramidal neurons. This layer is most conspicuous in the central parts of the entorhinal cortex. At other levels, the packing density of cells is not high and the smaller cells of the deeper part of this layer (Vb) intermingle with it; Finally, Layer VI—containing a very heterogeneous population of cells of different sizes and shapes. Cell density decreases toward the limit with the white matter. The cells of layer VI appear to blend, in a gradual way, both into the subjacent subcortical white matter and into the overlying layer V.

Regional organization

There have been several published attempts at subdividing the rat entorhinal cortex, and unfortunately there have been almost an equal number of different opinions concerning the number and terminology of the subfields. These have been discussed and reviewed by Menno Witter, Ricardo Insausti, and their colleagues (Insausti et al., 1997; Burwell and Witter, 2002). Nevertheless, (as Kanter et al. argue in Chapter 12) it is now generally accepted that the entorhinal cortex can be subdivided into two general areas, the lateral entorhinal area (LEA) and the medial entorhinal area (MEA; Figure 3.37). Layer II is more clearly demarcated in the LEA than in the MEA, and the cells are very densely packed and tend to be clustered in islands. The cells in layer II of the MEA are somewhat larger and do not show a distinct clustering into islands; the border between layers II and III is not as sharp as in the LEA. In both entorhinal areas, however, the overall differences in cell sizes between layers II and III facilitate the delineation of the two layers. The other cell layers, in particular layers IV–VI, can be better differentiated from each other in the MEA than in the LEA, and cells in the MEA generally show a more radial or columnar arrangement. The lamina dissecans of the MEA is sharply delineated, but it is less clear in the LEA.

It should also be stressed that the terms "lateral" and "medial entorhinal areas" do not relate in a simple manner to the cardinal transverse plane of the rat brain (Figure 3.37). Both the LEA and the MEA have a more or less triangular shape. The LEA occupies the rostrolateral part of the entorhinal cortex; its base is oriented rostrally and its tip caudolaterally, next to the rhinal fissure. The MEA occupies the remaining triangular area, which has its base caudally and its tip rostromedially such that the tip lies medial to the LEA. A different nomenclature has been proposed by Insausti and colleagues to accommodate the oblique orientation of the rat entorhinal cortex and address the need for subdemarcations of the LEA and MEA to bring the rodent more in line with that of the monkey and human (Insausti et al., 1997).

3.9.5.2 Neuron types

The cellular architecture of the rodent entorhinal cortex is extensively covered in Chapter 12 (see section 12.4.1). In order to reduce some redundancy, we refer the reader to this section of Chapter 12 in order to have a comprehensive coverage of this topic.

Intrinsic/associational connections

The entorhinal cortex contains a substantial system of associational connections. Chapter 12 provides a detailed description of connections arising from each of the cellular layers (section

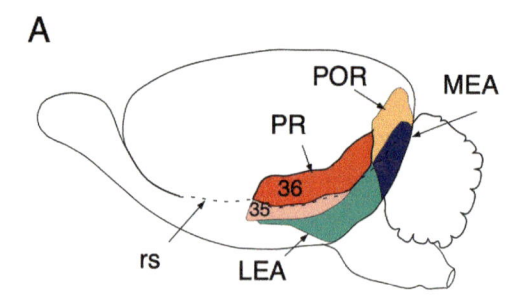

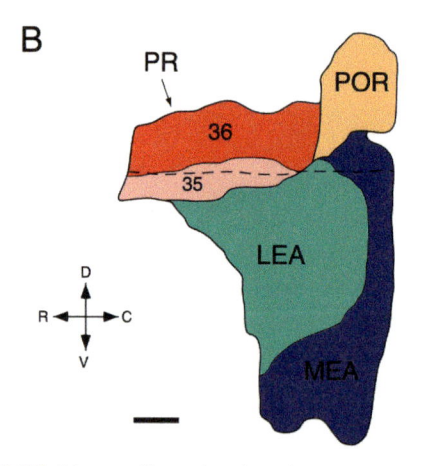

Figure 3.37 Diagram illustrating the relative position of the lateral (LEA) and medial (MEA) entorhinal cortex (area) as well as the perirhinal and postrhinal cortices. (A) Lateral view of the rat brain. (B) Unfolded map of the entorhinal, perirhinal, and postrhinal cortices. Scale bar is 1 mm. D—dorsal, V—ventral, R—rostral, C—caudal. (Adapted from Burwell and Amaral, 1998a.)

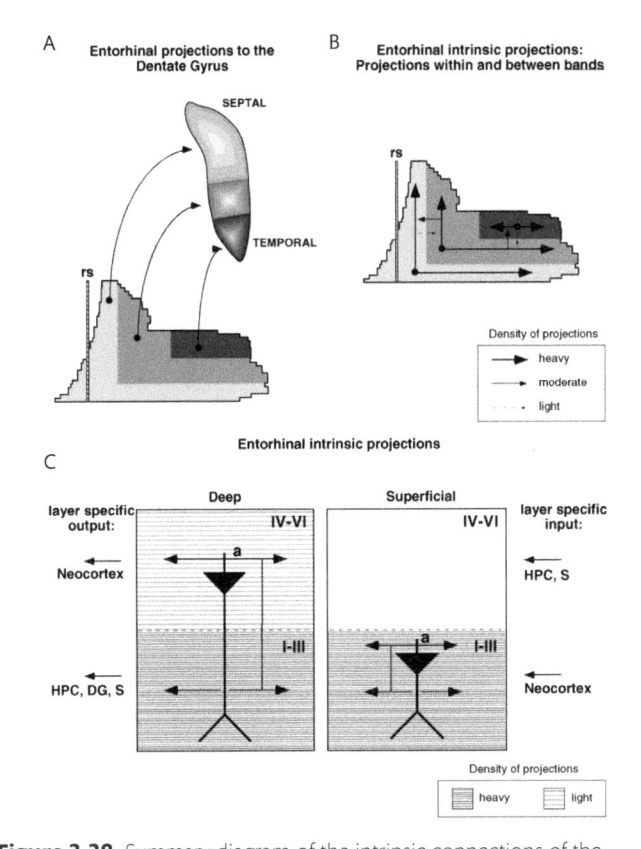

A Entorhinal projections to the Dentate Gyrus

B Entorhinal intrinsic projections: Projections within and between bands

Density of projections
→ heavy
→ moderate
⋯ light

Entorhinal intrinsic projections

C

Deep   Superficial

layer specific output: IV-VI   IV-VI   layer specific input:

Neocortex   HPC, S

I-III   I-III

HPC, DG, S   Neocortex

Density of projections
heavy   light

Figure 3.38 Summary diagram of the intrinsic connections of the entorhinal cortex. Relationship between the entorhinal cortex and the hippocampal formation and neocortex. (A) Organization of entorhinal projections to the dentate gyrus. Band of layer II cells located in the lateral and caudomedial portion of the entorhinal cortex (light gray) projects to the septal half of the dentate gyrus, a band in the mid-mediolateral entorhinal cortex (medium gray) projects to the third quarter of the dentate gyrus, and a band located in the most rostromedial entorhinal cortex (dark gray) projects to the temporal pole of the dentate gyrus. (B) Organization of entorhinal intrinsic projections: projections within and between bands. Each of these projection zones has substantial associational connections (large arrows) that remain largely within the zone of origin. Projections between each band are less prominent (small arrows). (C) Entorhinal intrinsic projections and entorhinal afferent and efferent projections. Entorhinal associational connections arise both from the deep and superficial layers of the entorhinal cortex (arrows within the boxes) and terminate mainly in the superficial layers. A less prominent associational connection within the deep layers is apparent primarily in lateral portions of the entorhinal cortex. (Adapted from Dolorfo and Amaral, 1998.)

12.4.2). Intra-entorhinal fibers are organized in three roughly rostrocaudally oriented bands, and connections that link different transverse (or mediolateral) regions of the entorhinal cortex are rather restricted (Dolorfo and Amaral, 1998) Associational connections originate in both superficial and deep layers. Projections originating from layers II and III tend to terminate mainly in the superficial layers, whereas projections originating from the deep layers terminate both in the deep and superficial layers (Quilichini et al., 2010).

The global organization of the associational connections in the entorhinal cortex can be best understood in relation to the topography of the entorhinal projections to other fields of the hippocampal formation (Figure 3.38). As we will describe shortly, different parts of the entorhinal cortex project to different septotemporal levels of

the dentate gyrus. The portions of the lateral and medial entorhinal areas that project to the septal half of the dentate gyrus, for example, are located laterally and caudally in the entorhinal cortex, close to the rhinal sulcus. Cells located in this region give rise to associational connections to other cells in the same region, but not in any substantial way to portions of the entorhinal cortex that project to other levels of the dentate gyrus. Thus, the associational connections would seem to be organized to integrate all of the information that comes into a particular portion of the entorhinal cortex and will be relayed to a particular septotemporal level of the dentate gyrus. There have been many advancements in our understanding of the intrinsic microcircuitry of the entorhinal cortex, and this topic is covered in detail in Chapter 12.

Commissural connections

Relatively strong commissural connections, arising from all portions of the entorhinal cortex, terminate predominantly in layers I and II of the homotopic area of the entorhinal cortex (Goldowitz et al., 1975; Hjorth-Simonsen and Zimmer, 1975; Ohara et al., 2019). The entorhinal cortex also gives rise to a commissural projection to other components of the contralateral hippocampal formation. The largest component of this projection is directed toward the dentate gyrus, but fields CA3 and CA1 of the hippocampus and the subiculum also receive a contralateral input. The crossed entorhinal projection is heaviest to septal portions of the hippocampal subfields and rapidly diminishes in strength at more temporal levels. The crossed projection arises primarily from layer III cells but also from the layer II calbindin cells.

Organization of the perforant and alvear pathways

As a reminder of our earlier description of the perforant path input to the dentate gyrus, hippocampus, and subiculum, both the lateral and medial entorhinal areas project to all three areas. The lateral and medial components of the perforant path terminate along the superficial-to-deep gradient in the molecular layer of the dentate gyrus and stratum lacunosum-moleculare of CA3 and along the transverse axis of CA1 and the subiculum (Figure 3.39) (Chapter 12, Figure 12.5). Layer II cells give rise to the projection to the dentate gyrus and CA3, and layer III cells project to CA1 and the subiculum. Although current usage often applies the term "perforant path" to all entorhinohippocampal projections, entorhinal fibers also reach CA1 via the alveus, i.e., the alvear pathway originally described by Ramón y Cajal. In the temporal portion of the hippocampus, most of the entorhinal fibers reach CA1 after perforating the subiculum (classical perforant pathway). At more septal levels, however, the number of entorhinal fibers that take the alvear pathway increases, and in the septal portion of the hippocampus, most of the entorhinal fibers reach CA1 via the alvear pathway. These fibers make a sharp turn in the alveus, perforate the pyramidal cell layer and terminate in the stratum lacunosum-moleculare. Part of this pathway terminates on inhibitory neurons and thus produces disynaptic inhibition of CA1 pyramidal cells (Empson and Heinemann, 1995a, 1995b). Both pathways demonstrate the same septotemporal organization of their projections. Thus, certain portions of the entorhinal cortex project to certain septotemporal levels of the other hippocampal fields.

Replicating earlier suggestions by Ruth and colleagues (Ruth et al., 1982; Ruth et al., 1988) and Witter (1989), Dolorfo and Amaral (1998) showed that cells located laterally and caudally in the entorhinal cortex project to septal levels of the hippocampal

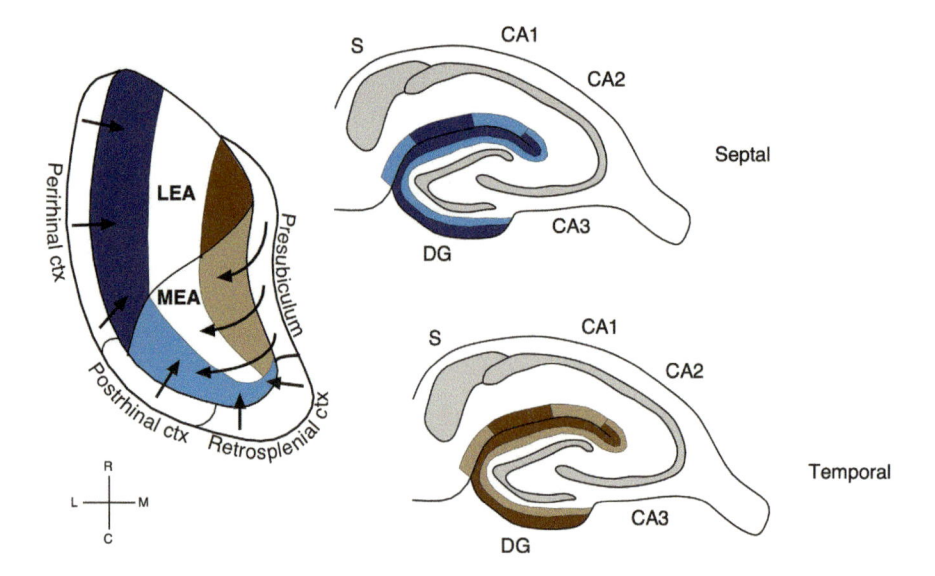

Figure 3.39 Laminar and topographic organization of the entorhinal projection to the dentate gyrus, the hippocampus, and the subiculum. The surface of the entorhinal cortex is represented on the left (the rhinal sulcus is to the left). The layer II entorhinal cortex projections to the dentate gyrus and the CA3–CA2 fields of the hippocampus terminate in a laminar fashion; the LEA projects superficially in the molecular layer and the stratum lacunosum-moleculare and the MEA projects deeper. There is a contrasting organization of the projections to CA1 and the subiculum. The layer III entorhinal cortex projections are organized topographically; the LEA projects to distal CA1 and proximal subiculum (i.e., at the CA1/subiculum border) and the MEA projects to proximal CA1 and distal subiculum. Laterally situated portions of the entorhinal cortex project to septal levels of the hippocampal formation, whereas progressively more medial portions of the entorhinal cortex project to more temporal levels of the hippocampal formation. R—rostral, C—caudal, M—medial, L—lateral.

fields, while cells located progressively more medially and rostrally project to more temporal levels of the hippocampal subfields (Figure 3.39). Thus, there may be three largely nonoverlapping domains of the entorhinal cortex, which project to three distinct levels of the dentate gyrus (Kerr et al., 2007). The laterally situated domain (encompassing cells of both the lateral and medial entorhinal areas) projects to the septal half of the dentate gyrus. Most of the cells in this domain project to all portions of the septal half of the dentate gyrus; thus, the projection is both divergent and convergent. The next domain is more medially situated and projects to the third-quarter of the dentate gyrus. The last domain is very medially and rostrally situated and projects to the temporal quarter of the dentate gyrus.

There are a number of functional implications of the organization of these projections. First and foremost, since the associational connections of the entorhinal cortex seem to respect this tripartite organization, it is reasonable to think of three functional, parallel systems encompassed within the entorhinohippocampal system. Second, one must be careful to bear in mind, when conducting stimulation or lesion experiments designed to evaluate the contributions of the medial and lateral perforant paths to hippocampal function, that the cells giving rise to the medial perforant path are actually located caudal (not medial) to the cells that give rise to the lateral perforant path.

Feedback projections from the hippocampus and subiculum

We have already mentioned that the dentate gyrus and the CA3 field of the hippocampus do not project back to the entorhinal cortex. Thus, the recipients of the layer II projection do not have any direct influence over the activities of the entorhinal cortex. It is only after the layer II and layer III projection systems are combined in CA1 and the subiculum that return projections to the

entorhinal cortex are generated. The return projections mainly terminate in the deep layers (V and VI) although some fibers ascend into layer I (Witter et al., 1988; Naber et al., 2001; Kloosterman et al., 2003). Within layer V, the projections preferentially target neurons in layer Vb (Surmeli et al., 2015). Projections from CA1 and the subiculum to the entorhinal cortex are also topographically organized (Figure 3.34). Septal portions of CA1 and the subiculum project chiefly to lateral parts of the entorhinal cortex, and more temporal parts of CA1 and the subiculum project to more medial parts of the entorhinal cortex. Moreover, the transverse location of the cells of origin in CA1 and the subiculum also determines whether these projections terminate in the medial or lateral entorhinal cortex. The projections from the proximal part of CA1 and the distal part of the subiculum distribute exclusively to the medial entorhinal cortex, whereas cells located in the distal part of CA1 and the proximal part of the subiculum project mainly to the lateral entorhinal cortex.

The important point about these return projections is that they are exactly in register, i.e., they are point-to-point reciprocal, with the entorhinal inputs to these areas (Figure 3.30). Thus, at the global level, all of the circuitry is available for reverberatory circuits to be established through the loop starting and ending at the entorhinal cortex. This remarkable topography confirms the critical role of the entorhinal cortex with respect to the input to, and output from, the hippocampal formation.

3.9.5.3 Extrinsic connections

Interconnections of the entorhinal cortex with neocortical regions

If the entorhinal cortex is viewed as the first step of processing in the hippocampal formation, it is reasonable to wonder what types

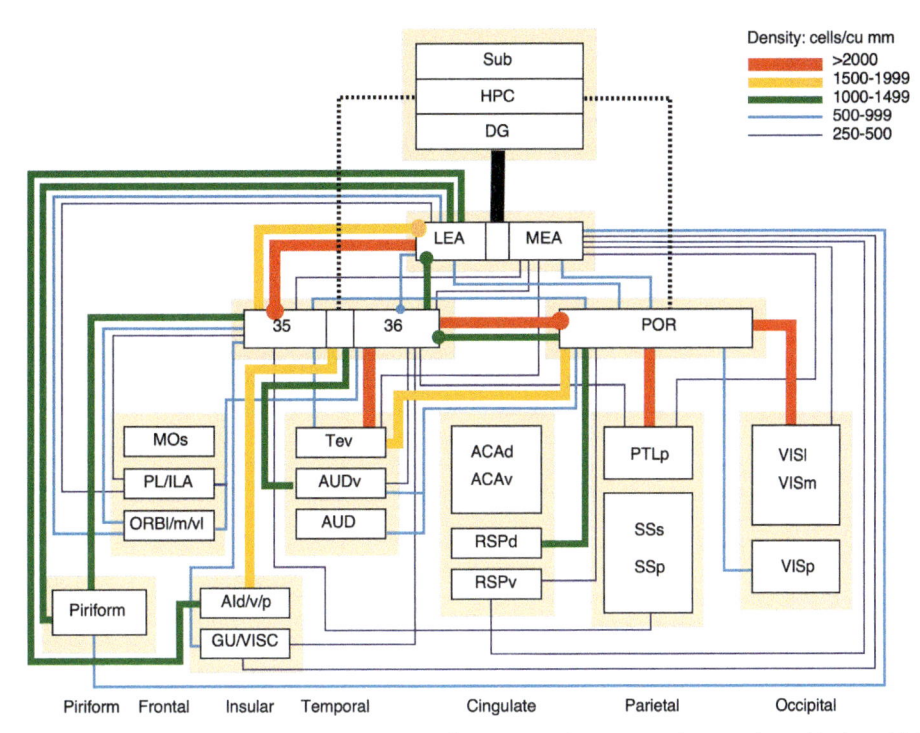

Figure 3.40 Pattern and strength of cortical and intrinsic connectivity of the rat parahippocampal region (entorhinal, perirhinal, and parahippocampal cortices). The thickness of the solid lines represents the relative strength of these connections based on densities of retrogradely labeled neurons. Open lines represent reported connections for which no comparable quantitative data are available. The weakest projections (< 250 labeled cells/mm³) are not shown in the figure. Adapted from (Burwell and Amaral, 1998b).

of information it receives. In other words, what is the "raw material" that the hippocampal formation uses to accomplish its purported function(s). This is an area in which there are substantial species differences. Keeping to the format that we have followed so far, we will give an overview of the inputs to the rat entorhinal cortex. However, doing so does a disservice to the significance of the connections between the entorhinal cortex and the neocortex, since these connections are so much more prominent in the monkey brain. Thus, in the comparison of the organization of the hippocampal formation in the rat, monkey, and human in a later portion of this chapter, we will return to an overview of the cortical inputs of the monkey entorhinal cortex.

Rebecca Burwell and colleagues have carried out a series of very thorough and quantitative analyses of the organization of cortical connections with the rat entorhinal cortex, and compared the results with inputs to the perirhinal and postrhinal cortices (Burwell and Amaral, 1998a; Agster and Burwell, 2009; Agster et al., 2016; also see Doan et al., 2019). They found many similarities in the complement of cortical inputs to the lateral and medial entorhinal areas (Figure 3.40). Both receive about one-third of their total input from the piriform cortex. They also receive roughly equal inputs from temporal and frontal regions. Some differences are observed in the proportions of insular, cingular, parietal, and occipital inputs. The LEA receives more input from the insular cortex (LEA 21%, MEA 6%). In contrast, the MEA receives more input from cingulate (LEA 3%, MEA 11%), parietal (LEA 3%, MEA 9%), and occipital (LEA 2%, MEA 12%) regions. Not all portions of the rat entorhinal cortex receive substantial cortical input. In fact, it is only the lateral and caudal parts of the entorhinal cortex (those projecting to septal levels of the dentate gyrus) that are heavily and directly innervated by the neocortex.

The neocortical inputs to the entorhinal cortex of the rat form two groups: those that terminate in the superficial layers (I–III), and those that terminate in the deep layers (IV–VI). The first category delivers information to the superficially located entorhinal neurons that are the source of the projections to the dentate gyrus, hippocampus, and the subiculum. The second group has greater influence on the deeply located cells of the entorhinal cortex, which, among other things, receive processed information from the other hippocampal fields and give rise to feedback projections to certain cortical regions. In general, the cortical afferents that reach the deep layers terminate rather diffusely, whereas those that terminate superficially have a more restricted mediolateral and/or rostrocaudal distribution.

A substantial input to the superficial layers of the entorhinal cortex originates from olfactory structures such as the olfactory bulb, the anterior olfactory nucleus, and the piriform cortex. These olfactory projections terminate throughout most of the rostrocaudal extent of the entorhinal cortex, mainly in layer I and the superficial portion of layer II. Only the most caudal portion of the rat medial entorhinal area does not receive any olfactory input. In addition to the principal cells of these layers, olfactory fibers also terminate on layer I GABAergic neurons that presumably interact with principal cells in layers II and III.

A second prominent cortical input to the superficial layers of the entorhinal cortex arises from the laterally adjacent perirhinal and postrhinal cortices (Furtak et al., 2007; Kerr et al., 2007; Agster and Burwell, 2009). The perirhinal and postrhinal cortices are polysensory convergence areas that receive inputs from a variety of unimodal and polymodal sensory cortices. The perirhinal cortex terminates mainly in the lateral entorhinal area, and the postrhinal cortex terminates heavily in the medial entorhinal area, but also

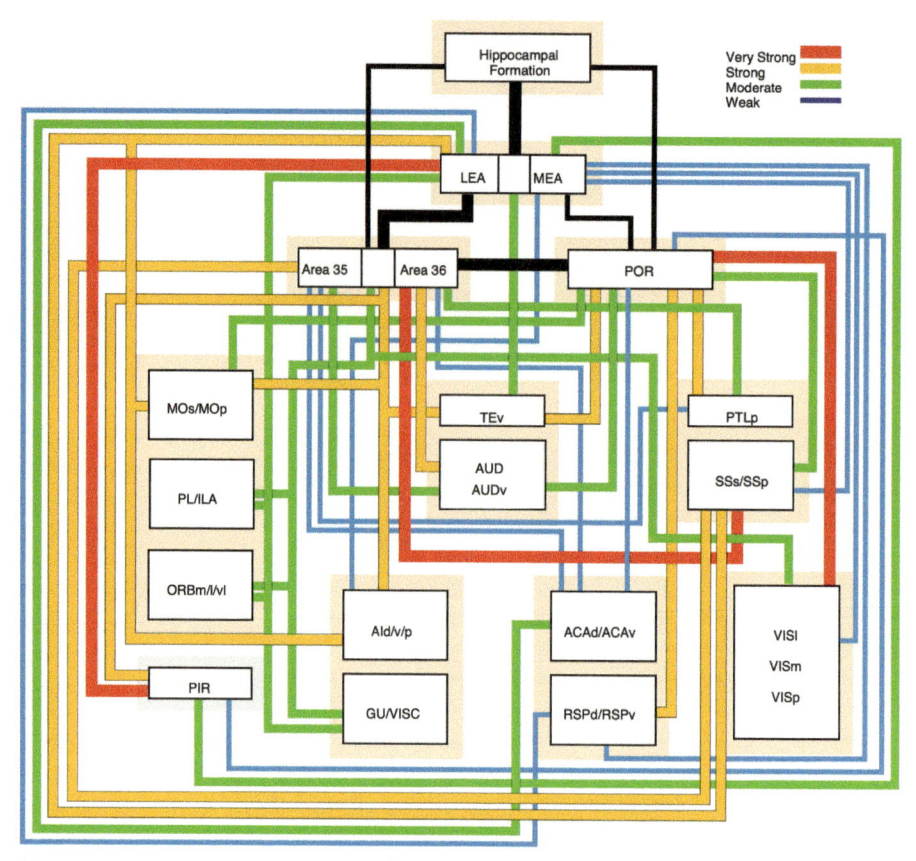

Figure 3.41 Summary of the cortical efferents of the perirhinal, postrhinal, and entorhinal cortices. The wiring diagram was simplified by combining some regions, yielding a total of 65 projections. The relative strength of projections is indicated by color and width of the connection lines. The heaviest 5% are designate very strong (red), the next 25% are strong (yellow), the next 30% are designated moderate (green), the next 15% are designate weak (blue). The bottom 25% of the projections was omitted from the diagram for simplification. The connections shown in black are adapted from other studies. (Adapted with permission from Agster and Burwell 2009.)

projects to the lateral and caudal part of the LEA (Burwell and Amaral, 1998ba, 1998b; Doan et al., 2019). In both cases, the projections terminate preferentially in layers I and III of the entorhinal cortex.

We shall address the issue of the perirhinal cortex more extensively in our discussion of the monkey entorhinal cortex. But it is important to give an overview of this area that provides a major input to the rat entorhinal cortex. The perirhinal cortex in the rat is made up of two areas, 35 and 36, which appear to receive slightly different complements of neocortical inputs (Burwell et al., 1995; Burwell, 2001; Furtak et al., 2007). Area 36 of the perirhinal cortex receives more, higher-level cortical input than does area 35. Most of this input comes from the ventral temporal associational area (Te$_v$), which is located dorsally adjacent to area 36. Other major inputs are from the postrhinal cortex and from the entorhinal cortex. The predominant inputs to area 35 arise from the piriform, entorhinal, and insular cortices. Area 35 receives over one-quarter of its input from the piriform cortex, and only slightly less from the lateral entorhinal area. About one-fifth of the total input arises from insular cortices. Interestingly, the perirhinal projections to the entorhinal cortex arise preferentially from area 35, and the intrinsic projections of the perirhinal cortex seem to be organized to funnel information into area 35, which, in turn, gives rise to the main perirhinal projections to the entorhinal cortex.

Cortical afferents to the deep layers of the entorhinal cortex arise from a variety of cortical areas. These include projections from the agranular insular cortex; from the medial prefrontal region; in particular the infralimbic, prelimbic, and anterior cingulate cortices; and from the retrosplenial cortex. Efferents originating heavily from neurons in layer Va as demonstrated for the medial entorhinal cortex (Surmeli et al., 2015) return projections to many of the cortical areas that provide inputs to the entorhinal cortex (Burwell and Amaral, 1998b; Kealy and Commins, 2011). There are projections to olfactory areas, originating predominantly from layers II, III and Va.

Cortical efferents of the entorhinal, perirhinal and postrhinal cortices largely reciprocate the cortical afferents to these regions (Figure 3.41) though the degree of reciprocity varies from region to region. The laminar organization of the efferent projections is consistent with feedback projections and the organization of these connections is detailed in (Agster and Burwell, 2009).

Other telencephalic connections: amygdala, claustrum, striatum

In addition to the cortical inputs just described, the entorhinal cortex receives a number of subcortical inputs. While some of these, like the monoaminergic and cholinergic inputs, may be viewed as largely modulatory, others, such as the input from the amygdaloid complex, might also provide additional sources of information. The subcortical telencephalic connections of the entorhinal cortex (as well as the perirhinal and postrhinal cortices) have been quantitatively studied by Burwell and colleagues (Agster et al., 2016; Tomas Pereira et al., 2016). These and additional studies are described in

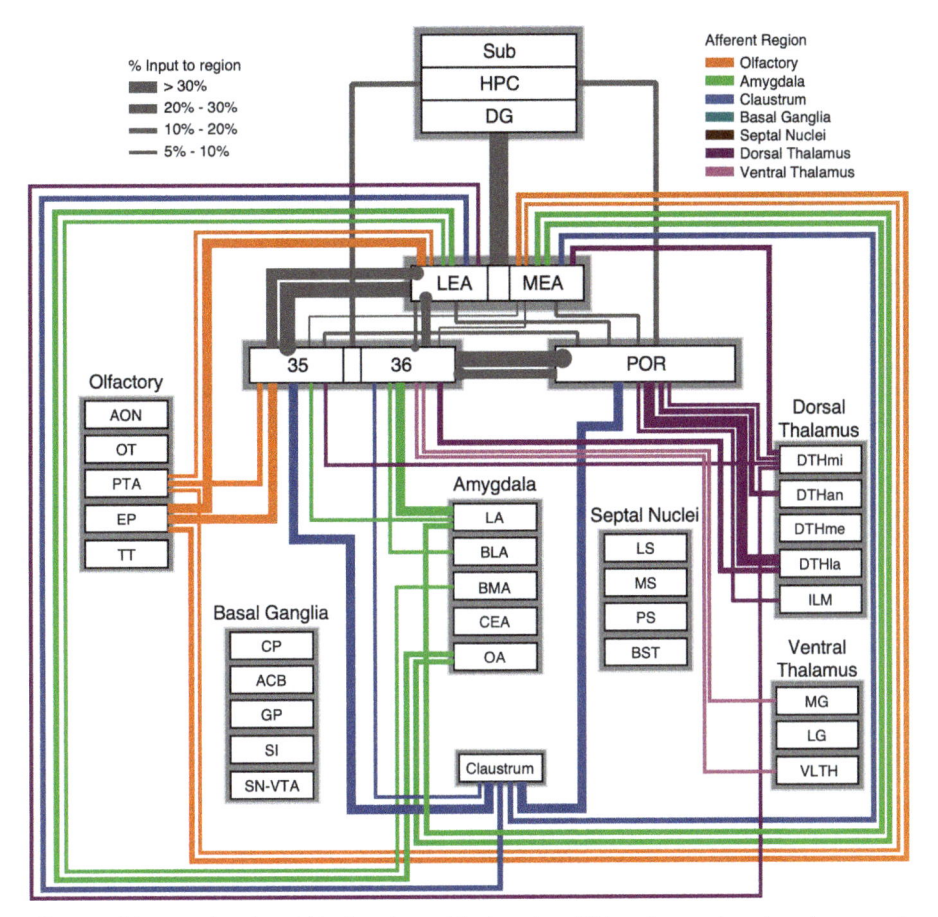

Figure 3.42 Subcortical afferents of the entorhinal, perirhinal, and postrhinal cortices. Wiring diagram based on the percentage measure representing the subcortical input to the perirhinal (PER) areas 35 and 36, POR, LEA, and MEA. Colors represent the afferent regions. Thickness of the bars represents the percentage of input to each target region. This measure is useful for comparing the pattern of inputs at the target regions. For example, PER area 35 receives a strong input from olfactory structures, whereas area 36 does not. Information for connections shown in gray are from prior studies. For simplicity, the weakest connections (<5%) are not shown. All basal ganglia connections were below 5%. (Illustration adapted with permission from Tomas Pereira, et al., 2016.)

Chapter 12. By way of summary we have included two illustrations (Figures 3.42 and 3.43), adapted from the work of the Burwell laboratory, that summarize the subcortical afferents and efferents, respectively.

Basal forebrain and hypothalamic connections

The entorhinal cortex receives its cholinergic innervation mainly from the septal nuclei. This projection is topographically organized such that cells in the horizontal limb of the nucleus of the diagonal band preferentially project to the most lateral part of the entorhinal cortex, whereas the medial septal nucleus and the vertical limb of the nucleus of the diagonal band project to more medial parts of the entorhinal cortex. Septal projections terminate densely in the cell-sparse lamina dissecans and less densely in layer II.

Like the hippocampus and the subiculum, but unlike the presubiculum and the parasubiculum, the entorhinal cortex projects back to the septal region. The projection originates from cells in layer Va although some layer II cells also contribute to these projections. The fibers from the entorhinal cortex preferentially terminate in the lateral septal complex.

The entorhinal cortex receives diffuse inputs from various structures in the hypothalamus. These include inputs from the supramammillary nucleus that terminate rather diffusely with some preference for layers III–VI, from the tuberomammillary nucleus, distributing diffusely throughout the entorhinal cortex, and from the lateral hypothalamic area reaching the deep layers of the entorhinal cortex.

Thalamic connections—nucleus reuniens and other midline nuclei

The major thalamic inputs to the entorhinal cortex originate in the nucleus reuniens and in the nucleus centralis medialis (Van der Werf et al., 2002; Cassel et al., 2013). The rhomboid, paraventricular, and parataenial nuclei also contribute minor projections. The nucleus reuniens fibers densely innervate the deep portion of layer I and layer III and give rise to a few collaterals that extend into layer II. Separate populations of nucleus reuniens cells project to the entorhinal cortex, CA1 and the subiculum. There is no evidence that the entorhinal cortex projects back to the thalamus (Scheel et al., 2020).

Brainstem inputs

The entorhinal cortex receives a dopaminergic input from cells located in the ventral tegmental area. The projection preferentially terminates in a restricted rostrolateral part of the lateral entorhinal

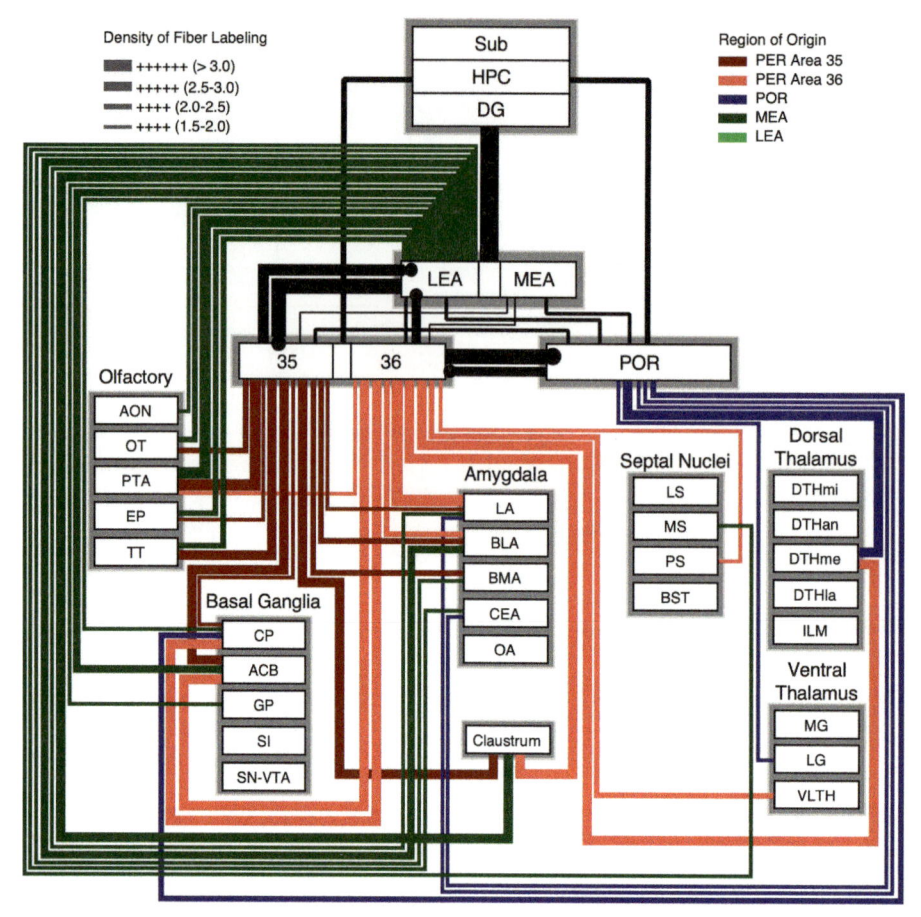

Figure 3.43 Subcortical efferents of the entorhinal, perirhinal and postrhinal cortices. Illustration adapted with permission from (Agster, Tomas Pereira et al. 2016). Wiring diagram representing subcortical output of the parahippocampal regions based on the densities of labeled cells in each subcortical structure. The projections are color coded according to their region of origin. The thickness of the lines indicates the relative strength of the projection.

area, where fibers are arranged in dense, columnar patches in layers I to III. The serotonergic innervation arises from the central, median, and dorsal raphe nuclei and terminates diffusely in all layers, but with a preference for the superficial layers. The noradrenergic locus coeruleus supplies the entorhinal cortex with a diffusely organized noradrenergic input that exhibits a slightly denser termination in layer I.

Before leaving this section on the morphology of neurons and connections of different fields of the rodent hippocampal formation, it is important to point out that the picture of hippocampal neuroanatomy will certainly get more complex as molecular techniques and sophisticated three-dimensional mapping techniques are employed. An example of this is the work of Qiu et al. (2024) in which the connectome of over 10,000 single neurons were mapped using sparse labeling with adenoassociated virus and sophisticated three-dimensional mapping and statistical techniques. Based on whole brain connectivity, they identified 43 projectome subtypes that could be associated with the location of the cell soma within a hippocampal field and features of the transcriptome. The dendritic and axonal morphology of the mapped neurons can be found online (https://mouse.digital-brain.cn/hipp). While this analysis has replicated most of the neuroanatomy that has been summarized in this section, it has also contributed unprecedented information related to the single cell heterogeneity of neurons in each of the hippocampal regions.

3.9.6 Chemical and molecular neuroanatomy

3.9.6.1 Transmitters and receptors

A detailed and comprehensive treatment of the chemical neuroanatomy of the hippocampal formation would demand a lengthy chapter of its own. We have already described the distribution of several systems defined by their neurotransmitter content (noradrenaline, serotonin, acetylcholine, and GABA), and a variety of reviews are available on the chemical neuroanatomy of the hippocampus (Swanson et al., 1987; Kobayashi and Amaral, 1999). We will thus restrict ourselves here to providing an overview of the diversity of neurochemical substances in the hippocampal formation.

A variety of peptides and other chemical makers have been shown to subdivide the population of GABAergic interneurons (Booker and Vida, 2018). Among the peptides that colocalize with particular populations of GABAergic interneurons are vasoactive intestinal peptide (VIP), somatostatin, neuropeptide Y, corticotropin releasing factor (CRF), substance P, cholecystokinin (CCK), galanin, and the opioid peptides dynorphin and enkephalin. It is worth commenting further on the distribution of the opioid peptides since, in addition to being localized to certain populations of interneurons, they are also observed within intrinsic excitatory pathways of the hippocampal formation. The fibers of the lateral perforant path, for example, are immunoreactive for Leu-enkephalin, whereas the mossy fibers of the dentate gyrus are positive for both enkephalins and dynorphin (Drake et al., 2007).

Another class of substances that mark certain subsets of GABAergic neurons selectively is the family of calcium-binding proteins including parvalbumin, calbindin, and calretinin (Drake et al., 2007; Houser, 2007). While parvalbumin immunoreactivity appears to be exclusively confined to a subset of GABAergic interneurons, the other calcium-binding proteins can be found both in interneurons and in principal neurons. And, while the precise function of the various calcium-binding proteins has not been well established, their existence has provided a useful anatomical tool. Although standard immunohistochemistry of GABAergic neurons with antibodies either to GAD or to GABA do not label dendrites very well, parvalbumin immunoreactive neurons are fully labeled in a Golgi-like fashion. Thus, even though parvalbumin does not label all GABAergic neurons, those that are labeled can be subjected to very precise analyses of their inputs. A more modern way to study classes of GABAergic neurons in the brain takes advantage of the ability to engineer mice who express Green Fluorescent Protein in their GABAergic neurons (Tamamaki et al., 2003).

3.9.6.2 Steroids

Neurons in the hippocampal formation have been shown to concentrate glucocorticoids and mineralcorticoids (McEwen and Wallach, 1973; McEwen et al., 2016; see Chapter 17). Studies using uptake of ^{3}H-corticosterone show that cells in CA2 and CA1 show the greatest uptake. There is slightly less uptake in CA3 cells and in cells of the polymorphic layer of the dentate gyrus; dentate granule cells also demonstrate some ^{3}H-corticosterone uptake. The amount of uptake in other fields of the hippocampal formation has not yet been described. What is perhaps most surprising is the fact that, in the rat, the hippocampus demonstrates the highest level of uptake of any brain region. The distribution of glucocorticoid receptor mRNA has also been evaluated in the tree shrew. Here the highest density of mRNA was observed in the pyramidal cells of the subiculum and in the granule cells of the dentate gyrus. In the hippocampus, higher densities of mRNA were observed in CA1 than in CA3. Mineralocorticoid receptor mRNA is also expressed in the tree shrew hippocampus. It is expressed most strongly in CA1 and less strongly in CA3; this contrasts with the pattern in the rat, where mineralocorticoid expression is higher in CA3. In situ hybridization has also been used in postmortem human brain tissue to study the distribution of glucocorticoid and mineralocorticoid receptors. Receptors for both steroids were highly expressed in cells of the dentate gyrus, CA3, and CA2. Lower levels of expression were observed in CA1. This is the opposite of the distribution observed in the rat and the tree shrew. As elaborated in Chapter 17, the glucocorticoids and mineralcorticoids receptors figure prominently in the literature of stress-induced alterations in the hippocampus.

Another class of steroid influencers of hippocampal function are the gonadal steroids. The discovery that estrogen receptors could be found outside of the hypothalamus, and in the hippocampus particularly, was an early accomplishment of Bruce McEwen (McEwen et al., 1968, reviewed in McEwen and Milner, 2017). This has led to a very intensive area of research across many laboratories that have studied the effects of estrogen, from molecular to behavioral, and across the life span (Hara et al., 2015; Luine and Frankfurt, 2020). Stimulation of estrogen receptors in the hippocampus has been shown to influence the number of dendritic spines in the CA1

region of the hippocampus, enhance memory performance, and even modulate the effects of other extrinsic transmitter systems on hippocampal neuron excitability. The interested reader is referred to the reviews referenced above to get an entry into this fascinating literature.

3.10 Comparative neuroanatomy of the mouse, rat, monkey, and human hippocampal formation

When one views a Nissl-stained section of the hippocampus in the rat, monkey, and human, it is immediately apparent that one is looking at the same brain region (Figures 3.2, 3.44). The densely packed granule cell layer is obvious in all three species, as is the progressively more complex lamination when one progresses from the dentate gyrus to the entorhinal cortex. On closer inspection, however, a number of differences make it clear that the hippocampal formation of the monkey or human is not simply a scaled-up version of the rat's. Some of the hippocampal fields, such as CA1 and the entorhinal cortex, are disproportionately larger in the primates. Based on Nissl-stained material for cell bodies, the entorhinal cortex appears to have many more subdivisions in the monkey and human than in the rat. And the laminar organization is much more distinct in the primate brain. In the following sections, we will review some of the similarities and differences in the organization and connections of the hippocampal formation in these three species. Of course, while we can address certain issues concerning cell number and distribution in the human brain, we are able to say very little about patterns of connectivity in the human hippocampal formation.

3.10.1 Neuron numbers

The number of neurons present in the various subdivisions of the hippocampal formation have been counted by several investigators but rarely has the same author analyzed the mouse, rat, monkey, and human hippocampal formation (but see van Dijk et al., 2016, as an exception). Moreover, there is a lot of variability in the estimates published in the literature and very few investigators have used modern stereological techniques to carry out these assessments. We have compiled a summary of current estimates of neuron number obtained with modern stereological techniques (Table 3.1). The data presented here are derived from published and unpublished work indicated in the legend of the table.

In our comparisons of the combined dentate gyrus and hippocampus in the rat, monkey, and human, the volume is about 10 times larger in monkeys than in rats, and 100 times larger in humans than in rats (rat: 32 mm^3, monkey: 340 mm^3; human: 3,300 mm^3). If, however, we compare the total number of neurons in the different hippocampal areas, we observe that certain regions are comparatively more developed than others in the monkey and human brain. In the dentate gyrus, there are approximately 10 times more granule cells in the monkey than in the rat, a ratio that parallels the overall volume differences. But there are only 15 times more dentate granule cells in humans as compared with rats, while the volume of the dentate gyrus plus the hippocampus is about 100 times larger in humans than in rats. In CA1, however, there are only three times more pyramidal cells in the monkey than in the rat, while there are 35 times more cells in humans than in rats.

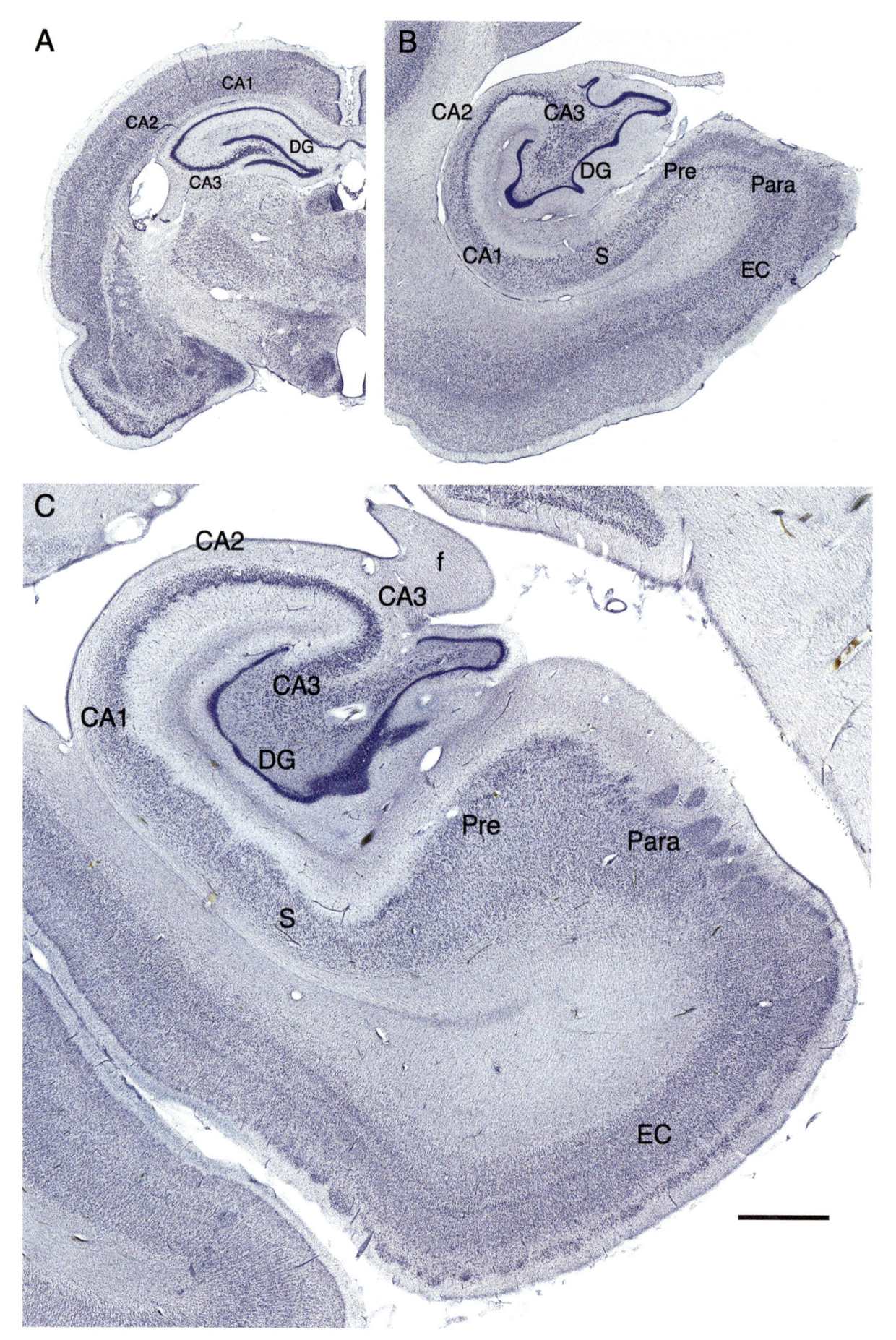

Figure 3.44 Nissl-stained coronal sections through the hippocampal formation of the rat (A), monkey (B) and human (C) presented at the same magnification. Scale bar in C is 2 mm and applies to all panels.

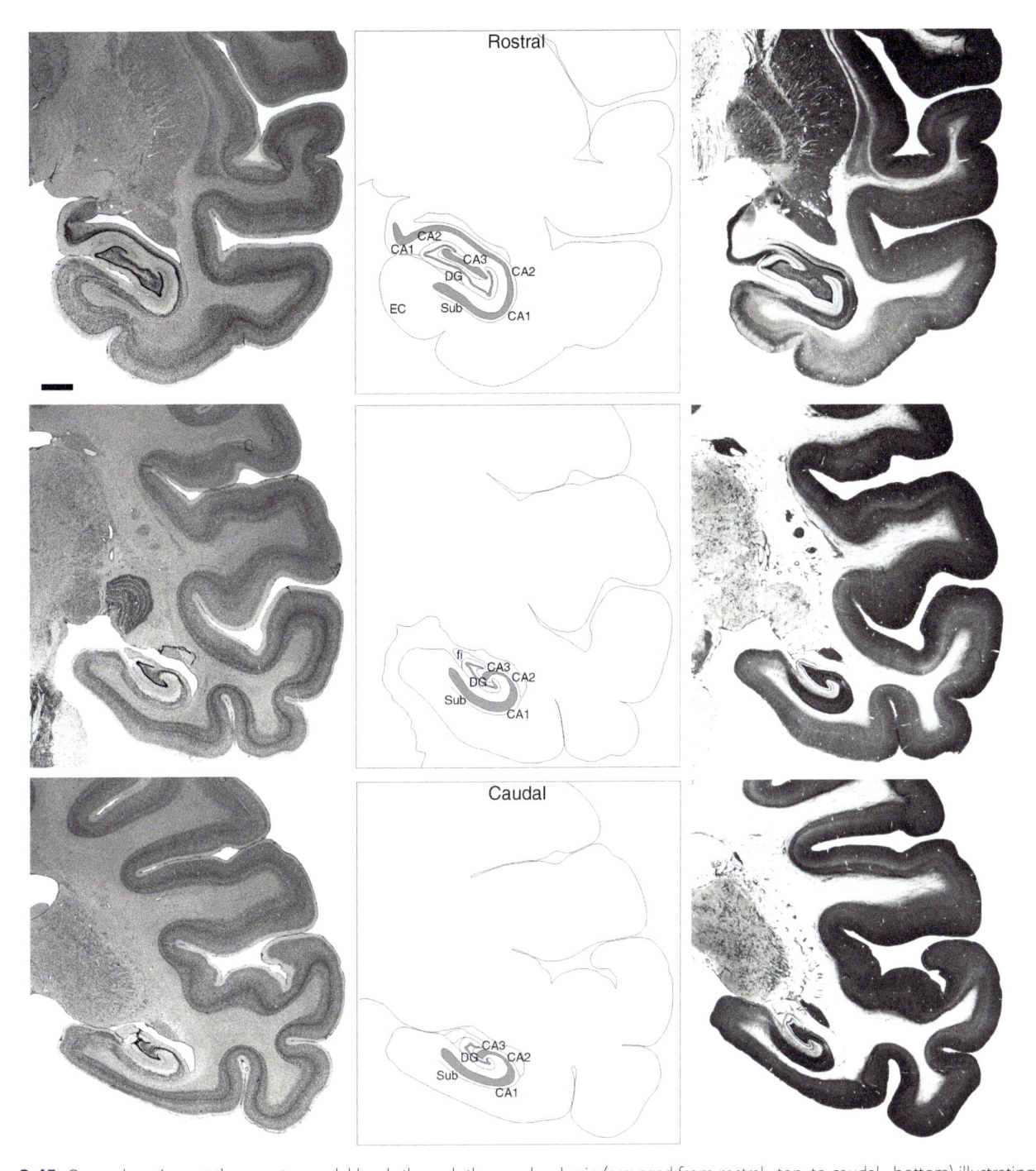

Figure 3.45 Coronal sections at three rostrocaudal levels through the monkey brain (arranged from rostral—top, to caudal—bottom) illustrating the position of the hippocampal formation. The three panels on the left are Nissl-stained sections; the three panels on the right are adjacent, Timm's sulfide-silver-stained section; the line drawings (middle column) highlight the different regions of the monkey hippocampal formation seen in the stained sections. Scale bar is 2 mm.

3.10.2 Comparison of the rodent and monkey hippocampal formation–connectivity and other features beyond neuron numbers

In monkeys, the hippocampal formation lies entirely within the temporal lobe (Figures 3.45–3.48) and lacks the pronounced "C" shape along its septotemporal axis, which is so characteristic in the rat. The region equivalent to the septal pole of the rat hippocampus is located caudally in the monkey and the equivalent of the temporal

pole is located rostrally (Figures 3.3, 3.4). Much of the entorhinal cortex is located rostral to the remainder of the hippocampal formation. In fact the rostral half of the entorhinal cortex lies ventral to the amygdaloid complex rather than the hippocampus.

3.10.2.1 Cytoarchitectonic organization

There are several cytoarchitectonic differences between the rat and monkey hippocampal formation. The polymorphic layer (or hilus) of

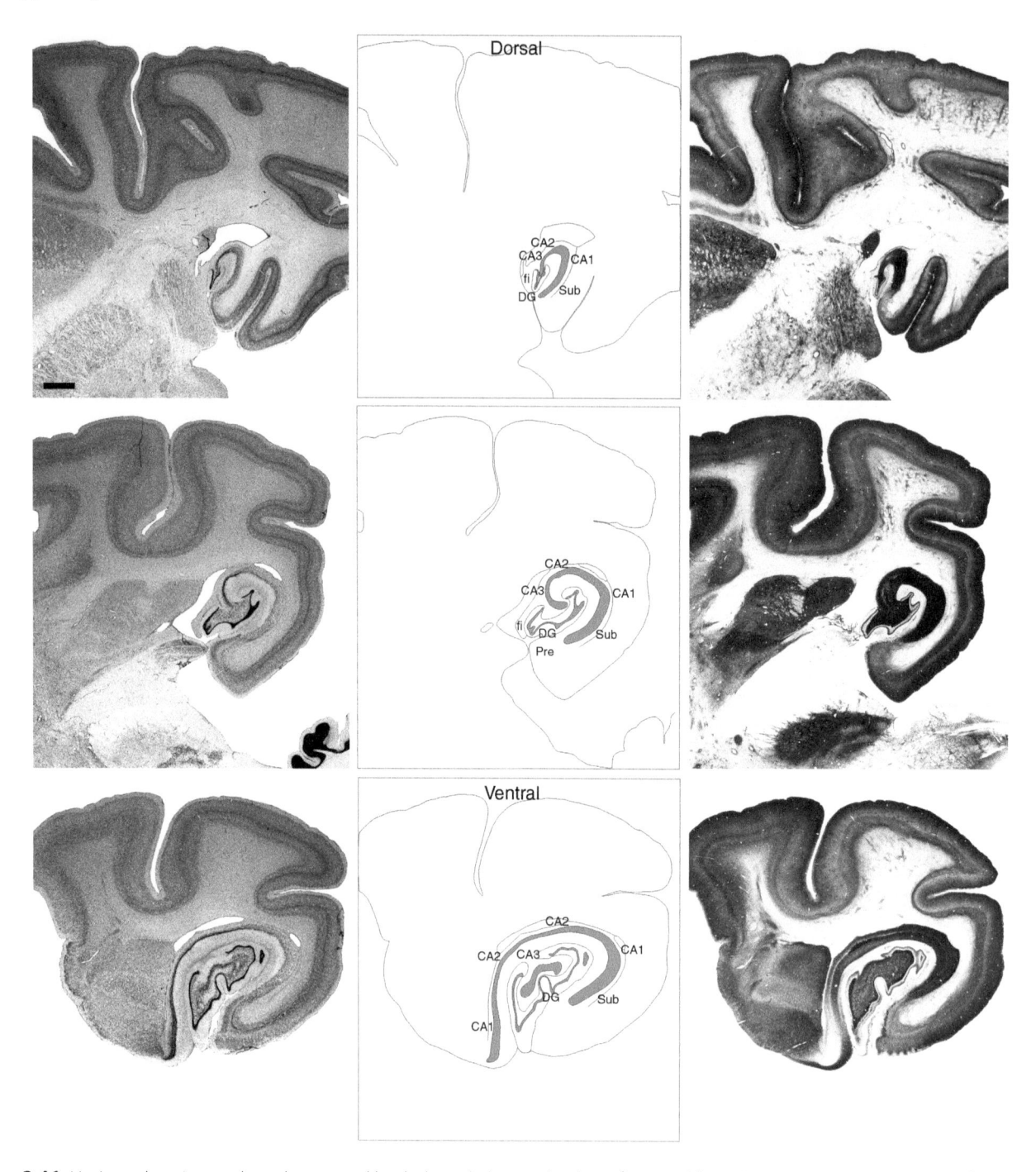

Figure 3.46 Horizontal sections at three dorsoventral levels through the monkey brain (arranged from dorsal—top, to ventral—bottom) illustrating the position of the hippocampal formation. The three panels on the left are Nissl-stained sections; the three panels on the right are adjacent, Timm's sulfide-silver-stained section; the line drawings (middle column) highlight the different regions of the monkey hippocampal formation seen in the stained sections. Scale bar is 2 mm.

the dentate gyrus is relatively reduced in the monkey and much of the territory enclosed within the blades of the granule cell layers is occupied by the CA3 field. This "hilar" portion of the CA3 region is so expansive that some authors have confused it for an enlarged polymorphic layer. Cells in this region bear the gold standard of inclusion in CA3, however, since they give rise to Schaffer collaterals to CA1.

The other obvious difference between the rat and monkey hippocampal formation is the much thicker pyramidal cell layer in the monkey CA1 (Figure 3.49). In the rat, this layer is tightly packed and is typically about 5 cells thick. In the monkey, the cell layer is much more diffusely organized and is 10–15 cells thick. As a result, the boundary between the pyramidal cell layer and the stratum radiatum is less clear, and so is the boundary between CA1 and the subiculum. And in the monkey, at least some of the Schaffer collaterals from CA3 terminate within the pyramidal cell layer, presumably on the apical dendrites of cells located deep in the layer or on the basal dendrites of neurons located superficially in the layer.

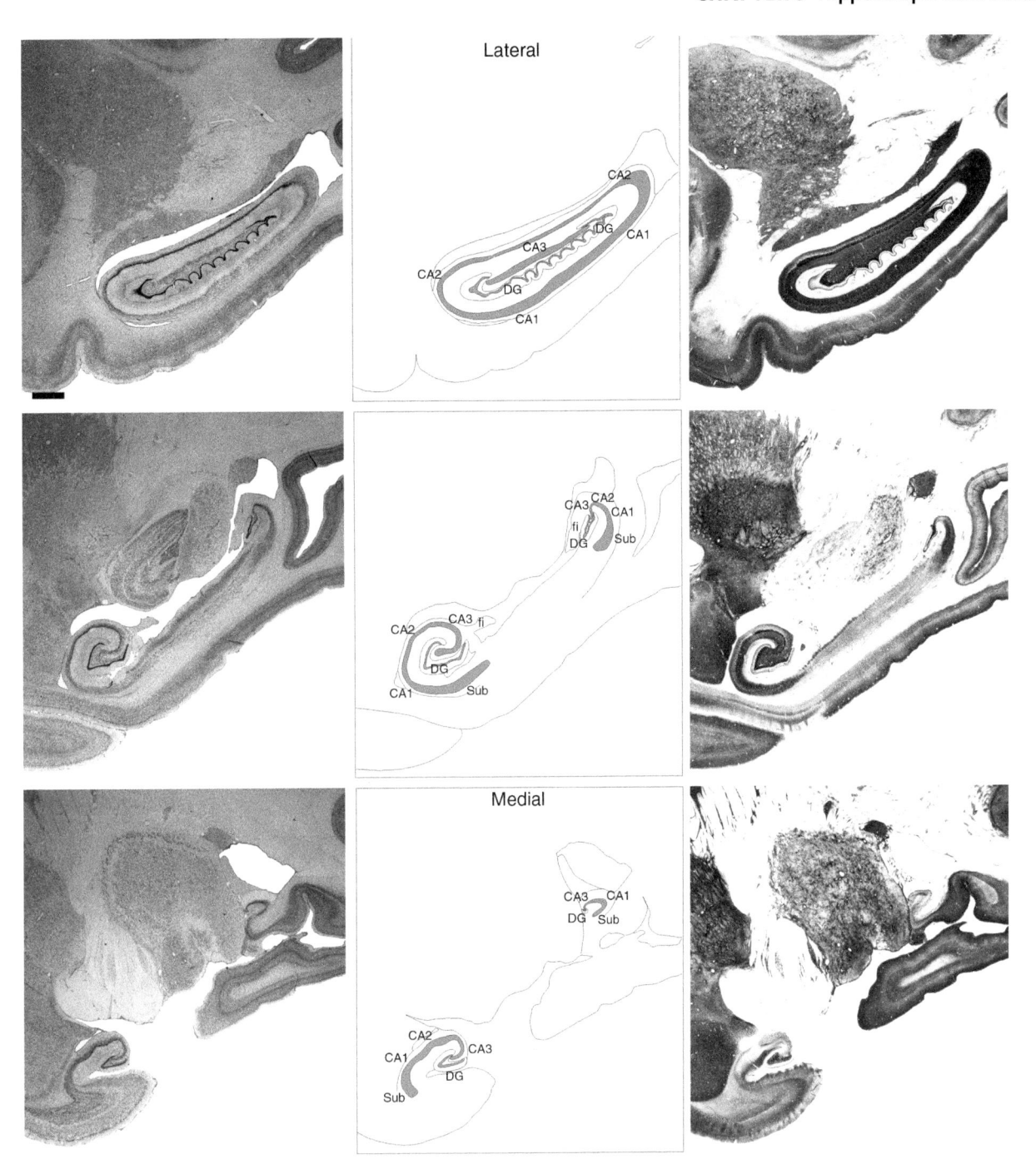

Figure 3.47 Sagittal sections at three mediolateral levels through the monkey brain (arranged from lateral—top, to medial—bottom) illustrating the position of the hippocampal formation. The three panels on the left are Nissl-stained sections; the three panels on the right are adjacent, Timm's sulfide-silver-stained section; the line drawings (middle column) highlight the different regions of the monkey hippocampal formation seen in the stained sections. Scale bar is 2 mm.

The entorhinal cortex exhibits major cytoarchitectonic differences between the rat and the monkey. The laminar organization of the monkey entorhinal cortex is much clearer than that in the rat. Throughout much of the entorhinal cortex, for example, there is a clear distinction between layers V and VI in the monkey, whereas these layers tend to blur together in the rat. The monkey entorhinal cortex is also much more differentiated than in the rat. As noted previously, the rat entorhinal cortex has typically been divided only into lateral and medial areas, whereas the monkey entorhinal cortex has been divided into seven distinct subdivisions.

3.10.2.2 Neuron types

There has been relatively little direct comparison of the morphology of similar neurons in the rat and monkey hippocampus. A few studies, using either the Golgi technique or intracellular staining techniques, have compared easily identified cell types. The granule cells of the monkey dentate gyrus have been examined with both the Golgi technique and intracellular filling techniques in the in vitro slice preparation (Duffy and Rakic, 1983; Seress and Mrzljak, 1987). Depending on which aspects of these studies one wishes

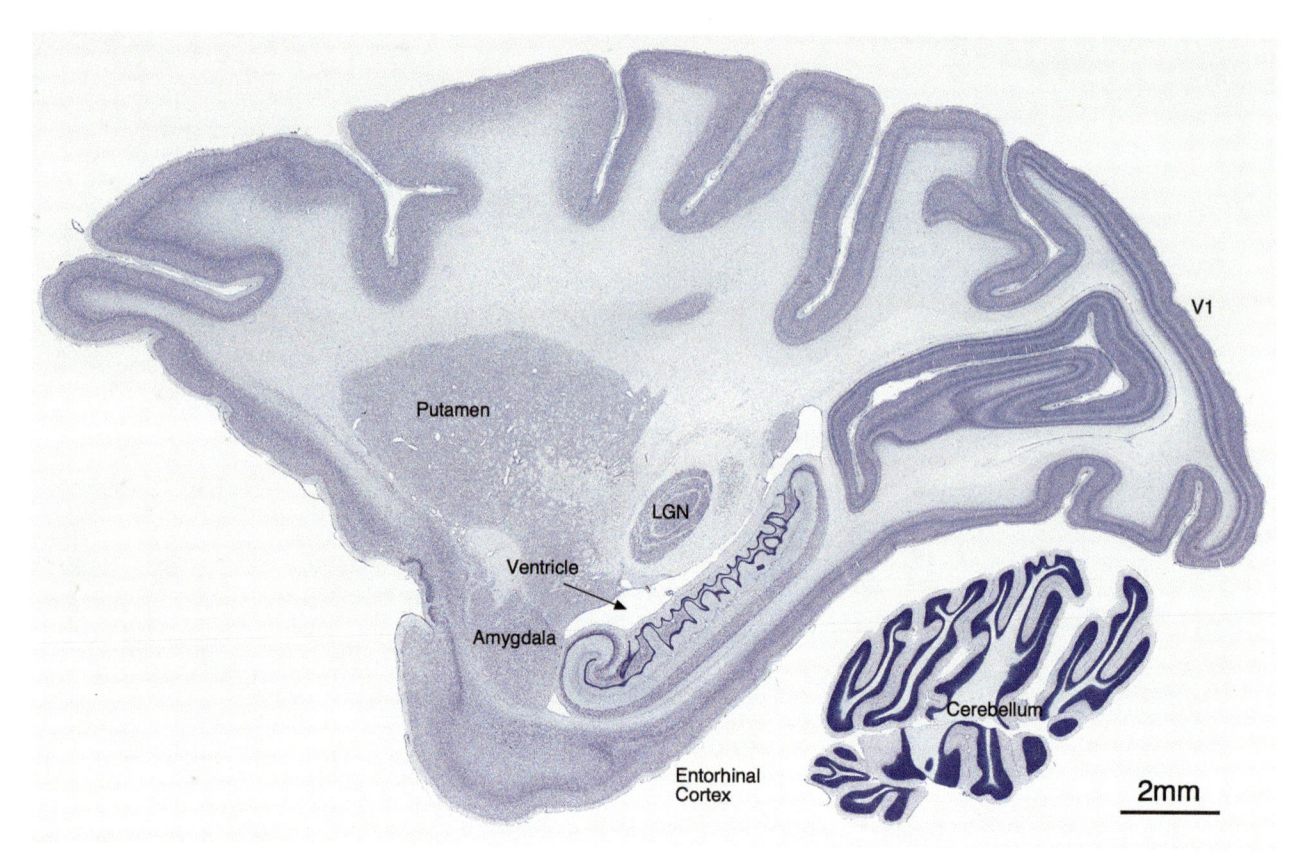

Figure 3.48 High resolution image of a Nissl-stained sagittal section through the macaque monkey hippocampal formation. The dentate gyrus and hippocampal fields are apparent in this image. It is also clear that the bulk of the hippocampus forms the ventral surface of the temporal horn of the lateral ventricle. The amygdala is immediately adjacent to the head of the hippocampal formation across the limit of the ventricle. The lateral geniculate nucleus (LGN) is labeled for reference.

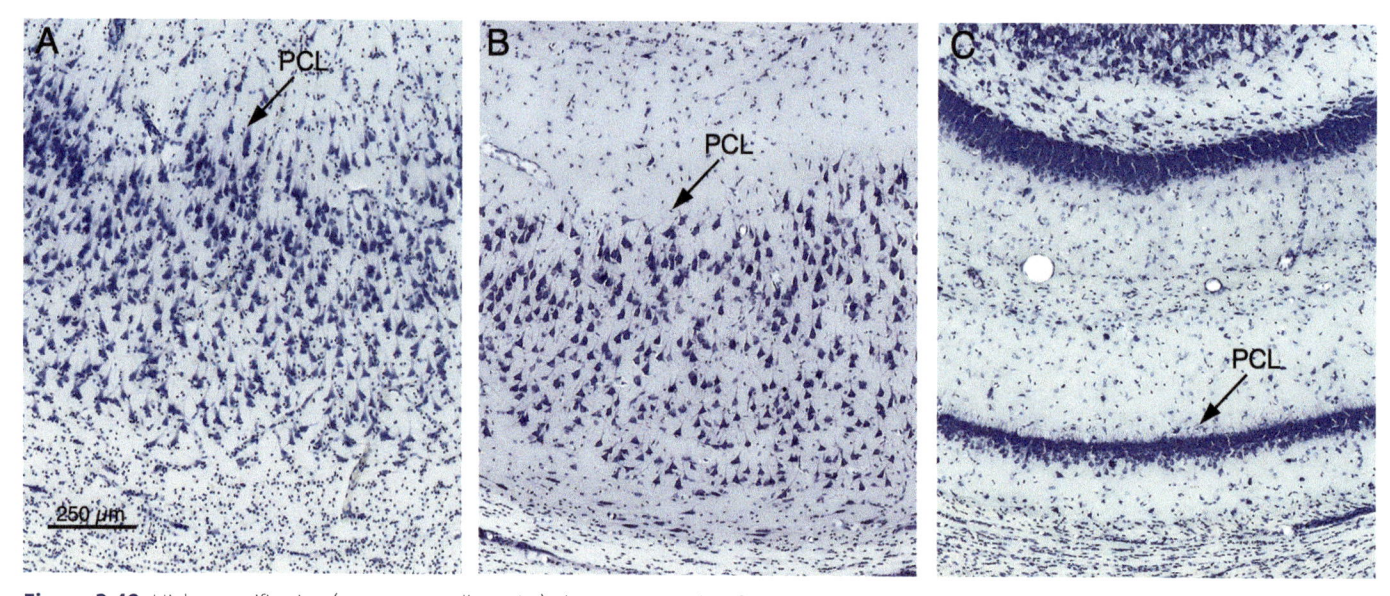

Figure 3.49 High-magnification (same across all species) photomicrographs of Nissl-stained coronal sections through the CA1 field of the hippocampus in the human (A), monkey (B), and rat (C). Note that the CA1 pyramidal cell layer in the rat (which is the darkly stained layer at the bottom of panel C) is about five cells thick. The monkey pyramidal cell layer is approximately 15 cells thick and shows some sublamination with the top half of the layer having a slightly higher density of neurons. The pyramidal cell layer in the human CA1 is even thicker and has a more laminated structure. Scale bar in A is 250 μm, applies to all panels.

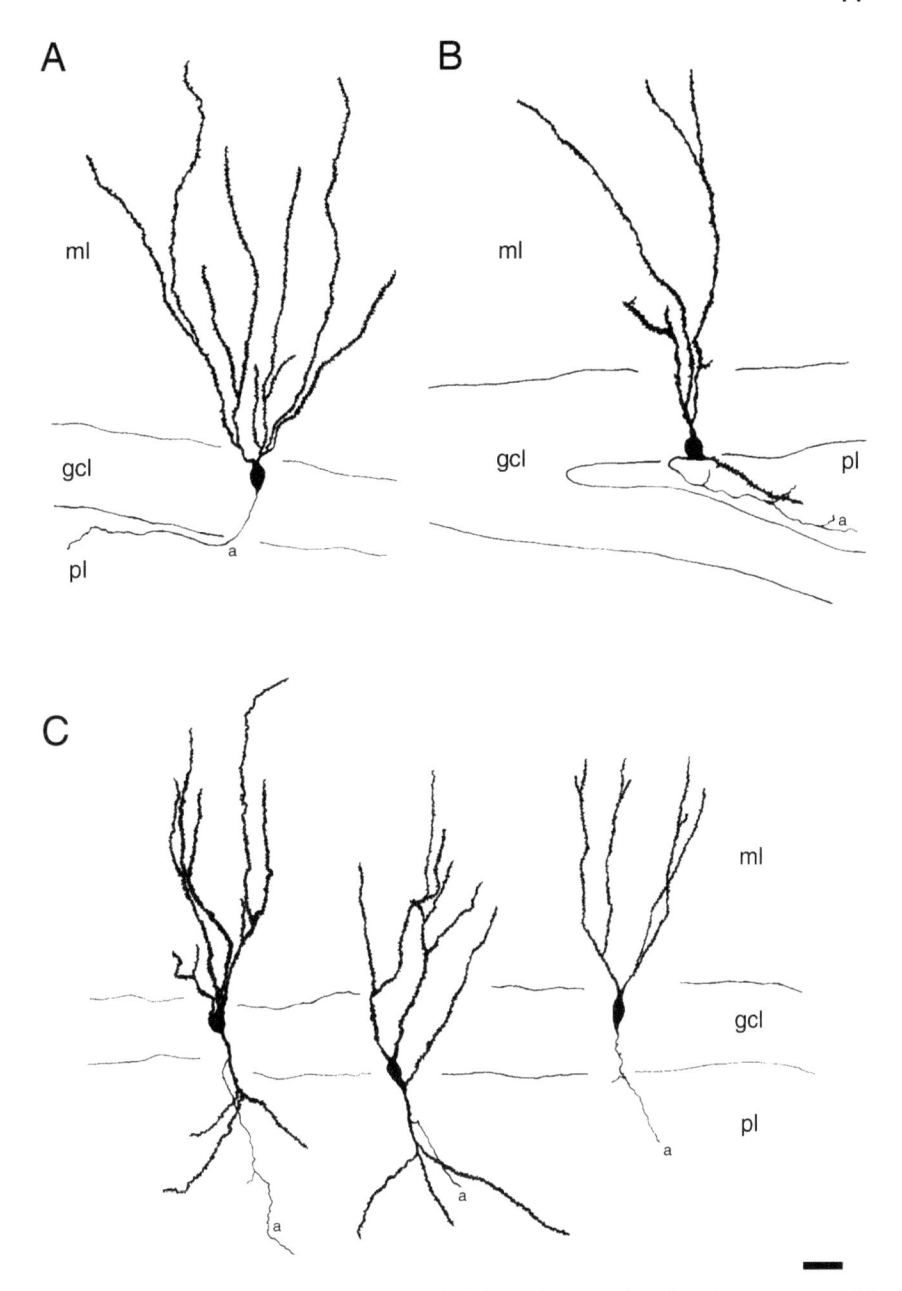

Figure 3.50 Camera lucida drawings of monkey and human granule cells. (A) Monkey granule cell in the upper part of the granule cell layer (gcl): The dendrites form a cone-like shape in the molecular layer (ml); the axon (a) originates from the base of the soma and extends into the polymorphic layer (pl). (B) Monkey granule cell in the deep part of the granule cell layer with a basal dendrite. Both apical and basal dendrites are fully covered with spines; the apical dendrites extend through the molecular layer, while the basal dendrites extend into the polymorphic layer; the axon originates from the base of the soma and extends into the polymorphic layer. (C) Three different types of human granule cells in the human dentate gyrus; the neuron on the right has dendrites in the molecular layer only, whereas the other two neurons have both apical dendrites extending into the molecular layer and basal dendrites extending into the polymorphic layer. Scale bar in C is 20 μm, applies to all panels. (Adapted with permission from Seress, 1987.)

to emphasize, it could be concluded that granule cells are basically similar in rats and monkeys, or that there have been substantial modifications of at least some granule cells. In general, dentate granule cells have the same unipolar apical dendritic tree in the monkey as in the rat. The total dendritic length of each granule cell is also relatively similar in the rat and the monkey. Seress and colleagues were the first to point out that at least some monkey granule cells have basal dendrites (Seress and Pokorny, 1981) (Figure 3.50), and a similar observation has been made by Scheibel and colleagues for human granule cells (Scheibel et al., 1974). This feature has never been reported for normal rat granule cells. Thus, it appears that there are some species differences in dentate granule cell morphology, but the functional significance of these differences is not yet clear.

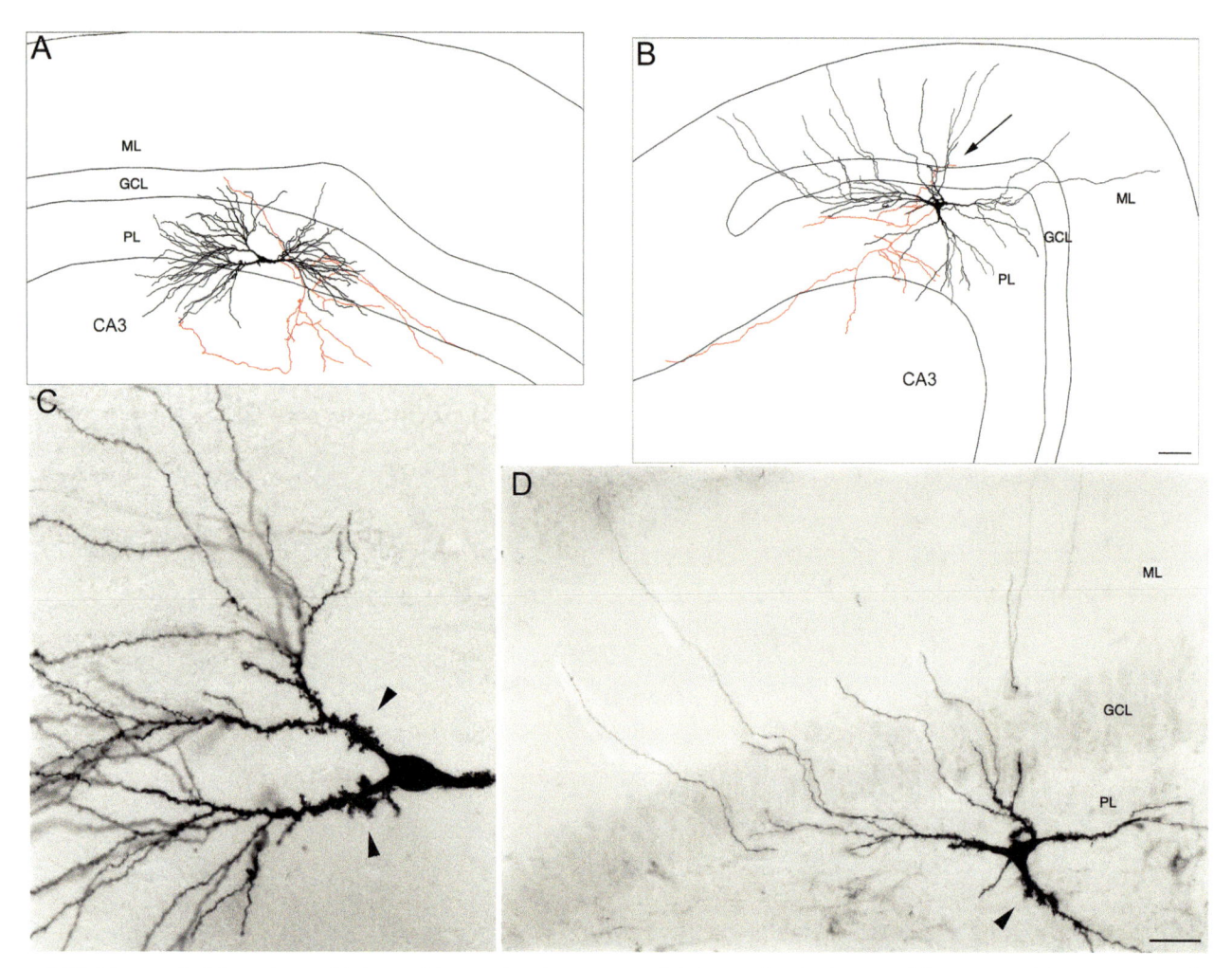

Figure 3.51 Mossy cell of the polymorphic layer of the monkey dentate gyrus. (A) Camera lucida drawing of the soma and dendritic arbor of an intracellularly labeled mossy cell. Note that the dendrites branch widely within the polymorphic layer and extend into the molecular layer, in contrast to what is observed in the rat. (B) Camera lucida drawing of the soma, dendrites and axonal plexus of a second mossy cell. Note that in this case, the dendrites ascend into the molecular layer of the dentate gyrus. (C) Photomicrograph of cell body and proximal dendrites of cell shown in panel A. Thorny excrescences are indicated with arrowheads. (D) Photomicrograph of cell body and proximal dendrites of neuron picture in panel B. Thorny excrescences are indicated with arrowheads. Scale bar is 100 μm. (Adapted from Buckmaster and Amaral, 2001.)

Another example of differences in an ostensibly similar cell type in the rat and the monkey has emerged from intracellular staining of mossy cells of the polymorphic region of the dentate gyrus (Buckmaster et al., 1992; Buckmaster and Amaral, 2001). In the rat, these cells give rise to the associational-commissural connections to the inner portion of the molecular layer, and its dendrites are generally confined to the polymorphic area, i.e., the dendrites extend neither into the molecular layer nor into the adjacent CA3 field. The mossy cell in the monkey is quite different. First, there appears to be at least two forms. One is very much like the rat mossy cell, with dendrites confined to the polymorphic cell layer and axons directed to the molecular layer. There is a second type, however, which extends much of its dendritic tree into the molecular layer (Figure 3.51). Moreover, many of these cells give rise to projections into the adjacent CA3 region. One implication of this altered morphology in the monkey is that these mossy cells are capable of receiving substantial perforant path innervation in the molecular layer of the dentate gyrus, whereas standard mossy cells are not (since the perforant path does not enter

the polymorphic layer). Moreover, in rats the granule cells are the only input from the dentate to CA3, whereas in the monkey the mossy cells appear to contribute an additional projection. These structural alterations suggest that there are at least some fundamental differences in the circuit characteristics of the dentate gyrus between the rat and the monkey. With greater direct comparisons, presumably other substantive species differences would arise. For example, Bautista et al. (2023) have noted distinct primate patterns of the distribution of inhibitory neurons in the macaque monkey entorhinal cortex.

3.10.2.3 Connections

Basic organization of the intrinsic hippocampal circuitry

To the extent that it has been examined, the basic principles of organization of the intrinsic circuitry of the monkey hippocampal formation resemble those observed in the rat (Kondo et al., 2008). So far, minor differences have been observed. In the monkey, for example, perforant path fibers arising from the rostral entorhinal area (the equivalent of the rat lateral entorhinal area) terminate, as in the rat, mainly in the outer third of the molecular layer of the dentate gyrus. But some terminations also continue in a decreasing gradient fashion into the middle third of the molecular layer (Witter and Amaral, 1991; Amaral et al., 2014). Projections from the caudal entorhinal cortex (the region equivalent to the rat medial entorhinal area) terminate in a similar fashion, heaviest in the middle third and gradually decreasing in the outer third of the molecular layer. Thus, the border between the lateral and medial entorhinal terminations is much less distinct in the monkey than in the rat.

Lack of commissural connections in the hippocampal formation of the monkey

One of the most striking connectional differences between the rat and the monkey relates to the organization of the commissural connections (Amaral et al., 1984; Demeter et al., 1985). In the rat, as we have reviewed, there are extensive commissural projections from the polymorphic layer of the dentate gyrus to the contralateral molecular layer of the dentate gyrus, and from the CA3 field of the hippocampus to the contralateral CA3 and CA1 fields. In the monkey, only the most rostral part of the dentate

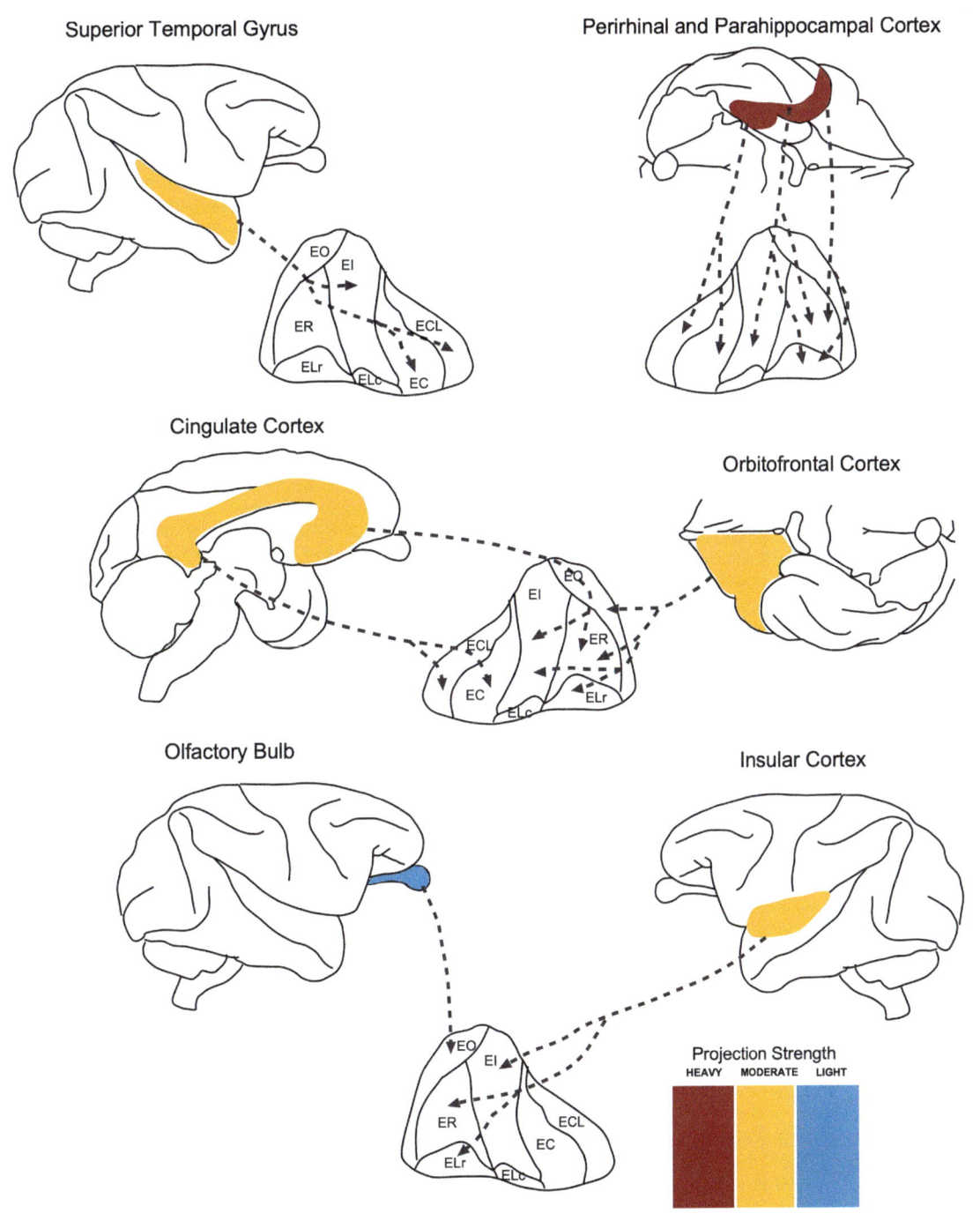

Figure 3.52 Summary diagram of the origin and topography of the major entorhinal cortical afferents in the macaque monkey. (Adapted with permission from Insausti et al., 1987, and Mohedano-Moriano et al., 2007.)

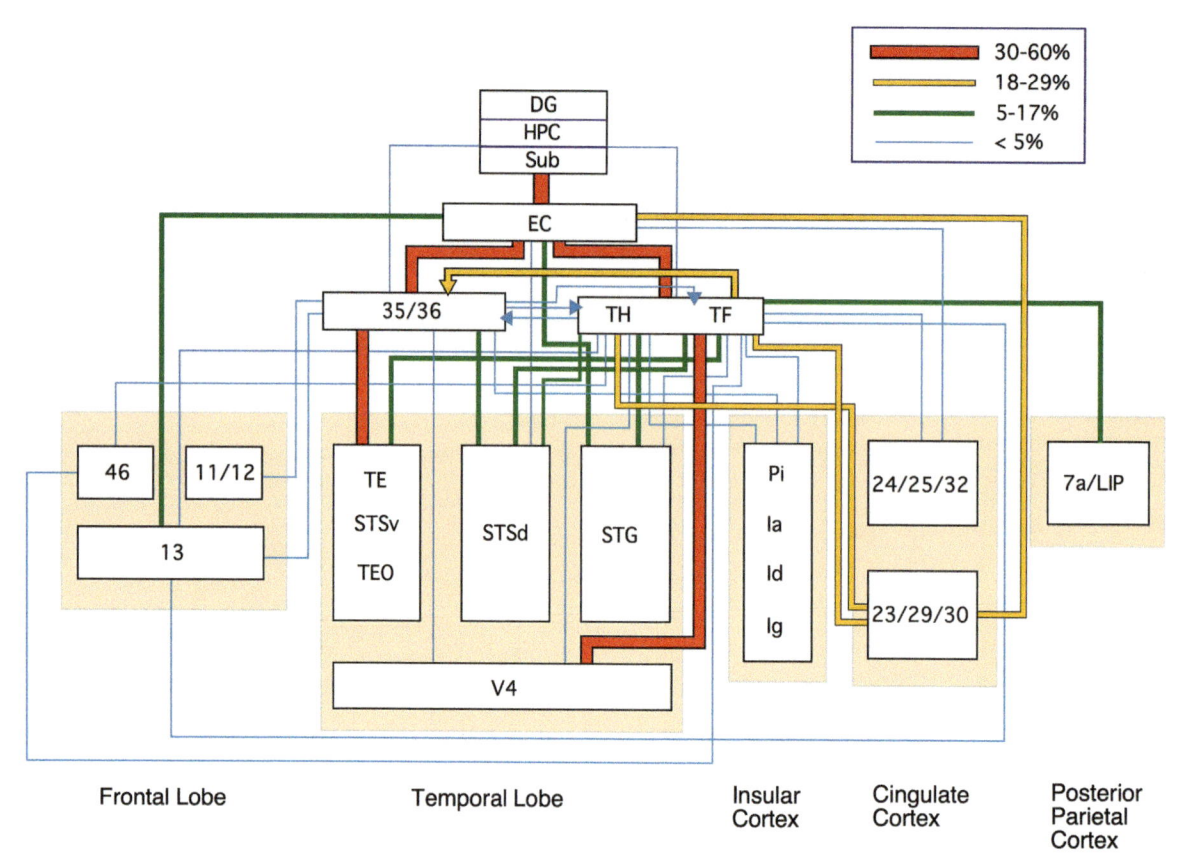

Figure 3.53 Summary diagram of the organization and strength of cortical inputs to the monkey entorhinal, perirhinal (areas 35 and 36), and parahippocampal (areas TF and TH) cortices. (Adapted from Suzuki and Amaral, 1994.)

gyrus and hippocampus (corresponding to the most temporal portion in the rat) demonstrates any commissural connections, and these are limited to the homotopic regions on the contralateral side. Interestingly, while the commissural connections of the dentate gyrus and hippocampus are largely absent, the connection originating in the presubiculum and terminating in layer III of the contralateral entorhinal cortex appears to be as robust in the monkey as in the rat.

Increased cortical interconnectivity of the monkey hippocampal formation

One major difference between the rat and monkey brain is the much greater amount of neocortex in the primate. Much of this neocortex is dedicated to visual processing, but there is also a substantial increase in the amount of association cortex, particularly in the frontal and temporal lobes. A substantial portion of this association cortex is polysensory, and most of the polysensory cortical regions are interconnected with the hippocampal formation via connections with the entorhinal cortex (Insausti et al., 1987; reviewed in Garcia and Buffalo, 2020). The more robust neocortical connectivity has given rise to the suggestion that processing in the primate hippocampal formation is more highly dependent on, and integrated with, processing of sensory information in the neocortex.

In the monkey temporal lobe, there is a massive expansion of the perirhinal and parahippocampal regions that border the hippocampal formation. Rostrally this region includes the perirhinal cortex, which comprises areas 35 and 36 of Brodmann. The

perirhinal cortex starts at a level through the rostral hippocampal formation and extends rostrally to reach the medial portion of the temporal polar cortex. The caudal continuation of the perirhinal cortex is the parahippocampal cortex that includes areas TF and TH of Bonin and Bailey (1947). Both of these regions are bordered laterally by the unimodal visual areas TE or TEO. The perirhinal and parahippocampal cortices are important contributors of the neocortical innervation of entorhinal cortex (Suzuki and Amaral, 1994; Suzuki, 1996; Miyashita, 2019).

The major inputs to the monkey entorhinal cortex are summarized in Figures 3.52 and 3.53. In both rats and monkeys, the entorhinal cortex provides the major interface for communication with the neocortex (Insausti et al., 1987; Mohedano-Moriano et al., 2007; Garcia and Buffalo, 2020; Bautista et al., 2023). As in the rat, the CA1 field of the hippocampus, subiculum, presubiculum, and parasubiculum project back to the entorhinal cortex in a topographical and laminar specific fashion (Witter and Amaral, 2020). For essentially all cortical regions, the return projections from the entorhinal cortex originate in layers V and VI (Munoz and Insausti, 2005), and terminate both deep and superficial in a manner typical of other cortical feedback projections. The laminar organization of the inputs to the entorhinal cortex varies according to the cortical area of origin. Projections from some regions, such as the perirhinal and parahippocampal cortices, terminate preferentially in layers I–III, which give rise to the perforant path projections. Projections from other cortical areas, such as the orbitofrontal and insular cortices, project to the deep layers of the entorhinal cortex that generate the major output pathways to the neocortex and other

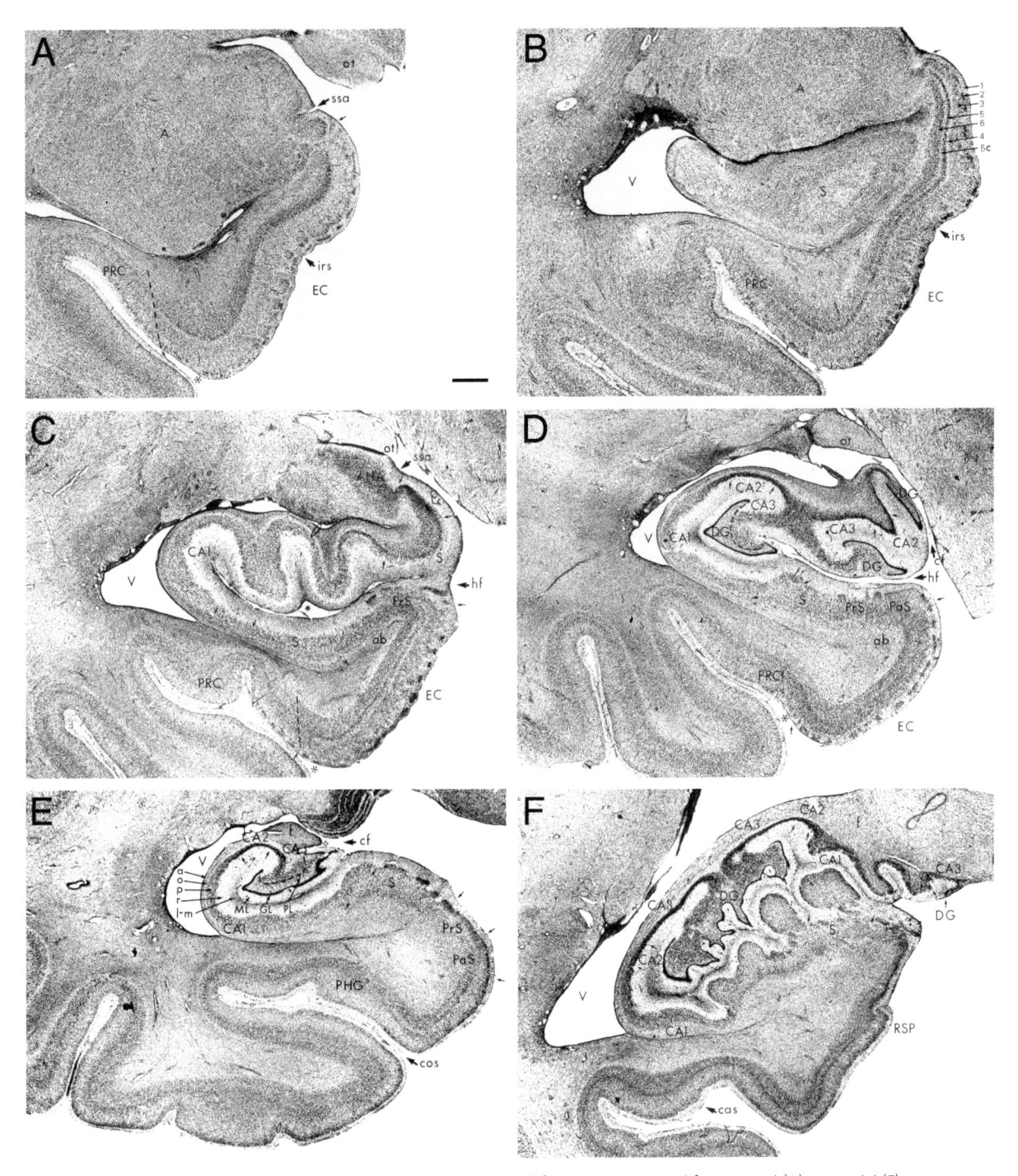

Figure 3.54 Nissl-stained coronal sections through the human hippocampal formation, arranged from rostral (A) to caudal (F).

regions. These latter connections, therefore, might preferentially be involved in modulating the output of the hippocampal formation. However, they may also contribute to the perforant pathway via some of the few layer V and VI neurons that contribute to this pathway, or through intrinsic deep to superficial connections within the entorhinal cortex.

While the perirhinal and parahippocampal cortices provide the major input to the hippocampal formation, other substantial inputs originate in the retrosplenial cortex (Kobayashi and Amaral, 2007), the polysensory region of the superior temporal gyrus (along the dorsal bank of the superior temporal gyrus), and the orbitofrontal cortex (mainly caudal area 13). The general rule is that the entorhinal cortex receives input only from cortical regions with demonstrated polysensory convergence. Thus, only olfactory input (which originates from all levels of the olfactory system including the olfactory bulb in the primate) has direct access to the hippocampal formation. The olfactory connection, however, provides another example of a difference between the rat and monkey hippocampal formation. While in the rat almost the entire entorhinal cortex receives a direct input from the olfactory bulb, in the monkey this is restricted to about 10% of the surface area of the entorhinal cortex.

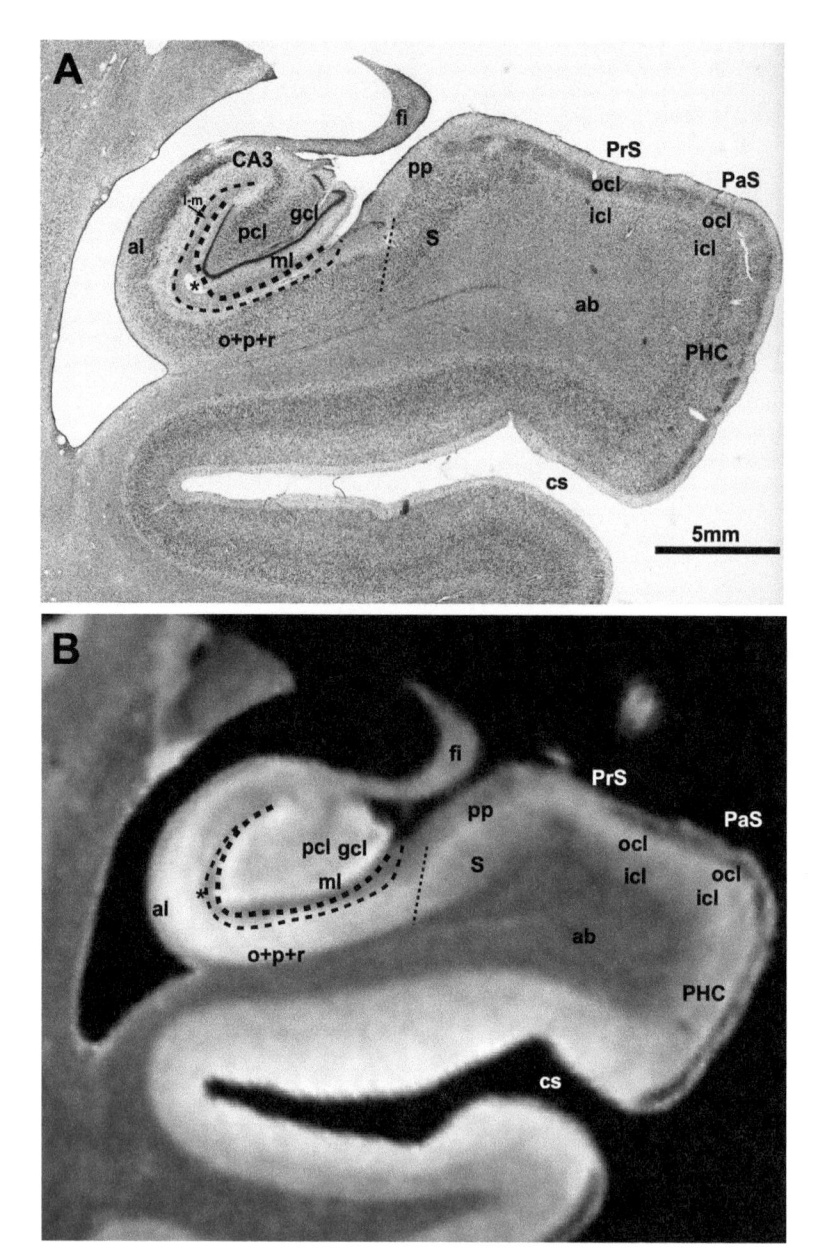

Figure 3.55 Comparison of Nissl-stained section through the postmortem hippocampus and an MRI scan of the same region.

Given this pattern of neocortical inputs to the monkey entorhinal cortex, the hippocampal formation can be viewed as the final stage in a cascade of neocortical sensory processing. From the unimodal association cortices, information converges on a few polysensory cortical regions that, in turn, project in a convergent fashion on the entorhinal cortex (Lavenex and Amaral, 2000; Bautista et al., 2023). The entorhinal cortex relays this information to the other hippocampal fields via the perforant and alvear pathways. Once the information processed by the hippocampal formation is returned to the deep layers of the entorhinal cortex, they return this highly processed information to many of the polysensory cortical regions that provide feedback projections to the unimodal sensory regions. It should be noted, however, that the projections from the perirhinal and parahippocampal cortices are not entirely reciprocal (Lavenex et al., 2002).

There are a number of implications of this cascade of projections into the entorhinal cortex and of the organization of the entorhinal

projections to the other hippocampal fields. One is that the information that the hippocampal formation is using has been highly preprocessed and integrated. Except for the olfactory input, very little elemental or unimodal sensory information is directed to the hippocampal formation. A second, related implication is that it is unlikely that there is appreciable segregation of sensory information processing in the hippocampal formation, i.e., visual information will not be processed separately from auditory information. In fact, the pattern of neuroanatomical connectivity would predict that the hippocampal formation carries out whatever functions it accomplishes with high level, multimodal representations of sensory experiences.

3.10.3 Comparison of the monkey and human hippocampal formation

At the risk of making points that may seem obvious, our understanding of the human hippocampus is necessarily primitive compared with that of the rat or the monkey. Since standard experimental tract-tracing studies cannot be done, novel approaches for mapping connections in the human brain will need to be developed. As we review below, forms of MRI such as diffusion-weighted imaging, are making inroads on defining hippocampal regions and pathways in the living human brain (Postans et al., 2020) Yet, the resolution still remains too low for direct comparison with tract-tracing studies in experimental animals. Perhaps the wizardry of molecular biology will someday provide new pathway-selective markers that will allow comparative studies of the rat, monkey, and human hippocampal formation. That being said, we will provide a short overview of the neuroanatomy of the human hippocampal formation (see also, Gonzalez-Arnay et al., 2024). Increasingly, investigators are attempting to use computational strategies to model the human hippocampal formation on the basis of experimental animal data (Gandolfi et al., 2023).

3.10.3.1 Cytoarchitectonic organization

The general appearance of the human hippocampal formation is reminiscent of the monkey hippocampal formation (Figures 3.2, 3.54). Yet, differences are also apparent. For example, the CA1 field of the hippocampus is even thicker in humans than in monkeys (Figure 3.49); in some regions, it is as much as 30 cells thick. In addition to being thicker, the CA1 pyramidal cell layer takes on a distinctly multilaminate appearance with cells of different size and shape predominating at different depths of the layer. Given evidence derived from rat studies that pyramidal cells at different levels within the layers receive and contribute different projections, (Masurkar et al., 2017), it can only be imagined how complex and subtle might be the laminar differences in connectivity and function of the human CA1. Unfortunately, there is little information concerning the exact morphological or neurochemical characteristics of these neurons; there is not even a comprehensive Golgi analysis of the neurons of the human dentate gyrus and hippocampus!

Another obvious difference is the cellular composition of the region enclosed within the limbs of the granule cell layer. There are far more cells in this region and the vast majority would appear to be cells of the CA3 field. The polymorphic layer of the dentate gyrus (the hilus) forms a very narrow band that lies just subjacent to the granule cell layer. Little is known about the morphology of cells in the human dentate gyrus. As indicated in the comparison between the rat and the monkey, however, there are clear differences in the morphology of certain cell types. As many as 30% of the granule cells in the human dentate gyrus have basal dendrites (Figure 3.50) an even larger number than in the monkey.

There are recent descriptive studies of the human subiculum, presubiculum, and parasubiculum (Insausti et al., 2017). There is also a review of the neuroanatomy of CA2 in the human brain (Insausti et al., 2023). The human entorhinal cortex has attracted considerably greater attention because of its vulnerability in Alzheimer's disease (see Chapter 20). While the same general regions identified in the monkey can be identified in the human, there is also evidence for additional fields in the human entorhinal cortex.

3.10.3.2 Connections

There is sparingly little information concerning the organization of connections in the human hippocampal formation. This is due to the fact that most neuroanatomical tracing techniques require the injection of tracers into the living brain. Some investigators have relied instead on techniques such as local application of the lipophilic dye DiI to map short pathways in human postmortem material (Lim, Blume, et al., 1997; Lim, Mufson, et al., 1997). They found that both the mossy fiber projection and the Schaffer collateral system (from CA3 to CA1) can be labeled over short distances by DiI, and they resemble the projections observed in the monkey. As important as these limited observations are, they highlight the fact that we do not currently know whether the neuroanatomical connections that have been described for the rat and the monkey are applicable to the human brain.

3.10.3.3 Critical comparison of the neuroanatomy of the rodent, monkey, and human hippocampal formation must await comparable quantitative data for each species

This chapter has dealt primarily with the rodent hippocampal formation since, as we pointed out at the beginning, much of the neuroanatomical information that is available is based on the mouse or rat and much of the electrophysiological and behavioral literature that is discussed throughout the rest of the book is also based on these species. With the dramatic increase in the use of noninvasive imaging of the human hippocampal formation, particularly in studies of memory, the need has grown for more detailed information about the neuroanatomical organization of the human hippocampal formation. This is also important as increasingly sophisticated models of hippocampus-related pathology are introduced, based primarily on rodent studies. A variety of models for temporal lobe epilepsy, for example, have been advanced based on cell degeneration and fiber sprouting in the rat hippocampus. But, if the fundamental circuit diagram of the rat hippocampal formation is different from that of the human, then models based on the rat may be misleading.

Unfortunately, the extent of the similarities and differences in the hippocampal formation of the rodent, monkey and human cannot currently be accurately gauged. Based on the few examples of established species differences described previously, it would not be surprising if substantial differences exist in the cellular morphology, connectivity, and chemical neuroanatomy of the hippocampal formation across species. The relevance of these differences to the normal function and the pathology of the hippocampal function will be an interesting future area of comparative neuroanatomy.

3.11 Neuroimaging studies of the hippocampal formation

3.11.1 Mouse and rat

Magnetic resonance imaging was first used to image the human brain in 1977 and its use for clinical diagnoses advanced rapidly as scanners were commercialized. Use of early MRI scanners for clinical research began in the mid-to-late 1980s. But use of MRI for animal models was delayed for some time. The main reason for this was the relatively low resolution of early scanners, which was adequate for the human brain but less so for experimental animals and particularly for the small brains of rodents. However, with the revolution in mouse genetics coupled with the creation of very high field MRI scanners (up to 21.0 T, [Ni, 2021]) the number of MRI studies with the mouse or rat as the subject has exploded.

Interest in imaging the mouse hippocampus started around 2000, and an early paper was published by Benveniste et al. (2000). We note that typical human MRI scanners have a magnet strength or 1.5 or 3.0 T and the higher the magnet strength the greater the potential resolution. But, human scanners do not typically use higher power magnets due to potential side effects like overheating the tissue under study. The Benveniste study employed a 9.4 T magnet. This postmortem study was carried out on brains removed from the animal after death. While the hippocampal formation could be detected and there was variation in intensity that roughly related to the layers of the hippocampus and dentate gyrus, the images provided a poor comparison with Nissl-stained sections. Some years later, Boretius et al. (2009) imaged living, anesthetized mice again using a 9.4 T scanner. They achieved a resolution of 30–40 μm in plane and 200–300 μm section thickness. By judicious selection of the imaging parameters, these investigators were able to detect hippocampal gray matter from white matter and thus could identify the pyramidal and granule cell layers. Interestingly, with manganese-enhanced MRI, it appears that the mossy fibers were highlighted but were mislabeled as CA3 pyramidal cells (their figure 9, lower right; also shown in Watanabe et al., 2013).

A departure from simply identifying regions within the hippocampus came from the work of Wu and Zhang (2016) who imaged living, anesthetized mice with a 11.7 T magnet and focused on diffusion weighted sequences that identify orientation of processes and fiber bundles. Perhaps the kindest thing that can be said about the results of these efforts is that because we already know the organization of hippocampal neuronal structure and its major pathways, one can get a crude sense of the organization as a result of output of the MRI. One would not be able to establish hippocampal connectivity on the basis of the imaging patterns though there is clearly some resemblance between the ground truth data and the imaging results.

Through the use of advanced scanning sequences and sophisticated analytic approaches, both the resolution and identification of hippocampal elements have improved. Wang et al. (2020) have achieved three-dimensional resolution of approximately 25 μm (the resolution of the light microscope is 0.25 μm). They are much better able to identify cellular layers, white matter, and the orientation of neurons and pathways. So, while the imaging of the mouse hippocampus has come a long way in 20 years, it is not the best tool for identifying neuroanatomical features of the mouse hippocampus.

But, there are several advantages to using MRI for investigating the mouse or rat hippocampus. First and foremost, MRI is non-invasive, so it is possible to carry out longitudinal studies. Qiu et al. (2013), for example, demonstrated that the volume of the hippocampus varies over the estrus cycle of the female mouse. It is also possible to achieve global perspectives of brain–behavior relationships using MRI. For example, Ellegood et al. (2015) explored the common brain alterations in 26 mouse models of autism carrying out MRI of mice and conducting quantitative measurements of several candidate brain regions. This would be a much more labor-intensive effort using standard histological techniques. Undoubtedly, other techniques such as functional MRI will be further developed to probe the mouse brain, especially of translational models, where the limits on resolution will not be as critical as reliability of findings (Ni, 2021).

3.11.2 Monkey

There has been far less effort to use MRI as a neuroanatomical tool probing the nonhuman primate hippocampus formation. That is not to say that MRI has not been used for research on nonhuman primates. MRI has been used for more than 30 years to define the boundaries of the hippocampal formation in order to produce lesions or place injections of tracer substances (Alvarez-Royo et al., 1991). There have been excellent nonhuman primate templates constructed and databases developed for analysis of nonhuman primate brain development (Shi et al., 2016). And some of this effort has been dedicated to analyzing the gross development of the hippocampal formation in the rhesus monkey (Payne et al., 2010; Hunsaker et al., 2014), including the development of automated segmentation tools (Hunsaker and Amaral, 2014). MRI has also been used to evaluate changes in hippocampal volume in the aging rhesus monkey (Kyle et al., 2019), which appear to be minimal. And, the effects of hippocampal lesions on brain organization and connectivity have also employed MRI techniques (Meng et al., 2014). There has been less of an attempt than in the mouse or the human, however, to define cytoarchitectonic fields or the organization of hippocampal layers. This is somewhat surprising, given the greater similarity of the monkey and human brains. But, perhaps this reflects the complexities and costs of using nonhuman primates in experimental research. It also reflects the fact that there is an ample supply of human participants in whom to probe hippocampal neuroanatomy using MRI.

3.11.3 Human

The human hippocampal formation has been a rich topic for both basic and clinical MRI research. A PubMed search in early 2022 of "human and hippocampus and MRI NOT animal" yields a result of 13,705 citations. Clearly, it is impossible to do justice to this literature in the brief summary that follows, and many of these papers relate to hippocampal function or pathology and are cited in other chapters of this book. In this section, we will briefly explore how useful MRI is for the neuroanatomical goals of studying the structure and connectivity of the human hippocampal formation for which experimental procedures are either not appropriate or not available, even for the postmortem brain.

3.11.3.1 How good is MRI at defining the volume of the human hippocampal formation?

Volumetric measurement of the hippocampus using MRI has provided the opportunity of conducting in vivo studies of neurodegenerative disorders (e.g., Alzheimer's disease) and psychiatric diseases, such as schizophrenia. Therefore, volumetric data on the whole or subportions of the hippocampal formation have been carried out since the early days of clinical use of MRI imaging (Jack et al., 1997; Juottonen et al., 1998). The accuracy of volumetric estimations of hippocampal structures have increased substantially, in part due to the increasing resolution of MRI scanners (Geuze et al., 2005) and the development of tools to carry out automatic segmentation of different portions of the hippocampal formation (Dale et al., 1999; Destrieux et al., 2010; Sakamoto et al., 2019). Reported values of the hippocampal volume range from 3,324 mm^3 (Pruessner et al., 2000) to 4,200 mm^3 (Morey et al., 2009), and values in between, 3,710 mm^3 (Wisse et al., 2012). Interestingly, postmortem stereological investigations yield the lower value of

2,840 mm³ (Chen et al., 2020). Differences in image resolution could account for differences among reports (reviewed in de Flores et al., 2015, who state, "high resolution neuroimaging is not *in vivo* histology"). This highlights the fact that MRI estimates of total hippocampal volume can vary depending on MRI strength, acquisition protocol, and segmentation procedures. But, in general, given adequate design of the study, modern MRI procedures can provide reliable estimates of total hippocampal volume.

3.11.3.2 How good is MRI at defining the boundaries between subdivisions of the human hippocampal formation?

Ex vivo studies

High resolution MRI can achieve a resolution of 200 μm × 200 μm × 200 μm, sufficient to reveal fine details of the hippocampal structure (Beaujoin et al., 2018; Yushkevich et al., 2021). It is important to remember that segmentation of the hippocampal fields is difficult even with histological sections at the microscopic scale (the so-called gold standard of hippocampal field discrimination). Research groups exploring MRI segmentation of the hippocampal formation often rely on histological validation of the segmentations performed on hippocampal MRI images. One approach is the introduction of matched high resolution in vivo and ex vivo MRI images with annotation of histologically delimited hippocampal fields. These studies are difficult to perform, and there are only a handful of them (Goubran et al., 2016; Wisse et al., 2017; Yushkevich et al., 2021).

Reports of ex vivo MRI with histological annotations are somewhat more abundant (e.g., de Flores et al., 2020; Yushkevich et al., 2021; Modo et al., 2023). However, all these efforts still lack enough resolution to unequivocally trace the boundaries of hippocampal

fields even with ex vivo high-resolution MRI scans. The resolution limits at detecting the layering of the hippocampus are shown in several reports (Goubran et al., 2016; Wisse et al., 2017; Beaujoin et al., 2018). In the Beaujoin et al. study, the hippocampal layers, i.e., alveus/oriens, pyramidal cell layer, and stratum radiatum/lacunosum-moleculare, are barely noticeable in T2 sequences. It is noteworthy that the delimitation of the transverse extent of the hippocampal fields in coronal sections could only be inferred from indirect estimation based on visible landmarks (Wisse et al., 2017). The interested reader is referred to the paper by Wisse et al. (2021), who discuss the problems with defining hippocampal layers from MRI scans that lack sufficient resolution and thus produce spurious results. Another take on this is the recent paper by Modo et al. (2023). Thus, while this may change in the future, currently it is fairly clear that in vivo MRI imaging techniques, particularly those that employ standard clinical scanners, are unable to reliably set the boundaries between the fields of the hippocampal formation.

3.11.3.3 How good is MRI at charting the pathways of the hippocampal formation?

Because of the limits of resolution described above, MRI studies of hippocampal fiber tracts have been limited to the most sizable fiber tracts of the hippocampus. For example, there are several reports evaluating the feasibility of visualizing the perforant path and the angular bundle (Augustinack et al., 2010; Zeineh et al., 2012; Beaujoin et al., 2018; Karat et al., 2023). A more complete account of the fibers encompassing the Papez circuit, that is, perforant path, fimbria-fornix, and mammillothalamic tract, is demonstrated by Choi et al. (2019), who used diffusion tensor weighted imaging at 7.0 T to chart this circuit more than 80 years after it was originally detailed by James Papez. Suffice it to say that while in vivo mapping of hippocampal pathways may have clinical value, thus far, these

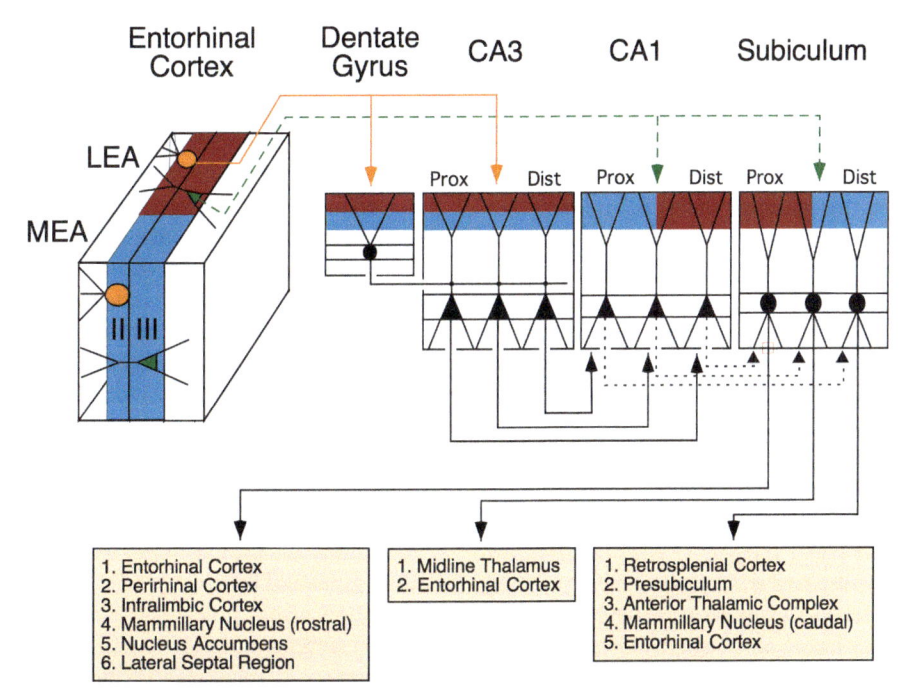

Figure 3.56 Summary diagram illustrating the transverse organization of the connections through the hippocampal formation. This figure highlights the possibility that information is segregated or "channeled" through the hippocampal formation and ultimately reaches different recipients of hippocampal output (Adapted from Amaral 1991).

hippocampus is the paper by Zheng et al. (2018) that reports the complete electron microscopic analysis of the 100,000-neuron brain of the adult fruit fly, *Drosophila melanogaster*. A video abstract of this paper is instructive (https://doi.org/10.1016/j.cell.2018.06.019#mmc8). This was a massive, multiyear project with more than 20 collaborators. The fly brain necessitated more than 7,000 sections to be produced, yielding approximately 21 million images and a dataset of 106 TB. This dataset is now being analyzed and provides the ability to map all connections between identified neurons. Of course, there is additional research that needs to be done to add the transmitter substance(s) of identified neurons. Similar approaches will ultimately be possible with the mouse hippocampus, or at least portions of it. And, we may ultimately achieve a realistic appreciation of all of the connections of the hippocampus—at least of the intrinsic connections.

Once we have a complete map of hippocampal circuitry, where does that lead the field? Well, in part, it would form the substrate for producing the ultimate digital model of the hippocampus that is currently based on crude quantitative data (Yu et al., 2020). This may be a useful link between static neuroanatomy and the goal that everyone is really aiming toward, which is understanding the function and dysfunction of the hippocampus leading to normal or altered behavior. Here, neuroanatomy is far ahead and will likely remain far ahead of efforts to understand the physiology of neurons and connections in the functioning experimental animal.

There are also challenges for the future of hippocampal neuroanatomy. With the limited information at hand, we already appreciate that there will be significant differences between the cellular and connectional neuroanatomy of the human hippocampal formation in relation to experimental animals. And here, the constraint is the development of tools to map neurons and connections in the human brain. The available tools are crude and unable to achieve the level of circuit analysis that is currently available for use in experimental animals. It would be unwise to anticipate that the neuroanatomy of the rodent or nonhuman primate hippocampal formation will simply scale up to the human brain. There will be differences which will need to be ascertained directly by analysis of the human brain. Thus, if an important goal of hippocampal neuroscience is to understand the function and dysfunction of the human hippocampal formation, neuroanatomical tools will need to be developed to map human hippocampal circuits with higher resolution than afforded by MRI and that can be carried out in the postmortem brain.

3.14 Conclusions

While this chapter has presented a substantial amount of neuroanatomical information, it has only begun to scratch the surface of what is available in the primary literature. However, because we have focused on general features and principles of organization, this should be more than adequate for delving into both the cellular and molecular aspects of hippocampal organization (Chapters 5 and 7) and the function of the hippocampal formation in the living organism (Chapters 11–13). The neuroanatomy of the hippocampal formation is unique and predicts that the behavioral functions that it subserves will undoubtedly be unique as well.

I, II, III, IV, V, VI	Cortical layers
A35	Area 35 of the perirhinal cortex
A36	Area 36 of the perirhinal cortex
A	axon
A	Amygdaloid complex
LA	Lateral nucleus
BLA	Basolateral nucleus
BMA	Basomedial nucleus
CEA	Central nucleus
OA	Olfactory amygdala
AAC	Axo-axonic cell
ab	Angular bundle
ACAd and ACAv	Dorsal and ventral anterior cingulate cortex
ACB	Nucleus accumbens
AId/v/p:	Agranular insular (dorsal, ventral, posterior) cortices
AON	Anterior olfactory nucleus
AUD, AUD v, p	Primary auditory cortex, ventral and posterior
al	Alveus
BC	Basket cell
Body	Body of the hippocampus
BST	Bed nucleus of the stria terminalis
CA1, CA2, CA3	Fields of the hippocampus
cas	Calcarine sulcus
CC, cc	Corpus callosum
CLA	Claustrum
CP	Caudate putamen
cs	Collateral sulcus
DG	dentate gyrus
Dig	Digitationes hippocampi
DTH	Dorsal thalamus
mi	midline group
an	anterior group
me	medial group
la	lateral group
ve	ventral group
EC	Entorhinal cortex
EC	Caudal division
ECL	Caudal limiting division
EI	Intermediate division
ELc, ELr	Lateral division (caudal and rostral)
EO	Olfactory division
EP	Endopiriform nucleus
FG	Fusiform gyrus
F, fi	Fimbria
fx	Fornix
GA	Gyrus ambiens
gcl	Granule cell layer of the dentate gyrus
GIL	Gyrus intralimbicus
GP	Globus pallidus
GSL	Gyrus semilunaris
GU	Gyrus uncinatus
GU	rodent gustatory area
Head	Head of the hippocampus
hf	Hippocampal fissure
HICAP	Hilar commissural–associational pathway associated cell

HIMPP	Hilar medial perforant pathway associated cell
HIPP, HIPP L	Hilar perforant pathway associated (like) cell
HP	Hilar projecting cell
HPC	Hippocampus
I	Insular cortex
Ia	Agranular insula
Id	Dysgraular insula
Ig	Granular insula
PI	Parainsula
Icl, ocl	Inner and outer cellular layers
ILA	infralimbic area
ILM	Intralaminar nuclei
irs	Intrarhinal sulcus
LEA	Lateral entorhinal area
LG, LGN	Lateral geniculate nucleus
LIP/7a	Posterior parietal cortex
LS	Lateral septum
LV	Lateral ventricle
LZ	Lateral hypothalamus
MB, MBO	Mammillary body
MEA	Medial entorhinal area
MEZ	Medial hypothalmus
MG	Medial geniculate
ml	Molecular layer of the dentate gyrus
MOCAP	molecular layer commissural–associational pathway associated cell
MOPP	Molecular layer perforant pathway associated cell
MO p, s	Primary and Secondary motor área
MS	Medial septem
NGFC,	Neurogliaform cell
oc	Optic chiasm
ot	Optic tract
OT	Olfactory tubercle
o+p+r	Stratum oriens, pramidale and radiatum
ORBI	l,m,v, vl Rodent orbital area (lateral, medial, ventral, ventrolateral)
Para, PaS, PaSub	Parasubiculum
PAR2	Parietal cortex, area 2
PCL, pcl	Pyramidal cell layer of the hippocampus
PCoA	Posterior cortical nucleus of the amygdala
PER, PR	Perirhinal cortex
Pir	Piriform cortex
PL/ILA	rodent medial prefrontal cortex
pl	Polymorphic cell layer of the dentate gyrus
PHC, PHG	Parahippocampal cortex, gyrus
PL	Prelimbic cortex
Pons	Pontine nuclei
pp	Perforant path
POR	Postrhinal cortex
PostSub	Postsubiculum
PTA	Piriform transition area
PTLp	Posterior parietal cortex
Pre, PrS	presubiculum
PRC	Perirhinal cortex
PS	Posterior septum
PVZ	Periventricular hypothalmus
rs	Rhinal sulcus
RSPd and RSPv	Retrosplenial cortex, dorsal and ventral
RT	Reticular nucleus
S, Sub	Subiculum
SI	Substantia innominata
sl	Stratum lucidum of the hippocampus
sl-m	Stratum lacunosum-moleculare of the hippocampus
SN/VTA	Substantia nigra/ventral tegmental area
so	Stratum oriens of the hippocampus
SP I	subiculum projecting cell I
SP II	subiculum projecting cell II
sr	Stratum radiatum of the hippocampus
SSp and SSs	Primary and supplementary somatosensory areas
SN	Substantia Nigra
spl	Splenium of the corpus callosum
STG	Superior temporal gyrus
STSd,STSv	Superior temporal sulcus (dorsal and ventral)
ssa	Sulcus semiannularis
Tail	Tail of the hippocampus
TC	Temporal cortex
TE/TEO	Inferotemporal visual cortex
Tev	Ventral temporal area
TE2, TE3	Temporal cortex 2 and 3
TF	Area TF of the parahipocampal cortex
TH	Area TH of the parahipocampal cortex
TML	Total molecular layer cell
TP	Temporal pole
TT	Taenia tecta
V	Ventricle
VLTH	Ventrolateral thalamus
VISC	Visceral granular insular cortex
VIS1 and VISm	Lateral and medial visual association cortex
VISp	Primary visual cortex
ZI	Zona incerta

REFERENCES

Acsady L, Kamondi A, Sik A, Freund T, Buzsaki G (1998) GABAergic cells are the major postsynaptic targets of mossy fibers in the rat hippocampus. *J Neurosci* **18**:3386–3403.

Aggleton JP, Christiansen K (2015) The subiculum: the heart of the extended hippocampal system. *Prog Brain Res* **219**:65–82.

Agster KL, Burwell RD (2009) Cortical efferents of the perirhinal, postrhinal, and entorhinal cortices of the rat. *Hippocampus* **19**:1159–1186.

Agster KL, Tomas Pereira I, Saddoris MP, Burwell RD (2016) Subcortical connections of the perirhinal, postrhinal, and entorhinal cortices of the rat: II. Efferents. *Hippocampus* **26**:1213–1230.

Allen GV, Hopkins DA (1989) Mamillary body in the rat: topography and synaptology of projections from the subicular complex, prefrontal cortex, and midbrain tegmentum. *J Comp Neurol* **286**:311–336.

Alvarez-Royo P, Clower RP, Zola-Morgan S, Squire LR (1991) Stereotaxic lesions of the hippocampus in monkeys: determination of surgical coordinates and analysis of lesions using magnetic resonance imaging. *J Neurosci Methods* **38**:223–232.

Amaral DG (1978) A Golgi study of cell types in the hilar region of the hippocampus in the rat. *J Comp Neurol* **182**:851–914.

Amaral DG (1991) Is there "channeling" of information through the intrinsic circuit of the rat hippocampus? *Brain Res Rev* **16**:193–220.

Amaral DG, Dent JA (1981) Development of the mossy fibers of the dentate gyrus: I. A light and electron microscopic study of the mossy fibers and their expansions. *J Comp Neurol* **195**:51–86.

Amaral DG, Dolorfo C, Alvarez-Royo P (1991) Organization of CA1 projections to the subiculum: a PHA-L analysis in the rat. *Hippocampus* 1:415–436.

Amaral DG, Insausti R, Cowan WM (1984) The commissural connections of the monkey hippocampal formation. *J Comp Neurol* 224:307–336.

Amaral DG, Insausti R, Cowan WM (1987) The entorhinal cortex of the monkey: I. Cytoarchitectonic organization. *J Comp Neurol* 264:326–355.

Amaral DG, Kondo H, Lavenex P (2014) An analysis of entorhinal cortex projections to the dentate gyrus, hippocampus, and subiculum of the neonatal macaque monkey. *J Comp Neurol* 522:1485–1505.

Amaral DG, Kurz, J. (1985) An analysis of the origins of the cholinergic and non-cholinergic septal projections to the hippocampal formation of the rat. *J Comp Neurol* 240:37–59.

Amaral DG, Witter MP (1989) The three dimensional organization of the hippocampal formation: a review of anatomical data. *Neuroscience* 31:571–591.

Andersen P, Bliss TVP, Skrede KK (1971) Lamellar organization of hippocampal excitatory pathways. *Experimental Brain Research* 13:222–238.

Augustinack JC, Helmer K, Huber KE, Kakunoori S, Zollei L, Fischl B (2010) Direct visualization of the perforant pathway in the human brain with ex vivo diffusion tensor imaging. *Front Hum Neurosci* 4:42.

Augustinack JC, Huber KE, Postelnicu GM, Kakunoori S, Wang R, van der Kouwe AJ, Wald LL, Stein TD, Frosch MP, Fischl B (2012) Entorhinal verrucae geometry is coincident and correlates with Alzheimer's lesions: a combined neuropathology and high-resolution ex vivo MRI analysis. *Acta Neuropathol* 123:85–96.

Bakst I, Avendaño, C., Morrison, JH, Amaral, DG (1986) An experimental analysis of the origins of the somatostatin immunoreactive fibers in the dentate gyrus of the rat. *J Neurosci* 6:1452–1462.

Barger N, Hanson KL, Teffer K, Schenker-Ahmed NM, Semendeferi K (2014) Evidence for evolutionary specialization in human limbic structures. *Front Hum Neurosci* 8:277.

Basu J, Siegelbaum SA (2015) The corticohippocampal circuit, synaptic plasticity, and memory. *Cold Spring Harb Perspect Biol* 7.

Bautista J, Garcia-Cabezas MA, Medalla M, Rosene DL, Zikopoulos B, Barbas H (2023) Pattern of ventral temporal lobe interconnections in rhesus macaques. *J Comp Neurol* 531:1963–1986.

Beaujoin J, Palomero-Gallagher N, Boumezbeur F, Axer M, Bernard J, Poupon F, Schmitz D, Mangin JF, Poupon C (2018) Post-mortem inference of the human hippocampal connectivity and microstructure using ultra-high field diffusion MRI at 11.7 T. *Brain Struct Funct* 223:2157–2179.

Benear SL, Ngo CT, Olson IR (2020) Dissecting the fornix in basic memory processes and neuropsychiatric disease: a review. *Brain Connect* 10:331–354.

Benveniste H, Kim K, Zhang L, Johnson GA (2000) Magnetic resonance microscopy of the C57BL mouse brain. *Neuroimage* 11:601–611.

Bienkowski MS (2023) Further refining the boundaries of the hippocampus CA2 with gene expression and connectivity: potential subregions and heterogeneous cell types. *Hippocampus* 33:150–160.

Bienkowski MS, Bowman I, Song MY, Gou L, Ard T, Cotter K, Zhu M, Benavidez NL, Yamashita S, Abu-Jaber J, Azam S, Lo D, Foster NN, Hintiryan H, Dong HW (2018) Integration of gene expression and brain-wide connectivity reveals the multiscale organization of mouse hippocampal networks. *Nat Neurosci* 21:1628–1643.

Bienkowski MS, Sepehrband F, Kurniawan ND, Stanis J, Korobkova L, Khanjani N, Clark K, Hintiryan H, Miller CA, Dong HW (2021)

Homologous laminar organization of the mouse and human subiculum. *Sci Rep* 11:3729.

Blackstad TW (1956) Commissural connections of the hippocampal region in the rat, with special reference to their mode of termination. *J Comp Neurol* 105:417–537.

Blackstad TW, Brink K, Hem J, Jeune B (1970) Distribution of hippocampal mossy fibers in the rat: an experimental study with silver impregnation methods. *J Comp Neurol* 138:433–450.

Bloss EB, Cembrowski MS, Karsh B, Colonell J, Fetter RD, Spruston N (2018) Single excitatory axons form clustered synapses onto CA1 pyramidal cell dendrites. *Nat Neurosci* 21:353–363.

Bobic Rasonja M, Oreskovic D, Knezovic V, Pogledic I, Pupacic D, Vuksic M, Brugger PC, Prayer D, Petanjek Z, Jovanov Milosevic N (2019) Histological and MRI study of the development of the human indusium griseum. *Cereb Cortex* 29:4709–4724.

Bonin G. v., and P. Bailey (1947) The neocortex of macaca mulatta. University of Illinois Press. Urbana.

Booker SA, Vida I (2018) Morphological diversity and connectivity of hippocampal interneurons. *Cell Tissue Res* 373:619–641.

Boretius S, Kasper L, Tammer R, Michaelis T, Frahm J (2009) MRI of cellular layers in mouse brain in vivo. *Neuroimage* 47:1252–1260.

Borhegyi Z, Leranth C (1997) Distinct substance P- and calretinin-containing projections from the supramammillary area to the hippocampus in rats—a species difference between rats and monkeys. *Experimental Brain Research* 115:369–374.

Botterill JJ, Gerencer KJ, Vinod KY, Alcantara-Gonzalez D, Scharfman HE (2021) Dorsal and ventral mossy cells differ in their axonal projections throughout the dentate gyrus of the mouse hippocampus. *Hippocampus* 31:522–539.

Bourne JN, Harris KM (2008) Balancing structure and function at hippocampal dendritic spines. *Annu Rev Neurosci* 31:47–67.

Braak H (1974) On the structure of the human archicortex: I. The cornu ammonis: a Golgi and pigmentarchitectonic study. *Cell Tissue Res* 152:349–383.

Braak H (1980) Architectonics of the Human Telencephalic Cortex. New York: Springer-Verlag.

Brodmann K (1909) Vergleichende Lokalisationslehre der Grosshirnrinde in ihren Prinzipien dargestellt auf Grund des Zellenbaues. Leipzig.

Buckmaster PS, Amaral, DG (2001) Intracellular recording and labeling of mossy cells and proximal CA3 pyramidal cells in macaque monkeys. *J Comp Neurol* 430:264–281.

Buckmaster PS, Strowbridge BW, Kunkel DD, Schmiege DL, Schwartzkroin PA (1992) Mossy cell axonal projections to the dentate gyrus molecular layer in the rat hippocampal slice. *Hippocampus* 2:349–362.

Buckmaster PS, Wenzel HJ, Kunkel DD, Schwartzkroin PA (1996) Axon arbors and synaptic connections of hippocampal mossy cells in the rat in vivo. *J Comp Neurol* 366:271–292.

Burwell RD (2001) Borders and cytoarchiture of the perirhinal and postrhinal cortices in the rat. *J Comp Neurol* 437:17–41.

Burwell RD, Amaral DG (1998a) Cortical afferents of the perirhinal, postrhinal, and entorhinal cortices of the rat. *J Comp Neurol* 398:179–205.

Burwell RD, Amaral DG (1998b) Perirhinal and postrhinal cortices of the rat: interconnectivity and connections with the entorhinal cortex. *J Comp Neurol* 391:293–321.

Burwell RD, Witter MP (2002) Basic Anatomy of the Parahippocampal Region in Monkeys and Rats. Oxford: Oxford University Press.

Burwell RD, Witter MP, Amaral DG (1995) Perirhinal and postrhinal cortices of the rat: a review of the neuroanatomical literature and comparison with findings from the monkey brain. *Hippocampus* 5:390–408.

Caballero-Bleda M, Witter MP (1993) Regional and laminar organization of projections from the presubiculum and parasubiculum to the entorhinal cortex: an anterograde tracing study in the rat. *J Comp Neurol* 328:115–129.

Canteras N, Swanson L (1992) Projections of the ventral subiculum to the amygdala, septum, and hypothalamus: a PHAL anterograde tract-tracing study in the rat. *J Comp Neurol* 324: 180–194.

Cassel JC, Pereira de Vasconcelos A, Loureiro M, Cholvin T, Dalrymple-Alford JC, Vertes RP (2013) The reuniens and rhomboid nuclei: neuroanatomy, electrophysiological characteristics and behavioral implications. *Prog Neurobiol* 111:34–52.

Cembrowski MS, Bachman JL, Wang L, Sugino K, Shields BC, Spruston N (2016) Spatial gene-expression gradients underlie prominent heterogeneity of CA1 pyramidal neurons. *Neuron* 89:351–368.

Cembrowski MS, Phillips MG, DiLisio SF, Shields BC, Winnubst J, Chandrashekar J, Bas E, Spruston N (2018) Dissociable structural and functional hippocampal outputs via distinct subiculum cell classes. *Cell* 173:1280–1292, e1218.

Cembrowski MS, Spruston N (2019) Heterogeneity within classical cell types is the rule: lessons from hippocampal pyramidal neurons. *Nat Rev Neurosci* 20:193–204.

Cembrowski MS, Wang L, Lemire AL, Copeland M, DiLisio SF, Clements J, Spruston N (2018) The subiculum is a patchwork of discrete subregions. *Elife* 7.

Chen F, Bertelsen AB, Holm IE, Nyengaard JR, Rosenberg R, Dorph-Petersen KA (2020) Hippocampal volume and cell number in depression, schizophrenia, and suicide subjects. *Brain Res* 1727:146546.

Choi SH, Kim YB, Paek SH, Cho ZH (2019) Papez circuit observed by in vivo human brain with 7.0T MRI super-resolution track density imaging and track tracing. *Front Neuroanat* 13:17.

Christiansen K, Dillingham CM, Wright NF, Saunders RC, Vann SD, Aggleton JP (2016) Complementary subicular pathways to the anterior thalamic nuclei and mammillary bodies in the rat and macaque monkey brain. *Eur J Neurosci* 43:1044–1061.

Claiborne BJ, Amaral DG, Cowan WM (1986) A light and electron microscopic analysis of the mossy fibers of the rat dentate gyrus. *J Comp Neurol* 246:435–458.

Claiborne BJ, Amaral DG, Cowan WM (1990) A quantitative three-dimensional analysis of granule cell dendrites in the rat dentate gyrus. *J Comp Neurol* 302:206–219.

Conrad LCA, Leonard CM, Pfaff DW (1974) Connections of the median and dorsal raphe nuclei in the rat: an autoradiographic and degeneration study. *J Comp Neurol* 156:179–206.

Cui Z, Gerfen CR, Young WS, 3rd (2013) Hypothalamic and other connections with dorsal CA2 area of the mouse hippocampus. *J Comp Neurol* 521:1844–1866.

Daitz HM, Powell TPS (1954) Studies of the connexions of the fornix system. *J Neurol Neurosurg Psychiatry* 17:75–82.

Dale AM, Fischl B, Sereno MI (1999) Cortical surface-based analysis: I. Segmentation and surface reconstruction. *Neuroimage* 9:179–194.

DeFelipe J, Fernandez-Gil MA, Kastanauskaite A, Bote RP, Presmanes YG, Ruiz MT (2007) Macroanatomy and microanatomy of the temporal lobe. *Semin Ultrasound CT MR* 28:404–415.

de Flores R, Berron D, Ding SL, Ittyerah R, Pluta JB, Xie L, Adler DH, Robinson JL, Schuck T, Trojanowski JQ, Grossman M, Liu W, Pickup S, Das SR, Wolk DA, Yushkevich PA, Wisse LEM (2020) Characterization of hippocampal subfields using ex vivo MRI, histology data: lessons for in vivo segmentation. *Hippocampus* 30:545–564.

de Flores R, La Joie R, Chetelat G (2015) Structural imaging of hippocampal subfields in healthy aging and Alzheimer's disease. *Neuroscience* 309:29–50.

Degro CE, Bolduan F, Vida I, Booker SA (2022) Interneuron diversity in the rat dentate gyrus: an unbiased in vitro classification. *Hippocampus* 32:310–331.

Deller T, Martinez A, Nitsch R, Frotscher M (1996a) A novel entorhinal projection to the rat dentate gyrus—direct innervation of proximal dendrites and cell bodies of granule cells and GABAergic neurons. *J Neurosci* 16:3322–3333.

Deller T, Nitsch R, Frotscher M (1996b) Heterogeneity of the commissural projection to the rat dentate gyrus—a phaseolus vulgaris leucoagglutinin tracing study. *Neuroscience* 75:111–121.

Demeter S, Rosene DL, Van Hoesen GW (1985) Interhemispheric pathways of the hippocampal formation, presubiculum and entorhinal and posterior parahippocampal cortices in the rhesus monkey: the structure and organization of the hippocampal commissures. *J Comp Neurol* 233:30–47.

Dent JA, Galvin NJ, Stanfield BB, Cowan WM (1983) The mode of termination of the hypothalamic projection to the dentate gyrus: an EM autoradiographic study. *Brain Res* 258:1–10.

Desmond NL, Levy WB (1985) Granule cell dendritic spine density in the rat hippocampus varies with spine shape and location. *Neurosci Lett* 54:219–224.

Destrieux C, Fischl B, Dale A, Halgren E (2010) Automatic parcellation of human cortical gyri and sulci using standard anatomical nomenclature. *Neuroimage* 53:1–15.

Diethorn EJ, Gould E (2023) Development of the hippocampal CA2 region and the emergence of social recognition. *Dev Neurobiol* 83:143–156.

Ding SL (2013) Comparative anatomy of the prosubiculum, subiculum, presubiculum, postsubiculum, and parasubiculum in human, monkey, and rodent. *J Comp Neurol* 521:4145–4162.

Ding SL, Royall JJ, Sunkin SM, Ng L, Facer BA, Lesnar P, Guillozet-Bongaarts A, McMurray B, Szafer A, Dolbeare TA, Stevens A, Tirrell L, Benner T, Caldejon S, Dalley RA, Dee N, Lau C, Nyhus J, Reding M, Riley ZL, et al. (2016) Comprehensive cellular-resolution atlas of the adult human brain. *J Comp Neurol* 524:3127–3481.

Ding SL, Van Hoesen GW (2010) Borders, extent, and topography of human perirhinal cortex as revealed using multiple modern neuroanatomical and pathological markers. *Hum Brain Mapp* 31:1359–1379.

Doan TP, Lagartos-Donate MJ, Nilssen ES, Ohara S, Witter MP (2019) Convergent projections from perirhinal and postrhinal cortices suggest a multisensory nature of lateral, but not medial, entorhinal cortex. *Cell Rep* 29:617–627, e617.

Dolleman-Van der Weel MJ, Witter MP (2000) Nucleus reuniens thalami innervates gamma aminobutyric acid positive cells in hippocampal field CA1 of the rat. *Neurosci Lett* 278:145–148.

Dolorfo CL, Amaral DG (1998) Entorhinal cortex of the rat: topographic organization of the cells of origin of the perforant path projection to the dentate gyrus. *J Comp Neurol* 398:25–48.

Dong HW, Swanson LW, Chen L, Fanselow MS, Toga AW (2009) Genomic-anatomic evidence for distinct functional domains in hippocampal field CA1. *Proc Natl Acad Sci U S A* 106:11794–11799.

Donovan MK, Wyss JM (1983) Evidence for some collateralization between cortical and diencephalic efferent axons of the rat subicular cortex. *Brain Res* 259:181–192.

Drake CT, Chavkin C, Milner TA (2007) Opioid systems in the dentate gyrus. *Prog Brain Res* 163:245–263.

Druckmann S, Feng L, Lee B, Yook C, Zhao T, Magee JC, Kim J (2014) Structured synaptic connectivity between hippocampal regions. *Neuron* 81:629–640.

Duffy CJ, Rakic P (1983) Differentiation of granule cell dendrites in the dentate gyrus of the rhesus monkey: a quantitative Golgi study. *J Comp Neurol* 214:224–237.

Duvernoy HM (1988) The Human Hippocampus. München: J.F. Bergman.

Ellegood J, Anagnostou E, Babineau BA, Crawley JN, Lin L, Genestine M, DiCicco-Bloom E, Lai JK, Foster JA, Penagarikano O, Geschwind DH, Pacey LK, Hampson DR, Laliberte CL, Mills AA, Tam E, Osborne LR, Kouser M, Espinosa-Becerra F, Xuan Z, et al. (2015) Clustering autism: using neuroanatomical differences in 26 mouse models to gain insight into the heterogeneity. *Mol Psychiatry* 20:118–125.

Empson RM, Heinemann U (1995a) Perforant path connections to area CA1 are predominantly inhibitory in the rat hippocampal-entorhinal cortex combined slice preparation. *Hippocampus* 5:104–107.

Empson RM, Heinemann U (1995b) The perforant path projection to hippocampal area CA1 in the rat hippocampal-entorhinal cortex combined slice. *J Physiol* 484 (Pt 3):707–720.

Espinoza C, Guzman SJ, Zhang X, Jonas P (2018) Parvalbumin (+) interneurons obey unique connectivity rules and establish a powerful lateral-inhibition microcircuit in dentate gyrus. *Nat Commun* 9:4605.

Eyre MD, Bartos M (2019) Somatostatin-expressing interneurons form axonal projections to the contralateral hippocampus. *Front Neural Circuits* 13:56.

Felleman DJ, Van Essen DC (1991) Distributed hierarchical processing in the primate cerebral cortex. *Cereb Cortex* 1:1–47.

Freund TF, Buzsaki G (1996) Interneurons of the hippocampus [review]. *Hippocampus* 6:347–470.

Fricke R, Cowan, WM (1978) An autoradiographic study of the commissural and ipsilateral hippocampo-dentate projections in the adult rat. *J Comp Neurol* 181:253–269.

Frotscher M, Seress L, Schwerdtfeger WK, Buhl EH (1991) The mossy cells of the fascia dentata: a comparative study of their fine structure and synaptic connections in rodents and primates. *J Comp Neurol* 312 (1):145-63. doi: 10.1002/cne.903120111. PMID: 1744242.

Funahashi M, Stewart M (1997) Presubicular and parasubicular cortical neurons of the rat—electrophysiological and morphological properties. *Hippocampus* 7:117–129.

Furtak SC, Wei SM, Agster KL, Burwell RD (2007) Functional neuroanatomy of the parahippocampal region in the rat: the perirhinal and postrhinal cortices. *Hippocampus* 17:709–722.

Gaarskjaer FB (1978a) Organization of the mossy fiber system of the rat studied in extended hippocampi: I. Terminal area related to number of granule and pyramidal cells. *J Comp Neurol* 178:49–72.

Gaarskjaer FB (1978b) Organization of the mossy fiber system of the rat studied in extended hippocampi: II. Experimental analysis of fiber distribution with silver impregnation methods. *J Comp Neurol* 178:73–88.

Gaarskjaer FB (1981) The hippocampal mossy fiber system of the rat studied with retrograde tracing techniques: correlation between topographic organization and neurogenetic gradients. *J Comp Neurol* 203:717–735.

Gandolfi D, Mapelli J, Solinas SMG, Triebkorn P, D'Angelo E, Jirsa V, Migliore M (2023) Full-scale scaffold model of the human hippocampus CA1 area. *Nat Comput Sci* 3:264–276.

Garcia AD, Buffalo EA (2020) Anatomy and function of the primate entorhinal cortex. *Annu Rev Vis Sci* 6:411–432.

Gaykema RPA, Luiten PGM, Nyakas C, Traber J (1990) Cortical projection patterns of the medial septum-diagonal band complex. *J Comp Neurol* 293:103–124.

Gertz SD, Lindenberg, R., Piavis, GW (1972) Structural variations in the rostral human hippocampus. *Johns Hopkins Med J* 130:367–376.

Geuze E, Vermetten E, Bremner JD (2005) MR-based in vivo hippocampal volumetrics:1. Review of methodologies currently employed. *Mol Psychiatry* 10:147–159.

Gloor P, Salanova, V., Olivier A., and Quesnay, L.F (1993) The human dorsal hippocampal commissure: an anatomically identifiable and functional pathway. *Brain* 116:1249–1273.

Gloveli T, Schmitz D, Empson RM, Dugladze T, Heinemann U (1997) Morphological and electrophysiological characterization of layer III cells of the medial entorhinal cortex of the rat. *Neuroscience* 77:629–648.

Goldowitz D, White WF, Steward O, Lynch G, Cotman C (1975) Anatomical evidence for a projection from the entorhinal cortex to the contralateral dentate gyrus of the rat. *Exp Neurol* 47:433–441.

Gomez-Isla, T, Price, JL, McKeel, DW, Jr. Morris, JC, Growdon, JH, Hyman BT (1996) Profound loss of layer II entorhinal cortex neurons occurs in very mild Alzheimer's disease. *J Neurosci* 16(14): 4491–4500.

González-Arnay E, Pérez-Santos I, Jiménez-Sánchez L, Cid E, Gal B, de la Prida LM, Cavada C. Immunohistochemical field parcellation of the human hippocampus along its antero-posterior axis. *Brain Struct Funct.* 2024 Mar;229(2):359–385. doi: 10.1007/s00429-023-02725-9. Epub 2024 Jan 5. PMID: 38180568; PMCID: PMC10917878.

Goubran M, Bernhardt BC, Cantor-Rivera D, Lau JC, Blinston C, Hammond RR, de Ribaupierre S, Burneo JG, Mirsattari SM, Steven DA, Parrent AG, Bernasconi A, Bernasconi N, Peters TM, Khan AR (2016) In vivo MRI signatures of hippocampal subfield pathology in intractable epilepsy. *Hum Brain Mapp* 37:1103–1119.

Greene JRT, Totterdell S (1997) Morphology and distribution of electrophysiologically defined classes of pyramidal and nonpyramidal neurons in rat ventral subiculum in vitro. *J Comp Neurol* 380: 395–408.

Groenewegen HJ, Vermeulen-Van Der Zee E, Te Kortschot A, Witter M (1987) Organization of the projections from the subiculum to the ventral striatum in the rat: a study using anterograde transport of Phaseolus Vulgaris leucoagglutinin. *Neuroscience* 23:103–120.

Guzman SJ, Schlogl A, Frotscher M, Jonas P (2016) Synaptic mechanisms of pattern completion in the hippocampal CA3 network. *Science* 353:1117–1123.

Haglund L, Swanson, LW, Kohler, C (1984) The projection of the supramammillary nucleus to the hippocampal formation: an immunohistochemical and anterograde transport study with the lectin PHA-L in the rat. *J Comp Neurol* 229:171–185.

Halasy K, Buhl EH, Lorinczi Z, Tamas G, Somogyi P (1996) Synaptic target selectivity and input of GABAergic basket and bistratified interneurons in the CA1 Area of the Rat Hippocampus. *Hippocampus* 6:306–329.

Han ZS, Buhl EH, Lorinczi Z, Somogyi P (1993) A high degree of spatial selectivity in the axonal and dendritic domains of physiologically identified local-circuit neurons in the dentate gyrus of the rat hippocampus. *Eur J Neurosci* 5:395–410.

Hara Y, Waters EM, McEwen BS, Morrison JH (2015) Estrogen effects on cognitive and synaptic health over the lifecourse. *Physiol Rev* 95:785–807.

Harding, AJ, Halliday GM, Kril JJ (1998) Variation in hippocampal neuron number with age and brain volume. *Cereb Cortex* 8:710–718.

Harris E, Witter MP, Weinstein G, Stewart M (2001) Intrinsic connectivity of the rat subiculum: I. Dendritic morphology and patterns of axonal arborization by pyramidal neurons. *J Comp Neurol* 435:490–505.

Harris KM, Jensen FE, Tsao B (1992) Three-dimensional structure of dendritic spines and synapses in rat hippocampus (CA1) at postnatal day 15 and adult ages: implications for the maturation of synaptic physiology and long-term potentiation. *J Neurosci* 12:2685–2705.

Hartig R, Glen D, Jung B, Logothetis NK, Paxinos G, Garza-Villarreal EA, Messinger A, Evrard HC (2021) The subcortical atlas of the rhesus macaque (SARM) for neuroimaging. *Neuroimage* 235:117996.

Hashimotodani Y, Karube F, Yanagawa Y, Fujiyama F, Kano M (2018) Supramammillary nucleus afferents to the dentate gyrus co-release glutamate and GABA and potentiate granule cell output. *Cell Rep* 25:2704–2715, e2704.

Haug F-MS (1976) Sulphide silver pattern and cytoarchitectonics of parahippocampal areas in the rat. In: Advances in Anatomy Embryology and Cell Biology (Brodal A, Hild W, van Limborgh J, et al., eds), vol 52, p 73. Berlin, Springer-Verlag.

Hausheer-Zarmakupi Z, Wolfer DP, Leisinger-Trigona MC, Lipp HP (1996) Selective breeding for extremes in open-field activity of mice entails a differentiation of hippocampal mossy fibers. *Behav Genet* 26:167–176.

Hawrylycz MJ, Lein ES, Guillozet-Bongaarts AL, Shen EH, Ng L, Miller JA, van de Lagemaat LN, Smith KA, Ebbert A, Riley ZL, Abajian C, Beckmann CF, Bernard A, Bertagnolli D, Boe AF, Cartagena PM, Chakravarty MM, Chapin M, Chong J, Dalley RA, et al. (2012) An anatomically comprehensive atlas of the adult human brain transcriptome. *Nature* 489:391–399.

Henze DA, Urban NN, Barrioneuvo G (2000) The multifarious hippocampal mossy fleer pathway: a review. *Neuroscience* 98:407–427.

Herkenham M (1978) The connections of the nucleus reuniens thalami: evidence for a direct thalamo-hippocampal pathway in the rat. *J Comp Neurol* 177:589–610.

Hjorth-Simonsen A, Jeune B (1972) Origin and termination of the hippocampal perforant path in the rat studied by silver impregnation. *J Comp Neurol* 144:215–232.

Hjorth-Simonsen A, Zimmer J (1975) Crossed pathways from the entorhinal area to the fascia dentata. *J Comp Neurol* 161:57–70.

Houser CR (2007) Interneurons of the dentate gyrus: an overview of cell types, terminal fields and neurochemical identity. *Prog Brain Res* 163:217–232.

Hunsaker MR, Amaral DG (2014) A semi-automated pipeline for the segmentation of rhesus macaque hippocampus: validation across a wide age range. *PLoS One* 9:e89456.

Hunsaker MR, Scott JA, Bauman MD, Schumann CM, Amaral DG (2014) Postnatal development of the hippocampus in the Rhesus macaque (Macaca mulatta): a longitudinal magnetic resonance imaging study. *Hippocampus* 24:794–807.

Huntgeburth SC, Petrides M (2016) Three-dimensional probability maps of the rhinal and the collateral sulci in the human brain. *Brain Struct Funct* 221:4235–4255.

Insausti R, Amaral DG (2012) Hippocampal Formation. San Diego: Academic Press.

Insausti R, Amaral DG, Cowan WM (1987) The entorhinal cortex of the monkey: II. Cortical afferents. *J Comp Neurol* 264:356–395.

Insausti R, Corcoles-Parada M, Ubero MM, Rodado A, Insausti AM, Munoz-Lopez M (2019) Cytoarchitectonic areas of the gyrus ambiens in the human brain. *Front Neuroanat* 13:21.

Insausti R, Herrero MT, Witter MP (1997) Entorhinal cortex of the rat: cytoarchitectonic subdivisions and the origin and distribution of cortical efferents. *Hippocampus* 7:146–183.

Insausti R, Juottonen K, Soininen H, Insausti AM, Partanen K, Vainio P, Laakso MP, Pitkanen A (1998) MR volumetric analysis of the human entorhinal, perirhinal, and temporopolar cortices. *Am J Neuroradiol* 19:659–671.

Insausti R, Munoz-Lopez M, Insausti AM (2023) The CA2 hippocampal subfield in humans: a review. *Hippocampus* 33:712–729.

Insausti R, Munoz-Lopez M, Insausti AM, Artacho-Perula E (2017) The human periallocortex: layer pattern in presubiculum, parasubiculum and entorhinal cortex: a review. *Front Neuroanat* 11:84.

Insausti R, Tunon T, Sobreviela T, Insausti AM, Gonzalo LM (1995) The human entorhinal cortex: a cytoarchitectonic analysis. *J Comp Neurol* 355:171–198.

Ishizuka N (2001) Laminar organization of the pyramidal cell layer of the subiculum in the rat. *J Comp Neurol* 435:89–110.

Ishizuka N, Cowan WM, Amaral DG (1995) A quantitative analysis of the dendritic organization of pyramidal cells in the rat hippocampus. *J Comp Neurol* 362:17–45.

Ishizuka N, Weber J, Amaral DG (1990) Organization of intrahippocampal projections originating from CA3 pyramidal cells in the rat. *J Comp Neurol* 295:580–623.

Jabès A, Banta Lavenex P, Amaral, DG, Lavenex, P (2011) Postnatal development of the hippocampal formation: A stereological study in macaque monkeys. *J Comp Neurol* 519(6):1051–1070.

Jack CR, Jr, Petersen RC, Xu YC, Waring SC, O'Brien PC, Tangalos EG, Smith GE, Ivnik RJ, Kokmen E (1997) Medial temporal atrophy on MRI in normal aging and very mild Alzheimer's disease. *Neurology* 49:786–794.

Jay TM, Witter MP (1991) Distribution of hippocampal CA1 and subicular efferents in the prefrontal cortex of the rat studied by means of anterograde transport of Phaseolus vulgaris-leucoagglutinin. *J Comp Neurol* 313:574–586.

Juottonen K, Laakso MP, Insausti R, Lehtovirta M, Pitkanen A, Partanen K, Soininen H (1998) Volumes of the entorhinal and perirhinal cortices in Alzheimer's disease. *Neurobiol Aging* 19:15–22.

Kaitz SS, Robertson RT (1981) Thalamic connections with limbic cortex: II. Corticothalamic projections. *J Comp Neurol* 195:527–545.

Karat BG, DeKraker J, Hussain U, Kohler S, Khan AR (2023) Mapping the macrostructure and microstructure of the in vivo human hippocampus using diffusion MRI. *Hum Brain Mapp* 44:5485–5503.

Kealy J, Commins S (2011) The rat perirhinal cortex: a review of anatomy, physiology, plasticity, and function. *Prog Neurobiol* 93:522–548.

Kempermann G, Brandon EP, Gage FH (1998a) Environmental stimulation of 129/SvJ mice causes increased cell proliferation and neurogenesis in the adult dentate gyrus. *Curr Biol* 8:939–942.

Kempermann G, Kuhn HG, Gage FH (1998b) Experience-induced neurogenesis in the senescent dentate gyrus. *J Neurosci* 18:3206–3212.

Kempermann G, Song H, Gage FH (2015) Neurogenesis in the adult hippocampus. *Cold Spring Harb Perspect Biol* 7:a018812.

Kerr KM, Agster KL, Furtak SC, Burwell RD (2007) Functional neuroanatomy of the parahippocampal region: the lateral and medial entorhinal areas. *Hippocampus* 17:697–708.

Kiss J, Csaki A, Bokor H, Shanabrough M, Leranth C (2000) The supramamillo-hippocampal and supramammillo-septal glutamatergic/aspartatergic projections in the rat: a combined. *Neuroscience* 97:657–669.

Kloosterman F, Witter Menno P, van Haeften T (2003) Topographical and laminar organization of subicular projections to the parahippocampal region of the rat. *J Comp Neurol* [print] 455:156–171.

Kobayashi Y, Amaral DG (1999) The hippocampal formation and perirhinal and parahippocampal cortices. In: Handbook of Chemical Neuroanatomy (B R, Björklund A, Hökfelt T, eds), pp 285–401. Amsterdam: Elsevier Science Publishers.

Kobayashi Y, Amaral DG (2007) Macaque monkey retrosplenial cortex: III. Cortical efferents. *J Comp Neurol* 502:810–833.

Kohara K, Pignatelli M, Rivest AJ, Jung HY, Kitamura T, Suh J, Frank D, Kajikawa K, Mise N, Obata Y, Wickersham IR, Tonegawa S (2014) Cell type-specific and genetic and optogenetic tools reveal hippocampal CA2 circuits. *Nat Neurosci* 17:269–279.

Kohler C (1985) Intrinsic projections of the retrohippocampal region in the rat brain: I. The subicular complex. *J Comp Neurol* **236**:504–522.

Kohler C, Steinbusch H (1982) Identification of serotonin and non-serotonin-containing neurons of the mid- brain raphe projecting to the entorhinal area and the hippocampal formation: a combined immunohistochemical and fluorescent retrograde tracing. *Neuroscience* 7:951–975.

Kondo H, Lavenex P, Amaral DG (2008) Intrinsic connections of the macaque monkey hippocampal formation: I. Dentate gyrus. *J Comp Neurol* **511**:497–520.

Kondo H, Lavenex P, Amaral DG (2009) Intrinsic connections of the macaque monkey hippocampal formation: II. CA3 connections. *J Comp Neurol* **515**:349–377.

Kyle CT, Stokes J, Bennett J, Meltzer J, Permenter MR, Vogt JA, Ekstrom A, Barnes CA (2019) Cytoarchitectonically-driven MRI atlas of nonhuman primate hippocampus: preservation of subfield volumes in aging. *Hippocampus* **29**:409–421.

Laatsch RH, Cowan WM (1967) Electron microscopic studies of the dentate gyrus of the rat: II. Degeneration of commissural afferents. *J Comp Neurol* **130**:241–262.

Lacaille JC, Mueller AL, Kunkel DD, Schwartzkroin PA (1987) Local circuit interactions between oriens/alveus interneurons and CA1 pyramidal cells in hippocampal slices: electrophysiology and morphology. *J Neurosci* 7:1979–1993.

Lavenex P, Amaral DG (2000) Hippocampal-neocortical interaction: a hierarchy of associativity. *Hippocampus* **10**:420–430.

Lavenex P, Suzuki WA, Amaral DG (2002) Perirhinal and parahippocampal cortices of the macaque monkey: projections to the neocortex. *J Comp Neurol* **447**:394–420.

Le Duigou C, Simonnet J, Telenczuk MT, Fricker D, Miles R (2014) Recurrent synapses and circuits in the CA3 region of the hippocampus: an associative network. *Front Cell Neurosci* 7:262.

Lein ES, Callaway EM, Albright TD, Gage FH (2005) Redefining the boundaries of the hippocampal CA2 subfield in the mouse using gene expression and 3-dimensional reconstruction. *J Comp Neurol* **485**:1–10.

Lein ES, Hawrylycz MJ, Ao N, Ayres M, Bensinger A, Bernard A, Boe AF, Boguski MS, Brockway KS, Byrnes EJ, Chen L, Chen L, Chen TM, Chin MC, Chong J, Crook BE, Czaplinska A, Dang CN, Datta S, Dee NR, et al. (2007) Genome-wide atlas of gene expression in the adult mouse brain. *Nature* **445**:168–176.

Lein ES, Zhao X, Gage FH (2004) Defining a molecular atlas of the hippocampus using DNA microarrays and high-throughput in situ hybridization. *J Neurosci* **24**:3879–3889.

Li X-G, Somogyi P, Ylinen A, Buzsaki G (1994) The hippocampal CA3 network: an in vivo intracellular labeling study. *J Comp Neurol* **339**:181–208.

Lim C, Blume HW, Madsen JR, Saper CB (1997) Connections of the hippocampal formation in humans: I. The mossy fiber pathway. *J Comp Neurol* **385**:325–351.

Lim C, Mufson EJ, Kordower JH, Blume HW, Madsen JR, Saper CB (1997) Connections of the hippocampal formation in humans: II. The endfolial fiber pathway. *J Comp Neurol* **385**:352–371.

Lin X, Amalraj M, Blanton C, Avila B, Holmes TC, Nitz DA, Xu X (2021) Noncanonical projections to the hippocampal CA3 regulate spatial learning and memory by modulating the feedforward hippocampal trisynaptic pathway. *PLoS Biol* **19**:e3001127.

Lin X, Cyrus N, Avila B, Holmes TC, Xu X (2023) Hippocampal CA3 inhibitory neurons receive extensive noncanonical synaptic inputs from CA1 and subicular complex. *J Comp Neurol* **531**:1333–1347.

Lipp HP, Schwegler H, Heimrich B, Cerbone A, Sadile AG (1987) Strain-specific correlations between hippocampal structural traits and habituation in a spatial novelty situation. *Behav Brain Res* **24**:111–123.

Lorente de Nó R (1934) Studies on the structure of the cerebral cortex: II. Continuation of the study of the ammonic system. *J Psychol Neurol* **46**:113–177.

Loughlin SE, Foote SL, Bloom FE (1986) Efferent projections of nucleus locus coeruleus: topographic organization of cells of origin demonstrated by three-dimensional reconstruction. *Neuroscience* **18**:291–306.

Luine V, Frankfurt M (2020) Estrogenic regulation of memory: the first 50 years. *Horm Behav* **121**:104711.

Magloczky Z, Acsady L, Freund TF (1994) Principal cells are the postsynaptic targets of supramammillary afferents in the hippocampus of the rat. *Hippocampus* **4**:322–334.

Mai J, Majtanik M, Paxinos G (2015) Atlas of the Human Brain. Academic Press.

Malik R, Dougherty KA, Parikh K, Byrne C, Johnston D (2016) Mapping the electrophysiological and morphological properties of CA1 pyramidal neurons along the longitudinal hippocampal axis. *Hippocampus* **26**:341–361.

Martin EA, Woodruff D, Rawson RL, Williams ME (2017) Examining hippocampal mossy fiber synapses by 3D electron microscopy in wildtype and kirrel3 knockout mice. *eNeuro* 4.

Masurkar AV, Srinivas KV, Brann DH, Warren R, Lowes DC, Siegelbaum SA (2017) Medial and lateral entorhinal cortex differentially excite deep versus superficial CA1 pyramidal neurons. *Cell Rep* **18**:148–160.

McEwen BS, Milner TA (2017) Understanding the broad influence of sex hormones and sex differences in the brain. *J Neurosci Res* **95**:24–39.

McEwen BS, Nasca C, Gray JD (2016) Stress effects on neuronal structure: hippocampus, amygdala, and prefrontal cortex. *Neuropsychopharmacology* **41**:3–23.

McEwen BS, Wallach G (1973) Corticosterone binding to hippocampus: nuclear and cytosol binding in vitro. *Brain Res* **57**:373–386.

McEwen BS, Weiss JM, Schwartz LS (1968) Selective retention of corticosterone by limbic structures in rat brain. *Nature* **220**:911–912.

McLardy T, Kilmer WL (1970) Hippocampal circuitry. *Am Psychol* **25**:563–566.

Meng Y, Payne C, Li L, Hu X, Zhang X, Bachevalier J (2014) Alterations of hippocampal projections in adult macaques with neonatal hippocampal lesions: a diffusion tensor imaging study. *Neuroimage* **102** Pt 2:828–837.

Merrill DA, Chiba AA, Tuszynski MH (2001) Conservation of neuronal number and size in the entorhinal cortex of behaviorally characterized aged rats. *J Comp Neurol* **438**(4):445–456.

Middleton SJ, McHugh TJ (2020) CA2: a highly connected intrahippocampal relay. *Annu Rev Neurosci* **43**:55–72.

Miyashita Y (2019) Perirhinal circuits for memory processing. *Nat Rev Neurosci* **20**:577–592.

Mizuseki K, Diba K, Pastalkova E, Buzsaki G (2011) Hippocampal CA1 pyramidal cells form functionally distinct sublayers. *Nat Neurosci* **14**:1174–1181.

Modo M, Sparling K, Novotny J, Perry N, Foley LM, Hitchens TK (2023) Mapping mesoscale connectivity within the human hippocampus. *Neuroimage* **282**:120406.

Mohedano-Moriano A, Pro-Sistiaga P, Arroyo-Jimenez MM, Artacho-Perula E, Insausti AM, Marcos P, Cebada-Sanchez S, Martinez-Ruiz J, Munoz M, Blaizot X, Martinez-Marcos A, Amaral DG, Insausti R (2007) Topographical and laminar distribution of cortical input to the monkey entorhinal cortex. *J Anat* **211**:250–260.

Morey RA, Petty CM, Xu Y, Hayes JP, Wagner HR, 2nd, Lewis DV, LaBar KS, Styner M, McCarthy G (2009) A comparison of automated segmentation and manual tracing for quantifying hippocampal and amygdala volumes. *Neuroimage* 45:855–866.

Mosko S, Lynch G, Cotman CW (1973) The distribution of septal projections to the hippocampus of the rat. *J Comp Neurol* 152:163–174.

Mulders WH, West MJ, Slomianka L(1997) Neuron numbers in the presubiculum, parasubiculum, and entorhinal area of the rat. *J Comp Neurol* 385(1):83–94.

Munoz M, Insausti R (2005) Cortical efferents of the entorhinal cortex and the adjacent parahippocampal region in the monkey (*Macaca fascicularis*). *Eur J Neurosci* 22:1368–1388.

Naber PA, da Silva FHL, Witter MP (2001a) Reciprocal connections between the entorhinal cortex and hippocampal fields CA1 and the subiculum are in register with the projections from CA1 to the subiculum. *Hippocampus* 11:99–104.

Naber PA, Witter MP (1998) Subicular efferents are organized mostly as parallel projections: a double-labeling, retrograde-tracing study in the rat. *J Comp Neurol* 393:284–297.

Naber PA, Witter MP, da Silva FHL (2001b) Evidence for a direct projection from the postrhinal cortex to the subiculum in the rat. *Hippocampus* 11:105–117.

Nafstad PHJ (1967) An electron microscope study on the termination of the perforant path fibres in the hippocampus and the fascia dentata. *Zeitschrift Fur Zellforschung Und Mikroskopische Anatomie* 76:532–542.

Ni R (2021) Magnetic resonance imaging in tauopathy animal models. *Front Aging Neurosci* 13:791679.

Nilssen ES, Doan TP, Nigro MJ, Ohara S, Witter MP (2019) Neurons and networks in the entorhinal cortex: a reappraisal of the lateral and medial entorhinal subdivisions mediating parallel cortical pathways. *Hippocampus* 29:1238–1254.

Ohara S, Gianatti M, Itou K, Berndtsson CH, Doan TP, Kitanishi T, Mizuseki K, Iijima T, Tsutsui KI, Witter MP (2019) Entorhinal layer II calbindin-expressing neurons originate widespread telencephalic and intrinsic projections. *Front Syst Neurosci* 13:54.

O'Reilly KC, Gulden Dahl A, Ulsaker Kruge I, Witter MP (2013) Subicular-parahippocampal projections revisited: development of a complex topography in the rat. *J Comp Neurol* 521:4284–4299.

Papp EA, Leergaard TB, Calabrese E, Johnson GA, Bjaalie JG (2014) Waxholm space atlas of the Sprague Dawley rat brain. *Neuroimage* 97:374–386.

Payne C, Machado CJ, Bliwise NG, Bache valier J (2010) Maturation of the hippocampal formation and amygdala in Macaca mulatta: a volumetric magnetic resonance imaging study. *Hippocampus* 20:922–935.

Pickel VM, Segal M, Bloom FE (1974) A radioautographic study of the efferent pathways of the nucleus locus coeruleus. *J Comp Neurol* 155:15–42.

Piguet O, Chareyron LJ, Banta Lavenex P, Amaral DG, Lavenex, P (2020) Postnatal development of the entorhinal cortex: A stereological study in macaque monkeys. *J Comp Neurol* 528(14):2308–2332.

Pikkarainen M, Ronkko S, Savander V, Insausti R, Pitkanen A (1999) Projections from the lateral, basal, and accessory basal nuclei of the amygdala to the hippocampal formation in rat. *J Comp Neurol* 403:229–260.

Pirker S, Schwarzer C, Wieselthaler A, Sieghart W, Sperk G (2000) GABA(A) receptors: immunocytochemical distribution of 13 subunits in the adult rat brain. *Neuroscience* 101:815–850.

Piskorowski RA, Chevaleyre V (2018) Memory circuits: CA2. *Curr Opin Neurobiol* 52:54–59.

Pitkänen A, Pikkarainen M, Nurminen N, Ylinen A (2000) Reciprocal connections between the amygdala and the hippocampal

formation, perirhinal cortex, and postrhinal cortex in rat: a review. *Ann N Y Acad Sci* 911.

Postans M, Parker GD, Lundell H, Ptito M, Hamandi K, Gray WP, Aggleton JP, Dyrby TB, Jones DK, Winter M (2020) Uncovering a role for the dorsal hippocampal commissure in recognition memory. *Cereb Cortex* 30:1001–1015.

Pruessner JC, Li LM, Serles W, Pruessner M, Collins DL, Kabani N, Lupien S, Evans AC (2000) Volumetry of hippocampus and amygdala with high-resolution MRI and three-dimensional analysis software: minimizing the discrepancies between laboratories. *Cereb Cortex* 10:433–442.

Pyapali GK, Sik A, Penttonen M, Buzsaki G, Turner DA (1998) Dendritic properties of hippocampal CA1 pyramidal neurons in the rat: intracellular staining in vivo and in vitro. *J Comp Neurol* 391:335–352.

Qiu LR, Germann J, Spring S, Alm C, Vousden DA, Palmert MR, Lerch JP (2013) Hippocampal volumes differ across the mouse estrous cycle, can change within 24 hours, and associate with cognitive strategies. *Neuroimage* 83:593–598.

Qiu S, Hu Y, Huang Y, Gao T, Wang X, Wang D, Ren B, Shi X, Chen Y, Wang X, Wang D, Han L, Liang Y, Liu D, Liu Q, Deng L, Chen Z, Zhan L, Chen T, Huang Y, et al. (2024) Whole-brain spatial organization of hippocampal single-neuron projectomes. *Science* 383:eadj9198.

Quilichini P, Sirota A, Buzsaki G (2010) Intrinsic circuit organization and theta-gamma oscillation dynamics in the entorhinal cortex of the rat. *J Neurosci* 30:11128–11142.

Raisman G, Cowan WM, Powell TPS (1965) The extrinsic afferent, commissural and association fibres of the hippocampus. *Brain* 88:963–997.

Rama S, Jensen TP, Rusakov DA (2019) Glutamate imaging reveals multiple sites of stochastic release in the CA3 giant mossy fiber boutons. *Front Cell Neurosci* 13:243.

Ramón y Cajal S (1893) Estructura del asta de Ammon y fascia dentata. *Ann Soc Esp Hist Nat* 22.

Ramón y Cajal S (1901–1902) Sobre un ganglio especial de la corteza esfeno-occipital. *Trab Lab Invest Biol Univ Madrid* 1:189–206.

Rapp PR, Gallagher M (1996) Preserved neuron number in the hippocampus of aged rats with spatial learning deficits. *Proc Natl Acad Sci U S A* 93:9926–9930.

Ribak CE, Seress L (1983) Five types of basket cell in the hippocampal dentate gyrus: a combined Golgi and electron microscopic study. *J Neurocytol* 12:577–597.

Ribak CE, Seress L, Amaral DG (1985) The development, ultrastructure and synaptic connections of the mossy cells of the dentate gyrus. *J Neurocytol* 14:835–857.

Ribak CE, Vaughn JE, Saito K (1978) Immunocytochemical localization of glutamic acid decarboxylase in neuronal somata following colchicine inhibition of axonal transport. *Brain Res* 140:315–332.

Rigby M, Grillo FW, Compans B, Neves G, Gallinaro J, Nashashibi S, Horton S, Pereira Machado PM, Carbajal MA, Vizcay-Barrena G, Levet F, Sibarita JB, Kirkland A, Fleck RA, Clopath C, Burrone J (2023) Multi-synaptic boutons are a feature of CA1 hippocampal connections in the stratum oriens. *Cell Rep* 42:112397.

Robert V, Cassim S, Chevaleyre V, Piskorowski RA (2018) Hippocampal area CA2: properties and contribution to hippocampal function. *Cell Tissue Res* 373:525–540.

Robertson RT, Kaitz SS (1981) Thalamic connections with limbic cortex: I. Thalamocortical projections. *J Comp Neurol* 195:501–525.

Rose M (1927) Die sog: Riechrinde beim Menschem und beim Aften: II. Teil des "Allocortex bei Tier und Mensch." *J Psychol Neurol* 34:261–401.

Rowland DC, Weible AP, Wickersham IR, Wu H, Mayford M, Witter MP, Kentros CG (2013) Transgenically targeted rabies virus demonstrates a major monosynaptic projection from hippocampal area CA2 to medial entorhinal layer II neurons. *J Neurosci* **33**:14889–14898.

Ruth RE, Collier TJ, Routtenberg A (1982) Topography between the entorhinal cortex and the dentate septotemporal axis in rats: I. Medial and intermediate entorhinal projecting cells. *J Comp Neurol* **209**:69–78.

Ruth RE, Collier TJ, Routtenberg A (1988) Topographical relationship between the entorhinal cortex and the septotemporal axis of the dentate gyrus in rats: II. Cells projecting from lateral entorhinal subdivisions. *J Comp Neurol* **270**:506–516.

Sakamoto R, Marano C, Miller MI, Lyketsos CG, Li Y, Mori S, Oishi K, Adni A (2019) Cloud-based brain magnetic resonance image segmentation and parcellation system for individualized prediction of cognitive worsening. *J Healthc Eng* **2019**:9507193.

Sammons RP, Vezir M, Moreno-Velasquez L, Cano G, Orlando M, Sievers M, Grasso E, Metodieva VD, Kempter R, Schmidt H, Schmitz D (2024) Structure and function of the hippocampal CA3 module. *Proc Natl Acad Sci U S A* **121**:e2312281120.

Sanchez-Bellot C, AlSubaie R, Mishchanchuk K, Wee RWS, MacAskill AF (2022) Two opposing hippocampus to prefrontal cortex pathways for the control of approach and avoidance behaviour. *Nat Commun* **13**:339.

Scharfman HE (2007) The CA3 "backprojection" to the dentate gyrus. *Prog Brain Res* **163**:627–637.

Scharfman HE (2016) The enigmatic mossy cell of the dentate gyrus. *Nat Rev Neurosci* **17**:562–575.

Scharfman HE (2018) Advances in understanding hilar mossy cells of the dentate gyrus. *Cell Tissue Res* **373**:643–652.

Scheel N, Wulff P, de Mooij-van Malsen JG (2020) Afferent connections of the thalamic nucleus reuniens in the mouse. *J Comp Neurol* **528**:1189–1202.

Scheibel ME, Crandall PH, Scheibel AB (1974) The hippocampal-dentate complex in temporal lobe epilepsy: a Golgi study. *Epilepsia* **15**:55–80.

Schlessinger AR, Cowan WM, Swanson LW (1978) The time of origin of neurons in Ammon's horn and the associated retrohippocampal fields. *Anat Embryol (Berl)* **154**(2):153–173.

Schultz C, Engelhardt M (2014) Anatomy of the hippocampal formation. *Front Neurol Neurosci* **34**:6–17.

Scorza CA, Araujo BH, Arida RM, Scorza FA, Torres LB, Amorim, HA, Cavalheiro EA (2010) Distinctive hippocampal CA2 subfield of the Amazon rodent Proechimys. *Neuroscience* **169**(3):965–973.

Seress L, Abraham H, Czeh B, Fuchs E, Leranth C (2008) Calretinin expression in hilar mossy cells of the hippocampal dentate gyrus of nonhuman primates and humans. *Hippocampus* **18**:425–434.

Seress L, Mrzljak, L. (1987) Basal dendrites of granule cells are normal features of the fetal and adult dentate gyrus of both monkey and human hippocampal formations. *Brain Res* **405**:169–174.

Seress L, Pokorny J (1981) Structure of the granular layer of the rat dentate gyrus: a light microscopic and golgi study. *J Anat* **133**:181–195.

Sheng M, Greenberg ME (1990) The regulation and function of c-fos and other immediate early genes in the nervous system. *Neuron* **4**:477–485.

Shi Y, Budin F, Yapuncich E, Rumple A, Young JT, Payne C, Zhang X, Hu X, Godfrey J, Howell B, Sanchez MM, Styner MA (2016) UNC-Emory infant atlases for macaque brain image analysis: postnatal brain development through 12 months. *Front Neurosci* **10**:617.

Shipley MT (1975) The topographical and laminar organization of the presubiculum's projection to the ipsi- and contralateral entorhinal cortex in the guinea pig. *J Comp Neurol* **160**:127–146.

Sik A, Penttonen M, Buzsaki G (1997) Interneurons in the hippocampal dentate gyrus—an in vivo intracellular study. *Eur J Neurosci* **9**:573–588.

Soriano E, Frotscher M (1989) A GABAergic axo-axonic cell in the fascia dentata controls the main excitatory hippocampal pathway. *Brain Res* **503**:170–174.

Sorra KE, Harris M (1993) Occurrence and three-dimensional structure of multiple synapses between individual radiatum axons and their target pyramidal cells in hippocampal area CA1. *J Neurosci* **13**:3736–3748.

Stephan H, Andy OJ (1970) The allocortex in primates. In: The Primate Brain (Noback CR, Montagna W, eds), vol 1, pp 109–135. New York: Appleton-Century-Crofts.

Stevens NA, Lankisch K, Draguhn A, Engelhardt M, Both M, Thome C (2024) Increased interhemispheric connectivity of a distinct type of hippocampal pyramidal cells. *J Neurosci* **44**.

Steward O, Scoville, SA (1976) Cells of origin of entorhinal cortical afferents to the hippocampus and fascia dentata of the rat. *J Comp Neurol* **169**:285–314.

Struble RG, Desmond NL, Levy WB (1978) Anatomical evidence for interlamellar inhibition in the fascia dentata. *Brain Res* **152**:580–585.

Sun Q, Sotayo A, Cazzulino AS, Snyder AM, Denny CA, Siegelbaum SA (2017) Proximodistal heterogeneity of hippocampal CA3 pyramidal neuron intrinsic properties, connectivity, and reactivation during memory recall. *Neuron* **95**:656–672, e653.

Sun Y, Grieco SF, Holmes TC, Xu X (2017) Local and long-range circuit connections to hilar mossy cells in the dentate gyrus. *eNeuro* **4**.

Surmeli G, Marcu DC, McClure C, Garden DLF, Pastoll H, Nolan MF (2015) Molecularly defined circuitry reveals input-output segregation in deep layers of the medial entorhinal cortex. *Neuron* **88**:1040–1053.

Suzuki WA (1996) Neuroanatomy of the monkey entorhinal, perirhinal and parahippocampal cortices: organization of cortical inputs and interconnections with amygdala and striatum. *Semin Neurosci* **8**:3–12.

Suzuki WA, Amaral DG (1994) Topographic organization of the reciprocal connections between the monkey entorhinal cortex and the perirhinal and parahippocampal cortices. *J Neurosci* **14**:1856–1877.

Swanson LW (1978) The anatomical organization of septo-hippocampal projections. In: Functions of the Septo-Hippocampal System (ed unknown), vol **58**, pp 25–48. Amsterdam: Elsevier North Holland.

Swanson LW, Cowan WM (1975) Hippocampus-hypothalamic connections: origin in subicular cortex, not Ammon's horn. *Science* **25**:303–304.

Swanson LW, Hartman BK (1975) The central adrenergic system: an immunofluorescence study of the location of cell bodies and their efferent connections in the rat utilizing dopamine-B- hydroxylase as a marker. *J Comp Neurol* **163**:467–506.

Swanson LW, Köhler, C., and Bjorklund, A. (1987) The limbic region: I. The septohippocampal system. In: Handbook of Chemical Neuroanatomy (Bjorklund A, Hokfelt T, Swanson LW, eds), vol **5**, part 1, pp 125–277.

Swanson LW, Sawchenko PE, Cowan WM (1981) Evidence for collateral projections by neurons in Ammon's horn, the dentate gyrus, and the subiculum: a multiple retrograde labeling study in the rat. *J Neurosci* **1**:548–559.

Swanson LW, Wyss JM, Cowan WM (1978) An autoradiographic study of the organization of intrahippocampal association pathways in the rat. *J Comp Neurol* **181**:681–716.

Tamamaki N, Abe K, Nojyo Y (1987) Columnar organization in the subiculum formed by axon branches originating from single CA1 pyramidal neurons in the rat hippocampus. *Brain Res* **412**:156–160.

Tamamaki N, Nojyo Y (1993) Projection of the entorhinal layer-II neurons in the rat as revealed by intracellular pressure-injection of neurobiotin. *Hippocampus* **3**:471–480.

Tamamaki N, Yanagawa Y, Tomioka R, Miyazaki J, Obata K, Kaneko T (2003) Green fluorescent protein expression and colocalization with calretinin, parvalbumin, and somatostatin in the GAD67-GFP knock-in mouse. *J Comp Neurol* **467**:60–79.

Tang Q, Burgalossi A, Ebbesen CL, Sanguinetti-Scheck JI, Schmidt H, Tukker JJ, Naumann R, Ray S, Preston-Ferrer P, Schmitz D, Brecht M (2016) Functional architecture of the rat parasubiculum. *J Neurosci* **36**:2289–2301.

Thompson CL, Pathak SD, Jeromin A, Ng LL, MacPherson CR, Mortrud MT, Cusick A, Riley ZL, Sunkin SM, Bernard A, Puchalski RB, Gage FH, Jones AR, Bajic VB, Hawrylycz MJ, Lein ES (2008) Genomic anatomy of the hippocampus. *Neuron* **60**:1010–1021.

Thompson SM, Robertson RT (1987) Organization of subcortical pathways for sensory projections to the limbic cortex: I. Subcortical projections to the medial limbic cortex in the rat. *J Comp Neurol* **265**:175–188.

Tomas Pereira I, Agster KL, Burwell RD (2016) Subcortical connections of the perirhinal, postrhinal, and entorhinal cortices of the rat: I. afferents. *Hippocampus* **26**:1189–1212.

Toni N, Schinder AF (2015) Maturation and functional integration of new granule cells into the adult hippocampus. *Cold Spring Harb Perspect Biol* **8**:a018903.

Van der Werf YD, Witter MP, Groenewegen HJ (2002) The intralaminar and midline nuclei of the thalamus: anatomical and functional evidence for participation in processes of arousal and awareness [review]. *Brain Res—Brain Res Rev* **39**:107–140.

van Dijk RM, Huang SH, Slomianka L, Amrein I (2016) Taxonomic separation of hippocampal networks: principal cell populations and adult neurogenesis. *Front Neuroanat* **10**:22.

van Groen T, Kadish I, Wyss JM (2002) Species differences in the projections from the entorhinal cortex to the hippocampus. *Brain Res Bull* **57**:553–556.

van Groen T, Miettinen P, Kadish I (2003) The entorhinal cortex of the mouse: organization of the projection to the hippocampal formation. *Hippocampus* **13**:133–149.

Van Groen T, Wyss JM (1988) Species differences in hippocampal commissural connections: studies in rat, guinea pig, rabbit, and cat. *J Comp Neurol* **267**:322–334.

Van Groen T, Wyss JM (1990) The connections of presubiculum and parasubiculum in the rat. *Brain Res* **518**:227–243.

van Strien NM, Cappaert NL, Witter MP (2009) The anatomy of memory: an interactive overview of the parahippocampal-hippocampal network. *Nat Rev Neurosci* **10**:272–282.

Vertes RP (2015) Major diencephalic inputs to the hippocampus: supramammillary nucleus and nucleus reuniens: circuitry and function. *Prog Brain Res* **219**:121–144.

Vertes RP, Fortin WJ, Crane AM (1999) Projections of the median raphe nucleus in the rat [review]. *J Comp Neurol* **407**:555–582.

Von Economo C (1929) The Cytoarchitectonics of the Human Cerebral Cortex. London; New York: Oxford University Press.

Walker MC, Ruiz A, Kullmann DM (2002) Do mossy fibers release GABA? *Epilepsia* **43**:196–202.

Wang N, White LE, Qi Y, Cofer G, Johnson GA (2020) Cytoarchitecture of the mouse brain by high resolution diffusion magnetic resonance imaging. *Neuroimage* **216**:116876.

Watanabe T, Frahm J, Michaelis T (2013) Cell layers and neuropil: contrast-enhanced MRI of mouse brain in vivo. *NMR Biomed* **26**:1870–1878.

West MJ, Slomianka L, Gundersen HJG (1991) Unbiased stereological estimation of the total number of neurons in the subdivisions of the rat hippocampus using the optical fractionator. *Anat Rec* **231**:482–497.

West, MJ, Slomianka L (1998) Total number of neurons in the layers of the human entorhinal cortex. *Hippocampus* **8**(1):69–82.

Wheeler DW, White CM, Rees CL, Komendantov AO, Hamilton DJ, Ascoli GA (2015) Hippocampome.org: a knowledge base of neuron types in the rodent hippocampus. *Elife* 4.

Wilson CO, Isokawa-Akesson M, Babb TL, Engel J, Jr., Cahan LD, Crandall PH (1987) Comparative view of local and interhemispheric limbic pathways in humans: an evoked potential analysis. In: Fundamental Mechanisms of Human Brain Function (Engel J, Jr, Ojemann GA, Lüders HO, Williamson PD, eds), pp 23–38. New York: Raven Press.

Wisse LE, Gerritsen L, Zwanenburg JJ, Kuijf HJ, Luijten PR, Biessels GJ, Geerlings MI (2012) Subfields of the hippocampal formation at 7 T MRI: in vivo volumetric assessment. *Neuroimage* **61**:1043–1049.

Wisse LEM, Chetelat G, Daugherty AM, de Flores R, la Joie R, Mueller SG, Stark CEL, Wang L, Yushkevich PA, Berron D, Raz N, Bakker A, Olsen RK, Carr VA (2021) Hippocampal subfield volumetry from structural isotropic 1 mm(3) MRI scans: a note of caution. *Hum Brain Mapp* **42**:539–550.

Wisse LEM, Daugherty AM, Olsen RK, Berron D, Carr VA, Stark CEL, Amaral RSC, Amunts K, Augustinack JC, Bender AR, Bernstein JD, Boccardi M, Bocchetta M, Burggren A, Chakravarty MM, Chupin M, Ekstrom A, de Flores R, Insausti R, Kanel P, et al. (2017) A harmonized segmentation protocol for hippocampal and parahippocampal subregions: why do we need one and what are the key goals? *Hippocampus* **27**:3–11.

Witter MP (1989) Connectivity of the rat hippocampus. In: Neurology and Neurobiology (Köhler C, ed), vol 52, pp 53–69. New York: Alan R. Liss.

Witter MP (2006) Connections of the subiculum of the rat: topography in relation to columnar and laminar organization. *Behav Brain Res* **174**:251–264.

Witter MP, Amaral, DG (1991) Entorhinal cortex of the monkey: V. Projections to the dentate gyrus, hippocampus, and subicular complex. *J Comp Neurol* **307**:437–459.

Witter MP, Amaral DG. The entorhinal cortex of the monkey: VI. Organization of projections from the hippocampus, subiculum, presubiculum, and parasubiculum. *J Comp Neurol.* 2021 Mar;529(4):828–852. doi: 10.1002/cne.24983. Epub 2020 Aug 4. PMID: 32656783; PMCID: PMC8933866.

Witter MP, Doan TP, Jacobsen B, Nilssen ES, Ohara S (2017) Architecture of the entorhinal cortex a review of entorhinal anatomy in rodents with some comparative notes. *Front Syst Neurosci* **11**:46.

Witter MP, Groenewegen HJ (1990) The subiculum: cytoarchitectonically a simple structure, but hodologically complex. In: Understanding the Brain through the Hippocampus (Storm-Mathisen J, Zimmer J, Ottersen OP, eds).

Witter MP, Groenewegen HJ, Lopes da Silva FH, Lohman AHM (1989) Functional organization of the extrinsic and intrinsic circuitry of the parahippocampal region. *Prog Neurobiol* **33**:161–253.

Witter MP, Holtrop R, van de Loosdrecht AA (1988) Direct projections from the periallocortical subicular complex to the fascia dentata in the rat. *Neurosci Res Commun* **2**:61–68.

Witter MP, Ostendorf RH, Groenewegen HJ (1990) Heterogeneity in the dorsal subiculum of the rat: distinct neuronal zones project to different cortical and subcortical targets. *Eur J Neurosci* 2:718–725.

Wouterlood FG, Saldana E, Witter MP (1990) Projection from the nucleus reuniens thalami to the hippocampal region: light and electron microscopic tracing study in the rat with the anterograde tracer *Phaseolus vulgaris*-leucoagglutinin. *J Comp Neurol* 296:179–203.

Wu D, Zhang J (2016) In vivo mapping of macroscopic neuronal projections in the mouse hippocampus using high-resolution diffusion MRI. *Neuroimage* 125:84–93.

Wyss JM, Swanson, LW, Cowan, WM (1979) Evidence for an input to the molecular layer and the stratum granulosum of the dentate gyrus from the supramammillary region of the hypothalamus. *Anat Embryol* 156:165–176.

Wyss JM, Swanson LW, Cowan WM (1980) The organization of the fimbria, dorsal fornix and ventral hippocampal commissure in the rat. *Anat Embryol (Berl)* 158:303–316.

Wyss JM, Van Groen T (1992) Connections between the retrosplenial cortex and the hippocampal formation in the rat: a review. *Hippocampus* 2:1–12.

Xu X, Sun Y, Holmes TC, Lopez AJ (2016) Noncanonical connections between the subiculum and hippocampal CA1. *J Comp Neurol* 524:3666–3673.

Yamawaki N, Li X, Lambot L, Ren LY, Radulovic J, Shepherd GMG (2019) Long-range inhibitory intersection of a retrosplenial thalamocortical circuit by apical tuft-targeting CA1 neurons. *Nat Neurosci* 22:618–626.

Yang S, Yang S, Moreira T, Hoffman G, Carlson GC, Bender KJ, Alger BE, Tang CM (2014) Interlamellar CA1 network in the hippocampus. *Proc Natl Acad Sci U S A* 111:12919–12924.

Yoder RM, Clark BJ, Taube JS (2011) Origins of landmark encoding in the brain. *Trends Neurosci* 34:561–571.

Yu GJ, Bouteiller JC, Berger TW (2020) Topographic organization of correlation along the longitudinal and transverse axes in rat hippocampal CA3 due to excitatory afferents. *Front Comput Neurosci* 14:588881.

Yushkevich PA, Munoz Lopez M, Iniguez de Onzono Martin MM, Ittyerah R, Lim S, Ravikumar S, Bedard ML, Pickup S, Liu W, Wang J, Hung LY, Lasserve J, Vergnet N, Xie L, Dong M, Cui S, McCollum L, Robinson JL, Schuck T, de Flores R, et al. (2021) Three-dimensional mapping of neurofibrillary tangle burden in the human medial temporal lobe. *Brain* 144:2784–2797.

Zeineh MM, Holdsworth S, Skare S, Atlas SW, Bammer R (2012) Ultra-high resolution diffusion tensor imaging of the microscopic pathways of the medial temporal lobe. *Neuroimage* 62:2065–2082.

Zeki S (2018) The rough seas of cortical cartography. *Trends Neurosci* 41:242–244.

Zhang L, Hernandez VS (2013) Synaptic innervation to rat hippocampus by vasopressin-immuno-positive fibres from the hypothalamic supraoptic and paraventricular nuclei. *Neuroscience* 228:139–162.

Zheng Z, Lauritzen JS, Perlman E, Robinson CG, Nichols M, Milkie D, Torrens O, Price J, Fisher CB, Sharifi N, Calle-Schuler SA, Kmecova L, Ali IJ, Karsh B, Trautman ET, Bogovic JA, Hanslovsky P, Jefferis G, Kazhdan M, Khairy K, et al. (2018) A complete electron microscopy volume of the brain of adult *Drosophila melanogaster*. *Cell* 174:730–743, e722.

4

Development of the Hippocampal Formation

Pierre Lavenex, David G. Amaral, Pamela Banta Lavenex, François Guillemot, Ricardo Insausti, and Noelia Urban

4.1 Overview

What are the fundamental issues regarding the development of the hippocampus? In this chapter, we have chosen to provide an overview of the basic principles governing hippocampal development, which are largely conserved across species. Although the production of the pyramidal neurons of the hippocampus continues until the last day of gestation in rodents and it is complete by midgestation in primates, the relative timeline of neuron production in different hippocampal regions follows the same pattern in different species. Similarly, research in both rodents and nonhuman primates has shown that GABAergic interneurons are born earlier than glutamatergic neurons, including the pyramidal cells of the hippocampus and the granule cells of the dentate gyrus. Since there is an increasing interest in translational research (as reflected in the last chapters of this book), we provide detailed information on the specific times when particular developmental processes take place in different species. This will hopefully help researchers in their choice of appropriately aged experimental animals when trying to model the normal and abnormal development of the human hippocampal formation. The basic organization of the hippocampal formation is provided in Chapter 3 and will not be repeated here.

We first present a comparative timeline of gestation and life span duration in mice, rats, macaque monkeys and humans (Table 4.1). Gestation lasts for 19–21 days in mice (*Mus musculus*), 21–23 days in rats (*Rattus norvegicus*), 167 ± 7 days in rhesus macaque monkeys (*Macaca mulatta*), and 268 ± 9 days (38 weeks and 2 days) in humans (*Homo sapiens*). At birth, infants of these different species exhibit different degrees of overall structural and functional brain maturation, which is also true for the hippocampal formation. We did not include a systematic comparison with precocial species, such as the guinea pig, that are also used in experimental research and only considered a couple of studies in which such comparison was deemed particularly meaningful. An important step in comparative and translational studies is thus to establish the ages at which typical developmental milestones are observed in different species. Therefore, we also describe the time of origin of neurons

and the establishment of major hippocampal connections, as well as some of the genetic and molecular processes that guide these developmental processes. In animal studies, experimental techniques including the use of extrinsic markers of cell division enable researchers to determine the ages at which certain populations of neurons are generated. In humans, the precise dating of neurogenesis is not possible, so the exact age at which neurons are generated cannot be established reliably. However, the appearance of recognizable cytoarchitectural, morphological, and neurochemical features may be used to infer the relative developmental profile of the human hippocampal formation. This information reveals that the relative temporal development of the different structures constituting the hippocampal formation is similar across species.

4.2 Early specification of hippocampal fields

4.2.1 Specification of the hippocampal primordium

The hippocampus originates from the dorsomedial part of the pallium (cortical mantle surrounding the lateral ventricles), which invaginates to form the telencephalic vesicles. The medial wall of the telencephalon gives rise to the choroid plexus and the cortical hem, a signaling center for hippocampus development and a source of Cajal-Retzius cells (Lun et al., 2015). The most ventral structures, the choroid plexus and the cortical hem, produce diffusible signaling molecules, including multiple bone morphogenetic proteins (BMPs) and Wingless/Integrated (WNT) molecules, which are crucial signals that specify hippocampal identity. The cortical hem is both necessary and sufficient to instruct hippocampal fate and is therefore considered an organizer of this region. The absence of the cortical transcription factor LHX2 is a requirement for the formation of the cortical hem (Mangale et al., 2008). This instructive role relies on the ability of the cortical hem to produce several WNT proteins, since elimination of WNT signaling impairs hippocampal specification (Grove et al., 1998). The cortical hem also produces Cajal-Retzius cells that guide the migration and dictate the final position of the future hippocampal neurons (Del Rio et al., 1995) and

Table 4.1 Life span and physical characteristics of the main species used to study the development of the hippocampal formation

	Mouse	Rat	Monkey	Human
Gestation	19–21 days	21–23 days	167 ± 7 days	268 ± 9 days
Eye opening	14 days	14 days	birth	birth
Weaning	21–28 days	21 days	292 days	639 days
Sexual maturity				
Female	42 days	50 days	3.4 y	13 y
Male	42 days	50 days	5.5 y	14 y
Average life span				
Wild	1–1.5 y	1–2 y	20 y	60–80 y
Captivity	2–3 y	2.5–3.5 y	25–30 y	
Body weight (adult)	20–40 g	300–500 g	5–10 kg	60–80 kg
Brain weight (adult)	0.5 g	2.5 g	80–100 g	1.3–1.4 kg
Brain/Body	1.8%	0.7%	1.2%	1.9%

Sources: (Silk et al., 1993; Sukow et al., 2001; Hopper et al., 2008; Jukic et al., 2013; Mattison et al., 2017; World Health Organization, 2020)

further contributes to the development of hippocampal connections (Del Rio et al., 1997).

4.2.2 Specification of the dentate gyrus and hippocampus proper

The dentate gyrus originates from the dentate neuroepithelium, the part of the ventricular zone of the medial pallium that is in direct contact with the cortical hem (Figure 4.1). The CA3, CA2, and CA1 fields of the hippocampus arise from the hippocampal neuroepithelium in a more dorsal ventricular zone. Hippocampal field identity is acquired very early during development (embryonic day 12.5 (E12.5) in the mouse), even before any known specific markers are expressed. The different hippocampal fields and the dentate gyrus later contain neurons with distinct morphologies, molecular markers, and connectivity, but the factors responsible for this patterning seem to be independent of surrounding signals. High levels of the proneural transcription factors Neurogenin1 and Neurogenin2 in progenitor cells promote the generation of projection neurons during hippocampal development. In the mouse, field specific markers such as the glutamate receptor subunit KA1 for CA1 can be detected by E14.5, as soon as CA1 neurons become postmitotic and before they reach their final position. Similarly, the expression of the POU-domain gene SCIP for CA3 can be identified from E15.5 (Tole et al., 1997). The transcription factor Prox1 is also detected in the dentate neuroepithelium from E14.5, before granule cell neurons migrate to their final destination. Prox1 is needed for the proliferation and specification of granule cells and is often used as a marker of dentate gyrus neurons because it is not expressed by hippocampal pyramidal neurons and is only expressed at low levels in some interneurons. Deletion of Prox1 changes dentate gyrus neurons into CA3 pyramidal neurons, even in postmitotic cells (Lavado and Oliver, 2007; Iwano et al., 2012; Rubin and Kessaris, 2013). Efforts to characterize gene expression throughout the brain, using large-scale in situ hybridization and single cell RNA-sequencing techniques, have identified many specific genetic markers for the different hippocampal structures (Thompson et al., 2008; Zeisel

et al., 2015). However, the specific contributions of each of these genes to the development of the hippocampus are unclear.

4.2.3 Early development of hippocampal fields in humans

The human hippocampus can be recognized at 9 weeks of gestation (Kostovic et al., 1993; Arnold and Trojanowski, 1996). Although there is no indication of dentate gyrus or hippocampal plate, a cingulate sulcus is present near the hem of the dorsal hippocampus, which is continuous with the ventral hippocampus.

At 10 weeks, the calbindin-positive hippocampal plate and the proliferating-cell-nuclear-antigen-positive (PCNA) dentate notch become visible (Gonzalez Arnay, 2015). The dorsal hem is replaced by the hippocampus primordium, which remains connected to the ventral hem. The primordium of the entorhinal cortex comprises a one-cell-thick layer made up of large neurons between a tapering cortical plate and a wider marginal zone (Kostovic et al., 1993; Šimić et al., 2022).

At 11 weeks, the future hippocampus can be recognized as a single cell layer between the cortical plate and the marginal zone at the ventral part of the telencephalic vesicle (Kostovic et al., 1993; Judas et al., 2005; Rados et al., 2006). As in other species, the majority of cells in the dentate neuroepithelium and hippocampal neuroepithelium express SOX2; dentate progenitors also express PAX6 (Zhong et al., 2020).

At 12 weeks, a hippocampal plate is visible at the level of the anterior limit of the choroid plexus. Calretinin-positive neurons represent the first sign of the dentate gyrus behind the anterior commissure. The ventral hippocampal primordium consists of a calbindin-positive hippocampal plate and a primitive dentate gyrus. Both hippocampal primordia are linked by a band of PCNA-positive cells, which connects the fimbria with the choroid plexus.

At 13–14 weeks, the primordium of the dentate gyrus is calretinin-positive, while the hippocampal plate is calbindin-positive (Abraham et al., 2009). The hilus of the dentate gyrus contains numerous Ki-67-positive proliferating cells, while the marginal zone is occupied by p73- and reelin-positive Cajal-Retzius cells (Seress, 2007).

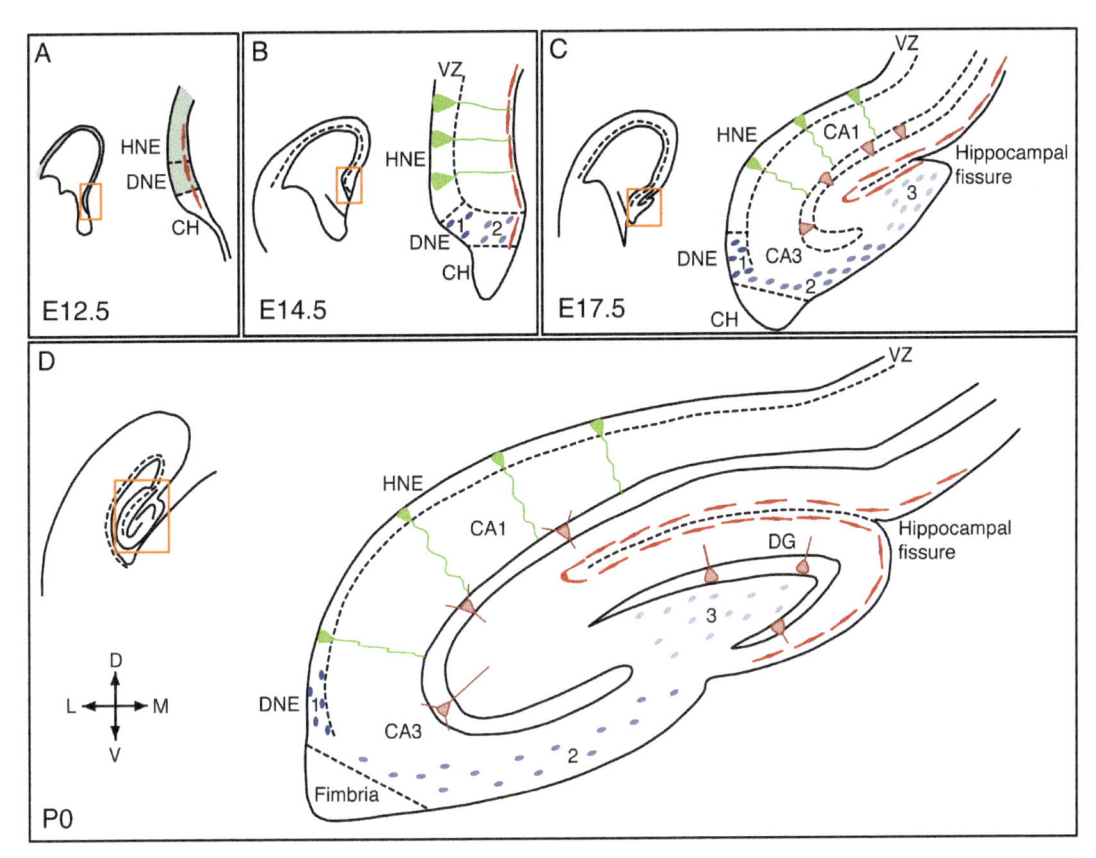

Figure 4.1 Development of the mouse hippocampus. (A) At embryonic day 12.5 (E12.5) the presumptive dentate neuroepithelium (DNE) is located between the hippocampal neuroepithelium (HNE) and the cortical hem (CH), which produces Cajal-Retzius cells (red) lining the pial surface. (B) At E14.5 dentate precursors of the primary matrix (1; dark blue cells) are located in the ventricular zone (VZ), and precursor cells start to migrate toward the pial surface forming the secondary matrix (2; medium blue cells). In the VZ of the HNE, radial glial precursors (green) will give rise to hippocampal neurons. (C) At E17.5 the hippocampal fissure is formed and dentate precursor cells migrate to and accumulate there, forming the tertiary matrix (3; light blue cells). Cajal-Retzius cells are also present and follow the hippocampal fissure. From the HNE, hippocampal neurons (red triangles) are born and migrate along radial glial cells toward their location in the hippocampal fields (CA1 and CA3 are shown). (D) At birth, granule neurons (red triangles) appear first in the suprapyramidal blade, below the hippocampal fissure. Precursor cells in the primary and secondary matrix will soon disappear, but cells in the tertiary matrix continue actively dividing and producing granule neurons through postnatal development. D, dorsal; M, medial; V, ventral; L, lateral. (Modified from Urban and Guillemot, 2014.)

In the entorhinal cortex, a cell-free stratum forms the prospective lamina dissecans, and up to five divisions can be observed based on the presence of cell islands and the two principal external and internal cell layers (Šimić et al., 2022).

At 15–16 weeks, the hippocampal plate shows an enlargement at its most anterior end. The hippocampal fissure deepens and shows capillaries mainly in the ventral hippocampus. Reelin- and p73-positive Cajal-Retzius cells accumulate at the fundus of the hippocampal fissure, with a maximal density anteriorly. The maturation of the dentate gyrus primordium, in particular ventrally, is indicated by the presence of vimentin- and GFAP-positive glial scaffolds. The junction between the dorsal and ventral hippocampus forms a cruciform shape, formed by the primordium of the dentate gyrus and prospective CA3 neurons entering the hilar region. Finally, a notch begins in the head of the hippocampus, where mitotic activity can be demonstrated by PCNA immunoreactivity. Very little is known about the prenatal development of the presubiculum and parasubiculum, except that they can be identified by 15 gestational weeks (Kostovic et al., 1989) and they may exhibit a development similar to that of the entorhinal cortex.

At 16–17.5 weeks, the cortical mantle shows the first signs of gyrification with the establishment of the lateral sulcus. The hippocampal plate contains calretinin-positive nonpyramidal cells, and the dentate gyrus contains only scattered neurons without any particular organization (Gonzalez Arnay, 2015).

Beginning at 17.5 weeks, there is a progressive obliteration of the hippocampal fissure, while the sulcus between the fimbria and the dentate gyrus deepens (Humphrey, 1967). The uncal pole of the hippocampus enlarges, and calretinin-immunostaining reveals a primordium of the dentate gyrus. Subpial Cajal-Retzius cells and prospective interneurons are also present in the hippocampal plate. PCNA-positive cells are present in the caudal part of the hippocampus, from where they migrate rostrally (Gonzalez Arnay, 2015).

Starting at about 20 weeks, this migration forms a stream that progressively colonizes the uncus, and forms the dentate gyrus located right above the hippocampal fissure. The most medial and anterior portion of the parahippocampal gyrus develops and forms the main constituents of the adult hippocampal head: the hippocampal amygdaloid transitional area, the subiculum, the CA fields, and the dentate gyrus. The bifurcation of the hippocampal fissure probably provides the structural basis for the digitations, which can be observed neatly individualized and in variable numbers at the dorsal surface of the hippocampal head.

At 21–25 weeks, the dorsal hippocampus is reduced to the induseum griseum, which is in continuation with the ventral hippocampus at very posterior levels and maintains a weak calretinin and calbindin immunoreactivity. In contrast, the ventral hippocampus shows an extended hippocampal fissure with an abundant population of calretinin-, reelin- and p73-positive cells, and abundant capillaries. Calretinin is expressed in neurons of the subiculum and prospective interneurons in the hilar region of the dentate gyrus. The main changes of the ventral hippocampus take place in the hippocampal head. The first indentations and evaginations of the dentate gyrus start along the longitudinal axis of the hippocampus, where CA1, CA3, and the dentate gyrus with a well-differentiated hilar region are clearly visible.

At 23 weeks, the granule cell layer of the dentate gyrus is not yet compact and expresses calbindin, the suprapyramidal blade showing stronger immunoreactivity. In addition, neurons closer to the molecular layer, which were born first, express denser calbindin immunoreactivity. In contrast, hilar cells are more mature and the number of proliferative cells decreases dramatically (Seress, 2001, 2007). The different fields of the hippocampus start to be recognizable. CA2 appears to be the most mature, while CA1 and the subiculum exhibit a relatively less compact deep layer, closer to the alveus (Arnold and Trojanowski, 1996a).

At 24 weeks, the basic cytoarchitectural features of the entorhinal cortex are clearly visible (Grateron et al., 2003), even though further myelination and synapse formation will continue into postnatal life (Hevner and Kinney, 1996; Insausti et al., 2010).

By 25 weeks, the major morphological constituents of the hippocampal formation are recognizable. The dorsal hippocampus is reduced to the induseum griseum. The transition with the tail of the hippocampus constitutes the most caudal portion of the dentate gyrus, the fasciola cinerea. In the hilus, PCNA-positive cells indicate the tertiary matrix of the dentate gyrus.

4.3 Neurogenesis and cell migration

While early patterning events are highly specific to the hippocampal primordium, the subsequent events of neuronal maturation and migration of hippocampal neurons greatly resemble that of cortical neurons. The dentate gyrus has a prolonged development compared with the hippocampal fields, and dentate gyrus neurons follow a more complex pattern of migration than hippocampal pyramidal neurons. This section outlines how the main projection neurons in the hippocampus are generated and discusses the mechanisms that direct their migration. It also presents the origin and integration of hippocampal interneurons, which originate in a different part of the telencephalon.

Table 4.2 offers a brief description of the time of neurogenesis (i.e., the birth date of neurons) in the hippocampal formation of mice, rats, monkeys, and humans. Given the increasing interest in translational research (as reflected in Chapters 18–20), it is important to establish the ages at which the same developmental processes take place in different species. We limit our description to the three most used species in preclinical studies, namely mice, rats, and macaque monkeys, as well as humans. Such fundamental knowledge about cell formation in the rodent and primate hippocampal formation dates back to the studies by Angevine (1965) for the mouse; Altman and colleagues (Altman and Das, 1965; Bayer and Altman, 1974) and

Cowan and colleagues (Schlessinger et al., 1975; Schlessinger et al., 1978) for the rat; and Rakic and Nowakowski (Nowakowski and Rakic, 1981; Rakic and Nowakowski, 1981) for the monkey. These studies were the first ones to describe the time course of the generation (i.e., birth date), sites of origin (i.e., stem cell location), and migratory pathways (i.e., to reach their final location) of the principal hippocampal neurons, including the pyramidal cells of the CA fields of the hippocampus and the granule cells of the dentate gyrus. More limited information has been obtained in humans, in particular by Seress and colleagues (Ribak et al., 1985; Seress, 2001; Seress et al., 2001) and Arnold and Trojanowski (1996). Single-cell transcriptome analysis of the prenatal development of the hippocampus has confirmed some of these early observations in humans (Zhong et al., 2020).

4.3.1 Pyramidal neurons

Pyramidal neurons of the hippocampus proper originate from progenitor cells in the ventricular neuroepithelial layers located below the ventricular wall along the CA1 primordium (Figure 4.2A). They are generated between embryonic days E10 and E18 in the mouse (with a peak at E14–E15), and between E16 and E20 in the rat (Table 4.2). CA3 pyramidal cells are generated with a peak of production at E17 in rats, whereas the peak of production of CA1 pyramidal cells is at E18 and E19. Except for the CA3 pyramidal cells, the route of migration is short because the hippocampus closely follows the curve of the ventricle. Newly born neurons adopt a multipolar shape, exit the ventricular zone, and migrate toward the pial surface. Initially they sojourn midway in the so-called intermediate zone, which will become stratum oriens in the adult. Future CA1 neurons form cell rows oriented perpendicular to the ventricular area, which migrate radially to form the CA1 pyramidal layer. From the ventricular germinal layer, early generated CA3 pyramidal cells take 3 to 4 days longer than CA1 cells to migrate to their final location. They first migrate tangentially along the ventricular wall in the prenatally existing intermediate zone, before moving radially to form the CA3 pyramidal cell layer. From the intermediate zone, hippocampal neurons adopt a bipolar shape and resume their migration toward the pial surface using the scaffold provided by radial glia. This radial migration is also controlled by Cajal-Retzius cells lining the pial surface, which govern the final position of the pyramidal cells in the hippocampal layers. The radial migration of hippocampal neurons resembles that of cortical neurons, with newer neurons being added closer to the pial surface. Thus, as is the case in the cortex, in which projection neurons are organized in several cell layers, recent studies have shown that hippocampal pyramidal neurons are organized in sublayers that are formed based on the time of birth of these neurons (Cembrowski and Spruston, 2019). Several genes implicated in the lamination of the cortex contribute to the laminar organization of the hippocampus: Reelin (RELN), cyclin-dependent kinase 5 (CDK5), Lissencephaly 1 (LIS1), alpha tubulin 1A (TUBA1A) and doublecortin (DCX, although the hippocampal defects in DCX mutant mice are relatively mild).

As mentioned above, while CA1 neurons have a very short migration path from the ventricular zone, CA3 neurons must migrate further to occupy their final position, especially those in the most proximal portion of CA3 (closer to the dentate gyrus). As a consequence, the later-generated CA1 pyramidal cells establish a distinct cellular layer earlier than the earlier-generated CA3 cells. It remains an open question whether the pyramidal neurons in CA1

Table 4.2 Timeline of neurogenesis in different hippocampal regions

	Mouse	Rat	Monkey	Human
Dentate gyrus				
Granule cells	E10-Postnatal	E14-Postnatal	E38-Postnatal	E70-Postnatal
Interneurons	E10–E16	E14–E18	E38–E50	
CA3				
Pyramidal cells	E10–E18 Peak: E13–E14	E16–E19 Peak: E17	E38–E62 Peak: E43–E48	E63–E105
Interneurons	E10–E16	E12.5–E15.5 Peak: E14	E38–E50	
CA2				
Pyramidal cells	E10–E15 Peak: E13–E14	E16–E19 Peak: E16–E17	E38–E56 Peak: E43–E48	E63–E105
Interneurons	E10–E16	E12.5–E15.5 Peak: E14	E38–E50	
CA1				
Pyramidal cells	E10–E18 Peak: E14–E15	E16–E20 Peak: E17–E19	E38–E70 Peak: E45–E50	E63–E105
Interneurons	E10–E16 Peak: E12.5	E12.5–E15.5 Peak: E14	E38–E45	
Subiculum				
Pyramidal cells superficial	E10–E15 Peak: E13–E14	E14–E18 Peak: E16–E17	E40–E56 Peak: E48–E50	
Interneurons	E10–E16	E12.5–E15.5 Peak: E14		
Pyramidal cells deep	E10–E15 Peak: E12	E15–E17 Peak: E16	E38–E50 Peak: E45–E48	
Interneurons		E12–E13		
Presubiculum				
Pyramidal cells superficial	E10–E16 Peak: E14–E15	E16–E19 Peak: E17–E18	E43–E70 Peak: E50–E62	
Pyramidal cells deep	E10–E15 Peak: E13–E14	E14–E17 Peak: E16	E38–E56 Peak: E48	
Parasubiculum				
Pyramidal cells superficial	E10–E15 Peak: E14–E15	E16–E19 Peak: E17–E18	E43–E75 Peak: E50–E62	
Pyramidal cells deep	E10–E15 Peak: E13–E14	E14–E17 Peak: E16	E38–E56 Peak: E48	
Entorhinal cortex				
Superficial layers			E45–E70 Peak: E56–E62	
Deep layers			E36–E56 Peak: E43–E48	
EC lateral				
Superficial layers	E10–E14.5 Peak: E13	E15–E17 Peak: E16		
Deep layers	E10–E14 Peak: E12.5	E14–E16 Peak: E14.5		
EC median				
Superficial layers	E10–E15 Peak: E14	E15–E17 Peak: E16		
Deep layers	E10–E14 Peak: E13	E14–E16 Peak: E15		

Mouse studies: (Angevine, 1965; Super et al., 1998a; Danglot et al., 2006; Tricoire et al., 2011)
Rat studies: (Schlessinger et al., 1975; Bayer, 1980; Amaral and Kurz, 1985; Bayer et al., 1993)
Monkey studies: (Rakic and Nowakowski, 1981)
Human studies: (Arnold and Trojanowski, 1996)

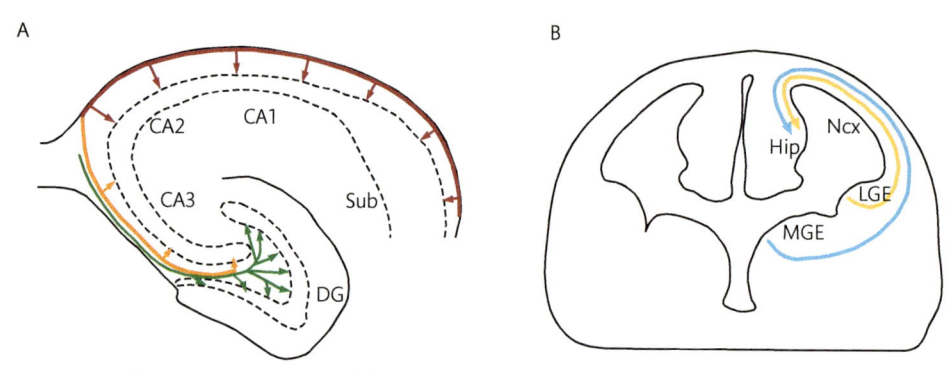

Figure 4.2 Migration trajectories of hippocampal neurons. (A) Pyramidal neurons of the hippocampus and subiculum originate from progenitor cells in the ventricular neuroepithelial layers located below the ventricular wall of the hippocampal primordium. Subicular and CA1 pyramidal neurons migrate radially to reach their final destinations. CA3 pyramidal migrate first tangentially in the intermediate zone, before moving radially to form the pyramidal cell layer. Granule cell neurons of the dentate gyrus originate from progenitor cells in different locations throughout development and postnatal life. (B) GABAergic interneurons of the hippocampus and the dentate gyrus originate from precursor cells located in the medial (MGE) and lateral (LGE)/caudal (CGE) ganglionic eminences. (Panel B, modified from Pleasure et al., 2000.)

and CA3 originate from the same segment but different cell populations within the hippocampal neuroepithelium. However, on E14.5 and E15.5 in the mouse, pyramidal cells already exhibit patterns of gene expression specific for CA3 and CA1 (Tole et al., 1997), which may be necessary for the appropriate regulation of migration and also contribute to their different adult morphological characteristics. Neurogenesis of CA3 pyramidal cells precedes that of CA1 pyramidal cells in all species studied to date (Table 4.2).

This developmental pattern was initially described by Altman and Bayer (1990) as the dentate-to-subicular neurogenetic gradient because the CA3 pyramidal cells situated close to the dentate gyrus are generated earlier than the CA1 pyramidal cells situated close to the subiculum. However, CA1 pyramidal cells reach their final position earlier than CA3 pyramidal cells. In rats, the CA1 pyramidal cell layer is completed by E20. At E21, the pyramidal cell layer begins to curve medially. This corresponds to the beginning of the morphogenesis of CA3, which is completed at E22, when the CA3 pyramidal cell layer extends medially toward the polymorphic layer of the dentate gyrus. The developmental pattern of the hippocampus proper was thus also described as reflecting a subicular-to-dentate morphogenetic gradient. However, since CA2 and subicular neurons are generated even earlier than CA3 neurons, the description of these two gradients may be too simplistic. In rodents, pyramidal neurons destined for the hippocampus are generated until the last days of gestation (Figure 4.3).

In monkeys, in contrast, all neurons destined for the hippocampus are generated by midgestation (Nowakowski and Rakic, 1981; Rakic and Nowakowski, 1981). The first neurons destined for the different hippocampal structures are generated almost simultaneously at E38, but cell division terminates at different times for neurons that will populate different structures (Figure 4.4). As in rodents, there is an inside-out spatiotemporal gradient in the generation of principal neurons in the entorhinal cortex, parasubiculum, presubiculum, subiculum, and hippocampus. Deeply located neurons are generated before superficially located neurons, which must therefore migrate through already established neurons to reach their final destinations. The production of neurons that form the subiculum and CA2 is the first to cease around E50 for the deeply located subicular neurons, and sometime between E56 and E65 for CA2 and the superficially located subicular neurons. The

production of neurons located in the deep layers of the entorhinal cortex ends around E56, whereas the production of neurons destined for the superficial layers continues until E70. Neuron production ends at E62 for CA3, and at E70 for CA1 (Table 4.2).

In humans, the ventricular zone of the hippocampal primordium at 9 weeks of gestation contains densely packed neuroblasts with mitotic cells along the ventricular border (Arnold and Trojanowski, 1996). Bipolar and pyramidal-shaped neurons are also found within the hippocampal plate that will become the pyramidal cell layer. Between 15 and 19 weeks of gestation, the subiculum has a more mature cytoarchitectural appearance than the hippocampus and the dentate gyrus (Arnold and Trojanowski, 1996). As is the case in the other species, there is an inside-out gradient of neuronal maturation, with deeper portions of the pyramidal cell layer maturing earlier than more superficial portions (Arnold and Trojanowski, 1996). This developmental pattern is confirmed by the distribution of PAX6-positive and HOPX-positive progenitors in the developing human hippocampus between 11 and 22 weeks of gestation (Zhong et al., 2020).

4.3.2 Granule cells

The formation of the granule cell layer of the dentate gyrus differs in many respects from the formation of the hippocampal pyramidal cell layer. In particular, neurogenesis in the dentate gyrus happens over a particularly long time, from around midgestation in rodents (E10.5 in mice and E14 in rats) and even earlier in primates (E38 in monkeys), to early postnatal development and throughout adult life (Table 4.2; see also Chapter 9). Nevertheless, neurogenesis of the dentate gyrus can be divided into a developmental period and an adult period, which exhibit different mechanisms of regulation. The developmental period involves the generation of the majority of the granule cells, their organization into the two blades of the dentate gyrus, and the establishment of afferent and efferent connections. This developmental period ends postnatally, but stem cells persist in the subgranular zone of the dentate gyrus and continue generating new granule cells that integrate into the granule cell layer throughout life (Frisen, 2016; Snyder, 2019).

In all species, the first granule cells of the dentate gyrus are generated at approximately the same time as the first pyramidal cells. There is a suprapyramidal-to-infrapyramidal gradient in the formation of

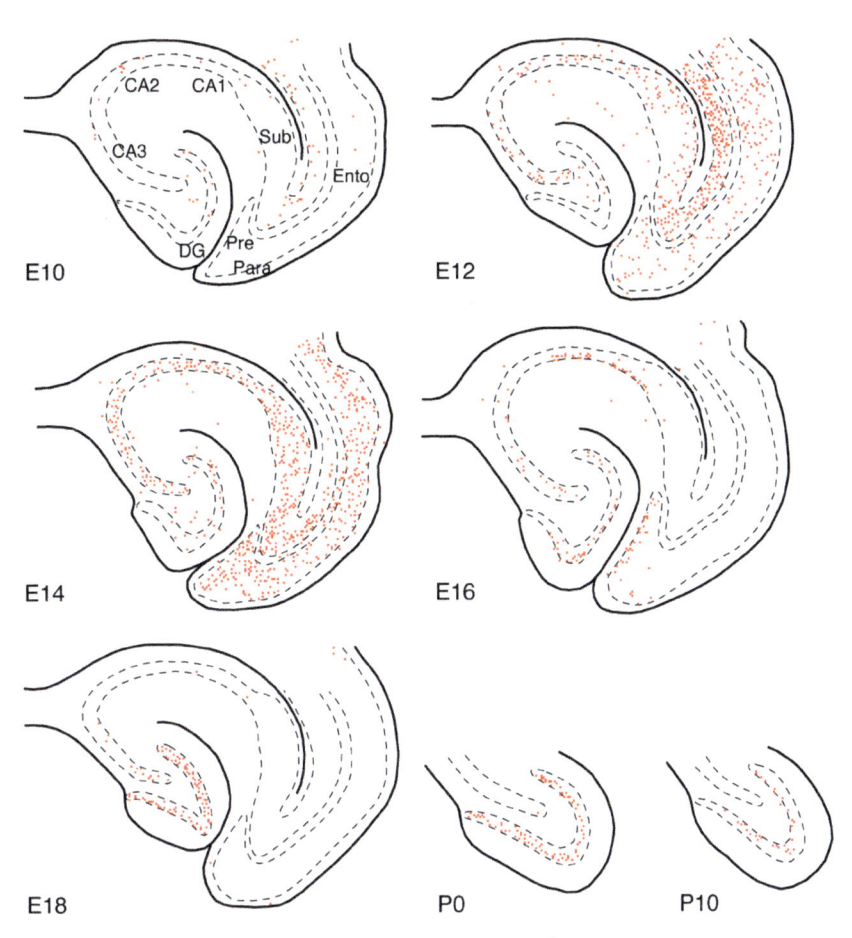

Figure 4.3 Neurons of the hippocampal formation labeled with a single injection of ³H-thymidine on different embryonic days, as seen in autoradiograms from animals killed postnatally. (Modified from Angevine, 1965.)

the two blades of the granule cell layer. The granule cells at the tip of the suprapyramidal blade are the first to be generated. In addition, the more superficially located neurons in the granule cell layer (closest to the molecular layer) are formed earlier than the neurons located more deeply (closest to the polymorphic layer). This implies that during development, as the population of granule cells increases, the newly generated neurons are progressively added to the deep portion of the granule cell layer, following an outside-in sequence of neuron addition (Angevine, 1965; Schlessinger et al., 1975), which contrasts with what is observed in the neocortex and the rest of the hippocampal formation (Figure 4.3) (Angevine, 1965; Schlessinger et al., 1978). There is also a temporal-to-septal gradient in the formation of granule cells, which is not observed for other cells in the hippocampal formation.

As noted above, the generation of granule cells lasts much longer during gestation than that of pyramidal neurons, and most importantly extends into the postnatal period in all species. The migration of postmitotic granule cells is also longer and much more complex than that of pyramidal neurons, as the origin of granule cells born at different times changes during development (Figure 4.1). The following sequence is observed in mice: First, from E10, granule cells originate from the dentate neuroepithelium, an area called the primary matrix, which is in direct contact with the cortical hem. Second, at E14.5 progenitor cells migrate away from the ventricular zone toward the hippocampal fissure, forming a new population of progenitors at the level of the secondary matrix. Finally, at E17.5,

progenitors migrate further toward the hippocampal fissure to form the tertiary matrix. This third neurogenic zone is located in the polymorphic layer, within the developing blades of the dentate gyrus, and is ultimately restricted to the subgranular zone by adulthood. The early postmitotic granule cells must thus migrate from the ventricular germinal layer along the already formed CA3 region through the narrow intermediate zone between the alveus and the future stratum oriens to form the granule cell layer of the dentate gyrus that surrounds the proximal portion of CA3.

In rats, only 20% of the granule cells are generated before birth (Schlessinger et al., 1975; Bayer, 1980); comparable estimates are not available in mice. The majority of granule cells found in the adult rat dentate gyrus are thus generated within the proliferative zone of the polymorphic layer, the tertiary matrix, with a peak of production in the first week of postnatal life. Schlessinger et al. (1975) suggested that the most likely source of this population of precursor cells was the neuroepithelial region adjoining the site of origin of the pyramidal cells of the future CA3. The origin of early glial fibers guiding cell migration toward the dentate primordium serves to accurately demarcate this region (Rickmann et al., 1987). From there, they must migrate to the region of the dentate primordium and set up a proliferative pool of cells. While it was suggested that the neural stem cells found in the subgranular zone of the adult dentate gyrus originate in the ventral hippocampus (Li et al., 2013), the prevalent view is that the same stem cells that give rise to developmentally born neurons transition to a radial glia-like fate to continue

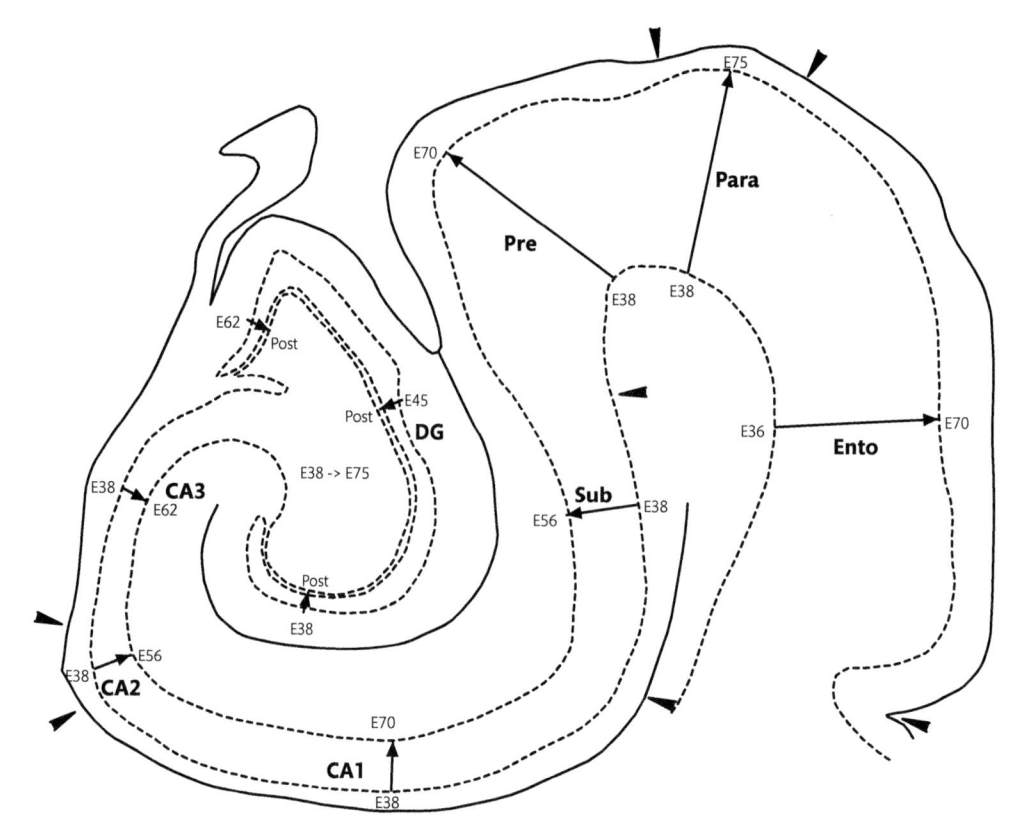

Figure 4.4 Summary of the time of origin of neurons in the rhesus monkey hippocampal formation. The age at the bottom of each arrow indicates the time that the first neurons are generated in a given region, and the age at the top of each arrow indicates the last time during development when neurons were labeled by an exposure to ^{3}H-thymidine. (Modified from Rakic and Nowakowski, 1981.)

generating neurons during adulthood (Berg et al., 2019). Thus, although the subgranular zone is most often considered in relation to adult neurogenesis, it originates as a neurogenic region during development (Hevner, 2016), and becomes clearly visible around birth in rodents and in the last quarter of gestation in primates. There is little variability in the morphological characteristics of granule cells found in adult individuals, even though the location of their cell bodies that depends on their birth date may impact the detailed organization of their dendritic arborization (Kerloch et al., 2019).

In monkeys, 60% of the dentate gyrus granule cells are generated before birth (Jabès et al., 2010, 2011). As in rodents, there is a mediolateral temporal gradient in the generation of granule cells (Figure 4.4). The granule cells destined for the suprapyramidal blade of the dentate gyrus are generated early, followed by those destined for the crest, and finally those destined for the infrapyramidal blade (Rakic and Nowakowski, 1981). However, granule cells generated after midgestation (E80) are distributed throughout the entire suprapyramidal to infrapyramidal extent of the dentate gyrus. Postnatal neurogenesis continues at a decreasing, though still substantial, rate during the first year after birth, with a peak of production within the first three postnatal months. In monkeys, more than 95% of the granule cells found in the mature dentate gyrus have been generated by 1 year of age (approximately 4 years of age for a human). New granule cells, however, are added to the dentate gyrus into young adulthood. Even in mature monkeys, there is ongoing cell proliferation, neurogenesis, and cell death in the context of an overall stable number of granule cells (Jabès et al., 2010). Importantly, the number of new neurons that could potentially be integrated into the granule cell layer of mature monkeys is about

1,300 per day or 0.02% of total neuron number (7.21 million). This daily rate of adult neurogenesis is about 10 times lower, in percentage of total neuron number, than that reported for 9- to 10-week-old rats, where 2,250 new neurons are generated per day, or 0.2% of total neuron number (Cameron and McKay, 2001). Given that monkeys live 20–30 years and rats 2–3 years (Havenaar et al., 1993), postnatal neurogenesis has a similar potential in rodents and primates. In both species, the entire population of granule cells could be renewed during an individual's lifetime.

In humans, the development of a cell layer in the primordial dentate gyrus can be observed as early as 10.5 gestational weeks, but it is only by 13.5 weeks that the granule cell layer becomes identifiable (Humphrey, 1967). If human developmental patterns follow the same relative timeline demonstrated with cell-birth marking techniques in rodents and nonhuman primates, this suggests that the first granule cells may be generated around 10 gestational weeks, at the time the first hippocampal neurons are born. Granule cell formation continues at significant levels for some time during the early postnatal period (Seress et al., 2001), with a relatively high rate during the first year of life (Sorrells et al., 2018), which corresponds to the first three postnatal months in monkeys (Rakic and Nowakowski, 1981; Jabès et al., 2010). All cytoarchitectonic layers of the dentate gyrus can be distinguished by the 24th gestational week. At this age, the suprapyramidal blade of the dentate gyrus is more differentiated than the infrapyramidal blade (Seress, 2001). This differential development of the two blades of the dentate gyrus is particularly evident at 15 gestational weeks, when the suprapyramidal blade is clearly visible and the infrapyramidal blade is not (Arnold and Trojanowski, 1996). This pattern is similar to what is observed in rodents and monkeys. At birth, the human granule cell layer includes approximately 70% of the granule cells found in adulthood (Seress, 2001), an estimate very close to what is found in monkeys. Radiocarbon analysis of DNA from neuronal hippocampal cells and mathematical modeling of ^{14}C data suggest that all dentate granule cell neurons may also turn over in the adult human hippocampus (Spalding et al., 2013; Bergmann et al., 2015), but the exact proportion of cells and whether different populations of cells may be replaced in different species remains to be investigated (Frisen, 2016; Snyder, 2019).

4.3.3 Regulation of developmental neurogenesis in the dentate gyrus

The molecular mechanisms that direct the development of the dentate gyrus and the generation of dentate granule cells during embryogenesis remain relatively poorly characterized in comparison to the cerebral cortex, even in the mouse, where almost all the relevant work has been conducted. Nevertheless, a number of signaling molecules and transcription factors have been shown to control the development of the dentate gyrus in mice (Table 4.3), including components of the WNT, BMP, and Notch signaling pathways, and the transcription factors Neurog2, NFIX, Tbr2, and Prox1 (Urban and Guillemot, 2014). During dentate gyrus development, BMPs promote the proliferation of neural precursors and Notch signaling prevents their differentiation, while WNT molecules promote both precursor proliferation and differentiation. The transcription factor Neurog2 acts as an effector of WNT signaling during the formation of the dentate gyrus and has an essential role in the proliferation and glutamatergic differentiation of dentate progenitors, as well as in the formation of a glial scaffold needed for their migration. Transcription factors of the Nuclear Factor 1 (NFI) family, like NFIX, are also essential for dentate gyrus formation. NFIX mutants present a decrease in the number of Prox1-positive granule neurons, as well as a disorganization of the glial scaffold and a defect in morphogenesis. Tbr2 promotes the proliferation and differentiation of intermediate progenitors in the dentate granule cell lineage, while Prox1 determines granule cell identity and promotes their differentiation.

4.3.4 Regulation of adult neurogenesis in the dentate gyrus

There is evidence for continued neurogenesis in the dentate gyrus of sexually mature individuals in both rodents and primates, including humans, that decreases with age (see Chapter 9). In contrast to what is observed during the embryonic and early postnatal periods, adult granule cell formation does not appear to follow any particular gradient. In the adult brain, proliferative granule cell progenitors are restricted to the subgranular zone, where neural stem cells are maintained in a quiescent state. The induction of quiescence during postnatal development is crucial to establishing and maintaining a pool of neural stem cells sufficient to support neurogenesis throughout life. If the quiescent stem cell pool is not properly formed or stem cells become excessively active, they subsequently become exhausted and neurogenesis declines rapidly. Exhaustion is caused mainly by the limited capacity of adult hippocampal stem cells to self-renew, as upon activation only a fraction of activated stem cells generate a new stem cell to replenish the pool (Zhou et al., 2018). As a result, hippocampal stem cell numbers and neurogenesis sharply decrease over time (Snyder, 2019). The main differences between embryonic and adult neurogenesis in the dentate gyrus are the very limited migration that adult-born neurons undergo and the frequency with which neural stem cells produce new neurons. Some rare neuronal types of the dentate gyrus, such as semilunar and hilar granule cells, are generated only during development (Kerloch et al., 2019).

The neurogenic process in the adult dentate gyrus is remarkably similar to the neurogenic process during development (Table 4.3). While the molecular identities of neural stem cells and granule cell neurons shift between the embryonic and adult dentate gyrus, intermediate progenitor cells, neuroblasts, and immature granule neurons have nearly identical transcriptional profiles at all ages

Table 4.3 Effects of the main pathways and transcription factors on the regulation of embryonic and adult hippocampal neurogenesis

Gene/Pathway	Development	Adulthood	Comparison
Wnt	Promotes the proliferation and differentiation of neural precursors	Promotes the activation of quiescent stem cells; enhances neuronal differentiation	Similar
BMPR-Ia	Promotes the proliferation of neural precursors	Maintains stem cells in a quiescent state	Different
Notch	Maintains the neural stem cells pool by preventing premature differentiation	Maintains the neural stem cells pool by preventing exit from quiescence	Similar
Neurog2	Determines the glutamatergic differentiation of neural stem cells	Expressed in glutamatergic neuronal precursors, but function not directly tested	-
Tbr2	Essential for the proliferation and differentiation of intermediate proliferating cells	Essential for the proliferation and differentiation of intermediate proliferating cells	Similar
Prox1	Promotes differentiation and determines granule cell identity	Expressed by granule neuron precursor cells; promotes differentiation	Similar
NFIX	Required for correct positioning of neural stem cells in the postnatal dentate gyrus	Not analyzed (only straight knockout analyzed at P20)	-
Tlx	No significant role in the development of the dentate gyrus	Essential for the proliferation of adult neural stem cells (only straight knockout tested)	Different
CcnD2	No significant role in the development of the dentate gyrus	Essential for the proliferation of adult neural stem cells (only straight knockout tested)	Different
Ascl1	No significant role in the development of the dentate gyrus	Essential for the proliferation of adult neural stem cells	Different

Source: (Urban and Guillemot, 2014)

(Hochgerner et al., 2018). Signaling genes in the WNT and Notch pathways and transcription factors like Tbr2 and Prox1, which are crucial factors for the generation and maturation of granule cells during development, have similar roles during adult neurogenesis. This suggests that the same genetic program involving the same key transcription factors drives the differentiation of intermediate progenitor cells into glutamatergic cells in the dentate gyrus from development to adulthood (Hodge et al., 2008).

However, this does not hold true for factors acting earlier in the granule cell lineage. In particular, analysis of mouse mutants for the transcription factors NFIX, Tlx, and Ascl1, and the cyclin CcnD2, provides strong evidence that the genetic programs that promote the early steps of neurogenesis in the dentate gyrus during development and in the adult are distinct (Kowalczyk et al., 2004; Niu et al., 2011; Martynoga et al., 2013; Andersen et al., 2014; Heng et al., 2014). The phenotypes of Tlx, Ascl1, and CcnD2 mutants are very similar, suggesting that these genes belong to a common regulatory pathway operating specifically during adult neurogenesis to promote stem cell activation. The loss of one of these genes in adult stem cells cannot be functionally compensated, whereas their loss during development has milder or no effects, suggesting that more robust, redundant regulatory mechanisms support embryonic and early postnatal neurogenesis than adult neurogenesis.

The quiescent state of neural stem cells is regulated by the same developmental signals that act during the formation of the dentate gyrus, but they often have very different effects on adult quiescent stem cells than in developmental proliferating progenitors. BMP, for example, works to induce hippocampal fate and promote the proliferation of neural progenitors during development, while in the adult brain it has a central role in maintaining the quiescence of adult neural stem cells (Mira et al., 2010). Similarly, the transcriptional regulator Id4 downstream of Notch2 and BMP4 maintains the quiescent state of adult stem cells, whereas it promotes the proliferation of embryonic neural progenitors, including in the hippocampal primordium (Blomfield et al., 2019; Zhang et al., 2019).

Other factors, which have important functions in adult hippocampal neurogenesis, were not studied specifically during dentate gyrus development. These include the transcriptional repressor REST, which is required to maintain neural stem cells in a transcriptional quiescent and undifferentiated state (Mukherjee et al., 2016), as well as several microRNAs. For instance, miR-132 plays important roles in dendrite maturation and in the function of newly generated neurons in the adult dentate gyrus, and miR-137 promotes stem cell proliferation in the adult hippocampus in vivo and in adult neural stem cell cultures (Szulwach et al., 2010). The methyl-CpG binding protein MBD1 can regulate the expression of several microRNAs in adult hippocampal stem cells. One of them is miR-184, which promotes proliferation and suppresses differentiation of hippocampal progenitors (Liu et al., 2010). Another is miR-195, which in turn can repress MBD1, in a feedback regulatory loop that regulates the balance between proliferation and differentiation of hippocampal stem cells (Liu et al., 2013). Mice heterozygous mutant for the gene DGCR8, which is part of the complex mediating the biogenesis of microRNAs, show reduced cell proliferation and neurogenesis in the hippocampus (Ouchi et al., 2013), providing further evidence for a role of microRNAs in the regulation of adult hippocampal neurogenesis.

The rate of generation of new neurons in the adult dentate gyrus is regulated by a surprisingly high number of stimuli, ranging from diet to exercise, to social interactions (Urban et al., 2019). These stimuli can act at several levels of the neurogenic process, from stem cell activation to proliferation of progenitors or survival and integration of the new neurons (see Chapter 9). Interestingly, in contrast to what was suggested by some early studies, modern design-based stereological studies of the number of neurons in the granule cell layer have revealed that granule cell number is essentially stable throughout adulthood under normal conditions. Given the complexity of the mechanisms regulating adult neurogenesis and cell survival, an increase or a decrease in granule cell number due to environmental or pathological conditions may be possible. However, the evidence so far has revealed that the influence of such factors on granule cell number appears limited to the developmental period.

4.3.5 Neurons of the polymorphic layer

There is little information regarding the development of individual classes of neurons found in the polymorphic layer of the dentate gyrus. Bayer (1980) reported that most cells found in the rat polymorphic layer are generated between E15 and E18, with a peak at E17, i.e., earlier than the neurons of the granule cell layer. The most prominent cells found in this layer are the mossy cells, which give rise to the associational connection to the ipsilateral molecular layer and the commissural projection to the contralateral dentate gyrus. The mossy cells are glutamatergic neurons that are most likely generated between E15 and E21 in rats. GABAergic interneurons located in the polymorphic layer are likely derived from stem cells located in the medial (MGE) and caudal (CGE) ganglionic eminences, as described in the next section. Cell proliferation observed at later ages in the rodent polymorphic layer represents the tertiary matrix for the generation of granule cells.

There is little published information regarding the specific time of birth of neurons found in the monkey polymorphic layer. The patterns of neurogenesis revealed by Rakic and Nowakowski (1981) in monkeys are consistent with the patterns described in rodents. However, to our knowledge, there is no study that distinguishes between GABAergic interneurons and glutamatergic mossy cells. Note also that the proliferative zone from which the dentate granule cells originate is much narrower in both monkeys and humans, as compared with rodents. Otherwise, the morphological characteristics of the development of the polymorphic layer appear similar across species. Ki-67-positive cells, an intrinsic marker of cell division, are found mostly in the polymorphic layer; fewer immunopositive cells are found in the molecular and granule cell layers. In humans, a large number of Ki-67-positive cells are detected in the polymorphic layer at the 13th week of gestation (Seress et al., 2001). At term (37–40 weeks), the dentate gyrus contains Ki-67-positive cells mostly in the polymorphic and granule cell layers, and fewer in the molecular layer. Some labeled cells appear to be glial elements in the molecular and polymorphic layers. Other labeled cells in the polymorphic and granule cell layers display chromatin characteristics typical of neurons, suggesting that those cells will likely become granule cells. Cell nuclei of large neurons in the polymorphic layer are never labeled, which indicates that these neurons were generated earlier during gestation.

4.3.6 GABAergic interneurons

Interneurons are often simply defined as GABAergic neurons contributing to the inhibitory activity of local circuits, and thus controlling the excitability of principal glutamatergic neurons. However, current views highlight the heterogeneity of hippocampal interneurons (Freund and Buzsaki, 1996; Somogyi and Klausberger, 2005; Danglot et al., 2006; Klausberger, 2009), which are considered integral components of the normal information processing within the hippocampal formation (Pelkey et al., 2017) (see Chapter 7). Hippocampal GABAergic interneurons differ from principal cells in both their morphological and developmental features. In contrast to the more uniform populations of granule cells and pyramidal neurons, hippocampal interneurons can be defined based on the location of their cell bodies, the organization of their dendritic trees, their axonal projections, or their immunoreactivity for different neuropeptides or calcium-binding proteins (see Chapter 3). Neuroanatomical classifications of interneurons can be complemented with information regarding their developmental origin, molecular profiles and electrophysiological characteristics, and the algorithmic roles they may play in information processing (as discussed in detail in Chapter 7). However, hippocampal interneurons cannot be easily grouped when all these criteria are considered. We therefore limit our description first to the developmental time of origin of GABAergic interneurons, mostly based on their locations in distinct regions/layers of the hippocampal formation.

GABAergic interneurons are generated earlier than principal neurons found in the dentate gyrus and the hippocampus (Table 4.2). And, despite the heterogeneity of the populations of interneurons found in the adult hippocampal formation, they all seem to derive from precursor cells located in the MGE and CGE (Figure 4.2), under the control of specific combinations of transcription factors (Pelkey et al., 2017); for example, NKX2.1 or LHX6 for interneurons derived from MGE and NR2F2 for interneurons derived from CGE (Pleasure et al., 2000). These cells thus need to migrate a much longer distance from their place of origin to their final destinations in the hippocampus than most cortical interneurons. This migration takes 2–3 days in mouse embryos. Interneurons derived from both MGE and CGE begin to reach the hippocampus fields at E14, while interneurons derived from the CGE start populating the dentate gyrus at E17. Upon their arrival, interneurons interact with projection neurons, and this interaction may be required for the final maturation of both cell types. The final positioning and differentiation of interneurons extend into postnatal ages.

Studies carried out in mice (Angevine, 1965), rats (Bayer, 1980), and monkeys (Rakic and Nowakowski, 1981) have shown that the production of neurons destined for the molecular and polymorphic layers of the dentate gyrus precedes the peak of production of granule cells (Table 4.2; Figures 4.3 and 4.4). Most neurons that ultimately reside in strata oriens, radiatum, and lacunosum-moleculare are generated earlier than the peak of production for the pyramidal neurons. Interneurons must travel tangentially over long distances to reach the hippocampus and migrate radially to reach their final locations. Interestingly, MGE produces parvalbumin-, somatostatin-, and nitric oxide synthase–expressing interneurons, which are preferentially located toward strata oriens and the pyramidal cell layer (Tricoire et al., 2011). CGE-derived interneurons contain cholecystokinin, calretinin, vasoactive intestinal peptide, and reelin, and are preferentially located in strata radiatum and lacunosum-moleculare. GABA itself may promote or arrest the radial migration of interneurons depending on cell maturity (Pelkey et al., 2017). This is due to the developmental regulation of expression of the K/Cl cotransporter KCC2, which extrudes chloride, and the Na-K-2Cl cotransporter, NKCC1, which accumulates chloride

intracellularly. Migrating interneurons initially express low levels of KCC2 and thus a higher intracellular chloride concentration, which allows GABA to increase motility via depolarization and activation of voltage-gated calcium channels. KCC2 expression increases as interneurons mature, which leads GABA to hyperpolarize the cell, and thus reduce calcium influx and stop radial migration.

The integration of interneurons in the dendritic layers of principal neurons initially suggested that GABAergic interneurons play a role in the morphogenesis of principal neurons and the proper laminar organization of the connectivity of hippocampal circuits. Indeed, commissural projections terminate transiently on GABAergic interneurons in stratum radiatum, before establishing synapses with the dendrites of pyramidal neurons. However, studies using DLX1/2 mutant mice, which lack GABAergic cells in the hippocampus, revealed that the elimination of interneurons does not have an impact on the laminar organization of the hippocampal commissural afferents (Pleasure et al., 2000). In contrast, the Cajal-Retzius cells, a type of pioneer neuron transiently present in the hippocampus during development and that subsequently die by apoptosis, appear to play a major role in the proper lamination and overall organization of hippocampal circuits (Frotscher, 1997; Anstotz et al., 2018).

In mice, the work by Angevine (1965) provides a comprehensive evaluation of the time of origin of hippocampal neurons. The birth dates of hippocampal interneurons can be inferred based on the locations of their cell bodies in the adult hippocampus. Since there are slight differences in the data reported in the graphical representations of the number of neurons and the illustrations showing the locations of the labeled neurons by Angevine, our summary in Table 4.2 is based on our interpretation of the illustrations (Figure 4.3). There is, to our knowledge, no double-labeling immunohistochemical study using exogenous cell-division markers that provides a comprehensive analysis of the time of origin of hippocampal GABAergic interneurons in mice.

In rats, the combined use of ^{3}H-thymidine autoradiography and glutamic acid decarboxylase (GAD)-like immunohistochemistry confirmed that GABAergic neurons are generated earlier than the principal cells of the hippocampal formation. In the dentate gyrus, the basket cells located at the base of the granule cell layer and the majority of other interneurons located in the polymorphic layer are generated before the interneurons found in the molecular layer. All interneurons of the dentate gyrus are generated well before the peak of production of granule cells. They have become postmitotic when it is estimated that less than 5% of the granule cells are born and well before a definitive molecular layer has formed (Amaral and Kurz, 1985). The peak of generation of GABAergic interneurons in the hippocampus and subiculum is around E14 in rats, that is well before the peak of generation of principal cells in CA3 (E17), CA2 (E16–E17), CA1 (E17–E19), and subiculum (deep E16, superficial E16–E17).

In monkeys, neurons generated at E38 are found in strata oriens, radiatum and lacunosum-moleculare of the hippocampus, the molecular layer of the subiculum, and the polymorphic and molecular layers of the dentate gyrus (Rakic and Nowakowski, 1981). There is an increase in the number of neurons generated at E40, which are found in strata radiatum and lacunosum-moleculare. Interneuron production appears to cease after E50. Similar to the developmental origin of interneurons described in rodents, primate interneurons also derive from distinct populations of precursor cells found in the ganglionic eminences (Hansen et al., 2013; Ma et al., 2013).

There is, to our knowledge, no specific information on the time of origin of hippocampal interneurons in humans. However, distinct subpopulations of GABAergic interneurons, which express different types of calcium-binding proteins, exhibit distinct temporal and regional patterns of development after midgestation, which are similar to those observed in monkeys and humans (Berger et al., 1993; Berger and Alvarez, 1994, 1996; Berger et al., 2001).

4.3.7 Cajal-Retzius cells

Although much is known about the molecular mechanisms guiding neuron migration that were unraveled with modern molecular techniques, it was initially postulated that neuronal migration may be guided by transient populations of neurons present in the marginal zone during development, such as the Cajal-Retzius cells. These cells extend long dendrites horizontally in the marginal zone, parallel to the pial surface (Retzius, 1893, 1894; Ramón y Cajal, 1911; Soriano and Del Rio, 2005). They synthesize and secrete reelin, which forms a component of the extracellular matrix and acts as a stop signal for migrating neurons. Early generated neurons are stopped as they approach the marginal zone, which has a high concentration of reelin. Late generated neurons migrate past the early generated neurons and approach the marginal zone to reach the stop signal provided by reelin. In this way the characteristic inside-out lamination of the cortex and hippocampus is formed. Because the marginal zone ultimately becomes layer I of the cortex, it remains an almost cell-free layer in normally developing mice. In reeler mutant mice, which do not produce reelin, layer I is densely filled with neurons. Early generated neurons migrate until they reach the pial surface, and later generated neurons accumulate beneath them. The normal inside-out lamination is reversed. Although this description is an oversimplification of the molecular mechanisms guiding neuronal migration, as it involves only one signaling molecule, it can explain the lamination of the reeler mouse hippocampus, in which a double pyramidal cell layer is formed. The marginal zone of the hippocampus proper corresponds to the stratum lacunosum-moleculare, which contains Cajal-Retzius cells and an extracellular matrix enriched in reelin. The absence of the stop signal allows some pyramidal cells to migrate into stratum radiatum and form a second pyramidal layer.

The marginal zone of the dentate gyrus corresponds to the outer portion of the molecular layer. If reelin acts as a stop signal and was the only mechanism guiding neuronal migration, one would expect granule cells to invade the molecular layer in reeler mice. However, the granule cells do not invade the molecular layer, and many granule cells are found in the polymorphic layer with their dendrites oriented in all directions. Other guiding mechanisms, such as the radial glial fibers required for neuronal migration (Rickmann et al., 1987), are dramatically altered in the dentate gyrus of reeler mice. In fact, astrocytes are found in lieu of radial glial cells in the developing dentate gyrus of reeler mice. This suggests that the gene RLN and its protein reelin may be involved in several other cellular processes important for the normal development of the brain, and the hippocampus in particular.

One important characteristic of the Cajal-Retzius cells is the fact that a large population of these cells are only transiently present during the development of the mammalian hippocampus (Super et al., 1998b; Soriano and Del Rio, 2005). Together with GABAergic interneurons generated before the principal cells, Cajal-Retzius cells are considered pioneer neurons forming layer-specific scaffolds that overlap with distinct hippocampal afferents at embryonic and early postnatal ages in mice. They may play a role in the proper lamination of the principal cell layers, as well as with the establishment and maturation of different hippocampal circuits (Glærum et al., 2024). Indeed, the protein reelin produced by the Cajal-Retzius cells has been shown to be one of the factors regulating the growth of entorhinal afferents in organotypic cultures (Del Rio et al., 1997), and the absence of Cajal-Retzius cells results in a reduction in latrophilin-2 that contributes to the topographical organization of hippocampal circuits (Pederick et al., 2021).

4.4 Development of hippocampal connections

The development of specific connections in the hippocampus, as in the rest of the brain, requires guidance of outgrowing axons to their proper target areas, followed by their restriction to a particular lamina and the formation of specific synapses with different cell types. The guidance of growing axons to their target areas involves both chemoattractant molecules that direct axons to a particular location and chemorepellent molecules that prevent invasion of adjacent sites. Multiple families of secreted and membrane-bound molecules exert attractive or repulsive actions in a highly site-specific and coordinated fashion. Functional interactions between guidance molecules increase the specificity and robustness, and also the complexity, of guidance mechanisms. The establishment of at least certain hippocampal connections follows a developmental program that may be independent of neuronal activity. This was shown, for example, by blocking electrical activity in entorhinal-hippocampal cocultures by application of the sodium channel blocker tetrodotoxin, which did not alter the development of the lamina-specific termination of entorhinal fibers or the differentiation of granule cell dendrites (Frotscher et al., 2000).

The hippocampus proper and the dentate gyrus both comprise only one layer of principal neurons but their main afferent and efferent projections are typically organized in several distinct layers that terminate in a nonoverlapping fashion. These projections interact with restricted dendritic segments of principal neurons that traverse the fields of axon terminals. Importantly, it is now clear that the development of hippocampal connections is not guided by the temporal profile of neurogenesis of principal cells. Indeed, guidance molecules, transient Cajal-Retzius cells, and GABAergic interneurons contribute to the laminar organization of specific hippocampal afferents and intrinsic connections. Furthermore, many axonal projections establish transient synaptic contacts with these two types of cells before connecting with principal glutamatergic neurons. Here, we briefly describe the major guidance molecules and the timeline of establishment of the major hippocampal connections in mice, rats, monkeys, and humans. We consider different steps in the establishment of these connections, including axon pathfinding, target recognition, and synapse formation.

4.4.1 Overall description of guidance molecules

A number of studies have provided clues about the signaling molecules that contribute to the guidance of entorhinal axons to their appropriate targets in the hippocampus and dentate gyrus, as well as for the establishment of other major hippocampal pathways. Soluble and membrane-bound molecules, which act as attractant or repellent signals, as well as different types of receptors expressed on different neuronal types contribute to the regulation of these processes. Here, we first provide a brief description of these different molecules.

Semaphorins. Semaphorins constitute a large family of guidance molecules that includes both transmembrane and secreted factors. Some of these semaphorins and their receptors, Neuropilin1, Neuropilin2, and the Plexins, are expressed in the hippocampus and act as repulsive guidance molecules for different hippocampal pathways. Sema3A is involved in the establishment of the entorhinal connections and mossy fibers. Sema3C is involved in the establishment of the septal connections. Sema3E-PlexinD1 signaling also contributes to the lamination of entorhinal axon terminals. Sema3F is involved in the establishment of intrahippocampal connections, acting via the Neuropilin2 and PlexinA3 receptors. Several other membrane-anchored semaphorins (Sema4B, Sema 5A, Sema 5B) are also expressed in the hippocampus and further restrict the growth of incoming fibers, thus helping to establish the laminar specificity of hippocampal projections.

Ephrins. Several ephrin receptors and their ligands also contribute to the formation of major hippocampal pathways. The Eph-A5 receptor is expressed by entorhinal fibers growing into the hippocampus, and one of its ligands, EphrinA3, is expressed in the dentate gyrus granule cell layer and the hippocampal pyramidal cell layer. Interaction of EphrinA3 with the Eph-A5 receptor in the dentate gyrus results in inhibition of entorhinal axons outgrowth into the inner molecular layer, therefore restricting the termination of the perforant path projections to the outer molecular layer (Stein et al., 1999). Disruption of Eph-A signaling by overexpression of a soluble Eph-A receptor also affects the mossy fiber infrapyramidal bundle which forms abnormally long projections that establish ectopic contacts and fails to retract to the proximal portion of CA3 (Martinez et al., 2005).

Netrin. Netrin1 exerts either chemoattractive or chemorepulsive effects on axons growing to or away from the ventral midline of the developing central nervous system. Netrin1 is expressed specifically in the target areas of hippocampal commissural fibers, while the Netrin1 receptor DDC is expressed in the areas sending the fibers. Netrin1 is involved in the attraction of axons to their termination zones in the contralateral hippocampus, and commissural axons fail to cross the midline in Netrin1-deficient mice (Barallobre et al., 2000). In these mice, ipsilateral entorhinohippocampal and CA3–CA1 associational projections also show an altered pattern of laminar termination. Netrin1 is expressed along the fimbria, where it chemoattracts both hippocamposeptal and septohippocampal fibers, and thus the same molecular cue serves in the establishment of these reciprocal connections.

Slit. The secreted repulsive molecules Slit1 and Slit2 are expressed by axons emanating from the entorhinal cortex, while their receptors Robo1 and Robo2 are expressed in the hippocampus and dentate gyrus. In the molecular layer of the dentate gyrus, Slit2 prevents Robo-expressing mossy fibers from growing to the distal dendritic segments of granule cells, suggesting a role in the laminar organization of the molecular layer. Robo expression could also prevent mossy fibers from crossing the Slit2-expressing midline (Nguyen Ba-Charvet et al., 1999). In addition, Robo2 plays a role in the formation of excitatory synapses on CA1 pyramidal neurons (Blockus et al., 2021).

Cadherin. Cadherin9 is required for the formation and differentiation of the dentate gyrus mossy fiber synapses onto CA3 neurons (Williams et al., 2011). Mossy fibers have the unique feature of making synapses on the proximal dendrites of CA3 pyramidal neurons, but not on CA2 or CA1 pyramidal neurons. This target specificity does not depend on selective axon growth toward CA3 pyramidal neurons but requires instead CA3-specific cell recognition cues. Cadherin9 is expressed by dentate granule cells and CA3 pyramidal neurons, and provides a bidirectional transsynaptic recognition cue for the establishment of synaptic contacts between the two cell types.

Teneurin. Teneurin-3 functions as a homophilic cell adhesion molecule, which mediates the recognition between axons and target cells, and is expressed in several hippocampal regions, including proximal CA1, distal subiculum, and the medial entorhinal cortex (Berns et al., 2018). It is required in both CA1 and subicular neurons for the precise targeting of the projections from the proximal portion of CA1 to the distal portion of the subiculum, which are also both interconnected with the medial entorhinal cortex. In parallel, expression of latrophilin-2 is required for the precise targeting of the projections from the distal portion of CA1 to the proximal portion of the subiculum, which are both interconnected with the lateral entorhinal cortex (Pederick et al., 2021). Thus, teneurin-3 and latrophilin-2 play complementary roles in the control of the assembly of complex and distributed functional circuits by matching expression and homophilic attraction.

In sum, several families of guidance molecules and their receptors direct the growth of the different hippocampal projections and ensure the establishment of specific connectivity. However, the experimental approaches employed so far have mainly addressed the role of individual factors. Yet, these different molecules most certainly act in concert, and it remains an open question how their interactions add specificity and provide robustness.

In the next sections, we describe the timing of establishment of specific hippocampal connections and add some details regarding the molecular mechanisms guiding these developmental processes: (1) the entorhinal connections to the dentate gyrus and hippocampus, (2) the dentate gyrus mossy fibers, (3) the commissural connections, (4) the septal connections, (5) the CA3 to CA1 connections, and (6) the CA1 to subiculum connections.

4.4.2 Entorhinal connections

As described in Chapters 3 and 12, the entorhinal cortex projects to the dentate gyrus, hippocampus, and subiculum. The lateral and medial components of the perforant path terminate along a superficial-to-deep gradient in the outer two-thirds of the molecular layer of the dentate gyrus and stratum lacunosum-moleculare of CA3, and along a transverse gradient in the stratum lacunosum-moleculare of CA1 and the molecular layer of the subiculum. Entorhinal cortex layer II neurons give rise to the projection to the dentate gyrus, CA3, and CA2, and layer III neurons project to CA1 and the subiculum. Although the term "perforant path" is often used to refer to all entorhinohippocampal projections, entorhinal fibers also reach CA1 via the alveus, i.e., the alvear pathway. These diverse, yet very specific, patterns of connectivity between the entorhinal cortex and the rest of the hippocampal formation must require the finely tuned regulation of expression of guidance molecules and cellular receptors for precise axonal pathfinding, discrete target layer recognition, and selective synapse formation.

In rats, the projections from the entorhinal cortex to the hippocampus and dentate gyrus form early in development, with the first entorhinal axons reaching the hippocampus between E16 (via the alvear path) and E17 (via the perforant path), and the dentate gyrus at P2 (Ceranik et al., 2000; JB Deng et al., 2007). In mice, the alvear pathway is observed as early as E15. The perforant path appears and entorhinal fibers arborize within stratum lacunosummoleculare at E17, and the first axons invading the outer molecular layer of the dentate gyrus are visible at E19 (Super and Soriano, 1994). From the very beginning, the entorhinal cortex projections reach the appropriate termination zones, when the definitive targets of entorhinal axons, the pyramidal cells in the hippocampus and the granule cells in the dentate gyrus are not yet fully developed. Transient Cajal-Retzius cells located in these termination zones project to the entorhinal cortex and provide a template that is used by the entorhinal axons to find their target layers in the hippocampus (Ceranik et al., 2000). Their role as pioneer neurons has been demonstrated by ablation of Cajal-Retzius cells in organotypic slice cultures of the dentate gyrus, which prevents entorhinal fibers from reaching the molecular layer (Del Rio et al., 1997). They also provide targets for incoming entorhinal fibers, which form transient synapses with these neurons. At birth, the entorhinal cortex projections to the molecular layer of the dentate gyrus are present and properly segregated as in the adult (Fricke and Cowan, 1977; Cowan et al., 1981; O'Reilly et al., 2015), even though the majority of the granule cells, their final targets, will be added postnatally.

Investigators have focused on repulsive guidance molecules expressed in the hippocampus that would prevent the entorhinal afferents from terminating in proximal layers close to the cell bodies of principal neurons (Brinks et al., 2004). Similarly, molecules specifically expressed in the entorhinal cortex were studied for their capacity to repel entorhinal axons, thereby directing them toward the hippocampus. In particular, repulsive effects of Sema3A on entorhinal fibers have been shown to act via the receptor Neuropilin1. As Sema3A is expressed by granule cells, this expression may also be involved in the termination of entorhinal fibers on distal granule cell dendrites. Neuropilin2, the receptor for Sema3F, is strongly expressed in the hippocampus, whereas the ligand is expressed in the developing entorhinal cortex. As Sema3F is repulsive for growing axons bearing its receptor, this particular pattern may be responsible for the lack of ingrowth of hippocampal and dentate axons into the entorhinal cortex. Similarly, Slit 1 and Slit 2 are expressed in the entorhinal cortex (Sasaki et al., 2020), and may repel axons of hippocampal neurons expressing their receptors Robo1 and Robo2. Ephrin-A3 also exerts repulsive effects on entorhinal axons, restricting their termination to the distal portion of the dendrites of hippocampal neurons (Stein et al., 1999). In addition, neurotrophic factors with attractive effects, pioneer neurons, and components of the extracellular matrix may also contribute to the guidance of entorhinal axons to their appropriate targets in the hippocampus and dentate gyrus.

As mentioned above, Cajal-Retzius cells project to the entorhinal cortex and provide a guiding scaffold for entorhinal axons to reach the hippocampus. Interestingly, the protein reelin secreted by the Cajal-Retzius cells does not play a role in axon guidance. Indeed, the entorhinohippocampal projection develops almost normally in reeler mutant mice, which lack reelin expression. Cajal-Retzius cells and their projections to the entorhinal cortex are present in these mutants and thus serve their normal function as a template for entorhinal axons. However, reelin contributes to the establishment of the branching pattern of entorhinal terminals in wild type mice, and in absence of reelin, entorhinal axons give rise to fewer collaterals and synapses. Thus, components of the extracellular matrix likely play an important part in the segregation of hippocampal afferents. For example, hyaluronic acid and proteoglycans contribute to target layer recognition of entorhinal fibers (Zhao et al., 2003). When hippocampal slices are treated with hyaluronidase and then cocultured with entorhinal cortex, entorhinal fibers invade the molecular layer but are no longer restricted to its outer two-thirds. Interestingly, no similar role of extracellular matrix components was found for the laminar specificity of commissural/associational fibers.

In sum, secreted molecules such as the semaphorins, membrane-bound receptors, extracellular matrix components, and a template formed by Cajal-Retzius cell axons are likely involved in the directed growth and layer-specific termination of entorhinal projections. The entorhinal axons reach their appropriate termination zone before the distal dendrites of pyramidal neurons and granule cells have grown into stratum lacunosum-moleculare and the outer molecular layer, respectively. A majority of Cajal-Retzius cells die after the entorhinohippocampal projection has formed, and the distal dendrites of pyramidal neurons and granule cells have grown into the entorhinal termination fields. At that time, entorhinal axons establish definitive synapses with the distal dendrites of pyramidal neurons and granule cells.

Experiments in which anterograde tracers were injected into the entorhinal cortex in 2-week-old macaque monkeys revealed that the three fiber bundles originating from the entorhinal cortex (the perforant path, the alvear pathway, and the commissural connection) are all established by this age (Amaral et al., 2014). Fundamental features of the laminar and topographic distribution of these pathways are also similar to those in adults. However, some of these projections are more extensive in the neonate than in the mature brain. The homotopic commissural projection from the entorhinal cortex, for example, originates from a larger region within the entorhinal cortex and terminates much more densely in layer I of the contralateral entorhinal cortex than in the adult. In sum, the overall topographical organization of the main cortical afferent pathways to the dentate gyrus and hippocampus are established by birth in monkeys.

In humans, robust reciprocal connections between the entorhinal cortex, hippocampus, and subiculum are present at 19 weeks of gestation (the earliest age evaluated in the study by Hevner and Kinney, 1996), and are topographically similar to those observed in adult primates. Specifically, projections to the hippocampus and subiculum originate from neurons in entorhinal cortex layers II and III, whereas reciprocal projections to the entorhinal cortex originate from pyramidal neurons in CA1 and the subiculum. In contrast, the perforant pathway projection to the dentate gyrus reaches only rudimentary stages of development by 22 weeks of gestation. The penetration and crossing of perforant path fibers through the hippocampal fissure can be seen at 23 weeks of gestation (Šimić et al., 2022).

4.4.3 Mossy fibers

The development of the mossy fibers has been studied in rats by Amaral and colleagues (Amaral and Dent, 1981; Cowan et al., 1981). The earliest mossy fibers are formed prenatally, when less than 20% of granule cells have been generated. At birth, Timm-stained preparations through the temporal portion of the hippocampal formation reveal a densely stained zone extending from the suprapyramidal granule cell layer, through the polymorphic layer, which forms a distinct band in the zone immediately superficial to the pyramidal cell layer of CA3. At this stage, the mossy fibers exhibit only small axonal expansions, but lack the swellings and protrusions that are characteristic of the fully developed mossy fiber expansions. They form both symmetric and asymmetric contacts with the primary dendritic shafts of hilar cells and CA3 pyramidal cells. Over the next 2 weeks, the mossy fiber projection expands in thickness within the stratum lucidum, extends rostrally toward the septal pole of the hippocampus, and forms a distinct infrapyramidal bundle of mossy fibers. The developmental pattern of mossy fibers parallels the suprapyramidal-to-infrapyramidal and temporal-to-septal gradients in the time of origin of the granule cells. Although the overall pattern of mossy fibers observed at 3 weeks of age is very similar to that observed in adult rats, this system continues to be modified with the addition of new granule cells, and the elaboration of individual mossy fibers, including a stereotyped pruning of the infrapyramidal bundle (Bagri et al., 2003).

The molecular mechanisms that govern the lamina-restricted projection of the dentate gyrus granule cells are not completely understood. However, semaphorins and their plexin receptors contribute to the proper organization of mossy fiber projections (Tawarayama et al., 2010). PlxnA4-expressing mossy fibers are prevented from entering the Sema6A-expressing suprapyramidal and infrapyramidal regions of CA3 but are permitted to grow into proximal parts of the regions, where the repulsive activity of Sema6A is suppressed by PlxnA2. In addition, Sema6B is expressed in CA3 and repels mossy fibers in a PlxnA4-dependent manner. In Sema6B-deficient mice, mossy fibers project to strata radiatum and oriens. The number of aberrant mossy fibers is increased in Sema6A-Sema6B double knockout mice, indicating that Sema6A and Sema6B function additively to guide the proper extension of mossy fibers. PlxnA2 does not suppress the Sema6B response, but itself promotes growth of mossy fibers. Thus, the balance between repulsion by Sema6A and Sema6B and attraction by PlxnA2 contributes to the definition of the hippocampal laminae that mossy fibers can innervate. Semaphorin 3F and its receptors neuropilin2 and plexin-A3 also seem to contribute to the pruning of collateral axons during postnatal development, and thus contribute to the refinement of mossy fiber projections (Bagri et al., 2003). The formation of the typical synaptic contacts between the mossy fibers and the dendrites of the CA3 pyramidal neurons, the so-called thorny excrescences (see Chapter 3), requires specific cell-surface molecular signals. Cadherin-9 encodes a type II cadherin expressed in both dentate granule cells and CA3 pyramidal neurons, it provides a bidirectional target recognition cue between these cells via homophilic binding (Williams et al., 2011).

4.4.4 Commissural connections

Commissural fibers, originating from CA3 pyramidal neurons and hilar mossy cells, project via the hippocampal commissure to the contralateral hippocampus and dentate gyrus. In the mouse hippocampus, the first commissural axons arrive in the contralateral hippocampus at E18 and in the dentate gyrus at P2 (Super and Soriano, 1994). This is considerably later than the arrival of the entorhinal axons. The commissural connections terminate on the proximal portion of dentate granule cells. Neither the time of arrival nor the presence of pioneer Cajal-Retzius cells or GABAergic interneurons plays a role in the proper lamination of the commissural afferents. Thus, it appears that the target cells, the principal neurons, which are already present at that time and have already grown a dendritic arbor may provide the appropriate guidance signals (Deller et al., 1999). Indeed, in reeler mice and knockout mice lacking the reelin receptors APOER2 or VLDR, the granule cells are more loosely distributed within the polymorphic and granule cell layers, and the commissural axons are distributed throughout these layers (Gebhardt et al., 2002). In contrast, the entorhinodentate projection forms normally in the outer molecular layer of these three lines of mutant mice. As with other commissural projections, Netrin1 and its receptor DCC may be important for the formation of the hippocampal commissure (Barallobre et al., 2000). Midline glial cells are also required for hippocampal commissural axons to cross the midline, as defects in midline glial structures in Nfia mutant mice result in the hippocampal commissure being reduced or absent (Shu et al., 2003).

4.4.5 Septal connections

The septohippocampal projection comprises two parts: a cholinergic component and a GABAergic component. The cells of origin of both components are located in the medial septal nucleus/diagonal band complex (see Chapter 3), and the ontogeny of these two fiber systems has not been entirely clarified. One study in rats suggested that both fiber systems reach the hippocampus at about the same time to establish synaptic contacts with distinct cell populations (Linke and Frotscher, 1993). In contrast, another study in mice suggested that the cholinergic system develops earlier than the GABAergic system (Super and Soriano, 1994). In adult animals, cholinergic septohippocampal afferents are thin, varicose axons with small axonal swellings; septal afferents at prenatal stages display these features. The view that most early septohippocampal fibers are cholinergic axons is also supported by the presence of acetylcholinesterase- and NGF receptor-positive fibers in the embryonic hippocampus (Milner et al., 1983; Koh and Loy, 1989). From P0, a distinct set of septohippocampal fibers is present, including thick axons following straight courses and displaying large boutons that form incipient basket-like arrangements (Super and Soriano, 1994). These morphological features correspond to those of the GABAergic septohippocampal fibers (Freund and Antal, 1988).

Overall, the hippocamposeptal projection is established earlier than the septohippocampal projection (Super and Soriano, 1994; Linke et al., 1995). The development of the septohippocampal projection may depend on the hippocamposeptal projection, which originates from nonpyramidal neurons and develops as early as E15 in mice and terminates in the medial septum at that age (Super and Soriano, 1994). Similarly in rats, the first hippocampal projection neurons are nonpyramidal neurons that may pave the way to the septum (Linke and Frotscher, 1993; Linke et al., 1995); hippocampal axons reach the septal region at E16 (Linke et al., 1995). Pyramidal cell axons follow this first cohort of axons into the medial septum. During the perinatal period, the hippocampal innervation of the lateral septum begins to form, which likely originates from pyramidal cells that are the main source of hippocamposeptal connections in the adult (Alonso and Kohler, 1982). Hippocampal projections run along the midline of the brain, approaching the medial septum. Axons to the lateral septum are first observed around E18/19, and the lateral septum is partly innervated by collaterals of axons that travel to the medial septum. The projection to the lateral septum becomes larger during early postnatal stages, whereas that to the medial septum is reduced. Projections from the subiculum preferentially target the lateral septum from the first postnatal days, and axonal distribution expands over the next 3 weeks (Tsamis et al., 2020).

Cells retrogradely labeled in the medial septum following injections into the hippocampus are first observed at E18 in the rat (Linke et al., 1995). At E19, the majority of the septal axons directed toward the hippocampal formation pass the hippocampus and grow further into the subicular complex and entorhinal cortex; collaterals of these fibers innervate the hippocampus (Linke and Frotscher, 1993). The general topography of the septohippocampal projection is rather diffuse at birth. Unlike the entorhinohippocampal and the hippocampal commissural projections, septohippocampal cholinergic fibers do not terminate in clearly demarcated layers, even in adulthood (Milner et al., 1983). Although a fairly adult pattern of the septohippocampal projection is reached by P10, including the projection reaching the dentate gyrus, many growth cones are still present. Moreover, there is an increase in the activity of both choline acetyltransferase (CAT) and acetylcholinesterase (AChE) until P21 in rats, when it reaches adult levels.

Cholinergic fibers are found in all layers of the hippocampal formation but are more concentrated in the cell body layers. They establish contacts with both principal neurons and interneurons, and their contacts are on cell bodies, dendritic shafts, and spines. In contrast, the GABAergic projection terminates almost exclusively on GABAergic interneurons. Inhibitory neurons afferent to inhibitory neurons may thus serve to disinhibit the activity of principal neurons. Several guidance molecules are likely involved in pathfinding and target recognition of septohippocampal fibers. For example, one of the semaphorins, Sema3C, repels the growth of septal fibers and its receptor, Neuropilin2, is expressed along the path of septal fibers, suggesting the involvement of this system in the formation of the septohippocampal projection (Steup et al., 2000). However, the development of the GABAergic septohippocampal pathway is normal in Sema3C-knockout mice (Rubio et al., 2011). Nevertheless, GABAergic septohippocampal fibers terminate preferentially onto Sema3C-positive interneurons, whereas cholinergic septohippocampal fibers terminate onto Sema3E and Sema-3A-positive pyramidal and granule cells (Pascual et al., 2005). Thus, class 3 secreted semaphorins likely contribute to the establishment of target-specific septohippocampal connections, yet redundant axonal guidance-related mechanisms certainly exist.

4.4.6 CA3 to CA1 connections

The axon guidance receptor Robo2 plays a role in establishing the cellular and subcellular specificity of excitatory projections from CA3 pyramidal neurons onto CA1 pyramidal neurons (Blockus et al., 2021). Whereas the expression of the Robo1 receptor is restricted to CA3, Robo2 receptor expression is restricted to strata oriens and radiatum of CA1, which are both recipient layers of CA3 and CA2 pyramidal neuron projections. Robo2 expression is

restricted to the postsynaptic element and is required for excitatory synapse formation from CA3 pyramidal neurons onto CA1 pyramidal neurons. Accordingly, conditional deletion of Robo2 expression from CA1 pyramidal neurons during development leads to a significant reduction in spine density in strata oriens and radiatum, but not in stratum lacunosum-moleculare, in which the entorhinal cortex projections terminate. In addition, the role of Robo2 in the establishment of synaptic connections between CA3 and CA1 pyramidal neurons is dependent on its ligand Slit and the presynaptic expression of the transmembrane protein Neurexin in CA3 pyramidal neurons. Although the exact nature of the interaction between these three proteins remains to be clarified, a Robo-Slit-Neurexin trans-synaptic complex appears necessary to promote excitatory synapse formation between CA3 and CA1 pyramidal neurons. Given that Robo1 expression is restricted to CA3, it would be interesting to determine whether it plays a similar role in the establishment of excitatory associational synapses between CA3 pyramidal neurons. It would also be interesting to determine the factors that prevent the establishment of excitatory synapses between CA1 pyramidal neurons, since CA1 intrinsic connections are very limited as compared with the massive projections from CA3 to CA3, CA2, and CA1. For example, whether cell-type-specific expression of different neurexin isoforms contribute to establishing this differential pattern of connectivity remains to be investigated (Gomez et al., 2021).

4.4.7 CA1 to subiculum connections

Two studies have also revealed the role of the evolutionarily conserved cell surface molecules teneurin-3 and latrophilin-2 in the establishment of parallel hippocampal networks between CA1 and the subiculum (Berns et al., 2018; Pederick et al., 2021). As discussed in Chapter 3, pyramidal cells located in the proximal portion of CA1 project to the distal portion of the subiculum, and both regions are more highly interconnected with the medial entorhinal cortex. In contrast, pyramidal cells located in the distal portion of CA1 project to the proximal portion of the subiculum and both regions are more highly interconnected with the lateral entorhinal cortex.

Although CA1 pyramidal neurons exhibit very similar structural characteristics along the transverse axis of the hippocampus, differences in gene expression contribute to the establishment of these patterns of connectivity (Figure 4.5). Teneurin-3 is most highly expressed in proximal CA1 and distal subiculum, as well as in other interconnected regions including the presubiculum, parasubiculum, medial mammillary nucleus, anteroventral thalamic nucleus, and medial entorhinal cortex (Berns et al., 2018). Conditional knockout expression of teneurin-3 reveals that a homophilic attraction mechanism contributes to the specificity of these connections. The lack of expression of teneurin-3 in CA1 pyramidal neurons leads to the distribution of proximal CA1 axons throughout the entire transverse axis of the subiculum. Similarly, the lack of expression of teneurin-3 in subicular neurons leads proximal CA1 neurons to avoid this area and to innervate nearby teneurin-3 expressing regions. Interestingly, although teneurin-3 is present in axons, dendrites, and neuronal somas, it is most prominently expressed in stratum lacunosum-moleculare of CA1 and the molecular layer of the subiculum, the recipient layers of direct projections from layer III neurons of the entorhinal cortex. Such layer-specific expression of teneurin-3 is thus fully consistent with

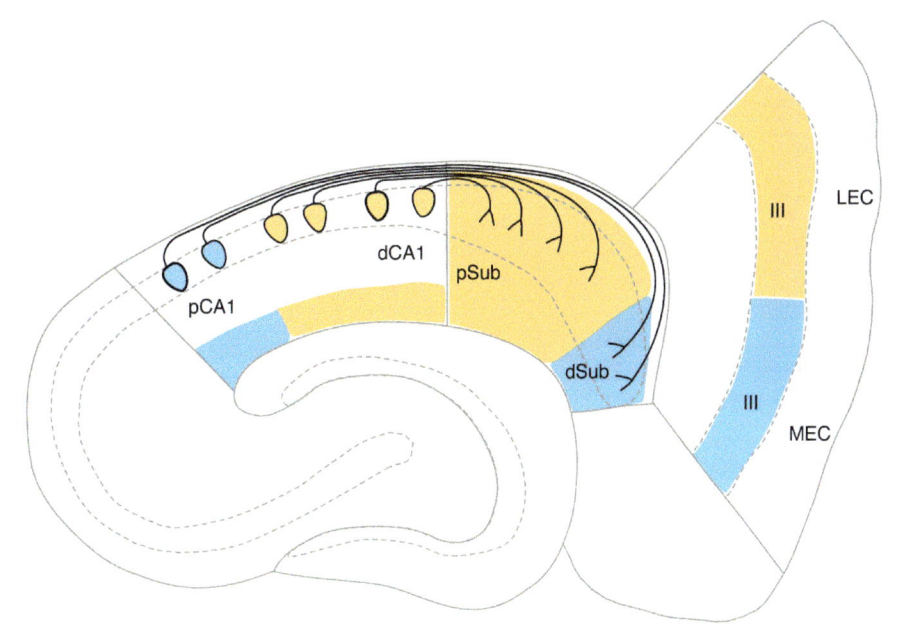

Figure 4.5 Latrophilin-2 and teneurin-3 instruct target selection of hippocampal axons through reciprocal repulsions. Teneurin-3-positive CA1 axons (blue) target the teneurin-3-positive distal subiculum via repulsion from latrophilin-2 in the proximal subiculum and attraction to teneurin-3 in the distal subiculum. Latrophilin-2-positive CA1 axons (yellow) target the latrophilin-2-positive proximal subiculum via repulsion from teneurin-3 in the distal subiculum. (Modified from Pederick et al., 2021.)

the mechanism of homophilic attraction that contributes to the specificity of the connections between multiple brain regions contributing to the same functional network.

The complementary pattern of expression of latrophilin-2 in the distal portion of CA1, the proximal portion of the subiculum, and the lateral entorhinal cortex contributes further to the establishment of these parallel hippocampal networks (Pederick et al., 2021). As was observed for teneurin-3, latrophilin-2 protein expression is confined to stratum lacunosum of CA1, layers I and II of the subiculum, and layer III of the lateral entorhinal cortex. In mice, latrophilin-2 and teneurin-3 proteins are first detected in the subiculum at postnatal day 2 and exhibit increasing expression in CA1 in the following days, reaching their highest expression levels by postnatal day 8. This pattern of protein expression follows the timing of target selection by CA1 axons in the subiculum. In contrast to teneurin-3, latrophilin-2 does not act through homophilic attraction. Instead, the interaction between latrophilin-2 and teneurin-3 results in heterophilic repulsion. First, latrophilin-2/teneurin-3 heterophilic repulsion and teneurin-3/teneurin-3 homophilic attraction contribute to guide proximal CA1 axons to target distal subiculum neurons. Second, teneurin-3/latrophilin-2 heterophilic repulsion contributes to guide distal CA1 axons expressing latrophilin-2 to target the latrophilin-2 expressing proximal subiculum (which lacks teneurin-3 expression). Finally, additional cell surface molecules may further subdivide the latrophilin-2 expressing regions to demarcate target specificity between mid-CA1 to midsubiculum projections and distal-CA1 to proximal subiculum projections.

4.5 Synapses and dendritic spines

Quantitative data on the development of synapses and dendritic spines was provided by electron microscopy and Golgi studies

performed more than 30 years ago. These studies were limited by the available quantitative analysis techniques and thus provided only estimates of the density of synapses or dendritic spines. There is little doubt that there is a general increase in synapse density during the early stages of development of hippocampal structures. However, it is difficult to determine the actual changes in synapse numbers and how much the reported changes in synaptic density are influenced by other factors. Nevertheless, many authors have reported that a peak in synapse density during early postnatal development is generally followed by a decrease. This peak of synaptic density was often interpreted as an overproduction or temporary increase in synapse numbers, followed by the elimination or pruning of synapses to reach adult values. This may well be the case. However, the quantitative information available to date is insufficient to support this conclusion for the hippocampal formation definitively. Indeed, a decrease in synapse density may be linked to an increase in the volume of the structure without changes in synapse numbers.

4.5.1 Granule cells

Consistent with the developmental patterns of neurogenesis discussed previously, the development of synapses in the molecular layer of the rat dentate gyrus is delayed in the infrapyramidal blade, as compared with the suprapyramidal blade (Crain et al., 1973). Interestingly, the relative proportion of asymmetric synapses (presumably excitatory) increases from birth to postnatal day 25, but it is unclear whether this observation results solely from an increase in asymmetric synapses or whether there is a simultaneous decrease in symmetric synapses. The major development of complex dendritic spines takes place after 11 postnatal days (Cotman et al., 1973). Four days after birth, synapses form on either large or small dendritic processes, but very rarely on spines. Some synapses contain abundant synaptic vesicles and an apparent fully differentiated asymmetric synaptic complex. Other synaptic endings contain flat synaptic vesicles and form symmetric synaptic contacts on large dendrites. At 11 postnatal days, synapses often form on small spine-like extensions of the dendritic shaft, which have a characteristic granular cytoplasm subjacent to the contact zone. Large dendritic shafts have both asymmetric and symmetric synaptic contacts. There are no myelinated fibers at this age. At 25 postnatal days, presynaptic profiles remain on average smaller than in young adult rats. Complex spines become more abundant and are found further out in the dendritic tree than at earlier ages, but they are still more numerous in the inner one-third of the molecular layer. In the outer molecular layer, synaptic contacts are most prevalent on relatively large to medium-sized dendritic shafts. By this age, myelinated axons appear throughout the molecular layer. In adults, most synapses, in particular asymmetric ones, form on spines or dendritic processes that look like spines. Only a few synaptic contacts exist on large dendritic shafts, and the majority of these contacts are symmetric (presumably inhibitory). Accordingly, the number of spines per 100 μm of dendritic length increases continuously from birth to 6 months of age in male Wistar rats (Wenzel et al., 1981). This finding is particularly important because many researchers consider 60-day-old rats to be adults, whereas significant morphological changes continue to happen thereafter. Note that 6-month-old rats are typically used as the young adult comparison group in studies on aging (see Chapter 15).

Steward and Falk (1986) generally confirmed these observations and further demonstrated that the presence of polyribosomes in the postsynaptic element is regulated developmentally. An inverse relationship is found between synapse density and the proportion of synapses with polyribosomes. Between 1 and 7 days of age, 60% of the spines with a synaptic contact contain polyribosomes. The proportion of spines with polyribosomes decreases to less than 25% at postnatal day 25 and remains relatively stable to reach about 21% at postnatal day 28, which is about twice as much as what is observed in adult animals (unspecified age; about 11%). While the proportion of synapses with polyribosomes is greatest between 1 and 7 postnatal days, the actual density of polyribosome-containing synapses is negligible at 1 day, increases to a peak at 7 days of age, and then decreases as synaptic density increases. Qualitatively, the most dramatic accumulations of polyribosomes are also found at 7 postnatal days, and therefore precedes the major development of dendritic spines which takes place after 11 days of age.

In monkeys, Rakic and colleagues reported similar changes in synaptic density and dendritic arborization in the molecular layer of the dentate gyrus. In a first study (Duffy and Rakic, 1983), Golgi-impregnated material was analyzed, but only fully impregnated granule cells that appear to be at the peak of their differentiation at a given age were selected for quantitative analysis. They reported a steady increase in total dendritic length and total number of spines per granule cells from E58 to postnatal day 150, which is followed by a decrease of both parameters in one monkey at postnatal day 315 and in two monkeys reportedly over 3 years of age. This subjective preselection of neurons may have impacted the results, since many granule cell neurons are still maturing within the granule cell layer past 1 year of age (Jabès et al., 2010). Furthermore, they used the Stensaas Golgi method that gives good results for fetal and neonatal brains but is less reliable in older ages (Seress, 1992). In a second study (Eckenhoff and Rakic, 1991), synaptic density was reported to increase exponentially from E60 to birth, and nearly linearly from birth to 152 postnatal days. Synaptic density decreases from postnatal day 152 to postnatal day 300, when it reaches adult levels. These results are also difficult to interpret, since they do not provide quantitative information on the actual number of synapses. The volume measurements reported in that study do not correspond to the quantitative estimates obtained with design-based stereological techniques (Jabès et al., 2010, 2011). When considering the changes in synapse density reported by Rakic and colleagues and the volumetric changes reported by Jabès and colleagues, there may indeed be a large increase in the number of synapses in the molecular layer between birth and 1 year of age, but it is unclear whether this represents an overproduction followed by an elimination to reach adult levels. Seress's conclusion that the postnatal dendritic development of granule cells in similar in rodents and primates seems very reasonable (Seress, 1992): the total dendritic length increases until it reaches the adult size without a significant regressive period; total dendritic length and the number of spines is higher in adults than in newborn monkeys.

4.5.2 Mossy cells

The mossy cells have an immature appearance at birth in rats, and on subsequent days their maturation lags somewhat behind that of the hippocampal pyramidal cells (Ribak et al., 1985). On postnatal day 1, the dendrites of the mossy cells have a very immature appearance, even less mature than those of the nearby CA3 pyramidal cells. Many of the dendrites bear growth cones primarily at their termini and have long, thin filipodia emanating from various points along their lengths. Many of the dendrites enter the molecular layer of the dentate gyrus, though this is rarely seen in the mature brain. At later stages, many of these dendrites appear to thin out progressively and it is possible that some of them are in the process of regression. However, it is also conceivable that these processes are present in the mature brain but are not visualized due to the inadequacies of the Golgi-staining process. On postnatal day 3, many dendritic growth cones and filipodial spines are still observed, but at later ages there appears to be a progressive decrease in these profiles. The filipodial spines are far less common on postnatal day 5, especially on the soma and proximal dendrites. There is no indication that these long spines may be the predecessors of the thorny excrescences. On day 5, a few typical spines are seen on the distal dendrites, and these often occur in patches. Typical pedunculate spines are first commonly seen on the distal dendrites around postnatal day 7, while thorny excrescences are first commonly seen between postnatal days 11 and 14. By postnatal day 21, the dendrites have attained a mature appearance, although the density of both typical spines and thorny excrescences is less than that found in adults.

In monkeys (Seress and Ribak, 1995b), the spine density on the distal dendrites of mossy cells is about one-third of the adult value in newborns. It reaches about 50% at one month, 75% between 3 and 7 months, and is close to 100% of the adult value at 1 year of age. In newborn monkeys, thorny excrescences are found essentially near the first branching of the primary dendrites. Distal dendrites display a few pedunculate spines, while a few somatic spines are also present. The number and complexity of thorny excrescences increases from birth to at least 3 months of age. Additional changes are difficult to detect using standard light microscopic techniques, and no other quantitative information is available.

In the newborn human, the somas of mossy cells have large numbers of spines and the proximal dendrites have spines with thin neck and round head and a few small, isolated, immature excrescences (Seress and Mrzljak, 1992). Distal dendrites are thinner than proximal dendrites and show a small number of pedunculate spines. Both proximal and distal dendrites have long filopodia. Mossy cells appear more mature in 3- to 7-month-old children, with frequent spines on the soma. Varicosities are rare on dendrites, and proximal dendrites have a few excrescences but no regular spines. The first large complex spines are observed on the proximal dendrites at 7 months of age. There is an increase in the number of large and complex spines on proximal dendrites and a decrease in the number of somal spines between 15 and 30 months of age. At 5 years of age, the complexity and size of the complex spines appear adult-like, but no quantitative information has been published. Proximal dendrites are covered by complex spines and distal dendrites display large numbers of small spines with thick necks and round heads. Nevertheless, many mossy cells appear less mature and display long filopodia on their dendrites that lack large excrescences. The number of mossy cells with elaborate and extensive large complex spines appears greater in adulthood.

4.5.3 CA3 pyramidal cells

In the rat, Amaral and Dent (1981) provided a detailed analysis of the development of mossy fibers using Timm and Golgi preparations. On the first postnatal day, the presence of mossy fibers is detectable in Timm-stained material within the hilus and incipient stratum lucidum. Over the next 2 weeks, the stained areas become more extensive, the size and density of the stained particles increase, and the particles become more intensely stained. These signs of progressive development of the mossy fibers appear to reflect, temporally and topographically, the developmental gradients followed by their parent granule cells. Golgi material confirms the presence of mossy fibers in the hilus on the first postnatal day and fascicles of mossy fibers are observed in CA3 stratum lucidum on postnatal day 3. Although these immature axons are devoid of large synaptic expansions, they exhibit prominent growth cones. Small expansions along the lengths of the axons appear on postnatal day 7 and reach approximately adult size and complexity by about postnatal day 14. The postsynaptic component of the mossy fiber synapse, the "thorny excrescence," is not visible on the proximal portion of the pyramidal cell dendrites until sometime after postnatal day 9.

At the electron microscopic level, small immature mossy fiber expansions make both symmetric and asymmetric contacts directly with dendritic shafts on the first postnatal day. These profiles are only one-tenth the size of mature expansions and grow rapidly between postnatal days 1 and 9. Around postnatal day 9, the thorny excrescences develop and the asymmetric synapses come to be associated with these spinous processes. Thus, it appears that mossy fibers establish contact with pyramidal cell dendrites early in the postnatal period, several days before there is any indication of spine development. Furthermore, the thorny excrescences develop after the more typical, pedunculate spines have appeared on the distal pyramidal cell dendrites. Finally, although the mossy fibers appear largely mature in 21-day-old rats, a more subtle and protracted development of the system continues long into adulthood.

In the monkey, the spine density of the dendritic segments of CA3 pyramidal cells located in strata oriens and lacunosum-moleculare at birth is about 50% of the adult value. It increases the most during the first 3 postnatal months to reach about 75% of the adult values at 3 months of age, and is close to the adult value by 1 year of age (Seress and Ribak, 1995a). The postnatal development of these neurons thus includes an initial 3-month period when thorny excrescences on proximal dendrites and pedunculate spines on distal dendrites grow rapidly in number and complexity. The rapid growth of thorny excrescences in light microscopic preparations coincides well with the appearance of the embedded postsynaptic spines within mossy fiber terminals in electron microscopic preparations, which suggests an increase in the number of synapses between mossy fiber terminals and pyramidal cells. After this rapid phase of growth, a slower development occurs between 3 months and 1 year of age. This latter phase is characterized by only small increases in the number of both postsynaptic spines associated with each large mossy fiber terminal and pedunculate spines on distal dendrites. At the same time, between birth and 3 months of age, numerous axons and axon terminals within large bundles of unmyelinated mossy fiber axons exhibit signs of degeneration in stratum lucidum. This process does not appear to be associated with granule cell death during postnatal development. Myelination of axons in strata oriens and lacunosum-moleculare continues during at least the first 9 postnatal months, while new spines are generated on both the apical and basal dendrites of pyramidal cells. It is important to note that there is no decrease in spine density during the postnatal period. Thus, spine density increases continuously from birth until at least 1 year of age and does not change significantly after that.

4.5.4 CA1 pyramidal cells

The differentiation of hippocampal pyramidal neurons similarly continues for a relatively long period during postnatal development in rodents. The dendritic arborization of CA1 hippocampal neurons expands the most within the first 15 postnatal days, but different parameters and specific regions of the dendritic tree follow different developmental profiles (Pokorny and Yamamoto, 1981). The number of dendritic branches located in strata oriens and lacunosum-moleculare is nearly adult-like 5 days after birth, whereas the number of dendritic branches in stratum radiatum becomes adult-like later, between 24 and 48 postnatal days. Similarly, the number of dendritic segments is nearly adult-like 15 days after birth in strata oriens and lacunosum-moleculare, whereas it becomes adult-like between 24 and 48 postnatal days in stratum radiatum. Accordingly, total dendritic length increases earlier in strata oriens and lacunosum-moleculare than in stratum radiatum.

The development of spines on the dendrites located in stratum radiatum reveals parallel maturational profiles (Kirov et al., 2004). At postnatal days P6–P7, there are only a few filopodia-like protrusions (presumed protospines) emerging from the dendrites. These protrusions are longer than at all other ages. At both P11–P12 and P15–P16, there is a mixture of dendritic spines and filopodial structures. By P20–P22, dendritic spines predominate and spine density is about 82% of the adult level. Interestingly, the normal development of these dendritic processes is dependent on synaptic transmission. Blocking synaptic transmission is associated with the elongation of dendritic protrusions at P6–P7, and an increase in dendritic spine density at P20–P22.

There is to our knowledge no published data on the development of synapses or dendritic spines of CA1 pyramidal neurons in monkeys or humans.

4.5.5 Molecular studies

As discussed above, the types of synapses found in various hippocampal circuits change during development. Axon terminals may reach their appropriate lamina and establish transient synaptic contacts with Cajal-Retzius cells or GABAergic interneurons prior to establishing contact with glutamatergic granule cells in the dentate gyrus and pyramidal cells in the hippocampus. Estimates of the number of excitatory or inhibitory synapses onto principal neurons or interneurons will thus provide important information about the establishment of hippocampal circuits, but it will not be sufficient to fully explain the functional changes taking place simultaneously. A well-known example is the excitatory/inhibitory shift of the actions of GABA during development observed in all species and brain structures studied (Ben-Ari et al., 2004). In addition, the subunit composition of individual receptors for different neurotransmitters has been shown to vary during development (Pickard et al., 2000; Sans et al., 2000; Travaglia et al., 2016b; McKay et al., 2018). For example, the different isoforms constituting the NMDA receptor vary throughout development and are associated with changes in the functional characteristics of NMDA receptors in the hippocampus (Le Bail et al., 2015). The developmental regulation of AMPA and NMDA receptor subunits is very complex, and likely contributes at least in part to the transition from non-specific synaptic activity necessary for brain development to the selective, input-specific synaptic plasticity underlying the emergence of memory (Lavenex et al., 2011; Favre et al., 2012a). However, these questions go well beyond the scope of the current chapter, and we refer the reader to Chapters 8–10 for more detailed information on the molecular mechanisms contributing to the structural and synaptic plasticity of hippocampal circuits.

4.5.6 Synapse and cell maturation

We have previously considered the molecules that regulate axon pathfinding and target recognition during development of the major hippocampal projection systems. The mechanisms controlling the maturation of the pre- and post-mitotic neurons and synaptogenesis have not been explored as extensively, but they appear to be largely similar in the hippocampus and other parts of the brain (Valnegri et al., 2015; Sudhof, 2018). We refer the reader to these previous expert reviews on the subject, as well as the other chapters of this book on structural and synaptic plasticity (Chapters 8–10). Here, only molecules that we previously discussed in the context of the regulation of neurogenesis, cell migration or the establishment of the major hippocampal connection systems will be considered.

Synapses are likely organized by transsynaptic cell-adhesion molecules that bidirectionally orchestrate their formation, remodeling, elimination, and function (Sudhof, 2018). Synapse formation will also be impacted by dendritic morphogenesis, which is regulated by three major classes of extrinsic factors: secreted cues, contact-mediated factors, and neuronal activity (Valnegri et al., 2015). The list of specific molecules involved in these processes keeps expanding, but a few examples will suffice to demonstrate the complexity of these processes. Neurotrophins stimulate activity-dependent dendritic growth. Diffusible secreted factors, such as semaphorins, that control axon guidance have also been implicated in dendrite patterning, including Sema3A in the regulation of apical dendrite formation in hippocampal CA1 pyramidal neurons (Nakamura et al., 2009). WNT proteins also appear to regulate dendrite growth and arborization in the mouse hippocampus, specifically in CA3 and CA1 but not in the dentate gyrus or CA2 (Rosso et al., 2005). Members of the ephrin ligand family and Eph receptors activate intracellular pathways that modulate neuronal morphology. For example, triple knockout of EphB1, EphB2, and EphB3 results in reduced dendrite number, length, and complexity in the mouse hippocampus (Hoogenraad et al., 2005), and it is now becoming clearer that distinct ephrin-B family members can regulate synapse formation through various mechanisms (Hruska and Dalva, 2012). Bone morphogenetic proteins (BMPs) also regulate the growth of pyramidal cell dendrites (Osorio et al., 2013). Contact-mediated regulators including cell adhesion molecules such as cadherins and protocadherins are crucial for dendrite tiling, self-avoidance, and arbor homeostasis (Valnegri et al., 2015). The effects of neuronal activity on dendrite morphogenesis are mediated by calcium signals via the activation of voltage-gated calcium channels (VGCCs) or glutamatergic NMDA receptors (NMDA-Rs) triggering calcium binding to calmodulin (CaM), which activates calcium/CaM-dependent protein kinases (CaMKs). Calcium-dependent signaling acts through CaM and CaMKs to positively and negatively regulate dendritic complexity, and via the activation of the mitogen-activated protein kinase (MAPK) to promote the extension and stabilization of dendritic filopodia. A number of intrinsic signals, including Foxo6, Neurogenin2, and NeuroD, also contribute to the regulation of dendrite morphogenesis (Puram and Bonni, 2013). Finally, epigenetic factors such as MECP2, which has been linked to Rett syndrome and autism, also contribute to the structural development of hippocampal neurons (Lagali et al., 2010). This very brief survey illustrates the need for more in-depth studies to decipher the role of multiple disease-related genes in hippocampal development and how the disturbance of these signaling pathways may underlie different facets of neurodevelopmental disorders.

4.6 In vitro models of early hippocampal development

In vitro approaches have been used for several decades to study the development and physiology of the hippocampus, and a number of these studies have already been considered in this chapter. Neurons and glial cells survive and differentiate well in culture systems, but cell-type-specific characteristics are better retained in slice cultures (Frotscher et al., 1995). Slice cultures have been particularly useful to confront different sets of afferent fibers with hippocampal target cells to examine the mechanisms determining the specificity of fiber–target interactions and to study the electrophysiological properties of hippocampal neurons. However, because the human hippocampus is different from that of rodents or even nonhuman primates (see Chapter 3), cell culture models generated from human pluripotent stem cells (hPSCs) have been developed to study its development and the etiology of diseases that affect the hippocampus.

The first study that reported the differentiation of hPSCs into human dentate gyrus stem-cell-like cells and ultimately to granule-like cells, used a protocol that recapitulates the expression pattern of key developmental genes during hippocampal neurogenesis (Yu et al., 2014). The in vitro–generated granule cells reach physiological maturity when maintained in long-term cocultures with human hippocampal astrocytes and can integrate morphologically and functionally in the host circuitry when transplanted in a mouse postnatal hippocampus. More recently, a protocol has been developed for the differentiation of hPSCs into human CA3 pyramidal neurons, which can mature in vitro and form an electrically active network (Sarkar et al., 2018). Cultures of pure neuronal subpopulations provide robust models to study neuronal specification during development. However, as they consist of relatively homogeneous populations of a single neuronal subtype, such cultures lack the cellular complexity needed to model neuronal circuits, which are composed of multiple neuronal subtypes. Such a limitation can be to some extent overcome by coculture experiments. In particular, the coculture of hPSC-derived human CA3 neurons and dentate gyrus granule cells results in the establishment of functional synapses between the two cell types (Sarkar et al., 2018).

Three-dimensional organoids represent a promising alternative to two-dimensional cultures or cocultures, as they contain multiple neuronal subtypes including neurons found in vivo in separate brain regions. Moreover, these cells can self-organize to form neuronal networks. hPSCs have been differentiated into dorsomedial telencephalic tissue (i.e., similar to the hippocampal primordium) capable, when maintained in long-term dissociated cultures, of generating hippocampal granule-like and pyramidal-like neurons, which form electrically active networks (Sarkar et al., 2018). Organoids have shortcomings that currently limit their use, including batch variability and low viability in very long-term cultures. However, this technology is progressing very rapidly, and these limitations may be overcome soon (Ciarpella et al., 2023). For example, it is possible to study the interactions taking place between different brain regions by cultivating together two organoids that have been patterned to differentiate into two distinct brain territories. Such cocultures, called "assembloids," have been used to model the migration of human cortical interneurons between organoids of dorsal and ventral telencephalic identities (Birey et al., 2017).

Although stem cell–derived neurons cultured in vitro and organoids do not become fully mature, the development of such techniques has the potential to greatly advance the analysis of human brain development.

4.7 Noninvasive MRI studies of postnatal development

Much of the motivation for investigating hippocampal development in animals is to better understand how this brain region functions in humans. In the previous sections of this chapter, we discussed the development of individual cells, pathways, and connections and described some of the molecular mechanisms that guide these processes. In the following sections, we consider the postnatal development of the hippocampus with a more integrative perspective incorporating information derived from molecular, structural, and functional studies. Here, we begin by describing noninvasive structural studies using magnetic resonance imaging (MRI). Although MRI provides the opportunity to directly compare the structure and functions of the hippocampal formation between humans and other animals commonly used in experimental research, such as nonhuman primates and rodents, to date there has been little direct comparison between species. Indeed, studies of hippocampal development using MRI have been hobbled by the difficulties associated with obtaining

high-quality images of very young brains when the hippocampus is going through its most dynamic phase of postnatal development. The smaller size of infant brains and the need for anesthesia have also limited analyses of early postnatal hippocampal development.

4.7.1 Interspecies comparisons

Several studies have used noninvasive MRI techniques to study the postnatal development of the hippocampus in humans and nonhuman primates, and their findings can be used to establish a comparative developmental timeline. MRI studies providing estimates of total hippocampal volume include a variety of cytoarchitectonic fields, generally comprising the dentate gyrus, the fields of the hippocampus proper, the subiculum, the presubiculum, and the parasubiculum. The entorhinal cortex is typically not included or is measured separately. A variety of analytical strategies have been used, starting with manual tracing of the hippocampus to automated segmentation programs. Here, we primarily consider studies that reported raw volumetric data (i.e., uncorrected for intracranial volume or other normalization procedures) derived from neuroanatomically informed, manual tracing of the whole hippocampus to define the postnatal volumetric profile of the hippocampus. We refer the reader to Chapter 3 for a discussion of some of the approaches being developed for the identification and segmentation of the hippocampal formation in MRI studies. Because we did not find any publication using MRI to study the development of the rodent hippocampus, we also present the volumetric development of the monkey and rat hippocampus derived from Nissl-stained sections from aldehyde-fixed postmortem brains to allow further interspecies comparisons.

As illustrated in Figure 4.6, the postnatal volumetric developmental profile of the hippocampus is very similar in humans (Uematsu et al., 2012; Narvacan et al., 2017), monkeys (Payne et al., 2010; Jabès et al., 2011; Hunsaker et al., 2014), and rats (unpublished data from the Lavenex laboratory). This comparative profile serves to establish that, with respect to overall hippocampal development, rhesus monkeys develop at approximately four times the speed of human children. Thus, a 6-month-old monkey would be roughly equivalent to a 2-year-old child, and a 2-year-old monkey to an 8-year-old child (Lavenex and Banta Lavenex, 2013). It can also be determined that the volume of the whole hippocampus reaches adult levels at about 2 years of age in monkeys and at about 8 years of age in humans. This is particularly important to consider in relation to the phenomenon of childhood amnesia, which is typically considered to end after 7 years of age (Bauer, 2006). The fact that the hippocampus reaches an adult-like volume does not mean that there are no additional structural or functional changes thereafter, but rather that most of the volumetric growth and maturation of some fundamental hippocampus-dependent functions have occurred by this time (Lavenex and Banta Lavenex, 2013). In monkeys, a similar developmental profile is observed based on estimates of hippocampal volume derived from MRI and Nissl-stained brain sections, even though differential shrinkage of perfusion-fixed tissue at different ages may lead to some differences in the growth curves established using these two different techniques. Nevertheless, both MRI and postmortem analyses indicate that the most dynamical period of hippocampal postnatal development is the first 3 to 6 months in monkeys, which is equivalent to the first 2 years in children. It is followed by slower but continued development until at least 2 years of age in monkeys, which is equivalent to about 8 years of age in humans.

In rats, we could not determine at what age the volume of the hippocampus plateaus based on published data. We therefore prepared Nissl-stained sections of brains perfusion-fixed with paraformaldehyde to obtain data comparable to those available for monkeys. The largest hippocampal growth takes place during the first 4 to 8 weeks, a period during which major changes in hippocampus-dependent functional processes are also known to take place (Wills et al., 2010; Langston et al., 2010). However, hippocampal volume continues to increase after 2 months of age, which is often described as adulthood in functional studies in rats. This developmental profile is consistent with the context of aging studies, in which young adult rats are considered to be at least six months of age (see Chapter 15).

4.7.2 MRI structural studies of the whole hippocampus in humans

The data presented in Figure 4.6 for humans are derived from two comprehensive studies (Uematsu et al., 2012; Narvacan et al., 2017), whose results are further supported by the results of less systematic studies. Giedd et al. (1996) were the first to publish a quantitative MRI study of the hippocampus in typically developing children between 4 and 18 years of age. Overall, they reported that the hippocampus was larger in males than in females, a finding that disappeared if controlled for total cerebral volume. They also noted that the right hippocampal volume appeared to increase in females, but not in males. However, the inclusion of a greater number of females below 8 years of age might have contributed to producing a spurious finding. Importantly, the slopes of the regression lines for the left and right hippocampus did not differ between sexes. They also reported that interindividual variability in hippocampal volume is very high, as can also be observed in Figure 4.6, which reports the findings of Uematsu et al. (2012) and Narvacan et al. (2017). Such high variability is found in nearly all structural MRI studies in humans and likely precludes the use of cross-sectional designs to study more subtle changes in hippocampal structure across postnatal development using MRI technology. Accordingly, longitudinal studies may be the only sound approach to further investigate these questions in humans, and such studies are particularly challenging in terms of financial and human resources.

In agreement with these data, Knickmeyer et al. (2008) and Pfluger et al. (1999) reported large increases in the volume of the human hippocampus within the first 2 years of postnatal life. Reinhardt et al. (2020) also reported a slower increase in overall hippocampal volume between 2 and 6 years of age in both typically developing children (boys and girls) and children with autism spectrum disorder. Schumann et al. (2004) did not find any age-related changes in overall hippocampal volume between 7.5 and 18.5 years of age in typically developing children and children with autism spectrum disorder. Note that Uematsu et al. (2012) used the same criteria to delineate the hippocampus, as initially described by Schumann et al. (2004). Other studies have also failed to find changes in overall hippocampal volume between 4 and 25 years of age (Gogtay et al., 2006) or between 8 and 31 years of age (Ostby et al., 2009).

It is important to note that several studies have reported hippocampal volumes that were corrected for intracranial or total cerebral volume. Although such normalization procedures may be useful to address specific research questions, we do not consider this approach to be appropriate to establish the fundamental processes underlying the normal postnatal development of the hippocampus. Indeed, if the reference volume changes whereas hippocampal volume does not, these normalization procedures will lead to erroneous conclusions with respect to the developmental processes taking place within the hippocampal formation itself. Nonetheless, we mention here a particularly large study by Lynch et al. (2019) that included 1,676 participants from 1 to 22 years of age. Both unadjusted and adjusted hippocampal volume increased with age, particularly during early development. However, their statistical analyses failed to distinguish between early development (before 8 years of age) and the following plateau that is reliably seen at later ages in other studies. Nevertheless, their data are consistent with earlier reports in demonstrating very high interindividual variability and the fact that the right hippocampal volume may be larger than the left. Also consistent was their finding that males had a larger hippocampus than females, although when adjusted for total cerebral volume females had a proportionately larger hippocampus. There were no age-by-sex interactions in growth.

4.7.3 MRI measurements of different regions or subfields

Analyses of different regions along the rostrocaudal axis of the hippocampal formation have also been motivated by findings from some functional MRI studies suggesting that different rostrocaudal portions may contribute to dissociable components of hippocampus-dependent memory functions (Poppenk et al., 2013; Ritchey et al., 2015). In these studies, the hippocampus is typically divided into an anterior "head," a middle "body," and a posterior "tail," and a series of rules have been adopted to demarcate these different regions of the hippocampal formation (Daugherty et al., 2015). The most influential analysis of developmental differences in different regions of the hippocampal formation was published by Gogtay et al. (2006). This study comprised 31 participants initially between 4 and 18 years of age who were scanned every 2 years for 6–10 years, thus covering ages from 4 to 25 years. They found no difference in total hippocampal volume between 4 and 25 years. However, a time-lapse sequence of hippocampal development was produced from the scans, which showed that some portions of the hippocampus may be expanding with age while other portions may be contracting. The posterior half of the hippocampus showed gradual gains in volume over this period (more so on the left) except for the posterior tip of the hippocampus, which showed a reduction over time. In the anterior half of the hippocampus, the front of the "head" showed a reduction in volume over time whereas the posterior part of the "head" increased in volume over time. The "body" of the hippocampus mainly increased in volume over time. Thus, whereas they reported developmental differences based on the anterior-posterior level of the hippocampus, these differences did not adhere to the so-called head, body, and tail demarcations. There were also some qualitative differences noticed when sex was evaluated. For females, the reduction at the posterior portion was more prominent, whereas the reduction at the anterior portion was less apparent. For males, the reduction was greater anteriorly and more minimal posteriorly. This type of volumetric shape analysis has been adopted by a number of recent studies, but it has produced variable results depending on whether the study was longitudinal or cross-sectional, and on other design features such as the hippocampal tracing techniques and the specific computations used

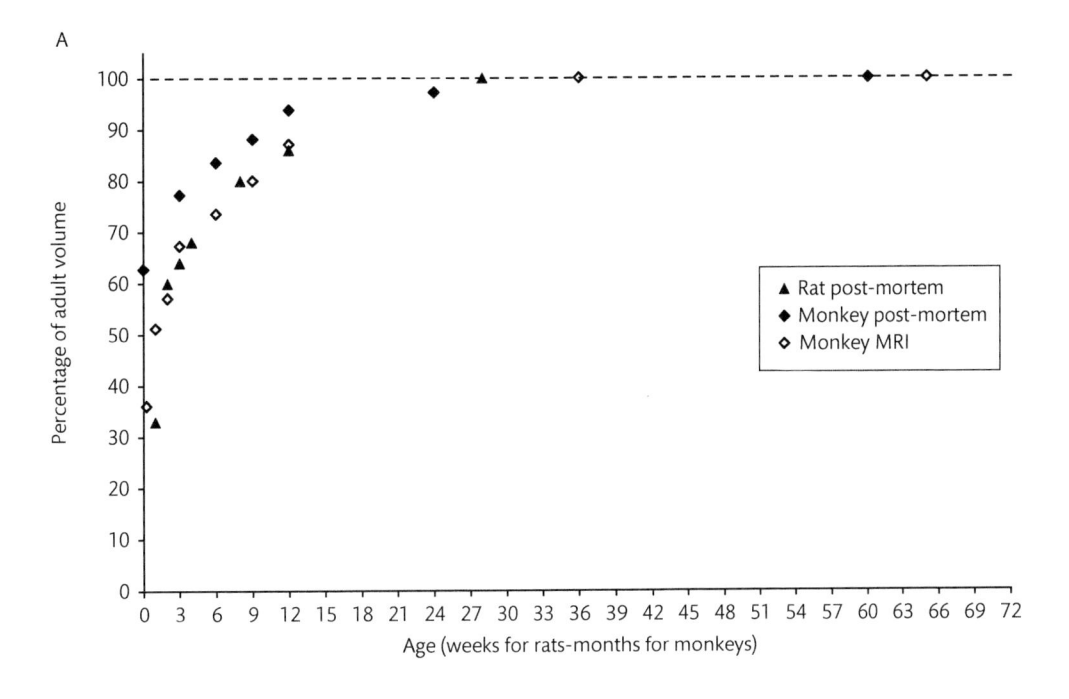

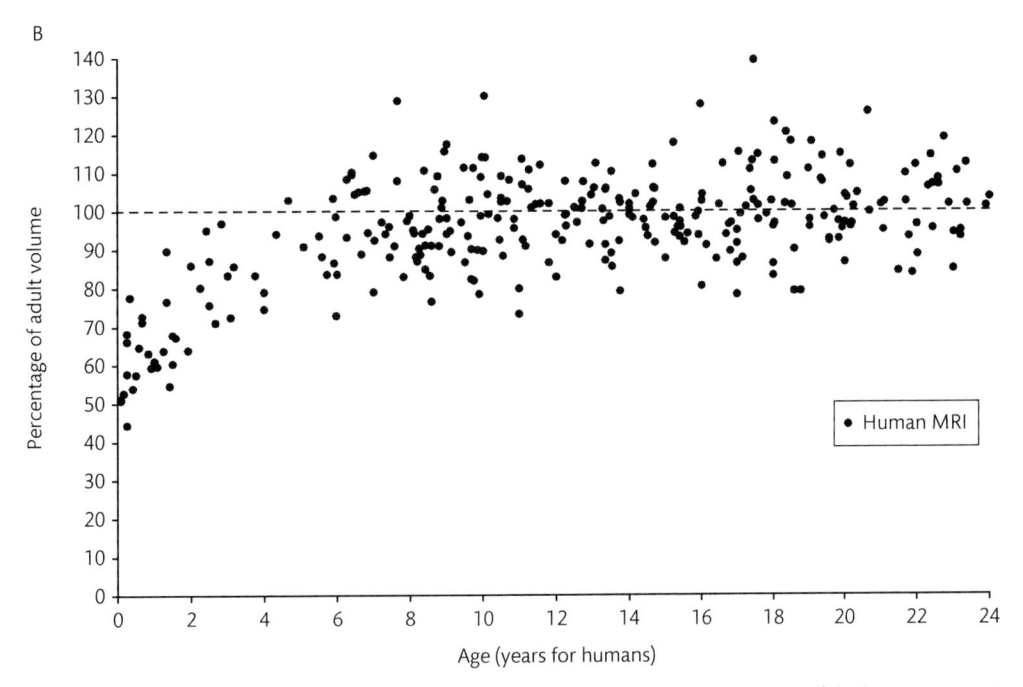

Figure 4.6 Postnatal volumetric development of the hippocampus. (A) Postnatal volumetric development of the hippocampus in rats and monkeys. Data for rats are derived from Nissl-stained sections of brains perfusion-fixed with paraformaldehyde (filled triangles; average value for four animals per age group; unpublished data from the Lavenex laboratory). Data for monkeys are derived from Nissl-stained sections of brains perfusion-fixed with paraformaldehyde (filled diamond; average value for four rhesus macaque monkeys per age group; Jabès et al., 2011), as well as from noninvasive MRI (empty diamond; average value for 24 rhesus macaque monkeys; Hunsaker et al., 2014). (B) Postnatal volumetric development of the hippocampus in humans, measured with noninvasive MRI technology. Each point represents the percentage of the average 20- to 30-year-old young adult volume for one individual. (Combined data from Narvacan et al., 2017, and Uematsu et al., 2012.)

to determine hippocampal shape. It is thus currently difficult to provide a definitive description of possible developmental changes in hippocampal shape or different regions along its longitudinal axis based on MRI studies.

Attempts at relating developmental changes in overall hippocampal volume to the emergence of episodic memory have not met with great success either. This is likely because the entire hippocampal volume is a relatively crude measure that ignores

important changes in functional subregions. Indeed, as suggested previously by animal studies (Lavenex and Banta Lavenex, 2013), changes in individual hippocampal subfields may better reveal the structural and functional changes underlying the development of mnemonic abilities. Although it is a daunting task even for trained neuroanatomists with high-resolution microscopes to draw accurate boundaries between adjacent fields in Nissl-stained sections (see Chapter 3), an international consortium of undaunted scientists is dedicated to developing strategies to demarcate hippocampal subfields in adult and eventually developing human brains using MRI technology. A 2019 progress report from this group indicated that important steps toward defining the boundaries of hippocampal subfields had taken place (Olsen et al., 2019). However, the group was still admittedly far from adopting a universally accepted and harmonized set of protocols for demarcating hippocampal subfields even from very high-resolution MRIs in adult individuals. Accordingly, recent attempts to evaluate subfield development in children have provided results that are yet too inconsistent to be discussed in the current chapter. Nevertheless, major efforts to demarcate subfields of the hippocampal formation are ongoing and increasingly sophisticated algorithms are being developed. Given the variability of the cytoarchitectonic organization and size of the hippocampal formation in adult individuals, it remains to be seen whether this goal is attainable for the developing brain. Since the immature brain has substantially different tissue characteristics, which change with maturation, a rigorous demarcation of the developing fields of the hippocampal formation with current MRI technology appears beyond the realm of practicality,

particularly given the difficulties in obtaining high-quality MRI scans from unanesthetized children.

4.8 Postmortem studies of postnatal development

Numerous studies have attempted to quantify the volumetric development of different subregions of the human hippocampal formation using MRI. However, as just discussed, one must be very cautious when interpreting these data because the different hippocampal subfields cannot yet be defined reliably with current MRI techniques. In contrast, detailed neuroanatomical studies in postmortem tissue enable a precise delineation of the boundaries of distinct hippocampal regions and layers (Figure 4.7), even if some neuroanatomists may be more willing to share a toothbrush than to adopt a common nomenclature (see Chapter 3). Moreover, such studies can also provide reliable information on the structural development of principal cell types. Unfortunately, no comprehensive study of the structural postnatal development of the hippocampus

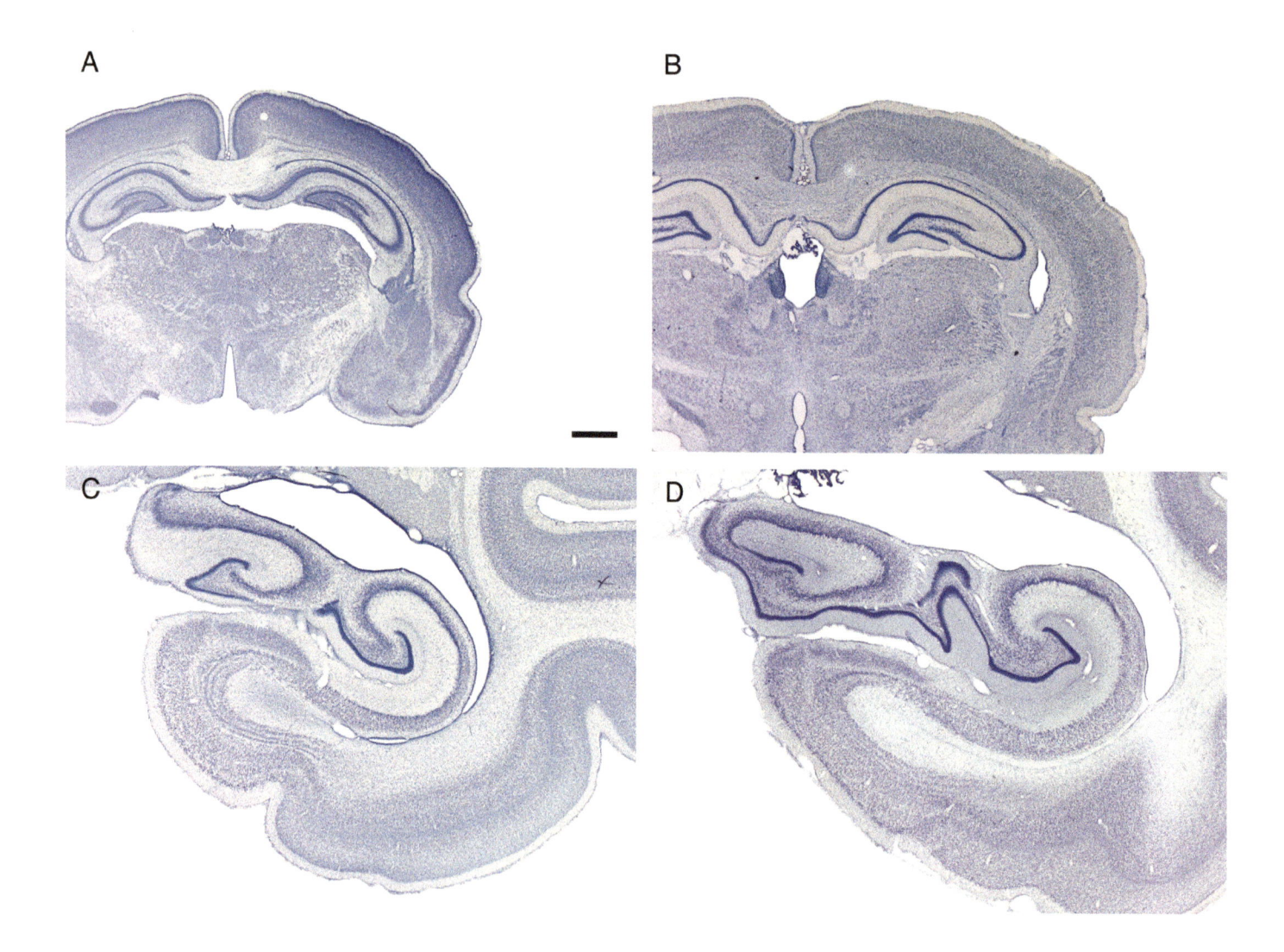

Figure 4.7 Nissl-stained coronal sections of the hippocampal formation. (A) 7-day-old rat. (B) 7-month-old rat. (C) 1-day-old monkey. (D) 5.4-year-old monkey. Scale bar in A: = 500 μm for panels A and B; = 1 mm for panels C and D.

has been carried out in rodents or humans. Especially in the case of human studies, nearly all reports on the structural postnatal development of the hippocampus provide only qualitative descriptions of a very limited number of cases at each postnatal age (and often just one case at given ages), thus precluding any generalization of their findings. However, since the relative development of different cell types and circuits appears to follow the same profile in different species, we can use the results of studies carried out in monkeys to provide a general framework describing the postnatal development of the hippocampal formation.

Historically, neuroanatomical data suggested that there is significant postnatal maturation of the primate hippocampal formation (Lavenex et al., 2007; Insausti et al., 2010). However, since much of this data was derived from largely qualitative reports, it was difficult to summarize and assimilate this information into a coherent, definitive picture. To rectify this, Lavenex, Banta Lavenex, Amaral, and colleagues have undertaken a series of systematic analyses of the postnatal structural and molecular development of the rhesus macaque monkey (*Macaca mulatta*) hippocampal formation. Their studies provide a coherent framework within which to integrate the piecemeal or qualitative information reported previously. In this section we summarize these findings regarding the postnatal development of distinct regions, layers, and putative functional circuits of the primate hippocampal formation. For this description, we follow the classical view of information flow through the hippocampal formation. However, these findings reveal that the sequential maturation of distinct hippocampal regions or layers does not follow this principal circuit but instead is characterized by the differential maturation of parallel hippocampal pathways (Lavenex and Banta Lavenex, 2013).

4.8.1 Dentate gyrus

As described previously, the dentate gyrus is far from mature at birth. Although granule cell neuron production decreases considerably after the first few postnatal months in monkeys, a substantial number of neurons continue to be generated throughout juvenile, adolescent (Nowakowski and Rakic, 1981; Rakic and Nowakowski, 1981; Eckenhoff and Rakic, 1988; Jabès et al., 2010), and adult life (Gould et al., 1999; Kornack and Rakic, 1999; Jabès et al., 2010). Indeed, about 40% of the total number of granule cells observed in adult (5- to 9-year-old) rhesus macaque monkeys (*Macaca mulatta*) are added to the granule cell layer postnatally (Jabès et al., 2010, 2011). Moreover, although 25% of these neurons are added in the first 3 months of postnatal life, the number of granule cells at 1 year of age still does not equal that of adults. This protracted period of neuron addition in the dentate gyrus is accompanied by a late maturation of the granule cell population, which continues after 1 year of age (equivalent to 4 years of age in humans). Specifically, there is a large population of small granule cells that is most prominent during the first 3 months after birth, and which gradually decreases over the 1st year. Nevertheless, there is still a greater number of small granule cells in 1-year-old monkeys than in 5- to 9-year-old monkeys, indicating that some developmental processes are not yet terminated at 1 year of age in monkeys. In parallel, although the mature-sized cell population exhibits a gradual increase in number between birth and 1 year of age, there are still fewer mature-sized cells in 1-year-old monkeys than in 5- to 9-year-olds. These data indicate that monkey granule cell neurons undergo a gradual but substantial structural

maturation from birth until beyond the 1st year after birth to achieve mature morphological characteristics.

As a result of these increases in granule cell number and soma size, the volume of the granule cell layer increases during the same postnatal period. At birth, the volume of the granule cell layer in Nissl-stained preparations is about 60% of that observed in 5- to 9-year-old monkeys. It increases linearly between birth and 1 year of age, when it reaches 88% of the volume observed in 5- to 9-year-old monkeys. Paralleling this gradual development of the granule cell layer, the molecular and polymorphic layers exhibit gradual increases in volume during the same postnatal period, suggesting a protracted development of the functional circuits to which the granule cells contribute.

These volumetric findings are consistent with the fact that the dendritic length and spine density of individual granule cells increase until at least the 5th postnatal month in monkeys (Duffy and Rakic, 1983; Seress, 1992). In rats, the number of dendritic spines per unit length increases between 2 and 7 months of age (Duffy and Teyler, 1978), which suggests a protracted postnatal development of the rat molecular layer, parallel to that observed volumetrically in monkeys. As described previously, entorhinal cortex fibers innervate the appropriate target zones in the dentate gyrus and hippocampus of 2-week-old monkeys (Amaral et al., 2014). However, no detailed quantitative analyses of these projections in infant and adult monkeys have been performed to evaluate the postnatal maturation of these projections. In humans, the myelination of these projections appears to occur largely during the postnatal period and is thought to continue even after the first decade of life (Abraham et al., 2010). Altogether, these data suggest that although the main afferent connections of the dentate gyrus are already present at birth in primates, they undergo important morphological maturation during postnatal life that might impact the functional properties of these pathways.

With respect to the late maturation of the granule cells, we can expect that their axons continue to mature and influence the development of their target cells in the polymorphic layer of the dentate gyrus and the CA3 field of the hippocampus during postnatal life. Indeed, the polymorphic layer exhibits a 25% increase in volume between 1 year and 5–9 years of age in monkeys, suggesting a protracted maturation of its cellular components (Jabès et al., 2010, 2011). Interestingly, the mossy cells, the major targets of the granule cell projections in the polymorphic layer, exhibit clear morphological changes in soma and dendritic structure until at least 9 months of age in monkeys (Seress and Ribak, 1995b) and at least 2.5 years of age in humans (Seress and Mrzljak, 1992). In addition, the number of spines per 100 μm of mossy cell dendrite appears to increase by about 10% between 1 year and 4–20 years of age in monkeys (Seress and Ribak, 1995b). Although the mossy cells and the axons of granule cells represent a major proportion of the polymorphic layer, there are a variety of other neuronal types and afferent projections targeting this area (Amaral and Lavenex, 2007; Amaral et al., 2007). Despite the early establishment of subcortical projections to the polymorphic layer of the dentate gyrus (Frotscher and Seress, 2007), myelination occurs relatively late in the polymorphic layer, as compared with other hippocampal regions in humans (Abraham et al., 2010).

In sum, the regions associated with the projections from the dentate gyrus to the polymorphic layer (and CA3, see 4.8.2) exhibit a slow and protracted development that continues beyond the 1st year of life in monkeys, and possibly persist for the first decade of life in humans. Detailed analyses of the postnatal maturation of the different cell types constituting the dentate gyrus will be necessary to provide a definitive answer regarding the functional consequences of this delayed maturation of distinct circuits within the dentate gyrus.

4.8.2 CA3

Located downstream from the dentate gyrus, the developmental increase in volume of CA3 generally parallels that of the dentate gyrus (Figure 4.8). Interestingly, however, the distal portion of CA3, which receives direct projections from entorhinal cortex layer II neurons, matures volumetrically earlier than the proximal portion of CA3 (Jabès et al., 2011). At the cellular level, the proximal CA3 pyramidal neurons exhibit significant changes in soma size within the first 3 to 6 postnatal months. In contrast, the size of distal CA3 pyramidal neurons does not vary during postnatal development, suggesting that they have already reached an adult-like size by birth. These quantitative data are in agreement with the description by Seress and Ribak (1995a) that the somas and dendrites of distal CA3 pyramidal neurons exhibit adult-like ultrastructural features at birth. To our knowledge, there is no published information on the ultrastructural characteristics of developing proximal CA3 pyramidal neurons.

Functionally, proximal and distal CA3 pyramidal neurons contribute to different hippocampal circuits. Proximal CA3 pyramidal cells typically display no or very few dendrites extending into stratum lacunosum-moleculare in 33- to 57-day-old rats (Ishizuka et al., 1995) or 10-month-old to 21-year-old monkeys (Buckmaster and Amaral, 2001), and therefore do not receive significant, direct inputs from the entorhinal cortex (Witter and Amaral, 1991). In contrast, the pyramidal neurons located in the proximal portion of CA3 receive large numbers of mossy fiber terminals on both their apical and basal dendrites and are thus under greater influence of the granule cells than distally located CA3 cells that receive only apical mossy fiber inputs (Amaral and Lavenex, 2007; Kondo et al., 2008). As described above, various aspects of the dentate gyrus structure mature late during postnatal development; this is also the case for the mossy fiber projections. Indeed, Timm-stained mossy fiber terminals, although visible at birth, become more heavily stained in 3-month-old and adult monkeys, and the width of CA3 stratum lucidum (in which the mossy fibers travel and terminate) continues to increase after 6 months of age. Accordingly, the volume of the endbulb (the zone of stratum lucidum located distally in CA3, where the mossy fibers bend rostrally and travel longitudinally) also continues to increase between 9 months and 1 year of age (Jabès et al., 2011). Consequently, the earlier structural maturation of distal CA3 pyramidal neurons, as compared with proximal CA3 pyramidal neurons, suggests a differential maturation of presumably distinct functional circuits within CA3: a relatively early-maturing system associated with projections arising from the entorhinal cortex (see 4.8.4 for CA1 and the subiculum) and a rather late-maturing system associated with mossy fiber projections arising from dentate granule cells.

4.8.3 CA2

Volumetric measurements reveal that CA2 develops earlier than the dentate gyrus and CA3 (Jabès et al., 2011). These findings are consistent with observations based on the immunohistochemical detection of nonphosphorylated high-molecular-weight neurofilament expression, a marker of structural maturity, suggesting an early maturation of CA2 (Lavenex et al., 2004). Interestingly, CA2 differs from the dentate gyrus, CA3, and CA1 based on its connectivity with subcortical structures (see Chapter 3). CA2 projects extensively to the other fields of the hippocampus, has no known projections toward the neocortex, and does not project extensively to subcortical structures. However, CA2 receives a particularly prominent innervation from the posterior hypothalamus, especially from the supramammillary area and the tuberomammillary nucleus. These projections terminate mainly in and around the CA2 pyramidal cell layer and mainly on principal cells, a region that exhibits early expression of nonphosphorylated high-molecular-weight neurofilament immunoreactivity. CA2 pyramidal neurons are also more strongly excited by entorhinal cortex inputs onto their distal dendrites in stratum lacunosum-moleculare than are CA3 and CA1 pyramidal neurons (Chevaleyre and Siegelbaum, 2010). CA2 neurons, in turn, make strong excitatory synaptic contacts with CA1 neurons and could contribute, together with direct inputs from entorhinal cortex layer III neurons to the CA1 stratum lacunosum-moleculare, to the firing of CA1 pyramidal neurons in the absence of excitatory inputs from CA3 pyramidal neurons. The early maturation of both subcortical and direct entorhinal cortex inputs to CA2 might explain why individual layers within CA2 do not exhibit a differential maturation (in contrast to what is observed in CA3, CA1, and the subiculum). In sum, CA2 might form distinct functional pathways that mature both structurally and functionally earlier than CA3, even though CA3 is itself the main source of intrahippocampal excitatory inputs to the adult CA2.

4.8.4 CA1

Volumetric analyses reveal that CA1 matures earlier than the dentate gyrus and CA3 (Jabès et al., 2011), despite the fact that the largest input to the CA1 pyramidal neurons comes from CA3 pyramidal neurons via the Schaffer collaterals. Furthermore, distinct layers within CA1 exhibit differential maturation. The most superficial layer of CA1, stratum lacunosum-moleculare in which the projections from the entorhinal cortex layer III neurons terminate, matures earlier than the deeper layers of CA1, strata oriens, pyramidale, and radiatum, in which the CA3 projections terminate. These findings in monkeys are consistent with reports of a tardy myelination of fibers in strata pyramidale and radiatum, as compared with stratum lacunosum-moleculare, in CA1 of humans (Abraham et al., 2010). Similarly, in rats the length and number of dendritic segments reach adult values as early as postnatal day 10 in CA1 stratum lacunosum-moleculare, whereas they continue to develop until postnatal day 48 in CA1 stratum radiatum (Pokorny and Yamamoto, 1981). Furthermore, axon terminals, spines, and synapses mature earlier in CA1 stratum lacunosum-moleculare than in stratum radiatum. Altogether these data suggest a differential maturation of distinct, putative functional circuits within CA1: a relatively early-maturing system associated with the entorhinal cortex projections reaching stratum lacunosum-moleculare and a rather late-maturing system associated with the Schaffer collateral projections from CA3 to strata radiatum, pyramidale, and oriens.

4.8.5 Subiculum

Volumetric measures indicate that the subiculum develops earlier than the dentate gyrus and CA3, and at about the same time as CA2

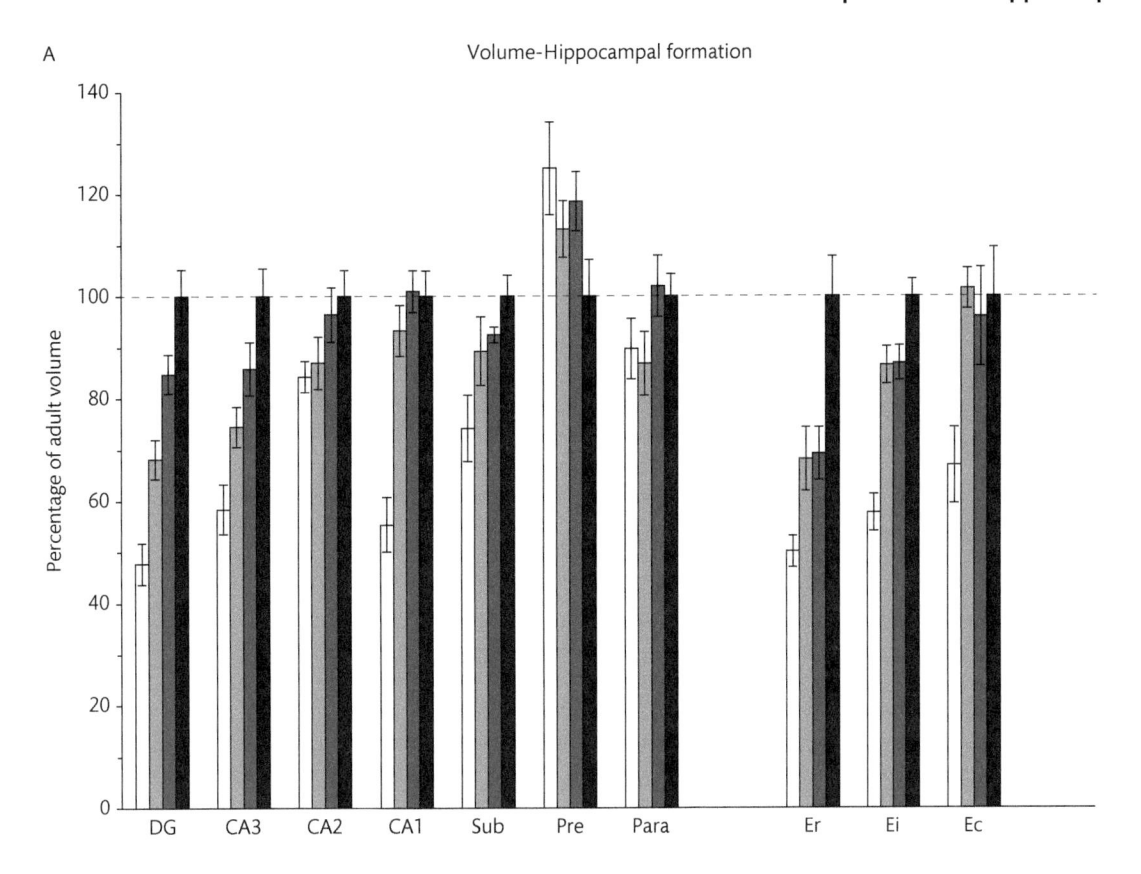

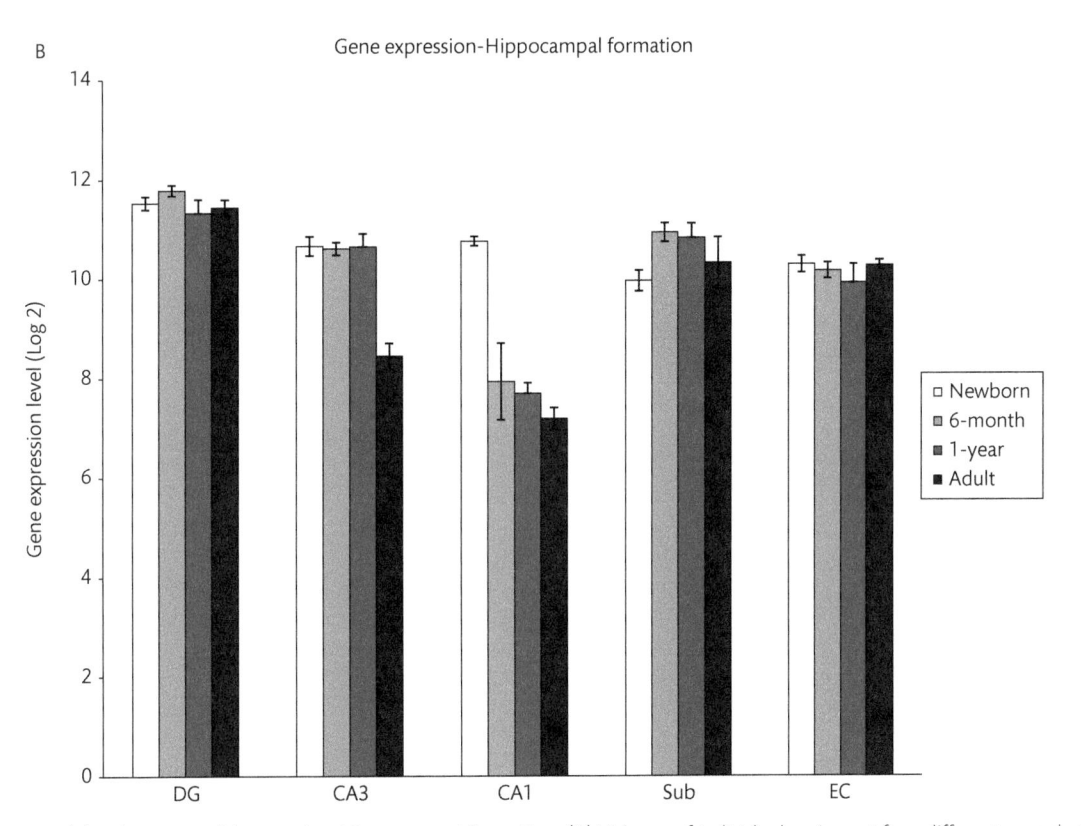

Figure 4.8 Postnatal development of the monkey hippocampal formation. (A) Volume of individual regions at four different ages during early postnatal development (expressed as percentage of the volume of the region observed in 5- to 10-year-old monkeys). (B) Microarray analysis of gene expression in the rhesus monkey hippocampal formation: GFAP gene expression decreased from birth to 6 months of age in CA1. GFAP gene expression decreased after 1 year of age in CA3. GFAP gene expression did not differ between CA3 and CA1 at birth, but it differed at all other ages. DG, dentate gyrus; CA3 and CA1, fields of the hippocampus; Sub, subiculum; EC, entorhinal cortex.

(Jabès et al., 2011). In addition, the subiculum is relatively more mature than CA1 until 6 months of age in monkeys (Figure 4.8). However, similar to what is observed in CA1, the molecular layer of the subiculum, in which projections from entorhinal cortex layer III neurons terminate, is overall more mature in the first postnatal year, as compared with the stratum pyramidale in which most of the CA1 projections terminate. Altogether, these data suggest a differential maturation of distinct, putative functional circuits within the subiculum: a relatively early-maturing system associated with the entorhinal cortex projections and a rather late-maturing system associated with the CA1 projections.

These volumetric data are consistent with the immunohistochemical detection of nonphosphorylated high-molecular-weight neurofilaments, which suggests an early maturation of the subiculum (Lavenex et al., 2004). Like CA2, the subiculum differs from the dentate gyrus, CA3 and CA1 based on its connectivity with subcortical structures. The subiculum is one of the two primary output structures of the hippocampal formation (the entorhinal cortex being the other) and the major source of efferent projections toward subcortical structures. The most prominent projections from the subiculum to subcortical structures reach the lateral septal nuclei, the nucleus accumbens, and the mammillary nuclei. Accordingly, these observations suggest that distinct functional pathways between the subiculum and subcortical structures mature both structurally and functionally earlier than the main excitatory pathways within the adult hippocampal formation.

4.8.6 Presubiculum and parasubiculum

The volumetric developmental profile of the presubiculum is unique (Figure 4.8). Unlike the other hippocampal fields, there is evidence for regressive events in the structural maturation of presubicular neurons and circuits, as suggested by decreases in the soma size of layer II neurons and the overall volume of layer I, from birth to 5–9 years of age (Jabès et al., 2011). However, the specific cellular changes that may contribute to this maturational profile are currently unknown. Volumetric measurements also suggest an early maturation of the parasubiculum, as compared with the rest of the hippocampal formation. Two unique features of the presubiculum and the parasubiculum, as compared with other hippocampal regions, are their reciprocal connections with the anterior thalamic nuclear complex and their heavy cholinergic innervation. Both structures also have reciprocal connections with the retrosplenial cortex (Kobayashi and Amaral, 2003, 2007). Functionally, experiments in rats have shown that the presubiculum and parasubiculum contain so-called head-direction cells, which exhibit adult-like firing properties as early as postnatal day 15 (Langston et al., 2010). Interestingly, functional projections from the presubiculum and parasubiculum to the medial entorhinal cortex are also observed as early as postnatal day 14–15 in rats (Canto et al., 2019). In monkeys, the caudal portion of the entorhinal (i.e., the equivalent of the medial entorhinal cortex in rats) exhibits an early structural maturation consistent with the developmental pattern observed in the presubiculum and parasubiculum (see 4.8.7). Accordingly, functional circuits including cells in the presubiculum, parasubiculum, retrosplenial cortex, and the caudal portion of the entorhinal cortex might contribute to the elaboration of a primitive spatial representation of the environment before other hippocampal circuits become functional (Langston et al., 2010;

Lavenex and Banta Lavenex, 2013). The exact nature of this representation remains to be determined.

4.8.7 Entorhinal cortex

As just discussed, distinct regions, layers, and cells of the hippocampal formation exhibit different profiles of structural development during early postnatal life. Consistent with these findings, the different layers and neurons of the seven subdivisions of the monkey entorhinal cortex exhibit different postnatal developmental profiles, which parallel the developmental profiles observed in the hippocampal structures with which they are interconnected (Piguet et al., 2020). This is particularly important because the entorhinal cortex constitutes the main gateway for bidirectional interaction between the neocortical areas comprised in the extended brain network subserving memory processes and the hippocampal formation. As a reminder, most neocortical inputs reaching the entorhinal cortex target preferentially its superficial layers II and III. In turn, entorhinal cortex layer II neurons project toward the dentate gyrus, CA3, and CA2, whereas layer III neurons project toward CA1 and the subiculum. In contrast, layer V and VI neurons receive reciprocal connections from CA1 and the subiculum, and project back to most of the neocortical areas that project to the entorhinal cortex.

Piguet et al. (2020) reported different developmental changes in neuronal soma size and volume of distinct layers in different subdivisions of the entorhinal cortex, and no changes in neuron number during early postnatal development. Specifically, they provided estimates of neuron number, neuronal soma size, and volume of the different layers and subdivisions of the monkey entorhinal cortex (Eo, Er, Elr, Ei, Elc, Ec, Ecl) at birth, 6 months, 1 year, and 5–9 years of age. Although soma size is not sufficient by itself to reflect the functional maturation of neurons, changes in neuronal soma size together with volumetric changes of individual layers provide information on the structural development of putative functional circuits to which these neurons contribute. As shown in the hippocampus (see 4.8.8), postnatal changes in the volume of individual layers or structures are correlated with functional changes revealed by genome-wide patterns of gene expression. In the monkey entorhinal cortex, layers I and II develop volumetrically early in most subdivisions. Layer III exhibits an early maturation between birth and 6 months of age in Ec and Ecl; a two-step/early maturation in Ei with a first increase in volume between birth and 6 months of age, followed by a second increase between 1 year and 5–9 years of age; and a late maturation after one year of age in Er. Layers V and VI exhibit an early maturation between birth and 6 months of age in Ec, a two-step and early maturation in Ei and Ecl, and a late maturation after 1 year of age in Er. Interestingly, neuronal soma size increases transiently at 6 months of age and decreases thereafter to reach adult size in most layers and subdivisions, except in layer II of Ei where neuronal soma size exhibits a two-step increase, in layer II of Ec and Ecl, where neuronal soma size does not differ between age groups, and in layer III of Ec and Ecl, where neuronal soma size decreases between birth and young adulthood.

Altogether, these findings support the theory that different hippocampal circuits exhibit distinct developmental profiles, which may subserve the emergence of different hippocampus-dependent memory processes (Lavenex and Banta Lavenex, 2013). In contrast, a study performed in mice reported that activity-dependent signals originating in layer II stellate cells of the medial entorhinal cortex contribute to some maturational processes of several hippocampal structures located downstream from it (Donato et al., 2017). However, these later findings do not appear to be consistent with the electrophysiological studies carried out in rats (Langston et al., 2010; Wills et al., 2010) showing that the functional maturation of discrete spatial cell types in different hippocampal structures follows the same developmental sequence as described by neuro-anatomical and gene expression studies targeting these regions in monkeys (Jabès et al., 2011; Lavenex et al., 2011; Favre et al., 2012b). Thus, it seems more likely that the stereotypic, sequential developmental patterns of maturation described in mice reflect the elaboration and/or strengthening of specific connections between neurons at different stages of hippocampal processing, rather than the functional maturation of hippocampal pathways (Cossart and Khazipov, 2022). This may be essential for the establishment of at-tractor network topologies contributing to the formation of grid patterns in the entorhinal cortex and may therefore not reflect the maturation of functional circuits supporting the emergence of dif-ferent hippocampus-dependent memory processes.

4.8.8 Evidence of postnatal maturation at the molecular level

Genome-wide analyses of gene expression in distinct regions of the monkey hippocampal formation from birth to young adulthood support the findings and interpretations of the neuroanatomical studies summarized above (Lavenex et al., 2011; Favre et al., 2012a, 2012b). Of particular interest is the fact that numerous genes ex-pressed in CA3 and CA1 exhibit a development-specific regulation that leads to a lower level of gene expression in older mature mon-keys, as compared with young developing monkeys. Most import-antly, the developmental changes observed at the gene-expression level confirm that CA1 matures earlier than CA3 (Figure 4.8B). Here, we consider further how the regulation of expression of sev-eral functional groups of genes might regulate synaptic plasticity in hippocampal circuits and thus contribute to the emergence of more selective and efficient memory processes (Lavenex and Banta Lavenex, 2013).

In a first study, Lavenex et al. (2011) reported that many genes associated with glycolysis and glutamate metabolism in astrocytes exhibit a lower expression level in CA1 of adult monkeys, as com-pared with other hippocampal regions. In addition, the expression of genes associated with glycolysis and glutamate metabolism in astrocytes reaches adult-like levels earlier during postnatal devel-opment in CA1 than in CA3, corroborating anatomical evidence revealing that CA1 matures earlier than the dentate gyrus and CA3 (Jabès et al., 2011). Accordingly, immunohistochemical analyses of the distribution of glial acidic fibrillary proteins revealed a differen-tial developmental profile of expression in CA1 and CA3, with levels in CA1 decreasing before those in CA3. In addition, the coverage of excitatory synapses by astrocytic processes undergoes a significant reduction in CA1 from birth to adulthood, as shown by electron microscopy analyses. Although at first glance decreased astrocytic coverage may seem maladaptive, and may indeed underlie the adult hippocampus's sensitivity to hypoxic/ischemic insult (Lavenex et al., 2011), decreased astrocytic coverage may also increase synaptic ef-ficacy in a manner that is advantageous for learning (Karlsson and Frank, 2008). Indeed, a reduction in glutamate clearance associ-ated with a relative decrease in astrocytic processes in the vicinity of synapses may affect transmitter release through modulation of presynaptic metabotropic glutamate receptors (Oliet et al., 2001).

Reduced glutamate clearance results in increased glutamate con-centration in the extracellular space (Tanaka et al., 1997; Bergles and Jahr, 1998), which in turn increases the activation of pre-synaptic metabotropic glutamate receptors (Scanziani et al., 1997), thus leading to a lower probability of glutamate release by the pre-synaptic terminal (Oliet et al., 2001). Presynaptic inhibition can be overcome by high-frequency bursts of afferent synaptic potentials (Grover et al., 2009), thus serving as a high-pass filter increasing the signal-to-noise ratio for information transmitted through these synapses (Oliet et al., 2001). Thus, the decreased astrocytic coverage of excitatory synapses observed in the adult CA1 could serve to en-sure that only the most salient information generates synaptic ac-tivity in the hippocampal circuits that contribute to learning and memory processes. A developmental decrease of astrocytic pro-cesses and functions may therefore contribute to the emergence of adult-like, selective memory function.

In a second study, Favre et al. (2012b) identified another important functional group involved in protein metabolism among the genes that were downregulated in CA1 and CA3 with age. This group of genes can be subdivided into two subgroups: one involved in protein synthesis and the other in protein degradation. The importance of protein synthesis in synaptic plasticity is well established. Indeed, as early as the 1960's, researchers showed that protein synthesis inhibi-tors impair memory performance, as well as long-term potentiation (LTP) and long-term depression (LTD) induction in CA1 (Flexner et al., 1963; Stanton and Sarvey, 1984). Demonstration of the role of protein degradation pathways in synaptic plasticity is more recent. For example, the proteasome inhibitor lactacystin, which prevents protein degradation, also leads to impaired memory performance and decreased LTP in CA1 (Lopez-Salon et al., 2001). From these experiments, it has become clear that the regulation of protein synthesis and degradation impacts synaptic plasticity, as well as learning and memory processes. Down regulation of both protein synthesis and protein degradation genes likely impacts the plasticity mechanisms that regulate synaptic transmission (Mabb and Ehlers, 2010). For example, the concomitant down regulation of genes in-volved in protein synthesis and protein degradation could reflect or underlie an increase in protein life span (i.e., if fewer proteins are degraded, fewer proteins need to be made). Increased protein life span might, in turn, lead to more stable and longer-lasting changes in the efficacy of synaptic transmission, which could be beneficial for learning and the maintenance of long-term memories. Again, as discussed above, the observed developmental changes in gene expression occur earlier in CA1, as compared with CA3. Finally, other functional groups of down regulated genes are preferen-tially expressed in neurons including genes involved in the MAPK signaling pathway, LTP, LTD, glutamate and GABA neurotrans-mitter pathways, regulation of dendritic processes and ion chan-nels (Favre et al., 2012b). The MAPK signaling pathway has been shown to be necessary for processes like LTP and is therefore es-sential for the mechanisms of synaptic plasticity (Peng et al., 2010). MAPK pathway overactivation in transgenic mice leads to deficits in hippocampal plasticity and hippocampal-dependent learning, which correlate with an increase in GABA release in the hippo-campus (Cui et al., 2008; Denayer et al., 2008; Peng et al., 2010). The relative overexpression of genes involved in the MAPK signaling pathway in young individuals, as compared with adults, might therefore be associated with lower learning and memory abilities in young individuals. The downregulation of the expression of genes involved in the MAPK signaling pathway with development would thus lead to improved hippocampal function, and to the concomitant improvements in learning and memory performance typically observed during normal postnatal development.

Several studies carried out in rodents have revealed that specific changes in gene expression contribute to critical steps in the functional maturation of the hippocampal formation (Travaglia et al., 2016a; Travaglia et al., 2016b; Guskjolen et al., 2018; Bessieres et al., 2020). In a first study, Travaglia et al. (2016a) quantified basal expression levels of a number of genes coding for genes associated with synaptic plasticity, glia, and connectivity in the dorsal portion of the rat hippocampus at postnatal days 17, 24, and 80. They found that the levels of numerous proteins known to be critical for the synaptic plasticity underlying memory formation (including immediate early genes, kinases, transcription factors, and AMPA glutamate receptor subunits) and/or their phosphorylation levels peak at postnatal day 17 and then decrease to reach adult levels. In contrast, the phosphorylation of calcium calmodulin kinase II-α and the extracellular signal-regulated kinases 2, and the levels of GluA1 and GluA2 increase from postnatal day 17 to postnatal day 24 to reach levels similar to those observed at postnatal day 80. It is difficult to directly compare the results of the studies performed in rats, which grouped several fields of the dorsal hippocampus, with those obtained in monkeys that analyzed separately distinct regions sampled at midrostrocaudal level of the hippocampus. However, both series of studies jointly point to the fact that the postnatal maturation of the hippocampal formation is characterized by specific changes in overall gene expression, which shifts from a highly plastic system to a less plastic system that would be more adapted to support long-term memory processes.

In a second study performed in rats, Travaglia et al. (2016b) reported a mGluR5-dependent developmental switch in the ratio of NMDA receptor subunit GluN2B/GluN2A expression, which could represent a critical mechanism by which excitatory synapses rapidly mature in response to experience during a critical developmental period. Interestingly, in this experiment, inhibitory avoidance training to context with a single footshock was tested at postnatal days 17 and 24. Training at postnatal day 17 produced significant freezing immediately after training, but memory expression was strongly decreased after 30 minutes and undetectable after 1 day. In contrast, training at postnatal day 24 produced significant freezing for at least 7 days. Contextual reminders presented between 1 and 16 days after conditioning failed to elicit freezing in postnatal day 17 trained rats, suggesting the absence of a memory trace resulting from inhibitory avoidance conditioning at postnatal day 17. However, when postnatal day 17 trained rats were presented with a reminder footshock delivered at postnatal day 26 in a new context, two days after a second test of inhibitory avoidance memory (i.e., exposure to the initial context without footshock), two-thirds of them exhibited a level of freezing, reflecting some memory of the initial inhibitory training experience (i.e., control rats did not). Although it is difficult to consider how exactly this type of fear conditioning in rats relates to the formation and free recall of episodic memory in humans (Bevandic et al., 2024), it does suggest that some latent memory trace acquired during initial conditioning was formed at postnatal day 17, even though rats would normally not exhibit any overt memory of this experience later in life. Additional experiments carried out in the same study showed that brain-derived neurotrophic factor (BDNF) and mGlur5-dependent processes influence the GluN2A/GluN2B ratio in the dorsal hippocampus. BDNF during conditioning at postnatal day 17 is necessary for the formation of a latent memory trace, which is dependent on GluN2B receptor activation, and the subsequent switch from GluN2B to GluN2A expression in the hippocampus. In this paradigm, after conditioning at postnatal day 17 the presentation of both context and footshock was necessary to reinstate contextual fear memories after postnatal day 24, whereas exposure to either context or footshock alone was insufficient. In contrast, postnatal day 24 trained rats exhibited initial learning and expression of inhibitory avoidance memory as well as retention after learning similar to that of adult rats. It is thus particularly interesting to consider that an increase in GluN2A/GluN2B gene expression ratio is also observed in the monkey hippocampus during postnatal development, and more specifically between birth and 6 months of age in CA1 and between 1 year and 5–9 years of age in CA3, as well as more gradually from birth to young adulthood in the dentate gyrus (Favre et al., 2012b). Altogether, these results suggest that although some latent memory trace may be established relatively early within hippocampal circuits, the offset of infantile amnesia (characterized by the absence of explicit free recall of information later in life) requires some maturational processes that happen at specific times in different hippocampal circuits during postnatal development.

In a third study, Bessieres et al. (2020) showed that different learning experiences at postnatal day 17 induce experience-specific latent memory traces in the hippocampus. They further demonstrated that hippocampal circuits are somewhat functional before rats can form long-lasting memories that will be accessible later in life. Importantly, however, they showed that the molecular signature of hippocampal function at early ages clearly differs from what is observed when long-lasting hippocampus-dependent memories can be formed and retrieved naturally. Various mechanisms, including differential regulation of immediate early genes expression, synaptic plasticity, and neuronal excitability markers, such as those described in the monkey studies discussed above, were also suggested to contribute to these developmental changes in memory processes.

Similarly, Guskjolen et al. (2018) have shown that the optogenetic reactivation of neuronal ensembles that were activated in the dentate gyrus during contextual fear conditioning in postnatal day 17 mice can induce freezing for up to 3 months after conditioning. In contrast to the results of the experiments in rats described above, mice trained at postnatal day 17 exhibited freezing behavior similar to that of postnatal day 60 mice 1 day after contextual fear conditioning. Nevertheless, they exhibited significant forgetting, as evidenced by reduced freezing after 15 days, and essentially no freezing after 30 or 90 days. Optogenetic stimulation of dentate granule cells activated during fear conditioning at postnatal day 17 (tagged via the immediate early gene Arc-dependent expression of channelrhodopsin-2) led to partial recovery of freezing and the activation of neurons in the dentate gyrus and downstream areas, including CA3, CA1, and the entorhinal cortex. Freezing was eliminated as soon as the optical stimulation of dentate granule cells was turned off. This study revealed that artificially reinstating patterns of encoding activity in the dentate gyrus and other hippocampal regions can lead to the expression of a memory that otherwise could not be naturally recovered via the sole presentation of reminder cues. It nevertheless confirmed that although some latent memory traces may be established relatively early within hippocampal circuits, the end of infantile amnesia requires specific modifications of these circuits during postnatal development.

4.9 A model linking hippocampal and memory development

The hippocampal formation, often considered as a whole functional unit, is the central component of a large brain network essential for the processing of spatial and episodic memories (Chapters 13, 14). Yet, it is now well established that different hippocampal structures and circuits contribute to different types of information processing (Chapter 16). Here, we consider the differential postnatal maturation of distinct hippocampal regions and layers and putative functional circuits from a global perspective that takes into consideration the work of many other researchers who have contributed to our current understanding of various hippocampal functions. The neuroanatomical and molecular data discussed above suggest that the differential maturation of distinct hippocampal circuits may underlie the emergence and maturation of different hippocampus-dependent memory processes, ultimately leading to the emergence of episodic memory concomitant with the maturation of all hippocampal circuits (Figure 4.9).

This model was initially proposed by Lavenex and Banta Lavenex (2013), and is based on the view that specific types of information processing are subserved by different hippocampal circuits, which can be summarized as follows: First, the dentate gyrus contributes to pattern separation, involving both spatial and nonspatial information (Kesner, 2007; Bakker et al., 2008; Borzello et al., 2023). Second, postnatal neurogenesis in the dentate gyrus contributes to the encoding of temporal associations, linking events that happened at the same time and distinguishing events that happened at different times (Aimone et al., 2006; Cai et al., 2016; Borzello et al., 2023). Varying levels of neurogenesis throughout postnatal development may impact encoding and forgetting of early memories (Jabès et al., 2010; Lavenex and Banta Lavenex, 2013; Akers et al., 2014). Third, CA3 contributes to both pattern completion and the rapid and flexible acquisition of spatial memories (Nakazawa et al., 2002; Rolls and Kesner, 2006). Fourth, CA1 contributes to the slow and gradual learning of the relations between more than two different items experienced simultaneously. Spatial and temporal aspects of memory become fully integrated within CA1 neuronal networks (Eichenbaum, 2017). Fifth, the subiculum, presubiculum and parasubiculum contribute to the integration of self-generated movement information (Rolls, 2006). As such, these structures can contribute to the process of path integration (O'Mara et al., 2001) and the elaboration or maintenance of spatial representations that subserve spatial navigation in absence of external information (Sharp, 1999). Sixth, as the main gateway between the hippocampus and the neocortex, the entorhinal cortex plays a pivotal role in memory processing. Here, we consider some of the functional distinctions proposed for the lateral (i.e., rostral in primates) and medial (i.e., caudal in primates) entorhinal cortex (Knierim et al., 2014; Tsao et al., 2018; Nilssen et al., 2019); see also Chapter 12 for more in-depth discussion. The lateral entorhinal cortex is thought to be particularly involved in emotional processing and the processing of individual items and locations based on a local frame of reference, and may provide the hippocampus with information about the content of an experience (Knierim et al., 2014; Nilssen et al.,

2019). In contrast, the medial entorhinal cortex is thought to be particularly involved in the processing of contextual information and locations based on a global frame of reference, and may provide the hippocampus with information about the context of an experience (Knierim et al., 2014; Nilssen et al., 2019). In addition, neurons in the lateral entorhinal cortex may provide a temporal signal that encodes time across multiple scales from seconds to hours, which may thus reflect the temporal structure of ongoing experience across different contexts (Tsao et al., 2018).

This model is heavily influenced by functional studies carried out in rodents and is thus naturally more focused on the development of spatial and episodic-like memory capacities. Nevertheless, the logic developed in this section can be revised or extended to other hippocampus-dependent processes as new data are gathered and integrated to provide a more comprehensive view of the development of various types of memories in humans and other animals. Research conducted by numerous groups has shown that this model is consistent with and can be used to understand the sequential development of different types of spatial capacities in children (Newcombe et al., 2000). Egocentric capacities emerge first in the newborn child and tend to dominate the child's spatial world for at least the first 6 months (Acredolo, 1978; Bremner, 1978; Acredolo and Evans, 1980). The use of cues or landmarks to remember spatial locations begins to appear between 8.5 and 12 months (Acredolo, 1978; Bremner, 1978; Acredolo and Evans, 1980; Bushnell et al., 1995; Lew et al., 2000). At the same time, children between 6 and 12 months of age demonstrate that they can use path integration (Acredolo, 1978; Rieser and Heiman, 1982; Bremner et al., 1994), whereas allocentric (viewpoint-independent) place learning does not begin to emerge until after 20 months of age and is only reliably expressed by a majority of children after 2 years of age (Newcombe et al., 1998; Ribordy et al., 2013). However, children's ability to solve complex allocentric spatial tasks, which require a high degree of spatial pattern separation improves gradually from 2 to 7 years of age (Ribordy et al., 2013; Ribordy Lambert et al., 2015), as does their ability to temporally distinguish separate events (Ribordy Lambert et al., 2017). Altogether, these improvements in spatial and temporal resolution processing evidenced in experimental studies performed in laboratory settings are consistent with age-related improvements in children's ability to create autobiographical memories that can be recalled later in life (Bauer, 2006).

4.9.1 Path integration

The studies reviewed above have shown that different hippocampal structures, regions, and layers that have direct interconnections exhibit similar developmental profiles. Accordingly, the caudal portion of the primate entorhinal cortex (medial portion in rodents) may contribute to a functional network including the subiculum, presubiculum, parasubiculum, and retrosplenial cortex that supports path integration abilities. These brain regions contain several cell types that contribute to spatial information processing, including place cells, head-direction cells, grid cells and boundary cells (Taube, 2007). During development, head-direction cells in the presubiculum and parasubiculum are the first to exhibit adult-like activity patterns (Langston et al., 2010), and functional projections from the presubiculum and parasubiculum to the medial entorhinal cortex are also observed as early as postnatal day 14–15 in rats (Canto et al., 2019). Hippocampal place cells evolve more gradually, whereas entorhinal cortex grid cells exhibit

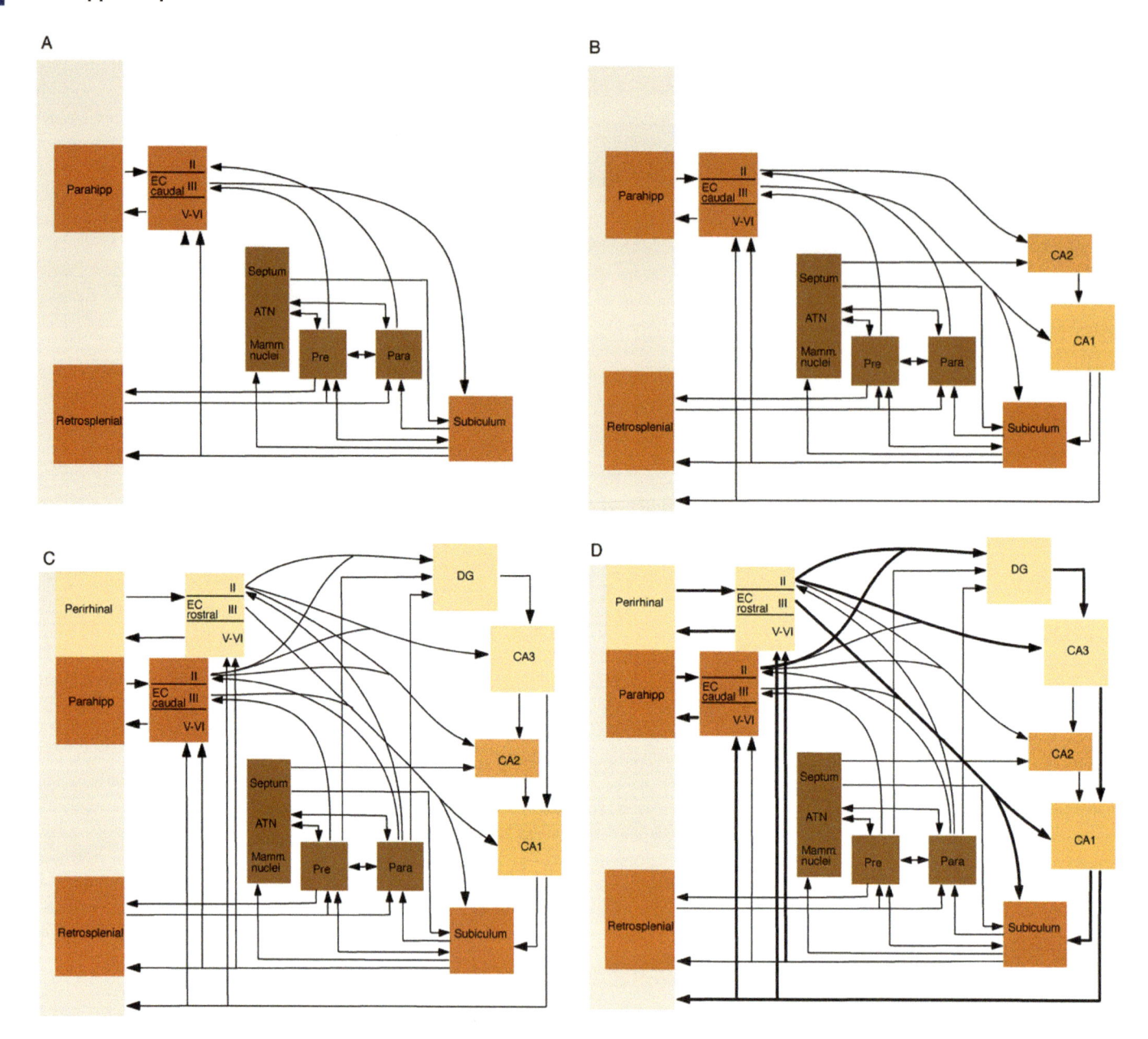

Figure 4.9 Hierarchical model of the postnatal maturation of the primate hippocampal formation. (A) The maturation of hippocampal circuits involving the subiculum, presubiculum, parasubiculum, and caudal entorhinal cortex might support path integration abilities before 1 year of age in children. (B) The maturation of hippocampal circuits involving the direct projections from the superficial layers of the entorhinal cortex to CA1 (and CA2) might support basic allocentric spatial memory abilities at 2 years of age in children. (C) The protracted maturation of hippocampal circuits involving the dentate gyrus and CA3 might support high-resolution allocentric spatial memory abilities after 3 years of age in children. (D) The more complete maturation of all hippocampal circuits might support episodic memory abilities after 7 years of age in children.

the slowest development (Langston et al., 2010; Wills et al., 2010). Interestingly, most neurons in layer III of the medial entorhinal cortex exhibit directional preferences at a very young age, as is the case in adult individuals (Langston et al., 2010). These neurons thus likely play a role in supporting path integration, which can be defined as a computational process by which an organism continually monitors its own movement (Taube, 2007), or an internal computation that transforms a sense of motion into a sense of location (Savelli and Knierim, 2019). It is important to understand that the term "path integration" does not implicitly denote the use of either an egocentric or allocentric frame of reference. Path integration can be used to support orientation and navigation

via either egocentric or allocentric strategies (Bostelmann et al., 2020). Accordingly, path integration may enable individuals to use an egocentric representation to successfully update their position and navigate in their environment before either visual scene information dependent on the parahippocampal cortex (Epstein, 2008; Epstein et al., 2017) or a basic allocentric spatial representations dependent on the functional maturation of CA1 becomes available during development (see 4.9.2). Accordingly, Piguet et al. (2020) proposed that the functional maturation of a discrete network including the subiculum, presubiculum, parasubiculum, and the caudal entorhinal cortex may underlie the emergence of egocentric path integration abilities in children between 6 and

12 months of age (Acredolo, 1978; Rieser and Heiman, 1982; Bremner et al., 1994).

4.9.2 Basic allocentric spatial memory

Research in rodents also demonstrated that CA1 place-cell activity and a basic allocentric representation of the environment can be subserved by the direct monosynaptic pathway from the entorhinal cortex to CA1. Mizumori et al. (1989) first showed that CA1 place-cell coding is maintained during reversible suppression of CA3 output to CA1, via inactivation of medial septum projections. Brun et al. (2002) later showed that CA1 place-cell coding persists following direct lesion of CA3 and that CA3-lesioned animals display place recognition. In contrast, specific lesion of the entorhinal cortex input to CA1 impairs CA1 place-cell coding (Brun et al., 2008). Finally, transgenic mice lacking NMDA receptors in CA3 pyramidal cells, thus functionally deafferenting CA1 from its CA3 inputs, exhibit essentially normal CA1 place cells and are capable of acquiring and remembering allocentric spatial memories experienced over repeated trials (Nakazawa et al., 2002; Nakazawa et al., 2003). Altogether, these experiments carried out in rodents indicate that CA1 place-cell activity and a basic allocentric representation of the environment acquired over repeated trials can be maintained by direct inputs from the entorhinal cortex to CA1. Accordingly, neuroanatomical studies in monkeys revealed that areas Ec and Ecl exhibit an early structural development between birth and 6 months of age (Piguet et al., 2020) that parallels what is observed in CA1 at the structural and molecular levels (Jabès et al., 2011; Lavenex et al., 2011; Favre et al., 2012a). Importantly, as described above, the early volumetric maturation of CA1 is primarily due to the early maturation of one specific layer, the stratum lacunosum-moleculare, in which the direct projections from the entorhinal cortex terminate. Given the proposed role of the rat medial entorhinal cortex (i.e., the caudal part of the primate entorhinal cortex) in the processing of contextual information and locations based on a global frame of reference (Knierim et al., 2014), it stands to reason that the maturation of the reciprocal connections between the caudal entorhinal cortex and CA1 may underlie the emergence of allocentric spatial processing, which is reliably observed in children from 2 years of age (Newcombe et al., 1998; Ribordy et al., 2013; Ribordy Lambert et al., 2017).

Note that bidirectional interaction between the hippocampus and the caudal entorhinal cortex may be critical to support this capacity. Indeed, grid cells found in the rat medial entorhinal cortex require an excitatory input from the hippocampus in order to maintain their normal firing pattern (Bonnevie et al., 2013). In the absence of hippocampal signal, grid cells become head-direction cells likely driven by direct inputs from the presubiculum. Similarly, Chareyron et al. (2017) have shown in monkeys that normal activation of the caudal entorhinal cortex (Ec and Ecl) during spatial exploration is dependent on the integrity of the hippocampus. These two studies, using different methodologies in different species, suggest that the primate caudal entorhinal cortex (i.e., medial entorhinal cortex in rodents) may not be fully functional in the absence of functional hippocampal circuits. Accordingly, the functional maturation of CA1 may itself contribute to the functional maturation of the caudal entorhinal cortex in support of basic allocentric spatial processing, beyond its earlier developing ability to support egocentric path integration via its interconnections with the subiculum, presubiculum, and parasubiculum. Such functional maturation

includes the ability to integrate visual scene information provided by the parahippocampal cortex, which may contribute to the construction of low-resolution, allocentric spatial representations of the environment.

4.9.3 Increased spatial memory precision and content

As described above, a direct projection from the entorhinal cortex to CA1 is thought to be able to subserve basic allocentric spatial processing. In contrast, computational models, in vivo studies carried out in rats, and imaging studies in humans support the theory that the dentate gyrus, together with its connections with CA3, subserve a process known as pattern separation (Kesner, 2007; Bakker et al., 2008; Borzello et al., 2023), which is necessary to discriminate individual items, episodes, or spatial locations that are very similar or close to one another (Gilbert et al., 1998; Kesner, 2007; Bakker et al., 2008; Morris et al., 2012). Accordingly, disrupting the CA3 input to CA1 results in decreased spatial tuning of CA1 place cells (Brun et al., 2002; Nakashiba et al., 2008). This suggests that the main trisynaptic hippocampal pathway (i.e., entorhinal cortex to dentate gyrus, dentate gyrus to CA3, CA3 to CA1) is necessary for high-resolution spatial discrimination (i.e., spatial pattern separation). The monkey dentate gyrus exhibits a protracted development and has not yet reached an adult volume at 1 year of age (i.e., 4 years of age in humans). Similarly, area Er of the entorhinal cortex, which projects to the distal dendritic portion of dentate granule cells, exhibits a protracted structural development that continues after 1 year of age (Piguet et al., 2020). This rostral portion of the entorhinal cortex (Er and the rostral part of Ei) receives significant projections from the amygdala and the perirhinal cortex and may be involved in the integration of emotional information, as well as in the processing of local features related to individual items and objects. Altogether, the maturation of the dentate gyrus, CA3 and the rostral entorhinal cortex may further contribute to the integration of spatial information about individual objects into a global representation of the environment, and thus contribute to increasing the precision of allocentric spatial representations. The fact that these regions exhibit a protracted development suggests that the processing capacities that they subserve exhibit a delayed emergence and continue to mature across an extended developmental timeline.

Early findings by Acredolo et al. (1975) are in agreement with the proposed theory that the improvements that occur in children's allocentric spatial memory after 2 years of age (i.e., after the basic capacity to learn and remember an allocentric representation of the environment has emerged) correspond to improvements in children's ability to more precisely calculate the spatial coordinates of individual locations based on distal environmental objects. It thus stands to reason that the gradual functional maturation of the rostral entorhinal cortex, dentate gyrus, and trisynaptic hippocampal pathway, may contribute to the improved spatial and temporal pattern separation abilities from 2 to 7 years of life in humans (Lavenex and Banta Lavenex, 2013; Ribordy Lambert et al., 2015, 2017). Accordingly, studies of both spatial and autobiographical episodic memories indicate that these forms of hippocampus-dependent memory mature significantly within the same age range (Acredolo et al., 1975; Herman and Siegel, 1978; Newcombe et al., 2000; Sluzenski et al., 2004; Bauer, 2006; Balcomb et al., 2011). Indeed, age-dependent maturation in spatial pattern separation capacities can explain the age-dependent improvements in children's performance in tasks such as the Morris search task (Overman et al.,

1996), the radial arm maze (Foreman et al., 1984; Aadland et al., 1985; Foreman et al., 1990; Overman et al., 1996), open-field tasks (Overman et al., 1996), and sandbox search tasks that test children's representation of multiple locations, relations between objects, and short-term retention of a spatial location (Sluzenski et al., 2004).

4.9.4 Episodic memory

The lack of autobiographical memories from our infancy has been hypothesized to result from the immaturity of the neurobiological substrates subserving these memories in adult individuals (Bauer, 2006; Newcombe et al., 2007), although concrete neurobiological evidence for these theories has been notably absent (Lavenex et al., 2007). It is now firmly established that from 2 years of age, children can solve a spatial task using a basic allocentric representation of the surrounding environment (Newcombe et al., 1998; Ribordy et al., 2013). The emergence of this capacity coincides temporally with the end of infantile amnesia, and likely coincides with the structural and functional maturation of the CA1 region of the hippocampus (Lavenex and Banta Lavenex, 2013). It is thus possible that mature CA1 processing confers the overall ability to form relational memories, including both spatial and episodic memories. Indeed, by 3.5 years of age, children are capable of solving a complex allocentric spatial task, which necessitates a high degree of spatial pattern separation in order to discriminate goal locations from closely apposed decoy locations over repeated trials (Ribordy et al., 2013). This capacity likely coincides with the structural and functional maturation of the dentate gyrus and trisynaptic hippocampal pathway. However, it has also been shown that the trisynaptic pathway is critical for rapid single-trial contextual learning (Nakashiba et al., 2008). The encoding of autobiographical memories, by definition, requires rapid, single-trial contextual learning. Structural findings in monkeys suggest that the impact of postnatal neurogenesis on hippocampal function differs in developing and mature individuals. Accordingly, Jabès et al. (2011) proposed that the immaturity of the dentate gyrus, with its concomitant high rate of neurogenesis, may underlie the phenomenon of childhood amnesia, the fact that as adults we have fewer memories from between 2 and 7 years of age than would be predicted by normal forgetting alone. They thus hypothesized that the gradual maturation of the trisynaptic hippocampal pathway subserves the gradual improvement, from 2 to 7 years of age, in our ability to create distinct, high-resolution, trial-unique autobiographical memories that can be recalled later in life.

Computational models and experimental studies in rodents also suggest that continued neurogenesis in the adult dentate gyrus plays a fundamental role in the temporal coding of events and the formation of episodic memories (Weisz and Argibay, 2009; W Deng et al., 2010; Cai et al., 2016). Newly generated immature neurons might contribute to the increased association of events occurring in close temporal proximity, whereas events that do not occur in close temporal proximity would be encoded by distinct groups of newly generated immature neurons. In conjunction with the reported role of the dentate gyrus in pattern separation, adult neurogenesis could help to disambiguate new events happening in familiar contexts and therefore contribute to the encoding of individual episodic memories (Aimone et al., 2009). This might explain the inability to form enduring episodic memories until the dentate gyrus has become sufficiently mature. Indeed, very high levels of plasticity are typically associated with the normal development of the brain (Knudsen, 2003; Hensch, 2004), and the dentate gyrus is likely no exception

(Josselyn and Frankland, 2012). Dentate gyrus circuits, and in particular the balance between highly plastic, immature neurons born later during development and less plastic, mature neurons born earlier during development, might not be optimally tuned to contribute to the separate encoding of distinct episodes until late postnatal development. The population of dentate gyrus granule cells, which continue to mature beyond 1 year of age in monkeys, might be too responsive to neuronal activity and undergoing continuous changes in synaptic plasticity that are important for normal development but are not optimal for learning and the establishment of long-term memories. This hypothesis is supported by the results of elegant studies carried out in two precocial species, guinea pigs and degus, which are characterized by longer gestation and reduced postnatal neurogenesis in the dentate gyrus (Akers et al., 2014). Indeed, unlike postnatal day 17 mice that show rapid forgetting, postnatal day 17 guinea pigs exhibit no change in spatial memory as a function of retention delay, and postnatal day 17 degus exhibit normal retention of a contextual fear memory for up to one month. These results indicate that some memories are persistent in precocial rodent species with low postnatal hippocampal neurogenesis. Although these results may also be influenced by differences in the maturation of other hippocampal circuits, it is interesting to note that Akers et al. (2014) also showed that increasing neurogenesis in both precocial species can induce forgetting, a compelling experimental evidence for the link between varying rates of neurogenesis and the maintenance of long-term memory.

As discussed above, the immaturity of the dentate gyrus may contribute to the phenomenon of childhood amnesia, possibly via both encoding and forgetting. In turn, the gradual maturation of the trisynaptic hippocampal pathway may subserve the gradual improvement from 2 to 7 years of age in our ability to create autobiographical memories that can be recalled later in life. In addition, several mechanisms have been proposed to explain how hippocampal networks may represent moments or epochs in temporally organized experiences (Eichenbaum, 2017), although there was no clear indication regarding a specific contribution of the entorhinal cortex to the representation of time in support of episodic memory. However, a study by Tsao et al. (2018) reported that neurons in the rat lateral entorhinal cortex may provide a temporal signal that encodes time across multiple scales, from seconds to hours, and may thus reflect the temporal structure of ongoing experience across different contexts. Accordingly, one may consider that the primate rostral entorhinal cortex may also contribute to the definition of the temporal component of episodic memory. Together with the protracted maturation of the trisynaptic pathway, which is critical for rapid, single-trial contextual learning in support of the encoding of episodic memories, the late maturation of rostral entorhinal circuits may also contribute to the gradual improvement during postnatal development in our ability to create spatiotemporally distinct autobiographical memories.

4.10 Conclusion

In this chapter, we have primarily focused on the structural development of the hippocampal formation, with the aim of providing a comprehensive description of the developmental periods and processes which contribute to the establishment of the main hippocampal circuits. We have focused on the general principles of hippocampal development that are valid across species in hope that it will serve as a general guide for how to investigate more pointed questions regarding the role of specific genes or regulatory pathways in the structural and functional maturation of the hippocampus. We believe that a better understanding of how the hippocampus is gradually built, and how genetic predispositions and individual experiences may influence these developmental processes in different species, will be key to furthering our understanding of the behavioral functions that it subserves in humans. Nothing in the hippocampus makes sense except in the light of development.

REFERENCES

Aadland J, Beatty WW, Maki RH (1985) Spatial memory of children and adults assessed in the radial maze. *Dev Psychobiol* 18:163–172.

Abraham H, Veszpremi B, Kravjak A, Kovacs K, Gomori E, Seress L (2009) Ontogeny of calbindin immunoreactivity in the human hippocampal formation with a special emphasis on granule cells of the dentate gyrus. *Int J Dev Neurosci* 27:115–127.

Abraham H, Vincze A, Jewgenow I, Veszpremi B, Kravjak A, Gomori E, Seress L (2010) Myelination in the human hippocampal formation from midgestation to adulthood. *Int J Dev Neurosci* 28:401–410.

Acredolo LP (1978) Development of spatial orientation in infancy. *Dev Psychol* 14:224–234.

Acredolo LP, Evans D (1980) Developmental changes in the effects of landmarks on infant spatial behavior. *Dev Psych* 16:312–318.

Acredolo LP, Pick HL, Olsen MG (1975) Environmental differentiation and familiarity as determinants of children's memory for spatial location. *Dev Psych* 11:495–501.

Aimone JB, Wiles J, Gage FH (2006) Potential role for adult neurogenesis in the encoding of time in new memories. *Nat Neurosci* 9:723–727.

Aimone JB, Wiles J, Gage FH (2009) Computational influence of adult neurogenesis on memory encoding. *Neuron* 61:187–202.

Akers KG, Martinez-Canabal A, Restivo L, Yiu AP, De Cristofaro A, Hsiang HL, Wheeler AL, Guskjolen A, Niibori Y, Shoji H, Ohira K, Richards BA, Miyakawa T, Josselyn SA, Frankland PW (2014) Hippocampal neurogenesis regulates forgetting during adulthood and infancy. *Science* 344:598–602.

Alonso A, Kohler C (1982) Evidence for separate projections of hippocampal pyramidal and non-pyramidal neurons to different parts of the septum in the rat brain. *Neurosci Lett* 31:209–214.

Altman J, Bayer SA (1990) Prolonged sojourn of developing pyramidal cells in the intermediate zone of the hippocampus and their settling in the stratum pyramidale. *J Comp Neurol* 301:343–364.

Altman J, Das GD (1965) Autoradiographic and histological evidence of postnatal hippocampal neurogenesis in rats. *J Comp Neurol* 124:319–336. Amaral DG, Dent JA (1981) Development of the mossy fibers of the dentate gyrus: I. A light and electron microscopic study of the mossy fibers and their expansions. *J Comp Neurol* 195:51–86.

Amaral DG, Kondo H, Lavenex P (2014) An analysis of entorhinal cortex projections to the dentate gyrus, hippocampus, and subiculum of the neonatal macaque monkey. *J Comp Neurol* 522:1485–1505.

Amaral DG, Kurz J (1985) The time of origin of cells demonstrating glutamic acid decarboxylase-like immunoreactivity in the hippocampal formation of the rat. *Neurosci Lett* 59:33–39.

Amaral DG, Lavenex P (2007) Hippocampal neuroanatomy. In: The Hippocampus Book (Andersen P, Morris RGM, Amaral DG, Bliss TV, O'Keefe J, eds), pp 37–114. Oxford: Oxford University Press.

Amaral DG, Scharfman HE, Lavenex P (2007) The dentate gyrus: fundamental neuroanatomical organization (dentate gyrus for dummies). *Prog Brain Res* 163:3–22.

Andersen J, Urban N, Achimastou A, Ito A, Simic M, Ullom K, Martynoga B, Lebel M, Goritz C, Frisen J, Nakafuku M, Guillemot F (2014) A transcriptional mechanism integrating inputs from extracellular signals to activate hippocampal stem cells. *Neuron* 83:1085–1097.

Angevine JB, Jr. (1965) Time of neuron origin in the hippocampal region: an autoradiographic study in the mouse. *Exp Neurol Suppl:Suppl* 2:1–70.

Anstotz M, Quattrocolo G, Maccaferri G (2018) Cajal-Retzius cells and GABAergic interneurons of the developing hippocampus: close electrophysiological encounters of the third kind. *Brain Res* 1697:124–133.

Arnold SE, Trojanowski JQ (1996) Human fetal hippocampal development: 1. Cytoarchitecture, myeloarchitecture, and neuronal morphologic features. *J Comp Neurol* 367:274–292.

Bagri A, Cheng HJ, Yaron A, Pleasure SJ, Tessier-Lavigne M (2003) Stereotyped pruning of long hippocampal axon branches triggered by retraction inducers of the semaphorin family. *Cell* 113:285–299.

Bakker A, Kirwan CB, Miller M, Stark CE (2008) Pattern separation in the human hippocampal CA3 and dentate gyrus. *Science* 319:1640–1642.

Balcomb F, Newcombe NS, Ferrara K (2011) Finding where and saying where: developmental relationships between place learning and language in the first year. *J Cogn Dev* 12:315–331.

Barallobre MJ, Del Rio JA, Alcantara S, Borrell V, Aguado F, Ruiz M, Carmona MA, Martin M, Fabre M, Yuste R, Tessier-Lavigne M, Soriano E (2000) Aberrant development of hippocampal circuits and altered neural activity in netrin 1-deficient mice. *Development* 127:4797–4810.

Bauer PJ (2006) Constructing a past in infancy: neuro-developmental account. *Trends Cogn Sci* 10:175–181.

Bayer SA (1980) Development of the hippocampal region in the rat: I. Neurogenesis examined with 3H-thymidine autoradiography. *J Comp Neurol* 190:87–114.

Bayer SA, Altman J (1974) Hippocampal development in the rat: cytogenesis and morphogenesis examined with autoradiography and low-level X-irradiation. *J Comp Neurol* 158:55–79.

Bayer SA, Altman J, Russo RJ, Zhang X (1993) Timetables of neurogenesis in the human brain based on experimentally determined patterns in the rat. *Neurotoxicology* 14:83–144.

Ben-Ari Y, Khalilov I, Represa A, Gozlan H (2004) Interneurons set the tune of developing networks. *Trends Neurosci* 27:422–427.

Berg DA, Su Y, Jimenez-Cyrus D, Patel A, Huang N, Morizet D, Lee S, Shah R, Ringeling FR, Jain R, Epstein JA, Wu QF, Canzar S, Ming GL, Song H, Bond AM (2019) A common embryonic origin of stem cells drives developmental and adult neurogenesis. *Cell* 177:654–668, e615.

Berger B, Alvarez C (1994) Neurochemical development of the hippocampal region in the fetal rhesus monkey: II. Immunocytochemistry of peptides, calcium-binding proteins, DARPP-32, and monoamine innervation in the entorhinal cortex by the end of gestation. *Hippocampus* 4:85–114.

Berger B, Alvarez C (1996) Neurochemical development of the hippocampal region in the fetal rhesus monkey, III: Calbindin-D28K, calretinin and parvalbumin with special mention of Cajal-Retzius cells and the retrosplenial cortex. *J Comp Neurol* 366:674–699.

Berger B, Alvarez C, Goldman-Rakic PS (1993) Neurochemical development of the hippocampal region in the fetal rhesus monkey: I. Early appearance of peptides, calcium-binding proteins, DARPP-32, and monoamine innervation in the entorhinal cortex during the first half of gestation (E47 to E90). *Hippocampus* 3:279–305.

Berger B, Esclapez M, Alvarez C, Meyer G, Catala M (2001) Human and monkey fetal brain development of the supramammillary-hippocampal projections: a system involved in the regulation of theta activity. *J Comp Neurol* 429:515–529.

Bergles DE, Jahr CE (1998) Glial contribution to glutamate uptake at Schaffer collateral-commissural synapses in the hippocampus. *J Neurosci* 18:7709–7716.

Bergmann O, Spalding KL, Frisen J (2015) Adult neurogenesis in humans. *Cold Spring Harb Perspect Biol* 7:a018994.

Berns DS, DeNardo LA, Pederick DT, Luo L (2018) Teneurin-3 controls topographic circuit assembly in the hippocampus. *Nature* 554:328–333.

Bessieres B, Travaglia A, Mowery TM, Zhang X, Alberini CM (2020) Early life experiences selectively mature learning and memory abilities. *Nat Commun* 11:628.

Bevandic J, Chareyron LJ, Bachevalier J, Cacucci F, Genzel L, Newcombe NS, Vargha-Khadem F, Olafsdottir HF (2024) Episodic memory development: bridging animal and human research. *Neuron* 112(7):1060–1080.

Birey F, Andersen J, Makinson CD, Islam S, Wei W, Huber N, Fan HC, Metzler KRC, Panagiotakos G, Thom N, O'Rourke NA, Steinmetz LM, Bernstein JA, Hallmayer J, Huguenard JR, Pasca SP (2017) Assembly of functionally integrated human forebrain spheroids. *Nature* 545:54–59.

Blockus H, Rolotti SV, Szoboszlay M, Peze-Heidsieck E, Ming T, Schroeder A, Apostolo N, Vennekens KM, Katsamba PS, Bahna F, Mannepalli S, Ahlsen G, Honig B, Shapiro L, de Wit J, Losonczy A, Polleux F (2021) Synaptogenic activity of the axon guidance molecule Robo2 underlies hippocampal circuit function. *Cell Rep* 37:109828.

Blomfield IM, Rocamonde B, Masdeu MDM, Mulugeta E, Vaga S, van den Berg DL, Huillard E, Guillemot F, Urban N (2019) Id4 promotes the elimination of the pro-activation factor Ascl1 to maintain quiescence of adult hippocampal stem cells. *Elife* 8:e48561.

Bonnevie T, Dunn B, Fyhn M, Hafting T, Derdikman D, Kubie JL, Roudi Y, Moser EI, Moser MB (2013) Grid cells require excitatory drive from the hippocampus. *Nat Neurosci* 16:309–317.

Borzello M, Ramirez S, Treves A, Lee I, Scharfman H, Stark C, Knierim JJ, Rangel LM (2023) Assessments of dentate gyrus function: discoveries and debates. *Nat Rev Neurosci* 24:502–517.

Bostelmann M, Lavenex P, Banta Lavenex P (2020) Children five-to-nine years old can use path integration to build a cognitive map without vision. *Cogn Psychol* 121:101307.

Bremner JG (1978) Egocentric versus allocentric spatial coding in nine-month-old infants: factors influencing the choice of code. *Dev Psychol* 14:346–355.

Bremner JG, Knowles L, Andreasen G (1994) Processes underlying young children's spatial orientation during movement. *J Exp Child Psychol* 57:355–376.

Brinks H, Conrad S, Vogt J, Oldekamp J, Sierra A, Deitinghoff L, Bechmann I, Alvarez-Bolado G, Heimrich B, Monnier PP, Mueller BK, Skutella T (2004) The repulsive guidance molecule RGMa is involved in the formation of afferent connections in the dentate gyrus. *J Neurosci* 24:3862–3869.

Brun VH, Leutgeb S, Wu HQ, Schwarcz R, Witter MP, Moser EI, Moser MB (2008) Impaired spatial representation in CA1 after lesion of direct input from entorhinal cortex. *Neuron* 57:290–302.

Brun VH, Otnass MK, Molden S, Steffenach HA, Witter MP, Moser MB, Moser EI (2002) Place cells and place recognition maintained by direct entorhinal-hippocampal circuitry. *Science* 296:2243–2246.

Buckmaster PS, Amaral DG (2001) Intracellular recording and labeling of mossy cells and proximal CA3 pyramidal cells in macaque monkeys. *J Comp Neurol* 430:264–281.

Bushnell EW, McKenzie BE, Lawrence DA, Connell S (1995) The spatial coding strategies of one-year-old infants in a locomotor search task. *Child Dev* 66:937–958.

Cai DJ et al. (2016) A shared neural ensemble links distinct contextual memories encoded close in time. *Nature* 534:115–118.

Cameron HA, McKay RDG (2001) Adult neurogenesis produces a large pool of new granule cells in the dentate gyrus. *J Comp Neurol* 435:406–417.

Canto CB, Koganezawa N, Lagartos-Donate MJ, O'Reilly KC, Mansvelder HD, Witter MP (2019) Postnatal development of functional projections from parasubiculum and presubiculum to medial entorhinal cortex in the rat. *J Neurosci* 39:8645–8663.

Cembrowski MS, Spruston N (2019) Heterogeneity within classical cell types is the rule: lessons from hippocampal pyramidal neurons. *Nat Rev Neurosci* 20:193–204.

Ceranik K, Zhao S, Frotscher M (2000) Development of the entorhino-hippocampal projection: guidance by Cajal-Retzius cell axons. *Ann N Y Acad Sci* 911:43–54.

Chareyron LJ, Banta Lavenex P, Amaral DG, Lavenex P (2017) Functional organization of the medial temporal lobe memory system following neonatal hippocampal lesion in rhesus monkeys. *Brain Struct Funct* 222:3899–3914.

Chevaleyre V, Siegelbaum SA (2010) Strong CA2 pyramidal neuron synapses define a powerful disynaptic cortico-hippocampal loop. *Neuron* 66:560–572.

Ciarpella F, Zamfir RG, Campanelli A, Pedrotti G, Di Chio M, Bottani E, Decimo I (2023) Generation of mouse hippocampal brain organoids from primary embryonic neural stem cells. *STAR Protoc* 4:102413.

Cossart R, Khazipov R (2022) How development sculpts hippocampal circuits and function. *Physiol Rev* 102:343–378.

Cotman C, Taylor D, Lynch G (1973) Ultrastructural changes in synapses in the dentate gyrus of the rat during development. *Brain Res* 63:205–213.

Cowan WM, Stanfield BB, Amaral DG (1981) Further observations on the development of the dentate gyrus. In: Studies in Developmental Neurobiology (Cowan WM, ed.), pp 395–435. Oxford: Oxford University Press.

Crain B, Cotman C, Taylor D, Lynch G (1973) A quantitative electron microscopic study of synaptogenesis in the dentate gyrus of the rat. *Brain Res* 63:195–204.

Cui Y, Costa RM, Murphy GG, Elgersma Y, Zhu Y, Gutmann DH, Parada LF, Mody I, Silva AJ (2008) Neurofibromin regulation of ERK signaling modulates GABA release and learning. *Cell* 135:549–560.

Danglot L, Triller A, Marty S (2006) The development of hippocampal interneurons in rodents. *Hippocampus* 16:1032–1060.

Daugherty AM, Yu Q, Flinn R, Ofen N (2015) A reliable and valid method for manual demarcation of hippocampal head, body, and tail. *Int J Dev Neurosci* 41:115–122.

Deller T, Drakew A, Frotscher M (1999) Different primary target cells are important for fiber lamination in the fascia dentata: a lesson from reeler mutant mice. *Exp Neurol* 156:239–253.

Del Rio JA, Heimrich B, Borrell V, Forster E, Drakew A, Alcantara S, Nakajima K, Miyata T, Ogawa M, Mikoshiba K, Derer P, Frotscher M, Soriano E (1997) A role for Cajal-Retzius cells and reelin in the development of hippocampal connections. *Nature* 385:70–74.

Del Rio JA, Martinez A, Fonseca M, Auladell C, Soriano E (1995) Glutamate-like immunoreactivity and fate of Cajal-Retzius cells in the murine cortex as identified with calretinin antibody. *Cereb Cortex* 5:13–21.

Denayer E, Ahmed T, Brems H, Van Woerden G, Borgesius NZ, Callaerts-Vegh Z, Yoshimura A, Hartmann D, Elgersma Y, D'Hooge R, Legius E, Balschun D (2008) Spred1 is required for synaptic plasticity and hippocampus-dependent learning. *J Neurosci* 28:14443–14449.

Deng JB, Yu DM, Wu P, Li MS (2007) The tracing study of developing entorhino-hippocampal pathway. *Int J Dev Neurosci* 25:251–258.

Deng W, Aimone JB, Gage FH (2010) New neurons and new memories: how does adult hippocampal neurogenesis affect learning and memory? *Nat Rev Neurosci* 11:339–350.

Donato F, Jacobsen RI, Moser MB, Moser EI (2017) Stellate cells drive maturation of the entorhinal-hippocampal circuit. *Science* 355(6330).

Duffy CJ, Rakic P (1983) Differentiation of granule cell dendrites in the dentate gyrus of the rhesus monkey: a quantitative Golgi study. *J Comp Neurol* 214:224–237.

Duffy CJ, Teyler TJ (1978) Development of potentiation in the dentate gyrus of rat: physiology and anatomy. *Brain Res Bull* 3:425–430.

Eckenhoff MF, Rakic P (1988) Nature and fate of proliferative cells in the hippocampal dentate gyrus during the life span of the rhesus monkey. *J Neurosci* 8:2729–2747.

Eckenhoff MF, Rakic P (1991) A quantitative analysis of synaptogenesis in the molecular layer of the dentate gyrus in the rhesus monkey. *Brain Res Dev Brain Res* 64:129–135.

Eichenbaum H (2017) On the integration of space, time, and memory. *Neuron* 95:1007–1018.

Epstein RA (2008) Parahippocampal and retrosplenial contributions to human spatial navigation. *Trends Cogn Sci* 12:388–396.

Epstein RA, Patai EZ, Julian JB, Spiers HJ (2017) The cognitive map in humans: spatial navigation and beyond. *Nat Neurosci* 20:1504–1513.

Favre G, Banta Lavenex P, Lavenex P (2012a) Developmental regulation of expression of schizophrenia susceptibility genes in the primate hippocampal formation. *Transl Psychiatry* 2:e173.

Favre G, Banta Lavenex P, Lavenex P (2012b) miRNA regulation of gene expression: a predictive bioinformatics analysis in the postnatally developing monkey hippocampus. *PLoS One* 7:e43435.

Flexner JB, Flexner LB, Stellar E (1963) Memory in mice as affected by intracerebral puromycin. *Science* 141:57–59.

Foreman N, Arber M, Savage J (1984) Spatial memory in preschool infants. *Dev Psychobiol* 17:129–137.

Foreman N, Warry R, Murray P (1990) Development of reference and working spatial memory in preschool children. *J Gen Psychol* 117:267–276.

Freund TF, Antal M (1988) GABA-containing neurons in the septum control inhibitory interneurons in the hippocampus. *Nature* 336:170–173.

Freund TF, Buzsaki G (1996) Interneurons of the hippocampus. *Hippocampus* 6:347–470.

Fricke R, Cowan WM (1977) An autoradiographic study of the development of the entorhinal and commissural afferents to the dentate gyrus of the rat. *J Comp Neurol* 173:231–250.

Frisen J (2016) Neurogenesis and gliogenesis in nervous system plasticity and repair. *Annu Rev Cell Dev Biol* 32:127–141.

Frotscher M (1997) Dual role of Cajal-Retzius cells and reelin in cortical development. *Cell Tissue Res* 290:315–322.

Frotscher M, Drakew A, Heimrich B (2000) Role of afferent innervation and neuronal activity in dendritic development and spine maturation of fascia dentata granule cells. *Cereb Cortex* 10:946–951.

Frotscher M, Heimrich B, Deller T, Nitsch R (1995) Understanding the cortex through the hippocampus: lamina-specific connections of the rat hippocampal neurons. *J Anat* 187:539–545.

Frotscher M, Seress L (2007) Morphological development of the hippocampus. In: The Hippocampus Book (Amaral DG, Andersen P, Bliss T, Morris RGM, O'Keefe J, eds), pp 115–131. New York: Oxford University Press.

Gebhardt C, Del Turco D, Drakew A, Tielsch A, Herz J, Frotscher M, Deller T (2002) Abnormal positioning of granule cells alters afferent fiber distribution in the mouse fascia dentata: morphologic evidence from reeler, apolipoprotein E receptor 2-, and very low density lipoprotein receptor knockout mice. *J Comp Neurol* 445:278–292.

Giedd JN, Vaituzis AC, Hamburger SD, Lange N, Rajapakse JC, Kaysen D, Vauss YC, Rapoport JL (1996) Quantitative MRI of the temporal lobe, amygdala, and hippocampus in normal human development: ages 4–18 years. *J Comp Neurol* 366:223–230.

Gilbert PE, Kesner RP, DeCoteau WE (1998) Memory for spatial location: role of the hippocampus in mediating spatial pattern separation. *J Neurosci* 18:804–810.

Glærum IL, Dunville K, Moan K, Krause M, Montaldo NP, Kirikae H, Nigro MJ, Sætrom P, van Loon B, Quattrocolo G (2024) Postnatal persistence of hippocampal Cajal-Retzius cells has a crucial role in the establishment of the hippocampal circuit. *Development* 151(1):dev202236. doi:10.1242/dev.202236. Epub 2024 Jan 9.

Gogtay N, Nugent TF, 3rd, Herman DH, Ordonez A, Greenstein D, Hayashi KM, Clasen L, Toga AW, Giedd JN, Rapoport JL, Thompson PM (2006) Dynamic mapping of normal human hippocampal development. *Hippocampus* 16:664–672.

Gomez AM, Traunmuller L, Scheiffele P (2021) Neurexins: molecular codes for shaping neuronal synapses. *Nat Rev Neurosci* 22:137–151.

Gonzalez Arnay E (2015) Estudio inmunohistoquimico del searrollo prenatal del hipocampo humano. In: Departamentao de anatomia, histologia y neurociencia. Madrid: Universidad autonoma de Madrid.

Gould E, Reeves AJ, Fallah M, Tanapat P, Gross CG, Fuchs E (1999) Hippocampal neurogenesis in adult Old World primates. *Proc Natl Acad Sci U S A* 96:5263–5267.

Grateron L, Cebada-Sanchez S, Marcos P, Mohedano-Moriano A, Insausti AM, Munoz M, Arroyo-Jimenez MM, Martinez-Marcos A, Artacho-Perula E, Blaizot X, Insausti R (2003) Postnatal development of calcium-binding proteins immunoreactivity (parvalbumin, calbindin, calretinin) in the human entorhinal cortex. *J Chem Neuroanat* 26:311–316.

Grove EA, Tole S, Limon J, Yip L, Ragsdale CW (1998) The hem of the embryonic cerebral cortex is defined by the expression of multiple Wnt genes and is compromised in Gli3-deficient mice. *Development* 125:2315–2325.

Grover LM, Kim E, Cooke JD, Holmes WR (2009) LTP in hippocampal area CA1 is induced by burst stimulation over a broad frequency range centered around delta. *Learn Mem* 16:69–81.

Guskjolen A, Kenney JW, de la Parra J, Yeung BA, Josselyn SA, Frankland PW (2018) Recovery of "lost" infant memories in mice. *Curr Biol* 28:2283–2290, e2283.

Hansen DV, Lui JH, Flandin P, Yoshikawa K, Rubenstein JL, Alvarez-Buylla A, Kriegstein AR (2013) Non-epithelial stem cells and cortical interneuron production in the human ganglionic eminences. *Nat Neurosci* 16:1576–1587.

Havenaar R, Meijer JC, Morton DB, Ritskes-Hoitinga J, Zwart P (1993) Biology and husbandry of laboratory animals. In: Principles of Laboratory Animal Science (Van Zutphen LFM, Baumans V, Beynen AC, eds), pp 17–74. Amsterdam: Elsevier Science.

Heng YH, McLeay RC, Harvey TJ, Smith AG, Barry G, Cato K, Plachez C, Little E, Mason S, Dixon C, Gronostajski RM, Bailey TL, Richards LJ, Piper M (2014) NFIX regulates neural progenitor cell differentiation during hippocampal morphogenesis. *Cereb Cortex* 24:261–279.

Hensch TK (2004) Critical period regulation. *Annu Rev Neurosci* 27:549–579.

Herman JF, Siegel AW (1978) The development of cognitive mapping of the large-scale environment. *J Exp Child Psychol* 26:389–406.

Hevner RF (2016) Evolution of the mammalian dentate gyrus. *J Comp Neurol* 524:578–594.

Hevner RF, Kinney HC (1996) Reciprocal entorhinal-hippocampal connections established by human fetal midgestation. *J Comp Neurol* 372:384–394.

Hochgerner H, Zeisel A, Lonnerberg P, Linnarsson S (2018) Conserved properties of dentate gyrus neurogenesis across postnatal development revealed by single-cell RNA sequencing. *Nat Neurosci* 21:290–299.

Hodge RD, Kowalczyk TD, Wolf SA, Encinas JM, Rippey C, Enikolopov G, Kempermann G, Hevner RF (2008) Intermediate progenitors in adult hippocampal neurogenesis: Tbr2 expression and coordinate regulation of neuronal output. *J Neurosci* 28:3707–3717.

Hoogenraad CC, Milstein AD, Ethell IM, Henkemeyer M, Sheng M (2005) GRIP1 controls dendrite morphogenesis by regulating EphB receptor trafficking. *Nat Neurosci* 8:906–915.

Hopper KJ, Capozzi DK, Newsome JT (2008) Effects of maternal and infant characteristics on birth weight and gestation length in a colony of rhesus macaques (*Macaca mulatta*). *Comp Med* 58:597–603.

Hruska M, Dalva MB (2012) Ephrin regulation of synapse formation, function and plasticity. *Mol Cell Neurosci* 50:35–44.

Humphrey T (1967) The development of the human hippocampal fissure. *J Anat* 101:655–676.

Hunsaker MR, Scott JA, Bauman MD, Schumann CM, Amaral DG (2014) Postnatal development of the hippocampus in the Rhesus macaque (*Macaca mulatta*): a longitudinal magnetic resonance imaging study. *Hippocampus* 24:794–807.

Insausti R, Cebada-Sanchez S, Marcos P (2010) Postnatal development of the human hippocampal formation. *Adv Anat Embryol Cell Biol* 206:1–86.

Ishizuka N, Cowan WM, Amaral DG (1995) A quantitative analysis of the dendritic organization of pyramidal cells in the rat hippocampus. *J Comp Neurol* 362:17–45.

Iwano T, Masuda A, Kiyonari H, Enomoto H, Matsuzaki F (2012) Prox1 postmitotically defines dentate gyrus cells by specifying granule cell identity over CA3 pyramidal cell fate in the hippocampus. *Development* 139:3051–3062.

Jabès A, Banta Lavenex P, Amaral DG, Lavenex P (2010) Quantitative analysis of postnatal neurogenesis and neuron number in the macaque monkey dentate gyrus. *Eur J Neurosci* 31:273–285.

Jabès A, Banta Lavenex P, Amaral DG, Lavenex P (2011) Postnatal development of the hippocampal formation: a stereological study in macaque monkeys. *J Comp Neurol* 519:1051–1070.

Josselyn SA, Frankland PW (2012) Infantile amnesia: a neurogenic hypothesis. *Learn Mem* 19:423–433.

Judas M, Rados M, Jovanov-Milosevic N, Hrabac P, Stern-Padovan R, Kostovic I (2005) Structural, immunocytochemical, and mr imaging properties of periventricular crossroads of growing cortical pathways in preterm infants. *AJNR Am J Neuroradiol* 26:2671–2684.

Jukic AM, Baird DD, Weinberg CR, McConnaughey DR, Wilcox AJ (2013) Length of human pregnancy and contributors to its natural variation. *Hum Reprod* 28:2848–2855.

Karlsson MP, Frank LM (2008) Network dynamics underlying the formation of sparse, informative representations in the hippocampus. *J Neurosci* 28:14271–14281.

Kerloch T, Clavreul S, Goron A, Abrous DN, Pacary E (2019) Dentate granule neurons generated during perinatal life display distinct morphological features compared with later-born neurons in the mouse hippocampus. *Cereb Cortex* 29:3527–3539.

Kesner RP (2007) A behavioral analysis of dentate gyrus function. *Prog Brain Res* 163:567–576.

Kirov SA, Goddard CA, Harris KM (2004) Age-dependence in the homeostatic upregulation of hippocampal dendritic spine number during blocked synaptic transmission. *Neuropharmacology* 47:640–648.

Klausberger T (2009) GABAergic interneurons targeting dendrites of pyramidal cells in the CA1 area of the hippocampus. *Eur J Neurosci* 30:947–957.

Knickmeyer RC, Gouttard S, Kang C, Evans D, Wilber K, Smith JK, Hamer RM, Lin W, Gerig G, Gilmore JH (2008) A structural MRI study of human brain development from birth to 2 years. *J Neurosci* 28:12176–12182.

Knierim JJ, Neunuebel JP, Deshmukh SS (2014) Functional correlates of the lateral and medial entorhinal cortex: objects, path integration and local-global reference frames. *Philos Trans R Soc Lond B Biol Sci* 369:20130369.

Knudsen EI (2003) Early experience and critical periods. In: Fundamental Neuroscience, Second Edition (Squire LR, Bloom FE, McConnell SK, Roberts JL, Spitzer NC, Zigmond MJ, eds), pp 555–573. London: Academic Press.

Kobayashi Y, Amaral DG (2003) Macaque monkey retrosplenial cortex: II. Cortical afferents. *J Comp Neurol* 466:48–79.

Kobayashi Y, Amaral DG (2007) Macaque monkey retrosplenial cortex: III. Cortical efferents. *J Comp Neurol* 502:810–833.

Koh S, Loy R (1989) Localization and development of nerve growth factor-sensitive rat basal forebrain neurons and their afferent projections to hippocampus and neocortex. *J Neurosci* 9:2999–0318.

Kondo H, Lavenex P, Amaral DG (2008) Intrinsic connections of the macaque monkey hippocampal formation: I. Dentate gyrus. *J Comp Neurol* 511:497–520.

Kornack DR, Rakic P (1999) Continuation of neurogenesis in the hippocampus of the adult macaque monkey. *Proc Natl Acad Sci U S A* 96:5768–5773.

Kostovic I, Petanjek Z, Judas M (1993) Early areal differentiation of the human cerebral cortex: entorhinal area. *Hippocampus* 3:447–458.

Kostovic I, Seress L, Mrzljak L, Judas M (1989) Early onset of synapse formation in the human hippocampus: a correlation with Nissl-Golgi architectonics in 15- and 16.5-week-old fetuses. *Neuroscience* 30:105–116.

Kowalczyk A, Filipkowski RK, Rylski M, Wilczynski GM, Konopacki FA, Jaworski J, Ciemerych MA, Sicinski P, Kaczmarek L (2004) The critical role of cyclin D2 in adult neurogenesis. *J Cell Biol* 167:209–213.

Lagali PS, Corcoran CP, Picketts DJ (2010) Hippocampus development and function: role of epigenetic factors and implications for cognitive disease. *Clin Genet* 78:321–333.

Langston RF, Ainge JA, Couey JJ, Canto CB, Bjerknes TL, Witter MP, Moser EI, Moser MB (2010) Development of the spatial representation system in the rat. *Science* 328:1576–1580.

Lavado A, Oliver G (2007) Prox1 expression patterns in the developing and adult murine brain. *Dev Dyn* 236:518–524.

Lavenex P, Banta Lavenex P (2013) Building hippocampal circuits to learn and remember: insights into the development of human memory. *Behav Brain Res* 254:8–21.

Lavenex P, Banta Lavenex P, Amaral DG (2004) Nonphosphorylated high-molecular-weight neurofilament expression suggests early maturation of the monkey subiculum. *Hippocampus* 14:797–801.

Lavenex P, Banta Lavenex P, Amaral DG (2007) Postnatal development of the primate hippocampal formation. *Dev Neurosci* **29**:179–192.

Lavenex P, Sugden SG, Davis RR, Gregg JP, Banta Lavenex P (2011) Developmental regulation of gene expression and astrocytic processes may explain selective hippocampal vulnerability. *Hippocampus* **21**:142–149.

Le Bail M, Martineau M, Sacchi S, Yatsenko N, Radzishevsky I, Conrod S, Ait Ouares K, Wolosker H, Pollegioni L, Billard JM, Mothet JP (2015) Identity of the NMDA receptor coagonist is synapse specific and developmentally regulated in the hippocampus. *Proc Natl Acad Sci U S A* **112**:E204–213.

Lew AR, Bremner JG, Lefkovitch LP (2000) The development of relational landmark use in six- to twelve-month-old infants in a spatial orientation task. *Child Develop* **71**:1179–1190.

Li G, Fang L, Fernandez G, Pleasure SJ (2013) The ventral hippocampus is the embryonic origin for adult neural stem cells in the dentate gyrus. *Neuron* **78**:658–672.

Linke R, Frotscher M (1993) Development of the rat septohippocampal projection: tracing with DiI and electron microscopy of identified growth cones. *J Comp Neurol* **332**:69–88.

Linke R, Pabst T, Frotscher M (1995) Development of the hippocamposeptal projection in the rat. *J Comp Neurol* **351**:602–616.

Liu C, Teng ZQ, McQuate AL, Jobe EM, Christ CC, von Hoyningen-Huene SJ, Reyes MD, Polich ED, Xing Y, Li Y, Guo W, Zhao X (2013) An epigenetic feedback regulatory loop involving microRNA-195 and MBD1 governs neural stem cell differentiation. *PLoS One* **8**:e51436.

Liu C, Teng ZQ, Santistevan NJ, Szulwach KE, Guo W, Jin P, Zhao X (2010) Epigenetic regulation of miR-184 by MBD1 governs neural stem cell proliferation and differentiation. *Cell Stem Cell* **6**:433–444.Lopez-Salon M, Alonso M, Vianna MR, Viola H, Mello e Souza T, Izquierdo I, Pasquini JM, Medina JH (2001) The ubiquitin-proteasome cascade is required for mammalian long-term memory formation. *Eur J Neurosci* **14**:1820–1826.

Lun MP, Monuki ES, Lehtinen MK (2015) Development and functions of the choroid plexus-cerebrospinal fluid system. *Nat Rev Neurosci* **16**:445–457.

Lynch KM, Shi Y, Toga AW, Clark KA, Pediatric Imaging, Neurocognition and Genetics Study (2019) Hippocampal shape maturation in childhood and adolescence. *Cereb Cortex* **29**:3651–3665.

Ma T, Wang C, Wang L, Zhou X, Tian M, Zhang Q, Zhang Y, Li J, Liu Z, Cai Y, Liu F, You Y, Chen C, Campbell K, Song H, Ma L, Rubenstein JL, Yang Z (2013) Subcortical origins of human and monkey neocortical interneurons. *Nat Neurosci* **16**:1588–1597.

Mabb AM, Ehlers MD (2010) Ubiquitination in postsynaptic function and plasticity. *Annu Rev Cell Dev Biol* **26**:179–210.

Mangale VS, Hirokawa KE, Satyaki PR, Gokulchandran N, Chikbire S, Subramanian L, Shetty AS, Martynoga B, Paul J, Mai MV, Li Y, Flanagan LA, Tole S, Monuki ES (2008) Lhx2 selector activity specifies cortical identity and suppresses hippocampal organizer fate. *Science* **319**:304–309.

Martinez A, Otal R, Sieber BA, Ibanez C, Soriano E (2005) Disruption of ephrin-A/EphA binding alters synaptogenesis and neural connectivity in the hippocampus. *Neuroscience* **135**:451–461.

Martynoga B, Mateo JL, Zhou B, Andersen J, Achimastou A, Urban N, van den Berg D, Georgopoulou D, Hadjur S, Wittbrodt J, Ettwiller L, Piper M, Gronostajski RM, Guillemot F (2013) Epigenomic enhancer annotation reveals a key role for NFIX in neural stem cell quiescence. *Genes Dev* **27**:1769–1786.

Mattison JA, Colman RJ, Beasley TM, Allison DB, Kemnitz JW, Roth GS, Ingram DK, Weindruch R, de Cabo R, Anderson RM (2017) Caloric restriction improves health and survival of rhesus monkeys. *Nat Commun* **8**:14063.

McKay S, Ryan TJ, McQueen J, Indersmitten T, Marwick KFM, Hasel P, Kopanitsa MV, Baxter PS, Martel MA, Kind PC, Wyllie DJA, O'Dell TJ, Grant SGN, Hardingham GE, Komiyama NH (2018) The developmental shift of NMDA receptor composition proceeds independently of GluN2 subunit-specific GluN2 C-terminal sequences. *Cell Rep* **25**:841–851, e844.

Milner TA, Loy R, Amaral DG (1983) An anatomical study of the development of the septo-hippocampal projection in the rat. *Brain Res* **284**:343–371.

Mira H, Andreu Z, Suh H, Lie DC, Jessberger S, Consiglio A, San Emeterio J, Hortiguela R, Marques-Torrejon MA, Nakashima K, Colak D, Gotz M, Farinas I, Gage FH (2010) Signaling through BMPR-IA regulates quiescence and long-term activity of neural stem cells in the adult hippocampus. *Cell Stem Cell* **7**:78–89.

Mizumori SJ, Barnes CA, McNaughton BL (1989) Reversible inactivation of the medial septum: selective effects on the spontaneous unit activity of different hippocampal cell types. *Brain Res* **500**:99–106.

Morris AM, Churchwell JC, Kesner RP, Gilbert PE (2012) Selective lesions of the dentate gyrus produce disruptions in place learning for adjacent spatial locations. *Neurobiol Learn Mem* **97**:326–331.

Mukherjee S, Brulet R, Zhang L, Hsieh J (2016) REST regulation of gene networks in adult neural stem cells. *Nat Commun* **7**:13360.

Nakamura F, Ugajin K, Yamashita N, Okada T, Uchida Y, Taniguchi M, Ohshima T, Goshima Y (2009) Increased proximal bifurcation of CA1 pyramidal apical dendrites in sema3A mutant mice. *J Comp Neurol* **516**:360–375.

Nakashiba T, Young JZ, McHugh TJ, Buhl DL, Tonegawa S (2008) Transgenic inhibition of synaptic transmission reveals role of CA3 output in hippocampal learning. *Science* **319**:1260–1264.

Nakazawa K, Quirk MC, Chitwood RA, Watanabe M, Yeckel MF, Sun LD, Kato A, Carr CA, Johnston D, Wilson MA, Tonegawa S (2002) Requirement for hippocampal CA3 NMDA receptors in associative memory recall. *Science* **297**:211–218.

Nakazawa K, Sun LD, Quirk MC, Rondi-Reig L, Wilson MA, Tonegawa S (2003) Hippocampal CA3 NMDA receptors are crucial for memory acquisition of one-time experience. *Neuron* **38**:305–315.Narvacan K, Treit S, Camicioli R, Martin W, Beaulieu C (2017) Evolution of deep gray matter volume across the human lifespan. *Hum Brain Mapp* **38**:3771–3790.

Newcombe NS, Drummey AB, Fox NA, Lie EH, Ottinger-Alberts W (2000) Remembering early childhood: how much, how, and why (or why not). *Curr Dir Psychol Sci* **9**:55–58.

Newcombe NS, Huttenlocher J, Bullock Drummey A, Wiley JG (1998) The development of spatial location coding: place learning and dead reckoning in the second and third years. *Cogn Dev* **13**:185–200.

Newcombe NS, Lloyd ME, Ratliff KR (2007) Development of episodic and autobiographical memory: a cognitive neuroscience perspective. *Adv Child Dev Behav* **35**:37–85.

Nguyen Ba-Charvet KT, Brose K, Marillat V, Kidd T, Goodman CS, Tessier-Lavigne M, Sotelo C, Chedotal A (1999) Slit2-mediated chemorepulsion and collapse of developing forebrain axons. *Neuron* **22**:463–473.

Nilssen ES, Doan TP, Nigro MJ, Ohara S, Witter MP (2019) Neurons and networks in the entorhinal cortex: a reappraisal of the lateral and medial entorhinal subdivisions mediating parallel cortical pathways. *Hippocampus* **29**:1238–1254.

Niu W, Zou Y, Shen C, Zhang CL (2011) Activation of postnatal neural stem cells requires nuclear receptor TLX. *J Neurosci* **31**:13816–13828.

Nowakowski RS, Rakic P (1981) The site of origin and route and rate of migration of neurons to the hippocampal region of the rhesus monkey. *J Comp Neurol* 196:126–154.

Oliet SH, Piet R, Poulain DA (2001) Control of glutamate clearance and synaptic efficacy by glial coverage of neurons. *Science* 292:923–926.

Olsen RK, Carr VA, Daugherty AM, et al. (2019) Progress update from the hippocampal subfields group. *Alzheimers Dement (Amst)* 11:439–449.

O'Mara SM, Commins S, Anderson M, Gigg J (2001) The subiculum: a review of form, physiology and function. *Prog Neurobiol* 64:129–155.

O'Reilly KC, Flatberg A, Islam S, Olsen LC, Kruge IU, Witter MP (2015) Identification of dorsal-ventral hippocampal differentiation in neonatal rats. *Brain Struct Funct* 220:2873–2893.

Osorio C, Chacon PJ, Kisiswa L, White M, Wyatt S, Rodriguez-Tebar A, Davies AM (2013) Growth differentiation factor 5 is a key physiological regulator of dendrite growth during development. *Development* 140:4751–4762.

Ostby Y, Tamnes CK, Fjell AM, Westlye LT, Due-Tonnessen P, Walhovd KB (2009) Heterogeneity in subcortical brain development: a structural magnetic resonance imaging study of brain maturation from 8 to 30 years. *J Neurosci* 29:11772–11782.

Ouchi Y, Banno Y, Shimizu Y, Ando S, Hasegawa H, Adachi K, Iwamoto T (2013) Reduced adult hippocampal neurogenesis and working memory deficits in the Dgcr8-deficient mouse model of 22q11.2 deletion-associated schizophrenia can be rescued by IGF2. *J Neurosci* 33:9408–9419.

Overman WH, Pate BJ, Moore K, Peuster A (1996) Ontogeny of place learning in children as measured in the radial arm maze, Morris search task, and open field task. *Behav Neurosci* 110:1205–1228.

Pascual M, Pozas E, Soriano E (2005) Role of class 3 semaphorins in the development and maturation of the septohippocampal pathway. *Hippocampus* 15:184–202.

Payne C, Machado CJ, Bliwise NG, Bachevalier J (2010) Maturation of the hippocampal formation and amygdala in Macaca mulatta: a volumetric magnetic resonance imaging study. *Hippocampus* 20:922–935.

Pederick DT, Lui JH, Gingrich EC, Xu C, Wagner MJ, Liu Y, He Z, Quake SR, Luo L (2021) Reciprocal repulsions instruct the precise assembly of parallel hippocampal networks. *Science* 372:1068–1073.

Pelkey KA, Chittajallu R, Craig MT, Tricoire L, Wester JC, McBain CJ (2017) Hippocampal GABAergic inhibitory interneurons. *Physiol Rev* 97:1619–1747.

Peng S, Zhang Y, Zhang J, Wang H, Ren B (2010) ERK in learning and memory: a review of recent research. *Int J Mol Sci* 11:222–232.

Pfluger T, Weil S, Weis S, Vollmar C, Heiss D, Egger J, Scheck R, Hahn K (1999) Normative volumetric data of the developing hippocampus in children based on magnetic resonance imaging. *Epilepsia* 40:414–423.

Pickard L, Noel J, Henley JM, Collingridge GL, Molnar E (2000) Developmental changes in synaptic AMPA and NMDA receptor distribution and AMPA receptor subunit composition in living hippocampal neurons. *J Neurosci* 20:7922–7931.

Piguet O, Chareyron LJ, Banta Lavenex P, Amaral DG, Lavenex P (2020) Postnatal development of the entorhinal cortex: a stereological study in macaque monkeys. *J Comp Neurol* 528:2308–2332.

Pleasure SJ, Anderson S, Hevner R, Bagri A, Marin O, Lowenstein DH, Rubenstein JL (2000) Cell migration from the ganglionic eminences is required for the development of hippocampal GABAergic interneurons. *Neuron* 28:727–740.

Pokorny J, Yamamoto T (1981) Postnatal ontogenesis of hippocampal CA1 area in rats: I. Development of dendritic arborisation in pyramidal neurons. *Brain Res Bull* 7:113–120.

Poppenk J, Evensmoen HR, Moscovitch M, Nadel L (2013) Long-axis specialization of the human hippocampus. *Trends Cogn Sci* 17:230–240.

Puram SV, Bonni A (2013) Cell-intrinsic drivers of dendrite morphogenesis. *Development* 140:4657–4671.

Rados M, Judas M, Kostovic I (2006) In vitro MRI of brain development. *Eur J Radiol* 57:187–198.

Rakic P, Nowakowski RS (1981) The time of origin of neurons in the hippocampal region of the rhesus monkey. *J Comp Neurol* 196:99–128.

Ramón y Cajal S (1911) Histologie du système nerveux de l'homme et des vertébrés. Paris: Maloine.

Reinhardt VP, Iosif AM, Libero L, Heath B, Rogers SJ, Ferrer E, Nordahl C, Ghetti S, Amaral D, Solomon M (2020) Understanding hippocampal development in young children with autism spectrum disorder. *J Am Acad Child Adolesc Psychiatry* 59:1069–1079.

Retzius G (1893) Die Cajalschen Zellen der Grosshirnrinde beim Menschen und bei Säugetieren. *Biol Unters* 5:1–9.

Retzius G (1894) Weitere Beiträge zur Kenntnis der Cajalschen Zellen der Grosshirnrinde des Menschen. *Biol Unters* 6:29–34.

Ribak CE, Seress L, Amaral DG (1985) The development, ultrastructure and synaptic connections of the mossy cells of the dentate gyrus. *J Neurocytol* 14:835–857.

Ribordy F, Jabes A, Banta Lavenex P, Lavenex P (2013) Development of allocentric spatial memory abilities in children from 18 months to 5 years of age. *Cogn Psychol* 66:1–29.

Ribordy Lambert F, Lavenex P, Banta Lavenex P (2015) Improvement of allocentric spatial memory resolution in children from 2 to 4 years of age. *Int J Behav Dev* 39:318–331.

Ribordy Lambert F, Lavenex P, Banta Lavenex P (2017) The "when" and the "where" of single-trial allocentric spatial memory performance in young children: insights into the development of episodic memory. *Dev Psychobiol* 59:185–196.

Rickmann M, Amaral DG, Cowan WM (1987) Organization of radial glial cells during the development of the rat dentate gyrus. *J Comp Neurol* 264:449–479.

Rieser JJ, Heiman ML (1982) Spatial self-reference systems and shortest-route behavior in toddlers. *Child Dev* 53:524–533.

Ritchey M, Libby LA, Ranganath C (2015) Cortico-hippocampal systems involved in memory and cognition: the PMAT framework. *Prog Brain Res* 219:45–64.

Rolls ET (2006) Neurophysiological and computational analyses of the primate presubiculum, subiculum and related areas. *Behav Brain Res* 174:289–303.

Rolls ET, Kesner RP (2006) A computational theory of hippocampal function, and empirical tests of the theory. *Prog Neurobiol* 79:1–48.

Rosso SB, Sussman D, Wynshaw-Boris A, Salinas PC (2005) Wnt signaling through Dishevelled, Rac and JNK regulates dendritic development. *Nat Neurosci* 8:34–42.

Rubin AN, Kessaris N (2013) PROX1: a lineage tracer for cortical interneurons originating in the lateral/caudal ganglionic eminence and preoptic area. *PLoS One* 8:e77339.

Rubio SE, Martinez A, Chauvet S, Mann F, Soriano E, Pascual M (2011) Semaphorin 3C is not required for the establishment and target specificity of the GABAergic septohippocampal pathway in vitro. *Eur J Neurosci* 34:1923–1933.

Sans N, Petralia RS, Wang YX, Blahos J, 2nd, Hell JW, Wenthold RJ (2000) A developmental change in NMDA receptor-associated proteins at hippocampal synapses. *J Neurosci* 20:1260–1271.

Sarkar A, Mei A, Paquola ACM, Stern S, Bardy C, Klug JR, Kim S, Neshat N, Kim HJ, Ku M, Shokhirev MN, Adamowicz DH, Marchetto MC, Jappelli R, Erwin JA, Padmanabhan K, Shtrahman M, Jin X, Gage FH (2018) Efficient generation of CA3 neurons from human pluripotent stem cells enables modeling of hippocampal connectivity in vitro. *Cell Stem Cell* 22:684–697 e689.

Sasaki T, Komatsu Y, Yamamori T (2020) Expression patterns of SLIT/ROBO mRNAs reveal a characteristic feature in the entorhinal-hippocampal area of macaque monkeys. *BMC Res Notes* 13:262.

Savelli F, Knierim JJ (2019) Origin and role of path integration in the cognitive representations of the hippocampus: computational insights into open questions. *J Exp Biol* 222.

Scanziani M, Salin PA, Vogt KE, Malenka RC, Nicoll RA (1997) Use-dependent increases in glutamate concentration activate pre-synaptic metabotropic glutamate receptors. *Nature* 385:630–634.

Schlessinger AR, Cowan WM, Gottlieb DI (1975) An autoradiographic study of the time of origin and the pattern of granule cell migration in the dentate gyrus of the rat. *J Comp Neurol* 159:149–175.

Schlessinger AR, Cowan WM, Swanson LW (1978) The time of origin of neurons in Ammon's horn and the associated retrohippocampal fields. *Anat Embryol (Berl)* 154:153–173.

Schumann CM, Hamstra J, Goodlin-Jones BL, Lotspeich LJ, Kwon H, Buonocore MH, Lammers CR, Reiss AL, Amaral DG (2004) The amygdala is enlarged in children but not adolescents with autism; the hippocampus is enlarged at all ages. *J Neurosci* 24:6392–6401.

Seress L (1992) Morphological variability and developmental aspects of monkey and human granule cells: differences between the rodent and primate dentate gyrus. *Epilepsy Res Suppl* 7:3–28.

Seress L (2001) Morphological changes of the human hippocampal formation from midgestation to early childhood. In: Handbook of Developmental Cognitive Neuroscience (Nelson CA, Luciana M, eds), pp 45–58. Cambridge, MA: MIT Press.

Seress L (2007) Comparative anatomy of the hippocampal dentate gyrus in adult and developing rodents, non-human primates and humans. *Prog Brain Res* 163:23–41.

Seress L, Abraham H, Tornoczky T, Kosztolanyi G (2001) Cell formation in the human hippocampal formation from mid-gestation to the late postnatal period. *Neuroscience* 105:831–843.

Seress L, Mrzljak L (1992) Postnatal development of mossy cells in the human dentate gyrus: a light microscopic Golgi study. *Hippocampus* 2:127–141.

Seress L, Ribak CE (1995a) Postnatal development of CA3 pyramidal neurons and their afferents in the Ammon's horn of rhesus monkeys. *Hippocampus* 5:217–231.

Seress L, Ribak CE (1995b) Postnatal development and synaptic connections of hilar mossy cells in the hippocampal dentate gyrus of rhesus monkeys. *J Comp Neurol* 355:93–110.

Sharp PE (1999) Complimentary roles for hippocampal versus subicular/entorhinal place cells in coding place, context, and events. *Hippocampus* 9:432–443.

Shu T, Butz KG, Plachez C, Gronostajski RM, Richards LJ (2003) Abnormal development of forebrain midline glia and commissural projections in Nfia knock-out mice. *J Neurosci* 23:203–212.

Silk J, Short J, Roberts J, Kusnitz J (1993) Gestation length in Rhesus macaques (*Macaca-mulatta*). *Int J Primatol* 14:95–104.

Šimić G, Krsnik Ž, Knezović V, Kelović Z, Mathiasen ML, Junaković A, Radoš M, Mulc D, Španić E, Quattrocolo G, Hall VJ, Zaborszky L, Vukšić M, Olucha Bordonau F, Kostović I, Witter MP, Hof PR (2022) Prenatal development of the human entorhinal cortex. *J Comp Neurol* 530:2711–2748.

Sluzenski J, Newcombe NS, Satlow E (2004) Knowing where things are in the second year of life: implications for hippocampal development. *J Cogn Neurosci* 16:1443–1451.

Snyder JS (2019) Recalibrating the relevance of adult neurogenesis. *Trends Neurosci* 42:164–178.

Somogyi P, Klausberger T (2005) Defined types of cortical interneurone structure space and spike timing in the hippocampus. *J Physiol* 562:9–26.

Soriano E, Del Rio JA (2005) The cells of Cajal-Retzius: still a mystery one century after. *Neuron* 46:389–394.

Sorrells SF, Paredes MF, Cebrian-Silla A, Sandoval K, Qi D, Kelley KW, James D, Mayer S, Chang J, Auguste KI, Chang EF, Gutierrez AJ, Kriegstein AR, Mathern GW, Oldham MC, Huang EJ, Garcia-Verdugo JM, Yang Z, Alvarez-Buylla A (2018) Human hippocampal neurogenesis drops sharply in children to undetectable levels in adults. *Nature*. 2018 Mar 15;555(7696):377–381.

Spalding KL, Bergmann O, Alkass K, Bernard S, Salehpour M, Huttner HB, Bostrom E, Westerlund I, Vial C, Buchholz BA, Possnert G, Mash DC, Druid H, Frisen J (2013) Dynamics of hippocampal neurogenesis in adult humans. *Cell* 153:1219–1227.

Stanton PK, Sarvey JM (1984) Blockade of long-term potentiation in rat hippocampal CA1 region by inhibitors of protein synthesis. *J Neurosci* 4:3080–3088.

Stein E, Savaskan NE, Ninnemann O, Nitsch R, Zhou R, Skutella T (1999) A role for the Eph ligand ephrin-A3 in entorhino-hippocampal axon targeting. *J Neurosci* 19:8885–8893.

Steup A, Lohrum M, Hamscho N, Savaskan NE, Ninnemann O, Nitsch R, Fujisawa H, Puschel AW, Skutella T (2000) Sema3C and netrin-1 differentially affect axon growth in the hippocampal formation. *Mol Cell Neurosci* 15:141–155.

Steward O, Falk PM (1986) Protein-synthetic machinery at postsynaptic sites during synaptogenesis: a quantitative study of the association between polyribosomes and developing synapses. *J Neurosci* 6:412–423.

Sudhof TC (2018) Towards an understanding of synapse formation. *Neuron* 100:276–293.

Sukow MA, Danneman P, Brayton C (2001) The Laboratory Mouse. Boca Raton: CRC Press.

Super H, Soriano E (1994) The organization of the embryonic and early postnatal murine hippocampus: II. Development of entorhinal, commissural, and septal connections studied with the lipophilic tracer DiI. *J Comp Neurol* 344:101–120.

Super H, Soriano E, Uylings HB (1998a) The functions of the preplate in development and evolution of the neocortex and hippocampus. *Brain Res Brain Res Rev* 27:40–64.

Super H, Martinez A, Del Rio JA, Soriano E (1998b) Involvement of distinct pioneer neurons in the formation of layer-specific connections in the hippocampus. *J Neurosci* 18:4616–4626.

Szulwach KE, Li X, Smrt RD, Li Y, Luo Y, Lin L, Santistevan NJ, Li W, Zhao X, Jin P (2010) Cross talk between microRNA and epigenetic regulation in adult neurogenesis. *J Cell Biol* 189:127–141.

Tanaka K, Watase K, Manabe T, Yamada K, Watanabe M, Takahashi K, Iwama H, Nishikawa T, Ichihara N, Kikuchi T, Okuyama S, Kawashima N, Hori S, Takimoto M, Wada K (1997) Epilepsy and exacerbation of brain injury in mice lacking the glutamate transporter GLT-1. *Science* 276:1699–1702.

Taube JS (2007) The head direction signal: origins and sensory-motor integration. *Annu Rev Neurosci* 30:181–207.

Tawarayama H, Yoshida Y, Suto F, Mitchell KJ, Fujisawa H (2010) Roles of semaphorin-6B and plexin-A2 in lamina-restricted projection of hippocampal mossy fibers. *J Neurosci* 30:7049–7060.

Thompson CL, Pathak SD, Jeromin A, Ng LL, MacPherson CR, Mortrud MT, Cusick A, Riley ZL, Sunkin SM, Bernard A, Puchalski RB, Gage FH, Jones AR, Bajic VB, Hawrylycz MJ, Lein ES (2008) Genomic anatomy of the hippocampus. *Neuron* 60:1010–1021.

Tole S, Christian C, Grove EA (1997) Early specification and autonomous development of cortical fields in the mouse hippocampus. *Development* 124:4959–4970.

Travaglia A, Bisaz R, Cruz E, Alberini CM (2016a) Developmental changes in plasticity, synaptic, glia and connectivity protein levels in rat dorsal hippocampus. *Neurobiol Learn Mem* 135:125–138.

Travaglia A, Bisaz R, Sweet ES, Blitzer RD, Alberini CM (2016b) Infantile amnesia reflects a developmental critical period for hippocampal learning. *Nat Neurosci* 19:1225–1233.

Tricoire L, Pelkey KA, Erkkila BE, Jeffries BW, Yuan X, McBain CJ (2011) A blueprint for the spatiotemporal origins of mouse hippocampal interneuron diversity. *J Neurosci* 31:10948–10970.

Tsamis KI, Lagartos Donato MJ, Dahl AG, O'Reilly KC, Witter MP (2020) Development and topographic organization of subicular projections to lateral septum in the rat brain. *Eur J Neurosci* 52(4):3140–3159. doi:10.1111/ejn.14696. Epub 2020 Feb 23.

Tsao A, Sugar J, Lu L, Wang C, Knierim JJ, Moser MB, Moser EI (2018) Integrating time from experience in the lateral entorhinal cortex. *Nature* 561:57–62.

Uematsu A, Matsui M, Tanaka C, Takahashi T, Noguchi K, Suzuki M, Nishijo H (2012) Developmental trajectories of amygdala and hippocampus from infancy to early adulthood in healthy individuals. *PLoS One* 7:e46970.

Urban N, Guillemot F (2014) Neurogenesis in the embryonic and adult brain: same regulators, different roles. *Front Cell Neurosci* 8:396.

Urban N, Blomfield IM, Guillemot F (2019) Quiescence of adult mammalian neural stem cells: A highly regulated rest. *Neuron* 104:834–848.

Valnegri P, Puram SV, Bonni A (2015) Regulation of dendrite morphogenesis by extrinsic cues. *Trends Neurosci* 38:439–447.

Weisz VI, Argibay PF (2009) A putative role for neurogenesis in neuro-computational terms: inferences from a hippocampal model. *Cognition* 112:229–240.

Wenzel J, Stender G, Duwe G (1981) [Development of neuron structure of the fascia dentata in the rat: neurohistologico-morphometric, ultrastructural and experimental study]. *J Hirnforsch* 22:629–683.

Williams ME, Wilke SA, Daggett A, Davis E, Otto S, Ravi D, Ripley B, Bushong EA, Ellisman MH, Klein G, Ghosh A (2011) Cadherin-9 regulates synapse-specific differentiation in the developing hippocampus. *Neuron* 71:640–655.

Wills TJ, Cacucci F, Burgess N, O'Keefe J (2010) Development of the hippocampal cognitive map in preweanling rats. *Science* 328:1573–1576.

Witter MP, Amaral DG (1991) Entorhinal cortex of the monkey: V. Projections to the dentate gyrus, hippocampus, and subicular complex. *J Comp Neurol* 307:437–459.

World Health Organization (2020) Life expectancy and healthy life expectancy. Data by WHO region. Retrieved at http://apps.who.int/gho/data/view.main.SDG2016LEXREGv?lang=en

Yu DX, Di Giorgio FP, Yao J, Marchetto MC, Brennand K, Wright R, Mei A, McHenry L, Lisuk D, Grasmick JM, Silberman P, Silberman G, Jappelli R, Gage FH (2014) Modeling hippocampal neurogenesis using human pluripotent stem cells. *Stem Cell Rep* 2:295–310.

Zeisel A, Munoz-Manchado AB, Codeluppi S, Lonnerberg P, La Manno G, Jureus A, Marques S, Munguba H, He L, Betsholtz C, Rolny C, Castelo-Branco G, Hjerling-Leffler J, Linnarsson S (2015) Brain structure: cell types in the mouse cortex and hippocampus revealed by single-cell RNA-seq. *Science* 347:1138–1142.

Zhang R, Boareto M, Engler A, Louvi A, Giachino C, Iber D, Taylor V (2019) Id4 downstream of Notch2 maintains neural stem cell quiescence in the adult hippocampus. *Cell Rep* 28:1485–1498 e1486.

Zhao S, Forster E, Chai X, Frotscher M (2003) Different signals control laminar specificity of commissural and entorhinal fibers to the dentate gyrus. *J Neurosci* 23:7351–7357.

Zhong S, Ding W, Sun L, Lu Y, Dong H, Fan X, Liu Z, Chen R, Zhang S, Ma Q, Tang F, Wu Q, Wang X (2020) Decoding the development of the human hippocampus. *Nature* 577:531–536.

Zhou Y, Bond AM, Shade JE, Zhu Y, Davis CO, Wang X, Su Y, Yoon KJ, Phan AT, Chen WJ, Oh JH, Marsh-Armstrong N, Atabai K, Ming GL, Song H (2018) Autocrine Mfge8 signaling prevents developmental exhaustion of the adult neural stem cell pool. *Cell Stem Cell* 23:444–452 e444.

5

Structural and Functional Properties of Hippocampal Neurons

Nelson Spruston, Rebecca Piskorowski, Vivien Chevaleyre, Mark D. Eyre, Chris J. McBain, and Marlene Bartos

5.1 Introduction

As detailed in Chapter 3, the hippocampus is extensively integrated with many brain regions. Its bidirectional interactions with sensory and motor areas suggest that it plays a key role of turning sensation into action. The hippocampus is not unique in this regard, but numerous studies in humans and other mammals suggest that it is essential for allowing animals to learn from experience to build models of the world that critically shape the sensorimotor transformation.

In this chapter, we explore the complex menagerie of excitatory and inhibitory neurons in the hippocampal formation. Ultimately, neural computations are performed by circuits, but these computations are shaped by the types of neurons they contain and their properties. For these reasons, we consider the properties of neurons throughout the hippocampal formation in the context of their local circuitry as well as inputs and outputs from other brain regions.

As most of what is known about the cellular properties of hippocampal neurons derives from studies in rodents, we focus this chapter on the hippocampal formation of the rat and mouse. Throughout the chapter, we do not always identify the species used in each study. Rather, we focus on concepts that are likely to apply in both rats and mice, as well as other mammalian species, including humans and other primates.

5.2 Circuitry

One way to conceptualize hippocampal circuitry is through its interactions with other cortical structures. The hippocampus is part of the telencephalon, a thick sheet of tissue that enwraps, but does not fully surround, other structures such as ventricles, fiber tracts, and the diencephalon. The hippocampal formation comprises a bulge at the caudal part of the cortical sheet. The major telencephalic input to the hippocampus is from the entorhinal cortex (EC) and the major telencephalic outputs are via CA1 and subiculum (SUB) "back" to EC and "forward" to retrosplenial cortex (RSC), prefrontal cortex (PFC), perirhinal cortex (PeRC), postrhinal cortex (PoRC), and

the amygdalar cortex (AMC) (Figure 5.1). Each of these structures has interactions with other sensory and motor areas. For example, RSC lies adjacent to visual cortex (lateral to RSC), anterior cingulate cortex, and somatomotor cortex (medial to RSC).

The telencephalic view is limited, however, because the hippocampus also has numerous bidirectional connections with diencephalic structures (Figure 5.1B–D). Considered together, the hippocampus appears to act as a hub that takes inputs from throughout the brain, processes them in a circuit shaped by previous experience, and feeds back to many other brain areas, some of which also provide input to the hippocampus, and others that do not.

The core of the hippocampus is often described as a feedforward *trisynaptic circuit* (Figure 5.1B). Although this is of historical significance, it is important to bear in mind that each component of the trisynaptic circuit—dentate gyrus (DG), CA3, and CA1—has many additional inputs and outputs (see also Chapter 3). For example, the trisynaptic concept ignores the important roles of hippocampal structures such as CA2 and subiculum, diminishes the critical role of CA3 recurrent (feedback) connections, and obscures the importance of the long-range recurrent circuit formed by the hippocampus and EC (Figure 5.1B). In this chapter, we comprehensively review the cellular composition of all areas of the hippocampal formation, including the DG, CA3, CA2, CA1, subiculum, presubiculum, parasubiculum, and EC (Figure 5.1C).

5.3 History

The silver-staining method developed by Camillo Golgi in the late 19th century allowed for the first detailed visualization of neuronal morphology. These images revealed the intricate branching patterns of dendrites, indicating that understanding the function of neurons would require understanding the purpose of these branches. Santiago Ramón y Cajal extensively utilized Golgi's method in the early 20th century, making significant contributions by carefully documenting the diversity of neuronal structure in various brain regions and species.

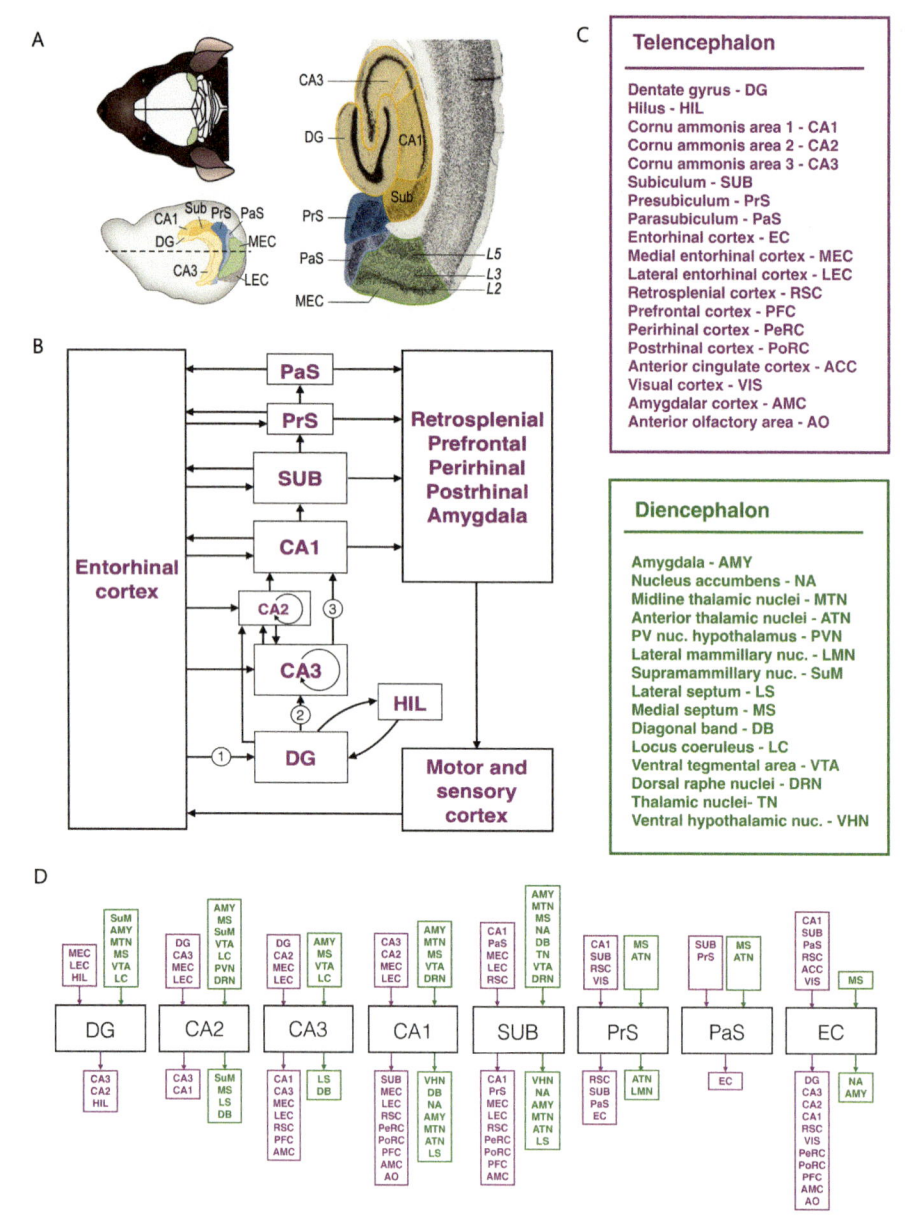

Figure 5.1 Anatomical overview of the hippocampal formation and its connections. (A) Left: cartoon of the position of the hippocampal formation (top, green; bottom, various colors) in the mouse brain. Right: histological horizontal section of the mouse brain illustrating different hippocampal regions considered in this chapter. (B) Diagram telencephalic hippocampal circuitry. (C) Lists of brain regions with direct hippocampal connections: telencephalon (purple), diencephalon (green). (D) Inputs (top) and outputs (bottom) of all hippocampal areas. (Source: (A) Tukker et al., 2022.)

The study of neuronal function began in the 1940s using sharp microelectrodes in live animals, brain slices, and dissociated neurons in culture. In the 1960s, some researchers deviated from the traditional method of recording from cell bodies and attempted to record directly from dendrites. The electrophysiological studies of this era revealed that functional diversity mirrored the structural diversity of neurons and their dendritic morphologies.

Beginning in the 1970s, the advent of the patch-clamp recording technique revolutionized detailed electrophysiological studies of neurons. It revealed that neurons contain diverse ion channels and receptors, activated by neurotransmitters and transmembrane potential, which can be modulated by physiological factors such as neuromodulators. In the early 1990s, patch-clamp electrodes were

placed directly on dendrites, resulting in unique electrophysiological signatures. Concurrently, the use of calcium-sensitive fluorophores allowed for assessment of neuronal function with subcellular precision. Overall, it became clear that the functional diversity of neurons is a result of a combination of structural and molecular diversity.

In the 21st century, advances in technology have further expanded our understanding of neuronal complexity and diversity. RNA-sequencing methods (RNA-seq) have provided an in-depth view of gene expression in different types of neurons, revealing diverse molecular fingerprints across the brain. Additionally, high-resolution, whole-brain imaging techniques have allowed for visualization and analysis of axon morphologies, even in neurons with extensive branching and long axon projections. These and other new methods continue to reveal a complex and diverse landscape of neuronal structure and function.

The hippocampus has been a central focus in cellular neuroscience, serving as a microcosm for important discoveries and lessons. Many major concepts in the field have been discovered first (or early) in the hippocampus. This chapter provides an overview of the conceptual advances in cellular neuroscience that stem from studies of neurons in the hippocampal formation. The work is organized by first examining the excitatory neurons in the major hippocampal subfields, followed by a focus on inhibitory interneurons. Rather than providing a comprehensive review of the thousands of papers in the field, the goal is to provide an overview of key advances and principles, while including enough background and references to allow readers to delve deeper into specific areas of interest. Due to the vastness of the literature, the chapter relies heavily on citations of review articles and pointers to other chapters in this book. Additionally, readers are encouraged to consult the chapter in the first edition, as it contains additional information and references not included in the new version. The literature has expanded significantly since the first edition was published, necessitating a complete rewrite of this chapter.

5.4 Cell types

Throughout this chapter, the concept of "cell types" is prevalent and important. On the surface, this may seem simple; for example, the differences between the principle (excitatory) neurons in the different hippocampal subfields (e.g., CA1, CA2, CA3, DG) reflect the existence of different principal cell types. It is apparent, however, that even within these subfields there is considerable diversity. At the simplest level, there are differences between excitatory neurons, inhibitory interneurons, and modulatory neurons. Within each of these broad classes, there are also differences not only between neurons found in different regions but also within the population residing in any given region. With the advent of high-dimensional analysis of gene expression, it has become clear that the number of ways to subdivide cell types may be limitless.

Arguably, there is no absolute answer to the question, "How many cell types are there?" We argue, therefore, that we must identify cell types pragmatically, based on a combination of data modalities, including gene expression, soma location, dendritic morphology, and axonal projections. This kind of multimodal, high-dimensional analysis of large populations of neurons has led to improvements in our understanding of the diversity of the complex structure and function of hippocampal neurons, offering conceptual insights that will likely apply to other areas of the brain.

As these pragmatic divisions of cells into groups emerge, it will be important to understand how their unique cellular and synaptic properties, as well as integration into circuits, enable computations that could not be performed by networks of neurons with simpler, more uniform properties. This endeavor is still in its infancy, but one that will ultimately be needed if we are to understand circuit function not only in terms of artificial neural networks but also from a biological perspective. For now, however, the field has mainly focused on the properties of neurons and synapses, which is the primary focus of this chapter.

5.5 CA1 pyramidal neurons

The pyramidal neurons in the CA1 region of the hippocampus are among the most extensively studied and well-understood neurons in the brain. This is due to a combination of interest in the hippocampus, which plays a critical role in explicit memory, and the accessibility of these neurons, which are organized in a tightly packed layer of cell bodies (stratum pyramidale) that is easily identifiable in histological analysis of the mammalian brain. Due to the large amount of knowledge about CA1 pyramidal neurons, this chapter begins by discussing the principles derived from hundreds of studies over the course of more than a century.

5.5.1 Dendritic morphology is stereotypical but variable

Pyramidal neurons, which are abundant in both archicortex and neocortex, are named for the triangular shape of the soma (Ramón y Cajal, 1995). Multiple primary branches emanate from the base of the triangle—the basal dendrites—and a larger primary dendrite emanates from the apex of the triangle—the apical dendrite. Each of these primary dendrites branches extensively, with almost all branches studded with dendritic spines, which are the sites of contact for most excitatory synaptic inputs.

CA1 dendritic trees have a stereotypical structure, with considerable variation on this theme (Figure 5.2). In some cells, the primary apical dendrite forms a major branch point hundreds of microns from the soma, at the boundary of stratum radiatum and stratum lacunosum-moleculare; in other cells, the primary apical dendrite branches closer to the soma, forming twin apical dendrites, each of which forms another branch at the border of stratum radiatum and stratum lacunosum-moleculare (Bannister and Larkman, 1995; Jarsky et al., 2008; Pyapali et al., 1998). Branches contained within stratum lacunosum-moleculare form the so-called apical tuft dendrites. Within stratum radiatum, dozens of smaller-diameter branches emanate from the primary apical dendrites, the so-called oblique dendrites. Within stratum oriens, basal dendrites usually consist of 2–5 primary dendrites, each of which branches extensively to form a structure that looks like the roots of a tree.

Systematic variation in the dendritic structure of CA1 pyramidal neurons has been observed along the major physical axes of the hippocampus. For example, CA1 neurons located more laterally (i.e., closer to CA3) contain more basal dendrites and fewer apical tuft dendrites, while those located more medially (i.e., closer to subiculum) contain more apical tuft dendrites and fewer basal dendrites (Graves et al., 2012). Similarly, CA1 pyramidal neurons in the dorsal hippocampus have more branches than their counterparts in the ventral hippocampus (Dougherty et al., 2012) and pyramidal cells in deep layers have larger basal dendritic trees than cells in superficial layers (SH Lee et al., 2014).

An important theme of this chapter is the relationship between structure and function. Synaptic inputs arriving onto different dendritic domains can differentially influence action potential firing. These differences may be exploited for the purpose of dendritic computation or compensated in the service of dendritic democracy (Häusser and Mel, 2003; London and Häusser, 2005; Spruston, 2008). A host of studies on CA1 pyramidal neurons have addressed this theme and are considered below.

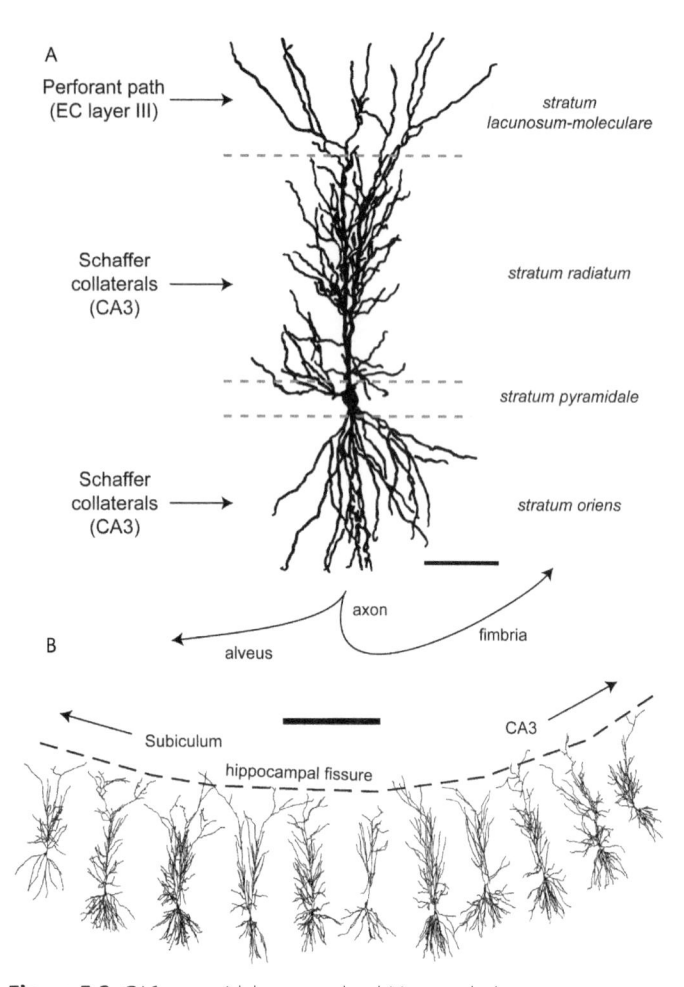

Figure 5.2 CA1 pyramidal neuron dendritic morphology.
(A) Camera lucida drawing of a CA1 pyramidal neuron, depicting major sources of excitatory input (left) and layers of hippocampal area CA1 (right). Scale bar = 100 μm. (B) Drawings of several CA1 pyramidal neurons illustrating structural diversity. Scale bar = 500 μm. (Sources: (A) Bannister and Larkman, 1995; (B) Pyapali et al., 1998.)

5.5.2 Myriad factors influence action potential firing in vivo

Intracellular recordings in awake rodents have provided insight into the mechanisms responsible for action potential firing in CA1 pyramidal neurons. These experiments have been conducted in freely running rats or in head-fixed mice running on a linear treadmill with cues along the track or on a spherical treadmill coupled to a virtual reality environment. Recordings have been obtained with either sharp microelectrodes or patch-clamp electrodes in the whole-cell configuration (A Lee and Brecht, 2018; Schmidt-Hieber and Nolan, 2017).

5.5.2.1 Spatially tuned firing in running animals

When animals are running, CA1 pyramidal neurons exhibit spatially modulated firing at a location referred to as the place field of the neuron (Figure 5.3A). Typically, a depolarizing "ramp" drives several action potentials as an animal traverses a few tens of centimeters of its environment in a few seconds (Epsztein et al., 2011; Harvey et al., 2009; D Lee et al., 2012). This depolarizing ramp has an amplitude of ~10–15 mV, taking the membrane potential (V_m) from the resting potential (V_{rest}, about -55 to -65 mV) to above the firing threshold (around -45 to -50 mV). This depolarization is accompanied by an increase in the theta oscillation

(~4–12 Hz), which is prominent in running animals (Harvey et al., 2009; Whishaw and Vanderwolf, 1973). Occasionally, CA1 pyramidal neurons in running animals undergo large depolarizations that elicit high-frequency firing followed by a period of depolarization-induced refractoriness to spiking (Bittner et al., 2015; Epsztein et al., 2011; D Lee et al., 2012). These so-called plateau potentials, which can last for hundreds of milliseconds, are mediated by activation of voltage-gated calcium (Ca_v) channels in dendrites and are powerful mediators of synaptic plasticity (Golding et al., 1999, 2002; Remy and Spruston, 2007; Takahashi and Magee, 2009; Wong and Prince, 1978). In vivo, even a single plateau potential can result in plasticity so powerful that it produces a new place field in a neuron (Figure 5.3B) (Bittner et al., 2015, 2017).

In running animals, action potential firing in CA1 pyramidal neurons is thought to reflect a code of the animal's environment in the context of behavioral task demands, thus positioning it to participate in the storage and retrieval of episodic memories and their behavioral manifestations (Eichenbaum, 2017; O'Keefe and Krupic, 2021; Ranganath, 2019). Recently, the long-standing question of the behavioral *consequences* of CA1 pyramidal neuron firing was addressed in two studies. The first showed that stimulation of neurons coding for the rewarded location on a linear track caused licking, even when stimulation occurred at other locations (Robinson et al., 2020). The second showed that SWRs were associated with a decrease in blood glucose, indicating a role for hippocampal activity in regulating body-wide metabolic functions (Tingley et al., 2021). These two studies undoubtedly signal a new era of research into the functional outcomes of hippocampal activity.

5.5.2.2 Sharp wave ripples in quiescent animals

In quiescent animals, the local field potential (LFP) alternates between seconds-long periods of large- and small-amplitude irregular activity (LIA and SIA), reflecting cortical up- and down-states. These states correspond to low arousal, pupil constriction, and depolarized V_m (during LIA) and moderate arousal, pupil microdilation, and hyperpolarized V_m (during SIA) (Hulse et al., 2017; Kajikawa et al., 2021). During LIA, CA1 pyramidal neurons occasionally fire action potentials during sharp wave ripple (SWR) events (Csicsvari et al., 2000; Hulse et al., 2016; Valero et al., 2017). These spikes are driven by depolarizations that are smaller (<10 mV) and briefer (~50–100 ms) than those observed in running animals. SWR depolarizations are accompanied by a high-frequency ripple oscillation (~120–200 Hz) at the peak of the depolarization (English et al., 2014; Gan et al., 2017; Hulse et al., 2016; Valero et al., 2015). Many CA1 cells depolarize in this manner during SWRs, but in most cases the depolarization remains below the firing threshold, resulting in sparse firing during SWRs (Figure 5.3B) (Csicsvari et al., 2000; Hulse et al., 2016; Kajikawa et al., 2022).

5.5.2.3 Multiple sources of excitatory synaptic input

What synaptic inputs are responsible for the membrane potential dynamics that drive firing in different behavioral states? Excitatory synaptic inputs to CA1 pyramidal neurons arise primarily from two sources: CA3 via the Schaffer collateral (SC) axons from CA3 and layer III of the EC via the perforant path (PP) and temporoammonic alvear (TA) pathways from layer III of the EC (Figure 5.2). The SC axons provide most of the excitatory synaptic inputs to CA1. These synapses number in the thousands for each neuron and are located on dendritic spines in basal dendrites in stratum oriens and apical

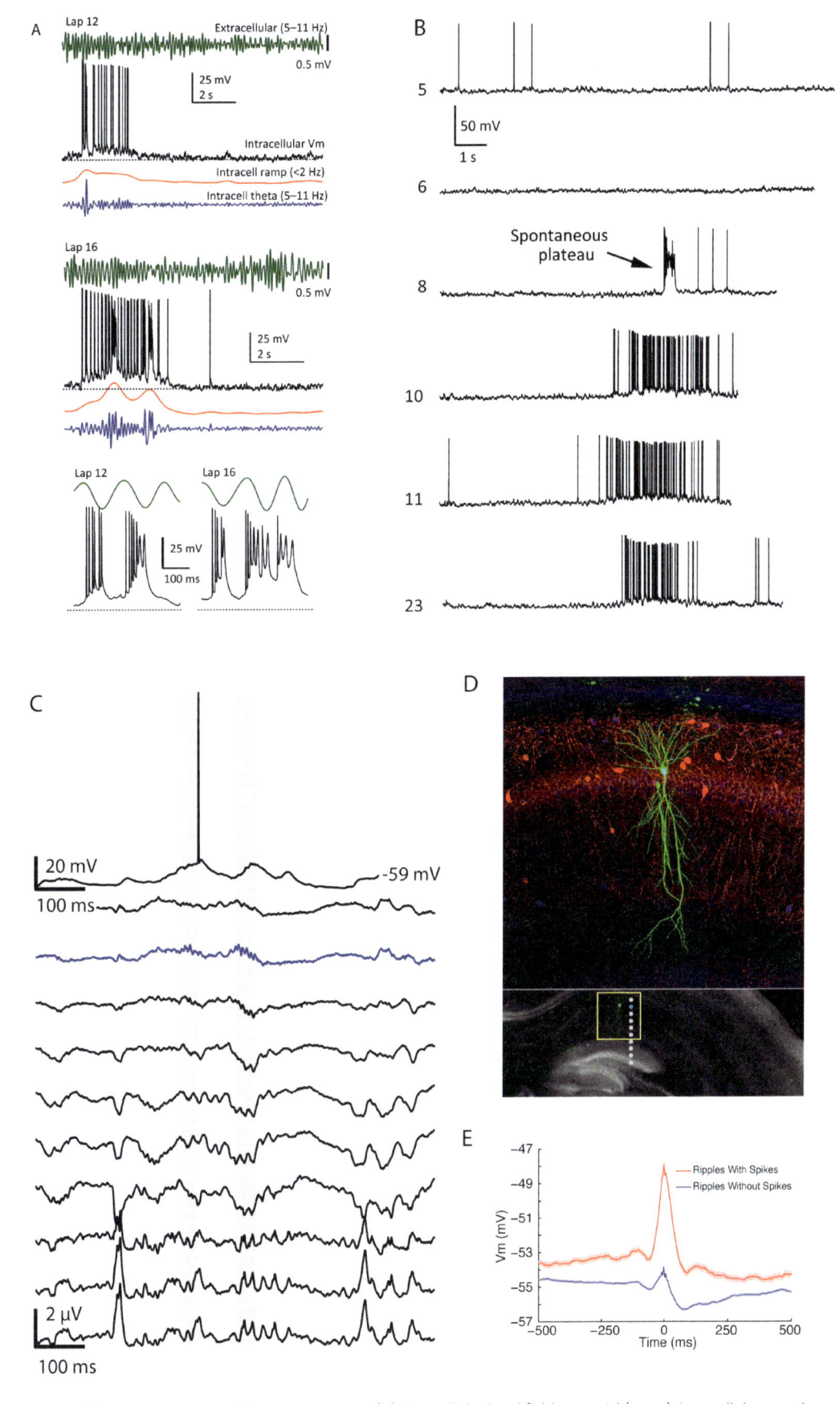

Figure 5.3 Action potential firing in CA1 pyramidal neurons in vivo. (A) Extracellular local field potential (green), intracellular membrane potential (V$_m$, black), and filtered intracellular V$_m$ (red and blue) of a CA1 pyramidal cell in a mouse running on a treadmill. Recordings are shown for two full laps (top, middle) and expanded portions of each (bottom). (B) Intracellular V$_m$ for six laps. The cell fired infrequently until a plateau potential occurred spontaneously on lap 8. The cell fired when the mouse was at the same position on the track on subsequent laps. (C) Intracellular V$_m$ recording from a CA1 pyramidal neuron (top trace) and extracellular local field potential recordings (other traces during LIA in an awake, untethered, but immobile mouse. Two ripples are apparent in the blue trace (highlighted by shading). Action potential firing occurs during the first ripple, but not the second. (D) Reconstructed CA1 pyramidal neuron following intracellular recording. Dots indicate the approximate location of LFP recordings in C. (E) Averaged intracellular V$_m$ during ripples for events with and without action potentials. (Source: (A, B) Bittner et al., 2015; (C, D) Kajikawa et al., 2022; (E) Hulse et al., 2016.)

dendrites in stratum radiatum (Bloss et al., 2016; Megías et al., 2001; Nicholson et al., 2006). PP/TA excitatory inputs from EC are fewer in number and are predominantly restricted to dendrites and spines of the apical tuft, in stratum lacunosum-moleculare. They can also depolarize CA1 neurons and contribute to their firing (Bloss et al., 2018; Jarsky et al., 2005; Milstein et al., 2015; Takahashi and Magee, 2009; Yeckel and Berger, 1995) but their depolarizing influence is considerably weaker than that of SC synapses. CA1 neurons also receive excitatory inputs from CA2 (see section later in this chapter), the midline thalamus (nucleus reuniens), and the central amygdala (Herkenham, 1978; Kemppainen et al., 2002; Krettek and Price, 1977; Pikkarainen et al., 1999; Weel and Witter, 1996; Weel et al., 1997).

The functional effects of excitatory synapses onto CA1 pyramidal neurons have primarily been determined by studying the SC and PP/TA inputs. Both exhibit short-term facilitation in response to pairs of presynaptic action potentials. Sustained firing of these inputs produces steady synaptic responses at ~1–10 Hz, but short-term depression at higher frequencies (Koutsoumpa and Papatheodoropoulos, 2021; Otmakhov et al., 1993).

5.5.2.4 Effects of inhibition on CA1 pyramidal neuron activity in vivo

Inhibition also shapes the CA1 response to circuit activation. Numerous types of inhibitory interneurons provide feedforward and feedback inhibition as well as disinhibition. How these excitatory and inhibitory inputs are coordinated to drive action potential firing depends on the behavioral state of the animal, which correlates closely with the activity of a variety of neuromodulatory inputs to the hippocampus. This topic is covered more extensively later in this chapter, with a focus on the key role of cholinergic input from the medial septum.

5.5.2.5 Integration of multiple synaptic inputs during different behavioral states

In running animals, many CA3 neurons are active, resulting in large and long-lasting depolarization of CA1 neurons as the animal runs through a neuron's place field (Mizuseki et al., 2012; X Zhao et al., 2020). During these events, the overall firing rate of CA1 neurons is also influenced by concurrent inhibition, which is strong but not spatially tuned (Grienberger et al., 2017). The contribution of PP/TA inputs during this form of firing is unclear. However, these excitatory inputs from EC provide important contributions to the generation of plateau potentials in vivo (Bittner et al., 2015), which likely occur in response to combined input from CA3 and EC, together with some disinhibition (Jarsky et al., 2005; Milstein et al., 2015; Soltesz, 1995; Takahashi and Magee, 2009).

In quiescent animals, firing in CA3 neurons is sparser and burst firing in a small population of CA3 neurons is believed to underlie the depolarization of CA1 neurons associated with SWRs (Csicsvari et al., 2000). An alternative model posits that some action potentials during SWRs may arise from firing in CA1 neurons connected via axonal gap junctions (Draguhn et al., 1998; Schmitz et al., 2001; Traub et al., 2012), resulting in high-frequency excitation phase locked to the ripple (Maier et al., 2011). In support of this model, one study observed spikelets associated with SWRs in vivo (Epsztein et al., 2010) and in slices, spontaneously occurring SWRs can occur in concert with spikes at membrane potentials well below the usual spike threshold (Bahner et al., 2011). However, spikes during SWRs in vivo usually (but not always) occur during membrane potential depolarization, reflecting brief excitation combined with strong inhibition, including phase-locked inhibition driving the ripple at the peak of the SWR, as well as longer-lasting inhibition that produces a post-SWR hyperpolarization (Buzsaki et al., 1992; English et al., 2014; Gan et al., 2017; Hulse et al., 2016; Kajikawa et al., 2022; Klausberger et al., 2003; Valero et al., 2015; Ylinen et al., 1995).

5.5.2.6 Variability of action potential firing in vivo

The firing properties of CA1 pyramidal neurons are variable. Many cells are silent (Thompson and Best, 1989), particularly in small environments, whereas in larger environments, some cells have only a single place field, and others have two or more place fields (Fenton et al., 2008; Rich et al., 2014). These differences may reflect a combination of discrete and continuous differences in gene expression (as described later in this chapter) and/or differences in modulatory state that affect excitability. In keeping with the latter view, depolarizing a cell by just a few millivolts via a small current injected through a patch-clamp electrode can convert a silent cell to a firing cell with distinct spatial modulation, i.e., a place cell (D Lee et al., 2012). This depolarization-mediated firing is not simply attributable to moving the membrane potential closer to firing threshold; rather, depolarization amplifies spatially modulated synaptic inputs via a mechanism involving persistently active voltage-gated sodium (Na_v) channels (C Hsu et al., 2018). Thus, even small effects on membrane potential can have a significant effect on action potential firing.

5.5.2.7 Spatial firing properties and synaptic plasticity

Multiple plasticity mechanisms may contribute to action potential firing in CA1 pyramidal neurons in vivo. In animals exploring novel environments, firing fields can appear suddenly (Cohen et al., 2017; Frank et al., 2004; Hill, 1978; Leutgeb et al., 2004; Sheffield et al., 2017; Wilson and McNaughton, 1993), suggesting that plasticity mechanisms that do not require action potential firing (Dudman et al., 2007; Golding et al., 2002; Remy and Spruston, 2007) may contribute to the appearance of some firing fields in novel environments. Plateau potentials can rapidly induce firing fields in cells that were previously silent via a novel form of synaptic potentiation that has a seconds-long timing window and does not require extensive repetition (Figure 5.3A) (Bittner et al., 2015, 2017). These induced firing fields can be simple place cells or cells with more complex dependencies on position and context, such as behavioral trajectory (X Zhao et al., 2022; X Zhao et al., 2020). In addition, a robust form of synaptic plasticity occurs in CA1 pyramidal neurons even in the absence of action potential firing (Golding et al., 2002; Hardie and Spruston, 2009; Remy and Spruston, 2007). This may explain the delayed appearance of some new place cells after an animal is placed in a novel environment (Sheffield and Dombeck, 2019). Not all place-cell firing requires synaptic plasticity, however, as most firing fields are apparent immediately in novel environments (Frank et al., 2004; Hill, 1978; Leutgeb et al., 2004; Wilson and McNaughton, 1993). Nevertheless, synaptic plasticity may alter the hippocampal map by creating new firing fields and modifying others. Consistent with this, NMDA receptors (GluNs) are not required for the formation of firing fields (Kentros et al., 1998; McHugh et al., 1996) but they are required for firing-field stability (Kentros et al., 1998). In addition, synaptic plasticity can result in changes in the rate and timing of action potentials, as well as the underlying synaptic input, as an animal traverses a place field multiple times (Cohen et al., 2017; Dong et al., 2021; Mehta, 2015; Sheffield and Dombeck, 2019).

5.5.3 Voltage-gated channels influence synaptic integration and action potential firing patterns

Individual neurons can be viewed as computing devices that execute complex input-output functions. They are continuously bombarded with synaptic inputs that activate excitatory, inhibitory, and modulatory receptors and effectors. The strength, temporal pattern, location, and voltage-gated channels activated by these inputs all contribute to determining whether a neuron fires a spike at a given time.

A wide range of voltage-gated channels play a role in shaping the way neurons respond to synaptic inputs and the dynamics of action potential firing during sustained depolarizations. Studies on CA1 pyramidal neurons have yielded a wealth of knowledge about these processes, leading to several key insights.

5.5.3.1 Voltage-gated channels are active near the resting potential

Several voltage-gated channels are sensitive to small changes in membrane potential near the resting potential. Thus, much of what is often referred to as passive membrane properties is likely to be mediated by channels that are open at the resting potential but nonetheless gated by changes in membrane potential. One example is the hyperpolarization-activated channels that are permeable to both sodium and potassium ions (i.e., cation channels). These so-called HCN channels are abundant in CA1 pyramidal neurons, including the dendrites. They are open at the resting potential and activated by hyperpolarization to mediate a current called I_h. Blocking HCN channels approximately doubles input resistance and produces a comparable slowing of EPSP decay (Golding et al., 2005; Magee, 1998; Yamada-Hanff and Bean, 2015). Upregulating HCN channels has the opposite effect (Poolos et al., 2002). Thus, HCN channels have a major influence on synaptic integration. For example, HCN channels have been shown to normalize the time course of EPSPs at different dendritic locations (Magee, 1999). Even after HCN channels are blocked, the input resistance of CA1 pyramidal neurons remains sensitive to the holding potential, suggesting that other voltage-sensitive channels are also open at rest in these neurons (Spruston and Johnston, 1992). Other examples of ion channels that are open and/or activated near the resting potential of CA1 pyramidal neurons are A-type voltage-gated potassium (K_v) channels, M-current, and voltage-gated sodium (Nav) channels (Carter et al., 2012; George et al., 2009; Hu et al., 2002, 2007; Shah et al., 2011; Yamada-Hanff and Bean, 2015).

Voltage-gated sodium channels that activate rapidly but inactivate slowly near the resting potential in CA1 pyramidal neurons produce a persistent sodium current (Crill, 1996; French et al., 1990), which has a substantial impact on synaptic integration and action potential firing (Carter et al., 2012; Y Park et al., 2013; Vervaeke et al., 2006a; Yamada-Hanff and Bean, 2015). In vivo, activation of persistent sodium current in CA1 neurons causes considerable amplification of EPSPs, especially when the neuron is already depolarized by a few millivolts from its normal resting potential (C Hsu et al., 2018). This effect is powerful enough for slight depolarization of a silent cell in vivo to produce firing in a specific place field as animals navigate in a maze or a virtual reality environment.

Persistent sodium current is likely to be mediated by opening of a small fraction of the same channels that are responsible for action potential firing, many of which are located in the axon (Colbert and Pan, 2002; Royeck et al., 2008).

5.5.3.2 Some voltage-gated channels are not uniformly distributed in CA1 dendrites

While Na_v channels have been shown to be present at approximately constant densities along the length of the apical dendrites of CA1 pyramidal neurons, other channels are expressed at highly nonuniform densities. The two best-studied examples are voltage-gated potassium (K_v) channels of the K_v4.2 subtype, which mediates A-type potassium current, and HCN channels, which mediate I_h.

K_v4.2 channels are responsible for a so-called delayed rectifier current in CA1 pyramidal cells, providing a major contribution to action-potential repolarization. These channels are present in the soma and proximal dendrites, but their density increases steadily along the length of the apical dendrites (Cai et al., 2004; Hoffman et al., 1997; Rhodes et al., 2004). As described later in this chapter, these channels have a major influence on the excitability of the dendritic tree (Hoffman et al., 1997; Losonczy and Magee, 2006; Losonczy et al., 2008; Weber et al., 2016).

HCN channels are also distributed nonuniformly in the dendrites of CA1 pyramidal neurons. Specifically, their density increases along the length of the apical dendrites, such that their density is very high in the distal apical dendrites (Bittner et al., 2012; Lörincz et al., 2002; Magee, 1998). Blocking HCN channels reduces voltage attenuation along CA1 apical dendrites (Magee, 1998). Therefore, a major function of these channels, along with their nonuniform distribution resulting in high density in distal dendrites, is to increase the electrical compartmentalization of CA1 pyramidal neurons. While this may be puzzling, as on the surface it would seem to diminish the importance of the most distal synapses, it may be the case that electrical compartmentalization is central to the computational properties of pyramidal neurons. In keeping with this observation, it appears that other channels that contribute to the resting conductance of dendritic membrane are also nonuniformly distributed in a manner that further promotes compartmentalization (Golding et al., 2005). Another important function of HCN channels is to normalize the amount of temporal summation for synaptic inputs arriving at different dendritic locations (Magee, 1999).

The dendrites of CA1 pyramidal neurons contain several subtypes of voltage-gated calcium channels, but their distributions are only partially understood (Magee and Johnston, 1995a). This is an important topic for future work. Another important topic is the distribution of channels in the basal dendrites. Because recording from these dendrites is more difficult, relatively little is known about their properties and the channels that mediate them. In addition, understanding the mechanisms of protein transport and its regulation that lead to nonuniform channel distribution is an important cell biological question.

5.5.3.3 Voltage- and calcium-sensitive ion channels influence action potential firing dynamics

When the net result of dendritic integration of synaptic inputs is that the PSP approaches the threshold for action potential firing, the resulting spiking pattern (if any) depends on many factors. In addition to the strength and time course of the PSP, voltage-gated ion channels that are active near the resting potential can shape the membrane potential in ways that promote or suppress action potential initiation. In addition, voltage-gated and calcium-sensitive channels are activated by action potentials, leading to changes in firing patterns during sustained, above-threshold PSPs.

The effects of ion channels on repetitive spiking are typically treated separately from their effects on synaptic integration by eliciting firing with repeated or sustained current injections (Figure 5.4). Typically, the voltage-gated and calcium-sensitive potassium channels that are activated by action potentials produce a fast afterhyperpolarization (AHP) that inhibits subsequent spiking, leading to a complete or partial refractory period. Similarly, during repeated spiking, slowly activating potassium currents can lead to spike-frequency accommodation (Schwartzkroin, 1977). Multiple types of voltage- and calcium-activated potassium channels contribute to these effects, with different currents having effects that operate over different time scales, thus producing fast, slow, and medium AHPs (Figure 5.4A) (Gu et al., 2005; Kaczorowski et al., 2007; Lancaster and Nicoll, 1987; Madison and Nicoll, 1984; Sahu and Turner, 2021). As described below, many of the channels that regulate patterns of action potential firing are also regulated by neuromodulatory systems.

In most CA1 pyramidal neurons, the fast AHP is either absent or followed by an afterdepolarization (ADP) mediated by a balance between R-type Ca_v channels ($Ca_v2.3$) and D-type potassium channels (K_v1). In most cells, the effect of Ca_v channels is large enough to overcome the effects of K_v channels, thus resulting in an ADP, which can in some cases drive a high-frequency burst of spikes (Figure 5.4B–C) (Metz et al., 2005, 2007; J Park et al., 2010). Bursting is terminated by inactivation of Ca_v channels and activation of K_v channels. However, these effects are relatively slow, allowing multiple spikes in a burst to have a cumulative effect on the currents underlying the ADP, thus resulting in a larger ADP after a burst of spikes. This larger, postburst ADP is increased by the action of glutamate and acetylcholine (ACh) acting on metabotropic glutamate and ACh receptors (mGluRs and mAChRs) (Figure 5.4D) (J Park and Spruston, 2012; J Park et al., 2010).

5.5.4 Dendritic properties and synaptic location influence synaptic integration

In addition to the effects of voltage- and calcium-gated channels on neuronal responses to synaptic inputs, the structure of the dendritic tree and the location of the synapses is another important set of factors. The influence of dendritic structure on synaptic integration has been studied extensively in CA1 pyramidal neurons.

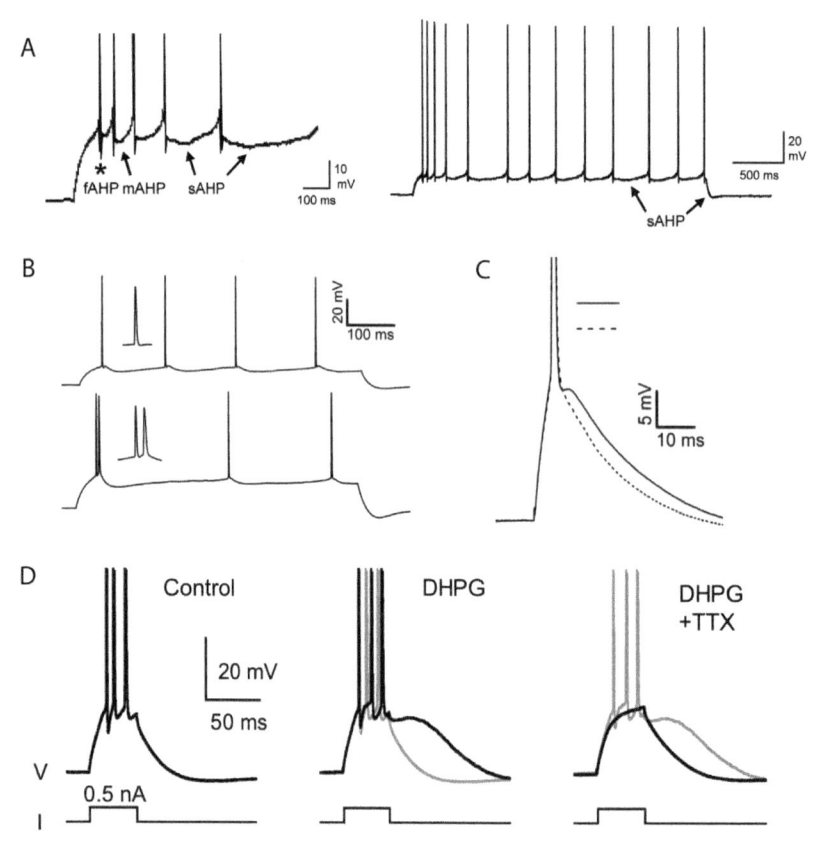

Figure 5.4 Spike-frequency adaptation and bursting in CA1 pyramidal neurons. (A) Left: A train of action potentials from a CA1 pyramidal neuron, indicating spike-frequency adaptation, and fast, medium, and slow afterhyperpolarization (fAHP, mAHP, sAHP). Right: A longer record of the same train of spikes showing the increasing length of the AHP, which contributes to spike-frequency adaptation. (B) V_m responses to a step current injection in two CA1 pyramidal cells: a regular spiking neuron (top) and a bursting neuron (bottom). Insets show single spikes and bursts at better temporal resolution. (C) V_m responses to 5 ms current injections that elicited single spikes in regular spiking (dashed line) and bursting (solid line) CA1 pyramidal cells, showing the larger postspike ADP in the bursting neuron. (D) V_m responses to 40 ms current injections, which elicited three action potentials followed by an ADP that was enhanced following application of the mGluR agonist DHPG. Blocking action potentials with TTX eliminated the ADP observed in the presence of DHPG. Gray traces are superimpositions of the previous example response. (Sources: (A) Sahu and Turner, 2021; (B, C) Metz et al., 2005; (D) Park et al., 2010.)

5.5.4.1 Distinct synaptic inputs onto different dendritic domains

Strikingly, synaptic inputs from different sources are localized on different compartments of the CA1 dendritic tree. SC axons innervate the basal and apical dendrites, with hundreds of microns separating the most proximal and distal synapses (Figure 5.2). Even more extreme, PP/TA axons form synapses exclusively on the apical tuft dendrites, several hundred microns from the soma. This large range of dendritic locations has important implications for synaptic integration and synaptic plasticity.

Different dendritic domains of CA1 pyramidal neurons also receive distinct inhibitory synaptic inputs. For example, inhibitory inputs from basket cells are mostly located on the soma and very proximal dendrites (Freund and Buzsáki, 1996; Halasy et al., 1996), while inputs from neurogliaform cells predominantly target distal apical dendrites. Overall, most of the dendritic inhibition onto CA1 pyramidal neurons is located on large apical and basal dendrites, relatively close to the soma, where it is well positioned to inhibit depolarization of the soma and axon initial segment. In addition, however, some interneuron subtypes selectively target more distal branches (Bloss et al., 2016; Gidon and Segev, 2012).

5.5.4.2 Effects of dendrites on synaptic integration

Importantly, many synaptic inputs are located at long distances (relative to dendritic diameter) from the action-potential initiation zone, which normally resides in the axon initial segment, which emanates from the soma or from a primary dendrite very close to the soma (Colbert and Johnston, 1996; Colbert and Pan, 2002). Dendrites have electrical properties that cause them to function as leaky cables. Thus, while an EPSP might be quite large when measured in a dendrite near the synapse, it is much smaller at the action-potential initiation zone in the axon (Magee and Cook, 2000). This is true for several reasons; the structure and membrane properties of dendrites are major factors.

Cable theory provides a framework for understanding how the physical structure, membrane properties (resistance and capacitance), and internal resistance collectively influence how much a synapse will influence the membrane potential at a distant location such as the cell body (Rall, 2011). These properties have all been constrained by experiments in CA1 pyramidal neurons, including simultaneous patch-clamp recordings from the soma and a primary apical dendrite, which allows for direct measurements of voltage attenuation between two locations (Golding et al., 2005; Magee and Cook, 2000). When combined with detailed morphological measurements of the lengths, diameter, and branching structure of the dendritic tree, this can be used to develop computational models that provide insight into how synapses affect membrane potential in different parts of the neuron. A major conclusion of these studies is that in the absence of active amplification of EPSP spread, the effect of a synapse on membrane potential in the axon initial segment depends greatly on its dendritic position. In fact, this effect is so large that activation of a single synapse at a distal dendritic location is expected to have a negligible effect on the membrane potential in the cell body or the axon initial segment. Thus, action potential firing must be driven by the concerted action of multiple excitatory synaptic inputs, estimated in CA1 neurons to be on the order of 10–100 synapses (Katz et al., 2009; Magee and Cook, 2000).

Although dendrites contain numerous voltage-gated channels, it is instructive to first consider how dendritic structure influences synaptic potentials in the simpler case of passive dendrites (Figure 5.5). This can be summarized with a few simple principles. (1) Synapses located on small structures such as dendritic spines or small-diameter dendrites (especially near sealed ends) will produce relatively large voltage changes for a small amount of charge entering the cell via synaptically gated receptors. (2) The change in membrane potential at the synapse (e.g., in a dendritic spine) can significantly reduce the driving force for transmembrane current flow, thus limiting the local impact of one or more synapses. In the extreme, a dendritic branch could be depolarized enough by N synapses that activation of N+ 1 synapses would produce a negligibly larger influx of current. (3) A localized voltage change in one part of the cell (e.g., at a synapse) causes charge to flow along the dendrite, which in turn changes the membrane potential at other locations, owing to the capacitance of the membrane. (4) Any deviation of the membrane potential from equilibrium (i.e., the resting potential) will produce a driving force for transmembrane ionic current. This produces a local decrease in the voltage change (i.e., moving closer to equilibrium), which in turn reduces longitudinal current within the dendrite. (5) Longitudinal current flow produces voltage changes that are proportional to the local input impedance. Therefore, current flowing from small structures (e.g., a small-diameter dendrite) to larger structures (e.g., a branch point formed by a larger dendrite) will produce a local voltage drop. The soma is a particularly large structure, resulting in a significant voltage drop from dendrites to the soma. By contrast, a voltage change produced at a large-diameter dendrite or branch point will attenuate much less as it spreads into smaller diameter dendrites, especially close to a sealed end, where input impedance is highest.

The net result of these principles is that synapses produce voltage changes that vary dramatically in space and time. A large local voltage change that rises quickly will decay rapidly as current flows longitudinally into dendrites, while at a distal location the membrane potential will be smaller, owing to loss of charge across intervening membrane, and will rise and fall more gradually owing to the membrane capacitance and the smaller driving force for longitudinal current. For example, a synapse in the apical tuft of a CA1 pyramidal neuron produces a 10 mV local EPSP lasting about 2 ms (full width at half maximal amplitude), while at the soma this would produce an EPSP at least 100x smaller (i.e., 0.1 mV or less) and 5–10x slower. This massive attenuation is observed for two reasons: (1) the high input impedance of small-diameter dendrites leads to large local synaptic potentials, which decrease in amplitude as current flows to larger-diameter branches, owing to their lower input impedance; (2) some charge is lost across the membrane resistance as current flows internally from the dendrite to the soma. Importantly, only the second factor influences the "efficacy cost" of placing a synapse on a distal dendrite—that is, the reduced depolarization at the soma (i.e., near the action potential initiation zone) caused by moving a synapse to a distal dendritic location. In the example above, the same synapse placed at the soma would produce an EPSP about 10x larger than when placed on an apical tuft dendrite (Golding et al., 2005; Spruston, 2008).

Dendritic spines also have very high input impedance, so very small synaptic currents will produce large membrane potentials in the spine head, regardless of the diameter of the parent dendrite. This results in efficient activation of GluN and other

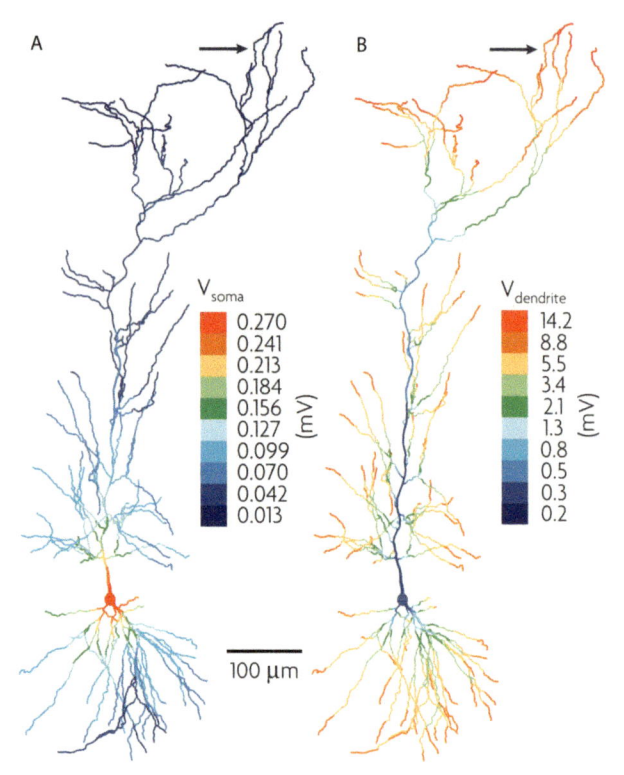

Figure 5.5 Attenuation of synaptic strength in CA1 pyramidal neurons. (A) Amplitude of the somatic EPSP for an excitatory synapse of fixed synaptic conductance (0.3 nS) simulated at each dendritic location in a model of a CA1 pyramidal neuron with passive dendrites. Synapses proximal to the soma produce somatic EPSP amplitudes of 0.2–0.3 mV (yellow/red on the linear color scale), but the amplitude falls off sharply as a function of distance. Synapses approximately 150 μm from the soma produce somatic EPSPs of approximately half of this unitary amplitude (0.1 mV; light blue on the scale), whereas synapses in distal dendrites produce somatic EPSPs of less than one-tenth of this unitary amplitude (less than 0.02 mV; dark blue on the scale). (B) Amplitude of the local EPSP in the same simulations. The amplitude in the main apical dendrite and in the soma is 0.2–0.3 mV (dark blue on the logarithmic color scale), but the local amplitude for synapses on smaller dendrites is considerably larger. Proximal basal, apical oblique, and tuft branches depolarize by a few millivolts (green/yellow on the scale), whereas the most distal branches depolarize by more than 10 mV (red on the scale). At the location marked by the arrow in parts A and B of the figure, the local synaptic potential is approximately 13 mV and the resultant somatic EPSP is approximately 0.014 mV (>900-fold attenuation). This voltage attenuation is largely a consequence of the small diameter, and thus the high impedance, of the distal dendrites, which causes large local EPSPs (almost 50-fold larger than the 0.27 mV EPSP for the somatic synapse). (Source: Spruston, 2008.)

voltage-sensitive channels that may reside in spines (Cornejo et al., 2022; Harnett et al., 2012). On all but the smallest diameter dendrites, there will be a substantial voltage drop from the spine head to the dendritic shaft, thus localizing electrical signals to the spine, which may be important for restricting activity-dependent plasticity to activated spines and not their inactive neighbors (Harnett et al., 2012).

All the factors discussed above have significant implications for using the voltage-clamp technique to study the biophysical properties of synapses (see Chapter 6). Even for synapses located on dendrites, a voltage-clamp imposed by a somatic electrode may fail to adequately detect or control voltage at the synapse. This results in considerable filtering of the measured synaptic current (Spruston

et al., 1993; S Williams and Mitchell, 2008). In addition, failure of the somatic electrode to control the synaptic membrane potential may fail to prevent activation of voltage-gated channels, which can further distort the measured current. These errors can be significant, even for synapses located a few tens of microns from the soma; for those located hundreds of microns from the soma, the errors can be extreme.

5.5.4.3 Dendritic voltage-gated channels produce dendritic spikes and promote plasticity

While the foregoing analysis implies that synapses are less efficient when located further from the axon initial segment, this is not necessarily the case, because dendrites contain voltage-gated channels, which further influence the process of synaptic integration. The dendrites of CA1 pyramidal neurons contain various types of voltage-gated sodium, calcium, and potassium channels, each of which is activated by depolarization. These channels contribute to the ability of CA1 pyramidal neurons to produce multiple types of dendritically initiated spikes—i.e., dendritic spikes (Figure 5.6A–C) (Andreasen and Nedergaard, 1996; Golding et al., 1999; Losonczy and Magee, 2006; Schwartzkroin and Slawsky, 1977; Spruston, 2008). Dendritic sodium spikes are brief (2–3 ms), while dendritic calcium spikes are considerably longer (tens to hundreds of ms). In addition, synapses contain GluNs, which act as glutamate-dependent voltage-gated channels that can also contribute to dendritic spikes. In neocortical pyramidal neurons, dendritic spikes that rely principally on GluN activation have been reported (Major et al., 2013). These dendritic NMDA-receptor mediated spikes appear to be less prevalent in CA1 pyramidal neurons, although they may exist in apical tuft dendrites (Wei et al., 2001). Certainly, GluNs are important contributors, along with AMPA receptors (GluA), to the glutamate-mediated synaptic excitation that drives dendritic sodium and calcium spikes (Harnett et al., 2012; Weber et al., 2016). Although dendritic spikes have mostly been studied in hippocampal slices in vitro, several in vivo studies indicate that these events are indeed engaged in the intact brain (Kamondi et al., 1998; Sheffield and Dombeck, 2015; Stuart and Spruston, 2015).

Unlike action potentials, which propagate actively over long distances in the axon, dendritic spikes attenuate as they spread from their site of initiation to other parts of the neuron (Gasparini et al., 2004; Golding and Spruston, 1998; Golding et al., 1999; Losonczy and Magee, 2006). Thus, their functional roles are complex. Dendritic calcium spikes exert a relatively strong influence over axonal action potential initiation, owing to their long duration, greater charge entry, and diminished attenuation over long distance. The longest types of dendritic calcium spikes—plateau potentials that last hundreds of milliseconds—can drive high-frequency bursts of action potentials in the axon (Epsztein et al., 2011; Golding et al., 1999; Takahashi and Magee, 2009; Wong and Prince, 1978). On the other hand, dendritic sodium spikes are generated in small-diameter branches and they produce smaller voltage changes in the soma; whether they are above or below threshold for action potential firing depends on the total number of activated synaptic inputs, their spatiotemporal pattern, and the number of dendritic branches engaged (Ariav et al., 2003; Gasparini and Magee, 2006; Gasparini et al., 2004; Golding and Spruston, 1998; Y Kim et al., 2015; Losonczy and Magee, 2006). Dendritic spikes in individual branches are also subject to plasticity, which can change the strength of the output from a dendritic branch to the soma (Losonczy et al., 2008).

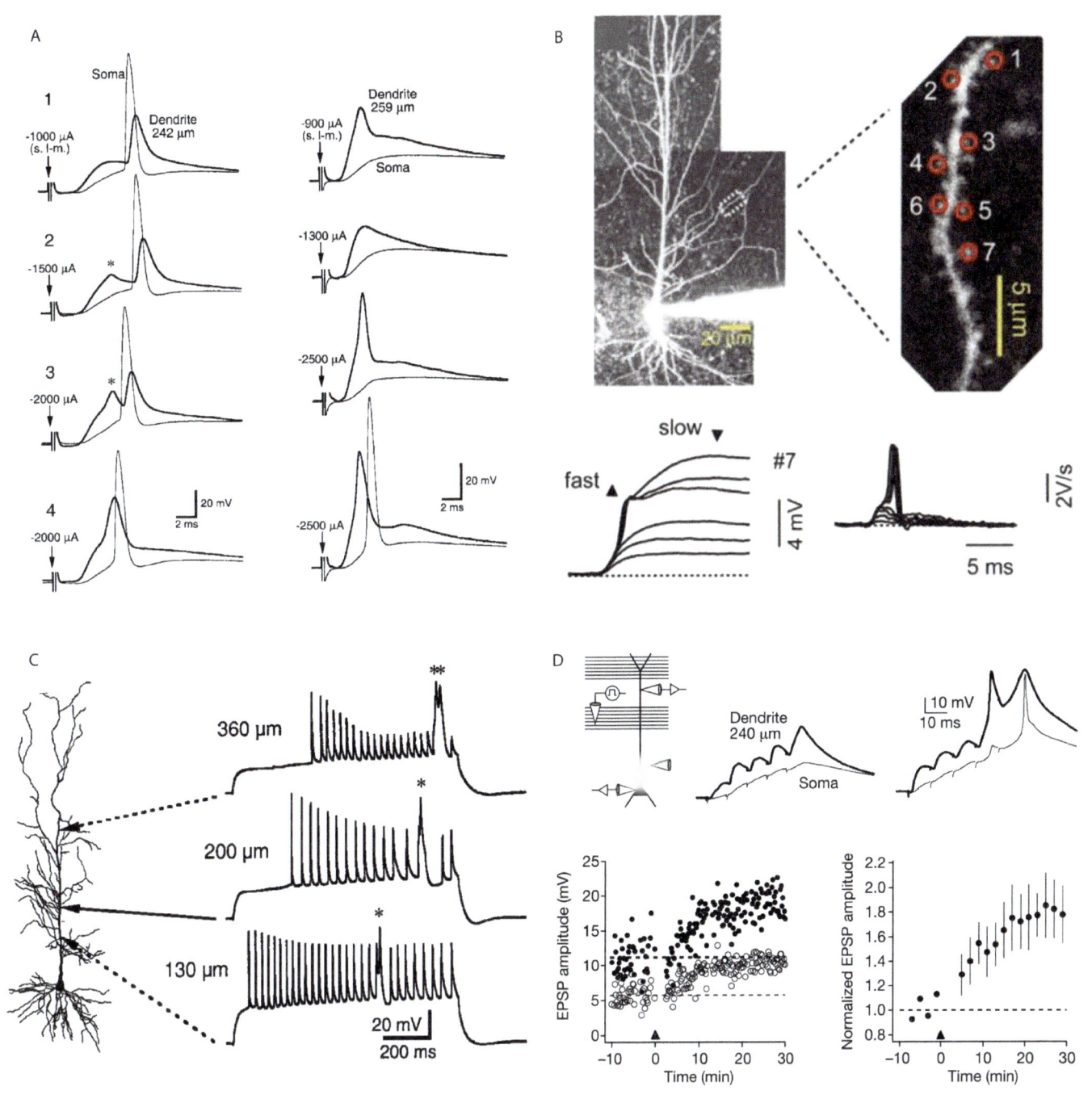

Figure 5.6 Dendritic spikes and dendritic spike–induced LTP in CA1 pyramidal neurons. (A) Paired recordings from the soma and apical dendrites of CA1 pyramidal neurons. Left: examples #1–4 are responses to stimulation of axons in stratum lacunosum-moleculare (s.l.-m.) at increasing stimulus intensity. At higher stimulus intensity, signs of dendritic spikes (*) are observed prior to somatic action potentials that subsequently propagate into the dendrites. On some responses to the highest intensity (example #4), larger dendritic spikes precede somatic action potentials that lack a backpropagating action potential, presumably because the larger dendritic spike results in inactivation of dendritic Na_v channels. Right: similar responses in a different recording. In some cases (examples #1 and #3) dendritic spikes are observed without somatic action potential firing. (B) Glutamate uncaging onto dendritic spines at the indicated locations. As larger numbers of locations are stimulated together, both fast and slow nonlinearities indicative of nonlinear dendritic responses are observed (bottom left). The fast response is evident from the first derivative of V_m (bottom right). (C) Dendritic recordings from three different cells at the locations corresponding approximately to those indicated on the cell shown (corresponding to middle trace). In each case, sufficiently strong dendritic current injection elicited one or more dendritic calcium spikes (*). (D) Theta-burst stimulation (TBS) of excitatory synaptic inputs from CA3 (shown) or EC results in LTP even when TTX is applied near the soma to prevent axonal action potentials and/or their backpropagation into the dendrites. Examples of two TBS responses are shown (top), as well as LTP induced in the same cell (bottom left) and summary data (bottom right). (Sources: (A) Golding and Spruston, 1998; (B) Losonczy and Magee, 2006; (C) Golding et al., 1999; (D) Golding et al., 2002.)

While dendritically initiated spikes may exert some influence over action potential initiation in the axon, they may also have a local function in the dendrites. Dendritic sodium, calcium, and NMDAR-mediated spikes all contribute to the induction of synaptic plasticity at excitatory synapses on CA1 pyramidal neurons, including synaptic inputs from CA3 and EC (Golding et al., 2002; Hardie and Spruston, 2009; Y Kim et al., 2015; S Williams et al., 2007). For example, in hippocampal slices in vitro, synaptically evoked dendritic spikes can result in long-term potentiation (LTP) of synaptic strength, even in the absence of action potential firing in the soma (Figure 5.6D) (Golding et al., 2002; Y Kim et al., 2015). Even a single dendritic calcium spike is sufficient to induce LTP at CA3-to-CA1 synapses (Remy and Spruston, 2007), and in awake mice in vivo, a single plateau potential can convert silent CA1 cells to place cells (Figure 5.3B) (Bittner et al., 2015, 2017). In addition, the occurrence of calcium transients localized to the dendrites of CA1 pyramidal neurons predicts the formation and stability of new place fields as animals navigate novel environments, suggesting an important role for spike-independent forms of synaptic plasticity (Sheffield and Dombeck, 2015; Sheffield et al., 2017).

5.5.4.4 Dendritic voltage-gated channels produce backpropagating action potentials

In addition to supporting the initiation of dendritic spikes, voltage-gated channels in dendrites play an important role in backpropagation of axonally initiated action potentials into the dendritic tree (Figure 5.7) (Magee and Johnston, 1995a, 1995b; Spruston et al., 1995). Dendritic Na_v channels allow for active propagation into

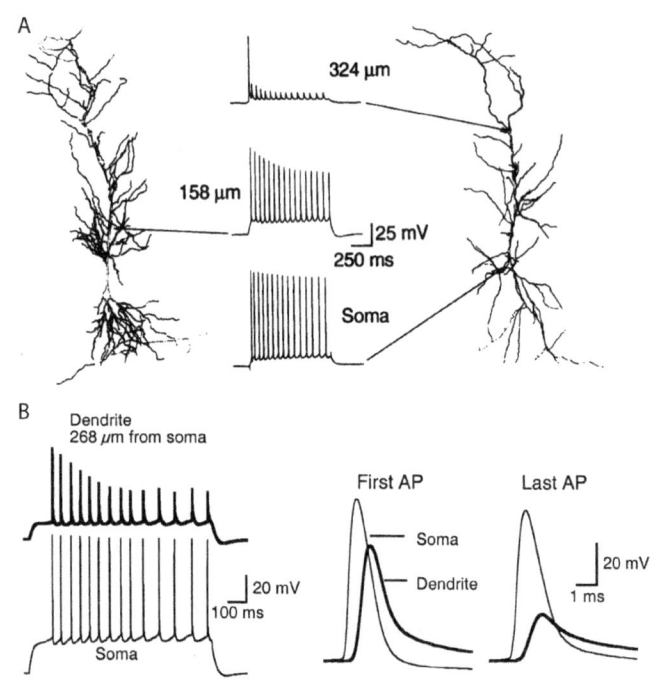

Figure 5.7 Activity-dependent action potential backpropagation in CA1 pyramidal neurons. (A) Trains of action potentials recorded in proximal apical dendrites (left cell) and distal apical dendrites (right cell, along with simultaneous somatic recording) illustrating activity-dependent amplitude of backpropagating action potentials. (B) Another recording showing that action potentials are recorded first in the soma and with a short delay in the simultaneous dendritic recording. (Source: Spruston et al., 1995.)

dendrites and K_v channels support active repolarization (Golding et al., 2001; Hoffman et al., 1997). Importantly, because the ratio of Na_v-to-K_v channels in dendrites is not as high as in the axon, backpropagating action potentials attenuate as they propagate into dendrites. Furthermore, under conditions of incomplete active regeneration, action potential propagation is prone to fail at branch points in the dendritic tree (Frick et al., 2003; Gasparini et al., 2007).

Action potential backpropagation in CA1 pyramidal neurons is even weaker during repetitive firing. Under these conditions, dendritic Na_v channels enter a prolonged inactivation state following activation (Colbert et al., 1997; H Jung et al., 1997; Mickus et al., 1999), causing backpropagating action potentials to attenuate (Andreasen and Lambert, 1995; Golding et al., 2001; Spruston et al., 1995).

Backpropagating action potentials can also induce synaptic plasticity at active synapses. When synaptic activation is repeatedly paired with backpropagating action potentials at sufficiently high rates, it leads to LTP of synaptic strength. Preventing action potentials from propagating back into the dendrites blocks this form of LTP (Magee and Johnston, 1997). Importantly, however, when EPSPs are paired with action potentials at lower rates, it leads to long-term depression (LTD) of synaptic strength (Christie et al., 1996). A key distinction is that high-frequency pairing of EPSPs and action potentials amplifies dendritic calcium signals more effectively than low-frequency pairing, thus leading to LTP instead of LTD (Johnston et al., 2003). The relative timing of synaptic activation and backpropagating action potentials has also been proposed to influence the magnitude and direction of synaptic plasticity at CA3–CA1 synapses, although separating this influence from the pairing frequency is difficult, and at low pairing rates LTD tends to occur regardless of the relative timing (Lisman and Spruston, 2010). Furthermore, when EPSPs are strong enough to elicit dendritic spikes, LTP is robustly induced in a manner that does not require backpropagating action potentials (Hardie and Spruston, 2009). Similarly, dendritic plateau potentials are powerful triggers of synaptic plasticity in vivo, likely independent of action potential backpropagation (Bittner et al., 2017). Thus, the role of backpropagating action potentials for LTP and LTD in behaving animals remains uncertain.

As mentioned above, $K_v4.2$ channels are expressed in CA1 dendrites, with their density increasing as a function of distance from the soma. As such, they play a key role in regulating dendritic excitability. The relatively low density of $K_v4.2$ channels allows excitatory inputs to drive action potential initiation in the axon, followed by backpropagation into the dendrites. For more distal synaptic inputs, however, their location further from the axon may limit their ability to drive action potential firing in the axon. At the same time, the high density of dendritic $K_v4.2$ channels limit the initiation of dendritic spikes. With stronger excitatory activation, dendritic sodium spikes can be initiated, but the relatively high density of dendritic potassium channels, largely attributable to $K_v4.2$, prevents these spikes from actively propagating into the soma. As a result, even when dendritic sodium spikes are measured in the dendrites, they can be followed by a backpropagating action potential (Golding and Spruston, 1998). With even stronger synaptic excitation, however, calcium channel activation is recruited, $K_v4.2$ channels inactivate, and calcium spikes (including plateau potentials) can drive high-frequency action potential firing in the axon (Golding et al., 1999; Hoffman et al., 1997). Thus, the nonuniform distribution of $K_v4.2$ channels, with their highest density in the apical dendrites, along with other types of dendritic potassium channels, has a major influence over action potential firing, backpropagation, dendritic spike initiation, and consequently synaptic plasticity (Johnston et al., 2000).

5.5.5 Synaptic structure and function vary across the dendritic tree

Synaptic ultrastructure has been studied extensively in CA1 pyramidal neurons. A key concept is that dendritic spines and synapses come in a variety of shapes and sizes (Figure 5.8). Across cell types, dendritic spines have been given qualitative descriptions such as simple, pedunculated, branched, racemose, thorny, etc. (Fiala et al., 2008). Similarly, postsynaptic densities have been described based on their shape and given names such as continuous, segmented, partitioned, and perforated (Nicholson et al., 2006). These names are useful descriptors, but they may not reflect a true distinction between functional classes. Rather, the diversity of spines and synapses likely reflects a continuum of sizes and shapes that arise from different functional stages ranging from nascent spines to structurally established spines with very few receptors, to well-established spines mediating strong synaptic responses (Ofer et al., 2021; Tønnesen et al., 2014).

5.5.5.1 Spine structure is variable

A diverse range of dendritic spines and postsynaptic densities has been observed in CA1 neurons (Harris, 1999; Harris et al., 1992, 2015, 2022; Nicholson et al., 2006). Most spines have long, thin necks, and a larger head, and as a result, dendritic spines are estimated to have very high input impedance, on the order of hundreds of MΩ, which likely amplifies local depolarization and therefore charge entry through GluNs (Cornejo et al., 2022; Harnett et al., 2012; Noguchi et al., 2005). The dimensions of spine necks and heads vary considerably, however, and are influenced by synaptic plasticity (Katz et al., 2009; Nägerl et al., 2004; Tønnesen et al., 2014). For example, LTP is believed to be mediated by an increase in the size of the spine head, along with an increase in currents mediated by glutamate-gated ionotropic (GluA) receptors (Bourne and Harris, 2007; Matsuzaki et al., 2004). In concert with this change, spine necks get shorter and wider. Several reasons have been proposed for these changes, including that these changes serve to normalize chemical and electrical compartmentalization (Svoboda et al., 1996; Tønnesen et al., 2014; Yuste and Bonhoeffer, 2001).

5.5.5.2 Spine size correlates with the number of synaptic vesicles and receptors

In general, the size of dendritic spines covaries with the area of the postsynaptic density and the number of glutamate-gated receptor channels (Matsuzaki et al., 2001; Nicholson and Geinisman, 2009; Takumi et al., 1999). Similarly, the size of postsynaptic structures correlates with the size of presynaptic structures such as the number of synaptic vesicles and active zones (Harris and Stevens, 1989; Harris and Sultan, 1995; Schikorski and Stevens, 1997). In CA1 pyramidal neurons, these measures exhibit a skewed distribution, with most synapses centered on a large peak of modest size and a smaller number of synapses that are substantially larger, and therefore likely stronger (Nicholson et al., 2006). This observation suggests that a minority population of the thousands of synaptic inputs onto any given pyramidal cell may provide most of the depolarization that drives action potential firing, while most presynaptic inputs to CA1 pyramidal neurons constitute a reserve pool that may be converted to strong synapses by activity-dependent synaptic plasticity. Importantly, LTP would have to be balanced by LTD for the observed skewed distribution to be maintained.

5.5.5.3 Spine structure varies across dendritic compartments

Significant differences in the distributions of synaptic ultrastructure and channel densities have been observed in different compartments of CA1 dendrites. For example, large, perforated postsynaptic densities are more abundant in the distal portions of the apical dendrites, including distal oblique and tuft branches, as well as in distal basal dendrites. These large, perforated postsynaptic densities contain more GluA and GluN channels than their smaller, nonperforated counterparts (Katz et al., 2009; Nicholson and Geinisman, 2009; Nicholson et al., 2006). However, in the smallest-diameter branches, while GluA density is high, GluN density is lower, likely reflecting the increased activation of GluN channels expected to result from the large local depolarization mediated by strong synapses on small, and therefore high-impedance, dendrites. Thus, the lower GluN density at synapses on the smallest dendrites may serve to normalize the amount of GluN activation resulting from the combined effects of activation by presynaptic glutamate release and relief of magnesium block owing to postsynaptic depolarization (Menon et al., 2013).

An additional, related observation is that a novel class of synapses called compound synapses is observed almost exclusively in the apical tuft dendrites (Bloss et al., 2018). These synapses constitute two presynaptic boutons from the same axon forming contacts onto two adjacent dendritic spines on the same neuron. This arrangement indicates a particularly strong form of synaptic connection on an electrotonically remote portion of the CA1 dendritic tree.

Collectively, these observations of synapse structure and receptor content likely explain physiological recordings suggesting that synaptic currents are larger at more distal dendritic locations and that synaptic potentials detected at the soma are, on average, less dependent on distance than would be predicted from passive cable theory (Bittner et al., 2012; Magee and Cook, 2000).

5.5.6 Inhibition influences synaptic integration

The vastly diverse population of hippocampal inhibitory interneurons is considered later in this chapter. Here we summarize some key principles regarding the effects of inhibition on synaptic integration in CA1 pyramidal neurons.

A significant fraction (10%–40%) of inhibitory synaptic inputs is located on the axon, soma, and proximal dendrites, where they are well positioned to influence action potential initiation in the axon initial segment (Bloss et al., 2016; Megías et al., 2001). This allows inhibition not only to curtail the effects of excitation, thus inhibiting firing rate, but also to influence temporal integration and spike timing. In a passive system, the postsynaptic potential (PSP) would have a slow component of decay that is governed by the membrane time constant, which is about 30–40 ms in CA1 pyramidal neurons (Golding et al., 2005). In practice, however, PSP decay is more rapid because of feedforward inhibition, which accelerates decay of the PSP. The net result is that temporal summation of PSPs is more limited, thus reducing the variance of spike times in response to trains of presynaptic action potentials when SCs are repeatedly activated (Pouille and Scanziani, 2001). This effect is consistent with the

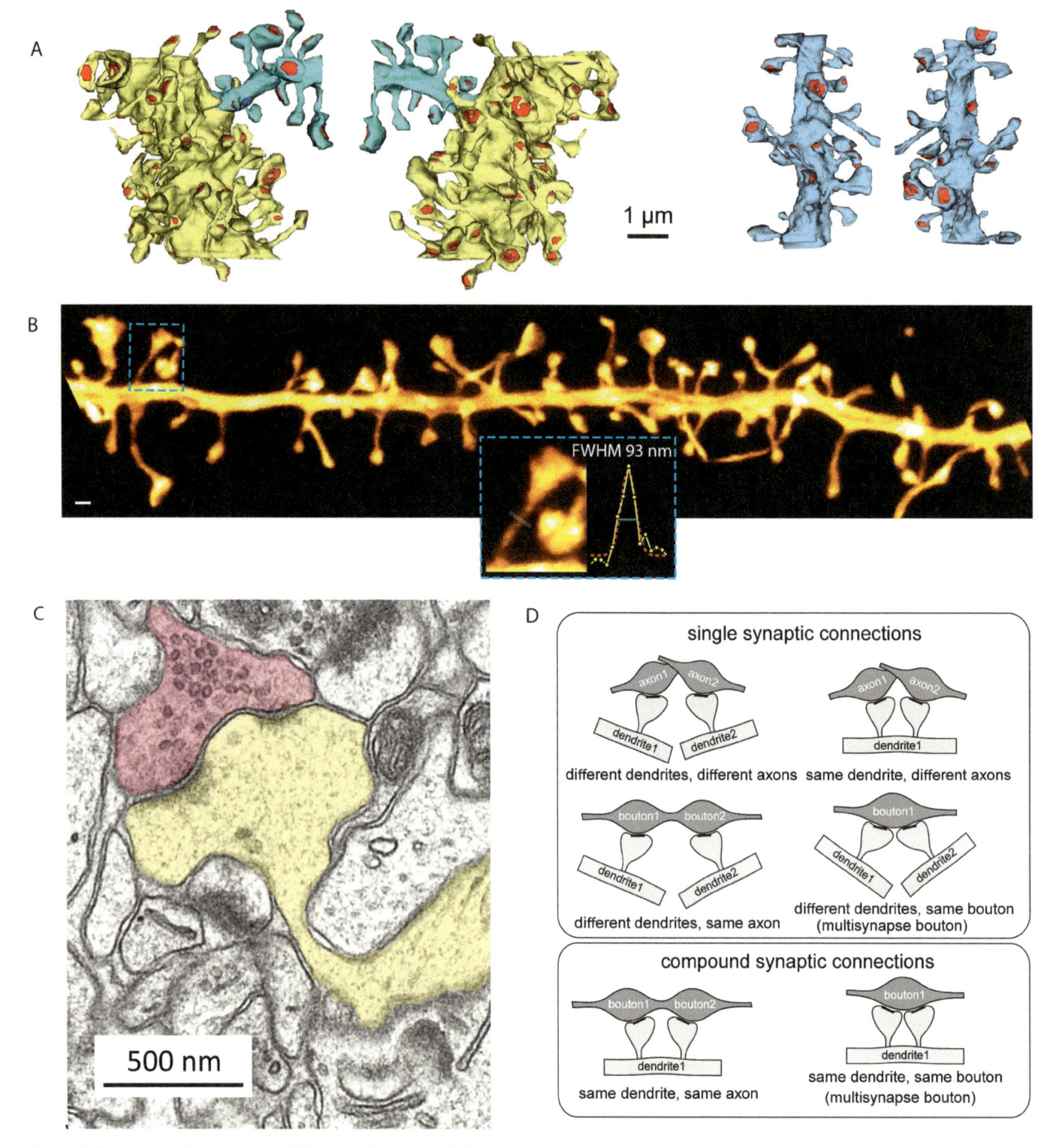

Figure 5.8 Synaptic ultrastructure in CA1 pyramidal neurons. (A) Dendritic segments and spines reconstructed from serial section electron micrographs. Main apical dendrite is yellow, oblique branches are blue, postsynaptic densities are red. Pairs of images are rotations of the same segments. (B) Image of a CA1 dendrite and spines obtained using super-resolution light microscopy. (C) Electron micrograph of a synapse on a CA1 pyramidal neuron showing a presynaptic terminal (pink) with multiple vesicles and a dendritic spine (yellow) with a perforated postsynaptic density. (D) Cartoons of synaptic arrangements observed in CA1. (Sources: (A) Courtesy of Kristen Harris, Masaaki Kuwajima, and Josef Spacek, Harris et al., 2015, 2022; (B) Tønnesen et al., 2014; (C, D) Bloss et al., 2018.)

influence of HCN channels, which also limit temporal summation, as noted above.

Most inhibitory synaptic input is dendritic, where it can exert multiple effects. In general, dendritic inhibition has been shown to reduce the amount of firing caused by a given excitatory input, whereas perisomatic inhibition has the additional effect of (not observed for dendritic inhibition) reducing the maximal firing rate (Pouille et al., 2013). More specifically, neuropeptide Y (NPY)-expressing interneurons innervate the apical oblique and primary apical tuft branches of the dendrites, where their activation is well suited to reduce the amount of depolarizing charge that reaches the soma and the axon. In contrast, somatostatin (SOM)-expressing interneurons are more biased toward terminal dendritic branches in the apical tuft (Bloss et al., 2016). While these distal inputs can also reduce the amount of current arriving at the soma, even from somewhat more proximal excitatory synapses (Gidon and Segev, 2012), they are particularly effective at inhibiting dendritic spike initiation (Bloss et al., 2016).

A combination of factors—including EPSP kinetics, the membrane time constant, short-term plasticity, and disynaptic inhibition of interneurons—cause feedback inhibition in CA1 pyramidal neurons to shift from perisomatic to more distal dendritic sources during sustained firing. While the significance of this shift is not entirely understood, it may serve to synchronize the firing of CA1 pyramidal neurons at the onset of a strong input but change the way synaptic inputs are integrated in the dendrites during sustained input (Pouille and Scanziani, 2004).

5.5.7 Dendritic computation in CA1 pyramidal neurons

Taken together, the features of CA1 pyramidal neurons described above suggest some important hypotheses about how synaptic inputs are integrated, and therefore what kinds of computations are performed in the dendrites of these neurons. Here, we provide a summary of some key principles. This topic is considered more extensively in Chapter 7, which focuses on computations performed by local circuits.

First, despite considerable electrical compartmentalization of the dendritic tree, synapses at all dendritic locations can contribute to action potential firing in the axon through cooperative interactions that benefit from the nonlinear properties of the neuron imparted by Na_v and Ca_v channels, as well as GluNs. Activation of the relatively strong synapses can trigger dendritically initiated spikes in individual dendritic branches (Ariav et al., 2003; Gasparini et al., 2004; Golding and Spruston, 1998; Losonczy and Magee, 2006). On their own, these dendritic spikes may not drive action potential firing in the axon, but they amplify the impact of activating synapses on a branch. When synapses on multiple dendrites are activated, they may produce sufficient axonal depolarization to produce action potential depolarization. Synapses on any branch, at any distance from the soma, may contribute to this multistage integrative process, both because more distal synapses have more GluA, on average, and because voltage-gated channels can amplify their impact. One hypothesis is that each pyramidal neuron constitutes a multilevel network, with individual dendritic branches operating as integrate-and-fire units and the soma/axon operating as an integrate-and-fire unit for input arriving from spiking dendritic branches (Jadi et al., 2014; Katz et al., 2009; Losonczy and Magee, 2006). This hypothesis has not yet been tested directly, owing to the difficulty of preventing branch spiking without interfering with other aspects of synaptic integration. However, experiments suggest that even the excitability of individual dendritic branches is a target of activity-dependent plasticity, with the contribution of local dendritic spikes increasing substantially following local downregulation of $K_v4.2$ channels (Losonczy et al., 2008).

Second, dendritic calcium spikes are a powerful mechanism by which voltage-gated channels in dendrites amplify the impact of distal dendritic synapses. In fact, considerable evidence supports the notion that these events occur in response to coincident activation of CA3–CA1 synapses in apical and basal dendrites together with

EC–CA1 synapses in the apical tuft dendrites (Figure 5.9) (Bittner et al., 2015; Jarsky et al., 2005; Takahashi and Magee, 2009). In some cases, dendritic calcium spikes cause plateau potentials, which drive bursts of action potentials in the axon, which have been shown to propagate and produce output to downstream targets (Apostolides et al., 2016).

Third, dendritic spikes are powerful signals for synaptic plasticity. Both sodium- and calcium-channel mediated spikes have been shown to induce LTP of SC synapses onto CA1 pyramidal neurons (Golding et al., 2002; Y Kim et al., 2015). While backpropagating action potentials can also induce synaptic plasticity (LTP and LTD) in CA1 neurons (Christie et al., 1996; Johnston et al., 2003; Magee and Johnston, 1997), dendritically initiated spikes are more robust inducers of plasticity (Hardie and Spruston, 2009); even a single dendritic calcium spike or plateau potential can induce LTP (Bittner et al., 2015; Remy and Spruston, 2007). Plateau potentials serve as powerful signals for a synaptic plasticity rule that has a time window of a few seconds (Bittner et al., 2017). Any synapse active in a 2–3 second window around the plateau potential is rapidly potentiated by a mechanism referred to as behavioral time scale plasticity (BTSP). This form of synaptic plasticity can lead to the conversion of a silent cell to a place cell, including place cells that depend on environmental and/or behavioral context (Bittner et al., 2015; X Zhao et al., 2022; X Zhao et al., 2020). Thus, weak synapses, which constitute most of the excitatory inputs to dendritic spines (Nicholson et al., 2006), may have little impact on action potential firing, but if they are potentiated by BTSP, they can contribute to the rapid formation of firing that reliably codes for the behavioral conditions that produced the plateau potential. Similarly, there is evidence that spikes localized to individual dendritic branches may contribute to plasticity that influences the firing properties of CA1 pyramidal neurons during behavior (Sheffield and Dombeck, 2015; Sheffield et al., 2017).

Fourth, as noted above and discussed in more detail later in this chapter, a wide variety of interneuron subtypes target different cellular compartments of CA1 pyramidal neurons. Each of these cellular domains is likely to be activated under different conditions, and their activation or inhibition (i.e., resulting in disinhibition) adds further complexity to the computations that may be performed by pyramidal neurons. In neocortical pyramidal neurons, while dendritic inhibition raised the threshold for eliciting dendritic spikes, somatic inhibition reduced the amplitude of somatically recorded dendritic spikes (Jadi et al., 2012). Similar principles are likely to hold in CA1 pyramidal neurons, with different types of inhibitory interneurons mediating different effects depending on cell-type-specific features of their dendritic inhibition (Bloss et al., 2016).

All these observations suggest that CA1 pyramidal neurons perform computations that involve coincidence detection. The number of excitatory inputs needed to produce an action potential in CA1 pyramidal neurons is likely in the range of ~15–100, based on unitary EPSPs of 0.2–0.7 mV (Magee and Cook, 2000; Otmakhov et al., 1993) and a voltage from V_{rest} to threshold of 10–20 mV. These estimates are based on the size of readily resolvable unitary EPSPs, which likely arise from a relatively small population of strong synapses; most individual synaptic inputs come from significantly weaker synapses, many of which may be undetectable in somatic recordings (Magee and Cook, 2000). Dendritic spikes and inhibition will also influence these estimates. Nevertheless, coincident activation of multiple CA3–CA1 synapses, likely leading to local

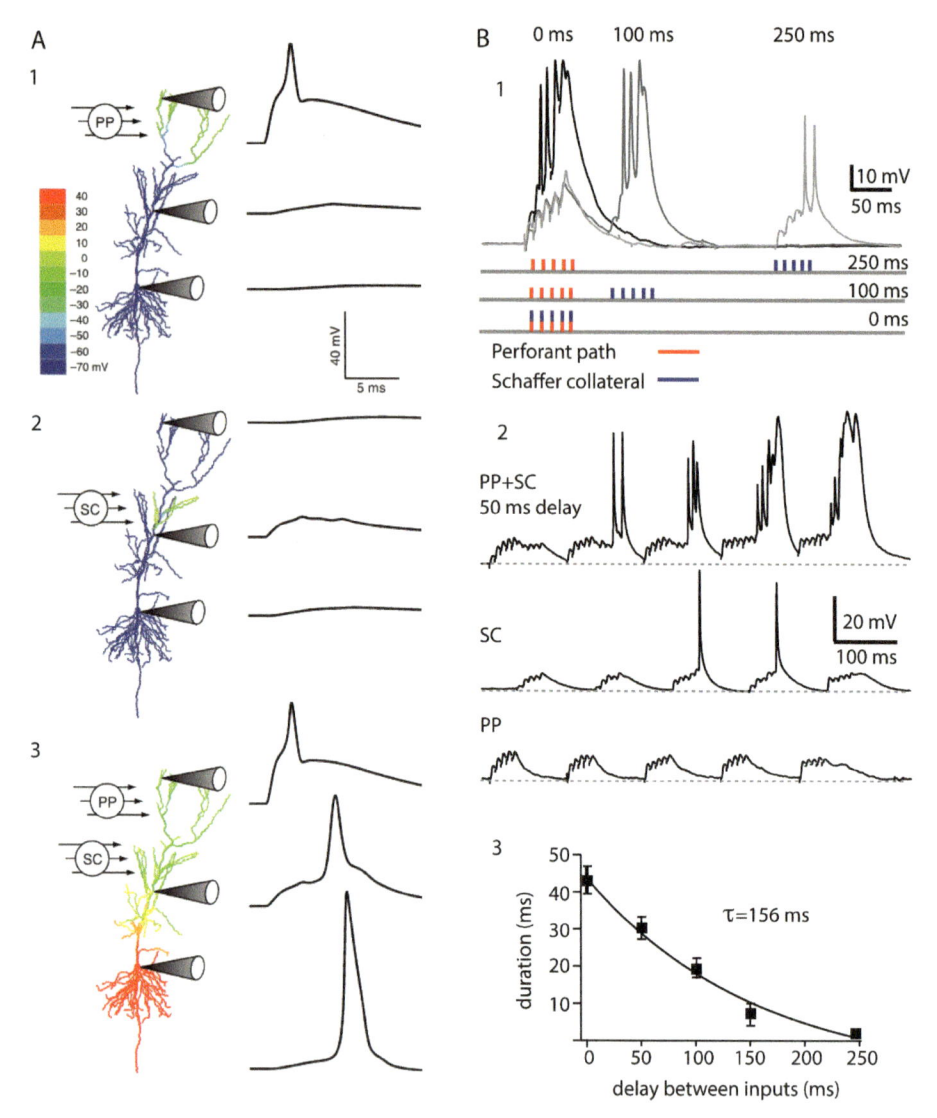

Figure 5.9 Dendritic coincidence detection in CA1 pyramidal neurons. (A) Simulations in a computational model of a CA1 pyramidal neuron showing responses to synaptic stimulation of perforant path (PP), Schaffer collateral (SC), or both inputs combined (panels 1–3). In each panel the V_m response is shown at the soma (bottom trace), the main apical dendrite (middle trace), and a distal apical tuft dendrite (top trace). Color code shows the peak local V_m response to synaptic stimulation. PP stimulation was simulated to evoke a distal dendritic sodium spike, which fails to propagate to the soma and axon. SC stimulation was simulated to produce a modest subthreshold response. Stimulation of both pathways together allows the dendritic sodium spike to elicit an axonal action potential (shown at the soma). (B) Somatic V_m responses in a CA1 pyramidal neuron in response to stimulation of PP, with or without stimulation of SC with varying delay. Panel 1: with PP-SC delays of 250, 100, or 0 ms, showing plateau potentials at 100 ms and 0 ms delay. Panel 2: Stimulation of PP + SC (top, 50 ms delay), SC alone (middle), or PP alone (bottom). Only coincident stimulation produces plateau potentials, which are strongest toward the end of a train of repeated PP + SC stimuli. Panel 3: Duration of the plateau potential as a function of the delay between PP and SC stimuli. (Sources: (A) Jarsky et al., 2005; (B) Takahashi and Magee, 2009.)

spikes in one or more branches, is certainly necessary to drive action potential firing. Coincident activation of synapses from CA3 axons and EC axons synapses together can also drive dendritic calcium spikes and plateau potentials (Jarsky et al., 2005; Takahashi and Magee, 2009), which can drive both action potential bursting and robust synaptic plasticity.

5.5.8 Neuromodulation

Neuromodulation strongly influences action potential firing and other aspects of CA1 pyramidal neuron function. Early electrophysiological studies of the CA1 region, using field potential recordings and intracellular recordings, were among the first to show that several modulatory neurotransmitters (e.g., histamine, dopamine, serotonin, norepinephrine, acetylcholine) could modify

the functional properties of mammalian neurons and their synaptic inputs (Andrade and Nicoll, 1987; Benardo and Prince, 1982a, 1982b; Cole and Nicoll, 1983, 1984; Haas and Greene, 1984, 1986; Hasselmo and Schnell, 1994; Madison and Nicoll, 1982; Otmakhova and Lisman, 1999; Ropert, 1988). These effects are mediated by neurotransmitters acting on G-protein-coupled receptors (GPCRs), which in turn mobilize intracellular signal-transduction pathways that ultimately modulate the activity of voltage- and neurotransmitter-gated ion channels as well as synaptic release machinery. Myriad studies have used hippocampal neurons (in slices or dissociated culture) to study the underlying molecular mechanisms in detail. We do not cover these studies here. Rather, we provide some examples of studies revealing how neuromodulation may shape the computational properties of CA1 pyramidal neurons.

5.5.8.1 Cholinergic modulation

Of the various neuromodulators influencing the function of CA1 pyramidal neurons, the best understood are the effects of ACh. In running animals, ACh is released from the terminals of axons from the medial septum, which innervate the hippocampus extensively. This results in a plethora of effects on cellular excitability, synaptic transmission, and synaptic plasticity in many cell types, including CA1 pyramidal neurons. Importantly, cholinergic modulation is necessary for the theta oscillations and place-coding properties observed in CA1 pyramidal neurons. In resting or sleeping animals, reduced cholinergic modulation is associated with a shift in the local field potential from theta oscillations to LIA and SIA, including SWRs (Hasselmo and McGaughy, 2004; Hulse et al., 2017; Hunt et al., 2018; Jarosiewicz et al., 2002; Kay and Frank, 2019). The effects of ACh on network and cellular activity in behaving animals is discussed in greater detail in Chapter 11. Here we review some key findings related to the effects of cholinergic modulation in CA1 pyramidal neurons, which has been studied mostly in slices (Dannenberg et al., 2017).

The effects of ACh on CA1 pyramidal neurons is mediated primarily by activation of the M1 type of muscarinic acetylcholine receptors (mAChRs) (Dannenberg et al., 2017). Early studies demonstrated that mAChR activation produced a small depolarization as well as reduction of spike-frequency accommodation, which was caused by modulation of the so-called M-current (Cole and Nicoll, 1984) and voltage- and calcium-activated potassium channels responsible for gradual hyperpolarizing effects such as the medium and slow AHP (Madison and Nicoll, 1984; Sahu and Turner, 2021). Yet another effect of mAChR activation is to enhance action potential backpropagation and dendritic calcium entry during trains of action potentials (Egorov et al., 1999; Hoffman and Johnston, 1999; Tsubokawa and Ross, 1997). Crucially, modulation of dendritic excitability by mAChRs can also be localized to individual dendritic branches, where pairing of mAChR activation with synaptic stimulation leads to branch-specific enhancement of dendritic spiking (Losonczy et al., 2008). The mechanism may complement the effects of neuromodulation on synaptic plasticity, a topic which is covered in depth in Chapter 10.

Cholinergic receptor activation also causes inhibition of excitatory synaptic transmission onto CA1 pyramidal neurons via activation of the M4 type of mAChRs, which reduces the strength of excitatory inputs from CA3 without affecting EC inputs (Dannenberg et al., 2017; Hasselmo and Schnell, 1994). Effects also vary across dendritic domains, with the effects on inhibition of SC excitation greater for synapses on mid-apical dendrites compared with basal or more distal apical dendrites (Leung and Péloquin, 2010).

5.5.8.2 Synergistic modulation by activation of multiple types of GPCRs

Some effects of cholinergic modulation on the excitability of CA1 pyramidal neurons are mimicked by activation of group I mGluRs. Remarkably, these effects are also synergistic, as coapplication of low concentrations of agonists for mAChRs and mGluRs, or synaptic stimulation to activate these receptors more naturally, produces increases in excitability that far exceed the expected effects of activating a proportionally larger number of receptors of either type on its own (Park and Spruston, 2012). In addition, coactivation of mAChRs and mGluRs can induce increases in excitability that are slow to develop and outlast the stimulation period by tens of minutes (Park and Spruston, 2012). The mechanisms of these synergistic and long-lasting effects require further exploration.

5.5.9 Pyramidal neuron properties vary along spatial dimensions of the hippocampus

There is growing evidence for considerable variation within the population of CA1 pyramidal neurons. This variation has been uncovered by studies comparing properties—including intrinsic physiological properties, gene expression, and integration into circuitry—along the three geometrical axes of the hippocampus. These three axes include the dorsal/ventral, proximal/distal, and superficial/deep axes (Cembrowski and Spruston, 2019). Transcriptional profiling using RNA-seq has proven to be a powerful approach for the study of molecular differences between cell types in the brain. Complemented by other approaches, such as in situ hybridization (ISH) and immunohistochemistry (IHC), a wealth of knowledge is beginning to emerge regarding the molecular basis of cellular diversity in the hippocampus. These approaches enable not only identification of cellular diversity but also expression of transgenes used to label or manipulate specific populations of cells to study function.

5.5.9.1 Gene expression

A comprehensive assessment of gene expression in a variety of hippocampal cell types indicated considerable variability between granule cells of the DG, mossy cells of the hilus, and pyramidal cells in CA3 and CA1 (Figure 5.10A) (Cembrowski, Wang, et al., 2016). In addition to differences across classes of cells, considerable differences in gene expression are also observed within cell classes.

In CA1, large differences in gene expression are observed between the dorsal and ventral regions of the hippocampus (Figure 5.10A–C). Specifically, 265 genes exhibited greater than twofold differential expression between CA1 pyramidal neurons in dorsal and ventral hippocampus (Figure 5.10B–C) (Cembrowski, Bachman, et al., 2016), confirming and extending the list of differentially expressed genes identified using in situ hybridization (ISH) (Dong et al., 2009).

Interestingly, analysis of the dorsal/ventral differences in gene expression in CA1 indicate that these differences occur along gradients, rather than reflecting discrete cell populations at different locations (Figure 5.10D). Consistent with this conclusion, a study involving single-cell RNA-seq of several hundred or several thousand hippocampal neurons similarly revealed prominently continuous variation in gene expression (Yao et al., 2021; Zeisel et al., 2015, 2018).

The concept of continuous gradients of gene expression may generalize to at least some other hippocampal areas. Large differences have been observed in gene expression between dorsal and ventral areas of CA3 and DG (Figure 5.10A). Although it is uncertain whether these gradients reflect continuous or discrete transcriptional variability in these regions, a noteworthy finding is that some genes exhibit differential dorsal-ventral expression across multiple cell types (Cembrowski, Wang, et al., 2016). On the other hand, as described later in this chapter, the situation appears to be different in the subiculum, where discrete cell types are observed along the dorsal-ventral axis (Cembrowski, Wang, et al., 2018). Similarly, morphological and physiological analysis of pyramidal neurons in superficial/deep and proximal/distal CA1 is also consistent with discrete variation.

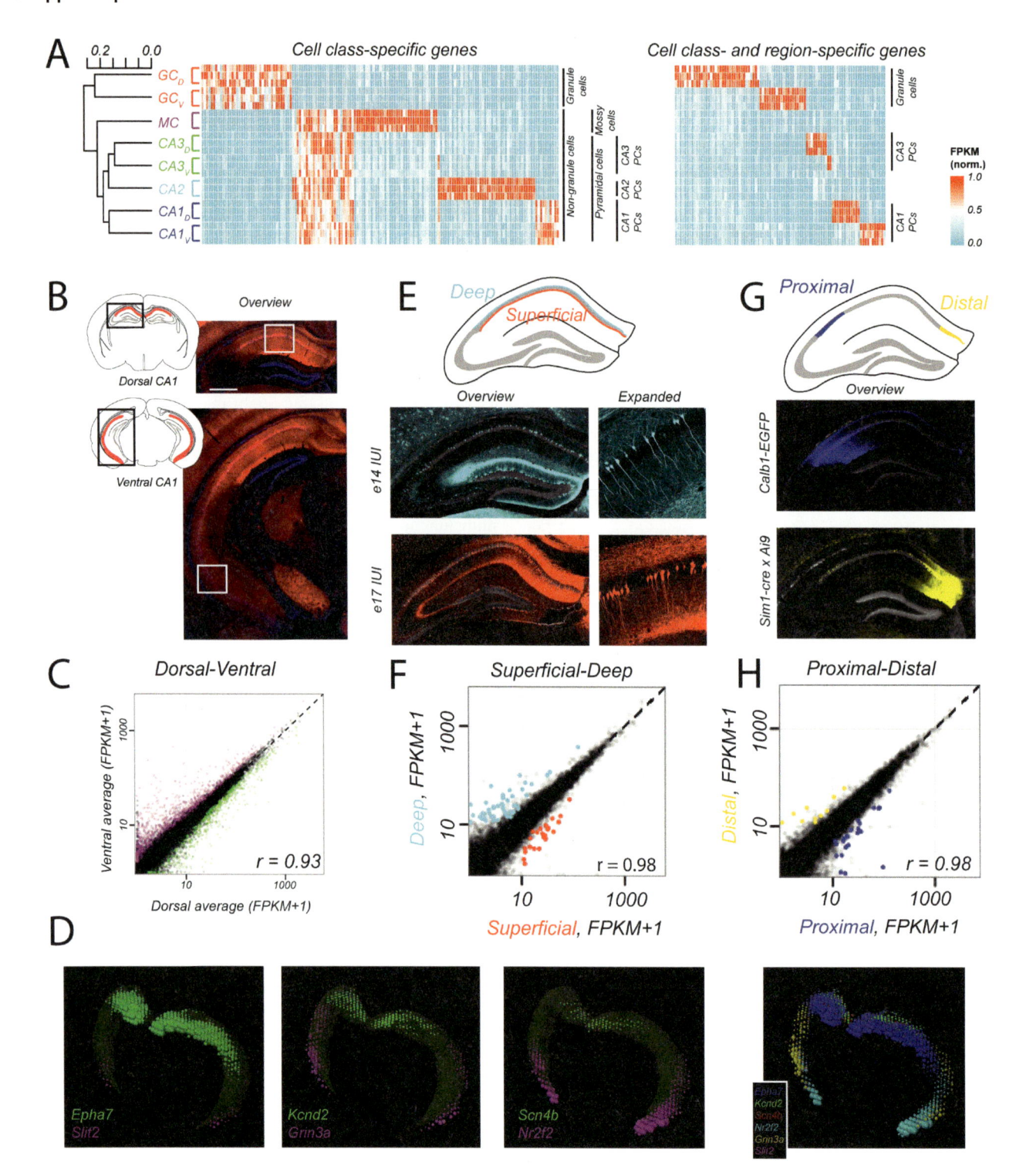

Figure 5.10 Diversity of gene expression in CA1 pyramidal neurons. (A) RNA-seq reveals groups of genes that clearly distinguish between major hippocampal cell classes (left) as well as dorsal-ventral regional differences within cell classes (right). (B) Dissection strategy for isolating labeled CA1 pyramidal cells in dorsal and ventral hippocampus. (C) Differential gene expression between these two groups. (D) Dorsal–ventral gradients of gene expression in CA1 pyramidal neurons. (E) Genetic labeling strategy for distinguishing pyramidal neurons in superficial and deep CA1. (F) Differential gene expression between these two groups. (G) Genetic labeling strategy for distinguishing pyramidal neurons in proximal and distal CA1. (H) Differential gene expression between these two groups. (Sources: (A) Hipposeq: Cembrowski et al., 2016a; (B–H) Cembrowski et al., 2016b.)

Differences in gene expression have also been observed between CA1 pyramidal neurons along other spatial dimensions. Early studies discovered that cells that lie deeper in the CA1 pyramidal cell layer can be distinguished from their more superficial counterparts based on calbindin, which is selectively expressed in superficial cells (Baimbridge et al., 1991; Slomianka et al., 2011). By taking advantage of the developmental gradient along this axis (deep cells are born earlier), RNA-seq determined that calbindin is just one of several dozen genes that are differentially expressed along this axis (Figure10E–F) (Cembrowski, Bachman, et al., 2016). Similarly, a few dozen genes were found to be differentially expressed in proximal/distal CA1 (Figure 5.10G–H) (Cembrowski, Bachman, et al., 2016).

Tools for exploring differences in gene expression along these three axes, as well as in other regions of the hippocampus are available online (Cembrowski, Wang, et al., 2016; Yao et al., 2021; Zeisel et al., 2018). Similarly, a comprehensive online atlas of hippocampal neuron morphologies is also available (Wheeler et al., 2015).

5.5.9.2 Morphology and physiology

Morphological differences have also been described for CA1 pyramidal neurons along the three axes of the hippocampus (Dougherty et al., 2012; Graves et al., 2012; S Lee et al., 2014). In keeping with studies of gene expression, many of the morphological and physiological properties of CA1 pyramidal neurons have been found to vary continuously along the dorsal/ventral axis (Figure 5.11A–B) (Malik et al., 2016). The functional significance of these differences is unclear, but given the impact of structure on function, as described above, the differences are likely to be meaningful.

Neurons in the deep layers of CA1 (i.e., closer to the alveus and ventricle) are more likely to form place cells and to remap across different environments, whereas cells in superficial layers are more likely to exhibit consistent firing properties across environments and they fire more during SWRs (Danielson, Zaremba, et al., 2016; Geiller et al., 2017; Mizuseki et al., 2011; Valero et al., 2015). In proximal CA1 cells (i.e., closer to CA2), where inputs are dominated by MEC, spatial information is greater than in more distal CA1 cells (i.e., closer to subiculum), where input is dominated by LEC (Henriksen et al., 2010). Based on this and related observations, it has been suggested that proximal and distal CA1 process information about the context and content of experiences, respectively (Knierim et al., 2014). Differences in the coding properties of CA1 neurons also exist along the dorsal/ventral axis (Cembrowski, Wang, et al., 2016; M Jung et al., 1994; Keinath et al., 2014). Differences in the excitability of CA1 pyramidal neurons across the superficial/deep axis are discernible (SH Lee et al., 2014).

Along the proximal/distal axis, CA1 pyramidal neurons have been shown to exhibit markedly different burst-firing properties (Jarsky et al., 2008). Analysis of the burst-firing properties and their modulation indicate that there are two distinct types of pyramidal neurons along the proximal/distal axis (Graves et al., 2012). As noted above, some CA1 pyramidal neurons exhibit regular spiking in response to sustained depolarization, while others exhibit bursting (Figure 5.4B). These two types of responses also exhibit interesting dynamics. In response to a train of brief current injections, regular spiking neurons respond initially with single spikes, but later produce bursts (i.e., late bursting). In contrast, bursting neurons respond initially with bursting, followed later by single spikes (i.e., early bursting) (Figure 5.11C). Late bursting cells are predominantly located in proximal CA1, while early bursting cells are predominantly located in distal CA1. These early- and late-bursting firing patterns, which are also observed in subiculum (Moore et al., 2009), correlate with differences in dendritic morphology and modulation by metabotropic glutamate receptors, suggesting the existence of distinct types of CA1 pyramidal neurons (Graves et al., 2012).

These two cell types are also differentially modulated by mAChRs and mGluRs. In late bursting cells, bursting is enhanced by activation of mGluR5 and decreased by activation of mGluR1 and mAChR. In early bursting cells, effects are the opposite. In both cell types, synergistic activation of mAChRs and mGluRs enhances bursting, but activation of mGluRs alone increases/decreases bursting in late/early bursting neurons, respectively. This countermodulation of bursting may regulate the balance between

strong activity in pyramidal neurons in proximal versus distal CA1 (Graves et al., 2012).

5.5.9.3 Axon projections

There is good evidence that different types of CA1 pyramidal neurons are differentially integrated into local and long-range circuitry (see Chapter 7). For example, deep layer pyramidal neurons receive more inhibitory inputs from local parvalbumin-expressing basket cells (PVBCs), whereas these same inhibitory interneurons receive stronger excitation from superficial pyramidal cells, suggesting a form of lateral inhibition of deep-layer cells by superficial cells (SH Lee et al., 2014). Inputs from the amygdala are primarily restricted to the distal (closer to subiculum) and ventral portions of CA1 (Pikkarainen et al., 1999). Inputs from lateral and medial entorhinal cortex (LEC and MEC) differentially innervate CA1 cells along both the superficial/deep and proximal/distal axes, with deep and proximal cells receiving the most input from MEC and superficial and distal cells receiving the most input from LEC (Knierim et al., 2014; Masurkar et al., 2017). LEC and MEC have been shown to carry different types of information about the environment and its content (Knierim et al., 2014). These two forms of information are combined in CA1, giving rise to neuronal receptive field properties that respond to a combination of spatial and contextual features (Eichenbaum, 2017; Henriksen et al., 2010; Wood et al., 2000; X Zhao et al., 2022; X Zhao et al., 2020). However, the distinct connectivity of amygdala, LEC, and MEC projections to cells in different regions of CA1, as well as differential connections with local-circuit interneurons, suggests that distinct CA1 neurons may process different kinds of information.

As CA1 pyramidal neurons constitute a major output of the hippocampus (see Chapter 3), determining how these outputs are assembled at the cellular level is an acute challenge that is amenable to recently developed whole-brain imaging technologies (Economo et al., 2016; Gong et al., 2016; Winnubst et al., 2019). While it is clear that individual cells project to different downstream targets (Arszovszki et al., 2014; Ciocchi et al., 2015; SH Lee et al., 2014), many more single-cell reconstructions of CA1 axon arborizations are needed. Furthermore, additional studies will be needed to link the properties of single-cell axonal projections to the differences in circuit integration, gene expression, morphology, and physiology discussed above.

5.5.9.4 Modular encoding

One prominent theory of hippocampal function is that it serves to bind together the what, where, and when of episodic experiences (Buzsáki and Tingley, 2018; Eichenbaum, 2017; Eichenbaum and Cohen, 2014; Lisman et al., 2017; Olsen et al., 2012; Sugar and Moser, 2019; Whittington et al., 2022), thus potentially linking the concepts of the hippocampal cognitive map and episodic memory (see Chapter 14). Determining how these processes are mediated by distinct types of cells defined by differences in gene expression, morphology, physiology, and circuit integration presents a fundamental challenge for the field.

5.6 CA3 pyramidal neurons

Pyramidal neurons in CA1 receive primary input from pyramidal neurons in area CA3. CA3 differs from CA1 in several ways, one of the most notable being the extensive interconnected network of pyramidal neurons. This has been proposed to be a crucial property that allows CA3 to contribute to associative memory as well as computations such as pattern separation and pattern completion.

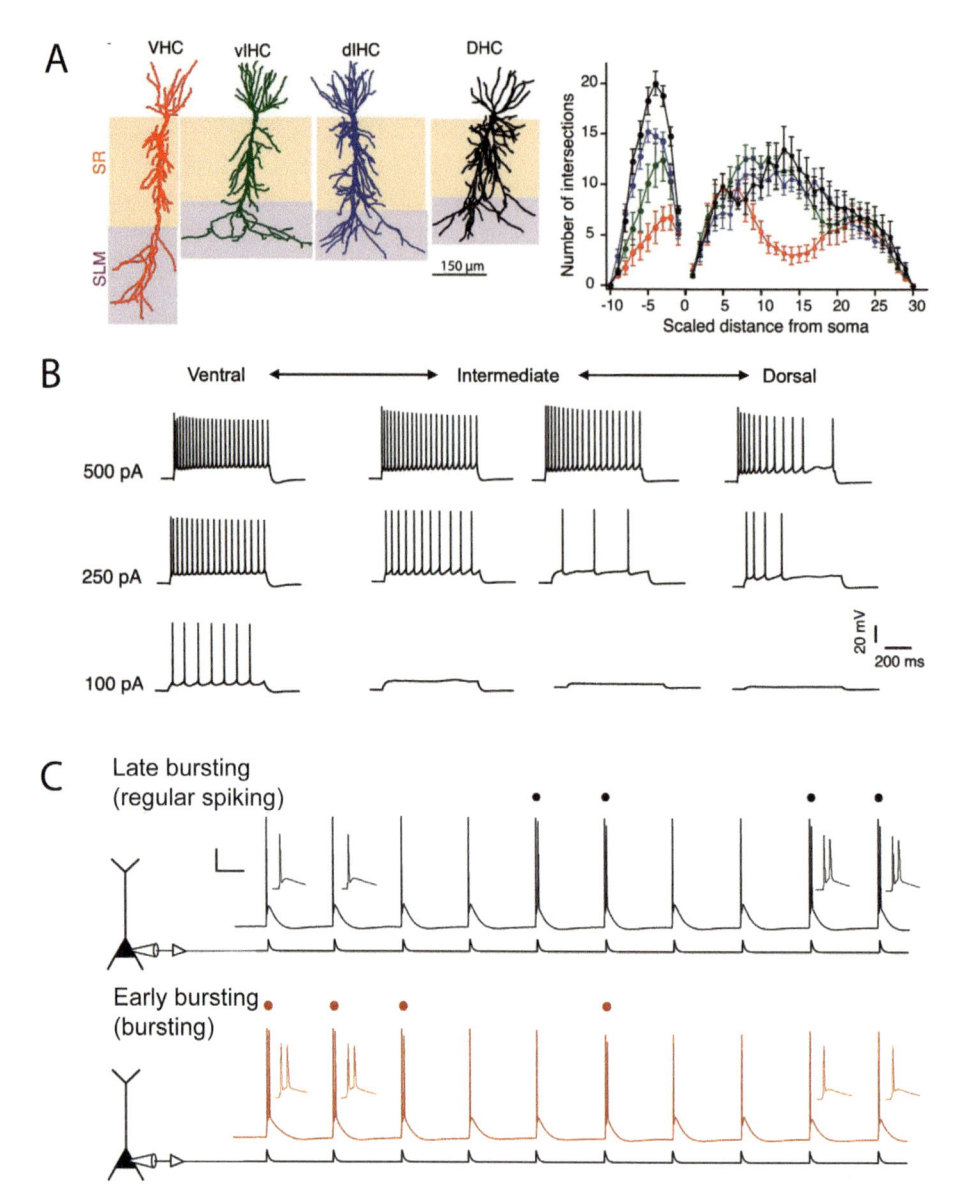

Figure 5.11 Diversity of morphology and physiology of CA1 pyramidal neurons. (A) Reconstructions of dendritic morphology (left) and Sholl plots of dendritic branching (right) for neurons from ventral hippocampus (VHC, red), dorsal hippocampus (DHC, black), and ventral and dorsal intermediate hippocampus (vIHC and dIHC, green and blue). (B) V_m responses to step current injections of different amplitudes (100, 250, 500 pA) from neurons at different positions along the ventral-dorsal axis. (C) A train of short current pulses produces first single spikes and then bursts (indicated by dots) in a regular spiking (or late bursting) neuron. The same stimulus produces first bursts and then single spikes in a bursting (or late spiking) neuron. Insets show the afterdepolarization (ADP) that sometimes drives a second spike to produce a burst. Late bursting (regular spiking) cells are most abundant closer to the CA2/CA1 border. Early bursting (bursting) cells are most abundant near the CA1/subiculum border. (Sources: (A,B) Malik et al., 2016; (C) Graves et al., 2012.)

In the following sections, we examine the unique properties of CA3 pyramidal neurons and their connections.

5.6.1 Distinctive dendritic morphology

Ramón y Cajal first noted the difference in size and shape of the dendritic arbors between areas CA1 and CA2/CA3 in 1904 (Ramón y Cajal, 1911). Subsequently, numerous anatomical studies that have noted several differences between pyramidal neurons in CA3 and CA1 (Figure 5.12A). Lorente de Nó observed that the principal cells in CA3 were heterogeneous along the proximal-distal hippocampal axis, and he subdivided this region into CA3a, CA3b, and CA3c (Lorente de No, 1934). While there are no definable borders between these three subregions, numerous aspects of CA3 morphology, physiology, and function vary gradually as a function of the somatic location along this axis (Figure 5.12B).

5.6.1.1 Dendritic arbors

CA3 pyramidal neurons have 1–3 primary apical dendrites that branch to thick secondary apical dendrites (Figure 5.12A). A fraction of these secondary dendrites branches further into thinner side dendrites that end in the deep upper third of stratum radiatum, nearer the pyramidal layer. The other secondary dendrites extend to the stratum lacunosum-moleculare, branching obliquely several times. The length of dendrites in the molecular layer is larger for distal and intermediate CA3 pyramidal neurons as compared with CA1 (Ishizuka et al., 1995). Both the size of the soma and the length of apical dendrites increase in a gradient along the proximodistal axis. The proximal CA3 cells that are nestled between the blades of the DG have relatively short apical dendrites, the apical dendritic length increases and is maximal in distal CA3 cells adjacent to CA2. These cells have very long and branched dendritic arbors that have numerous terminals in stratum lacunosum-moleculare (Ishizuka et al., 1995). The dendrites in this distal compartment form synapses with axons from layer 2 neurons in the MEC and LEC, which form the perforant path.

5.6.1.2 Thorny excrescences

With the Golgi-staining technique of the time, Ramón y Cajal was readily able to distinguish the presence of unique enlarged dendritic spine-like structures on the proximal dendrites of CA3 pyramidal neurons (Ramón y Cajal, 1911). He gave these structures the name *excrescensias*, and described them as thorn-shaped, predicting that they may serve as a specialized connection with the terminal originating from DG because they colocalize with the mossy fiber axonal projections. Later, in his analysis of the morphological structure of the hippocampus, Lorente de Nó noted that the size and organization of the extended dendritic arbors for CA2 and CA3 pyramidal neurons were indistinguishable and he chose to use the presence of thorny excrescences as a defining feature to differentiate these two regions (Figure 5.12C–D) (Lorente de Nó, 1934). Thorny excrescences are unique dendritic structures that are found on 80%–90% of CA3 pyramidal cells (Gonzales et al., 2001), with a smaller subpopulation of CA3 pyramidal cells receiving no input from the mossy fiber axons (Figure 5.12E) (Hunt et al., 2018). In area CA3, these structures are found in clusters in stratum lucidum. This means that for proximal CA3 neurons located between the blades of the DG, thorny excrescences are located on both the apical and basal dendrites near the soma, as the mossy fibers are located on both sides of the pyramidal layer in this region. For more distal CA3 pyramidal neurons (i.e., closer to CA2), the thorny excrescences are found on the primary apical dendrite running through stratum lucidum ~10–20 μm from the soma (Ishizuka et al., 1995). Thorny excrescences consist of 1–16 large spines that branch from the shaft of the proximal dendrite. A single CA3 neuron can have several dozen of these thorny excrescences (Chicurel and Harris, 1992). Three-dimensional reconstructions of these synapses have revealed that the postsynaptic structure contains mitochondria and microtubules as well as smooth endoplasmic reticulum and ribosomes. These large, branched spine-like structures are surrounded by a single large presynaptic mossy fiber bouton (~4–10 μm diameter) and extend all the way to the CA3 dendritic shaft. These specialized structures contain 15–30 active zones and associated postsynaptic densities (Chicurel and Harris, 1992; Rollenhagen et al., 2007; Wilke et al., 2013). From quantified measures of CA3 pyramidal neuron dendrites, the number of thorny excrescences decreases along the proximal-distal axis in CA3, consistent with changes in input from DG.

5.6.2 Synaptic inputs

CA3 pyramidal neurons receive excitatory synaptic input from several sources. The most prominent and unusual input is the mossy fiber synapse, while the most numerous are the recurrent collaterals between CA3 pyramidal neurons. Several extrahippocampal inputs, mediated by a variety of neurotransmitters, also innervate CA3.

5.6.2.1 Mossy fiber inputs constitute a conditional detonator synapse

The mossy fiber input is poised to provide a strong excitatory drive near the site of action potential generation of CA3 pyramidal cells, with several properties that have earned it the name conditional detonator synapse. At very low frequency, the release probability of this synapse is low due to poor coupling between calcium entry via voltage-activated calcium channels and the action of the vesicle release machinery (Vyleta and Jonas, 2014). Thus, under some circumstances, mossy fiber inputs produce small EPSPs that are far from action potential threshold. However, this synapse is capable of numerous forms of long- and short-term pre- and postsynaptic plasticity that can rapidly transform its synaptic strength. For instance, with short bursts of stimulation, a single granule cell is capable of firing action potentials in numerous CA3 pyramidal cells in vivo (Henze et al., 2002). Mossy fibers also synapse onto interneurons via en passant boutons and through small filopodial extensions from large mossy fiber boutons. The feedforward inhibition recruited by a mossy fibers is considerable: it has been shown that a single mossy fiber forms 5–10 times more synapses onto interneurons in CA3 than pyramidal cells (Acsády et al., 1998). The synaptic properties and plasticity of mossy fiber–interneuron synapses is diverse, as it is dictated by the postsynaptic target (McBain, 2008). However, this recruitment of feedforward inhibition plays an important role in how mossy fiber activity regulates the timing and excitability of the CA3 network. Thus, a combination of synaptic and cellular properties and local networks in area CA3 permit variable and scalable CA3 output in response to different patterns of granule cell input.

There is compelling evidence that mossy fibers can corelease both GABA and glutamate (Muenster-Wandowski et al., 2013). Following the induction of seizures or seizure-like activity, GABA and vesicular transporters are detected in mossy fiber boutons and granule cells, indicating that mossy fibers have the necessary machinery required for mixed neurotransmitter release (Gómez-Lira et al., 2002, 2005; Sloviter et al., 1996). Electron microscopic, histological, and mRNA studies have detected the presence of both excitatory and inhibitory neurotransmitters within single mossy fiber terminals as well as the presence of both postsynaptic glutamate and GABA receptors (Bergersen et al., 2003; Lamas et al., 2001; Zander et al., 2010). Additionally, electron microscopic, immunohistochemical, and single-cell mRNA analysis have shown the expression of vesicular glutamate transporter vGluT, the vesicular GABA transporter VGAT, and the GABA synthesizing enzymes GAD67 and GAD65 (Zander et al., 2010). Data from very young animals showed increased vGluT and vGAT colocalization. Electrophysiological recordings performed from acutely dissociated CA3 pyramidal neurons showed that direct mossy fiber terminal stimulation resulted in mixed neurotransmitter release at early postnatal stages and solely glutamatergic release in adults (Beltrán and Gutiérrez, 2012).

5.6.2.2 Direct input from entorhinal cortex

A major excitatory input to area CA3 comes from layer II of EC, which gives rise to the perforant path. Axons originating from both the MEC and LEC form synapses with CA3 dendrites in the stratum lacunosum-moleculare (Amaral and Witter, 1989; van Groen et al., 2003). The perforant path has been extensively studied in the DG, but less extensively in area CA3 (Witter, 2007a). This input is segregated such that LEC inputs terminate in the most superficial region of stratum lacunosum-moleculare while MEC inputs terminate in the deeper region of stratum lacunosum-moleculare bordering stratum radiatum (Witter, 2007a). Consistent with the distal-proximal gradient of dendritic length in CA3 pyramidal neurons, there is also a large diversity of synaptic strength of the perforant

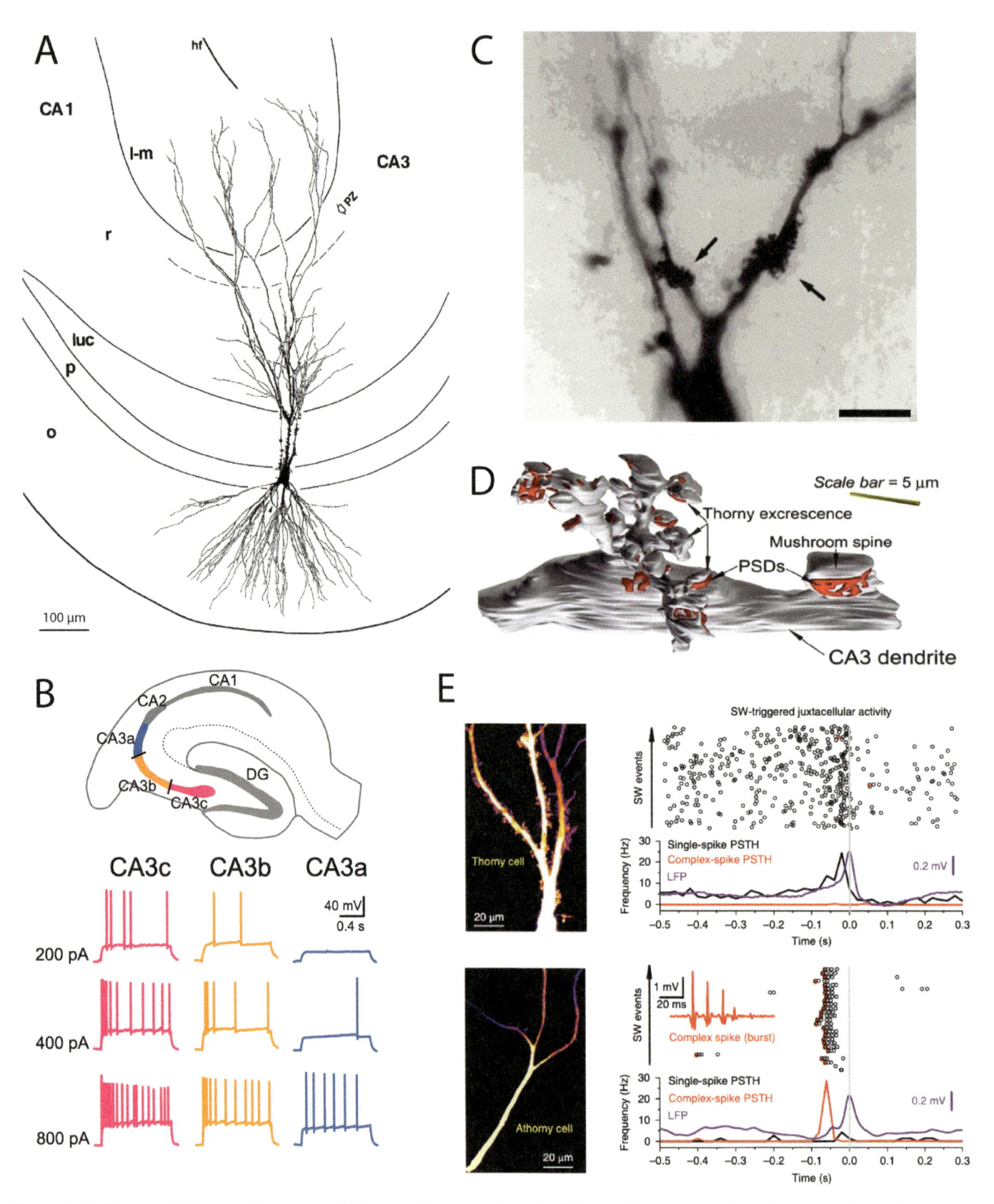

Figure 5.12 Diversity of CA3 pyramidal neurons. (A) The dendritic morphology of a CA3 pyramidal neuron as shown by a camera lucida drawing. Virtually all dendritic side branches in *stratum radiatum* are located in the deeper portions of stratum radiatum and there are few of these branches in the projection zone (PZ) indicated by a dashed line and open arrowhead. Branching of the dendritic tree recommences once the dendrites enter stratum lacunosum-moleculare (1-m). Large numbers of thorny excrescences are seen on the proximal apical dendrites of this neuron; there are also a few typical spines in the region of *stratum lucidum*. The axon of this neuron is marked with an arrowhead. (B) Action potential firing patters of CA3 pyramidal neurons vary along the proximal/distal CA3 axis. Neurons closest to the dentate gyrus, i.e., proximal CA3, have higher firing rates at equivalent current injections as compared to distal CA3 pyramidal neurons. The colors of the example traces correspond to the region of CA3 of the soma. (C) Photomicrographs of a labeled CA3 pyramidal neuron located in the proximal portion of field CA3 in a wholemount of a thick slice. The cell body was located deep within the slice. Clusters of thorny excrescences are visible on the apical branches (arrows). A relatively large cluster is visible on the right

path input. That is, proximal CA3 pyramidal cells have dendrites that do not enter the stratum lacunosum-moleculare, and thus have practically no synaptic inputs from EC. The length of dendrites that enter this distal layer gradually increases with a maximal amount in area CA2 (Ishizuka et al., 1995). Functional measurements in acute hippocampal slices revealed an increase in EPSPs along the proximal-distal gradient with electrical stimulation in stratum lacunosum-moleculare (Sun et al., 2017a).

5.6.2.3 Other synaptic inputs

Area CA3 also receives other inputs from extrahippocampal regions. One important input is from the septal complex, mainly the medial septal nucleus and the diagonal band of Broca (Amaral and Kurz, 1985). These fibers form cholinergic synapses on CA3 pyramidal cells, mostly in stratum oriens. Acetylcholine is known to be a powerful modulator of area CA3 with many diverse roles, acting through both nicotinic and muscarinic receptors. Cholinergic receptor activation leads to a 10–15 mV membrane potential depolarization of CA3 pyramidal neurons that results in phasic action potential firing that can either be lower-frequency bursts of APs or small clusters of APs at theta-frequency (Cobb et al., 1999; J Williams and Kauer, 1997). This AP firing results from changes in membrane excitability via reduced K_v7 conductance (i.e., M-current) following activation of M1-acetylcholine receptors (Vervaeke et al., 2006b). The properties and frequencies of the cholinergically induced burst firing of CA3 pyramidal cells are shaped by both excitatory and inhibitory synaptic transmission (J Williams and Kauer, 1997). Additionally, activation of nicotinic receptors has been shown to enhance glutamatergic transmission of the EC inputs to CA3 and DG (Radcliffe et al., 1999). Interestingly, activation of muscarinic acetylcholine receptors suppresses excitatory transmission at commissural/associational (C/A) inputs in stratum radiatum (Hasselmo et al., 1995; Vogt and Regehr, 2001) but not at cortical inputs (Hasselmo, 2006). In parallel, muscarinic receptor activation decreases neurotransmitter release from parvalbumin-expressing basket cells in area CA3 (Hájos et al., 1998; Szabó et al., 2010). In acute hippocampal slices, network activity resembling gamma oscillations can be induced by application of carbachol (Hájos and Paulsen, 2009; Hájos et al., 2004). In vivo, acetylcholine levels are high during periods of high theta rhythm (Marrosu et al., 1995) and may act to reduce sharp wave ripple activity, as optogenetic excitation of septal cholinergic inputs strongly suppress SWRs (Hunt et al., 2018; Vandecasteele et al., 2014). Lastly, area CA3 receives input from the amygdala (Kemppainen et al., 2002; Pitkänen et al., 2000) as well as the ventral tegmental area (Gasbarri et al., 1994; Swanson, 1982). The contribution of these inputs to CA3 pyramidal neuron physiology and function is currently unexplored.

5.6.3 Recurrent connectivity

A major source of excitatory synaptic input in area CA3 originates from other CA3 cells. This projection, referred to as commissural/associational (C/A) connections allows CA3 to function as an autoassociative network underlying memory storage and recall (Figure 5.13A) (Rolls, 1996). Each CA3 pyramidal neuron has a single myelinated axon that divides into several collaterals in stratum oriens. These fibers then project from the parent neuron to areas CA3 and CA1. It is estimated that at least 30%–70% of the approximately 30,000 to 60,000 synapses made by a CA3 axon terminate on other CA3 neurons (X Li et al., 1994; Wittner et al., 2007), forming a sparsely interconnected network (Figure 5.13B) (Guzman et al., 2016). The rest of the axons form synapses—again, bilaterally—in areas CA1 and CA2 via the Schaffer Collateral (SC) projection.

There is a gradient of axonal projection targets along the proximal-distal CA3 axis. In addition to forming the SC projections to stratum radiatum and stratum oriens of CA1, they also branch and project locally in stratum oriens of CA3. More distal CA3 neurons project more heavily to contra- and ipsilateral CA3 stratum radiatum and stratum oriens, making up the bulk of the C/A system. The most distal CA3 pyramidal neurons adjacent to CA2 have no Schaffer collaterals (Ishizuka et al., 1990) but rather only send extensive recurrent connections to CA3. There also exists an organization to the SC projections along the dorsal/ventral axis of the hippocampus. Ventral and proximal CA3 neurons project more to dorsal and distal CA1, while dorsal and proximal CA3 neurons project along the same dorsal/ventral axis. Ventral distal CA3 cells project in the same transverse plane to proximal CA1, and as the CA3 cells become more dorsal, they project increasingly to the ventral proximal CA1 (see Chapter 3).

Recent technological advances have allowed for complete morphological constructions of individual neurons and their entire axonal projection in the intact mouse brain (Winnubst et al., 2019). In this way, it is possible to examine and directly compare the axonal projections of a dorsal CA3 neuron that has expansive bilateral projections to CA1 and septum to a ventral CA3 neuron that has a very dense axonal arbor that projects locally, contributing to the associational system (Figure 5.13C). Including this and a previously published study (Ropireddy et al., 2011), however, the number of reconstructed axon arborizations is small, making quantitative comparisons impossible. Nevertheless, the available data support the notion that CA3 axons arborize extensively within CA3 and project extensively to CA1, in some cases bilaterally.

5.6.4 Firing properties in vivo

Electrophysiological recordings of CA3 pyramidal neuron activity in vivo before and after changes of the environment result in remapping of the CA3 ensemble activity (I Lee et al., 2004; Leutgeb

---

Figure 5.12 Continued

(arrow), and another large cluster is present in the middle of the tree (arrow). Scale bar = 25 μm. (D) A 3-dimensional reconstruction from 150 serial ultrathin sections of a 20 μm segment of dendrite from a CA3 neuron with thorny excrescences. The thorns show post-synaptic densities (PSD) in red and there is also a single mushroom spine with a PSD (scale bar 5 μm). (E) Cell-type-specific activity patterns during sharp-wave dynamics in vivo. Top left, morphology of a thorny CA3 neuron labeled following juxtacellular recordings. The presence of thorny excrescences is clear along the proximal apical dendritic region. Upper right, Summary of juxtacellular activity for the corresponding thorny CA3 cell from image. Top: SW-triggered raster plot of spiking activity (black circles). Bottom: SW-triggered activity for single spikes (black) and complex spikes (red) relative to the peak of the average SW LFP waveform (violet). Lower left, morphology of an athorny CA3 neuron, labeled following juxtacellular recording. The lack of thorny excrescences is clear along the proximal apical dendritic region. Lower right, Single-cell summary of juxtacellular recording for the corresponding athorny cell from the image. Top: SW-triggered raster plot of spiking activity (black circles). Bottom: SW-triggered activity for single spikes (black) and complex spikes (red) relative to the peak of the average SW LFP waveform (violet). Note the very few complex spikes emitted by the thorny cell while the athorny cell exhibits consistent complex spiking before SW onset. (Sources: (A) Ishizuka et al., 1995; (B) Sun et al., 2017a; (C) Gonzales et al., 2001; (D) https://www.physoc.org/abstracts/dendritic-and-synaptic-remodelling-in-mammalian-hippocampus-following-stress/; (E) Hunt et al., 2018.)

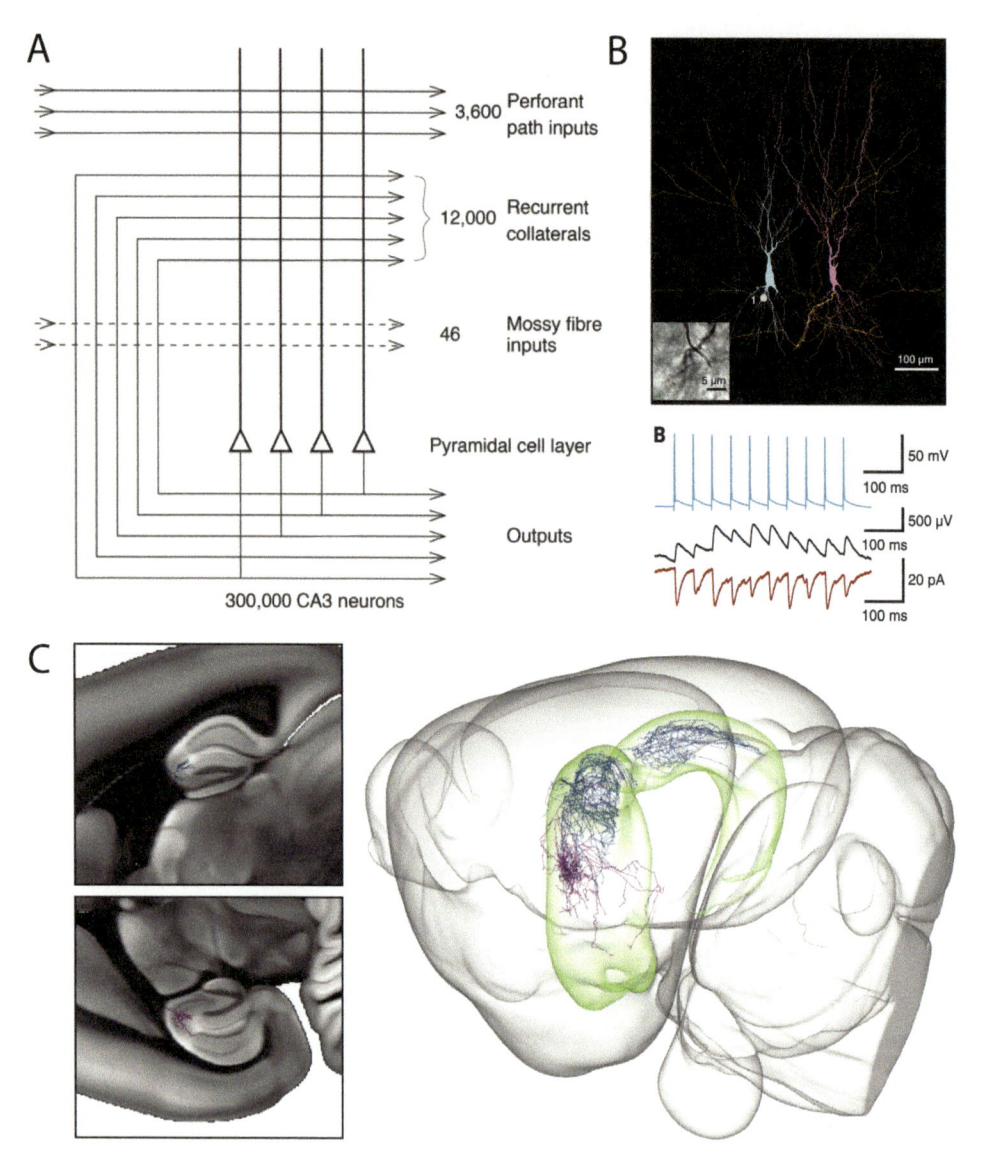

Figure 5.13 Connections of CA3 pyramidal neurons. (A) Illustration of the autoassociative network in CA3. This diagram shows the relative numbers of connections from the perforant path, recurrent collaterals, and mossy fiber inputs onto CA3 pyramidal neurons. (B) Microconnectivity of the CA3 cell network. A small number of morphological contacts and functional release sites per unitary connection. Left: digital reconstruction of a functionally connected CA3–CA3 pair based on the post hoc biocytin labeling. Soma and dendrites of presynaptic cell are shown in magenta, axon of presynaptic cell is in yellow, soma and dendrites of postsynaptic cell are in cyan. Gray dot indicates putative synaptic contact; inset shows light micrograph of the contact. Right: unitary EPSPs and EPSCs from the same morphologically reconstructed neuron. Upper traces represent presynaptic action potentials, center traces average unitary EPSPs, and bottom traces average unitary EPSCs. (C) Illustration of the highly recurrent connectivity of CA3 pyramidal neurons using reconstructed neurons from the MouseLight neuron browser database. Left: Position of reconstructed dendrites from a CA3 neuron in dorsal (left) and ventral (right) hippocampus. Dendrites (black) are overlaid on sagittal sections. Right: Dendrites and axons of the same two CA3 neurons were reconstructed using an automated two-photon block-face imaging microscope in brains from mice that had sparsely labeled populations of neurons. The main panel shows the two extensive axonal arbors or these neurons. The dorsal CA3 neuron (blue) projects extensively through the stratum radiatum of both ipsi- and contralateral CA1. The ventral neuron (magenta) projects only to local neighboring CA3 neurons, contributing to the associational recurrent network of CA3. (Sources: (A) Rolls, 2013; (B) Guzman et al., 2016; (C) http://ml-neuronbrowser. janelia.org ; Winnubst et al., 2019.)

et al., 2007, 2004; Neunuebel and Knierim, 2014; Rolls, 2013). Similarly, calcium imaging of CA3 ensembles show distinct populations of cells that code for dissimilar contexts (Rebola et al., 2017). This property of the CA3 network underlies the region's hallmark pattern-completion role in memory and learning (see Chapter 14).

The cellular physiology underlying CA3 pyramidal neuron function during exploration is emerging. Whole-cell recordings in vivo show that during locomotion and hippocampal theta oscillation, CA3 pyramidal neurons are quite different from CA1 in that they have a hyperpolarized membrane potential and low firing rate (Malezieux

et al., 2020). During quiescence, the membrane potential changes of CA3 pyramidal neurons behave in a very heterogeneous way, with many neurons hyperpolarizing at SWR onset (Kajikawa et al., 2022), contrasting with CA1 depolarization and firing during SWRs.

5.6.5 Diverse properties

There is mounting evidence from extracellular recordings in behaving mice and rats that different CA3 subregions participate in divergent ways during the encoding of spatial and contextual information. The properties of place cells display a functional gradient along the proximodistal axis with proximal CA3 neurons (i.e., closer to DG) playing a role in pattern separation while distal CA3 (i.e., closer to CA2) is more strongly involved with pattern completion (H Lee et al., 2020; H Lee et al., 2015; Lu et al., 2015). In vivo recordings have indicated that the input resistance of CA3 pyramidal cells varies along the proximodistal axis (Kowalski et al., 2016; Turner et al., 1995). Whole-cell recordings in acute hippocampal slices have measured a 3- to 5-fold gradient in input resistance from the proximal to distal CA3 cells, attributable in part to a proximodistal gradient of HCN channel expression, as well as to differences in dendritic morphology (Q Sun et al., 2017). Proximal cells near the DG have a compact somatodendritic compartment and very little to no detectible I_h. Thus, these cells are the most excitable of CA3 pyramidal neurons, with the highest firing rates. In contrast, distal CA3 cells have a lower input resistance and are appreciably less excitable, firing fewer action potentials in response to current step injections.

Consistent with predictions based on morphological data, the synaptic strength of the mossy fiber–CA3 synapse decreases in strength along the proximal-distal axis of CA3 (Q Sun et al., 2017). Neurons closest to DG have two sets of mossy fiber inputs from both the apical and basal stratum lucidum, thus receiving a stronger excitatory drive than CA3a neurons bordering CA2. In contrast, these neurons receive weaker excitation from perforant path than more distal CA3 neurons (Q Sun et al., 2017a), consistent with the gradient of dendritic length and terminals in the molecular layer.

Heterogeneity in the action potential firing properties of CA3 pyramidal cells has also been observed. A hallmark of CA3 activity is the complex spike burst, rapid firing that occurs during sharp wave ripples (Kowalski et al., 2016). In vitro slice studies revealed that a fraction of CA3 pyramidal cells generate bursts of action potentials when stimulated with depolarizing current injection (Wong and Prince, 1978). Deep cells, located closer to stratum oriens, are more likely to undergo this burst firing (Bilkey and Schwartzkroin, 1990). Some of this diversity in CA3 pyramidal neuron physiology may be linked to processes that occur during hippocampal development. It was observed that a fraction of early born CA3 pyramidal neurons localize to the deeper layer of the pyramidal layer and have a more depolarized resting membrane potential. By analyzing spontaneous network activity in the absence of inhibitory transmission, it was found that these early-born cells fire earlier than later-born cells, indicating that a single bursting CA3 pyramidal cell may be able to recruit network activity in the adult hippocampus (Marissal et al., 2012).

There is evidence that dendritic spikes underlie complex spike bursts in CA3 pyramidal neurons, as in CA1 pyramidal neurons. CA3 cells that fire regularly timed action potentials with current injection required paired proximal and distal dendritic depolarization to fire complex spike bursts, while other cells that showed a propensity to fire bursts of action potentials with current injection were found to fire complex bursts with correlated inputs localized to a single dendritic branch (Balind et al., 2019). Burst firing cells were more numerous in distal CA3 pyramidal cells, likely due to the gradient of HCN channels in the proximal-distal CA3 axis, as the amount of I_h correlated with the bursting rate. Interestingly, in proximal CA3 cells there is a high concentration of $K_v2.2$ channels that likely act to regulate bursting dynamics (Balind et al., 2019).

5.6.6 A small population of pyramidal neurons are not innervated by mossy fibers

A separate population of CA3 pyramidal cells with unique morphology and physiological properties has also been described (Figure 5.12E) (Hunt et al., 2018). These cells lack thorny excrescences and do not receive direct excitatory input from mossy fibers. These athorny cells are located in relatively distal CA3 with somata localized to the deep pyramidal layer. They have dendritic arbors with fewer secondary branches terminating in stratum radiatum and more dendritic length in stratum lacunosum-moleculare. These cells fire high-frequency bursts of action potentials (150 Hz) even just above the threshold for AP firing. Furthermore, in vivo juxtacellular recordings of sharp wave LFPs revealed that athorny and thorny CA3 cells fire at different phases of the sharp wave. Additionally, the two cell populations are affected in opposite ways by acetylcholine (ACh). This dual action of ACh may account for the desynchronization of the CA3 network activity observed with increased cholinergic tone. It has also been shown, by in silico modeling, that the athorny CA3 cells may serve as a feedforward sublayer, allowing for pattern completion in the CA3 network (Hunt et al., 2018).

5.6.7 Unique dendritic excitability

CA3 pyramidal neurons integrate excitatory input from the mossy fibers, the perforant path, as well as commissural/associational fibers. As in CA1 pyramidal neurons, CA3 neurons possess excitable dendrites that play a central role in integrating these different inputs and regulating synaptic plasticity. With advances in recordings from CA3 dendrites, several notable differences have been observed in dendritic excitability as compared with CA1 cells. One of the most striking is that action potentials in CA3 pyramidal neurons can backpropagate into the apical dendrite with minimal changes in decay time course, allowing for a very high frequency (up to 100 Hz) feedback signal to the dendrite that allows for optimal spike-timing-dependent plasticity at A/C synapses (S Kim et al., 2012). Dendritic NMDAR-mediated spikes in CA3 apical dendrites play a key role in LTP induction, both for subthreshold synaptic events paired with mossy fiber inputs, as well as when paired with backpropagating action potentials (Brandalise and Gerber, 2014; Brandalise et al., 2016). Dendritic spikes in the apical CA3 dendrites also display unique properties. The probability of spike initiation in dendrites increases to nearly 1 at distances >100 μm from the soma. This is likely due to a combination of passive cable properties as well as a more negatively shifted midpoint potential of the Na_v activation curve in these neurons (S Kim et al., 2012).

The thin basal dendrites of CA3 cells have unique excitability mechanisms. Simultaneous stimulation of several neighboring spines results in a strong supralinear summation of synaptic potentials that is mediated almost entirely by NMDAR activation (Makara and Magee, 2013). Interestingly, the dynamics of the NMDAR-mediated spike decay are regulated by G-protein-coupled inward rectifier potassium (GIRK) channels. The conductance of these channels is linked to numerous G-proteins and is tightly coupled to $GABA_B$ receptors in the dendrites of CA3 neurons (Kulik et al., 2006; Lüscher et al., 1997; Sodickson and Bean, 1996).

Morphologically distinct classes of CA3 pyramidal neurons have two distinct types of dendritic calcium spikes (Magó et al., 2021). The first are slow calcium spikes like those observed in CA1

blockade of inhibitory transmission increased CA3–CA1 transmission by ~2-fold but resulted in a 4- to 5-fold increase in the EPSP in CA2 (Piskorowski and Chevaleyre, 2013). Part of the feedforward inhibition is mediated by PV interneurons that efficiently control EPSP amplitude and action potential firing of CA2 pyramidal neurons (Nasrallah et al., 2019).

5.7.2.4 Entorhinal cortex

CA2 pyramidal cells receive synaptic input from EC at the distal dendritic compartment (Bartesaghi and Gessi, 2004; Chevaleyre and Siegelbaum, 2010; Cui et al., 2013; Hitti and Siegelbaum, 2014; Kohara et al., 2014). A distinguishing aspect of CA2 pyramidal neurons is that distal EC inputs are stronger than in CA1 and CA3 pyramidal neurons. Extracellular recordings in vivo reported that area CA2 is the first CA region to be active in response to stimulation of EC inputs to the hippocampus (Bartesaghi and Gessi, 2004). In slice recordings, mild electrical stimulation of distal cortical inputs is sufficient to make CA2 pyramidal neurons fire action potentials (Chevaleyre and Siegelbaum, 2010). This strong EC connection in area CA2 contrasts with distal CA1 cortical inputs, which have both high levels of feedforward inhibition as well as a large I_h current that prevents strong excitation of CA1 pyramidal neurons (Srinivas et al., 2017). The expression of HCN1 channels that mediates I_h at distal cortical inputs is much lower in stratum lacunosum-moleculare of CA2 compared with CA1, and EPSPs from distal inputs are less affected by block of I_h. Together with the intrinsic properties of CA2 pyramidal neurons, the large dendritic branching in stratum lacunosum-moleculare and the high density of spines in these dendrites provide efficient anatomical grounds for strong excitation by EC inputs (Srinivas et al., 2017).

5.7.3 Axon morphology and synaptic targets

CA2 pyramidal neurons project widely to intra- and extrahippocampal areas. Initially, unilateral injection of dye or AAV-GFP into area CA2 revealed ipsilateral and contralateral projections to areas CA1, CA2, and CA3 (Cui et al., 2013; Tamamaki et al., 1988). Later, the discovery of numerous genes selectively expressed in CA2 pyramidal neurons allowed for the development of transgenic mice that enabled more precise examination of CA2 axonal targets.

CA2 pyramidal neurons project to area CA1 in stratum oriens and stratum radiatum (Tamamaki et al., 1988). Paired whole-cell recordings between CA2 and CA1 pyramidal neurons in acute hippocampal slices directly demonstrated an excitatory monosynaptic connection from CA2 to CA1, which was several-fold stronger than the corresponding CA3 to CA1 connection (Chevaleyre and Siegelbaum, 2010). Multiple transgenic mouse lines have been shown to achieve selective expression in CA2 pyramidal neurons, thus allowing reporter or effector proteins to be selectively expressed in CA2. Axons identified in this way were shown to project to both the CA1 and CA3 subfields (Boehringer et al., 2017; Hitti and Siegelbaum, 2014). Further examination of the CA2 to CA1 projections showed that dorsal CA2 pyramidal neurons project to ventral proximal CA1 cells and the subiculum (Meira et al., 2018). Optogenetic experiments revealed that CA2 pyramidal neurons have a differential excitatory drive along the radial CA1 axis, providing the strongest excitation onto deep-layer CA1 pyramidal neurons (Kohara et al., 2014). CA2 pyramidal neurons were also shown to engage more feedforward inhibition onto deep CA1

pyramidal neurons than superficial pyramidal neurons (Nasrallah et al., 2019). A significant fraction of this inhibition is sensitive to the mu-opioid receptor agonist DAMGO, indicating that it is primarily mediated by PV interneurons. This is interesting, as deep CA1 pyramidal neurons receive more transmission from PV interneurons, and deep and superficial CA1 pyramidal neurons project to different cortical and limbic regions (SH Lee et al., 2014). It is currently unknown whether this scenario is also true for deep and superficial CA2 pyramidal neurons. CA2 pyramidal neurons also project to area CA3. Optogenetic experiments also showed that while area CA2 elicits direct excitation and feedforward inhibition in CA1 and CA3, the inhibitory drive of CA2 predominates in area CA3 (Boehringer et al., 2017). CA2 pyramidal neurons also project to extrahippocampal structures, such as SuM (Cui et al., 2013) and dorsal lateral septum (Cui et al., 2013; Leroy et al., 2018). In summary, by projecting to every CA subfield, CA2 pyramidal neurons are poised to act on the entire hippocampal network, as well as directly influencing other brain regions.

5.7.4 Resting potential and action potential firing properties

In addition to differences in morphology and synaptic inputs and outputs, the resting and active properties of CA2 cells are distinct from those of their neighbors in CA3 and CA1.

5.7.4.1 Resting membrane potential

In comparison to CA1 pyramidal neurons, it has been consistently reported that the resting membrane potential, V_{rest}, of CA2 pyramidal neurons is more hyperpolarized, with values ranging from -76 mV to -74 mV (Chevaleyre and Siegelbaum, 2010; Piskorowski et al., 2016; Robert et al., 2020; Srinivas et al., 2017; Q Sun et al., 2014, 2017; M Zhao et al., 2007). The mechanism allowing this relatively more hyperpolarized resting membrane potential is that CA2 pyramidal neurons express high levels of the two-pore leak potassium channel, TREK (Talley et al., 2001), which contributes to a lower input resistance (R_N) than both CA1 and CA3 pyramidal neurons (Chevaleyre and Siegelbaum, 2010; Piskorowski et al., 2016; Srinivas et al., 2017).

5.7.4.2 Action potential firing properties

The action potential firing properties of CA2 pyramidal neurons make them readily distinguishable from their neighbors in CA1. Given the much lower R_N, larger current injections are required to evoke action potential firing. The firing threshold is approximately -45 mV, with action potentials lacking the large slow AHP of CA1 pyramidal neurons (Antonio et al., 2014; Chevaleyre and Siegelbaum, 2010; Robert et al., 2020; Q Sun et al., 2017). The action potential firing frequency is also generally slower and shows less adaptation than areas CA1 and CA3. In CA1 pyramidal neurons the voltage-gated potassium channel K_v2 contributes significantly to shape their firing pattern (Liu and Bean, 2014), but it is largely absent in area CA2 (Palacio et al., 2017) representing one of the many molecular differences that may shape the specific firing properties of CA2 pyramidal neurons (Dudek et al., 2016).

5.7.4.3 Neuromodulation

While pyramidal neurons are generally silent under basal conditions in acute brain slices, spontaneous action potential firing can be triggered by neuromodulator application. For example, activation of oxytocinergic or cholinergic receptors depolarizes CA2 pyramidal neurons and induces occasional bursting activity (Robert et al., 2020; Tirko et al., 2018). The initial depolarization of the membrane potential involves the activation of the M-current by oxytocinergic and muscarinic receptors. While these bursts can be shaped by synaptic transmission, they can also occur without glutamatergic or GABAergic transmission (Robert et al., 2020).

5.7.4.4 Firing properties in vivo

There are several reports indicating that certain pyramidal neurons in area CA2/CA3a have unusual action potential firing properties in vivo. For individual CA2 neurons within place fields, the temporal firing patterns and theta modulation is comparable to CA1 and CA3 (Martig and Mizumori, 2011). However, when comparing CA2 pyramidal neuron firing activity during repeated visits to the same environment over several hours, major differences emerge. Instead of coding for environmental features or differences between environments, as is the case for CA1 and CA3, CA2 neurons alter their spatial firing pattern rapidly over time, indicating the firing patterns of these cells may not represent space like other hippocampal subfields (Mankin et al., 2015). Extracellular recordings during behavior have reported that around a third of CA2 pyramidal neurons, called N units, are not positively modulated during SWRs (Kay et al., 2016). In contrast to classical place cells that are activated when the animal is moving, N units are activated during periods of sleep or immobility and might thus encode a representation of space when the animal is stationary. There is evidence that activity of CA2 pyramidal neurons may play a role in the initiation of some SWRs (Oliva et al., 2016a). Some pyramidal neurons, called ramping cells, which are mostly located in the deep pyramidal layer, display an increase in their firing hundreds of milliseconds before initiation of the SWR. This is followed by a rapid increase in firing in superficial CA2 pyramidal neurons, called phasic cells, an activity associated with SWR that precedes the increase in activity in CA3 and then CA1.

Lastly, in vivo extracellular recordings in areas CA3 and CA2 have revealed that the probability of neurons firing in rapid spike-bursts increases along the CA2/CA3 proximodistal axis, with the probability being highest in CA2 (Oliva et al., 2016b). Furthermore, using juxtacellular recordings of CA2 and CA3 pyramidal neurons in vivo, the propensity to burst correlates with those cells that have the greatest fraction of their distal dendritic branches in stratum lacunosum-moleculare (L Ding et al., 2020). At the CA2/CA3a border region, there is a heterogeneous mix of cell types that can be challenging to identify as either CA2 or CA3 based on a fixed set of morphological or molecular criteria. Nonetheless, the unique contribution of this region to sharp waves and burst firing is becoming more evident.

5.7.5 Dendritic membrane properties

The passive membrane properties of dendrites combined with their morphology and branching location can strongly influence the propagation and integration of synaptic potentials along their dendritic arbor. This is particularly relevant for area CA2, as the pyramidal neurons in this region receive exceptionally strong synaptic drive from cortical inputs located at very distal dendrites. Using both modeling and direct recording techniques, distal synaptic inputs have been shown to efficiently propagate throughout CA2 pyramidal neuron dendrites (Srinivas et al., 2017). Furthermore, CA2 pyramidal neurons have active properties that further enable distal

inputs to drive action potential firing. The presence of dendritic spikes in CA2 in response to cortical input stimulation was first observed with in vivo recordings (Bartesaghi and Gessi, 2004). Dual recording of CA2 pyramidal neuron soma and dendrites in slices showed that stimulation of cortical axons resulted in the activation of sodium spikelets in distal dendrites. These sodium spikelets contribute to an efficient coupling between distal input and CA2 pyramidal neurons, where they were far more likely to elicit spikes than in neighboring CA1 pyramidal neurons (Q Sun et al., 2014).

5.7.6 Unique molecular composition, calcium-buffering proteins, and signaling cascades

Nearly 70 years after area CA2 was first identified, transcriptional profiling microarray experiments revealed the existence of several different proteins that could effectively demarcate the borders between area CA3, CA2, and CA1 (Figure 5.15A) (X Zhao et al., 2001). An extension of this work further defined the CA2 boundaries along the dorsal and ventral hippocampal axis (Lein et al., 2005). Since then, there is a growing list of unique proteins with neuronal relevance that are enriched in CA2 (Dudek et al., 2016). Furthermore, RNA-seq studies, in combination with in situ information from the Allen Brain Atlas (ABA), have provided a wealth of information about the functional molecular composition of the hippocampal subfields (Figure 5.15B) (Cembrowski, Wang, et al., 2016).

Another characteristic concerning the molecular composition of area CA2 is the unusual nature of the extracellular matrix (Figure 5.15C). In this region, there exists an exceptionally dense perineuronal net (PNN) (Celio, 1993; Seeger et al., 1994; Yamamoto et al., 1988). In contrast to CA1 and CA3, the PNN in area CA2 clearly enmeshes interneurons, pyramidal neurons, and astrocytic processes (Brückner et al., 2003; Yamamoto et al., 1988). Markers for PNN components aggrecan and neurocan are expressed in CA2 pyramidal neurons, are associated with glutamatergic synapses, and have been proposed to regulate synaptic plasticity of pyramidal neurons (Carstens et al., 2016) and inhibitory synapses (Domínguez et al., 2019). It is likely that this matrix is playing multiple roles in area CA2, although its specific roles are yet to be established.

5.7.7 Synaptic plasticity

As knowledge of the molecular composition of CA2 has facilitated studies of this area, studies of phenomena such as LTP have begun to paint a picture of interesting differences from plasticity in other hippocampal areas.

5.7.7.1 Reluctant LTP at Schaffer collateral synapses in CA2

One of the most remarkable cellular properties that differentiates CA2 pyramidal cells from CA1 and CA3 is the lack of activity-evoked postsynaptic LTP at SC synapses (Figure 5.16). Stimulation protocols frequently used to evoke robust LTP in area CA1, such as high-frequency stimulation or a pre/postsynaptic pairing-protocol, fail to induce LTP in area CA2 (Chevaleyre and Siegelbaum, 2010; M Zhao et al., 2007). This unusual phenomenon may be attributable to several factors acting in parallel. First, differences in calcium buffering in CA2 pyramidal neuron dendritic spines were revealed by imaging experiments in acute hippocampal slices, showing much lower calcium transients triggered by electrical stimulation. Second, increasing intracellular calcium concentration as well as preventing calcium extrusion in CA2 pyramidal

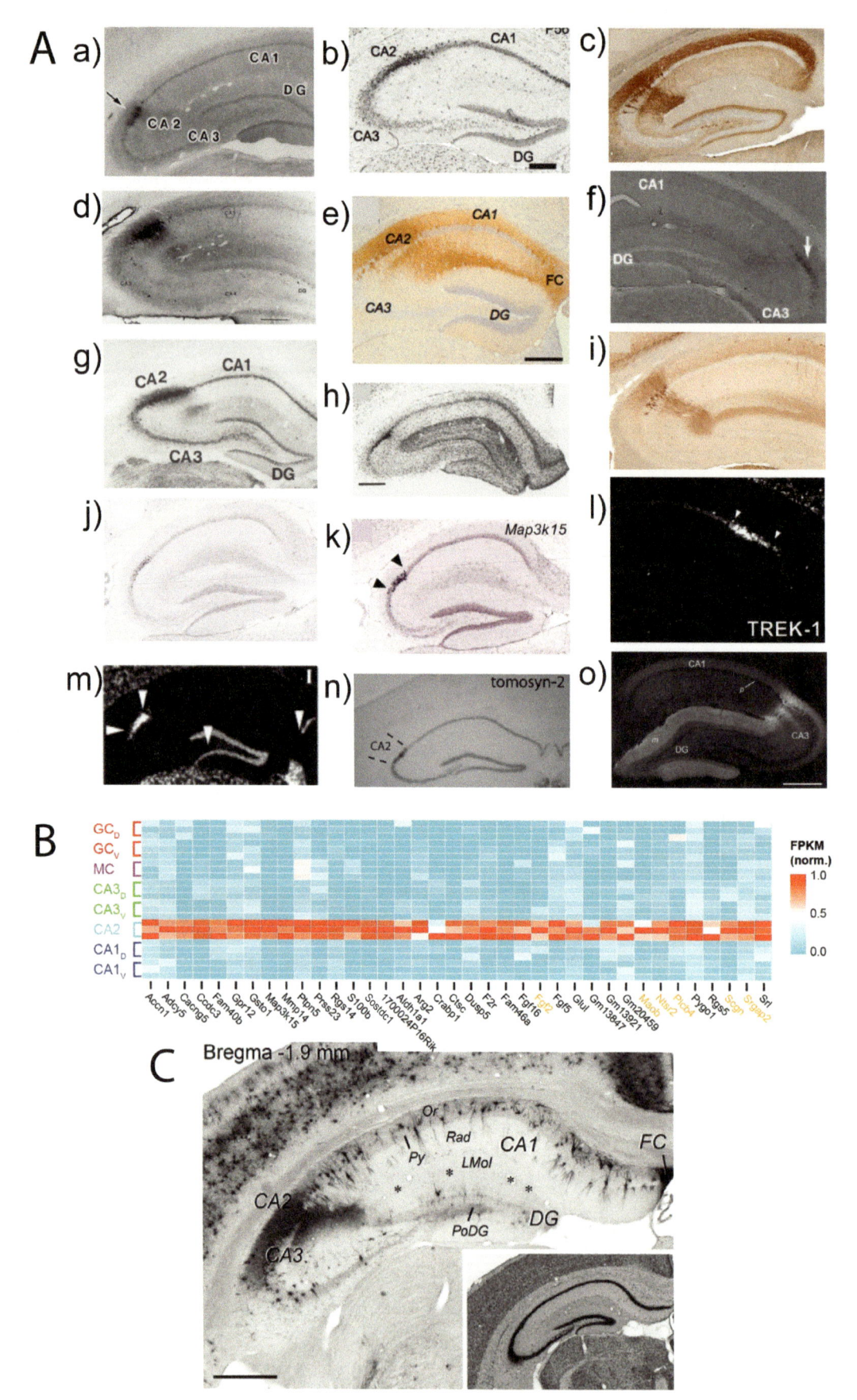

Figure 5.15 Molecular markers in CA2 pyramidal neurons. (A) A series of examples of proteins that are enriched or uniquely expressed in hippocampal area CA2. (a) Adenosine A1 Receptor (Ochiishi et al., 1999), (b) Adenylate cyclase 5 (Visel et al., 2006), (c) Amigo2 (GENSAT Brain Atlas of gene expression in EGFP Transgenic Mice. http://www.gensat.org (2003)). (d) mGluR4 (Phillips et al., 1997), (e) RGS-14 (Lee et al., 2010), (f) Striatal Enriched Protein Tyrosine phosphatase (STEP) (Venkitaramani et al., 2009), (g) Epidermal growth factor receptor (Tucker et al., 1993), (h) basic fibroblast growth factor (bFGF) (T Williams et al., 1996), (i) Cacng5 (GENSAT Brain Atlas of gene expression in EGFP Transgenic Mice. http://www.gensat.org (2003), (j) vasopressin 1b receptor (Young et al., 2006), (k) Map3k15 (Lein et al., 2007), (l) Two-pore domain potassium channel, TREK-1 (Talley et al., 2001), (m) Purkinje cell protein 4 (Lein et al., 2005), (n) Tomosyn-2 (Groffen et al., 2005), (o) Alpha actinin-2 (Wyszynski et al., 1998). (B) Heat map of replicate FPKM values for novel CA2 marker genes identified by RNA-seq. Orange names indicate genes with previously characterized neuronal relevance. (C) Extracellular matrix labeled by W. floribunda agglutinin staining reveals a highly unusual density of the perineuronal net in CA2 pyramidal cells and interneurons. Scale bar = 500 μm, inset shows Nissl-stain of the same coronal section. (Sources: (A) as listed above; (B) Cembrowski et al., 2016a; (C) Brückner et al., 2003.)

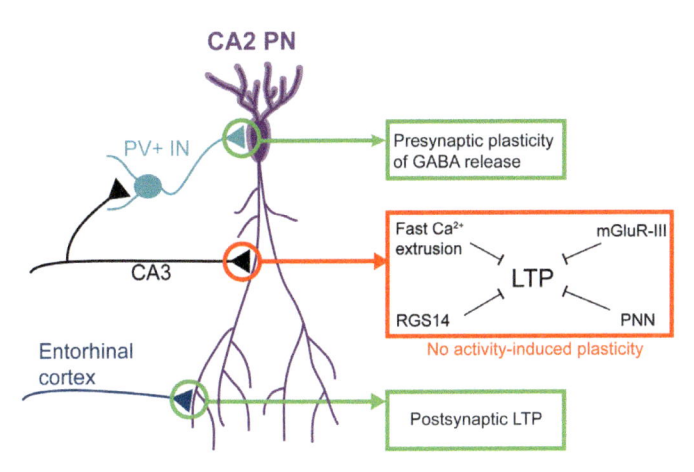

Figure 5.16 Synaptic plasticity at excitatory and inhibitory synapses onto CA2 pyramidal neurons. One of the main peculiarities of synaptic plasticity in area CA2 is that excitatory inputs from CA3 PN do not express activity-induced long-term potentiation (LTP). The machinery required for LTP induction is present, however the plasticity is prevented in basal conditions by a fast calcium extrusion, the regulatory G protein signaling protein (RGS14), mGluR-III, and the perineuronal net (PNN). In contrast to CA3–CA2 synapses, cortical inputs to CA2 PN do express LTP. Activation of oxytocin (OXT) receptors facilitate LTP induction with a weak tetanus and activation of neurokynin (NK1) receptors contributes to synaptic tagging/capture phenomena. Inhibitory transmission from parvalbumin-expressing (PV+) interneurons express iLTD mediated by activation of delta opioid receptors (DORs). The induction of this plasticity requires activation of the ErbB4 receptor by Neuregulin 1 (NRG1), a signaling maintained by PNN integrity.

neurons could enable NMDAR-dependent LTP at the SC-CA2 synapse (Simons et al., 2009). Third, CA2 pyramidal neurons are enriched in the signaling protein regulator of G-protein signaling 14 (RGS14), which acts to suppress postsynaptic LTP. RGS proteins play an important part in GPCR signaling pathways, and RGS14 is a scaffolding protein that links G-protein and mitogen-activated protein (MAP) kinase signaling cascades. Whole-cell recordings performed in hippocampal slices from RGS14 knockout (KO) mice revealed a nascent postsynaptic LTP following HFS stimulation. This LTP was similar to canonical LTP observed in area CA1, as it was prevented by blockade of NMDARs or inhibition of CaMK (Evans et al., 2018) and the ERK/MAP kinase pathways (SE Lee et al., 2010). Postsynaptic LTP at SC-CA2 synapses could also be revealed in slices after pharmacological blockade of group III mGluRs (Dasgupta et al., 2020). This LTP was dependent on both NMDAR activation and on the ERK/MAP kinase pathway. Together, these data show that the molecular pathways required for LTP induction are present in CA2 pyramidal neurons, but they are actively silenced by diverse mechanisms preventing LTP induction under baseline conditions.

5.7.7.2 Plasticity of direct inputs from entorhinal cortex

In contrast to SC-CA2 synapses, distal excitatory inputs from EC do display NMDAR-dependent LTP in area CA2. Just as the synaptic drive from distal cortical inputs is stronger in CA2 pyramidal neurons as compared with EC-CA1 synapses, the same tetanic stimulation of distal inputs resulted in larger LTP in area CA2 compared with area CA1 (Chevaleyre and Siegelbaum, 2010). One potential explanation of this observation could be the much lower concentration of HCN channels, which are not enriched in the

distal dendrites of CA2 pyramidal neurons (Srinivas et al., 2017). Oxytocin receptors that are strongly expressed in area CA2 might also contribute to the larger LTP at this synapse, as deletion or block of oxytocin receptors reduced LTP between distal inputs and CA2 pyramidal neurons when a weak tetanus was used, indicating a facilitatory action of these receptors (Lin et al., 2018).

5.7.7.3 Plasticity of inhibitory synapses

Inhibitory transmission in area CA2 is highly plastic. It has been found that GABA release from parvalbumin-expressing interneurons can undergo a long-term depression (LTD) following the activation of delta-opioid receptors (DORs) (Leroy et al., 2017; Piskorowski and Chevaleyre, 2013). An important consequence of this LTD of feedforward inhibition is that it enables CA3 inputs to drive action potential firing in CA2 pyramidal neurons (Nasrallah et al., 2015). This inhibitory plasticity appears to be necessary for normal social memory formation. Pharmacological blockade of DORs (Leroy et al., 2017) or targeted deletion of the DOR gene in area CA2 (Domínguez et al., 2019) in mice resulted in a compromised ability to discriminate between a novel and familiar conspecific.

5.7.8 Neuromodulation

Given that area CA2 receives multiple inputs from extrahippocampal structures including hypothalamic nuclei, it is not surprising that this region also expresses a unique set of receptors and is modulated by many neuromodulators.

5.7.8.1 Oxytocin and vasopressin

Receptors for oxytocin and vasopressin are strongly enriched in area CA2 and exert numerous effects on both synaptic transmission and the intrinsic properties of CA2 pyramidal neurons. Activation of both the oxytocin and the V1b vasopressin receptor induced a large increase in SC-CA2 transmission (Pagani et al., 2014). Oxytocin application was found to both increase excitatory transmission from cortical inputs and decrease GABA transmission onto CA2 pyramidal neurons (Lin et al., 2018). Application of an oxytocin agonist also directly modulated intrinsic properties of CA2 pyramidal neurons, causing the cells to depolarize and display repetitive burst firing (Tirko et al., 2018). Both oxytocin (Lin et al., 2018; Raam et al., 2017) and vasopressin receptors (Smith et al., 2016) in area CA2 have been implicated in regulating cellular processes allowing social memory formation.

5.7.8.2 Acetylcholine

Cholinergic receptors also have a strong effect on synaptic transmission and intrinsic properties of pyramidal neurons in area CA2. The activation of mAChRs by carbachol application decreased synaptic transmission at both SC and cortical inputs (Robert et al., 2020). This effect was mediated by activation of M1 and M3 muscarinic receptors, which caused a decrease in glutamate release. The involvement of M1/M3 receptors has been confirmed in the LTD of glutamatergic inputs mediated by carbachol, although nicotinic receptors might also play a role in the maintenance of the depression (Benoy et al., 2021). Following carbachol application, LTP at both SC- and distal inputs was facilitated (Benoy et al., 2021). Carbachol application strongly modulates the intrinsic properties of CA2 pyramidal neurons, causing a membrane potential depolarization, leading to repetitive burst firing (Robert et al., 2020). Furthermore, activation of nicotinic receptors increases spontaneous EPSPs onto

CA2 pyramidal neurons, an effect likely mediated through an in-direct decrease in GABA transmission (Pimpinella et al., 2021).

5.7.8.3 Adenosine

Excitatory transmission from SC inputs to CA2 pyramidal neurons is also strongly controlled by adenosine A1 receptors, which are highly expressed in area CA2 (Ochiishi et al., 1999). Application of A1 receptors antagonists such as DPCPX or caffeine induced a much larger increase in SC transmission in area CA2 compared with area CA1 (Muñoz and Solís, 2019; Simons et al., 2012). At least part of the increase in transmission likely resulted from an increase in glu-tamate release, and the increased sensitivity of area CA2 to A1 re-ceptor blockade might result from a more efficient coupling of these receptors to their downstream targets (Muñoz and Solís, 2019).

5.8 Dentate gyrus

Granule cells are the principal excitatory cells of the dentate gyrus. They are the most abundant cells in the hippocampus, numbering in the millions in humans, and ~1 million in rodents. Granule cells integrate input from EC and other brain regions and send their output exclusively to hippocampal area CA3. They play a central role in hippocampal memory processes including pattern separation, storage of engrams and grid-to-place code conversion (see Chapter 14).

5.8.1 Granule cell morphology

The morphology of dentate granule cells differs considerably from hippocampal pyramidal cells (Figure 5.17A–B). Granule cells have small round somata (typically ~10x18 μm) that are aligned in the granule cell layer and project a single conical dendritic tree into the molecular layer. Their dendrites branch abundantly near the soma, with numerous small-caliber higher-order dendrites that extend throughout the entire molecular layer to the hippocampal fissure. The majority of the synaptic inputs contact spines within the outer two-thirds of the molecular layer (Amaral et al., 2007). The axon of each granule cell originates from the basal side of the cell, passes through the hilus and into area CA3 via stratum lucidum. A typical granule cell forms 10–15 "giant" mossy fiber boutons in area CA3 (Figure 5.17C). Each CA3 pyramidal neurons receives input from approximately 50 granule cells (see above section of CA3 pyramidal neurons) (Amaral et al., 1990). Collateral axons also branch in the hilus where they form synapses with 11–18 mossy cells. A single granule cell also synapses onto approximately 100 to 150 inter-neurons in area CA3 and the dentate hilus (Acsády et al., 1998).

5.8.2 Excitatory and inhibitory synaptic inputs

Granule cells in the dentate gyrus receive input from multiple sources. The principal excitatory input is from EC. Additional ex-citatory inputs come from the mossy cells of the hilus and several extrahippocampal sources.

5.8.2.1 Entorhinal cortex

Axons from EC innervate the outermost two-thirds of the den-dritic compartment. This input, known as the perforant path, is the major input to the dentate gyrus, forming asymmetric synapses with nearly 85% of the spines on dentate granule cells (Amaral et al., 2007; Hjorth-Simonsen and Jeune, 1972). The most distal dendritic

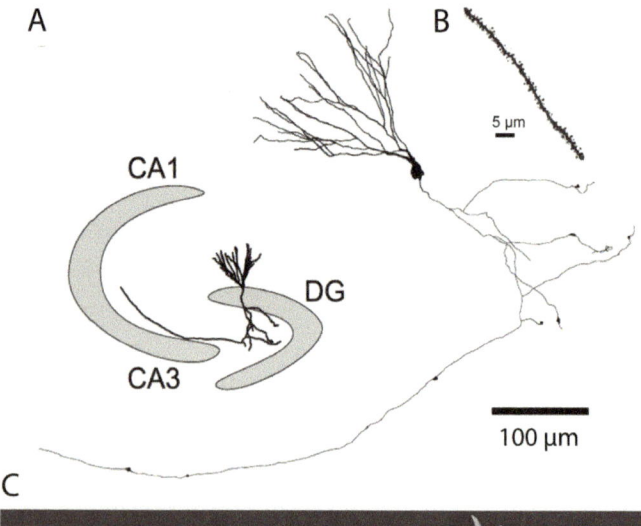

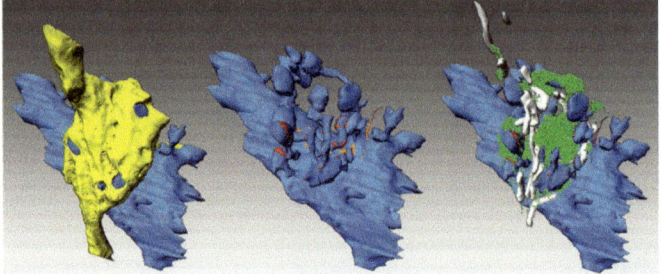

Figure 5.17 Morphology of dentate gyrus granule cells. (A) Granule cell was filled with biocytin during whole-cell recording and subsequently labeled with FITC–avidin. The inset shows the approximate position of the cell within the hippocampus. DG, Dentate gyrus. (B) A typical spine-bearing dendrite from a different cell at high magnification. (C) Three-dimensional reconstructions of an adult mossy fiber bouton (MFB) and its postsynaptic target dendrite. Left: Volume reconstructions of an en passant mossy fiber bouton (depicted in yellow) and its postsynaptic target dendrite (blue). Note, that the spiny excrescences were almost entirely covered by the nerve terminal. Middle: Distribution of the two membrane specializations, active zones (AZs; in red) and puncta adherentia (PA, regions thought to act in adhesion; in orange) on the postsynaptic target dendrite (blue). Note, that AZs were mainly located on the spiny excrescences, whereas PAs were exclusively found at the dendritic shaft. Right: Organization of the pool of synaptic vesicles (green dots) at an individual MFB. The pool was distributed throughout the entire nerve terminal. Mitochondria (in white) formed either cluster-like arrangements or bands associated with the pool of synaptic vesicles (green dots). (Sources: (A, B) Schmidt-Hieber et al., 2007; (C) Rollenhagen and Lübke, 2010.)

region receives input originating from LEC, whereas the medial dendritic region receives input from MEC. Thus, these two in-puts are called the lateral and medial perforant pathways (LPP and MPP). Histological studies have revealed significant differences in the chemical composition of these two pathways. These two inputs can be readily distinguished with the Timm staining method, with very intense heavy metal staining in the LPP, and near absence in the MPP. Furthermore, fibers of the LPP contain enkephalin while the MPP fibers stain readily for dynorphin, CCK, and mGluR2/3 receptors (Fredens et al., 1984; Witter, 2007b). Slice electrophysi-ology studies comparing the properties of the perforant path pro-jection cells have revealed that cells from the MEC and LEC have different intrinsic properties (van der Linden and da Silva, 1998; Wang and Lambert, 2003). For further details, see the description of entorhinal cortex neuron properties in the section 5.12, dedicated to the parahippocampal cortex.

5.8.2.2 Mossy cells (hilus)

Mossy cells provide a significant source of excitatory synaptic input to granule cells of the dentate gyrus. Synapses from mossy cell axons are limited to the inner portions of the molecular layer, thus positioning them to strongly influence action potential firing in dentate granule cells (Buckmaster et al., 1996). However, mossy cells also innervate inhibitory interneurons in the hilus, which in turn inhibit granule cells (Scharfman, 2016).

5.8.2.3 Supramammillary nucleus

Dentate granule cells also receive a hypothalamic input from the SuM. These fibers originate from large calretinin-positive cells and densely innervate the inner molecular layer of the dentate gyrus, contacting both dentate granule cells and interneurons (Haglund et al., 1984; Vertes and McKenna, 2000; Wyss et al., 1979). The SuM innervation to granule cells is highly unusual because the fibers possess both glutamate- and GABA-containing vesicles (Soussi et al., 2010), both of which are released following optogenetic activation of these fibers (Chen et al., 2020; Hashimotodani et al., 2018; Pedersen et al., 2017). While there is evidence that the glutamatergic transmission from this input is critical for modulating spatial memory (Y Li et al., 2020), the contribution of the GABAergic transmission is not yet understood.

5.8.2.4 Neuromodulatory inputs

As in other hippocampal areas, the dentate gyrus receives modulatory input from extrahippocampal areas. These include cholinergic input from MS and the diagonal band of Broca (Amaral and Kurz, 1985), dopamine and noradrenaline from LC (Wagatsuma et al., 2018), dopamine from VTA (Gasbarri et al., 1994), and serotonin from the raphe nuclei (McKenna and Vertes, 2001).

Input from MS and the diagonal band of Broca consists of multiple fiber types. Axons from these regions are sparsely distributed throughout the molecular layer and more densely innervate the polymorphic layer, the inner-third region closest to the granule cell soma. Both GABAergic and cholinergic cells project to the dentate gyrus, making this projection heterogeneous. Interestingly, the GABAergic terminals appear to specifically target interneurons in the dentate gyrus, while the cholinergic terminals form excitatory synapses onto granule cells (Amaral and Kurz, 1985; Swanson et al., 1978).

5.8.3 Granule cells are relatively inexcitable

A defining feature of dentate gyrus granule cells is that they fire sparsely compared with other principal cells in the hippocampus (Figure 5.18A). Electrophysiological and calcium imaging studies have shown that only a small fraction of granule cells fire action potentials in a given environment with a vast majority of cells staying silent (Figure 5.19) (Alme et al., 2010; Danielson, Kaifosh, et al., 2016; Diamantaki et al., 2016; GoodSmith et al., 2017; Hainmueller and Bartos, 2018; Neunuebel and Knierim, 2012; Pilz et al., 2016; Senzai and Buzsáki, 2017; X Zhang et al., 2020).

There are several aspects of granule cell physiology that render them relatively inexcitable, especially compared with hippocampal pyramidal cells. First, granule cells have a hyperpolarized membrane potential, reported to be ~-85 mV (Krueppel et al., 2011; Schmidt-Hieber et al., 2004, 2007). Furthermore, their action

potential threshold is nearly 10 mV more depolarized than that of CA3 pyramidal neurons (Kress et al., 2008; Krueppel et al., 2011). These features result in a large voltage difference that must be surmounted to trigger action potential firing. Furthermore, the frequency-dependent synaptic response properties of granule cells are different from CA1 pyramidal neurons. Granule cells lack a membrane potential resonance, indicating that there is no frequency of input timing that will favor membrane depolarization (Mishra and Narayanan, 2020). Thus, given similar synaptic input, granule cells are much less likely to fire action potentials compared with CA1. Compared with CA1 and CA3 pyramidal neurons, dentate granule cells have fewer excitatory voltage-activated channels in their dendrites and they exhibit strong dendritic voltage attenuation (Figure 5.18B–C) (S Kim et al., 2018; Krueppel et al., 2011; Schmidt-Hieber et al., 2007). Thus, synchronous synaptic inputs summate linearly in dentate granule cells over a wide range of frequencies, with only high-frequency inputs resulting in NMDAR-mediated spikes and nonlinear summation (S Kim et al., 2018). A relatively high K_v to Na_v channel-mediated current ratio imposes a strong distance-dependent attenuation of somatic action potentials, preventing backpropagating action potentials from depolarizing the dendritic compartment (S Kim et al., 2018; Krueppel et al., 2011; Schmidt-Hieber et al., 2007). In addition, an extensive network of GABAergic inhibitory interneurons controls the output and timing of these cells. In particular, the parvalbumin basket cells provide strong inhibition of perisomatic regions of these granule cells, synchronizing network activity during theta and gamma oscillations and sharp wave ripples (Bartos et al., 2002, 2007; Szabo et al., 2017). Taken together, dentate granule cells have numerous properties that allow them to serve as relatively linear integrators of synaptic input, allowing only precisely timed combinations of synaptic events to lead to action potential firing.

This combination of properties and circuitry allow granule cells to serve their unique role in sparse coding and engram formation (see Chapter 14). Intriguingly, the intrinsic excitability of engram granule cells is altered following re-exposure to training cues (Pignatelli et al., 2019). Specifically, dentate gyrus engram cells were labeled during fear conditioning and the next day the animals were exposed to the same contextual cues used for training. Whole-cell recordings of labeled granule cells (i.e., engram cells) revealed a transient increase in membrane resistance and a decrease in rheobase following cue exposure that lasted for about 1 hour. This enhanced excitability of the engram cells was due to a reduction in the $K_{ir}2.1$ conductance induced by synaptic activation of NMDA receptors during re-exposure to the contextual cues (Pignatelli et al., 2019). This phenomenon likely allows for the strengthening of synaptic inputs and synaptic plasticity at the mossy fiber-CA3 synapse even with repeated experience, enabling memory retrieval. These results were supported by whole-cell recordings of granule cells in awake, behaving mice, which found that both active and silent granule cells received spatially tuned input, and that action potential firing of the small subset of cells that fired action potentials was correlated with higher intrinsic excitability (X Zhang et al., 2020).

5.8.4 Semilunar granule cells

At first glance, semilunar granule cells appear to be displaced granule cells with somata in the molecular layer. However, these are a separate population of glutamatergic cells in the dentate gyrus that play an interesting functional role. Originally named

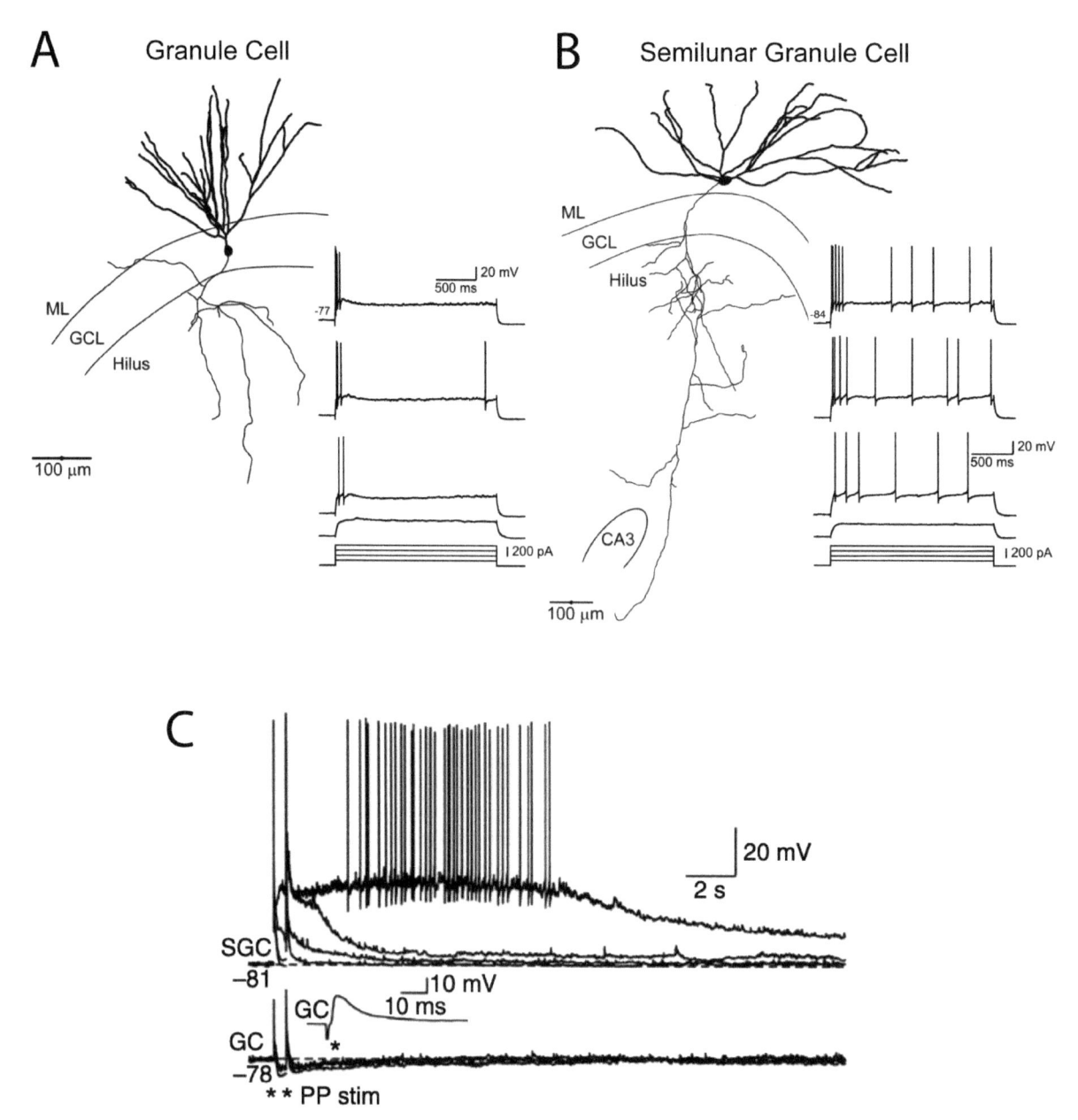

Figure 5.20 Semilunar granule cells in the dentate gyrus.. (A) Illustration of a fully reconstructed granule cell shows the typical location of the somata in the granule cell layer (GCL) and compact dendritic spread in the molecular layer (ML). The axon (mossy fiber, thin line) is seen projecting in the hilus, toward CA3. Inset, membrane voltage traces from a recorded granule cell demonstrating the highly adapting firing pattern in response to several current injection steps. (B) Reconstruction of a biocytin-filled semilunar granule cell shows the location of somata in the ML and demonstrates the wider dendritic span compared with the granule cell in A. Note the high degree of branching of the SGC axon (thin line) in the hilus and projection to CA3. Inset, current-clamp recordings from a semilunar granule cell demonstrating continuous firing during several depolarizing current injection steps. (C) Intracellular responses to graded perforant pathway stimulation in an SGC (top) and granule cell (bottom, not simultaneous with SGC). Monosynaptic granule cell EPSP shown in inset. (Sources: (A, B) Gupta et al., 2012; (C) Larimer and Strowbridge, 2010.)

5.8.5.2 Presynaptic voltage-gated channels

The presynaptic mossy fiber bouton is rich in voltage-gated ion channels. An important consequence of this excitability is that action potentials recorded at the presynaptic bouton are appreciably different than action potentials recorded at the soma. Specifically, the presence of dendrotoxin-sensitive K_v channels with gating kinetics that allow for rapid and complete reset of the membrane potential after action potential firing in mossy fiber boutons, resulting in action potentials that are approximately twice as fast and have a reduced afterdepolarization compared with somatic action potentials (Geiger and Jonas, 2000). While K_v channels shape the repolarizing phase of the action potential, the rising phase is shaped by a very large number of Na_v channels with rapid inactivation kinetics, which amplify the presynaptic action potentials and enhance calcium influx (Engel and Jonas, 2005). Furthermore, recordings at mossy fiber boutons have shown the presence of a K_V7 current that is open at rest, acting as a shunting current to oppose calcium influx through P/Q and N-type channels during and after action potential firing (Martinello et al., 2019).

5.8.6 Mossy fiber function

In vivo experiments have shown that high-frequency firing by a single granule cell can induce firing in CA3 cells (Henze et al., 2002). This observation led to the theory that the MF-CA3 synapse could operate as a conditional detonator, that is, a single granule cell could control the output of a CA3 cell. While a single EPSP or isolated action potential in a mossy fiber is unable to evoke firing (Jonas et al., 1993; S Kim et al., 2012; Mori et al., 2004), there is a remarkable level of facilitation, and a large and prolonged posttetanic potentiation, making the amount of neurotransmitter released at this synapse tightly linked to action potential firing frequency (Salin et al., 1996). This is particularly striking with natural stimulation patterns, such as those observed during granule cell place-cell burst-firing, that can lead to short-term facilitation increasing responses by 4- to 5-fold (Gundlfinger et al., 2010).

5.8.6.1 Properties of presynaptic release

The mossy fiber synapse is one of the few synapses large enough to permit electrophysiological recordings at the presynaptic bouton. Dual recordings at mossy fiber boutons and postsynaptic CA3 pyramidal neurons in the presence of several calcium chelators have demonstrated that coupling between vesicle release and calcium influx is "loose"; that is, release can be evoked even when the distance between the source of Ca^{2+} influx and release machinery is ~100 nm (Vyleta and Jonas, 2014). This coupling can explain both the very low release probability with a single action potential, as well as the striking facilitation at this synapse, because it is likely that the endogenous Ca^{2+} buffers in the terminal can be saturated with high-frequency events, allowing more neurotransmitter release.

One of the more striking findings is that subthreshold dendritic events in granule cells can play a role in information processing by affecting vesicle release from mossy fiber terminals. Specifically, stimulation of perforant path inputs led to forward-propagated excitatory presynaptic potentials at the mossy fiber bouton (Alle and Geiger, 2006). Action potentials occurring during presynaptic excitatory potentials exhibited enhanced neurotransmitter release that depended on the timing of the action potential relative to the rise and decay of the excitatory presynaptic potential.

5.8.6.2 Conditional detonator synapses

An important consequence of these forms of short-term plasticity at presynaptic mossy fiber terminals is that it allows for different modes of synaptic computation. In the "subdetonation" mode, there are several separate ways that granule cell activity can lead to CA3 action potential firing. Separate inputs from individual granule cells can summate spatially onto a single CA3 pyramidal neuron, or individual granule cells firing high-frequency bursts can result in CA3 firing. These effects lead to presynaptic plasticity at mossy fiber boutons that then allows for a transient period of "full detonation," that is, action potential generation in CA3 cells can be made more likely by a preceding single action potential from granule cells due to the short-term facilitation at the presynaptic terminal. This posttetanic potentiation (PTP) is a short-lived presynaptic phenomenon of this synapse, causing a transient depolarization that allows for a second action potential to result in enhanced synaptic vesicle release. Evidence for this computational switch was demonstrated by dual pre- and postsynaptic recordings in hippocampal slices before and after a 1 second pulse of 100 Hz firing of the presynapse (Vyleta et al., 2016). Whole-cell recordings of dentate granule cells

performed in awake mice during spatial navigation examined the natural activity patterns of granule cells (Vandael et al., 2020). Consistent with these cells being sparsely active (Alme et al., 2010; Pilz et al., 2016), granule cells fired at very low frequency most of the time. Sometimes, however, the cells would fire in bursts, and even bursts of bursts (i.e., "superbursts"). When these burst-firing patterns were used to stimulate the presynaptic mossy fiber bouton, PTP could be observed. Thus, while granule cells are generally inexcitable, they can fire in bursts during spatial navigation, resulting in a transient facilitation of glutamate release, which allows the mossy fiber synapses to behave as conditional detonator synapses, controlling the action potential firing of CA3 neurons.

5.8.7 Cellular properties of adult-born granule cells

As adult-born neurogenesis is more extensively covered in Chapter 9, here we present only a brief description of the cellular properties of newborn granule cells and how they integrate into the local network of the dentate gyrus.

Radial glia-like neural stem cells in the dentate gyrus give rise to dentate granule cells throughout life. These adult-born granule cells (abGCs) undergo a maturation process that in many ways resembles the neurodevelopmental processes that occur during development, albeit on a longer timeline. For the first 2–3 weeks following birth, immature abGCs are inexcitable, rarely firing action potentials and receiving little to no synaptic input (Espósito et al., 2005). At this stage, they are innervated by GABAergic synapses that are depolarizing at this stage in development, resulting in calcium signaling that promotes further maturation of glutamatergic synapses and survival of the abGCs (Chancey et al., 2013; Espósito et al., 2005; Ge et al., 2006; Jagasia et al., 2009; Overstreet-Wadiche et al., 2006). During this early period in development, mossy cells of the hilus (see below) form the first glutamatergic synapses onto abGCs as well as contributing bisynaptic feedforward inhibition (Chancey et al., 2014). During the first three postmitotic weeks, the majority of abGCs do not survive and undergo apoptosis (Biebl et al., 2000; Dayer et al., 2003), but the probability of survival is strongly influenced by elevated activity of the dentate gyrus network via stimulation, environmental enrichment or learning (Kitamura et al., 2010; Tashiro et al., 2007).

Between 4 and 8 weeks following mitosis, abGCs start to acquire inhibitory GABAergic input and activation via the perforant path (Dieni et al., 2016; Ge et al., 2006; Marín-Burgin et al., 2012). Interestingly, at this age, abGCs have a higher membrane resistance and less perisomatic inhibition, making them intrinsically more excitable than mature GCs (Brunner et al., 2014; Dieni et al., 2016; Mongiat et al., 2009; Schmidt-Hieber et al., 2004). The reduction in membrane resistance with age has been linked to increased expression of K_{ir} channel (Mongiat et al., 2009), as well as an increased expression of GIRK/$GABA_B$ coupled signaling in mature GCs (Gonzalez et al., 2018). LEC inputs onto distal dendrites in the outer molecular layer provide a stronger excitatory input to abGCs than the MEC inputs (Luna et al., 2019; Vivar et al., 2012; Woods et al., 2018). Additionally, the PP synapses of 4–6 week-old abGCs have a lower threshold for long-term plasticity than mature GCs (Schmidt-Hieber et al., 2004). This enhanced plasticity is dependent on the developmentally regulated expression of NR2B-containing NMDARs (Ge et al., 2007). Furthermore, in vivo studies demonstrated enhanced plasticity at MF-CA3 synapses formed by abGCs at the same age (Gu et al., 2012). During these weeks of maturation of synaptic inputs, the dendrites and spines of abGCs increase in size and number (Gonçalves et al., 2016; Lemaire et al., 2012; Toni et al., 2007; C Zhao et al., 2006). Over a period of weeks, the axon of the abGCs form synapses onto mossy cells and interneurons and form mossy fiber synapses with CA3 pyramidal neurons (Faulkner et al., 2008; G Sun et al., 2013; Toni et al., 2008).

5.9 Hilus

Numerous excitatory and inhibitory cell types are present in the polymorphic layer (hilus) between the dentate granule cells and the CA3 pyramidal neurons (Amaral, 1978). The most prominent and well-studied principal neurons in this region are the mossy cells. In addition, a population of spiny neurons in the hilus has also been identified that differs from mossy cells. These neurons, fewer in number than mossy cells, are distinguishable by a lack of thorny excrescences and the presence of axon collaterals that extend to the outer molecular layer of the dentate gyrus (Lübke et al., 1998). Though these neurons are spiny, it is not clear if they form excitatory or inhibitory synapses on their targets in the molecular layer.

5.9.1 Mossy cells

Mossy cells are glutamatergic interneurons that have soma and dendrites in the hilus of the dentate gyrus. These cells have a multipolar soma with 3–5 very thick dendrites that branch once or twice to produce long, thin extensions (Figure 5.21A,B). A notable feature of these cells is the presence of many enlarged spine-like structures that are similar in many ways to the thorny excrescences of CA3 pyramidal neurons. At lower magnification, these cells have a mossy appearance, hence their distinctive name (Amaral, 1978). These thorny excrescences are located on the soma and proximal dendrites mossy cells. While potentially a defining feature of these cells, there is a large amount of diversity in the morphological features of mossy cells, with some cells having numerous excrescences and others being smooth, yet with indistinguishable electrophysiological properties (Scharfman, 1993; Scharfman and Schwartzkroin, 1988). The expansive dendrites of mossy cells are located primarily in the hilus; however, some mossy cells have long thin dendrites that extend through the granule cell layer into the molecular layer (Blackstad et al., 2016; Buckmaster, 2012; Buckmaster and Amaral, 2001; Scharfman, 1991). In response to depolarizing current injections in slices, mossy cells fire regular trains of action potentials (Figure 5.21C).

Mossy cells have a unique transcriptional profile, as determined by RNA-seq. The expression of several dozen genes readily distinguishes them from neighboring granule cells in the dentate gyrus and pyramidal cells in CA3 (Figure 5.21D). Careful inspection of the Allen Institute ISH atlas to determine location of these differentially expressed genes revealed that many of them are differentially expressed along the dorsal-ventral axis (Cembrowski, Wang, et al., 2016).

5.9.2 Inputs to mossy cells and other hilar cells

Determining the synaptic inputs and outputs of mossy cells has been difficult. The dentate hilus does not have the laminar organization that allows selective stimulation of separate inputs in area CA1, for example. Thus, in order to determine which cells synapse onto other cells, simultaneous paired recordings of two or more cells had

been one of the best ways to determine connectivity and synapse properties in this region. Like the rest of the hippocampus, hilar mossy cells display a large amount of heterogeneity and numerous inputs, making the task of studying these cells challenging.

The primary input to mossy cells is the glutamatergic input from granule cells that form giant MF synapses on thorny excrescences. These inputs are similar to the MF synapses onto CA3 pyramidal neurons and have likewise been found to have properties resembling a detonator synapse (Scharfman et al., 1990). In vivo recordings, in which the activity of mossy cells and granule cells could be discriminated by the action potential waveform and bursting propensity, showed that granule cell firing reliably resulted in mossy cell firing (Senzai and Buzsáki, 2017). Furthermore, the granule cell to mossy cell synapse was shown both in slices and in vivo to exhibit robust frequency facilitation, similar to the giant MF synapses in CA3 (Scharfman et al., 1990; Senzai and Buzsáki, 2017).

Another major input to mossy cells is from a direct glutamatergic synapse from semilunar granule cells (P Williams et al., 2007). While this synapse is not as powerful as input from granule cells, paired recordings have shown a large EPSP in mossy cells with a very short latency following action potential firing in semi-lunar granule cells.

A fraction of mossy cells also receives direct excitatory input from the perforant path input onto dendritic branches that extend into the molecular layer (Blackstad et al., 2016; Buckmaster, 2012; Scharfman, 1991). Furthermore, mossy cells receive excitatory input from other ipsilateral mossy cells (Larimer and Strowbridge, 2008; Ma et al., 2021) as well as a potentially important input from CA3 pyramidal neurons (Scharfman, 2007; Y Sun et al., 2017). Lastly, mossy cells form selective reciprocal connections with hilar interneurons (Larimer and Strowbridge, 2008). The mossy cell to hilar interneuron synapse has a high failure rate but facilitates, whereas the inhibitory hilar interneuron to mossy cell synapse has a high probability of release and depresses on low-frequency paired stimulation. Thus, the strong preference for mossy cells to excite interneurons, and interneurons to inhibit mossy cells, may enable hilar networks to generate sparse representations of entorhinal input patterns (Larimer and Strowbridge, 2008).

Retrograde labeling studies have demonstrated that mossy cells in the hilus receive extrahippocampal inputs. The most well-characterized is a cholinergic input from the septal nucleus and diagonal band of Broca (Azevedo et al., 2019; Deller et al., 1999; Y Sun et al., 2017). Additional inputs were detected from the raphe nucleus and the SuM (Y Sun et al., 2017).

5.9.3 Outputs of mossy cells

Mossy cells have a complex axonal projection with potentially distinct local and distal targets. Locally, these cells project very densely through the ipsilateral hilus into the inner molecular layer, synapsing preferentially onto hilar interneurons in the hilus, with few synapses onto other mossy cells (Larimer and Strowbridge, 2008). Distal ipsilateral and contralateral mossy cell axons, which span more than half of the dorsal-ventral extent of the hippocampus, project extensively to the inner molecular layer, forming synapses onto granule cells and inhibitory interneurons (Amaral, 1978; Buckmaster et al., 1996; Scharfman, 2016; Scharfman et al., 1990). Even though they are excitatory cells, mossy cells provide an overall inhibitory drive to DG granule cells. Evidence for this first came from cell-specific silencing of mossy cell synaptic transmission that resulted in

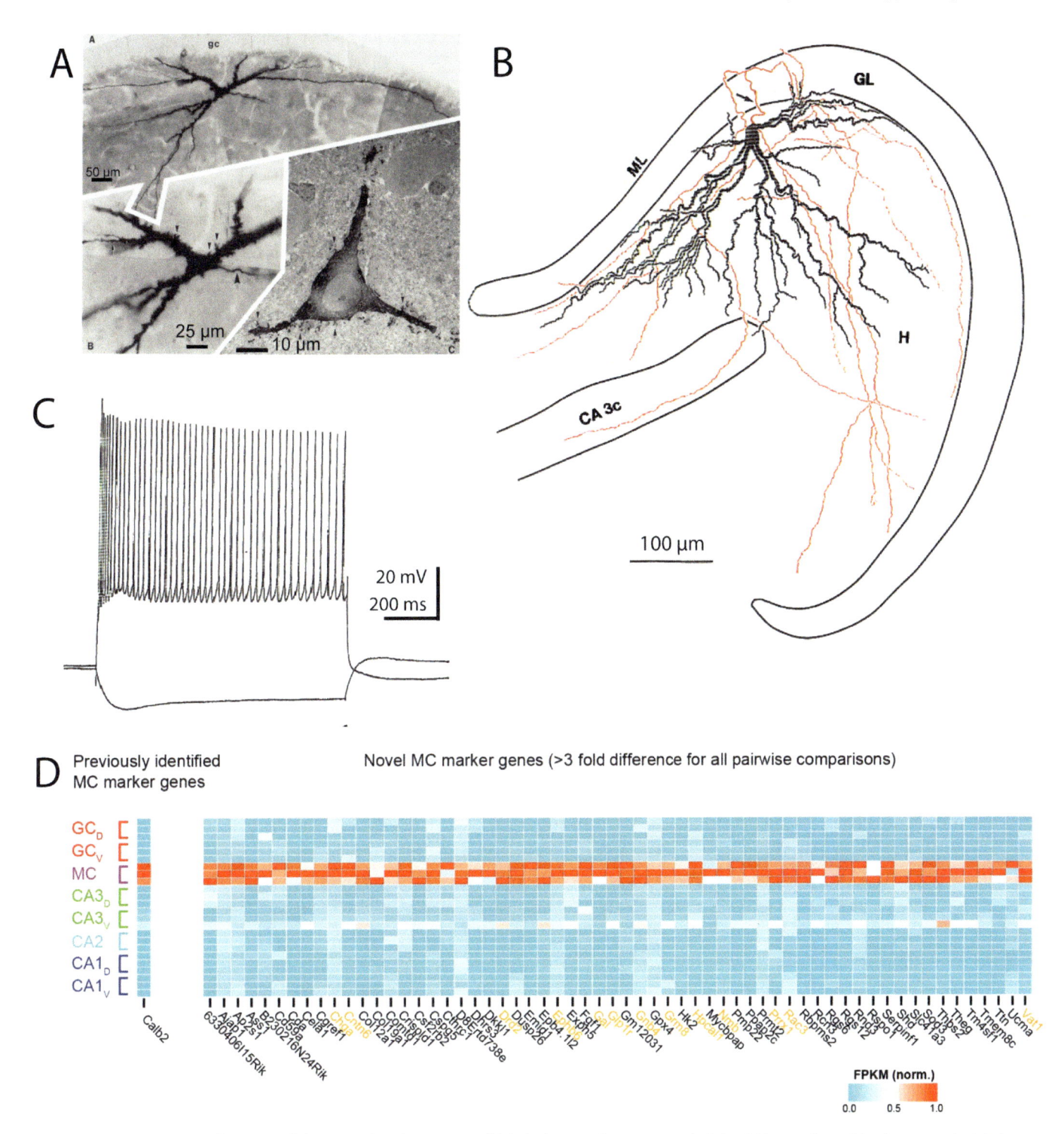

Figure 5.21 Mossy cells of the hilus. (A) Top: Multipolar mossy cell labeled in vivo has an extended dendritic tree, branching between the blades of the granule cell layer (gc; i.e., in the dentate hilus). Bottom left: The same cell body and proximal dendrites are covered with thorny excrescences (small arrowheads), whereas the distal dendrites have small spines (small arrow). Large arrowhead indicates the primary axon. Bottom right: Electron micrograph of an mossy cell filled in vitro. The multipolar mossy cell gives rise to three main dendrites. Arrowheads indicate thorny excrescences. (B) Complex dendritic and axonal morphology of a biocytin-filled and reconstructed hilar mossy cell. The axon (red) is restricted mainly to the hilus with some collaterals projecting to CA3c. Arrow: origin of the axon from the cell body. H, hilar region; GL, granule cell layer; ML, molecular layer. (C) Whole-cell recording of the mossy cell shown in (B). Responses to current injections of 1,000 pA (maximum firing rate) and -300 pA. (D) Gene expression properties of hilar mossy cells. Heat map of replicate FPKM values for the previously identified mossy cell marker gene *Calb2* and novel mossy cell marker genes identified by RNA-seq. Orange gene names indicates previously characterized neuronal relevance. (Sources: (A) Buckmaster et al., 1996; (B) Lübke et al., 1998; (C) Lübke et al., 1998; (D) Cembrowski et al., 2016a.)

transient hyperexcitability in the dentate gyrus (Jinde et al., 2012). Viral expression methods were later used to show more directly that pairing stimulation of the perforant path with mossy cell transmission resulted in a net reduction in granule cell AP firing (T Hsu et al., 2015).

Axonal projections differ between dorsal and ventral mossy cells. Specifically, the axons of ventral mossy cells are restricted largely to the inner molecular layer all along the septotemporal axis of the hippocampus, whereas the axons of dorsal mossy cells innervate the inner molecular layer in a pattern that depended upon the septotemporal location of the targeted area. More ventral regions are innervated only at very distal dendrites of the inner molecular layer, leaving a gap between the innervated area and the granule cells (Botterill et al., 2021). Thus, in the ventral hippocampus there are discrete lamina within the inner molecular layer with separation between axons arising from dorsal and ventral mossy cell axons.

5.9.4 Mossy cell activity in vivo

Several studies have shown that mossy cells have high levels of activity in awake, behaving animals, especially in comparison to dentate granule cells. Mossy cells have elevated c-Fos expression in the absence of any behavioral testing, consistent with high levels of spontaneous activity (Bernstein et al., 2019; Moretto et al., 2017). Recordings of mossy cells in vitro have shown that they exhibit a large number of spontaneous EPSPs with fairly high amplitude, which frequently results in action potential firing (Scharfman, 1993, 1995; Scharfman and Schwartzkroin, 1988). Additionally, in vivo recordings of neurons in the dentate gyrus of behaving rats revealed that mossy cell activity is spatially modulated but they often fire at multiple locations in the same environment (GoodSmith et al., 2017; Senzai and Buzsáki, 2017). In vivo calcium imaging studies showed that mossy cells were active at several spatially restricted locations while animals explored a virtual environment on a treadmill. In these experiments, confirmed mossy cells showed elevated activity during exploration (Danielson et al., 2017). The divergent properties of spatial encoding by granule cells and mossy cells is puzzling, given the high probability that a granule cell can excite mossy cells. However, this divergence likely comes from the different sets of inputs for granule cells and mossy cells, with each being tuned differently to environmental factors (Senzai and Buzsáki, 2017) and also by each being controlled differently by inhibitory interneurons.

5.9.5 Intrinsic excitability of mossy cells

The intrinsic properties of mossy cells support the hypothesis that these cells are highly excitable. First, they have a relatively depolarized resting membrane potential of ~-60 mV, which is 10–20 mV more depolarized than granule cells (Jinno et al., 2003; Lübke et al., 1998; Scharfman, 1995). Additionally, these cells have a high membrane resistance, allowing synaptic inputs to effectively depolarize the soma (Jinno et al., 2003; Lübke et al., 1998; Scharfman, 1995; Scharfman and Schwartzkroin, 1988). As with their axonal projection properties, mossy cells also show a dorsal/ventral difference in their intrinsic properties. Following blockade of glutamatergic and GABAergic transmission, ventral mossy cells exhibit membrane depolarization and intrinsic rhythmic bursting. This bursting was found to be mediated by a persistent sodium current that was not detected in dorsal mossy cells. Interestingly, if a GABA$_B$ receptor antagonist was not applied, the mossy cells did not depolarize,

indicating that a potassium current linked to GABA$_B$ receptor activation is participating in controlling the resting membrane potential of these cells (Jinno et al., 2003).

5.10   Subiculum

We began this chapter by considering CA1 pyramidal neurons, which constitute a major output of the hippocampus. The other major output is the subiculum, which contains as many axons (possibly more) that project from the hippocampus to other parts of the brain. Although there have been far fewer studies of pyramidal neurons in subiculum than in CA1, key concepts emerging from these studies mirror those from CA1, speaking to their generality. On the other hand, some key differences may offer insight into the circuit computations reflected in the various stages of information processing in the hippocampal formation.

5.10.1 Firing properties in vivo

Extracellular recordings in freely moving rats reveal that neurons in the subiculum fire more than their counterparts in CA1, thus producing less refined firing fields than the place fields observed in CA1. Nevertheless, the total amount of spatial information in the subiculum matches or exceeds that observed for a similar population of CA1 neurons (Sharp and Green, 1994). Many cells in the subiculum fire in relation to the animal's position relative to boundaries in the environment, including border cells, boundary vector cells, and vector field cells (Lever et al., 2009; Poulter et al., 2021; Sharp, 2006).

5.10.2 Regional differences

Significant differences have been observed between the functional properties of neurons in different parts of the subiculum. These include differences between dorsal and ventral subiculum, proximal and distal subiculum, and superficial versus deep layers.

5.10.2.1 Functional differences

Recordings indicate that dorsal subiculum contains more refined spatial information. In keeping with this observation, lesions reveal that the dorsal subiculum has a greater role in spatial functions, such as supporting navigation through learning, while the ventral subiculum appears to have a greater role in nonspatial or emotional functions (Aggleton and Christiansen, 2015; O'Mara et al., 2009). Accordingly, distinctly different properties—including action potential firing, functional plasticity, gene expression, and axon projection patterns—have been observed for the neurons in dorsal and ventral subiculum. Similarly, different properties have been observed for neurons in the proximal and distal portions of the subiculum (closer to and further from CA1, respectively) as well as across the layers of the subiculum. These regional differences constitute a major focus of the following sections.

5.10.2.2 Regional connectivity

Regional differences in the properties of pyramidal neurons in the subiculum are best understood in the context of their connections with hippocampal area CA1 and the medial and lateral parts of EC (MEC and LEC) (Figure 5.22A). Neurons in the subiculum receive most of their input from CA1 pyramidal neurons, which innervate the bulk of the dendritic tree, and EC, which innervates

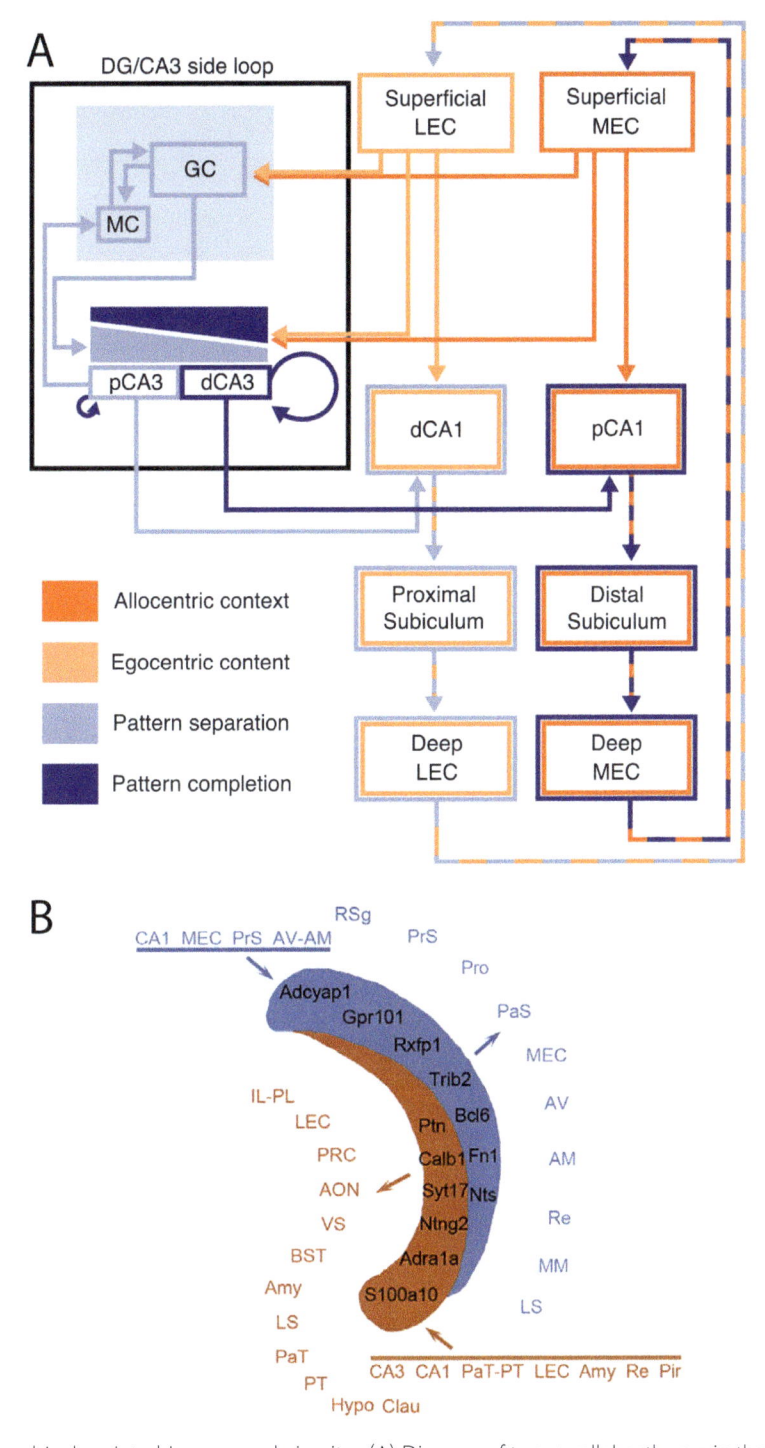

Figure 5.22 Integration of the subiculum into hippocampal circuitry. (A) Diagram of two parallel pathways in the hippocampal formation. (B) Schematic illustration of various marker genes in dorsal and ventral subiculum, as well as different downstream targets of the two areas. (Sources: (A) Lee et al., 2020; (B) Ding et al., 2020.)

the distal apical tuft dendrites. In the proximal subiculum (pSUB), which has also been called prosubiculum (S Ding, 2013), most of the hippocampal input comes from the distal CA1 (dCA1), whereas in the distal subiculum (dSUB), most of the hippocampal input comes from proximal CA1 (pCA1). The pCA1-to-dSUB circuit is bidirectionally connected with medial entorhinal cortex (MEC). By contrast, the dCA1-to-pSUB circuit is bidirectionally connected with lateral entorhinal cortex (LEC). These two pathways have

been proposed to constitute parallel processing streams that process allocentric and egocentric information, respectively (H Lee et al., 2020). Notably, pCA1-dSUB is more prominent in dorsal hippocampus while dCA1-pSUB is more prominent in the ventral hippocampus (Figure 5.22B) (S Ding et al., 2020; Wang et al., 2020), suggesting that these two streams may contribute differently to the complex functional distinctions observed along the dorsal-ventral axis of the hippocampus (Strange et al., 2014).

5.10.3 Morphology, synaptic inputs, and outputs

Principal neurons in the subiculum have stereotypical pyramidal morphologies. Inputs arrive from various sources, and outputs are divergent.

5.10.3.1 Morphology and synaptic inputs

Pyramidal neurons in the subiculum resemble those in other brain areas, including CA1. They have a triangular cell body with separate dendritic trees extending from the apical and basal parts of the cell body (Harris et al., 2001). The most prominent excitatory synaptic input is from axons of CA1 pyramidal neurons. In addition, as in other hippocampal pyramidal neurons, a direct excitatory input from EC innervates the most distal portions of the apical dendrites. Other sources of excitatory input include parasubiculum (PaS), retrosplenial cortex (RSC), superficial layers of MEC, the nucleus of the diagonal band (DB), nucleus accumbens (NA), and thalamus (Roy et al., 2017). Although it has not been studied, it may reasonably be presumed that these and other synaptic inputs would have diminished impact on depolarization of the soma, unless they are enhanced by active mechanisms such as dendritic spikes.

Local inhibitory interneurons also regulate the firing of pyramidal neurons in the subiculum. Although much less studied than in other areas of the hippocampus, evidence supports the notion that specific types of inhibitory interneurons target different cellular compartments, thus providing different contributions to the process of synaptic integration (Ferraguti et al., 2005; Menendez De La Prida, 2003).

Several neuromodulatory systems innervate the subiculum, including cholinergic, dopaminergic, noradrenergic, and serotonergic inputs. The impact of these systems has been studied far less than in other hippocampal regions, but there is evidence that both synaptic transmission and cellular excitability are modulated in a variety of ways by these systems. For example, dopamine receptor activation has been shown to depress excitatory synaptic transmission and lower the threshold for induction of LTP (Behr et al., 2000; Roggenhofer et al., 2013). Additional, cell-type-specific effects of mGluR and mAChR receptor activation are described below.

5.10.3.2 Projection targets

Pyramidal neurons in the subiculum project to many targets, both within and outside of the hippocampal formation (Roy et al., 2017; Winnubst et al., 2019). Intrahippocampal projections include considerable local collaterals in the subiculum, some projections back to CA1, and projections to EC (deep layers only). Longer-range projection targets include RSC, postrhinal cortex (PoRC), perirhinal cortex (PeRC), amygdalar cortex (AMC), hypothalamus, thalamus NA, lateral septum (LS), periaqueductal gray, and mammillary bodies (MBs). While studies based on retrograde labeling initially suggested that each individual neuron in the subiculum projects to just one of these targets (Naber and Witter, 1998), single-cell, whole-brain reconstructions indicate that at least a third of the cells project to two or more long-range projection targets (Figure 5.23) (Winnubst et al., 2019). An online database of over 1,100 single-cell axonal arborizations in the mouse brain (http://ml-neuronbrowser.janelia.org/) includes 87 reconstructed neurons in the subiculum; of these, about one-third project to EC, thus forming a closed loop with the structure providing the predominant excitatory input to the hippocampal formation (Figure 5.22). Only a small fraction of these cells includes projections to contralateral entorhinal cortex.

5.10.4 Evidence for multiple cell types in the subiculum

A plethora of evidence indicates that the subiculum contains several different types of principal neurons. In the dorsal subiculum alone, there are two readily distinguishable types based on physiological properties such as action potential firing, modulation, and plasticity; additional dorsal cell types have been distinguished based on morphology and gene expression. In ventral subiculum, gene expression profiling using scRNA-seq has revealed even greater cellular diversity.

5.10.4.1 Physiological and morphological properties

Numerous in vitro studies have demonstrated that pyramidal neurons in the subiculum respond to depolarizing current injections with either regular spiking or burst-firing patterns (Menendez De La Prida, 2006). This has been mostly studied in hippocampal slices from rodents, but one study showed the existence of regular spiking and burst-firing patterns in slices prepared from human neurosurgery patients (Wozny et al., 2005). Although early data suggested graded amounts of bursting (Staff et al., 2000), subsequent studies have shown that these two firing patterns reflect the existence of discrete cell types with differences in several electrophysiological properties, as well as differences in morphology, and modulation by mGluRs and mAChRs (Graves et al., 2012).

Pyramidal neurons in pSUB (i.e., closer to CA1) are more likely to exhibit regular spiking, while those in dSUB (i.e., further from CA1) more commonly exhibit burst firing (Jarsky et al., 2008). A study of retrogradely labeled neurons showed that the bursting phenotype correlated better with position along the proximal-distal axis than with projection type (Y Kim and Spruston, 2012). However, as neurons in pSUB and dSUB project to distinct targets (e.g., pSUB: LEC PFC, NA; dSUB: MEC RSC, VHN), a strong correlation exists between projection target and bursting. A third population of principal neurons is localized midway along the proximal-distal axis; other than local collaterals, these cells project exclusively to midline thalamic nuclei (Winnubst et al., 2019). By using a retrograde labeling strategy to distinguish between neurons in pSUB and dSUB, regular spiking neurons were found to be greatest in pSUB and bursting neurons more abundant in dSUB (Figure 5.24) (Cembrowski, Phillips, et al., 2018).

While the two classes of cell types in the subiculum are commonly referred to as regular spiking and bursting, both cell types in fact exhibit bursting, albeit with different dynamics. In response to multiple, brief depolarizing current pulses, regular spiking neurons initially fire single spikes, but later in a train of stimuli they begin to burst. In contrast, bursting neurons initially burst but switch to single spikes later in the train. This parallels the situation in CA1 pyramidal cells (Figure 5.11C) (Graves et al., 2012). Thus, the two cell types may more accurately be called early spiking late bursting (ESLB) and early bursting late spiking (EBLS) neurons (corresponding to regular spiking and bursting cells, respectively).

5.10.4.2 Differential modulation of distinct cell types in the dorsal subiculum

Remarkably, the amount of bursting exhibited by each of these cell types is subject to modulation with distinct features (Graves et al.,

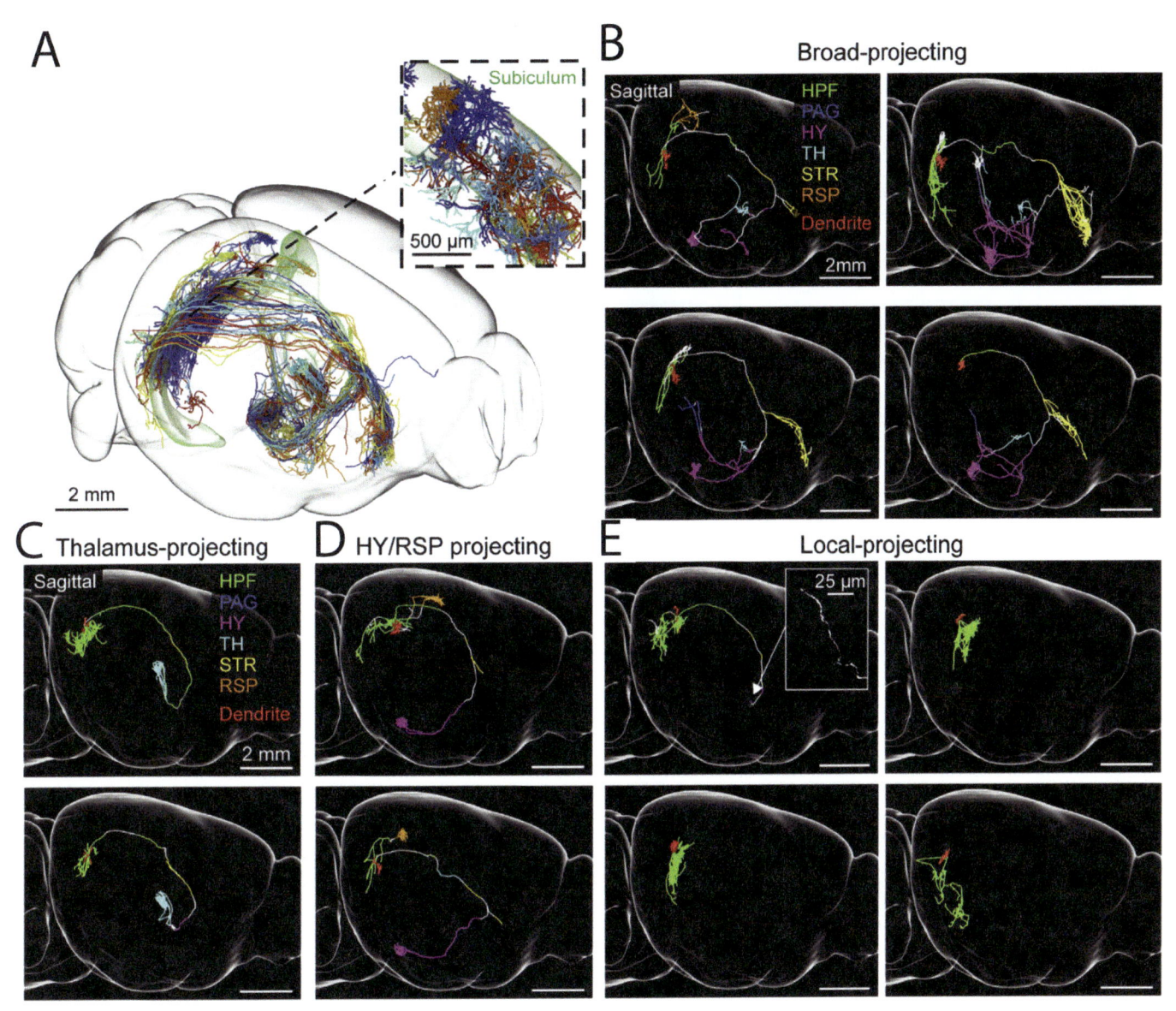

Figure 5.23 Projections of individually reconstructed axons from pyramidal cells in the subiculum. (A) Overlay of 73 reconstructed cells. Examples are shown from several putative projection classes. (B) Neurons projecting broadly to several target areas. (C) Neurons projecting to the thalamus. (D) Neurons projecting to the hypothalamus (HY) and retrosplenial cortex (RSP). (E) Neurons projecting locally within subiculum and/or with few branches to other targets. (Source: (A–E) Winnubst et al., 2019.)

2012; Moore et al., 2009). In both cell types, theta-burst stimulation (TBS) of axons in slices results in a long-lasting increase in the number of bursts in response to a train of brief current injections. This effect does not require activation of excitatory ionotropic glutamate receptors. Instead, it results from activation of metabotropic receptors, specifically mGluRs and mAChRs. The effects of activating these two classes of receptors are mechanistically distinct in the two cell types. In the ESLB cells, activation of mGluRs results in an increase in bursting. In the EBLS cells, however, increased bursting in response to TBS depends on synergistic activation of both mGluR and mAChR activation, as blocking either receptor type eliminates the effect, similar to the synergistic effect of mGluR and mAChR activation on bursting in CA1 pyramidal cells (Graves et al., 2012; Moore et al., 2009).

The modulatory effects of TBS stimulation on bursting are bidirectional in a manner that depends on cell type and mGluR subtypes.

In ESLB cells, blocking mGluR5 results in a TBS-induced decrease in spiking that requires synergistic activation of both mGluR1 and mAChR. In EBLS cells, blocking mGluR1 or mAChR activation produces a TBS-induced decrease in spiking that requires activation of mGluR5. In other words, these effects can be summarized as follows. ESLB cells: mGluR5-mediated increase and synergistic mGluR1/mAChR-mediated decrease. EBLS cells: mGluR5-mediated decrease and synergistic mGluR1/mAChR-mediated increase. Thus, in both cell types there is a synergistic interaction and the effects that increase bursting (mGluR5 in one case and mGluR1/mAChR in the other) are dominant when both pathways are activated (Graves et al., 2012). Importantly, the actions of these modulatory receptors are exactly opposite in the two cell types.

A puzzling aspect of these findings is that mGluR1 and mGluR5 are both thought to be coupled to the same G_q-protein-based intracellular signaling pathways. These observations suggest that this

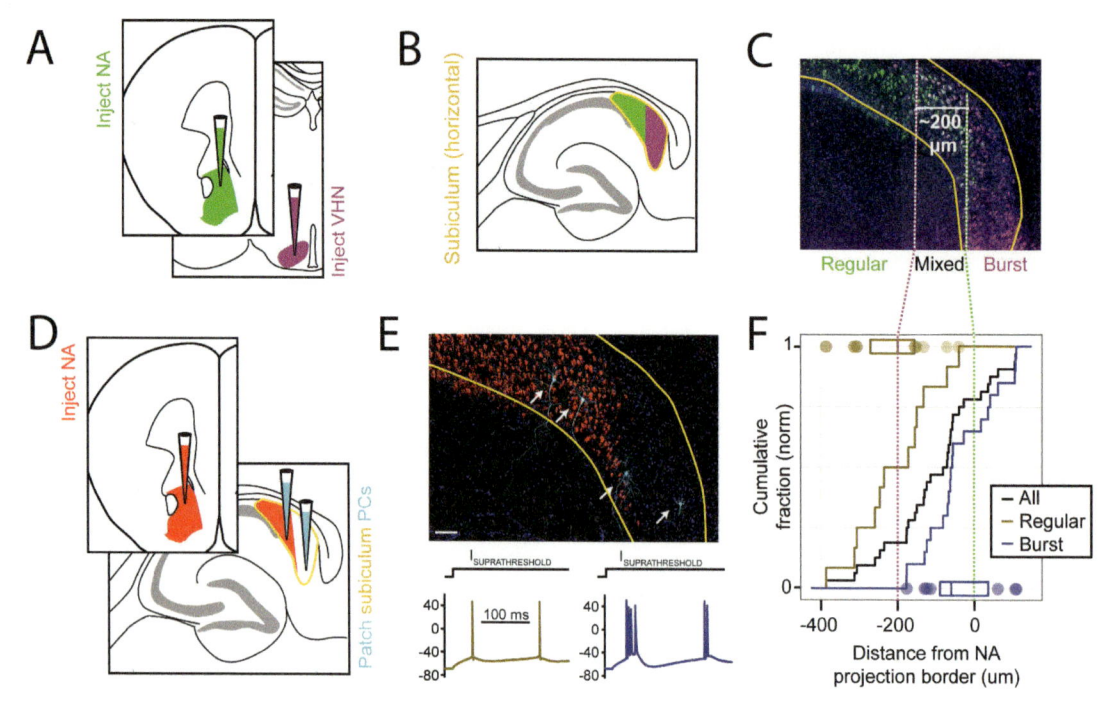

Figure 5.24 Bursting neurons are localized to distal portions of the subiculum. (A) Schematic of retrograde tracer injections in nucleus accumbens (NA) and ventral hypothalamic nuclei (VHN). (B) Schematic of tracers from NA and VHN. (C) Labeled neurons from NA (green), VHN (magenta), and DAPI-labeling of all cell bodies (blue). (D) Schematic of retrograde tracers from NA and patch-clamp recordings from labeled or unlabeled neurons in proximal and distal subiculum, respectively. (E) Neurons labeled from retrograde tracers in NA (red), DAPI-labeling of all cell bodies (blue), and filled neurons from patch-clamp recordings (cyan). (F) Cumulative fraction of regular-spiking and bursting neurons as a function of distance from the NA projection-labeled border. (Sources: (A–F) Cembrowski et al., 2018b.)

cannot be entirely true. Whether mGluR1 and mGluR5 mediated pathways can be activated separately is unclear, but the need for coactivation of mAChR to elicit the effects of mGluR1 activation is an interesting clue to this mystery.

5.10.4.3 Diverse forms of synaptic plasticity

The two types of neurons described above have also been shown to exhibit plasticity in their responses to synaptic input, both at CA1-subiculum and EC-subiculum synapses (Behr et al., 2009). As with the modulation described above, synaptic plasticity is strikingly different for CA1 inputs to the two cell types (Fidzinski et al., 2008). In both cell types, repetitive stimulation leads to both NMDA receptor-dependent LTD and mGluR-dependent LTP. At frequencies above ~4 Hz, LTP dominates in both cell types. At lower frequencies, however, LTD dominates in bursting cells and LTP dominates in regular spiking cells. In each case, pharmacologically inhibiting the dominant form of plasticity reveals the latent form of plasticity in the opposite direction (Fidzinski et al., 2008). In addition, in both cell types, these forms of plasticity were dependent on coactivation of mAChRs, and block of L-type calcium channels reversed the sign of the plasticity (Shor et al., 2009). These findings are reminiscent of the synergistic actions of mGluRs and mAChRs on the modulation and plasticity of action potential firing in these neurons. The complex signaling mechanisms responsible for these effects are poorly understood. The functional implications are also obscure, but the fact that plasticity can take an opposite form in the two cell types hints at the possibility of distinct computational roles and counterbalanced output to downstream targets of the hippocampal formation.

5.10.4.4 Gene expression reveals a patchwork of cell types

RNA-seq has been used to provide transcriptional profiles for principal cells throughout the subiculum. The resulting picture is one of significant cellular diversity. Microdissection of proximal and distal dorsal subiculum, followed by population-based RNA-seq, revealed differential expression of hundreds of genes between these two regions. Many of the differentially expressed genes have ontologies associated with various aspects of neuronal function. Others have more general functions, or in some cases unknown functions, but they are nevertheless useful markers of the two distinct cell types (Figure 5.25A,B) (Cembrowski, Phillips, et al., 2018). Electrophysiological recordings confirmed that regular spiking cells overlap predominantly with marker genes from the proximal subiculum and bursting cells overlap with marker genes from the distal subiculum (Cembrowski, Phillips, et al., 2018).

Single-cell RNA-seq (sc-RNA-seq) has revealed that in addition to the transcriptional diversity across these proximal and distal regions of the dorsal subiculum, distinct gene expression profiles are observed for additional cells throughout the full dorsal-ventral extent of the subiculum, with FISH and IHC validating these distinctions and permitting localization of the distinct cell types. Two studies constitute the most extensive transcriptional characterization of any region in the hippocampal formation, so they are considered here in detail (Cembrowski, Phillips, et al., 2018; Cembrowski, Wang, et al., 2018).

The first study, based on sc-RNA-seq from 1,150 cells, revealed eight distinct types of principal (excitatory) neurons (Figure 5.25C) (Cembrowski, Wang, et al., 2018). In dorsal subiculum, cells in the distal portion formed a single class expressing the marker gene *Fn1*

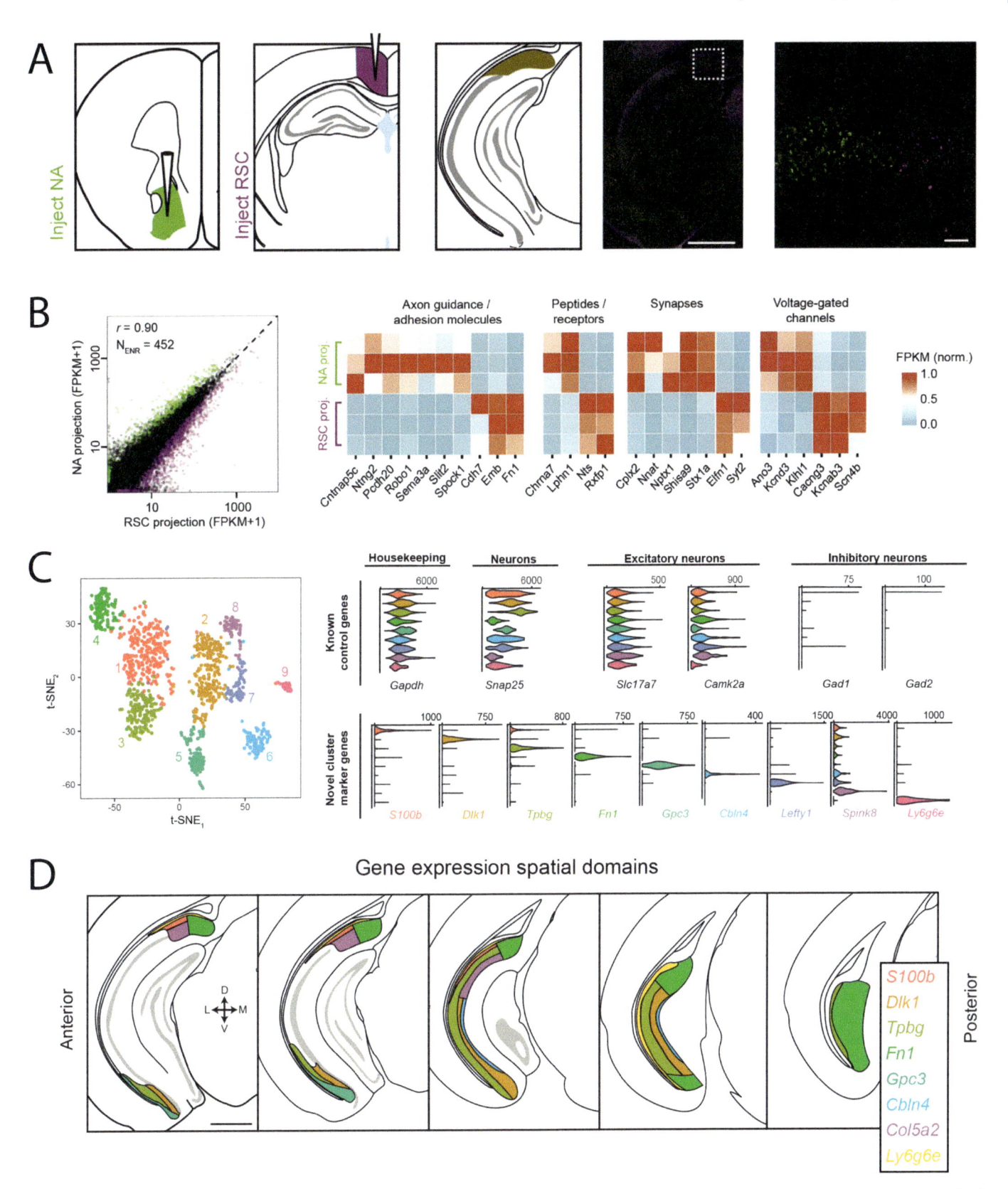

Figure 5.25 Gene expression in principal cells of the subiculum. (A) Left to right: Cartoons of retrograde tracer injections in nucleus accumbens (NA) and retrosplenial cortex (RSC). Cartoon of dorsal subiculum. Image of labeled coronal brain section. Expansion of dorsal subiculum (as shown by box to the left) showing cells labeled by NA (green) and RSC (magenta) injections. (B) Left: Expression levels of all genes, as determined by RNA-seq for NA- and RSC-labeled populations. Differentially expressed genes are labeled in color. Right: Examples of differentially expressed genes. (C) Left: t-SNE plot of 1103 cells analyzed by single-cell RNA-seq of principal cells in subiculum. Note: group 7 is from contamination by CA1 pyramidal cells. Right: Violin plots showing expression levels of selected genes for each of the color-coded groups in the t-SNE plot. (D) Cartoon representing localization of each of the eight groups of cells in the subiculum, as determined from analysis of cell type-specific genes in the Allen Institute in situ hybridization atlas. (Sources: (A–B) Cembrowski et al., 2018b; (C–D) Cembrowski et al., 2018a.)

(among others), whereas cells in the proximal portion could be further subdivided into two groups, expressing marker genes *S100b* and *Col5a2* respectively, and largely occupying discrete zones. In addition, a small population of cells expressing *Ly6g6e* spanned the proximal and distal regions and was restricted to the deepest layers of subiculum. Thus, there are at least four subtypes of principal cells in the dorsal subiculum. Of these four types, the distal and two proximal types (*Fn1, S100b, Col5a2*) are restricted to dorsal and intermediate portions of the subiculum, while the deep-layer cell type (*Ly6g6e*) extend further into the intermediate and ventral subiculum as well. A fifth cell type expressing *Tpbg* partially occupies proximal subiculum at relatively posterior locations and is also abundant at intermediate and ventral locations. Finally, three additional cell types, expressing *Dlk1* or *Cbln4* or *Gpc3*, occupy exclusively intermediate and ventral positions in the subiculum. Although key marker genes are used here to label these transcriptional cell types, these genes are expressed elsewhere in the brain, including other areas of the hippocampal formation, albeit at lower levels. Thus, care must be taken when using knowledge of gene expression to design strategies for cell-type-specific labeling for imaging or manipulating neural activity. For example, one effective strategy is to combine Cre lines with local injection of viruses carrying Cre-dependent transgenes (Cembrowski, Wang, et al., 2018; S Ding et al., 2020).

The second study, based on a larger sample of nearly 15,000 cells, arrived at conclusions largely consistent with the first study (S Ding et al., 2020). In both studies, the anatomical locations were determined by examining the expression of key marker genes in the Allen Institute in situ hybridization atlas (Lein et al., 2007). Notably, the second study used the terms prosubiculum and subiculum to describe the proximal and distal portions of the subiculum, respectively. In addition, they assigned the *Gpc3*-expressing cells to ventral CA1 and the hippocampal-amygdala transition area rather than the ventral subiculum annotation used in the first study. In the second study, the larger transcriptomic dataset identified 27 neuronal types in the subiculum complex. These transcriptionally defined clusters align with the eight transcriptional types described above. With few exceptions, the larger set of 27 transcriptomic clusters reflects a division of the eight cell types described above into smaller subgroups. This study also found that cells associated with the distal subiculum are more prominent in dorsal hippocampus, whereas cells mapping to proximal subiculum (prosubiculum) are more prominent in ventral hippocampus.

An even larger study of approximately 1.3 million cells in the neocortex and hippocampal formation arrived at similar conclusions to the two studies described above (Yao et al., 2021). They identified eight transcriptomic clusters in proximal subiculum (prosubiculum) and three in distal subiculum. An additional five clusters were mapped to "CA1-prosubiculum," reflecting the fact that a gradual transcriptomic gradient was observed along the proximal-distal axis, particularly in intermediate and ventral portions of the hippocampus. As in previous studies, a prominent dorsal-ventral gradient was identified in both CA1 and subiculum (Cembrowski, Bachman, et al., 2016; Cembrowski, Wang, et al., 2018; S Ding et al., 2020). In dorsal hippocampus, the difference in gene expression between CA1 and the distal subiculum was considerably greater than in the ventral hippocampus.

The distribution of differentially expressed genes identified by these studies has allowed the locations of transcriptional clusters

to be mapped to their location within the hippocampal formation (Figure 5.25D). Leveraging this knowledge, subsequent studies combining FISH with anterograde and retrograde tracer injections has led to insights into the relationship between transcriptionally defined cell types in the subiculum and their axonal projections. For example, neurons in the distal dorsal subiculum project to RSC, MEC, and VHN, among other regions, whereas neurons in proximal subiculum (prosubiculum) project to distinct targets such as IL, NA LEC, and others. These projections have been mapped in detail at the mesoscopic level (Bienkowski et al., 2018; Cembrowski, Phillips, et al., 2018; S Ding et al., 2020) and full axonal arborizations have been reconstructed for several dozen individual neurons in the dorsal subiculum (Figure 5.23) (Winnubst et al., 2019). Nevertheless, knowledge of the relationship between transcriptional cell types and their projections is incomplete, so additional work is needed.

Together, these studies and others provide important insights into cellular diversity in the subiculum. As in the CA1 region, cellular diversity of principal neurons can be identified along all three major axes: proximal-distal, superficial-deep, and dorsal-ventral. Although graded transcriptional variation may also occur in subiculum, it does not appear to be as prominent as it is in CA1, where distinct subtypes have not been identified along the dorsal-ventral axis (Cembrowski, Bachman, et al., 2016). In contrast, a larger number of transcriptionally distinct principal cell types occupy discrete zones within the subiculum (Cembrowski, Wang, et al., 2018). In both regions, however, transcriptional diversity is paralleled by differences in other features that follow naturally from differences in gene expression, such as morphology, connectivity, action potential firing patterns, and neuromodulation.

5.10.4.5 Functional implications of cellular diversity

A central challenge will be to determine how these substantively different cellular populations, along with their distinct functional properties and projections, contribute to the computational function of the hippocampal formation. Knowledge of gene expression and axon projections will likely play a critical role in this process. For example, an important concept that has considerable experimental support is that dorsal hippocampus—in particular pCA1 and dSUB—are involved in spatial navigation, whereas more ventral regions—in particular dCA1 and pSUB—are involved in more emotional aspects of hippocampal function (O'Mara et al., 2009). Rigorously testing this idea will require manipulation of cells proposed to be critical for these distinct functions (Cembrowski, Phillips, et al., 2018; Roy et al., 2017). This will require sophisticated methods, as the cells contributing to these distinct functions are too closely intertwined for spatial targeting alone to achieve separable manipulations. Such experiments will undoubtedly benefit from the ever-increasing body of knowledge about gene expression and axon projections, both of which can be exploited to achieve reversible, cell-type-specific manipulations of neural activity in behaving animals.

5.11 Parahippocampal cortex

The hippocampus is bidirectionally connected to the neocortex via the presubiculum (PrS), parasubiculum (PaS), and entorhinal cortex (EC) (Figure 5.26A). Collectively, these three structures, which can be distinguished based on a variety of features including molecular markers (Figure 5.26B–C), are considered periarchicortex, because they are transitional between the three-layered archicortex of hippocampus and the six-layered structure of neocortex. However, PrS and EC are also six-layered structures. EC provides the major source of excitatory input to the hippocampus. In addition, it receives outputs from CA1 and SUB, thus creating a long-range recurrent loop. PrS and PaS are parahippocampal areas lying in between SUB and EC. Although they do not provide much input to the hippocampus, like EC, they receive inputs from the hippocampus, which are integrated with other cortical and subcortical inputs before relaying output to numerous downstream targets (Figure 5.1 and Chapter 3).

Each of these parahippocampal areas contains an eclectic collection of cells with different inputs, outputs, and physiological properties. As a result, they also exhibit diverse response properties in vivo, including grid cells, head-direction cells, border cells, and boundary vector cells (Tukker et al., 2022) (see Chapter 12). Several studies have examined the functional organization of parahippocampal areas. The most common approaches include retrograde labeling IHC, electrophysiology, and expression of transgenic reporter proteins. In the following sections, we summarize what is known about the cellular organization of these systems.

5.11.1 Presubiculum

Presubiculum lies in between subiculum and entorhinal cortex. PrS is distinguishable from the neighboring subiculum by a few molecular characteristics. It exhibits stronger staining for AChE and vGluT2, whereas SUB has much stronger staining for GluR1 (Ishihara and Fukuda, 2016). PrS is also distinguishable from PaS, because layer 2 is much more densely packed in the latter structure (Simonnet and Fricker, 2018). It contains a diverse array of neurons, inputs, and outputs. Although neurons from PrS exhibit a variety of response properties in vivo (Boccara et al., 2010; Sharp, 1996; Simonnet and Fricker, 2018), it has been most extensively studied because of the large proportion of head-direction cells in the dorsal part of PrS, which is also known as postsubiculum (Taube et al., 1990).

5.11.1.1 Inputs to presubiculum

CA1 provides some direct excitatory input. Most input to PrS, however, comes from other cortical and subcortical structures. Importantly, PrS receives a strong input from anterior thalamic nuclei (ATN), a key source of head-direction signals in the mammalian brain (Peyrache et al., 2019). In addition, PrS receives inputs from retrosplenial cortex (RSC) and visual cortex (VIS). Thus, it has been proposed that PrS integrates high-level visual information with subcortical inputs, combining environmental landmarks with vestibular and path-integration signals to produce a robust representation of heading direction (Wang et al., 2020; Yoder et al., 2011).

5.11.1.2 Firing properties in vivo

Cells in layer 2 of PrS notably lack head-direction selectivity, likely because they do not receive input from ATN or from cells in deeper layers. The densely packed cells in layer 2 of PrS fall into two categories based on their expression of calbindin (Figure 5.27A–B). Cells expressing calbindin send their projections primarily to contralateral PrS, while those lacking calbindin project to ipsilateral RSC (Preston-Ferrer et al., 2016).

Pyramidal cells in layers 3–6 of PrS respond selectively to head direction (Figure 5.27C), a feature likely attributable in large part to input from head-direction cells in ATN. Most head-direction cells in PrS are pyramidal neurons, and at least some project to MEC (Preston-Ferrer et al., 2016; Tukker et al., 2022), where they are likely important for the formation of grid cells (Winter et al., 2015). Cells in the deepest layers of PrS (layers 4–6) may inherit this property, at least in part, from cells in more superficial layers. While projections from superficial to deep layers of PrS are observed, projections in the reverse direction (deep to superficial) are not (Funahashi and Stewart, 1997; Simonnet and Fricker, 2018).

5.11.1.3 Morphological and physiological properties

The morphological and physiological properties of neurons in PrS are diverse. In layers 2 and 3, both pyramidal and fusiform cells are present, and their firing properties are wide-ranging, including regular spiking and intrinsically bursting neurons (Abbasi and Kumar, 2013; Funahashi and Stewart, 1997; L Huang et al., 2017; Menendez de la Prida et al., 2003; Peng et al., 2017; Simonnet and Fricker, 2018). However, most of the cells in layer 3 are small pyramidal cells that exhibit regular spiking (Figure 5.27D,E), while deep-layer pyramidal cells exhibit synaptically evoked burst discharges that likely result from recurrent connectivity (Funahashi et al., 1999; Simonnet and Fricker, 2018). Although layer 4 was initially described as a cell-free layer, a recent study identified a population of medium-to-large pyramidal cells that occupy PrS layer 4 and project to LMN (L Huang et al., 2017; Simonnet and Fricker, 2018). Layer 5 contains medium-to-large pyramidal cells, while layer 6 contains a smaller population of pyramidal and fusiform cells (Simonnet et al., 2013). Layer 5 neurons have been found to fall into six categories based on axon projects to the following targets: RSC, SUB, PaS, RSC+PaS, RSC+SUB, MEC+SUB (Honda et al., 2011). Physiological studies of neurons labeled with retrograde tracers from multiple targets of PrS revealed that most of these long-range projecting neurons were regular spiking, with the notable exception of LMN-projecting neurons in layer 4, which exhibited strong intrinsic burst firing (L Huang et al., 2017; Yoder and Taube, 2011).

5.11.1.4 Mechanisms of head-direction selectivity

Models of head-direction selectivity are principally determined by network connectivity, but intrinsic membrane properties can also contribute. A simple model that produces firing corresponding to a single heading direction consists of a ring of neurons that are connected by excitatory connections to nearby neighbors and global inhibition (Hulse and Jayaraman, 2020). While such models produce firing at a single location, they require continuous excitation for heading direction to be sustained. The need for a continuous excitatory input can be obviated, however, if the intrinsic properties of the neurons support persistent firing. Accordingly, it has been shown that neurons in the dorsal PrS exhibit persistent firing following a brief depolarizing input in the presence of ACh (Figure 5.27F). This form of persistent firing is mediated by a calcium-activated nonselective cation current that is upregulated by cholinergic input acting on mAChRs (Yoshida and Hasselmo, 2009).

5.11.2 Parasubiculum

Parasubiculum is a narrow band of cells lying between PrS and MEC and curving over the top of the most mediodorsal parts of MEC (Figure 5.28A). PaS is readily distinguishable from PrS and

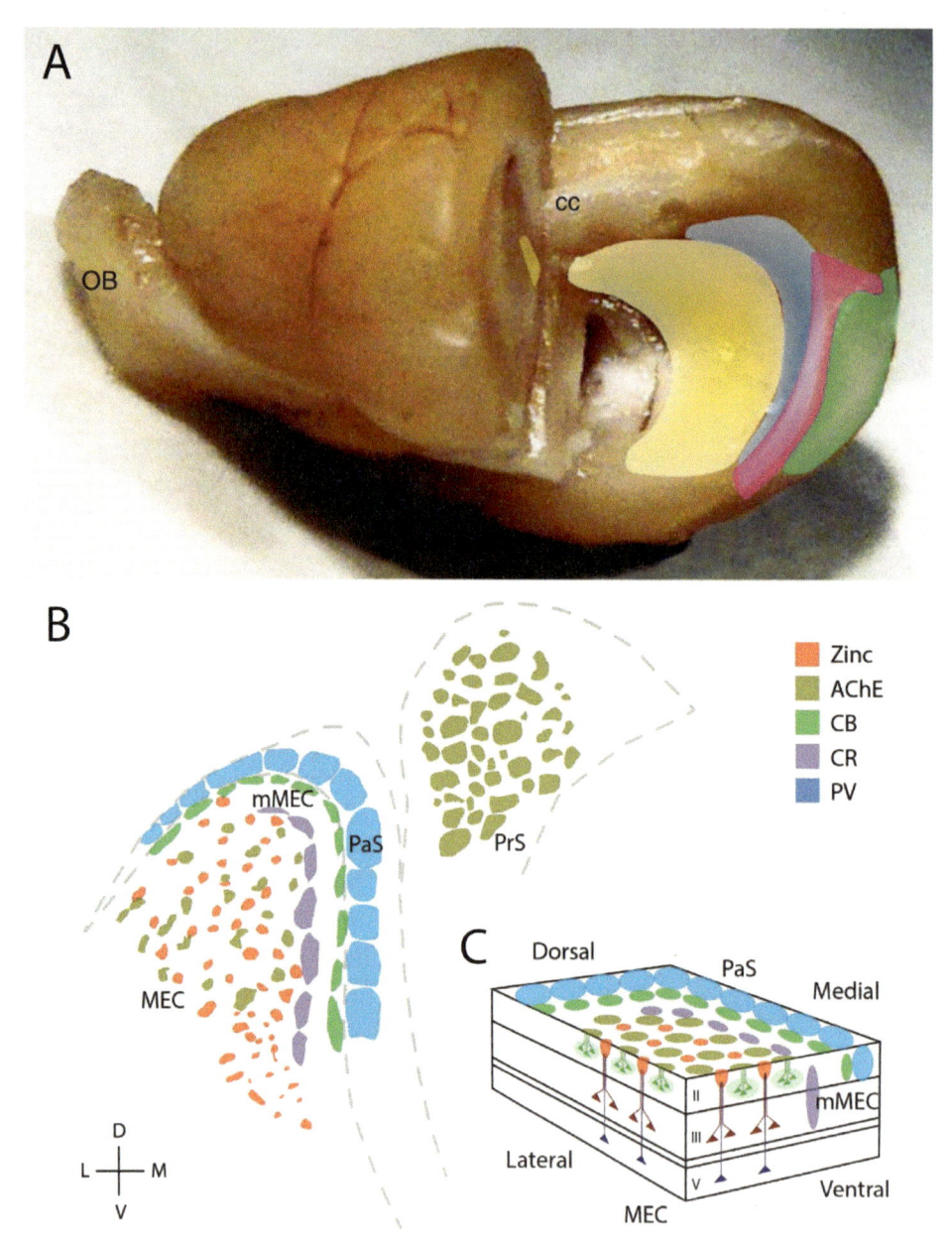

Figure 5.26 Anatomy and molecular organization of parahippocampal areas. (A) Photograph of the rat brain illustrating the location of hippocampal and parahippocampal areas in the right hemisphere (medial view with left hemisphere cut out). Outlines: hippocampus/subiculum (yellow), presubiculum (blue), parasubiculum (pink), and MEC (green). cc, corpus callosum; OB, olfactory bulb. (B) Cartoon of key marker-gene localization in the medial entorhinal cortex (MEC) and presubiculum. (C) Three-dimensional cartoon of panel B, showing how each marker is expressed in the different layers of the MEC and PaS. (Sources: (A) Boccara et al., 2010; (B, C) Ray et al., 2017.)

MEC based on a few molecular markers: cytochrome oxidase and AChE staining, Wfs1 staining (which is present in PaS and some layers of MEC, but absent in PrS), and calbindin (low in PaS and limited to inhibitory neurons in PaS but not in MEC) (Sammons et al., 2019; Tang et al., 2016). In addition, PaS is separated from MEC by a transitional zone, which contains PV-expressing inhibitory interneurons, calretinin-positive neurons, and narrow band of calbindin-positive neurons (Figure 5.28B) (Ray et al., 2017).

5.11.2.1 Inputs and outputs of parasubiculum

Major excitatory inputs to PaS include SUB, PrS, and ATN (Tang et al., 2016). The strong staining for AChE is indicative of considerable input from MS. Similarly, tracer injections indicate that

GABAergic neurons in MS also provide considerable input to PaS (Tang et al., 2016). In keeping with the role of MS in modulating theta oscillations, theta activity is stronger in PaS than in PrS or MEC (Boccara et al., 2010; Ebbesen et al., 2016). The principal output of PaS are patches of pyramidal cells in layer II of MEC (Burgalossi et al., 2011; Tang et al., 2016).

5.11.2.2 Response properties in vivo

Recordings from PaS in freely moving animals indicate that they tend to fire in bursts (Ebbesen et al., 2016) and about half of the cells are strongly selective for head direction (Taube, 1995). The remaining half consist of grid cells, border cells, and irregularly firing cells that nevertheless contain strong spatial information (Figure 5.28C).

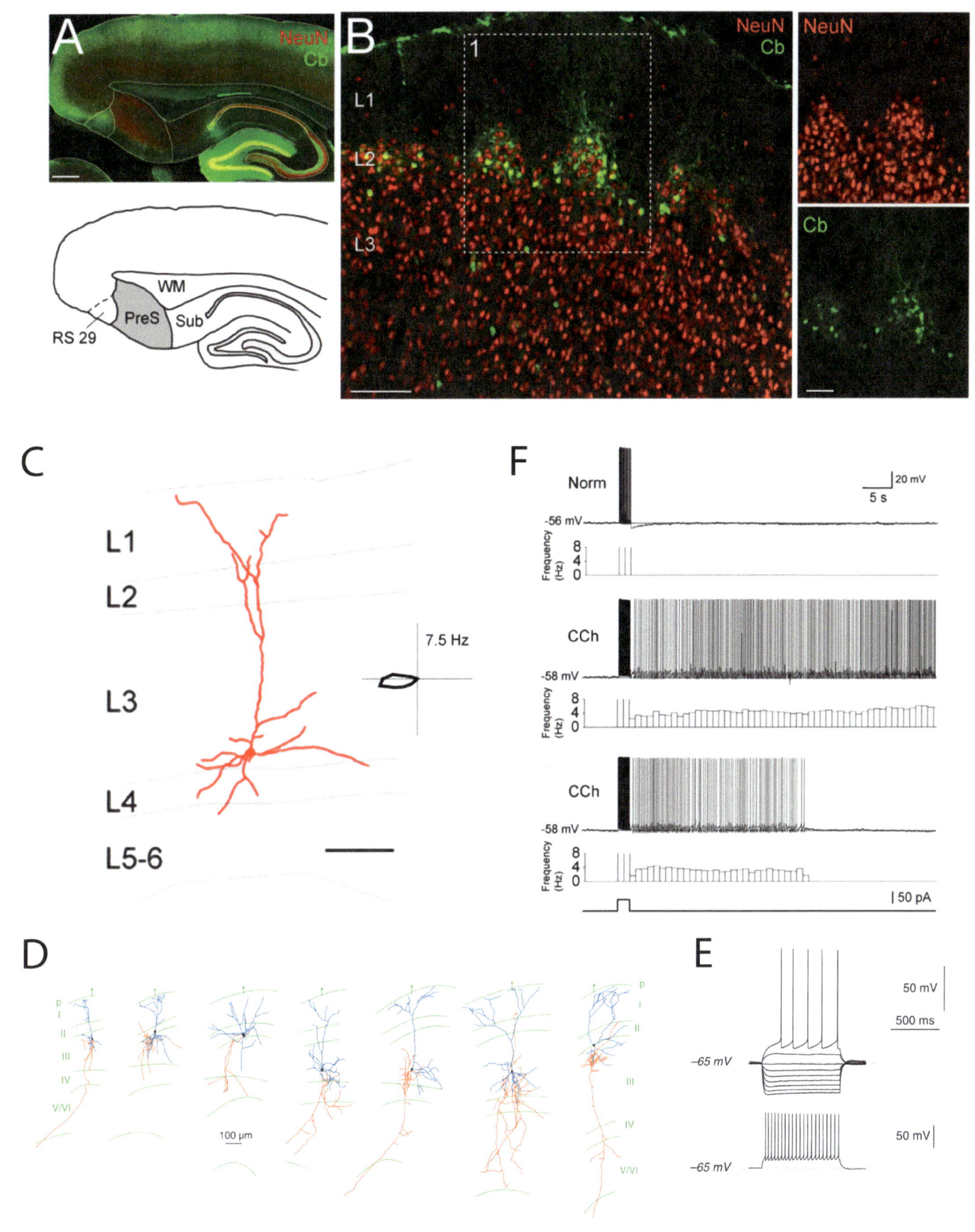

Figure 5.27 Organizational and functional properties of presubiculum. (A) Staining of the hippocampal formation for NeuN and calbindin (Cb). Scale bar = 500 μm. (B) Higher magnification view of presubiculum. Scale bar = 100 μm (left), 50 μm (right). (C) Reconstruction of a neuron labeled during a juxtacellular recording in vivo. Inset: head-direction selectivity of the illustrated cell. (D) Reconstructions of biocytin-filled pyramidal neurons in superficial layers of PrS. (E) Intracellular V$_m$ recorded from a pyramidal neuron in PrS in vitro. (F) Persistent firing of a presubiculum neuron recorded in vitro. (Sources: (A–C) Preston-Ferrer et al., 2016; (D–E) Simmonet and Fricker, 2018; (F) Yoshida and Hasselmo, 2009.)

Neurons in PaS are strongly modulated by theta rhythm (Boccara et al., 2010; Burgalossi et al., 2011; Tang et al., 2016).

5.11.2.3 Cellular organization and molecular markers

Although PaS has been described as a six-layered structure, the absence of fibers between the superficial and deep layers suggests that deep layers may actually belong to PrS or MEC, thus making PaS a relatively narrow sheet of cells sandwiched between six layered structures on either side. Another intriguing structural feature is that PaS consists of a small number of discrete patches of neurons that are synaptically connected by axons within the layer (Burgalossi et al., 2011; Tang et al., 2016).

Most VGAT-negative neurons (hence presumably excitatory) in PaS are pyramidal cells that express the marker gene *Wfs1*, thus distinguishing them from cells in the neighboring transition zone adjacent to MEC (Sammons et al., 2019). PaS also contains many VGAT-expressing neurons, which stain for various markers of inhibitory interneurons, including PV, VIP, SOM, and CCK (Ray and Brecht, 2016; Sammons et al., 2019). Notably, most reelin-expressing neurons in PaS also express VGAT, indicating that they are inhibitory (Sammons et al., 2019); this contrasts with the reelin-positive stellate cells in layer II of EC, which are excitatory (see below).

5.11.2.4 Physiological properties

A few studies have assessed the morphological and physiological properties of neurons in PrS and PaS. Current injection into pyramidal neurons in PaS neurons elicits regular spiking (Sammons et al., 2019). While repeated synaptic stimulation can produce large EPSPs and burst discharges, this occurs mostly in the deeper layers (Funahashi and Stewart, 1997), which may in fact be part of PrS or MEC, as noted above. Pyramidal neurons in PrS and PaS exhibit a measurable theta oscillation of the resting potential and a modest amount of sag in response to hyperpolarizing current injections (Funahashi and Stewart, 1997; Sammons et al., 2019). As expected from the strong interconnections between patches of pyramidal cells in PaS, local connections, including reciprocal connections, have been observed between excitatory cells in PaS slices (Sammons et al., 2021).

5.11.3 Entorhinal cortex

Entorhinal cortex is a six-layered structure containing several distinct types of principal neurons. It is perhaps best known for the presence of grid cells in MEC (Rowland et al., 2016). In addition, however, several other properties related to the cognitive map of space have also been observed in this region, including head-direction cells, border cells, object vector cells, speed cells, and cells exhibiting combinations of these properties (Tukker et al., 2022). Here we summarize what is known about the cellular organization of EC. A more extensive treatment can be found in Chapter 12.

5.11.3.1 Layer II stellate cells (ocean)

Layer II of EC (ECII) consists of pyramidal cells and stellate cells, both of which are believed to be excitatory neurons (Figure 5.29). Pyramidal cells are organized into roughly hexagonally arranged patches that are best characterized by expression of calbindin. Cells in these patches have also been called "island cells" because they are surrounded by stellate cells, which form an ocean of cells that are interspersed between the islands; both cell populations receive distinct cellular patterns of inhibition (Varga et al., 2010). Stellate cells, or "ocean cells," are best characterized by the expression of reelin (Kitamura, 2017). In between the islands are complementary patches of PCP4 and zinc-positive neuropil containing the dendrites of pyramidal cells in layers III and V (Figure 5.26C) (Ray et al., 2017; Varga et al., 2010).

The presence of zinc in between the islands indicates input to ECII stellate cells and the dendrites of ECIII pyramidal cells from zinc-containing glutamatergic terminals of neurons of PrS. In contrast, zinc staining is not observed in islands, indicating that ECII pyramidal cells do not receive inputs from PrS. Instead, islands receive inputs from neurons of the PaS (Ray et al., 2017; Tang et al., 2016). Thus, pyramidal cells in ECII and ECIII receive input from PaS and PrS, respectively, thus potentially forming parallel information-processing pathways. The presence of acetylcholinesterase (AChE) in ECII islands (Figure 5.26C) indicates that these pyramidal neurons receive input from cholinergic neurons in the medial septum. Island cells are also selectively innervated by CCK-expressing basket cells (Ray et al., 2017; Varga et al., 2010).

Stellate cells in ECII derive their name from their star-like appearance (Figure 5.29C). They have relatively large ovoid or trapezoid-shaped cell bodies, with numerous spine studded dendrites radiating out from the soma and spanning EC layers I to III. Dendritic branches often terminate in bouquets of about six dendritic spines (Klink and Alonso, 1997b). ECII stellate cells have been studied extensively, initially because of their unusual electrophysiological features, and later because of their grid-like firing properties.

In vivo recordings from freely moving animals have revealed that about one-quarter of ECII stellate cells are grid cells (Rowland et al., 2018). For each grid cell, the spacing of the firing fields in the grid depends on the location of the cell in EC. Specifically, cells located dorsally near the postrhinal border have shorter distances between firing fields than cells located more ventrally (Fyhn et al., 2004). In addition to grid cells, ECII stellate cells encode head direction, speed, and object borders (Domnisoru et al., 2013; Gu et al., 2018; Rowland et al., 2018; C Sun et al., 2015).

Recordings in vitro have identified a few unusual features of ECII stellate (ocean) cells (Figure 5.29C–D) (Alonso and Klink, 1993; Alonso and Llinás, 1989). They exhibit a large amount of sag in hyperpolarizing voltage responses, a feature characteristic of I_h, which is mediated by HCN channels. In addition, upon depolarization, they exhibit prominent oscillations in the theta-frequency range. Pharmacological studies have revealed that these intrinsic oscillations are mediated by interactions between persistent sodium current and HCN-mediated I_h (Alonso and Llinás, 1989; Dickson et al., 2000; Fan et al., 1994; Magistretti and Alonso, 1999a, 1999b; Magistretti et al., 1999; White et al., 1993). Several studies have demonstrated that these intrinsic oscillations are subject to modulation following activation of mAChRs (Gloveli et al., 1999; Klink and Alonso, 1997a; Shalinsky et al., 2002). Similar observations have been made in pyramidal neurons of PaS, where theta oscillations are strongest (Glasgow and Chapman, 2008).

Voltage clamp measurements of I_h in stellate cells along the dorsal/ventral axis revealed a correlation between the kinetics of current activation and deactivation and the membrane resonance, suggesting the hypothesis that I_h may contribute to the dorsal/ventral difference in subthreshold membrane oscillations and grid-cell firing distances (Giocomo and Hasselmo, 2008). In EC, immunohistochemical staining has shown the presence of hyperpolarizing-activated nonselective cation channel (HCN) subunits HCN1 and HCN2

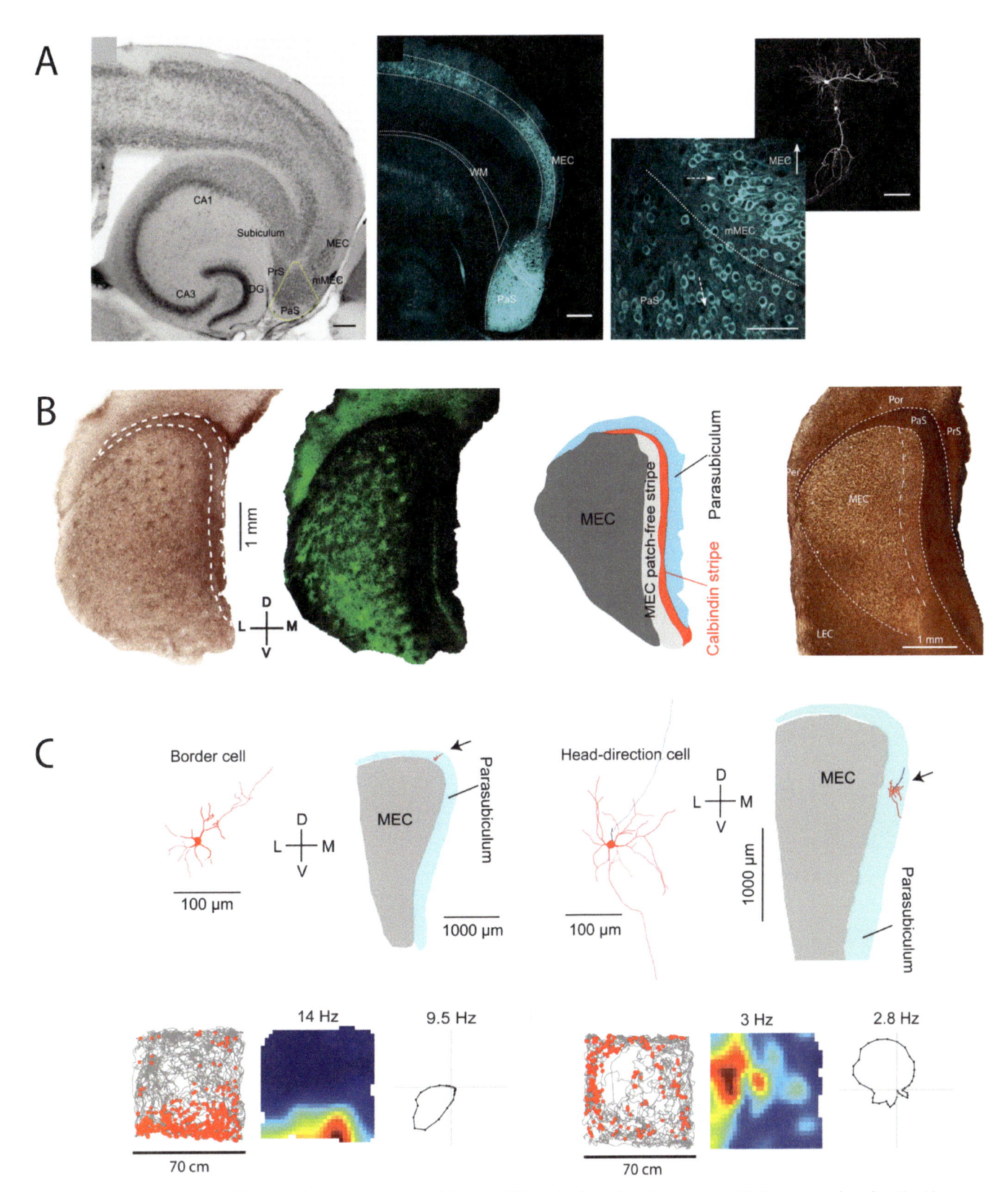

Figure 5.28 Organizational and functional properties of parasubiculum. (A) Left: horizontal section labeled with the neuronal marker NeuN. Scale bar, 200 μm. Middle: horizontal slice stained for WFS1, which is expressed at high levels in PaS and MEC layer II. Dotted lines outline the lateral and medial borders of the PaS, as well as MEC layer II and the fiber tract. WM, white matter. Scale bar, 200 μm. Right: closeup of WFS1 labeling in the PaS. Note the change in projection angle of apical dendrites of WFS1-expressing cells between the PaS and neighboring medialmost MEC (mMEC). Dashed arrows indicate the general projection direction of dendrites of PaS and mMEC neurons. Solid arrow indicates location of MEC. Inset, biocytin labeling of two filled neurons: one in the PaS and one in the mMEC. Scale bars, 100 μm. (B) Left: tangential section stained for acetylcholinesterase activity (dark precipitate). The shape of PaS is outlined by the white dashed line. Middle left: the same tangential section processed for calbindin immunoreactivity (green); the shape of the parasubiculum is negatively outlined by an absence of calbindin immunoreactivity. Middle, right: schematic of the parasubiculum (blue) and adjacent MEC subdivisions. Right: tangential section showing high levels of acetylcholinesterase in PaS. PrS, Presubiculum; LEC, lateral entorhinal cortex; PaS, parasubiculum; Por, postrhinal cortex; Per, perirhinal cortex. (C) Dendritic morphology, location, and functional properties of a border cell (left) and a head-direction cell (right) in PaS. Bottom plots: left, walking location (gray lines) in the square enclosure and spikes (red dots); middle, heat map of firing rate by location; right, polar plot of firing by head direction. (Sources: (A) Sammons et al., 2019; (B, C) Tang et al., 2016.)

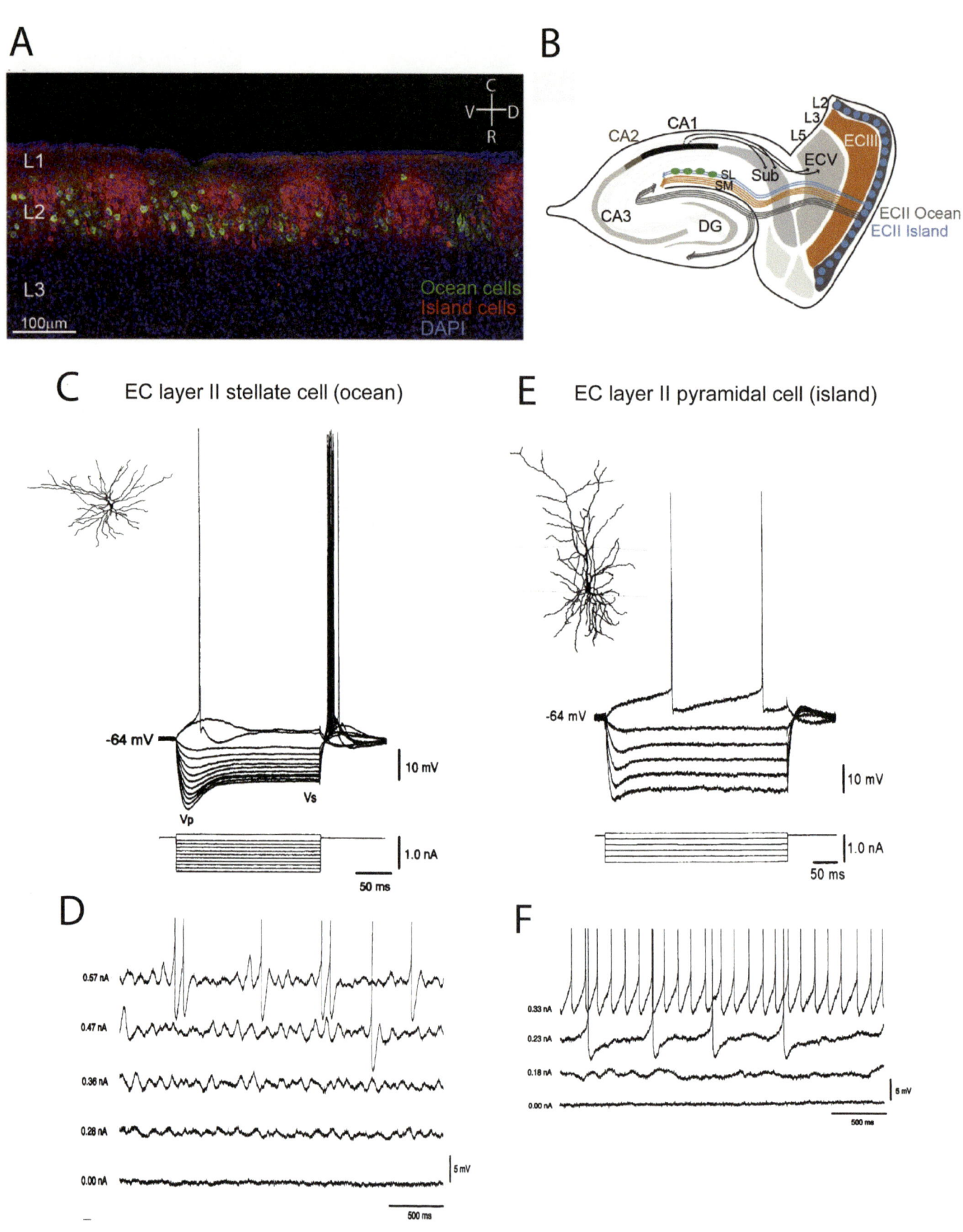

Figure 5.29 Organization of entorhinal cortex layer II. (A) Sagittal section of MEC illustrating major cell types in layer II (L2): island cells (WFS1 positive, red) and ocean cells (reelin positive, green). DAPI: nuclei staining (blue). D; dorsal, V; ventral, R; rostral, C; caudal. (B) Diagram of entorhinal-hippocampal circuit. Island cells (blue, ECIIi) directly project to stratum lacunosum (SL) of CA1 where they contact GABAergic interneurons (green). ECIII cells (orange) project to stratum moleculare (SM) of CA1 where they contact CA1 pyramidal cells. Ocean cells (gray, ECIIo) project to the dentate gyrus (DG), CA3, and CA2. Sub; subiculum. (C) Voltage-current relation of an EC layer II stellate cell. The response of the cell to hyperpolarizing and depolarizing current steps from the resting membrane potential. Inset, camera lucida reconstruction of a stellate cell. (D) Stellate cell subthreshold rhythmic voltage oscillations. Development of oscillations with increasing levels of depolarization. Note that at rest (0 nA, V_m = -64 mV), no membrane potential oscillations are present, but they clearly develop with current injection of 0.28 nA (V_m = -58 mV). (E) Voltage-current relationship of nonstellate cells. The responses of a pyramidal cell to injection of depolarizing and hyperpolarizing current pulses applied from the resting membrane potential. Inset, camera lucida reconstruction of a layer II pyramidal cell. (F) Subthreshold membrane voltage behavior of nonstellate cells with membrane depolarization. Note the absence of both the persistent rhythmic subthreshold oscillatory activity. (Sources: (A, B) Kitamura, 2017; (C–F) Alonso and Klink, 1993.)

(Notomi and Shigemoto, 2004). Furthermore, the kinetics of I_h is determined by the subunits as well as many intracellular signaling factors, such as the presence of cyclic nucleotides that can alter the gating of these channels (Chen et al., 2001; Wang et al., 2001). Recordings of stellate cells in slices from HCN1 knockout (KO) animals revealed membrane potential oscillations in these cells that were substantially slower than wild-type controls, as well as a lack of change along the dorsal-ventral axis (Giocomo and Hasselmo, 2009). In HCN1 KO mice, the grid-cell firing spacing was substantially increased for all cells, yet there still remained an increase in grid-cell firing distance along the dorsal-ventral axis, indicating that the potential presence of HCN2 or differences in synaptic input are contributing to the topographical organization of the grid-cell network (Giocomo et al., 2011). As a cautionary note, however, relating the intrinsic properties of neurons to higher-order properties such as network oscillations is complex and therefore challenging.

The stellate cells (ocean) of layer II are the primary source of the PP projection from EC to DG, CA2, and CA3 (Figure 5.29B) (van Groen et al., 2003; Steward and Scoville, 1976). Detailed reconstructions have revealed that the axonal arborization from a single layer II stellate cell is extensive, encompassing both the suprapyramidal and infrapyramidal blades of the dentate gyrus and encompassing more than two thirds of the septo-temporal extent of the dentate gyrus (Tamamaki, 1997; Tamamaki and Nojyo, 1993). The axons of layer II stellate cells also form synapses on CA3 pyramidal neurons. Importantly, many stellate-cell axons do not cross the hippocampal fissure; rather, they project along one side of the fissure to CA3 and bend around the fissure. Axon collaterals also branch and form synaptic connections within EC (superficial and deep layers) and subiculum (Germroth et al., 1991; Klink and Alonso, 1997b; Lingenhöhl and Finch, 1991; Tamamaki and Nojyo, 1993).

5.11.3.2 Layer II pyramidal cells (islands)

Pyramidal cells (islands) of layer II have both basal and apical dendrites, with spine density decreasing with distance from the soma (Figure 5.29E) (Tang et al., 2014). In vitro, several electrophysiological properties differ markedly from those of ECII stellate cells (Alonso and Klink, 1993). Namely, ECII pyramidal cells exhibit less sag in response to hyperpolarizing current injections, compared with ECII stellate cells, indicative of less HCN-mediated I_h. In addition, they do not exhibit the subthreshold oscillations that are observed in stellate cells in vitro (Figure 5.29E–F).

ECII pyramidal (island) cells receive strong input from PaS (Tang et al., 2016). Several other axon projections have been observed from ECII pyramidal cells. Approximately half of the cells project extensively to local superficial layers of the ipsilateral entorhinal cortex, ~30% projecting to the contralateral EC, 20% to hippocampal area CA1, and a small minority to the medial septum (Fuchs et al., 2016; Kanter et al., 2017; Kitamura et al., 2014; Ohara et al., 2019; Varga et al., 2010). ECII pyramidal cells that project to the hippocampus do not project to DG or CA3. Instead, they form a projection to CA1, which primarily targets inhibitory interneurons near the border of SR and SLM (Figure 5.29B) (Kitamura et al., 2014).

5.11.3.3 Layer III pyramidal cells

Layer III pyramidal neurons are the most numerous neuronal subtype in EC. These cells can readily be labeled by immunohistochemical staining for Purkinje cell protein 4 (PCP4)

(Tang et al., 2015) or oxidation resistance 1 gene (*Oxr1*) (Suh et al., 2011), revealing a uniform uninterrupted sheet of cells in layer III. The somata of these cells are pyramidal, with dendrites that extend into layer I, forming bundles that appear to avoid the calbindin-expressing clusters of layer II pyramidal cells (Figure 5.30) (Ray et al., 2017; Tang et al., 2015).

Zinc-positive terminals cluster in regions complementary to calbindin patches, localizing to PCP4-stained regions (Ray et al., 2017; Slomianka and Geneser, 1991). There is evidence from developmental studies that these zinc terminals arrive from the presubiculum (Slomianka and Geneser, 1997), and electrophysiological studies indicated that these inputs indeed selectively target layer III pyramidal neurons (Burgalossi et al., 2011; Canto and Witter, 2012).

ECIII pyramidal cells do not innervate DG or CA3. Instead, they form the direct, PP/TA projection from EC to CA1 (Figure 5.29B). Projections to CA1 are bilateral; in addition, they project to contralateral EC (Dickson et al., 1997; van Groen et al., 2003; Ohara et al., 2019; Steward and Scoville, 1976).

The intrinsic electrophysiological properties of ECIII pyramidal cells are uniform and independent of axonal targeting (Gloveli, Schmitz, Empson, and Heinemann, 1997; Tang et al., 2015). In brain slices, ECIII pyramidal cells exhibit regular spiking patterns in response to depolarization and they lack intrinsic oscillatory properties and pronounced I_h (Figure 5.30D) (Dickson et al., 1997; Gloveli, Schmitz, Empson, Dugladze, et al., 1997). With electrical stimulation, many ECIII pyramidal neurons display a broad excitatory postsynaptic potential that can last up to 3 seconds, whereas others have a fast EPSP followed by a prolonged inhibitory hyperpolarization (Gloveli, Schmitz, Empson, and Heinemann, 1997). In vivo, ECIII pyramidal cells exhibit spatial tuning, regular spiking at high firing rates, and weak modulation by theta rhythm (Ebbesen et al., 2016; Quilichini et al., 2010; Tang et al., 2015).

5.11.3.4 Theta oscillations and parallel processing in superficial layers

Theta oscillations are a prominent feature of the local field potential in EC, particularly in layer II, where theta is strongest in the islands (populated by pyramidal cells) and weaker in the ocean (populated by stellate cells) (Ray et al., 2014). Projections from PaS to ECII are strong, and likely also contribute to the theta oscillations observed there (Tang et al., 2016). Theta oscillations are enhanced by modulatory inputs arriving from MS.

Juxtacellular recordings in vivo have enabled comparison of the firing properties of morphologically identified cell types in ECII, ECIII, and PaS (Figure 5.31) (Ebbesen et al., 2016). Theta rhythmicity, theta locking, and theta-cycle skipping—the latter a property that may be essential for grid-cell periodicity (Brandon et al., 2013)—were all observed to be greatest in pyramidal cells of ECII and PaS. In contrast, fewer ECII stellate cells and ECIII pyramidal cells exhibited these properties, but they were more likely to exhibit phase precession on successive theta cycles. Similarly, functional imaging suggests that ECII pyramidal cells are modulated by running speed to a greater extent than ECII stellate cells (C Sun et al., 2015). These findings are inconsistent with the observation that intrinsic oscillations are greatest in ECII stellate cells (as described above), suggesting that relating the intrinsic membrane properties observed in vitro to the firing properties observed in vivo is a challenging problem.

The physiological properties of PaS(pyramidal)-ECII(pyramidal) and ECII(stellate)-ECIII(pyramidal) cells are mirrored by differences in connectivity. PaS pyramidal cells connect strongly to ECII pyramidal cells, whereas ECII stellate cells connect strongly to ECIII pyramidal cells. Together, these observations suggest that the two groups of cells may constitute parallel processing streams in the EC (Ebbesen et al., 2016). Intriguingly, the ECII(stellate)-ECIII(pyramidal) pathways excite all hippocampal subfields, whereas the PaS(pyramidal)-ECII(pyramidal) pathway drives inhibition of CA1 (Figure 5.29B).

The relative contributions of these cell types to the population of grid cells recorded in freely moving animals is uncertain. Grid cells are abundant in layer II of EC, but the relative contributions of ECII stellate cells and pyramidal cells is unclear (Domnisoru et al., 2013; C Sun et al., 2015; Tang et al., 2014). Conflicting results also make it inconclusive whether ECIII pyramidal cells exhibit grid-cell firing (Boccara et al., 2010; Sargolini et al., 2006; Tang et al., 2015).

5.11.3.5 Deep-layer pyramidal neurons

Cells in the deep layers of EC are functionally distinct from their counterparts in superficial layers in several ways. Layer IV is a cell-free layer, while layer V contains pyramidal neurons and polymorphic neurons, many of which show grid-like responses in vivo that are modulated by theta rhythm and by head direction (Dickson et al., 2000; Gerlei et al., 2021; Sargolini et al., 2006). In brain slices, the physiological properties of pyramidal and polymorphic cells are similar (Egorov, Heinemann, et al., 2002; Hamam et al., 2000, 2002), but distinctions between different types of pyramidal neurons have been made based on cytoarchitecture, morphology, gene expression, and connectivity.

ECV can be subdivided into two sublayers, called ECVa and ECVb, with distinct properties (Figure 5.32) (Gerlei et al., 2021). ECVa neurons are large pyramidal neurons that project to numerous cortical and subcortical targets (Sürmeli et al., 2015). They also form extensive reciprocal connections with other cells in ECVa, but rarely with ECVb cells. Most of the neurons in ECVb are relatively small and more densely packed pyramidal cells. They form reciprocal connections with other ECVb neurons and some connections with ECVa neurons. Their axons remain mostly within EC, extending superficially where they form connections in ECII and ECIII (Gerlei et al., 2021; Ohara et al., 2018).

Inputs from the dorsal hippocampus preferentially innervate ECVb, whereas inputs from the ventral hippocampus favor ECVa. Inputs from ECII stellate and ECIII pyramidal cells are restricted to ECVb neurons. While hippocampal inputs are restricted to basal dendrites, inputs from other areas, such as PrS, and within

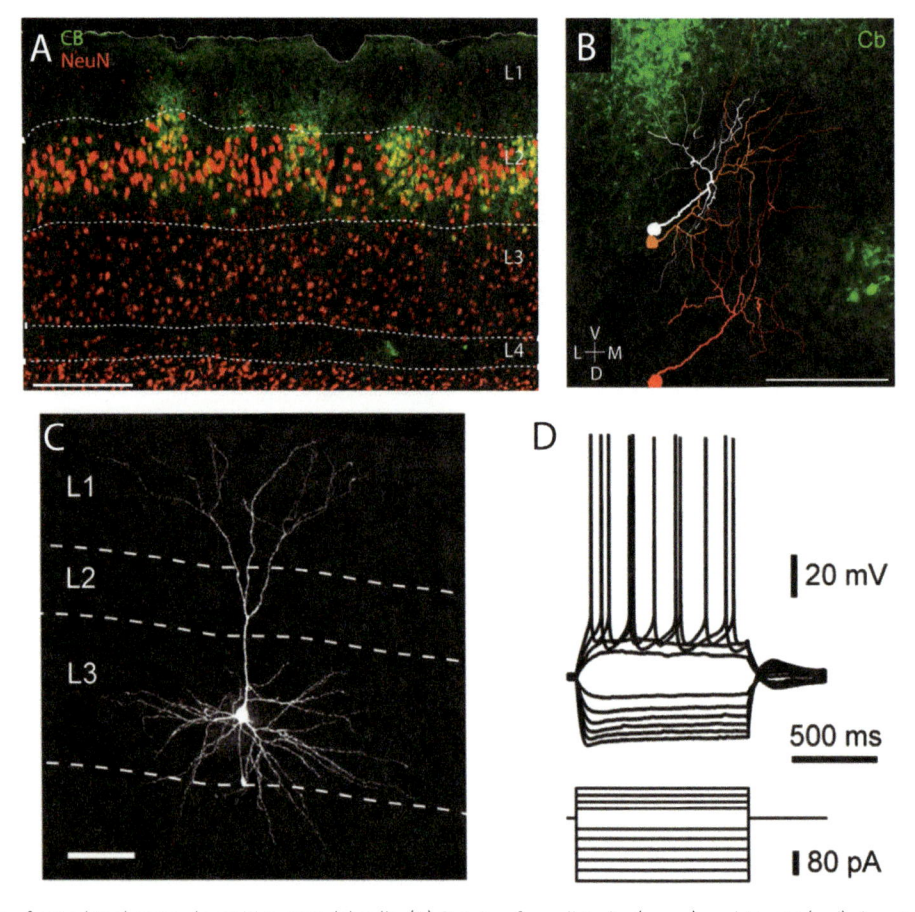

Figure 5.30 Properties of entorhinal cortex layer III pyramidal cells. (A) Staining for calbindin (green) and NeuN (red) showing the homogeneous and uniform distribution of neuronal somata in layer III of MEC. Note comparison of the modular organization of the adjacent layer II. Scale bar, 250 μm. (B) Reconstructions of the apical dendritic morphologies of three representative layer III pyramidal neurons, superimposed on the calbindin (Cb) staining in MEC layer II (tangential view). Note that the dendrites largely avoid the calbindin territories. Scale bar, 200 μm. (C) Dendritic morphology of a layer III pyramidal neuron in MEC. Scale bar, 100 μm. (D) V_m responses to current injection in a layer III pyramidal neuron in MEC in a slice preparation. (Source: (A–D) Tang et al., 2015.)

EC, target apical dendrites (Wouterlood et al., 2004), suggesting the possibility of complex mechanisms of dendritic integration and computation (Medinilla et al., 2013).

In addition to these differences in inputs and outputs, pyramidal neurons in ECVa and ECVb also differ in terms of gene expression and morphology. Neurons in ECVa express *Etv1*, whereas neurons in ECVb express *Ctip2* (Figure 5.32B) (Sürmeli et al., 2015). Morphologically, pyramidal neurons in ECVa and ECVb can be distinguished on the orientation of their basal dendrites, which are more horizontally oriented in ECVa (Figure 5.32C) (Hamam et al., 2002; Sürmeli et al., 2015).

Gene expression in EC has been assessed using a combination of RNA-seq, detailed analysis of the Allen Institute in situ hybridization (ISH) atlas, and immunohistochemistry (IHC). Approximately 700–800 genes exhibited layer-specific expression and a similar number exhibited differences along the dorsal-ventral axis. Genes distinguishing sublayers (e.g., ECVa and ECVb) as well as subgroups of cells within a layer (e.g., islands) were also identified using this approach (Ramsden et al., 2015; Sürmeli et al., 2015).

A striking property of layer V pyramidal cells in entorhinal cortex is their ability to integrate neural activity over long periods of time. During activation of mAChRs, stimuli lasting for a few seconds can lead to sustained action potential firing for several minutes (Figure 5.32D) (Egorov, Hamam, et al., 2002). Furthermore, repeated stimulation leads to sustained firing at higher frequencies. This unique form of neural integration, which is mediated by a calcium-activated, nonspecific cation current, has been proposed to contribute to the function of EC in working and long-term memory (Egorov, Heinemann, et al., 2002; Hasselmo and Brandon, 2008).

The ability to identify region- and cell-type- specific gene expression through approaches such as ISH, IHC, and RNA-seq is a powerful tool not only for investigating cellular diversity but also for exploring the role of specific cell types in circuit function and behavior. Excellent examples of this approach have been pursued in studies of MEC, including studies involving both cell-type specific imaging and manipulation in freely moving animals (Kitamura, 2017; Kitamura et al., 2015; C Sun et al., 2015). A major challenge for the field is to integrate these and similar studies in other brain regions (e.g., hippocampus, subiculum, amygdala, neocortex) into testable models of the contributions of various brain regions and cell types to processes related to spatial navigation and memory (Eichenbaum, 1999; Eichenbaum and Cohen, 2014; Kumaran and McClelland, 2012; Marr, 1971; McClelland et al., 1995; W Sun et al., 2021). An even greater challenge will be to relate the unique functional properties of various cell types and their synaptic connections to models and theories of brain function.

5.12 Local circuit inhibitory interneurons

Although pyramidal cells are considered the "workhorses" of information processing and representation, hippocampal circuits also comprise a smaller yet highly diverse set of GABAergic inhibitory interneurons that critically regulate the activity of pyramidal cells (see Chapters 7 and 10 for further discussion). GABAergic inhibitory interneurons represent ~10%–15% of the entire hippocampal neuronal population (Bezaire and Soltesz, 2013; Freund and Buzsáki, 1996; Pelkey et al., 2017), and they release the neurotransmitter GABA onto their targets. The postsynaptic effect of synaptically released GABA is mediated by $GABA_A$ and $GABA_B$ receptors, permeable to $Cl^-/HCO3^-$ or coupled via G proteins to potassium channels, respectively. Consequently, a shunt and/or hyperpolarization results in the reduced excitability of the target cell.

While traditional views posit that the primary function of inhibition is to regulate excitability of individual cells and to counterbalance excitation in neuronal networks, increasing evidence indicates that inhibition has more complex roles in cortical networks than previously assumed. Inhibition can determine not only if but also when, where, and how individual neurons become active. By providing timed rhythmic inhibitory output signals, interneurons synchronize pyramidal cell assemblies and thereby contribute to the processing and encoding of information. Moreover, interneurons synchronize and entrain the activity of neuronal populations at various oscillatory frequencies, and thereby support the transfer and binding of information across brain areas (Bartos et al., 2007). Finally, GABAergic inhibition can modulate transmission and plasticity of glutamatergic synapses, shut off specific subcellular domains of their target cells, promote "winner-takes-all" situations (de Almeida et al., 2009; Strüber et al., 2017), and sharpen the tuning of individual pyramidal cells (Hefft and Jonas, 2005; Isaacson and Scanziani, 2011; Royer et al., 2012). Thus, while pyramidal cell assemblies maintain the information content of neuronal representation, inhibitory interneurons play a crucial role in sculpting the activity of individual pyramidal cells, neuronal subnetworks, and their temporal dynamics.

As described earlier in this chapter, principal glutamatergic cells of both the hippocampal areas CA1-3 and the dentate gyrus (DG) have their cell bodies organized in highly structured lamina. In the CA1 region of the hippocampus, pyramidal neuron dendrites lie orthogonal to the cell body layer and span the entire subfield from the deep layers of the stratum oriens to the superficial layer of the stratum lacunosum-moleculare. This organization allows pyramidal cells to receive layer-specific synaptic inputs. In contrast, the cell bodies of interneurons do not show a similar layered organization. Their somata are scattered throughout all subfields and layers of the hippocampus, and their dendrites have divergent orientations and extents within their respective subfields. The positioning of their somata and the reach of their dendritic arbors determines which hippocampal pathways activate them, thereby providing either feedforward or feedback inhibition, or both (Figure 5.33A).

GABAergic interneurons are highly diverse and are characterized by distinct morphologies, molecular, intrinsic, and synaptic properties, target selectivity, connectivity, and activity profiles (Pelkey et al., 2017), all of which has given rise to their classification into various types (Figure 5.33B–C). Indeed, the diversity of GABAergic cell types has been proposed to provide a spatially and temporally fine-tuned control of activity of single cells, even at the level of their subcellular compartments (e.g., soma, proximal or distal dendritic tree, spines). Here we aim to relate interneuron characteristics to their functional role on the level of the individual cell, the microcircuit and selected hippocampus-related mnemonic functions. This is a crucial topic in interneuron neuroscience, because impaired inhibition has been implicated in deficient processing of information in various brain disease states including epilepsy, Alzheimer's disease, Rett syndrome, and depression (Lewis et al., 2005; Neumann et al., 2017; Sauer et al., 2015; Verret et al., 2012; see also Chapters 18–20).

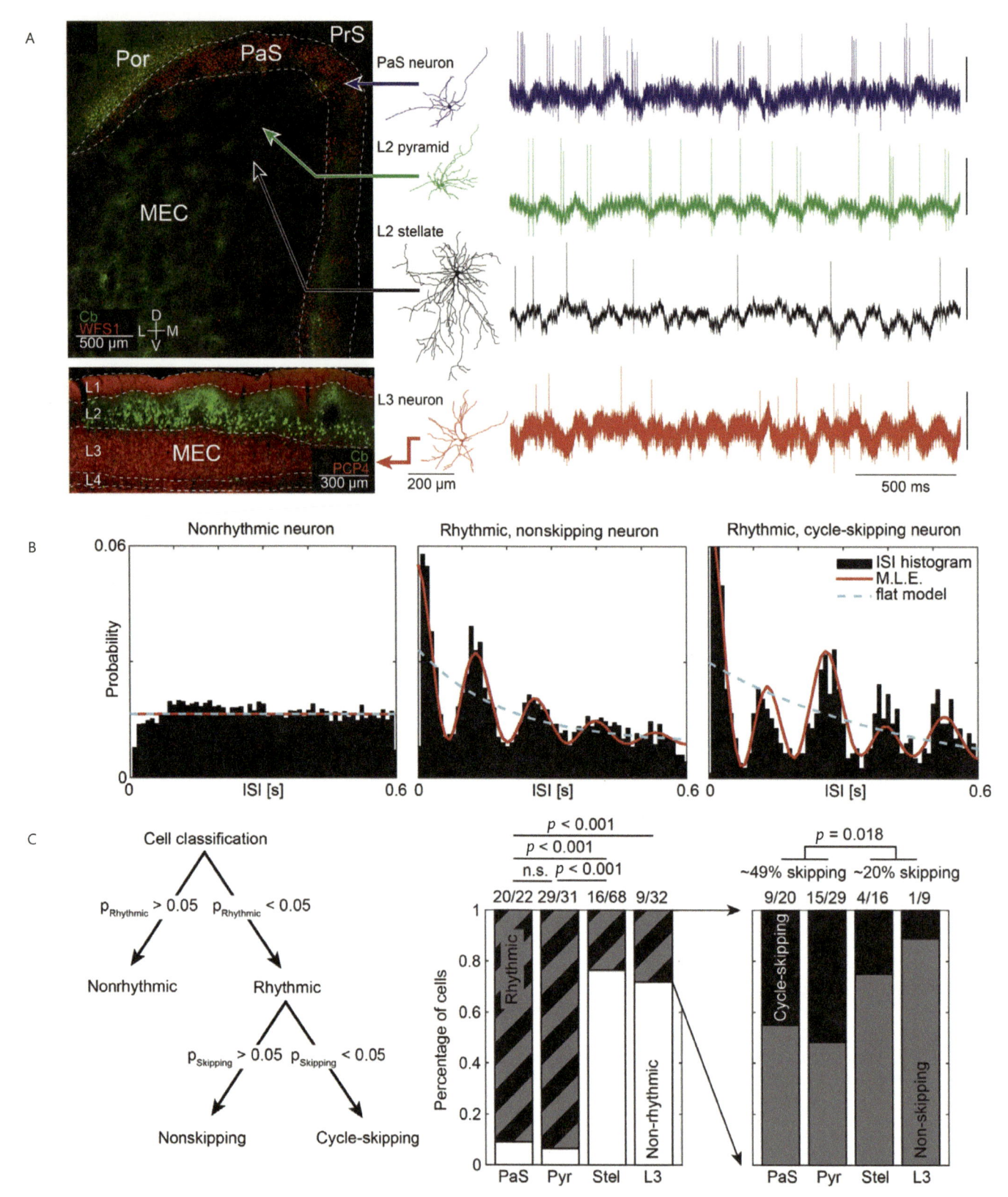

Figure 5.31 Firing properties of neurons in the superficial layers of entorhinal cortex. (A) Top left: tangential section of the parasubiculum (PaS) and layer II of medial entorhinal cortex (MEC) stained for calbindin (Cb, green) and WFS1 (red). Also visible are the presubiculum (PrS) and postrhinal cortex (Por). Bottom left: parasagittal section of the MEC stained for Cb (green) and PCP4 (red). Right: reconstructions of examples of the four neuron types (tangential sections, top view): a PaS neuron (blue), an MEC LII pyramidal neuron (green), an MEC LII stellate cell (black), and an MEC LIII neuron (red), corresponding to the anatomical cell types marked by arrows. Juxtacellular recording traces of the reconstructed cells. The spiking of the PaS neuron and the MEC LII pyramidal neuron exhibit bursting and theta-modulation. Scale bars, 1 mV. (B) Interspike interval (ISI) histograms (black bars) of nonrhythmic (left), rhythmic and nonskipping (middle), and rhythmic but theta cycle-skipping (right) neurons recorded with juxtacellular electrodes. Solid red lines show maximum likelihood estimates of the ISI, and dashed blue lines indicate a flat model (no rhythmicity or cycle skipping). Bin width, 1 ms. (C) Left: flow diagram of the cell classification procedure. Middle: comparison of the proportions of nonrhythmic and rhythmic neurons recorded in the PaS, identified and putative MEC LII pyramidal neurons, identified and putative MEC LII stellate cells, and MEC LIII neurons. Right: comparison of the proportions of rhythmic, non-cycle-skipping and rhythmic, theta cycle-skipping neurons recorded in the four neuron types. The generally rhythmic cell types (PaS and ECII pyramidal) have a larger proportion of theta cycle-skipping neurons than the generally nonrhythmic cell types (stellate and ECIII). (Source: (A–C) Ebbesen et al., 2016.)

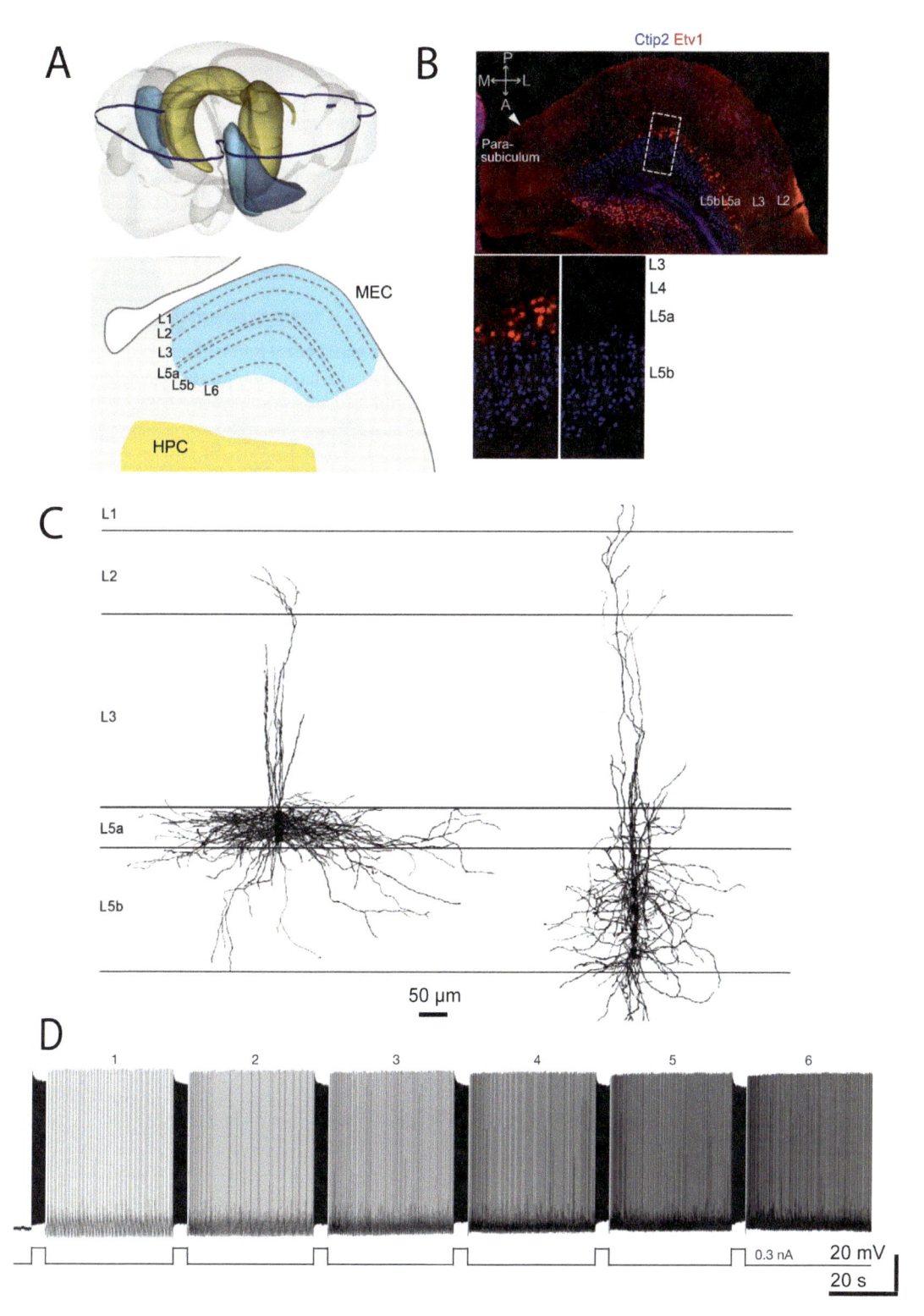

Figure 5.32 Properties of pyramidal neurons in the deep layers of entorhinal cortex. (A) Schematic of the mouse brain (top) showing the hippocampus (yellow), medial entorhinal cortex (MEC, light blue), and lateral entorhinal cortex (LEC, dark blue). The horizontal section (bottom) is from the plane highlighted in the top panel (dark blue outline). (B) Layer 5a and 5b are demarcated by neurons expressing the transcription factors Etv1 and Ctip2, respectively. (C) Superimposition of reconstructions of 10 nonresponsive (L5a, left) and 10 responsive neurons (L5b, right). Note the restricted spread of the basal dendrites into adjacent layers. (D) Intracellular recording from a layer 5 pyramidal neuron in a brain slice from EC bathed in 10 μM carbachol to activate mAChRs. Responses to repeated 4-second-long depolarizing current steps gives rise to distinct increases in stable discharge rate (1 to 6). (Sources: (A–B) Gerlei et al., 2021; (C) Sürmeli et al., 2015; (D) Egorov et al., 2002.)

of the inhibitory output synapse (e.g., soma, dendrite), the type and density of postsynaptic $GABA_A$ receptors ($GABA_A$Rs), and GABA reuptake mechanisms. Detailed investigations into the functional (e.g., rise time, peak amplitude, decay time constant) and dynamic properties (e.g., short- or long-term weight changes) of GABAergic synapses have been performed for some interneuron types, particularly for PVIs, cholecystokinin (CCK)-expressing interneurons (CCKIs), and neurogliaform interneurons (NGFIs). These interneuron types have transmitter-release profiles defined as synchronous (each action potential rapidly produces neurotransmitter release), asynchronous (upon axon terminal depolarization, the fusion of vesicles is subject to a variable delay), and a combination of phasic and tonic, respectively (Armstrong et al., 2011; Bartos et al., 2001, 2002; Daw et al., 2009; Hefft and Jonas, 2005; Szabadics et al., 2007).

5.12.1.4 Input properties

Temporally precise recruitment of interneurons by excitatory input synapses is considered a central aspect in controlling information processing in neuronal networks. Interneurons receive many thousands of glutamatergic inputs along their entire dendritic tree (Bezaire and Soltesz, 2013; Gulyás et al., 1999; Mátyás et al., 2004). Depending on the distribution of their dendritic arbors, interneurons can influence excitation from a broad range of defined input pathways. Because distinct excitatory pathways (e.g., SC and PP) likely have distinct roles in information processing within the circuit, the ability of interneurons to selectively influence these patterns undoubtedly influences network computation in myriad ways.

The effect of excitatory inputs on interneuron activity depends, however, on further factors including presynaptic release properties, the type and density of postsynaptic ionotropic and metabotropic glutamate receptors (iGluRs, mGluRs, respectively), and the integrative properties of interneuron dendrites (Geiger et al., 1997; Glickfeld and Scanziani, 2006; Isaac et al., 2007; Jonas et al., 2004). Furthermore, different interneurons express distinct subtypes of iGluRs and mGluRs, further influencing their physiological function. Finally, repetitive activation of convergent glutamatergic inputs produces short-term plasticity (facilitation or depression) of excitatory postsynaptic potentials (EPSPs), and repetitive activation at high frequencies for longer periods of time can induce long-term plasticity expressed as long-term potentiation (LTP) or long-term depression (LTD) of EPSPs (Kullmann and Lamsa, 2007). These forms of plasticity alter the efficiency of interneuron recruitment in the local circuit (Bartos et al., 2007). The molecular and cellular mechanisms underlying synaptic plasticity at interneuron inputs are highly diverse and vary in a cell-type-specific manner, thereby adding to the enormous diversity of interneurons (see Chapter 6).

5.12.1.5 Gene expression

The field of neuronal classification has been revolutionized by the emergence of genomic sequence analysis techniques (Fuzik et al., 2016; Gouwens et al., 2020; Harris et al., 2018; Zeisel et al., 2015). Originally, single cell reverse transcription polymerase chain reaction (RT-PCR) studies were employed that coupled whole-cell electrophysiological recordings with the harvesting of individual cell transcripts, which were then amplified using PCR. However, due to the small amounts of mRNA harvested from a single cell, only a small fraction of neuronally expressed genes encoding a single channel or receptor could be identified at any one time (Geiger

et al., 1995; Tricoire et al., 2010). For replicable genome-wide expression analysis, microarray-based techniques were developed and applied both on the level of single cells or populations of cells, sorted either manually or automatically based on a fluorescence molecule expressed in a neurochemically defined neuron population. Quantitative single-cell RNA sequencing (scRNA-seq) and single nuclei sequencing (snRNA-seq) have subsequently emerged as powerful tools in the neurosciences, because they allow the linkage of cell physiology to gene expression profiles from both the cell and nucleus from live and fixed tissue samples (Lein et al., 2017; Zeisel et al., 2015). Patch-seq is another method that combines single neuron whole-cell recordings, intracellular labelling, and in-depth transcriptional profiling of over 10,000 genes, allowing the identification of genetic, morphological, and physiological characterization of individual interneurons (Fuzik et al., 2016; Harris et al., 2018; Zeisel et al., 2015). Classification of interneuron types using single-cell transcriptomics has, for example, shown that the *Sncg* gene (gamma-synuclein) is selectively expressed in CCK-interneurons but not in PVIs, SOM-expressing interneurons (SOMIs) or non-CCK-containing, vasoactive intestinal polypeptide (VIP)-expressing cells (Gouwens et al., 2020; Tasic et al., 2016; Yao et al., 2021). Moreover, *Unc5b* (netrin receptor) is largely expressed in PV-AAIs and not in PV-BCs (Dudok, Klein, et al., 2021; Dudok, Szoboszlay, et al., 2021; Paul et al., 2017). AAIs in CA1 express the transcription factor *SATB1* (Yamada and Jinno, 2015), which has so far not been identified in AAIs of the DG. Thus, genetic access to interneuron types, together with the development of transgenic driver lines and in vivo recordings and imaging (Geiller et al., 2020; Hainmueller and Bartos, 2018; Ziv et al., 2013), has facilitated interrogation of long-standing questions on the dynamics and functional impact of the various interneuron types in the control of hippocampal circuit function.

5.13 Physiological properties of inhibitory interneurons

The complement of voltage- and ligand-gated ion channels in inhibitory and excitatory neurons in the hippocampus varies significantly. Different types of interneurons perform distinct functions, in part because they express distinct complements of channels. Here, we survey specific examples of interneuron types in which channels regulating passive membrane properties, excitability and action potential phenotype have been well characterized.

5.13.1 Passive membrane properties

Where studied, inhibitory interneurons possess resting membrane potentials (V_{rest}) slightly more depolarized than those obtained from principal cells. Estimates of interneuron V_{rest} have provided values spanning a wide range but typically lie 5–10 mV more depolarized than values obtained from pyramidal cells (Geiger et al., 1997; Hosp et al., 2014; Tricoire et al., 2010; Vida et al., 1998).

Interneurons generally have a higher input resistance (R_N) than principal cells, presumably due to their smaller somata and total dendritic length, but measured values of R_N are highly variable among interneuron types (Glickfeld and Scanziani, 2006; Nörenberg et al., 2010). Interneurons have a relatively fast membrane time constant (τ_m), ranging from ~7 ms in NGFCs to ~20 ms in CCK-BCs (Armstrong et al., 2011; Glickfeld and Scanziani, 2006; Hosp et al.,

2014; Pouille and Scanziani, 2004). Single-cell modeling based on somatodendritic recordings from DG BCs revealed a nonuniform membrane resistivity (R_m) across the soma, distal dendrites, and axon, and that the intracellular resistivity (R_i) is variable among individual BCs (Nörenberg et al., 2010).

The passive membrane parameters of various CA3 interneuron types have been determined (Chitwood et al., 1999); R_N values were significantly higher than those reported for BCs (~180 MΩ), but similar to stratum lucidum interneurons (~440 MΩ). Compartmental modeling of these cells indicates that although the total surface area of the interneurons and the physical length of their dendrites are considerably shorter than for CA1 pyramidal neurons, their electrotonic profiles are often surprisingly similar.

What are the functional consequences of these passive membrane properties on the integration of synaptic inputs? As EPSPs propagate from their induction site at distal dendrites to the soma, they will be attenuated and decelerated. This filtering depends on several factors such as synapse location, the architecture of the dendritic tree, the passive electrotonic profile, and the active membrane properties (Emri et al., 2001). For PV-BCs, the combination of a low R_N and a fast τ_m implies a low R_m. The combination of a low R_m with large-diameter PV-BC dendrites supports fast propagation of EPSPs (Geiger et al., 1997; Nörenberg et al., 2010). However, it also implies that interneuron dendrites conduct EPSPs with strong amplitude attenuation.

Indeed, as EPSPs propagate along dendrites to the soma, their amplitude declines, and their time course becomes governed by τ_m. Thus, a fast τ_m defines a narrow (~5 ms at BC-GC synapses in the DG) time window for temporal summation of EPSPs, and thereby supports coincidence detection, which could strongly modify synaptic properties (Geiger et al., 1997; Glickfeld and Scanziani, 2006; Nörenberg et al., 2010). In contrast, other interneuron types such as CCK-BCs, SOM-expressing CA1 OLM, or DG HIPP cells have higher R_N and longer τ_m (Cea-del Rio et al., 2010; Glickfeld and Scanziani, 2006; Hosp et al., 2014; Morin et al., 1996; Taverna et al., 2005), resulting in less attenuation, and thus a broader time window for temporal integration of converging inputs. A reduced attenuation of synaptic signals will be further supported by active membrane properties in CA1 OLM cells. Thus, interneurons are equipped with distinct passive membrane properties, which shape the spatiotemporal integration of EPSPs and the recruitment of different classes of inhibition within the local network.

5.13.2 Voltage-gated channels in inhibitory interneurons

The distinctive physiological properties of diverse GABAergic cells suggests that each type expresses a unique blend of ligand-gated and voltage-gated channels. However, only a few studies have examined the molecular composition of channels in identified interneuron types. Here, we discuss the physiological characteristics of the morphologically and/or neurochemically defined interneuron types that have been studied most extensively.

5.13.2.1 Action potential discharge patterns

PVIs—including BCs, BiCs, and AAIs—are called "fast-spiking" because they generate trains of action potentials at high frequencies (>100 Hz) in response to sustained depolarization. Their spike trains are nonadapting (constant interspike intervals) and nonaccommodating (stable peak action potential amplitude). In a

few cases, acceleration of train discharges was observed. Individual spikes are short (half-duration <0.5 ms), and followed by large, narrow AHPs. Small changes in input currents can cause large changes in discharge frequency.

In contrast, other interneuron types exhibit markedly different properties. For example, SOM-expressing OLM cells and CCK-BCs in CA1, as well as HICAPs in DG, show a lower discharge frequency resulting from spike-frequency adaptation. In these cells, individual spikes have a longer half-duration (>0.5 ms), which increases during trains of action potentials. NGFIs and Ivy cells discharge upon suprathreshold depolarization with a prolonged delay prior to the first spike. They possess broader spikes (>0.5 ms) and moderate spike-frequency adaptation. Finally, interneuron-preferring cells are characterized by a variety of discharge behaviors including irregular firing upon longer lasting current injections, bursting (3–4 spikes at the beginning of the depolarizing current injection) or a stuttering (bursts of spikes interleaved with silent periods) phenotype.

In addition to these activity patterns, a novel form of persistent firing has been observed in some interneuron types including PV-BCs, NGFIs, and Ivy cells (Chittajallu et al., 2020; Elgueta et al., 2015; Krook-Magnuson et al., 2011; Sheffield et al., 2011). Persistent firing emerges in the axons remote from the AIS, propagates retro-gradely to the soma, and can last for several minutes. In some cases, action potentials generated at remote axonal connections fail to propagate actively, resulting in spikelets observed at the soma (Sheffield et al., 2011). The mechanisms underlying the emergence of persistent firing are not fully clarified and may differ somewhat between cell types. In general, persistent firing does not require synaptic transmission (Sheffield et al., 2011), but does require activation of voltage-gated channels (Chittajallu et al., 2020; Elgueta et al., 2015; Sheffield et al., 2013). Intriguingly, persistent firing requires interactions between interneurons and astrocytes (Deemyad et al., 2018).

5.13.2.2 Voltage-gated potassium channels in inhibitory interneurons

The properties of interneuron action potentials suggest that they express voltage-gated ion channels distinct from their pyramidal neuron counterparts. For example, only certain types of K_v channels will support fast spiking. In recombinant systems, the potassium channel subunits $K_v3.1b$ and $K_v3.2$ confer currents that activate at highly depolarized potentials, show little inactivation during sustained depolarization, and deactivate rapidly upon repolarization (Rudy and McBain, 2001). Single-cell RT-PCR revealed high expression of $K_v3.1$ and $K_v3.2$ in hippocampal PVIs and recordings from PVIs revealed that large macroscopic potassium currents were dominated by $K_v3.2$ channels with fast kinetics (Martina et al., 1998). PVIs also express a slower delayed rectifier current and a rapid inactivating A-type current, mediated by $K_v4.2$ and $K_v4.3$ channels, as revealed by single cell RT-PCR analysis (Martina et al., 1998). However, the expression level of $K_v4.3$ is higher in other interneuron types, such as CCK- and calbindin (CB)-expressing cells and SOMIs (Bourdeau et al., 2007; Martina et al., 1998).

Similar to DG PVIs, macroscopic currents in CA1 OLM cells are mediated by a large-amplitude fast-delayed rectifier mediated by $K_v3.2$ and smaller contributions from a slow-delayed rectifier and rapidly inactivating A-type $K_v4.3$ channels (Lien et al., 2002). Dynamic-clamp experiments in which the artificial potassium conductances were added to real neurons revealed that K_v3-mediated currents act to keep action potentials brief by rapidly repolarizing the membrane potential and limiting the duration of the AHP (Lien et al., 2002). Moreover, high discharge frequencies are supported because K_v channels facilitate the recovery of Na_v channels from inactivation. In contrast, spike adaptation and action potential broadening, as observed in pyramidal cells, can be achieved by low-threshold inactivation K_v channels. Interestingly, PKA phosphorylation of $K_v3.2$ subunits triggered by histamine via H2 receptors reduces $K_v3.2$ function in PVIs and SOMIs, and thereby causes a broadening of action potentials and a reduction in the maximal discharge frequency (Atzori et al., 2000). Although both PVIs and OLM cells express $K_v3.2$ channels, the discharge frequency is higher in PVIs compared with OLM cells. This can be explained by subtle differences in the activation and inactivation properties of K_v channels (Lien et al., 2002; Martina et al., 1998). Thus, differential tuning of K_v3 channel properties (e.g., phosphorylation state, auxiliary subunits) could contribute to the different firing properties among interneuron types.

$K_v3.2$ channels cover the entire somatodendritic domain of all PVIs and 50% of SOMIs, whereas $K_v3.1b$ is only expressed in PVIs and not SOMIs (Du et al., 1996). The high density of K_v3 channels and their rapid gating kinetics allow them to rapidly repolarize the membrane after a depolarization. This results in a narrow time window for coincidence detection of multiple temporally and spatially converging synaptic inputs onto PVIs (Hu et al., 2010). Thus, EPSPs in PVIs trigger action potential generation at higher temporal precision than in pyramidal cells (Fricker and Miles, 2000).

The axons of PVIs express K_v3 as well as $K_v1.1$ and $K_v1.2$ channels, with the highest clustering of K_v3 channels at presynaptic sites (Cudmore et al., 2010; Rudy and McBain, 2001). $K_v1.1$ and $K_v1.2$ channels are enriched at the axon initial segment, with higher densities in interneurons than in pyramidal cells (Lorincz and Nusser, 2008). The low activation threshold of K_v1 channels and their slow gating characteristics define input-output conversion properties of PVIs (Hu et al., 2014). Indeed, longer-lasting events activate these channels and in turn suppresses action potential initiation. In contrast, fast EPSPs will bypass K_v1 channel activation and cause action potential generation with little delay (Hu et al., 2014). Thus, K_v1 channels add to the ability of fast coincidence detection of PVIs. Moreover, inactivation of these channels might cause delayed discharges upon long-lasting depolarization (Goldberg et al., 2008).

5.13.2.3 Voltage-gated sodium channels in inhibitory interneurons

Short-duration action potentials in interneurons depend on the reciprocal tuning of Na_v and K_v channel gating. Unlike pyramidal cells, PVI dendrites are almost devoid of Na_v channels. In PVIs, >95% of their Na_v channels are in the axon membrane, with the highest densities at the AIS close to the soma (distance ~20 μm). These are largely formed by the $Na_v1.1$ and $Na_v1.6$ subunits, with a lower contribution of $Na_v1.2$, $Na_v1.4$, and $Na_v1.7$ subunits (Hu and Jonas, 2014; Lorincz and Nusser, 2008). Single-cell modeling revealed that the rapid inactivation of Na_v channels, together with their fast recovery from inactivation, ensures short refractory periods, and together with the fast noninactivating delayed rectifier $K_v3.2$ channels allows the generation of the fast-spiking phenotype of PVIs (Hu et al., 2014, 2018). Indeed, inactivation of axonal Na_v channels is ~2-fold faster than that of somatic channels in hippocampal pyramidal cells and PVI somata (Hu et al., 2014). A further important criterion

for the fast-spiking phenotype is the high density of Na_v channels in PVI axons (Hu et al., 2014). Consistent with the high importance of fast interneuron discharges in the synchronization of neuronal networks at higher frequencies, reduced levels of $Na_v1.1$ in PVIs leads to reduced cortical gamma activity, altered network synchrony, and cognitive deficits in human amyloid-precursor-protein-transgenic mice (Verret et al., 2012).

In contrast to PVIs, OLM cells exhibit higher levels and uniform densities of Na_v channels across dendrites (Martina et al., 2000). Moreover, the peak Na_v conductance density in OLM dendrites is three times higher than that seen in dendrites of cortical pyramidal cells (Martina et al., 2000; Stuart and Sakmann, 1994). Simultaneous recordings from dendrites and the soma of OLM cells showed that long depolarizing stimuli close to threshold induced action potentials in the axon, whereas short stimuli shifted spike initiation to the somatodendritic domain (Martina et al., 2000). What could be the functional role of this shift? Dendritic action potential induction and its active propagation to distal dendrites (Martina et al., 2000) ensures reliable recruitment of OLM cells for the control of associative synaptic plasticity at their glutamatergic inputs (Topolnik et al., 2005). Moreover, OLM cell recruitment ensures reliable control of signaling at entorhinal cortex inputs onto pyramidal cell dendrites (Leao et al., 2012). This channel organization stands in marked contrast to the expression of voltage-gated channels in pyramidal cell dendrites, where dendritic action potentials are attenuated, dendritic spike induction is prevented, and where EPSPs are reduced by high densities of A-type K_v channels (Hoffman et al., 1997). However, whether a comparable organization of voltage-gated channels and dendritic initiation of action potentials exists in other interneuron types remains to be examined.

5.13.2.4 Voltage-gated calcium channels in inhibitory interneurons

Several types of Ca_v channels coexist in all neurons. While the identities and biophysical characteristics of Ca_v channels, as well as their role in shaping the physiological properties, have been examined extensively in principal cells, much less is known about them in GABAergic cells (Vinet and Sík, 2006). High-resolution antibody labeling shows that high-voltage-gated P/Q-type ($Ca_v2.1$) and N-type ($Ca_v2.2$) channels are widely expressed in almost all interneuron types, with the highest abundance at presynaptic release sites. Similarly, low-voltage-activated T-type ($Ca_v3.1$) channels, characterized by rapid inactivation, are uniformly expressed in interneurons, whereas high-voltage-activated longer-lasting L-type ($Ca_v1.2$ and $Ca_v1.3$) channels are abundant in SOMIs, calretinin (CR)-positive cells, and PVIs. However, detailed investigations of Ca_v channel subtypes in identified interneurons are lacking, making comparisons difficult.

PVIs rely on P/Q type Ca_v channels for transmitter release, whereas CCK-interneurons use predominantly N-type Ca_v channels (Hefft and Jonas, 2005). The generation of presynaptic action potentials at gamma frequencies evokes both synchronous and asynchronous IPSCs in target pyramidal cells of the DG and in CA1. However, N-type Ca_v channels trigger predominantly asynchronous GABA release from CCK cells, whereas P/Q-type Ca_v channels mediate predominantly synchronous release at PVI output synapses, as a result of differential coupling between Ca_v channels and exocytosis in the two cell types (Hefft and Jonas, 2005). Consequently, PVI terminals generate IPSCs with high temporal precision and thereby provide a stable inhibitory output to the hippocampal microcircuitry, whereas IPSCs mediated at CCKI-mediated synapses are characterized by less reliable inhibitory output (Daw et al., 2009; Hefft and Jonas, 2005).

Two-photon imaging of calcium signals revealed the activation of T-, L-, N-, and P/Q-type Ca_v channels by backpropagating action potentials in SOM-positive OLM dendrites (Topolnik et al., 2009). L-type Ca_v channels in these dendrites play a key role in the induction of an unusual form of dendritic plasticity. This form of plasticity requires the recruitment of mGluR5 in OLM cell dendrites by presynaptic glutamate release, mGluR5-induced calcium release from internal stores and protein-kinase C activation, and is expressed as the potentiation of L-type Ca_v channels (Topolnik et al., 2009). Given that these channels play a key role in the induction of Hebbian synaptic plasticity at excitatory inputs targeting OLM cells (Topolnik et al., 2009), L-type Ca_v channel regulation may represent a powerful mechanism shaping synaptic plasticity. The somatic and dendritic membrane of PVIs also express L-type Ca_vs (largely $Ca_v1.3$), but they are absent from the axonal membrane (Jiang and Swann, 2005). In contrast to OLM cells, L-type Ca_v channels do not contribute to the induction of associative Hebbian LTP at pyramidal cell-to-PVI synapses in the DG (Hainmueller et al., 2014). However, they facilitate CREB phosphorylation, which in turn increases the coupling between PVI excitation and gene transcription in CA1 (Cohen et al., 2016).

5.13.2.5 Hyperpolarization-activated cation channels

HCN channels producing I_h are expressed abundantly in neurons throughout the central nervous system and are assembled from four subunits, HCN1-4 (Magee, 1999; Santoro et al., 1998, 2000; S Williams and Stuart, 2000). Antibody labeling revealed that all four subunits are expressed in the axon and terminals of hippocampal GABAergic cells (Notomi and Shigemoto, 2004). Quantitative single-cell RT-PCR analysis suggests that HCN channels in DG PVIs are primarily formed by HCN1 and HCN2 subunits (Aponte et al., 2006). In principal cells, I_h current density increases with distance from the soma to distal dendrites (Magee, 1998b). Although it remained unclear whether similar distributions exist in GABAergic cells, single-cell models propose that HCN channels are dendritically expressed in OLM cells, but with density distributions opposite to the ones observed in pyramidal cell dendrites (Sekulić et al., 2015). Moreover, recordings from DG PVIs and their target pyramidal cells combined with the block of HCN channels indicated their expression in the soma, dendrites, axon, and presynaptic terminals of PVIs (Aponte et al., 2006).

HCN subunits assemble into homo- or heterotetrameric non-selective cation channels. Their presence is correlated with a *sag*, which can be evoked upon longer lasting intracellular hyperpolarizing current injections. The first demonstration that I_h currents exist in interneurons came from OLM cells in CA1 (Maccaferri and McBain, 1996). In these cells and other interneurons, I_h currents contribute to the resting conductance (Aponte et al., 2006; Maccaferri and McBain, 1996). The sag was particularly large in CA1 OLM cells and CCK-expressing interneurons (Tricoire et al., 2011). Upon activation, HCN-mediated conductances shift the membrane potential away from the resting potential to more depolarized values (reversal potential at ~-30 mV in DG PVIs and CA1 OLM cells). Upon depolarization, HCN channels deactivate and the membrane potential moves back toward the original V_{rest}

value. Moreover, in DG PVIs, HCN channels seem to regulate the reliability of action potential propagation along the axon and GABA release. Indeed, I_h block by ZD 7288 increased spike-propagation failures along PVI axons and reduced the miniature IPSC frequency. This effect can be largely explained by the hyperpolarization of the PVI membrane upon I_h block.

5.14 Inhibitory axons target specific cellular domains and cell types

One of the striking features of GABAergic cells is their remarkable anatomical diversity, particularly the laminar distribution of their dendritic processes and axonal arborizations, which allow predictions about the sources of their afferent inputs and postsynaptic target selectivity. Indeed, axonal specializations, including the domain-specificity of inhibitory output synapses and the number of synapses per cell, define the spatiotemporal control of interneuron types over the activity of their target cells.

5.14.1 Perisomatic inhibition

PV-expressing AAIs (Figures 5.34 and 5.35) make up ~4% of the total CA1 interneuron population (Bezaire and Soltesz, 2013). Their axons originate either at the soma or from a primary dendrite and target the AIS of up to 1,200 pyramidal cells (Buhl et al., 1994; Gulyás et al., 2010; Somogyi, 1977). Each axonal branch forms a characteristic cartridge composed of 2–10 boutons (Somogyi, 1977). In CA1, a single pyramidal cell is contacted by ~6 AAIs (Buhl et al., 1994). The somata of AAIs are typically restricted to the stratum pyramidale and its borders with the stratum oriens and stratum radiatum. The dendrites of AAIs arise from cell bodies and extend into stratum oriens or through stratum radiatum and into the stratum lacunosum-moleculare (Gulyás et al., 1999). This broad dendritic distribution among layers positions AAIs to receive excitatory inputs from the majority of afferent projections innervating the CA1 subfield (Buhl et al., 1994; XG Li et al., 1992). CA3 AAIs show similar anatomical characteristics as those in CA1 (Gulyás et al., 1993).

AAIs in the DG have somata located in the granule cell layer or at its border with the hilus (Doischer et al., 2008). Their axon collaterals target the AIS of GCs and also project into the hilar/CA3 area, where they may contact mossy cells and CA3 pyramidal cells. AAIs innervate the AIS of granule cells, but not interneurons. The AIS of principal cells possesses the highest density of Na_v channels on the neuronal surface and thus is responsible for action potential initiation (C Huang and Rasband, 2018). On the basis of in vitro studies, it has been suggested that chloride-conducting α2-subunit containing $GABA_A$ receptors may exert depolarizing, shunting (Szabadics et al., 2006), or hyperpolarizing effects (Dugladze et al., 2012; Glickfeld et al., 2009) on the AIS of pyramidal cells. The impact of GABA on the AIS under in vivo recordings conditions, however, indicates a predominantly inhibitory influence on neuronal activity (Cobb et al., 1995; Dudok, Klein, et al., 2021; Dudok, Szoboszlay, et al., 2021; Geiller et al., 2020).

The axons of PV-BCs selectively target the soma and proximal dendrites of pyramidal cells (~99%) and interneurons, forming multiple contacts often described as a *basket* (~1%; (Bartos et al., 2001, 2002; Halasy et al., 1996; Pawelzik et al., 2003; Sik et al., 1995); Figures 5.34 and 5.35). BCs make up ~14% of the total CA1

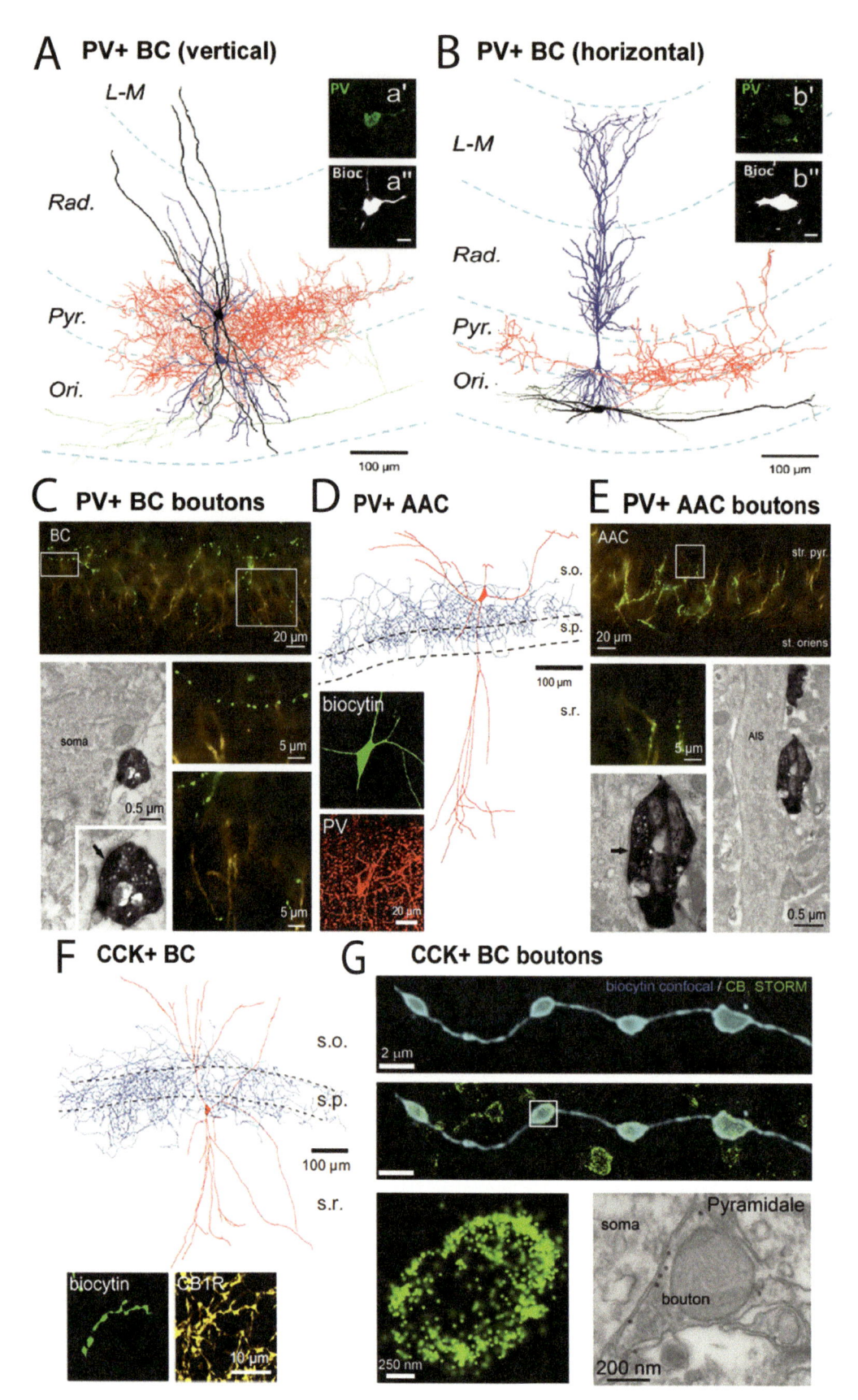

Figure 5.34 Interneuron subtypes innervating the perisomatic region of CA1 pyramidal cells. (A) Morphological reconstruction (soma/dendrites black, axon red) of a vertical basket cell (BC) filled with biocytin (Bioc) and immunoreactive for parvalbumin (PV, green). (B) Morphological reconstruction of a horizontal basket cell (soma/dendrites black, axon red) filled with biocytin; immunoreactive for parvalbumin. (C) Immunohistochemistry and electron microscopy images illustrating that PV + BC axon terminals (green) target pyramidal cell somata but avoid ankyrin G-immunoreactive axon initial segments. (D) Morphological reconstruction of a vertical axo-axonic cell (soma/dendrites red, axon blue) filled with biocytin; immunoreactive for PV. (E) Immunohistochemistry and electron microscopy images illustrating that PV-expressing axo-axonic cell output terminals (green) form cartridge-like structures and target ankyrin G-immunoreactive axon initial segments of pyramidal cells. (F) Morphological reconstruction of a vertical cholecystokinin (CCK) basket cell (soma/dendrites red, axon blue), whose biocytin-filled axon was immunoreactive for cannabinoid type-1 receptors (CB1R). (G) Super-resolution STORM images show intense CB1R immunolabeling within a segment of biocytin-filled axon, and an electron micrograph shows CB1R expression in perisomatic-targeting GABAergic terminals. (Sources: (A, B) Booker et al., 2017; (C, E) Gulyás et al., 2010; (D, F) Nissen et al., 2010; (G) Pelkey et al., 2017.)

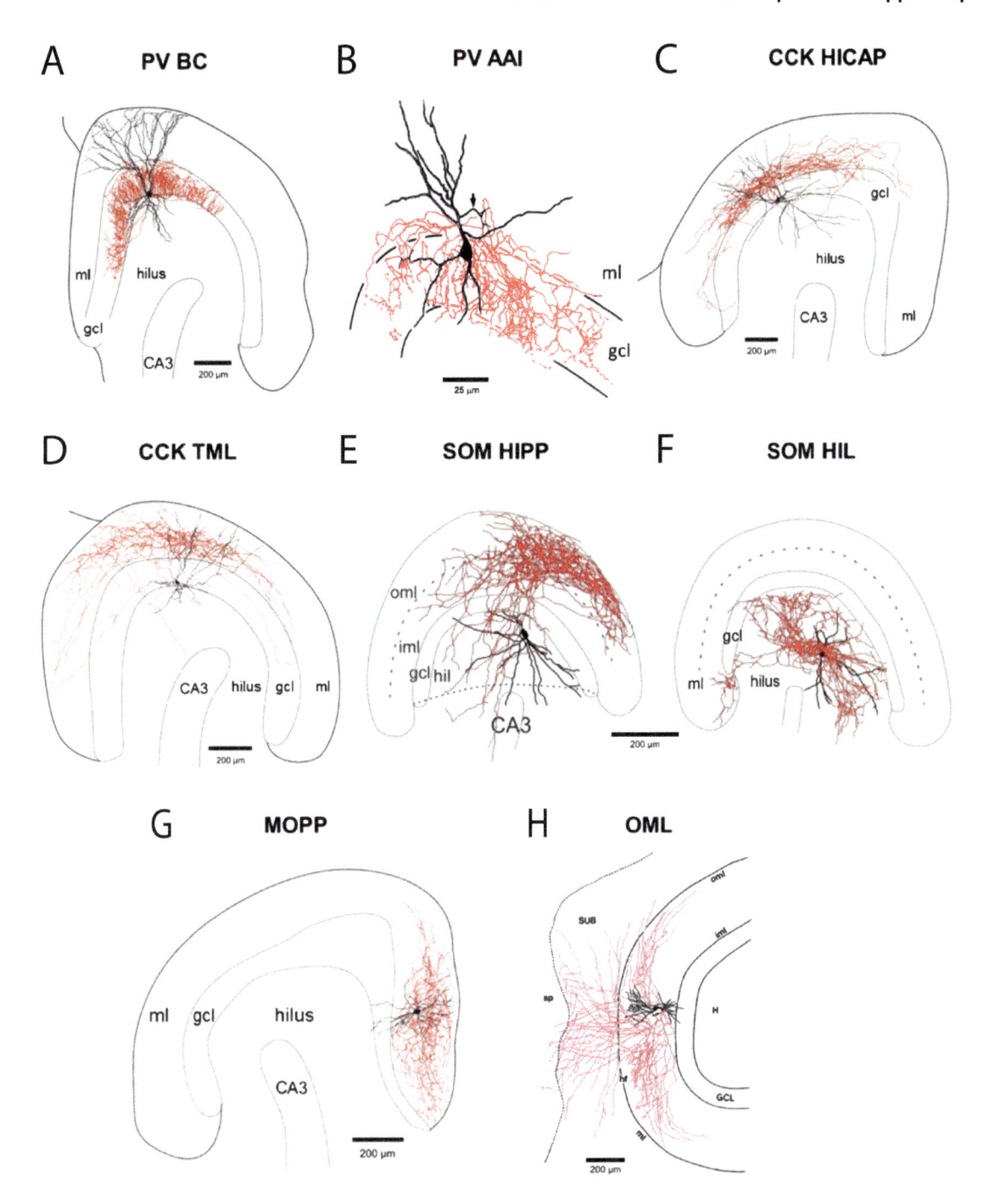

Figure 5.35 Morphological reconstructions of labeled interneurons in the dentate gyrus. (A) Basket cell (soma/dendrites black, axon red in all panels) with axon localized in the granule cell layer (gcl). (B) Putative axo-axonic cell. (C) Hilar commissural/associational path (HICAP) interneuron with axon collaterals restricted to the inner molecular layer. (D) total molecular layer cell (TML). (E) Hilar perforant-path-associated (HIPP) cell with axons largely distributed in the outer half of the molecular layer. Note, few axon fibers in the hilus. (F) Hilar interneuron (HIL) with axons largely distributed in the hilus. (G) Molecular layer perforant path (MOPP) cells with soma and dendrites in the outer half of the molecular layer. The axon also remains in the outer two thirds of the molecular layer. (H) Outer molecular layer (OML) cell with soma in OML and axons in OML and crossing the hippocampal fissure into subiculum. (Sources: (A, C, D, G) Hosp et al., 2014; (B) Soriano and Frotscher, 1989; (E, F) Yuan et al., 2017; (H) Ceranik et al., 1997.)

interneuron population (Bezaire and Soltesz, 2013) and ~25% of known anatomical and neurochemical interneuron types. Given their high numbers and the strong and functionally relevant inhibition they provide, PV-BCs are among the most studied interneuron type. PV-BCs are generally fast-spiking and have low input resistance (Bartos et al., 2001, 2002; Savanthrapadian et al., 2014).

Their cell bodies are located either in the stratum pyramidale or nearby parts of stratum radiatum or stratum oriens, and their dendrites extend into all layers of CA1 from the alveus to the stratum lacunosum-moleculare (Buhl et al., 1994; McBain et al., 1994; Sik et al., 1995). Like AAIs, BCs in the DG have their somata largely located in the granule cell layer or at its border with the hilus, with dendrites extending into the entire molecular layer and hilus. This large extent of BC dendrites (Doischer et al., 2008; Gulyás et al., 1999; Hosp et al., 2014) positions them to receive excitatory inputs from all major afferent pathways (Amaral, 1978; Gulyás et al., 1999; Sambandan et al., 2010). In the DG, PV-BC dendrites possess non-uniform passive membrane properties, with proximal dendrites possessing lower R_N than distal locations, which supports the strengthening of distal synaptic inputs (Elgueta and Bartos, 2019; Nörenberg et al., 2010). Collectively PV-BCs receive ~10 times more excitatory than inhibitory inputs (Halasy et al., 1996), pointing to their high excitability.

The axon arises from the soma of PV-BCs in CA1, but from either the soma or proximal apical dendrites of PV-BCs in the DG. The axon ramifies along the principal cell layer contacting cell bodies (CA1 ~53%; DG ~89%) and proximal dendrites (CA1 ~44%; DG ~7%) of pyramidal cells or GCs (Halasy and Somogyi, 1993; Halasy et al., 1996). The lateral extent of the axon can exceed ~700 μm (Strüber et al., 2017) forming ~10,000 synaptic contacts (Halasy et al., 1996; Sik et al., 1995). Paired recordings between presynaptic PV-BCs and CA1 pyramidal cells revealed selectivity in the microcircuit connectivity between these cell types (Figure 5.36A–B). Here, PV-BCs provide stronger inhibition to deep-layer pyramidal cells projecting to the amygdala than to those within the superficial layer connecting with the medial prefrontal cortex (SH Lee et al., 2014). In turn, PV-BCs receive more frequent inputs from superficial pyramidal cells, demonstrating a bias in target selectivity by both excitatory input and inhibitory output in CA1 (SH Lee et al., 2014) (see Chapter 7). In the DG, axon density declines exponentially with distance, and correlates with the number of PVI-mediated contacts, resulting in strong inhibition at closely spaced partners and weak inhibition at more distant target cells (Strüber et al., 2015). A distance-dependent decline in the time course of inhibitory signals was also observed, and is likely dictated by the subunit composition of postsynaptic $GABA_A$ receptor subunits (Strüber et al., 2015). Neuronal network modeling revealed that this form of distance-dependent inhibition supports local synchronization of pyramidal cells and the processing of complex afferent inputs in parallel neuronal centers (Strüber et al., 2017) (Figure 5.36C).

PV-BCs also innervate other interneurons via GABAergic synapses including PVIs, AAIs, CCK-BCs, and dendrite-targeting interneurons (Bartos et al., 2001; Karson et al., 2009; Savanthrapadian et al., 2014; Sik et al., 1995). Moreover, hippocampal PVIs are interconnected by gap junctions (Bartos et al., 2001; Meyer et al., 2002; Tamás et al., 2000). Computational work has proposed that mutual inhibitory synapses and gap junctions among PVIs support high synchronization of neuronal networks at high frequencies (Bartos et al., 2002, 2007; Wulff et al., 2009). Moreover, connexin-36 knockout mice showed reduced synchronization of neuronal network activity and reduced spatial reference memory, reinforcing the importance of gap junction coupling between interneurons in higher network functions (Allen et al., 2011).

A subgroup of hippocampal BCs express CCK (CCK-BCs) and, like PV-BCs, form perisomatic basket contacts (Figure 5.34). However, CCK-BCs target approximately half as many pyramidal cells as PV-BCs (Bezaire and Soltesz, 2013). CCK-BCs in CA1 can be further subdivided in those coexpressing VIP, which have somata located within the stratum radiatum, and those expressing vGluT3 at their axon terminals (Somogyi et al., 2004) with soma location in stratum pyramidale and stratum oriens (Daw et al.,

2009; Vida et al., 1998). The dendritic distribution of CCK-BCs is similar to that of PV-BCs. In contrast to PV-BCs, they receive twice as many GABAergic than glutamatergic inputs (Mátyás et al., 2004), suggesting a high inhibitory drive onto CCK-BCs, which correlates with the high density of extrasynaptic $GABA_B$ receptors at their dendrites (Booker et al., 2017). In the DG, axonal arbors of CCK-BCs are restricted to the outer third of the granule cell layer and inner molecular layer. They contact proximal dendrites of both GCs and interneurons with a preference for CCKIs and PVIs (Hefft and Jonas, 2005; Savanthrapadian et al., 2014). This particular synaptic location allows CCK-BCs in the DG to gate excitatory inputs originating from both ipsi- and contralateral mossy cells (Scharfman, 2016). The axonal distribution pattern is similar to those of hilar commissural-associational pathway-associated cells (HICAP), which ramify predominantly in the inner molecular layer (76%) and the outer third of the granule cell layer (23%; Halasy and Somogyi, 1993; Han et al., 1993; Hosp et al., 2014; Mott et al., 1997; Figure 5.35).

CCK-BCs are regular spiking cells that fire trains of action potentials at moderate frequencies (up to about half the rate of PV-BC fast-spiking cells), with marked spike-frequency adaptation during the train (Booker et al., 2017). In contrast to PV-BCs, which after a precise latency generate large amplitude and fast time course inhibitory postsynaptic currents (IPCS) onto postsynaptic pyramidal cells and interneurons (Bartos et al., 2001, 2002), CCK-BCs evoke IPSCs with marked temporal jitter, leading to asynchronous GABA release properties and temporally less-precise inhibition (Daw et al., 2009; Hefft and Jonas, 2005; Neu et al., 2007). In CA1, IPSC signaling is mediated by postsynaptic α1 and α2-containing $GABA_A$R subunits (Nyiri et al., 2001), which are predominantly located at PVI and CCKI basket synapses, respectively. CCK axon terminals express CB1 cannabinoid receptors (CB1Rs), and GABAergic transmission is modulated by retrograde endocannabinoid signaling (Neu et al., 2007).

5.14.2 Dendritic inhibition

Distal dendritic inhibition is provided by a diverse population of GABAergic cells (Bloss et al., 2016; Freund and Buzsáki, 1996; Hosp et al., 2014; Klausberger, 2009; Klausberger and Somogyi, 2008; Pelkey et al., 2017). With unique dendritic and axonal distributions, neurochemical marker content, and physiological properties, they inhibit pyramidal cells in a pathway-specific manner or across pathways, and occasionally project to distant target areas (Melzer et al., 2012).

With the development of genetic strategies, several studies of the functional role of dendritic inhibition have focused on SOMIs. One of the best-studied SOMIs is the OLM interneuron in CA1, which makes up ~5% of CA1 interneurons (Bezaire and Soltesz, 2013) (Figure 5.37). Their soma and horizontally arranged spiny dendrites are located in stratum oriens, whereas the axon crosses stratum pyramidale and radiatum, to broadly ramify in stratum lacunosum-moleculare (Freund and Buzsáki, 1996; Maccaferri and McBain, 1996; McBain et al., 1994; Sik et al., 1995). OLM cells receive excitatory inputs almost entirely from local pyramidal cells (Blasco-Ibáñez and Freund, 1995) and, once recruited, provide feedback inhibition to the distal dendrites of pyramidal neurons and interneurons by targeting both dendritic spines and shafts. Since the total length of their axons is high, ~63 mm in CA1 (Martina et al., 2000), but the lateral spread is low (<1 mm), a high density

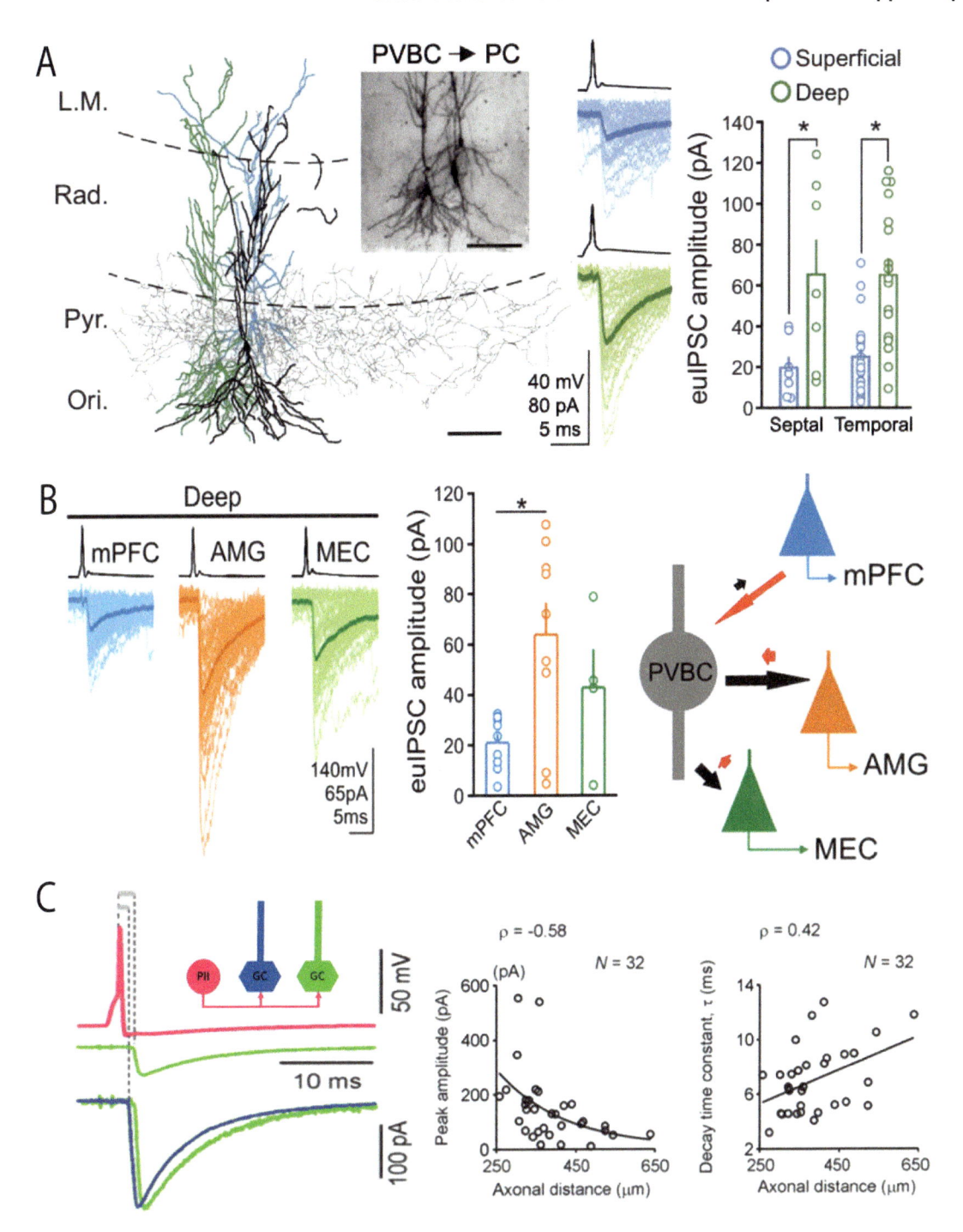

Figure 5.36 Pyramidal cells (PCs) and interneurons form subtype-specific microcircuits. (A) Paired whole-cell recordings in CA1 between a presynaptic PV-BC (black) and a neighboring PC located in the deep (green) and superficial pyramidal cell layer (blue). The probability of observing a connection from a PV-BC to either a deep or a superficial PC is the same; however, deep PCs demonstrate larger amplitude IPSCs. This finding is consistent along the entire axis of the hippocampus (septal to temporal poles). (B) Among the deep layer PC population, CA1 PV-BCs evoke larger amplitude IPSCs in PCs that project to the amygdala (AMG) than those projecting to the medial prefrontal cortex (mPFC). Left: example paired recordings. Center: Summary of data from all recorded pairs. Right: Schematic summary of the connectivity. Length of arrows is proportional to mean EPSC amplitudes times connection probability. Red arrows show inputs from PCs onto PVBCs, and that those from AMG- and MEC-projecting PCs are of very low amplitude and probability. (C) PV-expressing interneurons (PIIs) provide distance-dependent inhibition to DG granule cells (GCs). Left: representative sequential paired recording from one presynaptic PII and two postsynaptic GCs. The green GC is more distant from the PII than the blue GC (shown schematically). The action potential in the PII (upper trace) evokes an IPSC in the green GC (middle trace) that is small, as shown in the lower trace peak-scaled to the IPSC evoked in the blue GC. Note the difference in decay kinetics and onset latency (gray dashed lines). Center: mean uIPSC peak amplitudes decline exponentially with axonal distance. Right, decay time constants (τ) increase linearly with axonal distance. (Sources: (A, B) Lee et al., 2014; (C) Strüber et al., 2015.)

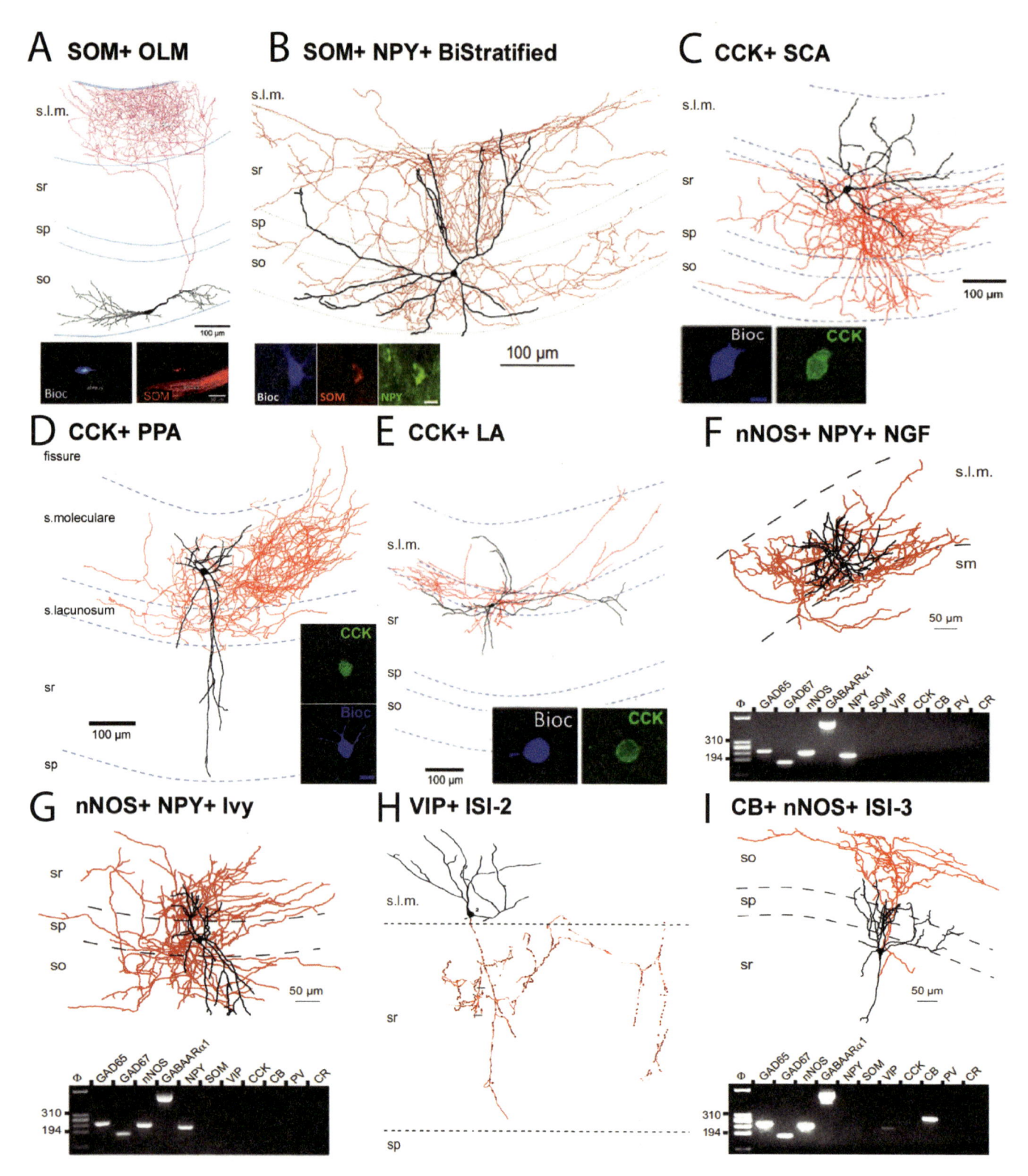

Figure 5.37 Interneuron types innervating the dendritic regions of CA1 pyramidal cells. (A) Morphological reconstruction of an OLM cell (dendrites black, axon red in all panels) filled with biocytin (Bioc, blue); immunoreactive for somatostatin (SOM, red). (B) Morphological reconstruction of a bistratified cell filled with biocytin; immunoreactive for SOM and neuropeptide Y (NPY, green). (C) Morphological reconstruction of a Schaffer Collateral–associated cell filled with biocytin; immunoreactive for cholecystokinin (CCK, green). (D) Morphological reconstruction of a perforant-path-associated cell filled with biocytin; immunoreactive for CCK. Note the axon collaterals that cross the hippocampal fissure into the dentate gyrus. (E) Morphological reconstruction of a stratum lacunosum–associated cell filled with biocytin; immunoreactive for CCK. (F) Morphological reconstruction of a neurogliaform cell filled with biocytin and expression profile determined by RT-PCR: GAD65, GAD67, nNOS, and NPY. (G) Morphological reconstruction of an Ivy cell filled with biocytin; RT-PCR expression: GAD65, GAD67, nNOS, and NPY. (H) Morphological reconstruction of a type 2 interneuron-selective cell; immunoreactive for vasoactive intestinal peptide (VIP). (I) Morphological reconstruction of a type 3 interneuron-selective cell filled with biocytin; RT-PCR expression GAD67, nNOS, and calbindin (CB). (Sources: (A) Martina et al., 2000; (B) Klausberger et al., 2004; (C–E) Booker et al., 2016; (F, G, I) Tricoire et al., 2010; (H) Acsády et al., 1996.)

of output synapses is expected. Their synapse location at distal dendritic shafts and spines allows OLM cells to gate excitatory inputs to CA1 from layer III entorhinal cortex, the thalamic nucleus reuniens, and the amygdala (Herkenham, 1978; Leao et al., 2012; Maccaferri and McBain, 1995). OLM cell dendrites express high densities of voltage-gated channels, which support both dendritic action potential generation and the boosting of dendritic excitatory signals.

Dendritically evoked spikes could be important for efficient OLM recruitment, whereas backpropagating action potentials may control synaptic plasticity at dendritic glutamatergic inputs (Martina et al., 2000). Due to the long electrotonic distance between distally evoked inhibitory signals and the pyramidal cell soma, as well as strong filtering by dendrites and spines, IPSCs detected at the pyramidal cell soma have small amplitudes and slow kinetic properties as compared with perisomatically evoked events (Maccaferri et al., 2000; Savanthrapadian et al., 2014). However, at local dendritic sites, OLM cell-mediated inhibition markedly reduces the amplitude of excitatory postsynaptic currents (EPSCs) and thereby inhibits long-lasting plasticity at PP inputs (Leao et al., 2012). Consequently, dendritic inhibition reduces extrahippocampal information flow to CA1. Since OLM cells also inhibit stratum radiatum and stratum lacunosum-moleculare interneurons (Leao et al., 2012; Maccaferri et al., 2000), they support the emergence of synaptic plasticity at SC inputs onto CA1 pyramidal cells. Thus, this specialized local connectivity allows OLM cells to strongly influence information flow from either intrahippocampal flow from CA3 or extrahippocampal entorhinal/thalamic inputs to CA1 (Leao et al., 2012; Siwani et al., 2018).

SOM-positive hilar perforant path-associated interneurons (HIPPs) function in a similar way to OLM cells in CA1. HIPPs are located within the DG (Hosp et al., 2014) (Figure 5.35). Their cell bodies and dendrites are confined to the hilus and are predominantly targeted by mossy fiber synapses originating from GCs (Yuan et al., 2017). Once activated, HIPP cells provide feedback inhibition to the distal apical dendrites of both GCs and PVIs (Elgueta and Bartos, 2019; Savanthrapadian et al., 2014). Interestingly, a small proportion of axon collaterals (<2%) is located within the hilus and forms perisomatic contacts to PVIs (Savanthrapadian et al., 2014). Mossy-fiber-mediated signals facilitate and thereby boost the recruitment of DG-SOMIs (Elgueta and Bartos, 2019). Thus, SOMIs in DG are functionally homologous to their CA1 counterparts. Interestingly, the specific somatodendritic membrane properties of DG-PVIs (high distal R_m) together with the strong hyperpolarization evoked by dendritic inhibitory signals allow DG-SOMIs to efficiently control the activity of PVIs (Elgueta and Bartos, 2019). In contrast, inhibition at GC distal dendrites has only a mild influence on their activity, which might be explained by the high proportion (~55%) of SOMI synapses located at GC spines (Buckmaster et al., 2002) and their very likely localized inhibitory effect on input signaling and synaptic plasticity.

Bistratified cells (BiCs) account for ~6% of the total interneuron population in CA1 (Bezaire and Soltesz, 2013) (Figure 5.37). Their cell bodies are largely located in the stratum pyramidale, but a small proportion has been found at the pyramidal cell borders with stratum oriens and radiatum, as well as the alveus (Tukker et al., 2007). BiCs with vertically oriented dendrites extend in the stratum oriens and stratum radiatum and thus receive their primary inputs from the Schaffer collaterals (Buhl et al., 1994). The axons of PV-BiCs cross the pyramidal cell layer to arborize in two main areas,

the stratum oriens and stratum radiatum, where they form synaptic contacts onto the basal and apical distal dendrites of pyramidal cells (Katona et al., 2014; Klausberger et al., 2004; Tukker et al., 2007). Thus, BiCs preferentially target dendrites (~80%), including spines (~20%), but rarely cell bodies (~4%). Moreover, BiCs preferentially contact pyramidal cells (>90%) rather than interneurons (<10%) including PV-BCs (Halasy et al., 1996). The axonal length is high (~79 mm) and forms a large number of synapses (~16,000) onto ~2,500 pyramidal cells (Sik et al., 1995), leading to high network connectivity. PV-BiC-mediated output synapses are anatomically smaller than those of PV-BCs (Halasy et al., 1996). These synapses produce fast IPSCs with small amplitude at pyramidal cells (Booker et al., 2013), likely caused by a low initial release probability and dendritic filtering. Antibody labeling revealed that PV-BiCs co-express neuropeptide Y (NPY) and SOM (Klausberger et al., 2004; Varga et al., 2014) in contrast to BCs and AAIs, which do not.

Distal dendritic inhibition is further provided by CCK-dendrite targeting inhibitory interneurons (CCK-DIIs), which make up ~5% of the total CA1 interneuron population. These cells have their cell bodies located across all CA layers, with enrichment in the stratum radiatum and at the border with stratum lacunosum-moleculare (Cea-del Rio et al., 2011; Vida et al., 1998). This group of cells falls into several morphologically distinct types. First, Schaffer collateral-associated (SCA) interneurons (SCAs; Figure 5.37) extend their axons throughout the stratum radiatum to target the basal dendrites of pyramidal cells (Vida et al., 1998). SCA interneurons also inhibit other interneurons in stratum pyramidale (Vida et al., 1998). They evoke small, strongly depressing IPSCs with high failure rates (Booker et al., 2017). Second, apical dendrite-targeting interneurons (ADIs) innervate the apical dendritic shaft of pyramidal cells (Klausberger et al., 2005). Third, perforant path-associated cells (PPAs; Figure 5.37) confine their axon to the stratum lacunosum-moleculare and target the distal apical tuft of pyramidal cells (Klausberger et al., 2005). Interestingly, PPAs also extend their axon into the stratum moleculare of the DG, where they target the distal dendrites of GCs.

An unusual form of dendritic inhibition is contributed by NGFIs and Ivy cells (Figure 5.37). Their small somata are typically found in the stratum lacunosum-moleculare of CA1-3 and the stratum moleculare of the DG (Armstrong et al., 2011; Fuentealba et al., 2008; Krook-Magnuson et al., 2011; Price et al., 2005). Their dendrites branch extensively and give rise to a locally ramifying axon, which forms a dense plexus. Indeed, with a total length of ~144 mm, NGFI axons are approximately ~3-fold more expansive than those of PV-BCs (Bezaire and Soltesz, 2013). NGFIs receive excitatory afferents from the entorhinal cortex and provide classical feedforward inhibition to their target cells. NGFIs make up a small cell population at ~9% of the total interneuron population in CA1 (Bezaire and Soltesz, 2013). In the DG, NGFI axons can cross the fissure and project to CA1 and/or the subiculum (Armstrong et al., 2011; Ceranik et al., 1997). NGFIs form small en passant output synapses characterized by a large synaptic cleft at dendritic shafts and spines of pyramidal cells (Fuentealba et al., 2010). However, a large proportion of synapses appear not to contact a discrete postsynaptic element (Oláh et al., 2009). NGFI-mediated inhibitory postsynaptic signals have two components, the first is mediated by GABA$_A$Rs and a second by GABA$_B$Rs (Armstrong et al., 2011; Price et al., 2005). IPSCs are of small amplitude (~20 pA) and possess very slow decay kinetics, in the range of several tens of milliseconds (Price et al., 2005). These features in combination with their dense axon are thought to enable NGFIs to transmit via volume conduction. The released GABA also binds at presynaptic $GABA_B$Rs, reducing GABA and glutamate release, thus mediating both homo- and heterosynaptic depression (Oláh et al., 2009; Price et al., 2005). In addition, NGFIs are strongly interconnected via electrical synapses, thereby forming extensive interneuron networks (Armstrong et al., 2011; Price et al., 2005). In the DG, NGFIs receive low-frequency spontaneous excitatory inputs, which can strongly facilitate. Once recruited, NGFIs provide inhibition onto both principal cells and interneurons (Armstrong et al., 2011; Price et al., 2005). NGFIs express the neuropeptide Y (NPY), reelin, neuronal nitric oxide synthase (nNOS), α-actin 2, and the COUP transcription factor 2 (COUPTF2).

Ivy cells are so-named because of the vine-like appearance of their axon (Fuentealba et al., 2008) (Figure 5.37). They form ~23% of the CA1 interneuron population and together with NGFIs represent the largest family of interneuron types in CA1 (~32%) (Bezaire and Soltesz, 2013). However, unlike NGFIs, their somata are not located in the stratum lacunosum-moleculare but reside throughout the strata radiatum, oriens, and pyramidale. Similar to NGFIs, their total axonal length is the highest among interneuron types (~177 mm) and is larger, by a factor of ~4, than the axon of PV-BCs (Bezaire and Soltesz, 2013). Like NGFIs, Ivy cells express NPY and nNOS, but not all of them express COUPTF2. However, a clearer distinction is that Ivy cells do not express reelin (Fuentealba et al., 2008, 2010). Ivy cells contact CA1 pyramidal cells with high probability (~80%) and generate IPSCs with high reliability, indicating a strong dendritic inhibitory effect on pyramidal cell dendrites in the stratum oriens and stratum radiatum.

5.14.3 Interneurons inhibiting other interneurons

A large proportion of calretinin (CR) and/or VIP-expressing interneurons selectively target other interneurons (Figures 5.33 and 5.37). Although most interneurons preferentially target pyramidal cells, they can also target interneurons of the same, or different, morphological, or neurochemical type with low connection probability (~10%). In contrast, interneuron selective interneurons (ISI) only contact the dendritic compartments of GABAergic cells and thereby provide disinhibition to the microcircuitry (Tyan et al., 2014). Based on their soma location, axonal distribution profile, and neurochemical marker content they can be subdivided in three types.

ISI-1 cells are CR-positive and have somata located in the strata radiatum, pyramidale, or oriens of CA1 (Gulyás et al., 1996). Their dendrites are distributed throughout the strata radiatum and lacunosum-moleculare of CA1 and are predominantly recruited by excitatory inputs derived from the SC, PP, and the collaterals of CA1 pyramidal cells. Once recruited, they preferentially disinhibit the apical dendrites of CA1 pyramidal cells. Their dendrites are markedly interconnected via zona adherentia and gap junctions, as well as chemical synapses, and they can potentially synchronize their inhibitory output.

ISI-2 cells express VIP and ~50% of them are positive for CR. Their somata and dendrites are located in the stratum radiatum and stratum lacunosum-moleculare of CA1 and thus are largely activated by SC and PP inputs. Their axons distribute throughout stratum radiatum to inhibit CR cells as well as CB-CCK-positive, dendrite-targeting cells and VIP-CCK-BCs.

ISI-3 cells, express both VIP and CR and locate their somata in the stratum pyramidale and stratum radiatum. Their axons are confined to the stratum oriens and preferentially inhibit OLM cells and BiCs (Tyan et al., 2014). Their IPSCs have small amplitudes and show no plastic changes at low frequencies (Tyan et al., 2014). Thus, their net activity is to disinhibit the most distal apical dendrites of CA1 pyramidal cells (Tyan et al., 2014). In the DG, ISIs inhibit HIPP cells and thus, similar to CA1, disinhibit the distal apical dendrites of GCs (Hajos et al., 1996).

5.14.4 Boundary and long-range inhibitory connections

In classical anatomical literature, GABAergic axons were termed "short axon cells." However, this terminology does not hold for BCs and Ivy cells, since the cumulative axon length of a single PV-BC in the DG is ~33 mm (Nörenberg et al., 2010), ~46 mm in CA1 (Sik et al., 1995), and, in the exceptional case of Ivy cells, ~177 mm (Bezaire and Soltesz, 2013). However, the lateral extent of the axon is local, generating a massively divergent yet local inhibitory output (Espinoza et al., 2018; Strüber et al., 2017). Several lines of evidence show that some classes of GABAergic cells can project over longer distances. Some long-range projecting interneurons (LPIs) are termed "boundary cells" (e.g., NGFI, Ivy cells, outer molecular layer [OML] interneurons in the DG) because their axons cross from the DG into neighboring hippocampal areas, such as CA1 and subiculum (Armstrong et al., 2011; Ceranik et al., 1997; Szabo et al., 2017) (Figure 5.35). Other LPIs project over even longer distances to remote brain regions. For example, DG hilar (HIL) interneurons ramify both locally within the hilus and project to the medial septum (Yuan et al., 2017). Moreover, some stratum oriens interneurons in CA3 and CA1 project to the DG (Jinno et al., 2007; Klausberger and Somogyi, 2008) and presumably relay a generalization of the activity in the CA areas back to the DG. A substantial fraction of LPIs expresses SOM. Single-cell labeling and retrograde tracing in vivo revealed that SOM-LPIs have somata located in various hippocampal layers including stratum oriens and stratum radiatum in CA1 (Gulyás et al., 2003; Jinno and Kosaka, 2002; Jinno et al., 2007; Katona et al., 2017; Takács et al., 2008; Yuan et al., 2017) or the hilus in the DG (Yuan et al., 2017). Another SOM-LPI population projects to the contralateral DG (Eyre and Bartos, 2019; Leranth et al., 1990). Similar to hippocampal SOMIs, a large fraction of SOM-LPIs express mGluR1α and the mAChR M2 (Jinno et al., 2007). In addition to ISIs that make local contacts within CA1, an ISI type expressing VIP and M2 receptors has been identified that targets local interneurons but also projects to the subiculum, where it contacts both principal and GABAergic cells (Francavilla et al., 2018), thus exhibiting region-specific target and functional preferences. LPIs are generally believed to synchronize neuronal rhythmic activity across brain regions, allowing coordinated neuronal discharges and thus, coordinated information processing.

In summary, interneurons provide compartment-selective inhibition. The differential activation of various cell types will consequently produce selective inhibition to the soma, AIS, or dendrites of pyramidal cells, granule cells, and interneurons. $GABA_A$ receptor-mediated signals will locally interact with excitatory ones, influence synaptic plasticity, and control synaptic integration of postsynaptic signals, as well as the initiation and backpropagation of action potentials.

5.15 Interneuron synapses and synaptic plasticity

Interneurons are integrated in complex neuronal networks and interconnected with principal and GABAergic cells. Excitatory signaling onto interneurons is mediated by iGluRs and mGluRs. Despite having many common features with glutamate receptors in principal cells, there are several differences and exceptions, which will be highlighted in the following sections. Glutamatergic inputs onto interneurons can undergo long-lasting potentiation and/or depression. However, different interneuron types possess distinct and nonoverlapping types of synaptic plasticity, which can be explained by cell type-specific cellular and molecular mechanisms. The high diversity of mechanisms and conditions of long-lasting changes in input efficacy adds to the enormous functional heterogeneity of interneuron types within neuronal networks.

5.15.1 Excitatory inputs

Hippocampal interneurons receive afferent excitatory input from several intrinsic and extrinsic sources. Most fast excitatory synaptic transmission is mediated by postsynaptic iGluRs called AMPA receptors (AMPARs). These are homomeric or heteromeric assemblies of four subunits: GluR1-4. The composition of the receptors determines their functional properties as well as the induction and expression of synaptic plasticity. AMPARs of pyramidal cells are mainly comprised of GluR1/2 or 2/3 subunits, which form calcium-impermeable receptors (CI-AMPARs) and show linear current-voltage relationships. In contrast, interneurons express both GluR2-lacking, calcium-permeable receptors (CP-AMPARs) and GluR2-containing, CI-AMPARs. Single-cell RT-PCR together with electrophysiological recordings has revealed that both CP- and CI-AMPARs can be expressed by single interneurons in CA3 stratum lucidum. For example, GC-mediated MF synapses target CA3 interneurons at synapses containing CP-AMPARs, whereas inputs from CA3 pyramidal cells target the same cell at synapses with CI-AMPARs (Tóth and McBain, 1998). Similarly, MF inputs targeting basal PVI dendrites innervate GluR2-lacking synapses, whereas PP inputs contacting apical dendrites of the same PVI innervate GluR2-containing synapses (Sambandan et al., 2010). PCR analysis of mRNA transcripts revealed that hippocampal interneurons, particularly PVIs, express higher levels of GluR1 and GluR4, but lower levels of GluR2 subunits compared with pyramidal cells (Jonas et al., 2004; Tsuzuki et al., 2001). Interestingly, the expression of AMPAR subunits depends on the developmental origin of GABAergic cells. SC inputs onto CA1 interneurons originating from the medial ganglionic eminence (MGE) express GluR2-lacking AMPARs (e.g., PVIs, SOMIs, nNOS cells), whereas those originating from the caudal ganglionic eminence (CGE) express GluR2-containing AMPARs (e.g., CCKIs, VIPs, CRs) (Matta et al., 2013).

AMPARs containing GluR1/4 and lacking GluR2 have fast kinetics, high calcium permeability, and large single-channel conductances (Geiger et al., 1995). Consequently, the time course of evoked EPSCs in interneurons is much faster than in postsynaptic pyramidal cells (Lawrence and McBain, 2003). For example, EPSCs at GC-CA3 synapses have a decay time constant of ~4.7 ms, whereas the decay for EPSCs at GC-BC synapses in the DG is ~0.8 ms (Geiger et al., 1995). Similarly, EPSCs at GC synapses onto CA3 stratum lucidum interneurons decay very rapidly with a time constant of

~1.7 ms (Walker et al., 2002). However, the fast kinetics at pyramidal cell output synapses on PV-BCs and stratum lucidum interneurons are not a general principal, because EPSCs at CA1 pyramidal-to-OLM cell synapses have a slower time course with a decay time constant of ~4.1 ms (Pouille and Scanziani, 2004). The fast time course of EPSCs plays a key role in the rapid and precise recruitment of PVIs (Hu et al., 2014; Pouille and Scanziani, 2004), which in turn supports temporally precise population activity of pyramidal cells and the generation of synchronous activity patterns in neuronal networks (Bartos et al., 2007; Fuchs et al., 2007).

NMDARs, like AMPARs, are iGluRs formed as tetrameric heterodimers assembled from five different subunit types (GluN1, GluN2A-D). Their subunit composition strongly varies among interneuron types, but all functional receptor isoforms are permeable to both sodium and calcium (von Engelhardt et al., 2015; Lei and McBain, 2002; Matta et al., 2013). NMDARs activate and deactivate much more slowly than AMPARs, on a time scale of hundreds of milliseconds, and have a several-fold larger single channel conductance (Bekkers and Stevens, 1989). Previous investigations indicated that the contribution of CP-AMPARs and NMDARs to interneuron excitation is inversely related: inputs containing CP-AMPARs typically display smaller NMDAR-mediated components than synapses containing CI-AMPARs (Kullmann and Lamsa, 2007; Laezza and Dingledine, 2004; Lei and McBain, 2002; Maccaferri and Dingledine, 2002). For example, MF inputs onto stratum lucidum interneurons in CA3 and SC inputs onto stratum radiatum interneurons in CA1 show small CP-AMPA/NMDA receptor-mediated current ratios (Maccaferri and Dingledine, 2002), whereas the ratio at CA3 pyramidal cell–stratum lucidum interneuron synapses can be large (Lei and McBain, 2002, 2004). Interestingly, interneurons that originate from the MGE, such as PVIs, have the smallest NMDAR-mediated component (Matta et al., 2013). In contrast, CGE-derived interneurons including CCKIs and VIPs have AMPA/NMDA amplitude ratios close to unity (Matta et al., 2013). At synapses with high NMDAR/AMPAR ratios, trains of EPSPs trigger trains of action potentials, whereas at synapses with low NMDAR/AMPAR ratios only single spikes are triggered (Lei and McBain, 2002). Despite their low abundance, selective ablation of NMDARs in PVIs during development leads to a reduction in the synchrony of fast network oscillations at theta (6–12 Hz) and gamma (30–100 Hz) frequencies, as well as alterations in both short- and long-term spatial memory (Korotkova et al., 2010).

5.15.2 Kainate receptors

Kainate receptors (KRs) are a third class of iGluRs formed by homo- or heteromeric tetramers (GluK1-5) and are expressed pre- and postsynaptically. KRs have been identified in various interneurons including OLMs, BiCs, and CA1 interneurons in stratum radiatum. Exogenous kainate application induces enhanced excitability and action potential generation (Cossart et al., 1998). In a few examples, EPSCs with slow kinetics could be observed in CA1 interneurons, primarily OLM cells (Cossart et al., 2002; Goldin et al., 2007). GluK1 antagonists reduced the frequency of theta oscillations, suggesting their important role in the entrainment of OLM cells (Goldin et al., 2007). Synchronous GABA release is reduced at CCKI output synapses via presynaptic modulation by GluK1-containing KRs, but this does not occur at PVI synapses contacting interneurons or pyramidal cells (Daw et al., 2010). Such a mechanism may act as a switch toward prolonged inhibition when pyramidal cell activity, and thus glutamate release, is high. Together with AMPARs and NMDARs, KRs will determine the integration of synaptic inputs and the time window of neuronal recruitment, whereas the calcium permeability of these receptors will determine input-specific plasticity changes (Kullmann and Lamsa, 2007; Sambandan et al., 2010).

5.15.3 Metabotropic glutamate receptors

mGluRs are broadly expressed both pre- and postsynaptically in GABAergic cells throughout the central nervous system and their activation influences interneuron excitability and transmitter release. However, only a few studies have addressed the role of mGluRs in defined interneuron types. The group I isoform mGluR1α is enriched in SOMIs, both in CA1 and DG (Baude et al., 1993; Ferraguti et al., 2004; Yuan et al., 2017), and it is also expressed in VIPs, CRs, and dendrite-targeting, CCK-expressing interneurons in CA1 (Ferraguti et al., 2004). Immunohistochemistry and quantitative electron microscopy revealed that mGluR1α and mGluR5 are coexpressed in DG as well as CA1-3 PVIs (Hainmueller et al., 2014). These receptors are expressed close to glutamatergic synapses and are thought to support the generation of theta oscillations and long-term plasticity. Group III members mGluR4, 7a, 7b and 8a are found at presynaptic GABAergic release sites targeting interneurons but not pyramidal cells, pointing to target cell specificity (Shigemoto et al., 1997). Their activation reduces transmitter release by diminishing calcium influx through presynaptic N-type Ca_v channels (Rudy and McBain, 2001). mGluR8 has a unique expression profile, as it is expressed at presynaptic GABAergic VIP-containing terminals targeting muscarinic M2 receptor-expressing interneurons (Ferraguti et al., 2005). Very little is known about the expression profile of group II mGluRs. Much more work is needed to assess the role of mGluRs in regulating excitability and synaptic transmission in specific interneuron types.

5.15.4 Synaptic plasticity at inputs onto interneurons

Synaptic plasticity at glutamatergic inputs onto pyramidal cells has been broadly accepted as a major cellular mechanism underlying learning and memory (Bliss and Collingridge, 1993; Hebb, 1949). Current theories suggest that during learning, synaptic weights are modified, allowing selected groups of cortical pyramidal cells to form new associations, leading to the formation of cell assemblies, which represent mnemonic information with their activity patterns and spike times. In the hippocampus, cell assemblies have been shown to form a complex cognitive map of the environment (see Chapter 11). Interneurons may assist in the network dynamics and the organization of pyramidal cell assemblies, because both rate remapping and global remapping involve changes in the firing frequency of pyramidal cells, which is regulated by inhibition. Indeed, several factors can promote connection changes onto interneurons and thus influence their recruitment. One factor is short-term plasticity. Repetitive activation of glutamatergic synapses causes short-term facilitation (STF) or depression (STD) of subsequent postsynaptic EPSPs. STF integrates synaptic inputs across broader time windows and enhances the probability of action potential generation, whereas STD narrows the time window for integration and coincidence detection of synaptic inputs during repetitive activation. In vitro whole-cell recordings revealed that these two forms of short-term plasticity at recurrent inputs onto PVIs and SOMIs lead to temporal segregation of perisomatic and dendritic inhibition in

the CA1 network (Pouille and Scanziani, 2004). The first integration window emerges after a short latency, which defines the spike timing of the cell, whereas the second window occurs after a longer latency, allowing integration of dendritically evoked EPSPs and temporal limitation of pyramidal cell activity (Pouille and Scanziani, 2001, 2004; Royer et al., 2012). In this way, interneurons can influence whether a pyramidal cell is recruited to, or removed from, an assembly of synchronously active pyramidal cells.

Another factor that promotes connection changes is long-lasting plasticity at pyramidal cell to interneuron synapses. Only a few examples of NMDAR-dependent long-lasting plasticity have been observed in interneurons. In CA1 stratum radiatum, a subset of interneurons express NMDAR-dependent long-term potentiation (LTP) and long-term depression (LTD) (Lamsa et al., 2005). However, other major types of interneuron plasticity depend on the activation of mGluRs and CP-AMPARs. A plethora of cellular and molecular mechanisms underlying the emergence of synaptic plasticity at interneuron inputs has been identified, indicating that the various interneuron types process distinct and nonoverlapping types of plasticity (Bartos et al., 2011; Kullmann and Lamsa, 2007; Laezza and Dingledine, 2004).

The conditions for the induction of synaptic plasticity in interneurons are different from those of pyramidal cells. For example, high-frequency stimulation of pyramidal cell inputs in CA3 onto stratum radiatum interneurons evokes LTD, which depends on CP-AMPARs and presynaptic mGluR7 (Pelkey et al., 2005). Moreover, stimulation of CP-AMPAR-mediated inputs at theta and gamma frequencies, which naturally emerge during environmental explorations, when paired with postsynaptic hyperpolarization, evokes LTP in CA1 feedback interneurons including PVIs, CCKIs, and SOM-OLM cells (Lamsa et al., 2007; Nissen et al., 2010). The hyperpolarization during the induction phase increases the driving force for calcium entry and the removal of the polyamine block, which is typical for CP-AMPARs. This form of NMDAR-independent LTP is termed "anti-Hebbian" and it can emerge either in quiescent interneurons (Figure 5.38) or during rhythmic neuronal network activity patterns under conditions where interneurons activate out of phase with respect to pyramidal cells. Anti-Hebbian plasticity thus may increase recruitment of interneurons, particularly PVIs, and pace spike timing in pyramidal cell associations. In contrast (Figure 5.38), associative Hebbian activation of presynaptic pyramidal cells drives PVIs at theta frequencies and causes the opposite, LTD (Camiré and Topolnik, 2014). This form of plasticity also requires the activation of CP-AMPARs and postsynaptic group I mGluRs (Camiré and Topolnik, 2014), and might be involved in the disconnection of PVIs from pyramidal cell assemblies representing a given information with their synchronized activity. Such a mechanism might support remapping of pyramidal cell associations.

In the DG, PVIs receive feedback MF-mediated inputs at their basal dendrites and feedforward PP-mediated inputs at their apical dendrites (Alle et al., 2001; Sambandan et al., 2010). Repeated activation of both inputs at gamma frequencies evokes Hebbian LTP at MF synapses but not PP inputs, in good correlation to the observed synapse-specific expression of CP-AMPARs at basal dendrites but CI-AMPARs at apical dendrites (Sambandan et al., 2010). This form of LTP is postsynaptically induced, requires a local calcium increase and the activation of CP-AMPARs, but is expressed presynaptically (Alle et al., 2001; Sambandan et al., 2010), implying the involvement

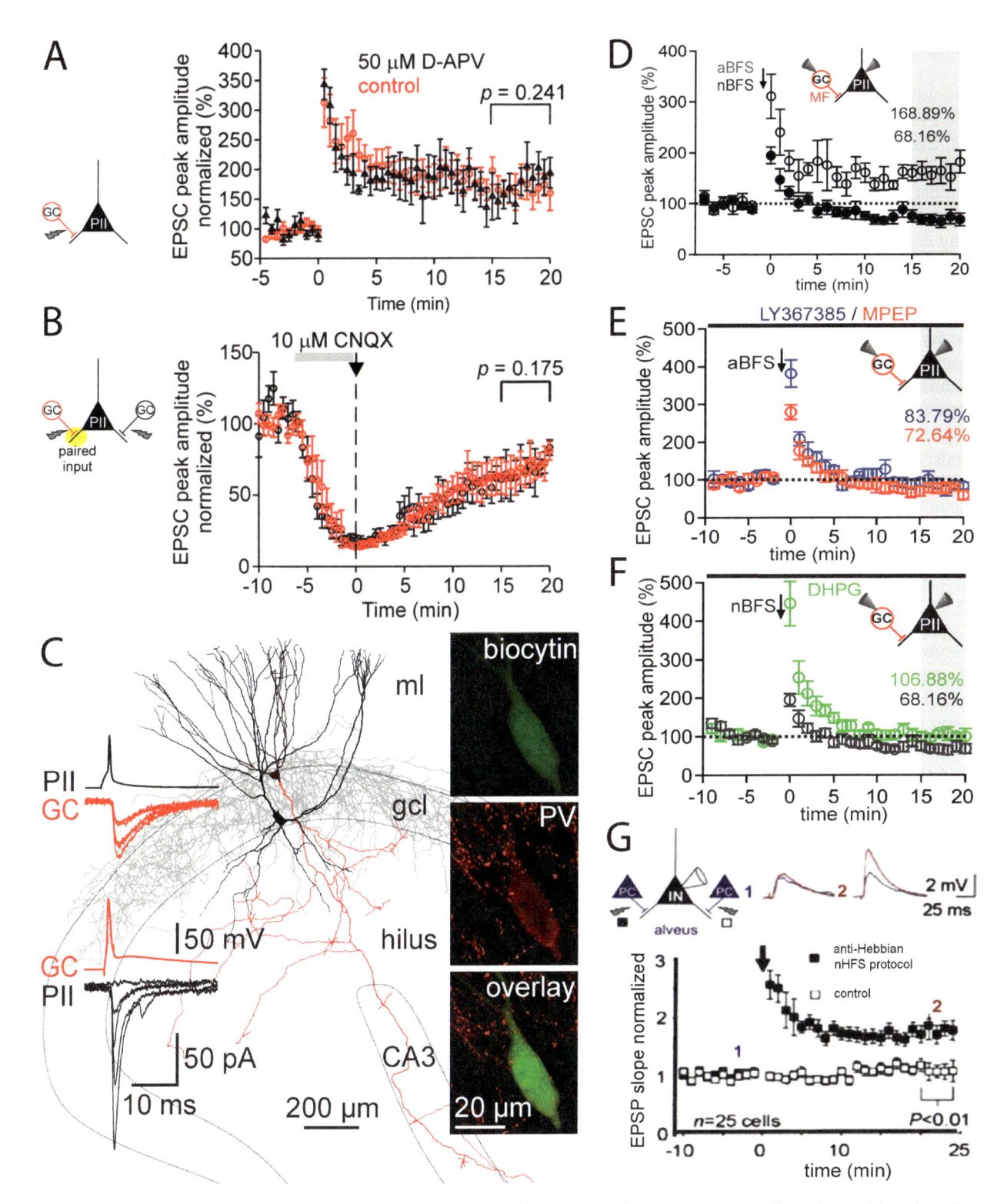

Figure 5.38 Plasticity of glutamatergic synaptic inputs onto interneurons. (A) Schematic of the experimental configuration. Hebbian-like LTP was evoked by an extracellular associative burst frequency stimulation (aBFS) at GC inputs (red circles) targeting a PV-expressing interneuron (PII) in the DG. In the presence of D-APV (50 μM) LTP is still observed, and thus is independent of NMDA receptors. (B) EPSCs amplitude plotted as a function of time for two independent GC inputs targeting a single PII. After a baseline period, 10 μM CNQX was washed in to block AMPARs. An aBFS was applied to one GC input (red circle, at $t = 0$, arrow). Washout of CNQX was started immediately after the pairing protocol. Recovery of the paired GC input (red circles) and the unpaired GC input (black circles) were similar, indicating that LTP was not induced and, thus, depends on AMPARs. (C) Reconstruction of a biocytin-filled and bidirectionally coupled GC-PII pair; GC axon in red. Insets indicate the reciprocal connection. Immunoreactivity for parvalbumin (PV) in the biocytin-filled interneuron is shown. (D) PII inputs show associative Hebbian-like LTP but not under conditions of nonassociative BFS (nBFS) at GC inputs. Application of an anti-Hebbian nBFS (at $t = 0$, arrow) evoked long-term depression (LTD) at GC-PII synapses. Amplitudes were normalized to the baseline and binned minute-wise. LTP was measured 15–20 min after induction (gray area). (E) An aBFS applied to GC-PII pairs induces posttetanic potentiation (PTP), followed by LTD in the presence of either LY367385 to block mGluR1α (blue, five pairs) or MPEP to block mGluR5 (red, five pairs). The black horizontal bar indicates the time of LY367385 or MPEP bath application. (F) Effect of the nBFS protocol on unitary EPSC amplitude in controls (black, 10 pairs) and in the presence of the group I agonist DHPG (5 μM; green, seven pairs), which abolished LTD induction. Group I mGluRs are specifically expressed at GC output synapses, indicating that LTD is expressed GC terminals. (G) Anti-Hebbian LTP occurs in interneurons with rectifying AMPARs in the feedback circuit. High-frequency presynaptic stimulation (HFS) paired with postsynaptic hyperpolarization evoked LTP in 25 out of 31 interneurons located in the oriens-alveus (NMDARs blocked with 100 μM APV). Insets, average EPSPs before and after LTP induction. (Sources: (A, B) Sambandan et al., 2010; (C–F) Hainmueller et al., 2014; (G) Lamsa et al., 2007.)

in the somatosensory cortex (Oláh et al., 2009) (Figure 5.39C). Phasic transmission refers to the fast release of transmitter and activation of GABA$_A$ receptors containing a γ subunit, meaning that they are also modulated by barbiturates and benzodiazepines. Tonic transmission instead relies on GABA$_A$ receptors that are located extrasynaptically on the postsynaptic membrane and are activated by the low background level of GABA that diffuses out of synapses to the extracellular space, termed "spillover." These GABA$_A$ receptors contain a δ instead of a γ subunit, which raises their affinity for GABA and their single channel open time, leading to a much more sustained conductance. Any GABA released from interneurons can activate both classes of receptor. However, in contrast to the fast IPSCs generated at PVI output synapses, paired recordings revealed that NGFIs generate IPSCs with small peak amplitudes and slow decay time constants in their target cells (Overstreet-Wadiche and McBain, 2015; Price et al., 2005). This slow inhibitory signaling is supported by morphological and physiological factors. First, the density of axon collaterals and boutons is high for NGFIs (compared with other interneuron types). Indeed, a bouton density of ~42 per 100 μm dendritic length was observed for DG and CA1 NGFIs, which is twice the density of CA1 PV-BCs (Sik et al., 1995). Second, the observed prolonged GABA release is supported by the fact that most NGFI boutons (~66,000 per cell) are not classical synapses, as they lack clear postsynaptic specializations (Overstreet-Wadiche and McBain, 2015). Thus, the combination of these two factors has been called "volume transmission," meaning that this spillover of GABA to extrasynaptic GABA$_A$Rs and GABA$_B$Rs, and the induction of long-lasting inhibitory postsynaptic signals, is a dominant feature of NGFI signaling (Oláh et al., 2009; Overstreet-Wadiche and McBain, 2015; Szabadics et al., 2007). However, NGFI-mediated GABA release therefore also lacks target cell specificity. What might be the potential role of slow NGFI-mediated inhibition in microcircuits? One potential functional scenario could be that desensitization of GABA$_A$ receptors during prolonged GABA exposure, together with presynaptically reduced GABA release via GABA$_B$R activation, may suppress feedforward inhibition and thereby support activation of pyramidal cells by excitatory inputs. The lack of presynaptic GABA$_B$Rs at PP terminals supports this hypothesis (Price et al., 2005).

The alignment of GABAergic fibers with excitatory projection pathways implies specific interactions with postsynaptic target cells but also with presynaptic glutamatergic and GABAergic partners. Indeed, spillover of GABA in CA3 can inhibit glutamate release at MF synapses targeting pyramidal cells via GABA$_B$Rs (Vogt and Nicoll, 1999). Moreover, activation of OLM cells in CA1 inhibits signaling from extrahippocampal inputs (from EC) onto CA1 pyramidal cells and at the same time supports intrahippocampal information flow (from CA3) by disinhibiting SC inputs, which can thereby control mnemonic functions within the hippocampus (Leao et al., 2012).

5.16 Interneuron microcircuit function

Interneurons predominantly contact principal cells, but several lines of evidence indicate that interneuron type-specific local circuitries exist to carry out specific microcircuit computations. Target cell specificity, connectivity motifs and topologies enable complex signal processing on the level of individual neurons and cell assemblies, including modulation of gain, offset, dynamic range, and synchronization, and thereby influence how neuronal populations are recruited according to the strength, number, and location of glutamatergic and GABAergic synaptic inputs.

5.16.1 Connectivity rules in microcircuits

As outlined above, interneurons show a high selectivity in the domain of the target cell they innervate and in the nature of the target neuron, resulting in the formation of distinct compositions of microcircuits. Interneurons also distinguish among defined types of target pyramidal cells and follow distinct local connectivity rules. To some degree, this is to be expected, because pyramidal cells segregate into different types based on their long-range projections to cortical and subcortical areas. PV-BCs target pyramidal cells with mean connection probabilities of ~20% (Bartos et al., 2001, 2002). However, in the DG they are more likely to target neighboring GCs (<100 μm distance; ~30% connection probability) with a higher number of synaptic release sites than distant GCs (>100 μm distance), giving rise to strong perisomatic inhibition to close neighbors and weak inhibition to more distant target cells (Strüber et al., 2015) (Figure 5.36C). Moreover, unidirectional inhibition is 10 times more frequent than reciprocal connections, demonstrating a prevalent lateral inhibition in this circuit (Espinoza et al., 2018). Distance-dependent lateral inhibition is assumed to support the formation of focal spots of strong local interconnected microcircuits for parallel processing of information (Strüber et al., 2015, 2017). Such a mechanisms may increase the computational capacity of neuronal networks (Espinoza et al., 2018; Strüber et al., 2017). The combination of strong local and broad lateral inhibition is efficient in suppressing weakly active GCs but keeping strongly active GCs unaffected, and thereby may implement a winner-take-all mechanism (Espinoza et al., 2018). Furthermore, CA1-PVIs generate larger amplitude IPSCs in pyramidal cells located in the deep pyramidal cell layer closer to stratum oriens preferentially projecting to the amygdala than to the PCs located in the superficial layer close to stratum radiatum (Figure 5.36A–B), which preferentially project to the prefrontal cortex (SH Lee et al., 2014). In turn, excitatory inputs onto CA1-PVIs arose more frequently from superficial pyramidal cells that target the prefrontal cortex, demonstrating the presence of specialized PVI-pyramidal cell microcircuits. These biased inhibitory and excitatory connections may be important in the information flow between the hippocampus and cortical brain regions, and in the coordination of behaviors.

5.16.2 Somatodendritic routing of inhibition

Cognitive processes emerge from the input-output transformations in hippocampal networks. These transformations are highly complex and depend on the connectivity patterns in any given neuronal circuit, as well as the input-output transformations on the level of individual cells in the network. Important building blocks in the input-output transformation of individual pyramidal cells are feedforward and feedback inhibition. In CA1, for example, stimulation of SCs excites both local pyramidal cells and BCs. Here, the feedforward, BC-mediated, short-latency disynaptic inhibition curtails synaptic excitation and leaves a short, 2 ms time-window for action potential generation, as discussed previously. In the DG, similarly rapid recruitment of BCs can be achieved by the recurrent mossy fiber inputs, thereby ensuring short-latency feedback inhibition to GCs (Geiger et al., 1997). During repetitive afferent activation of the alveus, BC-mediated IPSCs show multiple-pulse depression, whereas IPSCs evoked by dendrite-targeting inhibitory cells exhibit multiple-pulse facilitation in CA1 pyramidal cells. The contribution of the two inhibitory inputs results in the emergence of two integration windows, one emerging after a short latency that defines spike time, and a broader one, appearing after a longer latency, which allows integration of dendritically evoked EPSPs and limits the duration of pyramidal cell activity (Pouille and Scanziani, 2001, 2004; Royer et al., 2012). Similarly, repetitive afferent stimulation induces a first, short-latency, fast, PVI-mediated inhibitory signal in DG-GCs and a delayed, slow, dendritic HICAP- and HIPP-mediated inhibition onto GCs (Savanthrapadian et al., 2014). Thus, routing of inhibition from the soma to the dendrites controls spike precision as well as the duration of pyramidal cell activity, and, thereby, the transmission of contextual and spatial information among hippocampal areas.

5.16.3 Control of synaptic plasticity

Dendritic inhibition influences local voltage-gated conductances in pyramidal cells, shunts excitatory signals, influences the shape of calcium transients and the induction of long-lasting synaptic plasticity (Isaacson and Scanziani, 2011; Miles et al., 1996). Repetitive activation of PP at theta frequencies induces associative long-lasting potentiation of EPSPs at CA1 pyramidal cell and DG GC dendrites, which depends on postsynaptic NMDAR activation and an increase in dendritic intracellular calcium (Schmidt-Hieber et al., 2004; Weisskopf and Nicoll, 1995). Therefore, dendritic inhibition provided by, for example, SOM-expressing dendrite-targeting cells is optimally positioned to limit dendritic calcium signals and the induction of synaptic plasticity (Leao et al., 2012). This effect might be further supported by the strong hyperpolarizing effect of dendritic inhibition, which reduces the local membrane potential in GC dendrites and thereby increases the dynamic range of linear summation of individual EPSPs required for GC recruitment (Krueppel et al., 2011), an important requirement for the induction of associative synaptic plasticity (see Chapter 10).

5.16.4 Gain control

The location of synaptic inhibition strongly influences the gain control of pyramidal cell outputs (Pouille et al., 2009, 2013). The rate at which the discharge of a neuron responds to the strength of the excitatory input is termed "gain" and is an important property that describes a neuron's ability to integrate incoming signals (Carvalho and Buonomano, 2009). If excitation and inhibition arrive coincidently at the same dendritic compartment of CA1 pyramidal cells, the gain remains constant. With increasing inhibition, a stronger excitatory input is required to recruit the cell to fire: the ratio between excitation and inhibition is reduced, and thus gain is decreased. Interestingly, if the inhibitory input arrives at a perisomatic location, it alters the way excitatory signals propagate from the dendrites to the soma, and hence to the axon initial segment, where action potentials are generated. The membrane becomes leakier due to the inhibitory conductance, resulting in a rightward shift of the input-output function (e.g., a rise in the action potential threshold) and also a reduction in the maximal firing rate (Pouille et al., 2009, 2013).

5.16.5 Dynamic range

Since glutamatergic inputs control not only the activity of single neurons but also populations of pyramidal cells (divergence), and several pyramidal cells receive overlapping input (convergence), small changes in the number of active inputs may increase the population of active target pyramidal cells. The amplitude of EPSCs necessary to reach the threshold in CA1 pyramidal cells is dynamic and depends on the number of presynaptically active cells (Pouille et al., 2009). This normalization of the activation threshold is achieved by the concomitant recruitment of feedforward inhibition, which acts homogeneously across pyramidal cell populations. Feedforward inhibition ensures that the threshold of excitatory currents increases with stimulus strength, and that the maximum firing rate of the neuron is now due to a greater number of active inputs (Pouille et al., 2009). Such a mechanism may support sparse activity in the hippocampal network under conditions of strong afferent excitatory inputs. In combination with structural and functional differences in feedforward inhibition, such as distance-dependent inhibition (Strüber et al., 2017), concomitant inhibition will determine which pyramidal cells are recruited and which ones are not (Pouille et al., 2009).

5.17 Interneurons and network rhythms

A key factor in the transfer of information between neurons is synchronization during neuronal oscillations. Fast network activity patterns at theta (4–10 Hz), gamma (30–100 Hz), and sharp wave-associated ripple (SWRs, 100–200 Hz) frequencies are proposed to underlie the processing, encoding, and recall of information in mammals (Gray and Singer, 1989; Ribary et al., 1991). In the hippocampus, theta-gamma patterns typically coexist and emerge under certain behavioral conditions that correlate with cognitive tasks such as enhanced attention, working memory, and spatial learning (Buzsáki, 2001; Engel et al., 2001). SWRs occur during resting and slow-wave sleep, supporting offline replay and consolidation of previous experiences (Diba and Buzsáki, 2007; Wilson and McNaughton, 1994). Several lines of experimental and theoretical evidence indicate that inhibitory interneurons play a key role in the generation of fast network oscillations, including local inhibitory feedback in microcircuits, and mutual and long-range inhibition (Bartos et al., 2007; Buzsáki, 2001). In vivo evidence for the important role of interneurons in the generation of fast rhythmic network activity patterns came from intracellular recordings in CA1 in anaesthetized and awake rodents (Fuentealba et al., 2008; Katona et al., 2014; Klausberger et al., 2003, 2004, 2005; Varga et al., 2012, 2014; Ylinen et al., 1995), demonstrating that single spikes of pyramidal cells and identified interneurons were phase-locked to individual gamma cycles, as monitored with local field potentials.

The dominance of some interneuron types in the generation of certain oscillatory frequencies has been best examined for PVIs and SOMIs. The fast-spiking characteristics of perisomatic-inhibiting interneurons together with their rapid action potential conduction, the fast time course of synaptic inhibition, the broad divergence of the inhibitory output onto large pyramidal cell populations, as well as short feedback connections, allow PVIs to contribute to fast gamma and SWR activity patterns (Bartos et al., 2007). Accordingly, PVIs discharge during the ascending phase of individual gamma and ripple cycles in alternation with pyramidal cell discharges (Klausberger et al., 2005; Tukker et al., 2007; Varga et al., 2014) (Figure 5.40). Moreover, mutual inhibition among PVIs can support synchrony of oscillatory activity (Bartos et al., 2001, 2002). In contrast, the slower discharge characteristics of dendrite targeting SOMIs, together with the slow time course of inhibitory signals at

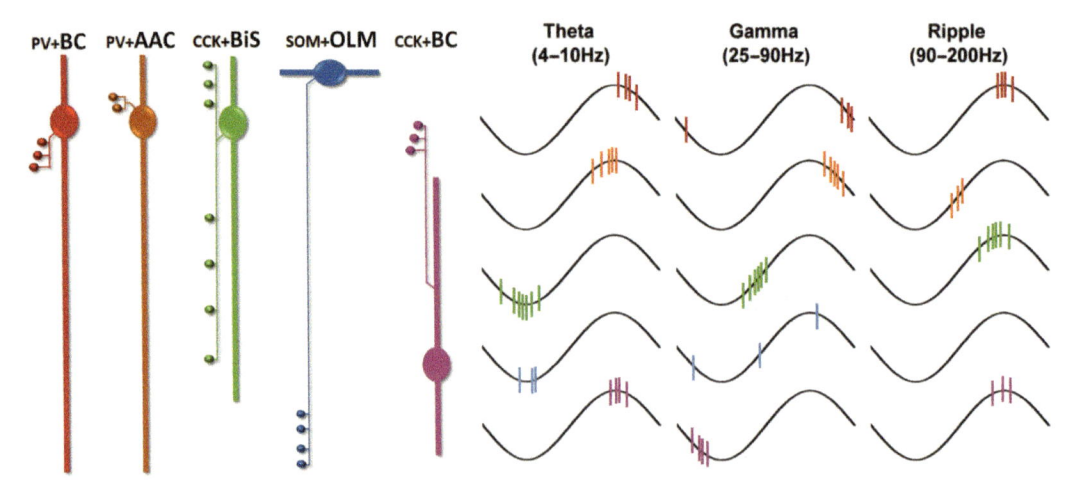

Figure 5.40 Phase coupling of interneuron types to fast network oscillations. Left: color-coded illustrations of major types of interneurons. Right: for each of three oscillation frequency bands (theta, gamma, ripple), the peak of firing activity of each interneuron category is depicted as a color-coded vertical bar on a single oscillation cycle. Note that the number, timing, and phase of spikes differs between Interneuron types; OLM cells have no phase preference during gamma oscillations, as shown by evenly distributed single spikes, and rarely fire during ripple events. See main text for further discussion.

their output synapses and the longer feedback connections, result in their preferred contribution to the generation of theta oscillations (Hu et al., 2014; Klausberger et al., 2005; Varga et al., 2012). Finally, long-range projecting interneurons may support the synchronization of network activity across hippocampal areas and more distant brain regions (Katona et al., 2017; Szabo et al., 2017).

5.18 Concluding remarks

Throughout this chapter, we have highlighted the extraordinary diversity of both excitatory and inhibitory cell types in the hippocampus. These neurons differ in their morphology, molecular composition, sources of synaptic inputs and targets of their outputs, and properties of input and output synapses, including differences in strength, kinetics, short- and long-term plasticity, and intrinsic membrane properties that govern the relationship between synaptic input and action potential firing. Furthermore, these properties are subject to changes based on behavioral and environmental conditions that influence neuromodulatory and hormonal effects on neurophysiology, as well as the effects of a lifetime of experience on the structure and functions of neurons and the circuits they constitute.

The hippocampus serves as a microcosm for this complexity, which exists at an even broader scale throughout the mammalian brain. In the 15 years since the publication of the first edition of this book, much has been discovered, and we eagerly anticipate further developments in the field. With the complexity of the brain, it is likely that there will be more to describe in the next 15 years. However, we hope that this will be complemented by progress in leveraging our understanding of this complexity to gain deeper insight into how biological brains enable intelligent behavior.

Acknowledgments

This chapter is dedicated to the memory of our beloved friend and colleague, Vivien Chevaleyre. The authors thank the following people for helpful input on the chapter: Michael Brecht, Mark Cembrowski, Csaba Földy, and Albert Lee. Support for the authors was provided by the following organizations: Howard Hughes Medical Institute, National Institute of Child Health and Human Development, Inserm, CNRS, L'Agence National de la Recherche, Federal Ministry of Education and Research, Germany (BMBF), German Research Foundation, European Research Council, Volkswagen Stiftung. We would also like to thank Laurel Royer (HHMI Janelia) and Pamela Clifford (NIH) for securing permissions to reproduce figures.

REFERENCES

Abbasi S, Kumar SS (2013) Electrophysiological and morphological characterization of cells in superficial layers of rat presubiculum: physiology and morphology of cells in presubiculum. *Journal of Comparative Neurology* 521:3116–3132.

Acsády L, Görcs TJ, Freund TF (1996) Different populations of vasoactive intestinal polypeptide-immunoreactive interneurons are specialized to control pyramidal cells or interneurons in the hippocampus. *Neuroscience* 73:317–334.

Acsády L, Kamondi A, Sík A, Freund T, Buzsáki G (1998) GABAergic cells are the major postsynaptic targets of mossy fibers in the rat hippocampus. *Journal of Neuroscience: Official Journal of the Society for Neuroscience* 18:3386–3403.

Acsády L, Katona I, Martínez-Guijarro FJ, Buzsáki G, Freund TF (2000) Unusual target selectivity of perisomatic inhibitory cells in the hilar region of the rat hippocampus. *Journal of Neuroscience: The Official Journal of the Society for Neuroscience* 20:6907–6919.

Aggleton JP, Christiansen K (2015) The subiculum: the heart of the extended hippocampal system. *Progress in Brain Research* 219:65–82.

Ali AB, Thomson AM (1998) Facilitating pyramid to horizontal oriens-alveus interneurone inputs: dual intracellular recordings in slices of rat hippocampus. *Journal of Physiology* 507:185–199.

Ali AB, Todorova M (2010) Asynchronous release of GABA via tonic cannabinoid receptor activation at identified interneuron synapses in rat CA1. *European Journal of Neuroscience* 31:1196–1207.

Alle H, Geiger JRP (2006) Combined analog and action potential coding in hippocampal mossy fibers. *Science* 311:1290–1293.

Alle H, Jonas P, Geiger JR (2001) PTP and LTP at a hippocampal mossy fiber-interneuron synapse. *Proceedings of the National Academy of Sciences of the United States of America* 98:14708–14713.

Allen K, Fuchs EC, Jaschonek H, Bannerman DM, Monyer H (2011) Gap junctions between interneurons are required for normal spatial coding in the hippocampus and short-term spatial memory. *Journal of Neuroscience* 31:6542–6552.

Alme CB, Buzzetti RA, Marrone DF, Leutgeb JK, Chawla MK, Schaner MJ, Bohanick JD, Khoboko T, Leutgeb S, Moser EI, et al. (2010) Hippocampal granule cells opt for early retirement. *Hippocampus* 20:1109–1123.

Alonso A, Klink R (1993) Differential electroresponsiveness of stellate and pyramidal-like cells of medial entorhinal cortex layer II. *Journal of Neurophysiology* 70:128–143.

Alonso A, Llinás RR (1989) Subthreshold Na+-dependent theta-like rhythmicity in stellate cells of entorhinal cortex layer II. *Nature* 342:175–177.

Amaral DG (1978) A golgi study of cell types in the hilar region of the hippocampus in the rat. *Journal of Comparative Neurology* 182:851–914.

Amaral DG, Ishizuka N, Claiborne B (1990) Neurons, numbers and the hippocampal network. *Progress in Brain Research* 83:1–11.

Amaral DG, Kurz J (1985) An analysis of the origins of the cholinergic and noncholinergic septal projections to the hippocampal formation of the rat. *Journal of Comparative Neurology* 240:37–59.

Amaral DG, Scharfman HE, Lavenex P (2007) The dentate gyrus: fundamental neuroanatomical organization (dentate gyrus for dummies). *Progress in Brain Research* 163:3–790.

Amaral D, Witter M (1989) The three-dimensional organization of the hippocampal formation: a review of anatomical data. *Neuroscience* 31:571–591.

Andrade R, Nicoll RA (1987) Pharmacologically distinct actions of serotonin on single pyramidal neurones of the rat hippocampus recorded in vitro. *Journal of Physiology* 394:99–124.

Andreasen M, Lambert JD (1995) Regenerative properties of pyramidal cell dendrites in area CA1 of the rat hippocampus. *Journal of Physiology* 483(Pt 2):421–441.

Andreasen M, Nedergaard S (1996) Dendritic electrogenesis in rat hippocampal CA1 pyramidal neurons: functional aspects of Na+ and Ca2+ currents in apical dendrites. *Hippocampus* 6:79–95.

Antonio AS, Liban K, Ikrar T, Tsyganovskiy E, Xu X (2014) Distinct physiological and developmental properties of hippocampal CA2 subfield revealed by using anti-Purkinje cell protein 4 (PCP4) immunostaining. *Journal of Comparative Neurology* 522:1333–1354.

Aponte Y, Lien C-C, Reisinger E, Jonas P (2006) Hyperpolarization-activated cation channels in fast-spiking interneurons of rat hippocampus. *Journal of Physiology* 574:229–243.

Apostolides PF, Milstein AD, Grienberger C, Bittner KC, Magee JC (2016) Axonal filtering allows reliable output during dendritic plateau-driven complex spiking in CA1 neurons. *Neuron* 89:770–783.

Ariav G, Polsky A, Schiller J (2003) Submillisecond precision of the input-output transformation function mediated by fast sodium dendritic spikes in basal dendrites of CA1 pyramidal neurons. *Journal of Neuroscience: The Official Journal of the Society for Neuroscience* 23:7750–7758.

Armstrong C, Szabadics J, Tamás G, Soltesz I (2011) Neurogliaform cells in the molecular layer of the dentate gyrus as feed-forward γ-aminobutyric acidergic modulators of entorhinal-hippocampal interplay. *Journal of Comparative Neurology* 519:1476–1491.

Arszovszki A, Borhegyi Z, Klausberger T (2014) Three axonal projection routes of individual pyramidal cells in the ventral CA1 hippocampus. *Frontiers in Neuroanatomy* 8:53.

Artinian J, Jordan A, Khlaifia A, Honoré E, La Fontaine A, Racine A-S, Laplante I, Lacaille J-C (2019) Regulation of hippocampal memory by mTORC1 in somatostatin interneurons. *Journal of*

Neuroscience: The Official Journal of the Society for Neuroscience 39:8439–8456.

Atzori M, Lau D, Tansey EP, Chow A, Ozaita A, Rudy B, McBain CJ (2000) H2 histamine receptor-phosphorylation of Kv3.2 modulates interneuron fast spiking. *Nature Neuroscience* 3:791–798.

Azevedo EP, Pomeranz L, Cheng J, Schneeberger M, Vaughan R, Stern SA, Tan B, Doerig K, Greengard P, Friedman JM (2019) A role of Drd2 hippocampal neurons in context-dependent food intake. *Neuron* 102:873–886, e5.

Bahner F, Weiss EK, Birke G, Maier N, Schmitz D, Rudolph U, Frotscher M, Traub RD, Both M, Draguhn A (2011) Cellular correlate of assembly formation in oscillating hippocampal networks in vitro. *Proceedings of the National Academy of Sciences* 108:E607–E616.

Baimbridge KG, Peet MJ, McLennan H, Church J (1991) Bursting response to current-evoked depolarization in rat CA1 pyramidal neurons is correlated with lucifer yellow dye coupling but not with the presence of calbindin-D28k. *Synapse* 7:269–277.

Balind SR, Magó Á, Ahmadi M, Kis N, Varga-Németh Z, Lőrincz A, Makara JK (2019) Diverse synaptic and dendritic mechanisms of complex spike burst generation in hippocampal CA3 pyramidal cells. *Nature Communications* 10:1859.

Bannister NJ, Larkman AU (1995) Dendritic morphology of CA1 pyramidal neurones from the rat hippocampus: I. Branching patterns. *Journal of Comparative Neurology* 360:150–160.

Bartesaghi R, Gessi T (2004) Parallel activation of field CA2 and dentate gyrus by synaptically elicited perforant path volleys. *Hippocampus* 14:948–963.

Bartesaghi R, Ravasi L (1999) Pyramidal neuron types in field CA2 of the guinea pig. *Brain Research Bulletin* 50:263–273.

Bartos M, Alle H, Vida I (2011) Role of microcircuit structure and input integration in hippocampal interneuron recruitment and plasticity. *Neuropharmacology* 60:730–739.

Bartos M, Elgueta C (2012) Functional characteristics of parvalbumin- and cholecystokinin-expressing basket cells. *Journal of Physiology* 590:669–681.

Bartos M, Vida I, Frotscher M, Geiger JR, Jonas P (2001) Rapid signaling at inhibitory synapses in a dentate gyrus interneuron network. *Journal of Neuroscience: The Official Journal of the Society for Neuroscience* 21:2687–2698.

Bartos M, Vida I, Frotscher M, Meyer A, Monyer H, Geiger JRP, Jonas P (2002) Fast synaptic inhibition promotes synchronized gamma oscillations in hippocampal interneuron networks. *Proceedings of the National Academy of Sciences* 99:13222.

Bartos M, Vida I, Jonas P (2007) Synaptic mechanisms of synchronized gamma oscillations in inhibitory interneuron networks. *Nature Reviews Neuroscience* 8:45–56.

Baude A, Nusser Z, Roberts JD, Mulvihill E, McIlhinney RA, Somogyi P (1993) The metabotropic glutamate receptor (mGluR1 alpha) is concentrated at perisynaptic membrane of neuronal subpopulations as detected by immunogold reaction. *Neuron* 11:771–787.

Behr J, Gloveli T, Schmitz D, Heinemann U (2000) Dopamine depresses excitatory synaptic transmission onto rat subicular neurons via presynaptic D1-like dopamine receptors. *Journal of Neurophysiology* 84:112–119.

Behr J, Wozny C, Fidzinski P, Schmitz D (2009) Synaptic plasticity in the subiculum. *Progress in Neurobiology* 89:334–342.

Bekkers JM, Stevens CF (1989) NMDA and non-NMDA receptors are co-localized at individual excitatory synapses in cultured rat hippocampus. *Nature* 341:230–233.

Beltrán JQ, Gutiérrez R (2012) Co-release of glutamate and GABA from single, identified mossy fibre giant boutons. *Journal of Physiology* 590:4789–4800.

Benardo LS, Prince DA (1982a) Dopamine action on hippocampal pyramidal cells. *Journal of Neuroscience: The Official Journal of the Society for Neuroscience* 2:415–423.

Benardo LS, Prince DA (1982b) Dopamine modulates a Ca2+-activated potassium conductance in mammalian hippocampal pyramidal cells. *Nature* 297:76–79.

Benoy A, Ibrahim MZB, Behnisch T, Sajikumar S (2021) Metaplastic reinforcement of long-term potentiation in hippocampal area CA2 by cholinergic receptor activation. *Journal of Neuroscience* 41:9082–9098.

Bergersen L, Ruiz A, Bjaalie JG, Kullmann DM, Gundersen V (2003) GABA and GABAA receptors at hippocampal mossy fibre synapses. *European Journal of Neuroscience* 18:931–941.

Bernstein HL, Lu Y-L, Botterill JJ, Scharfman HE (2019) Novelty and novel objects increase c-Fos immunoreactivity in mossy cells in the mouse dentate gyrus. *Neural Plasticity* 2019:1–16.

Bezaire MJ, Soltesz I (2013) Quantitative assessment of CA1 local circuits: knowledge base for interneuron-pyramidal cell connectivity. *Hippocampus* 23:751–785.

Biebl M, Cooper CM, Winkler J, Kuhn HG (2000) Analysis of neurogenesis and programmed cell death reveals a self-renewing capacity in the adult rat brain. *Neuroscience Letters* 291:17–20.

Bienkowski MS, Bowman I, Song MY, Gou L, Ard T, Cotter K, Zhu M, Benavidez NL, Yamashita S, Abu-Jaber J, et al. (2018) Integration of gene expression and brain-wide connectivity reveals the multiscale organization of mouse hippocampal networks. *Nature Neuroscience* 21:1628–1643.

Bilkey DK, Schwartzkroin PA (1990) Variation in electrophysiology and morphology of hippocampal CA3 pyramidal cells. *Brain Research* 514:77–83.

Bischofberger J, Engel D, Li L, Geiger JRP, Jonas P (2006) Patch-clamp recording from mossy fiber terminals in hippocampal slices. *Nature Protocols* 1:2075–2081.

Bittner KC, Andrasfalvy BK, Magee JC (2012) Ion channel gradients in the apical tuft region of CA1 pyramidal neurons. *PLoS One* 7:e46652.

Bittner KC, Grienberger C, Vaidya SP, Milstein AD, Macklin JJ, Suh J, Tonegawa S, Magee JC (2015) Conjunctive input processing drives feature selectivity in hippocampal CA1 neurons. *Nature Neuroscience* 18:1133–1142.

Bittner KC, Milstein AD, Grienberger C, Romani S, Magee JC (2017) Behavioral time scale synaptic plasticity underlies CA1 place fields. *Science* 357:1033–1036.

Blackstad JS, Osen KK, Scharfman HE, Storm-Mathisen J, Blackstad TW, Leergaard TB (2016) Observations on hippocampal mossy cells in mink (*Neovison vison*) with special reference to dendrites ascending to the granular and molecular layers. *Hippocampus* 26:229–245.

Blasco-Ibáñez JM, Freund TF (1995) Synaptic input of horizontal interneurons in stratum oriens of the hippocampal CA1 subfield: structural basis of feed-back activation. *European Journal of Neuroscience* 7:2170–2180.

Bliss TVP, Collingridge GL (1993) A synaptic model of memory: long-term potentiation in the hippocampus. *Nature* 361:31–39.

Bloss EB, Cembrowski MS, Karsh B, Colonell J, Fetter RD, Spruston N (2016) Structured dendritic inhibition supports branch-selective integration in CA1 pyramidal cells. *Neuron* 89:1016–1030.

Bloss EB, Cembrowski MS, Karsh B, Colonell J, Fetter RD, Spruston N (2018) Single excitatory axons form clustered synapses onto CA1 pyramidal cell dendrites. *Nature Neuroscience* 21:353–363.

Boccara CN, Sargolini F, Thoresen VH, Solstad T, Witter MP, Moser EI, Moser M-B (2010) Grid cells in pre- and parasubiculum. *Nature Neuroscience* 13:987–994.

Boehringer R, Polygalov D, Huang AJY, Middleton SJ, Robert V, Wintzer ME, Piskorowski RA, Chevaleyre V, McHugh TJ (2017) Chronic loss of CA2 transmission leads to hippocampal hyperexcitability. *Neuron* 94:642–655, e9.

Booker SA, Althof D, Gross A, Loreth D, Müller J, Unger A, Fakler B, Varro A, Watanabe M, Gassmann M, et al. (2017) KCTD12 auxiliary proteins modulate kinetics of GABAB receptor-mediated inhibition in cholecystokinin-containing interneurons. *Cerebral Cortex* 27:2318–2334.

Booker SA, Gross A, Althof D, Shigemoto R, Bettler B, Frotscher M, Hearing M, Wickman K, Watanabe M, Kulik Á, et al. (2013) Differential GABAB-receptor-mediated effects in perisomatic- and dendrite-targeting parvalbumin interneurons. *Journal of Neuroscience: The Official Journal of the Society for Neuroscience* 33:7961–7974.

Botterill JJ, Gerencer KJ, Vinod KY, Alcantara-Gonzalez D, Scharfman HE (2021) Dorsal and ventral mossy cells differ in their axonal projections throughout the dentate gyrus of the mouse hippocampus. *Hippocampus* 31:522–539.

Bourdeau ML, Morin F, Laurent CE, Azzi M, Lacaille J-C (2007) Kv4.3-mediated A-type K+ currents underlie rhythmic activity in hippocampal interneurons. *Journal of Neuroscience: The Official Journal of the Society for Neuroscience* 27:1942–1953.

Bourne J, Harris KM (2007) Do thin spines learn to be mushroom spines that remember? *Current Opinion in Neurobiology* 17:381–386.

Brandalise F, Carta S, Helmchen F, Lisman J, Gerber U (2016) Dendritic NMDA spikes are necessary for timing-dependent associative LTP in CA3 pyramidal cells. *Nature Communications* 7:13480.

Brandalise F, Gerber U (2014) Mossy fiber-evoked subthreshold responses induce timing-dependent plasticity at hippocampal CA3 recurrent synapses. *Proceedings of the National Academy of Sciences* 111:4303–4308.

Brandon MP, Bogaard AR, Schultheiss NW, Hasselmo ME (2013) Segregation of cortical head direction cell assemblies on alternating theta cycles. *Nature Neuroscience* 16:739–748.

Brückner G, Grosche J, Hartlage-Rübsamen M, Schmidt S, Schachner M (2003) Region and lamina-specific distribution of extracellular matrix proteoglycans, hyaluronan and tenascin-R in the mouse hippocampal formation. *Journal of Chemical Neuroanatomy* 26:37–50.

Brunner J, Neubrandt M, Van-Weert S, Andrási T, Borgmann FBK, Jessberger S, Szabadics J (2014) Adult-born granule cells mature through two functionally distinct states. *ELife* 3:e03104.

Buckmaster PS (2012) Mossy cell dendritic structure quantified and compared with other hippocampal neurons labeled in rats in vivo. *Epilepsia* 53:9–17.

Buckmaster PS, Amaral DG (2001) Intracellular recording and labeling of mossy cells and proximal CA3 pyramidal cells in macaque monkeys. *Journal of Comparative Neurology* 430:264–281.

Buckmaster PS, Wenzel HJ, Kunkel DD, Schwartzkroin PA (1996) Axon arbors and synaptic connections of hippocampal mossy cells in the rat in vivo. *Journal of Comparative Neurology* 366:270–292.

Buckmaster PS, Yamawaki R, Zhang GF (2002) Axon arbors and synaptic connections of a vulnerable population of interneurons in the dentate gyrus in vivo. *Journal of Comparative Neurology* 445:360–373.

Bucurenciu I, Kulik A, Schwaller B, Frotscher M, Jonas P (2008) Nanodomain coupling between Ca2+ channels and Ca2+ sensors promotes fast and efficient transmitter release at a cortical GABAergic synapse. *Neuron* 57:536–545.

Buhl EH, Han ZS, Lorinczi Z, Stezhka VV, Karnup SV, Somogyi P (1994) Physiological properties of anatomically identified axo-axonic cells in the rat hippocampus. *Journal of Neurophysiology* 71:1289–1307.

Burgalossi A, Herfst L, Heimendahl M von, Förste H, Haskic K, Schmidt M, Brecht M (2011) Microcircuits of functionally identified neurons in the rat medial entorhinal cortex. *Neuron* 70:773–786.

Buzsáki G (2001) Hippocampal GABAergic interneurons: a physiological perspective. *Neurochemical Research* 26:899–905.

Buzsaki G, Horvath Z, Urioste R, Hetke J, Wise K (1992) High-frequency network oscillation in the hippocampus. *Science* 256:1025–1027.

Buzsáki G, Tingley D (2018) Space and time: the hippocampus as a sequence generator. *Trends in Cognitive Sciences* 22:853–869.

Cai X, Liang CW, Muralidharan S, Muralidharan S, Kao JPY, Tang C-M, Thompson SM (2004) Unique roles of SK and Kv4.2 potassium channels in dendritic integration. *Neuron* 44:351–364.

Ramón y Cajal S (1995) Histology of the Nervous System of Man and Vertebrates. Oxford: Oxford University Press.

Camiré O, Topolnik L (2014) Dendritic calcium nonlinearities switch the direction of synaptic plasticity in fast-spiking interneurons. *Journal of Neuroscience: The Official Journal of the Society for Neuroscience* 34:3864–3877.

Canto CB, Witter MP (2012) Cellular properties of principal neurons in the rat entorhinal cortex: II. The medial entorhinal cortex. *Hippocampus* 22:1277–1299.

Capogna M, Pearce RA (2011) GABA A,slow: causes and consequences. *Trends in Neurosciences* 34:101–112.

Carstens KE, Phillips ML, Pozzo-Miller L, Weinberg RJ, Dudek SM (2016) Perineuronal nets suppress plasticity of excitatory synapses on CA2 pyramidal neurons. *Journal of Neuroscience* 36:6312–6320.

Carter BC, Giessel AJ, Sabatini BL, Bean BP (2012) Transient sodium current at subthreshold voltages: activation by EPSP waveforms. *Neuron* 75:1081–1093.

Carvalho TP, Buonomano DV (2009) Differential effects of excitatory and inhibitory plasticity on synaptically driven neuronal input-output functions. *Neuron* 61:774–785.

Cea-del Rio CA, Lawrence JJ, Erdelyi F, Szabo G, McBain CJ (2011) Cholinergic modulation amplifies the intrinsic oscillatory properties of CA1 hippocampal cholecystokinin-positive interneurons. *Journal of Physiology* 589:609–627.

Cea-del Rio CA, Lawrence JJ, Tricoire L, Erdelyi F, Szabo G, McBain CJ (2010) M3 muscarinic acetylcholine receptor expression confers differential cholinergic modulation to neurochemically distinct hippocampal basket cell subtypes. *Journal of Neuroscience: The Official Journal of the Society for Neuroscience* 30:6011–6024.

Celio MR (1993) Perineuronal nets of extracellular matrix around parvalbumin-containing neurons of the hippocampus. *Hippocampus* 3 Spec No:55–60.

Cembrowski MS, Bachman JL, Wang L, Sugino K, Shields BC, Spruston N (2016) Spatial gene-expression gradients underlie prominent heterogeneity of CA1 pyramidal neurons. *Neuron* 89:351–368.

Cembrowski MS, Phillips MG, DiLisio SF, Shields BC, Winnubst J, Chandrashekar J, Bas E, Spruston N (2018) Dissociable structural and functional hippocampal outputs via distinct subiculum cell classes. *Cell* 173:1280–1292, e18.

Cembrowski MS, Spruston N (2019) Heterogeneity within classical cell types is the rule: lessons from hippocampal pyramidal neurons. *Nature Reviews Neuroscience* 20:1–12.

Cembrowski MS, Wang L, Lemire AL, Copeland M, DiLisio SF, Clements J, Spruston N (2018) The subiculum is a patchwork of discrete subregions. *ELife* 7:65.

Cembrowski MS, Wang L, Sugino K, Shields BC, Spruston N (2016) Hipposeq: a comprehensive RNA-seq database of gene expression in hippocampal principal neurons. *ELife* 5:e14997.

Ceranik K, Bender R, Geiger JR, Monyer H, Jonas P, Frotscher M, Lübke J (1997) A novel type of GABAergic interneuron connecting the input and the output regions of the hippocampus. *Journal of Neuroscience: The Official Journal of the Society for Neuroscience* 17:5380–5394.

Chancey JH, Adlaf EW, Sapp MC, Pugh PC, Wadiche JI, Overstreet-Wadiche LS (2013) GABA depolarization is required for experience-dependent synapse unsilencing in adult-born neurons. *Journal of Neuroscience* 33:6614.

Chancey JH, Poulsen DJ, Wadiche JI, Overstreet-Wadiche L (2014) Hilar mossy cells provide the first glutamatergic synapses to adult-born dentate granule cells. *Journal of Neuroscience* 34:2349–2354.

Chen S, He L, Huang AJY, Boehringer R, Robert V, Wintzer ME, Polygalov D, Weitemier AZ, Tao Y, Gu M, et al. (2020) A hypothalamic novelty signal modulates hippocampal memory. *Nature* 586:270–274.

Chen S, Wang J, Siegelbaum SA (2001) Properties of hyperpolarization-activated pacemaker current defined by coassembly of HCN1 and HCN2 subunits and basal modulation by cyclic nucleotide. *Journal of General Physiology* 117:491–504.

Chevaleyre V, Siegelbaum SA (2010) Strong CA2 pyramidal neuron synapses define a powerful disynaptic cortico-hippocampal loop. *Neuron* 66:560–572.

Chicurel ME, Harris KM (1992) Three-dimensional analysis of the structure and composition of CA3 branched dendritic spines and their synaptic relationships with mossy fiber boutons in the rat hippocampus. *Journal of Comparative Neurology* 325:169–182.

Chittajallu R, Auville K, Mahadevan V, Lai M, Hunt S, Calvigioni D, Pelkey KA, Zaghloul KA, McBain CJ (2020) Activity-dependent tuning of intrinsic excitability in mouse and human neurogliaform cells. *ELife* 9:e57571.

Chitwood RA, Hubbard A, Jaffe DB (1999) Passive electrotonic properties of rat hippocampal CA3 interneurones. *Journal of Physiology* 515(Pt 3):743–756.

Christie BR, Magee JC, Johnston D (1996) The role of dendritic action potentials and Ca2+ influx in the induction of homosynaptic long-term depression in hippocampal CA1 pyramidal neurons. *Learning and Memory* 3:160–169.

Ciocchi S, Passecker J, Malagon-Vina H, Mikus N, Klausberger T (2015) Selective information routing by ventral hippocampal CA1 projection neurons. *Science* 348:560–563.

Cobb SR, Buhl EH, Halasy K, Paulsen O, Somogyi P (1995) Synchronization of neuronal activity in hippocampus by individual GABAergic interneurons. *Nature* 378:75–78.

Cobb SR, Bulters DO, Suchak S, Riedel G, Morris RG, Davies CH (1999) Activation of nicotinic acetylcholine receptors patterns network activity in the rodent hippocampus. *Journal of Physiology* 518:131–140.

Cobb SR, Halasy K, Vida I, Nyiri G, Tamás G, Buhl EH, Somogyi P (1997) Synaptic effects of identified interneurons innervating both interneurons and pyramidal cells in the rat hippocampus. *Neuroscience* 79:629–648.

Cohen JD, Bolstad M, Lee AK (2017) Experience-dependent shaping of hippocampal CA1 intracellular activity in novel and familiar environments. *ELife* 6:e23040.

Cohen SM, Ma H, Kuchibhotla KV, Watson BO, Buzsáki G, Froemke RC, Tsien RW (2016) Excitation-transcription coupling in parvalbumin-positive interneurons employs a novel CaM kinase-dependent pathway distinct from excitatory neurons. *Neuron* 90:292–307.

Colbert CM, Johnston D (1996) Axonal action-potential initiation and Na+ channel densities in the soma and axon initial segment of subicular pyramidal neurons. *Journal of Neuroscience* 16:6676–6686.

Colbert CM, Magee JC, Hoffman DA, Johnston D (1997) Slow recovery from inactivation of Na+ channels underlies the activity-dependent attenuation of dendritic action potentials in hippocampal CA1 pyramidal neurons. *Journal of Neuroscience: The Official Journal of the Society for Neuroscience* 17:6512–6521.

Colbert CM, Pan E (2002) Ion channel properties underlying axonal action potential initiation in pyramidal neurons. *Nature Neuroscience* 5:533–538.

Cole AE, Nicoll RA (1983) Acetylcholine mediates a slow synaptic potential in hippocampal pyramidal cells. *Science* 221:1299–1301.

Cole AE, Nicoll RA (1984) Characterization of a slow cholinergic post-synaptic potential recorded in vitro from rat hippocampal pyramidal cells. *Journal of Physiology* 352:173–188.

Cornejo VH, Ofer N, Yuste R (2022) Voltage compartmentalization in dendritic spines in vivo. *Science* 375:82–86.

Cossart R, Epsztein J, Tyzio R, Becq H, Hirsch J, Ben-Ari Y, Crépel V (2002) Quantal release of glutamate generates pure kainate and mixed AMPA/kainate EPSCs in hippocampal neurons. *Neuron* 35:147–159.

Cossart R, Esclapez M, Hirsch JC, Bernard C, Ben-Ari Y (1998) GluR5 kainate receptor activation in interneurons increases tonic inhibition of pyramidal cells. *Nature Neuroscience* 1:470–478.

Cossart R, Ikegaya Y, Yuste R (2005) Calcium imaging of cortical networks dynamics. *Cell Calcium* 37:451–457.

Crill WE (1996) Persistent sodium current in mammalian central neurons. *Annual Review of Physiology* 58:349–362.

Csicsvari J, Hirase H, Mamiya A, Buzsáki G (2000) Ensemble patterns of hippocampal CA3-CA1 neurons during sharp wave-associated population events. *Neuron* 28:585–594.

Cudmore RH, Fronzaroli-Molinieres L, Giraud P, Debanne D (2010) Spike-time precision and network synchrony are controlled by the homeostatic regulation of the D-type potassium current. *Journal of Neuroscience* 30:12885–12895.

Cui Z, Gerfen CR, Young WS (2013) Hypothalamic and other connections with dorsal CA2 area of the mouse hippocampus. *Journal of Comparative Neurology* 521:1844–1866.

Danielson NB, Kaifosh P, Zaremba JD, Lovett-Barron M, Tsai J, Denny CA, Balough EM, Goldberg AR, Drew LJ, Hen R, et al. (2016) Distinct contribution of adult-born hippocampal granule cells to context encoding. *Neuron* 90:101–112.

Danielson NB, Turi GF, Ladow M, Chavlis S, Petrantonakis PC, Poirazi P, Losonczy A (2017) In vivo imaging of dentate gyrus mossy cells in behaving mice. *Neuron* 93:552–559, e4.

Danielson NB, Zaremba JD, Kaifosh P, Bowler J, Ladow M, Losonczy A (2016a) Sublayer-specific coding dynamics during spatial navigation and learning in hippocampal area CA1. *Neuron* 91:652–665.

Dannenberg H, Young K, Hasselmo M (2017) Modulation of hippocampal circuits by muscarinic and nicotinic receptors. *Frontiers in Neural Circuits* 11:1–18.

Dasgupta A, Lim YJ, Kumar K, Baby N, Pang KLK, Benoy A, Behnisch T, Sajikumar S (2020) Group III metabotropic glutamate receptors gate long-term potentiation and synaptic tagging/capture in rat hippocampal area CA2. *ELife* 9:919–920.

Daw MI, Pelkey KA, Chittajallu R, McBain CJ (2010) Presynaptic kainate receptor activation preserves asynchronous GABA release despite the reduction in synchronous release from hippocampal cholecystokinin interneurons. *Journal of Neuroscience* 30:11202–11209.

Daw MI, Tricoire L, Erdélyi F, Szabó G, McBain CJ (2009) Asynchronous transmitter release from cholecystokinin-containing inhibitory interneurons is widespread and target-cell independent. *Journal of Neuroscience* 29:11112–11122.

Dayer AG, Ford AA, Cleaver KM, Yassaee M, Cameron HA (2003) Short-term and long-term survival of new neurons in the rat dentate gyrus. *Journal of Comparative Neurology* 460:563–572.

de Almeida L, Idiart M, Lisman JE (2009) A second function of gamma frequency oscillations: an E%-max winner-take-all mechanism selects which cells fire. *Journal of Neuroscience: The Official Journal of the Society for Neuroscience* 29:7497–7503.

Deemyad T, Lüthi J, Spruston N (2018) Astrocytes integrate and drive action potential firing in inhibitory subnetworks. *Nature Communications* 9:4336.

DeFelipe J, López-Cruz PL, Benavides-Piccione R, Bielza C, Larrañaga P, Anderson S, Burkhalter A, Cauli B, Fairén A, Feldmeyer D, et al. (2013) New insights into the classification and nomenclature of cortical GABAergic interneurons. *Nature Reviews Neuroscience* 14:202–216.

Deller T, Katona I, Cozzari C, Frotscher M, Freund TF (1999) Cholinergic innervation of mossy cells in the rat fascia dentata. *Hippocampus* 9:314–320.

Diamantaki M, Frey M, Berens P, Preston-Ferrer P, Burgalossi A (2016) Sparse activity of identified dentate granule cells during spatial exploration. *ELife* 5:e20252.

Diba K, Buzsáki G (2007) Forward and reverse hippocampal place-cell sequences during ripples. *Nature Neuroscience* 10:1241–1242.

Dickson CT, Magistretti J, Shalinsky M, Hamam B, Alonso A (2000) Oscillatory activity in entorhinal neurons and circuits. Mechanisms and function. *Annals of the New York Academy of Sciences* 911:127–150.

Dickson CT, Mena AR, Alonso A (1997) Electroresponsiveness of medial entorhinal cortex layer III neurons in vitro. *Neuroscience* 81:937–950.

Dieni CV, Panichi R, Aimone JB, Kuo CT, Wadiche JI, Overstreet-Wadiche L (2016) Low excitatory innervation balances high intrinsic excitability of immature dentate neurons. *Nature Communications* 7:11313.

Ding L, Chen H, Diamantaki M, Coletta S, Preston-Ferrer P, Burgalossi A (2020) Structural correlates of CA2 and CA3 pyramidal cell activity in freely-moving mice. *Journal of Neuroscience* 40:5797–5806.

Ding S-L (2013) Comparative anatomy of the prosubiculum, subiculum, presubiculum, postsubiculum, and parasubiculum in human, monkey, and rodent. *Journal of Comparative Neurology* 521:4145–4162.

Ding S-L, Yao Z, Hirokawa KE, Nguyen TN, Graybuck LT, Fong O, Bohn P, Ngo K, Smith KA, Koch C, et al. (2020) Distinct transcriptomic cell types and neural circuits of the subiculum and prosubiculum along the dorsal-ventral axis. *Cell Reports* 31:107648.

Doischer D, Hosp JA, Yanagawa Y, Obata K, Jonas P, Vida I, Bartos M (2008) Postnatal differentiation of basket cells from slow to fast signaling devices. *Journal of Neuroscience* 28:12956–12968.

Domínguez S, Rey CC, Therreau L, Fanton A, Massotte D, Verret L, Piskorowski RA, Chevaleyre V (2019) Maturation of PNN and ErbB4 signaling in area CA2 during adolescence underlies the emergence of PV interneuron plasticity and social memory. *Cell Reports* 29:1099–1112, e4.

Domnisoru C, Kinkhabwala AA, Tank DW (2013) Membrane potential dynamics of grid cells. *Nature* 495:199–204.

Dong C, Madar AD, Sheffield MEJ (2021) Distinct place cell dynamics in CA1 and CA3 encode experience in new environments. *Nature Communications* 12:2977.

Dong H-W, Swanson LW, Chen L, Fanselow MS, Toga AW (2009) Genomic-anatomic evidence for distinct functional domains in hippocampal field CA1. *Proceedings of the National Academy of Sciences of the United States of America* 106:11794–11799.

Dougherty KA, Islam T, Johnston D (2012) Intrinsic excitability of CA1 pyramidal neurones from the rat dorsal and ventral hippocampus. *Journal of Physiology* 590:5707–5722.

Draguhn A, Traub RD, Schmitz D, Jefferys JG (1998) Electrical coupling underlies high-frequency oscillations in the hippocampus in vitro. *Nature* 394:189–192.

Du J, Zhang L, Weiser M, Rudy B, McBain CJ (1996) Developmental expression and functional characterization of the potassium-channel subunit Kv3.1b in parvalbumin-containing interneurons of the rat hippocampus. *Journal of Neuroscience: The Official Journal of the Society for Neuroscience* 16:506–518.

Dudek SM, Alexander GM, Farris S (2016) Rediscovering area CA2: unique properties and functions. *Nature Reviews Neuroscience* 17:89–102.

Dudman JT, Tsay D, Siegelbaum SA (2007) A role for synaptic inputs at distal dendrites: instructive signals for hippocampal long-term plasticity. *Neuron* 56:866–879.

Dudok B, Klein PM, Hwaun E, Lee BR, Yao Z, Fong O, Bowler JC, Terada S, Sparks FT, Szabo GG, et al. (2021) Alternating sources of perisomatic inhibition during behavior. *Neuron* 109:997–1012, e9.

Dudok B, Szoboszlay M, Paul A, Klein PM, Liao Z, Hwaun E, Szabo GG, Geiller T, Vancura B, Wang B-S, et al. (2021) Recruitment and inhibitory action of hippocampal axo-axonic cells during behavior. *Neuron* 109:3838–3850, e8.

Dugladze T, Schmitz D, Whittington MA, Vida I, Gloveli T (2012) Segregation of axonal and somatic activity during fast network oscillations. *Science* 336:1458–1461.

Dupret D, O'Neill J, Csicsvari J (2013) Dynamic reconfiguration of hippocampal interneuron circuits during spatial learning. *Neuron* 78:166–180.

Ebbesen CL, Reifenstein ET, Tang Q, Burgalossi A, Ray S, Schreiber S, Kempter R, Brecht M (2016) Cell type-specific differences in spike timing and spike shape in the rat parasubiculum and superficial medial entorhinal cortex. *Cell Reports* 16:1005–1015.

Economo MN, Clack NG, Lavis LD, Gerfen CR, Svoboda K, Myers EW, Chandrashekar J (2016) A platform for brain-wide imaging and reconstruction of individual neurons. *ELife* 5:e10566.

Egorov AV, Gloveli T, Müller W (1999) Muscarinic control of dendritic excitability and Ca(2+) signaling in CA1 pyramidal neurons in rat hippocampal slice. *Journal of Neurophysiology* 82:1909–1915.

Egorov AV, Hamam BN, Fransén E, Hasselmo ME, Alonso AA (2002) Graded persistent activity in entorhinal cortex neurons. *Nature* 420:173–178.

Egorov AV, Heinemann U, Müller W (2002) Differential excitability and voltage-dependent Ca2+ signalling in two types of medial entorhinal cortex layer V neurons. *European Journal of Neuroscience* 16:1305–1312.

Eichenbaum H (1999) The hippocampus and mechanisms of declarative memory. *Behavioural Brain Research* 103:123–133.

Eichenbaum H (2017) On the integration of space, time, and memory. *Neuron* 95:1007–1018.

Eichenbaum H, Cohen NJ (2014) Can we reconcile the declarative memory and spatial navigation views on hippocampal function? *Neuron* 83:764–770.

Elgueta C, Bartos M (2019) Dendritic inhibition differentially regulates excitability of dentate gyrus parvalbumin-expressing interneurons and granule cells. *Nature Communications* 10:5561.

Elgueta C, Köhler J, Bartos M (2015) Persistent discharges in dentate gyrus perisoma-inhibiting interneurons require hyperpolarization-activated cyclic nucleotide-gated channel activation. *Journal of Neuroscience: The Official Journal of the Society for Neuroscience* 35:4131–4139.

Emri Z, Antal K, Gulyás AI, Megías M, Freund TF (2001) Electrotonic profile and passive propagation of synaptic potentials in three subpopulations of hippocampal CA1 interneurons. *Neuroscience* 104:1013–1026.

Engel AK, Fries P, Singer W (2001) Dynamic predictions: oscillations and synchrony in top-down processing. *Nature Reviews Neuroscience* 2:704–716.

Engel D, Jonas P (2005) Presynaptic action potential amplification by voltage-gated Na+ channels in hippocampal mossy fiber boutons. *Neuron* 45:405–417.

English DF, McKenzie S, Evans T, Kim K, Yoon E, Buzsáki G (2017) Pyramidal cell-interneuron circuit architecture and dynamics in hippocampal networks. *Neuron* 96:505–520, e7.

English DF, Peyrache A, Stark E, Roux L, Vallentin D, Long MA, Buzsáki G (2014) Excitation and inhibition compete to control spiking during hippocampal ripples: intracellular study in behaving mice. *Journal of Neuroscience* 34:16509–16517.

Epsztein J, Brecht M, Lee AK (2011) Intracellular determinants of hippocampal CA1 place and silent cell activity in a novel environment. *Neuron* 70:109–120.

Epsztein J, Lee AK, Chorev E, Brecht M (2010) Impact of spikelets on hippocampal CA1 pyramidal cell activity during spatial exploration. *Science* 327:474–477.

Erwin SR, Sun W, Copeland M, Lindo S, Spruston N, Cembrowski MS (2020) A sparse, spatially biased subtype of mature granule cell dominates recruitment in hippocampal-associated behaviors. *Cell Reports* 31:107551.

Espinoza C, Guzman SJ, Zhang X, Jonas P (2018) Parvalbumin + interneurons obey unique connectivity rules and establish a powerful lateral-inhibition microcircuit in dentate gyrus. *Nature Communications* 9:4605.

Espósito MS, Piatti VC, Laplagne DA, Morgenstern NA, Ferrari CC, Pitossi FJ, Schinder AF (2005) Neuronal differentiation in the adult hippocampus recapitulates embryonic development. *Journal of Neuroscience* 25:10074.

Evans PR, Parra-Bueno P, Smirnov MS, Lustberg DJ, Dudek SM, Hepler JR, Yasuda R (2018) RGS14 restricts plasticity in hippocampal CA2 by limiting postsynaptic calcium signaling. *ENeuro* 5:ENEURO.0353-17.2018.

Eyre MD, Bartos M (2019) Somatostatin-expressing interneurons form axonal projections to the contralateral hippocampus. *Frontiers in Neural Circuits* 13:56.

Fan S, Stewart M, Wong RK (1994) Differences in voltage-dependent sodium currents exhibited by superficial and deep layer neurons of guinea pig entorhinal cortex. *Journal of Neurophysiology* 71:1986–1991.

Faulkner RL, Jang M-H, Liu X-B, Duan X, Sailor KA, Kim JY, Ge S, Jones EG, Ming G, Song H, et al. (2008) Development of hippocampal mossy fiber synaptic outputs by new neurons in the adult brain. *Proceedings of the National Academy of Sciences* 105:14157–14162.

Fenton AA, Kao H-Y, Neymotin SA, Olypher A, Vayntrub Y, Lytton WW, Ludvig N (2008) Unmasking the CA1 ensemble place code by exposures to small and large environments: more place cells and multiple, irregularly arranged, and expanded place fields in the larger space. *Journal of Neuroscience* 28:11250–11262.

Ferraguti F, Cobden P, Pollard M, Cope D, Shigemoto R, Watanabe M, Somogyi P (2004) Immunolocalization of metabotropic glutamate receptor 1alpha (mGluR1alpha) in distinct classes of interneuron in the CA1 region of the rat hippocampus. *Hippocampus* 14:193–215.

Ferraguti F, Klausberger T, Cobden P, Baude A, Roberts JDB, Szucs P, Kinoshita A, Shigemoto R, Somogyi P, Dalezios Y (2005)

Metabotropic glutamate receptor 8-expressing nerve terminals target subsets of GABAergic neurons in the hippocampus. *Journal of Neuroscience: The Official Journal of the Society for Neuroscience* 25:10520–10536.

Fiala JC, Spacek J, Harris KM (2008) Chapter 1: Dendrite structure. In: Dendrites (Stuart G, Spruston N, Häusser M, eds), pp 1–34. Oxford: Oxford University Press.

Fidzinski P, Shor O, Behr J (2008) Target-cell-specific bidirectional synaptic plasticity at hippocampal output synapses. *European Journal of Neuroscience* 27:1111–1118.

Francavilla R, Villette V, Luo X, Chamberland S, Muñoz-Pino E, Camiré O, Wagner K, Kis V, Somogyi P, Topolnik L (2018) Connectivity and network state-dependent recruitment of long-range VIP-GABAergic neurons in the mouse hippocampus. *Nature Communications* 9:5043.

Frank LM, Stanley GB, Brown EN (2004) Hippocampal plasticity across multiple days of exposure to novel environments. *Journal of Neuroscience: The Official Journal of the Society for Neuroscience* 24:7681–7689.

Fredens K, Stengaard-Pedersen K, Larsson L-I (1984) Localization of enkephalin and cholecystokinin immunoreactivities in the perforant path terminal fields of the rat hippocampal formation. *Brain Research* 304:255–263.

French CR, Sah P, Buckett KJ, Gage PW (1990) A voltage-dependent persistent sodium current in mammalian hippocampal neurons. *Journal of General Physiology* 95:1139–1157.

Freund TF, Buzsáki G (1996) Interneurons of the hippocampus. *Hippocampus* 6:347–470.

Frick A, Magee J, Koester HJ, Migliore M, Johnston D (2003) Normalization of Ca2+ signals by small oblique dendrites of CA1 pyramidal neurons. *Journal of Neuroscience* 23:3243.

Fricker D, Miles R (2000) EPSP amplification and the precision of spike timing in hippocampal neurons. *Neuron* 28:559–569.

Fuchs EC, Neitz A, Pinna R, Melzer S, Caputi A, Monyer H (2016) Local and distant input controlling excitation in layer II of the medial entorhinal cortex. *Neuron* 89:194–208.

Fuchs EC, Zivkovic AR, Cunningham MO, Middleton S, Lebeau FEN, Bannerman DM, Rozov A, Whittington MA, Traub RD, Rawlins JNP, et al. (2007) Recruitment of parvalbumin-positive interneurons determines hippocampal function and associated behavior. *Neuron* 53:591–604.

Fuentealba P, Begum R, Capogna M, Jinno S, Márton LF, Csicsvari J, Thomson A, Somogyi P, Klausberger T (2008) Ivy cells: a population of nitric-oxide-producing, slow-spiking GABAergic neurons and their involvement in hippocampal network activity. *Neuron* 57:917–929.

Fuentealba P, Klausberger T, Karayannis T, Suen WY, Huck J, Tomioka R, Rockland K, Capogna M, Studer M, Morales M, et al. (2010) Expression of COUP-TFII nuclear receptor in restricted GABAergic neuronal populations in the adult rat hippocampus. *Journal of Neuroscience: The Official Journal of the Society for Neuroscience* 30:1595–1609.

Funahashi M, Harris E, Stewart M (1999) Re-entrant activity in a presubiculum-subiculum circuit generates epileptiform activity in vitro. *Brain Research* 849:139–146.

Funahashi M, Stewart M (1997) Presubicular and parasubicular cortical neurons of the rat: functional separation of deep and superficial neurons in vitro. *Journal of Physiology* 501(Pt 2):387–403.

Fuzik J, Zeisel A, Máté Z, Calvigioni D, Yanagawa Y, Szabó G, Linnarsson S, Harkany T (2016) Integration of electrophysiological recordings with single-cell RNA-seq data identifies neuronal subtypes. *Nature Biotechnology* 34:175–183.

Fyhn M, Molden S, Witter MP, Moser EI, Moser M-B (2004) Spatial representation in the entorhinal cortex. *Science* 305:1258–1264.

Gan J, Weng S, Pernía-Andrade AJ, Csicsvari J, Jonas P (2017) Phase-locked inhibition, but not excitation, underlies hippocampal ripple oscillations in awake mice in vivo. *Neuron* 93:308–314.

Gasbarri A, Packard MG, Campana E, Pacitti C (1994) Anterograde and retrograde tracing of projections from the ventral tegmental area to the hippocampal formation in the rat. *Brain Research Bulletin* 33:445–452.

Gasparini S, Losonczy A, Chen X, Johnston D, Magee JC (2007) Associative pairing enhances action potential back-propagation in radial oblique branches of CA1 pyramidal neurons. *Journal of Physiology* 580:787–800.

Gasparini S, Magee JC (2006) State-dependent dendritic computation in hippocampal CA1 pyramidal neurons. *Journal of Neuroscience: The Official Journal of the Society for Neuroscience* 26:2088–2100.

Gasparini S, Migliore M, Magee JC (2004) On the initiation and propagation of dendritic spikes in CA1 pyramidal neurons. *Journal of Neuroscience: The Official Journal of the Society for Neuroscience* 24:11046–11056.

Ge S, Goh ELK, Sailor KA, Kitabatake Y, Ming G, Song H (2006) GABA regulates synaptic integration of newly generated neurons in the adult brain. *Nature* 439:589–593.

Ge S, Yang C, Hsu K, Ming G, Song H (2007) A critical period for enhanced synaptic plasticity in newly generated neurons of the adult brain. *Neuron* 54:559–566.

Geiger JRP, Jonas P (2000) Dynamic control of presynaptic Ca2+ inflow by fast-inactivating K+ channels in hippocampal mossy fiber boutons. *Neuron* 28:927–939.

Geiger JR, Lübke J, Roth A, Frotscher M, Jonas P (1997) Submillisecond AMPA receptor-mediated signaling at a principal neuron-interneuron synapse. *Neuron* 18:1009–1023.

Geiger JR, Melcher T, Koh DS, Sakmann B, Seeburg PH, Jonas P, Monyer H (1995) Relative abundance of subunit mRNAs determines gating and Ca2+ permeability of AMPA receptors in principal neurons and interneurons in rat CNS. *Neuron* 15:193–204.

Geiller T, Fattahi M, Choi J-S, Royer S (2017) Place cells are more strongly tied to landmarks in deep than in superficial CA1. *Nature Communications* 8:14531.

Geiller T, Vancura B, Terada S, Troullinou E, Chavlis S, Tsagkatakis G, Tsakalides P, Ócsai K, Poirazi P, Rózsa BJ, et al. (2020) Large-scale 3D two-photon imaging of molecularly identified CA1 interneuron dynamics in behaving mice. *Neuron* 108:968–983, e9.

George MS, Abbott LF, Siegelbaum SA (2009) HCN hyperpolarization-activated cation channels inhibit EPSPs by interactions with M-type K(+) channels. *Nature Neuroscience* 12:577–584.

Gerlei KZ, Brown CM, Sürmeli G, Nolan MF (2021) Deep entorhinal cortex: from circuit organization to spatial cognition and memory. *Trends in Neurosciences* 44:876–887.

Germroth P, Schwerdtfeger WK, Buhl EH (1991) Ultrastructure and aspects of functional organization of pyramidal and nonpyramidal entorhinal projection neurons contributing to the perforant path. *Journal of Comparative Neurology* 305:215–231.

Gidon A, Segev I (2012) Principles governing the operation of synaptic inhibition in dendrites. *Neuron* 75:330–341.

Giocomo LM, Hasselmo ME (2008) Time constants of h current in layer II stellate cells differ along the dorsal to ventral axis of medial entorhinal cortex. *Journal of Neuroscience* 28:9414.

Giocomo LM, Hasselmo ME (2009) Knock-out of HCN1 subunit flattens dorsal–ventral frequency gradient of medial entorhinal neurons in adult mice. *Journal of Neuroscience* 29:7625.

Giocomo LM, Hussaini SA, Zheng F, Kandel ER, Moser M-B, Moser EI (2011) Grid cells use HCN1 channels for spatial scaling. *Cell* 147:1159–1170.

Glasgow SD, Chapman CA (2008) Conductances mediating intrinsic theta-frequency membrane potential oscillations in layer II parasubicular neurons. *Journal of Neurophysiology* 100:2746–2756.

Glickfeld LL, Roberts JD, Somogyi P, Scanziani M (2009) Interneurons hyperpolarize pyramidal cells along their entire somatodendritic axis. *Nature Neuroscience* 12:21–23.

Glickfeld LL, Scanziani M (2006) Distinct timing in the activity of cannabinoid-sensitive and cannabinoid-insensitive basket cells. *Nature Neuroscience* 9:807–815.

Gloveli T, Egorov AV, Schmitz D, Heinemann U, Müller W (1999) Carbachol-induced changes in excitability and [Ca2+]i signalling in projection cells of medial entorhinal cortex layers II and III. *European Journal of Neuroscience* 11:3626–3636.

Gloveli T, Schmitz D, Empson RM, Dugladze T, Heinemann U (1997) Morphological and electrophysiological characterization of layer III cells of the medial entorhinal cortex of the rat. *Neuroscience* 77:629–648.

Gloveli T, Schmitz D, Empson RM, Heinemann U (1997a) Frequency-dependent information flow from the entorhinal cortex to the hippocampus. *Journal of Neurophysiology* 78:3444–3449.

Goldberg EM, Clark BD, Zagha E, Nahmani M, Erisir A, Rudy B (2008) K+ channels at the axon initial segment dampen near-threshold excitability of neocortical fast-spiking GABAergic interneurons. *Neuron* 58:387–400.

Goldin M, Epsztein J, Jorquera I, Represa A, Ben-Ari Y, Crépel V, Cossart R (2007) Synaptic kainate receptors tune oriens–lacunosum moleculare interneurons to operate at theta frequency. *Journal of Neuroscience* 27:9560–9572.

Golding NL, Jung HY, Mickus T, Spruston N (1999) Dendritic calcium spike initiation and repolarization are controlled by distinct potassium channel subtypes in CA1 pyramidal neurons. *Journal of Neuroscience: The Official Journal of the Society for Neuroscience* 19:8789–8798.

Golding NL, Kath WL, Spruston N (2001) Dichotomy of action-potential backpropagation in CA1 pyramidal neuron dendrites. *Journal of Neurophysiology* 86:2998–3010.

Golding NL, Mickus TJ, Katz Y, Kath WL, Spruston N (2005) Factors mediating powerful voltage attenuation along CA1 pyramidal neuron dendrites. *Journal of Physiology* 568:69–82.

Golding NL, Spruston N (1998) Dendritic sodium spikes are variable triggers of axonal action potentials in hippocampal CA1 pyramidal neurons. *Neuron* 21:1189–1200.

Golding NL, Staff NP, Spruston N (2002) Dendritic spikes as a mechanism for cooperative long-term potentiation. *Nature* 418:326–331.

Gómez-Lira G, Lamas M, Romo-Parra H, Gutiérrez R (2005) Programmed and induced phenotype of the hippocampal granule cells. *Journal of Neuroscience* 25:6939.

Gómez-Lira G, Trillo E, Ramirez M, Asai M, Sitges M, Gutiérrez R (2002) The expression of GABA in mossy fiber synaptosomes coincides with the seizure-induced expression of GABAergic transmission in the mossy fiber synapse. *Experimental Neurology* 177:276–283.

Gonçalves JT, Bloyd CW, Shtrahman M, Johnston ST, Schafer ST, Parylak SL, Tran T, Chang T, Gage FH (2016) In vivo imaging of dendritic pruning in dentate granule cells. *Nature Neuroscience* 19:788–791.

Gong H, Xu D, Yuan J, Li X, Guo C, Peng J, Li Y, Schwarz LA, Li A, Hu B, et al. (2016) High-throughput dual-colour precision imaging for brain-wide connectome with cytoarchitectonic landmarks at the cellular level. *Nature Communications* 7:12142.

Gonzales RB, DeLeon Galvan CJ, Rangel YM, Claiborne BJ (2001) Distribution of thorny excrescences on CA3 pyramidal neurons in the rat hippocampus. *Journal of Comparative Neurology* 430:357–368.

Gonzalez JC, Epps SA, Markwardt SJ, Wadiche JI, Overstreet-Wadiche L (2018) Constitutive and synaptic activation of GIRK channels differentiates mature and newborn dentate granule cells. *Journal of Neuroscience* 38:6513.

GoodSmith D, Chen X, Wang C, Kim SH, Song H, Burgalossi A, Christian KM, Knierim JJ (2017) Spatial representations of granule cells and mossy cells of the dentate gyrus. *Neuron* 93:677–690, e5.

Gouwens NW, Sorensen SA, Baftizadeh F, Budzillo A, Lee BR, Jarsky T, Alfiler L, Baker K, Barkan E, Berry K, et al. (2020) Integrated morphoelectric and transcriptomic classification of cortical GABAergic cells. *Cell* 183:935–953, e19.

Graves AR, Moore SJ, Bloss EB, Mensh BD, Kath WL, Spruston N (2012) Hippocampal pyramidal neurons comprise two distinct cell types that are countermodulated by metabotropic receptors. *Neuron* 76:776–789.

Gray CM, Singer W (1989) Stimulus-specific neuronal oscillations in orientation columns of cat visual cortex. *Proceedings of the National Academy of Sciences of the United States of America* 86:1698–1702.

Grienberger C, Milstein AD, Bittner KC, Romani S, Magee JC (2017) Inhibitory suppression of heterogeneously tuned excitation enhances spatial coding in CA1 place cells. *Nature Neuroscience* 20:417–426.

Groffen AJA, Jacobsen L, Schut D, Verhage M (2005) Two distinct genes drive expression of seven tomosyn isoforms in the mammalian brain, sharing a conserved structure with a unique variable domain. *Journal of Neurochemistry* 92:554–568.

Gu N, Vervaeke K, Hu H, Storm JF (2005) Kv7/KCNQ/M and HCN/h, but not KCa2/SK channels, contribute to the somatic medium after-hyperpolarization and excitability control in CA1 hippocampal pyramidal cells. *Journal of Physiology* 566:689–715.

Gu Y, Arruda-Carvalho M, Wang J, Janoschka SR, Josselyn SA, Frankland PW, Ge S (2012) Optical controlling reveals time-dependent roles for adult-born dentate granule cells. *Nature Neuroscience* 15:1700–1706.

Gu Y, Lewallen S, Kinkhabwala AA, Domnisoru C, Yoon K, Gauthier JL, Fiete IR, Tank DW (2018) A map-like micro-organization of grid cells in the medial entorhinal cortex. *Cell* 175:736–750, e30.

Gulyás AI, Hájos N, Freund TF (1996) Interneurons containing calretinin are specialized to control other interneurons in the rat hippocampus. *Journal of Neuroscience: The Official Journal of the Society for Neuroscience* 16:3397–3411.

Gulyás AI, Hájos N, Katona I, Freund TF (2003) Interneurons are the local targets of hippocampal inhibitory cells which project to the medial septum. *European Journal of Neuroscience* 17:1861–1872.

Gulyás AI, Megías M, Emri Z, Freund TF (1999) Total number and ratio of excitatory and inhibitory synapses converging onto single interneurons of different types in the CA1 area of the rat hippocampus. *Journal of Neuroscience: The Official Journal of the Society for Neuroscience* 19:10082–10097.

Gulyás AI, Miles R, Sik A, Tóth K, Tamamaki N, Freund TF (1993) Hippocampal pyramidal cells excite inhibitory neurons through a single release site. *Nature* 366:683–687.

Gulyás AI, Szabó GG, Ulbert I, Holderith N, Monyer H, Erdélyi F, Szabó G, Freund TF, Hájos N (2010) Parvalbumin-containing fast-spiking basket cells generate the field potential oscillations induced by cholinergic receptor activation in the hippocampus. *Journal of Neuroscience* 30:15134–15145.

Gundlfinger A, Breustedt J, Sullivan D, Schmitz D (2010) Natural spike trains trigger short- and long-lasting dynamics at hippocampal mossy fiber synapses in rodents. *PLoS One* 5:1–9.

Gupta A, Elgammal FS, Proddutur A, Shah S, Santhakumar V (2012) Decrease in tonic inhibition contributes to increase in dentate semilunar granule cell excitability after brain injury. *Journal of Neuroscience* 32:2523–2537.

Gupta A, Proddutur A, Chang Y-J, Raturi V, Guevarra J, Shah Y, Elgammal FS, Santhakumar V (2020) Dendritic morphology and inhibitory regulation distinguish dentate semilunar granule cells from granule cells through distinct stages of postnatal development. *Brain Structure and Function* 225:2841–2855.

Guzman SJ, Schlögl A, Frotscher M, Jonas P (2016) Synaptic mechanisms of pattern completion in the hippocampal CA3 network. *Science* 353:1117–1123.

Haas HL, Greene RW (1984) Adenosine enhances afterhyperpolarization and accommodation in hippocampal pyramidal cells. *Pflugers Archiv: European Journal of Physiology* 402:244–247.

Haas HL, Greene RW (1986) Effects of histamine on hippocampal pyramidal cells of the rat in vitro. *Experimental Brain Research* 62:123–130.

Haglund L, Swanson LW, Köhler C (1984) The projection of the supramammillary nucleus to the hippocampal formation: an immunohistochemical and anterograde transport study with the lectin PHA-L in the rat. *Journal of Comparative Neurology* 229:171–185.

Hainmueller T, Bartos M (2018) Parallel emergence of stable and dynamic memory engrams in the hippocampus. *Nature* 558:292–296.

Hainmueller T, Krieglstein K, Kulik A, Bartos M (2014) Joint CP-AMPA and group I mGlu receptor activation is required for synaptic plasticity in dentate gyrus fast-spiking interneurons. *Proceedings of the National Academy of Sciences of the United States of America* 111:13211–13216.

Hajos N, Acsady L, Freund TF (1996) Target selectivity and neurochemical characteristics of VIP-immunoreactive interneurons in the rat dentate gyrus. *European Journal of Neuroscience* 8:1415–1431.

Hájos N, Pálhalmi J, Mann EO, Németh B, Paulsen O, Freund TF (2004) Spike timing of distinct types of GABAergic interneuron during hippocampal gamma oscillations in vitro. *Journal of Neuroscience* 24:9127–9137.

Hájos N, Papp EC, Acsády L, Levey AI, Freund TF (1998) Distinct interneuron types express m2 muscarinic receptor immunoreactivity on their dendrites or axon terminals in the hippocampus. *Neuroscience* 82:355–376.

Hájos N, Paulsen O (2009) Network mechanisms of gamma oscillations in the CA3 region of the hippocampus. *Neural Networks* 22:1113–1119.

Halasy K, Buhl EH, Lörinczi Z, Tamás G, Somogyi P (1996). Synaptic target selectivity and input of GABAergic basket and bistratified interneurons in the CA1 area of the rat hippocampus. *Hippocampus* 6:306–329.

Halasy K, Hajszan T, Kovács EG, Lam T-T, Leranth C (2004) Distribution and origin of vesicular glutamate transporter 2-immunoreactive fibers in the rat hippocampus. *Hippocampus* 14:908–918.

Halasy K, Somogyi P (1993) Subdivisions in the multiple GABAergic innervation of granule cells in the dentate gyrus of the rat hippocampus. *European Journal of Neuroscience* 5:411–429.

Hallermann S, Pawlu C, Jonas P, Heckmann M (2003) A large pool of releasable vesicles in a cortical glutamatergic synapse. *Proceedings of the National Academy of Sciences* 100:8975–8980.

Hamam BN, Amaral DG, Alonso AA (2002) Morphological and electrophysiological characteristics of layer V neurons of the rat lateral entorhinal cortex. *Journal of Comparative Neurology* 451:45–61.

Hamam BN, Kennedy TE, Alonso A, Amaral DG (2000) Morphological and electrophysiological characteristics of layer V neurons of the rat medial entorhinal cortex. *Journal of Comparative Neurology* 418:457–472.

Han Z, Buhl EH, Lörinczi Z, Somogyi P (1993) A high degree of spatial selectivity in the axonal and dendritic domains of physiologically identified local-circuit neurons in the dentate gyms of the rat hippocampus. *European Journal of Neuroscience* 5:395–410.

Hardie J, Spruston N (2009) Synaptic depolarization is more effective than back-propagating action potentials during induction of associative long-term potentiation in hippocampal pyramidal neurons. *Journal of Neuroscience: The Official Journal of the Society for Neuroscience* 29:3233–3241.

Harnett MT, Makara JK, Spruston N, Kath WL, Magee JC (2012) Synaptic amplification by dendritic spines enhances input cooperativity. *Nature* 491:599–602.

Harris E, Witter MP, Weinstein G, Stewart M (2001) Intrinsic connectivity of the rat subiculum: I. Dendritic morphology and patterns of axonal arborization by pyramidal neurons. *Journal of Comparative Neurology* 435:490–505.

Harris K, Stevens J (1989) Dendritic spines of CA 1 pyramidal cells in the rat hippocampus: serial electron microscopy with reference to their biophysical characteristics. *Journal of Neuroscience* 9:2982–2997.

Harris KD, Hochgerner H, Skene NG, Magno L, Katona L, Bengtsson Gonzales C, Somogyi P, Kessaris N, Linnarsson S, Hjerling-Leffler J (2018) Classes and continua of hippocampal CA1 inhibitory neurons revealed by single-cell transcriptomics. *PLoS Biology* 16:e2006387.

Harris KM (1999) Structure, development, and plasticity of dendritic spines. *Current Opinion in Neurobiology* 9:343–348.

Harris KM, Hubbard DD, Kuwajima M, Abraham WC, Bourne JN, Bowden JB, Haessly A, Mendenhall JM, Parker PH, Shi B, et al. (2022) Dendritic spine density scales with microtubule number in rat hippocampal dendrites. *Neuroscience* 489:84–97.

Harris KM, Jensen FE, Tsao B (1992) Three-dimensional structure of dendritic spines and synapses in rat hippocampus (CA1) at postnatal day 15 and adult ages: implications for the maturation of synaptic physiology and long-term potentiation. *Journal of Neuroscience: The Official Journal of the Society for Neuroscience* 12:2685–2705.

Harris KM, Spacek J, Bell ME, Parker PH, Lindsey LF, Baden AD, Vogelstein JT, Burns R (2015) A resource from 3D electron microscopy of hippocampal neuropil for user training and tool development. *Scientific Data* 2:150046.

Harris Km, Sultan P (1995) Variation in the number, location and size of synaptic vesicles provides an anatomical basis for the non-uniform probability of release at hippocampal CA1 synapses. *Neuropharmacology* 34:1387–1395.

Harvey CD, Collman F, Dombeck DA, Tank DW (2009) Intracellular dynamics of hippocampal place cells during virtual navigation. *Nature* 461:941–946.

Hashimotodani Y, Karube F, Yanagawa Y, Fujiyama F, Kano M (2018) Supramammillary nucleus afferents to the dentate gyrus co-release glutamate and GABA and potentiate granule cell output. *Cell Reports* 25:2704–2715, e4.

Hasselmo ME (2006) The role of acetylcholine in learning and memory. *Current Opinion in Neurobiology* 16:710–715.

Hasselmo ME, Brandon MP (2008) Linking cellular mechanisms to behavior: entorhinal persistent spiking and membrane potential oscillations may underlie path integration, grid cell firing, and episodic memory. *Neural Plasticity* 2008:658323.

Hasselmo ME, McGaughy J (2004) High acetylcholine levels set circuit dynamics for attention and encoding and low acetylcholine levels set dynamics for consolidation. *Progress in Brain Research* 145:207–231.

Hasselmo ME, Schnell E (1994) Laminar selectivity of the cholinergic suppression of synaptic transmission in rat hippocampal region CA1: computational modeling and brain slice physiology. *Journal of Neuroscience: The Official Journal of the Society for Neuroscience* 14:3898–3914.

Hasselmo M, Schnell E, Barkai E (1995) Dynamics of learning and recall at excitatory recurrent synapses and cholinergic modulation in rat hippocampal region CA3. *Journal of Neuroscience* 15:5249.

Häusser M, Mel B (2003) Dendrites: bug or feature? *Current Opinion in Neurobiology* 13:372–383.

Hebb D (1949) The Organization of Behavior. New York: Wiley.

Hefft S, Jonas P (2005) Asynchronous GABA release generates long-lasting inhibition at a hippocampal interneuron-principal neuron synapse. *Nature Neuroscience* 8:1319–1328.

Helton TD, Zhao M, Farris S, Dudek SM (2018) Diversity of dendritic morphology and entorhinal cortex synaptic effectiveness in mouse CA2 pyramidal neurons. *Hippocampus* 7:10300–10315.

Henriksen EJ, Colgin LL, Barnes CA, Witter MP, Moser M-B, Moser EI (2010) Spatial representation along the proximodistal axis of CA1. *Neuron* 68:127–137.

Henze DA, Wittner L, Buzsáki G (2002) Single granule cells reliably discharge targets in the hippocampal CA3 network in vivo. *Nature Neuroscience* 5:790–795.

Herkenham M (1978) The connections of the nucleus reuniens thalami: evidence for a direct thalamo-hippocampal pathway in the rat. *Journal of Comparative Neurology* 177:589–609.

Hill AJ (1978) First occurrence of hippocampal spatial firing in a new environment. *Experimental Neurology* 62:282–297.

Hitti FL, Siegelbaum SA (2014) The hippocampal CA2 region is essential for social memory. *Nature* 508:88–92.

Hjorth-Simonsen A, Jeune B (1972) Origin and termination of the hippocampal perforant path in the rat studied by silver impregnation. *Journal of Comparative Neurology* 144:215–231.

Hoffman DA, Johnston D (1999) Neuromodulation of dendritic action potentials. *Journal of Neurophysiology* 81:408–411.

Hoffman DA, Magee JC, Colbert CM, Johnston D (1997) K+ channel regulation of signal propagation in dendrites of hippocampal pyramidal neurons. *Nature* 387:869–875.

Honda Y, Furuta T, Kaneko T, Shibata H, Sasaki H (2011) Patterns of axonal collateralization of single layer V cortical projection neurons in the rat presubiculum. *Journal of Comparative Neurology* 519:1395–1412.

Horn ME, Nicoll RA (2018) Somatostatin and parvalbumin inhibitory synapses onto hippocampal pyramidal neurons are regulated by distinct mechanisms. *Proceedings of the National Academy of Sciences of the United States of America* 115:589–594.

Hosp JA, Strüber M, Yanagawa Y, Obata K, Vida I, Jonas P, Bartos M (2014) Morpho-physiological criteria divide dentate gyrus interneurons into classes. *Hippocampus* 24:189–203.

Hsu C-L, Zhao X, Milstein AD, Spruston N (2018) Persistent sodium current mediates the steep voltage dependence of spatial coding in hippocampal pyramidal neurons. *Neuron* 99:147–162, e8.

Hsu T-T, Lee C-T, Tai M-H, Lien C-C (2015) Differential recruitment of dentate gyrus interneuron types by commissural versus perforant pathways. *Cerebral Cortex* 26:2715–2727.

Hu H, Gan J, Jonas P (2014) Interneurons: fast-spiking, parvalbumin+ GABAergic interneurons: from cellular design to microcircuit function. *Science* 345:1255263.

Hu H, Jonas P (2014) A supercritical density of Na(+) channels ensures fast signaling in GABAergic interneuron axons. *Nature Neuroscience* 17:686–693.

Hu H, Martina M, Jonas P (2010) Dendritic mechanisms underlying rapid synaptic activation of fast-spiking hippocampal interneurons. *Science* 327:52–58.

Hu H, Roth FC, Vandael D, Jonas P (2018) Complementary tuning of Na+ and K+ channel gating underlies fast and energy-efficient action potentials in GABAergic interneuron axons. *Neuron* 98:156–165, e6.

Hu H, Vervaeke K, Storm JF (2002) Two forms of electrical resonance at theta frequencies, generated by M-current, h-current and persistent Na+ current in rat hippocampal pyramidal cells. *Journal of Physiology* 545:783–805.

Hu H, Vervaeke K, Storm JF (2007) M-channels (Kv7/KCNQ channels) that regulate synaptic integration, excitability, and spike pattern of CA1 pyramidal cells are located in the perisomatic region. *Journal of Neuroscience: The Official Journal of the Society for Neuroscience* 27:1853–1867.

Huang CY-M, Rasband MN (2018) Axon initial segments: structure, function, and disease. *Annals of the New York Academy of Sciences* 1420:46–61.

Huang L-W, Simonnet J, Nassar M, Richevaux L, Lofredi R, Fricker D (2017) Laminar localization and projection-specific properties of presubicular neurons targeting the lateral mammillary nucleus, thalamus, or medial entorhinal cortex. *Eneuro* 4:ENEURO.0370-16.2017.

Hulse BK, Jayaraman V (2020) Mechanisms underlying the neural computation of head direction. *Annual Review of Neuroscience* 43:31–54.

Hulse BK, Lubenov EV, Siapas AG (2017) Brain state dependence of hippocampal subthreshold activity in awake mice. *Cell Reports* 18:136–147.

Hulse BK, Moreaux LC, Lubenov EV, Siapas AG (2016) Membrane potential dynamics of CA1 pyramidal neurons during hippocampal ripples in awake mice. *Neuron* 89:800–813.

Hunt DL, Linaro D, Si B, Romani S, Spruston N (2018) A novel pyramidal cell type promotes sharp-wave synchronization in the hippocampus. *Nature Neuroscience* 21:985–995.

Isaac JTR, Ashby MC, McBain CJ (2007) The role of the GluR2 subunit in AMPA receptor function and synaptic plasticity. *Neuron* 54:859–871.

Isaacson JS, Scanziani M (2011) How inhibition shapes cortical activity. *Neuron* 72:231–243.

Ishihara Y, Fukuda T (2016) Immunohistochemical investigation of the internal structure of the mouse subiculum. *Neuroscience* 337:242–266.

Ishizuka N, Cowan WM, Amaral DG (1995) A quantitative analysis of the dendritic organization of pyramidal cells in the rat hippocampus. *Journal of Comparative Neurology* 362:17–45.

Ishizuka N, Weber J, Amaral D (1990) Organization of intrahippocampal projections originating from CA3 pyramidal cells in the rat. *Journal of Comparative Neurology* 295:580–623.

Jadi M, Polsky A, Schiller J, Mel BW (2012) Location-dependent effects of inhibition on local spiking in pyramidal neuron dendrites. *PLoS Computational Biology* 8:e1002550.

Jadi MP, Behabadi BF, Poleg-Polsky A, Schiller J, Mel BW (2014) An augmented two-layer model captures nonlinear analog spatial integration effects in pyramidal neuron dendrites. *Proceedings of the IEEE* 102:782–798.

Jagasia R, Steib K, Englberger E, Herold S, Faus-Kessler T, Saxe M, Gage FH, Song H, Lie DC (2009) GABA-cAMP response element-binding protein signaling regulates maturation and survival of newly generated neurons in the adult hippocampus. *Journal of Neuroscience* 29:7966.

Jarosiewicz B, McNaughton BL, Skaggs WE (2002) Hippocampal population activity during the small-amplitude irregular activity state in the rat. *Journal of Neuroscience* 22:1373–1384.

Jarsky T, Mady R, Kennedy B, Spruston N (2008) Distribution of bursting neurons in the CA1 region and the subiculum of the rat hippocampus. *Journal of Comparative Neurology* 506:535–547.

Jarsky T, Roxin A, Kath W, Spruston N (2005) Conditional dendritic spike propagation following distal synaptic activation of hippocampal CA1 pyramidal neurons. *Nature Neuroscience* 8:1667–1676.

Jiang M, Swann JW (2005) A role for L-type calcium channels in the maturation of parvalbumin-containing hippocampal interneurons. *Neuroscience* 135:839–850.

Jinde S, Zsiros V, Jiang Z, Nakao K, Pickel J, Kohno K, Belforte JE, Nakazawa K (2012) Hilar mossy cell degeneration causes transient dentate granule cell hyperexcitability and impaired pattern separation. *Neuron* 76:1189–1200.

Jinno S, Ishizuka S, Kosaka T (2003) Ionic currents underlying rhythmic bursting of ventral mossy cells in the developing mouse dentate gyrus. *European Journal of Neuroscience* 17:1338–1354.

Jinno S, Klausberger T, Márton LF, Dalezios Y, Roberts JDB, Fuentealba P, Bushong EA, Henze D, Buzsáki G, Somogyi P (2007) Neuronal diversity in GABAergic long-range projections from the hippocampus. *Journal of Neuroscience* 27:8790–8804.

Jinno S, Kosaka T (2002) Patterns of expression of calcium binding proteins and neuronal nitric oxide synthase in different populations of hippocampal GABAergic neurons in mice. *Journal of Comparative Neurology* 449:1–25.

Johnston D, Christie BR, Frick A, Gray R, Hoffman DA, Schexnayder LK, Watanabe S, Yuan, L-L (2003) Active dendrites, potassium channels and synaptic plasticity. *Philosophical Transactions of the Royal Society of London Series B, Biological Sciences* 358:667–674.

Johnston D, Hoffman DA, Magee JC, Poolos NP, Watanabe S, Colbert CM, Migliore M (2000) Dendritic potassium channels in hippocampal pyramidal neurons. *Journal of Physiology* 525(Pt 1):75–81.

Jonas P, Bischofberger J, Fricker D, Miles R (2004) Interneuron diversity series: fast in, fast out—temporal and spatial signal processing in hippocampal interneurons. *Trends in Neurosciences* 27:30–40.

Jonas P, Major G, Sakmann B (1993) Quantal components of unitary EPSCs at the mossy fibre synapse on CA3 pyramidal cells of rat hippocampus. *Journal of Physiology* 472:615–663.

Jung HY, Mickus T, Spruston N (1997) Prolonged sodium channel inactivation contributes to dendritic action potential attenuation in hippocampal pyramidal neurons. *Journal of Neuroscience: The Official Journal of the Society for Neuroscience* 17:6639–6646.

Jung M, Wiener S, McNaughton B (1994) Comparison of spatial firing characteristics of units in dorsal and ventral hippocampus of the rat. *Journal of Neuroscience* 14:7347–7356.

Kaczorowski CC, Disterhoft J, Spruston N (2007) Stability and plasticity of intrinsic membrane properties in hippocampal CA1 pyramidal neurons: effects of internal anions: stability and plasticity of membrane properties in CA1 pyramidal neurons. *Journal of Physiology* 578:799–818.

Kajikawa K, Hulse BK, Siapas AG, Lubenov EV (2021) Inhibition is the hallmark of CA3 intracellular dynamics around awake ripples. *BioRxiv preprint server for Biology* doi: https://doi.org/10.1101/2021.04.20.440699.

Kajikawa K, Hulse BK, Siapas AG, Lubenov EV (2022) Up–down states and ripples differentially modulate membrane potential dynamics across DG, CA3, and CA1 in awake mice. *ELife* 11:25.

Kamondi A, Acsády L, Buzsáki G (1998) Dendritic spikes are enhanced by cooperative network activity in the intact hippocampus. *Journal of Neuroscience: The Official Journal of the Society for Neuroscience* 18:3919–3928.

Kanter BR, Lykken CM, Avesar D, Weible A, Dickinson J, Dunn B, Borgesius NZ, Roudi Y, Kentros CG (2017) A novel mechanism for the grid-to-place cell transformation revealed by transgenic depolarization of medial entorhinal cortex layer II. *Neuron* 93:1480–1492, e6.

Karson MA, Tang A-H, Milner TA, Alger BE (2009) Synaptic cross talk between perisomatic-targeting interneuron classes expressing cholecystokinin and parvalbumin in hippocampus. *Journal of Neuroscience: The Official Journal of the Society for Neuroscience* 29:4140–4154.

Katona L, Lapray D, Viney TJ, Oulhaj A, Borhegyi Z, Micklem BR, Klausberger T, Somogyi P (2014) Sleep and movement differentiates actions of two types of somatostatin-expressing GABAergic interneuron in rat hippocampus. *Neuron* 82:872–886.

Katona L, Micklem B, Borhegyi Z, Swiejkowski DA, Valenti O, Viney TJ, Kotzadimitriou D, Klausberger T, Somogyi P (2017) Behavior-dependent activity patterns of GABAergic long-range projecting neurons in the rat hippocampus. *Hippocampus* 27:359–377.

Katz Y, Menon V, Nicholson DA, Geinisman Y, Kath WL, Spruston N (2009) Synapse distribution suggests a two-stage model of dendritic integration in CA1 pyramidal neurons. *Neuron* 63:171–177.

Kay K, Frank LM (2019) Three brain states in the hippocampus and cortex. *Hippocampus* 29:184–238.

Kay K, Sosa M, Chung JE, Karlsson MP, Larkin MC, Frank LM (2016) A hippocampal network for spatial coding during immobility and sleep. *Nature* 531:185–190.

Keinath AT, Wang ME, Wann EG, Yuan RK, Dudman JT, Muzzio IA (2014) Precise spatial coding is preserved along the longitudinal hippocampal axis: redundant hippocampal spatial coding and memory. *Hippocampus* 24:1533–1548.

Kemppainen S, Jolkkonen E, Pitkänen A (2002) Projections from the posterior cortical nucleus of the amygdala to the hippocampal formation and parahippocampal region in rat. *Hippocampus* 12:735–755.

Kentros C, Hargreaves E, Hawkins RD, Kandel ER, Shapiro M, Muller RV (1998) Abolition of long-term stability of new hippocampal place cell maps by NMDA receptor blockade. *Science* 280:2121–2126.

Kerr AM, Reisinger E, Jonas P (2008) Differential dependence of phasic transmitter release on synaptotagmin 1 at GABAergic and glutamatergic hippocampal synapses. *Proceedings of the National Academy of Sciences of the United States of America* 105:15581–15586.

Kim D, Jeong H, Lee J, Ghim J-W, Her ES, Lee S-H, Jung MW (2016) Distinct roles of parvalbumin- and somatostatin-expressing interneurons in working memory. *Neuron* 92:902–915.

Kim S, Guzman SJ, Hu H, Jonas P (2012) Active dendrites support efficient initiation of dendritic spikes in hippocampal CA3 pyramidal neurons. *Nature Neuroscience* 15:600–606.

Kim S, Kim Y, Lee S-H, Ho W-K (2018) Dendritic spikes in hippocampal granule cells are necessary for long-term potentiation at the perforant path synapse. *ELife* 7:e35269.

Kim Y, Hsu C-L, Cembrowski MS, Mensh BD, Spruston N (2015) Dendritic sodium spikes are required for long-term potentiation at distal synapses on hippocampal pyramidal neurons. *ELife* 4:372.

Kim Y, Spruston N (2012) Target-specific output patterns are predicted by the distribution of regular-spiking and bursting pyramidal neurons in the subiculum. *Hippocampus* 22:693–706.

Kitamura T (2017) Driving and regulating temporal association learning coordinated by entorhinal-hippocampal network. *Neuroscience Research* **121**:1–6.

Kitamura T, Pignatelli M, Suh J, Kohara K, Yoshiki A, Abe K, Tonegawa S (2014) Island cells control temporal association memory. *Science* **343**:896–901.

Kitamura T, Saitoh Y, Murayama A, Sugiyama H, Inokuchi K (2010) LTP induction within a narrow critical period of immature stages enhances the survival of newly generated neurons in the adult rat dentate gyrus. *Molecular Brain* **3**:13.

Kitamura T, Sun C, Martin J, Kitch LJ, Schnitzer MJ, Tonegawa S (2015) Entorhinal cortical ocean cells encode specific contexts and drive context-specific fear memory. *Neuron* **87**:1317–1331.

Klausberger T (2009) GABAergic interneurons targeting dendrites of pyramidal cells in the CA1 area of the hippocampus. *European Journal of Neuroscience* **30**:947–957.

Klausberger T, Magill PJ, Márton LF, Roberts JDB, Cobden PM, Buzsáki G, Somogyi P (2003) Brain-state- and cell-type-specific firing of hippocampal interneurons in vivo. *Nature* **421**:844–848.

Klausberger T, Márton LF, Baude A, Roberts JDB, Magill PJ, Somogyi P (2004) Spike timing of dendrite-targeting bistratified cells during hippocampal network oscillations in vivo. *Nature Neuroscience* **7**:41–47.

Klausberger T, Marton LF, O'Neill J, Huck JHJ, Dalezios Y, Fuentealba P, Suen WY, Papp E, Kaneko T, Watanabe M, et al. (2005) Complementary roles of cholecystokinin- and parvalbumin-expressing GABAergic neurons in hippocampal network oscillations. *Journal of Neuroscience* **25**:9782–9793.

Klausberger T, Somogyi P (2008) Neuronal diversity and temporal dynamics: the unity of hippocampal circuit operations. *Science* **321**:53–57.

Klink R, Alonso A (1997a) Ionic mechanisms of muscarinic depolarization in entorhinal cortex layer II neurons. *Journal of Neurophysiology* **77**:1829–1843.

Klink R, Alonso A (1997b) Morphological characteristics of layer II projection neurons in the rat medial entorhinal cortex. *Hippocampus* **7**:571–583.

Knierim JJ, Neunuebel JP, Deshmukh SS (2014) Functional correlates of the lateral and medial entorhinal cortex: objects, path integration and local-global reference frames. *Philosophical Transactions of the Royal Society B: Biological Sciences* **369**:20130369.

Kohara K, Pignatelli M, Rivest AJ, Jung H-Y, Kitamura T, Suh J, Frank D, Kajikawa K, Mise N, Obata Y, et al. (2014) Cell type-specific genetic and optogenetic tools reveal hippocampal CA2 circuits. *Nature Neuroscience* **17**:269–279.

Korotkova T, Fuchs EC, Ponomarenko A, Engelhardt J von, Monyer H (2010) NMDA receptor ablation on parvalbumin-positive interneurons impairs hippocampal synchrony, spatial representations, and working memory. *Neuron* **68**:557–569.

Koutsoumpa A, Papatheodoropoulos C (2021) Frequency-dependent layer-specific differences in short-term synaptic plasticity in the dorsal and ventral CA1 hippocampal field. *Synapse* **75**:e22199.

Kowalski J, Gan J, Jonas P, Pernía-Andrade AJ (2016) Intrinsic membrane properties determine hippocampal differential firing pattern in vivo in anesthetized rats. *Hippocampus* **26**:668–682.

Kraushaar U, Jonas P (2000) Efficacy and stability of quantal GABA release at a hippocampal interneuron-principal neuron synapse. *Journal of Neuroscience: The Official Journal of the Society for Neuroscience* **20**:5594–5607.

Kress GJ, Dowling MJ, Meeks JP, Mennerick S (2008) High threshold, proximal initiation, and slow conduction velocity of action potentials in dentate granule neuron mossy fibers. *Journal of Neurophysiology* **100**:281–291.

Krettek JE, Price JL (1977) The cortical projections of the mediodorsal nucleus and adjacent thalamic nuclei in the rat. *Journal of Comparative Neurology* **171**:157–191.

Krook-Magnuson E, Luu L, Lee S-H, Varga C, Soltesz I (2011) Ivy and neurogliaform interneurons are a major target of μ-opioid receptor modulation. *Journal of Neuroscience: The Official Journal of the Society for Neuroscience* **31**:14861–14870.

Krueppel R, Remy S, Beck H (2011) Dendritic integration in hippocampal dentate granule cells. *Neuron* **71**:512–528.

Kulik Á, Vida I, Fukazawa Y, Guetg N, Kasugai Y, Marker CL, Rigato F, Bettler B, Wickman K, Frotscher M, et al. (2006) Compartment-dependent colocalization of Kir3.2-containing K+ channels and GABAB receptors in hippocampal pyramidal cells. *Journal of Neuroscience* **26**:4289.

Kullmann DM, Lamsa KP (2007) Long-term synaptic plasticity in hippocampal interneurons. *Nature Reviews Neuroscience* **8**:687–699.

Kumaran D, McClelland JL (2012) Generalization through the recurrent interaction of episodic memories: a model of the hippocampal system. *Psychological Review* **119**:573–616.

Laezza F, Dingledine R (2004) Voltage-controlled plasticity at GluR2-deficient synapses onto hippocampal interneurons. *Journal of Neurophysiology* **92**:3575–3581.

Lamas M, Gómez-Lira G, Gutiérrez R (2001) Vesicular GABA transporter mRNA expression in the dentate gyrus and in mossy fiber synaptosomes. *Molecular Brain Research* **93**:209–214.

Lamsa K, Heeroma JH, Kullmann DM (2005) Hebbian LTP in feed-forward inhibitory interneurons and the temporal fidelity of input discrimination. *Nature Neuroscience* **8**:916–924.

Lamsa KP, Heeroma JH, Somogyi P, Rusakov DA, Kullmann DM (2007) Anti-Hebbian long-term potentiation in the hippocampal feedback inhibitory circuit. *Science* **315**:1262–1266.

Lancaster B, Nicoll RA (1987) Properties of two calcium-activated hyperpolarizations in rat hippocampal neurones. *Journal of Physiology* **389**:187–203.

Larimer P, Strowbridge BW (2008) Nonrandom local circuits in the dentate gyrus. *Journal of Neuroscience* **28**:12212.

Larimer P, Strowbridge BW (2010) Representing information in neuronal cell assemblies: persistent activity in the dentate gyrus mediated by semilunar granule cells. *Nature Neuroscience* **13**:213–222.

Lawrence JJ, Grinspan ZM, McBain CJ (2004) Quantal transmission at mossy fibre targets in the CA3 region of the rat hippocampus. *Journal of Physiology* **554**:175–193.

Lawrence JJ, McBain CJ (2003) Interneuron diversity series: containing the detonation–feedforward inhibition in the CA3 hippocampus. *Trends in Neurosciences* **26**:631–640.

Leao RN, Mikulovic S, Leão KE, Munguba H, Gezelius H, Enjin A, Patra K, Eriksson A, Loew LM, Tort ABL, et al. (2012) OLM interneurons differentially modulate CA3 and entorhinal inputs to hippocampal CA1 neurons. *Nature Neuroscience* **15**:1524–1530.

Lee AK, Brecht M (2018) Elucidating neuronal mechanisms using intracellular recordings during behavior. *Trends in Neurosciences* **41**:385–403.

Lee D, Lin B-J, Lee AK (2012) Hippocampal place fields emerge upon single-cell manipulation of excitability during behavior. *Science* **337**:849–853.

Lee H, GoodSmith D, Knierim JJ (2020) Parallel processing streams in the hippocampus. *Current Opinion in Neurobiology* **64**:127–134.

Lee H, Wang C, Deshmukh SS, Knierim JJ (2015) Neural population evidence of functional heterogeneity along the CA3 transverse axis: pattern completion versus pattern separation. *Neuron* **87**:1093–1105.

Lee I, Rao G, Knierim JJ (2004) A double dissociation between hippocampal subfields: differential time course of CA3 and CA1 place cells for processing changed environments. *Neuron* 42:803–815.

Lee SE, Simons SB, Heldt SA, Zhao M, Schroeder JP, Vellano CP, Cowan DP, Ramineni S, Yates CK, Feng Y, et al. (2010) RGS14 is a natural suppressor of both synaptic plasticity in CA2 neurons and hippocampal-based learning and memory. *The Proceedings of the National Academy of Sciences U S A* 107:16994–16998.

Lee S-H, Marchionni I, Bezaire M, Varga C, Danielson N, Lovett-Barron M, Losonczy A, Soltesz I (2014) Parvalbumin-positive basket cells differentiate among hippocampal pyramidal cells. *Neuron* 82:1129–1144.

Lei S, McBain CJ (2002) Distinct NMDA receptors provide differential modes of transmission at mossy fiber-interneuron synapses. *Neuron* 33:921–933.

Lei S, McBain CJ (2004) Two loci of expression for long-term depression at hippocampal mossy fiber-interneuron synapses. *Journal of Neuroscience* 24:2112–2121.

Lein ES, Belgard TG, Hawrylycz M, Molnár Z (2017) Transcriptomic perspectives on neocortical structure, development, evolution, and disease. *Annual Review of Neuroscience* 40:629–652.

Lein ES, Callaway EM, Albright TD, Gage FH (2005) Redefining the boundaries of the hippocampal CA2 subfield in the mouse using gene expression and 3-dimensional reconstruction. *Journal of Comparative Neurology* 485:1–10.

Lein ES, Hawrylycz MJ, Ao N, Ayres M, Bensinger A, Bernard A, Boe AF, Boguski MS, Brockway KS, Byrnes EJ, et al. (2007) Genome-wide atlas of gene expression in the adult mouse brain. *Nature* 445:168–176.

Lemaire V, Tronel S, Montaron M-F, Fabre A, Dugast E, Abrous DN (2012) Long-lasting plasticity of hippocampal adult-born neurons. *Journal of Neuroscience* 32:3101.

Leranth C, Malcolm AJ, Frotscher M (1990) Afferent and efferent synaptic connections of somatostatin-immunoreactive neurons in the rat fascia dentata. *Journal of Comparative Neurology* 295:111–122.

Leroy F, Brann DH, MeiraT, Siegelbaum SA (2017) Input-timing-dependent plasticity in the hippocampal CA2 region and its potential role in social memory. *Neuron* 95:1089–1102, e5.

Leroy F, Park J, Asok A, Brann DH, Meira T, Boyle LM, Buss EW, Kandel ER, Siegelbaum SA (2018) A circuit from hippocampal CA2 to lateral septum disinhibits social aggression. *Nature* 564:213–218.

Leung LS, Péloquin P (2010) Cholinergic modulation differs between basal and apical dendritic excitation of hippocampal CA1 pyramidal cells. *Cerebral Cortex* 20:1865–1877.

Leutgeb JK, Leutgeb S, Moser M-B, Moser EI (2007) Pattern separation in the dentate gyrus and CA3 of the hippocampus. *Science* 315:961–966.

Leutgeb S, Leutgeb JK, Treves A, Moser M-B, Moser EI (2004) Distinct ensemble codes in hippocampal areas CA3 and CA1. *Science* 305:1295–1298.

Lever C, Burton S, Jeewajee A, O'Keefe J, Burgess N (2009) Boundary vector cells in the subiculum of the hippocampal formation. *Journal of Neuroscience: The Official Journal of the Society for Neuroscience* 29:9771–9777.

Lewis DA, Hashimoto T, Volk DW (2005) Cortical inhibitory neurons and schizophrenia. *Nature Reviews Neuroscience* 6:312–324.

Li X, Somogyi P, Ylinen A, Buzsáki G (1994) The hippocampal Ca3 network—an in-vivo intracellular labeling study. *Journal of Comparative Neurology* 339:181–208.

Li XG, Somogyi P, Tepper JM, Buzsáki G (1992) Axonal and dendritic arborization of an intracellularly labeled chandelier cell in the CA1 region of rat hippocampus. *Experimental Brain Research* 90:519–525.

Li Y, Bao H, Luo Y, Yoan C, Sullivan HA, Quintanilla L, Wickersham I, Lazarus M, Shin Y-YI, Song J (2020) Supramammillary nucleus synchronizes with dentate gyrus to regulate spatial memory retrieval through glutamate release. *ELife* 9:604–623.

Lien C-C, Martina M, Schultz JH, Ehmke H, Jonas P (2002) Gating, modulation and subunit composition of voltage-gated K(+) channels in dendritic inhibitory interneurones of rat hippocampus. *Journal of Physiology* 538:405–419.

Lin Y-T, Hsieh T-Y, Tsai T-C, Chen C-C, Huang C-C, Hsu K-S (2018) Conditional deletion of hippocampal CA2/CA3a oxytocin receptors impairs the persistence of long-term social recognition memory in mice. *Journal of Neuroscience: The Official Journal of the Society for Neuroscience* 38:1218–1231.

Lingenhöhl K, Finch DM (1991) Morphological characterization of rat entorhinal neurons in vivo: soma-dendritic structure and axonal domains. *Experimental Brain Research Experimentelle Hirnforschung Expérimentation Cérébrale* 84:57–74.

Lisman J, Buzsáki G, Eichenbaum H, Nadel L, Ranganath C, Redish AD (2017) Viewpoints: how the hippocampus contributes to memory, navigation and cognition. *Nature Neuroscience* 20:1434–1447.

Lisman J, Spruston N (2010) Questions about STDP as a general model of synaptic plasticity. *Frontiers in Synaptic Neuroscience* 2:140.

Liu PW, Bean BP (2014) Kv2 channel regulation of action potential repolarization and firing patterns in superior cervical ganglion neurons and hippocampal CA1 pyramidal neurons. *Journal of Neuroscience* 34:4991–5002.

London M, Häusser M (2005) Dendritic computation. *Annual Review of Neuroscience* 28:503–532.

Lorente de Nó R (1934) Studies on the structure of the cerebral cortex: II. Continuation of the study of the ammonic system. *Journal f. Psychologie and Neurologie* 46:113–175.

Lörincz A, Notomi T, Tamás G, Shigemoto R, Nusser Z (2002) Polarized and compartment-dependent distribution of HCN1 in pyramidal cell dendrites. *Nature Neuroscience* 5:1185–1193.

Lorincz A, Nusser Z (2008) Cell-type-dependent molecular composition of the axon initial segment. *Journal of Neuroscience: The Official Journal of the Society for Neuroscience* 28:14329–14340.

Losonczy A, Magee JC (2006) Integrative properties of radial oblique dendrites in hippocampal CA1 pyramidal neurons. *Neuron* 50:291–307.

Losonczy A, Makara JK, Magee JC (2008) Compartmentalized dendritic plasticity and input feature storage in neurons. *Nature* 452:436–441.

Lovett-Barron M, Turi GF, Kaifosh P, Lee PH, Bolze F, Sun X-H, Nicoud J-F, Zemelman BV, Sternson SM, Losonczy A (2012) Regulation of neuronal input transformations by tunable dendritic inhibition. *Nature Neuroscience* 15:423-30.

Lu L, Igarashi KM, Witter MP, Moser EI, Moser M-B (2015) Topography of place maps along the CA3-to-CA2 axis of the hippocampus. *Neuron* 87:1078–1092.

Lübke J, Frotscher M, Spruston N (1998) Specialized electrophysiological properties of anatomically identified neurons in the hilar region of the rat fascia dentata. *Journal of Neurophysiology* 79:1518–1534.

Luna VM, Anacker C, Burghardt NS, Khandaker H, Andreu V, Millette A, Leary P, Ravenelle R, Jimenez JC, Mastrodonato A, et al. (2019) Adult-born hippocampal neurons bidirectionally modulate entorhinal inputs into the dentate gyrus. *Science* 364:578–583.

Lüscher C, Jan LY, Stoffel M, Malenka RC, Nicoll RA (1997) G protein-coupled inwardly rectifying K+ channels (GIRKs) mediate postsynaptic but not presynaptic transmitter actions in hippocampal neurons. *Neuron* 19:687–695.

Ma Y, Bayguinov PO, McMahon SM, Scharfman HE, Jackson MB (2021) Direct synaptic excitation between hilar mossy cells revealed with a targeted voltage sensor. *Hippocampus* 31:1215–1232.

Maccaferri G, David J, Roberts B, Szucs P, Cottingham CA, Somogyi P (2000) Cell surface domain specific postsynaptic currents evoked by identified GABAergic neurones in rat hippocampus in vitro. *Journal of Physiology* 524:91–116.

Maccaferri G, Dingledine R (2002) Control of feedforward dendritic inhibition by NMDA receptor-dependent spike timing in hippocampal interneurons. *Journal of Neuroscience: The Official Journal of the Society for Neuroscience* 22:5462–5472.

Maccaferri G, McBain CJ (1995) Passive propagation of LTD to stratum oriens-alveus inhibitory neurons modulates the temporoammonic input to the hippocampal CA1 region. *Neuron* 15:137–145.

Maccaferri G, McBain CJ (1996) Long-term potentiation in distinct subtypes of hippocampal nonpyramidal neurons. *Journal of Neuroscience: The Official Journal of the Society for Neuroscience* 16:5334–5343.

Madison DV, Nicoll RA (1982) Noradrenaline blocks accommodation of pyramidal cell discharge in the hippocampus. *Nature* 299:636–638.

Madison DV, Nicoll RA (1984) Control of the repetitive discharge of rat CA 1 pyramidal neurones in vitro. *Journal of Physiology* 354:319–331.

Magee J (1999) Dendritic Ih normalizes temporal summation in hippocampal CA1 neurons. *Nature Neuroscience* 2:508–514.

Magee JC (1998) Dendritic hyperpolarization-activated currents modify the integrative properties of hippocampal CA1 pyramidal neurons. *Journal of Neuroscience: The Official Journal of the Society for Neuroscience* 18:7613–7624.

Magee JC, Cook E (2000) Somatic EPSP amplitude is independent of synapse location in hippocampal pyramidal neurons. *Nature Neuroscience* 3:895–903.

Magee JC, Johnston D (1995a) Characterization of single voltage-gated Na+ and Ca2+ channels in apical dendrites of rat CA1 pyramidal neurons. *Journal of Physiology* 487:67–90.

Magee JC, Johnston D (1995b) Synaptic activation of voltage-gated channels in the dendrites of hippocampal pyramidal neurons. *Science* 268:301–304.

Magee JC, Johnston D (1997) A synaptically controlled, associative signal for Hebbian plasticity in hippocampal neurons. *Science* 275:209–213.

Magistretti J, Alonso A (1999a) Biophysical properties and slow voltage-dependent inactivation of a sustained sodium current in entorhinal cortex layer-II principal neurons: a whole-cell and single-channel study. *Journal of General Physiology* 114:491–509.

Magistretti J, Alonso A (1999b) Slow voltage-dependent inactivation of a sustained sodium current in stellate cells of rat entorhinal cortex layer II. *Annals of the New York Academy of Sciences* 868:84–87.

Magistretti J, Ragsdale DS, Alonso A (1999) High conductance sustained single-channel activity responsible for the low-threshold persistent Na(+) current in entorhinal cortex neurons. *Journal of Neuroscience: The Official Journal of the Society for Neuroscience* 19:7334–7341.

Magó Á, Kis N, Lükő B, Makara JK (2021) Distinct dendritic Ca2+ spike forms produce opposing input-output transformations in rat CA3 pyramidal cells. *ELife* 10:e74493.

Maier N, Güldenagel M, Söhl G, Siegmund H, Willecke K, Draguhn A (2002) Reduction of high-frequency network oscillations (ripples) and pathological network discharges in hippocampal slices from connexin 36-deficient mice. *Journal of Physiology* 541:521–528.

Maier N, Tejero-Cantero Á, Dorrn AL, Winterer J, Beed PS, Morris G, Kempter R, Poulet JFA, Leibold C, Schmitz D (2011) Coherent phasic excitation during hippocampal ripples. *Neuron* 72:137–152.

Major G, Larkum ME, Schiller J (2013) Active properties of neocortical pyramidal neuron dendrites. *Annual Review of Neuroscience* 36:1–24.

Makara JK, Magee JC (2013) Variable dendritic integration in hippocampal ca3 pyramidal neurons. *Neuron* 80:1438–1450.

Malezieux M, Kees AL, Mulle C (2020) Theta oscillations coincide with sustained hyperpolarization in CA3 pyramidal cells, underlying decreased firing. *Cell Reports* 32:107868.

Malik R, Dougherty KA, Parikh K, Byrne C, Johnston D (2016) Mapping the electrophysiological and morphological properties of CA1 pyramidal neurons along the longitudinal hippocampal axis. *Hippocampus* 26:341–361.

Mankin EA, Diehl GW, Sparks FT, Leutgeb S, Leutgeb JK (2015) Hippocampal CA2 activity patterns change over time to a larger extent than between spatial contexts. *Neuron* 85:190–201.

Marín-Burgin A, Mongiat LA, Pardi MB, Schinder AF (2012) Unique processing during a period of high excitation/inhibition balance in adult-born neurons. *Science* 335:1238–1242.

Marissal T, Bonifazi P, Picardo MA, Nardou R, Petit LF, Baude A, Fishell GJ, Ben-Ari Y, Cossart R (2012) Pioneer glutamatergic cells develop into a morpho-functionally distinct population in the juvenile CA3 hippocampus. *Nature Communications* 3:1316.

Marr D (1971) Simple memory: a theory for archicortex. *Philosophical Transactions of the Royal Society of London Series B, Biological Sciences* 262:23–81.

Marrosu F, Portas C, Mascia MS, Casu MA, Fà M, Giagheddu M, Imperato A, Gessa GL (1995) Microdialysis measurement of cortical and hippocampal acetylcholine release during sleep-wake cycle in freely moving cats. *Brain Research* 671:329–332.

Martig AK, Mizumori SJY (2011) Ventral tegmental area disruption selectively affects CA1/CA2 but not CA3 place fields during a differential reward working memory task. *Hippocampus* 21:172–184.

Martina M, Schultz JH, Ehmke H, Monyer H, Jonas P (1998) Functional and molecular differences between voltage-gated K+ channels of fast-spiking interneurons and pyramidal neurons of rat hippocampus. *Journal of Neuroscience: The Official Journal of the Society for Neuroscience* 18:8111–8125.

Martina M, Vida I, Jonas P (2000) Distal initiation and active propagation of action potentials in interneuron dendrites. *Science* 287:295–300.

Martinello K, Giacalone E, Migliore M, Brown DA, Shah MM (2019) The subthreshold-active KV7 current regulates neurotransmission by limiting spike-induced Ca2+ influx in hippocampal mossy fiber synaptic terminals. *Communications Biology* 2:145.

Masurkar AV, Srinivas KV, Brann DH, Warren R, Lowes DC, Siegelbaum SA (2017) Medial and lateral entorhinal cortex differentially excite deep versus superficial CA1 pyramidal neurons. *Cell Reports* 18:148–160.

Matsuzaki M, Ellis-Davies GC, Nemoto T, Miyashita Y, Iino M, Kasai H (2001) Dendritic spine geometry is critical for AMPA receptor expression in hippocampal CA1 pyramidal neurons. *Nature Neuroscience* 4:1086–1092.

Matsuzaki M, Honkura N, Ellis-Davies GCR, Kasai H (2004) Structural basis of long-term potentiation in single dendritic spines. *Nature* 429:761–766.

Matta JA, Pelkey KA, Craig MT, Chittajallu R, Jeffries BW, McBain CJ (2013) Developmental origin dictates interneuron AMPA and NMDA receptor subunit composition and plasticity. *Nature Neuroscience* 16:1032–1041.

Mátyás F, Freund TF, Gulyás AI (2004) Convergence of excitatory and inhibitory inputs onto CCK-containing basket cells in the CA1 area of the rat hippocampus. *European Journal of Neuroscience* 19:1243–1256.

McBain CJ (2008) Differential mechanisms of transmission and plasticity at mossy fiber synapses. *Progress in Brain Research* 169:225–240.

McBain CJ, DiChiara TJ, Kauer JA (1994) Activation of metabotropic glutamate receptors differentially affects two classes of hippocampal interneurons and potentiates excitatory synaptic transmission. *Journal of Neuroscience: The Official Journal of the Society for Neuroscience* 14:4433–4445.

McClelland JL, McNaughton BL, O'Reilly RC (1995) Why there are complementary learning systems in the hippocampus and neocortex: insights from the successes and failures of connectionist models of learning and memory. *Psychological Review* 102:419–457.

McHugh TJ, Blum KI, Tsien JZ, Tonegawa S, Wilson MA (1996) Impaired hippocampal representation of space in CA1-specific NMDAR1 knockout mice. *Cell* 87:1339–1349.

McKenna JT, Vertes RP (2001) Collateral projections from the median raphe nucleus to the medial septum and hippocampus. *Brain Research Bulletin* 54:619–630.

Medinilla V, Johnson O, Gasparini S (2013) Features of proximal and distal excitatory synaptic inputs to layer V neurons of the rat medial entorhinal cortex: excitatory inputs to entorhinal layer V neurons. *Journal of Physiology* 591:169–183.

Megías M, Emri Z, Freund TF, Gulyás AI (2001) Total number and distribution of inhibitory and excitatory synapses on hippocampal CA1 pyramidal cells. *Neuroscience* 102:527–540.

Mehta MR (2015) From synaptic plasticity to spatial maps and sequence learning: place field plasticity. *Hippocampus* 25:756–762.

Meira T, Leroy F, Buss EW, Oliva A, Park J, Siegelbaum SA (2018) A hippocampal circuit linking dorsal CA2 to ventral CA1 critical for social memory dynamics. *Nature Communications* 9:1–14.

Melzer S, Michael M, Caputi A, Eliava M, Fuchs EC, Whittington MA, Monyer H (2012) Long-range-projecting GABAergic neurons modulate inhibition in hippocampus and entorhinal cortex. *Science* 335:1506–1510.

Menendez De La Prida L (2003) Control of bursting by local inhibition in the rat subiculum in vitro. *Journal of Physiology* 549:219–230.

Menendez De La Prida L (2006) Functional features of the rat subicular microcircuits studied in vitro. *Behavioural Brain Research* 174:198–205.

Menendez de la Prida L, Suarez F, Pozo MA (2003) Electrophysiological and morphological diversity of neurons from the rat subicular complex in vitro. *Hippocampus* 13:728–744.

Menon V, Musial TF, Liu A, Katz Y, Kath WL, Spruston N, Nicholson DA (2013) Balanced synaptic impact via distance-dependent synapse distribution and complementary expression of AMPARs and NMDARs in hippocampal dendrites. *Neuron* 80:1451–1463.

Mercer A, Eastlake K, Trigg HL, Thomson AM (2012) Local circuitry involving parvalbumin-positive basket cells in the CA2 region of the hippocampus. *Hippocampus* 22:43–56.

Metz AE, Jarsky T, Martina M, Spruston N (2005) R-type calcium channels contribute to afterdepolarization and bursting in hippocampal CA1 pyramidal neurons. *Journal of Neuroscience: The Official Journal of the Society for Neuroscience* 25:5763–5773.

Metz AE, Spruston N, Martina M (2007) Dendritic D-type potassium currents inhibit the spike afterdepolarization in rat hippocampal CA1 pyramidal neurons: dendritic D-type potassium currents inhibit afterdepolarization. *Journal of Physiology* 581:175–187.

Meyer AH, Katona I, Blatow M, Rozov A, Monyer H (2002) In vivo labeling of parvalbumin-positive interneurons and analysis of electrical coupling in identified neurons. *Journal of Neuroscience: The Official Journal of the Society for Neuroscience* 22:7055–7064.

Mickus T, Jung HY, Spruston N (1999) Slow sodium channel inactivation in CA1 pyramidal cells. *Annals of the New York Academy of Sciences* 868:97–101.

Miles R (1990) Variation in strength of inhibitory synapses in the CA3 region of guinea-pig hippocampus in vitro. *Journal of Physiology* 431:659–676.

Miles R, Tóth K, Gulyás AI, Hájos N, Freund TF (1996) Differences between somatic and dendritic inhibition in the hippocampus. *Neuron* 16:815–823.

Milstein AD, Bloss EB, Apostolides PF, Vaidya SP, Dilly GA, Zemelman BV, Magee JC (2015) Inhibitory gating of input comparison in the CA1 microcircuit. *Neuron* 87:1274–1289.

Mishra P, Narayanan R (2020) Heterogeneities in intrinsic excitability and frequency-dependent response properties of granule cells across the blades of the rat dentate gyrus. *Journal of Neurophysiology* 123:755–772.

Mizuseki K, Diba K, Pastalkova E, Buzsáki G (2011) Hippocampal CA1 pyramidal cells form functionally distinct sublayers. *Nature Neuroscience* 14:1174–1181.

Mizuseki K, Royer S, Diba K, Buzsáki G (2012) Activity dynamics and behavioral correlates of CA3 and CA1 hippocampal pyramidal neurons. *Hippocampus* 22:1659–1680.

Mongiat LA, Espósito MS, Lombardi G, Schinder AF (2009) Reliable activation of immature neurons in the adult hippocampus. *PLoS One* 4:1–11.

Moore SJ, Cooper DC, Spruston N (2009) Plasticity of burst firing induced by synergistic activation of metabotropic glutamate and acetylcholine receptors. *Neuron* 61:287–300.

Moretto JN, Duffy ÁM, Scharfman HE (2017) Acute restraint stress decreases c-fos immunoreactivity in hilar mossy cells of the adult dentate gyrus. *Brain Structure and Function* 222:2405–2419.

Mori M, Abegg MH, Gähwiler BH, Gerber U (2004) A frequency-dependent switch from inhibition to excitation in a hippocampal unitary circuit. *Nature* 431:453–456.

Morin F, Beaulieu C, Lacaille JC (1996) Membrane properties and synaptic currents evoked in CA1 interneuron subtypes in rat hippocampal slices. *Journal of Neurophysiology* 76:1–16.

Mott DD, Dingledine R (2003) Interneuron diversity series: interneuron research—challenges and strategies. *Trends in Neurosciences* 26:484–488.

Mott DD, Turner DA, Okazaki MM, Lewis DV (1997) Interneurons of the dentate-hilus border of the rat dentate gyrus: morphological and electrophysiological heterogeneity. *Journal of Neuroscience: The Official Journal of the Society for Neuroscience* 17:3990–4005.

Muenster-Wandowski A, Gómez-Lira G, Gutierrez R (2013) Mixed neurotransmission in the hippocampal mossy fibers. *Frontiers in Cellular Neuroscience* 7:210.

Muñoz M-D, Solís JM (2019) Characterisation of the mechanisms underlying the special sensitivity of the CA2 hippocampal area to adenosine receptor antagonists. *Neuropharmacology* 144:9–18.

Naber PA, Witter MP (1998) Subicular efferents are organized mostly as parallel projections: a double-labeling, retrograde-tracing study in the rat. *Journal of Comparative Neurology* 393:284–297.

Nägerl UV, Eberhorn N, Cambridge SB, Bonhoeffer T (2004) Bidirectional activity-dependent morphological plasticity in hippocampal neurons. *Neuron* 44:759–767.

Nasrallah K, Piskorowski RA, Chevaleyre V (2015) Inhibitory plasticity permits the recruitment of CA2 pyramidal neurons by CA3(1,2,3). *ENeuro* 2:1–12.

Nasrallah K, Therreau L, Robert V, Huang AJY, McHugh TJ, Piskorowski RA, Chevaleyre V (2019) Routing hippocampal information flow through parvalbumin interneuron plasticity in area CA2. *Cell Reports* 27:86–98, e3.

Neu A, Földy C, Soltesz I (2007) Postsynaptic origin of CB1-dependent tonic inhibition of GABA release at cholecystokinin-positive basket cell to pyramidal cell synapses in the CA1 region of the rat hippocampus. *Journal of Physiology* 578:233–247.

Neumann AR, Raedt R, Steenland HW, Sprengers M, Bzymek K, Navratilova Z, Mesina L, Xie J, Lapointe V, Kloosterman F, et al. (2017) Involvement of fast-spiking cells in ictal sequences during spontaneous seizures in rats with chronic temporal lobe epilepsy. *Brain: A Journal of Neurology* 140:2355–2369.

Neunuebel JP, Knierim JJ (2012) Spatial firing correlates of physiologically distinct cell types of the rat dentate gyrus. *Journal of Neuroscience* 32:3848–3858.

Neunuebel JP, Knierim JJ (2014) CA3 retrieves coherent representations from degraded input: direct evidence for CA3 pattern completion and dentate gyrus pattern separation. *Neuron* 81:416–427.

Nicholson DA, Geinisman Y (2009) Axospinous synaptic subtype-specific differences in structure, size, ionotropic receptor expression, and connectivity in apical dendritic regions of rat hippocampal CA1 pyramidal neurons. *Journal of Comparative Neurology* 512:399–418.

Nicholson DA, Trana R, Katz Y, Kath WL, Spruston N, Geinisman Y (2006) Distance-dependent differences in synapse number and AMPA receptor expression in hippocampal CA1 pyramidal neurons. *Neuron* 50:431–442.

Nissen W, Szabo A, Somogyi J, Somogyi P, Lamsa KP (2010) Cell type-specific long-term plasticity at glutamatergic synapses onto hippocampal interneurons expressing either parvalbumin or CB1 cannabinoid receptor. *Journal of Neuroscience* 30:1337–1347.

Noguchi J, Matsuzaki M, Ellis-Davies GCR, Kasai H (2005) Spine-neck geometry determines NMDA receptor-dependent Ca2+ signaling in dendrites. *Neuron* 46:609–622.

Nörenberg A, Hu H, Vida I, Bartos M, Jonas P (2010) Distinct non-uniform cable properties optimize rapid and efficient activation of fast-spiking GABAergic interneurons. *Proceedings of the National Academy of Sciences of the United States of America* 107:894–899.

Notomi T, Shigemoto R (2004) Immunohistochemical localization of Ih channel subunits, HCN1-4, in the rat brain. *Journal of Comparative Neurology* 471:241–276.

Nyiri G, Freund TF, Somogyi P (2001) Input-dependent synaptic targeting of α2-subunit-containing GABAA receptors in synapses of hippocampal pyramidal cells of the rat. *European Journal of Neuroscience* 13:428–442.

Ochiishi T, Saitoh Y, Yukawa A, Saji M, Ren Y, Shirao T, Miyamoto H, Nakata H, Sekino Y (1999) High level of adenosine A1 receptor-like immunoreactivity in the CA2/CA3a region of the adult rat hippocampus. *Neuroscience* 93:955–967.

Ofer N, Berger DR, Kasthuri N, Lichtman JW, Yuste R (2021) Ultrastructural analysis of dendritic spine necks reveals a continuum of spine morphologies. *Developmental Neurobiology* 81:746–757.

Ohara S, Gianatti M, Itou K, Berndtsson CH, Doan TP, Kitanishi T, Mizuseki K, Iijima T, Tsutsui K-I, Witter MP (2019) Entorhinal layer II calbindin-expressing neurons originate widespread telencephalic and intrinsic projections. *Frontiers in Systems Neuroscience* 13:54.

Ohara S, Onodera M, Simonsen ØW, Yoshino R, Hioki H, Iijima T, Tsutsui K-I, Witter MP (2018) Intrinsic projections of layer Vb neurons to layers Va III, II in the lateral and medial entorhinal cortex of the rat. *Cell Reports* 24:107–116.

Okamoto K, Ikegaya Y (2019) Recurrent connections between CA2 pyramidal cells. *Hippocampus* 29:305–312.

O'Keefe J, Krupic J (2021) Do hippocampal pyramidal cells respond to nonspatial stimuli? *Physiological Reviews* 101:1427–1456.

Oláh S, Füle M, Komlósi G, Varga C, Báldi R, Barzó P, Tamás G (2009) Regulation of cortical microcircuits by unitary GABA-mediated volume transmission. *Nature* 461:1278–1281.

Oliva A, Fernández-Ruiz A, Buzsáki G, Berényi A (2016a) Role of hippocampal CA2 region in triggering sharp-wave ripples. *Neuron* 91:1342–1355.

Oliva A, Fernández-Ruiz A, Buzsáki G, Berényi A (2016b) Spatial coding and physiological properties of hippocampal neurons in the cornu ammonis subregions. *Hippocampus* 26:1593–1607.

Olsen RK, Moses SN, Riggs L, Ryan JD (2012) The hippocampus supports multiple cognitive processes through relational binding and comparison. *Frontiers in Human Neuroscience* 6:146.

O'Mara SM, Sanchez-Vives MV, Brotons-Mas JR, O'Hare E (2009) Roles for the subiculum in spatial information processing, memory, motivation and the temporal control of behaviour. *Progress in Neuro-Psychopharmacology and Biological Psychiatry* 33:782–790.

Oren I, Nissen W, Kullmann DM, Somogyi P, Lamsa KP (2009) Role of ionotropic glutamate receptors in long-term potentiation in rat hippocampal CA1 oriens-lacunosum moleculare interneurons. *Journal of Neuroscience* 29:939–950.

Otmakhov N, Shirke AM, Malinow R (1993) Measuring the impact of probabilistic transmission on neuronal output. *Neuron* 10:1101–1111.

Otmakhova NA, Lisman JE (1999) Dopamine selectively inhibits the direct cortical pathway to the CA1 hippocampal region. *Journal of Neuroscience: The Official Journal of the Society for Neuroscience* 19:1437–1445.

Overstreet-Wadiche LS, Bensen AL, Westbrook GL (2006) Delayed development of adult-generated granule cells in dentate gyrus. *Journal of Neuroscience* 26:2326.

Overstreet-Wadiche L, McBain CJ (2015) Neurogliaform cells in cortical circuits. *Nature Reviews Neuroscience* 16:458–468.

Pagani JH, Zhao M, Cui Z, Avram SKW, Caruana DA, Dudek SM, Young WS (2014) Role of the vasopressin 1b receptor in rodent aggressive behavior and synaptic plasticity in hippocampal area CA2. *Molecular Psychiatry* 20:490–499.

Palacio S, Chevaleyre V, Brann DH, Murray KD, Piskorowski RA, Trimmer JS (2017) Heterogeneity in Kv2 channel expression shapes action potential characteristics and firing patterns in CA1 versus CA2 hippocampal pyramidal neurons. *ENeuro* 4:ENEURO.0267-17.2017.

Park JY, Remy S, Varela J, Cooper DC, Chung S, Kang H-W, Lee J-H, Spruston N (2010) A post-burst after depolarization is mediated by group i metabotropic glutamate receptor-dependent upregulation of Ca(v)2.3 R-type calcium channels in CA1 pyramidal neurons. *PLoS Biology* 8:e1000534.

Park JY, Spruston N (2012) Synergistic actions of metabotropic acetylcholine and glutamate receptors on the excitability of hippocampal CA1 pyramidal neurons. *Journal of Neuroscience: The Official Journal of the Society for Neuroscience* 32:6081–6091.

Park YY, Johnston D, Gray R (2013) Slowly inactivating component of Na+ current in peri-somatic region of hippocampal CA1 pyramidal neurons. *Journal of Neurophysiology* 109:1378–1390.

Paul A, Crow M, Raudales R, He M, Gillis J, Huang ZJ (2017) Transcriptional architecture of synaptic communication delineates GABAergic neuron identity. *Cell* 171:522–539, e20.

Pawelzik H, Hughes DI, Thomson AM (2003) Modulation of inhibitory autapses and synapses on rat CA1 interneurones by GABA(A) receptor ligands. *Journal of Physiology* 546:701–716.

Pedersen NP, Ferrari L, Venner A, Wang JL, Abbott SBG, Vujovic N, Arrigoni E, Saper CB, Fuller PM (2017) Supramammillary glutamate neurons are a key node of the arousal system. *Nature Communications* 8:1–16.

Pelkey KA, Chittajallu R, Craig MT, Tricoire L, Wester JC, McBain CJ (2017) Hippocampal GABAergic inhibitory interneurons. *Physiological Reviews* 97:1619–1747.

Pelkey KA, Lavezzari G, Racca C, Roche KW, McBain CJ (2005) mGluR7 is a metaplastic switch controlling bidirectional plasticity of feedforward inhibition. *Neuron* 46:89–102.

Peng Y, Barreda Tomás FJ, Klisch C, Vida I, Geiger JRP (2017) Layer-specific organization of local excitatory and inhibitory synaptic connectivity in the rat presubiculum. *Cerebral Cortex* 27:2435–2452.

Perez Y, Morin F, Lacaille JC (2001) A Hebbian form of long-term potentiation dependent on mGluR1a in hippocampal inhibitory interneurons. *Proceedings of the National Academy of Sciences of the United States of America* 98:9401–9406.

Petilla Interneuron Nomenclature Group, Ascoli GA, Alonso-Nanclares L, Anderson SA, Barrionuevo G, Benavides-Piccione R, Burkhalter A, Buzsáki G, Cauli B, Defelipe J, et al. (2008) Petilla terminology: nomenclature of features of GABAergic interneurons of the cerebral cortex. *Nature Reviews. Neuroscience* 9:557–568.

Peyrache A, Duszkiewicz AJ, Viejo G, Angeles-Duran S (2019) Thalamocortical processing of the head-direction sense. *Progress in Neurobiology* 183:101693.

Phillips T, Makoff A, Brown S, Rees S, Emson P (1997) Localization of mGluR4 protein in the rat cerebral cortex and hippocampus. *Neuroreport* 8:3349–3354.

Pignatelli M, Ryan TJ, Roy DS, Lovett C, Smith LM, Muralidhar S, Tonegawa S (2019) Engram cell excitability state determines the efficacy of memory retrieval. *Neuron* 101:274–284, e5.

Pikkarainen M, Rönkkö S, Savander V, Insausti R, Pitkänen A (1999) Projections from the lateral, basal, and accessory basal nuclei of the amygdala to the hippocampal formation in rat. *Journal of Comparative Neurology* 403:229–260.

Pilz G-A, Carta S, Stäuble A, Ayaz A, Jessberger S, Helmchen F (2016) Functional imaging of dentate granule cells in the adult mouse hippocampus. *Journal of Neuroscience* 36:7407–7414.

Pimpinella D, Mastrorilli V, Giorgi C, Coemans S, Lecca S, Lalive AL, Ostermann H, Fuchs EC, Monyer H, Mele A, et al. (2021) Septal cholinergic input to CA2 hippocampal region controls social novelty discrimination via nicotinic receptor-mediated disinhibition. *ELife* 10:e65580.

Piskorowski RA, Chevaleyre V (2013) Delta-opioid receptors mediate unique plasticity onto parvalbumin-expressing interneurons in area CA2 of the hippocampus. *Journal of Neuroscience* 33:14567–14578.

Piskorowski RA, Nasrallah K, Diamantopoulou A, Mukai J, Hassan SI, Siegelbaum SA, Gogos JA, Chevaleyre V (2016) Age-dependent specific changes in area CA2 of the hippocampus and social memory deficit in a mouse model of the 22q11.2 deletion syndrome. *Neuron* 89:163–176.

Pitkänen A, Pikkarainen M, Nurminen N, Ylinen A (2000) Reciprocal connections between the amygdala and the hippocampal formation, perirhinal cortex, and postrhinal cortex in rat. A review. *Annals of the New York Academy of Sciences* 911:369–391.

Poolos NP, Migliore M, Johnston D (2002) Pharmacological upregulation of h-channels reduces the excitability of pyramidal neuron dendrites. *Nature Neuroscience* 5:767–774.

Pouille F, Marin-Burgin A, Adesnik H, Atallah BV, Scanziani M (2009) Input normalization by global feedforward inhibition expands cortical dynamic range. *Nature Neuroscience* 12:1577–1585.

Pouille F, Scanziani M (2001) Enforcement of temporal fidelity in pyramidal cells by somatic feed-forward inhibition. *Science* 293:1159–1163.

Pouille F, Scanziani M (2004) Routing of spike series by dynamic circuits in the hippocampus. *Nature* 429:717–723.

Pouille F, Watkinson O, Scanziani M, Trevelyan AJ (2013) The contribution of synaptic location to inhibitory gain control in pyramidal cells. *Physiological Reports* 1:e00067.

Poulter S, Lee SA, Dachtler J, Wills TJ, Lever C (2021) Vector trace cells in the subiculum of the hippocampal formation. *Nature Neuroscience* 24:266–275.

Preston-Ferrer P, Coletta S, Frey M, Burgalossi A (2016) Anatomical organization of presubicular head-direction circuits. *ELife* 5:e14592.

Price CJ, Cauli B, Kovacs ER, Kulik A, Lambolez B, Shigemoto R, Capogna M (2005) Neurogliaform neurons form a novel inhibitory network in the hippocampal CA1 area. *Journal of Neuroscience: The Official Journal of the Society for Neuroscience* 25:6775–6786.

Pyapali GK, Sik A, Penttonen M, Buzsaki G, Turner DA (1998) Dendritic properties of hippocampal CA1 pyramidal neurons in the rat: Intracellular staining in vivo and in vitro. *Journal of Comparative Neurology* 391:335–352.

Que L, Lukacsovich D, Luo W, Földy C (2021) Transcriptional and morphological profiling of parvalbumin interneuron subpopulations in the mouse hippocampus. *Nature Communications* 12:108.

Quilichini P, Sirota A, Buzsáki G (2010) Intrinsic circuit organization and theta–gamma oscillation dynamics in the entorhinal cortex of the rat. *Journal of Neuroscience* 30:11128.

Raam T, McAvoy KM, Besnard A, Veenema A, Sahay A (2017) Hippocampal oxytocin receptors are necessary for discrimination of social stimuli. *Nature Communications* 8:2001.

Radcliffe KA, Fisher JL, Gray R, Dani JA (1999) Nicotinic modulation of glutamate and GABA synaptic transmission in hippocampal neurons. *Annals of the New York Academy of Sciences* 868:591–610.

Rall W (2011) Core conductor theory and cable properties of neurons. In: Comprehensive Physiology (Kandel ER, ed.), pp 39–97. Bethesda, MD: American Physiology Society, John Wiley & Sons.

Ramón y Cajal S (1911) Histologie du système nerveux de l'homme & des vertébrés. A. Maloine.

Ramsden HL, Sürmeli G, McDonagh SG, Nolan MF (2015) Laminar and dorsoventral molecular organization of the medial entorhinal cortex revealed by large-scale anatomical analysis of gene expression. *PLOS Computational Biology* 11:e1004032.

Ranganath C (2019) Time, memory, and the legacy of Howard Eichenbaum. *Hippocampus* 29:146–161.

Ray S, Brecht M (2016) Structural development and dorsoventral maturation of the medial entorhinal cortex. *ELife* 5:e13343.

Ray S, Burgalossi A, Brecht M, Naumann RK (2017) Complementary modular microcircuits of the rat medial entorhinal cortex. *Frontiers in Systems Neuroscience* 11:20.

Ray S, Naumann R, Burgalossi A, Tang Q, Schmidt H, Brecht M (2014) Grid-layout and theta-modulation of layer 2 pyramidal neurons in medial entorhinal cortex. *Science* 343:891–896.

Rebola N, Carta M, Mulle C (2017) Operation and plasticity of hippocampal CA3 circuits: implications for memory encoding. *Nature Reviews Neuroscience* 18:208–220.

Remy S, Spruston N (2007) Dendritic spikes induce single-burst long-term potentiation. *Proceedings of the National Academy of Sciences* 104:17192–17197.

Rhodes KJ, Carroll KI, Sung MA, Doliveira LC, Monaghan MM, Burke SL, Strassle BW, Buchwalder L, Menegola M, Cao J, et al. (2004) KChIPs and Kv4 subunits as integral components of A-type potassium channels in mammalian brain. *Journal of Neuroscience* 24:7903–7915.

Ribary U, Ioannides AA, Singh KD, Hasson R, Bolton JP, Lado F, Mogilner A, Llinás R (1991) Magnetic field tomography of coherent thalamocortical 40-Hz oscillations in humans. *Proceedings of the National Academy of Sciences of the United States of America* 88:11037–11041.

Rich PD, Liaw H-P, Lee AK (2014) Large environments reveal the statistical structure governing hippocampal representations. *Science* 345:814–817.

Robert V, Therreau L, Chevaleyre V, Lepicard E, Viollet C, Cognet J, Huang AJ, Boehringer R, Polygalov D, McHugh TJ, et al. (2021) Local circuit allowing hypothalamic control of hippocampal area CA2 activity and consequences for CA1. *ELife* 10:e63352.

Robert V, Therreau L, Davatolhagh MF, Bernardo-Garcia FJ, Clements KN, Chevaleyre V, Piskorowski RA (2020) The mechanisms shaping CA2 pyramidal neuron action potential bursting induced by muscarinic acetylcholine receptor activation. *Journal of General Physiology* 152:e201912462.

Robinson NTM, Descamps LAL, Russell LE, Buchholz MO, Bicknell BA, Antonov GK, Lau JYN, Nutbrown R, Schmidt-Hieber C, Häusser M (2020) Targeted activation of hippocampal place cells drives memory-guided spatial behavior. *Cell* 183:1586–1599, e10.

Roggenhofer E, Fidzinski P, Shor O, Behr J (2013) Reduced threshold for induction of LTP by activation of dopamine D1/D5 receptors at hippocampal CA1–subiculum synapses. *PLoS One* 8:e62520.

Rollenhagen A, Lübke J (2010) The mossy fiber bouton: the "common" or the "unique" synapse? *Frontiers in Synaptic Neuroscience* 2:2.

Rollenhagen A, Satzler K, Rodriguez EP, Jonas P, Frotscher M, Lübke JHR (2007) Structural determinants of transmission at large hippocampal mossy fiber synapses. *Journal of Neuroscience* 27:10434–10444.

Rolls ET (1996) A theory of hippocampal function in memory. *Hippocampus* 6:601–620.

Rolls ET (2013) The mechanisms for pattern completion and pattern separation in the hippocampus. *Frontiers in Systems Neuroscience* 7:74.

Ropert N (1988) Inhibitory action of serotonin in CA1 hippocampal neurons in vitro. *Neuroscience* 26:69–81.

Ropireddy D, Scorcioni R, Lasher B, Buzsáki G, Ascoli GA (2011) Axonal morphometry of hippocampal pyramidal neurons semiautomatically reconstructed after in vivo labeling in different CA3 locations. *Brain Structure and Function* 216:1–15.

Roth BL (2016) DREADDs for Neuroscientists. *Neuron* 89:683–694.

Rovira-Esteban L, Hájos N, Nagy GA, Crespo C, Nacher J, Varea E, Blasco-Ibáñez JM (2020) Semilunar granule cells are the primary source of the perisomatic excitatory innervation onto parvalbumin-expressing interneurons in the dentate gyrus. *ENeuro* 7:ENEURO.0323-19.2020.

Rowland DC, Obenhaus HA, Skytøen ER, Zhang Q, Kentros CG, Moser EI, Moser M-B (2018) Functional properties of stellate cells in medial entorhinal cortex layer II. *ELife* 7:e36664.

Rowland DC, Roudi Y, Moser M-B, Moser EI (2016) Ten years of grid cells. *Annual Review of Neuroscience* 39:19–40.

Roy DS, Kitamura T, Okuyama T, Ogawa SK, Sun C, Obata Y, Yoshiki A, Tonegawa S (2017) Distinct neural circuits for the formation and retrieval of episodic memories. *Cell* 170:1000–1012, e19.

Royeck M, Horstmann M-T, Remy S, Reitze M, Yaari Y, Beck H (2008) Role of axonal NaV1.6 sodium channels in action potential initiation of CA1 pyramidal neurons. *Journal of Neurophysiology* 100:2361–2380.

Royer S, Zemelman BV, Losonczy A, Kim J, Chance F, Magee JC, Buzsáki G (2012) Control of timing, rate and bursts of hippocampal place cells by dendritic and somatic inhibition. *Nature Neuroscience* 15:769–775.

Rudy B, McBain CJ (2001) Kv3 channels: voltage-gated K+ channels designed for high-frequency repetitive firing. *Trends in Neurosciences* 24:517–526.

Sahu G, Turner RW (2021) The molecular basis for the calcium-dependent slow afterhyperpolarization in CA1 hippocampal pyramidal neurons. *Frontiers in Physiology* 12:759707.

Salin PA, Scanziani M, Malenka RC, Nicoll RA (1996) Distinct short-term plasticity at two excitatory synapses in the hippocampus. *Proceedings of the National Academy of Sciences* 93:13304.

Sambandan S, Sauer J-F, Vida I, Bartos M (2010) Associative plasticity at excitatory synapses facilitates recruitment of fast-spiking interneurons in the dentate gyrus. *Journal of Neuroscience: The Official Journal of the Society for Neuroscience* 30:11826–11837.

Sammons RP, Parthier D, Stumpf A, Schmitz D (2019) Electrophysiological and molecular characterization of the parasubiculum. *Journal of Neuroscience* 39:8860–8876.

Sammons RP, Tzilivaki A, Schmitz D (2021) Local microcircuitry of PaS shows distinct and common features of excitatory and inhibitory connectivity. *Cerebral Cortex* 32:76–92.

Santoro B, Chen S, Luthi A, Pavlidis P, Shumyatsky GP, Tibbs GR, Siegelbaum SA (2000) Molecular and functional heterogeneity of hyperpolarization-activated pacemaker channels in the mouse CNS. *Journal of Neuroscience: The Official Journal of the Society for Neuroscience* 20:5264–5275.

Santoro B, Liu DT, Yao H, Bartsch D, Kandel ER, Siegelbaum SA, Tibbs GR (1998) Identification of a gene encoding a hyperpolarization-activated pacemaker channel of brain. *Cell* 93:717–729.

Sargolini F, Fyhn M, Hafting T, McNaughton BL, Witter MP, Moser M-B, Moser EI (2006) Conjunctive representation of position, direction, and velocity in entorhinal cortex. *Science* 312:758–762.

Sauer J-F, Strüber M, Bartos M (2015) Impaired fast-spiking interneuron function in a genetic mouse model of depression. *ELife* 4:e04979.

Savanthrapadian S, Meyer T, Elgueta C, Booker SA, Vida I, Bartos M (2014) Synaptic properties of SOM- and CCK-expressing cells in dentate gyrus interneuron networks. *Journal of Neuroscience: The Official Journal of the Society for Neuroscience* 34:8197–8209.

Scharfman H (1991) Dentate hilar cells with dendrites in the molecular layer have lower thresholds for synaptic activation by perforant path than granule cells. *Journal of Neuroscience* 11:1660.

Scharfman HE (1993) Characteristics of spontaneous and evoked EPSPs recorded from dentate spiny hilar cells in rat hippocampal slices. *Journal of Neurophysiology* 70:742–757.

Scharfman HE (1995) Electrophysiological diversity of pyramidal-shaped neurons at the granule cell layer/hilus border of the rat dentate gyrus recorded in vitro. *Hippocampus* 5:287–305.

Scharfman HE (2007) The CA3 "backprojection" to the dentate gyrus. *Progress in Brain Research* 163:627–637.

Scharfman HE (2016) The enigmatic mossy cell of the dentate gyrus. *Nature Reviews Neuroscience* 17:562–575.

Scharfman HE, Kunkel DD, Schwartzkroin PA (1990) Synaptic connections of dentate granule cells and hilar neurons: results of paired intracellular recordings and intracellular horseradish peroxidase injections. *Neuroscience* 37:693–707.

Scharfman H, Schwartzkroin P (1988) Electrophysiology of morphologically identified mossy cells of the dentate hilus recorded in guinea pig hippocampal slices. *Journal of Neuroscience* 8:3812.

Schikorski T, Stevens CF (1997) Quantitative ultrastructural analysis of hippocampal excitatory synapses. *Journal of Neuroscience* 17:5858–5867.

Schmidt-Hieber C, Jonas P, Bischofberger J (2004) Enhanced synaptic plasticity in newly generated granule cells of the adult hippocampus. *Nature* 429:184–187.

Schmidt-Hieber C, Jonas P, Bischofberger J (2007) Subthreshold dendritic signal processing and coincidence detection in dentate gyrus granule cells. *Journal of Neuroscience* 27:8430–8441.

Schmidt-Hieber C, Nolan MF (2017) Synaptic integrative mechanisms for spatial cognition. *Nature Neuroscience* 20:1483–1492.

Schmitz D, Schuchmann S, Fisahn A, Draguhn A, Buhl EH, Petrasch-Parwez E, Dermietzel R, Heinemann U, Traub RD (2001) Axo-axonal coupling: a novel mechanism for ultrafast neuronal communication. *Neuron* 31:831–840.

Schwartzkroin PA (1977) Further characteristics of hippocampal CA1 cells in vitro. *Brain Research* 128:53–68.

Schwartzkroin PA, Slawsky M (1977) Probable calcium spikes in hippocampal neurons. *Brain Research* 135:157–161.

Seeger G, Brauer K, Härtig W, Brückner G (1994) Mapping of perineuronal nets in the rat brain stained by colloidal iron hydroxide histochemistry and lectin cytochemistry. *Neuroscience* 58:371–388.

Sekulić V, Chen T-C, Lawrence JJ, Skinner FK (2015) Dendritic distributions of I h channels in experimentally-derived multi-compartment models of oriens-lacunosum/moleculare (O-LM) hippocampal interneurons. *Frontiers in Synaptic Neuroscience* 7:2.

Senzai Y, Buzsáki G (2017) Physiological properties and behavioral correlates of hippocampal granule cells and mossy cells. *Neuron* 93:691–704, e5.

Shah MM, Migliore M, Brown DA (2011) Differential effects of Kv7 (M-) channels on synaptic integration in distinct subcellular compartments of rat hippocampal pyramidal neurons. *Journal of Physiology* 589:6029–6038.

Shalinsky MH, Magistretti J, Ma L, Alonso AA (2002) Muscarinic activation of a cation current and associated current noise in entorhinal-cortex layer-II neurons. *Journal of Neurophysiology* 88:1197–1211.

Sharp PE (1996) Multiple spatial/behavioral correlates for cells in the rat postsubiculum: multiple regression analysis and comparison to other hippocampal areas. *Cerebral Cortex* 6:238–259.

Sharp PE (2006) Subicular place cells generate the same "map" for different environments: comparison with hippocampal cells. *Behavioural Brain Research* 174:206–214.

Sharp PE, Green C (1994) Spatial correlates of firing patterns of single cells in the subiculum of the freely moving rat. *Journal of Neuroscience: The Official Journal of the Society for Neuroscience* 14:2339–2356.

Sheffield ME, Dombeck DA (2019) Dendritic mechanisms of hippocampal place field formation. *Current Opinion in Neurobiology* 54:1–11.

Sheffield MEJ, Adoff MD, Dombeck DA (2017) Increased prevalence of calcium transients across the dendritic arbor during place field formation. *Neuron* 96:490–504.

Sheffield MEJ, Best TK, Mensh BD, Kath WL, Spruston N (2011) Slow integration leads to persistent action potential firing in distal axons of coupled interneurons. *Nature Neuroscience* 14:200–207.

Sheffield MEJ, Dombeck DA (2015) Calcium transient prevalence across the dendritic arbour predicts place field properties. *Nature* 517:200–204.

Sheffield MEJ, Edgerton GB, Heuermann RJ, Deemyad T, Mensh BD, Spruston N (2013) Mechanisms of retroaxonal barrage firing in hippocampal interneurons. *Journal of Physiology* 591:4793–4805.

Shigemoto R, Kinoshita A, Wada E, Nomura S, Ohishi H, Takada M, Flor PJ, Neki A, Abe T, Nakanishi S, et al. (1997) Differential presynaptic localization of metabotropic glutamate receptor subtypes in the rat hippocampus. *Journal of Neuroscience: The Official Journal of the Society for Neuroscience* 17:7503–7522.

Shor OL, Fidzinski P, Behr J (2009) Muscarinic acetylcholine receptors and voltage-gated calcium channels contribute to bidirectional synaptic plasticity at CA1-subiculum synapses. *Neuroscience Letters* 449:220–223.

Sik A, Penttonen M, Ylinen A, Buzsáki G (1995) Hippocampal CA1 interneurons: an in vivo intracellular labeling study. *Journal of Neuroscience: The Official Journal of the Society for Neuroscience* 15:6651–6665.

Simonnet J, Eugène E, Cohen I, Miles R, Fricker D (2013) Cellular neuroanatomy of rat presubiculum. *European Journal of Neuroscience* 37:583–597.

Simonnet J, Fricker D (2018) Cellular components and circuitry of the presubiculum and its functional role in the head direction system. *Cell and Tissue Research* 373:541–556.

Simons SB, Caruana DA, Zhao M, Dudek SM (2012) Caffeine-induced synaptic potentiation in hippocampal CA2 neurons. *Nature Neuroscience* 15:23–25.

Simons SB, Escobedo Y, Yasuda R, Dudek SM (2009) Regional differences in hippocampal calcium handling provide a cellular mechanism for limiting plasticity. *Proceedings of the National Academy of Sciences of the United States of America* 106:14080–14084.

Siwani S, França ASC, Mikulovic S, Reis A, Hilscher MM, Edwards SJ, Leão RN, Tort ABL, Kullander K (2018) OLMα2 cells bidirectionally modulate learning. *Neuron* 99:404–412, e3.

Slomianka L, Amrein I, Knuesel I, Sørensen JC, Wolfer DP (2011) Hippocampal pyramidal cells: the reemergence of cortical lamination. *Brain Structure and Function* 216:301–317.

Slomianka L, Geneser FA (1991) Distribution of acetylcholinesterase in the hippocampal region of the mouse: I. Entorhinal area, parasubiculum, retrosplenial area, and Presubiculum. *Journal of Comparative Neurology* 303:339–354.

Slomianka L, Geneser FA (1997) Postnatal development of zinc-containing cells and neuropil in the hippocampal region of the mouse. *Hippocampus* 7:321–340.

Sloviter RS (1991) Feedforward and feedback inhibition of hippocampal principal cell activity evoked by perforant path stimulation: GABA-mediated mechanisms that regulate excitability in vivo. *Hippocampus* 1:31–40.

Sloviter RS, Dichter MA, Rachinsky TL, Dean E, Goodman JH, Sollas AL, Martin DL (1996) Basal expression and induction of glutamate decarboxylase GABA in excitatory granule cells of the rat and monkey hippocampal dentate gyrus. *Journal of Comparative Neurology* 373:593–618.

Smith AS, Avram SKW, Cymerblit-Sabba A, Song J, Young WS (2016) Targeted activation of the hippocampal CA2 area strongly enhances social memory. *Molecular Psychiatry* 21:1–8.

Sodickson DL, Bean BP (1996) GABAB receptor-activated inwardly rectifying potassium current in dissociated hippocampal CA3 neurons. *Journal of Neuroscience* 16:6374.

Soltesz I (1995) Brief history of cortico-hippocampal time with a special reference to the direct entorhinal input to CA1. *Hippocampus* 5:120–124.

Somogyi J, Baude A, Omori Y, Shimizu H, El Mestikawy S, Fukaya M, Shigemoto R, Watanabe M, Somogyi P (2004) GABAergic basket cells expressing cholecystokinin contain vesicular glutamate transporter type 3 (VGLUT3) in their synaptic terminals in hippocampus and isocortex of the rat. *European Journal of Neuroscience* 19:552–569.

Somogyi P, Klausberger T (2005) Defined types of cortical interneurone structure space and spike timing in the hippocampus. *J Physiology* 562:9–26.

Somogyi P (1977) A specific "axo-axonal" interneuron in the visual cortex of the rat. *Brain Research* 136:345–350.

Soriano E, Frotscher M (1989) A GABAergic axo-axonic cell in the fascia dentata controls the main excitatory hippocampal pathway. *Brain Research* 503:170–174.

Soussi R, Zhang N, Tahtakran S, Houser CR, Esclapez M (2010) Heterogeneity of the supramammillary-hippocampal pathways: evidence for a unique GABAergic neurotransmitter phenotype and regional differences. *European Journal of Neuroscience* 32:771–785.

Spruston N (2008) Pyramidal neurons: dendritic structure and synaptic integration. *Nature Reviews Neuroscience* 9:206–221.

Spruston N, Jaffe DB, Williams SH, Johnston D (1993) Voltage- and space-clamp errors associated with the measurement of electrotonically remote synaptic events. *Journal of Neurophysiology* 70:781–802.

Spruston N, Johnston D (1992) Perforated patch-clamp analysis of the passive membrane properties of three classes of hippocampal neurons. *Journal of Neurophysiology* 67:508–529.

Spruston N, Schiller Y, Stuart GJ, Sakmann B (1995) Activity-dependent action potential invasion and calcium influx into hippocampal CA1 dendrites. *Science* 268:297–300.

Srinivas KV, Buss EW, Sun Q, Santoro B, Takahashi H, Nicholson DA, Siegelbaum SA (2017) The dendrites of CA2 and CA1 pyramidal neurons differentially regulate information flow in the cortico-hippocampal circuit. *Journal of Neuroscience* 37:3276–3293.

Staff NP, Jung HY, Thiagarajan T, Yao M, Spruston N (2000) Resting and active properties of pyramidal neurons in subiculum and CA1 of rat hippocampus. *Journal of Neurophysiology* 84:2398–2408.

Steward O, Scoville SA (1976) Cells of origin of entorhinal cortical afferents to the hippocampus and fascia dentata of the rat. *Journal of Comparative Neurology* 169:347–370.

Strange BA, Witter MP, Lein ES, Moser EI (2014) Functional organization of the hippocampal longitudinal axis. *Nature Reviews Neuroscience* 15:655–669.

Strüber M, Jonas P, Bartos M (2015) Strength and duration of perisomatic GABAergic inhibition depend on distance between synaptically connected cells. *Proceedings of the National Academy of Sciences of the United States of America* 112:1220–1225.

Strüber M, Sauer J-F, Jonas P, Bartos M (2017) Distance-dependent inhibition facilitates focality of gamma oscillations in the dentate gyrus. *Nature Communications* 8:758.

Stuart GJ, Sakmann B (1994) Active propagation of somatic action potentials into neocortical pyramidal cell dendrites. *Nature* 367:69–72.

Stuart GJ, Spruston N (2015) Dendritic integration: 60 years of progress. *Nature Neuroscience* 18:1713–1721.

Sugar J, Moser M (2019) Episodic memory: neuronal codes for what, where, and when. *Hippocampus* 29:1190–1205.

Suh J, Rivest AJ, Nakashiba T, Tominaga T, Tonegawa S (2011) Entorhinal cortex layer III input to the hippocampus is crucial for temporal association memory. *Science* 334:1415–1420.

Sun C, Kitamura T, Yamamoto J, Martin J, Pignatelli M, Kitch LJ, Schnitzer MJ, Tonegawa S (2015) Distinct speed dependence of entorhinal island and ocean cells, including respective grid cells. *Proceedings of the National Academy of Sciences* 112:9466.

Sun GJ, Sailor KA, Mahmood QA, Chavali N, Christian KM, Song H, Ming G (2013) Seamless reconstruction of intact adult-born neurons by serial end-block imaging reveals complex axonal guidance and development in the adult hippocampus. *Journal of Neuroscience* 33:11400.

Sun Q, Sotayo A, Cazzulino AS, Snyder AM, Denny CA, Siegelbaum SA (2017a). Proximodistal heterogeneity of hippocampal CA3 pyramidal neuron intrinsic properties, connectivity, and reactivation during memory recall. *Neuron* 95:656–672, e3.

Sun Q, Srinivas KV, Sotayo A, Siegelbaum SA (2014) Dendritic Na(+) spikes enable cortical input to drive action potential output from hippocampal CA2 pyramidal neurons. *ELife* 3:7750.

Sun W, Advani M, Spruston N, Saxe A, Fitzgerald JE (2021) Organizing memories for generalization in complementary learning systems. *Neuroscience* 26:1438–1448.

Sun Y, Grieco SF, Holmes TC, Xu X (2017b). Local and long-range circuit connections to hilar mossy cells in the dentate gyrus. *Eneuro* 4:ENEURO.0097-17.2017.

Sürmeli G, Marcu DC, McClure C, Garden DLF, Pastoll H, Nolan MF (2015) Molecularly defined circuitry reveals input-output segregation in deep layers of the medial entorhinal cortex. *Neuron* 88:1040–1053.

Svoboda K, Tank DW, Denk W (1996) Direct measurement of coupling between dendritic spines and shafts. *Science* 272:716–719.

Swanson LW (1982) The projections of the ventral tegmental area and adjacent regions: a combined fluorescent retrograde tracer and immunofluorescence study in the rat. *Brain Research Bulletin* 9:321–353.

Swanson LW, Wyss JM, Cowan WM (1978) An autoradiographic study of the organization of intrahippocampal association pathways in the rat. *Journal of Comparative Neurology* 181:681–715.

Szabadics J, Tamás G, Soltesz I (2007) Different transmitter transients underlie presynaptic cell type specificity of GABAA,slow and GABAA,fast. *Proceedings of the National Academy of Sciences of the United States of America* 104:14831–14836.

Szabadics J, Varga C, Molnár G, Oláh S, Barzó P, Tamás G (2006) Excitatory effect of GABAergic axo-axonic cells in cortical microcircuits. *Science* 311:233–235.

Szabo GG, Du X, Oijala M, Varga C, Parent JM, Soltesz I (2017) Extended interneuronal network of the dentate gyrus. *Cell Reports* 20:1262–1268.

Szabó GG, Holderith N, Gulyás AI, Freund TF, Hájos N (2010) Distinct synaptic properties of perisomatic inhibitory cell types and their different modulation by cholinergic receptor activation in the CA3 region of the mouse hippocampus. *European Journal of Neuroscience* 31:2234–2246.

Takács VT, Freund TF, Gulyás AI (2008) Types and synaptic connections of hippocampal inhibitory neurons reciprocally connected with the medial septum. *European Journal of Neuroscience* 28:148–164.

Takahashi H, Magee JC (2009) Pathway interactions and synaptic plasticity in the dendritic tuft regions of CA1 pyramidal neurons. *Neuron* 62:102–111.

Takeuchi T, Duszkiewicz AJ, Sonneborn A, Spooner PA, Yamasaki M, Watanabe M, Smith CC, Fernández G, Deisseroth K, Greene RW, et al. (2016) Locus coeruleus and dopaminergic consolidation of everyday memory. *Nature* 537:357–362.

Takumi Y, Ramírez-León V, Laake P, Rinvik E, Ottersen OP (1999) Different modes of expression of AMPA and NMDA receptors in hippocampal synapses. *Nature Neuroscience* 2:618–624.

Talley EM, Solorzano G, Lei Q, Kim D, Bayliss DA (2001) CNS distribution of members of the two-pore-domain (KCNK) potassium channel family. *Journal of Neuroscience* 21:7491–7505.

Tamamaki N (1997) Organization of the entorhinal projection to the rat dentate gyrus revealed by DiI anterograde labeling. *Experimental Brain Research Experimentelle Hirnforschung Expérimentation Cérébrale* 116:250–258.

Tamamaki N, Abe K, Nojyo Y (1988) Three-dimensional analysis of the whole axonal arbors originating from single CA2 pyramidal neurons in the rat hippocampus with the aid of a computer graphic technique. *Brain Research* 452:255–272.

Tamamaki N, Nojyo Y (1993) Projection of the entorhinal layer II neurons in the rat as revealed by intracellular pressure-injection of neurobiotin. *Hippocampus* 3:471–480.

Williams SR, Mitchell SJ (2008) Direct measurement of somatic voltage clamp errors in central neurons. *Nature Neuroscience* 11:790–798.

Williams SR, Stuart GJ (2000) Site independence of EPSP time course is mediated by dendritic I(h) in neocortical pyramidal neurons. *Journal of Neurophysiology* 83:3177–3182.

Williams SR, Wozny C, Mitchell SJ (2007). The back and forth of dendritic plasticity. *Neuron* 56:947–953.

Williams TE, Meshul CK, Cherry NJ, Tiffany NM, Eckenstein FP, Woodward WR (1996) Characterization and distribution of basic fibroblast growth factor-containing cells in the rat hippocampus. *Journal of Comparative Neurology* 370:147–158.

Wilson MA, McNaughton BL (1993) Dynamics of the hippocampal ensemble code for space. *Science* 261:1055–1058.

Wilson MA, McNaughton BL (1994) Reactivation of hippocampal ensemble memories during sleep. *Science* 265:676–679.

Winnubst J, Bas E, Ferreira TA, Wu Z, Economo MN, Edson P, Arthur BJ, Bruns C, Rokicki K, Schauder D, et al. (2019) Reconstruction of 1,000 projection neurons reveals new cell types and organization of long-range connectivity in the mouse brain. *Cell* 179:268–281, e13.

Winter SS, Clark BJ, Taube JS (2015) Disruption of the head direction cell network impairs the parahippocampal grid cell signal. *Science* 347:870–874.

Witter MP (2007a) Intrinsic and extrinsic wiring of CA3: indications for connectional heterogeneity. *Learning and Memory* 14:705–713.

Witter MP (2007b) The perforant path: projections from the entorhinal cortex to the dentate gyrus. *Progress in Brain Research* 163:43–61.

Wittner L, Henze D, Zaborszky L, Buzsaki G (2007) Three-dimensional reconstruction of the axon arbor of a CA3 pyramidal cell recorded and filled in vivo. *Brain Structure & Function* 212:75–83.

Wittner L, Huberfeld G, Clémenceau S, Eross L, Dezamis E, Entz L, Ulbert I, Baulac M, Freund TF, Maglóczky Z, et al. (2009) The epileptic human hippocampal cornu ammonis 2 region generates spontaneous interictal-like activity in vitro. *Brain: A Journal of Neurology* 132:3032–3046.

Wong RK, Prince DA (1978) Participation of calcium spikes during intrinsic burst firing in hippocampal neurons. *Brain Research* 159:385–390.

Wood ER, Dudchenko PA, Robitsek RJ, Eichenbaum H (2000) Hippocampal neurons encode information about different types of memory episodes occurring in the same location. *Neuron* 27:623–633.

Woods NI, Vaaga CE, Chatzi C, Adelson JD, Collie MF, Perederiy JV, Tovar KR, Westbrook GL (2018) Preferential targeting of lateral entorhinal inputs onto newly integrated granule cells. *Journal of Neuroscience* 38:5843.

Wouterlood FG, van Haeften T, Eijkhoudt M, Baks-te-Bulte L, Goede PH, Witter MP (2004) Input from the presubiculum to dendrites of layer-V neurons of the medial entorhinal cortex of the rat. *Brain Research* 1013:1–12.

Wozny C, Knopp A, Lehmann T-N, Heinemann U, Behr J (2005) The subiculum: a potential site of ictogenesis in human temporal lobe epilepsy. *Epilepsia* 46(Suppl 5):17–21.

Wu X, Morishita W, Beier KT, Heifets BD, Malenka RC (2021) 5-HT modulation of a medial septal circuit tunes social memory stability. *Nature* 599:96–101.

Wulff P, Ponomarenko AA, Bartos M, Korotkova TM, Fuchs EC, Bähner F, Both M, Tort ABL, Kopell NJ, Wisden W, et al. (2009) Hippocampal theta rhythm and its coupling with gamma oscillations require fast inhibition onto parvalbumin-positive interneurons. *The Proceedings of the National Academy of Sciences U S A* 106:3561–3566.

Wyss JM, Swanson LW, Cowan WM (1979) Evidence for an input to the molecular layer and the stratum granulosum of the dentate gyrus from the supramammillary region of the hypothalamus. *Anatomy and Embryology* 156:165–176.

Wyszynski M, Kharazia V, Shanghvi R, Rao A, Beggs AH, Craig AM, Weinberg R, Sheng M (1998) Differential regional expression and ultrastructural localization of alpha-actinin-2, a putative NMDA receptor-anchoring protein, in rat brain. *Journal of Neuroscience: The Official Journal of the Society for Neuroscience* 18:1383–1392.

Yamada J, Jinno S (2015) Subclass-specific formation of perineuronal nets around parvalbumin-expressing GABAergic neurons in Ammon's horn of the mouse hippocampus. *Journal of Comparative Neurology* 523:790–804.

Yamada-Hanff J, Bean BP (2015) Activation of *I* h and TTX-sensitive sodium current at subthreshold voltages during CA1 pyramidal neuron firing. *Journal of Neurophysiology* 114:2376–2389.

Yamamoto M, Marshall P, Hemmendinger LM, Boyer AB, Caviness VS (1988) Distribution of glucuronic acid-and-sulfate-containing glycoproteins in the central nervous system of the adult mouse. *Neuroscience Research* 5:273–298.

Yao Z, van Velthoven CTJ, Nguyen TN, Goldy J, Sedeno-Cortes AE, Baftizadeh F, Bertagnolli D, Casper T, Chiang M, Crichton K, et al. (2021b) A taxonomy of transcriptomic cell types across the isocortex and hippocampal formation. *Cell* 184:3222–3241, e26.

Yeckel MF, Berger TW (1995) Monosynaptic excitation of hippocampal CA1 pyramidal cells by afferents from the entorhinal cortex. *Hippocampus* 5:108–114.

Ylinen A, Bragin A, Nádasdy Z, Jandó G, Szabó I, Sik A, Buzsáki G (1995) Sharp wave-associated high-frequency oscillation (200 Hz) in the intact hippocampus: network and intracellular mechanisms. *Journal of Neuroscience: The Official Journal of the Society for Neuroscience* 15:30–46.

Yoder RM, Clark BJ, Taube JS (2011) Origins of landmark encoding in the brain. *Trends in Neurosciences* 34:561–571.

Yoder RM, Taube JS (2011) Projections to the anterodorsal thalamus and lateral mammillary nuclei arise from different cell populations within the postsubiculum: implications for the control of head direction cells. *Hippocampus* 21:1062–1073.

Yoshida M, Hasselmo ME (2009) Persistent firing supported by an intrinsic cellular mechanism in a component of the head direction system. *Journal of Neuroscience* 29:4945–4952.

Young WS, Li J, Wersinger SR, Palkovits M (2006) The vasopressin 1b receptor is prominent in the hippocampal area CA2 where it is unaffected by restraint stress or adrenalectomy. *Neuroscience* 143:1031–1039.

Yuan M, Meyer T, Benkowitz C, Savanthrapadian S, Ansel-Bollepalli L, Foggetti A, Wulff P, Alcami P, Elgueta C, Bartos M (2017) Somatostatin-positive interneurons in the dentate gyrus of mice provide local- and long-range septal synaptic inhibition. *ELife* 6:e21105.

Yuste R, Bonhoeffer T (2001) Morphological changes in dendritic spines associated with long-term synaptic plasticity. *Annual Review of Neuroscience* 24:1071–1089.

Zander J-F, Münster-Wandowski A, Brunk I, Pahner I, Gómez-Lira G, Heinemann U, Gutiérrez R, Laube G, Ahnert-Hilger G (2010) Synaptic and vesicular coexistence of VGLUT and VGAT in selected excitatory and inhibitory synapses. *Journal of Neuroscience* 30:7634–7645.

Zeisel A, Hochgerner H, Lönnerberg P, Johnsson A, Memic F, van der Zwan J, Häring M, Braun E, Borm LE, La Manno G, et al. (2018) Molecular architecture of the mouse nervous system. *Cell* 174:999–1014, e22.

Zeisel A, Muñoz-Manchado AB, Codeluppi S, Lönnerberg P, La Manno G, Juréus A, Marques S, Munguba H, He L, Betsholtz C, et al. (2015) Brain structure. Cell types in the mouse cortex and hippocampus revealed by single-cell RNA-seq. *Science* 347:1138–1142.

Zhang L, Hernández VS (2013) Synaptic innervation to rat hippocampus by vasopressin-immuno-positive fibres from the hypothalamic supraoptic and paraventricular nuclei. *Neuroscience* 228:139–162.

Zhang X, Schlögl A, Jonas P (2020) Selective routing of spatial information flow from input to output in hippocampal granule cells. *Neuron* 107:1212–1225, e7.

Zhao C, Teng EM, Summers RG, Ming G, Gage FH (2006) Distinct morphological stages of dentate granule neuron maturation in the adult mouse hippocampus. *Journal of Neuroscience* 26:3.

Zhao M, Choi Y-S, Obrietan K, Dudek SM (2007) Synaptic plasticity (and the lack thereof) in hippocampal CA2 neurons. *Journal of Neuroscience: The Official Journal of the Society for Neuroscience* 27:12025–12032.

Zhao X, Hsu C-L, Spruston N (2022) Rapid synaptic plasticity contributes to a learned conjunctive code of position and choice-related information in the hippocampus. *Neuron* 110:96–108, e4.

Zhao X, Lein ES, He A, Smith SC, Aston C, Gage FH (2001) Transcriptional profiling reveals strict boundaries between hippocampal subregions. *Journal of Comparative Neurology* 441:187–196.

Zhao X, Wang Y, Spruston N, Magee JC (2020) Membrane potential dynamics underlying context-dependent sensory responses in the hippocampus. *Nature Neuroscience* 23:881–891.

Ziv Y, Burns LD, Cocker ED, Hamel EO, Ghosh KK, Kitch LJ, Gamal AE, Schnitzer MJ (2013) Long-term dynamics of CA1 hippocampal place codes. *Nature Neuroscience* 16:264–266.

6

Synaptic Function

Dimitri M. Kullmann and Kirill E. Volynski

6.1 Overview: structure and function

Ever since Sherrington coined the term "synapse" (from the Greek "hold together"), this structure has attracted intense interest for several reasons. First, the information passing through the synapses supplied by an individual neuron reflects the outcome of its integrative functions. Second, with some notable exceptions it acts as a one-way "valve," transmitting information from the pre- to the postsynaptic neuron. Third, different forms of plasticity of synaptic transmission are implicated in fast computation and information processing in the brain, and are the leading candidate cellular substrates of memory formation and storage. This chapter reviews the fundamental operation of synaptic transmission and addresses some of the ways that individual synapses in the hippocampus are specialized to transmit and process signals and encode a history of their recent activity. It also provides the physiological context to Chapter 8, which examines the function of many of the molecules underlying synaptic transmission. The mechanisms of induction and expression of long-term changes in synaptic strength are addressed in Chapter 10.

Although the hippocampus has provided extensive information on the mechanisms by which neurons communicate with one another, the fundamental principles underlying synaptic transmission were originally elucidated at the mammalian or arthropod neuromuscular junction. Indeed, many of the mechanisms underlying the trafficking of presynaptic vesicles are shared with other intracellular membrane-bound compartments and are even present in prokaryotes. We therefore start by summarizing some general features that are shared with other synapses. We then examine the various types of hippocampal synapse (classified anatomically) to see how their functional properties differ and how these distinct characteristics shed light on their roles.

For the purpose of this chapter, a synapse is taken to represent the specialized structural and functional unit that is composed of one or more contiguous synaptic specializations occurring at the interface between two neurons (the presynaptic and postsynaptic partners). Thus, a single synapse can contain multiple neurotransmitter release sites and postsynaptic specializations where receptors detect the released neurotransmitter. However, a pair of pre- and postsynaptic neurons can also be connected via more than one synapse. Although this definition of a synapse is primarily morphological, it should be borne in mind that major insights into synaptic function have relied principally on electrophysiological, pharmacological, optical, and biochemical methods, often in the absence of histological reconstruction of the underlying elements.

Not all communication between neurons is via synapses: some neurotransmitters are released from axonal varicosities in the absence of postsynaptic specialization. The fact that receptors are sometimes relatively remote from the site of release of their endogenous ligands (e.g., monoamines, peptides, acetylcholine) has been taken as evidence that two distinct forms of signaling exist: (1) "point-to-point" or "wiring" transmission at synapses and (2) a more diffuse "spillover," "extrasynaptic," or "volume" transmission mediated by diffusion of neuroactive substances through the extracellular space. As is argued below, the distinction between these concepts is blurred by the existence of numerous types of receptors at variable distances from the release sites of their endogenous agonists. Neurons can also exert effects on their neighbors via mechanisms that do not involve neurotransmitters at all, for instance via field effects or gap junctions. "Electrical" synapses consisting of gap junctions act as relatively low-impedance pathways that permit the passive flow of electrical signals among connected neurons (Connors and Long, 2004; Pereda, 2014). They can also permit ions to flow down their electrochemical gradients, thereby dissipating their local accumulation and depletion. Finally, not all hippocampal synapses are formed between neurons: morphological and electrophysiological evidence supports the existence of excitatory synapses between hippocampal neurons and a subset of oligodendrocyte precursors (Bergles et al., 2000).

6.1.1 Synaptic ultrastructure

The stages of synaptic transmission can be broken down into neurotransmitter release from a presynaptic specialization, diffusion of the neurotransmitter across the synaptic cleft, and activation of postsynaptic receptors (Figure 6.1). These phenomena must be understood in the context of the detailed ultrastructure of the synapse.

The electron micrograph in Figure 6.2 illustrates some features of hippocampal synapses. The pre- and postsynaptic elements are separated by a synaptic cleft. This cleft is often narrower (~ 20–40 nm) than the gap separating nonsynaptic membranes and appears relatively dense, reflecting the presence of a "basal substance" containing intercellular adhesion molecules. These molecules, some of which are described in detail in Chapter 8, are thought to contribute

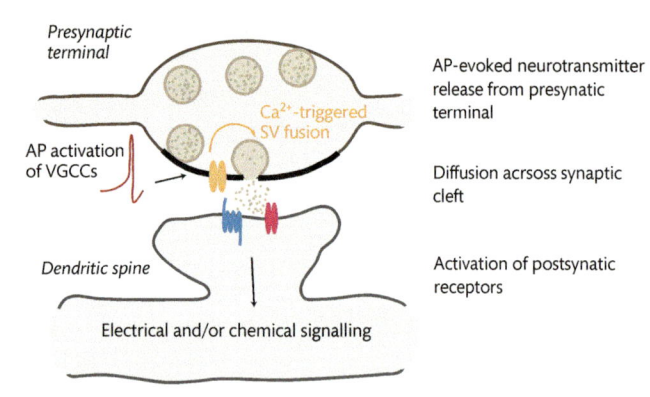

Presynaptic terminal

AP activation of VGCCs

Ca^{2+}-triggered SV fusion

Dendritic spine

AP-evoked neurotransmitter release from presynatic terminal

Diffusion acrsoss synaptic cleft

Activation of postsynatic receptors

Electrical and/or chemical signalling

Figure 6.1 Key stages of synaptic transmission. When an action potential reaches a presynaptic terminal (or, more generally, a presynaptic bouton) it depolarizes the presynaptic membrane, leading to activation of VGCCs located in the vicinity of release-ready vesicles docked at the active zone. Ca^{2+} influx into the terminal activates vesicular release sensors and triggers fusion of synaptic vesicles ("SV fusion") with the plasma membrane, and release of neurotransmitters into the synaptic cleft. Neurotransmitter molecules diffuse across the synaptic cleft and activate postsynaptic ionotropic and metabotropic receptors, resulting in downstream electrical and chemical signaling in the postsynaptic cell. The whole process occurs on a timescale of a few milliseconds.

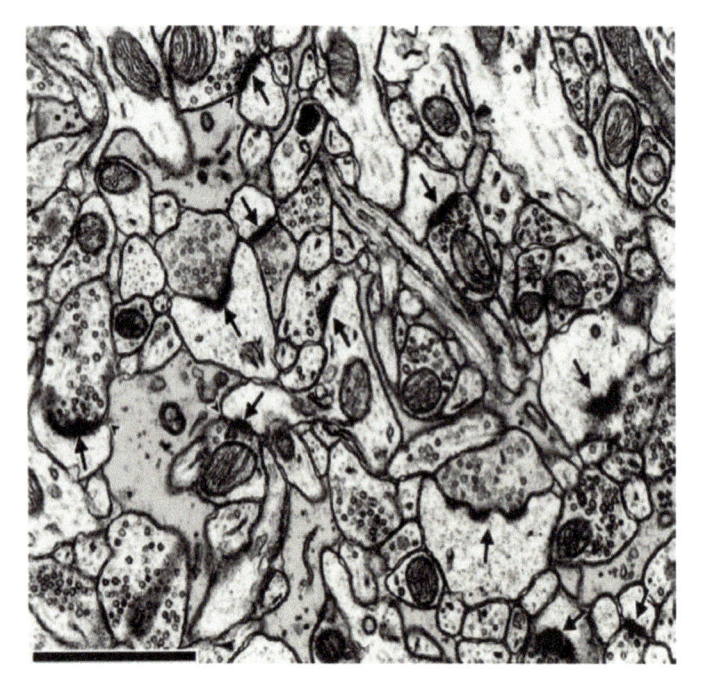

Figure 6.2 Fine structure of the hippocampal neuropil. Arrows point to individual asymmetrical (glutamatergic) synapses in a section taken from the stratum radiatum of CA1 in the rat. The presynaptic boutons contain numerous vesicles, which are frequently clustered close to membrane specializations (the active zone). A proportion of "docked" vesicles are in contact with the presynaptic membrane and are thought to represent the readily releasable pool of synaptic vesicles that are immediately ready for exocytosis. The electron-dense area is the postsynaptic density, which distinguishes these synapses from numerically less abundant symmetrical (inhibitory) synapses (see Figure 6.14). Astrocyte profiles, lacking vesicles and postsynaptic densities, contact the synaptic perimeter in some cases (arrowheads). Scale bar = 1 μm. (Source: Ventura and Harris, 1999, with permission.)

to the formation, stabilization, and plasticity of synapses (see also Chapter 10).

The presynaptic element is readily identified in electron micrographs by the presence of vesicles containing neurotransmitter molecules. It is generally agreed that synaptic vesicles are the morphological counterpart of the "quanta" that make up postsynaptic signals (see below). These synaptic vesicles are generally of uniform diameter (~ 45 nm) and are aggregated near a membrane specialization that can be identified ultrastructurally as a thickening. This specialization is termed the active zone (AZ), which is the site of exocytosis; and the thickening reflects the presence of multiple membrane-associated proteins (the cytomatrix of the AZ) that mediate and regulate synaptic vesicle exo- and endocytosis. Among them are proteins that recruit synaptic vesicles and voltage-gated Ca^{2+} channels (VGCCs) to the release sites, proteins that mediate synaptic vesicle fusion, transsynaptic cell adhesion proteins that coordinate the precise alignment of the pre- and postsynaptic specializations, and proteins involved in sorting of synaptic vesicle proteins during endocytosis (Imig et al., 2014; Michel et al., 2015; Biederer et al., 2017). In addition, endoplasmic reticulum and mitochondria, whose functions include acting as Ca^{2+} buffers, are frequently present presynaptically, reflecting the importance of controlling the cytoplasmic Ca^{2+} concentration and the energetic demands of transmitter release (principally represented by the work required for transmitter synthesis, vesicular packaging, exocytosis, and reuptake) (Devine and Kittler, 2018).

On the postsynaptic side, there is also an increased membrane density visible in electron micrographs. Synapses with obvious postsynaptic thickening are known as asymmetrical, or type I, synapses (Gray, 1959). The "postsynaptic density" (PSD) is a relatively detergent-resistant structure containing glutamate receptors and associated macromolecules (discussed in Chapter 8). Some synapses lack this specialization and are therefore known as "symmetrical," or type II, synapses. Such synapses are principally GABAergic and are concentrated around the soma and axonal initial segment of principal neurons but are also found on dendrites and on inhibitory neurons.

In addition to the pre- and postsynaptic elements that make up a synapse, astrocyte processes commonly occur in close proximity to the synaptic cleft. They have a critical role in clearing neurotransmitter from the extracellular space. They also buffer extracellular ion transients and provide for the energetic demands of synaptic transmission. Although astrocyte processes are often thought of as an obligatory partner, making up the third element of a "tripartite" synapse, their presence at excitatory and inhibitory synapses is much more haphazard in the hippocampus than in other regions of the brain, such as the cerebellar cortex. Indeed, many synapses in the hippocampus are not contacted by an obvious astrocytic process at all (Ventura and Harris, 1999).

6.2 Presynaptic release of neurotransmitters

Anatomical, biochemical, and electrophysiological methods have converged on the following general account of neurotransmitter exocytosis (Südhof, 2013; Kaeser and Regehr, 2014) (Figure 6.1). When an action potential invades the nerve terminal, it depolarizes the presynaptic membrane, leading to transient (~1–2 ms) activation of presynaptic VGCCs, which are concentrated in and around the AZ. Ca^{2+} influx leads to a brief local increase in the intracellular Ca^{2+} concentration in the immediate vicinity of the VGCCs. This is known as a Ca^{2+} nano- or microdomain, which can reach 10–100 μM and then collapses on a timescale of milliseconds through buffering, diffusion, and extrusion of Ca^{2+} ions. This signal activates vesicular Ca^{2+} release sensors and triggers exocytosis of vesicles docked at the AZ. The majority of neurotransmitter release at central synapses occurs with high temporal precision, completing within less than several milliseconds of action potential invasion, and is therefore defined as fast or "synchronous." However, a significant proportion of vesicular exocytosis also occurs on a longer timescale of several tens to hundreds of milliseconds and is defined as "asynchronous" release. The relative importance of synchronous and asynchronous neurotransmitter release varies among different types of synapses, and the differential synapse-specific kinetics of exocytosis are thought to be important for information processing in the brain (Hefft and Jonas, 2005; Luo and Südhof, 2017; Volynski and Krishnakumar, 2018). Synaptic vesicles can also fuse with the presynaptic membrane in the absence of action potentials, albeit at a very low rate. The postsynaptic signals generated by such spontaneous exocytosis are often known as miniature postsynaptic currents or potentials, or "minis". This chapter primarily focuses on action potential-evoked neurotransmitter release. As for spontaneous release, we refer the reader to recent reviews describing the underlying mechanisms and possible physiological functions or this mode of exocytosis (Kavalali, 2015; Schneggenburger and Rosenmund, 2015). As we discuss below, it is generally agreed that synchronous and asynchronous modes of neurotransmitter exocytosis rely principally on the same core vesicular fusion machinery but are regulated by different Ca^{2+} signals and release sensors. Synaptic vesicle exocytosis is balanced by endocytosis that leads to the retrieval of vesicular proteins from the plasma membrane and to the formation of functional vesicles that are re-filled with neurotransmitters. In the next sections, we will consider the molecular mechanisms that underlie the major stages of the synaptic vesicle cycle and the different modes of transmitter release.

6.2.1 Vesicular fusion machinery

Considerable effort has gone into dissecting the molecular identity of the proteins underlying regulated synaptic vesicle exocytosis

(Jahn and Fasshauer, 2012; Südhof, 2013; Kaeser and Regehr, 2014; Rizo, 2022).

At the core of the synaptic vesicle fusion machinery are the SNARE proteins. The acronym derives from the identification of proteins that interact with NSF (N-ethylmaleimide-sensitive factor): SNAPs (soluble NSF adaptor proteins), hence SNAREs for SNAP REceptors (Söllner et al., 1993).

Synaptic vesicle fusion is mediated by a complex of three SNAREs: syntaxin 1 and SNAP-25 (synaptosomal-associated protein, 25kDa), which are anchored to the presynaptic plasma membrane, and vesicle-associated membrane protein (VAMP, also called synaptobrevin), associated with the synaptic vesicle membrane. SNARE proteins are actually central to the trafficking of all intracellular membrane-bound vesicles, and fall into two categories, v-SNARES on the transport vesicles (e.g., synaptic vesicles) and t-SNAREs on the target membrane (e.g., presynaptic membrane). The specificity of interaction between different types of v- and t-SNAREs determining how the contents of membrane-bound compartments are sorted and trafficked. Formation of the complex between v- and t-SNAREs provides the energy required for vesicular fusion (Söllner et al., 1993) (Figure 6.3). The α-helices of v- and t-SNAREs anchored in the two fusing membranes initially form a partially assembled trans-SNARE complex. Progressive assembly of this complex generates an inward force that pulls the two membranes together (Südhof and Rothman, 2009). A demonstration of the principal roles of SNAREs in synaptic vesicle exocytosis comes from in vitro fusion assays, whereby recombinant v- and t-SNARE proteins reconstituted into separate lipid bilayer vesicles can be shown to assemble into SNARE-pins (SNARE complexes linking two membranes), followed by fusion of the docked membranes (Weber et al., 1998).

6.2.2 The readily releasable pool of vesicles

In contrast to the constitutive trafficking of intracellular organelles, synaptic vesicle exocytosis is coordinated with action potential firing, generally with millisecond precision. This synchrony relies on a pool of presynaptic vesicles that are docked at the AZ in close proximity (20–100 nm) to VGCCs. Some of these vesicles are ready to fuse immediately after sensing action potential-associated Ca^{2+} influx and therefore are called the readily releasable pool (RRP)

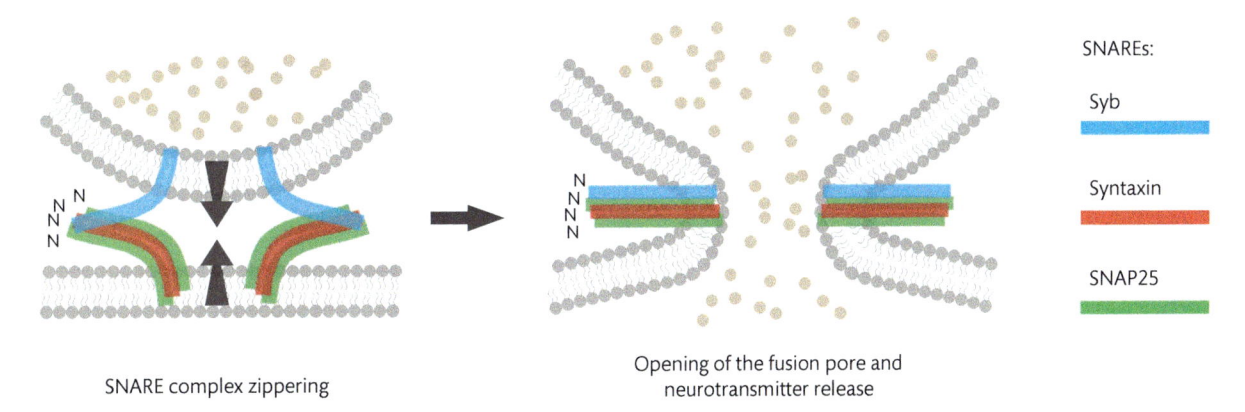

SNARE complex zippering

Opening of the fusion pore and neurotransmitter release

SNAREs:

Syb

Syntaxin

SNAP25

Figure 6.3 The zippering model of SNARE-catalyzed membrane fusion. Three alpha helices anchored in the target membrane (two copies of SNAP-25 and one of syntaxin) assemble with the fourth alpha helix anchored in the vesicular membrane (Synaptobrevin, Syb) to form a partially assembled trans-SNARE complex or SNAREpin. Zippering begins at the N-termini and progresses toward the C-termini, bringing the membranes together, until the membranes fuse and the SNAREs enter a low-energy state (the cis-SNARE complex). (Adapted from Südhof and Rothman, 2009.)

of vesicles (Rosenmund and Stevens, 1996; Kaeser and Regehr, 2014, 2017).

The current consensus is that RRP vesicles contain partially assembled ("primed" or "half-zippered") SNARE complexes (SNARE-pins) that are clamped in this state by two key molecules: the adapter protein complexin, and the Ca^{2+} release sensor synaptotagmin. Ca^{2+} binding to synaptotagmin molecules leads to release of the clamp, allowing SNARE-pins to fully zipper, thus synchronizing synaptic vesicle fusion to action potential-evoked Ca^{2+} influx (Südhof and Rothman, 2009; Jahn and Fasshauer, 2012; Kaeser and Regehr, 2014; Brunger et al., 2018; Volynski and Krishnakumar, 2018) (Figure 6.4).

The RRP is coordinated by a large multiprotein complex consisting of RIM proteins (Rab3-interacting molecules), RIM-BP (RIM binding protein), and Munc13. RIMs are multidomain proteins that are integral components of the cytomatrix at the presynaptic active zone. The RIM family contains seven members (encoded by four genes, *RIM1-4*) that bind most of the other AZ-enriched proteins and thus provide a molecular template for the spatial organization of the presynaptic release machinery (Mittelstaedt et al., 2010; Südhof, 2012; Michel et al., 2015). Figure 6.4 summarizes how RIM proteins are thought to promote formation of the RRP and regulate transmitter release. First, RIMs mediate vesicular docking by binding to the small GTP-binding proteins Rab3 and Rab27 that are located on the vesicles (Gracheva et al., 2008; Mittelstaedt et al., 2010; Südhof, 2012). Second, RIMs interact with and activate the multidomain protein Munc13, which acts as a priming factor. Munc13 is normally present as an inactive dimer. Binding of a RIM to the "C2A" domain of Munc13 breaks the Munc13 dimer and recruits Munc13 molecules to the active zone (L Deng et al., 2011). Third, RIMs and RIM-BPs bind to each other and to VGCCs. In this way VGCCs and RRP vesicles are brought into close proximity (less than 100 nm) (Han et al., 2011; Kaeser et al., 2011). The key role of RIMs in orchestrating transmitter release is underlined by the finding that their genetic deletion prevents most transmitter release by impairing synaptic vesicle priming, dislocating VGCCs from the active zone, and reducing presynaptic Ca^{2+} influx (L Deng et al., 2011; Han et al., 2011; Kaeser et al., 2011).

Interestingly, in contrast to in vitro reconstitution experiments, vesicle fusion at live synapses requires so-called SM proteins (Sec1/Munc18-like proteins) in addition to SNARE proteins (Südhof and Rothman, 2009; Südhof, 2013). Munc-18 is a multidomain cytosolic protein that was first identified because of its interaction with the synaptic t-SNARE syntaxin (Hata et al., 1993). This interaction was shown to negatively regulate the priming of synaptic vesicles (Dulubova et al., 1999). Prior to synaptic vesicle priming, the t-SNARE syntaxin-1 is present in the presynaptic membrane in an inactive ("closed") conformation bound to Munc18. In this closed conformation, the SNARE motif of syntaxin is hidden from interaction with the other SNAREs, namely SNAP25 and synaptobrevin. Munc13 acts as a critical priming factor. Binding of Munc13 to the syntaxin-1/Munc18 complex catalyzes a conformational switch, activates syntaxin by exposing its SNARE motif, and thus initiates formation of the SNARE-pin (Augustin et al., 1999; Richmond et al., 2001; Varoqueaux et al., 2002; Ma et al., 2013). Paradoxically, genetic deletion of Munc-18, or of its yeast homologue Sec1p, completely abolishes vesicular fusion (Grote et al., 2000; Verhage et al., 2000).

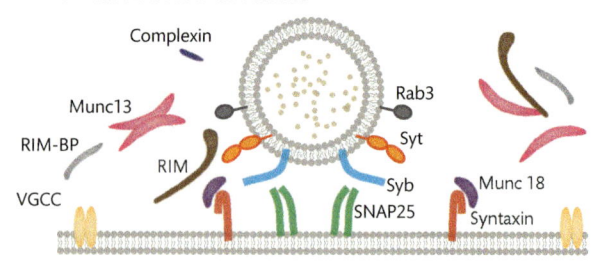

Major presynatpic proteins involved in formation of RRP of vesicles

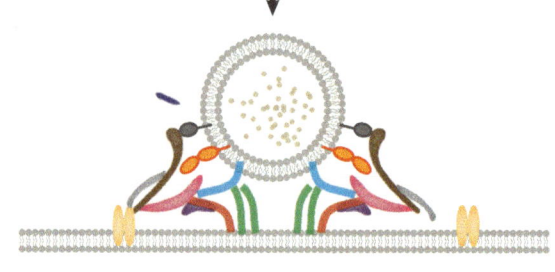

Step 1. Vesicle docking and activation of syntaxin by Munc 13

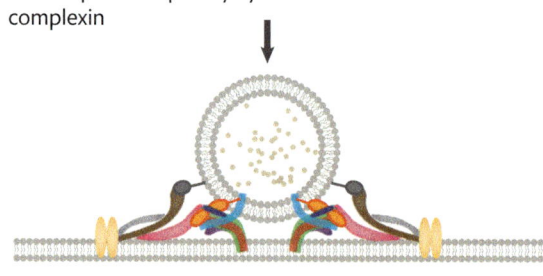

Step 2. Vesicle priming - formation of SNARE-pins clamped by Syt and complexin

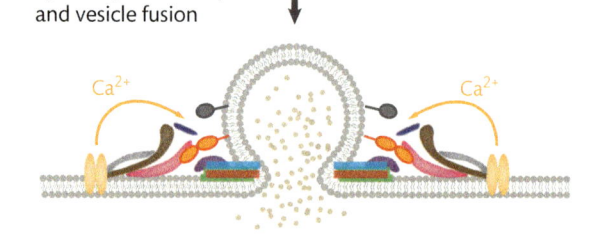

Step 3. Ca^{2+}- triggered removal of the Syt/complexin clamp and vesicle fusion

Figure 6.4 Formation of RRP vesicles. Major presynaptic proteins that are involved in the formation of RRP of vesicles: RIM, RIM-BP, VGCC, Munc13, Munc18, Rab3, synaptotagmin (Syt), complexin and the SNARE proteins SNAP 25, Syntaxin and Synaptobrevin (Syb).

Step 1. Synaptic vesicles are docked at the active zone via the interaction of RIM, Rab3 and Munc13. VGCC are tethered to docked synaptic vesicles via their interaction with RIM and RIM-BP proteins. At rest the SNARE binding motif is inhibited by binding to Munc18. The syntaxin/Munc18 complex is activated by Munc13 leading to opening of the syntaxin SNARE binding site.

Step 2. During vesicle priming, partially assembled SNARE complexes are formed (SNARE-pins) and arrested (clamped) in this state by binding to synaptotagmin (Syt) and complexin molecules (see Figure. 6-6 below that describes the structural organization of clamped SNARE-pins).

Step 3. Ca^{2+} binding by synaptotagmin molecules leads to removal of the fusion clamp, full SNARE zippering and synaptic vesicle fusion with the presynaptic membrane.

It was later demonstrated that in addition to binding of monomeric syntaxin, Munc18 also binds to SNARE-pins via a distinct structural motif (Dulubova et al., 2007). This binding appears to be a prerequisite for facilitating the final stage of synaptic vesicle fusion; however, precisely how Munc18 promotes exocytosis remains unknown. Among hypotheses are that Munc18 binding to SNARE-pins catalyzes lipid mixing between the fusing membranes (Südhof, 2013) and that Munc18 spatially organizes partially assembled SNARE-pins around the fusion site (Südhof and Rothman, 2009). Finally, complexin and synaptotagmin molecules bind to partially assembled SNARE-pins and clamp them in a half-zippered state until the arrival of the Ca^{2+} signal (Südhof, 2013; Kaeser and Regehr, 2014; Brunger et al., 2018; Volynski and Krishnakumar, 2018).

In addition to RIMs, Munc13, Munc18, complexins and synaptotagmins, other presynaptic proteins have also been shown to contribute to the assembly and regulation of the RRP. These include CAPS (Ca^{2+}-dependent activator protein in secretion) (Jockusch et al., 2007) and ELKS—thus named because it is rich in glutamate (E), leucine (L), lysine (K), and serine (S) residues (Held et al., 2016).

In general, the number of RRP vesicles estimated using functional electrophysiological and imaging assays correlates with the number of docked vesicles at the AZ visualized using electron microscopy at different synapses, consistent with the principle that the RRP represents a subpopulation of docked vesicles (Südhof, 2013; Kaeser and Regehr, 2017). The ratio between fully primed RRP vesicles and morphologically docked vesicles, however, varies among synapses and also changes dynamically during repetitive neuronal activity (Miki et al., 2018; Neher and Brose, 2018).

Assuming that all vesicles within the RRP are equivalent, the average number of vesicles released per action potential can be expressed as $N_{rel} = m \times p_v$, where m is the RPP size and p_v is the average release probability of individual RRP vesicles. The relative probability of observing $0, 1, \ldots, m$ vesicles on a given trial is then described by a binomial distribution. Both the RRP size and the vesicular release probability vary extensively, not only among different types of synapses but also among synapses supplied by a single axon.

6.2.3 Presynaptic Ca^{2+} dynamics shapes the efficacy and kinetics of evoked neurotransmitter release

As mentioned above, at many synapses synchronous release of neurotransmitter is essentially complete within a millisecond of action potential arrival. This temporal precision depends on, first, the fast activation kinetics of VGCCs and their close proximity to the RRP vesicles at the AZ, resulting in a very rapid increase in the local cytoplasmic Ca^{2+} concentration (Figure 6.5), and second, the fast binding kinetics and activation of vesicular Ca^{2+} release sensors (synaptotagmins).

We will next consider the factors determining action potential-evoked presynaptic Ca^{2+} dynamics at vesicular release sites in greater detail. The VGCCs expressed at a given synapse clearly have a critical role. Of the various pharmacologically and biophysically defined classes, P/Q- and N-type channels (also known as $Ca_V2.1$ and $Ca_V2.2$, respectively) account for most of the Ca^{2+} influx that triggers evoked exocytosis (Dolphin and Lee, 2020). A third class of Ca^2 channels, R-type ($Ca_V2.3$), has a relatively smaller role at most synapses. Because of their high voltage threshold, all three types are mostly closed at resting potentials. They open rapidly on depolarization, but because their closure lags slightly behind action

potential repolarization, they are still able to carry Ca^{2+} flux when the presynaptic membrane potential has returned close to the resting value. The bulk of the Ca^{2+} influx triggering exocytosis therefore occurs during repolarization, at which time the inward driving force for Ca^{2+} ions is maximal. Interestingly, whereas both N- and P/Q-type channels contribute to triggering glutamate release at individual synapses, many GABAergic terminals appear to fall into two classes: those that rely mainly on N-type channels and those that predominantly use P/Q-type channels (Poncer et al., 1997). Some synapses equipped with N-type VGCCs are powerfully inhibited by neurotransmitters acting via presynaptic G-protein-coupled receptors such as endocannabinoids.

The relative localization of VGCCs and RRP vesicles is another key factor that determines the Ca^{2+} concentration profile determining exocytosis. The small size of the presynaptic AZ (~ 200–300 nm) makes it difficult to simultaneously visualize RRP vesicles and Ca^{2+} channels at central synapses. Nevertheless, freeze-fracture immunogold electron microscopy studies have demonstrated that $Ca_V2.1$ VGCCs, at both glutamatergic and GABAergic synapses, are nonrandomly distributed in the AZ, with a substantial proportion of channels located in small clusters (~ 40–80 nm), each containing tens of channels (Holderith et al., 2012; Althof et al., 2015; Nakamura et al., 2015). The number of such clusters correlates with the number of docking sites at the AZ (Miki et al., 2017). Interestingly, single fluorescence particle tracking experiments have shown that many VGCCs diffuse freely in the presynaptic membrane (Schneider et al., 2015), implying that the coupling distance between VGCCs and RRP vesicles is a dynamic parameter.

The average coupling distance can be estimated using a combination of electrophysiological recordings, pharmacological manipulations and computational modeling. The distinct properties of two Ca^{2+} chelators have proved especially useful: 1,2-bis(o-aminophenoxy)ethane-N,N,N′,N′-tetraacetic acid (BAPTA) has much faster binding kinetics than ethylene glycol-bis(β-aminoethyl ether)-N,N,N′,N′-tetraacetic acid (EGTA). Both chelators are available as acetoxymethyl esters to aid their intracellular accumulation. The principle underlying the use of EGTA/BAPTA to dissect Ca^{2+}-exocytosis coupling is illustrated in Figure 6.5. If RRP vesicles are located in close proximity to VGCCs (within ~10–20 nm), only the fast chelator BAPTA is able to intercept Ca^{2+} ions on their way to the vesicular release sensor and therefore inhibit neurotransmitter release. On the other hand, if VGCCs and RRP vesicles are separated by a greater distance (typically more than ~ 70–90 nm) then both BAPTA and EGTA are able to suppress the local Ca^{2+} transient seen by Ca^{2+} sensors, and therefore both chelators inhibit exocytosis (Eggermann et al., 2011). Synapses can thus be classified into two types: those with "tight" VGCC-release sensor coupling, where synchronous release is inhibited by millimolar concentrations of BAPTA but not EGTA, and those with "loose" coupling, where synchronous release is efficiently inhibited by both fast and slow chelators applied in the millimolar range. Based on this classification, transmitter release is triggered by "Ca^{2+} nanodomains" at synapses with tight coupling and by "Ca^{2+} microdomains" at synapses with loose coupling. GABAergic synapses between parvalbumin-positive interneurons and hippocampal granule cells exhibit tight coupling (Bucurenciu et al., 2008), while glutamatergic synapses between hippocampal mossy fiber boutons and CA3 pyramidal cells exhibit loose coupling (Vyleta and Jonas, 2014). Interestingly, the coupling distance can vary among synapses supplied by a single axon,

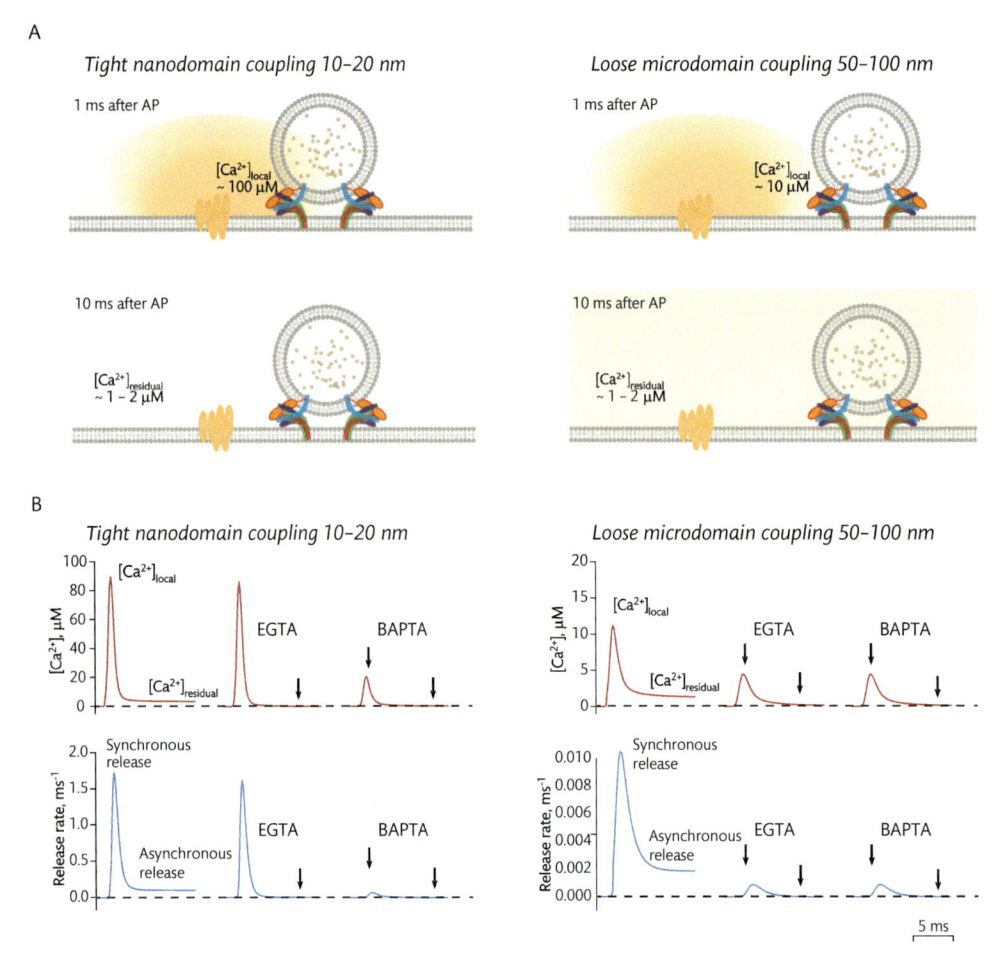

Figure 6.5 Presynaptic Ca^{2+} dynamics and action potential-evoked release. (A) Schematic representation of Ca^{2+} dynamics at vesicular release sites with tight nanodomain (left) and loose microdomain (right) coupling. During activation of VGCCs (top, ~ 0.5–1 ms after an action potential) the local Ca^{2+} concentration at release sites ([Ca^{2+}]$_{local}$) transiently reaches ~ 100 μM at synapses with tight coupling but only 10 – 20 μM at synapses with loose coupling. After VGCC closure, Ca^{2+} nano/microdomains around VGCCs quickly collapse and Ca^{2+} ions equilibrate throughout the presynaptic terminal. The global presynaptic Ca^{2+} concentration ([Ca^{2+}]$_{residual}$) does not return immediately to its resting value but instead remains elevated within the range of 1–2 μM for tens to hundreds of milliseconds. For simplicity only SNARE proteins, synaptotagmin, complexin, and VGCC are shown on the diagrams. (B) Schematic traces depicting the effects of slow (EGTA) and fast (BAPTA) Ca^{2+} buffers on Ca^{2+} dynamics at release sites and on synchronous and asynchronous exocytosis. EGTA inhibits the increase in [Ca^{2+}]$_{local}$ and therefore synchronous release only at synapses with loose coupling, whilst BAPTA suppresses [Ca^{2+}]$_{local}$ and synchronous release at both types of synapses. Both EGTA and BAPTA effectively suppress [Ca^{2+}]$_{residual}$ and asynchronous release.

contributing to a target-cell-specific adjustment of synaptic strength (Rozov et al., 2001). Furthermore, it is likely that at many synapses (e.g., between Schaffer collaterals and CA1 pyramidal cells) there is substantial heterogeneity among RRP vesicles in individual boutons, with some vesicles loosely and others tightly coupled to VGCCs (Mendonça et al., 2022).

The coupling distance is directly linked to the release probability of RRP vesicles (p_v). Vesicles at synapses with tight coupling normally have much higher p_v than those at synapses with loose coupling, with implications for short-term synaptic plasticity, as discussed below. Another difference is that far fewer VGCCs contribute to triggering exocytosis at synapses with tight than with loose coupling (Bucurenciu et al., 2010; Vyleta and Jonas, 2014; Chamberland et al., 2018). Furthermore, tight coupling increases the rate and precision of synchronous release (Bucurenciu et al., 2010) and decreases the ratio between synchronous and asynchronous release (see below).

Based on fluorescence imaging and computational modeling, it has been estimated that the local Ca^{2+} concentration

at release sites ([Ca^{2+}]$_{local}$) transiently reaches ~ 100 μM at synapses with tight coupling but only 10–20 μM at synapses with loose coupling (Helmchen et al., 1997; Bollmann et al., 2000; Schneggenburger and Neher, 2000; Scott and Rusakov, 2006; Bucurenciu et al., 2010; Eggermann and Jonas, 2011; Eggermann et al., 2011; Ermolyuk et al., 2013; Nakamura et al., 2015; Chamberland et al., 2018) (Figure 6.5). The curve relating transmitter release to extracellular Ca^{2+} is sigmoid, with a steep slope indicating a 2.3–3.5 power relationship at physiological Ca^{2+} concentrations (~ 1–2 mM). The vesicular release machinery itself has an even steeper (4.2–4.4 power) dependency on the intracellular Ca^{2+} concentration, as measured at the calyx of Held, a large glutamatergic synapse in the auditory brainstem that allows direct patch clamp access to the presynaptic terminal (Schneggenburger and Forsythe, 2006). The difference between the dependence of release on extracellular and intracellular Ca^{2+} is accounted for by nonlinear properties of Ca^{2+} diffusion and buffering, and saturation of permeation via VGCCs.

Presynaptic VGCCs close within ~ 1 to 2 ms of membrane repolarization following an action potential. This is followed by a rapid collapse of Ca^{2+} nano/microdomains around VGCCs as Ca^{2+} ions equilibrate throughout the presynaptic terminal (Figure 6.5) (Matveev et al., 2004; Kaeser and Regehr, 2014; Timofeeva and Volynski, 2015). However, the bulk intraterminal Ca^{2+} concentration does not return immediately to its resting value (~ 20–50 nM), but instead remains elevated (~ 1–2 μM) before slowly decreasing through binding to endogenous buffers, sequestration in presynaptic organelles such as mitochondria, and extrusion by transporters. The slow decay rate of presynaptic Ca^{2+} is determined by the initial magnitude of Ca^{2+} influx, the presynaptic terminal morphology, and the efficiency and abundance of endogenous Ca^{2+} buffers and transporters. Typically, the residual Ca^{2+} concentration ($[Ca^{2+}]_{residual}$) decays on a timescale of tens to hundreds of milliseconds following a single action potential, but may take seconds or even tens of seconds after a high-frequency burst of activity. The elevated presynaptic Ca^{2+} concentration has two important consequences. First, it underlies the delayed asynchronous component of action-potential-evoked transmitter release (Figure 6.5). Second, it has a key role in shaping short-term synaptic plasticity (see section 6.3.3 below).

Asynchronous release is potentiated during and after bursts of presynaptic neuronal firing (in line with the prominent increase of $[Ca^{2+}]_{residual}$). Delayed asynchronous release has an important role in shaping communication between neurons by modulating the probability of postsynaptic neuron firing (Hefft and Jonas, 2005; Luo and Südhof, 2017; Deng et al., 2020). The balance between synchronous and asynchronous varies among different types of synapses. For example, cholecystokinin (CCK)-expressing interneurons in the dentate gyrus release GABA in a highly asynchronous manner, in contrast to parvalbumin (PV)-positive interneurons (Hefft and Jonas, 2005). Furthermore, the balance between synchronous and asynchronous release can be differentially tuned among synaptic outputs of a single pyramidal cell and depends in part on the identity of the postsynaptic target cells (Deng et al., 2020; Mendonça et al., 2022).

6.2.4 Synaptotagmins–presynaptic Ca^{2+} release sensors

Synchronous and asynchronous release modes are synergistically regulated by synaptotagmin Ca^{2+} sensor family members with distinct molecular properties. Among the synaptotagmins, four isoforms act as the main regulators of presynaptic release of neurotransmitters. Synaptotagmins 1, 2, and 9 (Syt1, Syt2, and Syt9) act as Ca^{2+} sensors for fast synchronous release. These isoforms have a relatively low Ca^{2+} affinity (~ 10–20 μM in the presence of membranes) and are therefore only activated within Ca^{2+} nano/microdomains ($[Ca^{2+}]_{local}$ in the range of 10–100 μM, see above) (Sugita et al., 2002; Xu et al., 2007). The slower high-affinity synaptotagmin 7 (Syt7, affinity ~1.5–5 μM) is also activated by the global elevation of $[Ca^{2+}]_{residual}$ and therefore has been implicated in the regulation of delayed asynchronous release and short-term synaptic plasticity (Bacaj et al., 2013; Jackman et al., 2016; Huson and Regehr, 2020).

Syt1, Syt2, and Syt9 isoforms are expressed at different types of synapses but have broadly similar molecular properties (Xu et al., 2007) (Figure 6.6). They are intrinsic vesicle proteins with a small luminal domain, a transmembrane domain, and a larger cytoplasmic part that contains two Ca^{2+}-binding C2A and C2B domains. Each C2 domain can bind 2–3 Ca^{2+} ions (Südhof, 2013). Syt7 has a similar domain organization but is primarily located in the presynaptic membrane and is ubiquitously expressed by neurons in the central nervous system (CNS) (Sugita et al., 2001). Upon Ca^{2+} binding, the surface loops adjacent to the Ca^{2+} binding sites on both C2A and C2B domains partially insert into the target membrane (Bai et al., 2004; Grushin et al., 2019). This membrane insertion is required for triggering of synaptic vesicle exocytosis (Rhee et al., 2005; Paddock et al., 2008, 2011). The C2A and C2B domains have distinct functions. While Ca^{2+} binding to the C2A domain of Syt1 facilitates synchronous release, activation of the C2B domain is absolutely essential (Mackler et al., 2002; Shin et al., 2009). In contrast, Ca^{2+} activation of the Syt7 C2A domain is critical for its role in the regulation of asynchronous release and short-term synaptic plasticity (Bacaj et al., 2013; Jackman et al., 2016).

Precisely how synaptotagmins trigger synaptic vesicle exocytosis remains the subject of debate. A prevailing view is that Ca^{2+} binding and membrane loop insertion of the C2 domains leads to the release of the fusion clamp and fast zippering of the SNARE complex, leading to fusion of the vesicular and presynaptic membranes on a submillisecond time scale (Südhof, 2013; Brunger et al., 2018; Volynski and Krishnakumar, 2018; Grushin et al., 2019). The crystal structure of SNARE/complexin/Syt1 provides direct insights into the possible structural organization of the clamped SNARE-pin architecture and suggests that each SNAREpin binds two synaptotagmin molecules (Figure 6.7) (Zhou et al., 2017; Brunger et al., 2018).

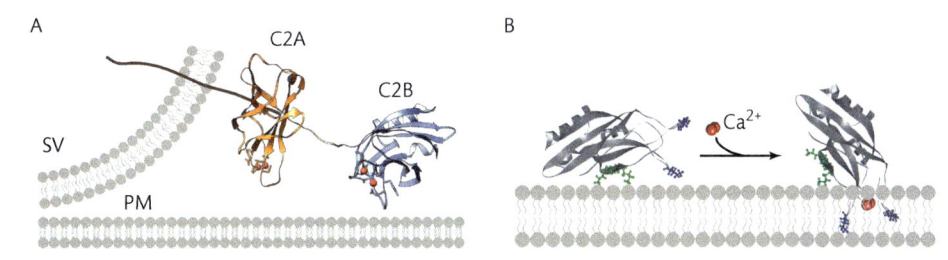

Figure 6.6 Domain structure and Ca^{2+} activation of synaptotagmins. (A) Syt1 is an intrinsic synaptic vesicle protein consisting of a small luminal domain, a transmembrane domain and a larger cytoplasmic part that contains two Ca^{2+}-binding C2A and C2B domains. Each C2 domain can bind 2–3 Ca^{2+} ions (red spheres). Structure of C2 domains is adapted from Lyubimov et al. (2016). (B) Molecular model showing Ca^{2+} activation of Syt1 C2B domain (updated from Bai et al., 2004). Upon binding of Ca^{2+} (red spheres) the adjacent surface loops (blue structures) partially insert into the target membrane which leads to reversal of the exocytosis clamp and synaptic vesicle fusion.

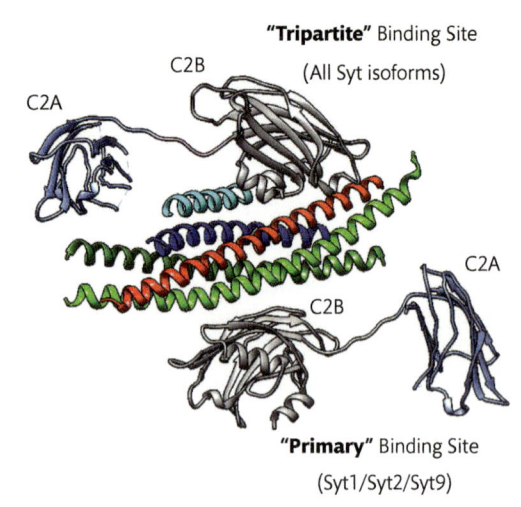

"Tripartite" Binding Site
(All Syt isoforms)

"Primary" Binding Site
(Syt1/Syt2/Syt9)

Figure 6.7 Structure of the SNARE complex in association with Synaptotagmin 1 and complexin. Two Syt1 molecules can bind to a single SNARE complex. Both Syt1 interactions are mediated by its C2B domain: Complexin (Cpx)-independent interfacing with the SNAP25 helices (green), termed the "primary" binding site, and Cpx-dependent, involving portions of helices derived from complexin (cyan), syntaxin (red) and VAMP2 (blue), termed the "tripartite" binding site. The "primary" interface is exclusively found on the low Ca^{2+} affinity fast release sensors (Syt1, Syt2 and Syt9), while the "tripartite" binding site is conserved among all synaptotagmin isoforms (including Syt7) and several other C2 domain proteins. The model is adapted from the crystal structure (Zhou et al., 2017) (PDB ID: 5W5C).

Although the energy of assembly of two or three SNAREpins is sufficient to trigger membrane fusion (Hua and Scheller, 2001; Sinha et al., 2011), under physiological conditions coordinated clamping and activation of a larger number of SNAREpins probably occurs, explaining the high Ca^{2+} cooperativity of exocytosis. Indeed, energetic considerations imply that simultaneous activation of multiple SNARE complexes on a given RRP vesicle is required to sustain the rate of synchronous release (Shi et al., 2012; Acuna et al., 2014). Furthermore, recent cryoelectron tomography analysis of docked synaptic-like vesicles in endocrine cells and cultured hippocampal neurons has revealed the presence of exactly six structures symmetrically arranged at the vesicle–plasma interface. These are likely to represent SNAREpins with bound regulatory proteins (X Li et al., 2019; Radhakrishnan et al., 2021).

6.2.5 Synaptic vesicle recycling and refilling with neurotransmitters

Once fusion has occurred, SNARE proteins must be dissociated and made available for another round of exocytosis. This step involves the soluble ATPase NSF and α-SNAP. The requirement for ATP hydrolysis probably reflects the energetically unfavorable reversal of the formation of the core complex (Chen and Scheller, 2001; Jahn et al., 2003). The vesicle membrane, together with the membrane-associated proteins (including the vesicular ATPase and transporters, v-SNAREs, and synaptotagmin) must also be endocytosed if full fusion has occurred.

In most nonneuronal cells endocytosis is predominantly a constitutive process. In contrast, synaptic vesicle endocytosis is tightly regulated by neuronal activity and is spatiotemporally coupled to exocytosis (Soykan et al., 2016; Xie et al., 2017; Maritzen and Haucke, 2018). Several modes of membrane retrieval have been

described at nerve terminals (Soykan et al., 2016; Kaempf and Maritzen, 2017; Watanabe and Boucrot, 2017; Gan and Watanabe, 2018) (Figure 6.8). These include a "kiss-and-run" mechanism, whereby the fusion pore opens only transiently, and full fusion, whereby the vesicle collapses followed by diffusion of vesicular proteins in the plasma membrane. After full fusion, vesicle membranes can be retrieved via clathrin-mediated endocytosis (CME) or clathrin-independent endocytosis (CIE) followed by reformation of synaptic vesicles by clathrin coats budding from endosomes. Finally, another mode of vesicle retrieval has been reported after intense presynaptic activity: fusion of multiple synaptic vesicles is followed by activity-dependent bulk endocytosis from distal sites. The balance between different modes of endocytosis depends on

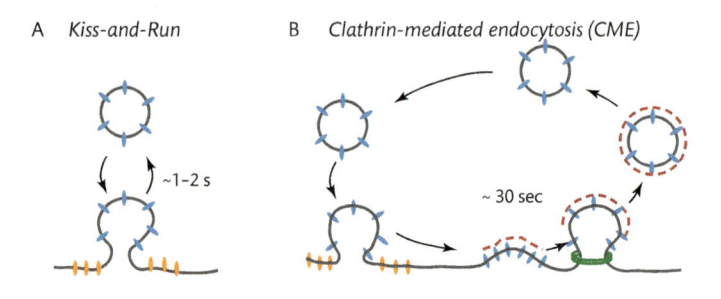

A   *Kiss-and-Run*   B   *Clathrin-mediated endocytosis (CME)*

~1-2 s   ~ 30 sec

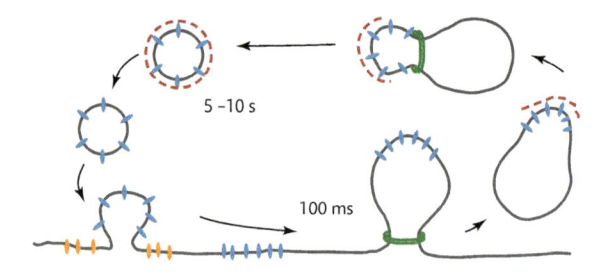

C   *Ultrafast endocytosis (UFE) and Clathrin-dependent SV reformation*

5 - 10 s

100 ms

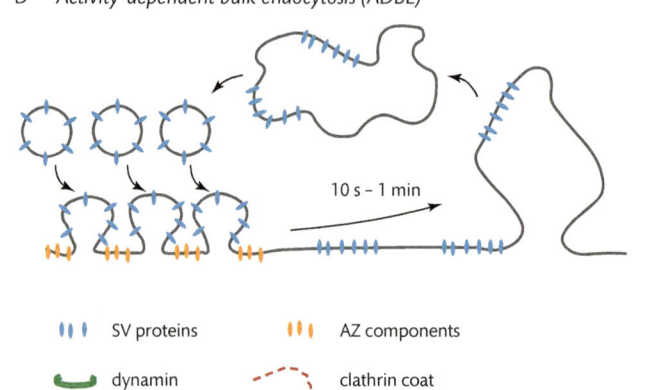

D   *Activity-dependent bulk endocytosis (ADBE)*

10 s – 1 min

SV proteins   AZ components

dynamin   clathrin coat

Figure 6.8 Modes of synaptic vesicle recycling. (a) Kiss-and-Run, transient opening and closure of the fusion pore. (b) Full fusion followed by diffusion of vesicular proteins to distal sites and clathrin mediated endocytosis (CME). (c) Full fusion followed by clathrin-independent ultrafast endocytosis at the periactive zone and clathrin/AP-2-mediated synaptic vesicle reformation from endosomal-like vacuoles. (d) Fusion of multiple vesicles followed by bulk membrane internalization at distal sites. At a later stage vesicles can be reformed from bulk endosomes. (The diagram is adapted from Soykan et al., 2016; Watanabe and Boucrot, 2017.)

the pattern of activity and temperature. Under physiological conditions, the CIE pathway predominates, operating on multiple timescales—from hundreds of milliseconds (ultrafast endocytosis, UFE) to tens of seconds (Kaempf and Maritzen, 2017; Watanabe and Boucrot, 2017; Gan and Watanabe, 2018).

Presynaptic terminals sort and recycle individual synaptic vesicle membrane proteins with high precision and efficiency (Takamori et al., 2006; Gauthier-Kemper et al., 2015; Kaempf and Maritzen, 2017). Indeed, alterations in vesicle protein composition compromise neurotransmission (Koo et al., 2015; Kaempf and Maritzen, 2017). Vesicle proteins disperse after exocytosis and then recluster at the periactive zone, assisted by the endocytosis adaptor proteins (Gimber et al., 2015; Kaempf and Maritzen, 2017), and then undergo either CIE or CME. The precise molecular mechanisms of clustering and sorting of vesicle proteins on the presynaptic membrane prior to endocytosis however remain poorly understood. Finally, coupling of exo- and endocytosis depends on preceding activity and is thought to be regulated by both an increase of $[Ca^{2+}]_{residual}$ and vesicle protein concentration on the presynaptic membrane (Maritzen and Haucke, 2018).

Neurotransmitter molecules are translocated from the cytoplasm into vesicles by specific transporters, which exploit a proton gradient formed by vesicular ATPases. The two principal vesicular amino acid neurotransmitters differ slightly in their uptake mechanisms. A family of proteins (VGLUT1-3, encoded by *SLC17A7*, *SLC17A7* and *SLC17A7*, respectively) mediate glutamate uptake by exchanging for protons, but also allow chloride ions that were taken up during endocytosis to escape into the cytoplasm (Martineau et al., 2017). In the case of GABA, vesicular uptake is mediated by VGAT (*SLC32A1*), with evidence for both GABA/H^+ exchange and GABA/Cl^- cotransport (Farsi et al., 2016).

6.3 Neurotransmitter diffusion and activation of postsynaptic receptors

Following release, neurotransmitter molecules diffuse across the cleft to activate postsynaptic receptors. Because the synaptic cleft spans only approximately 20 nm, the time taken by neurotransmitter molecules to reach the nearest possible postsynaptic receptors is negligible: assuming that neurotransmitter molecules diffuse freely in the extracellular space, they should reach most of the receptors in the synaptic cleft within 100 ps. However, although many receptors occur in the postsynaptic membrane opposite the active zone, others are further away. Several classes of receptors (considered in detail below) show distinct patterns of localization: in the presynaptic membrane within the synaptic cleft or in a perisynaptic halo around the synapse, either pre- or postsynaptically. To assess the functional role of these types of receptor, it is important to understand how the endogenous ligands reach them following release from presynaptic varicosities. The factors that determine the activation of these receptors are as follows.

- Amount of neurotransmitter released
- Temporal profile of release
- Distance from release site to receptors
- Diffusion coefficient (or diffusivity) of the neurotransmitter in the cleft and in the extracellular medium
- Diffusional obstacles

- Neurotransmitter transporters, their affinity and kinetics, and other binding sites
- Kinetics of the receptors

Astrocytes have an important role in determining receptor activation, because they frequently extend processes that contact the perimeter of the synaptic cleft and because they express transporters and receptors on their surface, which buffer and/or sequester the neurotransmitter molecules. A further role of astrocytes in the case of glutamate, is to convert it enzymatically to glutamine (see below).

6.3.1 Receptors and receptor activation

Receptors fall into two distinct classes: ionotropic and metabotropic. Ionotropic receptors, also known as ligand-gated ion channels, contain binding sites for neurotransmitters. Docking of one or more transmitter molecules causes the channel to open, allowing charged ions to travel down their electrochemical gradients. In the case of metabotropic receptors, ligand binding triggers an intracellular biochemical cascade beginning with dissociation of GTP-binding proteins (G proteins), hence their alternative name G-protein-coupled receptors (GPCRs). The identity of the G protein subunits that interact with a given metabotropic receptor, and of their downstream targets, determines the effect of ligand binding on neuronal excitability and other signaling cascades.

Ionotropic receptors generally occur postsynaptically, although they can also occur in axons and presynaptic membranes (MacDermott et al., 1999). Excitatory depolarizing signals mediated by ionotropic receptors take the form principally of an influx of Na^+ ions, accompanied by variable amounts of Ca^{2+} influx. K^+ ions are also able to permeate, but generally flow in the opposite direction. Glutamate receptors (see below) are the main mediators of postsynaptic depolarizing signals in the hippocampus. The postsynaptic ion flux constitutes the excitatory postsynaptic current (EPSC), whose size is determined by the membrane potential, the reversal potential for each ion species, its permeability through the receptor, and the mean number of receptor channels opening. The EPSC depolarizes the postsynaptic membrane, and gives rise to an excitatory postsynaptic potential (EPSP), which summates with other EPSPs and can lead to the opening of voltage-gated ion channels and activate regenerative currents. Such currents, mainly mediated by voltage-dependent Na^+ and Ca^{2+} channels, can depolarize the postsynaptic membrane to reach the threshold to trigger an action potential. Although the action potential is an all-or-nothing event, normally initiated in the axon initial segment, in many neurons regenerative depolarizing currents can also arise in dendrites (see Chapter 5).

Inhibitory ionotropic signals are mediated principally by $GABA_A$ receptors. Although glycine receptors also contribute to inhibition in spinal and brainstem neurons, they are not known to have an important role in the hippocampus. Inhibitory postsynaptic currents (IPSCs) are carried by Cl^- and HCO_3^- ions flowing down their electrochemical gradients. Because the permeability of $GABA_A$ receptors for Cl^- is greater than that for HCO_3^-, and the equilibrium potential for Cl^- is relatively negative, the IPSC generally hyperpolarizes the neuron, giving rise to an inhibitory postsynaptic potential (IPSP). Synaptic inhibition has two effects on neuronal excitability. First, it drives the membrane potential away from the threshold for activating regenerative depolarizing currents; and, second, by lowering the membrane resistivity it shunts EPSCs that would normally depolarize the neuron.

Although IPSPs and EPSPs contribute to the excitability of the neuron, they do not sum linearly because of several factors, addressed in Chapter 5. Briefly, voltage- and time-dependent electrical properties of dendrites cause synaptic currents to dissipate or amplify as they propagate, the results of which depend strongly on the initial spatial profile of the membrane voltage, on the geometric distribution of active synapses, and on the density and kinetics of a set of voltage-gated ion channels.

Metabotropic receptors (GPCRs) occur both pre- and postsynaptically, and have highly diverse effects depending on their G-protein coupling. Most such receptors exert their actions over a slower timescale, lasting up to seconds. Several hundred distinct GPCRs occur in the brain, and for many the endogenous ligands are not known. Such GPCRs are known as orphan receptors. G proteins, which mediate the immediate downstream consequences of GPCR activation, are heterotrimeric assemblies consisting of a $G\alpha$ subunit and a tightly bound $G\beta$-γ complex (Oldham and Hamm, 2006). In the resting state, GPCRs are bound on their intracellular aspect to both a $G\alpha$ subunit, which in turn binds a guanosine diphosphate (GDP) molecule, and to the $G\beta$-γ subunit complex. Agonist binding to GPCRs leads to an intracellular conformational change that leads to guanine triphosphate (GTP) being exchanged for GDP, and dissociation of both the $G\alpha$ subunit and the $G\beta$-γ complex. GPCRs can be classified into different classes according to their $G\alpha$ subunits, which themselves belong to different families. The $G\alpha_s$ family leads to activation of adenylate cyclase, while the $G\alpha_{i/o}$ family have the opposite effect (inhibition of adenylate cyclase). The $G\alpha_q$ family acts on phospholipase C-β (PLC). Another class of $G\alpha$ subunits activates small GTPases. The $G\beta$-γ complex also has downstream effects on signaling, in particular by modulating ion channels, and reassembly with the $G\alpha$ subunit also inhibits the actions of the latter.

As a general principle, activation of presynaptic GPCRs (mainly belonging to the $G\alpha_{i/o}$ class, usually shortened to $G_{i/o}$-coupled receptors) depresses neurotransmitter release (Huang and Thathiah, 2015). This effect is mediated in large part through $G_{\beta-\gamma}$-mediated modulation of presynaptic Ca^{2+} channels but also through an effect on SNARE proteins.

Postsynaptic GPCRs have numerous actions. The effector mechanisms include opening of G-protein-coupled inwardly rectifying K^+ (GIRK) channels, mediated by $G\beta$-γ subunits (Huang and Thathiah, 2015). This would normally hyperpolarize and therefore inhibit neurons. However, G_q-coupled receptors, such as muscarinic M1 and M3 receptors, typically have a net pro-excitatory effect: PLC, activated by the $G_{\alpha q}$ subunit, cleaves phosphatidylinositol 4,5 bisphosphate (PIP_2) to generate diacylglycerol (DAG) and inositol 1,4,5-trisphosphate (IP_3). The reduction in PIP_2 concentration leads to closure of M-type K^+ channels, resulting in membrane depolarization (Brown and Passmore, 2009), while IP_3 triggers Ca^{2+} release from intracellular stores, which itself may lead to regenerative Ca^{2+} release and more remote effects such as modulation of gene transcription (Berridge, 2016).

Receptor activation must eventually terminate. The most important mechanism that underlies this is rapid dissipation of the neurotransmitter pulse by diffusion into the large extracellular space, which can drop the concentration 100-fold within a few milliseconds. Neurotransmitter molecules are ultimately cleared by specific transporter proteins. Acetylcholine, ATP, and some neuroactive peptides can also be broken down by extracellular enzymes.

Although a complete neurotransmitter transport cycle takes tens or hundreds of milliseconds, some transporters (in particular for glutamate) are present in high concentrations close to synapses, and are able to quench a large fraction of neurotransmitter molecules diffusing out of the synaptic cleft (Danbolt, 2001). Neurotransmitter molecules dissociate from their receptors, thus returning them to an unbound state, leading to deactivation. Nevertheless, some receptors remain bound for several hundred milliseconds, long after the concentration of free neurotransmitters in the extracellular space has collapsed, because they bind neurotransmitter molecules with very high affinity. A further mechanism that contributes to the termination of receptor activation is desensitization: In the continued presence of agonist molecules, ionotropic receptors generally enter a closed state that is conformationally different from the unbound state. Desensitization of metabotropic receptors arises through several mechanisms, including phosphorylation by G-protein-coupled receptor kinases (GRKs). GRK-phosphorylated receptors then bind β-arrestin, which uncouples GPCRs from G proteins (Carmona-Rosas et al., 2018). Another phenomenon involves internalization.

6.3.2 Quantal transmission

The conventional view of synaptic function—originating from studies by Katz and coworkers at the neuromuscular junction—is that transmission is quantized; that is, repeated presynaptic action potentials give rise to postsynaptic signals that fluctuate from trial to trial among discrete levels. These discrete levels occur at integral multiples (0, 1, 2, . . .) of an underlying unit, the "quantum."

The quantal description of neurotransmission not only gives a powerful insight into the biophysics of transmitter release and receptor activation but also provides a shortcut for investigating the mechanisms of synaptic signaling modulation. Thus, factors that reduce or increase the presynaptic release of transmitter almost universally affect the average number of quanta released across a population of release sites (the quantal content m, which is the product of the number of available quanta n, and their average release probability p). Factors that modulate the state of the postsynaptic receptors alter the size of the response to an individual package of neurotransmitter (the quantal amplitude Q).

This model of transmission has received only partial support from studies in the CNS. As already hinted above, if exocytosis is incomplete or the neurotransmitter is discharged slowly, a single vesicle may give a graded postsynaptic effect, even if it originally contained a fixed amount of neurotransmitter. Moreover, nonuniformities in the distribution of receptors available to detect transmitter released at different synapses, or in the degree of distortion that the postsynaptic signals undergo as they propagate to the cell body, are likely to conceal any quantal structure in the amplitude fluctuations of postsynaptic signals recorded at the soma. Finally, unlike the neuromuscular junction, where a single presynaptic end-plate has a large number of relatively uniform, well-separated release sites, most hippocampal synapses probably contain only one or a few release sites (Schikorski and Stevens, 1997), which probably interact nonlinearly. Nevertheless, recordings of synaptic signals have reported large trial-to-trial fluctuations in the size of the postsynaptic response to activation of a single or a small number of presynaptic axons. In some cases, it has even been possible to discern clustering of postsynaptic response amplitudes at integral multiples of the unit value, perhaps reflecting the fortuitous case where underlying release events gave similar responses, and where they summed relatively linearly across the various active synapses or release sites (Kullmann and Nicoll, 1992). These cases probably represent only a small number of recordings but have helped shed light on the parameters that underlie transmission.

The more general finding is that, although transmission is stochastic and can even fail on occasion, EPSCs, EPSPs, IPSCs, and IPSPs tend not to cluster systematically at preferred amplitudes. It has nevertheless been possible to extract some information on the mechanisms of modulation of synaptic strength from examining the trial-to-trial variability of such signals. This application of quantal analysis relies on making a few assumptions, but some of them have been found to be reasonably robust. For instance, if it is assumed that failures of transmission reflect cases where the presynaptic action potential did not trigger exocytosis, it may be possible to use the frequency of such failures as an indirect witness of the state of the presynaptic terminal. That is, if a physiological or pharmacological event decreases the rate at which presynaptic action potentials elicit postsynaptic responses, it may be inferred that the presynaptic release probability has decreased. Other approaches rely on estimating the coefficient of variation of the postsynaptic signal. These approaches, however, must be used with caution. They have been at the center of a controversy surrounding the mechanisms of expression of long-term potentiation (see Chapter 10), and some of the disagreements can be attributed to unjustified assumptions about the underlying mechanisms.

6.3.3 Short-term plasticity

Implicit in the outline of quantal transmission given above is the assumption that action potentials repeatedly invading a presynaptic terminal trigger neurotransmitter release with a constant probability. In fact, synapses show numerous forms of memory of their activation history. Long-term potentiation and depression (LTP and LTD, respectively) persist for hours if not longer and are considered in detail in Chapter 10. There are, however, other forms of use-dependent plasticity that last up to a few minutes and that may play an equally important role in the second-to-second traffic of information through synapses. Phenomenologically, they are divided into increases and decreases in transmission: facilitation, augmentation, and potentiation on the one hand, and depression on the other (Zucker and Regehr, 2002). There is some redundancy in these terms. "Facilitation" describes the enhancement of transmission often seen following a preceding action potential. If the synapse is stimulated twice in rapid succession and the second response is larger than the first, the phenomenon is often referred to as "paired pulse facilitation." "Augmentation" refers to a gradual increase in synaptic strength with repeated stimulation. "Potentiation" (often referred to as posttetanic potentiation to distinguish it from long-term potentiation) requires a high-frequency train of stimuli for its induction and persists for up to a few minutes after the end of the train. (The "tetanus" that gives its name to posttetanic potentiation refers to the postsynaptic response observed during the high-frequency train, in which consecutive responses merge together, and which resembles the sustained muscle contraction that occurs when inhibition of motoneurons is compromised by tetanus toxin.)

Many synapses do not show these facilitatory phenomena and, instead, depress when repeatedly stimulated. At some hippocampal synapses early facilitation gives way to later depression with prolonged trains of stimulation.

These distinct patterns of short-term plasticity result from a large number of processes occurring principally in the presynaptic terminals (Zucker and Regehr, 2002). The following is an incomplete list of events that contribute to short-term plasticity.

1. Facilitation/augmentation/potentiation
   - If the presynaptic free Ca^{2+} concentration has not returned to baseline levels or if the occupancy of Ca^{2+} buffers is high, successive action potentials may give rise to larger increments of Ca^{2+}, thereby enhancing exocytosis.
   - High-affinity Ca^{2+} sensors (including Syt7) detect a slow buildup of residual Ca^{2+} in the presynaptic varicosity and contribute to triggering exocytosis.
   - Some presynaptic protein kinases activated with repeated Ca^2 influx may phosphorylate proteins involved in making vesicles available for exocytosis or in triggering exocytosis itself.

2. Depression
   - The RRP may become depleted.
   - Repeated depolarizing pulses inactivate presynaptic voltage-dependent Ca^{2+} channels, reducing the amount of Ca^{2+} entry following successive action potentials.
   - Depletion of extracellular Ca^{2+} from the restricted synaptic cleft may transiently reduce Ca^{2+} availability.
   - Presynaptic autoreceptors activated by released neurotransmitters decrease further transmitter release during subsequent action potentials.

The above list focuses on presynaptic mechanisms that contribute to short-term plasticity. However, postsynaptic mechanisms also contribute. In particular, depolarizing synaptic potentials can summate, leading to activation of regenerative currents in the postsynaptic dendrite. Interactions with dendritic action potentials further complicate the relation between voltage signals measured at the soma and presynaptic transmitter release: Orthodromically or antidromically propagating action potentials can either amplify or shunt synaptic potentials, depending on many variables, such as their temporal relation and the distribution of voltage-gated channels (Stuart and Häusser, 2001). Nonlinearities in the secondary message cascade may also amplify metabotropic receptor-mediated signals. Another postsynaptic mechanism contributing to the facilitation of some glutamatergic signals is relief from voltage-dependent block of the ion channel by polyamines (Rozov et al., 1998). Conversely, at some synapses desensitization of receptors can contribute to use-dependent depression of neurotransmission (Brenowitz and Trussell, 2001). However, it has also been argued that lateral mobility of receptors may limit the impact of such desensitization (Heine et al., 2008).

Because principal neurons frequently discharge in bursts of action potentials, the degree of postsynaptic facilitation or depression during such bursts may contain much of the information transmitted through the network. Indeed, it has been argued that lasting changes in short-term plasticity are of greater importance for information encoding than synaptic strength per se (defined as the size of an EPSP or IPSP evoked after an interval sufficiently long for short-term plasticity phenomena to have dissipated) (Markram and Tsodyks, 1996). However, because short-term plasticity is mediated predominantly through use-dependent alteration in release probability, the information contained in a facilitating or depressing burst is inevitably corrupted by the stochastic nature of transmitter release. That is, the degree of facilitation or depression at a synapse can be reliably detected by the network only by averaging out the response to a stereotyped sequence of action potentials repeatedly delivered to the presynaptic neuron. This has led to an almost diametrically opposite view of the importance of bursts: Because high-probability synapses generally depress and low-probability synapses usually facilitate, the function of bursts is to cancel out the effects of the initial release probability and minimize the sampling error arising from stochastic release. Thus, it is argued that the most important modifiable parameter relevant to information transmission is the quantal amplitude (Lisman, 1997). Against this background, there has been considerable interest in the long-term consequences of particular timing patterns of pre- and postsynaptic action potentials. Notably, it has been reported at several cortical synapses that if presynaptic glutamate release occurs shortly before a postsynaptic action potential it can lead to persistent enhancement of transmission. If, on the other hand, the presynaptic stimulus lags behind the postsynaptic action potential, it can be followed by depression of transmission (Bi and Poo, 2001). The mechanisms underlying these phenomena and their relevance to learning are further considered in Chapter 10.

6.4 Glutamatergic synaptic transmission

The main excitatory transmitter in the hippocampus, as elsewhere in the mammalian CNS, is glutamate. Following exocytosis, glutamate is taken up into neurons and glia, although this process takes place at a much slower rate than passive diffusion away from the release site (see below). Of the glutamate transporters, the most abundant in the rodent hippocampus is EAAT2 (excitatory amino acid transporter 2, encoded by *SLC1A2*), followed by EAAT1 (*SLC1A3*) and EAAT3 (*SLC1A1*) (Danbolt, 2001). In the hippocampus, EAAT2 and EAAT1 are almost exclusively expressed in

astrocytes. EAAT3 is principally expressed in neurons although at a relatively low level, so it probably contributes relatively little to clearing glutamate following exocytosis. However, it has been proposed to supply glutamate for GABA synthesis in inhibitory boutons (Sepkuty et al., 2002).

Glutamate taken up into astrocytes is decarboxylated by glutamine synthetase (Figure 6.9). The intracellular concentration of glutamate in astrocytes is thereby kept low, which is necessary to make continued uptake of glutamate energetically favorable. The energy required for uptake of glutamate comes from the cotransport of three Na^+ ions down their electrochemical gradient. In addition, flux measurements have shown that one H^+ ion accompanies glutamate, and one K^+ ion is countertransported (Zerangue and Kavanaugh, 1996). Because the net movement of glutamate is dictated by the electrochemical gradients for these other species, it is possible to reverse uptake; moreover, evidence exists that such reversed uptake can take place during ischemia, when extracellular K^+ builds up and cells become depolarized because of ATP depletion (Rossi et al., 2000). Because the extracellular accumulation of glutamate can exacerbate depolarization of neurons by acting at glutamate receptors, there is the possibility of triggering a positive feedback loop. This cascade may underlie part of the "excitotoxic" role of glutamate in stroke.

Astrocytic glutamine, formed from decarboxylation of glutamate, can enter metabolic pathways in astrocytes, but it can also diffuse passively down its concentration gradient into the extracellular space, a phenomenon facilitated by several transporters. From here it is taken up into presynaptic terminals, where it can be converted back to glutamate and repackaged into vesicles.

6.4.1 Glutamate receptors

The three major classes of ionotropic glutamate receptors (Table 6.1) take their names from agonists that activate them in a relatively selective fashion (Hansen et al., 2021). At most excitatory

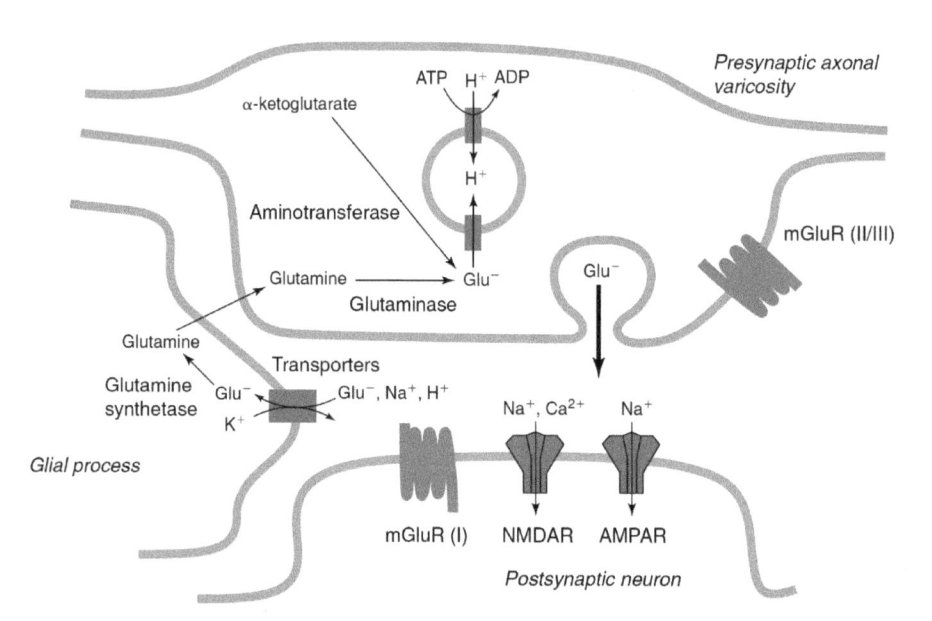

Figure 6.9 Glutamate–glutamine cycle. The excitatory neurotransmitter glutamate is synthesized from a-ketoglutarate, which is produced by the Krebs cycle, and recycled from glutamine. Following release, glutamate is taken up by glial cells, where it is rapidly decarboxylated to form glutamine. Glutamine can diffuse across the extracellular space back to presynaptic varicosities. The diagram also shows the arrangement of several types of glutamate receptors: AMPA and NMDA receptors tend to be located opposite release sites, and group I metabotropic receptors [mGluR (I)] tend to be located in a perisynaptic distribution. Group II and III metabotropic receptors tend to be located presynaptically.

Table 6.1 Ionotropic glutamate receptors

Receptor type	Agonists	Subunits	Permeant ions
AMPA (α-amino-3-hydroxy-5-methyl-4-soxazolepropionic acid)	Glutamate, AMPA, kainate	GluA1-4	Na^+, K^+ (Ca^{2+})
Kainate	Glutamate, kainate	GluK1-5	Na^+, K^+ (Ca^{2+})
NMDA (N-methyl-D-aspartic acid)	Glutamate, glycine, D-serine (endogenous co-agonists), NMDA	GluN1, GluN2A-D, GluN3A-B	Na^+, K^+ Ca^{2+}

hippocampal synapses, EPSCs are mediated by AMPA and NMDA receptors, which have strikingly different biophysical and pharmacological properties. Kainate receptors have a relatively poorly understood role in synaptic transmission. All three receptor types are multimeric, made up of four homologous pore-forming subunits. These subunits are encoded by several genes that undergo alternative splicing, which contribute to defining their kinetic properties. The importance of the molecular variability of the subunits making up each class of receptors is considered further in Chapter 8. Here, we concentrate on the major pharmacological and biophysical differences that exist among the various receptors.

6.4.1.1 AMPA receptors

AMPA receptors are composed of different combinations of four subunits (GluA1-4, encoded by *GRIA1-4*). Each subunit has a large extracellular N-terminus, three transmembrane domains and an intracellular C-terminus. A loop dives into the membrane from the intracellular side between the first and second membrane-spanning domains and lines the conduction pore, where it acts as an ion-selectivity filter. The ligand-binding domain is composed of the proximal N-terminus and part of the extracellular loop between the second and third transmembrane domains.

AMPA receptors occur at the majority of excitatory synapses in the hippocampus and gate a cation-selective channel. At resting membrane potentials, Na^+ influx accounts for most of the current, but the channel is also permeable to other small monovalent cations, so K^+ efflux can also occur at depolarized potentials. Most AMPA receptors in pyramidal neurons of the adult hippocampus (at least in rodents) are thought to be GluA1/2 or GluA2/3 heterotetramers (Schwenk et al., 2014). Parvalbumin-positive interneurons tend to express GluA2-lacking receptors (mainly GluA1/4 and GluA3/4 heterotetramers).

AMPA receptors are optimally activated by a brief transient of glutamate. When a membrane patch taken from the soma or proximal dendrite of a hippocampal neuron is exposed to a pulse of 1 mM glutamate (roughly corresponding to the synaptic glutamate transient; see below) a current is generated with a submillisecond risetime. This reflects both very fast binding kinetics and a high opening probability: the peak probability that a bound receptor is in the open state has been estimated at approximately 0.6 (Jonas et al., 1993).

Native AMPA receptors deactivate rapidly following clearance of synaptic glutamate (with a time constant of 2.3–3.0 ms). Deactivation is probably sufficient to explain the termination of AMPA receptor-mediated EPSCs, on the grounds that glutamate is cleared from the synaptic cleft faster than this. If glutamate is not cleared, however, AMPA receptors close rapidly and enter a desensitized state from which they recover relatively slowly. The time course of desensitization depends on the subunit composition of the receptors and is affected by alternative splicing of the subunit mRNA (so-called flip and flop variants), but it usually proceeds with a decay time constant of the order of 5–10 ms) (Hansen et al., 2021). AMPA receptors can even desensitize in the presence of slowly rising glutamate concentrations that are insufficient to open them. This form of desensitization may be an adaptation that prevents excessive receptor activation under pathological conditions where extracellular glutamate accumulates. Some degree of desensitization also occurs with extremely brief (millisecond) exposure to the agonist, so if a second pulse is applied after a short delay, a smaller response is obtained.

Depending on their subunit composition, AMPA receptors can also show significant permeability to Ca^{2+} ions. This permeability is determined by the presence or absence of a critical amino acid (arginine, R) in a pore-lining segment of the GluA2 subunit. This subunit undergoes posttranscriptional RNA editing, resulting in a change of the codon at this position from glutamine (Q), encoded by the genomic sequence, to arginine (Sommer et al., 1991). The presence of the edited form of GluA2 ensures that the receptor is impermeable to Ca^{2+}, which is the case for most of the glutamate receptors in principal cells. If the GluA2 subunit is absent, the receptor has significant Ca^{2+} permeability. Such receptors are present in some hippocampal interneurons (Geiger et al., 1995).

"Q/R editing" has several other consequences for AMPA receptor function (Hansen et al., 2021). If the edited (R) form of GluA2 is present in the receptor, its conductance is relatively small and is independent of the transmembrane voltage. If the edited GluA2 is absent from the receptor, the current–voltage relation becomes highly nonlinear (Figure 6.10). That is, the receptor functions as a rectifier, with a conductance that increases with the transmembrane potential difference. This transition between low- and high-conductance states is due to blockade of the receptor by intracellular polyamine molecules, which enter the ion channel but can be expelled in a voltage-dependent manner.

The single-channel conductance of native receptors varies broadly, from <1 pS to approximately 30 pS, depending not only the presence of edited GluA2 but also on the identity of other subunits (Hansen et al., 2021). Bound receptors do not remain open continuously. In common with other ligand-gated ion channels, they flicker between open and closed states; and even in their open state they fluctuate among distinct preferred conductance levels.

Cryoelectron microscopy studies have revealed how movement of the ligand-binding domain is coupled to channel opening (Twomey et al., 2017; Zhao et al., 2019). Both the opening probability and the conductance of the channel can be modulated by phosphorylation of residues in the C-terminus, phenomena that have implications for the mechanisms of long-term synaptic plasticity (see Chapter 10). Finally, AMPA receptors interact with several other proteins that modulate their trafficking and kinetics, of

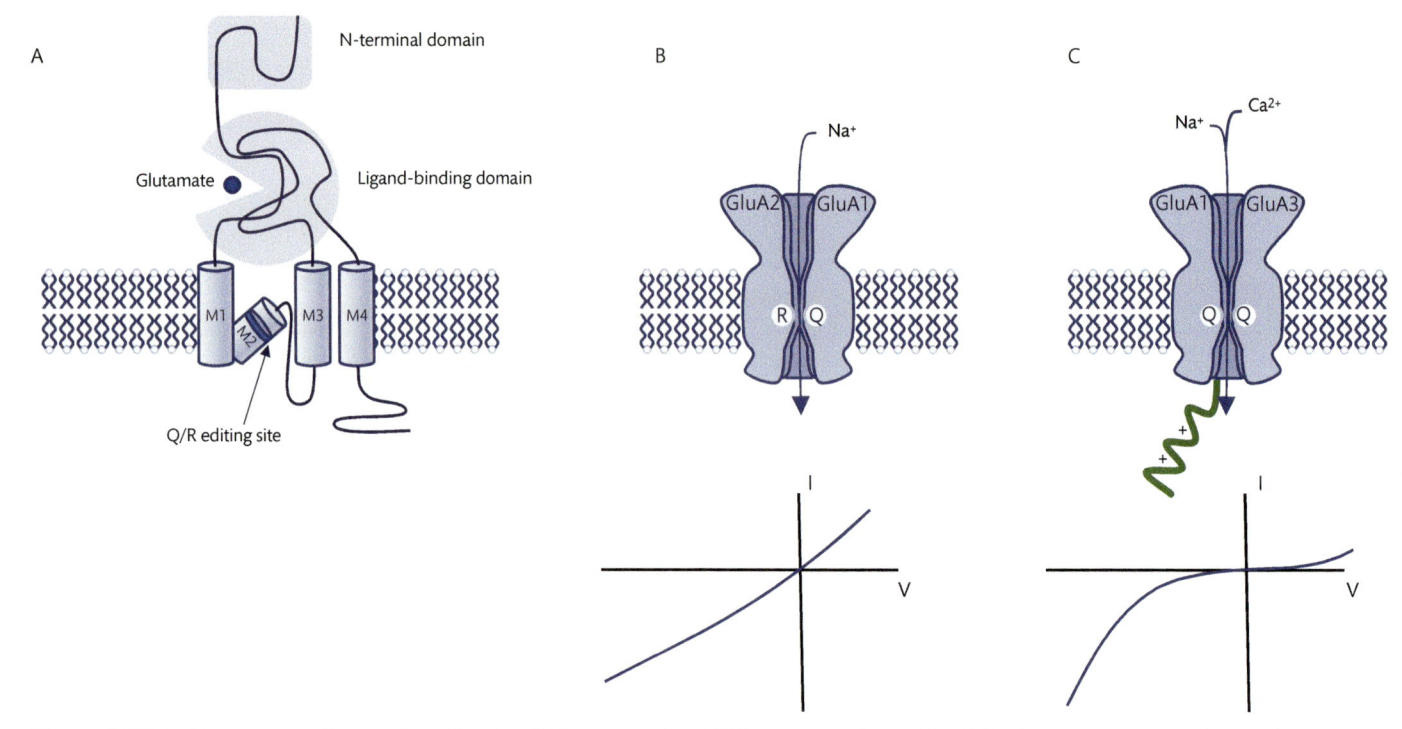

Figure 6.10 AMPA receptor editing and rectification. (A) Structure of an AMPA receptor subunit. The Q/R editing site corresponds to a glutamine codon of *GRIA2* that undergoes posttranscriptional editing to an arginine. (B) AMPA receptors incorporating an edited GluA2 subunit are impermeable to Ca^{2+} ions (top) and exhibit an approximately linear current-voltage (I–V) relationship (bottom schematic). (C) AMPA receptors devoid of edited GluA2 (e.g., GluA1–GluA3 heterotetramers) are permeable to Ca^{2+} and exhibit inward rectification due to voltage-dependent insertion of polyamines (indicated schematically in green) into the cytoplasmic orifice of the channel.

which TARPs (transmembrane AMPAR regulatory proteins) have received the most attention (Greger et al., 2017).

6.4.1.2 Kainate receptors

Kainate receptors share many features with AMPA receptors (Hansen et al., 2021; Mayer, 2021). They too are heterotetrameric, made up of different combinations of subunits that exist in five subtypes: GluK1-5, encoded by *GRIK1-5*. Although GluK1-3 can assemble as homotetrameric receptors, GluK4 and GluK5 do not, and only contribute to functional receptors when coassembled with GluK1, GluK2, or GluK3. GluK1 and GluK2 undergo Q/R editing with similar consequences as for GluA2, although the proportion of edited subunits in the brain is considerably below 100%.

The biophysical properties of recombinant kainate receptors are similar to those of AMPA receptors. That is, they open and desensitize rapidly, and they have single-channel conductances, rectification properties, and Ca^{2+} permeabilities that depend on Q/R editing. However, synaptic kainate receptor-mediated signals exhibit very slow kinetics. Furthermore, although kainate receptors are abundant in the hippocampus, synaptic responses mediated by them are very small and generally require trains of high-frequency stimuli to be detected. The auxiliary protein Neto1 has been shown to modulate kainate receptors, providing a possible explanation for the distinct properties of recombinant and native receptors (Straub et al., 2011; Tang et al., 2011).

Evidence has emerged for a role of presynaptic kainate receptors in modulating transmitter release (Chittajallu et al., 1996; Rodríguez-Moreno et al., 1997), axon excitability (Semyanov and Kullmann, 2001), and synaptic plasticity (Nair et al., 2021). Surprisingly, kainate receptors at various synapses, activated by different concentrations of agonists, either enhance or depress transmitter release (Schmitz et al., 2001). The mechanisms underlying these phenomena are incompletely understood and may include depolarization, Ca^{2+} influx via permeable receptors, and coupling to a metabotropic cascade (Falcón-Moya and Rodríguez-Moreno, 2021).

6.4.1.3 NMDA receptors

NMDA receptors are also homologous with AMPA and kainate receptors (Hansen et al., 2021). They exist as heteroteramers with two obligatory GluN1 subunits (encoded by *GRIN1*), and two other subunits drawn from GluN2A-D (encoded by *GRIN2A-B*) or, less commonly, GluN3A or GluN3B (*GRIN3A* or *GRIN3B*). The GluN1 subunit does not bind glutamate but, instead, contains a binding site for another amino acid, glycine or D-serine, which acts as a coagonist (see below). GluN2A-B or GluN3A/B subunits, on the other hand, contain the glutamate-binding site. Their expression is tightly regulated in different regions of the brain and at different stages of development. NMDA receptors also differ in composition depending on their subcellular location. Thus, although NMDA receptors are concentrated at synapses, a proportion of mainly GluN2B subunit-containing receptors is present in extrasynaptic membranes (Tovar and Westbrook, 2002).

NMDA receptors have several striking properties that mark them out as distinct from AMPA and kainate receptors.

First, they have very slow kinetics and can continue to mediate an ion flux for several hundreds of milliseconds after the glutamate pulse has terminated. The slow kinetics are explained by an extremely slow receptor unbinding rate (Hansen et al., 2021). That is, upon glutamate binding to NMDA receptors, they remain bound for a long time, during which time the channel can undergo repeated opening and closing events. Reflecting the very slow dissociation rate, the apparent potency of glutamate at NMDA receptors is much higher than at AMPA receptors.

Second, in order to open, both the glutamate binding site and the so-called strychnine-insensitive glycine site must be occupied (Johnson and Ascher, 1987). There remains some uncertainty whether the ambient extracellular glycine and/or D-serine concentration in the brain is sufficient to ensure that this site is saturated. Alternatively, it has been proposed that D-serine has a physiological role in dynamically modulating NMDA receptor function (Henneberger et al., 2010).

Third, NMDA receptors are highly permeable to Ca^{2+} ions as well as monovalent cations (Ascher and Nowak, 1988). Ca^2 influx via NMDA receptors has a central role in the induction of long-term synaptic plasticity (see Chapter 10). Accompanying the high Ca^2 permeability of NMDA receptors is a relatively high single-channel conductance (40–50 pS), which is greater than that of most AMPA receptors (Jahr and Stevens, 1987).

Finally, extracellular Mg^2 ions block the channel pore in a voltage-dependent manner (Mayer et al., 1984; Nowak et al., 1984). Thus, at resting membrane potentials (more negative than approximately –50 mV), NMDA receptors are unable to mediate an ion flux even if both coagonist sites are bound. However, membrane depolarization relieves the Mg^{2+} blockade. The voltage-dependence explains the role of NMDA receptors as synaptic coincidence detectors: Ca^{2+} influx occurs only if there is a conjunction of presynaptic glutamate release and postsynaptic depolarization, a situation that arises when pre- and postsynaptic activity occur together (Wigström and Gustafsson, 1986). The significance of this phenomenon for long-term modification of synaptic strength is addressed in Chapter 10.

6.4.2 Colocalization of glutamate receptors

Both AMPA and NMDA receptors are present at a much higher density at synapses than in extrasynaptic membranes (Nusser et al., 1998). However, some synapses may be devoid of AMPA receptors, especially early in postnatal development.

Reflecting the colocalization of AMPA and NMDA (and possibly kainate) receptors, EPSCs generally show several kinetically distinct components, which can be distinguished with pharmacological and electrophysiological manipulations (Hestrin et al., 1990). At most hippocampal synapses, at negative membrane potentials, the EPSC has fast kinetics and is fully blocked by specific AMPA receptor antagonists. This EPSC is analogous to the fast synaptic current carried by acetylcholine receptors at the neuromuscular junction, which "short-circuits" the transmembrane potential. At depolarized membrane potentials (above -50 mV), a slower NMDA receptor-mediated component of the EPSC emerges, which accounts for a substantial fraction of the charge transfer because of the very slow NMDA receptor kinetics. Both AMPA and NMDA receptor-mediated components disappear near 0 mV because this represents the reversal potential for the mixture of monovalent cations that account for the bulk of the current. However, Ca^{2+} influx still occurs at this membrane potential because the reversal potential for Ca^{2+} is positive. If the neuron is held at a positive membrane potential, the dual-component EPSC appears again, although it is now an outward current (Figure 6.11).

Kainate receptors generally do not contribute appreciably to fast EPSCs recorded in principal neurons. Nevertheless, a small and slow current mediated by these receptors can be detected in some neurons in response to high-frequency trains of presynaptic action potentials (especially in CA3 pyramidal neurons in response to mossy fiber stimulation, and in some interneurons) (Castillo et al., 1997; Vignes and Collingridge, 1997).

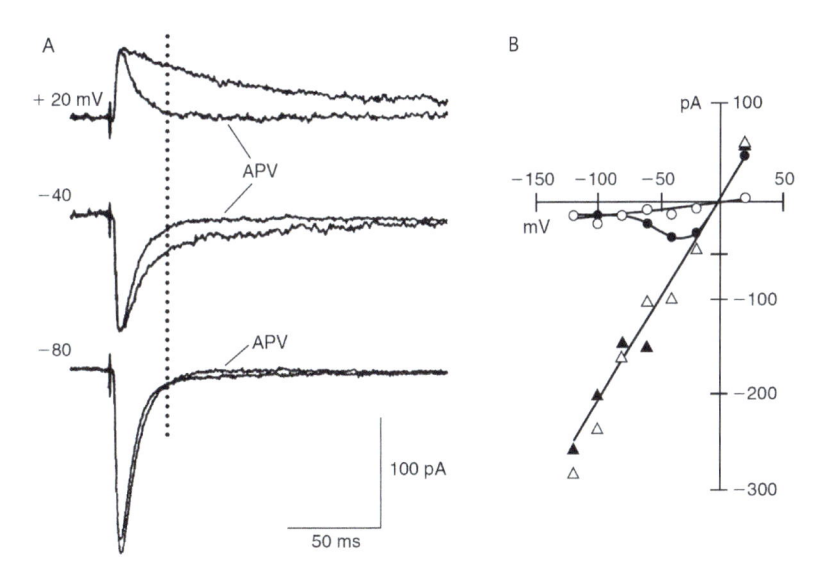

Figure 6.11 Dual-component glutamatergic transmission at hippocampal synapses. (A) EPSCs recorded in a pyramidal neuron at various voltages. As the postsynaptic cell is depolarized, a slow component appears. This slow current is abolished by the NMDA receptor blocker aminophosphonovalerate (APV). (B) Current-voltage (I–V) relation is plotted for the peak of the EPSCs (triangles) and for a later time point indicated by the vertical dotted line in A. Filled symbols, control conditions; open symbols, in the presence of APV. The I–V relation of the APV-sensitive component (circles, measured at a time shown by the dotted line in A) shows a region of negative slope (that is, increasing conductance as the cell is depolarized) characteristic of voltage-dependent relief of blockade of NMDA receptors by Mg^2 ions. In contrast, the peak of the EPSC (triangles) has an approximately linear I–V relation because the AMPA receptors in pyramidal neurons mainly contain edited GluA2 subunits. (Source: Hestrin et al., 1990, with permission.)

Table 6.2 Metabotropic glutamate receptors

Group	Subtypes	Transduction mechanisms	Agonists
I	mGluR1,5	Phospholipase C	Glutamate (S)-3,5-dihydroxyphenylglycine (DHPG)
II	mGluR2,3	Adenylyl cyclase	Glutamate (2S,1'R;2'R,3'R)-2-(2,3-Dicarboxycyclopropyl)glycine (DCG-IV)
III	mGluR4,6-8	Adenylyl cyclase	Glutamate L-Amino-phosphonobutyrate (L-AP4)

6.4.3 Metabotropic glutamate receptors

Metabotropic glutamate receptors (mGluRs), in common with other GPCRs, have an extracellular N-terminus, seven transmembrane segments, and an intracellular C-terminus. Glutamate binding stabilizes them in the active state (Gregory and Goudet, 2021). Metabotropic glutamate receptors fall into three classes, although eight genes have been identified (Table 6.2).

Group I receptors (mGluR1 and 5, encoded by *GRM1* and *GRM5*) are generally localized to postsynaptic membranes and tend to occur in a halo around the synaptic cleft (Baude et al., 1993). They are coupled via $G\alpha_q$ to phospholipase C, and their activation leads to an increase in both inositol trisphosphate and diacylglycerol. Activation of these receptors triggers Ca^{2+} release from intracellular stores and can elicit a slow depolarization (Crépel et al., 1994; Guérineau et al., 1994).

Group II (mGluR2 and 3, encoded by *GRM2* and *GRM3*) and group III (mGluR4, 6, 7, 8, encoded by *GRM4* and *GRM6-7*) receptors are $G\alpha_{i/o}$-coupled and tend to be located in presynaptic membranes. At mossy fibers, mGluR2 receptors are located relatively far from glutamate release sites—in axonal membranes—implying that they detect only glutamate molecules that have escaped from the synaptic cleft (Yokoi et al., 1996). Group III receptors, on the other hand, tend to be located in synapses, that is, very close to or even within active zones (Shigemoto et al., 1996, 1997). Both types are negatively coupled to adenylate cyclase. The distinction between group II and group III receptors is principally pharmacological: L-2-amino-4-phosphonobutyric acid (L-AP4) is a selective agonist at group III, but not group II, receptors (Gregory and Goudet, 2021).

The physiological roles of metabotropic receptors are not fully understood. The perisynaptic postsynaptic group I receptors preferentially respond to trains of action potentials that result in the prolonged presence of glutamate in their vicinity. Prolonged activation of group I mGluRs by intermediate frequency stimuli can also elicit a form of NMDA receptor-independent long-term depression (see Chapter 10). As for group II receptors, their predominantly extrasynaptic and presynaptic location implies that they detect the extracellular buildup of glutamate. They may therefore act as autoreceptors that regulate neurotransmitter release as a function of the volume-averaged excitatory traffic (Scanziani et al., 1997). The intrasynaptic presynaptic location of some group III receptors prompts speculation that they act as autoreceptors on a smaller spatial scale. However, they are also present at some GABAergic terminals (Shigemoto et al., 1997), which are not known to release glutamate. They can detect glutamate released from neighboring synapses (Semyanov and Kullmann, 2000), so their role may be akin to that of group II receptors.

6.4.4 Receptor targeting and anchoring

How glutamate receptors are trafficked and targeted to postsynaptic densities is considered from a molecular perspective in Chapter 8. AMPA receptor insertion plays a major part in synapse maturation and long-term potentiation (further considered in Chapter 10). Briefly, this takes place in two stages. First, glutamate receptors in intracellular trafficking vesicles undergo exocytosis, using a membrane fusion process akin to that outlined above governing presynaptic neurotransmitter release. This occurs on a relatively slow timescale, and uses a distinct set of SNARE proteins (Jurado et al., 2013), although postsynaptic synaptotagmin-1 (a "fast" Ca^{2+} sensor) and synaptotagmin-7 (which has a high Ca^{2+} affinity and is therefore considered a "slow" sensor), have been implicated in synapse strengthening during long-term potentiation (D Wu et al., 2017). Second, AMPA receptors are anchored at postsynaptic densities through an interaction with the scaffolding protein PSD-95, mediated in large part by TARPs (see Chapter 8). Recent evidence points to an important role of the extracellular N-terminal domain of AMPA receptors in binding to TARPs (Watson et al., 2021).

NMDA receptors are also anchored to a large number of scaffolding, signaling, and transduction proteins. This anchoring is mediated via an interaction between the C-termini of GluN2 subunits and several so-called PDZ domain proteins, in particular PSD-95 and SAP97 (Kornau et al., 1995). Some group I metabotropic glutamate receptors are also anchored via a PDZ domain protein, Homer (Brakeman et al., 1997).

6.5 GABAergic synaptic transmission

The major inhibitory transmitter GABA (γ-aminobutyric acid) is synthesized by decarboxylation of glutamate. Two isoforms of glutamic acid decarboxylase exist (Lee et al., 2019). GAD67 (encoded by *GAD1*) is widespread in the cytoplasm, whereas GAD65 (*GAD2*) is more closely associated with presynaptic terminals of GABAergic neurons. The expression of GAD65 varies in response to changes in neuronal activity, implying that it may have a regulatory role in GABAergic transmission. Uptake into vesicles is facilitated by the vesicular GABA transporter VGAT, which can also mediate vesicular glycine transport. Following exocytosis, GABA diffuses out of the synaptic cleft and is mainly taken up by three transporters: GAT1-3, encoded by *SLC6A1*, *SLC6A13* and *SLC6A11*, respectively (Scimemi, 2014) (Figure 6.12). These transporters are located not only in astrocytes but also, in the case of GAT2, in interneurons and principal cells. GABA uptake is electrogenic; that is, the amino acid is transported together with two Na^+ ions (and possibly one Cl^- ion) (Kavanaugh et al., 1992). This stoichiometry

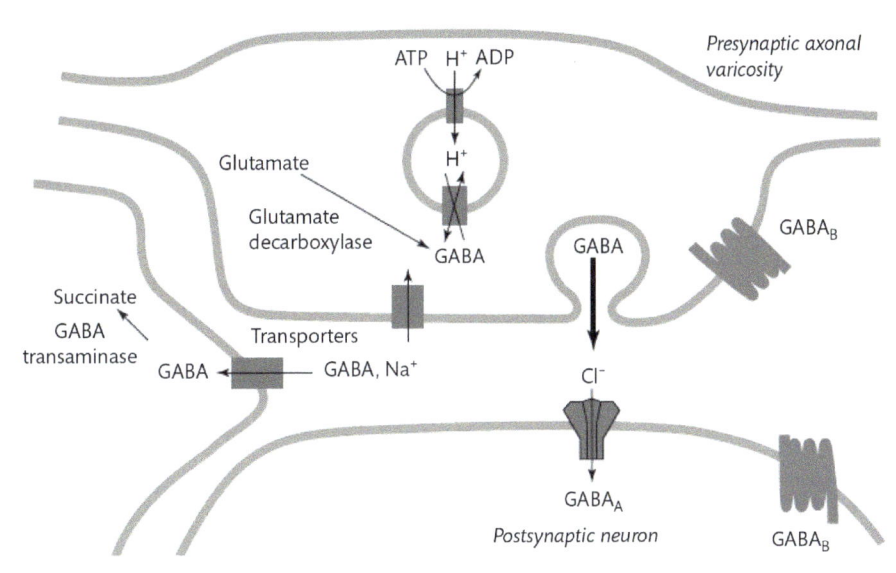

Figure 6.12 GABA cycle. The inhibitory neurotransmitter GABA is synthesized from glutamate via the action of two enzymes, GAD-65 and GAD-67. Following release, GABA is taken up by both neurons and glial cells. GABA can be converted back to glutamate or to succinate by the mitochondrial enzyme GABA transaminase. The diagram also shows the arrangement of GABA$_A$ and GABA$_B$ receptors. Ionotropic GABA$_A$ receptors tend to be located opposite release sites, although extrasynaptic receptors also occur in dentate granule cells. GABA$_B$ receptors occur both pre- and postsynaptically.

normally ensures that GABA is taken up into cells because the driving force provided by the Na$^+$ electrochemical gradient is sufficient to overcome the gradient for GABA. However, because the transport stoichiometry is less electrogenic than for glutamate, the equilibrium concentration of GABA in the extracellular space may be higher. Indeed, high-affinity GABA receptors are tonically active in the absence of presynaptic activity (Semyanov et al., 2004).

GABA receptors are divided into ionotropic (GABA$_A$) and metabotropic (GABA$_B$) receptors (Table 6.3). GABA$_C$ receptors are ionotropic receptors with an unusual pharmacological profile and are made up of ρ subunits. Because they are not known to have a major role in the hippocampus, they are not considered here.

6.5.1 GABA$_A$ receptors

GABA$_A$ receptors are heteropentameric, and are structurally homologous to nicotinic cholinergic receptors. They consist of subunits drawn from seven families: α1-6 (*GABRA1-6*), β1-3 (*GABRB1-3*), γ1-3 (*GABRG1-3*), δ (*GABRD*), ε (*GABRE*), π (*GABRP*), and θ (*GABRQ*) (Olsen and Sieghart, 2008). Of these, α6, ε, π, and θ appear to be excluded from the rodent hippocampus or to occur at very low levels. The remaining subunits show differential distributions at a macroscopic level. Thus, α1, α2, α4, β3, γ2, and δ are present in the dentate gyrus, while in the hippocampus proper, the principal subunits are α1, α2, α5, β3, and γ2, with relatively lower levels of α4, β1, β2, γ3, and δ. α1 and γ1 are present only at very low levels in the hippocampal formation (Sperk et al., 1997).

Most hippocampal GABA$_A$ receptors probably contain two α subunits and two β subunits, together with either a γ subunit or a δ subunit but not both. α subunits in particular have important roles in determining the affinity for GABA and the sensitivity to numerous modulatory agents such as Zn^{2+} ions and exogenous molecules such as ethanol, benzodiazepines, barbiturates and general anesthetics (Olsen and Sieghart, 2008). γ subunits also affect the binding of several of these agents and, in addition, mediate anchoring of GABA$_A$ receptors to synapses via an indirect interaction with gephyrin, a scaffolding protein that is important in the formation and stabilization of both GABAergic and glycinergic synapses (Essrich et al., 1998). δ-containing receptors tend not to be confined to synapses but have a high affinity for GABA and are insensitive to benzodiazepines. They mediate a large fraction of GABA$_A$ receptor-dependent tonic inhibition in dentate granule cells (Nusser and Mody, 2002).

GABA$_A$ receptor-mediated IPSCs have a fast onset, although their decay is generally slower than that of AMPA receptor-mediated EPSCs. Their single-channel conductance is highly variable, ranging from <1 to >30 pS, depending on their subunit composition.

Depending on the subunit composition, benzodiazepines enhance the affinity of GABA$_A$ receptors for the agonist, resulting in a prolongation and potentiation of IPSCs. Although barbiturates have a superficially similar effect on IPSC kinetics, they act by increasing the proportion of the time that GABA-liganded channels remain open. The effects on GABAergic transmission account

Table 6.3 GABA receptors

Receptor type	Subunits	Effector	Agonists	Antagonists	Modulators
GABA$_A$	α1-5, β1-3, γ1-3, δ	Channel permeable to Cl$^-$, HCO$_3^-$	GABA Muscimol	Picrotoxin Bicuculline SR95531	Benzodiazepines, barbiturates, Zn^{2+}, ethanol, neurosteroids
GABA$_B$	GBR1 GBR2	$G_{\alpha i/o}$, $G_{\beta/\gamma}$	GABA Baclofen	Saclofen CGP35348	

for their usefulness as sedative, anxiolytic, and antiepileptic agents. Combined genetic and pharmacological manipulation of the receptors has suggested that α1-containing receptors preferentially mediate the sedative effects of systemic benzodiazepines, while α2- and α3-containing receptors contribute to anxiolytic effects (Rudolph and Möhler, 2006).

GABA$_A$ receptors are permeable only to anions. The current is carried overwhelmingly by Cl$^-$ ions, but receptors are also permeable to HCO$_3^-$. Because neurons are normally depolarized relative to the Cl$^-$ reversal potential, GABA$_A$ receptor-mediated IPSCs are generally hyperpolarizing. The situation is different in neurons at early stages of development (Ben-Ari et al., 1989), when the intracellular Cl$^-$ concentration is relatively high because the principal extrusion mechanism (the K$^+$/Cl$^-$ cotransporter KCC2) is not expressed abundantly (Rivera et al., 1999). The electrochemical gradient then dictates that Cl$^-$ ions flow out of the cell, making the current depolarizing. Somewhat confusingly, this is usually referred to as a "depolarizing IPSC." Such depolarizing GABAergic signals can, under some conditions, bring neurons to firing threshold and trigger Ca^2 influx, and they may have an important role in the early stages of neural circuit formation. Prolonged and intense activation of GABA$_A$ receptors in the adult brain can also result in a shift in the reversal potential for GABA, because the outward Cl$^-$ transport mediated by KCC2 is overwhelmed by the inward Cl- flux via GABA$_A$ receptors (Staley et al., 1995). Extracellular K$^+$ also accumulates through the action of KCC2, further contributing to neuronal depolarization (Kaila et al., 1997). Although depolarizing responses can be achieved experimentally by iontophoretic application of GABA and occurs during seizures, it is not clear whether they occur with synaptic activity under physiological conditions in adult animals, which generally activates only a small proportion of the receptors on a neuron and for a short time.

6.5.2 GABA$_B$ receptors

GABA$_B$ receptors occur as heterodimers composed of GBR$_1$ and GBR$_2$ (encoded by *GABBR1/2*) (Pin and Bettler, 2016), both of which can undergo alternative splicing. GABA$_B$ receptors are G$_{i/o}$-coupled, and are widespread at both pre- and postsynaptic elements of synapses and also in extrasynaptic membranes (Fritschy et al., 1999). The GABA$_B$ receptor agonist baclofen powerfully depresses the synaptic release of both glutamate and GABA, reflecting the widespread distribution of presynaptic GABA$_B$ receptors.

On the postsynaptic side, the GABA$_B$-triggered cascade leads to the opening of G-protein-gated inward-rectifying K$^+$ (GIRK) channels. Activation of these channels causes a slow IPSP, lasting several hundred milliseconds. This is easily distinguished from the GABA$_A$ receptor-mediated IPSP, not only because of its slow kinetics but also because it is independent of the Cl$^-$ reversal potential.

In contrast to GABA$_A$ receptor-mediated IPSCs, it has proved difficult to elicit GABA$_B$ receptor-mediated synaptic responses by activating single presynaptic neurons. This observation most likely reflects a requirement for GABA to be released from multiple presynaptic terminals in order to activate the receptors (Scanziani, 2000). This argument suggests that uptake mechanisms are insufficient to isolate GABAergic terminals functionally from one another, at least as far as high affinity GABA$_B$ receptors are concerned. An exception to the rule that multiple cells need to be activated is that single neurogliaform cells can generate prominent GABA$_B$ receptor-mediated IPSCs in their targets (Tamás et al.,

2003). The unusual signaling properties of these interneurons are addressed below.

6.6 Other neurotransmitters

In comparison with glutamate and GABA, other neurotransmitters are present at fewer synapses or exert more subtle effects on neurons. Some of them carry a diffuse signal in the extracellular space and may therefore have roles in determining the overall state of the hippocampal circuitry. Relatively less is known about the mechanisms underlying their release and postsynaptic actions.

6.6.1 Purinergic transmission

ATP is thought to be coreleased with other neurotransmitters, and acts on trimeric ionotropic P2X receptors (encoded by *P2X1-7*). These channels are cation-selective. In the presence of broad-spectrum antagonists of amino acid receptors, a fast depolarizing purinergic postsynaptic current has been reported in response to extracellular stimulation in hippocampal neurons (Pankratov et al., 1998). However, to detect such a current it is necessary to stimulate many presynaptic fibers synchronously, and at a very low frequency, implying that the receptors desensitize easily. The physiological or pathological role of this class of receptors is not known. ATP undergoes extracellular enzymatic degradation by ectonucloeotidases, which eventually results in the formation of adenosine. Adenosine is probably also released by neurons directly, and extracellular adenosine accumulation occurs under conditions of metabolic stress. Presynaptic G$_{i/o}$-coupled A1 adenosine receptors are widespread on excitatory terminals, where they depress glutamate release (L Wu and Saggau, 1994). This phenomenon contributes to the potent depressant effect of hypoxia on excitatory synaptic transmission. GABA release is relatively less sensitive to adenosine (Yoon and Rothman, 1991). Postsynaptic G$_s$-coupled A$_{2A}$ receptors have been implicated in GABAergic synapse stabilization (Gomez-Castro et al., 2021).

6.6.2 Monoaminergic transmission

Among other small molecules that act as neurotransmitters are the monoamines noradrenaline (norepinephrine), dopamine (DA), serotonin (5-HT), and histamine (Nicoll et al., 1990).

Norepinephrine acts at specific G-protein coupled receptors, of which 9 types exist. α$_{1A,B,D}$ receptors are G$_q$-coupled, α$_{2A-C}$ are G$_{i/o}$-coupled, and β$_{1-3}$ are G$_s$-coupled (Altosaar et al., 2021). α1 and α2 receptors are mainly expressed in the vasculature in the hippocampus, but β receptors are widely expressed in neurons. Their activation increases the frequency of action potential firing and reduces spike frequency adaptation during continued depolarizing current injection (Madison and Nicoll, 1982). Norepinephrine is released by afferents originating in brainstem nuclei, most importantly the locus coeruleus, and has been implicated in facilitating long-term potentiation. Serotonin activates both ionotropic depolarizing 5-HT$_3$ receptors and several metabotropic receptors, of which 13 types exist, grouped into the 5-HT$_1$ and 5-HT$_5$ G$_{i/o}$-coupled family, the 5-HT$_2$ G$_q$-coupled family, and the 5-HT$_4$, 5-HT$_6$, and 5-HT$_7$ G$_s$-coupled receptors (Andrade et al., 2019). Serotonin is released from afferents from raphe nuclei and has diverse neuromodulatory actions, of which GIRK channel activation is prominent. Ionotropic 5-HT$_3$ receptors modulate interneuron migration (Murthy et al.,

2014), and distinguish a heterogeneous subtype of interneurons from parvalbumin- and somatostatin-positive interneurons (Rudy et al., 2011). Histamine acts at metabotropic receptors: H1 receptors couple to G_q, H2 receptors couple to G_s, and H3 and H4 receptors both couple to $G_{i/o}$ (Chazot et al., 2021). Histamine has been reported to enhance NMDA receptor-mediated currents (Bekkers, 1993).

The hippocampus receives dopaminergic projections from both the substantia nigra pars compacta and the ventral tegmental area. Dopamine acts at two groups of metabotropic receptors (Beaulieu et al., 2019). D1-like receptors (D1 and D5) are G_s-coupled, whereas D2-like receptors (D2, D3, D4) are $G_{i/o}$-coupled. Transcripts for all of these receptors can be detected in the hippocampus. Exogenous dopamine hyperpolarizes a proportion of pyramidal neurons, an action that is principally mediated by D1 receptors. However, synaptically released dopamine has complex actions on the hippocampal circuitry mediated by multiple receptors (Rosen et al., 2015).

6.6.3 Cholinergic transmission

Acetylcholine is also released from extrinsic afferents, although in this case their cell bodies lie in diencephalic structures, in particular the medial septal nuclei and the nucleus of the diagonal band (see Chapter 3). Some cholinergic afferent projections also release GABA, and it has been proposed that the two transmitters are present in distinct populations of presynaptic vesicles (Takács et al., 2018). A population of intrinsic cholinergic interneurons also exists in the hippocampus. Acetylcholine acts on both depolarizing ionotropic (nicotinic) and metabotropic (muscarinic) receptors.

Nicotinic receptors are pentameric, and several types occur in the hippocampus: homomeric receptors (mainly α7 homopentamers), and heteromeric receptors containing the β2 subunit (mainly α4β2) (Gotti et al., 2021). These receptors can be distinguished by their affinity for acetylcholine, by their desensitization kinetics, and by selective agonists and antagonists. Homopentameric α7 receptors have a lower affinity for the endogenous agonist than do α4β2 receptors, desensitize fast, and are inhibited by methyllacaconitine (MLA) and a-bungarotoxin. Activation of these receptors by exogenous agonist application has been shown to enhance evoked glutamate and GABA release (McGehee et al., 1995). This observation implies that they are located presynaptically, a conclusion supported by immunohistochemical evidence for colocalization with both glutamatergic and GABAergic terminals in the hippocampus (Fabian-Fine et al., 2001). However, they also occur postsynaptically, and by analogy with NMDA receptors, their high Ca^{2+} permeability implies a role that goes beyond mere depolarization (Wanaverbecq et al., 2007). Heteromeric α4β2 receptors have a relatively higher affinity for acetylcholine and nicotine, desensitize slowly, and are antagonized by dihydro-β-erythroidine and mecamylamine.

Four muscarinic GPCRs (M1-4) are found in the hippocampus. M1 and M3 receptors are G_q-coupled, while M2 and M4 receptors are $G_{i/o}$-coupled (Birdsall et al., 2021). Somatodendritic M1 and M3 receptors typically depolarize neurons by inhibiting the tonically active M-type K^+ current, thereby facilitating burst-firing of neurons. This current is mediated at least in part by heteromultimeric K^+ channels containing Kv7.2 and Kv7.3 subunits (Brown and Passmore, 2009). Among other consequences of muscarinic receptor activation are activation of GIRK channels (Seeger and Alzheimer, 2001),

and inhibition of another population of "SK" potassium channels expressed on dendritic spines, thereby facilitating NMDA receptor opening (Buchanan et al., 2010). M2 and M4 receptors are mainly expressed presynaptically, where they inhibit transmitter release (Behrends and ten Bruggencate, 1993). Although prominent on cholinergic terminals, they also exist on noncholinergic axons.

In contrast to the amino acids glutamate and GABA, several of the transmitters considered in this section tend not to subserve conventional point-to-point (or "wiring") transmission. Instead, they act in large part by diffusing a relatively long distance from the axonal varicosities where they are released. Indeed, some such varicosities exist in the absence of identifiable postsynaptic structures. These transmitters are frequently described as neuromodulators, whose main role is to regulate the excitability of the circuitry. The involvement of the cholinergic projection to the hippocampus in setting the theta rhythm is an important example of such a phenomenon.

6.6.4 Peptidergic transmission

A large number of peptides occur in axonal varicosities and bind to specific receptors in the hippocampus (Hökfelt et al., 1980). They include the opioid peptides, somatostatin, neuropeptide Y, galanin and cholecystokinin. Of these, the opioid peptides (enkephalins, endorphins, dynorphin, endomorphins) have been studied most extensively. They act at several $G_{i/o}$-coupled receptors with distinct pharmacological profiles (δ, k, μ), although there is evidence that these receptors can heterodimerize (Jordan and Devi, 1999).

Peptides are mainly contained in dense-core vesicles, which occur in GABAergic synapses and at mossy fiber synapses. They probably act diffusely to modulate either pre- or postsynaptic metabotropic receptors in the vicinity of the site where they are released (Weisskopf et al., 1993).

6.6.5 Other molecules

Some molecules have an uncertain status as neurotransmitters in the hippocampus. Glycine receptors occur in the hippocampus, where they open Cl^- conductance. However, glycinergic synaptic transmission has not been demonstrated (in contrast to the spinal cord).

The Zn^{2+} ion is associated with synaptic vesicles of glutamatergic synapses throughout the hippocampus but is especially prominent in mossy fibers. Exogenous Zn^{2+} inhibits $GABA_A$ and NMDA receptors, as well as glutamate uptake, but there is some uncertainty as to what extent these effects are shared by synaptic release of Zn^{2+} (Vogt et al., 2000; Kay, 2003; Ruiz et al., 2004).

Nitric oxide (NO) does not appear to function as a synaptic neurotransmitter in the conventional sense. It is synthesized in neurons expressing nitric oxide synthase (in particular ivy cells, neurogliaform cells, and interneuron-targeting interneurons that express VIP and calretinin) in a Ca^{2+}-dependent manner and does not require packaging into vesicles to exert its effects. Instead NO diffuses through membranes to its targets, which include soluble guanylyl cyclase. Its functional role remains poorly understood (Esplugues, 2002).

Products of lipid metabolism also have a role in intercellular communication. Notable among these products are arachidonic acid (AA), and the endocannabinoids anandamide and 2-arachidonylglycerol. Both AA and the endocannabinoids are synthesized in a Ca^{2+}-dependent manner and are potential retrograde messengers. Anandamide and 2-arachidonylglycerol act at presynaptic $G_{i/o}$-coupled CB1 receptors to depress neurotransmitter release (Abood et al., 2019). The role of endocannabinoid signaling in modulation of inhibition is considered further below.

6.7 Special features of individual hippocampal synapses

As discussed below, the functional properties of synapses between different neuron types differ extensively. The underlying developmental mechanisms are incompletely understood, but are likely to result from the combinatorial logic of transsynaptic interactions involving isoforms of cadherins, protocadherins, neurexins, neuregulins, leucine-rich repeat proteins, and immunoglobulin superfamily proteins (de Wit and Ghosh, 2016; Exposito-Alonso et al., 2020). Some of these proteins are involved in the close apposition of presynaptic release sites with postsynaptic receptor domains (Biederer et al., 2017).

6.7.1 Small excitatory spine synapses

In contrast to the neuromuscular junction, hippocampal synapses usually occur at axonal varicosities (the widely used term "terminal" is thus misleading). These varicosities occur at regular intervals along many axons. Their spacing is approximately 4 μm for Schaffer collaterals and associational/commissural fibers and approximately 5 μm for mossy fibers (Shepherd and Harris, 1998) (see Chapter 3).

The most abundant type of synapse in the hippocampus is the small glutamatergic synapse made on dendritic spines. This subserves transmission from the perforant path to dentate granule cells, as well as associational/commissural projections to CA3 pyramidal neurons and Schaffer collateral transmission to CA1 pyramidal neurons. The monosynaptic temporoammonic projection to the distal dendrites of CA1 pyramidal neurons has broadly similar biophysical properties, although glutamatergic excitation results in highly nonlinear postsynaptic integration because of the high impedance of the apical dendrites (Golding et al., 1999; Takahashi and Magee, 2009). Similar synapses relay excitatory signals from CA1 pyramidal neurons to subicular pyramidal cells and from the latter to the entorhinal cortex. Just over half of the presynaptic varicosities in CA1 appear to contain mitochondria. The postsynaptic densities range widely in area: between approximately 0.05 μm^2 and 0.5 μm^2 (Harris and Sultan, 1995). Dendritic spines in the rat dentate gyrus measure up to 0.8 μm in diameter and approximately 1 μm in length (Trommald and Hulleberg, 1997), and generally receive only one presynaptic bouton. However, the presynaptic varicosity is sometimes in synaptic contact with more than one spine (Sorra and Harris, 1993). Spines are thought to represent principally biochemical compartments. The degree to which electrical signals are compartmentalized by spines remains a subject of debate (Cornejo et al., 2022). Spine necks are often innervated by GABAergic or dopaminergic synapses in the neocortex or striatum, respectively. However, this is a rare occurrence in the rodent hippocampus, and the overwhelming majority of spines only receive one glutamatergic synapse.

The synaptic cleft is often closely apposed by an astrocytic process, although this is highly variable: many glutamatergic synapses in CA1 are not contacted by astrocytes, and when they are, only part of the perimeter of the synaptic cleft is bounded by an astrocytic process (Ventura and Harris, 1999). Because astrocytes express abundant glutamate transporters, this implies that there may be considerable variability in the spatiotemporal profile of glutamate in the vicinity of the synapse following exocytosis (Rusakov et al., 2011).

Both AMPA and NMDA receptors are localized to the postsynaptic density (Nusser et al., 1998; Takumi et al., 1999). Whether kainate receptors are also present is less clear. Indeed, glutamatergic EPSCs at Schaffer collateral–CA1 synapses are entirely blocked by antagonists of AMPA and NMDA receptors, leaving little room for the involvement of postsynaptic kainate receptors (Castillo et al., 1997; Vignes and Collingridge, 1997). The AMPA receptors at small spine synapses on principal neurons have a low permeability to Ca^{2+} and are nonrectifying, reflecting the presence of edited GluA2 subunits in almost all receptors (Jonas et al., 1994). Most AMPA receptors are thought to be GluA1/2 and GluA2/3 heteromers (Wenthold et al., 1996). Ca^2 influx, however, occurs as an indirect consequence of AMPA receptor activation because the consequent depolarization allows Ca^{2+}-permeable NMDA receptors to open. In addition, the depolarization allows voltage-gated Ca^2 channels in the dendritic spine and nearby region of the dendrite to open. A further source of Ca^{2+} is from intracellular stores, triggered by second messengers including inositol trisphosphate and Ca^2 itself (Emptage et al., 1999). Some of the disagreement about the relative importance of the various sources of Ca^{2+} probably reflects differences in recording methods: Although whole-cell recordings allow voltage control of the dendrite, they may interfere with intracellular Ca^{2+} homeostasis. Intracellular microelectrode recordings, though minimizing this source of error, sacrifice voltage control.

Although AMPA and NMDA receptors both contribute to EPSCs evoked by simultaneous stimulation of numerous presynaptic fibers, EPSCs evoked by action potentials in single presynaptic axons sometimes lack an AMPA receptor-mediated component (Kullmann, 1994; Isaac et al., 1995; Liao et al., 1995). Such EPSCs are evoked only under conditions where the postsynaptic neuron is depolarized or Mg^{2+} ions are omitted from the extracellular solution to reveal the NMDA receptor-mediated component. This observation has led to the hypothesis that AMPA receptors are absent or nonfunctional at a proportion of synapses, which are consequently often referred to as "silent synapses." Immunohistochemical studies provide support for this hypothesis: some small and/or immature synapses appear not to stain for AMPA receptors (Nusser et al., 1998; Takumi et al., 1999). In contrast, NMDA receptor density appears to be more uniform across synapses of different size (Racca et al., 2000). Taken together with the observation that the proportion of silent synapses diminishes with age (Hanse et al., 2013), it is tempting to conclude that synaptic maturation develops by an initial expression of NMDA receptors, followed later by insertion of AMPA receptors. This phenomenon may share mechanisms in common with long-term potentiation (see Chapter 10).

Alternative explanations for silent synapses exist: Because NMDA receptors have a higher affinity for glutamate than AMPA receptors (Patneau and Mayer, 1990), they might respond to a relatively low and prolonged pulse of glutamate that is insufficient to activate AMPA receptors. Such a glutamate profile could arise by diffusion from neighboring synapses ("spillover") (Asztely et al., 1997; Kullmann and Asztely, 1998). Thus, the NMDA receptors of the recorded cell might be acting as bystanders, eavesdropping on the excitatory traffic through many synapses formed on neighboring cells.

In favor of this model is the observation that raising the recording temperature from room temperature (thereby enhancing glutamate uptake) reduces the discrepancy between the number of quanta detected by NMDA and AMPA receptors. Conversely, blocking glutamate uptake pharmacologically increases the ratio of NMDA to AMPA receptor-mediated signaling, consistent with an exacerbation of crosstalk among synapses.

Another possible explanation for selective activation of NMDA receptors is that the glutamate released from the presynaptic terminal to activate AMPA receptors is insufficient. This could occur if release took place via a "fusion pore." That is, glutamate could slowly escape from a vesicle via a small, possibly flickering, opening to the synaptic cleft. Evidence for this phenomenon comes in part from the observation that enhancing the affinity of AMPA receptors for glutamate with pharmacological tools can unsilence such a "whispering" synapse (Choi et al., 2000).

The various explanations for silent synapses (absence of functional AMPA receptors, spillover, fusion pore release) are not mutually exclusive. These issues have attracted attention because they have implications for the interpretation of changes in quantal parameters during long-term potentiation or depression (Kullmann, 2003) (see Chapter 10).

Synapses exhibit considerable variability, both in structure and in function. It has been suggested that quantal parameters are positively correlated across different synapses (Schikorski and Stevens, 1997). Thus, synapses with large presynaptic elements tend to have many docked vesicles (as well as more vesicles in total), large active zones and PSDs, and large postsynaptic spines. If multivesicular release occurs, it should do so preferentially at such synapses and give rise to large postsynaptic signals. Conversely, small synapses, some of which are possibly devoid of AMPA receptors, may not contribute appreciably to the excitatory traffic impinging on the postsynaptic neuron.

Even though a pyramidal neuron has 10,000 to 30,000 spine synapses, it has been estimated that only 16 to 26 need to fire synchronously to bring it to action potential threshold (Otmakhov et al., 1993). Clearly, fewer large quanta are required than small ones, and dendritic nonlinearities further complicate this equation.

Dentate granule cells are much smaller and have fewer total spines than pyramidal neurons, although they have the same spine density per unit length of dendrite (Trommald and Hulleberg, 1997). The two extrinsic excitatory projections to granule cells show a striking difference in their short-term plasticity when two presynaptic stimuli are delivered in rapid succession. Lateral perforant path synapses exhibit marked facilitation of the second EPSC compared with the first EPSC ("paired pulse facilitation"). This behavior is essentially the same as at Schaffer collateral synapses on CA1 pyramidal neurons. In contrast, medial perforant path synapses show less pronounced paired pulse facilitation or even depression (McNaughton, 1980). This phenomenon is seen under conditions where inhibitory transmission is blocked, and it appears to reflect intrinsic differences between the glutamatergic synapses in the two pathways. Indeed, medial perforant path synapses appear to have a higher initial release probability than lateral perforant path synapses (Min et al., 1998). Medial and lateral perforant path synapses also show several differences in sensitivity to neurotransmitters acting on presynaptic receptors (Dahl and Sarvey, 1989; Kahle and Cotman, 1989; Macek et al., 1996).

6.7.2 Mossy fiber synapses

Mossy fibers are the thin, unmyelinated axons of dentate granule cells. They form several distinct types of synapse (Henze et al., 2000). Those formed on CA3 pyramidal neurons are in many ways unique (Figure 6.13). First, they are much larger than any other synapses in the hippocampus, with a diameter up to 10 μm. Second, the large presynaptic element (volume approximately 50 μm³) contains numerous dense-core vesicles in addition to the small clear vesicles that predominate in other glutamatergic terminals. These dense-core vesicles are thought to contain dynorphin, Zn^{2+}, and other molecules, many of which are released in an activity-dependent manner. Although mossy fibers are excitatory, they contain abundant GABA (Sandler and Smith, 1991), raising the possibility that they may also package this neurotransmitter in some vesicles and release it following action potential invasion. Indeed, this possibility has some experimental support (Walker et al., 2001; Gutiérrez, 2002). Third, the postsynaptic element is a highly branched structure ("thorny excrescence") akin to a large, complex spine, occurring in the proximal part of the apical dendrite of the CA3 pyramidal neuron. These structures are also found in relatively small numbers in the proximal basal dendrites. The postsynaptic excrescence invaginates the presynaptic terminal. Mossy fiber synapses on CA3 pyramidal neurons can contain between 3 and 80 active zones, each of which

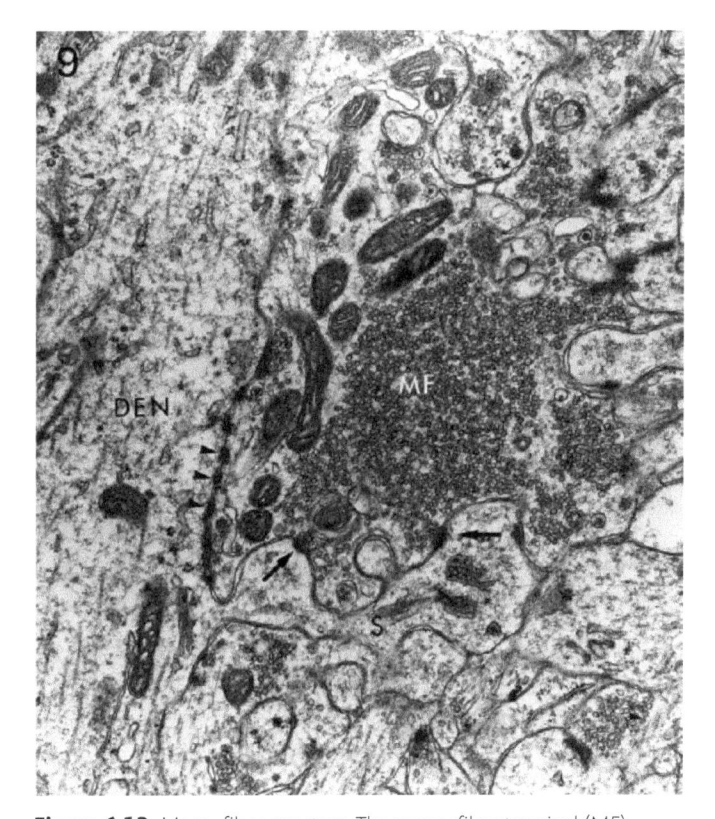

Figure 6.13 Mossy fiber structure. The mossy fiber terminal (MF) contains numerous small (approximately 40 nm diameter) vesicles as well as mitochondria and larger vesicles, some of which are dense-cored. Some vesicles are found close to membrane specializations (arrows) that represent release sites in contact with a postsynaptic complex spine (S) belonging to a CA3 pyramidal neuron. DEN, dendrite. Arrowheads point to puncta adherentia, symmetrical membrane specializations often seen at synapses. (Source: Amaral and Dent, 1981, with permission.)

is apposed to a PSD. Mossy fiber boutons have been estimated to contain approximately 2,000 Ca^{2+} channels, of which P/Q-type are the most abundant, with a smaller contribution from N- and R-type channels (L Li et al., 2007).

Although mossy fiber synapses on CA3 pyramidal neurons are large and complex, this projection is sparse: Each mossy fiber makes only about 14 synapses in CA3 (see Chapter 3). Moreover, at low frequencies unitary mossy fiber EPSCs evoked in individual CA3 pyramidal neurons have a peak amplitude corresponding to a synaptic conductance of approximately 1 nS and consist of approximately 5 quanta (Jonas et al., 1993). This conductance is only approximately fivefold larger than at the far more abundant glutamatergic input to CA3 pyramidal neurons, the associational-commissural fibers.

Mirroring their anatomical complexity, mossy fiber–CA3 synapses show many physiological and pharmacological peculiarities. EPSCs contain a kainate receptor-mediated component in addition to the AMPA receptor-mediated component (Castillo et al., 1997; Vignes and Collingridge, 1997), whereas the NMDA component is relatively small (Jonas et al., 1993). The kainate component is generally thought to be carried by GluK2-containing receptors (Mulle et al., 1998).

Mossy fiber EPSCs exhibit very pronounced facilitation with modest increases in granule cell discharge frequency (Regehr et al., 1994), and a brief train of action potentials in a single mossy fiber can bring a CA3 pyramidal neuron to firing threshold in vivo (Henze et al., 2002). It has been proposed that the likelihood of generating postsynaptic firing is best predicted by the total number of presynaptic action potentials in a burst rather than its frequency (Chamberland et al., 2018). This phenomenon most likely reflects an interplay between Ca^{2+} dynamics and buffering at release sites (Scott and Rusakov, 2006; Chamberland et al., 2018), although autoreceptors also have a role (see below). Following even more intense trains of presynaptic high-frequency action potentials in (e.g., 100 Hz for 1 second), transmission at mossy fibers can remain elevated for hours (Henze et al., 2000). This form of long-term potentiation is distinct from that seen at other spine synapses in the hippocampus in that it is not dependent on NMDA receptors.

Transmission at mossy fiber synapses can be profoundly depressed by activation of several classes of presynaptic receptors, including group II (and in some species group III) metabotropic glutamate receptors (Kamiya et al., 1996) and $GABA_B$ and opioid receptors (Weisskopf et al., 1993). Presynaptic kainate receptors have a paradoxical function: With low concentrations of agonists, probably corresponding to that achieved with synaptic glutamate release, they facilitate transmission, whereas with higher concentrations transmission is depressed (Schmitz et al., 2003). Presynaptic kainate autoreceptors have been shown to contribute to frequency-dependent facilitation of transmission. Presynaptic $GABA_A$ receptors also facilitate transmission, are tonically active and detect spillover of GABA from neighboring synapses (Ruiz et al., 2010). Direct patch clamp recordings from mossy fiber boutons have revealed that $GABA_A$ receptors have a depolarizing action, explained by a relatively high intracellular Cl^- concentration. This depolarization broadens presynaptic action potentials, most likely by inactivating K^+ channels, leading to an enhanced activation of Ca^{2+} channels and consequent increase in neurotransmitter release probability (Ruiz et al., 2010).

A second type of mossy fiber synapse is formed on glutamatergic mossy cells of the dentate hilus. The presynaptic varicosities are also large and contain pleomorphic vesicles. Numerically far more important are small synapses on other hilar interneurons (Acsády et al., 1998). They have a very different shape in that the presynaptic element is a filopodial extension off the shaft of the mossy fiber itself, which makes a single contact with the target interneuron. These synapses are much smaller than the synapses on CA3 pyramidal neurons and probably contain only a single release site. Although they are highly susceptible to presynaptic modulation via metabotropic glutamate receptors, many mossy fiber synapses on interneurons appear not to exhibit marked frequency-dependent facilitation or NMDA receptor-independent LTP (Maccaferri et al., 1998). However, this conclusion may not apply universally to the interneuronal targets of mossy fibers: short- and long-term potentiation have been reported in identified basket cells in response to high-frequency trains of stimuli delivered to single presynaptic granule cells (Alle et al., 2001) (see Chapter 10).

The fourth type of synapse formed by mossy fibers is on the proximal dendrites of other granule cells. Although this projection is normally sparse, it increases following intense seizure activity, in common with the infrapyramidal projection to CA3 ("mossy fiber sprouting").

6.7.3 Other glutamatergic synapses on interneurons

Excitatory synapses on interneurons made by pyramidal neurons are generally small and are made directly on the soma and dendrites (Box 6.3). From limited ultrastructural and electrophysiological data obtained in parallel, they contain a single release site (Gulyás et al., 1993). Recent studies in human tissue resected at surgery however suggest that multiple release sites are the norm (Molnár et al., 2016). Two important pharmacological features distinguish them from small spine synapses on principal neurons. First, at some synapses, especially those made on parvalbumin-positive interneurons, the AMPA receptors are permeable to Ca^{2+} (Jonas et al., 1994), which can be explained by the absence of the Q/R-edited GluA2 subunit that confers Ca^{2+} impermeability at other receptors. Another highly variable property of glutamatergic synapses at interneurons is that some have a kainate receptor-mediated component (Cossart et al., 1998; Frerking et al., 1998). In contrast to mossy fiber–CA3 synapses, interneurons are enriched in GluK1.

The kinetics of AMPA receptor-mediated EPSCs vary extensively among the various excitatory synapses in the hippocampus. In general, the rise times and decay time constants are slow in pyramidal neurons, intermediate in granule cells, and fast in interneurons (Geiger et al., 1997). Although this matches the passive membrane time constants of the various neurons, the difference persists once the cable properties of the neurons have been taken into account. That is, the different kinetics appear to be an intrinsic property of the neurons and/or synapses and, indeed, appear to reflect the subunit composition and splice variants of AMPA receptors expressed in each neuron (Lambolez et al., 1996).

Glutamatergic synapses supplied by the same axon can exhibit markedly different properties such as the degree of facilitation or depression, implying a retrograde signal from the target neuron that specifies some of the properties of the presynaptic terminal (Reyes et al., 1998). Another difference between synapses is the expression of presynaptic group III metabotropic glutamate receptors. As already mentioned, these receptors are present at mossy fiber synapses in some species (for instance in guinea pigs) but not at Schaffer collateral synapses on CA1 pyramidal neurons. However, excitatory transmission to interneurons is highly sensitive to agonists of group III metabotropic receptors (Scanziani et al., 1998). Small synapses on pyramidal neurons, in contrast, are insensitive. This differential sensitivity to group III agonists parallels the distribution of some subtypes of group III receptors imaged with high-resolution immunohistochemical methods. For instance, mGluR7 appears to be expressed in presynaptic active zones apposed to interneurons and not at active zones apposed to pyramidal neurons (Shigemoto et al., 1996).

Finally, glutamatergic synapses to interneurons exhibit several forms of long-term plasticity, including LTP dependent on group I mGluRs and Ca^{2+}-permeable AMPA receptors (Kullmann and Lamsa, 2011).

6.7.4 Inhibitory synapses

GABAergic inhibition of principal neurons has an essential role in regulating the transmission of information through the hippocampal formation (see Box 6.4). The wide range of interneuron morphologies is summarized in Chapter 3, and their intrinsic properties and circuit functions are considered in Chapters 5 and 7. Not all interneurons are GABAergic: Mossy cells in the dentate hilus and giant spiny interneurons in the stratum radiatum are glutamatergic and more akin to pyramidal neurons. There are also intrinsic cholinergic interneurons in the hippocampus. Because relatively little is known about synapses made by glutamatergic and cholinergic interneurons, this section restricts its attention to GABAergic signaling (Figure 6.14). Complementing the variability of interneuron morphology, GABAergic synapses fall into various types depending on their location on the target neuron: axo-axonic, perisomatic, and dendritic. Axo-axonic synapses on principal neurons are exclusively made by parvalbumin-positive interneurons, while perisomatic synapses are innervated by both parvalbumin-positive and cholecystokinin-positive interneurons. As for dendritic synapses, these tend to be made by somatostatin-positive interneurons as well as ivy cells, neurogliaform cells, and other members of the 5-HT3 interneuron family.

Axo-axonic synapses occur 50 to 70 μm from the soma of the target neuron. Situated at the strategic point for action potential initiation, these synapses exert extremely powerful control over the

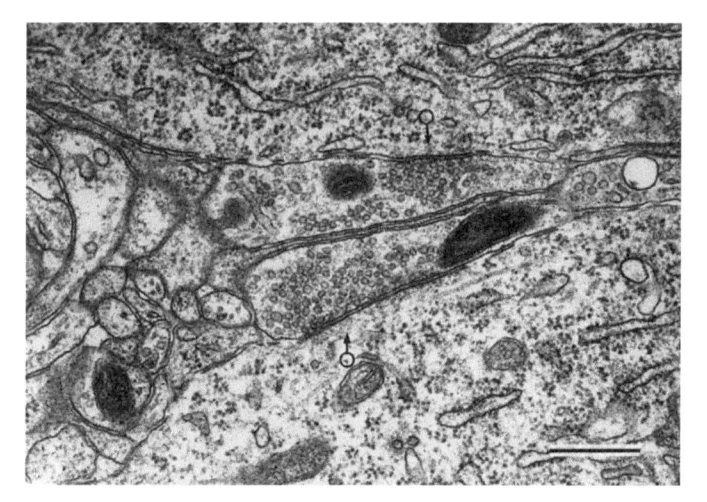

Figure 6.14 Inhibitory synapse structure. The arrows point to two symmetrical synapses on neighboring CA1 pyramidal cell bodies. Bar = 0.5 μm. (Source: Harris and Landis, 1986, with permission.)

discharge of target cells. They yield large-amplitude IPSCs with fast kinetics and activity-dependent depression. Early reports that α2-containing $GABA_A$ receptors are selectively enriched at axo-axonic synapses have not been borne out (Kerti-Szigeti and Nusser, 2016).

Paradoxically, for a synapse optimally located to censor the output of principal neurons, the $GABA_A$ reversal potential in proximal axons appears to be relatively depolarized compared with somatodendritic compartments (Khirug et al., 2008). It has even been proposed that neocortical chandelier cells, which are homologous with hippocampal axo-axonic cells, can trigger action potentials in downstream pyramidal neurons (Szabadics et al., 2006).

Axo-somatic synapses are made by basket cells, whose axon collaterals form clusters of boutons surrounding the soma of the target neuron (see Chapter 3). Basket cells mediate powerful inhibition of principal neurons by release of GABA from the multiple synapses. Interestingly, axo-somatic synapses made two subtypes of basket cells exhibit markedly different properties. Those made by cholecystokinin-positive cells exhibit paired pulse facilitation, with prominent asynchronous release, rely on loose coupling of VGCCs to release sensors, predominantly express presynaptic N-type VGCCs, and are powerfully inhibited by endocannabinoids, while synapses made by parvalbumin-positive interneurons exhibit paired pulse depression, with highly synchronized GABA exocytosis relying on tight coupling, and express P/Q-type VGCCs (Armstrong and Soltesz, 2012; Pelkey et al., 2017).

Dendritic GABAergic inhibitory synapses on pyramidal cells are made by a variety of interneurons whose cell bodies are found in the strata oriens, radiatum, and lacunosum-moleculare. Synapses formed on the distal dendrites are thought to control the excitability of the postsynaptic neuron relatively indirectly. They are unlikely to hyperpolarize the cell body effectively because they are electrically remote, but they may be highly effective in shunting locally evoked EPSCs (Staley and Mody, 1992).

GABAergic IPSCs in pyramidal neurons have highly variable kinetics. Some IPSCs with exceptionally slow decay time constants (30 ms or longer), known as $GABA_{A-Slow}$ IPSCs (Pearce, 1993), are thought to result from release of a cloud of GABA that persists in the extracellular space for a relatively long time. The presynaptic neurons giving rise to this unusual mode of signaling are at least in part neurogliaform cells (Overstreet-Wadiche and McBain, 2015). Their axonal boutons are very small, and some do not form conventional synapses, implying that they signal through a form of volume transmission, activating both $GABA_A$ and $GABA_B$ receptors relatively diffusely.

In contrast to glutamatergic synapses, GABA release is relatively resistant to adenosine (Yoon and Rothman, 1991). Surprisingly, GABAergic synapses on interneurons are as sensitive to group III metabotropic glutamate agonists as glutamatergic synapses even though only the latter actually release the endogenous agonist. These receptors can detect glutamate spillover from neighboring excitatory synapses (Semyanov and Kullmann, 2000).

6.7.5 Tonic inhibition

Some $GABA_A$ receptors are active even in the absence of presynaptic activity, a phenomenon known as "tonic" inhibition (to distinguish it from "phasic" inhibition represented by the occurrence of IPSCs) (Semyanov et al., 2004). Tonic $GABA_A$ receptor-mediated inhibition has been reported in numerous cell types, including interneurons, and it has been proposed that this reflects a homeostatic role in regulating circuit excitability (Semyanov et al., 2003). Pharmacological and genetic dissection of tonic inhibition has revealed contributions from δ-containing and α5-containing receptors, which have a relatively high affinity for ambient GABA, and which are at least in part located to extrasynaptic membranes (Brickley and Mody, 2012; Hannan et al., 2020). A component of tonic inhibition reflects the spontaneous opening of receptors in the unbound state (Wlodarczyk et al., 2013).

Inhibitory synapses are also made among interneurons. These synapses appear to show use-dependent depression similar to that seen at most GABAergic synapses on principal cells, although the kinetics of the IPSCs are generally faster (Bartos et al., 2001). Parvalbumin-positive basket cells are also coupled by gap junctions (Fukuda and Kosaka, 2000). Genetic deletion of connexin 36 perturbs γ frequency oscillations, possibly because of impaired electrical coupling among these interneurons (Hormuzdi et al., 2001).

6.8 Unresolved issues

There are numerous unresolved issues surrounding synaptic function that cannot be listed completely here. Many are fundamental questions concerning transmitter release, such as the mechanisms by which synaptotagmin transduces the Ca^{2+} surge to trigger exocytosis, how the degree of filling of a vesicle affects its readiness for release, and whether and under what conditions exocytosis can take place via a fusion pore. Other important questions concern postsynaptic mechanisms. Some of these questions, such as the targeting and clustering of glutamate receptors at synapses, have attracted intense interest because of their potential role in the development and plasticity of excitatory transmission. They are taken up in greater detail in Chapter 7. Other areas, such as the detailed postsynaptic signaling cascades, leading to effects as remote as nuclear transcription, are discussed, in the context of LTP, in Chapter 10.

As in so many areas of neuroscience, insights at a molecular level are outpacing progress at a more macroscopic level. For instance, although the involvement of cholinergic mechanisms in theta rhythms is on a relatively secure footing, this understanding remains at a qualitative level. Many critical parameters remain far from established: What is the temporal profile of acetylcholine release? Where are the target receptors in relation to the sites of release? How many individual terminals cooperate to activate muscarinic and nicotinic receptors? Which of the numerous actions of these receptors actually take place in vivo?

Similar questions occur for each of the other neurotransmitters described here. Most of this chapter has concentrated on fast ionotropic signaling by glutamate and GABA; this is because, to a great extent, electrophysiological methods are so powerful in detecting and quantifying EPSP/Cs and IPSP/Cs. More diffuse types of signaling mediated by metabotropic receptors or even by extrasynaptic actions at ionotropic receptors may be of similar or even greater importance for understanding the roles of these transmitters in intercellular signaling. As for the monoamines and peptides, they are considered less important only on the grounds that the releasing axons are relatively sparse. However, not until their actions have been put on a sound quantitative footing similar to that of the amino acid neurotransmitters will it be possible to know if this ranking is correct.

Acknowledgments

Our thanks to the editors for helpful input to this chapter.

REFERENCES

Abood M, et al. (2019) Cannabinoid receptors (version 2019.4) in the IUPHAR/BPS Guide to Pharmacology Database. *IUPHAR/ BPS Guide to Pharmacology CITE 2019(4)*. doi: 10.2218/gtopdb/ F13/2019.4.

Acsády L, Kamondi A, Sik A, Freund T, Buzsáki G (1998) GABAergic cells are the major postsynaptic targets of mossy fibers in the rat hippocampus. *J Neurosci* 18:3386–3403.

Acuna C, Guo Q, Burré J, Sharma M, Sun J, Südhof TC (2014) Microsecond dissection of neurotransmitter release: SNARE-complex assembly dictates speed and $Ca^{2}+$ sensitivity. *Neuron* 82:1088–1100.

Alle H, Jonas P, Geiger JRP (2001) PTP and LTP at a hippocampal mossy fiber-interneuron synapse. *PNAS* 98:14708–14713.

Althof D, Baehrens D, Watanabe M, Suzuki N, Fakler B, Kulik Á (2015) Inhibitory and excitatory axon terminals share a common nano-architecture of their Cav2.1 (P/Q-type) Ca(2+) channels. *Front Cell Neurosci* 9:315.

Altosaar K, et al. (2021) Adrenoceptors in GtoPdb v.2021.3. *IUPHAR/ BPS Guide to Pharmacology CITE 2021(3)*. doi: 10.2218/gtopdb/ F4/2021.3.

Amaral DG, Dent JA (1981) Development of the mossy fibers of the dentate gyrus: I. A light and electron microscopic study of the mossy fibers and their expansions. *J Comp Neurol* 195:51–86.

Andrade R, et al. (2019) 5-Hydroxytryptamine receptors (version 2019.4) in the IUPHAR/BPS Guide to Pharmacology Database. *IUPHAR/BPS Guide to Pharmacology CITE 2019(4)*. doi: 10.2218/ gtopdb/F1/2019.4.

Armstrong C, Soltesz I (2012) Basket cell dichotomy in microcircuit function. *J Physiol* 590:683–694.

Ascher P, Nowak L (1988) The role of divalent cations in the N-methyl-D-aspartate responses of mouse central neurones in culture. *J Physiol* 399:247–266.

Asztely F, Erdemli G, Kullmann DM (1997) Extrasynaptic glutamate spillover in the hippocampus: dependence on temperature and the role of active glutamate uptake. *Neuron* 18:281–293.

Augustin I, Rosenmund C, Südhof TC, Brose N (1999) Munc13-1 is essential for fusion competence of glutamatergic synaptic vesicles. *Nature* 400:457–461.

Bacaj T, Wu D, Yang X, Morishita W, Zhou P, Xu W, Malenka RC, Südhof TC (2013) Synaptotagmin-1 and synaptotagmin-7 trigger synchronous and asynchronous phases of neurotransmitter release. *Neuron* 80:947–959.

Bai J, Tucker WC, Chapman ER (2004) PIP2 increases the speed of response of synaptotagmin and steers its membrane-penetration activity toward the plasma membrane. *Nat Struct Mol Biol* 11:36–44.

Bartos M, Vida I, Frotscher M, Geiger JRP, Jonas P (2001) Rapid signaling at inhibitory synapses in a dentate gyrus interneuron network. *J Neurosci* 21:2687–2698.

Baude A, Nusser Z, Roberts JD, Mulvihill E, McIlhinney RA, Somogyi P (1993) The metabotropic glutamate receptor (mGluR1 alpha) is concentrated at perisynaptic membrane of neuronal subpopulations as detected by immunogold reaction. *Neuron* 11:771–787.

Beaulieu J-M, et al. (2019) Dopamine receptors (version 2019.4) in the IUPHAR/BPS Guide to Pharmacology Database. *IUPHAR/*

BPS Guide to Pharmacology CITE 2019(4). doi: 10.2218/gtopdb/F20/2019.4.

Behrends JC, ten Bruggencate G (1993) Cholinergic modulation of synaptic inhibition in the guinea pig hippocampus in vitro: excitation of GABAergic interneurons and inhibition of GABA-release. *J Neurophysiol* 69:626–629.

Bekkers JM (1993) Enhancement by histamine of NMDA-mediated synaptic transmission in the hippocampus. *Science* 261:104–106.

Ben-Ari Y, Cherubini E, Corradetti R, Gaiarsa JL (1989) Giant synaptic potentials in immature rat CA3 hippocampal neurones. *J Physiol* 416:303–325.

Bergles DE, Roberts JD, Somogyi P, Jahr CE (2000) Glutamatergic synapses on oligodendrocyte precursor cells in the hippocampus. *Nature* 405:187–191.

Berridge MJ (2016) The inositol trisphosphate/calcium signaling pathway in health and disease. *Physiol Rev* 96:1261–1296.

Bi G, Poo M (2001) Synaptic modification by correlated activity: Hebb's postulate revisited. *Annu Rev Neurosci* 24:139–166.

Biederer T, Kaeser PS, Blanpied TA (2017) Transcellular nanoalignment of synaptic function. *Neuron* 96:680–696.

Birdsall NJM, et al. (2021) Acetylcholine receptors (muscarinic) in GtoPdb v.2021.3. *IUPHAR/BPS Guide to Pharmacology CITE 2021(3)*. doi: 10.2218/gtopdb/F2/2021.3.

Bollmann JH, Sakmann B, Borst JG (2000) Calcium sensitivity of glutamate release in a calyx-type terminal. *Science* 289:953–957.

Brakeman PR, Lanahan AA, O'Brien R, Roche K, Barnes CA, Huganir RL, Worley PF (1997) Homer: a protein that selectively binds metabotropic glutamate receptors. *Nature* 386:284–288.

Brenowitz S, Trussell LO (2001) Minimizing synaptic depression by control of release probability. *J Neurosci* 21:1857–1867.

Brickley SG, Mody I (2012) Extrasynaptic GABAA receptors: their function in the CNS and implications for disease. *Neuron* 73:23–34.

Brown DA, Passmore GM (2009) Neural KCNQ (Kv7) channels. *Br J Pharmacol* 156:1185–1195.

Brunger AT, Choi UB, Lai Y, Leitz J, Zhou Q (2018) Molecular mechanisms of fast neurotransmitter release. *Annu Rev Biophys* 47:469–497.

Buchanan KA, Petrovic MM, Chamberlain SEL, Marrion NV, Mellor JR (2010) Facilitation of long-term potentiation by muscarinic M1 receptors is mediated by inhibition of SK channels. *Neuron* 68:948–963.

Bucurenciu I, Bischofberger J, Jonas P (2010) A small number of open Ca2+ channels trigger transmitter release at a central GABAergic synapse. *Nat Neurosci* 13:19–21.

Bucurenciu I, Kulik A, Schwaller B, Frotscher M, Jonas P (2008) Nanodomain coupling between Ca2+ channels and Ca2+ sensors promotes fast and efficient transmitter release at a cortical GABAergic synapse. *Neuron* 57:536–545.

Carmona-Rosas G, Alcántara-Hernández R, Hernández-Espinosa DA (2018) Dissecting the signaling features of the multi-protein complex GPCR/β-arrestin/ERK1/2. *Eur J Cell Biol* 97:349–358.

Castillo PE, Malenka RC, Nicoll RA (1997) Kainate receptors mediate a slow postsynaptic current in hippocampal CA3 neurons. *Nature* 388:182–186.

Chamberland S, Timofeeva Y, Evstratova A, Volynski K, Tóth K (2018) Action potential counting at giant mossy fiber terminals gates information transfer in the hippocampus. *Proc Natl Acad Sci U S A* 115:7434–7439.

Chazot P, et al. (2021) Histamine receptors in GtoPdb v.2021.3. *IUPHAR/BPS Guide to Pharmacology CITE 2021(3)*. doi: 10.2218/gtopdb/F33/2021.3.

Chen YA, Scheller RH (2001) SNARE-mediated membrane fusion. *Nat Rev Mol Cell Biol* 2:98–106.

Chittajallu R, Vignes M, Dev KK, Barnes JM, Collingridge GL, Henley JM (1996) Regulation of glutamate release by presynaptic kainate receptors in the hippocampus. *Nature* 379:78–81.

Choi S, Klingauf J, Tsien RW (2000) Postfusional regulation of cleft glutamate concentration during LTP at "silent synapses." *Nat Neurosci* 3:330–336.

Connors BW, Long MA (2004) Electrical synapses in the mammalian brain. *Annu Rev Neurosci* 27:393–418.

Cornejo VH, Ofer N, Yuste R (2022) Voltage compartmentalization in dendritic spines in vivo. *Science* 375:82–86.

Cossart R, Esclapez M, Hirsch JC, Bernard C, Ben-Ari Y (1998) GluR5 kainate receptor activation in interneurons increases tonic inhibition of pyramidal cells. *Nat Neurosci* 1:470–478.

Crépel V, Aniksztejn L, Ben-Ari Y, Hammond C (1994) Glutamate metabotropic receptors increase a Ca(2+)-activated nonspecific cationic current in CA1 hippocampal neurons. *J Neurophysiol* 72:1561–1569.

Dahl D, Sarvey JM (1989) Norepinephrine induces pathway-specific long-lasting potentiation and depression in the hippocampal dentate gyrus. *Proc Natl Acad Sci U S A* 86:4776–4780.

Danbolt NC (2001) Glutamate uptake. *Prog Neurobiol* 65:1–105.

de Wit J, Ghosh A (2016) Specification of synaptic connectivity by cell surface interactions. *Nat Rev Neurosci* 17:4–4.

Deng L, Kaeser PS, Xu W, Südhof TC (2011) RIM proteins activate vesicle priming by reversing autoinhibitory homodimerization of Munc13. *Neuron* 69:317–331.

Deng S, Li J, He Q, Zhang X, Zhu J, Li L, Mi Z, Yang X, Jiang M, Dong Q, Mao Y, Shu Y (2020) Regulation of recurrent inhibition by asynchronous glutamate release in neocortex. *Neuron* 105:522–533, e4.

Devine MJ, Kittler JT (2018) Mitochondria at the neuronal presynapse in health and disease. *Nat Rev Neurosci* 19:63–80.

Dolphin AC, Lee A (2020) Presynaptic calcium channels: specialized control of synaptic neurotransmitter release. *Nat Rev Neurosci* 21:213–229.

Dulubova I, Khvotchev M, Liu S, Huryeva I, Südhof TC, Rizo J (2007) Munc18-1 binds directly to the neuronal SNARE complex. *Proc Natl Acad Sci U S A* 104:2697–2702.

Dulubova I, Sugita S, Hill S, Hosaka M, Fernandez I, Südhof TC, Rizo J (1999) A conformational switch in syntaxin during exocytosis: role of munc18. *EMBO J* 18:4372–4382.

Eggermann E, Bucurenciu I, Goswami SP, Jonas P (2011) Nanodomain coupling between Ca^2+ channels and sensors of exocytosis at fast mammalian synapses. *Nat Rev Neurosci* 13:7–21.

Eggermann E, Jonas P (2011) How the "slow" Ca(2+) buffer parvalbumin affects transmitter release in nanodomain-coupling regimes. *Nat Neurosci* 15:20–22.

Emptage N, Bliss TV, Fine A (1999) Single synaptic events evoke NMDA receptor-mediated release of calcium from internal stores in hippocampal dendritic spines. *Neuron* 22:115–124.

Ermolyuk YS, Alder FG, Surges R, Pavlov IY, Timofeeva Y, Kullmann DM, Volynski KE (2013) Differential triggering of spontaneous glutamate release by P/Q-, N- and R-type Ca2+ channels. *Nat Neurosci* 16:1754–1763.

Esplugues JV (2002) NO as a signalling molecule in the nervous system. *Br J Pharmacol* 135:1079–1095.

Essrich C, Lorez M, Benson JA, Fritschy JM, Lüscher B (1998) Postsynaptic clustering of major GABAA receptor subtypes requires the gamma 2 subunit and gephyrin. *Nat Neurosci* 1:563–571.

Exposito-Alonso D, Osório C, Bernard C, Pascual-García S, Del Pino I, Marín O, Rico B (2020) Subcellular sorting of neuregulins controls the assembly of excitatory-inhibitory cortical circuits. *Elife* 9:e57000.

Fabian-Fine R, Skehel P, Errington ML, Davies HA, Sher E, Stewart MG, Fine A (2001) Ultrastructural distribution of the alpha7 nicotinic acetylcholine receptor subunit in rat hippocampus. *J Neurosci* 21:7993–8003.

Falcón-Moya R, Rodríguez-Moreno A (2021) Metabotropic actions of kainate receptors modulating glutamate release. *Neuropharmacology* 197:108696.

Farsi Z, Preobraschenski J, van den Bogaart G, Riedel D, Jahn R, Woehler A (2016) Single-vesicle imaging reveals different transport mechanisms between glutamatergic and GABAergic vesicles. *Science* 351:981–984.

Frerking M, Malenka RC, Nicoll RA (1998) Synaptic activation of kainate receptors on hippocampal interneurons. *Nat Neurosci* 1:479–486.

Fritschy JM, Meskenaite V, Weinmann O, Honer M, Benke D, Mohler H (1999) GABAB-receptor splice variants GB1a and GB1b in rat brain: developmental regulation, cellular distribution and extrasynaptic localization. *Eur J Neurosci* 11:761–768.

Fukuda T, Kosaka T (2000) Gap junctions linking the dendritic network of GABAergic interneurons in the hippocampus. *J Neurosci* 20:1519–1528.

Gan Q, Watanabe S (2018) Synaptic vesicle endocytosis in different model systems. *Front Cell Neurosci* 12:171.

Gauthier-Kemper A, Kahms M, Klingauf J (2015) Restoring synaptic vesicles during compensatory endocytosis. *Essays Biochem* 57:121–134.

Geiger JR, Lübke J, Roth A, Frotscher M, Jonas P (1997) Submillisecond AMPA receptor-mediated signaling at a principal neuron-interneuron synapse. *Neuron* 18:1009–1023.

Geiger JR, Melcher T, Koh DS, Sakmann B, Seeburg PH, Jonas P, Monyer H (1995) Relative abundance of subunit mRNAs determines gating and Ca2+ permeability of AMPA receptors in principal neurons and interneurons in rat CNS. *Neuron* 15:193–204.

Gimber N, Tadeus G, Maritzen T, Schmoranzer J, Haucke V (2015) Diffusional spread and confinement of newly exocytosed synaptic vesicle proteins. *Nat Commun* 6:8392.

Golding NL, Jung HY, Mickus T, Spruston N (1999) Dendritic calcium spike initiation and repolarization are controlled by distinct potassium channel subtypes in CA1 pyramidal neurons. *J Neurosci* 19:8789–8798.

Gomez-Castro F, et al. (2021) Convergence of adenosine and GABA signaling for synapse stabilization during development. *Science* 374:eabk2055.

Gotti C, Marks MJ, Millar NS, Wonnacott S (2021) Nicotinic acetylcholine receptors (nACh) in GtoPdb v.2021.3. *IUPHAR/BPS Guide to Pharmacology CITE 2021(3)*. doi: 10.2218/gtopdb/F76/2021.3.

Gracheva EO, Hadwiger G, Nonet ML, Richmond JE (2008) Direct interactions between C. elegans RAB-3 and Rim provide a mechanism to target vesicles to the presynaptic density. *Neurosci Lett* 444:137–142.

Gray EG (1959) Axo-somatic and axo-dendritic synapses of the cerebral cortex: an electron microscope study. *J Anat* 93:420–433.

Greger IH, Watson JF, Cull-Candy SG (2017) Structural and functional architecture of AMPA-type glutamate receptors and their auxiliary proteins. *Neuron* 94:713–730.

Gregory KJ, Goudet C (2021) International union of basic and clinical pharmacology: CXI. Pharmacology, signaling, and physiology of metabotropic glutamate receptors. *Pharmacol Rev* 73:521–569.

Grote E, Carr CM, Novick PJ (2000) Ordering the final events in yeast exocytosis. *J Cell Biol* 151:439–452.

Grushin K, Wang J, Coleman J, Rothman JE, Sindelar CV, Krishnakumar SS (2019) Structural basis for the clamping and Ca2+ activation of SNARE-mediated fusion by synaptotagmin. *Nat Commun* 10:2413.

Guérineau NC, Gähwiler BH, Gerber U (1994) Reduction of resting K+ current by metabotropic glutamate and muscarinic receptors in rat CA3 cells: mediation by G-proteins. *J Physiol* 474:27–33.

Gulyás AI, Miles R, Sík A, Tóth K, Tamamaki N, Freund TF (1993) Hippocampal pyramidal cells excite inhibitory neurons through a single release site. *Nature* 366:683–687.

Gutiérrez R (2002) Activity-dependent expression of simultaneous glutamatergic and GABAergic neurotransmission from the mossy fibers in vitro. *J Neurophysiol* 87:2562–2570.

Han Y, Kaeser PS, Südhof TC, Schneggenburger R (2011) RIM determines Ca2+ channel density and vesicle docking at the presynaptic active zone. *Neuron* 69:304–316.

Hannan S, Minere M, Harris J, Izquierdo P, Thomas P, Tench B, Smart TG (2020) GABAAR isoform and subunit structural motifs determine synaptic and extrasynaptic receptor localisation. *Neuropharmacology* 169:107540.

Hanse E, Seth H, Riebe I (2013) AMPA-silent synapses in brain development and pathology. *Nat Rev Neurosci* 14:839–850.

Hansen KB, Wollmuth LP, Bowie D, Furukawa H, Menniti FS, Sobolevsky AI, Swanson GT, Swanger SA, Greger IH, Nakagawa T, et al. (2021) Structure, function, and pharmacology of glutamate receptor ion channels. *Pharmacol Rev* 73:298–487.

Harris KM, Landis DM (1986) Membrane structure at synaptic junctions in area CA1 of the rat hippocampus. *Neuroscience* 19:857–872.

Harris KM, Sultan P (1995) Variation in the number, location and size of synaptic vesicles provides an anatomical basis for the non-uniform probability of release at hippocampal CA1 synapses. *Neuropharmacology* 34:1387–1395.

Hata Y, Slaughter CA, Südhof TC (1993) Synaptic vesicle fusion complex contains unc-18 homologue bound to syntaxin. *Nature* 366:347–351.

Hefft S, Jonas P (2005) Asynchronous GABA release generates long-lasting inhibition at a hippocampal interneuron-principal neuron synapse. *Nat Neurosci* 8:1319–1328.

Heine M, Groc L, Frischknecht R, Béïque J-C, Lounis B, Rumbaugh G, Huganir RL, Cognet L, Choquet D (2008) Surface mobility of postsynaptic AMPARs tunes synaptic transmission. *Science* 320:201–205.

Held RG, Liu C, Kaeser PS (2016) ELKS controls the pool of readily releasable vesicles at excitatory synapses through its N-terminal coiled-coil domains. *Elife* 5:e14862.

Helmchen F, Borst JG, Sakmann B (1997) Calcium dynamics associated with a single action potential in a CNS presynaptic terminal. *Biophys J* 72:1458–1471.

Henneberger C, Papouin T, Oliet SHR, Rusakov DA (2010) Long-term potentiation depends on release of D-serine from astrocytes. *Nature* 463:232–236.

Henze DA, Urban NN, Barrionuevo G (2000) The multifarious hippocampal mossy fiber pathway: a review. *Neuroscience* 98:407–427.

Henze DA, Wittner L, Buzsáki G (2002) Single granule cells reliably discharge targets in the hippocampal CA3 network in vivo. *Nat Neurosci* 5:790–795.

Hestrin S, Sah P, Nicoll RA (1990) Mechanisms generating the time course of dual component excitatory synaptic currents recorded in hippocampal slices. *Neuron* 5:247–253.

Holderith N, Lorincz A, Katona G, Rózsa B, Kulik A, Watanabe M, Nusser Z (2012) Release probability of hippocampal glutamatergic terminals scales with the size of the active zone. *Nat Neurosci* **15**:988–997.

Hormuzdi SG, Pais I, LeBeau FEN, Towers SK, Rozov A, Buhl EH, Whittington MA, Monyer H (2001) Impaired electrical signaling disrupts gamma frequency oscillations in connexin 36-deficient mice. *Neuron* **31**:487–495.

Hua Y, Scheller RH (2001) Three SNARE complexes cooperate to mediate membrane fusion. *Proc Natl Acad Sci U S A* **98**:8065–8070.

Huang Y, Thathiah A (2015) Regulation of neuronal communication by G protein-coupled receptors. *FEBS Letters* **589**:1607–1619.

Huson V, Regehr WG (2020) Diverse roles of synaptotagmin-7 in regulating vesicle fusion. *Curr Opin Neurobiol* **63**:42–52.

Imig C, Min S-W, Krinner S, Arancillo M, Rosenmund C, Südhof TC, Rhee J, Brose N, Cooper BH (2014) The morphological and molecular nature of synaptic vesicle priming at presynaptic active zones. *Neuron* **84**:416–431.

Isaac JT, Nicoll RA, Malenka RC (1995) Evidence for silent synapses: implications for the expression of LTP. *Neuron* **15**:427–434.

Jackman SL, Turecek J, Belinsky JE, Regehr WG (2016) The calcium sensor synaptotagmin 7 is required for synaptic facilitation. *Nature* **529**:88–91.

Jahn R, Fasshauer D (2012) Molecular machines governing exocytosis of synaptic vesicles. *Nature* **490**:201–207.

Jahn R, Lang T, Südhof TC (2003) Membrane fusion. *Cell* **112**:519–533.

Jahr CE, Stevens CF (1987) Glutamate activates multiple single channel conductances in hippocampal neurons. *Nature* **325**:522–525.

Jockusch WJ, Speidel D, Sigler A, Sørensen JB, Varoqueaux F, Rhee J-S, Brose N (2007) CAPS-1 and CAPS-2 are essential synaptic vesicle priming proteins. *Cell* **131**:796–808.

Johnson JW, Ascher P (1987) Glycine potentiates the NMDA response in cultured mouse brain neurons. *Nature* **325**:529–531.

Jonas P, Major G, Sakmann B (1993) Quantal components of unitary EPSCs at the mossy fibre synapse on CA3 pyramidal cells of rat hippocampus. *J Physiol (Lond)* **472**:615–663.

Jonas P, Racca C, Sakmann B, Seeburg PH, Monyer H (1994) Differences in Ca2+ permeability of AMPA-type glutamate receptor channels in neocortical neurons caused by differential GluR-B subunit expression. *Neuron* **12**:1281–1289.

Jordan BA, Devi LA (1999) G-protein-coupled receptor heterodimerization modulates receptor function. *Nature* **399**:697–700.

Jurado S, Goswami D, Zhang Y, Molina AJM, Südhof TC, Malenka RC (2013) LTP requires a unique postsynaptic SNARE fusion machinery. *Neuron* **77**:542–558.

Kaempf N, Maritzen T (2017) Safeguards of neurotransmission: endocytic adaptors as regulators of synaptic vesicle composition and function. *Front Cell Neurosci* **11**:320.

Kaeser PS, Deng L, Wang Y, Dulubova I, Liu X, Rizo J, Südhof TC (2011) RIM proteins tether Ca2+ channels to presynaptic active zones via a direct PDZ-domain interaction. *Cell* **144**:282–295.

Kaeser PS, Regehr WG (2014) Molecular mechanisms for synchronous, asynchronous, and spontaneous neurotransmitter release. *Annu Rev Physiol* **76**:333–363.

Kaeser PS, Regehr WG (2017) The readily releasable pool of synaptic vesicles. *Curr Opin Neurobiol* **43**:63–70.

Kahle JS, Cotman CW (1989) Carbachol depresses synaptic responses in the medial but not the lateral perforant path. *Brain Res* **482**:159–163.

Kaila K, Lamsa K, Smirnov S, Taira T, Voipio J (1997) Long-lasting GABA-mediated depolarization evoked by high-frequency stimulation in pyramidal neurons of rat hippocampal slice is attributable to a network-driven, bicarbonate-dependent K+ transient. *J Neurosci* **17**:7662–7672.

Kamiya H, Shinozaki H, Yamamoto C (1996) Activation of metabotropic glutamate receptor type 2/3 suppresses transmission at rat hippocampal mossy fibre synapses. *J Physiol* **493**(Pt 2):447–455.

Kavalali ET (2015) The mechanisms and functions of spontaneous neurotransmitter release. *Nat Rev Neurosci* **16**:5–16.

Kavanaugh MP, Arriza JL, North RA, Amara SG (1992) Electrogenic uptake of gamma-aminobutyric acid by a cloned transporter expressed in Xenopus oocytes. *J Biol Chem* **267**:22007–22009.

Kay AR (2003) Evidence for chelatable zinc in the extracellular space of the hippocampus, but little evidence for synaptic release of Zn. *J Neurosci* **23**:6847–6855.

Kerti-Szigeti K, Nusser Z (2016) Similar GABAA receptor subunit composition in somatic and axon initial segment synapses of hippocampal pyramidal cells Bartos M, ed. *eLife* **5**:e18426.

Khirug S, Yamada J, Afzalov R, Voipio J, Khiroug L, Kaila K (2008) GABAergic depolarization of the axon initial segment in cortical principal neurons is caused by the Na-K-2Cl cotransporter NKCC1. *J Neurosci* **28**:4635–4639.

Koo SJ, Kochlamazashvili G, Rost B, Puchkov D, Gimber N, Lehmann M, Tadeus G, Schmoranzer J, Rosenmund C, Haucke V, Maritzen T (2015) Vesicular synaptobrevin/VAMP2 levels guarded by AP180 control efficient neurotransmission. *Neuron* **88**:330–344.

Kornau HC, Schenker LT, Kennedy MB, Seeburg PH (1995) Domain interaction between NMDA receptor subunits and the postsynaptic density protein PSD-95. *Science* **269**:1737–1740.

Kullmann DM (1994) Amplitude fluctuations of dual-component EPSCs in hippocampal pyramidal cells: implications for long-term potentiation. *Neuron* **12**:1111–1120.

Kullmann DM (2003) Silent synapses: what are they telling us about long-term potentiation? *Philos Trans R Soc Lond B Biol Sci* **358**:727–733.

Kullmann DM, Asztely F (1998) Extrasynaptic glutamate spillover in the hippocampus: evidence and implications. *Trends Neurosci* **21**:8–14.

Kullmann DM, Lamsa KP (2011) LTP and LTD in cortical GABAergic interneurons: emerging rules and roles. *Neuropharmacology* **60**:712–719.

Kullmann DM, Nicoll RA (1992) Long-term potentiation is associated with increases in quantal content and quantal amplitude. *Nature* **357**:240–244.

Lambolez B, Ropert N, Perrais D, Rossier J, Hestrin S (1996) Correlation between kinetics and RNA splicing of alpha-amino-3-hydroxy-5-methylisoxazole-4-propionic acid receptors in neocortical neurons. *Proc Natl Acad Sci U S A* **93**:1797–1802.

Lee S-E, Lee Y, Lee GH (2019) The regulation of glutamic acid decarboxylases in GABA neurotransmission in the brain. *Arch Pharm Res* **42**:1031–1039.

Li L, Bischofberger J, Jonas P (2007) Differential gating and recruitment of P/Q-, N-, and R-type Ca2+ channels in hippocampal mossy fiber boutons. *J Neurosci* **27**:13420–13429.

Li X, Radhakrishnan A, Grushin K, Kasula R, Chaudhuri A, Gomathinayagam S, Krishnakumar SS, Liu J, Rothman JE (2019) Symmetrical organization of proteins under docked synaptic vesicles. *FEBS Lett* **593**:144–153.

Liao D, Hessler NA, Malinow R (1995) Activation of postsynaptically silent synapses during pairing-induced LTP in CA1 region of hippocampal slice. *Nature* **375**:400–404.

Lisman JE (1997) Bursts as a unit of neural information: making unreliable synapses reliable. *Trends Neurosci* **20**:38–43.

Luo F, Südhof TC (2017) Synaptotagmin-7-mediated asynchronous release boosts high-fidelity synchronous transmission at a central synapse. *Neuron* **94**:826–839, e3.

Lyubimov AY, Uervirojnangkoorn M, Zeldin OB, Zhou Q, Zhao M, Brewster AS, Michels-Clark T, Holton JM, Sauter NK, Weis WI,

Semyanov A, Walker MC, Kullmann DM, Silver RA (2004) Tonically active GABA A receptors: modulating gain and maintaining the tone. *Trends Neurosci* 27:262–269.

Sepkuty JP, Cohen AS, Eccles C, Rafiq A, Behar K, Ganel R, Coulter DA, Rothstein JD (2002) A neuronal glutamate transporter contributes to neurotransmitter GABA synthesis and epilepsy. *J Neurosci* 22:6372–6379.

Shepherd GM, Harris KM (1998) Three-dimensional structure and composition of CA3-->CA1 axons in rat hippocampal slices: implications for presynaptic connectivity and compartmentalization. *J Neurosci* 18:8300–8310.

Shi L, Shen Q-T, Kiel A, Wang J, Wang H-W, Melia TJ, Rothman JE, Pincet F (2012) SNARE proteins: one to fuse and three to keep the nascent fusion pore open. *Science* 335:1355–1359.

Shigemoto R, Kinoshita A, Wada E, Nomura S, Ohishi H, Takada M, Flor PJ, Neki A, Abe T, Nakanishi S, Mizuno N (1997) Differential presynaptic localization of metabotropic glutamate receptor subtypes in the rat hippocampus. *J Neurosci* 17:7503–7522.

Shigemoto R, Kulik A, Roberts JD, Ohishi H, Nusser Z, Kaneko T, Somogyi P (1996) Target-cell-specific concentration of a metabotropic glutamate receptor in the presynaptic active zone. *Nature* 381:523–525.

Shin O-H, Xu J, Rizo J, Südhof TC (2009) Differential but convergent functions of Ca2+ binding to synaptotagmin-1 C2 domains mediate neurotransmitter release. *Proc Natl Acad Sci U S A* 106:16469–16474.

Sinha R, Ahmed S, Jahn R, Klingauf J (2011) Two synaptobrevin molecules are sufficient for vesicle fusion in central nervous system synapses. *Proc Natl Acad Sci U S A* 108:14318–14323.

Söllner T, Whiteheart SW, Brunner M, Erdjument-Bromage H, Geromanos S, Tempst P, Rothman JE (1993) SNAP receptors implicated in vesicle targeting and fusion. *Nature* 362:318–324.

Sommer B, Köhler M, Sprengel R, Seeburg PH (1991) RNA editing in brain controls a determinant of ion flow in glutamate-gated channels. *Cell* 67:11–19.

Sorra KE, Harris KM (1993) Occurrence and three-dimensional structure of multiple synapses between individual radiatum axons and their target pyramidal cells in hippocampal area CA1. *J Neurosci* 13:3736–3748.

Soykan T, Maritzen T, Haucke V (2016) Modes and mechanisms of synaptic vesicle recycling. *Curr Opin Neurobiol* 39:17–23.

Sperk G, Schwarzer C, Tsunashima K, Fuchs K, Sieghart W (1997) GABA(A) receptor subunits in the rat hippocampus: I. immunocytochemical distribution of 13 subunits. *Neuroscience* 80:987–1000.

Staley KJ, Mody I (1992) Shunting of excitatory input to dentate gyrus granule cells by a depolarizing GABAA receptor-mediated postsynaptic conductance. *J Neurophysiol* 68:197–212.

Staley KJ, Soldo BL, Proctor WR (1995) Ionic mechanisms of neuronal excitation by inhibitory GABAA receptors. *Science* 269:977–981.

Straub C, Hunt DL, Yamasaki M, Kim KS, Watanabe M, Castillo PE, Tomita S (2011) Distinct functions of kainate receptors in the brain are determined by the auxiliary subunit Neto1. *Nat Neurosci* 14:866–873.

Stuart GJ, Häusser M (2001) Dendritic coincidence detection of EPSPs and action potentials. *Nat Neurosci* 4:63–71.

Südhof TC (2012) The presynaptic active zone. *Neuron* 75:11–25.

Südhof TC (2013) Neurotransmitter release: the last millisecond in the life of a synaptic vesicle. *Neuron* 80:675–690.

Südhof TC, Rothman JE (2009) Membrane fusion: grappling with SNARE and SM proteins. *Science* 323:474–477.

Sugita S, Han W, Butz S, Liu X, Fernández-Chacón R, Lao Y, Südhof TC (2001) Synaptotagmin VII as a plasma membrane Ca(2+) sensor in exocytosis. *Neuron* 30:459–473.

Sugita S, Shin O-H, Han W, Lao Y, Südhof TC (2002) Synaptotagmins form a hierarchy of exocytotic Ca(2+) sensors with distinct Ca(2+) affinities. *EMBO J* 21:270–280.

Szabadics J, Varga C, Molnár G, Oláh S, Barzó P, Tamás G (2006) Excitatory effect of GABAergic axo-axonic cells in cortical microcircuits. *Science* 311:233–235.

Takács VT, Cserép C, Schlingloff D, Pósfai B, Szőnyi A, Sos KE, Környei Z, Dénes Á, Gulyás AI, Freund TF, Nyiri G (2018) Co-transmission of acetylcholine and GABA regulates hippocampal states. *Nat Commun* 9:2848.

Takahashi H, Magee JC (2009) Pathway interactions and synaptic plasticity in the dendritic tuft regions of CA1 pyramidal neurons. *Neuron* 62:102–111.

Takamori S, et al. (2006) Molecular anatomy of a trafficking organelle. *Cell* 127:831–846.

Takumi Y, Ramírez-León V, Laake P, Rinvik E, Ottersen OP (1999) Different modes of expression of AMPA and NMDA receptors in hippocampal synapses. *Nat Neurosci* 2:618–624.

Tamás G, Simon AL, Szabadics J (2003) Identified sources and targets of slow inhibition in the neocortex. *Science* 299:1902–1905.

Tang M, Pelkey KA, Ng D, Ivakine E, McBain CJ, Salter MW, McInnes RR (2011) Neto1 is an auxiliary subunit of native synaptic kainate receptors. *J Neurosci* 31:10009–10018.

Timofeeva Y, Volynski KE (2015) Calmodulin as a major calcium buffer shaping vesicular release and short-term synaptic plasticity: facilitation through buffer dislocation. *Front Cell Neurosci* 9:239.

Tovar KR, Westbrook GL (2002) Mobile NMDA receptors at hippocampal synapses. *Neuron* 34:255–264.

Trommald M, Hulleberg G (1997) Dimensions and density of dendritic spines from rat dentate granule cells based on reconstructions from serial electron micrographs. *J Comp Neurol* 377:15–28.

Twomey EC, Yelshanskaya MV, Grassucci RA, Frank J, Sobolevsky AI (2017) Channel opening and gating mechanism in AMPA-subtype glutamate receptors. *Nature* 549:60–65.

Varoqueaux F, Sigler A, Rhee J-S, Brose N, Enk C, Reim K, Rosenmund C (2002) Total arrest of spontaneous and evoked synaptic transmission but normal synaptogenesis in the absence of Munc13-mediated vesicle priming. *Proc Natl Acad Sci U S A* 99:9037–9042.

Ventura R, Harris KM (1999) Three-dimensional relationships between hippocampal synapses and astrocytes. *J Neurosci* 19:6897–6906.

Verhage M, Maia AS, Plomp JJ, Brussaard AB, Heeroma JH, Vermeer H, Toonen RF, Hammer RE, van den Berg TK, Missler M, Geuze HJ, Südhof TC (2000) Synaptic assembly of the brain in the absence of neurotransmitter secretion. *Science* 287:864–869.

Vignes M, Collingridge GL (1997) The synaptic activation of kainate receptors. *Nature* 388:179–182.

Vogt K, Mellor J, Tong G, Nicoll R (2000) The actions of synaptically released zinc at hippocampal mossy fiber synapses. *Neuron* 26:187–196.

Volynski KE, Krishnakumar SS (2018) Synergistic control of neurotransmitter release by different members of the synaptotagmin family. *Curr Opin Neurobiol* 51:154–162.

Vyleta NP, Jonas P (2014) Loose coupling between Ca2+ channels and release sensors at a plastic hippocampal synapse. *Science* 343:665–670.

Walker MC, Ruiz A, Kullmann DM (2001) Monosynaptic GABAergic signaling from dentate to CA3 with a pharmacological and physiological profile typical of mossy fiber synapses. *Neuron* 29:703–715.

Wanaverbecq N, Semyanov A, Pavlov I, Walker MC, Kullmann DM (2007) Cholinergic axons modulate GABAergic signaling among hippocampal interneurons via postsynaptic alpha 7 nicotinic receptors. *J Neurosci* 27:5683–5693.

Watanabe S, Boucrot E (2017) Fast and ultrafast endocytosis. *Curr Opin Cell Biol* 47:64–71.

Watson JF, Pinggera A, Ho H, Greger IH (2021) AMPA receptor anchoring at CA1 synapses is determined by N-terminal domain and TARP γ8 interactions. *Nat Commun* 12:5083.

Weber T, Zemelman BV, McNew JA, Westermann B, Gmachl M, Parlati F, Söllner TH, Rothman JE (1998) SNAREpins: minimal machinery for membrane fusion. *Cell* 92:759–772.

Weisskopf MG, Zalutsky RA, Nicoll RA (1993) The opioid peptide dynorphin mediates heterosynaptic depression of hippocampal mossy fibre synapses and modulates long-term potentiation. *Nature* 365:188.

Wenthold RJ, Petralia RS, Blahos J II, Niedzielski AS (1996) Evidence for multiple AMPA receptor complexes in hippocampal CA1/CA2 neurons. *J Neurosci* 16:1982–1989.

Wigström H, Gustafsson B (1986) Postsynaptic control of hippocampal long-term potentiation. *J Physiol (Paris)* 81:228–236.

Wlodarczyk AI, Sylantyev S, Herd MB, Kersanté F, Lambert JJ, Rusakov DA, Linthorst ACE, Semyanov A, Belelli D, Pavlov I, Walker MC (2013) GABA-independent GABAA receptor openings maintain tonic currents. *J Neurosci* 33:3905–3914.

Wu D, Bacaj T, Morishita W, Goswami D, Arendt KL, Xu W, Chen L, Malenka RC, Südhof TC (2017) Postsynaptic synaptotagmins mediate AMPA receptor exocytosis during LTP. *Nature* 544:316–321.

Wu LG, Saggau P (1994) Adenosine inhibits evoked synaptic transmission primarily by reducing presynaptic calcium influx in area CA1 of hippocampus. *Neuron* 12:1139–1148.

Xie Z, Long J, Liu J, Chai Z, Kang X, Wang C (2017) Molecular mechanisms for the coupling of endocytosis to exocytosis in neurons. *Front Mol Neurosci* 10:47.

Xu J, Mashimo T, Südhof TC (2007) Synaptotagmin-1, -2, and -9: Ca(2+) sensors for fast release that specify distinct presynaptic properties in subsets of neurons. *Neuron* 54:567–581.

Yokoi M, Kobayashi K, Manabe T, Takahashi T, Sakaguchi I, Katsuura G, Shigemoto R, Ohishi H, Nomura S, Nakamura K, Nakao K, Katsuki M, Nakanishi S (1996) Impairment of hippocampal mossy fiber LTD in mice lacking mGluR2. *Science* 273:645–647.

Yoon KW, Rothman SM (1991) Adenosine inhibits excitatory but not inhibitory synaptic transmission in the hippocampus. *J Neurosci* 11:1375–1380.

Zerangue N, Kavanaugh MP (1996) Flux coupling in a neuronal glutamate transporter. *Nature* 383:634–637.

Zhao Y, Chen S, Swensen AC, Qian W-J, Gouaux E (2019) Architecture and subunit arrangement of native AMPA receptors elucidated by cryo-EM. *Science* 364:355–362.

Zhou Q, Zhou P, Wang AL, Wu D, Zhao M, Südhof TC, Brunger AT (2017) The primed SNARE-complexin-synaptotagmin complex for neuronal exocytosis. *Nature* 548:420–425.

Zucker RS, Regehr WG (2002) Short-term synaptic plasticity. *Annu Rev Physiol* 64:355–405.

7

Local Circuits

Andres D. Grosmark, Aaron D. Milstein, Attila Losonczy, and Ivan Soltesz

7.1 Overview

The diversity of local circuit architectures across the subregions of the hippocampus provides a rich platform to investigate the relationship between neuronal network structure and function. For example, while principal cells in cornu ammonis area 1 (CA1) integrate distinct feedforward (FF) excitatory input streams (from cornu ammonis area 3 [CA3] and entorhinal cortex layer III [ECIII]), CA3 pyramidal cells (PCs) integrate not only FF inputs (from the dentate gyrus [DG] and entorhinal cortex layer II [ECII] but also feedback [FB] inputs from other CA3 PCs). The DG represents yet another basic circuit variant, with FF (ECII) and FB integration being accomplished by two different principal cell types: granule cells (GCs) and mossy cells (MCs). In this chapter, we will review evidence for unique functional and computational roles for the diverse excitatory and inhibitory cell types and circuit motifs found in the hippocampus. In doing so, we will primarily focus on the DG, CA1, and CA3 networks to illustrate the overarching principles of local circuit organization and function, while recognizing that similar basic mechanisms and fundamental rules of local circuit operation are likely at play in other, less well studied areas of the hippocampal formation (e.g., the subiculum and CA2) as well. Entorhinal local circuits are discussed in a separately in Chapter 12.

7.1.1 Dentate gyrus

7.1.1.1 Summary of local circuits in the dentate gyrus

The DG is typically regarded as the primary input region of the hippocampus, which is presumed to act as a preprocessor for incoming cortical information, preparing it for subsequent processing in the downstream CA3 region. In particular, computational theories of hippocampal functions have argued that the local circuit architecture and dynamics of the DG lend themselves to decorrelation of input patterns from the EC, a process termed pattern separation (Marr, 1971; McNaughton and Morris, 1987; McNaughton and Nadel, 1990; Treves and Rolls, 1994; Rolls and Kesner, 2006; Myers and Scharfman, 2009; Yassa and Stark, 2011; Knierim and Neunuebel, 2016). Specifically, this computational function is proposed to be aided by the FF circuit with no direct recurrent excitatory connections among its major principal cells, the GCs, and by the strong lateral inhibition from GABA (gamma-aminobutyric acid)-ergic interneurons (INs). Some salient features of the DG circuitry include the following (Figure 7.1A,B):

- GCs mediate FF integration: they receive glutamatergic excitatory input from the EC and, in turn, send excitatory output to CA3 via the mossy fibers (MFs).
- Hilar MCs, which mediate FB integration, receiving excitatory inputs from a relatively small number of GCs and providing highly distributed excitatory output to a large number of GCs.
- Inhibitory control over GC and MC activity implemented via FB and FF inhibition from GABAergic INs.
- Adult neurogenesis, which the DG is one of the few brain regions to exhibit.

7.1.1.2 Principal cells in the dentate gyrus

The two excitatory principal cell types of the DG—the GCs and hilar MCs—while sharing a common developmental origin (G Li et al., 2008), are characterized by several highly divergent properties. GCs are the main output principal cells of the DG and are the most numerous cell types in the hippocampus: the number of GCs in the DG in one brain hemisphere of the rat is estimated to be approximately one million (Boss et al., 1985; West et al., 1991; Dyhrfjeld-Johnsen et al., 2007). Cell bodies of GCs form a tightly packed GC layer (GCL), while the monopolar dendrites of GCs are found in the molecular layers (MLs) and their axons extend from the soma into the hilus and CA3. The DG receives specific afferents that arise primarily from excitatory stellate cells in layer 2 (LII) of the medial and lateral EC, and terminate in the middle and outer molecular layers (MML and OML) of the DG, respectively (Witter, 2007). The commissural/associational (C/A) inputs from hilar MCs (see below) form synapses in the inner molecular layer (IML). While most GCs are located in the GCL, there are smaller subsets that reside in the IML (semilunar GCs; Williams et al., 2007; Larimer and Strowbridge, 2010) and in the hilus (ectopic GCs; Scharfman et al., 2007; Scharfman and Pierce, 2012). Some GCs are also found in the CA3 region (Szabadics et al., 2010). Finally, GC progenitors (stem cells) are located in the DG subgranular zone (Kempermann et al., 2015).

The other principal glutamatergic cells of the DG are the MCs (Ratzliff et al., 2002; Scharfman and Myers, 2012; Scharfman, 2016), which are far less numerous (30,000 MCs in the rat), and located in the hilus, where they receive inputs primarily from MFs of GCs onto large complex spines (thorny excrescences) (Scharfman, 1992, 1999; Frotscher et al., 1994; Buckmaster and Jongen-Relo, 1999; Dyhrfjeld-Johnsen et al., 2007). In contrast to GCs, MCs

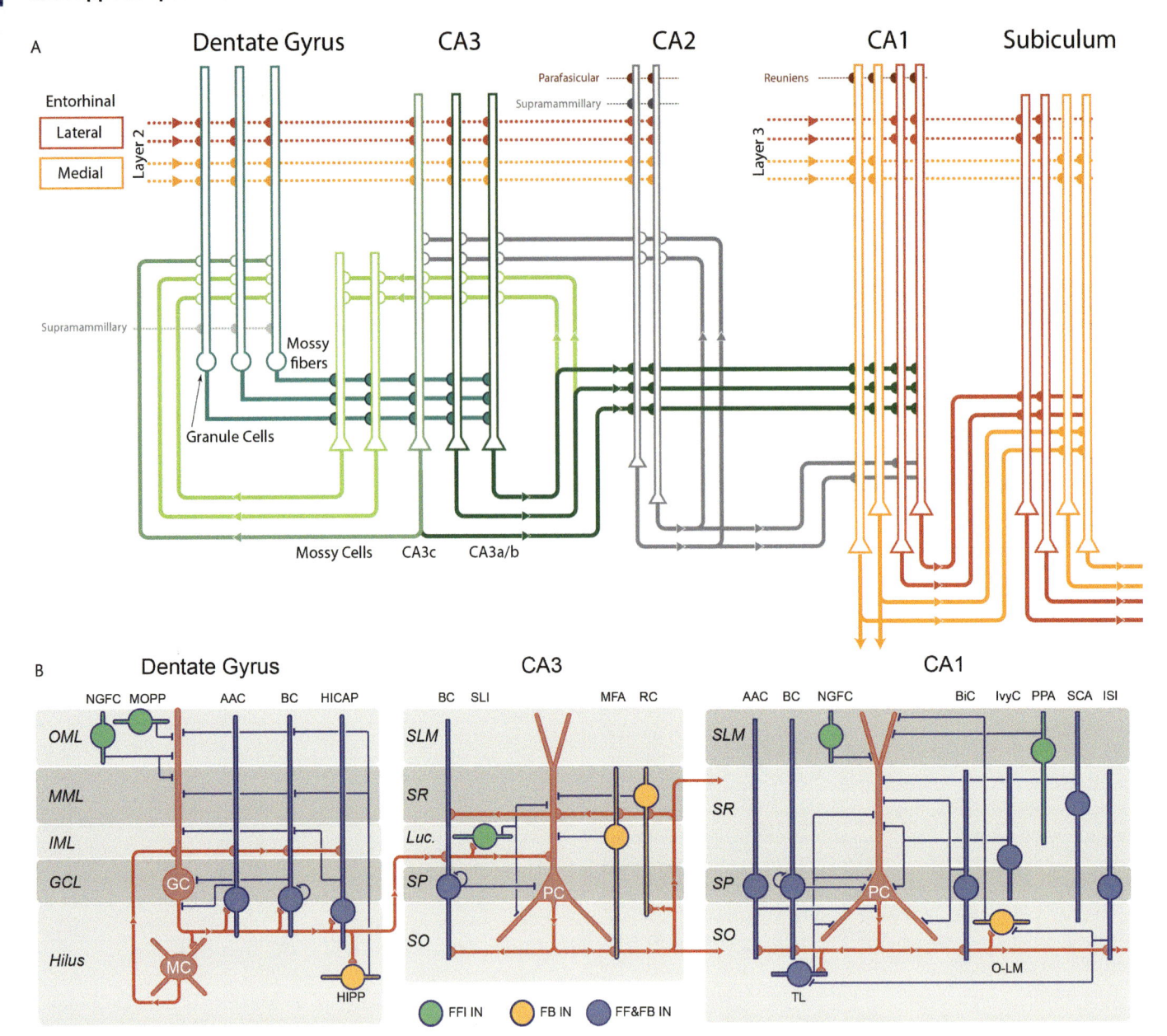

Figure 7.1 Global and local hippocampal circuit anatomy. (A) Simplified schematic of global excitatory connectivity to and within the hippocampus. External excitatory inputs are shown by dashed lines, while intrinsic hippocampal connectivity is shown in solid lines (neuromodulatory inputs are not shown). The main excitatory cell types of the dentate gyrus are the numerous GCs and the recurrently connected MCs. The DG receives extrinsic excitatory inputs from the lateral and medial entorhinal cortices (LEC and MEC, respectively) as well as the supramammillary hypothalamic nucleus. The main excitatory cell type in the CA3, CA2, and CA1 subregions is the PC. The CA3 and CA2 subregions are notable for their high level of recurrent connectivity and CA3 receives strong FF excitatory inputs from GCs' MFs (note that CA2 also receives MF inputs in mice). In addition to its external EC and recurrent CA3 inputs, the CA2 subregion also receives afferents from the parafasicular nucleus of the thalamus as well as from the supramammillary nucleus. The downstream CA1 region uniquely receives external input from the nucleus reuniens of the thalamus and together with the subiculum is considered the main output structure of the hippocampal formation. (B) A schematic of the local circuit organization and major GABAergic IN types of hippocampal subregions. Note that all hippocampal subregions contain INs that provide primarily feedforward (FF) or feedback (FB) inhibition to principal cells as well INs that can act as both FF and FB elements (FF&FB). In all subregions, multiple types of INs are specialized to inhibit perisomatic or dendritic compartments of principal cells. Most INs subtypes identified in CA1 are also present in CA3 (not indicated, except BCs). Most IN interconnectivity is not shown, and only one type of IN-specific IN is indicated. Dentate gyrus layers: GCL: granule cell layer; MML: medial molecular layer; IML: inner molecular layer. CA3/CA1 layers: SLM: lacunosum-moleculare; SR: strat. radiatum; Luc.: strat. lucidum; SP: strat. pyramidale; SO: strat. oriens. GC: granule cell; MC: mossy cell; NGFC: neurogliaform cell; MOPP: molecular layer perforant path cell; AAC: axo-axonic cell; BC: basket cell; HICAP: hilar commissural/associational path associated cell; HIPP: hilar perforant path cell; CA3PC: CA3 pyramidal cell; SLI: spiny lucidum IN; MFA: MF associated cell; RC: radiatum cell; CA1PC: CA1 pyramidal cell; BiC: bistratified cell; IvyC: Ivy cell; PPA: perforant path associated cell; SCA: Schaffer collateral-associated cell; ISI: IN-specific IN; TL: trilaminar cell; O-LM: oriens-lacunosum-moleculare IN. (Source: Panel A was a previously unpublished figure produced shortly before his passing by the late John Lisman [with advice from I.S.] and is included with minimal modifications here as a tribute to him from the authors.)

provide FB associational and FB commissural inputs to GCs across a large extent of the longitudinal axis of the DG (Scharfman and Schwartzkroin, 1988; Buckmaster et al., 1992; Soltesz et al., 1993). Individual MCs contact other MCs and INs within the ipsilateral hilus (Buckmaster et al., 1996; Wenzel et al., 1997; Y Sun et al., 2017), and also send axons ipsilaterally and contralaterally to the IML, where they extensively innervate dendrites of GCs and INs. Thus, the overall net impact of MCs on GCs could either be excitatory via direct connections or indirectly inhibitory via disynaptic inhibition (Scharfman, 1995b; Buckmaster et al., 1996; Scharfman and Bernstein, 2015; Bui et al., 2018; Scharfman, 2018). There is evidence that this varies depending on anatomical distance to the targets of MCs (local vs. long-range), and may become biased toward excitation by the selective long-term potentiation (LTP) of MC–GC synapses (Hashimotodani et al., 2017).

7.1.1.3 Granule cell projection to CA3 pyramidal cells and hilar mossy cells

The main efferent projection from the DG to other hippocampal areas primarily arises from GCs that project to the hilus and CA3. The axons of GCs, called MFs, form giant presynaptic boutons that innervate elaborate clusters of postsynaptic spines called thorny excrescences, which are expressed on both MG GCs and CA3 PCs. GCs also form more typical synapses onto hilar and CA3 INs via small boutons that arise from hilar collaterals and from filamentous extensions from the giant boutons. GCs contribute to FB inhibition within the DG by recruiting GABAergic INs located in the DG hilus, while also contributing to FF inhibition within CA3 by activating inhibitory neurons in the CA3 stratum lucidum (Luc.) (Figure 7.1B). In general, the MF system is considered "lamellar" in the proximal (CA3c-b) subregions of the CA3, running parallel to the transverse axis of the hippocampus, while it follows the longitudinal axis in the distal CA3a subregion and in area CA2 (Amaral and Witter, 1989; Acsady et al., 1998). GCs project sparsely to CA3 PCs (300,000 per hemisphere in the rat), with each GC innervating about 10–15 CA3 PCs (West et al., 1991; Acsady et al., 1998) and with each CA3 PC receiving MF input from approximately 50 GCs, so that the pairwise connection probability between dentate GCs and CA3 PCs is approximately 0.005%. These large en passant MF boutons terminate exclusively onto CA3 PCs or hilar MCs with large thorny excrescences located on their proximal dendrites. Besides this proximal dendritic location, other structural properties also suggest that these MF synapses are highly efficient: a single MF bouton communicates with its postsynaptic partner at 18–45 synaptic release sites (Chicurel and Harris, 1992; Wilke et al., 2013) containing large vesicle pools (Geiger and Jonas, 2000; Hallermann et al., 2003; Rollenhagen et al., 2007). Synaptic transmission at MF boutons is also characterized by several unique features related to short-term adaptation, including low initial release probability and prominent presynaptic paired-pulse facilitation due to loose coupling between presynaptic voltage-gated Ca^{2+} channels and release sensors. These features contribute to strong frequency-dependent facilitation and posttetanic potentiation at these synapses (Griffith, 1990; Salin et al., 1996; Toth et al., 2000; Nicoll and Schmitz, 2005; Vyleta and Jonas, 2014). MF–MC synapses exhibit both long- and short-term plasticity phenomena that are generally similar to the MF synapses onto CA3 PCs (Lysetskiy et al., 2005). Together, the probability of single spike transmission at these synapses is low, but transmission in response to spike trains in GCs is

robust. Collectively, these features have led to the characterization of the MF terminals on CA3 PCs and MCs as "conditional detonator synapses" for their function in effectively activating a sparse subset of CA3 PCs or MCs contingent on repeated presynaptic activation (Geiger and Jonas, 2000; Henze et al., 2002; Bischofberger et al., 2006; Pelkey et al., 2006). Nevertheless, GC burst-firing has also been shown to elicit presynaptic LTP that increases basal release probability and reduces the range of presynaptic facilitation (Gundlfinger et al., 2007; Gundlfinger et al., 2010; Mistry et al., 2011), while posttetanic potentiation has also been shown to switch MF synapses to "full detonators" for tens of seconds (Vyleta et al., 2016), implying that under certain behavioral conditions single unitary MF excitatory postsynaptic potentials (EPSPs) can trigger spikes in CA3 PCs or MCs.

7.1.1.4 Interneurons in the dentate gyrus

In addition to GCs and MCs, GABAergic INs are also critical constituents of the DG circuitry (Halasy and Somogyi, 1993b; Han et al., 1993; Freund and Buzsaki, 1996; Acsady et al., 1998; Pelkey et al., 2017; Booker and Vida, 2018), providing both FF and FB inhibition to principal cells (Figure 7.1B). The INs in the DG are heterogeneous, with marked differences in the diversity of IN subtypes in the DG compared with the CA1-3 regions, albeit with similarities in their principles. Akin to the CA1–3 regions, DG INs are most commonly classified by the location of their cell bodies and dendrites, their neurochemical marker profiles, and their axon projections. This classification scheme emphasizes the specificity of IN terminal fields to sublayers of the DG and subcellular domain-specific innervation of target cells (mostly GCs), but the nomenclature is distinct from the CA3 regions. Accordingly, previous morphological studies and reviews have identified at least four types of DG INs (Amaral et al., 2007; Houser, 2007; Hosp et al., 2014), while more recent classifications consider at least nine types with distinct anatomical and neurochemical properties (Booker and Vida, 2018). For example, parvalbumin-expressing (PV+) basket cells (PV+ BC) and PV+ axo-axonic cells (AACs) innervate the cell bodies and axon initial segment of the GCs, respectively (Amaral, 1978; Seress and Pokorny, 1981; Ribak and Seress, 1983; Soriano and Frotscher, 1989; Han et al., 1993; E Buhl, Han, et al., 1994; Koh et al., 1995; Scharfman, 1995a; Doischer et al., 2008; Norenberg et al., 2010; Hosp et al., 2014). These perisomatic-targeting INs in DG participate in FF and, to a lesser extent, in FB inhibition onto GCs with high connection probability (>50%; Doischer et al., 2008) as well as onto other INs, including strong mutual inhibition between PV+ BCs (Doischer et al., 2008; Savanthrapadian et al., 2014).

Several GABAergic IN subtypes innervate GC dendrites (Figure 7.1B). The most common of these cells are the somatostatin-expressing (SOM+) HIPP cells (hilar IN with perforant path-associated terminals), which innervate dendritic areas of GCs matching the LII EC inputs in the outer two-thirds of the ML (Halasy and Somogyi, 1993a; Han et al., 1993; Sik et al., 1997; Savanthrapadian et al., 2014). As the horizontal-oriented dendrites of HIPP cells are restricted to the hilus, these cells are considered as predominantly FB INs, innervating GC dendrites, and to lesser extent other INs, including other HIPP cells (Sik et al., 1997; Savanthrapadian et al., 2014; Yuan et al., 2017). The IML is innervated by a population of CCK+ INs called HICAP cells, characterized by cell bodies in the hilus and axons targeting the commissural/associational pathway from MCs (Soriano and Frotscher, 1989; Halasy and Somogyi, 1993a; Han et al., 1993; Hosp et al., 2014; Savanthrapadian et al., 2014). These INs have vertically oriented dendrites both in the hilus and ML, indicating that they can participate in both FF and FB inhibitory circuits, innervating both GCs (Hefft and Jonas, 2005) and other INs (Savanthrapadian et al., 2014). The third main type of dendrite-targeting INs is the molecular layer perforant path (MOPP) IN with cell body in the OML and axon terminals in the OML and MML (Halasy and Somogyi, 1993a; Han et al., 1993), producing FF inhibition of GCs via perforant path activation (Y Li et al., 2013). In addition to these major classes, other IN types have been described in the DG that innervate GC dendrites as well as MCs and other INs (for example, neurogliaform cells [NGFCs] and IN-specific INs [ISIs]; Freund and Buzsaki, 1996; Gulyas et al., 1996; Armstrong et al., 2011). One notable feature of some INs in the DG/hilar region is that their axon collaterals cross the hippocampal fissure and arborize in CA1 (e.g., NGFCs; Armstrong et al., 2011; Markwardt et al., 2011), or in the subiculum (e.g., OML cells; Ceranik et al., 1997), or project outside the hippocampal formation (e.g., SOM+ hilar INs projecting to the medial septum; Yuan et al., 2017), indicating that these INs can influence multiple regions.

7.1.1.5 Granule cell projections onto GABAergic interneurons

In contrast to the strong innervation of CA3 PCs and hilar MCs by large complex MF boutons containing multiple release sites, GABAergic INs located in the CA3 Luc. are innervated by small en passant boutons and filopodia that emanate from large MF boutons and form single-release sites directly onto IN dendrites (Acsady et al., 1998; Frotscher et al., 2006; Wilke et al., 2013). MFs target about 10 times as many INs as principal cells, providing the basis for strong and widespread FF inhibitory control of CA3 PCs via disynaptic inhibition. A diverse population of GABAergic INs has been shown to participate in FF inhibition (Figure 7.1B) with cell-type-specific short-term plasticity properties, including PV+ BCs and AACs, cholecystokinin-expressing (CCK+) BCs, and spiny lucidum INs (Szabadics and Soltesz, 2009; Szabo et al., 2010; Neubrandt et al., 2017; Neubrandt et al., 2018). Furthermore, the probability of FF inhibition between individual GCs and CA3 PCs has been shown to be independent of the direct excitation (Neubrandt et al., 2018). Therefore, this strong and randomly distributed FF inhibition may help to prevent runaway excitation, ensure tight spike timing of CA3 PCs (Mori et al., 2007; Torborg et al., 2010), and aid hippocampal signal sparsification, supporting precise memory encoding and retrieval (Ruediger et al., 2011; Restivo et al., 2015). Indeed, the strength of the FF MF drive onto INs is modifiable by a plethora of activity- and experience-dependent plasticity mechanisms ranging from seconds-long potentiation following MF bursts (Neubrandt et al., 2018), through various forms of target cell-dependent presynaptic long-term depression and potentiation (Maccaferri et al., 1998; Pelkey et al., 2006; Pelkey and McBain, 2008; Pelkey et al., 2008; McBain and Kauer, 2009), to learning-related structural plasticity, which manifests as an increased filopodial growth from MF boutons onto FF INs (Ruediger et al., 2011; Donato et al., 2013).

7.1.2 CA3

7.1.2.1 Connectivity of CA3 pyramidal cells

The CA3 circuit architecture is traditionally depicted as receiving three major afferent inputs innervating nonoverlapping dendritic domains of its main principal cell type, the CA3 PC: the strong FF MF input from the DG GCs onto thorny excrescences located on proximal apical dendrites of CA3 PCs in the Luc. (see above; Chicurel and Harris, 1992; Wilke et al., 2013), the direct FF cortical input from LII EC stellate cells onto the distal dendritic tuft in the stratum lacunosum-moleculare (SLM), and associational and commissural inputs from other CA3 PCs (A/C, depending on the origin of inputs from either ipsilateral or contralateral CA3) onto small-diameter apical and basal dendrites in stratum radiatum (SR) (Witter, 2007) (Figure 7.1A,B). Among these, the extensive excitatory recurrent interconnectivity between CA3 PCs is the main characteristic feature of the CA3 circuit: a single CA3 PC (~300,000 cells per hemisphere; Amaral et al., 1990; Ishizuka et al., 1990) may cover approximately two-thirds of the longitudinal extent of the hippocampus and may give rise to 30,000–60,000 axon terminals (X Li et al., 1994; Sik et al., 1997), forming a huge recurrent autoassociative network. This hallmark property of the CA3 local circuit architecture has long inspired computational models of memory because this recurrent circuit is ideally suited to work as an attractor network in which patterns of activity can be rapidly stored and reconstructed as attractor states (Marr, 1971; McNaughton and Morris, 1987; Treves and Rolls, 1994; Lisman, 1999; Rolls, 2007; Bush et al., 2010; Savin et al., 2014; Kesner and Rolls, 2015) formed primarily through autoassociative Hebbian plastic changes of synaptic weights among CA3 PCs (Nakazawa et al., 2002; Nakashiba et al., 2008; Mishra et al., 2016; Rebola et al., 2017). Due to these autoassociative properties of the CA3 network, activity patterns stored in ensembles of strongly interconnected CA3 PCs can be reactivated and completed even in response to partial ensemble activation by external sources, a process called pattern completion (McClelland and Rumelhart, 1985; McNaughton and Morris, 1987; O'Reilly and McClelland, 1994; Rolls and Treves, 1994; Rolls and Kesner, 2006). Pattern reactivation is thought to primarily occur during network synchronization events that manifest as high-frequency oscillations in the hippocampal EEG termed sharp wave ripples (SWRs, see also section 7.4.3 below). The CA3 recurrent network, in particular the distal CA3a region together with CA2, have been strongly implicated in the generation of SWRs (Buzsaki, 2015; A Oliva et al., 2016), during which hippocampal ensembles are reactivated, supporting memory consolidation and hippocampal-dependent cognitive functions (Carr et al., 2011; Buzsaki, 2015).

For successful and efficient pattern completion, the CA3 pyramidal network has often been conceptualized and modeled as a network of highly interconnected neurons, where connectivity among homogeneous populations of CA3 PCs is random and close to all-to-all (McNaughton and Morris, 1987; Lisman, 1999; Rolls, 2013). However, recent studies have provided several major updates to this traditional depiction of the CA3 PC network. First, a recent functional connectivity analysis (Guzman et al., 2016) using simultaneous recordings from multiple CA3 PC in acute brain slices found that connectivity among CA3 PCs is not random but highly enriched in disynaptic connectivity motifs, such as reciprocal, convergent, divergent, and chain connections. Indeed, CA3 network models found that incorporating sparse and nonrandom connectivity supports efficient memory storage and retrieval (Dubreuil and Brunel, 2016; Guzman et al., 2016).

Second, recent investigations into detailed morphological, molecular, and physiological properties of CA3 PCs have uncovered prominent phenotypic diversity within this cell population that was heretofore characterized as monolithic (Bilkey and Schwartzkroin, 1990; Witter, 2007; Deguchi et al., 2011; Marissal et al., 2012; H Lee et al., 2015; Lu et al., 2015), in agreement with mounting evidence indicating that heterogeneity exists among hippocampal PCs (Soltesz and Losonczy, 2018; see also section 7.5 below). Notably, a study by Hunt and colleagues (Hunt et al., 2018) found that the CA3 PC population includes not only classically described regular-spiking PCs with thorny excrescences and strong MF inputs but also includes "athorny" CA3 PCs that are devoid of MF inputs. These athorny cells occupy a distinct cytoarchitectural position in CA3 (deep sublayer in CA3a and CA3b) and exhibit prominent burst firing. Intriguingly, this study also indicated a key role for athorny CA3 cell bursts as triggers of sharp waves (Hunt et al., 2018), suggesting that this CA3 PC subtype may promote full pattern reactivation (pattern completion) through the generation of SWRs.

Third, as single unitary EPSPs in the CA3–CA3 recurrent network are unable to fire a postsynaptic CA3 cell, multiple convergent inputs are required for efficient synaptic signaling between CA3 PCs. This circuit connectivity architecture enables synaptic weights at the A/C inputs to CA3 cells to be modifiable by several traditional long-term plasticity mechanisms, including NMDA-type glutamate receptor (NMDAR)–dependent Hebbian LTP (Zalutsky and Nicoll, 1990; Debanne et al., 1998; Tsukamoto et al., 2003; McBain, 2008; Rebola et al., 2017). However, a recent study in acute slices has also demonstrated that spike-timing-dependent plasticity (STDP) at CA3–CA3 A/C synapses shows noncanonical induction rules with broad and symmetrical curves, indicating that STDP at CA3–CA3 synapses occurs independently of temporal order, which may be particularly important for the reliability and generalizability of information stored in the CA3 autoassociative network (Mishra et al., 2016).

Lastly, convergent input integration onto CA3 PCs may result in nonlinear summation of temporally and spatially correlated synaptic inputs onto CA3 PC dendrites. Indeed, active dendritic mechanisms such as dendritic spikes mediated by NMDARs (Makara and Magee, 2013) or voltage-gated Na$^+$ channels (VGNas) (S Kim et al., 2012) have been shown to amplify coincident inputs onto CA3 cells. Recent computational models suggest that the dendritic properties of hippocampal PCs, which favor nonlinear interactions between proximal and distal inputs, may represent an important cellular mechanism for the enhancement of the number of memories that can be stored and recalled in the hippocampus (Kaifosh and Losonczy, 2016).

7.1.2.2 GABAergic control of CA3 pyramidal cells

Information processing performed by CA3 PCs and synchronization of network activity are under the control of a diverse types of CA3 GABAergic INs mediating both FF (see section 7.1.1.5 above) and FB inhibition. Most types of INs are not exclusive to CA3 but are found in other CA subfields and are characterized by the same general organizational principle of coalignment of their axonal fields with specific excitatory afferents within different layers (Vida and Frotscher, 2000; Hajos et al., 2004; Losonczy et al., 2004; Lasztoczi et al., 2011; Hajos et al., 2013; Papp et al., 2013; Tukker et al., 2013; Schlingloff et al., 2014; Szabo et al., 2014) (Figure 7.1B). Nevertheless, many detailed aspects of CA3 GABAergic circuits and their potential region-specific attributes remain unknown.

7.1.3 CA2

Hippocampal area CA2, located between CA1 and CA3 but anatomically smaller than those areas, may superficially appear to effectively be a subregion of area CA3. Indeed, CA2's cellular composition is similar to that observed in CA3, with PCs forming the main excitatory cell type and similar classes of INs observed in both regions (see M Jones and McHugh, 2011; Dudek et al., 2016; Robert et al., 2018). CA2's layered structure is also analogous to that observed in CA3, with SO, SR, and SLM input layers surrounding a densely packed SP layer. Finally, CA2 PCs are recurrently connected with each other and with the more numerous CA3 PCs and thus CA3 and CA2 together constitute the primary excitatory recurrent circuit of the hippocampus (Lorente De Nó, 1934; Tamamaki et al., 1988; Mercer et al., 2007; Cui et al., 2013). However, despite these cellular, anatomical, and circuit-level similarities between the CA3 and CA2 regions, both early and recent research has demonstrated significant differences between the two regions, which taken together support the classification of CA2 as an anatomically and functionally distinct hippocampal region.

Firstly, CA2 pyramidal neurons express a unique set of genes (X Zhao et al., 2001; Kohara et al., 2014a; San Antonio et al., 2014; Dudek et al., 2016). Notably, however, many of these genes are not expressed in the ventralmost portion of CA2 (Lein et al., 2004), suggesting the presence of CA2 circuit diversity along the hippocampal longitudinal axis, though this anatomically organized diversity remains relatively understudied. While the types of INs found in the CA2 region are generally similar to those in the CA1 or CA3 regions (though see Mercer et al., 2007; Mercer, Botcher, et al., 2012; Mercer, Eastlake, et al., 2012), INs are significantly more numerous in CA2 as compared with these other regions, with PV+, Reelin+ and Calbindin+ INs particularly enriched (Piskorowski and Chevaleyre, 2013; Botcher et al., 2014). Therefore, the influence of inhibition in sculpting circuit activity is thought to be even more robust in CA2 than in other CA circuits. The CA2 circuit is further distinguished from CA3 through its distinctive anatomical connectivity patterns. CA2 receives a unique set of ascending hypothalamic excitatory and neuromodulatory projections including from the paraventricular nucleus and, reciprocally, from the supramammillary nucleus (Haglund et al., 1984; Vertes and McKenna, 2000; Cui et al., 2013; Benoy et al., 2018). Like CA3, CA2 receives DG input, but unlike CA3, DG synapses onto CA2 PCs lack postsynaptic thorny excrescences and input at these synapses is generally not able to drive CA2 PC spiking activity (Kohara et al., 2014a; Llorens-Martín et al., 2015; Q Sun et al., 2017). Notably, unlike other Schaffer collateral synapses, CA3 inputs to CA2 do not undergo LTP, and under normal physiological conditions this input instead recruits strong FF inhibition leading to a net hyperpolarization of CA2 PCs (M Zhao et al., 2007; Chevaleyre and Siegelbaum, 2010; SE Lee et al., 2010; Carstens et al., 2016; Carstens and Dudek, 2019). Consistent with its large complement of INs, CA2 Schaffer collateral plasticity is instead mediated through disinhibitory local circuits. In particular, tetanizing Schaffer collateral stimulation leads to delta opioid receptor-dependent long-term depression of the CA3-recruited PV+ FF inhibition onto CA2 PCs, and this disinhibition in turn facilitates the CA3-driven spiking of CA2 PCs (Piskorowski and Chevaleyre, 2013; Nasrallah et al., 2015; Nasrallah et al., 2019). While DG and Schaffer collateral inputs to CA2 tend to weakly drive CA2 PCs while recruiting robust local inhibition, EC LII input onto CA2 PCs at the CA2 SLM is unusually strong and dynamic, being able to effectively drive CA2 PC spiking and undergoing NMDA-mediated LTP (Bartesaghi and Gessi, 2004; Chevaleyre and Siegelbaum, 2010). The relative strength of EC input onto CA2 has been attributed to the density of PP synapses onto CA2 PCs, the unique branching morphology of the apical dendrites that reach the CA2 SLM, as well as the active electrical properties of these dendrites, which promote the generation and propagation of sodium spikes from the SLM to the PC cell bodies (Bartesaghi and Ravasi, 1999; Piskorowski and Chevaleyre, 2012; Q Sun et al., 2014).

Within the CA2, local circuits may also be stratified along the superficial-deep axis, with a recent report demonstrating the presence of a group of deep-located "ramping" PCs showing elevated firing before CA1 SWR events switching to firing suppression during the SWR events themselves (A Oliva et al., 2016). These neurons were contrasted to the superficially located CA2 "phasic" neurons, which showed robust firing immediately prior to and during CA1 SWRs. However, circuit determinants of this anatomically organized functional heterogeneity remain unknown. Unlike CA3 projections to CA1 which predominately terminate in the SR layer and preferentially synapse onto superficial CA1 PCs, CA2 input to CA1 preferentially terminates in the SO and is stronger onto deep CA1 PCs (Tamamaki et al., 1988; Shinohara et al., 2012; Kohara et al., 2014a). However, a recent study suggests that this preferential recruitment of deep CA1 PCs by CA2 may be counterbalanced by elevated CA2-ellicited FF inhibition onto these deep cells (Nasrallah et al., 2019)—consequently, the functional implications of the distinct recruitment profiles of CA3 and CA2 on the CA1 circuit remain unclear.

7.1.4 CA1

7.1.4.1 Connectivity of CA1 pyramidal cells

The hippocampal CA1 region is the main output node of hippocampus, with its PCs (~310,000 per hemisphere in the rat; West et al., 1991; Bezaire and Soltesz, 2013) constituting the main projection neuron population of the hippocampus (Swanson et al., 1981; Witter et al., 1989; Witter, 2007). The layered structure of the CA1 region results from the orderly organization of CA1 PCs. The somata of CA1 PCs are located in the stratum pyramidale (SP), giving rise to a large diameter primary apical dendrite extending into SR, with fine oblique dendrites; and basal dendrites that extend within the stratum oriens (SO). The apical dendrite forms an elaborate tuft in the SLM. CA1 PC axons emanate from the soma or a proximal dendrite (Thome et al., 2014), cross SO where they form local synapses primarily onto INs, and project out of the hippocampus along a fiber bundle called the alveus. Below we briefly survey some salient organizational features of CA1 local circuits (Figure 7.1A,B):

- CA1 PCs receive their major FF excitatory drive from CA3 PCs via ipsilateral Schaffer collaterals and contralateral commissural fibers to the SR and SO layers (Schaffer, 1892; Amaral and Witter, 1989; Witter, 2007).
- CA1 PCs also receive weaker modulatory excitatory inputs from multiple sources: the temporoammonic pathway originating from LIII cells in the medial and lateral ECs and synapsing onto the distal dendritic tufts in the SLM (Steward and Scoville, 1976), from the axons of CA2 pyramids synapsing in SO (Kohara et al., 2014b), and from the amygdala, prefrontal cortex, and anterior cingulate cortex (Pitkanen et al., 2000; Rajasethupathy et al., 2015).

- The recurrent connectivity between CA1 PCs is sparse and local collaterals CA1 pyramids are strongly biased to innervate INs (Takacs et al., 2012).
- CA1 PCs are under control of diverse subtypes of CA1 GABAergic INs that provide FF and FB inhibition onto perisomatic and dendritic compartments of the CA1 pyramids, as detailed in section 7.3 below (Freund and Buzsaki, 1996; Klausberger and Somogyi, 2008; Pelkey et al., 2017).
- CA1 PCs exhibit prominent within-cell-type heterogeneity (Soltesz and Losonczy, 2018) as detailed in section 7.5 below.

While the quantitative circuit anatomy and connectivity of CA1 is one of the best characterized among cortical circuits (Amaral and Witter, 1989; Bezaire and Soltesz, 2013), the actual nature of canonical computations supported by the specific CA1 circuit architecture positioned downstream of the DG–CA3 circuit remains less understood. Computational models suggest that area CA1 can take the highly decorrelated activity patterns from CA3 and combine it with information carried by inputs from other (e.g., cortical) sources, resulting in a highly context-dependent and information-rich output from the hippocampus (McClelland and Goddard, 1996; Kaifosh and Losonczy, 2016). Indeed, the low connection probability between CA1 PCs (Knowles and Schwartzkroin, 1981; Deuchars and Thomson, 1996) as well as strong recurrent inhibition may support such context-dependent processing of similar activity patterns without risking memory interference as might occur in the more recurrently connected CA3 region.

7.1.5 Subiculum

Similar to cornu ammonis (CA) cortical circuits, the dominant excitatory cell type of the subiculum are PCs. However, subicular PCs are distinguishable from their CA counterparts in several important aspects. First, the subicular cell layer is significantly less densely packed than the CA pyramidal layers. Second, subicular cells send extensive long-range connections to both cortical and subcortical targets, and individual axons making up this wide connectivity show less collateralization than is observed from CA1 axons (Naber and Witter, 1998). This low collateralization in turn results in a marked segregation of outputs such that individual subicular PCs project to one or few downstream targets, with the cells' output targets segregated both by their intrinsic cellular properties and by their anatomical location within the subiculum (Witter et al., 1990; Canteras and Swanson, 1992; Naber and Witter, 1998; O'Mara et al., 2001; Y Kim and Spruston, 2012). Consequently, the subiculum is seen as supporting widespread and functionally divergent hippocampal outputs to much of the rest of the brain, including the hippocampus' primary output to many subcortical structures (Witter and Amaral, 2004; Aggleton and Christiansen, 2015; Matsumoto et al., 2019). Finally, subicular circuits differ from CA circuits in that the subiculum more robustly displays the anatomically organized intra-PC heterogeneity, which has only more recently began to come into focus in the CA fields (Cembrowski and Spruston, 2019).

Consistent with the allocortical structure observed in CA fields, the subiculum is generally divided into three layers with a deep polymorphic layer continuous with the CA1 SO, a loosely packed PC layer, and a superficial molecular layer (O'Mara, 2005; Matsumoto et al., 2019; though see Ishihara and Fukuda, 2016, for a more detailed cytoarchitectural analysis). As with other hippocampal regions, intrasubicular heterogeneity is partially organized along the proximodistal, dorsoventral, and superficial-deep anatomical axes (Y Kim and Spruston, 2012; Cembrowski, Phillips, et al., 2018). For example, though the entire subiculum receives EC LIII input, intrahippocampal input to the subiculum shows a columnar "inside-out" segregation such that the proximal (to CA1) subiculum receives CA1 afferents from the adjacent distal (to CA3) CA1, while the distal subiculum receives proximal CA1 afferents (Amaral et al., 1991; Witter and Amaral, 2004). Notably, the subiculum also sends both excitatory and inhibitory backprojections into CA1 (see X Xu et al., 2016) and onto adult-born GCs of the DG (Deshpande et al., 2013), though the precise anatomical distribution or functional implications of these subicular projections is not yet fully understood. Importantly, numerous extrahippocampal subicular efferents are partially segregated along the subiculum's anatomical axes (Naber and Witter, 1998; Witter and Amaral, 2004). This divergent connectivity, together with a pronounced degree of spatial clustering in the varied genetic expression patterns observed both across and within the three main subicular anatomical axes support the view that the subiculum is composed of an overlapping patchwork of functionally distinct subregions (Cembrowski, Wang, et al., 2018). This heterogeneity in turn complicates efforts to establish a singular canonical model of subicular local circuit wiring. For instance, while inhibitory circuits are generally thought to resemble their CA counterparts (Greene and Totterdell, 1997; Menendez de la Prida, 2006; Knopp et al., 2008), the intersubicular heterogeneity of these inhibitory circuits and thus their relationship to the established diversity of subicular excitatory circuits remains unclear.

Subicular pyramidal projection neurons can be further divided into subclasses displaying distinctive gene expression profiles and spiking properties. Two such classes are the intrinsically bursting (IB) cells and the regular spiking (RS) PCs (Stewart and Wong, 1993; Taube, 1993; Behr et al., 1996). IB cells respond to intracellular depolarization by immediately firing multiple action potentials (Menendez de la Prida et al., 2003; Graves et al., 2012), express the glutamate transporter VGLUT2 (Wozny et al., 2018) and discharge robustly in response to CA1 SWRs (Böhm et al., 2015; Eller et al., 2015). Conversely, following depolarization, RS cells emit single action potentials and show spike-frequency adaptation. IB cells are enriched in the deep and distal regions of the subiculum, while RS cells are relatively enriched in the superficial and medial subiculum (Greene and Totterdell, 1997; Staff et al., 2000; Jarsky et al., 2008; Y Kim and Spruston, 2012). Notably, PCs in subicular slices have been shown to form recurrent connections—however, while RS cells laterally project to both IB and RS cells, IB cell's recurrent projections are limited to other IB cell's (Böhm et al., 2015). The subiculum therefore hosts a unique local circuit featuring a combination of feedforward and recurrent excitatory motifs, however, the functional implications of this subcircuit remain largely unknown.

7.2 Elementary computations performed by local circuits

What types of computations are performed by the local neuronal circuits that constitute each subregion of the hippocampus? How do differences in circuit function relate to observed diversity in cell types and circuit wiring? In this section we survey evidence that the local circuits of the hippocampus implement a set of fundamental operations to transform their inputs into processed outputs.

Elementary local circuit motifs (Figure 7.2A) include FB inhibition (local excitatory neurons recruit disynaptic inhibition from local INs) and FF inhibition (afferent excitatory inputs recruit disynaptic inhibition onto local excitatory neurons), disinhibition (an IN-selective IN selectively targets local inhibitory neurons, reducing inhibition of local excitatory neurons), lateral inhibition (local excitatory neurons recruit inhibitory neurons that preferentially target other local excitatory neurons), recurrent excitation (local excitatory neurons recruit disynaptic excitation from other local excitatory neurons) and global FB inhibition (local excitatory neurons recruit disynaptic inhibition from local INs that nonselectively targets the population of local excitatory neurons). The elementary computations generated by such local circuit elements are discussed below, with select examples graphically illustrated in Figure 7.2B.

7.2.1 Gain modulation

One measure of neuronal excitability is the relationship between the total amount of excitatory input (typically measured as current, I), and output firing rate (f), referred to as an f-I curve. In different neuronal cell types, these relationships are typically estimated as linear beyond a certain threshold (rheobase), sigmoidal, or saturating. As the total number of active excitatory inputs to a neuron (or their firing rates or synaptic weights) increases, its action potential output increases. However, in the context of a neuronal circuit, afferent excitatory input also drives local GABAergic INs, resulting in disynaptic inhibition that reduces excitability (Figures 2A and 3). If neurons were perfect linear integrators of idealized synaptic currents arriving in a single compartment, synaptic inhibition would simply increase the amount of excitatory current required to reach a target firing rate, or "right-shift" the f-I curve. This effect of synaptic inhibition is also called "subtractive gain modulation" or simply "subtractive inhibition" (Figure 7.3A). However, in reality, synaptic inputs activate voltage-dependent conductances in separate neuronal compartments (axon, soma, proximal or distal dendrites), resulting in not only subtractive but also divisive effects of inhibition, which manifest as changes in the slope or saturation of the f-I curve (Figure 7.3A) (Losonczy et al., 2010; Pouille et al., 2013). Circuits in all hippocampal subregions contain the FF disynaptic inhibitory circuit motif required for these gain control operations. While gain modulation is a general effect of all synaptic inhibition and therefore not associated with particular cell types, hippocampal INs that respond rapidly to FF excitation such as fast-spiking perisomatic-targeting, axo-axonic, and dendrite-targeting bistratified INs (BiCs) are particularly effective at keeping pace with rapid fluctuations in input and dynamically adjusting postsynaptic excitability (Price et al., 2005; Pouille et al., 2009; Muller and Remy, 2014). Because of its importance, we will return to the topic of subtractive and divisive gain control in order to discuss it more detail in section 7.3.2 below.

7.2.2 Output normalization

For a given pattern of FF input to a neuronal network, the above-mentioned gain control operation can dynamically adjust the excitability of individual neurons in the population, limiting the number of neurons recruited and their output firing rates. However, as the size of the active neuronal population increases, recruitment of local inhibitory INs by recurrent excitatory collaterals provides an additional important mechanism to constrain the total amount of network output (Renno-Costa et al., 2019). Interestingly, many (but not all) of the hippocampal INs dedicated to FB control are

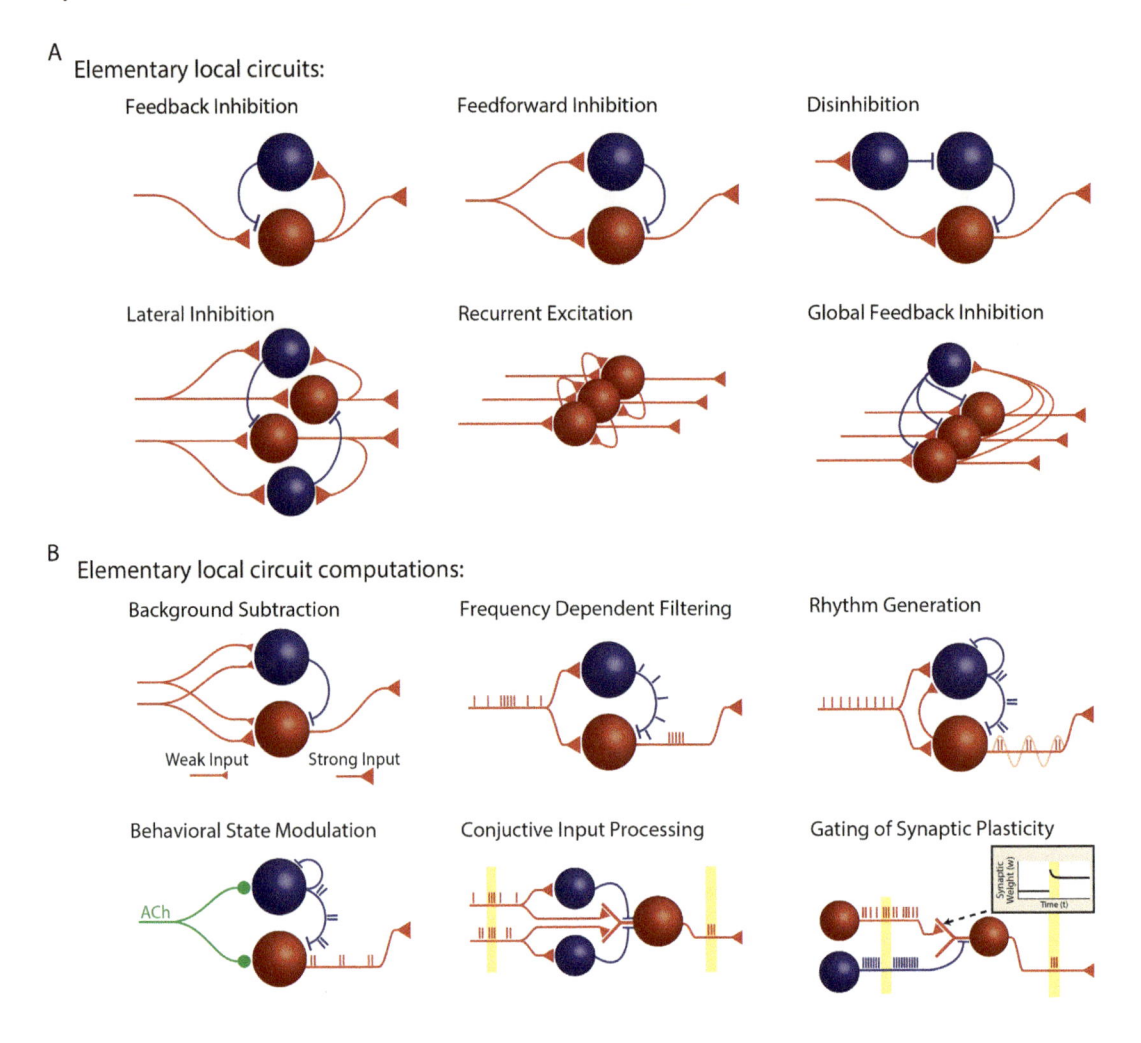

Figure 7.2 Elementary local circuits and computations. (A) Diagrams depict common local circuit wiring motifs found throughout hippocampal regions. Feedback inhibition: local excitatory neurons recruit disynaptic inhibition from local interneurons. Feedforward inhibition: afferent inputs recruit disynaptic inhibition onto local excitatory neurons. Disinhibition: An interneuron-selective interneuron targets local inhibitory neurons, reducing inhibition of local excitatory neurons. Lateral inhibition: local excitatory neurons recruit local inhibitory neurons that preferentially target other local excitatory neurons. Recurrent excitation: local excitatory neurons recruit disynaptic excitation from other local excitatory neurons. Global feedback inhibition: local excitatory neurons recruit disynaptic inhibition from local interneurons that nonselectively targets the population of local excitatory neurons. (B) Diagrams depict elementary computations performed by specific local circuit motifs. Background subtraction: weak afferent inputs onto local excitatory neurons are canceled by feedforward inhibition, but strong afferent inputs overcome inhibition and drive excitatory output. Frequency-dependent filtering: low-frequency afferent inputs onto local excitatory interneurons are canceled by feedforward inhibition, but high-frequency inputs selectively facilitate to overcome inhibition and drive excitatory output. Rhythm generation: in the presence of nonrhythmic afferent input, reciprocal interactions between local excitatory and inhibitory neurons generate oscillatory output. Behavioral state modulation: the oscillatory state of a local circuit is regulated by an afferent neuromodulatory input. Conjunctive input processing: output of a local excitatory neuron is preferentially driven by coincidence of afferent inputs arriving from two distinct sources. Gating of synaptic plasticity: afferent inputs onto local excitatory neurons only undergo activity-dependent synaptic plasticity under conditions when local inhibition is reduced. (Source: (A) modified with permission from Braganza and Beck, 2018.)

dendrite-targeting, such as oriens-lacunosum-moleculare (O-LM) neurons in CA1 and CA3 (Muller and Remy, 2014), and HIPP neurons in DG (Halasy and Somogyi, 1993a). While this mechanism is inherently slower to respond than rapid onset FF inhibition (~3 ms), FB modulation is still able to act on the timescales of gamma (~15–30 ms) and theta (~125 ms) oscillations in the hippocampus (C Varga et al., 2012). This canonical circuit operation normalizes network output so that the total number of active neurons in a population, and the distribution of their firing rates, can remain in a similar target range whether multiple distinct input patterns are presented either in isolation or in combination (Ohshiro et al., 2011).

7.2.3 Background subtraction

Hippocampal excitatory neurons called "place cells" selectively fire when an animal traverses through a restricted set of physical locations while navigating a spatial environment. However, even at locations outside a "place field," place cells receive a constant barrage of excitatory inputs. Another critical role of local circuit processing is to amplify the "signal" carried by the relevant inputs to a sparse subset of active neurons, and to suppress potentially large amplitude fluctuations arising from irrelevant inputs, or background "noise" (Grienberger et al., 2017) (Figure 7.2B). One important mechanism for individual neurons to discriminate between two sets of inputs that fire at similar rates is through synapse-specific changes

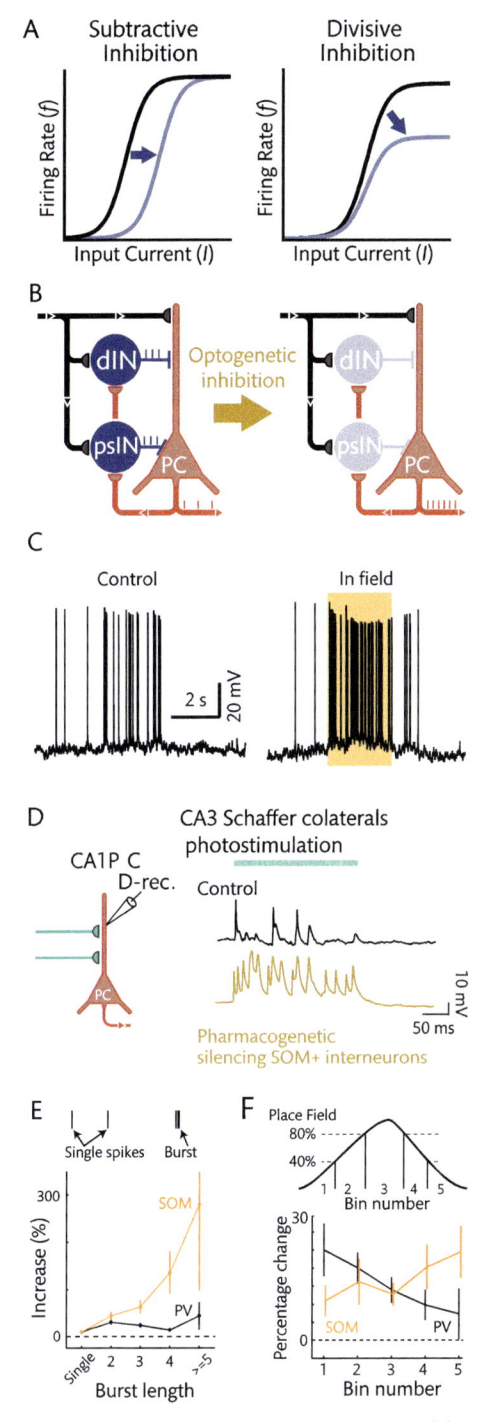

Figure 7.3 Effects of inhibition and disinhibition on CA1 PCs. (A) Subtractive inhibition results in a simple rightward shift in the input-output (I-f) curve of a cell or elementary local circuit. In contrast, the interaction of synaptic inputs with various voltage-dependent conductances often bring about divisive inhibition that manifests itself as a change in the slope or saturation of the I-f curve. (B) Schematic of IN cell-type specific manipulations in local circuits (dIN, dendritic-targeting INs; psIN, perisomatic-targeting INs). (C) Optogenetic inhibition of GABAergic CA1 INs within the in vivo spatial firing filed of a CA1 PC during head-fixed spatial exploration resulted in an increased firing rate within the cell's place field (traces show intracellular voltage recordings (Grienberger et al., 2017). (D) Pharmacogenetic silencing of SOM + dendrite-targeting INs in CA1 in vitro increased dendritic spiking in a CA1 PC evoked by CA3 Schaffer collateral stimulation (D-rec, dendritic recording (Lovett-Barron et al., 2012). (E) Optogenetic inhibition of SOM + INs, but not of PV + INs, in vivo increased burst spiking in CA1 pyramidal cells (burst length is expressed as the number of action potentials in a burst). (F) PC place fields were divided into five bins from place field entry to place field exit. Silencing PV + INs alters CA1 PC firing mostly upon place field entry, while silencing somatostatin-expressing dendrite-targeting IN affects firing mostly at the end of a place field (Royer et al., 2012).

in efficacy (also referred to as strength or weight; see chapter 10 for details on long-term synaptic plasticity). Excitatory inputs that have previously undergone long-term depression (LTD) weakly depolarize postsynaptic dendrites, while inputs that have previously undergone LTP cause large amplitude depolarizations. In turn, increased membrane depolarization activates voltage-dependent ion channels such as NMDARs, sodium channels, and calcium channels, which amplify strongly weighted synaptic inputs by further contributing depolarizing current (Losonczy and Magee, 2006; Takahashi and Magee, 2009; Krueppel et al., 2011; S Kim et al., 2012; Makara and Magee, 2013). Synaptic inhibition generated by local INs is more effective at suppressing these synaptic amplification mechanisms at less depolarized voltages (Muller et al., 2012), thus preferentially suppressing noisy background inputs active at positions outside a place field, while allowing the inputs active inside a place field to cross threshold for voltage-dependent amplification (Grienberger et al., 2017).

7.2.4 Ensemble selection

Plastic changes in synaptic weights, as mentioned above, serve as a memory mechanism to ensure that the same, stable subpopulation of neurons robustly responds upon each presentation of the same behaviorally relevant pattern of inputs. This process of recruiting a particular subset of a population to participate in the currently active neuronal representation is called "ensemble selection." What about when an input pattern is only partially complete, or corrupted by a source of noise? This fundamental computation, also called "pattern completion," has been extensively studied theoretically (Marr, 1971; Hopfield, 1982; de Almeida et al., 2007), and is thought to depend on local recurrent excitatory FB connections such as those between PCs in CA3 and MCs in DG (Guzman et al., 2016; Scharfman, 2016). According to this scheme, while the particular subset of afferent inputs to a circuit layer, their firing rates, and their postsynaptic strengths will initially determine which ensemble of postsynaptic neurons is selected, then this active group of neurons within the circuit layer will iteratively recruit additional partners to "fill out" missing components of the representation. Specifically, strong bidirectional connections between neurons that share feature selectivity (often referred to as "autoassociative" connections) comprise a strong reinforcing circuit motif that can enable ensemble selection and stored memory retrieval (de Almeida et al., 2007).

7.2.5 Frequency-dependent filtering

Each connection between cell types in the hippocampus can exhibit distinct neurotransmitter release probabilities and short-term dynamics. For example, the same axon from a CA3 PC can synapse onto a CA1 PC with low initial release probability that facilitates during a high-frequency train of action potentials, and separately synapse onto a CA1 IN with a high initial release probability that depresses during a train (H Sun et al., 2005). A CA1 IN, in turn, can then form either depressing or facilitating inhibitory synapses onto the PC (Figure 7.4), resulting in monosynaptic excitation and disynaptic inhibition (Figures 7.2 and 7.5) with different dynamics. Depending on the IN cell type and the timing of afferent inputs, these dynamic circuit elements can enable selective responses to particular input frequencies (Klyachko and Stevens, 2006). By combining facilitating excitation with depressing inhibition, a circuit can implement a high-pass filter (Figure 7.2B). The addition of a separate facilitating inhibitory element can then implement a high

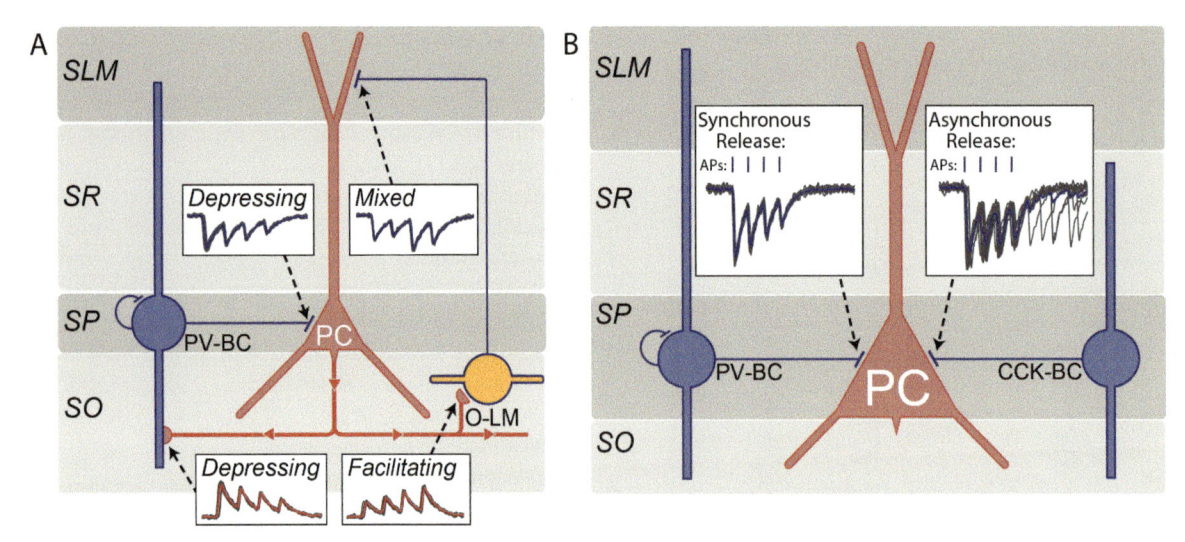

Figure 7.4 Cell type-specific differences in synaptic transmitter release dynamics in hippocampal local circuits. (A) CA1 PCs' excitatory synapses exhibit prominent short-term depression on parvalbumin-expressing basket cells (PV-BC), while excitatory synapses onto somatostatin-expressing O-LM IN *(O-LM)* show short-term facilitation. GABAergic output synapses from BC onto CA1 PCs show short-term depression, while synapses of O-LM cells onto CA1 PCs show a mixed facilitation-depression response. Postsynaptic membrane potential responses (EPSPs and IPSPs) are shown. (B) Action potential–evoked GABA rerelease from PV-BCs has short latency and high synchrony across synapses, while GABA release from cholecystokinin-expressing basket cells (CCK-BC) show high jitter and a prominent asynchronous release component following presynaptic action potentials. Inhibitory postsynaptic potentials (IPSPs) are shown.

frequency cutoff, resulting in a bandpass filter. Late onset facilitating inhibition is also effective at limiting the duration of response and implementing restricted temporal windows for synaptic integration. An extreme example of high-pass filtering is the MF synapse from DG GCs to CA3 PCs, which is referred to as a "conditional detonator" and which is only able to drive its target to spike upon sufficient facilitation of release probability during a high-frequency burst of action potentials (Vyleta et al., 2016; Chamberland et al., 2018). Interestingly, target-selective changes in short-term release probability dynamics can persist for multiple seconds, potentially allowing different modes of information processing for signals modulated at different timescales (Neubrandt et al., 2018).

7.2.6 Rhythm generation

When populations of neurons in a local circuit receive synchronous inputs, and generate synchronous outputs (Figure 7.2B), extracellular electrodes can detect large fluctuations in extracellular current and voltage, referred to as the "local field potential" (LFP). Such recordings in the hippocampus exhibit prominent oscillations that vary with behavioral state. In the awake state, animals engaged in spatial navigation exhibit prominent hippocampal population oscillations in the theta (~4–10 Hz) and gamma (~30–80 Hz) bands (Buzsaki, 2002; Buzsaki and Wang, 2012; Lisman and Jensen, 2013). When an awake animal stops locomoting, and during slow-wave sleep, hippocampal circuits are comparatively desynchronized and aperiodic, but intermittently emit hypersynchronous bursts of firing lasting ~100 ms called sharp waves. Coincident with these sharp wave events, a high frequency oscillation called a "ripple" (~110–200 Hz) is prominently detected in the CA1 SP layer (Buzsaki, 2015) as part of the SWR complex. During each of these types of population oscillations, each specific neuronal cell type emits spikes at a characteristic time point (or phase) relative to each cycle or period of the oscillation (Mizuseki et al., 2009; C Varga et al., 2012; Szabo et al., 2017). Multiple different mechanisms operating at different scales

have been shown to influence hippocampal rhythms, including extrinsic pacing by long-range projections from the medial septum (Vandecasteele et al., 2014; Y Wang et al., 2015), subcellular filtering by specific ion channels and the cable properties of neuronal dendrites (Hu et al., 2009; Vaidya and Johnston, 2013), and local circuit interactions (Stark et al., 2013; Stark et al., 2014). Interestingly, cell-type specific diversity in synaptic connectivity, intrinsic excitability, and synaptic signaling is sufficient to generate theta and gamma oscillations in the CA1 local circuit even in the absence of any oscillatory structure in the input to the circuit (Goutagny et al., 2009; Bezaire et al., 2016) (see section 7.4.1 below). Region-specific differences in local circuit architecture may support different types of rhythms—SWRs have been shown to originate in CA2/CA3 (A Oliva et al., 2016), and gamma oscillations are particularly prominent in the GCL of the DG (Csicsvari et al., 2003). Proposed computational roles for rhythmic activity in neuronal circuits include (1) segregation of active neurons into discrete coactive ensembles, (2) enforcement of permissive windows for spike timing to enhance downstream integration and plasticity, (3) representation of ordered sequences, and (4) modulating signaling between distinct downstream brain regions by varying oscillation frequency or phase (Buzsaki, 2002; Lisman and Buzsaki, 2008).

7.2.7 Behavioral state modulation

As mentioned above, theta oscillations and SWRs occur during specific behavioral states. Interestingly, specific hippocampal cell types are either up- or down-regulated during these events and during the transitions between behavioral states (Figure 7.2B). For example, CA3 BCs increase their firing rate during sharp waves, whereas AACs in CA3 decrease their firing rates up to hundreds of milliseconds before sharp wave onset (Hajos et al., 2013; Szabo et al., 2017). Interestingly, stimulation of cholinergic input from the medial septum increases theta oscillations and prevents sharp waves (Vandecasteele et al., 2014). Thus, specific elements of a local

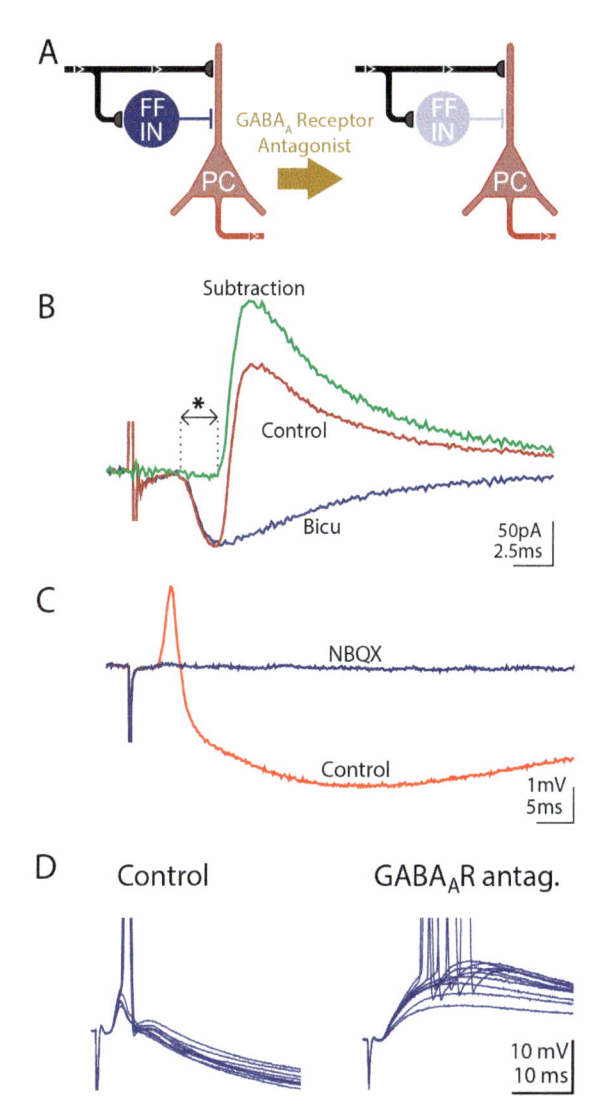

Figure 7.5 Role of feedforward inhibition in coincidence detection. (A) Schematics of feedforward inhibition. (B, C) Feedforward inhibition is responsible for coincidence detection. Whole-cell current recording from a CA1 PC on CA3-Schaffer collateral stimulation. Current traces recorded in control condition (red trace) and bicuculline (blue trace) and their algebraic difference (green trace). Under current-clamp conditions, stimulation of this feedforward inhibitory circuit triggered an early EPSP (blue trace) and a later IPSP (green trace) (B), both of which were blocked by the AMPA receptor antagonist NBQX confirming that the EPSP-IPSP sequence was being driven by glutamatergic afferents (C). (D) Voltage responses recorded in a CA1 PC in response to stimulation of two Schaffer collateral pathways under control or in the presence of a GABA-A receptor antagonist, illustrating that inhibitory input enforced a narrow temporal window for coincidence detection, which was lost in the absence of inhibitory control. (Modified with permission from Pouille and Scanziani, 2001.)

circuit can selectively receive extrinsic inputs that signal behavioral state transitions, and locally broadcast the signal to enact a local change in network dynamics.

7.2.8 Conjunctive input processing

A general circuit wiring principle shared throughout the hippocampus and cortex is that multiple distinct input pathways carrying different types of information converge onto single neurons, but segregate onto specific subcompartments of their neuronal dendrites

(Figure 7.2B) (Petreanu et al., 2009). How do local circuits detect coincidence of different inputs? In hippocampal area CA1, the distal dendrites of PCs primarily receive inputs from layer 3 (LIII) of EC and from the reuniens nucleus of the thalamus, whereas their more proximal apical dendrites primarily receive inputs from area CA3 (Wouterlood et al., 1990; Kajiwara et al., 2008). While synaptic inputs arriving onto distal dendrites are strongly attenuated along the path to the cell body, PCs increase the somatic impact of distal excitatory synapses by increasing their expression of AMPA-type glutamate receptors (Magee and Cook, 2000; Bittner et al., 2012). Thus, either proximal or distal dendritic inputs in isolation are capable of eliciting action potentials in CA1 PCs (Milstein et al., 2015). However, when high-frequency inputs at both proximal and distal input pathways are activated within the timescale of a theta cycle (~100 ms), voltage-dependent activation of NMDARs and calcium channels are recruited to generate a long, slow dendritic depolarization called a "plateau potential." These events result in high-frequency burst firing at the soma and axon, and can induce potent long-term plasticity at both CA3 and LIII EC inputs (Dudman et al., 2007; Takahashi and Magee, 2009; Bittner et al., 2015; Milstein et al., 2015; Bittner et al., 2017). In addition, some classes of interneurons in feedforward inhibitory circuits also perform active coincidence detection of distal and proximal inputs (Figure 7.6) with the result of further distinguishing circuit responses to simultaneous as opposed to asynchronous inputs (Milstein et al., 2015).

This mechanism for detecting coincidence of activity across multiple input pathways expands the information processing capabilities of a neuronal circuit, and enables some neurons to selectively respond to complex combinations of stimuli and context (Ranganathan et al., 2018). Also called "calcium spikes" or "complex spikes," these computationally relevant cellular events are heavily regulated by dendrite-targeting inhibition provided by the local circuit (Royer et al., 2012; Milstein et al., 2015; Grienberger et al., 2017; Schulz et al., 2018). While nonlinear integration dependent on NMDARs has also been observed in area CA3 and DG (Krueppel et al., 2011; S Kim et al., 2012; Makara and Magee, 2013; S Kim et al., 2018) whether these events depend on interactions between proximal and distal input pathways has yet to be determined. Interestingly, an operation of this type in CA3 and/or DG would result in very different associations due to differences in the spatial organization of inputs in those regions. While in CA1 inputs from LIII of either medial or lateral EC are segregated along the transverse axis of the hippocampus and arrive onto different PCs (Igarashi et al., 2014), in DG, all granule cells receive inputs from LII of both medial and lateral EC (Witter, 1993). Furthermore, in DG, the proximal input is an excitatory FB input from dentate MCs (Scharfman, 2016), while in CA3, the excitatory FB inputs from other CA3 PCs impinge on distal dendrites (Rebola et al., 2017). An input comparison between an extrinsic FF pathway containing information about the environment and a local FB pathway containing information recalled from memory could theoretically enable stored memories to be updated to reflect changes in the environment (Kaifosh and Losonczy, 2016).

7.2.9 Gating of synaptic plasticity

As mentioned above, large dendritic depolarizations recruit NMDARs and voltage-gated calcium channels (VGCCs), which further depolarize dendrites in a FB loop. The resulting calcium influx and downstream signaling induces plastic changes in the

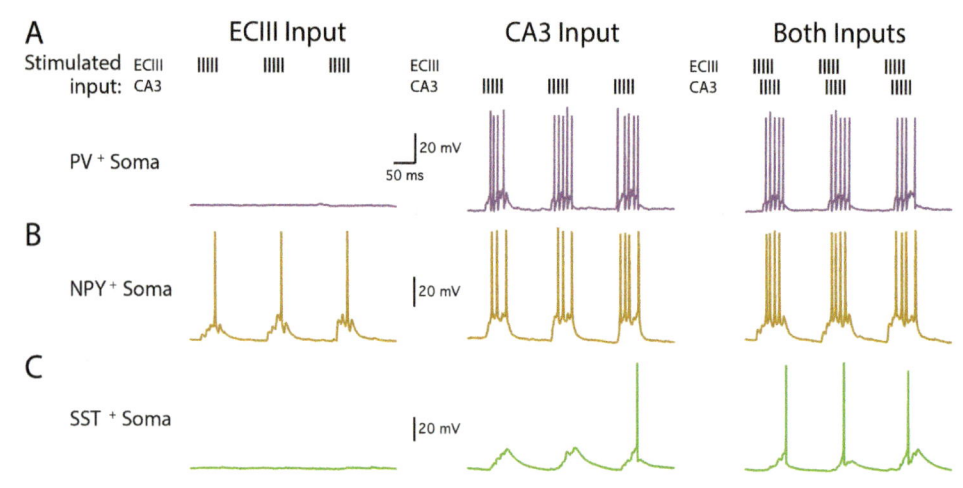

Figure 7.6 Inhibitory circuits integrate inputs from multiple pathways. (A) In vitro recordings were performed from CA1 IN soma during the electrical stimulation of either EC layer 3 (EC3) inputs (left column), CA3 inputs (middle column), or both inputs (right column). Parvalbumin-expressing INs (PV⁺) did not respond to EC3-input stimulation but responded equally robustly to CA3 and simultaneous CA3/EC3 input stimulation. (B) Neuropeptide Y-expressing dendrite-targeting INs (NPY⁺) responded weakly to EC3 input, moderately to CA3 input, and most robustly to conjunctive EC3/CA3 input. (C) Finally, somatostatin-expressing (SST⁺) INs recorded in the CA1 oriens layer showed no response to EC3 input, and a weak, mostly subthreshold, response to CA3 input. (Source: Milstein et al., 2015.)

strengths of excitatory synapses, providing a synaptic basis for learning and memory. These depolarizations are negatively modulated by dendrite-targeting inhibitory INs, thus providing a circuit mechanism to regulate whether or not learning can occur (Artinian and Lacaille, 2018). Importantly, hippocampal INs are a primary target of neuromodulatory inputs that signal attention, stimulus salience, and reward (V Varga et al., 2009; Lovett-Barron et al., 2014; Zaremba et al., 2017; Turi et al., 2019). In particular, learning-related activation of local inhibitory neurons that target other GABAergic INs can have a disinhibitory effect on local excitatory neurons and promote synaptic plasticity (Letzkus et al., 2015; Artinian and Lacaille, 2018).

7.3 Functional specificity and subcellular target selectivity of inhibition

In this section, building on the preceding discussions about the elementary computations performed by local circuits, we aim to describe some of the key organizational features of local circuits from the particular perspective of the inhibitory INs within the hippocampus. Decades of investigations into anatomical, physiological, molecular, and developmental properties of hippocampal INs—GABAergic non-PCs—has uncovered an astounding diversity of these cells and parsed them into distinct cell types in each hippocampal region (see chapter 5; Freund and Buzsaki, 1996; Klausberger and Somogyi, 2008; Petilla Interneuron Nomenclature et al., 2008; Pelkey et al., 2017; Booker and Vida, 2018). General organizational principles are informative in considering how INs are integrated into local circuits, interact with principal cells and each other, and participate in network operations. Below we focus on four general features of inhibitory circuit architecture in the hippocampus.

7.3.1 Perisomatic and dendritic inhibition

A well-established organizational principle of local circuit inhibitory architecture is the prominent subcellular target selectivity of

INs. That INs are embedded in a highly layered structure within each of the major hippocampal areas (CA1-3, DG) greatly facilitated the early recognition and classification of INs based on their axonal distribution and target selectivity. Seminal early studies established (Halasy and Somogyi, 1993b; Han et al., 1993; E Buhl, Halasy, et al., 1994; Freund and Buzsaki, 1996) that hippocampal INs selectively innervate distinct subcellular compartments of principal neurons, such as the soma, the axon initial segment, and the dendrites. Accordingly, hippocampal INs have been broadly divided into perisomatic-targeting and dendrite-targeting INs.

In order to understand the role of particular INs embedded within hippocampal microcircuits, it is necessary to consider a number of aspects simultaneously, including both anatomical properties (number and location of inhibitory synapses) as well as the functional and dynamic properties of their output synapses. All perisomatic and most dendritic INs target principal cells via multiple synaptic contacts, and the properties of GABA release exhibit presynaptic cell-type-specific differences (Elfant et al., 2008; McBain and Kauer, 2009; Ma et al., 2012). GABAergic INs exert their inhibitory actions on postsynaptic target cells by activation of fast ionotropic GABA$_A$ receptors (GABA$_A$Rs) and slow metabotropic GABA$_B$ receptors (GABA$_B$Rs) (Olsen and Sieghart, 2009). GABA$_A$Rs are primarily localized at synapses (although certain subunit isoforms are preferentially found at the extrasynaptic membranes, generating a substantial tonic inhibitory current) (Glykys and Mody, 2007) and are highly permeable to chloride and bicarbonate. Consequently, the direction and magnitude of GABA$_A$R-mediated changes in membrane potential depends on the intracellular concentrations of chloride and bicarbonate as well as the membrane potential of the postsynaptic neuron. Since the chloride reversal potential is only slightly negative relative to the resting membrane potential in PCs in the adult hippocampus, the effect of postsynaptic GABA$_A$R conductance on neuronal excitability is not primarily to hyperpolarize the membrane potential, but rather to decrease the effective input resistance of the membrane, thereby increasing the amount of excitatory current required to depolarize the membrane, an effect referred to as *shunting* inhibition.

7.3.1.1 Perisomatic inhibition in local circuits

While the somata and axon initial segments of hippocampal principal cells are devoid of excitatory inputs and are exclusively targeted by GABAergic synapses, they represent only about 8% of total inhibition received by CA1 PCs (Megias et al., 2001; Bezaire et al., 2016). Of broadly defined perisomatic-targeting INs (see chapter 5), the two main types of BCs (the PV+ and CCK+ BCs) innervate the cell body and the proximal dendrites of principal cells (Ribak and Seress, 1983; Somogyi et al., 2004; Glickfeld and Scanziani, 2006; Armstrong and Soltesz, 2012; Turi et al., 2019), while axo-axonic cells (AACs) selectively innervate the axon initial segment (Somogyi et al., 1985; E Buhl, Han, et al., 1994). Based on the available experimental literature and meta-analysis of the data (Bezaire and Soltesz, 2013), the cell body of a CA1 PC is estimated to receive a total of ~92 GABAergic synapses from ~17 PV+ and ~13 CCK+ BCs, while its axon initial segment receives a total of ~25–34 GABAergic boutons from ~6 AACs (E Buhl, Han, et al., 1994; Bezaire and Soltesz, 2013). Through their direct influence on the site of action potential initiation, perisomatic INs are well positioned to precisely regulate axosomatic action potential initiation, timing, and synchronization of PC assemblies (Cobb et al., 1995; Bartos et al., 2001; Jonas et al., 2004; Somogyi and Klausberger, 2005; Hu et al., 2014). Among these cells, PV+ fast-spiking BCs and AACs appear particularly well suited for high-fidelity, rapid and reliable regulation of axosomatic voltage dynamics of principal cells (Cobb et al., 1995; Bartos et al., 2001; Pouille and Scanziani, 2001; Bartos et al., 2002; Armstrong and Soltesz, 2012). Their roles as powerful and high-fidelity regulators of neuronal spiking output are further aided by their short-duration, nonadapting spiking profiles, as well as by high-probability and synchronous GABA release due to tight coupling of P/Q type VGCCs with the presynaptic release machinery (termed "nanodomain coupling"; Eggermann et al., 2011). Notably, hippocampal PV+ BCs are also interconnected via GABAergic synapses and gap junctions, which could further promote their synchronized inhibitory effect on target principal cells (Traub et al., 2001; Bartos et al., 2007). Various in vitro and in vivo experiments have demonstrated that inhibition from fast-spiking PV+ INs can strongly synchronize principal cells spiking in the gamma (~30–80 Hz) range (Bartos et al., 2002; Bartos et al., 2007). AACs selectively innervate the axon initial segment of principal cells (E Buhl, Han, et al., 1994) and their effect on principal cell membrane potential and output firing remain contentious as reports suggest that under some conditions in vitro they can promote spike initiation in principal cells of the neocortex and hippocampus (Szabadics et al., 2006; Woodruff et al., 2009). While CCK+ BCs, which can be found in two distinct, nonoverlapping subtypes based on vGluT3+ or VIP+ expression (Cope et al., 2002; Somogyi et al., 2004; Turi et al., 2019), also form multiple contacts on the soma and proximal dendrites of principal cells (Foldy et al., 2010), these cells have a regular spiking pattern and a low initial probability of GABA release, which is partially regulated by presynaptic CB1 cannabinoid receptors at their axon terminals (I Katona et al., 1999; R Wilson and Nicoll, 2001; Neu et al., 2007; Daw et al., 2009; Jonas and Hefft, 2010). They produce prominent asynchronous GABA$_A$R-mediated responses on connected principal cells due to the weak coupling between the presynaptic GABA release machinery and N-type VGCCs (termed

"microdomain coupling"; Hefft and Jonas, 2005; Daw et al., 2009; Jonas and Hefft, 2010) (Figure 7.4B). Furthermore, these different classes of perisomatic inhibitory cell types in the hippocampus exhibit distinct modulation and dynamics depending on behavioral state (see section 7.4 in this chapter), thus enabling state-dependent modulation of principal cell firing.

7.3.1.2 Dendritic inhibition in local circuits

The other, more diverse group of hippocampal INs predominantly innervates dendrites of principal neurons. In contrast to the nearly exclusive GABAergic innervation of the somata and axon initial segments, GABAergic and glutamatergic synapses intermingle on principal neuron dendrites. As functionally distinct excitatory input pathways are anatomically segregated on nonoverlapping proximal and distal dendritic subcompartments of hippocampal principal cells, these input pathways can be independently regulated by coaligned dendritic inhibition within these dendritic subcompartments in a layer-specific manner. Proximal dendrites of principal neurons receive intrahippocampal glutamatergic afferents: hilar MC collaterals in DG, MF and recurrent collaterals from other principal cells in CA3, and CA3 Schaffer collaterals in CA1 (Figure 7.1). For example, a CA1 PC receives approximately 30,000 excitatory synapses onto its dendrites, of which ~28,000 are from CA3 Schaffer collaterals inputs located on proximal apical and basal dendrites, and ~2000 synapses are from EC and nucleus reuniens inputs and are located on distal apical dendrites (Megias et al., 2001). This convergent excitation is balanced by ~200–1000 GABAergic synapses on proximal dendrites and ~300 on distal tuft dendrites (Megias et al., 2001; Bloss et al., 2016). Despite this lower relative density of GABAergic synapses, 92% of all inhibitory synapses are located on PC dendrites (Megias et al., 2001).

In the CA1 area, at least 12 IN subtypes have been classified as dendrite-targeting, and they can be grouped by whether they primarily innervate proximal or distal dendrites of principal cells (Klausberger, 2009) (Figure 7.1B). Proximal dendrites of CA1 PCs receive coaligned inhibition from at least four major dendrite-targeting IN types: the PV+/SOM+/Neuropeptide Y(NPY+) BiC (E Buhl et al., 1996; Maccaferri et al., 2000; Pawelzik et al., 2002; Klausberger et al., 2004), the CCK+ Schaffer collateral associated cell (SCA) primarily innervating thin oblique and basal dendrites (Cossart et al., 1998; Vida et al., 1998; Cope et al., 2002; Pawelzik et al., 2002), the CCK+ apical dendrite innervating cell (ADI), primarily innervating the main apical shaft (Klausberger et al., 2005), and the nitric oxide synthase (NOS+)/NPY+ Ivy cell (IvyC; Fuentealba, Begum, et al., 2008). Distal dendrites of PCs receive extrahippocampal glutamatergic inputs from the ECs and the nucleus reuniens and are also selectively innervated by multiple distinct INs classes: the SOM+ O-LM IN (McBain et al., 1994; Sik et al., 1995; Maccaferri and McBain, 1996), the CCK+ perforant path-associated cell (PPA; Hajos and Mody, 1997; Cossart et al., 1998; Vida et al., 1998; Pawelzik et al., 2002; Klausberger et al., 2005), and the NPY+ NGFC (Khazipov et al., 1995; Vida et al., 1998; Price et al., 2005; Zsiros and Maccaferri, 2005; Price et al., 2008).

Although there are notable differences in the layer-specific organization between the CA and DG areas, available evidence indicates that clear similarities exist among both perisomatic- and dendrite-targeting INs in the CA and DG (Figure 7.1B) (Halasy and Somogyi, 1993b; Han et al., 1993; Buckmaster and Schwartzkroin, 1995; Mott et al., 1997). For example, the proximal dendrites of GCs in the IML of the DG receive intrahippocampal excitatory inputs via the C/A path from contralateral and ipsilateral hilar MCs, and also receive coaligned inhibition from CCK+ hilar commissural associational path-associated (HICAP) INs. Similar to O-LM cells, SOM+ hilar perforant path-associated (HIPP) cells send axon arborizations to the OML where they coalign with the perforant path from EC. Finally, NOS+/NPY+ NGFCs have been described in the DG ML as well (Halasy and Somogyi, 1993a; Han et al., 1993; Armstrong et al., 2011), where they form a major subclass of the MOPP cells (Halasy and Somogyi, 1993a; Han et al., 1993) that are ML INs with axons restricted to the outer two-thirds of the ML, the termination zone of the perforant path fibers.

Similar to their perisomatic counterparts, dendrite-targeting INs have been shown to innervate target principal cells via multiple (~5–10) synapses (Halasy and Somogyi, 1993a; E Buhl, Halasy, et al., 1994a; Maccaferri et al., 2000), resulting in a total estimated convergence of ~80 dendrite-targeting INs onto a CA1 PC (Bezaire and Soltesz, 2013). While it has been shown that some INs preferentially innervate thick apical (e.g., ADIs) or thin radial oblique and basal dendrites (e.g., SCAs), the fine-scale subcellular connectivity along individual dendritic branches is still poorly characterized. However, a recent study using large-volume array tomography and transmission electron microscopy showed that molecularly defined INs in CA1 can be highly selective in their connectivity to specific dendritic branch types and exhibit precisely targeted connectivity along individual branches (Bloss et al., 2016). Specifically, SOM+ O-LM INs were found to preferentially innervate the branch ends of terminal tuft dendrites, NOS+ NGFCs were found to primarily target intermediate segments of tuft dendrites, and NPY+ INs (primarily BiCs) were found to preferentially innervate the origin of terminal branches in proximal apical oblique and basal dendrites, while synapses from NOS+ IvyCs appeared to be randomly distributed on the terminal branches of apical oblique and basal dendrites. These intriguing observations strongly suggest that pathway-selective inhibitory control of input-output transformations of individual principal cell dendrites may operate in a branch-selective manner, as has been previously predicted by computational models (Gidon and Segev, 2012; Jadi et al., 2012; Yang et al., 2016).

How is this remarkable subcellular domain-specificity of hippocampal INs established and maintained? While the embryonic origin and developmental maturation of various hippocampal IN types have now been characterized in detail (see Chapter 4) (Kepecs and Fishell, 2014; Pelkey et al., 2017), the genetic and molecular mechanisms whereby even broadly defined perisomatic or dendritic inhibitory connectivity are established and maintained remain poorly understood. Nevertheless, recent studies have started to provide insights into this process by demonstrating that cell-type-specific patterns of expression of transcription factors and synaptic proteins discriminate between INs that target the axon, soma, or dendrites of PCs (Favuzzi et al., 2019). Activity-dependent gene programs, in particular, gene networks regulated by the immediate early gene transcription factor NPAS4, have also been implicated in controlling domain-specific GABAergic synapse formation in the mouse hippocampus (Y Lin et al., 2008; Bloodgood et al., 2013). Specifically, it has been recently shown that NPAS4 coordinates the redistribution of GABAergic synapses formed on CA1 PCs, such that NPAS4 increases GABAergic synapse number on the cells body while decreasing GABAergic synapse number on apical dendrites, with CCK+ BCs being the major targets of NPAS4-dependent transcriptional regulation in CA1 (Hartzell et al., 2018).

7.3.1.3 Postsynaptic effects of perisomatic and dendrite-targeting interneurons in local circuits

The GABA$_A$Rs receptors that mediate the majority of fast inhibitory synaptic transmission in the brain are heteropentameric ion channels. Different cell types in the hippocampus can express distinct variants of each of the subunits that comprise these receptors, resulting in a large diversity of GABA$_A$R subtypes with distinct pharmacology (Olsen and Sieghart, 2009). For example, CA1 PCs express at least 14 GABA$_A$R subunits. While GABA$_A$Rs containing alpha1-3, beta2/3, and gamma2 subunits were found to be the most abundant in the hippocampus (Nusser et al., 1995; Klausberger et al., 2002; Fritschy et al., 2012), light microscopic immunofluorescence and electron microscopic immunogold studies into their detailed subcellular distribution revealed that INs targeting distinct subcellular compartments of hippocampal principal cells could act on distinct GABA$_A$R subtypes. For example, PV+ and CCK+ BCs have been suggested to act via partially distinct GABA$_A$R populations, (alpha1-containing and alpha2-containing GABA$_A$Rs, respectively), while output synapses of AACs contain high densities of GABA$_A$Rs with alpha2 subunits (Nusser et al., 1995; Nyiri et al., 2001; Klausberger et al., 2002; Fritschy et al., 2012). Note, however, that recent results suggest that perisomatic GABA synapses on CA1 and CA3 PCs have unimodal distributions with alpha1 and alpha2 subunits present at every synapse, and that alpha2 density is the same between synapses with presynaptic N-type or P/Q-type calcium channels (Kerti-Szigeti and Nusser, 2016). This notion is also supported by observations that the kinetics of the unitary inhibitory postsynaptic currents (IPSCs) from the two BC types appear to be similar (Szabo et al., 2010). Pharmacological studies in vitro also indicate that GABA$_A$R-mediated synaptic responses produced by distinct IN types display differential pharmacological sensitivities (Pawelzik et al., 1999; Thomson et al., 2000). Furthermore, NGFCs and IvyCs evoke slow GABA$_A$R-mediated responses on hippocampal principal cells (Vida et al., 1998; Price et al., 2005; Fuentealba, Begum, et al., 2008; Price et al., 2008; Armstrong et al., 2011), which is partially attributable to the presence of alpha5 and delta subunit-containing GABA$_A$Rs at their output synapses (Zarnowska et al., 2009; Karayannis et al., 2010). However, there are several other unique features of GABAergic transmission at the output synapses of IvyCs and NGFCs that have been implicated in the generation of slow dendritic GABAergic inhibition produced by these cells (Szabadics et al., 2007). These features include the extremely compact and dense axonal arborization of these cells with a high proportion of presynaptic axon terminals that do not appear to couple to a postsynaptic element (Vida et al., 1998) and support unitary volume transmission by activating extrasynaptic GABA$_A$Rs and GABA$_B$Rs in both principal cells and local INs (Vida et al., 1998; Price et al., 2005; Price et al., 2008; Armstrong et al., 2011; Booker et al., 2013).

Postsynaptic GABA$_B$Rs are predominantly extrasynaptic and, in most neurons, primarily activate G-protein-coupled inward rectifying potassium channels (GIRK), producing slow membrane hyperpolarization and inhibiting neural excitability (Vida et al., 1998; Kulik et al., 2003; Booker et al., 2013; Craig et al., 2013). GABA$_B$Rs are also found presynaptically and reduce neurotransmitter release via activation of GIRKs channels and/or inhibition of voltage-gated Ca^{2+} channels (Lei and McBain, 2003). Activation of presynaptic or postsynaptic $GABA_B$Rs in vitro has been shown to generally require strong electrical stimulation and release of GABA from multiple neurons resulting in GABA spillover (Isaacson et al., 1993; Scanziani, 2000). As described above, volume transmission from NGFCs is one major source of GABA activating $GABA_B$Rs in the hippocampus even after a single presynaptic action potential, and appears to be a common and generalized circuit motif across cortical regions (Vida et al., 1998; Tamas et al., 2003; Szabadics et al., 2007; Olah et al., 2009). Notably, several types of hippocampal INs also express postsynaptic $GABA_B$Rs, which regulate their somatodendritic excitability in a cell-type-specific manner (Booker, Althof, Degro, et al., 2017; Booker, Althof, Gross, et al., 2017; Booker and Vida, 2018). For example, postsynaptic $GABA_B$R-mediated signaling was preferentially observed in perisomatic-versus dendritic-targeting of PV+ and CCK+ INs in CA1 (Booker et al., 2013; Booker, Althof, Degro, et al., 2017).

7.3.2 Subtractive and divisive inhibition

In section 7.2.1, we have discussed the elementary computational aspects of gain control, a question that we can now revisit in more depth from the particular perspective of dendritic and somatic interneuronal inputs. A central question in this regard is: do perisomatic and dendritic INs have discernible effects on the input-output transformations carried out by principal neurons? The overall anatomical segregation and subcellular compartment-selective inhibition produced by perisomatic and dendritic INs strongly suggest a functional dissociation, whereby dendritic INs are ideally positioned to locally regulate integration and plasticity of dendritic excitatory inputs due to the spatial proximity of their output synapses to excitatory inputs on dendrites. Indeed, experiments both in vitro and in vivo have extensively demonstrated that dendritic inhibition recruited by local or long-range excitatory afferents can effectively regulate the integration and plasticity of excitatory inputs, and control active signal propagation in dendrites of hippocampal principal cells (Miles et al., 1996; Tsubokawa and Ross, 1996; Kanemoto et al., 2011; Lovett-Barron et al., 2012; Muller et al., 2012; Royer et al., 2012; Pouille et al., 2013; Lovett-Barron et al., 2014; Milstein et al., 2015; Basu et al., 2016; Sheffield et al., 2017).

Importantly, the effect of dendritic inhibition should be interpreted within the context of the active properties of principal cell dendrites. Decades of research on dendritic properties have shown that principal cell dendrites possess specific complements of voltage-gated ion channels that can amplify or attenuate synaptic signals, integrate inputs nonlinearly, and support active backpropagation of somatic action potentials into dendrites (Magee, 2000; Hausser and Mel, 2003; Spruston, 2008). In particular, CA PCs (Magee, 2000; Golding et al., 2001; Losonczy and Magee, 2006; Remy and Spruston, 2007; Spruston, 2008; S Kim et al., 2012) and, to a lesser degree, dendrites of GCs (Krueppel et al., 2011; S Kim et al., 2018) can sustain local dendritic spikes mediated by VGNas, VGCCs, or NMDARs, which undergo complex spatiotemporal interactions (Jarsky et al., 2005). Dendritic inhibition provided by SOM+ INs has been shown to effectively suppress dendritic electrogenesis and regulate input integration in CA1 PCs in response to optogenetic stimulation of CA3 Schaffer collaterals in vitro (Lovett-Barron et al., 2012) (Figure 7.3). More recently, NPY+ INs were found to play a critical role in suppressing dendritic plateau potentials and burst-firing output from CA1 PCs during dual pathway (CA3 and EC) integration

(Milstein et al., 2015) (Figure 7.6). Together, these studies demonstrate that inhibiting active dendrites of principal cells can effectively alter neuronal excitability by modulating the slope or gain of the f-I curve (divisive inhibition), whereas inhibition of passive dendrites would predict a subtractive shift of the f-I curve (see section 7.2.1 and Figure 7.3A above) (Holt and Koch, 1997; Pouille et al., 2013). However, as dendritic spike initiation in PCs in vitro was found to generally require some degree of input cooperativity (spatial clustering and temporal synchrony; Losonczy and Magee, 2006; Harnett et al., 2012; S Kim et al., 2012; Makara and Magee, 2013; Druckmann et al., 2014; Kastellakis et al., 2015) or conjunctive multipathway integration (Takahashi and Magee, 2009; Basu et al., 2013; Bittner et al., 2015; Milstein et al., 2015), our detailed understanding of which hippocampal behavioral states are conducive to dendritic electrogenesis in vivo, and the mechanism whereby distinct dendrite-targeting IN types can regulate this process in vivo remains far from complete (Royer et al., 2012; Grienberger et al., 2017; Sheffield et al., 2017).

How does perisomatic inhibition regulate principal cell input-output transformations? In vitro recordings showed that perisomatic GABAergic conductances could exert a divisive effect on the subthreshold input-output relation and on the suprathreshold f-I curve of CA1 PCs (Losonczy et al., 2010; Pouille et al., 2013). Furthermore, when considering the recruitment of neurons throughout the network, perisomatic FF inhibition (see section 7.3.3 below) can divisively control the dynamic range of the network as a whole (Pouille et al., 2009). However, it is also important to consider the complexity of the network architecture; for instance, dendrite-targeting INs are themselves modulated by INs targeting PC somata, and disinhibition (see section 7.3.4 below) resulting from this IN–IN connectivity can effectively cancel out the effect the of perisomatic inhibition on the firing rate of CA1 PCs (Lovett-Barron et al., 2012).

7.3.3 Feedforward and feedback inhibition

7.3.3.1 Anatomical substrates of hippocampal feedforward and feedback inhibition

The hippocampus shows a prominent laminar organization with a layer-specific distribution of afferent excitatory input pathways and local axon collaterals of principal cells. Embedded in this laminar structure, INs can receive inputs from only a subset of these excitatory inputs. For example, an average IN in CA1 receives ~8,000–17,000 synapses from CA3 Schaffer collaterals, ~1,400 synapses from the EC, and ~2,200 synapses from local collaterals of CA1 PCs (Gulyas, Megias, et al., 1999; Matyas et al., 2004; Takacs et al., 2012; Bezaire and Soltesz, 2013). Therefore, another informative classification of local circuit architecture considers the relative contribution of excitatory drive that INs receive from local collaterals (FB excitation) or from extrinsic afferents (FF excitation). In general, most INs receive multiple convergent inputs and participate in both FF and FB inhibition. However, some INs are preferentially embedded in FF or FB circuits. For example, as mentioned above in sections 7.1.1–7.1.3, O-LM cells in the CA together with their DG equivalent, the SOM+ HIPP cells, are considered primarily FB INs with their glutamatergic excitation almost exclusively originating from local collaterals (Blasco-Ibanez and Freund, 1995; Maccaferri, 2005; S Kim, 2014) (Figure 7.1B), and in turn, they provide FB inhibition onto the distal dendrites of principal neurons. Conversely, other INs with dendritic arborization restricted to hippocampal dendritic layers (e.g., NGFCs in CA1 and DG) primarily receive FF excitation from the ECs or upstream hippocampal areas.

The dendritic distribution of INs is generally correlated with the sources of their excitatory input and therefore to the type of inhibition (e.g., FF or FB) they mediate. For example, AACs with vertical dendrites are thought to receive all major excitatory input pathways, while radial dendrites of BiCs generally do not invade the SLM in CA1, and a subpopulation of BiCs have dendrites that do not even invade SR (C Varga et al., 2014). Furthermore, all the above-mentioned INs (BCs, AACs, BiCs), also contain a subset of cells located in CA1 SO with horizontal dendritic morphologies, indicating that these cells represent a predominantly FB subtype (Maccaferri et al., 2000; Losonczy et al., 2002; Pawelzik et al., 2002; Ganter et al., 2004; C Varga et al., 2014; Booker and Vida, 2018). Finally, while O-LM cells with cell bodies and horizontally oriented dendrites located in SO are also found in CA3, there are also SOM+ distal dendrite-targeting INs in CA3 with multipolar dendrites and with cell bodies located in CA3 SR (Gulyas et al., 1993; AA Oliva et al., 2000), which may suggest that the dendritic morphology and localization of SOM+ O-LM cells are governed by local recurrent inputs, as provided by CA3 PCs in the SR of CA3. While the dendritic distribution of INs largely determines the relative contribution of local and extrinsic excitatory inputs, other intracellular signaling networks have also been strongly implicated in the control of target-cell-selective synapse specification on INs (Sylwestrak and Ghosh, 2012; Schreiner et al., 2014; Traunmuller et al., 2016; Stachniak et al., 2019).

7.3.3.2 Functional roles of feedforward and feedback inhibition in local circuits

Both FF and FB inhibitory circuit motifs have been implicated in supporting a diverse array of synaptic, cellular, and local circuit computations. They control electrical activity in specific subcellular domains, regulate the timing and precision of action potentials in their target neurons, balance overall excitation and inhibition in large neuronal populations, and contribute to the generation of network oscillations. As most INs receive multiple convergent inputs and participate in both FF and FB inhibition, depending on the relative strength and timing of excitation from local and extrinsic sources, they can serve dynamically changing functions in these cellular and local circuit operations.

Excitatory afferent-targeting of INs (e.g., AACs) typically promote FF inhibition of principal cells. In most local circuits, FF excitation from afferent inputs effectively recruits INs and generates short-latency disynaptic inhibition onto principal cells. FF inhibition narrows the time window for excitatory input integration and action potential generation (Pouille and Scanziani, 2001; Pouille et al., 2009), thereby increasing the temporal precision of principal cell firing (Figure 7.5). At the local circuit level, FF inhibition has been shown to serve as a mechanism to expand the dynamic range of activity in principal cell assemblies (Pouille et al., 2009). During hippocampal network oscillations in vivo, FF inhibition has been implicated in maintaining temporal sequences of principal cell firing (Diba and Buzsaki, 2008). While fast-spiking PV+ BCs are likely to play a particularly important role in FF perisomatic inhibition in the hippocampus, other IN types, including CCK+ INs, may also be involved (Basu et al., 2013; Basu et al., 2016).

Hippocampal INs can participate in FB inhibitory circuits in two canonical ways. Reciprocal coupling between principal neurons

and INs where principal neurons provide excitatory drive onto INs that then target the very same principal neuron, provides anatomical and functional bases for FB *recurrent* inhibition (see above). In FB *lateral* inhibition, principal neurons receive inhibition from INs that were excited by other principal neurons within the local circuit. Both recurrent and lateral FB inhibition have been implicated in several functions in hippocampal local circuits. For example, FB recruitment of INs can limit the duration and the spread of excitation in the local principal neuron population and thus promote "winner-takes-all" dynamics, where the most active subset of principal cells can effectively suppress firing of the remaining weakly excited principal neurons. This sparsification mechanism provided by FB inhibition may play a particularly important role in the DG, where it can contribute to the generation of sparse and orthogonalized representations during pattern separation in vivo (de Almeida et al., 2009a; de Almeida et al., 2009b; Espinoza et al., 2018).

7.3.3.3 Biased structural connectivity and temporal dynamics in excitatory-inhibitory local circuits

Several important further questions arise in considering the overall influence of INs within local FF and FB circuits. First, what is the spatial extent of efferent connectivity of INs? While INs had been in the past referred to as "short axon" cells, the length and extent of their three-dimensional axonal arborization is in fact widespread, and depending on the cell type, can extend along both transverse (0.5–2.5 mm) and longitudinal axes (0.8–2.6 mm) and inhibit large numbers of principal cells (e.g., in CA1: 500–1,800, [Bezaire and Soltesz, 2013) spanning across hippocampal subregions (Sik et al., 1994; Ceranik et al., 1997; Hajos and Mody, 1997; Lasztoczi et al., 2011; L Katona et al., 2017; Szabo et al., 2017). This massive divergence of interneuronal outputs raises a second related question: do INs contact principal cells randomly and with uniform properties of synaptic transmission (sometimes referred to as "blanket inhibition"), or alternatively are there also topographical and target-specific rules governing their connectivity? Recent studies indicate that at least some INs are not randomly and uniformly connected within hippocampal local circuits. For example, inhibition at the output synapses of PV+ BCs in the DG displays distance-dependent topographical scaling, where inhibitory strength declines and signal duration increases with distance along individual axons due to differential expression of postsynaptic GABA$_A$-R subtypes (Espinoza et al., 2018). Furthermore, PV+ BCs in the CA1 region display intriguing target-cell-specificity: they receive stronger excitatory inputs from superficial PCs (cell bodies further from SO) but provide more powerful output to deep CA1 PCs (cell bodies closer to SO) (Lee et al., 2014). Finally, recent studies indicate that mature and adult-born GCs are differentially connected to FB INs (Temprana et al., 2015; Alvarez et al., 2016). While most of these studies have thus far focused on PV+ INs, it is possible that biased microcircuit connectivity rules also apply to other hippocampal IN types.

The efficacy and precision of the recruitment of INs by excitatory inputs are primarily determined by the properties of excitatory afferent synapses and by the intrinsic integrative properties of INs. As described above, most INs receive a large number of convergent FF and FB excitatory synaptic inputs (Takacs et al., 2012; Bezaire and Soltesz, 2013) and principal cells often contact INs via multiple synapses (Gulyas et al., 1993; Ali et al., 1998; Biro et al., 2006), and in turn, INs innervate postsynaptic cells through multiple contacts. For example, disynaptic inhibition mediated by fast-spiking PV+

INs in the CA1 (Pouille and Scanziani, 2001) and the DG (Geiger et al., 1997) show short-latency (<2 ms) recruitment of these cells by convergent activation of Schaffer collaterals and MFs, respectively. This rapid and reliable recruitment of PV+ INs is further aided by the subtype composition of the glutamate receptors expressed at their afferent synapses (Geiger et al., 1995; Geiger et al., 1997). A further consideration is the intrinsic properties of INs, especially the active properties of their dendrites that can further influence excitatory integration on these cells. While compared with principal cells dendritic properties of INs remain less characterized, there is some evidence that nonlinear properties of dendrites of some INs can also contribute to active input processing and output spike generation (Martina, 2000; Norenberg et al., 2010; Chiovini et al., 2014).

In addition to the absolute synaptic strength of input and output synapses of interneurons, short-term plasticity at these synapses also strongly modulates dynamic recruitment of interneurons onto local networks. Importantly, short-term plasticity of inputs from a single presynaptic cell type can vary depending on the cell type of the postsynaptic target (Salin et al., 1996; Losonczy et al., 2002; Blackman et al., 2013) (Figure 7.4A). This property can enable local circuits to dynamically route inhibition to different subcellular domains depending on the rate and timing of trains of inputs (Pouille and Scanziani, 2004; Milstein et al., 2015). For example, whereas PCs in CA1 contact perisomatic PV+ BCs with high initial release probability and depressing synapses, they contact other interneurons, including dendrite-targeting SOM+ interneurons, with low initial release probability and facilitating synapses (Gulyas et al., 1993; Ali et al., 1998; Losonczy et al., 2002). When activated by a train of repeated inputs, this results in the initial recruitment of "onset transient" perisomatic FB inhibition, followed by "late persistent" FB dendritic inhibition recruited through facilitating recurrent excitation (Pouille and Scanziani, 2004). It has also been shown in the CA1 that while both proximal (CA3) and distal (EC/reuniens) excitatory inputs firing at low frequencies are balanced out by rapid-onset FF inhibition, high-frequency bursts at these inputs cause presynaptic facilitation at excitatory inputs, transiently favoring excitation over inhibition (Milstein et al., 2015). This high-pass filtering is then further amplified postsynaptically by supralinear input summation in PC dendrites. Thus, target-cell-type-specific short-term dynamics provides a network-level mechanism to adaptively filter spatiotemporal patterns of synaptic input.

7.3.4 Disinhibitory local circuit motifs

While several major classes of hippocampal INs primarily target principal cells, this target selectivity is far from being exclusive. Each of the IN subtypes characterized thus far, with the apparent exception of AACs (E Buhl, Halasy, et al., 1994; C Varga et al., 2014), also innervates other INs at varying degrees, with an estimated 1%–10% of INs' targets being other INs (Bezaire and Soltesz, 2013). Conversely, ~6%–36% of synapses onto INs were found to be GABAergic. Both homotypic (within the same IN class) and heterotypic (between different INs classes) IN–IN connections have been observed in the hippocampus. Furthermore, hippocampal INs also receive long-range GABAergic inputs from cortical and subcortical sources, such as from EC and the medial septum (see also section 7.7 below, (Freund and Antal, 1988; Borhegyi et al., 2004; Melzer et al., 2012; Caputi et al., 2013; Kaifosh et al., 2013; Basu et al., 2016; Szonyi et al., 2019). Therefore, such IN interactions can lead to the removal of inhibition (disinhibition) (Figure 7.2A) from

distinct subcompartments of principal cells, which can result in a dynamic shift of inhibition impinging on principal cell populations. Among these IN interactions, inhibition originating from PV+ INs are among the best characterized and they can manifest in different forms. PV+ INs homotypically inhibit each other in CA1 and DG via fast kinetic, alpha1-subunit-containing GABA$_A$Rs (Cobb et al., 1995; Cobb et al., 1997; Bartos et al., 2002; Daw et al., 2009; Savanthrapadian et al., 2014; Kohus et al., 2016). This temporally precise inhibition among PV+ BCs has been implicated in the generation of coordinated network activity, in particular in the gamma (~30–80 Hz) frequency band (see section 7.4.2 below) (Bartos et al., 2001; Bartos et al., 2002; Bartos et al., 2007). In addition, PV+ BCs are also interconnected within-class via gap junctions that can further promote synchronization of the PV+ BCs (Bartos et al., 2001; Bartos et al., 2002; Bartos et al., 2007). PV+ BCs also target other INs, including CCK+ INs (Acsady et al., 2000; Karson et al., 2009; Savanthrapadian et al., 2014) and SOM+ BiCs and O-LM cells in CA1 (Lovett-Barron et al., 2012). This latter disinhibitory circuit motif has been implicated in redistributing inhibition between perisomatic and dendritic compartments of CA1 PCs (Lovett-Barron et al., 2012). Finally, some PV+ INs in the EC project to CA1 where they specifically target CCK INs (Melzer et al., 2012; Caputi et al., 2013; Basu et al., 2016). The resulting disinhibition has been shown to be permissive for plasticity of CA3 synapses onto CA1 PCs (Basu et al., 2016). In addition to PV+ INs, other hippocampal INs have also been shown to be homotypically interconnected (e.g, CCK–CCK (Daw et al., 2009; Savanthrapadian et al., 2014) or heterotypically (e.g., CCK-to-PV, [Karson et al., 2009). For instance, SOM+ FB O-LM cells have also been implicated in gating of information transfer in CA1 via their disinhibitory influence on FF INs (Elfant et al., 2008; Leao et al., 2012).

In addition to disinhibitory circuit motifs formed by INs that primarily target principal cells, distinct subsets of GABAergic hippocampal INs, so-called IN-specific INs (ISIs), selectively and preferentially innervate other INs, providing an additional cellular basis for disinhibition of PCs. Anatomical and, more recently, in vitro physiological properties of hippocampal ISI INs have been characterized in CA1 (Acsady, Arabadzisz, et al., 1996; Acsady, Gorcs, et al., 1996; Gulyas et al., 1996; Chamberland and Topolnik, 2012; Tyan et al., 2014; Francavilla et al., 2015; Francavilla et al., 2018; Turi et al., 2019). These studies indicate that CA1 ISIs can be further subdivided (ISI 1–3) based on their anatomical location and neurochemical marker profile. Type 1 ISIs express calretinin (CR) but not vasoactive intestinal polypeptide (VIP), located in throughout the CA1 SO/SP/SR layers. These INs were found to innervate each other via chemical and dendrodendritic electrical synapses and also to inhibit CB+ dendrite-targeting INs and CCK+/VIP+ BCs. Therefore, activation of ISI-1 INs may preferentially disinhibit Schaffer collateral-recipient dendrites of CA1 PCs. Type 2 ISIs express VIP (Francavilla et al., 2018), and typically located at the border of SR and SLM. These cells also primarily innervate dendrite-targeting CB+ INs, and in turn, provide disinhibition of proximal dendrites of CA1 PCs. VIP and CR coexpressing ISI-3 cells are typically located in SP and SR with their main axonal arborization in SO, where they primarily innervate SOM+ O-LM cells and to lesser extent PV+ BCs (Chamberland and Topolnik, 2012; Tyan et al., 2014). Thus, recruitment of ISI-3 cells is expected to disinhibit the apical tuft of CA1 PCs. A similar ISI-3 circuit motif has also been identified in the DG, where VIP+ INs primarily target SOM+

HIPP cells (Hajos et al., 1996). Targeting of SOM+ INs by VIP+ ISIs appears to be a common and generalized circuit motif across cortical regions and has been implicated in a multitude of neocortical functions, including sensorimotor integration, attention, memory-guided behaviors, and cortical gain control (Letzkus et al., 2011; S Lee et al., 2013; Pi et al., 2013; Fu et al., 2014; Zhang et al., 2014; Fu et al., 2015; Kuchibhotla et al., 2016; Kamigaki and Dan, 2017). While some recent studies have implicated VIP+ disinhibitory circuits in supporting spatial learning in the hippocampus (Donato et al., 2013; Turi et al., 2019), the roles of disinhibitory motifs in regulating hippocampal circuit function and behavior in vivo remain incompletely understood.

7.4 Local circuits underlying network dynamics

The remarkable richness of the local circuit features discussed above highlights the fact that the neuronal circuits of the hippocampus support multiple modes of information processing, similar to many other brain structures (Carr and Frank, 2012). In the hippocampus, the multiple modes of information processing often manifest themselves in the form of ensemble network oscillations of different frequencies correlated with distinct behavioral states (Buzsaki and Draguhn, 2004). For example, hippocampal theta-frequency (~4–10 Hz) rhythms occur during active exploration and running, as well as during REM sleep, whereas the considerably faster transient ripple oscillations (~120–250 Hz) take place during awake immobility and slow-wave sleep. The hippocampal rhythms, typically recorded in electroencephalograms (EEGs) and local field potentials (LFPs), are thus linked to normal cognition and are also known to be disrupted in various disorders, making it even more essential to understand the mechanisms underlying their generation. An important clue about the synaptic-cellular bases of hippocampal rhythms came from the demonstration in the early 1990s that gamma (~30–80 Hz) oscillations preferentially occur at specific phases of the slower theta rhythm (a phenomenon now known as cross-frequency coupling) and that perisomatic, $GABA_A$ receptor-dependent inhibitory inputs to CA1 and CA3 PCs play key mechanistic roles in the generation of both rhythms (Soltesz and Deschenes, 1993). The identification of the mechanisms underlying the generation of oscillations in the hippocampus and elsewhere is challenging for several reasons, including the complex anatomical connectivity and cellular diversity of the brain (Figure 7.7) (Cohen and Gulbinaite, 2014), the fact that many of the hippocampal rhythms exists in multiple forms with different pharmacological sensitivities, and the complexity of interactions between various hippocampal and extrahippocampal brain structures (Ferguson et al., 2017). Here, we focus specifically on the involvement of local circuits in rhythm generation, and the computations associated with the three major rhythms of the hippocampal formation: the theta, gamma, and ripple oscillations.

7.4.1 Theta rhythm

The theta rhythm was discovered more than 80 years ago in the rabbit (Jung and Kornmüller, 1938; Colgin, 2013), and research in the subsequent decades has revealed that theta exists in many other species as well, including rats, cats, and humans (Green and Arduini, 1954; Grastyan et al., 1959; Vanderwolf, 1969; Lega et al., 2012). Theta oscillation occurs during active exploration and REM sleep, and is often observed during behaviors associated with intake

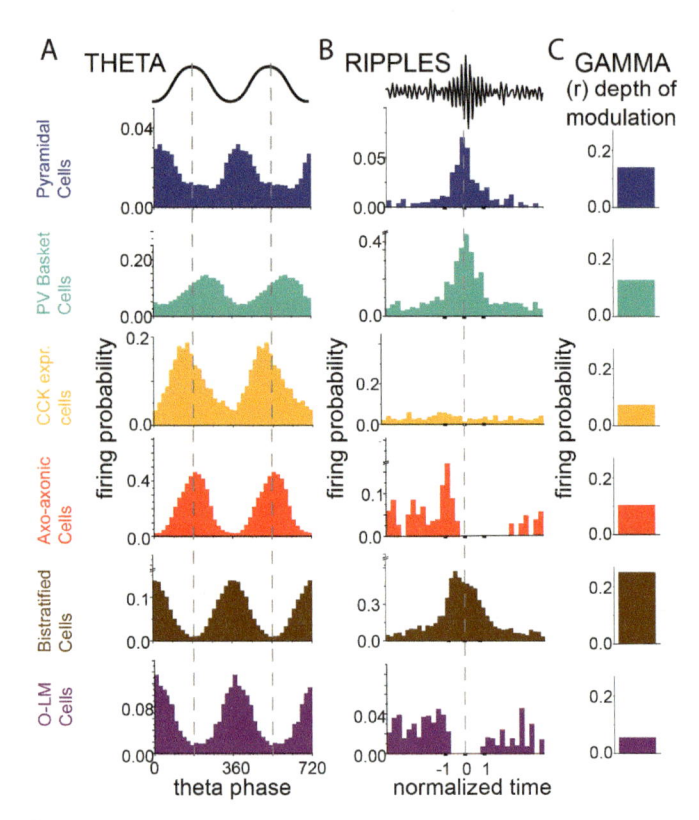

Figure 7.7 Discrete oscillatory bands recruit distinct IN types within CA1. In vivo juxtacellular recording together with simultaneous LFP recordings were carried out during different oscillatory regimes in hippocampal area CA1. Post hoc anatomical and immunocytochemical identification of the recorded neurons revealed that PCs and several IN types are differentially recruited by distinct oscillations. These differences in recruitment are observed both in the diversity of preferred phases of firing of different cells relative to the ongoing oscillation as well in the relative strength of neuronal recruitment at this phase (modulation depth). (A) During theta states PCs tended to fire near the trough of individual theta cycles, while most INs, except for BiCs and OL-M cells, showed the opposite phase preference. (B) PV + BCs and BiCs were the cells most strongly recruited by sharp wave ripple events, while conversely, axo-axonic cells were inhibited. (C) Among the oscillations examined, PCs showed the strongest phase modulation by gamma oscillations, which also strongly modulated the activity of PV + BCs and BiCs. (Source: Klausberger and Somogyi, 2008.)

of stimuli (Colgin, 2013), including whisking (Berg and Kleinfeld, 2003) and sniffing in rats (Macrides et al., 1982) and eye saccades in humans (Otero-Millan et al., 2008). Theta exists in two pharmacologically distinct forms, categorized based on sensitivity to the cholinergic antagonist atropine (Buzsaki, 2002; Colgin, 2013; Colgin, 2016), with the atropine-resistant theta typically occurring during exploration, with the atropine-sensitive form being observed during behavioral immobility (Kramis et al., 1975) and during urethane anesthesia, which decreases EC inputs to the hippocampus (Ylinen, Soltesz, et al., 1995). The hippocampal theta rhythm in humans is generally linked to similar behavioral states as it is in rodents (Lega et al., 2012), although some differences have been also reported (Qasim and Jacobs, 2016). There is now general agreement that theta rhythms are important for different types of learning and memory as well as synaptic plasticity (Colgin, 2013, 2016), although exactly how theta plays a role in these processes is not understood. Several possible explanations have been put forward, including roles for theta in the packaging or "chunking" of information (Dragoi and Buzsaki, 2006; Kepecs et al., 2006; Gupta et al., 2012), creating the appropriate timing to induce alterations in synaptic signals (Larson et al., 1986), and facilitating interareal interactions (Seidenbecher et al., 2003; M Jones and Wilson, 2005). All hippocampal regions can display theta oscillations, as can several closely connected extrahippocampal regions including the medial septum and the medial entorhinal cortex (MEC) (Buzsaki, 2002; Colgin, 2013), and several of such extrahippocampal brain regions exhibit increased theta coupling to the hippocampus during spatial memory processing, including the medial prefrontal cortex (J Kim et al., 2011), striatum (DeCoteau et al., 2007), and lateral amygdala (Seidenbecher et al., 2003). Multisite silicone probe recordings along the long axis of the hippocampus revealed that theta oscillations are not perfectly synchronized throughout the hippocampus, but they are traveling waves that propagate along the septotemporal axis (Lubenov and Siapas, 2009). Therefore, theta oscillations do not simply function as a "global clock" imposed on the anatomical extent of the hippocampus, but they appear to pattern hippocampal activity across anatomical space as well as, similar to how time on Earth is organized in a progression of local time zones. Such spatiotemporal patterning may be particularly important for the organization of the ongoing communications between the hippocampus and the various target regions innervated by CA1 PCs. Because the septal and temporal parts of the hippocampus project to distinct areas (e.g., the retrosplenial cortex and the mPFC, respectively), traveling waves may ensure that these targets receive CA1 peak input in a particular order (Lubenov and Siapas, 2009).

The theta rhythm, similarly to the gamma and ripple oscillations discussed in subsequent sections below, is typically recorded as the LFP signal using a small electrode placed within the hippocampal nervous tissue. It is important to appreciate that any excitable membrane (e.g., axon, soma, dendrite, spine, axon terminal) and any type of transmembrane current (e.g., ion fluxes through voltage-gated channels, synaptic currents, oscillations) can contribute to the extracellular field. The amplitude, shape, and frequency of the LFP waveform depend on the relative contribution, spatial density, and temporal coordination of the various sources as well as the distance of the recording LFP electrode from these current sources (Buzsaki et al., 2012). In most physiological situations, it is the synaptic activity that is considered to be the most important source of the extracellular current flow. A major component of the latter results from the activation of AMPARs and NMDARs by glutamate that leads to a net influx of cations from the extra- to the intracellular space, giving rise to a so-called local extracellular sink. In order to achieve electroneutrality, the extracellular sink needs to be balanced by an extracellular source, which is an opposing ion flux from the intra- to the extracellular space called a passive or return current. It should be noted that GABA$_A$ receptor-mediated transmembrane currents can be substantial and also contribute significantly to the LFP signals, particularly under conditions when the neuron is active and its membrane is depolarized away from the Cl$^-$ equilibrium potential (Buzsaki et al., 2012).

In terms of the involvement of local circuits in the generation of theta, a key question is whether the hippocampal circuitry is capable of generating the theta oscillations or whether theta is purely driven by and inherited from extrahippocampal areas. Of the external drivers, the medial septum has been known for many years to play a key role, since its lesion or inactivation in vivo disrupts

hippocampal theta (Soltesz and Deschenes, 1993; Brazhnik and Fox, 1999; Borhegyi et al., 2004; V Varga et al., 2008; Hangya et al., 2009; Colgin, 2013). The primacy of the medial septum in theta generation is underlined by the observation that the medial septum transitions to the theta state about 500 ms before theta appears in the hippocampus itself (Bland et al., 1999). Medial septal GABA cells fire rhythmically at theta frequencies (Hangya et al., 2009), and the GABAergic septohippocampal projection selectively terminates on hippocampal GABAergic INs (Freund and Antal, 1988). The other major septohippocampal projection originates from cholinergic neurons of the medial septum that do not fire rhythmically (Simon et al., 2006) and innervate both hippocampal principal cells and INs. Therefore, a basic form of theta may emerge from the slow muscarinic-receptor (mAChR)-mediated depolarization (Madison et al., 1987) of principal cells produced by cholinergic septohippocampal inputs that is modulated at the theta frequency by the rhythmic disinhibitory signal from the GABAergic septohippocampal afferents (Buzsaki, 2002). In addition to the central role played by the medial septum, CA1 receives theta-frequency inputs from both intrahippocampal sources such as CA3 and extrahippocampal areas, including EC. Accordingly, current source density analysis of the LFP signal from freely moving rats revealed multiple current dipoles (sink and source pairs) during theta, including current sinks in the SR and SLM layers reflecting CA3 and EC inputs, respectively (Kamondi et al., 1998; Buzsaki, 2002).

The presence of robust extrinsic rhythm generators does not exclude the possibility that local circuits within the hippocampus by themselves can generate some form of theta oscillation, and theoretical studies had suggested that the hippocampus may possess the minimal circuitry required for theta-frequency ensemble oscillations (Traub et al., 1989; White et al., 2000). Indeed, Goutagny et al. (2009) showed that the whole hippocampus in an in vitro preparation spontaneously generates low-frequency theta in CA1, even when input fibers from CA3 and entorhinal cortex (EC) are transected (Goutagny et al., 2009) (Figure 7.8). These theta oscillations were stable and dependent on both GABA$_A$ and AMPA receptors (AMPARs), and blockade of transmission across the septotemporal axis revealed multiple atropine-resistant theta oscillators in CA1. There was remarkable similarity between results from studies carried out in vivo (Royer et al., 2012; Stark et al., 2013) and the isolated hippocampal preparation (Goutagny et al., 2009; Amilhon et al., 2015), including the sparse firing of principal cells at rest, the phasic firing of PV cells, the reversed polarity of intracellularly recorded theta oscillations at around the presumed equilibrium potential for GABA$_A$-dependent inhibitory postsynaptic potentials (IPSPs) (Soltesz and Deschenes, 1993), and the fact that optogenetic silencing of PV but not SOM cells eliminated the theta rhythm (Royer et al., 2012; Stark et al., 2013; Amilhon et al., 2015). The inactivation experiments conducted in the isolated hippocampal preparation (Figure 7.8) (Goutagny et al., 2009; Amilhon et al., 2015) indicated that the minimum circuitry required for CA1 theta rhythmicity may be contained within about 1mm^3, which has been estimated to correspond to approximately 30,000 PCs and 500 PV cells (Ferguson et al., 2013; Ferguson et al., 2015; Ferguson et al., 2017). Taken together, these results showed that the local circuit in CA1 is capable of generating a form of atropine-resistant theta.

Another highly characteristic feature of the hippocampal theta rhythm is the fact that distinct interneuronal subtypes fire at different phases of the theta oscillation (Fuentealba, Begum, et al.,

2012; Bieri et al., 2014; Schomburg et al., 2014) and to potentially support distinct modes of CA1 spatial and mnemonic processing (Bieri et al., 2014; Yamamoto et al., 2014; Zheng et al., 2015). While likely involving the recruitment of a distinct subpopulation of INs (Colgin et al., 2009; Lasztoczi and Klausberger, 2014), the specific circuit mechanisms supporting fast gamma oscillations in CA1 remain unclear. This knowledge gap is partly attributable to the more recent discovery of fast as compared with slow CA1 gamma, the suppression and/or disconnection of EC afferents to CA1 in many anesthetized and in vitro recording preparations (Ylinen, Bragin, et al., 1995), and the relatively weaker efficacy of fast gamma in entraining CA1 neural activity (Belluscio et al., 2012; Schomburg et al., 2014). Therefore, it is likely that the majority of mechanistic studies of gamma oscillations to date pertain to slow gamma mechanisms.

Local inhibitory subcircuits are strongly implicated in the generation of slow gamma. In anesthetized rats the intracellular gamma oscillations of hippocampal excitatory cells were found to be associated with inhibitory postsynaptic potentials (IPSCs) (Soltesz and Deschenes, 1993; Pernia-Andrade and Jonas, 2014) and to reverse in polarity at the equilibrium potential of GABA$_A$-mediated Cl$^-$ currents (Soltesz and Deschenes, 1993; Penttonen et al., 1998). Moreover, in CA1, individual INs show a much greater degree of phase-locked spiking to gamma than do nearby PCs (Csicsvari et al., 2003; Hajos et al., 2004; Colgin et al., 2009), with BiCs cells and PV+ BCs displaying the strongest gamma modulation (Tukker et al., 2007). While several types of INs have been implicated in gamma generation (Freund and Buzsaki, 1996; Tukker et al., 2007; Klausberger and Somogyi, 2008; Lasztoczi and Klausberger, 2014; Veit et al., 2017), evidence suggests PV+ BCs play a particularly prominent role. The pattern of extracellular current sources and sinks during slow gamma oscillations (Csicsvari et al., 2003; Belluscio et al., 2012; Schomburg et al., 2014) is consistent with that of PV+ BC-mediated perisomatic inhibition (Penttonen et al., 1998; Mann, Suckling, et al., 2005). Furthermore, the biophysical and synaptic characteristics of PV+ BCs make them particularly fast and reliable transmitters of afferent activity (Buzsaki et al., 1983; Gulyas et al., 1993; Lien and Jonas, 2003; Tateno and Robinson, 2009) and therefore well suited for fast timescale network synchronization, as consistent with theoretical models (Hajos and Paulsen, 2009; Buzsaki and Wang, 2012). Finally, the biophysics of PV+ BCs appear to facilitate a pronounced resonance at slow gamma frequency in response to stochastic input (Pike et al., 2000; Cardin et al., 2009; Sohal et al., 2009), suggesting biophysical "tuning" for activity at this frequency. In CA1 the significant phase delay (approximately 90° or 5.5 ms) (Csicsvari et al., 2003; Tukker et al., 2007) between PC and IN spiking during gamma oscillations is consistent with excitatory-inhibitory (E-I) models of gamma generation in which cycles of excitation and FB or FF inhibition produce gamma rhythmicity (H Wilson and Cowan, 1972; Ermentrout and Kopell, 1998; Borgers and Kopell, 2003; Geisler et al., 2005; Mann, Radcliffe, et al., 2005). A recent theoretical study demonstrated that while FB inhibition is sufficient to generate gamma-frequency oscillations, in the absence of FF inhibition, gamma frequency varies widely with the total of amount of afferent excitation (Renno-Costa et al., 2019). This suggests that FF inhibition serves to normalize local circuit activity to the amount of input, providing additional stability to high-frequency network oscillations.

Notably, excitatory-inhibitory phase delays are shorter within the CA3 region (approximately 50° or 3.1 ms) (Csicsvari et al., 2003),

suggesting that the mechanisms of gamma generation may differ between the CA3 and CA1 regions. Moreover, other theoretical models (I-I models) (X-J Wang and Rinzel, 1992; Van Vreeswijk et al., 1994; XJ Wang and Buzsaki, 1996; Bartos et al., 2007) and experimental evidence (Whittington et al., 1995; Hormuzdi et al., 2001; D Buhl et al., 2003) suggest that synaptic and/or electrical coupling between inhibitory neurons may serve as an alternative or cooperative mechanism for gamma-band neural synchronization. How these diverse potential mechanisms of gamma synchronization cooperate or compete to generate distinct gamma-band oscillations across and within brain regions remains an open question for further research.

7.4.3 Sharp wave ripples

Sharp wave ripples are prominent short-lived (40–100 ms) CA1 region LFP events characterized by a fast (110–200 Hz) "ripple" oscillation in the CA1 SP and a large amplitude negative LFP deflection reflecting a current sink in the SR layer of CA1 (Buzsaki et al., 1983; Buzsaki, 1986, 2015). SWRs are the LFP correlates of hippocampal CA synchronous population burst events, which occur spontaneously during non-theta-associated behaviors including quiescence, slow-wave sleep, and reward consumption (Buzsaki et al., 1983). While they are thought to play a critical role in the hippocampal-dependent consolidation of memories across a range of extrahippocampal structures, the formation and evolution of SWR population events are determined by local hippocampal subcircuits. The first such subcircuit is the recurrent CA3/CA2 network, which is strongly implicated in SWR event generation: (1) SWR events persist after EC lesions (Suzuki and Smith, 1988; Ylinen, Soltesz, et al., 1995) and after medial septal and fimbria-fornix lesions (Buzsaki et al., 1983; Suzuki and Smith, 1988) but are suppressed by functional CA3 lesions (Nakashiba et al., 2009; Davoudi and Foster, 2019), (2) in vivo and in vitro unit recordings reveal that CA3/CA2 activity precedes CA1 SWR events (Csicsvari et al., 2000; Sullivan et al., 2011; A Oliva et al., 2016), and (3) SWR-associated patterns of extracellular sources and sinks in the CA1 region are similar to those evoked by direct Schaffer collateral stimulation (Buzsaki et al., 1983; Ylinen, Bragin, et al., 1995; Sullivan et al., 2011; Sasaki et al., 2018). While initiated in the CA3/CA2 recurrent network, the timing and content of SWR population bursts are biased by the activity of the network's DG and EC afferents (Sirota et al., 2003; Sullivan et al., 2011; Yamamoto and Tonegawa, 2017), with the latter recently implicated in the generation of learning-related multi-SWR "bursts" in postlearning quiet waking episodes (Yamamoto and Tonegawa, 2017). During theta states, recurrent excitation within the CA3/CA2 network is suppressed through the activation of presynaptic muscarinic and endocannabinoid (CB1) receptors (Robbe et al., 2006; Maier et al., 2012; Vandecasteele et al., 2014). The release of such neuromodulatory suppression during low-acetylcholine "offline" states promotes the buildup of self-reinforcing excitation in recurrently connected CA3/CA2 assemblies, resulting in SWR events. Consistent with this model of SWR event generation, SWR events most often begin in the most strongly recurrently connected hippocampal regions, CA2, CA3a, and distal CA3b, before propagating to the less recurrently connected proximal CA3b, CA3c regions, which in turn more effectively recruit the CA1 region (Amaral et al., 1990; X Li et al., 1994; Csicsvari et al., 2000; Wittner et al., 2007). Recent evidence further suggests that localized subcircuits of excitatory cells within the recurrent CA3/CA2 networks may be preferentially involved in SWR generation. A recently identified subpopulation of bursty, athorny CA3 PCs, lacking DG afferents and enriched in the deep layers (that is, near the SO) of CA3a and distal CA3b, was described to immediately precede and likely promote the formation of CA3 SWR events (Hunt et al., 2018). Another in vivo study identified a subpopulation of extracellularly recorded CA2, putatively excitatory, mostly superficially located cells, which fire immediately prior to CA3 and/or CA1 SWR events, primarily during quiet waking but not slow-wave sleep, suggesting that the specific subcircuits driving SWR event generation may vary by behavioral state (A Oliva et al., 2016).

While driven by recurrent excitation, population SWR events engage, and are in turn shaped by, specific fast timescale synchrony-promoting local inhibitory subcircuits (Figure 7.10) (Cutsuridis and Taxidis, 2013; Gan et al., 2017). SWR events most strongly recruit PV+ BCs and PV+ BiCs, while most AACs are inhibited and SOM+ INs show a bimodal distribution of SWR-modulation (Klausberger et al., 2003; Klausberger et al., 2004; C Varga et al., 2012; Hajos et al., 2013; Tukker et al., 2013; C Varga et al., 2014). Recent studies have implicated local circuits consisting of reciprocally interconnected PV+ BCs (Klausberger et al., 2003; Tukker et al., 2013; Valero et al., 2015): (1) PV+ BCs (along with PV+ BiCs) sharply increase their firing rates within SWRs and their spiking is phase-locked to individual local fast ripple-oscillation peaks; (2) optogenetic silencing of PV+ neurons strongly attenuates fast-frequency ripple oscillations, both in vitro (Schlingloff et al., 2014) and in vivo (Stark et al., 2014); and (3) genetically targeted optogenetic stimulation of PV+ cells in vitro (though not in a different CA1 in vivo preparation; Stark et al., 2014) elicit ripple oscillations, even after the pharmacological blockade of excitatory glutamatergic transmission (Schlingloff et al., 2014). However, while it is clear that PV+ BCs play a central role in SWR-formation, alternative, or potentially complementary, intrinsic mechanisms have been proposed to contribute to this timing (Draguhn et al., 1998; Maier et al., 2003; Chiovini et al., 2014).

SWR-associated population bursts show a skewed distribution of magnitude and anatomical extent along the hippocampal septotemporal axis, with a minority of particularly strong events extending across a large portion of the entire hippocampus (Mizuseki and Buzsaki, 2013; Patel et al., 2013). The more numerous lower amplitude events are typically spatially restricted and may terminate locally or travel along the septotemporal axis at 0.35 m/s, consistent with the conductance delays along the unmyelinated axons comprising the CA3/CA2 recurrent network (Patel et al., 2013). Notably, SWR co-occurrence and travel are partially dissociated between the temporal pole and the more septal and intermediate regions of the hippocampus, likely reflecting the unique makeup of temporal hippocampal afferents as well as the reduced interconnectivity between the temporal and more septal CA3/CA2 recurrent networks (Strange et al., 2014). However, regardless of the anatomical extent of the underlying SWR-associated population burst event and consistent with their dependence on local IN circuits, fast ripple oscillations remain phase-coherent only over short distances (Ylinen, Bragin, et al., 1995; Csicsvari et al., 1999; Csicsvari et al., 2000; Patel et al., 2013). Indeed, while elicited by CA3/CA2 SWR-events, not only are CA1 fast ripple oscillations not phase coherent with their upstream CA3/CA2 ripples but also they typically occur at a higher intrinsic frequency (Buzsaki et al., 1992; Csicsvari et al., 2000), likely reflecting the higher degree of excitatory convergence from CA3/CA2 to CA1 than within the CA3/CA2 recurrent network (Buzsaki et al., 1992). In turn, within the CA1 network superficial (that is near SR) PCs are more strongly recruited by SWR-events than are deep PCs, while INs generally show the opposite depth relationship (Mizuseki et al., 2011; Stark et al., 2014). The relatively weaker recruitment of deep PCs can thus likely be explained by more robust FF inhibition and weaker CA3 Schaffer collateral excitation unto these cells as compared with the superficial PCs (Valero et al., 2015).

7.4.4 Gap junctions

While it is generally accepted that fast chemical synaptic transmission serves as the primary vehicle for neuronal communication in hippocampal circuits, there is a growing body of experimental evidence and modeling work implicating important roles of electrical communication via gap junctions in pacing and

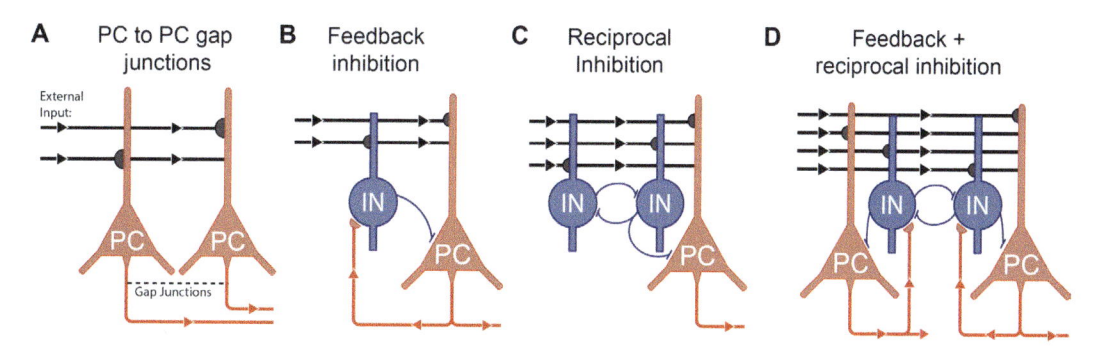

Figure 7.10 Proposed local circuit models for the generation of fast oscillations. The speed at which network synchronization can occur during fast oscillations such as gamma and the CA1 ripple oscillation suggest local network mechanisms are likely involved in their generation. (A) One such proposed network mechanism is the synchronization of PC (PC) output by electrical coupling effected by putative gap junctions between PC axons. However, the presence and function of these putative gap junctions remain controversial. (B) A second proposed network motif is simple feedback inhibition (also referred to as "PC-IN gamma" or "PING" motifs) in which cycles of excitation and feedback inhibition result in rhythmic principal cell output. (C) Conversely, in reciprocally inhibited circuits (also referred to as "ING" motifs) the cycles of inhibition and disinhibition are imposed by lateral connections between INs, such as those found between nearby PV+ basket cells, which are in turn driven by FF input. Since GABA_A transmission is generally faster than glutamate-mediated transmission, reciprocally inhibiting circuits may play an important role in the pacemaking of very fast oscillations such as ripples. (D) Consistent with this role, recent research suggests that the combination of reciprocal inhibition together with FB inhibition, particularly as mediated through networks of interconnected PV + BCs, is critical for the fast time-scale PC synchronization observed during CA1 ripples. (Source: after Stark et al., 2014.)

synchronizing hippocampal network activity. Connexin proteins form ion-permeant channels between neurons and mediate fast, bidirectional interneuronal communication and electrical coupling (Alcami and Pereda, 2019). Gap junctions have prominent low-pass filtering properties, so that rapid events, such as action potentials and fast synaptic currents are severely attenuated, while slower depolarizations/hyperpolarizations, including spike afterhyperpolarizations (AHPs), are transmitted more efficiently. Nevertheless, these filtered action potential "spikelets" can still promote coordinated spiking across coupled neurons.

Similar to neocortical circuits (Galarreta and Hestrin, 1999, 2001, 2002; Tamas et al., 2000; Fukuda and Kosaka, 2003; Connors and Long, 2004; Hestrin and Galarreta, 2005; Fukuda et al., 2006), the most convincing anatomical, physiological, and molecular evidence to date suggests the presence and functional role for gap junctions specifically between GABAergic INs in the adult hippocampus (Kosaka, 1983; Katsumaru et al., 1988; Fukuda and Kosaka, 2000; Venance et al., 2000; Hormuzdi et al., 2001; Meyer et al., 2002; Zsiros and Maccaferri, 2005; Hamzei-Sichani et al., 2012). Electrical synapses between hippocampal INs are predominantly composed of connexin-36, formed homotypically (between cells of the same class or subtype), and located either at dendrodendritic or somatodendritic contacts. Among these homotypic connections, electrical coupling between fast-spiking PV+ INs is the best characterized anatomically and functionally. Given the key role of fast-spiking PV+ cells in synchronizing network activity, especially in gamma range (see section 7.4.2 above), it is thus predicted that electrical coupling between PV+ INs can facilitate coordinated inhibitory synaptic transmission onto downstream principal cells, thus entraining synchronous network oscillatory activity. Indeed, Cx36 knockout mice exhibit lower hippocampal gamma (Hormuzdi et al., 2001) and impaired spatial memory, and place cells recorded from these mice exhibit reduced spatial selectively and theta phase precession (Allen et al., 2011). While these effects are most readily attributable to deletion of Cx36 between PV+ cells, homotypic connections among other hippocampal IN subtypes may also contribute. For example, extensive gap junctional coupling between IS-1 INs has been described (see section 7.3.4 above) via long dendrodendritic junctions among multiple dendrites (Gulyas et al., 1996), which can serve to synchronize the activity of these disinhibitory INs on their downstream targets.

The presence and functional role of potential coupling between hippocampal principal cells remains much less established. Based primarily on in vitro electrophysiological experimental results and modeling, axonal gap junctions between hippocampal PCs have been implicated in setting hippocampal network oscillations, especially at ripple (~200 Hz) frequency (Draguhn et al., 1998; Traub and Bibbig, 2000; Traub et al., 2018). According to this model of ripple generation, PCs excite each other both antidromically and orthodromically by their gap-junction-coupled axonal plexus, where ripples are generated, while INs simply inherit the rhythm. Nevertheless, no direct ultrastructural evidence has been observed for presence of gap junctions or Cx36 between hippocampal PCs, and loss of function of Cx36 in mice did not impact SWRs (Hormuzdi et al., 2001), suggesting that neuronal gap junctions between hippocampal neurons may not be essential for SWRs.

In summary, gap junctions provide hippocampal circuits with ability to synchronize neuronal populations, but the precise contributions

and mechanisms of electrical coupling between neurons to network synchronization requires future investigation.

7.5 Parallel processing and output selectivity

Conventionally, hippocampal circuit operations have been interpreted in a framework of random synaptic connections between homogeneous populations of functionally equivalent principal neurons in each hippocampal area. However, heterogeneity within the hippocampal principal cell population, in particular within CA1 and CA3 PCs is increasingly recognized and includes developmental, molecular, anatomical, and functional differences (Grosmark and Buzsaki, 2016; Soltesz and Losonczy, 2018; Valero and de la Prida, 2018; Cembrowski and Spruston, 2019). Multimodal within-cell-type heterogeneity has been described along all major axes of the hippocampus (transverse, longitudinal, and radial), and can in principle support the formation of several distinct nonuniform parallel circuit modules in the hippocampus that are independently controlled and affect different behaviors. Indeed, recent studies indicate that distinct subpopulations of principal cells differentially participate in network activities and produce structurally and functionally dissociable hippocampal output (Soltesz and Losonczy, 2018; Valero and de la Prida, 2018; Cembrowski and Spruston, 2019). Together these studies demonstrate that subpopulations of CA1 PCs can route distinct behavior-contingent information selectively to different target areas. While the hippocampal circuit architecture can, in principle, contain several parallel circuits, the main question from the perspective of local circuits is whether these parallel information channels represent uniform or nonuniform computational modules. Uniform modules would perform similar transformations on different afferent signals and send processed information to different downstream targets. Alternatively, the nature of the input-output transformation itself could be different, with nonuniform modules constituting the parallel circuits.

7.5.1 Heterogeneity of CA1 pyramidal cells and associated local circuits

The most detailed evidence for structural and functional heterogeneity of principal cells and their associated microcircuits is currently available in the CA1 region, where PCs exhibit topographically organized differences in terms of their anatomical, physiological, developmental, and molecular properties (Figure 7.11) (Igarashi et al., 2014; Grosmark and Buzsaki, 2016; Mallory and Giocomo, 2018; Soltesz and Losonczy, 2018; Valero and de la Prida, 2018; Cembrowski and Spruston, 2019). A particularly well-characterized subdivision between deep and superficial PCs exists along the radial axis of CA1, which is reflected in radial differences in the timing of neurogenesis and associated differences in genetic programs, molecular, structural, and physiological properties, as well as in connectivity (Soltesz and Losonczy, 2018; Valero and de la Prida, 2018; Cembrowski and Spruston, 2019). Recent studies have revealed asymmetric connectivity between radial CA1 PC subpopulations and PV+ BCs, which provided a compelling piece of evidence for the existence of spatially biased excitatory-inhibitory microcircuits in the hippocampus (SH Lee et al., 2014; Valero et al., 2015). Specifically, PV+ BCs provide unitary synaptic currents almost three times larger in deep compared with superficial CA1PCs in both the dorsal and ventral hippocampus (SH Lee

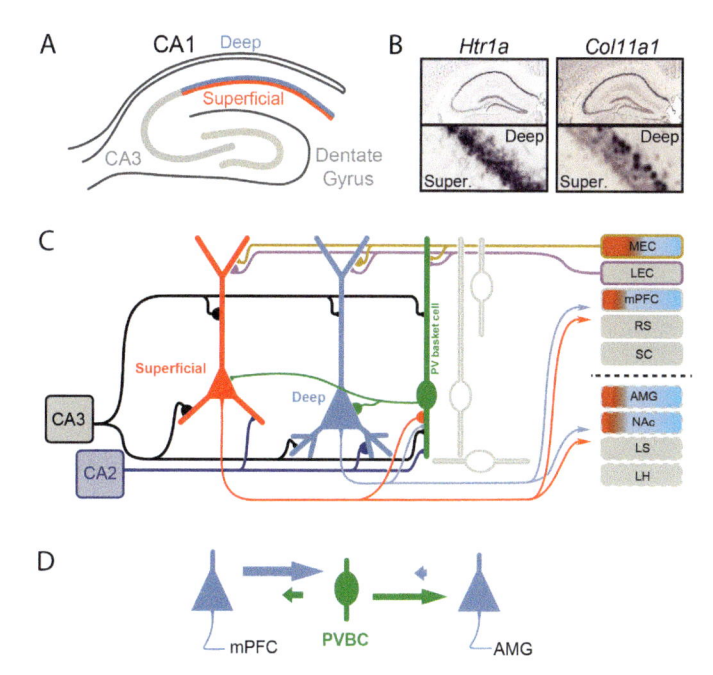

Figure 7.11 CA1 PC heterogeneity along the superficial/deep hippocampal axis. (A) A schematic of a coronal section of the dorsal hippocampus shows that the deep (blue) and superficial (red) sublayers of CA1 (note that the deep sublayer is located dorsally in dorsal CA1, reflecting its inversion with respect to the neocortex). (B) RNA sequencing (data not shown) and in situ hybridization revealed distinct genetic profiles of deep versus superficial CA1 PCs; note the distinct deep-superficial expression profiles of the two example genes (Cembrowski et al., 2016). (C) Functional and anatomical studies have revealed that compared with superficial cells, deep CA1 PCs generally receive stronger feedforward excitation from MEC and CA2 regions while superficial CA1 PCs receive stronger CA3 and LEC input. Deep CA1 PCs are also more strongly inhibited by local PV + BCs—the extent of superficial-deep differential innervation by other IN subtypes remains unclear. Superficial and deep cells may also differently innervate long-range CA1 targets (mPFC, medial prefrontal cortex; RS, retrosplenial cortex; SC, subicular complex; AMG, amygdala; NAc, nucleus accumbens; LS, lateral septum; LH, lateral hypothalamus). While similar numbers of deep and superficial CA1 efferents to MEC have been observed, projections to the mPFC, AMG, and NAc preferentially arise from the deep CA1 sublayer (this bias is shown in the coloring of the boxes on the right of the panel). (D) Notably, unique local CA1 circuit motifs have also been observed between PCs based on their distinct long-range projections. In particular, mPFC-targeting CA1 PCs strongly drive, but are more weakly inhibited by, local PV + BCs. In turn, PV + BCs strongly inhibit but are weakly driven by AMG-projecting CA1 PCs (Soltesz and Losonczy, 2018).

et al., 2014; Valero et al., 2015). The larger synaptic currents exert more effective control of action potential discharges and originate from a denser PV+ BCs innervation of the deep PCs. Notably, the differences extend to local recurrent excitatory connections as well, with superficial PCs innervating PV+ BCs with three times higher probability compared with deep cells. Thus, PV+ BCs receive more excitation from superficial PCs but deliver stronger inhibition to deep PCs. The biased inhibitory and excitatory microcircuit organization between the heterogeneous PCs and PV+ BCs sets up preferential lateral inhibition from the superficial to the deep layer. These biased local microcircuits could thus dynamically regulate routing of information between subcircuits of PCs, possibly depending on area-specific activity patterns and computational tasks. Recent studies also demonstrated differential afferent

connectivity of heterogeneous CA1 PC subpopulations that would further support the formation of parallel nonuniform subcircuits (Kohara et al., 2014b; Y Li et al., 2017; Masurkar et al., 2017). For example, CA2 PCs provide stronger excitatory inputs onto deep CA1 PCs compared with superficial CA1 PCs in the dorsal hippocampus (Kohara et al., 2014b). Among extrahippocampal afferents, the medial and lateral ECs (MEC and LEC, respectively) provide dual input streams into the hippocampus, with MEC and LEC projecting to different parts of CA1 along the proximodistal axis (Masurkar et al., 2017). Furthermore, the MEC preferentially targets deep CA1 PCs in proximal CA1 (toward CA2), while the LEC preferentially excites superficial PCs in distal CA1 (toward subiculum) (Masurkar et al., 2017).

In addition to distinct afferents, heterogeneous CA1 PCs also differ in terms of their efferent connectivity. For example, anxiety-related firing was selectively increased in CA1 PCs projecting to the prefrontal cortex, neurons targeting the nucleus accumbens exhibited prominent goal-directed firing, while triple-projecting neurons—targeting the prefrontal cortex, amygdala, and nucleus accumbens—were most active during tasks and SWR-related high-frequency oscillations (Ciocchi et al., 2015). Ventral hippocampal CA1 PCs preferentially located in the deep sublayer and which project to the nucleus accumbens shell play a necessary and sufficient role in social memory, CA1 PCs projecting to the basal amygdala mediate contextual fear behavior, whereas CA1 PCs projecting to the central amygdala mediate context-dependent cue fear memory retrieval (Okuyama et al., 2016; C Xu et al., 2016).

Intriguingly, CA1 PCs with distinct projection targets are differentially interconnected with local inhibitory circuits. Specifically, deep-layer amygdala-projecting CA1 PCs were found to receive inhibitory inputs three times larger than those onto deep-layer mPFC-projecting CA1 PCs, and in turn, the differentially projecting CA1 PCs from the same (deep) layer provide highly biased innervation to PV+ BCs, so that the CA1 PC population that receives less PV+ BC inhibition provides stronger excitation onto these INs (Lee et al., 2014) (Figure 7.11D).

7.5.2 Heterogeneity of CA2/3 pyramidal cells and granule cells from a local circuit perspective

Temporal origin and sublayer organization are also critical determinants in area CA3. Gene expression in CA3 PCs displays prominent laminar specificities within the discrete molecular subdomains that have been identified along the dorsal-ventral axis in CA3 (Thompson et al., 2008). A recent study uncovered a subpopulation of early-generated CA3 PCs with characteristic morphophysiological features and preferential location in the deeper part of CA3, which is able to synchronize network activity in the adult hippocampus (Marissal et al., 2012). Marked gradients of intrinsic membrane properties and synaptic connectivity have also been reported along the proximodistal axis of CA3 (from CA3c, proximal to DG, to CA3a, distal from DG): decreasing gradients of intrinsic excitability and DG MF synaptic input strength were countered by increasing gradients of recurrent excitation (being most prominent in the CA3b subregions) and direct synaptic excitation from the EC (Makara and Magee, 2013; Q Sun et al., 2017; Raus Balind et al., 2019). Intriguingly, a rare and deep CA3 PC subtype has recently been discovered with specialized morphology, anatomy, physiology, and a potential key role for initiating SWRs (see section 7.4.3 above) (Hunt et al., 2018).

Although the functional organization of within-cell-type heterogeneity of hippocampal principal cells and their associated microcircuits is best described in the CA1 and CA3 areas, available evidence suggests that within-cell-type multimodal heterogeneity is also present elsewhere in the hippocampal formation. For example, multimodal heterogeneity has been identified within CA2 PCs, where deep CA2 PCs play distinct roles in initiating SWRs (Dudek et al., 2016; Kay et al., 2016; A Oliva et al., 2016). Furthermore, subicular PCs can be divided into distinct classes based on morphological, electrophysiological, extrahippocampal projections, and plasticity properties, and a recent study uncovered coherent multimodal heterogeneity across the proximal-distal axis of the dorsal subiculum with dissociable roles in hippocampus-dependent learning (Cembrowski, Phillips, et al., 2018a; Cembrowski and Spruston, 2019). Finally, the question of principal cell heterogeneity is especially relevant in the DG, where there is compelling evidence for developmental programs parsing GCs into molecularly, functionally distinct subpopulations, which are defined by the timing of their neurogenesis (Kempermann et al., 2015) and appear to be differentially interconnected with inhibitory circuit motifs (Temprana et al., 2015; Alvarez et al., 2016). More work will be needed to better define the detailed relationships between heterogeneous subpopulations of PCs and their biased inhibitory circuit motifs.

7.6 Neuromodulation of local circuits

While the cellular composition and synaptic connectivity of hippocampal local circuits are the primary determinants of local circuit function, neuronal response properties and synaptic connections are also subject to neuromodulation originating from diverse long-range and local sources. By acting primarily through metabotropic signaling pathways, neuromodulators can profoundly alter intrinsic neuronal excitability, glutamatergic and GABAergic synaptic transmission, and functional and structural synaptic plasticity in local circuits (Marder, 2012). Thus, neuromodulators can dynamically adjust circuit functions and provide them with great flexibility in responding to, processing, and storing information. Below we summarize some salient features of local circuit neuromodulation in the hippocampus:

- Major sources of hippocampal neuromodulation are ascending afferent modulatory systems, originating from various subcortical nuclei (see section 7.6.1) with differential innervation of hippocampal regions both in terms of subregions and the longitudinal axis of the hippocampus, where these regions perform distinct tasks and are differentially innervated by neuromodulators.
- Subcortical modulatory afferents can cotransmit multiple neuromodulators and can corelease neuromodulators with glutamate or GABA.
- Local release of neuropeptides from INs represents another distinct source of neuromodulation (see section 7.6.2).
- Neuromodulators can act via point-to-point synaptic transmission or via nonsynaptic release of transmitters with divergent spatiotemporal transmitter profiles of release.
- Principal cells and INs are both subject to neuromodulation and exhibit cell-type and subcellular domain-specific receptor distribution.

- Individual neuromodulators can act on different receptor subtypes, including subtypes of G-protein-coupled metabotropic receptors and ionotropic receptors for certain neuromodulators (e.g., acetylcholine and serotonin).
- Modulatory signaling through the same receptor in different neurons can recruit cell-type-selective signaling pathways.

Cell-type-specific differences in receptor expression and intracellular downstream signaling provide divergence and specificity to neuromodulatory actions in local circuits. The net effect of neuromodulators on local circuits is, however, often difficult to decipher. Most neuromodulators act on multiple receptor subtypes, which may have ostensibly opposing effects, or may take place over different timescales. These receptors often exhibit differing affinity for their cognate ligands, meaning that the spatiotemporal profile of neuromodulator concentrations may determine the direction of modulation via activation of distinct receptors. Second, these receptors are differentially expressed in distinct cell types and subcellular compartments, including presynaptic axon terminals, where they can modulate short-term synaptic release dynamics, and postsynaptic somata and dendrites, where they can alter neuronal excitability. Finally, multiple neuromodulatory systems can also exhibit crosstalk through the expression of neuromodulator receptors on their presynaptic terminals, and through activation of overlapping cellular signaling pathways (e.g., G-proteins and modulation of voltage-gated K^+ channels).

7.6.1 Ascending subcortical modulatory systems

7.6.1.1 Acetylcholine

Cholinergic neuromodulation of the hippocampal formation plays a critical role in learning, attention, and oscillatory dynamics (Teles-Grilo Ruivo and Mellor, 2013; Dannenberg et al., 2017). Acetylcholine (ACh) affects hippocampal circuits via metabotropic muscarinic (mAChRs) and ionotropic nicotinic (nAChRs) receptors, and cholinergic afferents to the hippocampus arise from the basal forebrain medial septum and diagonal band of Broca (MSDB) complex. Cholinergic axons ramify extensively in all hippocampal layers and target both principal cells and INs (Drever et al., 2011). Early anatomical studies found that the vast majority (~90%) of cholinergic axons in the hippocampus lack synaptic junctional specializations (Umbriaco et al., 1995), suggesting that diffuse "volume" transmission of ACh prevails in the hippocampus. The latter view, however, has recently been challenged by findings that most cholinergic terminals form synapses, and also that these synapses cotransmit ACh with GABA (Takács et al., 2012).

Metabotropic ACh signaling in the hippocampus is mediated by multiple mAChRs, including Gq-coupled M1 and M3 and Gi/o-coupled M2 and M4 mAChRs. A complex interplay between these receptors leads to diverse response profiles in different subpopulations of hippocampal INs and PCs. The most prominent effects of muscarinic activation on PCs are mediated through M1/M3-receptor-mediated increase of postsynaptic excitability and NMDAR activity through the inhibition of K^+ channels including voltage-activated Kv7 (Petrovic et al., 2012), Kv4.2 (Losonczy et al., 2008), and Ca^{2+}-activated SK channels (Giessel and Sabatini, 2010), and conversion of spike afterhyperpolarization (AHP) to afterdepolarization (ADP), which lowers spike threshold (Vogt and Regehr, 2001; Gulledge and Kawaguchi, 2007; Dasari and Gulledge, 2011). In addition, mAChR activation (primarily M1 and M4) has been shown to suppress recurrent glutamatergic transmission between CA3 PCs and CA3 Schaffer collateral inputs to CA1, while transmission at more distal EC inputs onto these cells are thought to be relatively preserved (Hasselmo, 2006; Dasari and Gulledge, 2011). In contrast to the predominantly slow depolarizing effect of mAChR activation on principal cells, the responses of INs to cholinergic stimulation are much more diverse (McQuiston and Madison, 1999a; Widmer et al., 2006), including hyperpolarization, depolarization, or biphasic responses. Nonetheless, SOM+ O-LM cells, CCK+ BC and PV+ BCs all show increased firing frequency due to conversion of AHP to ADP, which is mediated by M1/M3 mAChR activation through the recruitment of the nonselective cation current I_{CAT} and inhibition of I_M and I_{AHP} (Lawrence et al., 2006; Cea-del Rio et al., 2010; Cea-del Rio et al., 2012). The most prominent effect of mAChR activation on GABAergic synaptic transmission is a presynaptic M2-mediated suppression of GABA release from axon terminals of PV+ BCs (Hefft et al., 2002; Chiang et al., 2010; Szabo et al., 2010; Lawrence et al., 2015).

Ionotropic nAChRs are most prominently expressed on hippocampal IN subtypes, primarily on CCK+ and VIP+ cells, where they can evoke large inward currents with rapid kinetics (S Jones and Yakel, 1997; McQuiston and Madison, 1999b; Frazier et al., 2003; Alkondon and Albuquerque, 2004; Albuquerque et al., 2009; McQuiston, 2014). A striking effect of nAChR activation within local circuits is the stimulation of transmitter release from certain glutamatergic and GABAergic terminals independently of presynaptic action potentials. For example, activation of presynaptic alpha7 nAChRs at MF terminals in CA3 leads to a robust enhancement of synaptic transmission (R Gray et al., 1996), which is in part mediated through action potential-independent synaptic release (Sharma and Vijayaraghavan, 2003; Sharma et al., 2008). Similarly, GABA release from perisomatic-targeting INs, presumably PV+ BCs, is robustly enhanced by alpha3/alpha4 nAChRs activation (MacDermott et al., 1999). In summary, cholinergic modulation of IN activity can have strong influences on network dynamics in the hippocampus. In vivo evidence for this was given recently by an imaging study (Lovett-Barron et al., 2014) in which aversive stimuli were shown to activate SOM+ O-LM cells in CA1 via MSDB cholinergic input and M1 mAChRs activation, leading to inhibition of the distal dendrites of CA1 principal cells, which was necessary for successful fear learning.

7.6.1.2 Dopamine and noradrenaline

The two major subcortical sources of subcortical catecholaminergic modulation of hippocampal local circuits are the afferents from the midbrain ventral tegmental area (VTA) releasing dopamine (DA) (Gasbarri, Packard, et al., 1994; Gasbarri, Verney, et al., 1994; Gasbarri et al., 1997; Edelmann and Lessmann, 2018) and afferents from the brainstem locus coeruleus (LC) releasing noradrenaline (NA) (Hortnagl et al., 1991; Milner et al., 2000; Walling et al., 2012). Notable recent work also suggests that DA may also be released in the hippocampus by LC fibers, where it is stored in these afferents as a precursor (Smith and Greene, 2012; McNamara and Dupret, 2017), and DA antagonists have been shown to effectively block the functional effects of LC stimulation in the hippocampus (Kempadoo et al., 2016; Takeuchi et al., 2016). At the behavioral level, NA/DA release from LC/VTA afferents is strongly associated with novelty, salience, or unexpected uncertainty (Yu and Dayan, 2005; Sara, 2009), and evidence indicates a role of NA/

DA in encoding and retrieval of novel and salient information in the hippocampus (Murchison et al., 2004; Kempadoo et al., 2016; Takeuchi et al., 2016; Wagatsuma et al., 2018).

The effect of DA and NA are mediated exclusively by metabotropic receptors that alter intrinsic excitability and synaptic strength mainly in excitatory circuit motifs. NA influences local circuits in all hippocampal subregions via alpha1-AR, alpha2-AR, and beta1-ARs. NA has been found to largely decrease the intrinsic excitability of PCs via alpha2-AR-mediated GIRK activation and occasionally also through beta1-ARs (Madison and Nicoll, 1986; Lacaille and Schwartzkroin, 1988). The most consistent downstream effect of NA appears to be on excitatory synapses in local circuits, where beta1-ARs enhance basal transmission, lowering the threshold for the induction, and helping the maintenance, of NMDAR-dependent Hebbian LTP (Huang and Kandel, 1996; Gelinas and Nguyen, 2005; Hu et al., 2007; Palacios-Filardo and Mellor, 2019), so that the EC drive to CA3 is increased via the DG, which may in turn promote information storage in hippocampal local circuits.

Overall, DA receptors are expressed more strongly in the DG than in CA3/CA1 (Ginsberg and Che, 2005), leading to the notion that DA modulation of hippocampal function is primarily mediated by changes to DG function. DA enhances GC excitability via D1Rs (Hamilton et al., 2010) and MC excitability via D2Rs (Etter and Krezel, 2014). In addition, DA facilitates basal synaptic transmission and long-term plasticity at select FF excitatory pathways, such as MFs and medial perforant path inputs to GCs, respectively (Kobayashi and Suzuki, 2007). Another well-established role of DA is to support the persistence of long-term plasticity (Hansen and Manahan-Vaughan, 2014; Wieschholleck and Manahan-Vaughan, 2014). Although dopaminergic modulation of hippocampal INs is much less well characterized, recent studies show long-term plasticity of FF inhibitory circuits in CA1 is regulated by D4 receptors that are selectively expressed on PV+ INs (Rosen et al., 2015), while PV+ BCs in CA3 are subject to D1/D5-mediated regulation of structural plasticity (Karunakaran et al., 2016).

7.6.1.3 Serotonin

Serotonergic (5-HT) modulation of local circuits provides an example for dual-action subcortical neuromodulation via distinct spatiotemporal release profiles of neuromodulators and of corelease of neuromodulators with other transmitters. Local circuits in all hippocampal subregions receive strong subcortical serotonergic innervation from the median and dorsal raphe nuclei (Tork, 1990; Gulyas, Acsady, et al., 1999; Leranth and Hajszan, 2007). Of the known 14 subtypes of 5-HT receptors, all but one (5-HT3R) are G-protein-coupled, with many of these confirmed to be functionally expressed in the hippocampus. The dorsal raphe fibers are thought to predominantly release from varicosities at nonsynaptic sites, indirectly targeting metabotropic G-protein coupled 5-HTRs (mostly 5-HT1A, 5-HT2A, 5-HT2C, 5-HT4 and 5-HT7). In contrast, ionotropic 5-HT3Rs were found to be predominantly localized at classic synapses that are clustered around the cell body and dendrites of INs formed by large boutons of thick axons originating from the median raphe. Several salient features of this fast subcortical serotonergic neuromodulation have been established. First, early in vitro recordings demonstrated that some hippocampal INs are excited by exogenous application of 5-HT via a depolarizing inward current, which was found to be G-protein independent (McMahon and Kauer, 1997). Later, optogenetic activation of median raphe afferents in CA1 and CA3 (V Varga et al., 2009) was used to demonstrate that median raphe nuclei projections can rapidly recruit INs through corelease of 5-HT and glutamate that activates postsynaptic 5-HT3R and ionotropic AMPAR glutamate receptors, respectively. These data suggest that, unlike other subcortical inputs into the hippocampus, the median raphe projections can trigger a rapid modulation of ongoing activity via ionotropic receptors (Nitz and McNaughton, 1999; Yoshida et al., 2019). Finally, more recent studies have also uncovered that although a highly heterogeneous population of hippocampal INs, including VIP+, SST+, CCK+, CR+ INs, express 5-HT3Rs, these INs have shared developmental origins, as they are all derived from the caudal ganglionic eminence (S Lee et al., 2010; Pelkey et al., 2017). This differential 5-HT3Rs-expression based on developmental origin appears to apply even within a classically defined IN subtype, as it has been shown that SST+ O-LM cells derived from CGE, but not those derived from MGE, express 5-HT3Rs, which may differentiate their roles in promoting network oscillations (Chittajallu et al., 2013).

Multiple different subtypes of metabotropic 5-HTRs are expressed both in principal cells and INs, postsynaptically and presynaptically, suggesting a complex role for serotonergic signaling in local circuits. One major metabotropic effect of 5-HT is the robust dampening of neuronal excitability via 5-HT1AR-mediated activation of GIRK channels on principal cells and INs (Andrade and Nicoll, 1987; Beck et al., 1992; Schmitz et al., 1997), whereas 5-HT2ARs mediate strong depolarization in a subset of INs located at the border of the SR and SLM layers in CA1 (Wyskiel and Andrade, 2016).

7.6.2 Neuropeptides

Some modulatory neuropeptides are released from subcortical hypothalamic afferents into the hippocampus, including oxytocin, vasopressin, and histamine, and peptidergic control of hippocampal circuit activity and hippocampal functions related to social, anxiety, and fear behaviors have been recognized (YT Lin and Hsu, 2018; Cilz et al., 2019). Among these, oxytocinergic afferents of the paraventricular nucleus arborize extensively in the hippocampus and oxytocin receptors have been detected in hippocampal neurons, primarily in INs. The effect of oxytocin on local circuit dynamics has been studied recently in CA1 in vitro; (Owen et al., 2013), where oxytocin was found to increase the spontaneous firing of PV+ BCs. This enhancement in spontaneous FF inhibition, however, was found to also induce a marked use-dependent depression of evoked IPSCs from these cells, thereby leading to a sharpening of spike fidelity and timing of FF excitation onto CA1 PCs, and an increase in signal-to-noise in the local circuit.

Another form of peptidergic modulation of hippocampal circuits is mediated by the opioid system acting on opioid receptors (OPRs)—mu (MOPR), delta (DOPR), and kappa (KOPR)—and their respective endogenous ligands—endorphins, enkephalins, and dynorphin. Endogenous opioids are synthetized and released both from long-range afferents and local cells into the hippocampus (Drake et al., 2007). Enkephalins are primarily contained in the MFs, in the lateral perforant path and in a subset of INs. DOPRs and MOPRs are predominantly localized perisomatically, dendritically, and presynaptically on different classes of INs (Drake and Milner, 2002), where activation of these receptors leads to an inhibition of voltage-gated Ca^{2+} channels and activation of voltage-gated K^+ channels (Al-Hasani and Bruchas, 2011). Thus, the action

of enkephalin/DOPR and the endorphin/MOPR in hippocampal local circuits is primarily disinhibitory: MOPR and DOPR activation reduces GABAergic release, causing disinhibition of principal cells and thereby facilitating synaptic plasticity (Madison and Nicoll, 1988; Lupica, 1995; Morris and Johnston, 1995; Drake et al., 2007). Furthermore, MOPR and DOPR expression appears to be complementary on select subtypes of perisomatic- and dendrite-targeting INs, respectively. Specifically, GABA release from PV+ baskets, but not from CCK+ BCs is inhibited by MOPR activation (Svoboda et al., 1999; Glickfeld et al., 2008), while DOPR activation reduces FB inhibition onto CA1 PCs by inhibiting GABA release from O-LM cells (Svoboda et al., 1999). MOPRs are also expressed on the most abundant IN class in the CA1, the dendritically targeting, NGFC family of cells that includes the IvyCs and NGFCs (Krook-Magnuson et al., 2011). MOPR activation has been shown to effectively hyperpolarize IvyCs and NGFCs, resulting in inhibition of the ability of these cells to display persistent firing (Krook-Magnuson et al., 2011), which is a state of continued firing in the absence of continued input (Sheffield et al., 2011). In addition, MOPRs may potentially affect other unusual properties of NGFCs such as GABAergic volume transmission (Olah et al., 2009). KOPRs are most abundantly expressed in the DG, where dynorphins are detected in the GCs, in which the dynorphin/KOPR system plays a role in regulating perforant path inputs, GC intrinsic excitability and MF output. Although KOPRs are also expressed in some, mainly SOM+ and NPY+, INs (Halasy et al., 2000; Racz and Halasy, 2002), their functional role in regulating inhibitory local circuits in the hippocampus remains unexplored.

Finally, neuropeptide release from local circuit GABAergic INs represents another major potential source of peptidergic neuromodulation. In addition to GABA, many INs also synthesize and store neuropeptides in dense core vesicles at presynaptic terminals, and IN subtype-specific expression of neuropeptides—such as SOM CCK, VIP, and NPY—has long been utilized to classify these cells (Freund and Buzsaki, 1996; Klausberger and Somogyi, 2008; Pelkey et al., 2017). Thus activity-dependent neuropeptide release from GABAergic INs represents another potential source of local circuit neuromodulation. Nevertheless, much less is known about the patterns of neuronal activity required for the release of neuropeptides from GABAergic terminals or about the downstream effects of these neuropeptides on intrinsic excitability and synaptic connectivity in local circuits. Recent studies, however, have begun to decipher several cell-type-specific regulatory functions of local neuropeptide release. For example, CCK has been shown to act as a cell-type-selective modulator of CCK+ and PV+ BC classes. In particular, CCK suppresses GABA transmission from CCK+ BCs onto CA1 PCs, but it strongly increases the output of PV+ BCs through a depolarizing action (Foldy et al., 2007). Intriguingly, while CCK has been shown to act via metabotropic CCK2 receptors on both cell types, it engages highly divergent intracellular pathways: CCK2 receptors on PCs use Gq–PLC pathway to trigger CB-mediated signaling, while CCK2 receptors on PV+ BCs are coupled to ryanodine receptor-mediated intracellular calcium release that leads to activation of nonselective cationic conductances and thus to depolarization of the PV+ BCs (SY Lee et al., 2011). Furthermore, VIP release from VIP+ INs in area CA3 has also recently been implicated in regulating the activity levels of PV+ INs, and consequently, network plasticity during learning (Donato et al., 2013).

7.6.3 Neuromodulation of local circuit function and behavioral state

While it is a challenging task to decipher overall circuit effects of neuromodulators in the hippocampus, a few organizational principles have emerged for understanding aspects of hippocampal neuromodulation. The first common function of separate neuromodulatory systems, in particular those of subcortical origin, appears to be a strong facilitation of long-term synaptic plasticity in the hippocampus, primarily via enhancing NMDAR-activity. The second common mechanism of diverse neuromodulators is the reconfiguring of IN networks and inhibitory transmission in the hippocampus. Third, and most importantly, it is well established that multiple different neuromodulatory systems exhibit coordinated activity during different behavioral states associated with active/quiet awake and rapid eye movement (REM)/slow-wave sleep (SWS) (Buzsaki, 2002; Teles-Grilo Ruivo and Mellor, 2013; Atherton et al., 2015; Buzsaki, 2015). Thus, during different behavioral states, both principal cell and IN intrinsic properties and synaptic weights at afferent and efferent pathways in the hippocampus are adjusted in a subtype-dependent manner by neuromodulation, which leads to different network activity states that are thought to support specific hippocampal circuit functions, including memory encoding, consolidation, and recall. The most complete framework of how behavioral state-dependent neuromodulation can control hippocampal circuit dynamics conducive to learning that has been proposed so far relates to the MSDBB-hippocampal cholinergic system. Hippocampal ACh levels show variation throughout the sleep–wake cycle, with ACh high during REM sleep and active wakefulness but low levels during quiet wakefulness and SWS (Marrosu et al., 1995; Steriade, 2004). According to this proposed model (Hasselmo, 2006; Sil'kis, 2010; Hummos et al., 2014), high ACh levels during awake exploration and REM sleep favor the encoding of novel information by potentiating FF afferent input synapses in the hippocampus via nAChR-mediated enhancement of MF and perforant path inputs. At the same time, ACh depolarizes INs and inhibits synaptic potentials at CA3 recurrent and Schaffer collateral synapses via mAChRs, resulting in suppression of recurrent excitation associated with retrieval of information. In contrast, when ACh levels are low, such as during quite wakefulness and SWS, recurrent excitatory hippocampal activity leads to retrieval and consolidation of previously stored information, supporting memory consolidation during SWRs. Consistent with this model, administration of ACh shifts SWR frequencies to gamma frequencies in vitro (Fischer et al., 2014), indicative of a switch from retrieval to encoding states, and optogenetic stimulation of MS cholinergic neurons has been found to decrease the probability of SWR occurrence in CA1 (Vandecasteele et al., 2014) and in CA3 (Hunt et al., 2018). Intriguingly, this later study in CA3 also found that ACh selectively suppressed the bursting propensity of athorny CA3 PCs (see section 7.1.2.1 above), suggesting a key role of athorny CA3 PCs in triggering SWRs (see section 7.4.3 above).

7.7 Multiscale GABAergic systems

Although GABAergic cells are most often thought of as being local circuit neurons, it is now clear that the hippocampal GABAergic system as a whole in fact constitutes a spatially multiscale system for delivering the neurotransmitter GABA at both local and distant output sites. There are three spatial scales that are currently recognized, each with its own dedicated GABAergic cells. First is the case of the classical, genuinely local circuit INs (see Chapter 5), where the vast majority of the output GABAergic synapses remain in the same well-defined brain area where the parent cell body is located (e.g., most typical CA1 INs). Second, at the other extreme, are those GABAergic cells whose output synapses are in a different brain area from where the parent cell body of origin is located (Caputi et al., 2013). These latter cells are the long-distance projecting GABA neurons, e.g., the entorhinohippocampal GABAergic cells, or the CA1-to-septum projecting GABAergic cells (Toth et al., 1993; Basu et al., 2016), that are dedicated to deliver GABA at distant brain areas where they typically synapse on other GABA cells, eliciting disinhibition (see section 7.7.1 below). More recently, a third class of GABAergic neurons, referred to as boundary-crossing neurons, has been recognized as a distinct category in the hippocampus (Szabo et al., 2017). These cells are GABAergic cells that extend their influence from the local networks to the immediately adjacent circuits, comprising a mesoscale (i.e., between local circuit and genuinely long-distance) INal system.

7.7.1 Boundary-crossing mesoscale inhibition

Numerous reports exist in the literature of anecdotal observations indicating that some of the axons of hippocampal INs sometimes seem to cross the classically defined boundaries of distinct areas such as the CA1, CA3, and the DG (Sik et al., 1994; Ceranik et al., 1997; Hajos and Mody, 1997; Szabadics and Soltesz, 2009; Armstrong et al., 2011; Lasztoczi et al., 2011; Szabo et al., 2014; L Katona et al., 2017). For example, some NGFCs in the DG not only seem to innervate the OML/MML but also have axons also in the adjacent CA1 or subiculum (Armstrong et al., 2011). Do these anecdotal observations indicate an accidental spillover of axons of otherwise bona fide "local circuit" INs across areal boundaries to neighboring hippocampal areas that constitute no more than a negligible minority of GABAergic projections?

A recent study employing dual retroviral and rabies strategy showed that these boundary-crossing projections may constitute a surprisingly robust GABAergic system that exists at the mesoscale (Szabo et al., 2017). In the case of GCs of the DG, retrograde transsynaptic labeling revealed nonprincipal presynaptic cells located outside of the DG, in both the CA1 and CA3 regions. Subsequent immunocytochemical analysis showed that the relative numerical abundance of PV and SOM cells that are located in the CA1 and CA3 regions was about 20% of the total presynaptic PV/SOM population innervating DG GCs (Szabo et al., 2017). Therefore, GC-innervating GABAergic INs with cell bodies located in the CA regions constitute a numerically significant population. Furthermore, such boundary-crossing INs in the CA regions with synaptic innervation of GCs included not just PV and SOM cells but also CB1-expressing as well as NOS-expressing cells, indicating that the "extended" interneuronal network of the DG constitutes a sophisticated, robust interneuronal network whose diversity is comparable to that of the major interneuronal classes that are known to innervate principal cells in hippocampal networks. Juxtacellular recordings in vivo also revealed that these boundary-crossing INs in the CA1 and CA3 relay patterns of activity, such as the SWRs generated within the CA regions back to GCs, forming a retrograde

GABAergic circuit that fundamentally extends the canonical "local circuit" interneuronal network (Szabo et al., 2017). The retrograde channeling of SWR-related activity from the downstream CA areas back to the DG may provide a significant regulatory pathway associated with the bidirectional DG-CA3 interplay hypothesized to play key roles in SWR-associated episodic memory sequencing and replay (Lisman et al., 2005).

Future quantitative studies with similar transsynaptic tracing techniques will be necessary to determine if the sizable contribution of boundary-crossing INs from adjacent areas also applies to the CA1 and other hippocampal regions. The possibility that a significant percentage of GABAergic inputs to hippocampal principal cells may not originate from the local INs present in a given anatomically defined circuit such as the CA1 has important implications for currently ongoing efforts to create data-driven, full-scale biophysical models of individual areas of the hippocampus (Bezaire et al., 2016). For example, in the case of the CA1 network, about 39% of GABAergic synaptic contacts on PCs could not be assigned to any of the known CA1 IN classes (Bezaire and Soltesz, 2013), indicating that it is likely that boundary-crossing, mesoscale GABAergic systems may need to be taken into account when assessing GABAergic inhibition impinging on hippocampal principal cells.

7.7.2 Long-distance GABAergic projections

While INs were previously regarded as exclusively local circuit elements, a view reflected in their name, mounting evidence suggests that long-range projecting INs (LRPIs) are common, if not ubiquitous, elements of cortical circuit architecture (Jinno, 2009; Caputi et al., 2013). The most direct evidence for LRPIs comes from studies performing bulk retrograde and anterograde tracing or single cell filling combined with post hoc cellular identification by immunocytochemistry, and more recently complemented by genetic targeting of IN subtypes. While these techniques do not generally allow for a complete quantitative accounting of all LRPI subtypes or the relative density of their projections in distal networks, they have illuminated the role of hippocampal LRPIs in supporting certain unique circuit motifs. In particular, hippocampal LRIPs (long range inhibitory projections) often target the same regions as do their neighboring excitatory cells (for instance, subiculum or EC projecting INs in CA1 [Ino et al., 1990; Jinno et al., 2007; Fuentealba, Tomioka, et al., 2008; Melzer et al., 2012; Basu et al., 2016), though they may also target upstream regions (CA3 and hilar projecting INs in CA1 [Sik et al., 1994], or project contralaterally (commissural projecting DG INs; Ribak and Seress, 1983; Goodman and Sloviter, 1992). Moreover, the majority of characterized LRIPs either originating in or targeting the hippocampus preferentially synapse onto other INs, and many are heavily myelinated (Jinno et al., 2007). Consequently, LRIPs are, as a class, thought to mediate fas-timescale long-range disinhibition, and, therefore play an important role in interregional oscillatory coupling (Figure 7.12) (Melzer et al., 2012; Caputi et al., 2013; Unal et al., 2018). Indeed, consistent with this hypothesis using a combination of genetically targeted optogenetic and electrophysiological techniques in vitro, it was found that stimulation of either entorhinohippocampal or hippocampoentorhinal LRPIs increased theta frequency oscillations through disinhibition in the targeted region (Melzer et al., 2012). A subsequent study utilizing a combined optogenetic, chemogenetic, electrophysiological, and

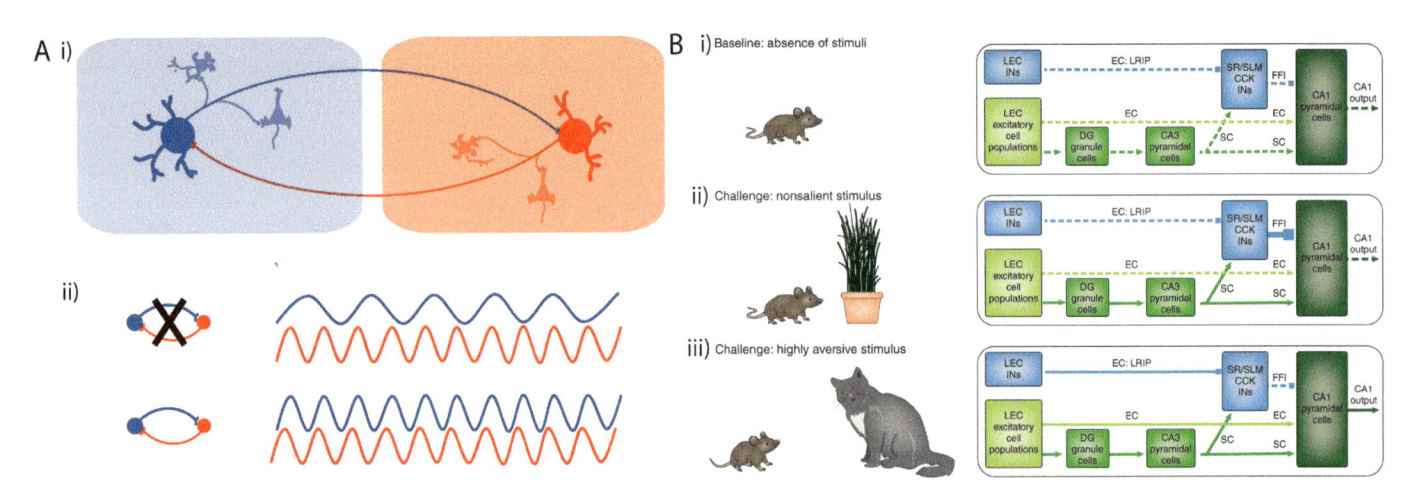

Figure 7.12 LRIPs promote long-range synchronization and information gating. (A, i) Long-range projecting inhibitory projections (LRIPs) project between regions (here shown in blue and red) where they typically synapse onto other INs, sometimes reciprocally as is shown in the schematic. In addition to their long-range projections, LRIPs often also make local synaptic contacts, promoting the synchronization of activity between their local and distal targets. (A, ii) Therefore, when LRIP connections are inhibited the local and distal networks may become desynchronized, while the enhancement of LRIP connectivity promotes the synchronization of local and distal and networks, which in turn can promote long-range spike-transmission by aligning the periods of maximal depolarization between these regions (Caputi et al., 2013). In a recent study in mice (Basu et al., 2016), LRIPs arising from the lateral entorhinal cortex (LEC) were found to target SR and LM-located feedforward CCK INs in area CA1. (B, i) Under baseline conditions LEC LRIP INs fired at a low rate (boxes show schematic of LEC-CA1 connectivity). (B, ii) When the animals were presented with a nonsalient stimulus, hippocampal-projecting LEC excitatory cells responded with elevated firing, recruiting DG GCs and then CA3 PCs through the trisynaptic pathway and directly exciting CA1 PCs. In turn, CA3 PCs recruited CA1 CCK cells, thus providing feedforward inhibition onto the CA1 PCs, attenuating the excitatory effect of their distally located LEC excitatory input. (B, iii) In contrast, when a salient, aversive stimulus was presented, both the LEC excitatory cells and the CA1-projecting LEC LRIPs were recruited. In this condition LEC-LRIPs inhibited CA1 CCK cells, thus disinhibiting the LEC to CA1 PC excitatory connection. Consequently, LEC LRIPs were found to play a role in gating the flow of information between LEC and CA1 through long-range disinhibition such that the activity associated with salient stimuli was preferentially propagated along the hippocampal network (Alexander and Soltesz, 2016).

calcium imaging approach further described that the disruption of the long-range inhibitory input from the EC to the hippocampus resulted in (1) reduced local CA1 disinhibition and PC excitability, (2) a reduction of cooperative Perforant-path/Schaffer-collateral fine-timescale input-timing-dependent plasticity onto CA1 PCs, and (3) a behavioral impairment of contextual and object memory discrimination (Figure 7.12) (Basu et al., 2016). However, perhaps the most thoroughly characterized group of hippocampal LRIPs are those involved in the reciprocal inhibitory connectivity between the hippocampus and GABAergic cells in the medial septum (MS), a basal forebrain structure implicated in hippocampal rhythmogenesis (Yoder and Pang, 2005; Muller and Remy, 2018). While medial septal INs projecting to the hippocampus appear to be uniformly PV positive (Freund, 1989; Ylinen, Soltesz, et al., 1995; Caputi et al., 2013; though see Unal et al., 2015), the hippocampal LRIPs with which they are often reciprocally connected are heterogeneous, and often project to other extrahippocampal targets, in addition to forming local connections (Alonso and Kohler, 1982; Schwerdtfeger and E Buhl, 1986; Miles et al., 1996; Jinno et al., 2007). Notably, while MS GABAergic projections target all hippocampal regions and several IN subtypes, individual MS LRIPs terminate in one or two hippocampal regions and target specific IN subtypes within these regions (Unal et al., 2018) and, like their hippocampal IN targets (L Katona et al., 2017; Unal et al., 2018), MS LRPIs show distinct network-state-dependent modulation patterns as well as distinct theta-phase preferences (Joshi et al., 2017; Unal et al., 2018). Consequently, the reciprocal MS-hippocampal GABAergic dialogue may support fast disinhibition of specific hippocampal interneuronal subcircuits, rapidly changing the local distribution of inhibition in a state-dependent manner (Somogyi et al., 2014).

7.8 Conclusion

The hippocampus contains a wide variety of local circuits. Some of these circuits, such as feedback and feedforward inhibitory and disinhibitory circuits, form nearly ubiquitous motifs observed across all hippocampal areas, while others such as the granule cell-mossy cell circuit, are observed only in specific regions. Moreover, even for widespread circuit motifs important details of the circuitry involved vary across regions, sublayers, and cell types. While some of this diversity has been established to support known hippocampal computational functions, the functions of other well identified local circuits remain to be uncovered.

REFERENCES

Acsady L, Arabadzisz D, Freund TF (1996) Correlated morphological and neurochemical features identify different subsets of vasoactive intestinal polypeptide-immunoreactive interneurons in rat hippocampus. Neuroscience 73:299–315.

Acsady L, Gorcs TJ, Freund TF (1996) Different populations of vasoactive intestinal polypeptide-immunoreactive interneurons are specialized to control pyramidal cells or interneurons in the hippocampus. Neuroscience 73:317–334.

Acsady L, Kamondi A, Sik A, Freund T, Buzsaki G (1998) GABAergic cells are the major postsynaptic targets of mossy fibers in the rat hippocampus. J Neurosci 18:3386–3403.

Acsady L, Katona I, Martinez-Guijarro FJ, Buzsaki G, Freund TF (2000) Unusual target selectivity of perisomatic inhibitory cells in the hilar region of the rat hippocampus. J Neurosci 20:6907–6919.

Aggleton JP, Christiansen K (2015) The subiculum: the heart of the extended hippocampal system. Prog Brain Res 219.

Albuquerque EX, Pereira EF, Alkondon M, Rogers SW (2009) Mammalian nicotinic acetylcholine receptors: from structure to function. Physiol Rev 89:73–120.

Alcami P, Pereda AE (2019) Beyond plasticity: the dynamic impact of electrical synapses on neural circuits. Nat Rev Neurosci 20:253–271.

Alexander A, Soltesz I (2016) Hippogate: a break-in from entorhinal cortex. Nat Neurosci 19:530–532.

Al-Hasani R, Bruchas MR (2011) Molecular mechanisms of opioid receptor-dependent signaling and behavior. Anesthesiology 115:1363–1381.

Ali AB, Deuchars J, Pawelzik H, Thomson AM (1998) CA1 pyramidal to basket and bistratified cell EPSPs: dual intracellular recordings in rat hippocampal slices. J Physiol 507(Pt 1):201–217.

Alkondon M, Albuquerque EX (2004) The nicotinic acetylcholine receptor subtypes and their function in the hippocampus and cerebral cortex. Prog Brain Res 145:109–120.

Allen K, Fuchs EC, Jaschonek H, Bannerman DM, Monyer H (2011) Gap junctions between interneurons are required for normal spatial coding in the hippocampus and short-term spatial memory. J Neurosci 31:6542–6552.

Alonso A, Kohler C (1982) Evidence for separate projections of hippocampal pyramidal and non-pyramidal neurons to different parts of the septum in the rat brain. Neurosci Lett 31:209–214.

Alvarez DD, Giacomini D, Yang SM, Trinchero MF, Temprana SG, Buttner KA, Beltramone N, Schinder AF (2016) A disynaptic feedback network activated by experience promotes the integration of new granule cells. Science 354:459–465.

Amaral DG (1978) A Golgi study of cell types in the hilar region of the hippocampus in the rat. J Comp Neurol 182:851–914.

Amaral DG, Dolorfo C, Alvarez-Royo P (1991) Organization of CA1 projections to the subiculum: a PHA-L analysis in the rat. Hippocampus 1.

Amaral DG, Ishizuka N, Claiborne B (1990) Neurons, numbers and the hippocampal network. Prog Brain Res 83:1–11.

Amaral DG, Scharfman HE, Lavenex P (2007) The dentate gyrus: fundamental neuroanatomical organization (dentate gyrus for dummies). Prog Brain Res 163:3–22.

Amaral DG, Witter MP (1989) The three-dimensional organization of the hippocampal formation: a review of anatomical data. Neuroscience 31:571–591.

Amilhon B, Huh CY, Manseau F, Ducharme G, Nichol H, Adamantidis A, Williams S (2015) Parvalbumin interneurons of hippocampus tune population activity at theta frequency. Neuron 86:1277–1289.

Andrade R, Nicoll RA (1987) Pharmacologically distinct actions of serotonin on single pyramidal neurones of the rat hippocampus recorded in vitro. J Physiol 394:99–124.

Armstrong C, Soltesz I (2012) Basket cell dichotomy in microcircuit function. J Physiol 590:683–694.

Armstrong C, Szabadics J, Tamas G, Soltesz I (2011) Neurogliaform cells in the molecular layer of the dentate gyrus as feed-forward gamma-aminobutyric acidergic modulators of entorhinal-hippocampal interplay. J Comp Neurol 519:1476–1491.

Artinian J, Lacaille JC (2018) Disinhibition in learning and memory circuits: new vistas for somatostatin interneurons and long-term synaptic plasticity. Brain Res Bull 141:20–26.

Atherton LA, Dupret D, Mellor JR (2015) Memory trace replay: the shaping of memory consolidation by neuromodulation. Trends Neurosci 38:560–570.

Bagur S, Benchenane K (2018) The theta rhythm mixes and matches gamma oscillations cycle by cycle. *Neuron* **100**:768–771.

Bartesaghi R, Gessi T (2004). Parallel activation of field CA2 and dentate gyrus by synaptically elicited perforant path volleys. *Hippocampus*, 14(8):948–963.

Bartesaghi R, Ravasi L (1999). Pyramidal neuron types in field CA2 of the guinea pig. *Brain research bulletin*, 50(4):263–273.

Bartos M, Vida I, Frotscher M, Geiger JR, Jonas P (2001) Rapid signaling at inhibitory synapses in a dentate gyrus interneuron network. *J Neurosci* **21**:2687–2698.

Bartos M, Vida I, Frotscher M, Meyer A, Monyer H, Geiger JR, Jonas P (2002) Fast synaptic inhibition promotes synchronized gamma oscillations in hippocampal interneuron networks. *Proc Natl Acad Sci U S A* **99**:13222–13227.

Bartos M, Vida I, Jonas P (2007) Synaptic mechanisms of synchronized gamma oscillations in inhibitory interneuron networks. *Nat Rev Neurosci* **8**:45–56.

Basu J, Srinivas KV, Cheung SK, Taniguchi H, Huang ZJ, Siegelbaum SA (2013) A cortico-hippocampal learning rule shapes inhibitory microcircuit activity to enhance hippocampal information flow. *Neuron* **79**:1208–1221.

Basu J, Zaremba JD, Cheung SK, Hitti FL, Zemelman BV, Losonczy A, Siegelbaum SA (2016) Gating of hippocampal activity, plasticity, and memory by entorhinal cortex long-range inhibition. *Science* **351**:aaa5694.

Beck SG, Choi KC, List TJ (1992) Comparison of 5-hydroxytryptamine1A-mediated hyperpolarization in CA1 and CA3 hippocampal pyramidal cells. *J Pharmacol Exp Ther* **263**:350–359.

Behr J, Empson RM, Schmitz D, Gloveli T, Heinemann U (1996) Electrophysiological properties of rat subicular neurons in vitro. *Neurosci Lett*, 220(1):41–44.

Belluscio MA, Mizuseki K, Schmidt R, Kempter R, Buzsaki G (2012) Cross-frequency phase-phase coupling between theta and gamma oscillations in the hippocampus. *J Neurosci* **32**:423–435.

Benoy A, Dasgupta A, Sajikumar S (2018) Hippocampal area CA2: an emerging modulatory gateway in the hippocampal circuit. *Exp Brain Res* **236**:919–931.

Berg RW, Kleinfeld D (2003) Rhythmic whisking by rat: retraction as well as protraction of the vibrissae is under active muscular control. *J Neurophysiol* **89**:104–117.

Bezaire MJ, Raikov I, Burk K, Vyas D, Soltesz I (2016) Interneuronal mechanisms of hippocampal theta oscillations in a full-scale model of the rodent CA1 circuit. *Elife* **5**:e18566.

Bezaire MJ, Soltesz I (2013) Quantitative assessment of CA1 local circuits: knowledge base for interneuron-pyramidal cell connectivity. *Hippocampus* **23**:751–785.

Bieri KW, Bobbitt KN, Colgin LL (2014) Slow and fast gamma rhythms coordinate different spatial coding modes in hippocampal place cells. *Neuron* **82**:670–681.

Bilkey DK, Schwartzkroin PA (1990) Variation in electrophysiology and morphology of hippocampal CA3 pyramidal cells. *Brain Res* **514**:77–83.

Biro AA, Holderith NB, Nusser Z (2006) Release probability-dependent scaling of the postsynaptic responses at single hippocampal GABAergic synapses. *J Neurosci* **26**:12487–12496.

Bischofberger J, Engel D, Frotscher M, Jonas P (2006) Timing and efficacy of transmitter release at mossy fiber synapses in the hippocampal network. *Pflugers Arch* **453**:361–372.

Bittner KC, Andrasfalvy BK, Magee JC (2012) Ion channel gradients in the apical tuft region of CA1 pyramidal neurons. *PLoS One* **7**:e46652.

Bittner KC, Grienberger C, Vaidya SP, Milstein AD, Macklin JJ, Suh J, Tonegawa S, Magee JC (2015) Conjunctive input processing drives feature selectivity in hippocampal CA1 neurons. *Nat Neurosci* **18**:1133–1142.

Bittner KC, Milstein AD, Grienberger C, Romani S, Magee JC (2017) Behavioral time scale synaptic plasticity underlies CA1 place fields. *Science* **357**:1033–1036.

Blackman AV, Abrahamsson T, Costa RP, Lalanne T, Sjostrom PJ (2013) Target-cell-specific short-term plasticity in local circuits. *Front Synaptic Neurosci* **5**:11.

Bland BH, Oddie SD, Colom LV (1999) Mechanisms of neural synchrony in the septohippocampal pathways underlying hippocampal theta generation. *J Neurosci* **19**:3223–3237.

Blasco-Ibanez JM, Freund TF (1995) Synaptic input of horizontal interneurons in stratum oriens of the hippocampal CA1 subfield: structural basis of feed-back activation. *Eur J Neurosci* **7**:2170–2180.

Bloodgood BL, Sharma N, Browne HA, Trepman AZ, Greenberg ME (2013) The activity-dependent transcription factor NPAS4 regulates domain-specific inhibition. *Nature* **503**:121–125.

Bloss EB, Cembrowski MS, Karsh B, Colonell J, Fetter RD, Spruston N (2016) Structured dendritic inhibition supports branch-selective integration in CA1 pyramidal cells. *Neuron* **89**:1016–1030.

Böhm C, Peng Y, Maier N, Winterer J, Poulet J. F, Geiger JR, Schmitz D (2015). Functional diversity of subicular principal cells during hippocampal ripples. *J Neurosci*, 35(40):13608–13618.

Booker SA, Althof D, Degro CE, Watanabe M, Kulik A, Vida I (2017) Differential surface density and modulatory effects of presynaptic GABAB receptors in hippocampal cholecystokinin and parvalbumin basket cells. *Brain Struct Funct* **222**:3677–3690.

Booker SA, Althof D, Gross A, Loreth D, Muller J, Unger A, Fakler B, Varro A, Watanabe M, Gassmann M, et al. (2017) KCTD12 auxiliary proteins modulate kinetics of GABAB receptor-mediated inhibition in cholecystokinin-containing interneurons. *Cereb Cortex* **27**:2318–2334.

Booker SA, Gross A, Althof D, Shigemoto R, Bettler B, Frotscher M, Hearing M, Wickman K, Watanabe M, Kulik A, et al. (2013) Differential GABAB-receptor-mediated effects in perisomatic- and dendrite-targeting parvalbumin interneurons. *J Neurosci* **33**:7961–7974.

Booker SA, Vida I (2018) Morphological diversity and connectivity of hippocampal interneurons. *Cell Tissue Res* **373**:619–641.

Borgers C, Kopell N (2003) Synchronization in networks of excitatory and inhibitory neurons with sparse, random connectivity. *Neural Comput* **15**:509–538.

Borhegyi Z, Varga V, Szilagyi N, Fabo D, Freund TF (2004) Phase segregation of medial septal GABAergic neurons during hippocampal theta activity. *J Neurosci* **24**:8470–8479.

Boss BD, Peterson GM, Cowan WM (1985) On the number of neurons in the dentate gyrus of the rat. *Brain Res* **338**:144–150.

Botcher NA, Falck JE, Thomson AM, Mercer A (2014) Distribution of interneurons in the CA2 region of the rat hippocampus. *Frontiers in neuroanatomy* **8**:104.

Braganza O, Beck H (2018) The circuit motif as a conceptual tool for multilevel neuroscience. *Trends Neurosci* **41**:128–136.

Bragin A, Jando G, Nadasdy Z, Hetke J, Wise K, Buzsaki G (1995) Gamma (40–100 Hz) oscillation in the hippocampus of the behaving rat. *J Neurosci* **15**:47–60.

Brazhnik ES, Fox SE (1999) Action potentials and relations to the theta rhythm of medial septal neurons in vivo. *Exp Brain Res* **127**:244–258.

Buckmaster PS, Jongen-Relo AL (1999) Highly specific neuron loss preserves lateral inhibitory circuits in the dentate gyrus of kainate-induced epileptic rats. *J Neurosci* **19**:9519–9529.

Buckmaster PS, Schwartzkroin PA (1995) Interneurons and inhibition in the dentate gyrus of the rat in vivo. *J Neurosci* **15**:774–789.

Buckmaster PS, Strowbridge BW, Kunkel DD, Schmiege DL, Schwartzkroin PA (1992) Mossy cell axonal projections to the dentate gyrus molecular layer in the rat hippocampal slice. *Hippocampus* **2**:349–362.

Buckmaster PS, Wenzel HJ, Kunkel DD, Schwartzkroin PA (1996) Axon arbors and synaptic connections of hippocampal mossy cells in the rat in vivo. *J Comp Neurol* **366**:271–292.

Buhl DL, Harris KD, Hormuzdi SG, Monyer H, Buzsaki G (2003) Selective impairment of hippocampal gamma oscillations in connexin-36 knock-out mouse in vivo. *J Neurosci* **23**:1013–1018.

Buhl EH, Halasy K, Somogyi P (1994) Diverse sources of hippocampal unitary inhibitory postsynaptic potentials and the number of synaptic release sites. *Nature* **368**:823–828.

Buhl EH, Han ZS, Lorinczi Z, Stezhka VV, Karnup SV, Somogyi P (1994) Physiological properties of anatomically identified axo-axonic cells in the rat hippocampus. *J Neurophysiol* **71**:1289–1307.

Buhl EH, Szilagyi T, Halasy K, Somogyi P (1996) Physiological properties of anatomically identified basket and bistratified cells in the CA1 area of the rat hippocampus in vitro. *Hippocampus* **6**:294–305.

Bui AD, Nguyen TM, Limouse C, Kim HK, Szabo GG, Felong S, Maroso M, Soltesz I (2018) Dentate gyrus mossy cells control spontaneous convulsive seizures and spatial memory. *Science* **359**:787–790.

Bush D, Philippides A, Husbands P, O'Shea M (2010) Dual coding with STDP in a spiking recurrent neural network model of the hippocampus. *PLoS Comput Biol* **6**:e1000839.

Buzsaki G (1986) Hippocampal sharp waves: their origin and significance. *Brain Res* **398**:242–252.

Buzsaki G (2002) Theta oscillations in the hippocampus. *Neuron* **33**:325–340.

Buzsaki G (2015) Hippocampal sharp wave-ripple: a cognitive biomarker for episodic memory and planning. *Hippocampus* **25**:1073–1188.

Buzsaki G, Anastassiou CA, Koch C (2012) The origin of extracellular fields and currents—EEG, ECoG, LFP and spikes. *Nat Rev Neurosci* **13**:407–420.

Buzsaki G, Draguhn A (2004) Neuronal oscillations in cortical networks. *Science* **304**:1926–1929.

Buzsaki G, Horvath Z, Urioste R, Hetke J, Wise K (1992) High-frequency network oscillation in the hippocampus. *Science* **256**:1025–1027.

Buzsaki G, Leung LW, Vanderwolf CH (1983) Cellular bases of hippocampal EEG in the behaving rat. *Brain Res* **287**:139–171.

Buzsaki G, Wang XJ (2012) Mechanisms of gamma oscillations. *Annu Rev Neurosci* **35**:203–225.

Canteras NS, Swanson LW (1992) Projections of the ventral subiculum to the amygdala, septum, and hypothalamus: a PHAL anterograde tract-tracing study in the rat. *Journal of Comparative Neurology* **324**(2):180–194.

Caputi A, Melzer S, Michael M, Monyer H (2013) The long and short of GABAergic neurons. *Curr Opin Neurobiol* **23**:179–186.

Cardin JA, Carlen M, Meletis K, Knoblich U, Zhang F, Deisseroth K, Tsai LH, Moore CI (2009) Driving fast-spiking cells induces gamma rhythm and controls sensory responses. *Nature* **459**:663–667.

Carr MF, Frank LM (2012) A single microcircuit with multiple functions: state dependent information processing in the hippocampus. *Curr Opin Neurobiol* **22**:704–708.

Carr MF, Jadhav SP, Frank LM (2011) Hippocampal replay in the awake state: a potential substrate for memory consolidation and retrieval. *Nat Neurosci* **14**:147–153.

Carstens KE, Dudek SM (2019) Regulation of synaptic plasticity in hippocampal area CA2. *Current opinion in neurobiology*, **54**:194–199.

Carstens KE, Phillips ML, Pozzo-Miller L, Weinberg RJ, Dudek SM (2016) Perineuronal nets suppress plasticity of excitatory synapses on CA2 pyramidal neurons. *J Neurosci*, **36**(23):6312–6320.

Cea-del Rio CA, Lawrence JJ, Tricoire L, Erdelyi F, Szabo G, McBain CJ (2010) M3 muscarinic acetylcholine receptor expression confers differential cholinergic modulation to neurochemically distinct hippocampal basket cell subtypes. *J Neurosci* **30**:6011–6024.

Cea-del Rio CA, McBain CJ, Pelkey KA (2012) An update on cholinergic regulation of cholecystokinin-expressing basket cells. *J Physiol* **590**:695–702.

Cembrowski MS, Bachman JL, Wang L, Sugino K, Shields BC, Spruston N (2016) Spatial gene-expression gradients underlie prominent heterogeneity of CA1 pyramidal neurons. *Neuron* **89**:351–368.

Cembrowski MS, Phillips MG, DiLisio SF, Shields BC, Winnubst J, Chandrashekar J, Bas E, Spruston N (2018) Dissociable structural and functional hippocampal outputs via distinct subiculum cell classes. *Cell* **174**:1036.

Cembrowski MS, Spruston N (2019) Heterogeneity within classical cell types is the rule: lessons from hippocampal pyramidal neurons. *Nat Rev Neurosci* **20**:193–204.

Cembrowski MS, Wang L, Lemire AL, Copeland M, DiLisio SF, Clements J, Spruston N (2018) The subiculum is a patchwork of discrete subregions. *Elife*, **7**:e37701.

Ceranik K, Bender R, Geiger JR, Monyer H, Jonas P, Frotscher M, Lubke J (1997) A novel type of GABAergic interneuron connecting the input and the output regions of the hippocampus. *J Neurosci* **17**:5380–5394.

Chamberland S, Timofeeva Y, Evstratova A, Volynski K, Toth K (2018) Action potential counting at giant mossy fiber terminals gates information transfer in the hippocampus. *Proc Natl Acad Sci U S A* **115**:7434–7439.

Chamberland S, Topolnik L (2012) Inhibitory control of hippocampal inhibitory neurons. *Front Neurosci* **6**:165.

Chance FS (2012) Hippocampal phase precession from dual input components. *J Neurosci* **32**:16693–16703a.

Chevaleyre V, Siegelbaum SA (2010) Strong CA2 pyramidal neuron synapses define a powerful disynaptic cortico-hippocampal loop. *Neuron* **66**(4):560–572.

Chiang PH, Yeh WC, Lee CT, Weng JY, Huang YY, Lien CC (2010) M(1)-like muscarinic acetylcholine receptors regulate fast-spiking interneuron excitability in rat dentate gyrus. *Neuroscience* **169**:39–51.

Chicurel ME, Harris KM (1992) Three-dimensional analysis of the structure and composition of CA3 branched dendritic spines and their synaptic relationships with mossy fiber boutons in the rat hippocampus. *J Comp Neurol* **325**:169–182.

Chiovini B, Turi GF, Katona G, Kaszas A, Palfi D, Maak P, Szalay G, Szabo MF, Szabo G, Szadai Z, et al. (2014) Dendritic spikes induce ripples in parvalbumin interneurons during hippocampal sharp waves. *Neuron* **82**:908–924.

Chittajallu R, Craig MT, McFarland A, Yuan X, Gerfen S, Tricoire L, Erkkila B, Barron SC, Lopez CM, Liang BJ, et al. (2013) Dual origins of functionally distinct O-LM interneurons revealed by differential 5-HT(3A)R expression. *Nat Neurosci* **16**:1598–1607.

Cilz NI, Cymerblit-Sabba A, Young WS (2019) Oxytocin and vasopressin in the rodent hippocampus. *Genes Brain Behav* **18**:e12535.

Ciocchi S, Passecker J, Malagon-Vina H, Mikus N, Klausberger T (2015) Brain computation: selective information routing by ventral hippocampal CA1 projection neurons. *Science* **348**:560–563.

Cobb SR, Buhl EH, Halasy K, Paulsen O, Somogyi P (1995) Synchronization of neuronal activity in hippocampus by individual GABAergic interneurons. *Nature* **378**:75–78.

Cobb SR, Halasy K, Vida I, Nyiri G, Tamas G, Buhl EH, Somogyi P (1997) Synaptic effects of identified interneurons innervating both interneurons and pyramidal cells in the rat hippocampus. *Neuroscience* **79**:629–648.

Cohen MX, Gulbinaite R (2014) Five methodological challenges in cognitive electrophysiology. *Neuroimage* **85**(Pt 2):702–710.

Colgin LL (2013) Mechanisms and functions of theta rhythms. *Annu Rev Neurosci* **36**:295–312.

Colgin LL (2015) Theta-gamma coupling in the entorhinal-hippocampal system. *Curr Opin Neurobiol* **31**:45–50.

Colgin LL (2016) Rhythms of the hippocampal network. *Nat Rev Neurosci* **17**:239–249.

Colgin LL, Denninger T, Fyhn M, Hafting T, Bonnevie T, Jensen O, Moser MB, Moser EI (2009) Frequency of gamma oscillations routes flow of information in the hippocampus. *Nature* **462**:353–357.

Colgin LL, Moser EI (2010) Gamma oscillations in the hippocampus. *Physiology (Bethesda)* **25**:319–329.

Connors BW, Long MA (2004) Electrical synapses in the mammalian brain. *Annu Rev Neurosci* **27**:393–418.

Cope DW, Maccaferri G, Marton LF, Roberts JD, Cobden PM, Somogyi P (2002) Cholecystokinin-immunopositive basket and Schaffer collateral-associated interneurones target different domains of pyramidal cells in the CA1 area of the rat hippocampus. *Neuroscience* **109**:63–80.

Cossart R, Esclapez M, Hirsch JC, Bernard C, Ben-Ari Y (1998) GluR5 kainate receptor activation in interneurons increases tonic inhibition of pyramidal cells. *Nat Neurosci* **1**:470–478.

Craig MT, Mayne EW, Bettler B, Paulsen O, McBain CJ (2013) Distinct roles of GABAB1a- and GABAB1b-containing GABAB receptors in spontaneous and evoked termination of persistent cortical activity. *J Physiol* **591**:835–843.

Csicsvari J, Hirase H, Czurko A, Mamiya A, Buzsaki G (1999) Fast network oscillations in the hippocampal CA1 region of the behaving rat. *J Neurosci* **19**: Rc20.

Csicsvari J, Hirase H, Mamiya A, Buzsaki G (2000) Ensemble patterns of hippocampal CA3-CA1 neurons during sharp wave-associated population events. *Neuron* **28**:585–594.

Csicsvari J, Jamieson B, Wise KD, Buzsaki G (2003) Mechanisms of gamma oscillations in the hippocampus of the behaving rat. *Neuron* **37**:311–322.

Cui Z, Gerfen CR, Young 3rd WS (2013) Hypothalamic and other connections with dorsal CA2 area of the mouse hippocampus. *Journal of comparative neurology* **521**(8):1844–1866.

Cutsuridis V, Taxidis J (2013) Deciphering the role of CA1 inhibitory circuits in sharp wave-ripple complexes. *Front Syst Neurosci* **7**:13.

Dannenberg H, Young K, Hasselmo M (2017) Modulation of hippocampal circuits by muscarinic and nicotinic receptors. *Front Neural Circuits* **11**:102.

Dasari S, Gulledge AT (2011) M1 and M4 receptors modulate hippocampal pyramidal neurons. *J Neurophysiol* **105**:779–792.

Davoudi H, Foster DJ (2019) Acute silencing of hippocampal CA3 reveals a dominant role in place field responses. *Nat Neurosci* **22**:337–342.

Daw MI, Tricoire L, Erdelyi F, Szabo G, McBain CJ (2009) Asynchronous transmitter release from cholecystokinin-containing inhibitory

interneurons is widespread and target-cell independent. *J Neurosci* **29**:11112–11122.

de Almeida L, Idiart M, Lisman JE (2007) Memory retrieval time and memory capacity of the CA3 network: role of gamma frequency oscillations. *Learn Mem* **14**:795–806.

de Almeida L, Idiart M, Lisman JE (2009a) The input-output transformation of the hippocampal granule cells: from grid cells to place fields. *J Neurosci* **29**:7504–7512.

de Almeida L, Idiart M, Lisman JE (2009b) A second function of gamma frequency oscillations: an E%-max winner-take-all mechanism selects which cells fire. *J Neurosci* **29**:7497–7503.

Debanne D, Gahwiler BH, Thompson SM (1998) Long-term synaptic plasticity between pairs of individual CA3 pyramidal cells in rat hippocampal slice cultures. *J Physiol* **507**(Pt 1):237–247.

DeCoteau WE, Thorn C, Gibson DJ, Courtemanche R, Mitra P, Kubota Y, Graybiel AM (2007) Oscillations of local field potentials in the rat dorsal striatum during spontaneous and instructed behaviors. *J Neurophysiol* **97**:3800–3805.

Deguchi Y, Donato F, Galimberti I, Cabuy E, Caroni P (2011) Temporally matched subpopulations of selectively interconnected principal neurons in the hippocampus. *Nat Neurosci* **14**:495–504.

Deshpande, A., Bergami, M., Ghanem, A., Conzelmann, K. K., Lepier, A., Götz, M., Berninger, B. (2013). Retrograde monosynaptic tracing reveals the temporal evolution of inputs onto new neurons in the adult dentate gyrus and olfactory bulb. *Proceedings of the National Academy of Sciences*, **110**(12), E1152–E1161.

Deuchars J, Thomson AM (1996) CA1 pyramid-pyramid connections in rat hippocampus in vitro: dual intracellular recordings with biocytin filling. *Neuroscience* **74**:1009–1018.

Diba K, Buzsaki G (2008) Hippocampal network dynamics constrain the time lag between pyramidal cells across modified environments. *J Neurosci* **28**:13448–13456.

Doischer D, Hosp JA, Yanagawa Y, Obata K, Jonas P, Vida I, Bartos M (2008) Postnatal differentiation of basket cells from slow to fast signaling devices. *J Neurosci* **28**:12956–12968.

Donato F, Rompani SB, Caroni P (2013) Parvalbumin-expressing basket-cell network plasticity induced by experience regulates adult learning. *Nature* **504**:272–276.

Dragoi G, Buzsaki G (2006) Temporal encoding of place sequences by hippocampal cell assemblies. *Neuron* **50**:145–157.

Draguhn A, Traub RD, Schmitz D, Jefferys JG (1998) Electrical coupling underlies high-frequency oscillations in the hippocampus in vitro. *Nature* **394**:189–192.

Drake CT, Chavkin C, Milner TA (2007) Opioid systems in the dentate gyrus. *Prog Brain Res* **163**:245–263.

Drake CT, Milner TA (2002) Mu opioid receptors are in discrete hippocampal interneuron subpopulations. *Hippocampus* **12**:119–136.

Drever BD, Riedel G, Platt B (2011) The cholinergic system and hippocampal plasticity. *Behav Brain Res* **221**:505–514.

Druckmann S, Feng L, Lee B, Yook C, Zhao T, Magee JC, Kim J (2014) Structured synaptic connectivity between hippocampal regions. *Neuron* **81**:629–640.

Dubreuil AM, Brunel N (2016) Storing structured sparse memories in a multi-modular cortical network model. *J Comput Neurosci* **40**:157–175.

Dudek SM, Alexander GM, Farris S (2016) Rediscovering area CA2: unique properties and functions. *Nat Rev Neurosci* **17**:89–102.

Dudman JT, Tsay D, Siegelbaum SA (2007) A role for synaptic inputs at distal dendrites: instructive signals for hippocampal long-term plasticity. *Neuron* **56**:866–879.

Dyhrfjeld-Johnsen J, Santhakumar V, Morgan RJ, Huerta R, Tsimring L, Soltesz I (2007) Topological determinants of epileptogenesis in large-scale structural and functional models of the dentate gyrus derived from experimental data. *J Neurophysiol* 97:1566–1587.

Edelmann E, Lessmann V (2018) Dopaminergic innervation and modulation of hippocampal networks. *Cell Tissue Res* 373:711–727.

Eggermann E, Bucurenciu I, Goswami SP, Jonas P (2011) Nanodomain coupling between Ca2+ channels and sensors of exocytosis at fast mammalian synapses. *Nat Rev Neurosci* 13:7.

Elfant D, Pal BZ, Emptage N, Capogna M (2008) Specific inhibitory synapses shift the balance from feedforward to feedback inhibition of hippocampal CA1 pyramidal cells. *Eur J Neurosci* 27:104–113.

Eller J, Zarnadze S, Bäuerle P, Dugladze T, Gloveli T (2015) Cell type-specific separation of subicular principal neurons during network activities. *PLoS One* 10(4):e0123636.

Ermentrout GB, Kopell N (1998) Fine structure of neural spiking and synchronization in the presence of conduction delays. *Proc Natl Acad Sci U S A* 95:1259–1264.

Espinoza C, Guzman SJ, Zhang X, Jonas P (2018) Parvalbumin(+) interneurons obey unique connectivity rules and establish a powerful lateral-inhibition microcircuit in dentate gyrus. *Nat Commun* 9:4605.

Etter G, Krezel W (2014) Dopamine D2 receptor controls hilar mossy cells excitability. *Hippocampus* 24:725–732.

Favuzzi E, Deogracias R, Marques-Smith A, Maeso P, Jezequel J, Exposito-Alonso D, Balia M, Kroon T, Hinojosa AJ, et al. (2019) Distinct molecular programs regulate synapse specificity in cortical inhibitory circuits. *Science* 363:413–417.

Fell J, Klaver P, Lehnertz K, Grunwald T, Schaller C, Elger CE, Fernandez G (2001) Human memory formation is accompanied by rhinal-hippocampal coupling and decoupling. *Nat Neurosci* 4:1259–1264.

Ferguson KA, Chatzikalymniou AP, Skinner FK (2017) Combining theory, model, and experiment to explain how intrinsic theta rhythms are generated in an in vitro whole hippocampus preparation without oscillatory inputs. *eNeuro* 4.

Ferguson KA, Huh CY, Amilhon B, Manseau F, Williams S, Skinner FK (2015) Network models provide insights into how oriens-lacunosum-moleculare and bistratified cell interactions influence the power of local hippocampal CA1 theta oscillations. *Front Syst Neurosci* 9:110.

Ferguson KA, Huh CY, Amilhon B, Williams S, Skinner FK (2013) Experimentally constrained CA1 fast-firing parvalbumin-positive interneuron network models exhibit sharp transitions into coherent high frequency rhythms. *Front Comput Neurosci* 7:144.

Fernandez-Ruiz A, Oliva A, Nagy GA, Maurer AP, Berenyi A, Buzsaki G (2017) Entorhinal-CA3 dual-input control of spike timing in the hippocampus by theta-gamma coupling. *Neuron* 93:1213–1226, e1215.

Fischer V, Both M, Draguhn A, Egorov AV (2014) Choline-mediated modulation of hippocampal sharp wave-ripple complexes in vitro. *J Neurochem* 129:792–805.

Foldy C, Lee SH, Morgan RJ, Soltesz I (2010) Regulation of fast-spiking basket cell synapses by the chloride channel ClC-2. *Nat Neurosci* 13:1047–1049.

Foldy C, Lee SY, Szabadics J, Neu A, Soltesz I (2007) Cell type-specific gating of perisomatic inhibition by cholecystokinin. *Nat Neurosci* 10:1128–1130.

Francavilla R, Luo X, Magnin E, Tyan L, Topolnik L (2015) Coordination of dendritic inhibition through local disinhibitory circuits. *Front Synaptic Neurosci* 7:5.

Francavilla R, Villette V, Luo X, Chamberland S, Munoz-Pino E, Camire O, Wagner K, Kis V, Somogyi P, Topolnik L (2018) Connectivity and network state-dependent recruitment of long-range VIP-GABAergic neurons in the mouse hippocampus. *Nat Commun* 9:5043.

Frazier CJ, Strowbridge BW, Papke RL (2003) Nicotinic receptors on local circuit neurons in dentate gyrus: a potential role in regulation of granule cell excitability. *J Neurophysiol* 89:3018–3028.

Freund TF (1989) GABAergic septohippocampal neurons contain parvalbumin. *Brain Res* 478:375–381.

Freund TF, Antal M (1988) GABA-containing neurons in the septum control inhibitory interneurons in the hippocampus. *Nature* 336:170–173.

Freund TF, Buzsaki G (1996) Interneurons of the hippocampus. *Hippocampus* 6:347–470.

Fries P, Reynolds JH, Rorie AE, Desimone R (2001) Modulation of oscillatory neuronal synchronization by selective visual attention. *Science* 291:1560–1563.

Fritschy JM, Panzanelli P, Tyagarajan SK (2012) Molecular and functional heterogeneity of GABAergic synapses. *Cell Mol Life Sci* 69:2485–2499.

Frotscher M, Jonas P, Sloviter RS (2006) Synapses formed by normal and abnormal hippocampal mossy fibers. *Cell Tissue Res* 326:361–367.

Frotscher M, Soriano E, Misgeld U (1994) Divergence of hippocampal mossy fibers. *Synapse* 16:148–160.

Fu Y, Kaneko M, Tang Y, Alvarez-Buylla A, Stryker MP (2015) A cortical disinhibitory circuit for enhancing adult plasticity. *Elife* 4:e05558.

Fu Y, Tucciarone JM, Espinosa JS, Sheng N, Darcy DP, Nicoll RA, Huang ZJ, Stryker MP (2014) A cortical circuit for gain control by behavioral state. *Cell* 156:1139–1152.

Fuentealba P, Begum R, Capogna M, Jinno S, Marton LF, Csicsvari J, Thomson A, Somogyi P, Klausberger T (2008) Ivy cells: a population of nitric-oxide-producing, slow-spiking GABAergic neurons and their involvement in hippocampal network activity. *Neuron* 57:917–929.

Fuentealba P, Klausberger T, Karayannis T, Suen WY, Huck J, Tomioka R, Rockland K, Capogna M, Studer M, Morales M, et al. (2010) Expression of COUP-TFII nuclear receptor in restricted GABAergic neuronal populations in the adult rat hippocampus. *J Neurosci* 30:1595–1609.

Fuentealba P, Tomioka R, Dalezios Y, Marton LF, Studer M, Rockland K, Klausberger T, Somogyi P (2008) Rhythmically active enkephalin-expressing GABAergic cells in the CA1 area of the hippocampus project to the subiculum and preferentially innervate interneurons. *J Neurosci* 28:10017–10022.

Fukuda T, Kosaka T (2000) Gap junctions linking the dendritic network of GABAergic interneurons in the hippocampus. *J Neurosci* 20:1519–1528.

Fukuda T, Kosaka T (2003) Ultrastructural study of gap junctions between dendrites of parvalbumin-containing GABAergic neurons in various neocortical areas of the adult rat. *Neuroscience* 120:5–20.

Fukuda T, Kosaka T, Singer W, Galuske RA (2006) Gap junctions among dendrites of cortical GABAergic neurons establish a dense and widespread intercolumnar network. *J Neurosci* 26:3434–3443.

Galarreta M, Hestrin S (1999) A network of fast-spiking cells in the neocortex connected by electrical synapses. *Nature* 402:72–75.

Galarreta M, Hestrin S (2001) Electrical synapses between GABA-releasing interneurons. *Nat Rev Neurosci* 2:425–433.

Galarreta M, Hestrin S (2002) Electrical and chemical synapses among parvalbumin fast-spiking GABAergic interneurons in adult mouse neocortex. *Proc Natl Acad Sci U S A* 99:12438–12443.

Gan J, Weng SM, Pernia-Andrade AJ, Csicsvari J, Jonas P (2017) Phase-locked inhibition, but not excitation, underlies hippocampal ripple oscillations in awake mice in vivo. *Neuron* 93:308–314.

Ganter P, Szucs P, Paulsen O, Somogyi P (2004) Properties of horizontal axo-axonic cells in stratum oriens of the hippocampal CA1 area of rats in vitro. *Hippocampus* 14:232–243.

Gasbarri A, Packard MG, Campana E, Pacitti C (1994) Anterograde and retrograde tracing of projections from the ventral tegmental area to the hippocampal formation in the rat. *Brain Res Bull* 33:445–452.

Gasbarri A, Sulli A, Packard MG (1997) The dopaminergic mesencephalic projections to the hippocampal formation in the rat. *Prog Neuropsychopharmacol Biol Psychiatry* 21:1–22.

Gasbarri A, Verney C, Innocenzi R, Campana E, Pacitti C (1994) Mesolimbic dopaminergic neurons innervating the hippocampal formation in the rat: a combined retrograde tracing and immunohistochemical study. *Brain Res* 668:71–79.

Geiger JR, Jonas P (2000) Dynamic control of presynaptic Ca(2+) inflow by fast-inactivating K(+) channels in hippocampal mossy fiber boutons. *Neuron* 28:927–939.

Geiger JR, Lubke J, Roth A, Frotscher M, Jonas P (1997) Submillisecond AMPA receptor-mediated signaling at a principal neuron-interneuron synapse. *Neuron* 18:1009–1023.

Geiger JR, Melcher T, Koh DS, Sakmann B, Seeburg PH, Jonas P, Monyer H (1995) Relative abundance of subunit mRNAs determines gating and Ca2+ permeability of AMPA receptors in principal neurons and interneurons in rat CNS. *Neuron* 15:193–204.

Geisler C, Brunel N, Wang XJ (2005) Contributions of intrinsic membrane dynamics to fast network oscillations with irregular neuronal discharges. *J Neurophysiol* 94:4344–4361.

Gelinas JN, Nguyen PV (2005) Beta-adrenergic receptor activation facilitates induction of a protein synthesis-dependent late phase of long-term potentiation. *J Neurosci* 25:3294–3303.

Gidon A, Segev I (2012) Principles governing the operation of synaptic inhibition in dendrites. *Neuron* 75:330–341.

Giessel AJ, Sabatini BL (2010) M1 muscarinic receptors boost synaptic potentials and calcium influx in dendritic spines by inhibiting postsynaptic SK channels. *Neuron* 68:936–947.

Ginsberg SD, Che S (2005) Expression profile analysis within the human hippocampus: comparison of CA1 and CA3 pyramidal neurons. *J Comp Neurol* 487:107–118.

Glickfeld LL, Atallah BV, Scanziani M (2008) Complementary modulation of somatic inhibition by opioids and cannabinoids. *J Neurosci* 28:1824–1832.

Glickfeld LL, Scanziani M (2006) Distinct timing in the activity of cannabinoid-sensitive and cannabinoid-insensitive basket cells. *Nat Neurosci* 9:807–815.

Glykys J, Mody I (2007) Activation of GABAA receptors: views from outside the synaptic cleft. *Neuron* 56:763–770.

Golding NL, Kath WL, Spruston N (2001) Dichotomy of action-potential backpropagation in CA1 pyramidal neuron dendrites. *J Neurophysiol* 86:2998–3010.

Goodman JH, Sloviter RS (1992) Evidence for commissurally projecting parvalbumin-immunoreactive basket cells in the dentate gyrus of the rat. *Hippocampus* 2:13–21.

Goutagny R, Jackson J, Williams S (2009) Self-generated theta oscillations in the hippocampus. *Nat Neurosci* 12:1491–1493.

Grastyan E, Lissak K, Madarasz I, Donhoffer H (1959) Hippocampal electrical activity during the development of conditioned reflexes. *Electroencephalography and Clinical Neurophysiology* 11:409–430.

Graves AR, Moore SJ, Bloss EB, Mensh BD, Kath WL, Spruston N (2012) Hippocampal pyramidal neurons comprise two distinct cell types that are countermodulated by metabotropic receptors. *Neuron* 76(4):776–789.

Gray CM (1994) Synchronous oscillations in neuronal systems: mechanisms and functions. *J Comput Neurosci* 1:11–38.

Gray R, Rajan AS, Radcliffe KA, Yakehiro M, Dani JA (1996) Hippocampal synaptic transmission enhanced by low concentrations of nicotine. *Nature* 383:713–716.

Green JD, Arduini AA (1954) Hippocampal electrical activity in arousal. *J Neurophysiol* 17:533–557.

Greene JRT, Totterdell S (1997) Morphology and distribution of electrophysiologically defined classes of pyramidal and nonpyramidal neurons in rat ventral subiculum in vitro. *Journal of Comparative Neurology* 380(3):395–408.

Grienberger C, Milstein AD, Bittner KC, Romani S, Magee JC (2017) Inhibitory suppression of heterogeneously tuned excitation enhances spatial coding in CA1 place cells. *Nat Neurosci* 20:417–426.

Griffith WH (1990) Voltage-clamp analysis of posttetanic potentiation of the mossy fiber to CA3 synapse in hippocampus. *J Neurophysiol* 63:491–501.

Grosmark AD, Buzsaki G (2016) Diversity in neural firing dynamics supports both rigid and learned hippocampal sequences. *Science* 351:1440–1443.

Gulledge AT, Kawaguchi Y (2007) Phasic cholinergic signaling in the hippocampus: functional homology with the neocortex? *Hippocampus* 17:327–332.

Gulyas AI, Acsady L, Freund TF (1999) Structural basis of the cholinergic and serotonergic modulation of GABAergic neurons in the hippocampus. *Neurochem Int* 34:359–372.

Gulyas AI, Hajos N, Freund TF (1996) Interneurons containing calretinin are specialized to control other interneurons in the rat hippocampus. *J Neurosci* 16:3397–3411.

Gulyas AI, Megias M, Emri Z, Freund TF (1999) Total number and ratio of excitatory and inhibitory synapses converging onto single interneurons of different types in the CA1 area of the rat hippocampus. *J Neurosci* 19:10082–10097.

Gulyas AI, Miles R, Sik A, Toth K, Tamamaki N, Freund TF (1993) Hippocampal pyramidal cells excite inhibitory neurons through a single release site. *Nature* 366:683–687.

Gundlfinger A, Breustedt J, Sullivan D, Schmitz D (2010) Natural spike trains trigger short- and long-lasting dynamics at hippocampal mossy fiber synapses in rodents. *PLoS One* 5:e9961.

Gundlfinger A, Leibold C, Gebert K, Moisel M, Schmitz D, Kempter R (2007) Differential modulation of short-term synaptic dynamics by long-term potentiation at mouse hippocampal mossy fibre synapses. *J Physiol* 585:853–865.

Gupta AS, van der Meer MA, Touretzky DS, Redish AD (2012) Segmentation of spatial experience by hippocampal theta sequences. *Nat Neurosci* 15:1032–1039.

Guzman SJ, Schlogl A, Frotscher M, Jonas P (2016) Synaptic mechanisms of pattern completion in the hippocampal CA3 network. *Science* 353:1117–1123.

Haglund L, Swanson LW, Köhler C (1984) The projection of the supramammillary nucleus to the hippocampal formation: an immunohistochemical and anterograde transport study with the lectin PHA-L in the rat. *Journal of Comparative Neurology* 229(2):171–185.

Hajos N, Acsady L, Freund TF (1996) Target selectivity and neurochemical characteristics of VIP-immunoreactive interneurons in the rat dentate gyrus. *Eur J Neurosci* 8:1415–1431.

Hajos N, Karlocai MR, Nemeth B, Ulbert I, Monyer H, Szabo G, Erdelyi F, Freund TF, Gulyas AI (2013) Input-output features of anatomically identified CA3 neurons during hippocampal sharp wave/ripple oscillation in vitro. *J Neurosci* 33:11677–11691.

Hajos N, Mody I (1997) Synaptic communication among hippocampal interneurons: properties of spontaneous IPSCs in morphologically identified cells. *J Neurosci* 17:8427–8442.

Hajos N, Palhalmi J, Mann EO, Nemeth B, Paulsen O, Freund TF (2004) Spike timing of distinct types of GABAergic interneuron during hippocampal gamma oscillations in vitro. *J Neurosci* 24:9127–9137.

Hajos N, Paulsen O (2009) Network mechanisms of gamma oscillations in the CA3 region of the hippocampus. *Neural Netw* 22:1113–1119.

Halasy K, Racz B, Maderspach K (2000) Kappa opioid receptors are expressed by interneurons in the CA1 area of the rat hippocampus: a correlated light and electron microscopic immunocytochemical study. *J Chem Neuroanat* 19:233–241.

Halasy K, Somogyi P (1993a) Distribution of GABAergic synapses and their targets in the dentate gyrus of rat: a quantitative immunoelectron microscopic analysis. *J Hirnforsch* 34:299–308.

Halasy K, Somogyi P (1993b) Subdivisions in the multiple GABAergic innervation of granule cells in the dentate gyrus of the rat hippocampus. *Eur J Neurosci* 5:411–429.

Hallermann S, Pawlu C, Jonas P, Heckmann M (2003) A large pool of releasable vesicles in a cortical glutamatergic synapse. *Proc Natl Acad Sci U S A* 100:8975–8980.

Hamilton TJ, Wheatley BM, Sinclair DB, Bachmann M, Larkum ME, Colmers WF (2010) Dopamine modulates synaptic plasticity in dendrites of rat and human dentate granule cells. *Proc Natl Acad Sci U S A* 107:18185–18190.

Hamzei-Sichani F, Davidson KG, Yasumura T, Janssen WG, Wearne SL, Hof PR, Traub RD, Gutierrez R, Ottersen OP, Rash JE (2012) Mixed electrical-chemical synapses in adult rat hippocampus are primarily glutamatergic and coupled by connexin-36. *Front Neuroanat* 6:13.

Han ZS, Buhl EH, Lorinczi Z, Somogyi P (1993) A high degree of spatial selectivity in the axonal and dendritic domains of physiologically identified local-circuit neurons in the dentate gyrus of the rat hippocampus. *Eur J Neurosci* 5:395–410.

Hangya B, Borhegyi Z, Szilagyi N, Freund TF, Varga V (2009) GABAergic neurons of the medial septum lead the hippocampal network during theta activity. *J Neurosci* 29:8094–8102.

Hansen N, Manahan-Vaughan D (2014) Dopamine D1/D5 receptors mediate informational saliency that promotes persistent hippocampal long-term plasticity. *Cereb Cortex* 24:845–858.

Harnett MT, Makara JK, Spruston N, Kath WL, Magee JC (2012) Synaptic amplification by dendritic spines enhances input cooperativity. *Nature* 491:599–602.

Harris KD, Csicsvari J, Hirase H, Dragoi G, Buzsaki G (2003) Organization of cell assemblies in the hippocampus. *Nature* 424:552–556.

Harris KD, Henze DA, Hirase H, Leinekugel X, Dragoi G, Czurko A, Buzsaki G (2002) Spike train dynamics predicts theta-related phase precession in hippocampal pyramidal cells. *Nature* 417:738–741.

Hartzell AL, Martyniuk KM, Brigidi GS, Heinz DA, Djaja NA, Payne A, Bloodgood BL (2018) NPAS4 recruits CCK basket cell synapses and enhances cannabinoid-sensitive inhibition in the mouse hippocampus. *Elife* 7:e35927.

Harvey CD, Collman F, Dombeck DA, Tank DW (2009) Intracellular dynamics of hippocampal place cells during virtual navigation. *Nature* 461:941–946.

Hashimotodani Y, Nasrallah K, Jensen KR, Chavez AE, Carrera D, Castillo PE (2017) LTP at hilar mossy cell-dentate granule cell synapses modulates dentate gyrus output by increasing excitation/inhibition balance. *Neuron* 95:928–943, e923.

Hasselmo ME (2006) The role of acetylcholine in learning and memory. *Curr Opin Neurobiol* 16:710–715.

Hausser M, Mel B (2003) Dendrites: bug or feature? *Curr Opin Neurobiol* 13:372–383.

Hefft S, Jonas P (2005) Asynchronous GABA release generates long-lasting inhibition at a hippocampal interneuron-principal neuron synapse. *Nat Neurosci* 8:1319–1328.

Hefft S, Kraushaar U, Geiger JR, Jonas P (2002) Presynaptic short-term depression is maintained during regulation of transmitter release at a GABAergic synapse in rat hippocampus. *J Physiol* 539:201–208.

Henze DA, Wittner L, Buzsaki G (2002) Single granule cells reliably discharge targets in the hippocampal CA3 network in vivo. *Nat Neurosci* 5:790–795.

Hestrin S, Galarreta M (2005) Electrical synapses define networks of neocortical GABAergic neurons. *Trends Neurosci* 28:304–309.

Holt GR, Koch C (1997) Shunting inhibition does not have a divisive effect on firing rates. *Neural Comput* 9:1001–1013.

Hopfield JJ (1982) Neural networks and physical systems with emergent collective computational abilities. *Proc Natl Acad Sci U S A* 79:2554–2558.

Hormuzdi SG, Pais I, LeBeau FE, Towers SK, Rozov A, Buhl EH, Whittington MA, Monyer H (2001) Impaired electrical signaling disrupts gamma frequency oscillations in connexin 36-deficient mice. *Neuron* 31:487–495.

Hortnagl H, Berger ML, Sperk G, Pifl C (1991) Regional heterogeneity in the distribution of neurotransmitter markers in the rat hippocampus. *Neuroscience* 45:261–272.

Hosp JA, Struber M, Yanagawa Y, Obata K, Vida I, Jonas P, Bartos M (2014) Morpho-physiological criteria divide dentate gyrus interneurons into classes. *Hippocampus* 24:189–203.

Houser CR (2007) Interneurons of the dentate gyrus: an overview of cell types, terminal fields and neurochemical identity. *Prog Brain Res* 163:217–232.

Howard MW, Rizzuto DS, Caplan JB, Madsen JR, Lisman J, Aschenbrenner-Scheibe R, Schulze-Bonhage A, Kahana MJ (2003) Gamma oscillations correlate with working memory load in humans. *Cereb Cortex* 13:1369–1374.

Hu H, Gan J, Jonas P (2014) Interneurons. Fast-spiking, parvalbumin (+) GABAergic interneurons: from cellular design to microcircuit function. *Science* 345:1255263.

Hu H, Real E, Takamiya K, Kang MG, Ledoux J, Huganir RL, Malinow R (2007) Emotion enhances learning via norepinephrine regulation of AMPA-receptor trafficking. *Cell* 131:160–173.

Hu H, Vervaeke K, Graham LJ, Storm JF (2009) Complementary theta resonance filtering by two spatially segregated mechanisms in CA1 hippocampal pyramidal neurons. *J Neurosci* 29:14472–14483.

Huang YY, Kandel ER (1996) Modulation of both the early and the late phase of mossy fiber LTP by the activation of beta-adrenergic receptors. *Neuron* 16:611–617.

Hummos A, Franklin CC, Nair SS (2014) Intrinsic mechanisms stabilize encoding and retrieval circuits differentially in a hippocampal network model. *Hippocampus* 24:1430–1448.

Hunt DL, Linaro D, Si B, Romani S, Spruston N (2018) A novel pyramidal cell type promotes sharp-wave synchronization in the hippocampus. *Nat Neurosci* 21:985–995.

Igarashi KM, Ito HT, Moser EI, Moser MB (2014) Functional diversity along the transverse axis of hippocampal area CA1. *FEBS Lett* 588:2470–2476.

Ino T, Matsuzaki S, Shinonaga Y, Ohishi H, Ogawa-Meguro R, Mizuno N (1990) Direct projections of non-pyramidal neurons of Ammon's horn to the amygdala and the entorhinal cortex. *Neurosci Lett* 115:161–166.

Isaacson JS, Solis JM, Nicoll RA (1993) Local and diffuse synaptic actions of GABA in the hippocampus. *Neuron* 10:165–175.

Ishihara Y, Fukuda T (2016) Immunohistochemical investigation of the internal structure of the mouse subiculum. *Neuroscience* 337:242–266.

Ishizuka N, Weber J, Amaral DG (1990) Organization of intrahippocampal projections originating from CA3 pyramidal cells in the rat. *J Comp Neurol* 295:580–623.

Izhikevich EM (2006) Polychronization: computation with spikes. *Neural Comput* 18:245–282.

Izhikevich EM (2010) Hybrid spiking models. *Philos Trans A Math Phys Eng Sci* 368:5061–5070.

Jadi M, Polsky A, Schiller J, Mel BW (2012) Location-dependent effects of inhibition on local spiking in pyramidal neuron dendrites. *PLoS Comput Biol* 8:e1002550.

Jaramillo J, Kempter R (2017) Phase precession: a neural code underlying episodic memory? *Curr Opin Neurobiol* 43:130–138.

Jaramillo J, Schmidt R, Kempter R (2014) Modeling inheritance of phase precession in the hippocampal formation. *J Neurosci* 34:7715–7731.

Jarsky T, Mady R, Kennedy B, Spruston N (2008) Distribution of bursting neurons in the CA1 region and the subiculum of the rat hippocampus. *Journal of Comparative Neurology* 506(4):535–547.

Jarsky T, Roxin A, Kath WL, Spruston N (2005) Conditional dendritic spike propagation following distal synaptic activation of hippocampal CA1 pyramidal neurons. *Nat Neurosci* 8:1667–1676.

Jensen O, Lisman JE (1996) Theta/gamma networks with slow NMDA channels learn sequences and encode episodic memory: role of NMDA channels in recall. *Learn Mem* 3:264–278.

Jensen O, Lisman JE (2000) Position reconstruction from an ensemble of hippocampal place cells: contribution of theta phase coding. *J Neurophysiol* 83:2602–2609.

Jinno S (2009) Structural organization of long-range GABAergic projection system of the hippocampus. *Front Neuroanat* 3:13.

Jinno S, Klausberger T, Marton LF, Dalezios Y, Roberts JD, Fuentealba P, Bushong EA, Henze D, Buzsaki G, Somogyi P (2007) Neuronal diversity in GABAergic long-range projections from the hippocampus. *J Neurosci* 27:8790–8804.

Jonas P, Bischofberger J, Fricker D, Miles R (2004) Interneuron Diversity series: Fast in, fast out—temporal and spatial signal processing in hippocampal interneurons. *Trends Neurosci* 27:30–40.

Jonas P, Hefft S (2010) GABA release at terminals of CCK-interneurons: synchrony, asynchrony and modulation by cannabinoid receptors (commentary on Ali and Todorova). *Eur J Neurosci* 31:1194–1195.

Jones MW, McHugh TJ (2011) Updating hippocampal representations: CA2 joins the circuit. *Trends in neurosciences* 34(10):526–535.

Jones MW, Wilson MA (2005) Theta rhythms coordinate hippocampal-prefrontal interactions in a spatial memory task. *PLoS Biol* 3:e402.

Jones S, Yakel JL (1997) Functional nicotinic ACh receptors on interneurones in the rat hippocampus. *J Physiol* 504(Pt 3):603–610.

Joshi A, Salib M, Viney TJ, Dupret D, Somogyi P (2017) Behavior-dependent activity and synaptic organization of septo-hippocampal GABAergic neurons selectively targeting the hippocampal CA3 area. *Neuron* 96:1342–1357, e1345.

Jung R, Kornmüller AE (1938) Eine methodik der ableitung iokalisierter potentialschwankungen aus subcorticalen hirngebieten. *Eur Arch Psychiatry Clin Neurosci* 109:1–30.

Kaifosh P, Losonczy A (2016) Mnemonic functions for nonlinear dendritic integration in hippocampal pyramidal circuits. *Neuron* 90:622–634.

Kaifosh P, Lovett-Barron M, Turi GF, Reardon TR, Losonczy A (2013) Septo-hippocampal GABAergic signaling across multiple modalities in awake mice. *Nat Neurosci* 16:1182–1184.

Kajiwara R, Wouterlood FG, Sah A, Boekel AJ, Baks-te Bulte LT, Witter MP (2008) Convergence of entorhinal and CA3 inputs onto pyramidal neurons and interneurons in hippocampal area CA1—an anatomical study in the rat. *Hippocampus* 18:266–280.

Kamigaki T, Dan Y (2017) Delay activity of specific prefrontal interneuron subtypes modulates memory-guided behavior. *Nat Neurosci* 20:854–863.

Kamondi A, Acsady L, Wang XJ, Buzsaki G (1998) Theta oscillations in somata and dendrites of hippocampal pyramidal cells in vivo: activity-dependent phase-precession of action potentials. *Hippocampus* 8:244–261.

Kanemoto Y, Matsuzaki M, Morita S, Hayama T, Noguchi J, Senda N, Momotake A, Arai T, Kasai H (2011) Spatial distributions of GABA receptors and local inhibition of Ca2+ transients studied with GABA uncaging in the dendrites of CA1 pyramidal neurons. *PLoS One* 6:e22652.

Karayannis T, Elfant D, Huerta-Ocampo I, Teki S, Scott RS, Rusakov DA, Jones MV, Capogna M (2010) Slow GABA transient and receptor desensitization shape synaptic responses evoked by hippocampal neurogliaform cells. *J Neurosci* 30:9898–9909.

Karson MA, Tang AH, Milner TA, Alger BE (2009) Synaptic cross talk between perisomatic-targeting interneuron classes expressing cholecystokinin and parvalbumin in hippocampus. *J Neurosci* 29:4140–4154.

Karunakaran S, Chowdhury A, Donato F, Quairiaux C, Michel CM, Caroni P (2016) PV plasticity sustained through D1/5 dopamine signaling required for long-term memory consolidation. *Nat Neurosci* 19:454–464.

Kastellakis G, Cai DJ, Mednick SC, Silva AJ, Poirazi P (2015) Synaptic clustering within dendrites: an emerging theory of memory formation. *Prog Neurobiol* 126:19–35.

Katona I, Sperlagh B, Sik A, Kafalvi A, Vizi ES, Mackie K, Freund TF (1999) Presynaptically located CB1 cannabinoid receptors regulate GABA release from axon terminals of specific hippocampal interneurons. *J Neurosci* 19:4544–4558.

Katona L, Micklem B, Borhegyi Z, Swiejkowski DA, Valenti O, Viney TJ, Kotzadimitriou D, Klausberger T, Somogyi P (2017) Behavior-dependent activity patterns of GABAergic long-range projecting neurons in the rat hippocampus. *Hippocampus* 27:359–377.

Katsumaru H, Kosaka T, Heizmann CW, Hama K (1988) Gap junctions on GABAergic neurons containing the calcium-binding protein parvalbumin in the rat hippocampus (CA1 region). *Exp Brain Res* 72:363–370.

Kay K, Sosa M, Chung JE, Karlsson MP, Larkin MC, Frank LM (2016) A hippocampal network for spatial coding during immobility and sleep. *Nature* 531:185–190.

Kempadoo KA, Mosharov EV, Choi SJ, Sulzer D, Kandel ER (2016) Dopamine release from the locus coeruleus to the dorsal hippocampus promotes spatial learning and memory. *Proc Natl Acad Sci U S A* 113:14835–14840.

Kempermann G, Song H, Gage FH (2015) Neurogenesis in the adult hippocampus. *Cold Spring Harb Perspect Biol* 7:a018812.

Kepecs A, Fishell G (2014) Interneuron cell types are fit to function. *Nature* 505:318–326.

Kepecs A, Uchida N, Mainen ZF (2006) The sniff as a unit of olfactory processing. *Chem Senses* 31:167–179.

Kerti-Szigeti K, Nusser Z (2016) Similar GABAA receptor subunit composition in somatic and axon initial segment synapses of hippocampal pyramidal cells. *Elife* 5:e18426.

Kesner RP, Rolls ET (2015) A computational theory of hippocampal function, and tests of the theory: new developments. *Neurosci Biobehav Rev* 48:92–147.

Khazipov R, Congar P, Ben-Ari Y (1995) Hippocampal CA1 lacunosum-moleculare interneurons: modulation of monosynaptic GABAergic IPSCs by presynaptic GABAB receptors. *J Neurophysiol* 74:2126–2137.

Kim J, Delcasso S, Lee I (2011) Neural correlates of object-in-place learning in hippocampus and prefrontal cortex. *J Neurosci* 31:16991–17006.

Kim S (2014) Action potential modulation in CA1 pyramidal neuron axons facilitates OLM interneuron activation in recurrent inhibitory microcircuits of rat hippocampus. *PLoS One* 9:e113124.

Kim S, Guzman SJ, Hu H, Jonas P (2012) Active dendrites support efficient initiation of dendritic spikes in hippocampal CA3 pyramidal neurons. *Nat Neurosci* 15:600–606.

Kim S, Kim Y, Lee SH, Ho WK (2018) Dendritic spikes in hippocampal granule cells are necessary for long-term potentiation at the perforant path synapse. *Elife* 7:e35269.

Kim Y, Spruston N (2012) Target-specific output patterns are predicted by the distribution of regular-spiking and bursting pyramidal neurons in the subiculum. *Hippocampus* 22(4):693–706.

Klausberger T (2009) GABAergic interneurons targeting dendrites of pyramidal cells in the CA1 area of the hippocampus. *Eur J Neurosci* 30:947–957.

Klausberger T, Magill PJ, Marton LF, Roberts JD, Cobden PM, Buzsaki G, Somogyi P (2003) Brain-state- and cell-type-specific firing of hippocampal interneurons in vivo. *Nature* 421:844–848.

Klausberger T, Marton LF, Baude A, Roberts JD, Magill PJ, Somogyi P (2004) Spike timing of dendrite-targeting bistratified cells during hippocampal network oscillations in vivo. *Nat Neurosci* 7:41–47.

Klausberger T, Marton LF, O'Neill J, Huck JH, Dalezios Y, Fuentealba P, Suen WY, Papp E, Kaneko T, Watanabe M, et al. (2005) Complementary roles of cholecystokinin- and parvalbumin-expressing GABAergic neurons in hippocampal network oscillations. *J Neurosci* 25:9782–9793.

Klausberger T, Roberts JD, Somogyi P (2002) Cell type- and input-specific differences in the number and subtypes of synaptic GABA(A) receptors in the hippocampus. *J Neurosci* 22:2513–2521.

Klausberger T, Somogyi P (2008) Neuronal diversity and temporal dynamics: the unity of hippocampal circuit operations. *Science* 321:53–57.

Klyachko VA, Stevens CF (2006) Excitatory and feed-forward inhibitory hippocampal synapses work synergistically as an adaptive filter of natural spike trains. *PLoS Biol* 4:e207.

Knierim JJ, Neunuebel JP (2016) Tracking the flow of hippocampal computation: Pattern separation, pattern completion, and attractor dynamics. *Neurobiol Learn Mem* 129:38–49.

Knopp A, Frahm C, Fidzinski P, Witte OW, Behr J (2008) Loss of GABAergic neurons in the subiculum and its functional implications in temporal lobe epilepsy. *Brain* 131(6):1516–1527.

Knowles WD, Schwartzkroin PA (1981) Axonal ramifications of hippocampal Ca1 pyramidal cells. *J Neurosci* 1:1236–1241.

Kobayashi K, Suzuki H (2007) Dopamine selectively potentiates hippocampal mossy fiber to CA3 synaptic transmission. *Neuropharmacology* 52:552–561.

Koh DS, Geiger JR, Jonas P, Sakmann B (1995) Ca(2+)-permeable AMPA and NMDA receptor channels in basket cells of rat hippocampal dentate gyrus. *J Physiol* 485(Pt 2):383–402.

Kohara K, Pignatelli M, Rivest A, Jung HY, Kitamura T, Suh J, Frank D, Kajikawa K, Mise N, Obata Y, et al.(2014a) Cell type-specific genetic and optogenetic tools reveal hippocampal CA2 circuits. *Nat Neurosci* 17:269–279.

Kohara K, Pignatelli M, Rivest AJ, Jung HY, Kitamura T, Suh J, Frank D, Kajikawa K, Mise N, Obata Y, W et al. (2014b) Cell type-specific genetic and optogenetic tools reveal hippocampal CA2 circuits. *Nat Neurosci* 17:269–279.

Kohus Z, Kali S, Rovira-Esteban L, Schlingloff D, Papp O, Freund TF, Hajos N, Gulyas AI (2016) Properties and dynamics of inhibitory synaptic communication within the CA3 microcircuits

of pyramidal cells and interneurons expressing parvalbumin or cholecystokinin. *J Physiol* 594:3745–3774.

Kosaka T (1983) Neuronal gap junctions in the polymorph layer of the rat dentate gyrus. *Brain Res* 277:347–351.

Kramis R, Vanderwolf CH, Bland BH (1975) Two types of hippocampal rhythmical slow activity in both the rabbit and the rat: relations to behavior and effects of atropine, diethyl ether, urethane, and pentobarbital. *Exp Neurol* 49:58–85.

Krook-Magnuson E, Luu L, Lee SH, Varga C, Soltesz I (2011) Ivy and neurogliaform interneurons are a major target of mu-opioid receptor modulation. *J Neurosci* 31:14861–14870.

Krook-Magnuson E, Varga C, Lee SH, Soltesz I (2012) New dimensions of interneuronal specialization unmasked by principal cell heterogeneity. *Trends Neurosci* 35:175–184.

Krueppel R, Remy S, Beck H (2011) Dendritic integration in hippocampal dentate granule cells. *Neuron* 71:512–528.

Kuchibhotla KV, Gill JV, Lindsay GW, Papadoyannis ES, Field RE, Sten TAH, ... Froemke RC (2017) Parallel processing by cortical inhibition enables context-dependent behavior. *Nat Neurosci* 20(1):62–71.

Kulik A, Vida I, Lujan R, Haas CA, Lopez-Bendito G, Shigemoto R, Frotscher M (2003) Subcellular localization of metabotropic GABA(B) receptor subunits GABA(B1a/b) and GABA(B2) in the rat hippocampus. *J Neurosci* 23:11026–11035.

Lacaille JC, Schwartzkroin PA (1988) Intracellular responses of rat hippocampal granule cells in vitro to discrete applications of norepinephrine. *Neurosci Lett* 89:176–181.

Larimer P, Strowbridge BW (2010) Representing information in cell assemblies: persistent activity mediated by semilunar granule cells. *Nat Neurosci* 13:213–222.

Larson J, Wong D, Lynch G (1986) Patterned stimulation at the theta frequency is optimal for the induction of hippocampal long-term potentiation. *Brain Res* 368:347–350.

Lasztoczi B, Klausberger T (2014) Layer-specific GABAergic control of distinct gamma oscillations in the CA1 hippocampus. *Neuron* 81:1126–1139.

Lasztoczi B, Tukker JJ, Somogyi P, Klausberger T (2011) Terminal field and firing selectivity of cholecystokinin-expressing interneurons in the hippocampal CA3 area. *J Neurosci* 31:18073–18093.

Lawrence JJ, Grinspan ZM, Statland JM, McBain CJ (2006) Muscarinic receptor activation tunes mouse stratum oriens interneurones to amplify spike reliability. *J Physiol* 571:555–562.

Lawrence JJ, Haario H, Stone EF (2015) Presynaptic cholinergic neuromodulation alters the temporal dynamics of short-term depression at parvalbumin-positive basket cell synapses from juvenile CA1 mouse hippocampus. *J Neurophysiol* 113:2408–2419.

Leao RN, Mikulovic S, Leao KE, Munguba H, Gezelius H, Enjin A, Patra K, Eriksson A, Loew LM, Tort AB, et al. (2012) OLM interneurons differentially modulate CA3 and entorhinal inputs to hippocampal CA1 neurons. *Nat Neurosci* 15:1524–1530.

Lee H, Wang C, Deshmukh SS, Knierim JJ (2015) Neural population evidence of functional heterogeneity along the CA3 transverse axis: pattern completion versus pattern separation. *Neuron* 87:1093–1105.

Lee S, Hjerling-Leffler J, Zagha E, Fishell G, Rudy B (2010) The largest group of superficial neocortical GABAergic interneurons expresses ionotropic serotonin receptors. *J Neurosci* 30:16796–16808.

Lee S, Kruglikov I, Huang ZJ, Fishell G, Rudy B (2013) A disinhibitory circuit mediates motor integration in the somatosensory cortex. *Nat Neurosci* 16:1662–1670.

Lee SE, Simons SB, Heldt SA, Zhao M, Schroeder JP, Vellano CP, ... Hepler JR (2010) RGS14 is a natural suppressor of both synaptic plasticity in CA2 neurons and hippocampal-based learning and memory. *Proceedings of the National Academy of Sciences* 107(39):16994–16998.

Lee SH, Marchionni I, Bezaire M, Varga C, Danielson N, Lovett-Barron M, Losonczy A, Soltesz I (2014) Parvalbumin-positive basket cells differentiate among hippocampal pyramidal cells. *Neuron* 82:1129–1144.

Lee SY, Foldy C, Szabadics J, Soltesz I (2011) Cell-type-specific CCK2 receptor signaling underlies the cholecystokinin-mediated selective excitation of hippocampal parvalbumin-positive fast-spiking basket cells. *J Neurosci* 31:10993–11002.

Lega BC, Jacobs J, Kahana M (2012) Human hippocampal theta oscillations and the formation of episodic memories. *Hippocampus* 22:748–761.

Lei S, McBain CJ (2003) GABA B receptor modulation of excitatory and inhibitory synaptic transmission onto rat CA3 hippocampal interneurons. *J Physiol* 546:439–453.

Lein ES, Zhao X, Gage FH (2004) Defining a molecular atlas of the hippocampus using DNA microarrays and high-throughput in situ hybridization. *Journal of Neuroscience* 24(15):3879–3889.

Leranth C, Hajszan T (2007) Extrinsic afferent systems to the dentate gyrus. *Prog Brain Res* 163:63–84.

Letzkus JJ, Wolff SB, Luthi A (2015) Disinhibition, a circuit mechanism for associative learning and memory. *Neuron* 88:264–276.

Letzkus JJ, Wolff SB, Meyer EM, Tovote P, Courtin J, Herry C, Luthi A (2011) A disinhibitory microcircuit for associative fear learning in the auditory cortex. *Nature* 480:331–335.

Leung LS (2011) A model of intracellular theta phase precession dependent on intrinsic subthreshold membrane currents. *J Neurosci* 31:12282–12296.

Li G, Berger O, Han SM, Paredes M, Wu NC, Pleasure SJ (2008) Hilar mossy cells share developmental influences with dentate granule neurons. *Dev Neurosci* 30:255–261.

Li XG, Somogyi P, Ylinen A, Buzsaki G (1994) The hippocampal CA3 network: an in vivo intracellular labeling study. *J Comp Neurol* 339:181–208.

Li Y, Stam FJ, Aimone JB, Goulding M, Callaway EM, Gage FH (2013) Molecular layer perforant path-associated cells contribute to feedforward inhibition in the adult dentate gyrus. *Proc Natl Acad Sci U S A* 110:9106–9111.

Li Y, Xu J, Liu Y, Zhu J, Liu N, Zeng W, ... Zhang X (2017) A distinct entorhinal cortex to hippocampal CA1 direct circuit for olfactory associative learning. *Nature neuroscience* 20(4):559–570.

Lien CC, Jonas P (2003) Kv3 potassium conductance is necessary and kinetically optimized for high-frequency action potential generation in hippocampal interneurons. *J Neurosci* 23:2058–2068.

Lin Y, Bloodgood BL, Hauser JL, Lapan AD, Koon AC, Kim TK, Hu LS, Malik AN, Greenberg ME (2008) Activity-dependent regulation of inhibitory synapse development by Npas4. *Nature* 455:1198–1204.

Lin YT, Hsu KS (2018) Oxytocin receptor signaling in the hippocampus: role in regulating neuronal excitability, network oscillatory activity, synaptic plasticity and social memory. *Prog Neurobiol* 171:1–14.

Lisman J (2005) The theta/gamma discrete phase code occuring during the hippocampal phase precession may be a more general brain coding scheme. *Hippocampus* 15:913–922.

Lisman J, Buzsaki G (2008) A neural coding scheme formed by the combined function of gamma and theta oscillations. *Schizophr Bull* 34:974–980.

Lisman JE (1999) Relating hippocampal circuitry to function: recall of memory sequences by reciprocal dentate-CA3 interactions. *Neuron* 22:233–242.

Lisman JE, Jensen O (2013) The theta-gamma neural code. *Neuron* 77:1002–1016.

Lisman JE, Talamini LM, Raffone A (2005) Recall of memory sequences by interaction of the dentate and CA3: a revised model of the phase precession. *Neural Netw* 18:1191–1201.

Llorens-Martín M, Jurado-Arjona J, Avila J, Hernández F (2015) Novel connection between newborn granule neurons and the hippocampal CA2 field. *Experimental neurology* 263:285–292.

Lopes-Dos-Santos V, van de Ven GM, Morley A, Trouche S, Campo-Urriza N, Dupret D (2018) Parsing hippocampal theta oscillations by nested spectral components during spatial exploration and memory-guided behavior. *Neuron* 100:940–952, e947.

Lorente De Nó R (1934) Studies on the structure of the cerebral cortex: II. Continuation of the study of the ammonic system. *Journal für Psychologie und Neurologie* 46:113–177.

Losonczy A, Biro AA, Nusser Z (2004) Persistently active cannabinoid receptors mute a subpopulation of hippocampal interneurons. *Proc Natl Acad Sci U S A* 101:1362–1367.

Losonczy A, Magee JC (2006) Integrative properties of radial oblique dendrites in hippocampal CA1 pyramidal neurons. *Neuron* 50:291–307.

Losonczy A, Makara JK, Magee JC (2008) Compartmentalized dendritic plasticity and input feature storage in neurons. *Nature* 452:436–441.

Losonczy A, Zemelman BV, Vaziri A, Magee JC (2010) Network mechanisms of theta related neuronal activity in hippocampal CA1 pyramidal neurons. *Nat Neurosci* 13:967–972.

Losonczy A, Zhang L, Shigemoto R, Somogyi P, Nusser Z (2002) Cell type dependence and variability in the short-term plasticity of EPSCs in identified mouse hippocampal interneurones. *J Physiol* 542:193–210.

Lovett-Barron M, Kaifosh P, Kheirbek MA, Danielson N, Zaremba JD, Reardon TR, Turi GF, Hen R, Zemelman BV, Losonczy A (2014) Dendritic inhibition in the hippocampus supports fear learning. *Science* 343:857–863.

Lovett-Barron M, Turi GF, Kaifosh P, Lee PH, Bolze F, Sun XH, Nicoud JF, Zemelman BV, Sternson SM, Losonczy A (2012) Regulation of neuronal input transformations by tunable dendritic inhibition. *Nat Neurosci* 15:423–430, S421–423.

Lu L, Igarashi KM, Witter MP, Moser EI, Moser MB (2015) Topography of place maps along the CA3-to-CA2 axis of the hippocampus. *Neuron* 87:1078–1092.

Lubenov EV, Siapas AG (2009) Hippocampal theta oscillations are travelling waves. *Nature* 459:534–539.

Lupica CR (1995) Delta and mu enkephalins inhibit spontaneous GABA-mediated IPSCs via a cyclic AMP-independent mechanism in the rat hippocampus. *J Neurosci* 15:737–749.

Lysetskiy M, Foldy C, Soltesz I (2005) Long- and short-term plasticity at mossy fiber synapses on mossy cells in the rat dentate gyrus. *Hippocampus* 15:691–696.

Ma Y, Hu H, Agmon A (2012) Short-term plasticity of unitary inhibitory-to-inhibitory synapses depends on the presynaptic interneuron subtype. *J Neurosci* 32:983–988.

Maccaferri G (2005) Stratum oriens horizontal interneurone diversity and hippocampal network dynamics. *J Physiol* 562:73–80.

Maccaferri G, McBain CJ (1996) The hyperpolarization-activated current (Ih) and its contribution to pacemaker activity in rat CA1 hippocampal stratum oriens-alveus interneurones. *J Physiol* 497(Pt 1):119–130.

Maccaferri G, Roberts JD, Szucs P, Cottingham CA, Somogyi P (2000) Cell surface domain specific postsynaptic currents evoked by identified GABAergic neurones in rat hippocampus in vitro. *J Physiol* 524(Pt 1):91–116.

Maccaferri G, Toth K, McBain CJ (1998) Target-specific expression of presynaptic mossy fiber plasticity. *Science* 279:1368–1370.

MacDermott AB, Role LW, Siegelbaum SA (1999) Presynaptic ionotropic receptors and the control of transmitter release. *Annu Rev Neurosci* 22:443–485.

Macrides F, Eichenbaum HB, Forbes WB (1982) Temporal relationship between sniffing and the limbic theta rhythm during odor discrimination reversal learning. *J Neurosci* 2:1705–1717.

Madison DV, Lancaster B, Nicoll RA (1987) Voltage clamp analysis of cholinergic action in the hippocampus. *J Neurosci* 7:733–741.

Madison DV, Nicoll RA (1986) Actions of noradrenaline recorded intracellularly in rat hippocampal CA1 pyramidal neurones, in vitro. *J Physiol* 372:221–244.

Madison DV, Nicoll RA (1988) Enkephalin hyperpolarizes interneurones in the rat hippocampus. *J Physiol* 398:123–130.

Magee JC (2000) Dendritic integration of excitatory synaptic input. *Nat Rev Neurosci* 1:181–190.

Magee JC (2001) Dendritic mechanisms of phase precession in hippocampal CA1 pyramidal neurons. *J Neurophysiol* 86:528–532.

Magee JC, Cook EP (2000) Somatic EPSP amplitude is independent of synapse location in hippocampal pyramidal neurons. *Nat Neurosci* 3:895–903.

Maier N, Morris G, Schuchmann S, Korotkova T, Ponomarenko A, Bohm C, Wozny C, Schmitz D (2012) Cannabinoids disrupt hippocampal sharp wave-ripples via inhibition of glutamate release. *Hippocampus* 22:1350–1362.

Maier N, Nimmrich V, Draguhn A (2003) Cellular and network mechanisms underlying spontaneous sharp wave-ripple complexes in mouse hippocampal slices. *J Physiol* 550:873–887.

Makara JK, Magee JC (2013) Variable dendritic integration in hippocampal CA3 pyramidal neurons. *Neuron* 80:1438–1450.

Mallory CS, Giocomo LM (2018) Heterogeneity in hippocampal place coding. *Curr Opin Neurobiol* 49:158–167.

Mann EO, Radcliffe CA, Paulsen O (2005) Hippocampal gamma-frequency oscillations: from interneurones to pyramidal cells, and back. *J Physiol* 562:55–63.

Mann EO, Suckling JM, Hajos N, Greenfield SA, Paulsen O (2005) Perisomatic feedback inhibition underlies cholinergically induced fast network oscillations in the rat hippocampus in vitro. *Neuron* 45:105–117.

Marder E (2012) Neuromodulation of neuronal circuits: back to the future. *Neuron* 76:1–11.

Marissal T, Bonifazi P, Picardo MA, Nardou R, Petit LF, Baude A, Fishell GJ, Ben-Ari Y, Cossart R (2012) Pioneer glutamatergic cells develop into a morpho-functionally distinct population in the juvenile CA3 hippocampus. *Nat Commun* 3:1316.

Markwardt SJ, Dieni CV, Wadiche JI, Overstreet-Wadiche L (2011) Ivy/neurogliaform interneurons coordinate activity in the neurogenic niche. *Nat Neurosci* 14:1407–1409.

Marr D (1971) Simple memory: a theory for archicortex. *Philos Trans R Soc Lond B Biol Sci* 262:23–81.

Marrosu F, Portas C, Mascia MS, Casu MA, Fa M, Giagheddu M, Imperato A, Gessa GL (1995) Microdialysis measurement of cortical and hippocampal acetylcholine release during sleep-wake cycle in freely moving cats. *Brain Res* 671:329–332.

Martina M (2000) Distal initiation and active propagation of action potentials in interneuron dendrites. *Science* 287:295–300.

Masurkar AV, Srinivas KV, Brann DH, Warren R, Lowes DC, Siegelbaum SA (2017) Medial and lateral entorhinal cortex differentially excite deep versus superficial CA1 pyramidal neurons. *Cell Rep* 18:148–160.

Matyas F, Freund TF, Gulyas AI (2004) Immunocytochemically defined interneuron populations in the hippocampus of mouse strains used in transgenic technology. *Hippocampus* 14:460–481.

McBain CJ (2008) New directions in synaptic and network plasticity—a move away from NMDA receptor mediated plasticity. *J Physiol* 586:1473–1474.

McBain CJ, DiChiara TJ, Kauer JA (1994) Activation of metabotropic glutamate receptors differentially affects two classes of hippocampal interneurons and potentiates excitatory synaptic transmission. *J Neurosci* 14:4433–4445.

McBain CJ, Kauer JA (2009) Presynaptic plasticity: targeted control of inhibitory networks. *Curr Opin Neurobiol* 19:254–262.

McClelland JL, Goddard NH (1996) Considerations arising from a complementary learning systems perspective on hippocampus and neocortex. *Hippocampus* 6:654–665.

McClelland JL, Rumelhart DE (1985) Distributed memory and the representation of general and specific information. *J Exp Psychol Gen* 114:159–197.

McMahon LL, Kauer JA (1997) Hippocampal interneurons are excited via serotonin-gated ion channels. *J Neurophysiol* 78:2493–2502.

McNamara CG, Dupret D (2017) Two sources of dopamine for the hippocampus. *Trends Neurosci* 40:383–384.

McNaughton BL, Morris RGM (1987) Hippocampal synaptic enhancement and information storage within a distributed memory system. *Trends Neurosci* 10:408–415.

McNaughton BL, Nadel L (1990) Hebb-Marr networks and the neurobiological representation of action in space. In: Neuroscience and Connectionist Theory, pp 1–63. Hillsdale, NJ: Lawrence Erlbaum Associates.

McQuiston AR (2014) Acetylcholine release and inhibitory interneuron activity in hippocampal CA1. *Front Synaptic Neurosci* 6:20.

McQuiston AR, Madison DV (1999a) Muscarinic receptor activity induces an afterdepolarization in a subpopulation of hippocampal CA1 interneurons. *J Neurosci* 19:5703–5710.

McQuiston AR, Madison DV (1999b) Nicotinic receptor activation excites distinct subtypes of interneurons in the rat hippocampus. *J Neurosci* 19:2887–2896.

Megias M, Emri Z, Freund TF, Gulyas AI (2001) Total number and distribution of inhibitory and excitatory synapses on hippocampal CA1 pyramidal cells. *Neuroscience* 102:527–540.

Melzer S, Michael M, Caputi A, Eliava M, Fuchs EC, Whittington MA, Monyer H (2012) Long-range-projecting GABAergic neurons modulate inhibition in hippocampus and entorhinal cortex. *Science* 335:1506–1510.

Menendez De La Prida L (2006) Functional features of the rat subicular microcircuits studied in vitro. *Behavioural brain research* 174(2):198–205.

Menendez De La Prida L, Suarez F, Pozo MA (2003) Electrophysiological and morphological diversity of neurons from the rat subicular complex in vitro. *Hippocampus* 13(6):728–744.

Mercer A, Botcher NA, Eastlake K, Thomson AM (2012) SP–SR interneurones: a novel class of neurones of the CA2 region of the hippocampus. *Hippocampus* 22(8):1758–1769.

Mercer A, Eastlake K, Trigg HL, Thomson AM (2012) Local circuitry involving parvalbumin-positive basket cells in the CA2 region of the hippocampus. *Hippocampus* 22(1):43–56.

Mercer A, Trigg HL, Thomson AM (2007) Characterization of neurons in the CA2 subfield of the adult rat hippocampus. *Journal of Neuroscience* 27(27): 7329–7338.

Meyer AH, Katona I, Blatow M, Rozov A, Monyer H (2002) In vivo labeling of parvalbumin-positive interneurons and analysis of electrical coupling in identified neurons. *J Neurosci* 22:7055–7064.

Miles R, Toth K, Gulyas AI, Hajos N, Freund TF (1996) Differences between somatic and dendritic inhibition in the hippocampus. *Neuron* 16:815–823.

Milner TA, Shah P, Pierce JP (2000) Beta-adrenergic receptors primarily are located on the dendrites of granule cells and interneurons but also are found on astrocytes and a few presynaptic profiles in the rat dentate gyrus. *Synapse* 36:178–193.

Milstein AD, Bloss EB, Apostolides PF, Vaidya SP, Dilly GA, Zemelman BV, Magee JC (2015) Inhibitory gating of input comparison in the CA1 microcircuit. *Neuron* 87:1274–1289.

Mishra RK, Kim S, Guzman SJ, Jonas P (2016) Symmetric spike timing-dependent plasticity at CA3-CA3 synapses optimizes storage and recall in autoassociative networks. *Nat Commun* 7:11552.

Mistry R, Dennis S, Frerking M, Mellor JR (2011) Dentate gyrus granule cell firing patterns can induce mossy fiber long-term potentiation in vitro. *Hippocampus* 21:1157–1168.

Mizuseki K, Buzsaki G (2013) Preconfigured, skewed distribution of firing rates in the hippocampus and entorhinal cortex. *Cell Rep* 4:1010–1021.

Mizuseki K, Diba K, Pastalkova E, Buzsaki G (2011) Hippocampal CA1 pyramidal cells form functionally distinct sublayers. *Nat Neurosci* 14:1174–1181.

Mizuseki K, Sirota A, Pastalkova E, Buzsaki G (2009) Theta oscillations provide temporal windows for local circuit computation in the entorhinal-hippocampal loop. *Neuron* 64:267–280.

Montgomery SM, Buzsaki G (2007) Gamma oscillations dynamically couple hippocampal CA3 and CA1 regions during memory task performance. *Proc Natl Acad Sci U S A* 104:14495–14500.

Mori M, Gahwiler BH, Gerber U (2007) Recruitment of an inhibitory hippocampal network after bursting in a single granule cell. *Proc Natl Acad Sci U S A* 104:7640–7645.

Morris BJ, Johnston HM (1995) A role for hippocampal opioids in long-term functional plasticity. *Trends Neurosci* 18:350–355.

Mott DD, Turner DA, Okazaki MM, Lewis DV (1997) Interneurons of the dentate-hilus border of the rat dentate gyrus: morphological and electrophysiological heterogeneity. *J Neurosci* 17:3990–4005.

Muller C, Beck H, Coulter D, Remy S (2012) Inhibitory control of linear and supralinear dendritic excitation in CA1 pyramidal neurons. *Neuron* 75:851–864.

Müller C, Remy S (2014) Dendritic inhibition mediated by O-LM and bistratified interneurons in the hippocampus. *Frontiers in synaptic neuroscience* 6:23.

Muller C, Remy S (2018) Septo-hippocampal interaction. *Cell Tissue Res* 373:565–575.

Murchison CF, Zhang XY, Zhang WP, Ouyang M, Lee A, Thomas SA (2004) A distinct role for norepinephrine in memory retrieval. *Cell* 117:131–143.

Myers CE, Scharfman HE (2009) A role for hilar cells in pattern separation in the dentate gyrus: a computational approach. *Hippocampus* 19:321–337.

Naber PA, Witter MP (1998) Subicular efferents are organized mostly as parallel projections: a double-labeling, retrograde-tracing study in the rat. *Journal of comparative neurology* 393(3):284–297.

Nakashiba T, Buhl DL, McHugh TJ, Tonegawa S (2009) Hippocampal CA3 output is crucial for ripple-associated reactivation and consolidation of memory. *Neuron* 62:781–787.

Nakashiba T, Young JZ, McHugh TJ, Buhl DL, Tonegawa S (2008) Transgenic inhibition of synaptic transmission reveals role of CA3 output in hippocampal learning. *Science* 319:1260–1264.

Nakazawa K, Quirk MC, Chitwood RA, Watanabe M, Yeckel MF, Sun LD, Kato A, Carr CA, Johnston D, Wilson MA, Tonegawa S (2002) Requirement for hippocampal CA3 NMDA receptors in associative memory recall. *Science* 297:211–218.

Nasrallah K, Piskorowski RA, Chevaleyre V (2015) Inhibitory plasticity permits the recruitment of CA2 pyramidal neurons by CA3. *Eneuro* 2(4).

Nasrallah K, Therreau L, Robert V, Huang AJ, McHugh TJ, Piskorowski RA, Chevaleyre V (2019) Routing hippocampal information flow through parvalbumin interneuron plasticity in area CA2. *Cell reports* 27(1):86–98.

Neu A, Foldy C, Soltesz I (2007) Postsynaptic origin of CB1-dependent tonic inhibition of GABA release at cholecystokinin-positive basket cell to pyramidal cell synapses in the CA1 region of the rat hippocampus. *J Physiol* 578:233–247.

Neubrandt M, Olah VJ, Brunner J, Marosi EL, Soltesz I, Szabadics J (2018) Single bursts of individual granule cells functionally rearrange feedforward inhibition. *J Neurosci* 38:1711–1724.

Neubrandt M, Olah VJ, Brunner J, Szabadics J (2017) Feedforward inhibition is randomly wired from individual granule cells onto CA3 pyramidal cells. *Hippocampus* 27:1034–1039.

Nicoll RA, Schmitz D (2005) Synaptic plasticity at hippocampal mossy fibre synapses. *Nat Rev Neurosci* 6:863–876.

Nitz DA, McNaughton BL (1999) Hippocampal EEG and unit activity responses to modulation of serotonergic median raphe neurons in the freely behaving rat. *Learn Mem* 6:153–167.

Norenberg A, Hu H, Vida I, Bartos M, Jonas P (2010) Distinct non-uniform cable properties optimize rapid and efficient activation of fast-spiking GABAergic interneurons. *Proc Natl Acad Sci U S A* 107:894–899.

Nusser Z, Roberts JD, Baude A, Richards JG, Sieghart W, Somogyi P (1995) Immunocytochemical localization of the alpha 1 and beta 2/3 subunits of the GABAA receptor in relation to specific GABAergic synapses in the dentate gyrus. *Eur J Neurosci* 7:630–646.

Nyiri G, Freund TF, Somogyi P (2001) Input-dependent synaptic targeting of alpha(2)-subunit-containing GABA(A) receptors in synapses of hippocampal pyramidal cells of the rat. *Eur J Neurosci* 13:428–442.

Ohshiro T, Angelaki DE, DeAngelis GC (2011) A normalization model of multisensory integration. *Nat Neurosci* 14:775–782.

O'Keefe J, Recce ML (1993) Phase relationship between hippocampal place units and the EEG theta rhythm. *Hippocampus* 3:317–330.

Okuyama T, Kitamura T, Roy DS, Itohara S, Tonegawa S (2016) Ventral CA1 neurons store social memory. *Science* 353:1536–1541.

Olah S, Fule M, Komlosi G, Varga C, Baldi R, Barzo P, Tamas G (2009) Regulation of cortical microcircuits by unitary GABA-mediated volume transmission. *Nature* 461:1278–1281.

Oliva A, Fernandez-Ruiz A, Buzsaki G, Berenyi A (2016) Role of hippocampal CA2 region in triggering sharp-wave ripples. *Neuron* 91:1342–1355.

Oliva AA, Jr., Jiang M, Lam T, Smith KL, Swann JW (2000) Novel hippocampal interneuronal subtypes identified using transgenic mice that express green fluorescent protein in GABAergic interneurons. *J Neurosci* 20:3354–3368.

Olsen RW, Sieghart W (2009) GABA A receptors: subtypes provide diversity of function and pharmacology. *Neuropharmacology* 56:141–148.

O'Mara S (2005) The subiculum: what it does, what it might do, and what neuroanatomy has yet to tell us. *Journal of anatomy* 207(3):271–282.

O'Mara SM, Commins S, Anderson M, Gigg J (2001) The subiculum: a review of form, physiology and function. *Progress in neurobiology* 64(2):129–155.

O'Reilly RC, McClelland JL (1994) Hippocampal conjunctive encoding, storage, and recall: avoiding a trade-off. *Hippocampus* 4:661–682.

Otero-Millan J, Troncoso XG, Macknik SL, Serrano-Pedraza I, Martinez-Conde S (2008) Saccades and microsaccades during visual fixation, exploration, and search: foundations for a common saccadic generator. *J Vis* 8:21 21–18.

Owen SF, Tuncdemir SN, Bader PL, Tirko NN, Fishell G, Tsien RW (2013) Oxytocin enhances hippocampal spike transmission by modulating fast-spiking interneurons. *Nature* **500**:458–462.

Palacios-Filardo J, Mellor JR (2019) Neuromodulation of hippocampal long-term synaptic plasticity. *Curr Opin Neurobiol* **54**:37–43.

Papp OI, Karlocai MR, Toth IE, Freund TF, Hajos N (2013) Different input and output properties characterize parvalbumin-positive basket and Axo-axonic cells in the hippocampal CA3 subfield. *Hippocampus* **23**:903–918.

Patel J, Schomburg EW, Berenyi A, Fujisawa S, Buzsaki G (2013) Local generation and propagation of ripples along the septotemporal axis of the hippocampus. *J Neurosci* **33**:17029–17041.

Pawelzik H, Bannister AP, Deuchars J, Ilia M, Thomson AM (1999) Modulation of bistratified cell IPSPs and basket cell IPSPs by pentobarbitone sodium, diazepam and Zn2+: dual recordings in slices of adult rat hippocampus. *Eur J Neurosci* **11**:3552–3564.

Pawelzik H, Hughes DI, Thomson AM (2002) Physiological and morphological diversity of immunocytochemically defined parvalbumin- and cholecystokinin-positive interneurones in CA1 of the adult rat hippocampus. *J Comp Neurol* **443**:346–367.

Pelkey KA, Chittajallu R, Craig MT, Tricoire L, Wester JC, McBain CJ (2017) Hippocampal GABAergic inhibitory interneurons. *Physiol Rev* **97**:1619–1747.

Pelkey KA, McBain CJ (2008) Target-cell-dependent plasticity within the mossy fibre-CA3 circuit reveals compartmentalized regulation of presynaptic function at divergent release sites. *J Physiol* **586**:1495–1502.

Pelkey KA, Topolnik L, Lacaille JC, McBain CJ (2006) Compartmentalized Ca(2+) channel regulation at divergent mossy-fiber release sites underlies target cell-dependent plasticity. *Neuron* **52**:497–510.

Pelkey KA, Topolnik L, Yuan XQ, Lacaille JC, McBain CJ (2008) State-dependent cAMP sensitivity of presynaptic function underlies metaplasticity in a hippocampal feedforward inhibitory circuit. *Neuron* **60**:980–987.

Penttonen M, Kamondi A, Acsady L, Buzsaki G (1998) Gamma frequency oscillation in the hippocampus of the rat: intracellular analysis in vivo. *Eur J Neurosci* **10**:718–728.

Pernia-Andrade AJ, Jonas P (2014) Theta-gamma-modulated synaptic currents in hippocampal granule cells in vivo define a mechanism for network oscillations. *Neuron* **81**:140–152.

Petilla Interneuron Nomenclature G, Ascoli GA, Alonso-Nanclares L, Anderson SA, Barrionuevo G, Benavides-Piccione R, Burkhalter A, Buzsaki G, Cauli B, Defelipe J, et al. (2008) Petilla terminology: nomenclature of features of GABAergic interneurons of the cerebral cortex. *Nat Rev Neurosci* **9**:557–568.

Petreanu L, Mao T, Sternson SM, Svoboda K (2009) The subcellular organization of neocortical excitatory connections. *Nature* **457**:1142–1145.

Petrovic MM, Nowacki J, Olivo V, Tsaneva-Atanasova K, Randall AD, Mellor JR (2012) Inhibition of postsynaptic Kv7/KCNQ/M channels facilitates long-term potentiation in the hippocampus. *PLoS One* **7**:e30402.

Pi HJ, Hangya B, Kvitsiani D, Sanders JI, Huang ZJ, Kepecs A (2013) Cortical interneurons that specialize in disinhibitory control. *Nature* **503**:521–524.

Pike FG, Goddard RS, Suckling JM, Ganter P, Kasthuri N, Paulsen O (2000) Distinct frequency preferences of different types of rat hippocampal neurones in response to oscillatory input currents. *J Physiol* **529**(Pt 1):205–213.

Piskorowski RA, Chevaleyre V (2012) Synaptic integration by different dendritic compartments of hippocampal CA1 and CA2 pyramidal neurons. *Cellular and Molecular Life Sciences* **69**:75–88.

Piskorowski RA, Chevaleyre V (2013) Delta-opioid receptors mediate unique plasticity onto parvalbumin-expressing interneurons in area CA2 of the hippocampus. *Journal of Neuroscience* **33**(36):14567–14578.

Pitkanen A, Pikkarainen M, Nurminen N, Ylinen A (2000) Reciprocal connections between the amygdala and the hippocampal formation, perirhinal cortex, and postrhinal cortex in rat. A review. *Ann N Y Acad Sci* **911**:369–391.

Pouille F, Marin-Burgin A, Adesnik H, Atallah BV, Scanziani M (2009) Input normalization by global feedforward inhibition expands cortical dynamic range. *Nat Neurosci* **12**:1577–1585.

Pouille F, Scanziani M (2001) Enforcement of temporal fidelity in pyramidal cells by somatic feed-forward inhibition. *Science* **293**:1159–1163.

Pouille F, Scanziani M (2004) Routing of spike series by dynamic circuits in the hippocampus. *Nature* **429**:717–723.

Pouille F, Watkinson O, Scanziani M, Trevelyan AJ (2013) The contribution of synaptic location to inhibitory gain control in pyramidal cells. *Physiol Rep* **1**:e00067.

Price CJ, Cauli B, Kovacs ER, Kulik A, Lambolez B, Shigemoto R, Capogna M (2005) Neurogliaform neurons form a novel inhibitory network in the hippocampal CA1 area. *J Neurosci* **25**:6775–6786.

Price CJ, Scott R, Rusakov DA, Capogna M (2008) GABA(B) receptor modulation of feedforward inhibition through hippocampal neurogliaform cells. *J Neurosci* **28**:6974–6982.

Qasim SE, Jacobs J (2016) Human hippocampal theta oscillations during movement without visual cues. *Neuron* **89**:1121–1123.

Racz B, Halasy K (2002) Kappa opioid receptor is expressed by somatostatin- and neuropeptide Y-containing interneurons in the rat hippocampus. *Brain Res* **931**:50–55.

Rajasethupathy P, Sankaran S, Marshel JH, Kim CK, Ferenczi E, Lee SY, … Deisseroth K (2015) Projections from neocortex mediate top-down control of memory retrieval. *Nature* **526**(7575):653–659.

Ranganathan GN, Apostolides PF, Harnett MT, Xu NL, Druckmann S, Magee JC (2018) Active dendritic integration and mixed neocortical network representations during an adaptive sensing behavior. *Nat Neurosci* **21**:1583–1590.

Ratzliff A, Santhakumar V, Howard A, Soltesz I (2002) Mossy cells in epilepsy: rigor mortis or vigor mortis? *Trends Neurosci* **25**: 140–144.

Raus Balind S, Mago A, Ahmadi M, Kis N, Varga-Nemeth Z, Lorincz A, Makara JK (2019) Diverse synaptic and dendritic mechanisms of complex spike burst generation in hippocampal CA3 pyramidal cells. *Nat Commun* **10**:1859.

Rebola N, Carta M, Mulle C (2017) Operation and plasticity of hippocampal CA3 circuits: implications for memory encoding. *Nat Rev Neurosci* **18**:208–220.

Remy S, Spruston N (2007) Dendritic spikes induce single-burst long-term potentiation. *Proc Natl Acad Sci U S A* **104**:17192–17197.

Renno-Costa C, Teixeira DG, Soltesz I (2019) Regulation of gamma-frequency oscillation by feedforward inhibition: a computational modeling study. *Hippocampus* **29**:957–970.

Restivo L, Niibori Y, Mercaldo V, Josselyn SA, Frankland PW (2015) Development of adult-generated cell connectivity with excitatory and inhibitory cell populations in the hippocampus. *J Neurosci* **35**:10600–10612.

Ribak CE, Seress L (1983) Five types of basket cell in the hippocampal dentate gyrus: a combined Golgi and electron microscopic study. *J Neurocytol* **12**:577–597.

Robbe D, Montgomery SM, Thome A, Rueda-Orozco PE, McNaughton BL, Buzsaki G (2006) Cannabinoids reveal importance of spike timing coordination in hippocampal function. *Nat Neurosci* **9**:1526–1533.

Robert V, Cassim S, Chevaleyre V, Piskorowski RA (2018) Hippocampal area CA2: properties and contribution to hippocampal function. *Cell and tissue research* **373**:525–540.

Rollenhagen A, Satzler K, Rodriguez EP, Jonas P, Frotscher M, Lubke JH (2007) Structural determinants of transmission at large hippocampal mossy fiber synapses. *J Neurosci* **27**:10434–10444.

Rolls ET (2007) An attractor network in the hippocampus: theory and neurophysiology. *Learn Mem* **14**:714–731.

Rolls ET (2013) A quantitative theory of the functions of the hippocampal CA3 network in memory. *Front Cell Neurosci* **7**:98.

Rolls ET, Kesner RP (2006) A computational theory of hippocampal function, and empirical tests of the theory. *Prog Neurobiol* **79**:1–48.

Rolls ET, Treves A (1994) Neural networks in the brain involved in memory and recall. *Prog Brain Res* **102**:335–341.

Rosen ZB, Cheung S, Siegelbaum SA (2015) Midbrain dopamine neurons bidirectionally regulate CA3-CA1 synaptic drive. *Nat Neurosci* **18**:1763–1771.

Royer S, Zemelman BV, Losonczy A, Kim J, Chance F, Magee JC, Buzsaki G (2012) Control of timing, rate and bursts of hippocampal place cells by dendritic and somatic inhibition. *Nat Neurosci* **15**:769–775.

Ruediger S, Vittori C, Bednarek E, Genoud C, Strata P, Sacchetti B, Caroni P (2011) Learning-related feedforward inhibitory connectivity growth required for memory precision. *Nature* **473**:514–518.

Salin PA, Scanziani M, Malenka RC, Nicoll RA (1996) Distinct short-term plasticity at two excitatory synapses in the hippocampus. *Proc Natl Acad Sci U S A* **93**:13304–13309.

San Antonio A, Liban K, Ikrar T, Tsyganovskiy E, Xu X (2014) Distinct physiological and developmental properties of hippocampal CA2 subfield revealed by using anti-Purkinje cell protein 4 (PCP4) immunostaining. *Journal of Comparative Neurology* **522**(6):1333–1354.

Sara SJ (2009) The locus coeruleus and noradrenergic modulation of cognition. *Nat Rev Neurosci* **10**:211–223.

Sasaki T, Piatti VC, Hwaun E, Ahmadi S, Lisman JE, Leutgeb S, Leutgeb JK (2018) Dentate network activity is necessary for spatial working memory by supporting CA3 sharp-wave ripple generation and prospective firing of CA3 neurons. *Nat Neurosci* **21**:258–269.

Savanthrapadian S, Meyer T, Elgueta C, Booker SA, Vida I, Bartos M (2014) Synaptic properties of SOM- and CCK-expressing cells in dentate gyrus interneuron networks. *J Neurosci* **34**:8197–8209.

Savin C, Dayan P, Lengyel M (2014) Optimal recall from bounded metaplastic synapses: predicting functional adaptations in hippocampal area CA3. *PLoS Comput Biol* **10**:e1003489.

Scanziani M (2000) GABA spillover activates postsynaptic GABA(B) receptors to control rhythmic hippocampal activity. *Neuron* **25**:673–681.

Schaffer K (1892) Beitrag zur Histologie der Ammonshornformation. *Arch Mikr Anat* **39**:611–632.

Scharfman H, Goodman J, McCloskey D (2007) Ectopic granule cells of the rat dentate gyrus. *Dev Neurosci* **29**:14–27.

Scharfman HE (1992) Blockade of excitation reveals inhibition of dentate spiny hilar neurons recorded in rat hippocampal slices. *J Neurophysiol* **68**:978–984.

Scharfman HE (1995a) Electrophysiological diversity of pyramidal-shaped neurons at the granule cell layer/hilus border of the rat dentate gyrus recorded in vitro. *Hippocampus* **5**:287–305.

Scharfman HE (1995b) Electrophysiological evidence that dentate hilar mossy cells are excitatory and innervate both granule cells and interneurons. *J Neurophysiol* **74**:179–194.

Scharfman HE (1999) The role of nonprincipal cells in dentate gyrus excitability and its relevance to animal models of epilepsy and temporal lobe epilepsy. *Adv Neurol* **79**:805–820.

Scharfman HE (2016) The enigmatic mossy cell of the dentate gyrus. *Nat Rev Neurosci* **17**:562–575.

Scharfman HE (2018) Advances in understanding hilar mossy cells of the dentate gyrus. *Cell Tissue Res* **373**:643–652.

Scharfman HE, Bernstein HL (2015) Potential implications of a monosynaptic pathway from mossy cells to adult-born granule cells of the dentate gyrus. *Front Syst Neurosci* **9**:112.

Scharfman HE, Myers CE (2012) Hilar mossy cells of the dentate gyrus: a historical perspective. *Front Neural Circuits* **6**:106.

Scharfman HE, Pierce JP (2012) New insights into the role of hilar ectopic granule cells in the dentate gyrus based on quantitative anatomic analysis and three-dimensional reconstruction. *Epilepsia* **53**(Suppl 1):109–115.

Scharfman HE, Schwartzkroin PA (1988) Electrophysiology of morphologically identified mossy cells of the dentate hilus recorded in guinea pig hippocampal slices. *J Neurosci* **8**:3812–3821.

Schlingloff D, Kali S, Freund TF, Hajos N, Gulyas AI (2014) Mechanisms of sharp wave initiation and ripple generation. *J Neurosci* **34**:11385–11398.

Schmitz D, Empson RM, Gloveli T, Heinemann U (1997) Serotonin blocks different patterns of low Mg2+-induced epileptiform activity in rat entorhinal cortex, but not hippocampus. *Neuroscience* **76**:449–458.

Schomburg EW, Fernandez-Ruiz A, Mizuseki K, Berenyi A, Anastassiou CA, Koch C, Buzsaki G (2014) Theta phase segregation of input-specific gamma patterns in entorhinal-hippocampal networks. *Neuron* **84**:470–485.

Schreiner D, Nguyen TM, Scheiffele P (2014) Polymorphic receptors: neuronal functions and molecular mechanisms of diversification. *Curr Opin Neurobiol* **27**:25–30.

Schulz JM, Knoflach F, Hernandez MC, Bischofberger J (2018) Dendrite-targeting interneurons control synaptic NMDA-receptor activation via nonlinear alpha5-GABAA receptors. *Nat Commun* **9**:3576.

Schwerdtfeger WK, Buhl E (1986) Various types of non-pyramidal hippocampal neurons project to the septum and contralateral hippocampus. *Brain Res* **386**:146–154.

Seidenbecher T, Laxmi TR, Stork O, Pape HC (2003) Amygdalar and hippocampal theta rhythm synchronization during fear memory retrieval. *Science* **301**:846–850.

Seress L, Pokorny J (1981) Structure of the granular layer of the rat dentate gyrus: a light microscopic and Golgi study. *J Anat* **133**:181–195.

Sharma G, Grybko M, Vijayaraghavan S (2008) Action potential-independent and nicotinic receptor-mediated concerted release of multiple quanta at hippocampal CA3-mossy fiber synapses. *J Neurosci* **28**:2563–2575.

Sharma G, Vijayaraghavan S (2003) Modulation of presynaptic store calcium induces release of glutamate and postsynaptic firing. *Neuron* **38**:929–939.

Sheffield ME, Best TK, Mensh BD, Kath WL, Spruston N (2011) Slow integration leads to persistent action potential firing in distal axons of coupled interneurons. *Nat Neurosci* **14**:200–207.

Sheffield MEJ, Adoff MD, Dombeck DA (2017) Increased prevalence of calcium transients across the dendritic arbor during place field formation. *Neuron* **96**:490–504, e495.

Shinohara Y, Hosoya A, Yahagi K, Ferecskó AS, Yaguchi K, Sík A, ... Hirase H (2012) Hippocampal CA3 and CA2 have distinct bilateral innervation patterns to CA1 in rodents. *European Journal of Neuroscience* **35**(5):702–710.

Sik A, Penttonen M, Buzsaki G (1997) Interneurons in the hippocampal dentate gyrus: an in vivo intracellular study. *Eur J Neurosci* **9**:573–588.

Sik A, Penttonen M, Ylinen A, Buzsaki G (1995) Hippocampal CA1 interneurons: an in vivo intracellular labeling study. *J Neurosci* 15:6651–6665.

Sik A, Ylinen A, Penttonen M, Buzsaki G (1994) Inhibitory CA1-CA3-hilar region feedback in the hippocampus. *Science* 265:1722–1724.

Sil'kis IG (2010) Paradoxical sleep as a tool for understanding the hippocampal mechanisms of contextual memory. *Neurosci Behav Physiol* 40:5–19.

Simon AP, Poindessous-Jazat F, Dutar P, Epelbaum J, Bassant MH (2006) Firing properties of anatomically identified neurons in the medial septum of anesthetized and unanesthetized restrained rats. *J Neurosci* 26:9038–9046.

Singer W (1993) Synchronization of cortical activity and its putative role in information processing and learning. *Annu Rev Physiol* 55:349–374.

Sirota A, Csicsvari J, Buhl D, Buzsaki G (2003) Communication between neocortex and hippocampus during sleep in rodents. *Proc Natl Acad Sci U S A* 100:2065–2069.

Smith CC, Greene RW (2012) CNS dopamine transmission mediated by noradrenergic innervation. *J Neurosci* 32:6072–6080.

Sohal VS, Zhang F, Yizhar O, Deisseroth K (2009) Parvalbumin neurons and gamma rhythms enhance cortical circuit performance. *Nature* 459:698–702.

Soltesz I, Bourassa J, Deschenes M (1993) The behavior of mossy cells of the rat dentate gyrus during theta oscillations in vivo. *Neuroscience* 57:555–564.

Soltesz I, Deschenes M (1993) Low- and high-frequency membrane potential oscillations during theta activity in CA1 and CA3 pyramidal neurons of the rat hippocampus under ketamine-xylazine anesthesia. *J Neurophysiol* 70:97–116.

Soltesz I, Losonczy A (2018) CA1 pyramidal cell diversity enabling parallel information processing in the hippocampus. *Nat Neurosci* 21:484–493.

Somogyi J, Baude A, Omori Y, Shimizu H, El Mestikawy S, Fukaya M, Shigemoto R, Watanabe M, Somogyi P (2004) GABAergic basket cells expressing cholecystokinin contain vesicular glutamate transporter type 3 (VGLUT3) in their synaptic terminals in hippocampus and isocortex of the rat. *Eur J Neurosci* 19:552–569.

Somogyi P, Freund TF, Hodgson AJ, Somogyi J, Beroukas D, Chubb IW (1985) Identified axo-axonic cells are immunoreactive for GABA in the hippocampus and visual cortex of the cat. *Brain Res* 332:143–149.

Somogyi P, Katona L, Klausberger T, Lasztoczi B, Viney TJ (2014) Temporal redistribution of inhibition over neuronal subcellular domains underlies state-dependent rhythmic change of excitability in the hippocampus. *Philos Trans R Soc Lond B Biol Sci* 369:20120518.

Somogyi P, Klausberger T (2005) Defined types of cortical interneurone structure space and spike timing in the hippocampus. *J Physiol* 562:9–26.

Soriano E, Frotscher M (1989) A GABAergic axo-axonic cell in the fascia dentata controls the main excitatory hippocampal pathway. *Brain Res* 503:170–174.

Spruston N (2008) Pyramidal neurons: dendritic structure and synaptic integration. *Nat Rev Neurosci* 9:206–221.

Stachniak TJ, Sylwestrak EL, Scheiffele P, Hall BJ, Ghosh A (2019) Elfn1-induced constitutive activation of mGluR7 determines frequency-dependent recruitment of somatostatin interneurons. *J Neurosci* 39:4461–4474.

Staff NP, Jung HY, Thiagarajan T, Yao M, Spruston N (2000) Resting and active properties of pyramidal neurons in subiculum and CA1 of rat hippocampus. *Journal of neurophysiology* 84(5):2398–2408.

Stark E, Eichler R, Roux L, Fujisawa S, Rotstein HG, Buzsaki G (2013) Inhibition-induced theta resonance in cortical circuits. *Neuron* 80:1263–1276.

Stark E, Roux L, Eichler R, Senzai Y, Royer S, Buzsaki G (2014) Pyramidal cell-interneuron interactions underlie hippocampal ripple oscillations. *Neuron* 83:467–480.

Steriade M (2004) Acetylcholine systems and rhythmic activities during the waking—sleep cycle. *Prog Brain Res* 145:179–196.

Steward O, Scoville SA (1976) Cells of origin of entorhinal cortical afferents to the hippocampus and fascia dentata of the rat. *J Comp Neurol* 169:347–370.

Stewart MARK, Wong RK (1993) Intrinsic properties and evoked responses of guinea pig subicular neurons in vitro. *Journal of neurophysiology* 70(1):232–245.

Strange BA, Witter MP, Lein ES, Moser EI (2014) Functional organization of the hippocampal longitudinal axis. *Nat Rev Neurosci* 15:655–669.

Sullivan D, Csicsvari J, Mizuseki K, Montgomery S, Diba K, Buzsaki G (2011) Relationships between hippocampal sharp waves, ripples, and fast gamma oscillation: influence of dentate and entorhinal cortical activity. *J Neurosci* 31:8605–8616.

Sun HY, Lyons SA, Dobrunz LE (2005) Mechanisms of target-cell specific short-term plasticity at Schaffer collateral synapses onto interneurones versus pyramidal cells in juvenile rats. *J Physiol* 568:815–840.

Sun Q, Sotayo A, Cazzulino AS, Snyder AM, Denny CA, Siegelbaum SA (2017) Proximodistal heterogeneity of hippocampal CA3 pyramidal neuron intrinsic properties, connectivity, and reactivation during memory recall. *Neuron* 95:656–672, e653.

Sun Q, Srinivas KV, Sotayo A, Siegelbaum SA (2014) Dendritic Na+ spikes enable cortical input to drive action potential output from hippocampal CA2 pyramidal neurons. *Elife* 3:e04551.

Sun Y, Grieco SF, Holmes TC, Xu X (2017) Local and long-range circuit connections to hilar mossy cells in the dentate gyrus. *Eneuro* 4(2).

Suzuki SS, Smith GK (1988) Spontaneous EEG spikes in the normal hippocampus: IV. Effects of medial septum and entorhinal cortex lesions. *Electroencephalogr Clin Neurophysiol* 70:73–83.

Svoboda KR, Adams CE, Lupica CR (1999) Opioid receptor subtype expression defines morphologically distinct classes of hippocampal interneurons. *J Neurosci* 19:85–95.

Swanson LW, Sawchenko PE, Cowan WM (1981) Evidence for collateral projections by neurons in Ammon's horn, the dentate gyrus, and the subiculum: a multiple retrograde labeling study in the rat. *J Neurosci* 1:548–559.

Sylwestrak EL, Ghosh A (2012) Elfn1 regulates target-specific release probability at CA1-interneuron synapses. *Science* 338:536–540.

Szabadics J, Soltesz I (2009) Functional specificity of mossy fiber innervation of GABAergic cells in the hippocampus. *J Neurosci* 29:4239–4251.

Szabadics J, Tamas G, Soltesz I (2007) Different transmitter transients underlie presynaptic cell type specificity of GABAA,slow and GABAA,fast. *Proc Natl Acad Sci U S A* 104:14831–14836.

Szabadics J, Varga C, Brunner J, Chen K, Soltesz I (2010) Granule cells in the CA3 area. *J Neurosci* 30:8296–8307.

Szabadics J, Varga C, Molnar G, Olah S, Barzo P, Tamas G (2006) Excitatory effect of GABAergic axo-axonic cells in cortical microcircuits. *Science* 311:233–235.

Szabo GG, Du X, Oijala M, Varga C, Parent JM, Soltesz I (2017) Extended interneuronal network of the dentate gyrus. *Cell Rep* 20:1262–1268.

Szabo GG, Holderith N, Gulyas AI, Freund TF, Hajos N (2010) Distinct synaptic properties of perisomatic inhibitory cell types and their different modulation by cholinergic receptor activation in the CA3 region of the mouse hippocampus. *Eur J Neurosci* 31:2234–2246.

Szabo GG, Papp OI, Mate Z, Szabo G, Hajos N (2014) Anatomically heterogeneous populations of CB1 cannabinoid receptor-expressing interneurons in the CA3 region of the hippocampus show homogeneous input-output characteristics. *Hippocampus* 24:1506–1523.

Szőnyi A, Sos KE, Nyilas R, Schlingloff D, Domonkos A, Takács VT, ... Nyiri G (2019) Brainstem nucleus incertus controls contextual memory formation. *Science* 364:(6442):eaaw0445.

Takacs VT, Klausberger T, Somogyi P, Freund TF, Gulyas AI (2012) Extrinsic and local glutamatergic inputs of the rat hippocampal CA1 area differentially innervate pyramidal cells and interneurons. *Hippocampus* 22:1379–1391.

Takács VT, Cserép C, Schlingloff D, Pósfai B, Szőnyi A, Sos KE, ... Nyiri G (2018) Co-transmission of acetylcholine and GABA regulates hippocampal states. *Nature communications* 9(1):2848.

Takahashi H, Magee JC (2009) Pathway interactions and synaptic plasticity in the dendritic tuft regions of CA1 pyramidal neurons. *Neuron* 62:102–111.

Takeuchi T, Duszkiewicz AJ, Sonneborn A, Spooner PA, Yamasaki M, Watanabe M, Smith CC, Fernandez G, Deisseroth K, Greene RW, Morris RG (2016) Locus coeruleus and dopaminergic consolidation of everyday memory. *Nature* 537:357–362.

Tamamaki N, Abe K, Nojyo Y (1988) Three-dimensional analysis of the whole axonal arbors originating from single CA2 pyramidal neurons in the rat hippocampus with the aid of a computer graphic technique. *Brain research* 452(1–2):255–272.

Tamas G, Buhl EH, Lorincz A, Somogyi P (2000) Proximally targeted GABAergic synapses and gap junctions synchronize cortical interneurons. *Nat Neurosci* 3:366–371.

Tamas G, Lorincz A, Simon A, Szabadics J (2003) Identified sources and targets of slow inhibition in the neocortex. *Science* 299:1902–1905.

Tateno T, Robinson HP (2009) Integration of broadband conductance input in rat somatosensory cortical inhibitory interneurons: an inhibition-controlled switch between intrinsic and input-driven spiking in fast-spiking cells. *J Neurophysiol* 101:1056–1072.

Taube JS (1993) Electrophysiological properties of neurons in the rat subiculum in vitro. *Experimental brain research* 96:304–318.

Teles-Grilo Ruivo LM, Mellor JR (2013) Cholinergic modulation of hippocampal network function. *Front Synaptic Neurosci* 5:2.

Temprana SG, Mongiat LA, Yang SM, Trinchero MF, Alvarez DD, Kropff E, Giacomini D, Beltramone N, Lanuza GM, Schinder AF (2015) Delayed coupling to feedback inhibition during a critical period for the integration of adult-born granule cells. *Neuron* 85:116–130.

Thome C, Kelly T, Yanez A, Schultz C, Engelhardt M, Cambridge SB, Both M, Draguhn A, Beck H, Egorov AV (2014) Axon-carrying dendrites convey privileged synaptic input in hippocampal neurons. *Neuron* 83:1418–1430.

Thompson CL, Pathak SD, Jeromin A, Ng LL, MacPherson CR, Mortrud MT, Cusick A, Riley ZL, Sunkin SM, Bernard A, et al. (2008) Genomic anatomy of the hippocampus. *Neuron* 60:1010–1021.

Thomson AM, Bannister AP, Hughes DI, Pawelzik H (2000) Differential sensitivity to Zolpidem of IPSPs activated by morphologically identified CA1 interneurons in slices of rat hippocampus. *Eur J Neurosci* 12:425–436.

Thurley K, Leibold C, Gundlfinger A, Schmitz D, Kempter R (2008) Phase precession through synaptic facilitation. *Neural Comput* 20:1285–1324.

Torborg CL, Nakashiba T, Tonegawa S, McBain CJ (2010) Control of CA3 output by feedforward inhibition despite developmental changes in the excitation-inhibition balance. *J Neurosci* 30:15628–15637.

Tork I (1990) Anatomy of the serotonergic system. *Ann N Y Acad Sci* 600:9–34; discussion 34–35.

Toth K, Borhegyi Z, Freund TF (1993) Postsynaptic targets of GABAergic hippocampal neurons in the medial septum-diagonal band of Broca complex. *J Neurosci* 13:3712–3724.

Toth K, Suares G, Lawrence JJ, Philips-Tansey E, McBain CJ (2000) Differential mechanisms of transmission at three types of mossy fiber synapse. *J Neurosci* 20:8279–8289.

Traub RD, Bibbig A (2000) A model of high-frequency ripples in the hippocampus based on synaptic coupling plus axon-axon gap junctions between pyramidal neurons. *J Neurosci* 20:2086–2093.

Traub RD, Kopell N, Bibbig A, Buhl EH, LeBeau FE, Whittington MA (2001) Gap junctions between interneuron dendrites can enhance synchrony of gamma oscillations in distributed networks. *J Neurosci* 21:9478–9486.

Traub RD, Miles R, Wong RK (1989) Model of the origin of rhythmic population oscillations in the hippocampal slice. *Science* 243:1319–1325.

Traub RD, Whittington MA, Gutierrez R, Draguhn A (2018) Electrical coupling between hippocampal neurons: contrasting roles of principal cell gap junctions and interneuron gap junctions. *Cell Tissue Res* 373:671–691.

Traunmuller L, Gomez AM, Nguyen TM, Scheiffele P (2016) Control of neuronal synapse specification by a highly dedicated alternative splicing program. *Science* 352:982–986.

Treves A, Rolls ET (1994) Computational analysis of the role of the hippocampus in memory. *Hippocampus* 4:374–391.

Tsubokawa H, Ross WN (1996) IPSPs modulate spike backpropagation and associated [Ca2+]i changes in the dendrites of hippocampal CA1 pyramidal neurons. *J Neurophysiol* 76:2896–2906.

Tsukamoto M, Yasui T, Yamada MK, Nishiyama N, Matsuki N, Ikegaya Y (2003) Mossy fibre synaptic NMDA receptors trigger non-Hebbian long-term potentiation at entorhino-CA3 synapses in the rat. *J Physiol* 546:665–675.

Tukker JJ, Fuentealba P, Hartwich K, Somogyi P, Klausberger T (2007) Cell type-specific tuning of hippocampal interneuron firing during gamma oscillations in vivo. *J Neurosci* 27:8184–8189.

Tukker JJ, Lasztoczi B, Katona L, Roberts JD, Pissadaki EK, Dalezios Y, Marton L, Zhang L, Klausberger T, Somogyi P (2013) Distinct dendritic arborization and in vivo firing patterns of parvalbumin-expressing basket cells in the hippocampal area CA3. *J Neurosci* 33:6809–6825.

Turi GF, Li WK, Chavlis S, Pandi I, O'Hare J, Priestley JB, ... Losonczy A (2019) Vasoactive intestinal polypeptide-expressing interneurons in the hippocampus support goal-oriented spatial learning. *Neuron* 101(6):1150–1165.

Tyan L, Chamberland S, Magnin E, Camire O, Francavilla R, David LS, Deisseroth K, Topolnik L (2014) Dendritic inhibition provided by interneuron-specific cells controls the firing rate and timing of the hippocampal feedback inhibitory circuitry. *J Neurosci* 34:4534–4547.

Umbriaco D, Garcia S, Beaulieu C, Descarries L (1995) Relational features of acetylcholine, noradrenaline, serotonin and GABA axon terminals in the stratum radiatum of adult rat hippocampus (CA1). *Hippocampus* 5:605–620.

Unal G, Crump MG, Viney TJ, Eltes T, Katona L, Klausberger T, Somogyi P (2018) Spatio-temporal specialization of GABAergic septo-hippocampal neurons for rhythmic network activity. *Brain Struct Funct* 223:2409–2432.

Unal G, Joshi A, Viney TJ, Kis V, Somogyi P (2015) Synaptic targets of medial septal projections in the hippocampus and extrahippocampal cortices of the mouse. *J Neurosci* **35**:15812–15826.

Vaidya SP, Johnston D (2013) Temporal synchrony and gamma-to-theta power conversion in the dendrites of CA1 pyramidal neurons. *Nat Neurosci* **16**:1812–1820.

Valero M, Cid E, Averkin RG, Aguilar J, Sanchez-Aguilera A, Viney TJ, Gomez-Dominguez D, Bellistri E, de la Prida LM (2015) Determinants of different deep and superficial CA1 pyramidal cell dynamics during sharp-wave ripples. *Nat Neurosci* **18**:1281–1290.

Valero M, de la Prida LM (2018) The hippocampus in depth: a sublayer-specific perspective of entorhinal-hippocampal function. *Curr Opin Neurobiol* **52**:107–114.

Van Vreeswijk C, Abbott LF, Ermentrout GB (1994) When inhibition not excitation synchronizes neural firing. *J Comput Neurosci* **1**:313–321.

Vandecasteele M, Varga V, Berenyi A, Papp E, Bartho P, Venance L, Freund TF, Buzsaki G (2014) Optogenetic activation of septal cholinergic neurons suppresses sharp wave ripples and enhances theta oscillations in the hippocampus. *Proc Natl Acad Sci U S A* **111**:13535–13540.

Vanderwolf CH (1969) Hippocampal electrical activity and voluntary movement in the rat. *Electroencephalogr Clin Neurophysiol* **26**:407–418.

Varga C, Golshani P, Soltesz I (2012) Frequency-invariant temporal ordering of interneuronal discharges during hippocampal oscillations in awake mice. *Proc Natl Acad Sci U S A* **109**:E2726–2734.

Varga C, Oijala M, Lish J, Szabo GG, Bezaire M, Marchionni I, ... Soltesz I (2014) Functional fission of parvalbumin interneuron classes during fast network events. *Elife* **3**:e04006.

Varga V, Hangya B, Kranitz K, Ludanyi A, Zemankovics R, Katona I, Shigemoto R, Freund TF, Borhegyi Z (2008) The presence of pacemaker HCN channels identifies theta rhythmic GABAergic neurons in the medial septum. *J Physiol* **586**:3893–3915.

Varga V, Losonczy A, Zemelman BV, Borhegyi Z, Nyiri G, Domonkos A, Hangya B, Holderith N, Magee JC, Freund TF (2009) Fast synaptic subcortical control of hippocampal circuits. *Science* **326**:449–453.

Veit J, Hakim R, Jadi MP, Sejnowski TJ, Adesnik H (2017) Cortical gamma band synchronization through somatostatin interneurons. *Nat Neurosci* **20**:951–959.

Venance L, Rozov A, Blatow M, Burnashev N, Feldmeyer D, Monyer H (2000) Connexin expression in electrically coupled postnatal rat brain neurons. *Proc Natl Acad Sci U S A* **97**:10260–10265.

Vertes RP, McKenna JT (2000) Collateral Projections from the Supramammillary Nucleus to the Medial Septum and Hippocampus. New York: Synapse. p 38.

Vida I, Frotscher M (2000) A hippocampal interneuron associated with the mossy fiber system. *Proc Natl Acad Sci U S A* **97**:1275–1280.

Vida I, Halasy K, Szinyei C, Somogyi P, Buhl EH (1998) Unitary IPSPs evoked by interneurons at the stratum radiatum-stratum lacunosum-moleculare border in the CA1 area of the rat hippocampus in vitro. *J Physiol* **506**(Pt 3):755–773.

Vogt KE, Regehr WG (2001) Cholinergic modulation of excitatory synaptic transmission in the CA3 area of the hippocampus. *J Neurosci* **21**:75–83.

Vyleta NP, Borges-Merjane C, Jonas P (2016) Plasticity-dependent, full detonation at hippocampal mossy fiber–CA3 pyramidal neuron synapses. *Elife* **5**:e17977.

Vyleta NP, Jonas P (2014) Loose coupling between Ca2+ channels and release sensors at a plastic hippocampal synapse. *Science* **343**:665–670.

Wagatsuma A, Okuyama T, Sun C, Smith LM, Abe K, Tonegawa S (2018) Locus coeruleus input to hippocampal CA3 drives single-trial learning of a novel context. *Proc Natl Acad Sci U S A* **115**:E310–E316.

Walling SG, Brown RA, Miyasaka N, Yoshihara Y, Harley CW (2012) Selective wheat germ agglutinin (WGA) uptake in the hippocampus from the locus coeruleus of dopamine-beta-hydroxylase-WGA transgenic mice. *Front Behav Neurosci* **6**:23.

Wang X-J, Rinzel J (1992) Alternating and synchronous rhythms in reciprocally inhibitory model neurons. *Neural Comput* 84–97.

Wang XJ, Buzsaki G (1996) Gamma oscillation by synaptic inhibition in a hippocampal interneuronal network model. *J Neurosci* **16**:6402–6413.

Wang Y, Romani S, Lustig B, Leonardo A, Pastalkova E (2015) Theta sequences are essential for internally generated hippocampal firing fields. *Nat Neurosci* **18**:282–288.

Wenzel HJ, Buckmaster PS, Anderson NL, Wenzel ME, Schwartzkroin PA (1997) Ultrastructural localization of neurotransmitter immunoreactivity in mossy cell axons and their synaptic targets in the rat dentate gyrus. *Hippocampus* **7**:559–570.

West MJ, Slomianka L, Gundersen HJ (1991) Unbiased stereological estimation of the total number of neurons in the subdivisions of the rat hippocampus using the optical fractionator. *Anat Rec* **231**:482–497.

White JA, Banks MI, Pearce RA, Kopell NJ (2000) Networks of interneurons with fast and slow gamma-aminobutyric acid type A (GABAA) kinetics provide substrate for mixed gamma-theta rhythm. *Proc Natl Acad Sci U S A* **97**:8128–8133.

Whittington MA, Traub RD, Jefferys JG (1995) Synchronized oscillations in interneuron networks driven by metabotropic glutamate receptor activation. *Nature* **373**:612–615.

Widmer H, Ferrigan L, Davies CH, Cobb SR (2006) Evoked slow muscarinic acetylcholinergic synaptic potentials in rat hippocampal interneurons. *Hippocampus* **16**:617–628.

Wiescholleck V, Manahan-Vaughan D (2014) Antagonism of D1/D5 receptors prevents long-term depression (LTD) and learning-facilitated LTD at the perforant path-dentate gyrus synapse in freely behaving rats. *Hippocampus* **24**:1615–1622.

Wilke SA, Antonios JK, Bushong EA, Badkoobehi A, Malek E, Hwang M, Terada M, Ellisman MH, Ghosh A (2013) Deconstructing complexity: serial block-face electron microscopic analysis of the hippocampal mossy fiber synapse. *J Neurosci* **33**:507–522.

Williams PA, Larimer P, Gao Y, Strowbridge BW (2007) Semilunar granule cells: glutamatergic neurons in the rat dentate gyrus with axon collaterals in the inner molecular layer. *J Neurosci* **27**:13756–13761.

Wilson HR, Cowan JD (1972) Excitatory and inhibitory interactions in localized populations of model neurons. *Biophys J* **12**:1–24.

Wilson RI, Nicoll RA (2001) Endogenous cannabinoids mediate retrograde signalling at hippocampal synapses. *Nature* **410**:588–592.

Witter MP (1993) Organization of the entorhinal-hippocampal system: a review of current anatomical data. *Hippocampus* **3**(Spec No):33–44.

Witter MP (2007) The perforant path: projections from the entorhinal cortex to the dentate gyrus. *Prog Brain Res* **163**:43–61.

Witter MP, Amaral DG (2004) Hippocampal Formation: The Rat Nervous System. Elsevier. pp 635–704.

Witter MP, Groenewegen HJ, Lopes da Silva FH, Lohman AH (1989) Functional organization of the extrinsic and intrinsic circuitry of the parahippocampal region. *Prog Neurobiol* **33**:161–253.

Witter MP, Ostendorf RH, Groenewegen HJ (1990) Heterogeneity in the dorsal subiculum of the rat. Distinct neuronal zones project to different cortical and subcortical targets. *European Journal of Neuroscience* **2**(8):718–725.

Wittner L, Henze DA, Zaborszky L, Buzsaki G (2007) Three-dimensional reconstruction of the axon arbor of a CA3 pyramidal cell recorded and filled in vivo. *Brain Struct Funct* 212:75–83.

Woodruff A, Xu Q, Anderson SA, Yuste R (2009) Depolarizing effect of neocortical chandelier neurons. *Front Neural Circuits* 3:15.

Wouterlood FG, Saldana E, Witter MP (1990) Projection from the nucleus reuniens thalami to the hippocampal region: light and electron microscopic tracing study in the rat with the anterograde tracer Phaseolus vulgaris-leucoagglutinin. *J Comp Neurol* 296:179–203.

Wozny C, Beed P, Nitzan N, Pössnecker Y, Rost BR, Schmitz D (2018) VGLUT2 functions as a differential marker for hippocampal output neurons. *Frontiers in Cellular Neuroscience* 12:337.

Wyskiel DR, Andrade R (2016) Serotonin excites hippocampal CA1 GABAergic interneurons at the stratum radiatum-stratum lacunosum moleculare border. *Hippocampus* 26:1107–1114.

Xu C, Krabbe S, Grundemann J, Botta P, Fadok JP, Osakada F, Saur D, Grewe BF, Schnitzer MJ, Callaway EM, et al. (2016) Distinct hippocampal pathways mediate dissociable roles of context in memory retrieval. *Cell* 167:961–972, e916.

Xu X, Sun Y, Holmes TC, López AJ (2016) Noncanonical connections between the subiculum and hippocampal CA1. *Journal of Comparative Neurology* 524(17):3666–3673.

Yamamoto J, Suh J, Takeuchi D, Tonegawa S (2014) Successful execution of working memory linked to synchronized high-frequency gamma oscillations. *Cell* 157:845–857.

Yamamoto J, Tonegawa S (2017) Direct medial entorhinal cortex input to hippocampal CA1 is crucial for extended quiet awake replay. *Neuron* 96:217–227, e214.

Yang GR, Murray JD, Wang XJ (2016) A dendritic disinhibitory circuit mechanism for pathway-specific gating. *Nat Commun* 7:12815.

Yassa MA, Stark CE (2011) Pattern separation in the hippocampus. *Trends Neurosci* 34:515–525.

Ylinen A, Bragin A, Nadasdy Z, Jando G, Szabo I, Sik A, Buzsaki G (1995) Sharp wave-associated high-frequency oscillation (200 Hz) in the intact hippocampus: network and intracellular mechanisms. *J Neurosci* 15:30–46.

Ylinen A, Soltesz I, Bragin A, Penttonen M, Sik A, Buzsaki G (1995) Intracellular correlates of hippocampal theta rhythm in identified pyramidal cells, granule cells, and basket cells. *Hippocampus* 5:78–90.

Yoder RM, Pang KC (2005) Involvement of GABAergic and cholinergic medial septal neurons in hippocampal theta rhythm. *Hippocampus* 15:381–392.

Yoshida K, Drew MR, Mimura M, Tanaka KF (2019) Serotonin-mediated inhibition of ventral hippocampus is required for sustained goal-directed behavior. *Nat Neurosci* 22:770–777.

Yu AJ, Dayan P (2005) Uncertainty, neuromodulation, and attention. *Neuron* 46:681–692.

Yuan M, Meyer T, Benkowitz C, Savanthrapadian S, Ansel-Bollepalli L, Foggetti A, ... & Bartos M (2017) Somatostatin-positive interneurons in the dentate gyrus of mice provide local-and long-range septal synaptic inhibition. *Elife* 6:e21105.

Zalutsky RA, Nicoll RA (1990) Comparison of two forms of long-term potentiation in single hippocampal neurons. *Science* 248:1619–1624.

Zaremba JD, Diamantopoulou A, Danielson NB, Grosmark AD, Kaifosh PW, Bowler JC, Liao Z, Sparks FT, Gogos JA, Losonczy A (2017) Impaired hippocampal place cell dynamics in a mouse model of the 22q11.2 deletion. *Nat Neurosci* 20:1612–1623.

Zarnowska ED, Keist R, Rudolph U, Pearce RA (2009) GABAA receptor alpha5 subunits contribute to GABAA,slow synaptic inhibition in mouse hippocampus. *J Neurophysiol* 101:1179–1191.

Zhang S, Xu M, Kamigaki T, Hoang Do JP, Chang WC, Jenvay S, Miyamichi K, Luo L, Dan Y (2014) Selective attention: long-range and local circuits for top-down modulation of visual cortex processing. *Science* 345:660–665.

Zhao M, Choi YS, Obrietan K, Dudek SM (2007) Synaptic plasticity (and the lack thereof) in hippocampal CA2 neurons. *Journal of Neuroscience: The Official Journal of the Society for Neuroscience* 27(44):12025–12032.

Zhao X, Lein ES, He A, Smith SC, Aston C, Gage FH (2001) Transcriptional profiling reveals strict boundaries between hippocampal subregions. *J Comp Neurol* 441(3):187–196.

Zhao M, Choi YS, Obrietan K, Dudek SM (2007) Synaptic plasticity (and the lack thereof) in hippocampal CA2 neurons. *Journal of Neuroscience* 27(44):12025–12032.

Zhao X, Lein ES, He A, Smith SC, Aston C, Gage FH (2001) Transcriptional profiling reveals strict boundaries between hippocampal subregions. *Journal of Comparative Neurology* 441(3):187–196.

Molecular Mechanisms of Synaptic Function in the Hippocampus

Paul G. Donlin-Asp, Anne-Sophie Hafner, and Erin M. Schuman

8.1 Overview

Proteins are the main effectors of cellular function in all cells, including neurons. The complement of proteins expressed in a particular cell is called the proteome. The proteome of an individual cell defines both its identity and its state, as changes in protein composition drive all long-lasting changes in neurons, including those that occur during development and plasticity. For example, NMDA-type glutamate receptor (NMDAR) composition is altered in hippocampal neurons after birth as GluN2B-containing receptors are progressively replaced by GluN2A-containing receptors (Monyer et al., 1994). In addition, AMPA-type glutamatergic receptors (AMPARs) are added and removed at excitatory postsynaptic sites in response to activity in order to adapt synaptic strength (Matsuzaki et al., 2001). In neurons, the proteome present in a synaptic compartment reflects the type of synapse (e.g., excitatory or inhibitory) as well as its history (e.g., recently potentiated, depressed, exposed to a neuromodulator, etc.). Rough estimates of the total number of proteins in a mature neuron predict that about 40×10^9 proteins are present in a single neuron coded from only ~4500 differentially expressed genes (Sharma et al., 2015).

As described in Chapters 3 and 5, neurons have unique complex, polarized morphologies that includes three major compartments: a dendritic arbor, a soma, and an axon. Axons typically terminate in presynaptic boutons that makes close contact with the dendrite or cell-body of another neuron at synapses. Each compartment has distinct functions, and these are reflected by the compartment's proteome. The axons and dendrites constitute the majority of a neuron's volume (Ishizuka et al., 1995; Ascoli et al., 2007). Moreover, dendrites and axons are branched, creating a network of compartments in which protein content may be differentially regulated. This chapter addresses the different mechanisms neurons use to address, maintain, and regulate proteins within individual synapses.

In this chapter, one aim is to describe the mechanisms involved in supplying synaptic proteins. We discuss dendrites and axons in two separate sections. We start by describing the cellular mechanisms currently known to target proteins to synaptic compartments. First focusing on the postsynaptic compartment, we explore the regulation of the synaptic proteome by outlining what is known about the dendritic transcriptome, local translation machinery, and protein homeostasis. In the second part of the chapter, we dive into the recently expanding field of the role of local protein synthesis within the axon. We finish the main part of the chapter with a discussion of the links between synaptic proteome deregulation and neurological disease. Most of the data discussed in this chapter have been obtained from studies performed on hippocampal neurons from rats or mice. Finally, at the end, we discuss the unresolved issues concerning mRNA targeting, mRNA half-lives, and local versus global proteome remodeling in axons and dendrites.

8.2 The postsynaptic proteome

Synaptic plasticity is the process by which synapses are modified in response to activity. Such modifications may be structural, making them bigger or smaller, or they may be functional, stronger or weaker, or they may be both. We begin with the postsynaptic compartment because the most research has been done on this side of the synaptic equation. Later, we will consider the presynaptic side.

During synaptic plasticity, proteins in the postsynaptic compartment are rearranged and new proteins are added to or removed from the synaptic pool. These changes can be local using nearby machineries to synthesize and degrade proteins, or alternatively, involve the capture of proteins that were produced in the soma and then moved into the dendrites. We note that the two mechanisms are not mutually exclusive. In this section, we first review the transport machinery involved in the addressing of proteins to postsynaptic compartments. Then we give a detailed overview of the local modulation to the synaptic proteome and transcriptome induced during synaptic plasticity in the hippocampus.

8.2.1 Targeting of postsynaptic proteins

The targeting of postsynaptic proteins involves the delivery of cargo (proteins) from the soma or dendrites into and out of the postsynaptic density. This trafficking function occurs during ongoing cellular homeostasis and in response to signals that indicate the need for changes in synaptic function or structure. When a neuron has established most of its connectivity within a network, a large part of its metabolism is focused on maintaining the function of synapses in the face of protein turnover. During plasticity, synaptic proteomes are remodeled. Upon long-term plasticity induction, one idea is that activated synapses are "tagged" or marked in order for the plasticity-related-protein products to be captured and preferentially incorporated into those synapses. The molecular identity of the tags, however, remains unknown. This phenomenon proposed by Frey and Morris in 1997 is known as synaptic tagging and capture (STC) (Frey and Morris, 1997). The concept of synaptic tagging is discussed at length in Chapter 10. The insertion of new proteins in response to activity is also driven by the activation of local signals. Some of these signals include the transient elevation of second-messengers such as Ca^{2+} (Bloodgood and Sabatini, 2005; Hangen et al., 2018) or the activation of intracellular signaling cascades like those that include CaMKII or Rho GTPase activity (Tashiro and Yuste, 2004; Opazo et al., 2010; Hanus et al., 2014; Hafner et al., 2015).

Dendritic spines are actin-rich compartments that protrude from the microtubule-rich dendritic shafts. Surprisingly, dendrites contain polarized microtubules with both plus-end-out and minus-end-out (Baas et al., 1988; Kleele et al., 2014; Yau et al., 2016), as observed using nanometric tracking of motor proteins (Tas et al., 2017) (see Figure 8.1A). This bidirectional organization allows cargo to move in both directions using the same motor proteins (i.e., kinesin, dynein). A consequence of this is that cargo such as neurotransmitter receptors will move in both anterograde and retrograde directions (Hanus et al., 2014; Hangen et al., 2018). Interestingly, in the case of the AMPA-type glutamate receptors (AMPARs), one report indicated a bias toward anterograde transport in distal dendrites mediated by the phosphorylation of the intracellular C-terminus of the GluA1 subunit (Hangen et al., 2018).

8.2.2 How are cargo deposited at synaptic sites?

Neuronal activity can influence the mobility of cargos (see Figure 8.1B). If neuronal activity is blocked, for example, some cargos become highly mobile and tend to cover long dendritic distances. In contrast, a transient increase in Ca^{2+} or activation of CaMKII quickly induces the arrest of mobile cargo (Hanus et al., 2014). This strong response is mediated by the direct phosphorylation of the kinesin motor-protein KIF17 by CaMKII. Phosphorylation of KIF17 results in the detachment of cargo from microtubules, thus directly preventing motion. When cargo are released from microtubules, they become accessible for actin-based transport. Actin transport, using myosin as a molecular motor, is used for local transport in spines and covers typically small distances of a few microns (van der Berg and Hoogenraad, 2012). We note that microtubule entries into spines have been reported to occur in response to synapse-specific calcium transients (Merriam et al., 2013). This process requires concomitant local actin polymerization and is promoted by drebrin, a protein known to mediate interactions between F-actin (polymerized actin) and microtubules (Merriam et al., 2013). In addition to mediating the indirect release of cargos from microtubules, Ca^{2+} also drives rapid actin remodeling in the spine (Chazeau et al., 2014; Mikhaylova et al., 2018). Essential F-actin regulators are present in the spine

such as the GTPase Rac1 or the WAVE-complex-promoting actin elongation and nucleation respectively (Soderling et al., 2003; Tashiro and Yuste, 2004). Such actin dynamics underlie structural synaptic plasticity (Cingolani and Goda, 2008), are essential for LTP expression in area CA1 (Krucker et al., 2000), and likely promote protein rearrangement inside, and flow within the spine (Hotulainen and Hoogenraad, 2010). Simultaneously, synaptic activity and long-term plasticity induce changes in the spine neck diameter and length (Bloodgood and Sabatini, 2005; Tønnesen et al., 2014). Shorter and wider spine necks can, in principal, promote the exchange of molecules between the dendrite and the spine by lowering diffusion barriers.

8.2.3 How is local synaptic remodeling regulated?

The mechanisms underlying protein addition and exchange during spine remodeling depend on the protein type: membrane proteins like neurotransmitter receptors are first associated with intracellular vesicles, whereas cytoplasmic proteins like kinases and scaffolding proteins (e.g., CaMKII, PSD-95) usually diffuse freely. Transmembrane proteins are trafficked to the plasma membrane via exocytosis, and then diffuse at the cell surface before they are tethered at the synapse (Opazo and Choquet, 2011). As an example, consider the AMPARs that mediate fast excitatory transmission (Chapter 6) and are highly regulated at synapses during plasticity. During steady-state synaptic transmission, AMPARs continuously exchange between an intracellular pool, the cell surface, and the postsynaptic density (PSD), maintaining a steady equilibrium of such receptors over time. Long-term synaptic plasticity promotes the endocytosis of additional receptors from the cell surface dendritic shafts and spines during long-term depression (LTD), and exocytosis during long-term potentiation (LTP) (Triller and Choquet, 2003; Shepherd and Huganir, 2007; Triller et al., 2008; Newpher and Ehlers, 2008; Choquet and Triller, 2013). Thus, activity disturbs the steady-state equilibrium by depleting or favoring the intracellular pool, but thereby creates a new equilibrium set-point. In addition, in LTP, the local trapping of AMPARs in the PSD is also increased through the phosphorylation of its auxiliary subunit stargazin by CaMKII. In parallel, increased Ca^{2+} concentration in spines mediated by NMDARs activates CaMKII and increases its affinity for this receptor, predominantly located at the PSD, in turn recruiting CaMKII to this subcellular compartment (Merrill et al., 2005; Shen et al., 2000; Otmakhov et al., 2004; Shen and Meyer, 1999). While the AMPAR, a transmembrane protein complex, and CamKII, a cytosolic holoenzyme, take very different routes to the synapse, their local trapping in the PSD are both mediated by molecular interactions resulting in a local increase in their protein concentrations.

8.2.4 From what source do synaptic proteins originate?

Initially, it was thought that production of proteins in neurons occurred exclusively in the cell body (Lasek et al., 1973). Accordingly, each synthesized protein would then travel from this "central" compartment to its final destination in the dendrite or axon. This idea has an appealing simplicity, but it requires that all proteins destined for extrasomatic sites must be efficiently targeted individually or in small groups over long distances to reach synaptic compartments. And that is not easy. Interestingly,

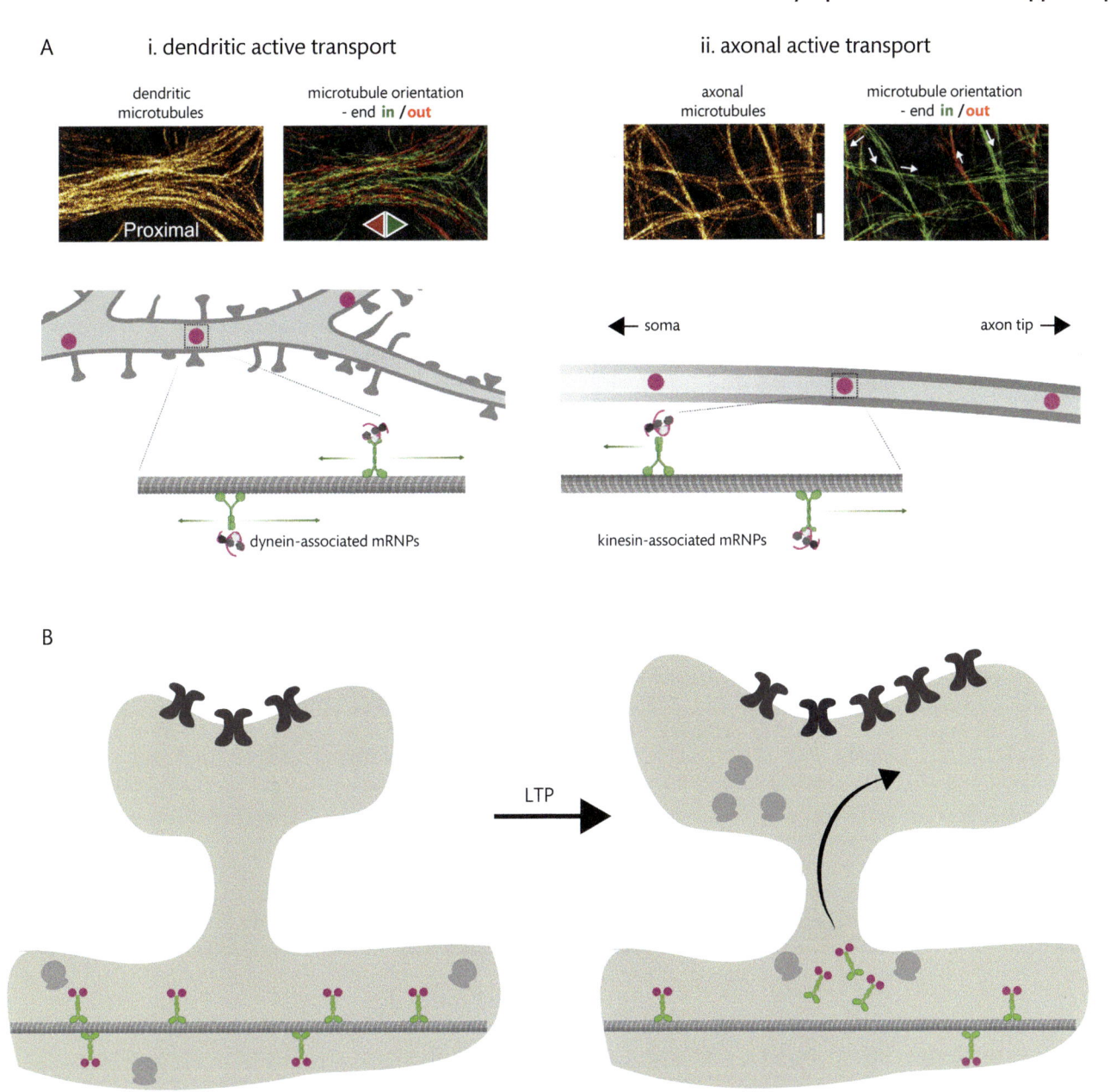

Figure 8.1 Translation machinery in neuronal processes. (A) Schematic representation of a neuron transcribing mRNA in its nucleus. The mRNAs are then exported into the cytoplasm, where the translation machinery can translate them into proteins. (i) Electron micrographs and 3D reconstructions endoplasmic reticulum compartments (ER) in dendrites (green on the left images) and ER-bound ribosomes (red on the right reconstructions). (Modified from Cui-wang et al., 2012.) (ii) Electron micrographs and 3D reconstructions showing polyribosomes (black arrows on the left image, black dots on right image) within and near dendritic spines. (Modified from Ostroff et al., 2018.) (iii) Super-resolution images obtained using expansion microscopy showing ongoing translation at the pre- and the postsynapse. (Data from Hafner et al., 2019.) (B) Nonexhaustive list of synaptically localized mRNA coding for key synaptic proteins of the pre- and the postsynaptic compartments. (Data extracted from Cajigas et al., 2012; Tushev et al., 2018; and Hafner et al., 2019.)

computational models relying on an exclusively somatic source of proteins fail to capture the reality of protein distribution within neurons (Bressloff and Earnshaw, 2007; Bressloff and Newby, 2013). A unique and central source of protein produces protein distributions that follow an exponential decay from the soma to the tip of dendrites whereas most protein in neurons do not exhibit this pattern. As such, based on morphological constrains and fast protein demands, there is an emerging consensus that many of the proteins that inhabit synapses arise, at least in part, from local sources (Holt and Schuman, 2013).

Gene expression is a multistep mechanism divided in two main processes. The first process is known as transcription resulting in the production of messenger RNAs (mRNAs). Transcription occurs exclusively in the neuronal nucleus (except for a small number of mitochondrially encoded genes). The second process is known as mRNA translation, resulting in the production of proteins. Gene expression is controlled and regulated by the respective rates and turnovers of the products of these two processes.

The evidence for the presence of mRNA and protein synthesis machinery within dendritic and axonal compartments, and the resulting local synthesis of protein have accumulated in recent years. In fact, producing proteins in these subcellular compartments could confer distinct advantages. For instance, a single mRNA molecule can be translated multiple times, resulting in multiple of copies of a particular protein. As such, local translation could dramatically (but inexpensively) increase the local concentration of a specific protein and, in turn, favor its synaptic incorporation. Spatially controlling the production of proteins in axons and dendrites might also provide an explanation for how neurons achieve the fine targeting of synaptic proteins to specific dendrites and synapses in a highly adaptable fashion. Notably, a recent computational model incorporating mRNA and protein turnover as well as local protein synthesis and local modulation of mRNA translation upon activity was able to (1) reproduce a variety of measured protein distributions and (2) achieve fast and highly localized changes in protein concentration in line with proteome remodeling dynamics observed at synapses during plasticity (Fonkeu et al., 2019). We shall below review evidence for both somatic and local protein synthesis in dendrites.

8.2.5 Transcriptional regulation

Altered gene expression is an essential component for the conversion of short-term memory into long-term memory (Kandel, 2001). Widespread changes occur within the transcriptome in response to synaptic plasticity (West and Greenberg, 2011). A number of the synaptic-plasticity-regulated transcripts, including the immediate early gene *Arc*, are known to exhibit activity-dependent localization. Retrograde signaling from the dendrite to the nucleus is also important in synaptic plasticity (Deisseroth et al., 1996; Herbst and Martin, 2017; Brigidi et al., 2019). Examples of retrograde signaling include the transport of importins to the soma from the dendrite and axonal compartments (required for nuclear import) (Thompson et al., 2004; Lai et al., 2008), as well as the transport of the transcription factor CREB and the transcription associated factor CRTC1 (Ch'Ng et al., 2012). Together, these changes likely contribute to the sustained changes in transcriptional programs seen during plasticity.

Plasticity likely alters both the somatic and dendritic transcriptomes. Such changes would allow for proteome remodeling by changing the pool of mRNAs available for translation. Furthermore, the potential processing and regulation of the existing transcriptome occurs as well. Recently, posttranscriptional RNA modifications (such as m6A) have been described (Merkurjev et al., 2018). Interestingly, intron-containing mRNAs as well as components of the spliceosome have been detected outside of the nucleus (Bell et al., 2010), potentially providing a ready-to-be processed pool of mRNAs at required sites. Activity-driven processing has been reported for microRNAs (miRNAs) (Sambandan et al., 2017), providing high spatiotemporal control over degradation or silencing of particular transcripts during neuronal activity. The CPEB family of proteins, responsible for cytoplasmic mRNA polyadenylation, are found throughout the cell including the dendrites. In response to synaptic activity, they can drive the elongation of mRNA poly(A) tail, thus increasing local mRNA stability (L Wu et al., 1998; Ivshina et al., 2014). Interestingly, activity can also lead to the local shortening of the 3' untranslated regions of mRNA (Tushev et al., 2018). Taken together, these data indicate there is active remodeling of the local transcriptome in dendrites in response to synaptic demands.

8.2.6 RNA transport and localization

Following transcription, mRNAs are rapidly translocated from the nucleus to the cytoplasm (see Figure 8.2A). Within the cytoplasm, transcripts can be localized to particular subcellular domains or compartments. The localization of an mRNA defines the subcellular environment where the concentration of the synthesized protein can be upregulated to favor domain-specific incorporation. Localizing mRNAs thereby creates an unevenness in the distribution of proteins in cells. This mechanism has been shown to be important to establish or maintain cell polarity, regulate gene expression, or sequester the activity of proteins. Historically, the subcellular localization of mRNAs has been studied during embryonic development (Martin and Ephrussi, 2009). Strikingly, in Drosophila embryos, up to ~70% of the transcriptome is localized in specific subcellular compartments (Lécuyer et al., 2007).

mRNAs are very large, often 10 times larger than the protein they code for. They are also sensitive to degradation by various nucleases. To prevent their degradation en route, mRNAs are transported within the neuron in protective macromolecular structures called granules (Krichevsky and Kosik, 2001). These granules are also enriched in ribosomal proteins but are unable to incorporate metabolic labeling such as radioactive amino acids. As such, they are described as translationally "incompetent"—an odd term for a macromolecular structure heralding so much potential. Importantly, following neuronal depolarization, some mRNAs, can rapidly shift from the RNA granule fraction to a competent place—such as to translationally active polysomes (Krichevsky and Kosik, 2001).

Using microarray approaches, the dendritic transcriptome was originally described as ~ 285 mRNAs (Poon et al., 2006; Zhong et al., 2006). Shortly thereafter, a high-throughput *in situ* hybridization assay performed by the Allen Brain Project identified ~68 mRNAs in the synaptic CA1 neuropil (i.e., stratum radiatum and lacunosum-moleculare) (Lein et al., 2007). The era of RNAseq ushered in depth and breadth to our understanding of local transcriptomes. For example, using RNAseq and microdissection of the CA1 region, ~2,550 unique mRNAs (more than half of the CA1 pyramidal neurons transcriptome) were detected in the synaptic neuropil (Cajigas et al., 2012) (see Figure 8.2B). Many of the detected transcripts code for proteins with known postsynaptic localization and function including PSD-95 or CaMKIIa. The gene ontology terms associated with the neuropil transcriptome span processes like neuronal ion channel clustering, regulation of synaptic plasticity, and RNA localization, suggesting that local protein synthesis plays a broad role in the supply of synaptic proteins. Interestingly, about 30% of the transcripts found in the dendrites code for transmembrane proteins (Cajigas et al., 2012). However, the synthesis of transmembrane proteins requires not only mRNAs and ribosomes but also additional secretory organelles (Hanus and Ehlers, 2008; Hanus et al., 2016).

Pursuing this critical issue of the source of proteins, many dendritic hippocampal mRNA species have been demonstrated to play a role in plasticity. For example, the dendritic localization of the mRNA encoding for key synaptic proteins like CaMKII alpha subunit (CaMKIIa) have been observed with sequencing, as described above, but also in early in situ hybridization studies (Burgin et al., 1990; Mayford et al., 1996). Notably, in a transgenic mouse in which the 3'UTR elements that drive CaMKIIa mRNA dendritic localization were deleted, there was an 85% loss in synaptic CaMKIIa

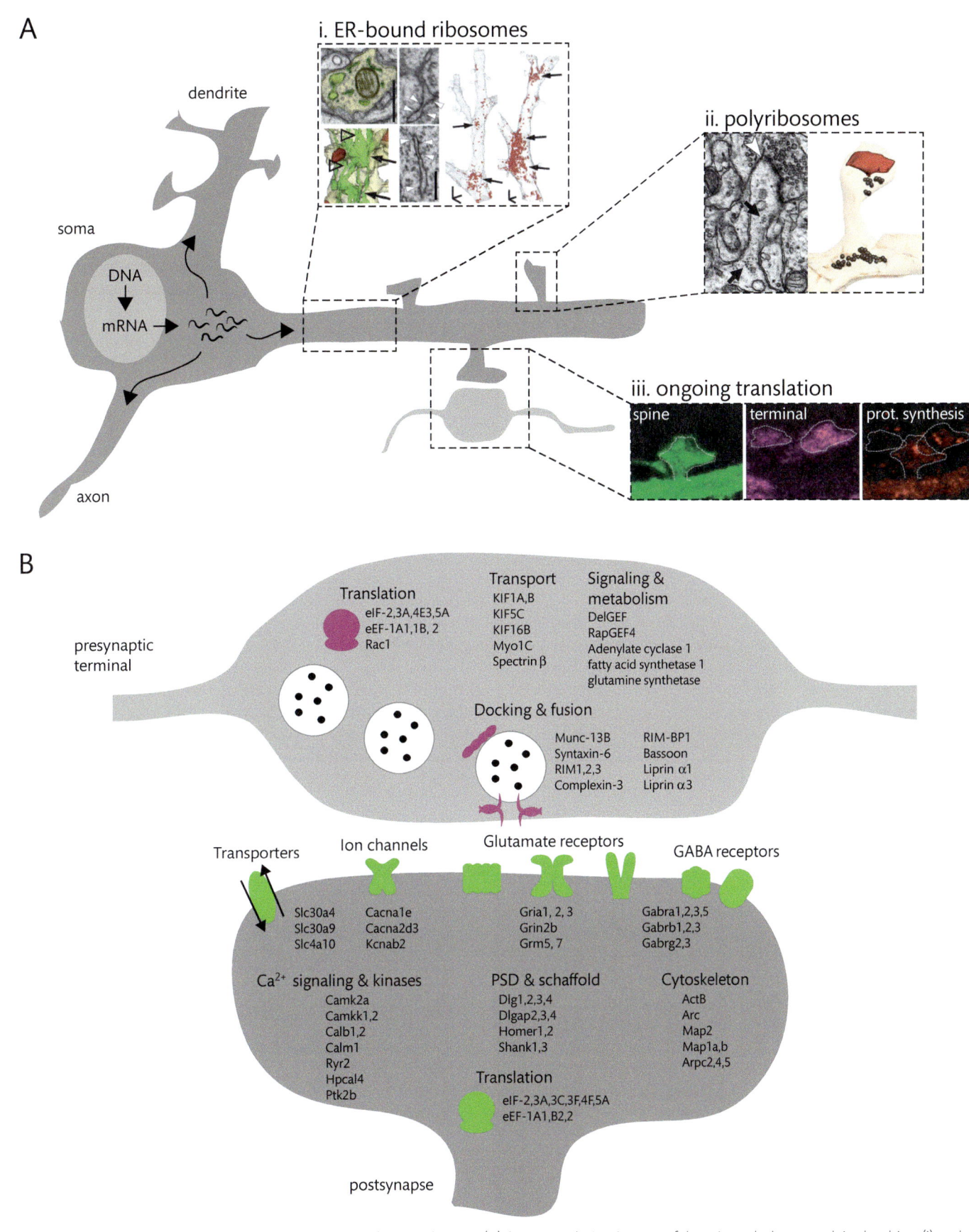

Figure 8.2 Cargo active transport mechanisms in dendrites and axons. (A) Super-resolution images of the microtubule network in dendrites (i) and in axons (ii) (top). (Modified from Tas et al., 2017.) Schematic representations of cargo transport by molecular motors in dendrites (i) and in axons (ii). (B) Scheme illustrating the delivery of cargo to potentiated synapses via the dissociation of kinesin motors from microtubules. Concomitantly ribosomes accumulate at the bottom and in the spine head of potentiated spines to allow the local production of additional proteins.

protein and an impairment the late phase of LTP (Miller et al., 2002). Using a computational framework to capture the spatial profile of CaMKIIa mRNAs and proteins, Fonkeu and colleagues estimated that ~60% of CaMKIIa protein in neurons is produced from local mRNAs in dendrites (Fonkeu et al., 2019). This suggests that local mRNA translation could be an important source of supply for this and other synaptic proteins.

8.2.7 Local translational machinery

The synthesis of proteins requires both mRNAs and ribosomes. Ribosomes are ribonucleoprotein nanomachines that translate the genetic information copied from DNA to mRNA into protein. The mammalian ribosome is composed of four rRNAs and ~80 ribosomal proteins organized in two subunits. Both the small and the large subunits are assembled independently in the nucleus and then exported to the cytoplasm. Upon binding of the small subunit to an mRNA the large subunit associates with this complex to form a full ribosome and initiates translation (Lafontaine, 2015). Despite compelling evidence that ribosomes are localized in dendrites, the underlying mechanisms for ribosome translocation remains poorly understood. In the neuronal cytoplasm a majority of ribosomes are associated with mRNA and engaged in their translation (Krichevsky and Kosik, 2001). A single mRNA associates with one or multiple ribosomes simultaneously, resulting in structures known as monosomes or polysomes, respectively. The number of ribosomes loaded onto an mRNA is generally thought to reflect the efficiency of translation.

Where have ribosomes been observed in neurons? Individual ribosomes, which appear as a singular round structure in electron micrographs, are extremely difficult to detect with certainty. Polyribosomes which often have a circular beaded appearance or a "beads-on-a-string" signature are easier to detect. An early study detected polyribosomes in and near dendritic spines in dentate gyrus granule cells (Steward and Fass, 1983; Steward and Levy, 1982). An electron microscopy analysis of the stratum radiatum of the CA1 region of the hippocampus reveal that ~12% of dendritic spines contain polyribosomes and there are more than two polyribosomes per micron of the dendritic shaft—while there is only one spine per micron (Ostroff et al., 2002) (see Figure 8.2A). Interesting, following LTP induction this number goes up to ~39% in spines with a clear coincident depletion of polyribosomes in dendritic shafts, suggesting their movement between these two compartments (Ostroff et al., 2002; Ostroff et al., 2018) (see Figure 8.2B). The positioning of polyribosomes beneath the postsynaptic density within the confined environment of the dendritic spine can increase the efficiency of protein incorporation at the activated synapse following translation.

The endoplasmic reticulum (ER) is often referred as the "cell within the cell." In neurons, the ER has been observed for decades in both axons and dendrites of hippocampus neurons using electron microscopy (Shute and Lewis, 1966; Broadwell and Cataldo, 1984; Spacek and Harris, 1998; Ramírez and Couve, 2011; Cui-wang et al., 2012). This single and continuous membrane-bound organelle is responsible for processing membrane and secreted proteins as well as lipid biogenesis. Rough ER, characterized by the abundant ribosomes studding the surface, is present in soma and dendrites. The complexity of ER membranes and tubules is maximal in mature neurons at the base of spines and at branch points (Cui-wang et al., 2012) (see Figure 8.2A). Interestingly, the density of ribosomes at the surface of the ER is also particularly high in mature dendrites at the base of spines and at branch points (Cui-wang et al., 2012), suggesting that those are hubs of transmembrane protein synthesis.

After their synthesis in the rough ER, transmembrane proteins traffic through the Golgi apparatus (GA) for further maturation (e.g., glycosylation). While in most cells the GA network is exclusively located in perinuclear regions, in neurons the GA also includes discrete structures dispersed in dendrites known as Golgi outposts (Pierce et al., 2001; Horton et al., 2005; Hanus and Ehlers, 2008). Such Golgi outposts are defined by their immunoreactivity for the Golgi matrix protein GM130 and/or in electron microscopy by a characteristic mini-Golgi stack ultrastructure. Additionally, Hanus and colleagues reported that many surface-expressed transmembrane proteins carry immature N-glycans, a signature of Golgi bypass or Golgi hypofunction (Hanus et al., 2016). This phenomenon, known as unconventional secretory processing, may allow dendrites lacking Golgi membranes to target membrane proteins to the surface. Interestingly, the proteins exported to the surface in these conditions have specific properties (e.g., stability) when compared with their counterparts carrying mature glycans (Hanus et al., 2016).

8.2.8 Local protein degradation

Finally, protein degradation is a crucial component governing protein turnover, serving various functions. The ubiquitin proteasome system (UPS) and the lysosome system are used for cytosolic and transmembrane protein degradation (Tai and Schuman, 2008). Both lysosomes and proteasomes are detected in dendrites. The UPS regulates the degradation of synaptic proteins of the PSD (Ehlers, 2003). Synaptic activity influences the ubiquitination and turnover of some PSD proteins, important for the control of synapse function and maintenance (Ehlers, 2003). Activity also enhances the recruitment of the proteasome into dendritic spines (Bingol and Schuman, 2006). Similarly, lysosome localization in dendrites is also highly regulated by activity (Goo et al., 2017). There is also ample evidence for a role of the UPS in learning and memory. For instance in rats, bilateral infusion of the proteasome inhibitor Lactacystin (administrated 4-7 h after training) to the CA1 region of the hippocampus caused full retrograde amnesia for a one-trial inhibitory avoidance training, indicating that the ubiquitin-proteasome cascade is crucial for long-term memory in the behaving animal (Lopez-Salon et al., 2003). Also in mouse, the absence of the ubiquitin ligase APC/C-Cdh1, involved in the targeting of proteins to the proteasome, blocks mGluR-dependent LTD in the hippocampus (Huang et al., 2015).

8.2.9 Regulation of the proteome during plasticity

Early work using inhibitors found that blocking protein synthesis impaired learning (Flexner et al., 1962), indicating a vital role for this process in learning and memory. Work on LTP found that the early phase of LTP, or E-LTP, was insensitive to translational inhibition (Frey et al., 1996) while the late phase, or L-LTP, was sensitive to translational and transcriptional inhibition (Frey et al., 1988). Very few studies have characterized the changes in the synaptic proteome during synaptic plasticity. However, one study revealed that ~300 individual proteins change at the level of translation during homeostatic up- or downscaling (Schanzenbächer et al., 2016). An earlier study had shown that a similar number of proteins were altered within the isolated hippocampal neuropil during dopaminergic stimulation (Hodas et al., 2012).

A defining characteristic of local protein synthesis is its dynamic nature. It is regulated by various forms of synaptic plasticity and neuronal activity itself (Jones et al., 2018). For instance, the neurotrophin BDNF induces long-lasting protein-synthesis-dependent plasticity at CA3–CA1 hippocampal synapses. CA1 dendrites isolated from their cell bodies still exhibited protein-synthesis-dependent plasticity (Kang and Schuman, 1996). Similarly, activation of group 1 metabotropic glutamate receptors (mGluRs) or paired-pulse low-frequency stimulation can induce a form of LTD that requires dendritic, but not somatic, protein synthesis (Huber et al., 2000). Moreover, isolated hippocampal dendritic fields can support protein-synthesis-dependent forms of LTP (Cracco et al., 2005; Y Huang and Kandel, 2005; Vickers et al., 2005), and localized application of protein synthesis inhibitors on CA1 pyramidal neuron dendrites inhibits late-phase LTP (Bradshaw et al., 2003). Some forms of homeostatic scaling (Sutton et al., 2004; Sutton et al., 2006) also require dendritic protein synthesis.

What has remained less defined is where in the dendrite (spines or shaft) local protein synthesis can occur. While the signaling pathways linked to the neurotrophin receptors are found within spines, the downstream signals themselves may propagate out from individual spines into the local dendritic environment (Rangaraju et al., 2017). If local protein synthesis functions to modulate the local proteome, one would expect a localized response for translation. Supporting this, tetanic stimulation induces an enrichment of polyribosomes within spines (Ostroff et al., 2002; Ostroff et al., 2012; Ostroff et al., 2018), suggestive of increased spine protein synthesis. Single molecule imaging studies of protein synthesis have described increases in spine translation (Tatavarty et al., 2012; Ifrim et al., 2015) for both PSD-95 and Arc. Additionally, recent work with metabolic labeling found a high number of spines (~60%) incorporate metabolic labeling within a short pulse (5 min) and that this number can be enhanced with various forms of synaptic plasticity (Hafner et al., 2019). These data suggest that spines themselves may be important sites for protein synthesis, but unlikely the exclusive site, as ribosomes and mRNA are found throughout the dendrite.

8.3 The presynaptic proteome

Similar to the postsynaptic compartment, the axonal proteome is dynamic in response to neuronal activity and synaptic plasticity. Regulating the proteome of the axon is an exceptional feat for the neuron, given the scale over which an axon projects (from millimeters up to a meter for motoneurons). As discussed in the following section, the neuron accomplishes this feat with unique structural organization of the axon and specialized transport mechanisms to meet the presynaptic demands.

8.3.1 Axonal organization and axonal transport

In the early developing neuron, one of the neurites rapidly differentiates into an axon (Goldberg, 2003). As it grows, the developing axon encounters guidance cues from the surrounding tissue that regulate its growth, path chosen, and synapse formation. Growth is mediated by the axonal cytoskeleton, which comprises intermediate filaments, actin, and microtubules. The organization of axonal microtubule polarity is distinct from dendrites: most microtubule plus-ends point away from the soma, whereas in the dendrite they show mixed polarity with plus/minus-ends pointing to and from

the soma equally (Burton and Paige, 1981). The uniform polarity of axons is maintained by direct transport of polymerized microtubules along the existing microtubule core network (Wang and Brown, 2002).

Early studies demonstrated the importance of microtubules in axonal transport: disruption of the microtubule cytoskeleton blocked axonal transport (Kreutzberg, 1969). Not long after, two distinct types of transport were described based on the kinetics of cargo distribution—fast axonal transport and slow axonal transport (Brady, 1985; Lasek and Brady, 1985; Vale, Reese, et al., 1985; Vale, Schnapp, et al., 1985; Sleigh et al., 2019). Fast axonal transport remains the best studied of the two (Maday et al., 2014). Reaching transport speeds of up to 1 μm/s (up to 400 mm/day), fast axonal transport is employed to move synaptic vesicles, organelles, and mRNAs down the axon (Hall and Hedgecock, 1991; Falzone et al., 2009). The second method of anterograde axonal transport, slow axonal transport, is used for cytoskeleton polymers and soluble cytosolic proteins, but is less understood. At speeds less than 0.1 μm/s (covering less than 8 mm/day), the regulation and purpose of this slow system transport remains elusive due to the difficulty of studying it in real time. Axonal cargo also exhibits retrograde transport (Schnapp and Reese, 1989). Due to the polarity of the microtubules, this is achieved using dynein-mediated transport (Hirokawa et al., 1990). Given that any cargo, such as a synaptic vesicle, can associate with both kinesins and dynein at the same time, it remains unknown how the neuron regulates cargo directionality in real-time (Maday et al., 2014).

Targeting cargo axonally (or dendritically) presents a unique challenge for the neuron. While some kinesin proteins are found highly enriched in the axon, such as the Kif5 family (Hirokawa et al., 2010), these motors alone are unlikely to be sufficient to achieve the asymmetric distribution of cargo throughout the neuron. Likely, additional sorting and targeting mechanisms contribute to axonal versus dendritic cargo targeting (Maeder et al., 2014). The axon initial segment (AIS) may play a role in this regard, serving as a sieve to filter out nonaxonal cargos. The exact mechanism for this remains unclear, however it likely requires the interplay of kinesins decoding microtubule-encoded cues (Jacobson et al., 2006) in the axon. Additional work has implicated the septins within the dendrite serving a similar function to filter out and prevent axonal cargos from entering into the dendrite (Karasmanis et al., 2018).

8.3.2 Transcriptomes and proteomes of the growing axon

Over the past decades, the fundamental biology of local protein synthesis in axonal growth and guidance as well as regeneration has been characterized in detail (Campbell and Holt, 2001; Sahoo et al., 2018; Cioni et al., 2018; Terenzio et al., 2018) in a variety of neuronal systems (discussed at length below). However, less attention has been given to a role in mature axons, despite very early evidence for an intrinsic capacity for protein synthesis in mature axons (Koenig, 1967; Morgan and Austin, 1968). Recent breakthroughs have illustrated the importance of local protein synthesis in mature axon terminals for both synaptic function (Scarnati et al., 2018) and plasticity (Younts et al., 2016; Hafner et al., 2019). In this section, we will discuss both of these topics. Given the focus of this book on the hippocampus, it should be noted that much of the work in understanding the axonal transcriptome and translatome has been conducted using nonhippocampal neurons. The principles from all of these various neurons remains the same, hence the importance of their discussion in this context. When notable work pertaining to the hippocampus or hippocampal neurons is discussed, it is noted.

The earliest evidence for RNA localization in axons was from work in developing axons (Bassell et al., 1994) and from invertebrate axons (Landry et al., 1992; Dirks et al., 1993; Gioio et al., 1994). The localization of mRNAs within developing axons, especially the growth cone, lead to the possibility of local translation being important in axonal growth and guidance (See Figure 8.3A–C). The growth cone, located at the distal tip of the developing axon, processes the environmental

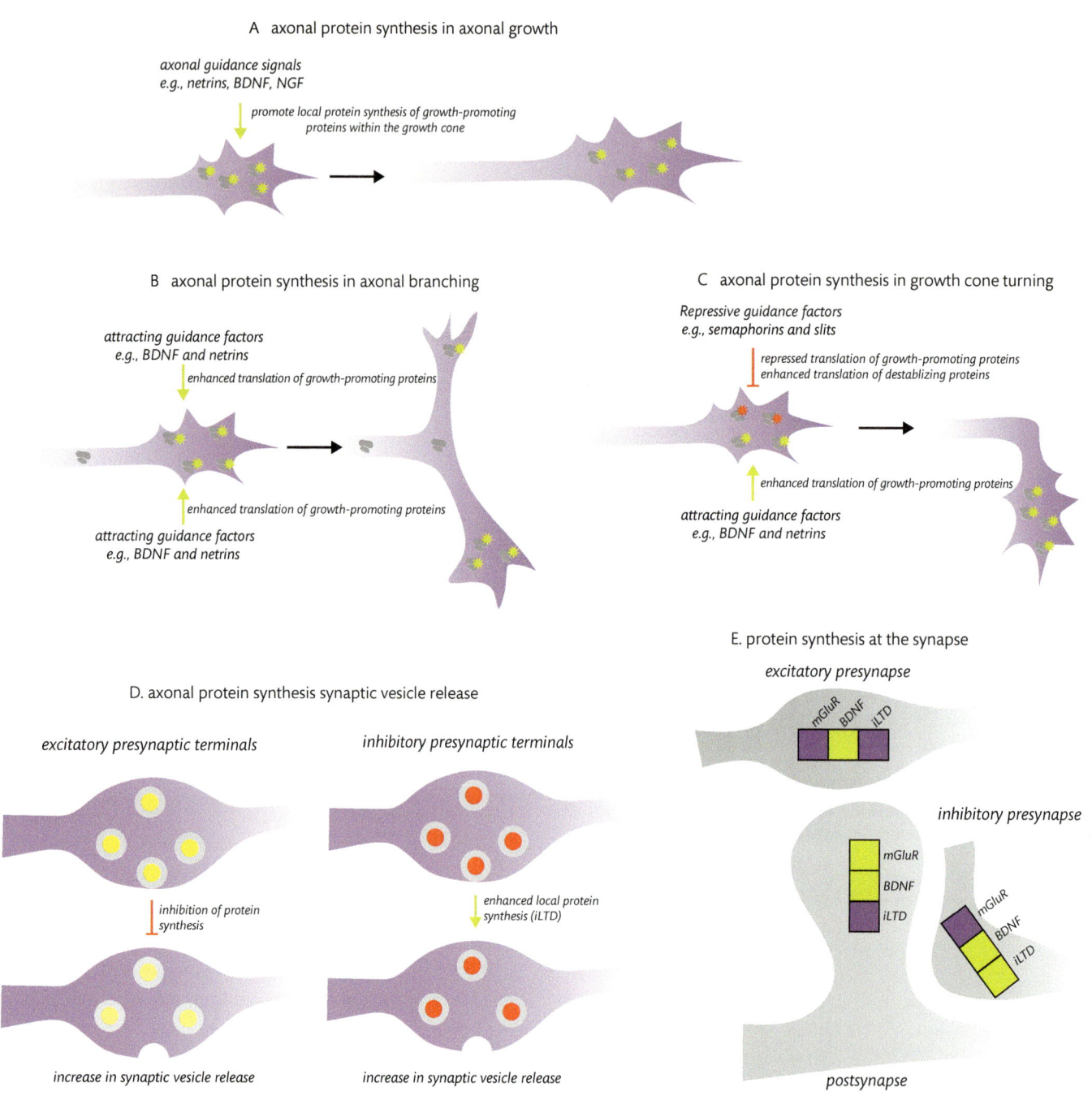

Figure 8.3 Roles of protein synthesis in axons. (A) In growing axons, growth-promoting factors (such as netrins, BDNF, and NGF) enhance ongoing translation of growth-promoting proteins such as GAP-43 in the axonal growth cone. These enhance the outgrowth of the growing axon. (B) Growth factors involved with axonal outgrowth can also lead to the translation of proteins such as Beta actin, which leads to establishment and outgrowth of axonal branches. (C) Gradients of repressive (orange line) and attracting growth factors (green arrow) can lead to asymmetric translation of growth promoting (green translational event) and growth-repressing proteins (orange translational event) in the axonal growth cone—leading to polarization of axonal outgrowth and eventual turning of the growth cone toward the attracting cues. (D) In the calyx of Held, inhibition of protein synthesis enhances the spontaneous release of vesicles suggesting that active protein synthesis may limit the pool of releasable presynaptic vesicles. While at inhibitory presynaptic terminals endocannabinoid stimulation enhances local translation and is necessary for the expression of endocannabinoid-mediated inhibitory LTD (iLTD). (E) Excitatory and inhibitory pre- and excitatory postsynapses can be engaged simultaneously or separately at the translational level during different forms of protein-synthesis dependent forms of synaptic plasticity. Scheme shows differential upregulation of translation (green boxes) relative to the baseline state (purple boxes).

cues autonomously—without consulting the cell body. In the retina, axons that have been physically isolated from their cell bodies in vivo remain capable of responding to guidance cues and of finding their path (Harris et al., 1987; Campbell and Holt, 2001). This is made possible by the localization of mRNAs that are transported and enriched in the tip of growing axons.

8.3.3 Which RNAs are involved?

Early work completed prior to the age of transcriptomics focused on a limited selection of RNAs, including β-actin mRNA (Bassell et al., 1998), growth associated protein 43 (Gap43) (Kruger et al., 1992), and neuritin/cpg15 (Akten et al., 2011). These mRNAs encode proteins known to be involved in both axonal growth and branching. The assumption, which has largely held true, is that the localized transcriptome of the developing axon supports the growth and survival of the axon. Such a functional role has been reported for β-actin mRNA in developing axons, where its local translation drives axonal branching (Donnelly et al., 2013) and predicts longer-lived branching events in developing axons (Wong et al., 2017). Additionally, Gap43 mRNA localization facilitates axonal growth (Donnelly et al., 2013), consistent with the known function for its encoded protein. Local translation in growth cones is also activated by guidance cues. For instance, Netrin1 or BDNF attractive cues induce an asymmetric translation of β-actin mRNA in growth cones resulting in a change of direction of the growing axon (Campbell and Holt, 2001; Zhang et al., 2001; Yao et al., 2006). In contrast, the repulsive cues SLIT2 or SEMA3A induce an asymmetric translation of mRNAs coding for proteins that promote actin filament disassembly (Deglincerti et al., 2015).

Extracellular cues outside the growing axon are also critical. These result in downstream translational responses via the direct coupling of receptors in the plasma membrane with downstream signaling cascades, which in turn regulate translation. Given this tight relationship between receiving a signaling cue and the underlying translational output, one would expect rather rapid responses at the translational level. Recent results suggest just this: changes in the proteome occur within minutes of stimulation (Cagnetta et al., 2018). Recent work has also indicated that axonal RNAs are transported along with late endosomes, and suggests this interaction serves as a platform for local translation of factors responsible for axonal integrity and survival (Cioni et al., 2018). This is consistent with previous reports of endosome association of septin mRNA, suggesting that endosomes may function as both transport and as translational platforms.

To date, only a few studies have directly examined the axonal transcriptome in hippocampal neurons (Taylor et al., 2005; Baleriola et al., 2014). Using microfluidic devices to isolate the soma and axons, Baleriola et al. found ~3,000 transcripts within the axonal transcriptome. Of interest, a sizable fraction of the transcriptome changed on long-term application of Aβ peptide, indicating a possible pathogenic response causing alterations in RNA homeostasis (transcription and degradation) in Alzheimer's disease. With the recent characterization of a vGLUT1+ presynaptic transcriptome (Hafner et al., 2019), dysregulation of these target mRNAs may play a role in the pathogenesis of Alzheimer's disease.

One existing pitfall of the studies examining much of the axonal transcriptomes is their reliance on cultured neuron systems, whose axonal transcriptomes may not reflect the complex growth environments encountered in vivo. Recent work, utilizing sparse viral labeling, isolation, and fluorescence sorting of growth cones from the cerebral cortex, provided a first characterization of the transcriptome of the growth cone in vivo (Poulopoulos et al., 2019). Among the enriched transcripts, the authors found an overrepresentation of mTOR-regulated transcripts, consistent with previous work demonstrating an important role for mTOR signaling in axonal growth (Terenzio et al., 2018). All these studies converge in their description of a developing axon transcriptome that is enriched for cytoskeletal and signaling molecule mRNAs, which makes sense: guidance cues activate signaling pathways that in turn remodel local cytoskeleton to orchestrate and implement growth decisions.

8.3.4 Local translation machinery in axons

The presence of ribosomes and polyribosomes in mammalian axonal growth cones has been repeatedly documented (Jung et al., 2012). In contrast, while postulated for a long time (Alvarez et al., 2000), only recently have ribosomes been detected in mature nonpathological axons and terminals from excitatory and inhibitory neurons (Hafner et al., 2019; Scarnati et al., 2018; Shigeoka et al., 2016; Younts et al., 2016). In fact, over 80% of excitatory terminals isolated from adult mouse hippocampus contain ribosomes (Hafner et al., 2019). In addition, it has been suggested that axons could use an external supply of ribosomes. Indeed, ribosomal proteins tagged with GFP in Schwann cells were observed in neighboring neuronal axons in the peripheral nervous system. Ribosomal transfer was increased when the axons are injured (Court et al., 2011). Recently, using a similar strategy, ribosome transfer was also observed in the CA1 region of adult hippocampus slices (Müller et al., 2018).

Despite evidence from the 1960s showing presynaptic incorporation of isotope-labeled amino acids within both synaptosomes and severed axons (Koenig, 1967; Morgan and Austin, 1968; Autilio et al., 1968), the presence of mRNAs in mature axons and their local translation have been repeatedly questioned (see, for instance, Südhof, 2018). With the advent of cell-type-specific ribosome tagging (i.e., RiboTag) (Sanz et al., 2009), characterizing cell-type- or cell-compartment-specific translatomes became possible. A translatome describes the full complement of mRNAs engaged with ribosomes, or in the process of translation. Using RiboTag labeling of ribosomes in retinal ganglion cells and taking advantage of the remote location of the axonal projections in the optic tectum, a recent study isolated the first mature axonal translatome (Shigeoka et al., 2016). Shigeoka et al. identified differences in the translatome over various developmental stages, including phases of axonal growth and maintenance. Intriguingly, the overlap between developing and mature axons was rather low, indicating a fundamental functional switch in which mRNAs are translated. Another study detected similar translatome changes as axons switch from active growth toward maturation (Zhang et al., 2016). Conceptually, this makes sense, as a developing axon and an established axon have distinct functional properties and needs.

While the above studies nicely describe the transcriptome and translatome of a few types of mature axons as a whole, they lack information on where exactly the axon transcripts localize. Importantly, if the presynaptic translation needs are similar to that of the postsynaptic compartment, RNAs and ribosomes should localize to the presynaptic bouton itself. Recent work characterized the localized transcriptome in excitatory presynaptic compartments (Hafner et al.,

2019)(see Figure 8.2B). To unravel the local presynaptic transcriptome in vGLUT1+ excitatory presynaptic terminals, Hafner and colleagues isolated these terminals by coupling biochemical fractionation with fluorescence-sorting (Biesemann et al., 2014; Hafner et al., 2019). The authors used the adult mouse forebrain (thus including the hippocampus) for their transcriptomic analysis. They identify 468 unique mRNAs enriched in vGLUT1+ presynaptic excitatory terminals. Among the most enriched transcripts in this local transcriptome were transcripts coding for many well-known presynaptic proteins including Bassoon, Rim1-3, Syntaxin-6, and signaling molecules like DelGEF and RapGEF4 (see Figure 8.2B). The gene ontology terms associated with the presynaptic transcriptome spanned components like the presynaptic active zone, ribosomes, and mitochondrial membrane. Strikingly, none of the transcripts coding for the proteins that inhabit synaptic vesicles were detected. A presynaptic bouton contains on average 200 synaptic vesicles, so at least 200 copies of each of the associated proteins must be present. In contrast, a bouton contains only ~40 copies of the active zone protein RIM1. Thus, one could argue that local translation is favored in cases where protein copy numbers are low, and the addition of a few molecules can have a big impact. Taken together, the above-described studies show that excitatory terminals contain a rich, diverse, yet selective population of transcripts for protein synthesis and local proteome remodeling. Interestingly, about 8% of the transcripts found in the excitatory presynaptic boutons code for transmembrane (Hafner et al., 2019) proteins that require additional secretory organelles for their synthesis.

As mentioned above, the ER has been observed for decades in both axons and dendrites of hippocampus neurons using electron microscopy (Broadwell and Cataldo, 1984; Ramírez and Couve, 2011; Cui-wang et al., 2012). Interestingly, the membrane thickness of axonal ER measured in the hippocampus is remarkably similar to that of the somatic rough ER (~70 nm) (Broadwell and Cataldo, 1984). However, rough ER (highly enriched for ribosomes) has not yet been observed in axons. Similarly, Golgi outposts have not been observed in axons. But as described above, neurons display unconventional secretory processing that allows membrane proteins to traffic directly from the ER membrane to the cell surface (Hanus et al., 2016). While it has not yet been observed in axons, it is possible that a similar phenomenon occurs there as well.

Finally, lysosomes and proteasomes have been detected in growing and mature axons (Parton et al., 1992) suggesting the ability of this compartment to locally regulate protein turnover. Interestingly, the disruption of lysosomal proteolysis slows the axonal transport of lysosomes and other membranous organelles like late endosomes and induces their accumulation within dystrophic axonal swellings (Lee et al., 2011). This result suggests that lysosomes are essential for axonal maintenance.

8.3.5 Local translation in mature axons

Local protein synthesis is regulated by various forms of synaptic plasticity and neuronal activity itself (Jones et al., 2018). Recent studies suggest a similar regulation in the presynaptic compartment. For example, an inverse relationship between activity and axonal protein synthesis has been observed in the calyx of Held, in which the inhibition of protein synthesis enhances the spontaneous release of vesicles (Scarnati et al., 2018) (see Figure 8.3D). This suggests active protein synthesis may limit the pool of releasable presynaptic vesicles. In addition, endocannabinoid stimulation enhances local translation in inhibitory terminals (Younts et al.,

2016) (see Figure 8.3D). This increase in translation is necessary for the expression of endocannabinoid-mediated inhibitory LTD (iLTD) (Younts et al., 2016). Expanding on this, Hafner et al. demonstrated that both inhibitory and excitatory presynaptic terminals as well as postsynaptic spines are enriched for both poly(A) RNA and ribosomes and are translationally active (see Figures 8.2A, 8.3E). Furthermore, the pre- and postsynapse can be engaged simultaneously or separately at the translational level during different forms of plasticity (Hafner et al., 2019). These patterns are seen in both hippocampal and cortical neuron cultures, suggesting a global role for plasticity regulated translation in the brain.

8.4 Dysregulation of local proteomes in diseases

8.4.1 Fragile X syndrome

Over the past few decades, many studies have reported that disruption of protein synthesis homeostasis contributes significantly to disease pathology. For example, Fragile X syndrome (FXS) was the first disease identified with translational dysregulation at its core. FXS is the leading genetic cause of autism and intellectual disability. At the cellular level, FXS neurons exhibit widespread immature spines (Irwin et al., 2000) and an exaggerated protein-synthesis-dependent mGluR-LTD (Huber et al., 2002). The disease results from loss of expression of the fragile X mRNA binding protein (FMRP), an mRNA-binding protein. FMRP's known function is to inhibit translation by stalling ribosomes on mRNAs (Darnell et al., 2011). As a result, the loss of FMRP is believed to result in widespread translational dysregulation in neurons (see Figure 8.4A).

FMRP's translational inhibition mechanism is reversible and has been linked to mGluR1/5-dependent signaling pathways (Richter et al., 2015). Genetic knockout of mGluR1/5 receptors in mice dampens the severity of FXS mouse symptoms (Dolen et al., 2007). This has led to the so called "mGluR" hypothesis of FXS. It was speculated that downstream translational targets regulated by mGluR signaling through FMRP are no longer translated in a regulated fashion, contributing to the underlying synaptic defects in the disease. Ongoing work needs to address whether mGluR signaling is the primary driver of FXS pathology, as mGluR antagonists so far have had little therapeutic effect in FXS patients. Nevertheless, it is clear that protein-synthesis dysregulation is an important feature of the disease. Evidence exists that this deregulation can occur locally within the dendrite (Muddashetty et al., 2007; Tatavarty et al., 2012; Ifrim et al., 2015), consistent with both pre- (Akins et al., 2017) and postsynaptic localization of FMRP (Antar et al., 2005). Additionally, recent work revealed that FMRP mRNA targets include transcription factors (Korb et al., 2017), indicating that widespread changes to the transcriptome may also contribute to FXS symptoms.

8.4.2 Axonopathies

A number of axonopathies display alterations in axonal protein synthesis homeostasis (Khalil et al., 2018) (See Figure 8.4B). Many studies have focused on diseases affecting the exceptionally long axons of the spinal motor neurons, such as spinal muscular atrophy (SMA) (Fallini et al., 2016) and amyotrophic lateral sclerosis (ALS) (Lopez-Erauskin et al., 2018). Increasing evidence points to a role in the brain as well. In fact, ALS has causative and symptomatic overlap with a CNS neurodegenerative disease called frontotemporal dementia (FTD)

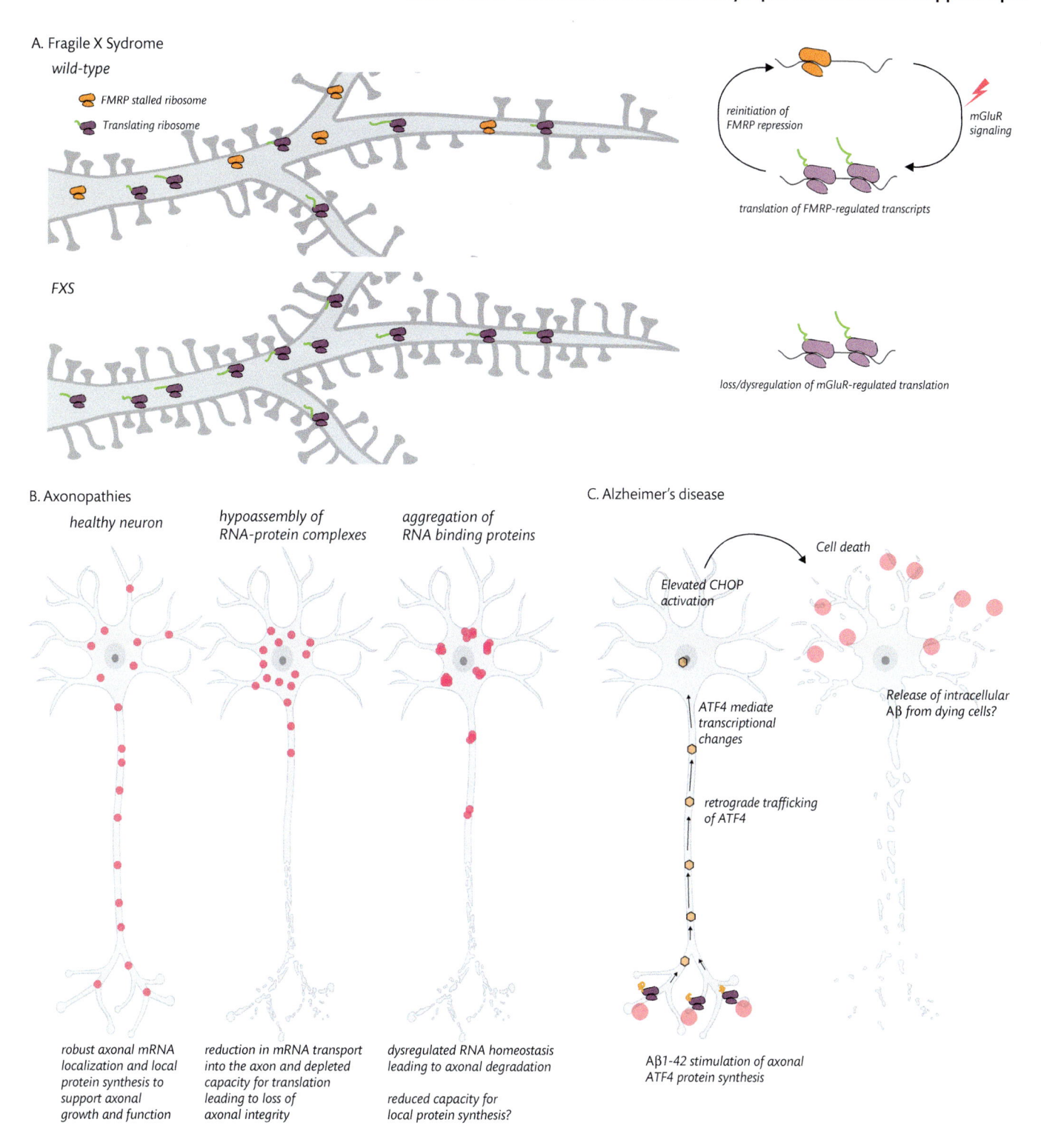

Figure 8.4 Translational dysregulation in neurodevelopmental and degenerative diseases. (A) The RNA-binding protein FMRP regulates the translation of approximately ~10% of the neuronal transcriptome. Functioning as a translational repressor, it keeps its targets translationally silenced until it is removed from mRNA during mGluR signaling, allowing translation of its target mRNAs. One of FMRP's mRNA targets is its own mRNA, allowing for accumulation of new FMRP protein and eventual re-repression of FMRP target mRNAs. In Fragile X syndrome (FXS), FMRP protein is lost, resulting in dysregulation of mGluR-regulated translation. (B) In normal developing and mature axons, mRNAs populate the axon with transcripts encoding for a number of growth and survival promoting factors. In diseases such as spinal muscular atrophy (SMA) growing evidence points to hypoassembly of mRNA and protein associated complexes leading to a reduction in mRNA transport into the axon, leading to eventual axonal degeneration and cell death. In diseases such as frontotemporal dementia (FTD) and amyotrophic lateral sclerosis (ALS) a number of causative mutations of the disease are in RNA-binding proteins important for localization and homeostasis regulation of mRNAs, such as TDP-43. These mutant proteins are prone to forming cytosolic aggregates within cells, possibly leading to dysregulation of mRNA regulation, transport, and homeostasis in cells. (C) Soluble Aβ peptides has been shown to stimulate the local translation of the transcription factor ATF4. Once translated in the axon, ATF4 is retrogradely trafficked to the soma, where it promotes the transcription of stress related genes, including CHOP. Prolonged elevation of CHOP leads to cell death and release of internalized Aβ peptides, promoting its spread through distal regions of the brain. (This figure was assembled using BioRender.)

(Ferrari et al., 2011). It is clear that similar pathogenic mechanisms (e.g., altered axonal protein synthesis) are likely to contribute to both neurodegenerative diseases. In recent work on an ALS/FTD causative mutations of the protein FUS (Fused-in-Sarcoma), hippocampal axonal protein synthesis was decreased as a result of the overexpression of mutant FUS in vitro (Lopez-Erauskin et al., 2018). Furthermore, overexpression of a mutant FUS resulted in progressive cognitive impairments and degeneration within the hippocampus, suggesting that axonal protein synthesis may play a role in FTD pathogenesis.

Apart from defects in axonal protein synthesis, axonal transport and the cytoskeleton are frequent hits in neurodegenerative diseases. Exome sequencing studies of rare ALS cases have identified mutations within TUBA4A (Smith et al., 2014), Kif5A (Nicolas et al., 2018) and Profilin 1 (Wu et al., 2012) as causative mutations for ALS. The axonal microtubule bundling protein tau is implicated in both FTD and Alzheimer's disease (Hutton et al., 1998). These diseases further highlight the importance of trafficking for the function and maintenance of the axon.

8.4.3 Alzheimer's disease

It has been reported that the pathological spread of Aβ in Alzheimer's disease can trigger translation of the transcription factor ATF4 in axons (Baleriola et al., 2014) (see Figure 8.4C). The abnormal expression of this transcription factor resulted in retrograde signaling to the cell body that eventually led to cell death. Also, the authors found a sizable (~800) number of transcripts that are uniquely enriched upon Aβ treatment, suggesting widespread transcriptome changes within the axon may facilitate both axonal degeneration and spread of the disease. There is also evidence for ATF4 RNA upregulation in postmortem brain samples from Alzheimer's patients, indicating that this may be a key disease mechanism.

8.5 Unresolved questions

8.5.1 Targeting signal mRNA and ribosomes in distal compartments

The first studies showing mRNA localization in dendrites date back to the early 1990s (Kleiman et al., 1990; Burgin et al., 1990).

While our understanding of the scope of this phenomenon has progressed significantly, the mechanisms underlying the process of mRNA localization remain poorly understood (see Figure 8.5A). This discrepancy arises because we have failed to identify many consensus RNA sequences across mRNA species that drive the mRNAs to defined subcellular localizations. While a few classical RNA-binding proteins (RBPs), such as the zipcode-binding protein family (ZBP1, IMP1/2/3) have a consensus sequence (Chao et al., 2010); it has become increasingly clear that RNA secondary structure, rather than the sequence itself, is likely a major determinant of RBP interaction with mRNA. As an example, FMRP exhibits preferences for G-quadraplex structures (Zhang et al., 2014), rather than classical RNA sequences. Indeed, recent work assessing 78 individual RBPs found a preference for motifs and structure rather than defined sequence elements (Dominguez et al., 2018). Indeed, the complexity of the associated elements with mRNA is steadily increasing, with over 1,000 RBPs now documented (Castello et al., 2016, Perez-Perri et al., 2018). Targeting of mRNAs to distal sites likely requires the complex interplay with a number of transacting factors, including RBPs and microRNAs. The combinatorial code represented by the binding of these factors is likely to determine the localization of the mRNA.

Interestingly, related to recognition motifs, Tushev et al. revealed a surprising diversity in neuronal mRNA 3′ untranslated regions (UTRs) in the rat hippocampal neuropil (Tushev et al., 2018). The analysis revealed that mRNAs localized in the CA1 neuropil tend to possess longer 3'UTRs, and more miRNA and RBP binding sites, than those detected in the CA1 somata layer. The author extracted the half-lives of the different transcripts and found that the longer 3'UTR isoforms tend to have longer half-lives. These results suggest mRNAs in dendrites might be longer-lived, explaining how an otherwise labile message can accumulate in dendrites and axons. Still remaining to be determined, is how neurons achieve the sorting of presynaptic versus dendritic transcripts.

8.5.2 Short-lived mRNA?

One of the most fascinating questions is how mRNA, which has a far shorter half-life than protein (hours versus days), can be transported and reach distal targets intact (see Figure 8.5B). It is important to note that, due to detection limits for both RNA and

Figure 8.5 Unresolved questions in the field. (A) Previous work on a number of localized mRNAs, such as Beta-actin mRNA, lead to a popularized idea that single defined "zipcode" sequences within mRNAs likely drive subcellular localization of mRNAs. With thousands of localized mRNAs now known in distal sites, it is increasingly likely that rather than individual defined RNA sequences directing mRNA localization there is instead a complex interplay between RNA structure and the RNA-binding proteins that coat these mRNAs, which defines where these RNAs localize. This "RBP code" has yet to be resolved. Furthermore, how ribosomes themselves populate distal sites is still unclear. With notable examples such as FMRP-stalling ribosomes, it is entirely possible that ribosomes are entirely transported on mRNA in a stalled state, activated and accumulating at distal sites in an activity dependent fashion. Alternatively, and untested, is the possibility that ribosomes could be directly transported in an RNA-independent fashion. (B) With mRNA's half-life being on the order of hours, how can distal dendritic and axonal sites be successfully populated with mRNA? One possibility is that distally localized mRNA could have a significantly longer half-life, due to either stabilization of the mRNA or sequestration of RNA degradation machinery. While direct compartment measurements have yet to be directly assessed, mRNA isoforms that are localized are known to exhibit longer half-lives than their non-localized counterparts (~10.5 hours vs. ~8.5 hours; Tuschev et al., 2018). (C) Surprisingly, the transcriptome in dendrites (Cajigas et al., 2012), the translatome in growing axons (Shigeoka et al., 2016), and the transcriptome in excitatory presynaptic compartments (Hafner et al., 2019) all are enriched in ribosomal proteins and more generally in regulators of translation. This suggests that translation may have a regulatory feedback loop, which can fine-tune itself in response to the needs of a particular compartment over time. The exact functional role for the translation of these factors has yet to be fully elucidated. (D) The final pressing question concerns how much the local proteome is remodeled independently from the global proteome. It remains unknown how rapidly the transcriptome could be modified in response to synaptic plasticity, and if normal cellular transport machinery (see Figure 8.2) would be capable of rapid adaptation. Recent work suggests two possible more rapid ways to modulate the local transcriptome, via cell-to-cell communication. These involve Arc capsids transferring mRNA (and potentially ribosomes) between cells and direct transfer of ribosomes (and potentially mRNAs) from glia to neuronal processes. The advantage to both is that this would allow nearly immediate adaptation of a local translatome, populating both mRNAs and ribosomes at distal sites. But it still remains unknown whether such rapid adaptions are required, as it still is untested how much proteomic remolding actually is driven by local translational changes versus more global (somatic) changes that are the shuttled directly to the required sites.

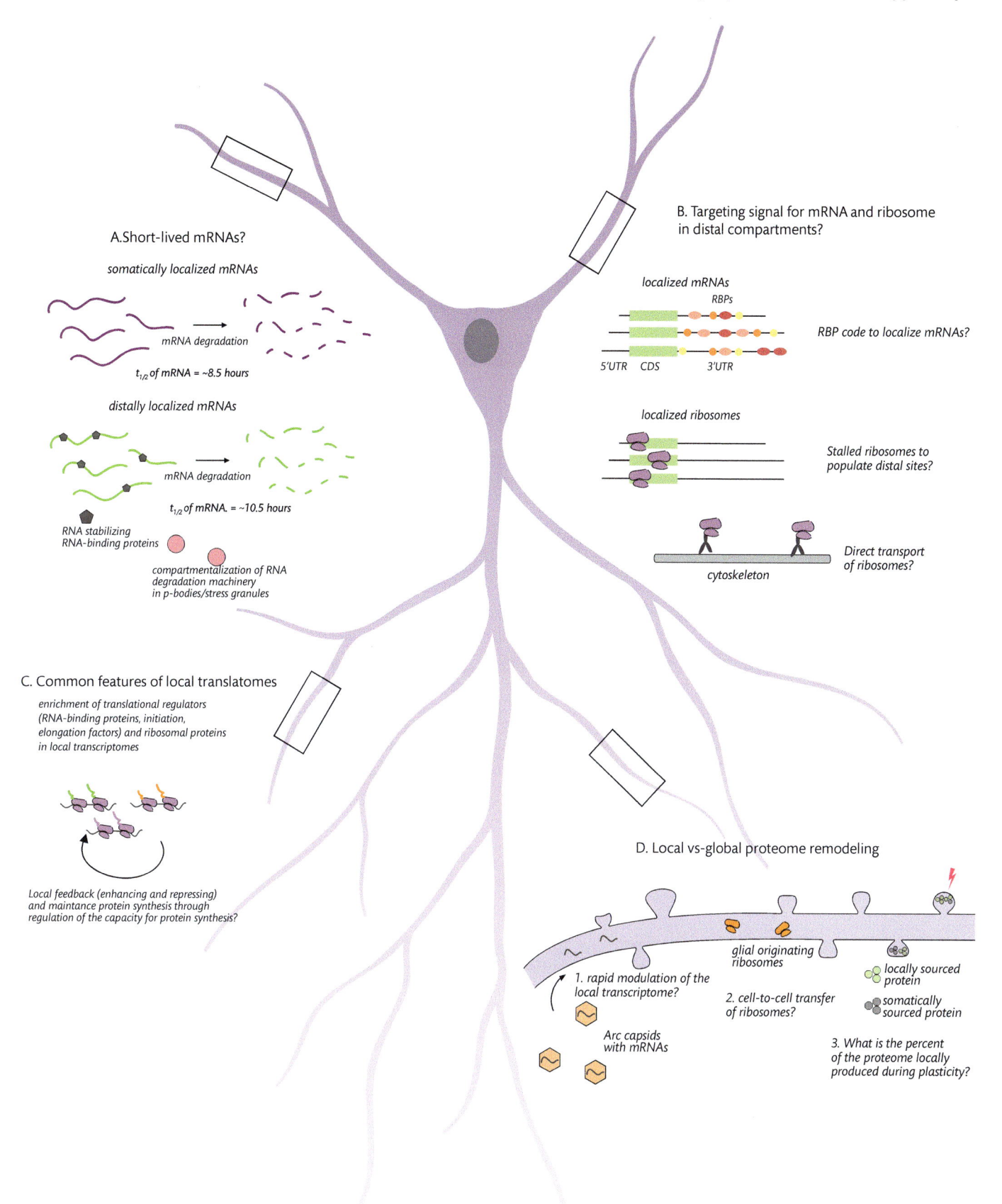

A. Short-lived mRNAs?

somatically localized mRNAs

mRNA degradation

$t_{1/2}$ of mRNA = ~8.5 hours

distally localized mRNAs

mRNA degradation

$t_{1/2}$ of mRNA. = ~10.5 hours

RNA stabilizing
RNA-binding proteins

compartmentalization of RNA
degradation machinery
in p-bodies/stress granules

B. Targeting signal for mRNA and ribosome
in distal compartments?

localized mRNAs

RBPs

RBP code to localize mRNAs?

5'UTR   CDS   3'UTR

localized ribosomes

Stalled ribosomes to
populate distal sites?

Direct transport
of ribosomes?

cytoskeleton

C. Common features of local translatomes

enrichment of translational regulators
(RNA-binding proteins, initiation,
elongation factors) and ribosomal proteins
in local transcriptomes

Local feedback (enhancing and repressing)
and maintance protein synthesis through
regulation of the capacity for protein synthesis?

D. Local vs-global proteome remodeling

glial originating
ribosomes

locally sourced
protein

somatically
sourced protein

1. rapid modulation of the
local transcriptome?

2. cell-to-cell transfer
of ribosomes?

Arc capsids
with mRNAs

3. What is the percent
of the proteome locally
produced during plasticity?

Figure 8.5 Continued

protein, existing half-life measurements are based on total (soma/dendrite/axon) samples. This raises an intriguing possibility: might mRNA half-life distally be simply much longer than "bulk" mRNA population? How might this occur? RNA degradation machinery is, in part, compartmentalized in the cell into structures called p-bodies (Luo et al., 2018). To be degraded, it is believed that mRNAs must be targeted to p-bodies. While p-bodies are found in dendrites (Cougot et al., 2008) and axons (Melemedjian et al., 2014), they are functionally segregated from the transporting mRNA pool in these regions. This segregation might confer some level of passive stability that prolongs mRNA half-lives. Additionally, classes of mRNA-binding proteins exist that confer additional stability to mRNAs. One such class of proteins, the ELAV family, has four members in the mammalian genome HuR/B/C/D (Hinman and Lou, 2008). Strikingly, HuB/C/D are only expressed in neurons, where they are readily detected in both axons and dendrites.

8.5.3 Common features of local transcriptomes

One surprising result of all transcriptomic studies is the large number of mRNAs that are present outside of the neuron soma: growing axons 1,000–4,500 mRNAs (Zivraj et al., 2010), dendrites >2,500 mRNAs (Cajigas et al., 2012), and already ~450 mRNAs identified in excitatory terminals (Hafner et al., 2019). Surprisingly, the transcriptome in dendrites (Cajigas et al., 2012), the translatome in growing axons (Shigeoka et al., 2016) and the transcriptome in excitatory presynaptic compartments (Hafner et al., 2019) share interesting features. All are enriched in ribosomal proteins and more generally in regulators of translation (see Figure 8.5C). This suggests that translation can promote itself perhaps to maintain translation when the activating signal has already vanished. The presence of transcripts coding for ribosomal proteins remains puzzling. Indeed, the biogenesis of ribosomes in eukaryotic cells occurs within the nucleus: the ribosomal RNAs of both subunits assemble with ribosomal proteins in the nucleolus before exiting the nucleus and finally stay in the cytoplasm. One hypothesis is that synthesizing ribosomal proteins in distal compartments constitutes a repair mechanism for damaged ribosomes or a means to specialize ribosomes. Recent evidence supports such a role, finding that intra-axonally synthesized ribosomal proteins incorporate into axonally localized ribosomes independent of the nucleolus (Shigeoka et al., 2019). Another common feature is the abundance of transcripts coding for signaling molecules. This is in line with experimental data showing that local protein synthesis participates in the propagation of signals via intracellular pathways. Both presynaptic and dendritic transcriptomes include mRNAs that code for proteins that are exclusively pre- or postsynaptic. Indeed, the vGLUT1+ enriched presynaptic transcriptome is enriched for mRNAs encoding proteins of the active zone while the dendritic transcriptome is enriched for mRNAs proteins of the PSD. Interestingly, they both contain mRNAs that code for cytosolic and transmembrane proteins.

8.5.4 Local versus global proteome remodeling

The ample evidence for plasticity-regulated translation in both the pre- and postsynaptic compartment raises the potential for crosstalk of proteomic remodeling at the synapse (see Figure 8.5D). Such crosstalk could couple changes in the pre- and postsynaptic proteomes, allowing coherent synaptic scaling or downscaling

depending on the synaptic needs. Recent work on the immediate early gene *Arc* found that local encapsulated mRNAs (including *Arc* transcript) could shuttle this across the synapse into neighboring neurons (Pastuzyn et al., 2018). These kinds of cross-neuronal transcriptome conversations could speed up proteomic changes during activity. Much like the transfer of ribosomes from glial cells to axons (Müller et al., 2018), it brings a new perspective on how neurons deal with providing goods to distant compartments.

Finally, the most pressing and open-ended unresolved issue is what is the contribution of pre- or postsynaptic translation to the long-lasting molecular and behavioral changes induced by synaptic plasticity? While we know widespread changes to the proteome occur in response to activity (Kahne et al., 2012) and during synaptic scaling or downscaling (Schanzenbacher et al., 2016; Schanzenbacher et al., 2018); we still don't understand how much of these proteomic changes are indeed local. Furthermore, how might local proteomic changes influence downstream behavior and learning and memory? In part, this limitation is brought about by lack of spatial control in our ability to perturb the local synthesis, relying on translational inhibitors of knockout animals of localization elements of individual mRNAs to disrupt translation. Until further refined tools are developed, allowing us to specifically block translation in either dendrites or axons, this will remain our greatest unresolved question.

REFERENCES

Akins MR, Berk-Rauch HE, Kwan KY, Mitchell ME, Shepard KA, Korsak LI, Stackpole EE, Warner-Schmidt JL, Sestan N, Cameron HA, et al. (2017) Axonal ribosomes and mRNAs associate with fragile X granules in adult rodent and human brains. *Hum Mol Genet* 26:192–209.

Akten B, Kye MJ, Hao le T, Wertz MH, Singh S, Nie D, Huang J, Merianda TT, Twiss JL, Beattie CE, et al. (2011) Interaction of survival of motor neuron (SMN) and HuD proteins with mRNA cpg15 rescues motor neuron axonal deficits. *Proc Natl Acad Sci U S A* 108:10337–10342.

Alvarez J, Giuditta A, Koenig E (2000) Protein synthesis in axons and terminals: significance for maintenance, plasticity and regulation of phenotype: with a critique of slow transport theory. *Prog Neurobiol* 62:1–62.

Antar LN, Dictenberg JB, Plociniak M, Afroz R, Bassell GJ (2005) Localization of FMRP-associated mRNA granules and requirement of microtubules for activity-dependent trafficking in hippocampal neurons. *Genes Brain Behav* 4:350–359.

Ascoli GA, Donohue DE, Halavi M (2007) NeuroMorpho.Org: a central resource for neuronal morphologies. *J Neurosci* 27:9247–9251.

Autilio LA, Appel SH, Pettis P, Gambetti PL (1968) Biochemical studies of synapses in vitro: I. Protein synthesis. *Biochemistry* 7:2615–2622.

Baas PW, Deitch JS, Black MM, Banker GA (1988) Polarity orientation of microtubules in hippocampal neurons: uniformity in the axon and nonuniformity in the dendrite. *Proc Natl Acad Sci U S A* 85:8335–8339.

Baleriola J, Walker CA, Jean YY, Crary JF, Troy CM, Nagy PL, Hengst U (2014) Axonally synthesized ATF4 transmits a neurodegenerative signal across brain regions. *Cell* 158:1159–1172.

Bassell GJ, Singer RH, Kosik KS (1994) Association of poly(A) mRNA with microtubules in cultured neurons. *Neuron* 12:571–582.

Bassell GJ, Zhang H, Byrd AL, Femino AM, Singer RH, Taneja KL, Lifshitz LM, Herman IM, Kosik KS (1998) Sorting of beta-actin mRNA, protein to neurites and growth cones in culture. *J Neurosci* 18:251–265.

Bell TJ, Miyashiro KY, Sul JY, Buckley PT, Lee MT, McCullough R, Jochems J, Kim J, Cantor CR, Parsons TD, et al. (2010) Intron retention facilitates splice variant diversity in calcium-activated big potassium channel populations. *Proc Natl Acad Sci U S A* 107:21152–21157.

Biesemann C, Gronborg M, Luquet E, Wichert SP, Bernard V, Bungers SR, Cooper B, Varoqueaux F, Li L, et al. (2014) Proteomic screening of glutamatergic mouse brain synaptosomes isolated by fluorescence activated sorting. *EMBO J* 33:157–170.

Bingol B, Schuman EM (2006) Activity-dependent dynamics and sequestration of proteasomes in dendritic spines. *Nature* 441:1144–1148.

Bloodgood BL, Sabatini BL (2005) Neuronal activity regulates diffusion across the neck of dendritic spines. *Science* 310:866–869.

Bradshaw KD, Emptage NJ, Bliss TV (2003) A role for dendritic protein synthesis in hippocampal late LTP. *Eur J Neurosci* 18:3150–3152.

Brady ST (1985) A novel brain ATPase with properties expected for the fast axonal transport motor. *Nature* 317:73–75.

Bressloff PC, Earnshaw BA (2007) Diffusion-trapping model of receptor trafficking in dendrites. *Phys Rev E Stat Nonlin Soft Matter Phys* 75:041915.

Bressloff PC, Newby JM (2013) Stochastic models of intracellular transport. *Rev Mod Phys* 85:135–196.

Brigidi GS, Hayes MGB, Delos Santos NP, Hartzell AL, Texari L, Lin PA, Bartlett A, Ecker JR, Benner C, Heinz S, et al. (2019) Genomic decoding of neuronal depolarization by stimulus-specific NPAS4 heterodimers. *Cell* 179:373–391.

Broadwell RD, Cataldo AM (1984) The neuronal endoplasmic-reticulum its cyto-chemistry and contribution to the endomembrane system: 2. Axons and terminals. *J Comp Neurol* 230:231–248.

Burgin KE, Waxham MN, Rickling S, Westgate SA, Mobley WC, Kelly PT (1990) In situ hybridization histochemistry of Ca2+/calmodulin-dependent protein kinase in developing rat brain. *J Neurosci* 10:1788–1798.

Burton PR, Paige JL (1981) Polarity of axoplasmic microtubules in the olfactory nerve of the frog. *Proc Natl Acad Sci U S A* 78:3269–3273.

Cagnetta R, Frese CK, Shigeoka T, Krijgsveld J, Holt CE (2018) Rapid cue-specific remodeling of the nascent axonal proteome. *Neuron* 99:29–46, e24.

Cajigas IJ, Tushev G, Will TJ, tom Dieck S, Fuerst N, Schuman EM (2012) The local transcriptome in the synaptic neuropil revealed by deep sequencing and high-resolution imaging. *Neuron* 74:453–466.

Campbell DS, Holt CE (2001) Chemotropic responses of retinal growth cones mediated by rapid local protein synthesis and degradation. *Neuron* 32:1013–1026.

Castello A, Horos R, Strein C, Fischer B, Eichelbaum K, Steinmetz LM, Krijgsveld J, Hentze MW (2016) Comprehensive identification of RNA-binding proteins by RNA interactome capture. *Methods Mol Biol* 1358:131–139.

Chao JA, Patskovsky Y, Patel V, Levy M, Almo SC, Singer RH (2010) ZBP1 recognition of beta-actin zipcode induces RNA looping. *Genes Dev* 24:148–158.

Chazeau A, Mehidi A, Nair D, Gautier JJ, Leduc C, Chamma I, Kage F, Kechkar A, Thoumine O, Rottner K, et al. (2014) Nanoscale segregation of actin nucleation and elongation factors determines dendritic spine protrusion. *EMBO J* 33:2745–2764.

Ch'ng TH, Uzgil B, Lin P, Avliyakulov NK, O'Dell TJ, Martin KC (2012) Activity-dependent transport of the transcriptional coactivator CRTC1 from synapse to nucleus. *Cell* 150:207–221.

Choquet D, Triller A (2013) The dynamic synapse. *Neuron* 80:691–703.

Cingolani LA, Goda Y (2008) Differential involvement of beta3 integrin in pre- and postsynaptic forms of adaptation to chronic activity deprivation. *Neuron Glia Biol* 4:179–187.

Cioni JM, Koppers M, Holt CE (2018) Molecular control of local translation in axon development and maintenance. *Curr Opin Neurobiol* 51:86–94.

Cougot N, Bhattacharyya SN, Tapia-Arancibia L, Bordonne R, Filipowicz W, Bertrand E, Rage F (2008) Dendrites of mammalian neurons contain specialized P-body-like structures that respond to neuronal activation. *J Neurosci* 28:13793–13804.

Court FA, Midha R, Cisterna BA, Grochmal J, Shakhbazau A, Hendriks WT, Van Minnen J (2011) Morphological evidence for a transport of ribosomes from Schwann cells to regenerating axons. *Glia* 59:1529–1539.

Cracco JB, Serrano P, Moskowitz SI, Bergold PJ, Sacktor TC (2005) Protein synthesis-dependent LTP in isolated dendrites of CA1 pyramidal cells. *Hippocampus* 15:551–556.

Cui-Wang T, Hanus C, Cui T, Helton T, Bourne J, Watson D, Harris KM, Ehlers MD (2012) Local zones of endoplasmic reticulum complexity confine cargo in neuronal dendrites. *Cell* 148:309–321.

Darnell JC, Van Driesche SJ, Zhang C, Hung KY, Mele A, Fraser CE, Stone EF, Chen C, Fak JJ, Chi SW, et al. (2011) FMRP stalls ribosomal translocation on mRNAs linked to synaptic function and autism. *Cell* 146:247–261.

Deglincerti A, Liu Y, Colak D, Hengst U, Xu G, Jaffrey SR (2015) Coupled local translation and degradation regulate growth cone collapse. *Nat Commun* 6:6888.

Deisseroth K, Bito H, Tsien RW (1996) Signaling from synapse to nucleus: postsynaptic CREB phosphorylation during multiple forms of hippocampal synaptic plasticity. *Neuron* 16:89–101.

Dirks RW, van Dorp AG, van Minnen J, Fransen JA, van der Ploeg M, Raap AK (1993) Ultrastructural evidence for the axonal localization of caudodorsal cell hormone mRNA in the central nervous system of the mollusc Lymnaea stagnalis. *Microsc Res Tech* 25:12–18.

Dolen G, Osterweil E, Rao BS, Smith GB, Auerbach BD, Chattarji S, Bear MF (2007) Correction of fragile X syndrome in mice. *Neuron* 56:955–962.

Dominguez D, Freese P, Alexis MS, Su A, Hochman M, Palden T, Bazile C, Lambert NJ, Van Nostrand EL, Pratt GA, et al. (2018) Sequence, Structure, and Context Preferences of Human RNA Binding Proteins. *Mol Cell* 70:854–867, e899.

Donnelly CJ, Park M, Spillane M, Yoo S, Pacheco A, Gomes C, Vuppalanchi D, McDonald M, Kim HH, Merianda TT, et al. (2013) Axonally synthesized beta-actin and GAP-43 proteins support distinct modes of axonal growth. *J Neurosci* 33:3311–3322.

Ehlers MD (2003) Activity level controls postsynaptic composition and signaling via the ubiquitin-proteasome system. *Nat Neurosci* 6:231–242.

Fallini C, Donlin-Asp PG, Rouanet JP, Bassell GJ, Rossoll W (2016) Deficiency of the survival of motor neuron protein impairs mRNA localization and local translation in the growth cone of motor neurons. *J Neurosci* 36:3811–3820.

Falzone TL, Stokin GB, Lillo C, Rodrigues EM, Westerman EL, Williams DS, Goldstein LS (2009) Axonal stress kinase activation and tau misbehavior induced by kinesin-1 transport defects. *J Neurosci* 29:5758–5767.

Ferrari R, Kapogiannis D, Huey ED, Momeni P (2011) FTD, ALS: a tale of two diseases. *Curr Alzheimer Res* 8:273–294.

Flexner JB, Flexner LB, Stellar E, De La Haba G, Roberts RB (1962) Inhibition of protein synthesis in brain and learning and memory following puromycin. *J Neurochem* 9:595–605.

Fonkeu Y, Kraynyukova N, Hafner AS, Kochen L, Sartori F, Schuman EM, Tchumatchenko T (2019) How mRNA localization and protein synthesis sites influence dendritic protein distribution and dynamics. *Neuron* 103:1109–1122, e1107.

Frey U, Frey S, Schollmeier F, Krug M (1996) Influence of actinomycin D, a RNA synthesis inhibitor, on long-term potentiation in rat hippocampal neurons in vivo and in vitro. *J Physiol* 490 (Pt 3): 703–711.

Frey U, Krug M, Reymann KG, Matthies H (1988) Anisomycin, an inhibitor of protein synthesis, blocks late phases of LTP phenomena in the hippocampal CA1 region in vitro. *Brain Res* 452:57–65.

Frey U, Morris RG (1997) Synaptic tagging and long-term potentiation. *Nature* 385:533–536.

Gioio AE, Chun JT, Crispino M, Capano CP, Giuditta A, Kaplan BB (1994) Kinesin mRNA is present in the squid giant axon. *J Neurochem* 63:13–18.

Goldberg JL (2003) How does an axon grow? *Genes Dev* 17:941–958.

Goo MS, Sancho L, Slepak N, Boassa D, Deerinck TJ, Ellisman MH, Bloodgood BL, Patrick GN (2017) Activity-dependent trafficking of lysosomes in dendrites and dendritic spines. *J Cell Biol* 216:2499–2513.

Hafner AS, Donlin-Asp PG, Leitch B, Herzog E, Schuman EM (2019) Local protein synthesis is a ubiquitous feature of neuronal pre- and postsynaptic compartments. *Science* 364(6441):eaau3644. doi:10.1126/science.aau3644. PMID: 31097639.

Hafner AS, Penn AC, Grillo-Bosch D, Retailleau N, Poujol C, Philippat A, Coussen F, Sainlos M, Opazo P, Choquet D (2015) Lengthening of the stargazin cytoplasmic tail increases synaptic transmission by promoting interaction to deeper domains of PSD-95. *Neuron* 86:475–489.

Hall DH, Hedgecock EM (1991) Kinesin-related gene unc-104 is required for axonal transport of synaptic vesicles in C. elegans. *Cell* 65:837–847.

Hangen E, Cordelieres FP, Petersen JD, Choquet D, Coussen F (2018) Neuronal activity and intracellular calcium levels regulate intracellular transport of newly synthesized AMPAR. *Cell Rep* 24:1001–1012, e1003.

Hanus C, Ehlers MD (2008) Secretory outposts for the local processing of membrane cargo in neuronal dendrites. *Traffic* 9:1437–1445.

Hanus C, Ehlers MD (2016) Specialization of biosynthetic membrane trafficking for neuronal form and function. *Curr Opin Neurobiol* 39:8–16.

Hanus C, Geptin H, Tushev G, Garg S, Alvarez-Castelao B, Sambandan S, Kochen L, Hafner AS, Langer JD, Schuman EM (2016) Unconventional secretory processing diversifies neuronal ion channel properties. *Elife* 5:e20609.

Hanus C, Kochen L, Tom Dieck S, Racine V, Sibarita JB, Schuman EM, Ehlers MD (2014) Synaptic control of secretory trafficking in dendrites. *Cell Rep* 7:1771–1778.

Harris WA, Holt CE, Bonhoeffer F (1987) Retinal axons with and without their somata, growing to and arborizing in the tectum of Xenopus embryos: a time-lapse video study of single fibres in vivo. *Development* 101:123–133.

Herbst WA, Martin KC (2017) Regulated transport of signaling proteins from synapse to nucleus. *Curr Opin Neurobiol* 45:78–84.

Hinman MN, Lou H (2008) Diverse molecular functions of Hu proteins. *Cell Mol Life Sci* 65:3168–3181.

Hirokawa N, Niwa S, Tanaka Y (2010) Molecular motors in neurons: transport mechanisms and roles in brain function, development, and disease. *Neuron* 68:610–638.

Hirokawa N, Sato-Yoshitake R, Yoshida T, Kawashima T (1990) Brain dynein (MAP1C) localizes on both anterogradely and retrogradely transported membranous organelles in vivo. *J Cell Biol* 111:1027–1037.

Hodas JJ, Nehring A, Hoche N, Sweredoski MJ, Pielot R, Hess S, Tirrell DA, Dieterich DC, Schuman EM (2012) Dopaminergic modulation of the hippocampal neuropil proteome identified by bioorthogonal noncanonical amino acid tagging (BONCAT). *Proteomics* 12:2464–2476.

Holt CE, Schuman EM (2013) The central dogma decentralized: new perspectives on RNA function and local translation in neurons. *Neuron* 80:648–657.

Horton AC, Racz B, Monson EE, Lin AL, Weinberg RJ, Ehlers MD (2005) Polarized secretory trafficking directs cargo for asymmetric dendrite growth and morphogenesis. *Neuron* 48:757–771.

Hotulainen P, Hoogenraad CC (2010) Actin in dendritic spines: connecting dynamics to function. *J Cell Biol* 189:619–629.

Huang J, Ikeuchi Y, Malumbres M, Bonni A (2015) A Cdh1-APC/FMRP ubiquitin signaling link drives mGluR-dependent synaptic plasticity in the mammalian brain. *Neuron* 86:726–739.

Huang YY, Kandel ER (2005) Theta frequency stimulation induces a local form of late phase LTP in the CA1 region of the hippocampus. *Learn Mem* 12:587–593.

Huber KM, Gallagher SM, Warren ST, Bear MF (2002) Altered synaptic plasticity in a mouse model of fragile X mental retardation. *Proc Natl Acad Sci U S A* 99:7746–7750.

Huber KM, Kayser MS, Bear MF (2000) Role for rapid dendritic protein synthesis in hippocampal mGluR-dependent long-term depression. *Science* 288:1254–1257.

Hutton M, Lendon CL, Rizzu P, Baker M, Froelich S, Houlden H, Pickering-Brown S, Chakraverty S, Isaacs A, Grover A, et al. (1998) Association of missense and 5'-splice-site mutations in tau with the inherited dementia FTDP-17. *Nature* 393:702–705.

Ifrim MF, Williams KR, Bassell GJ (2015) Single-molecule imaging of PSD-95 mRNA translation in dendrites and its dysregulation in a mouse model of fragile X syndrome. *J Neurosci* 35:7116–7130.

Irwin SA, Galvez R, Greenough WT (2000) Dendritic spine structural anomalies in fragile-X mental retardation syndrome. *Cereb Cortex* 10:1038–1044.

Ishizuka N, Cowan WM, Amaral DG (1995) A quantitative analysis of the dendritic organization of pyramidal cells in the rat hippocampus. *J Comp Neurol* 362:17–45.

Ivshina M, Lasko P, Richter JD (2014) Cytoplasmic polyadenylation element binding proteins in development, health, and disease. *Annu Rev Cell Dev Biol* 30:393–415.

Jacobson C, Schnapp B, Banker GA (2006) A change in the selective translocation of the Kinesin-1 motor domain marks the initial specification of the axon. *Neuron* 49:797–804.

Jones KJ, Templet S, Zemoura K, Kuzniewska B, Pena FX, Hwang H, Lei DJ, Haensgen H, Nguyen S, Saenz C, et al. (2018) Rapid, experience-dependent translation of neurogranin enables memory encoding. *Proc Natl Acad Sci U S A* 115:E5805–E5814.

Jung H, Yoon BC, Holt CE (2012) Axonal mRNA localization and local protein synthesis in nervous system assembly, maintenance and repair. *Nat Rev Neurosci* 13:308–324.

Kahne T, Kolodziej A, Smalla KH, Eisenschmidt E, Haus UU, Weismantel R, Kropf S, Wetzel W, Ohl FW, Tischmeyer W, et al. (2012) Synaptic proteome changes in mouse brain regions upon auditory discrimination learning. *Proteomics* 12:2433–2444.

Kandel ER (2001) The molecular biology of memory storage: a dialog between genes and synapses. *Biosci Rep* 21:565–611.

Kang H, Schuman EM (1996) A requirement for local protein synthesis in neurotrophin-induced hippocampal synaptic plasticity. *Science* 273:1402–1406.

Karasmanis EP, Phan CT, Angelis D, Kesisova IA, Hoogenraad CC, McKenney RJ, Spiliotis ET (2018) Polarity of neuronal membrane traffic requires sorting of kinesin motor cargo during entry into dendrites by a microtubule-associated septin. *Dev Cell* 46:518–524.

Khalil B, Morderer D, Price PL, Liu F, Rossoll W (2018) mRNP assembly, axonal transport, and local translation in neurodegenerative diseases. *Brain Res* 1693:75–91.

Kleele T, Marinkovic P, Williams PR, Stern S, Weigand EE, Engerer P, Naumann R, Hartmann J, Karl RM, Bradke F, et al. (2014) An assay to image neuronal microtubule dynamics in mice. *Nat Commun* 5:4827.

Kleiman R, Banker G, Steward O (1990) Differential subcellular localization of particular mRNAs in hippocampal neurons in culture. *Neuron* 5:821–830.

Koenig E (1967) Synthetic mechanisms in the axon: IV. In vitro incorporation of [3H]precursors into axonal protein and RNA. *J Neurochem* 14:437–446.

Korb E, Herre M, Zucker-Scharff I, Gresack J, Allis CD, Darnell RB (2017) Excess translation of epigenetic regulators contributes to fragile X syndrome and is alleviated by Brd4 inhibition. *Cell* 170:1209–1223, e1220.

Kreutzberg GW (1969) Neuronal dynamics and axonal flow: IV. Blockage of intra-axonal enzyme transport by colchicine. *Proc Natl Acad Sci U S A* 62:722–728.

Krichevsky AM, Kosik KS (2001) Neuronal RNA granules: a link between RNA localization and stimulation-dependent translation. *Neuron* 32:683–696.

Krucker T, Siggins GR, Halpain S (2000) Dynamic actin filaments are required for stable long-term potentiation (LTP) in area CA1 of the hippocampus. *Proc Natl Acad Sci U S A* 97:6856–6861.

Kruger L, Bendotti C, Rivolta R, Samanin R (1992) GAP-43 mRNA localization in the rat hippocampus CA3 field. *Brain Res Mol Brain Res* 13:267–272.

Lafontaine DL (2015) Noncoding RNAs in eukaryotic ribosome biogenesis and function. *Nat Struct Mol Biol* 22:11–19.

Lai KO, Zhao Y, Ch'ng TH, Martin KC (2008) Importin-mediated retrograde transport of CREB2 from distal processes to the nucleus in neurons. *Proc Natl Acad Sci U S A* 105:17175–17180.

Landry C, Crine P, DesGroseillers L (1992) Differential expression of neuropeptide gene mRNA within the LUQ cells of Aplysia californica. *J Neurobiol* 23:89–101.

Lasek RJ, Brady ST (1985) Attachment of transported vesicles to microtubules in axoplasm is facilitated by AMP-PNP. *Nature* 316:645–647.

Lasek RJ, Dabrowski C, Nordlander R (1973) Analysis of axoplasmic RNA from invertebrate giant axons. *Nat New Biol* 244:162–165.

Lecuyer E, Yoshida H, Parthasarathy N, Alm C, Babak T, Cerovina T, Hughes TR, Tomancak P, Krause HM (2007) Global analysis of mRNA localization reveals a prominent role in organizing cellular architecture and function. *Cell* 131:174–187.

Lee S, Sato Y, Nixon RA (2011) Lysosomal proteolysis inhibition selectively disrupts axonal transport of degradative organelles and causes an Alzheimer's-like axonal dystrophy. *J Neurosci* 31:7817–7830.

Lein ES, Hawrylycz MJ, Ao N, Ayres M, Bensinger A, Bernard A, Boe AF, Boguski MS, Brockway KS, Byrnes EJ, et al. (2007) Genome-wide atlas of gene expression in the adult mouse brain. *Nature* 445:168–176.

Lopez-Erauskin J, Tadokoro T, Baughn MW, Myers B, McAlonis-Downes M, Chillon-Marinas C, Asiaban JN, Artates J, Bui AT, Vetto AP, et al. (2018) ALS/FTD-linked mutation in FUS suppresses intra-axonal protein synthesis and drives disease without nuclear loss-of-function of FUS. *Neuron* 100:816–830, e817.

Lopez Salon M, Pasquini L, Besio Moreno M, Pasquini JM, Soto E (2003) Relationship between beta-amyloid degradation and the 26S proteasome in neural cells. *Exp Neurol* 180:131–143.

Luo Y, Na Z, Slavoff SA (2018) P-bodies: composition, properties, and functions. *Biochemistry* 57:2424–2431.

Maday S, Twelvetrees AE, Moughamian AJ, Holzbaur EL (2014) Axonal transport: cargo-specific mechanisms of motility and regulation. *Neuron* 84:292–309.

Maeder CI, Shen K, Hoogenraad CC (2014) Axon and dendritic trafficking. *Curr Opin Neurobiol* 27:165–170.

Martin KC, Ephrussi A (2009) mRNA localization: gene expression in the spatial dimension. *Cell* 136:719–730.

Matsuzaki M, Ellis-Davies GC, Nemoto T, Miyashita Y, Iino M, Kasai H (2001) Dendritic spine geometry is critical for AMPA receptor expression in hippocampal CA1 pyramidal neurons. *Nat Neurosci* 4:1086–1092.

Mayford M, Bach ME, Huang YY, Wang L, Hawkins RD, Kandel ER (1996) Control of memory formation through regulated expression of a CaMKII transgene. *Science* 274:1678–1683.

Melemedjian OK, Mejia GL, Lepow TS, Zoph OK, Price TJ (2014) Bidirectional regulation of P body formation mediated by eIF4F complex formation in sensory neurons. *Neurosci Lett* 563:169–174.

Merkurjev D, Hong WT, Iida K, Oomoto I, Goldie BJ, Yamaguti H, Ohara T, Kawaguchi SY, Hirano T, Martin KC, et al. (2018) Author correction: synaptic N(6)-methyladenosine (m(6)A) epitranscriptome reveals functional partitioning of localized transcripts. *Nat Neurosci* 21:1493.

Merriam EB, Millette M, Lumbard DC, Saengsawang W, Fothergill T, Hu X, Ferhat L, Dent EW (2013) Synaptic regulation of microtubule dynamics in dendritic spines by calcium, F-actin, and drebrin. *J Neurosci* 33:16471–16482.

Merrill MA, Chen Y, Strack S, Hell JW (2005) Activity-driven postsynaptic translocation of CaMKII. *Trends Pharmacol Sci* 26:645–653.

Mikhaylova M, Bar J, van Bommel B, Schatzle P, YuanXiang P, Raman R, Hradsky J, Konietzny A, Loktionov EY, Reddy PP, et al. (2018) Caldendrin directly couples postsynaptic calcium signals to actin remodeling in dendritic spines. *Neuron* 97:1110–1125, e1114.

Miller S, Yasuda M, Coats JK, Jones Y, Martone ME, Mayford M (2002) Disruption of dendritic translation of CaMKIIalpha impairs stabilization of synaptic plasticity and memory consolidation. *Neuron* 36:507–519.

Monyer H, Burnashev N, Laurie DJ, Sakmann B, Seeburg PH (1994) Developmental and regional expression in the rat brain and functional properties of four NMDA receptors. *Neuron* 12:529–540.

Morgan IG, Austin L (1968) Synaptosomal protein synthesis in a cell-free system. *J Neurochem* 15:41–51.

Muddashetty RS, Kelic S, Gross C, Xu M, Bassell GJ (2007) Dysregulated metabotropic glutamate receptor-dependent translation of AMPA receptor and postsynaptic density-95 mRNAs at synapses in a mouse model of fragile X syndrome. *J Neurosci* 27:5338–5348.

Muller K, Schnatz A, Schillner M, Woertge S, Muller C, von Graevenitz I, Waisman A, van Minnen J, Vogelaar CF (2018) A predominantly glial origin of axonal ribosomes after nerve injury. *Glia* 66:1591–1610.

Newpher TM, Ehlers MD (2008) Glutamate receptor dynamics in dendritic microdomains. *Neuron* 58:472–497.

Nicolas A, Kenna KP, Renton AE, Ticozzi N, Faghri F, Chia R, Dominov JA, Kenna BJ, Nalls MA, Keagle P, et al. (2018) Genome-wide analyses identify KIF5A as a novel Als gene. *Neuron* 97:1268–1283, e12ss66.

Opazo P, Choquet D (2011) A three-step model for the synaptic recruitment of AMPA receptors. *Mol Cell Neurosci* 46:1–8.

Opazo P, Labrecque S, Tigaret CM, Frouin A, Wiseman PW, De Koninck P, Choquet D (2010) CaMKII triggers the diffusional trapping of surface AMPARs through phosphorylation of stargazin. *Neuron* 67:239–252.

Ostroff LE, Cain CK, Jindal N, Dar N, Ledoux JE (2012) Stability of presynaptic vesicle pools and changes in synapse morphology in the amygdala following fear learning in adult rats. *J Comp Neurol* 520:295–314.

Ostroff LE, Fiala JC, Allwardt B, Harris KM (2002) Polyribosomes redistribute from dendritic shafts into spines with enlarged synapses during LTP in developing rat hippocampal slices. *Neuron* 35:535–545.

Ostroff LE, Watson DJ, Cao G, Parker PH, Smith H, Harris KM (2018) Shifting patterns of polyribosome accumulation at synapses over the course of hippocampal long-term potentiation. *Hippocampus* 28:416–430.

Otmakhov N, Tao-Cheng JH, Carpenter S, Asrican B, Dosemeci A, Reese TS, Lisman J (2004) Persistent accumulation of calcium/calmodulin-dependent protein kinase II in dendritic spines after induction of NMDA receptor-dependent chemical long-term potentiation. *J Neurosci* 24:9324–9331.

Parton RG, Simons K, Dotti CG (1992) Axonal and dendritic endocytic pathways in cultured neurons. *J Cell Biol* 119:123–137.

Pastuzyn ED, Day CE, Kearns RB, Kyrke-Smith M, Taibi AV, McCormick J, Yoder N, Belnap DM, Erlendsson S, Morado DR, et al. (2018) The neuronal gene arc encodes a repurposed retrotransposon gag protein that mediates intercellular RNA transfer. *Cell* 173:275.

Perez-Perri JI, Rogell B, Schwarzl T, Stein F, Zhou Y, Rettel M, Brosig A, Hentze MW (2018) Discovery of RNA-binding proteins and characterization of their dynamic responses by enhanced RNA interactome capture. *Nat Commun* 9:4408.

Pierce JP, Mayer T, McCarthy JB (2001) Evidence for a satellite secretory pathway in neuronal dendritic spines. *Curr Biol* 11:351–355.

Poon MM, Choi SH, Jamieson CA, Geschwind DH, Martin KC (2006) Identification of process-localized mRNAs from cultured rodent hippocampal neurons. *J Neurosci* 26:13390–13399.

Poulopoulos A, Murphy AJ, Ozkan A, Davis P, Hatch J, Kirchner R, Macklis JD (2019) Subcellular transcriptomes and proteomes of developing axon projections in the cerebral cortex. *Nature* 565:356–360.

Ramirez OA, Couve A (2011) The endoplasmic reticulum and protein trafficking in dendrites and axons. *Trends Cell Biol* 21:219–227.

Rangaraju V, Tom Dieck S, Schuman EM (2017) Local translation in neuronal compartments: how local is local? *EMBO Rep* 18:693–711.

Richter JD, Bassell GJ, Klann E (2015) Dysregulation and restoration of translational homeostasis in fragile X syndrome. *Nat Rev Neurosci* 16:595–605.

Sahoo PK, Lee SJ, Jaiswal PB, Alber S, Kar AN, Miller-Randolph S, Taylor EE, Smith T, Singh B, Ho TS, et al. (2018) Axonal G3BP1 stress granule protein limits axonal mRNA translation and nerve regeneration. *Nat Commun* 9:3358.

Sambandan S, Akbalik G, Kochen L, Rinne J, Kahlstatt J, Glock C, Tushev G, Alvarez-Castelao B, Heckel A, et al. (2017) Activity-dependent spatially localized miRNA maturation in neuronal dendrites. *Science* 355:634–637.

Sanz E, Yang L, Su T, Morris DR, McKnight GS, Amieux PS (2009) Cell-type-specific isolation of ribosome-associated mRNA from complex tissues. *Proc Natl Acad Sci U S A* 106:13939–13944.

Scarnati MS, Kataria R, Biswas M, Paradiso KG (2018) Active presynaptic ribosomes in the mammalian brain, and altered transmitter release after protein synthesis inhibition. *Elife* 7:e36697.

Schanzenbacher CT, Langer JD, Schuman EM (2018) Time- and polarity-dependent proteomic changes associated with homeostatic scaling at central synapses. *Elife* 7:e33322.

Schanzenbacher CT, Sambandan S, Langer JD, Schuman EM (2016) Nascent proteome remodeling following homeostatic scaling at hippocampal synapses. *Neuron* 92:358–371.

Schnapp BJ, Reese TS (1989) Dynein is the motor for retrograde axonal transport of organelles. *Proc Natl Acad Sci U S A* 86:1548–1552.

Sharma K, Schmitt S, Bergner CG, Tyanova S, Kannaiyan N, Manrique-Hoyos N, Kongi K, Cantuti L, Hanisch UK, Philips MA, et al. (2015) Cell type- and brain region-resolved mouse brain proteome. *Nat Neurosci* 18:1819–1831.

Shen K, Meyer T (1999) Dynamic control of CaMKII translocation and localization in hippocampal neurons by NMDA receptor stimulation. *Science* 284:162–166.

Shen K, Teruel MN, Connor JH, Shenolikar S, Meyer T (2000) Molecular memory by reversible translocation of calcium/calmodulin-dependent protein kinase II. *Nat Neurosci* 3:881–886.

Shepherd JD, Huganir RL (2007) The cell biology of synaptic plasticity: AMPA receptor trafficking. *Annu Rev Cell Dev Biol* 23:613–643.

Shigeoka T, Jung H, Jung J, Turner-Bridger B, Ohk J, Lin JQ, Amieux PS, Holt CE (2016) Dynamic axonal translation in developing and mature visual circuits. *Cell* 166:181–192.

Shigeoka T, Koppers M, Wong HH, Lin JQ, Cagnetta R, Dwivedy A, de Freitas Nascimento J, van Tartwijk FW, Strohl F, Cioni JM, et al. (2019) On-site ribosome remodeling by locally synthesized ribosomal proteins in axons. *Cell Rep* 29:3605–3619, e3610.

Shute CC, Lewis PR (1966) Electron microscopy of cholinergic terminals and acetylcholinesterase-containing neurones in the hippocampal formation of the rat. *Z Zellforsch Mikrosk Anat* 69:334–343.

Sleigh JN, Rossor AM, Fellows AD, Tosolini AP, Schiavo G (2019) Axonal transport and neurological disease. *Nat Rev Neurol* 15:691–703.

Smith BN, Ticozzi N, Fallini C, Gkazi AS, Topp S, Kenna KP, Scotter EL, Kost J, Keagle P, Miller JW, et al. (2014) Exome-wide rare variant analysis identifies TUBA4A mutations associated with familial ALS. *Neuron* 84:324–331.

Soderling SH, Langeberg LK, Soderling JA, Davee SM, Simerly R, Raber J, Scott JD (2003) Loss of WAVE-1 causes sensorimotor retardation and reduced learning and memory in mice. *Proc Natl Acad Sci U S A* 100:1723–1728.

Spacek J, Harris KM (1998) Three-dimensional organization of cell adhesion junctions at synapses and dendritic spines in area CA1 of the rat hippocampus. *J Comp Neurol* 393:58–68.

Steward O, Fass B (1983) Polyribosomes associated with dendritic spines in the denervated dentate gyrus: evidence for local regulation of protein synthesis during reinnervation. *Prog Brain Res* 58:131–136.

Steward O, Levy WB (1982) Preferential localization of polyribosomes under the base of dendritic spines in granule cells of the dentate gyrus. *J Neurosci* 2:284–291.

Sudhof TC (2018) Towards an understanding of synapse formation. *Neuron* 100:276–293.

Sutton MA, Ito HT, Cressy P, Kempf C, Woo JC, Schuman EM (2006) Miniature neurotransmission stabilizes synaptic function via tonic suppression of local dendritic protein synthesis. *Cell* 125:785–799.

Sutton MA, Wall NR, Aakalu GN, Schuman EM (2004) Regulation of dendritic protein synthesis by miniature synaptic events. *Science* 304:1979–1983.

Tai HC, Schuman EM (2008) Ubiquitin, the proteasome and protein degradation in neuronal function and dysfunction. *Nat Rev Neurosci* 9:826–838.

Tas RP, Chazeau A, Cloin BMC, Lambers MLA, Hoogenraad CC, Kapitein LC (2017) Differentiation between oppositely oriented microtubules controls polarized neuronal transport. *Neuron* 96:1264–1271, e1265.

Tashiro A, Yuste R (2004) Regulation of dendritic spine motility and stability by Rac1 and Rho kinase: evidence for two forms of spine motility. *Mol Cell Neurosci* 26:429–440.

Tatavarty V, Ifrim MF, Levin M, Korza G, Barbarese E, Yu J, Carson JH (2012) Single-molecule imaging of translational output from individual RNA granules in neurons. *Mol Biol Cell* 23:918–929.

Taylor AM, Blurton-Jones M, Rhee SW, Cribbs DH, Cotman CW, Jeon NL (2005) A microfluidic culture platform for CNS axonal injury, regeneration and transport. *Nat Methods* 2:599–605.

Terenzio M, Koley S, Samra N, Rishal I, Zhao Q, Sahoo PK, Urisman A, Marvaldi L, Oses-Prieto JA, Forester C, et al. (2018) Locally translated mTOR controls axonal local translation in nerve injury. *Science* 359:1416–1421.

Thompson KR, Otis KO, Chen DY, Zhao Y, O'Dell TJ, Martin KC (2004) Synapse to nucleus signaling during long-term synaptic plasticity; a role for the classical active nuclear import pathway. *Neuron* 44:997–1009.

Tonnesen J, Katona G, Rozsa B, Nagerl UV (2014) Spine neck plasticity regulates compartmentalization of synapses. *Nat Neurosci* 17:678–685.

Triller A, Choquet D (2003) Synaptic structure and diffusion dynamics of synaptic receptors. *Biol Cell* 95:465–476.

Triller A, Choquet D (2008) New concepts in synaptic biology derived from single-molecule imaging. *Neuron* 59:359–374.

Tushev G, Glock C, Heumuller M, Biever A, Jovanovic M, Schuman EM (2018) Alternative 3' UTRs modify the localization, regulatory potential, stability, and plasticity of mRNAs in neuronal compartments. *Neuron* 98:495–511, e496.

Vale RD, Reese TS, Sheetz MP (1985) Identification of a novel force-generating protein, kinesin, involved in microtubule-based motility. *Cell* 42:39–50.

Vale RD, Schnapp BJ, Reese TS, Sheetz MP (1985) Movement of organelles along filaments dissociated from the axoplasm of the squid giant axon. *Cell* 40:449–454.

van den Berg R, Hoogenraad CC (2012) Molecular motors in cargo trafficking and synapse assembly. *Adv Exp Med Biol* 970:173–196.

Vickers CA, Dickson KS, Wyllie DJ (2005) Induction and maintenance of late-phase long-term potentiation in isolated dendrites of rat hippocampal CA1 pyramidal neurones. *J Physiol* 568:803–813.

Wang L, Brown A (2002) Rapid movement of microtubules in axons. *Curr Biol* 12:1496–1501.

West AE, Greenberg ME (2011) Neuronal activity-regulated gene transcription in synapse development and cognitive function. *Cold Spring Harb Perspect Biol* 3(6):a005744.

Wong HH, Lin JQ, Strohl F, Roque CG, Cioni JM, Cagnetta R, Turner-Bridger B, Laine RF, Harris WA, Kaminski CF, et al. (2017) RNA docking and local translation regulate site-specific axon remodeling in vivo. *Neuron* 95:852–868, e8s58.

Wu CH, Fallini C, Ticozzi N, Keagle PJ, Sapp PC, Piotrowska K, Lowe P, Koppers M, McKenna-Yasek D, Baron DM, et al. (2012) Mutations in the profilin 1 gene cause familial amyotrophic lateral sclerosis. *Nature* 488:499–503.

Wu L, Wells D, Tay J, Mendis D, Abbott MA, Barnitt A, Quinlan E, Heynen A, Fallon JR, Richter JD (1998) CPEB-mediated cytoplasmic polyadenylation and the regulation of experience-dependent translation of alpha-CaMKII mRNA at synapses. *Neuron* 21:1129–1139.

Yao J, Sasaki Y, Wen Z, Bassell GJ, Zheng JQ (2006) An essential role for beta-actin mRNA localization and translation in Ca2+-dependent growth cone guidance. *Nat Neurosci* 9:1265–1273.

Yau KW, Schatzle P, Tortosa E, Pages S, Holtmaat A, Kapitein LC, Hoogenraad CC (2016) Dendrites in vitro and in vivo contain microtubules of opposite polarity and axon formation correlates with uniform plus-end-out microtubule orientation. *J Neurosci* 36:1071–1085.

Younts TJ, Monday HR, Dudok B, Klein ME, Jordan BA, Katona I, Castillo PE (2016) Presynaptic protein synthesis is required for long-term plasticity of GABA release. *Neuron* 92:479–492.

Zhang HL, Eom T, Oleynikov Y, Shenoy SM, Liebelt DA, Dictenberg JB, Singer RH, Bassell GJ (2001) Neurotrophin-induced transport of a beta-actin mRNP complex increases beta-actin levels and stimulates growth cone motility. *Neuron* 31:261–275.

Zhang KX, Tan L, Pellegrini M, Zipursky SL, McEwen JM (2016) Rapid changes in the translatome during the conversion of growth cones to synaptic terminals. *Cell Rep* 14:1258–1271.

Zhang Y, Gaetano CM, Williams KR, Bassell GJ, Mihailescu MR (2014) FMRP interacts with G-quadruplex structures in the 3'-UTR of its dendritic target Shank1 mRNA. *RNA Biol* 11:1364–1374.

Zhong J, Zhang T, Bloch LM (2006) Dendritic mRNAs encode diversified functionalities in hippocampal pyramidal neurons. *BMC Neurosci* 7:17.

Zivraj KH, Tung YC, Piper M, Gumy L, Fawcett JW, Yeo GS, Holt CE (2010) Subcellular profiling reveals distinct and developmentally regulated repertoire of growth cone mRNAs. *J Neurosci* 30:15464–15478.

9

Adult Neurogenesis

Matthew Shtrahman, Sarah L. Parylak, Tomohisa Toda, and Fred H. Gage

9.1 Introduction

The field of adult neurogenesis began with the now historic experiments by Altman et al. more than half a century ago demonstrating that new neurons are generated in the hippocampal dentate gyrus (DG) of adult rats (Altman, 1962, 1963). Subsequent work has shown that adult-born dentate granule cells (DGCs) are generated throughout most of the mammalian class, likely including humans (section 9.7). Despite 50 years of research and substantial progress in this field, the implications of adult neurogenesis for hippocampal function and disease are still not fully understood. However, many of the key molecular signals orchestrating the generation of adult-born DGCs have been established. They guide a developmental program in which new neurons are generated from adult stem cells in the dentate subgranular zone and mature in an activity-dependent manner to form functional connections with the existing hippocampal circuitry. In addition to synaptic activity, these programs respond to environmental cues, including those that alter the specialized environment of the neurogenic niche within the subgranular zone, further contributing to their enhanced plasticity. Much of this work has been made possible by the development of tools that label adult-born DGCs, manipulate their activity, and alter levels of neurogenesis. Using these approaches, we are now beginning to understand the impact that adult-born neurons have on the sparse firing in the DG and their role in pattern separation and the formation of episodic memories. Extensive work also continues in human subjects, with the goal of developing noninvasive tools for monitoring neurogenesis and understanding how this process is altered with aging and in various disease states. In the future, we may be able to harness the regenerative potential of this neurogenic niche to enhance memory and mood and treat psychiatric and neurological disorders.

9.2 A brief history of the discovery of adult hippocampal neurogenesis

9.2.1 First evidence of cellular proliferation in the adult brain

A century ago, the consensus in the field of neuroscience was that new neurons are generated only during development and not in the adult mammalian brain. Based on detailed anatomical observations, the pioneers of neuroanatomy concluded that structural development of the mammalian brain reached its plateau soon after birth (Ramón y Cajal, 1928; 1999). Even then, there were scattered reports implying the existence of mitotic cells in the adult mammalian brain (Hamilton, 1901; Allen, 1912; Sugita, 1918; Bryans, 1959). However, as Ramón y Cajal pointed out in his own work (Ramón y Cajal, 1928), these studies were not able to present clear evidence for adult-born "neurons" rather than other cell types, such as glial cells. In the 1960s, Joseph Altman presented the possibility of newborn neurons in the adult brain using [^{3}H]-thymidine autoradiography (section 9.5.1, Figure 9.1). Altman found evidence of newborn cells in the granule cell layer of the DG, the olfactory bulb (OB), and the neocortex, using adult rat and cat brains (Altman, 1962, 1963; Altman and Das, 1965, 1966). Based on the location of these putative adult-born neurons within centers of cognitive and memory function, he hypothesized that adult-born neurons likely have functional importance for learning and memory. However due to technical concerns and limitations, his findings were not fully appreciated for decades; the evidence specifically identifying newborn cells as neurons was not definitive and was presumably not strong enough to challenge prevailing ideas about adult neurogenesis.

In the late 1970s and 1980s, Michael Kaplan and his colleagues used electron microscopy to show that [^{3}H]-thymidine positive cells with structural features of neurons, including synaptic vesicles, were found in the DG and OB of the adult rat brain (Kaplan and Hinds, 1977; Kaplan and Bell, 1984; Kaplan, 1985). Using the same methods, they also showed evidence of mitotic cells in the subventricular zone (SVZ) in adult monkey brains (Kaplan, 1983). However, Kaplan's and Altman's ideas faced a major setback when another pioneer in the study of brain development, Pasko Rakic, presented contradictory results using the same methods. He used [^{3}H]-thymidine to label dividing cells in the adult primate brain and did not find any clear evidence of adult-born "neurons" (Rakic, 1985a, 1985b; Eckenhoff and Rakic, 1988), and concluded at that time that all neurons in the primate brain are generated during embryonic and perinatal periods. Rakic and colleagues argued that adult neurogenesis found in the rodent brain could be a feature specific to rodents and that the structural stability of the primate brain, including the absence of adult neurogenesis, contributes to primates' advanced social and cognitive abilities. Thus, the work of Kaplan and others was not sufficient to overturn the almost-century-old

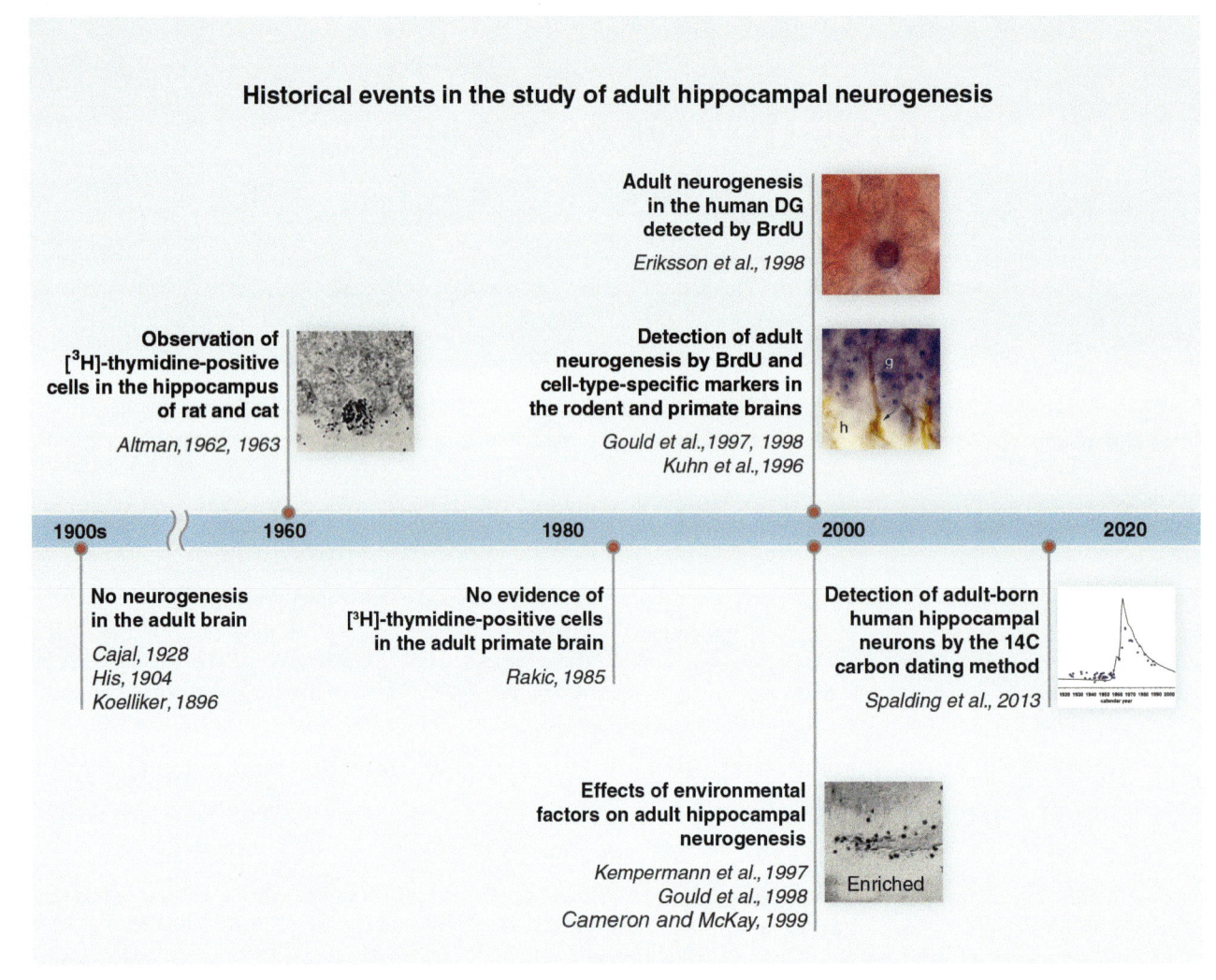

Figure 9.1 Timeline of major milestones in the history of adult neurogenesis.

dogma, and like Altman before him, Kaplan left the field frustrated (Kempermann, 2012).

9.2.2 Rediscovery of adult hippocampal neurogenesis

It was not until the late 1980s and early 1990s that several new approaches were introduced that revived the debate on adult neurogenesis. Using a retrograde axonal tracer injected into the mossy fiber layer, Stanfield and Trice demonstrated that [3H]-thymidine labeled newly generated cells that extend mossy fiber axons (Stanfield and Trice, 1988). This finding supports the conclusion that newly generated cells in the DG are neuronal cells with extensive axonal projections. In parallel, using the songbird as a model, Nottebohm's group showed that a number of new neurons are seasonally generated in the adult songbird brain and that they receive synaptic inputs and respond to sensory inputs (Goldman and Nottebohm, 1983; Paton and Nottebohm, 1984; Burd and Nottebohm, 1985; Barnea and Nottebohm, 1994). Gould's group combined [3H]-thymidine autoradiography with immunohistochemistry for cell-type-specific markers and found that about 70%–80% of [3-H]-positive cells express neuron-specific enolase (NSE), while some of them express glial fibrillary acidic protein (GFAP) (Cameron, Wooley, McEwen, et al., 1993). Their findings strongly supported the idea that adult-born cells could differentiate into either neurons or glial cells. They

also found that levels of adult neurogenesis could be regulated by adrenal steroids using the same approach (Cameron and Gould, 1994), a finding that also influenced later studies.

It was the advent of the synthetic thymidine analogue 5-bromo-3'-deoxyuridine (BrdU, section 9.5.1), which incorporates into the newly synthesized DNA of proliferating cells and can be readily detected by immunohistochemistry (Gratzner, 1982; Nowakowski et al., 1989), that finally elevated adult neurogenesis toward wide acceptance. BrdU could be colabeled with several newly developed neuron-specific markers such as NeuN, polysialylated neuronal cell adhesion molecule (PSA-NCAM), and NSE (Marangos et al., 1980; Mullen et al., 1992; Seki and Arai, 1993). This approach in combination with stereology, multicolor immunofluorescence, and confocal microscopy definitively determined whether adult-generated cells developed into neurons or other cell types (Kuhn et al., 1996; Kempermann et al., 1997a). Using these methods, adult hippocampal neurogenesis has been repeatedly observed in the rodent brain (Parent and Lowenstein, 1997; Kempermann, Kuhn, et al., 1998; van Praag et al., 1999). Later, the same methods were applied to nonhuman primates by Rakic and a colleague. They found evidence for the generation of new neurons in the DG of adult primates (Kornack and Rakic, 1999), which they had failed to find using autoradiography as described above. The capstone of this line of experimentation was the discovery of adult-born neurons in the human brain using BrdU (Eriksson et al., 1998), and subsequent experiments confirming these findings using a carbon dating method (Spalding et al., 2013) (Figure 9.1). These studies are discussed in more detail in section 9.7.

At the same time, tissue culture approaches to isolate somatic stem cells from the adult hippocampus were developed. Several groups have established protocols for isolating neural stem cells from embryonic and adult brain tissues (Reynolds and Weiss, 1992; Ray et al., 1993; Ray and Gage, 1994; Palmer et al., 1995). Isolated neural stem cells are able to proliferate and differentiate into neurons or glia in vitro, indicating that isolated adult neural stem cells possess capabilities for self-renewal and multipotency. Isolation of neural stem cells was further demonstrated from adult human brain tissue (Roy et al., 2000; Palmer et al., 2001). Thus, in vitro studies have provided important evidence for the existence of neural stem cells in the adult brain and have been integral in establishing experimental studies of adult hippocampal neurogenesis.

Over the last three decades, evidence of adult hippocampal neurogenesis has been reported across many species with few exceptions (Barnea and Nottebohm, 1996; Gould et al., 1997; Gould et al., 1998; Gould et al., 1999; Patzke et al., 2015; Hevner, 2016), indicating the importance of adult hippocampal neurogenesis for cognitive function and plasticity throughout much of recent evolution. A number of studies have identified genetic (Kempermann et al., 1997a; Kempermann et al., 2006; Gonçalves, Schafer, et al., 2016), epigenetic (Hsieh and Zhao, 2016; Yao et al., 2016), and environmental factors (Kempermann et al., 1997b, Kempermann, Brandon, et al., 1998; Toda et al., 2018) that dynamically modulate adult hippocampal neurogenesis, indicating that it is a tightly regulated process that has consequences for hippocampal function in cognitive and social abilities, a finding that we explore in the remainder of the chapter.

9.3 Key cellular and molecular factors in the development of adult-born DGCs

9.3.1 Overview of stem cells and neurogenesis

Classically, stemness is defined by two attributes: (1) the ability of a cell to undergo self-renewal, to divide to produce more stem cells, and (2) multipotency, the ability to differentiate into more than one possible cell type. Stem cells provide a dramatic form of plasticity that literally shapes us during development and, to a more limited extent, during adulthood. These cells also support maintenance, repair, and regeneration of nearly all tissues. However, these vital properties do not come without a cost. The potential for self-renewal is thought to be finite, and each cell division requires DNA replication that introduces errors into our somatic genome (Fuchs and Chen, 2013). These errors are not only potentially deleterious for the function of the cell and its progeny but also leads to increased risk of neoplasm, which can be lethal for the organism. These challenges place a fundamental limitation on self-renewal and likely the life span of an organism. Nature attempts to balance these risks through a division of labor. There exists a population of quiescent stem cells that serves as a master template and rarely undergoes cell division, presumably preserving their finite capacity for self-renewal and limiting the number of times their DNA is copied. Their progeny

are referred to as "intermediate progenitors" or "transient amplifying" cells. As these names imply, transient amplifying cells take on the brunt of the responsibility for expanding the pool of progenitors and subsequently differentiate to feed the mature cell population to match physiological demand. This strategy is often observed in self-renewing cell populations throughout the body, including the stem cells of the adult DG, as discussed below.

In the subgranular zone (SGZ) of the DG, there exist quiescent Type I radial glia-like stem cells (Kunze et al., 2009) that are capable of generating dentate granule neurons (Figure 9.2) and astrocytes (Suh et al., 2007), making them multipotent. They can undergo either symmetric or asymmetric division (Figure 9.3). Symmetric division serves to renew the stem cell population producing two Type I stem cells. During the more common asymmetric division (Kronenberg et al., 2003), one daughter cell repopulates the quiescent stem cell pool, while the other differentiates into a Type II transient amplifying cell. Although they are sometimes lumped together with Type I cells in the term "neural stem cells," Type II and III cells are not multipotent with the possible exception of Type IIa cells, (Suh et al., 2007); therefore, they are not considered true stem cells using the definition of stemness described above. The terms "neural precursors" or "neural progenitor cells" (NPCs) are often used when referring to these populations as a whole, although usage of these terms can vary. As discussed in detail in section 9.4, Type II cells respond to neuronal activity and other environmental cues to fine-tune their population through a mix of cell division and apoptosis to meet the demands of the network, and thus form a critical point of regulation. However, cell division and apoptosis are typically well balanced under normal conditions such that each Type II cell forms a small number of postmitotic neurons on average (Kempermann and Kronenberg, 2003; Berg et al., 2015; Figure 9.3) and any mutations incurred during their expansion are not widely distributed to progeny throughout the network.

9.3.2 Subgranular zone is a neurogenic niche

The SGZ and its characteristic components including stem cells, vasculature, and support cells, form postnatally during the second week of life in the mouse (Nicola et al., 2015). This laminar structure forms a thin band a few cells thick, lying between the dentate granule cell layer and the hilus (Figure 9.2). Evidence indicates that niches like the SGZ are critical for maintaining stemness, which is not a cell autonomous property but is rather an aggregate feature of stem cells and the specialized environment in which they reside. For example, Shihabuddin et al. showed that proliferating cells isolated from the spinal cord could differentiate into astrocytes, oligodendrocytes, and neurons upon treatment with fibroblast growth factor-2 (FGF2) in vitro (Shihabuddin et al., 2000). Transplanting these expanded cells back into the spinal cord produced glial progeny only. However, transplanting them into the SGZ niche resulted in the development of dentate granule neurons (Suhonen et al., 1996; Shihabuddin et al., 2000). Thus, while stem cells may have intrinsic features that impart stemness, the specialized environment of the niche is necessary for supporting cell division and can direct their fate. In particular, the neurogenic permissive niche of the adult SGZ has cellular and molecular components that influence the quiescence, proliferation, and differentiation of its resident stem cells. Importantly, the niche also provides cues of both local and distal origin to modulate stem cell characteristics to meet the demands of the hippocampal circuit (section 9.4).

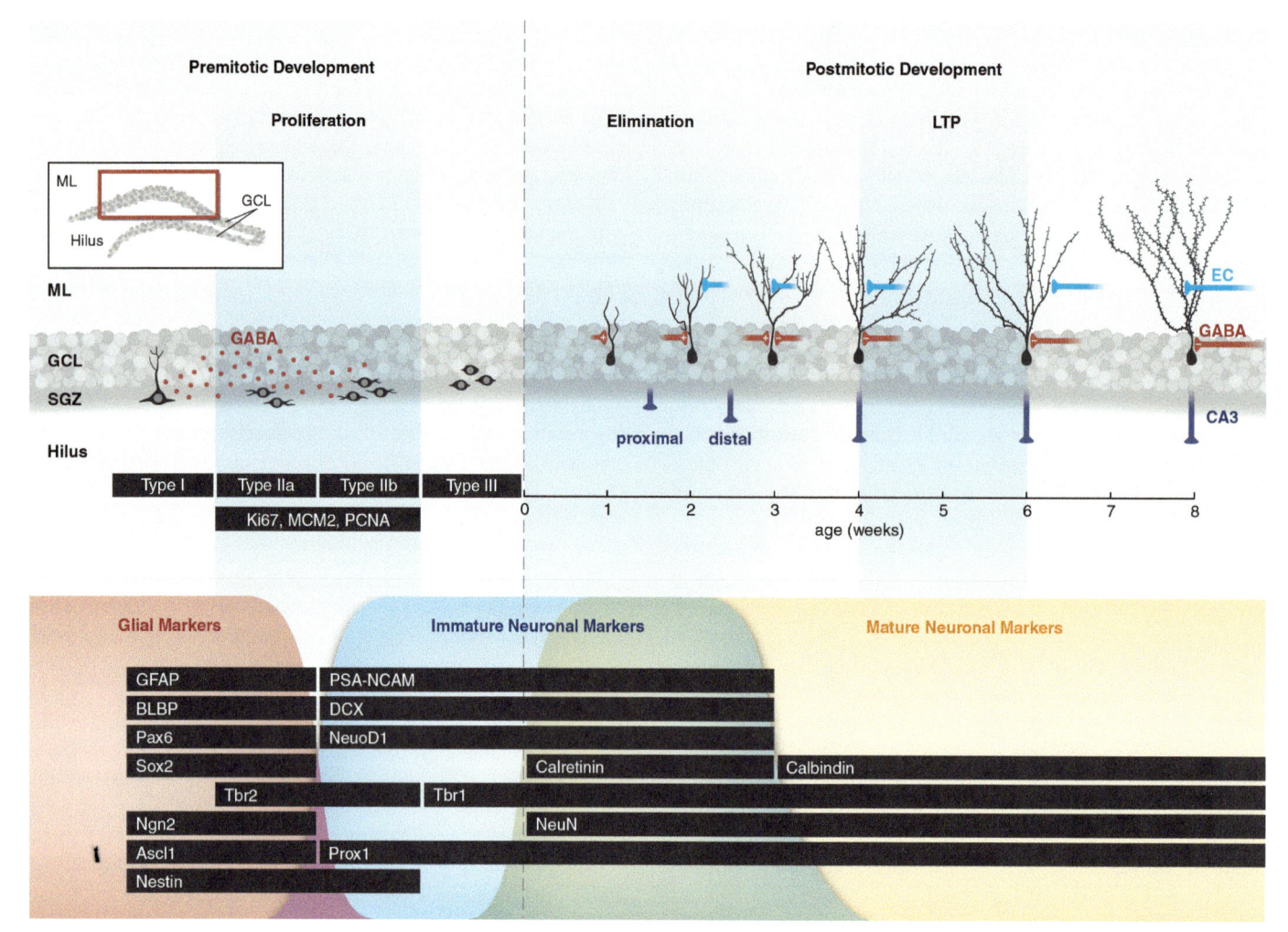

Figure 9.2 Development stages of adult-born DGCs. The developmental stages of adult-born neurons are depicted progressing from left to right with the vertical dotted line marking the transition from premitotic to postmitotic development. The SGZ is a stem cell niche that sits just below the GCL, where Type I radial glial-like cells and their progeny reside. Cells in this region sense aggregate network activity through extrasynaptic GABA that diffuses from inhibitory interneuron synapses innervating nearby mature DGCs. Type I cells are neural stem cells defined by their trianguloid cell body, single radial process that extends perpendicular to the GCL, and expression of glial markers such as GFAP. Largely through asymmetric division, these cells produce Type II cells, which have short processes that are oriented parallel to the GCL. Most proliferation occurs at this stage. In addition to expressing markers of cell division (Ki67, PCNA, and MCM2), Type II cells express the transcription factor Tbr2. Type II cells can be divided into two distinct stages: Type IIa cells, which inherit glia markers from their Type I precursors, subsequently differentiate into Type IIb cells, which begin to express immature neuronal markers, such as DCX, and are committed to a neuronal fate. Type III neuroblasts often have short or absent processes and begin to migrate out of the SGZ into the GCL. They are defined histologically by the expression of immature neuronal markers (DCX, PSA-NCAM) and lack of expression of both early NPC (Nestin) and postmitotic (NeuN) markers. As Type III cells exit the cell cycle, they begin to express "mature" or postmitotic neuronal markers such as NeuN as early as 1 day after their last mitotic event. This also marks the start of a critical period, where approximately 50% of adult-born cells die in the first few weeks (see Figure 9.3). Early postmitotic neurons continue to migrate within the GCL and within the 1st week extend an apical dendrite and axon (mossy fiber). At 1 week of age, the first GABAergic synapses onto adult-born DGCs can be identified, whose activity elicits low-amplitude excitatory potentials. The relative strength of synaptic connections are depicted in the schematic by their length. By day 10, mossy fibers reach the proximal portion of CA3 forming functional synapses onto pyramidal cells in this region. At 2 weeks, the first glutamatergic inputs from the entorhinal cortex (EC) are detected and the immature dendritic arbor continues to develop. At approximately day 16, functional mossy fibers synapses can be measured in the distal aspect of CA3 and the first dendritic spines can be observed. At 3 weeks of age, the expression of immature neuronal markers such as DCX, PSA-NCAM, and calretinin drop significantly and calbindin expression begins. Also, around this time the reversal potential for GABA-induced currents equals the resting potential of adult-born DGCs, marking the switch from excitatory to inhibitory GABAergic inputs. By 4 weeks of age, ~5% or less adult-born DGCs still express immature markers (6% of 4-week-old cells express calretinin [(Brandt et al., 2003] and 2% express DCX [Brown et al., 2003]). DGCs also reach peak excitability around this age. The strength of both glutamatergic and GABAergic synaptic inputs continues to increase over the next few weeks until reaching mature levels around 7 and 8 weeks of age, respectively. In particular, weeks 4 to 6 mark a period of heightened synaptic plasticity (LTP). At 8 weeks of age, adult-born DGCs are functionally and morphologically indistinguishable from mature DGCs born during perinatal development. *Note:* For clarity, the transition between histological markers is depicted by discrete borders of the dark gray bars. However, these transitions are continuous and in many cases ~5% or less of cells continue to express markers beyond the depicted borders into the next developmental stage. For example, 3% of Sox2 expressing cells also express DCX (Brown, 2003). *Abbreviations:* molecular layer (ML), granule cell layer (GCL), subgranular zone (SGZ), entorhinal cortex (EC), long-term plasticity (LTP).

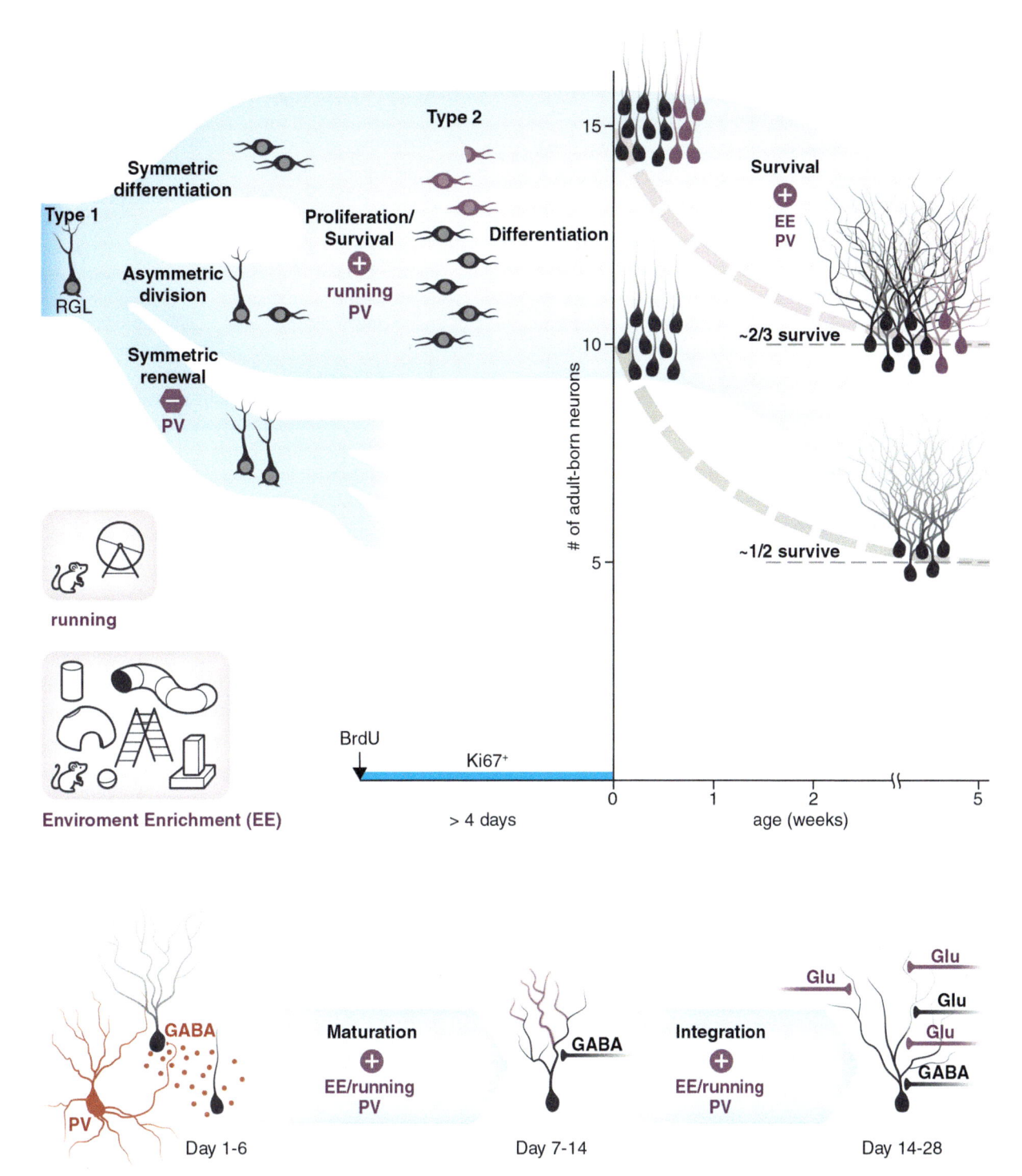

Figure 9.3 Running and environmental enrichment (EE) modulate the number of adult-born DGCs and their integration into the dentate gyrus. *Top:* **Gray cells** represent the average number of Type II cells and neurons generated from a single activated Type I radial glia-like cell (RGL) as measured from lineage tracing constructed using in vivo two-photon imaging in mice under **standard housing conditions** (Type III neuroblasts could not be distinguished from immature neurons using this approach) (Fig. S3 in Pilz et al., 2018). A Type I RGL can either undergo symmetric renewal where it generates 2 RGLs, asymmetric division creating 1 RGL and 1 Type II cell, or symmetric differentiation creating 2 Type II cells. In most lineages, Type II cells undergo symmetric differentiation during the final division, generating two neurons. Day 0 marks the last cell division observed under imaging, which is more accurate than "birthdating" with proliferative markers such as BrdU or Mo-MLV, as Type II cells can continue to proliferate for days (Pilz et al., 2018) after being tagged (Song et al., 2013). Under standard housing conditions, each RGL generates 5 Type II cells and each Type II cell generates 2 immature neurons, totaling 10 immature neurons on average. Approximately 1/2 of immature neurons survive to reach maturity, generating 5 mature neurons on average for each RGL over the course of the imaging experiment (2 months). Thus, consistent with previous studies, each Type II cell generates approximately a single mature neuron on average (Berg et al., 2015). **Running** and exposure to an enriched environment (**EE**) modulates different developmental phases of adult neurogenesis via GABAergic transmission from PV interneurons (Fabel, 2009; Song et al., 2012, 2013). Activation of PV interneurons **attenuates symmetric division of Type I RGLs**. In addition, running **enhances proliferation and survival of Type II cells** and as a result increase the number of postmitotic neuronal progeny by approximately 50% (Kronenberg et al., 2006; Hodge et al., 2008; Fabel, 2009). Extrapolating from the number of cells generated at baseline, running yields an additional **2.5 Type II cells** and **5 immature postmitotic neurons** generated by each RGL on average. Exposure to an EE **enhances the fraction of surviving adult-born neurons** from ~1/2 to ~2/3. When combined with running, this doubles the number of predicted mature neurons generated from a single Type I RGL cell to 10 mature neurons on average.
Bottom: Early postmitotic neurons (Day 1–6) sense activation of the dentate gyrus during combined running and EE through extrasynaptic GABA that is released from PV interneurons providing negative feedback onto mature DGCs. This results in adult-born DGCs exhibiting **more complex dendritic arbors** at Days 7–14 and **increased glutamatergic innervation** from entorhinal cortex at Days 14–28 (Alvarez et al., 2016).

The cellular components of the neurogenic zone include a variety of cell types, including glia, vascular endothelial cells, pericytes, neurons, and the stem cells themselves. Collectively, they promote neurogenesis through direct cell contact or secretion of growth factors. For example, in the SGZ, Type I radial glia-like stem cells are coupled via gap junctions. Transgenic mice that lack the gap junction protein connexin in GFAP+ Type I cells exhibit reduced numbers of Type I cells, dividing (Ki67+ and BrdU+) cells in the SGZ, and Prox1+ granule neurons during adulthood (Kunze et al., 2009). In addition, Type I cells make intimate contacts with immature neurons within the SGZ and provide a scaffold for their dendrites to reach the molecular layer (Shapiro et al., 2005; Plümpe et al., 2006). Thus, stem cells are not only a source for DGCs but also serve as structural, autocrine, and paracrine components of the niche, facilitating adult neurogenesis.

In addition to neurons, these Type I cells can also differentiate into astrocytes that may exert their own influence on developing granule neurons in the adult hippocampus. H. Song et al. demonstrated that primary cultured astrocytes from the adult hippocampus promote neurogenesis in FGF-2 dependent stem cells by cellular contacts and diffusible factors in vitro (Song et al., 2002; Barkho et al., 2006). In contrast, co-culturing FGF-2 dependent stem cells with hippocampal neurons, including DGCs, or astrocytes from the spinal cord resulted in gliogenesis. Soluble factors such as Sonic hedgehog (Shh), a fundamental factor guiding normal brain development and patterning, is expressed by astrocytes and likely plays a role in the above observations. Inhibition of Shh signaling by small molecules attenuates proliferation of precursor cells in the DG (Lai et al., 2003). Also, elimination or overexpression of Smo, a downstream effector of Shh, resulted in a decreased or expanded granule cell population, respectively (Machold et al., 2003; Han et al., 2008). Thus, astrocytes, in part via Shh secretion, contribute to the neurogenic permissiveness of the SGZ.

In addition to the factors described above, both astrocytes and Type I cells in the adult hippocampus secrete a variety of Wnt glycoproteins that bind to the Frizzled (Fz) family of receptors expressed on the surface of neural stem and progenitor cells and neurons (Lie et al., 2005; Wexler et al., 2009). In the "canonical" downstream Wnt pathway, Wnt binding stabilizes the intracellular transcription factor β-catenin, which is constitutively degraded in the absence of Wnt activation. This increase in β-catenin facilitates its entry into the nucleus, where it binds and forms a complex with transcription factors belonging to the T-cell factor/lymphoid enhancer (TCF/LEF) family. Together they bind enhancer elements of Wnt target genes, activating their transcription. During adult neurogenesis, Wnt activation is thought to promote both the proliferation and differentiation of adult neural progenitor cells, enhancing adult neurogenesis in the hippocampus (Lie et al., 2005). This is in part thought to be mediated by activation of NeuroD1, which induces differentiation and commitment of NPCs toward the neuronal fate. The NeuroD1 promoter contains TCF-LEF binding sites that activate NeuroD1 transcription and overlap with Sox2 binding cites that repress it, allowing for bidirectional regulation (Kuwabara et al., 2009).

Both astrocytes and Type I cells in the SGZ make close contact with vascular endothelial cells with processes known as endfeet that terminate onto blood vessels (Filippov et al., 2003). Therefore, the vascular system and its connections within the SGZ are thought to be among the critical components of the neurogenic niche (Palmer et al., 2000; Palmer et al., 2001). Interestingly, vascular endothelial growth factor (VEGF) is a potent activator of angiogenesis and neurogenesis in the SGZ, where Nestin+ cells express VEGF and regulate the proliferation of Type I cells (Kirby et al., 2015). In addition, transient amplifying cells in the SGZ express VEGF receptor 2 (Jin et al., 2002; Schänzer et al., 2006), which may contribute to augmentation of neurogenesis by exercise and exposure to an enriched environment (Cao et al., 2004; Fabel, 2009) (section 9.4.1). In addition, Licht et al. showed that VEGF overexpression in the hippocampus resulted in enhanced in vivo long-term potentiation (LTP) and memory during context-dependent fear conditioning (Licht et al., 2011). Many questions regarding neurovascular coupling in the SGZ remain, including the exact sources of VEGF and to what extent stem cells in this region are exposed to intravascular contents. The latter question has important implications for aging-related decline in neurogenesis. In particular, heterochronic parabiosis experiments, in which the circulatory systems from an old and a young animal are connected, indicate that systemic factors in the serum are critical determinants of brain aging. Blood from young mice can enhance neurogenesis, whereas blood from old mice leads to decreased proliferation of NPCs and a subsequent decrease in mature DGCs (Villeda et al., 2011; Katsimpardi et al., 2014; Smith et al., 2015). B2M, CCL11, CCL2, and other factors have been isolated from aged humans and have been shown to recapitulate many of the above effects of aged blood on adult neurogenesis in vivo and in in vitro models (Smith et al., 2018). Thus, soluble constituents in the blood can have deleterious or rejuvenating effects on the niche.

Increasing evidence indicates that microglia and immune cells also make critical contributions to support neurogenesis and the neurogenic niche (Gemma and Bachstetter, 2013). Under physiological conditions ramified microglia, with their extended process, survey the SGZ and DG for apoptotic precursor cells and immature neurons eliminated during premitotic and post mitotic development. After brain injury, microglia become activated, taking on an amoeboid morphology and actively clear cells through phagocytosis. In contrast to injury, clearance of apoptotic cells during neurogenesis does not result in the initiation of the inflammatory cascade. In addition to clearance, microglia are thought to influence proliferation, differentiation, and survival of immature neurons and their precursors. For example, microglia secrete insulin-like growth factor 1 (IGF-1) and brain-derived neurotrophic factor (BDNF), which are known to augment neurogenesis (Åberg et al., 2000; Nakajima et al., 2001; Ziv et al., 2006; Ziv and Schwartz, 2008). Also, microglia-conditioned medium has been shown to promote enhanced proliferation of precursor cells and differentiation toward neuronal fate in vitro, further suggesting a potential supportive role of microglia in vivo (Aarum et al., 2003; Morgan et al., 2004). Receptor-mediated cellular contacts and signaling between microglia and developing neurons may also be important for proper neuronal development. The neuronal protein fraktaline (neurotactin) interacts with the microglia receptor CX3CR1 to maintain neurogenesis (Bachstetter et al., 2011). Loss of CX3CR1 leads to impairment of LTP, contextual fear conditioning (CFC), and performance on the Morris watermaze (MWM) (Rogers et al., 2011), and administration of exogenous fraktaline reversed attenuation of neurogenesis observed in aging (Bachstetter et al., 2011).

Finally, neurogenesis and the function of stem cells in the SGZ is strongly influenced by the region's extracellular matrix (ECM), a complex acellular scaffold consisting of water, polysaccharides, and proteins, particularly proteoglycans, present throughout the brain and other organs. The ECM not only determines a tissue's stiffness and elasticity but also is involved in tissue-specific biochemical signaling that affects important cellular functions including proliferation and differentiation (Frantz et al., 2010). In the SGZ, a number of ECM components are thought to play important roles in neurogenesis and synaptic plasticity. In fact, ECM components in the DG and the enzymes that degrade them, matrix metalloproteinases (MMP), have been implicated in the maintenance and the pathological impairment of hippocampus-dependent memories, respectively (Dityatev et al., 2010; Castellano et al., 2017; Tajerian et al., 2018). Noteworthy ECM components in the SGZ include reelin, a serine protease expressed throughput the brain during development, which has been implicated in regulating neuronal migration. It was originally identified through loss-of-function mutations in the Reeler mouse, whose phenotype includes ataxia, impaired cortical lamination, and cerebellar hypoplasia (Fatemi, 2001). More recent work shows that loss of reelin results in reduced stem cell proliferation and altered differentiation, resulting in decreased numbers of DGCs and increased gliogenesis in the DG (Zhao et al., 2007; Sibbe et al., 2015). Laminins, a major family of trimeric ECM proteins in the SGZ niche, are thought to enhance proliferation of neural progenitor cells. Like reelin, laminin is a glycoprotein that also regulates the balance between neurogenesis and gliogenesis, primarily though the neurogenesis promoting receptor B1-integrin expressed by neural stem cells (Porcheri et al., 2014; Brooker et al., 2016). B1-integrin has multiple important ligand partners in the ECM including tenascin-R. Knockout of tenascin-R leads to enhanced neurogenesis and increased numbers of mature dentate granule neurons during adulthood (Xu et al., 2014). Although the mechanism is not fully elucidated, it has been suggested that the increased numbers of hilar interneurons in tenascin-R knockout animals facilitates survival of adult-born DGCs, despite reduced proliferation of NPCs in the SGZ in these animals (Tozuka et al., 2005; Xu et al., 2014).

9.3.3 Premitotic development and differentiation

NPC development in the SGZ can be divided into a series of stages or cellular programs that are defined by their characteristic morphology, function, potency, and gene expression patterns. As with cataloging neuronal subtypes, defining progenitor cell types is fraught with challenges as there is often no simple one-to-one correspondence between the above characteristics, nor clear discrete boundaries between cell types. Despite these limitations, characterizing progenitor cell types (Figure 9.2) has utility for understanding how adult neurogenesis is regulated and its effects on memory (sections 9.4 and 9.6).

Type I radial glia-like, or radial astrocyte-like cells, as they are sometimes referred to, share multiple characteristics with mature astrocytes. First, they are morphologically similar to astrocytes, with specialized processes that make intimate contacts with neurons and endothelial cells (see section 9.3.2 above). These precursor cells are also electrophysiologically similar to astrocytes, with similar currents and passive membrane properties (Filippov et al., 2003; Fukuda et al., 2003; Kempermann, 2012). Type I cells also share a number of astrocyte markers including glial fibrillary acidic protein (GFAP), glutamate aspartate transporter (GLAST), and brain lipid-binding protein (BLBP). However, unlike mature astrocytes, Type I cells have a single prominent apical projection that extends from a trianguloid cell body toward the granule cell

layer, providing guidance for migrating immature DGCs and their dendrites. They express stem cell factors that promote self-renewal and multipotency such as Sox2 (also expressed in a subset of mature astrocytes) and Pax6, and they lack expression of the mature astrocyte marker S100B (Maekawa et al., 2005; Steiner et al., 2006). Most, but not all, Type I cells express the intermediate filament Nestin (Filippov et al., 2003; Steiner et al., 2006; DeCarolis et al., 2013). Likewise, a subset of Type I cells express the proneuronal transcription factor Ascl1 (Mash 1) (Kim et al., 2011; Anderson and Strowbridge, 2014; Bottes et al., 2021), indicating that Type I cells may not be a homogeneous cell population (Lugert et al., 2010; DeCarolis et al., 2013). This is further complicated by the fact that the stage at which adult neural stem cells lose expression of GFAP and other astrocyte markers is not entirely resolved (Steiner et al., 2006; H Liu et al., 2010; Lugert et al., 2010). Regardless of these heterogeneities, Type I cells are largely quiescent, with only approximately 2% to 6% of these cells undergoing cell division at any time (Kronenberg et al., 2003; J Song et al., 2012).

Type II cells are largely delineated by expression of the transcription factor Tbr2, whose expression is not observed in cells with radial glia-like morphology and is rarely seen in cells not expressing GFP in the SGZ of Nestin-GFP mice (Type III cells and neurons) (Hodge and Hevner, 2011). Type II cells are heterogeneous in their morphology, gene expression, and potency and are commonly subdivided into two putative subtypes, IIa and IIb (Kronenberg et al., 2003; Kempermann et al., 2004; Steiner et al., 2006). When Type I cells undergo asymmetric division, they produce a single Type II-a daughter cell. While Type II-a cells continue to express many of the same glial markers seen in Type I cells (Steiner et al., 2006), they can be distinguished morphologically by their dense chromatin and short tangential processes that tend to orient parallel to the granule cell layer, in contrast to the perpendicular radial process of Type I cells (Figure 9.2). Type IIa cells are thought to exhibit some level of multipotency (Suh et al., 2007), but are highly proliferative unlike their Type I parent cells (Kronenberg et al., 2003; H Liu et al., 2010). Type II-a cells begin to lose expression of glial markers and increase levels of expression of Ascl1, which is thought to facilitate their differentiation into neurons (Beckervordersandforth et al., 2015). It is likely that neuronal fate is set with the transition from Type IIa to Type IIb cells, where the switch from a multipotent glia-like precursor cell to a unipotent cell expressing neuron-specific markers such as doublecortin (DCX), Prox1, PSA-NCAM, and NeuroD takes place (Figure 9.2) (Kronenberg et al., 2003; Steiner et al., 2006, 2008; Z Gao et al., 2009). This transition requires the expression of transcription factors, such as Sox21 and Tbr2, that actively suppress the expression of Sox2 and Pax6 (Beckervordersandforth et al., 2015). Thus, there is little or no overlap of glial cell markers with neuronal markers in Type IIb cells. Importantly, Type II cells also express GABA receptors that respond to tonic GABA release from local parvalbumin (PV)-expressing interneurons, which modulates their proliferation and survival in response to activity (Tozuka et al., 2005; J Song et al., 2013), and augments neurogenesis after exercise (van Praag et al., 1999; Hodge et al., 2008).

Type III or "neuroblast-like" cells often lack the horizontal astrocyte-like processes of Type II cells and can exhibit a short single apical dendrite. Type III cells are capable of migrating out of the SGZ, but typically remain in the inner portion of the granule cell layer. Type III cells are premitotic and therefore lack NeuN expression; but, under physiological conditions Type III cells neither exhibit significant proliferative capacity, nor serve as a critical regulation point for adult neurogenesis (Kronenberg et al., 2003). However, the number of Type III cells and their migration is altered by seizures (Jessberger et al., 2005). Type III cells can be distinguished from their Type IIb precursors by the lack of Nestin expression, and although somewhat unwieldy, can be defined by their Nestin-DCX+ NeuN- (or Nestin-DCX+ Ki67+) expression profile (Figure 9.2).

9.3.4 Postmitotic maturation

Whether all cells exit the cell cycle at the neuroblast-like stage or whether an earlier exit is permissible is not known. Regardless, the last mitotic event marks the birth date of the immature neurons, which express NeuN as early as 1 day after terminal mitosis (Brandt et al., 2003; Kempermann, 2012). However, measuring the birthdate, which is typically marked by administration of BrdU or Moloney murine leukemia virus (Mo-MLV), is often imprecise and a source of confusion (section 9.5). These agents label dividing cells, which in the SGZ are predominantly composed of Type II cells (section 9.3.3). Type II cells can divide multiple times and often take more than 4 days to differentiate into postmitotic neurons (J Song et al., 2013; Pilz et al., 2018). Thus, experiments requiring precise birthdating should be cautious when using these approaches.

In addition to NeuN, early immature granule neurons can also be distinguished from Type III cells by expression of the calcium-binding protein calretinin, which continues expression for the first 3–4 weeks of postmitotic development (Brandt et al., 2003) (Figure 9.2). DCX, which displays a broad window of expression starting with Type IIb transient amplifying cells, continues to be expressed postmitotically for approximately 3 weeks (Brown et al., 2003). During these early weeks immature neurons (expressing calretinin, DCX, PSA-NCAM) complete their migration into the inner granule cell layer (Kempermann and Kronenberg, 2003; Espósito et al., 2005; E Mathews et al., 2010) and their dendritic and axonal arbors begin to form. This period is also an important for selective survival and competition between immature neurons, approximately half of which undergo programmed cell death during the first few days to weeks after birth (Pilz et al., 2018). Despite not having formed proper synaptic connections, early immature DGCs, like progenitor cells, can sense network activity via activation of receptors by extrasynaptic GABA release from local interneurons that depolarizes early immature neurons (Espósito et al., 2005; Ge et al., 2006; Overstreet-Wadiche, 2006b). As early as day 7, bona fide GABAergic synaptic contacts begin to form onto immature DGCs and remain excitatory (depolarizing) until neurons reach 3–4 weeks of age (Ge et al., 2006). However, GABAergic synaptic inputs at 4 weeks are still relatively weak compared with mature levels (Espósito et al., 2005; Marin-Burgin et al., 2012) and do not reach maturity until at least 6 and 8 weeks of age for PV- and somatostatin (SOM)-expressing cells, respectively (Groisman et al., 2020). In comparison to GABAergic synaptic innervation, the first glutamatergic synaptic inputs, originating predominantly from the entorhinal cortex, are delayed. Both evoked and spontaneous glutamatergic synaptic inputs can be first measured beginning between 14 and 19 days of age (Espósito et al., 2005; Ge et al., 2006; Mongiat et al., 2009). Early on, these inputs primarily activate NMDA receptors, which together with coincident excitatory GABAergic input (Heigele et al., 2016), appears to be important for activity-dependent survival of immature DGCs (Tashiro et al., 2006; Kempermann, 2012; Toni

and Schinder, 2016) (Figure 9.3). This coincident input also triggers AMPA receptor insertion, strengthening glutamatergic inputs onto immature DGCs, which reach maximum strength after 7 weeks of age (Mongiat et al., 2009).

Within the first few days of birth, DGCs begin to extend axons or "mossy fibers" toward the hilus, first reaching CA3 at approximately day 10 (Stanfield and Trice, 1988; Hastings and Gould, 1999; Markakis and Gage, 1999; Toni et al., 2008; Kempermann, 2012). Adult mossy fibers continue to grow at the rate of 70 µm/day, populating the distal CA3 pyramidal cell layer early in week 3 (~16 days) (Zhao, 2006), after which they show continued growth and maturation for weeks (Faulkner et al., 2008; Toni et al., 2008). Although the strength of DGC to CA3 pyramidal cell synapses reaches mature levels at 4 weeks of age (Gu et al., 2012), mossy fiber boutons do not reach their full size and complexity until DGCs are 2 months of age. In comparison, the development of mossy fiber synapses onto inhibitory neurons is considerably delayed, reaching maturation at 6 weeks and greater than 8 weeks of age for PV- and SOM-expressing interneurons, respectively (Groisman et al., 2020). Meanwhile, the development of the dendritic arbor lags slightly behind that of the axonal arbor. The first dendrites reach the middle of the molecular layer by day 14, spanning the full thickness of the molecular layer around day 21 (compared with ~16 days for mossy fibers to reach distal CA3). The earliest dendritic spines become visible on day 16 and continue to mature along with the dendritic arbor over weeks (Zhao, 2006). Interestingly, the expansion and pruning of the dendritic arbor is regulated in a homeostatic fashion to limit excessive branching and promote a similar dendritic tree structure among adult-born DGCs (Gonçalves, Bloyd, et al., 2016).

After exiting the cell cycle, immature neurons begin to mature and undergo extensive changes in their intrinsic electrical properties. Early in postmitotic development (~1 week), DGCs express few ion channels, including inward-rectifying K^+ channels, resulting in a high input resistance (~4 GΩ) and thus a low threshold for generating an action potential under current clamp (Espósito et al., 2005; Mongiat et al., 2009). However even with suprathreshold current injection, only a single broad and low amplitude action potential can be generated, corresponding to the small number of voltage-gated channels (Na^+ and K^+ currents < 1 nA) observed in these early postmitotic cells. It is not until 3 weeks of age that multiple action potentials can be elicited in response to prolonged depolarization (Mongiat et al., 2009), although with a higher current threshold for generating the first spike. The number of spikes that can be generated in response to current injection peaks at ~4 weeks of age, when voltage-gated Na^+ (and K^+) current amplitudes (~3 to 5 nA) are close to values measured in mature neurons (~3.5 to 6 nA), but input resistance is still elevated (~500 MΩ at 4 weeks vs ~200 MΩ in mature neurons). Combined with the fact that 4-week-old DGCs experience limited feedforward and feedback synaptic inhibition, explains why these cells are hyperexcitable and preferentially recruited by inputs from entorhinal cortex compared with mature neurons (Espósito et al., 2005; Marin-Burgin et al., 2012; Dieni et al., 2013; Temprana et al., 2015). Lastly, long-term potentiation (LTP) of both excitatory inputs and outputs of immature DGCs peaks at 4 to 6 weeks of age and is enhanced compared with mature DGCs, further amplifying the excitability and impact of immature neurons at this age on the hippocampal network (Ge et al., 2007; Gu et al., 2012). After 8 weeks, adult born neurons are mature and indistinguishable physiologically from perinatal born neurons.

9.4 Environment and experience modulate the development of adult-born DGCs

Soon after the rediscovery of adult hippocampal neurogenesis, a series of studies revealed that adult hippocampal neurogenesis is highly regulated by experience, biochemical signals, and the environment. In particular, physical activity, enriched environment, stress, diet, aging, and other factors were shown to influence the proliferation, survival, and development of NPCs and immature neurons. This work established a foundation for future studies investigating how changes in structure and functional plasticity in newborn DGCs contribute to cognitive function in the hippocampus.

9.4.1 Enriched environment and running

The first clear evidence for the regulation of adult hippocampal neurogenesis by environmental factors was demonstrated in rodents that were exposed to an enriched environment (EE), which consisted of an enlarged home cage equipped with novel toys and allowing opportunities for enhanced social interaction (Figure 9.3). Exposure to EE significantly increased the number of adult-born cells and improved spatial learning (Kempermann et al., 1997b). While it had been previously shown that an EE induces structural and functional changes in the brain (Rosenzweig et al., 1962; Fiala et al., 1978; Bartoletti et al., 2004), the significant addition of new neurons in the adult in response to environmental stimuli was striking and unexpected. The resulting increase in the total number of adult-born neurons could be explained by augmenting one or more steps during neurogenesis: activation of quiescent Type I neural stem cells, increased proliferation or differentiation of NPCs or neuroblasts, and enhanced survival or integration of immature neurons (section 9.3). Clarification was provided by subsequent studies showing that voluntary physical exercise selectively increases the number of proliferating NPCs, whereas environmental enrichment promotes the survival of newborn neurons (van Praag et al., 1999; Suh et al., 2007; Hodge et al., 2008). Running can also induce activation of Type I neural stem cells (Lugert et al., 2010; Gebara et al., 2016). Following differentiation from neuroblasts, the time course of neuronal maturation and integration is also modulated by physical activity or exposure to an EE (Piatti et al., 2011; Gonçalves, Schafer, et al., 2016). These findings indicated that different types of environmental stimuli could modulate distinct maturation steps during adult hippocampal neurogenesis. Although the mechanisms for this modulation are not fully known, several signals that mediate the effect of environmental stimuli have been described and are discussed below.

EEss are thought to affect gene expression in the brain (Rampon et al., 2000), particularly the expression of neurotrophic factors. Both environmental enrichment and voluntary physical activity induce expression of brain-derived neurotrophic factor (BDNF), which is important in regulating neurogenesis (Neeper et al., 1995; Rossi et al., 2006; Kobilo et al., 2011) and for the integration of newborn neurons (Bergami et al., 2008; L Wang et al., 2015). Importantly, there is a critical period for the effects of environmental stimuli on the survival and integration of adult-born DGCs, which is largely restricted to the first 3 weeks after the birth of adult-born neurons (Tashiro et al., 2007).

In addition to EE and running, hippocampus-dependent associative learning, including spatial navigation learning and trace eyeblink conditioning, was also reported to increase adult neurogenesis in rats (Gould, 1999). Later studies demonstrated increased survival of adult-born DGCs born 7–13 days before the first day of MWM training and decreased survival of cells born 1–4 days prior to the first day of MWM (Drapeau et al., 2007; Dupret et al., 2007), suggesting developmental stage-dependent effects of learning on adult neurogenesis. Similarly, in mice, the numbers of surviving cells born 1–2 weeks before training was increased (Kee et al., 2007). However, other studies using the same strain of rats as above showed the opposite relationship, where DGCs born 8–10 days and 1–3 days before training on MWM exhibited increased and decreased survival, respectively (Ambrogini et al., 2000; Ambrogini et al., 2004). Furthermore, other mouse studies reported no effects of spatial learning on the proliferation or survival of adult-born cells (van Praag et al., 1999; Trinchero et al., 2015). Some have suggested that in addition to species and strain differences, variation in the level of difficulty of the task (Epp et al., 2011) or other experimental parameters may contribute to these discordant observations. Further studies are necessary to resolve the precise contribution of learning to adult neurogenesis.

Ultimately, sensory inputs during EE and other salient experiences activate neural activity in the hippocampus through the release of glutamate, gamma-aminobutyric acid (GABA), and other neurotransmitters. Recent studies have revealed how their downstream signaling cascades play crucial roles in the survival and integration of adult-born neurons (Ge et al., 2006: Ge et al., 2007; Tashiro et al., 2007). Silencing mature DGCs using optogenetic tools during exposure to a novel environment prevents the environmentally induced increase in integration of immature DGCs (Kirschen et al., 2017), suggesting that novelty-induced neural activity in mature DGCs plays a key role in the integration of immature DGCs. Glutamatergic inputs acting through NMDA receptors are essential for the survival of immature DGCs (Cameron et al., 1995; Tashiro et al., 2006) and for the neurogenic effects of physical activity (Kitamura et al., 2003). Although the entorhinal cortex is the primary source of glutamatergic input onto these neurons, the exact source of innervation leading to NMDA receptor-dependent integration of immature neurons is not known.

Intriguingly, GABAergic inputs from PV interneurons impart varying effects at different points in the development and maturation of adult-born neurons and their precursors. GABAergic tonic inputs from PV interneurons inhibit the activation of Type I quiescent neural stem cells (Song et al., 2012), suggesting that GABAergic signaling is essential for the maintenance of Type I quiescent neural stem cells. On the other hand, GABAergic inputs from PV interneurons onto neural progenitors and newborn DGCs enhance their survival and maturation, respectively (Song et al., 2013). It is likely that this signaling pathway also mediates the effect of EE on DGCs (Alvarez et al., 2016). Thus, similar GABAergic signals seem to have distinct roles in the regulation of adult hippocampal neurogenesis depending on their targets.

The medial septum imposes the generation of rhythmic firing patterns in the hippocampus during physical activity and receives inputs from many other brain regions (Vanderwolf, 1969; Teitelbaum et al., 1975; Yoder and Pang, 2005). Cholinergic neurons are often considered the primary driver of the output of the medial septum, delivering innervation to other brain regions and facilitating their synchronization. However, optogenetic experiments demonstrate that the activity of PV interneurons in the DG is regulated by long-range GABAergic interneurons from the medial septum, and this in turn affects the maintenance of quiescent neural stem cells (Bao et al., 2017). Thus, the medial septum may mediate physical activity-induced changes in the hippocampus and regulate adult neurogenesis through long-range innervation from GABAergic neurons. Interestingly, the medial septum also receives long-range innervation from inhibitory neurons located in CA1 (Müller and Remy, 2018). Thus, there appears to be a complex regulatory loop modulating adult hippocampal neurogenesis, the details and implications of which are still not fully understood (see also the following section for the functional roles of adult-born DGCs).

9.4.2 Aging, stress, and hormonal regulation

The decline of neurogenesis with age was first described by Altman (Altman and Das, 1965) and age is among the most prominent physiological modulators of neurogenesis. With age, the rate of proliferation and the total number of Type I quiescent neural stem cells and newborn cells decreases, and this decrease is observed across species (Kuhn et al., 1996; Aizawa et al., 2009; Amrein et al., 2011; Encinas et al., 2011; Spalding et al., 2013; Patzke et al., 2015; Dennis et al., 2016; see section 9.7.1 and Boldrini et al., 2018; Kempermann et al., 2018; Sorrells et al., 2018; Moreno-Jiménez et al., 2019, for discussion of the effects of aging on human adult hippocampal neurogenesis). In early studies, both stress and its mediator, corticosteroids and activation of the hypothalamic-pituitary-adrenal (HPA) axis, were identified as negative regulators of adult hippocampal neurogenesis (Gould et al., 1992; Gould et al., 1997; Gould et al., 1998; Cameron and Gould, 1994). Reducing corticosteroid levels could restore the rate of cell proliferation and the total numbers of newborn cells in old animals to levels exceeding those observed in young animals (Cameron and McKay, 1999). This finding was striking because it demonstrates that the age-dependent decline of adult hippocampal neurogenesis is highly reversible. Aging is one of the most significant risk factors for cognitive decline and neurodegenerative disorders, and the levels of adult hippocampal neurogenesis are linked to cognitive abilities both in rodents and nonhuman primates (Aizawa et al., 2009; Clelland et al., 2009; Sahay et al., 2011; Nakashiba et al., 2012; McAvoy et al., 2016; Meyers et al., 2016). Importantly, environmental stimuli can also stimulate the generation of adult-born cells even at older ages (Kempermann, Brandon, et al., 1998; Kempermann et al., 2002; van Praag et al., 2005; Kronenberg et al., 2006), and the addition of as little as 100 adult-born neurons in old mice can reverse cognitive decline to some extent (Berdugo-Vega et al., 2020). Thus, a series of experiments have demonstrated that even in advanced age, increasing adult hippocampal neurogenesis could have the potential to enhance cognitive ability and provide therapeutic benefit.

During aging, the ratio of gliogenesis increases at the expense of neurogenesis (Kempermann, Kuhn, et al., 1998; Spalding et al., 2013). These alterations appear to be due to both cell intrinsic changes in adult neural stem cells and stem cell extrinsic changes, including changes in metabolic status, transcriptional and epigenetic regulation, hormonal regulation, and neurotrophic signaling (Kuhn et al., 1996; Cameron and McKay, 1999; Villeda et al., 2011, 2014; Silva-Vargas et al., 2013; Kuipers et al., 2015; Moore et al., 2015; Nicola et al., 2015; Yousef et al., 2015; Corenblum et al., 2016; H Zhang et al., 2016; Beckervordersandforth et al., 2017; Castellano et al., 2017). One interesting study found that activated quiescent neural stem cells became astrocytes after several rounds of cell division, which raises the possibility of a "disposable" neural stem cell

model (Encinas et al., 2011). This observation indicates that the reduction of adult hippocampal neurogenesis during aging is a unidirectional process due to the depletion of the adult neural stem cell pool. In contrast, Bonaguidi et al. showed that neural stem cells can undergo activation, return to quiescence, and reactivate with limited depletion by glial differentiation (Bonaguidi et al., 2011). Since Type I quiescent neural stem cells seem to be a heterogeneous population (Jhaveri et al., 2015), distinct radial glia-like populations may respond differently to changing environmental cues during aging. Further investigation of Type I quiescent neural stem cells using in vivo imaging and single-cell strategies, including single-cell RNA-sequencing, proteomics, and genetics, will be instrumental in revealing the nature of the heterogeneity of Type I quiescent neural stem cells (Shin et al., 2015; Shah et al., 2016; Artegiani et al., 2017; Dulken et al., 2017; Hochgerner et al., 2018; X Wang et al., 2018). Indeed, in vivo imaging has revealed the existence of heterogeneous stem cell populations with a range of self-renewal capabilities (Pilz et al., 2018; Bottes et al., 2021). Furthermore, an elegant study demonstrated that the self-renewal capability of Type I quiescent neural stem cells changes during aging to ensure the maintenance of stem cell pools (Harris et al., 2021), reconciling contradictory results from previous studies. The age-dependent changes of Type I quiescent neural stem cells occurs as early as 5 months in mice at the transcriptional level (Ibrayeva et al., 2021), and epigenetic aging may underlie these age-dependent changes in the quiescent state and self-renewal capability of adult neural stem cells (Bedrosian et al., 2021; bin Imtiaz et al., 2021). Further investigations are needed to determine the origin of the intriguing phenomenon of stem cell aging.

Changes in the neurogenic niche (section 9.3.2) also impact adult hippocampal neurogenesis. Recent studies found that the expression levels of *Bmp4* and *Bmp6* as well as *Dkk1*, a Wnt antagonist, are increased during aging in the hippocampus (Seib et al., 2013; Yousef et al., 2015; Meyers et al., 2016), and that attenuation of BMP signaling or the loss of *Dkk1* reversed the reduced proliferation of NPCs. Furthermore, balanced BMP signaling plays a critical role in the maintenance of quiescent neural stem cells (Mira et al., 2010). Taken together, these findings suggest that the balance between BMP and Wnt signaling levels is a critical factor in maintaining the local environment of the neurogenic niche. Conversely, unbalanced BMP-Wnt signaling is a feature of the aging neurogenic niche, which contributes to impaired cognitive function (Yousef et al., 2015; McAvoy et al., 2016; Meyers et al., 2016). This work also suggests that cognitive decline with aging can be reversed at least in part by increasing adult neurogenesis in the hippocampus via manipulation of the BMP-Wnt pathways.

Intriguingly, adult hippocampal neurogenesis not only modulates cognitive ability but also impacts emotional regulation and stress resilience, which could be relevant to mental disorders such as anxiety and depression (Miller and Hen, 2015; Yun et al., 2016; Anacker and Hen, 2017; Toda et al., 2018). As mentioned earlier, adult hippocampal neurogenesis is affected by chronic or acute stress from the perinatal period to adulthood (Cameron and Gould, 1994; Gould et al., 1997; Lemaire et al., 2000; Czeh et al., 2001; Lu et al., 2003; Pham et al., 2003; Mirescu et al., 2004; Lehmann et al., 2013). In addition, unpredictable mild stress that induces depression-like behavior in rodent models also decreased adult neurogenesis (Mineur et al., 2007). Increased adult hippocampal neurogenesis could attenuate the levels of anxiety in response to chronic stress (Hill et al., 2015) (section 9.8.2). In rodent models, adult-born neurons buffer the stress responses, and depletion of adult-born neurons augments stress responses and increases anxiety and depression-like behavior, probably through the dysregulation of the HPA axis (Revest et al., 2009; Snyder et al., 2011; Lehmann et al., 2013). An acute stress response activates the HPA axis and induces the secretion of glucocorticoid hormones from the adrenal cortex. A majority of Type I quiescent neural stem cells, transient amplifying cells (Type IIa, but not Type IIb), neuroblasts, and mature neurons express glucocorticoid receptors (GRs) (Cameron, Wooley, and Gould, 1993; Garcia et al., 2004), providing a route by which different stages of hippocampal neurogenesis can be affected by stress through GRs. An excess application of corticosterone or acute stress through the activation of GRs inhibits proliferation, differentiation, and survival (Cameron and Gould, 1994; Wong and Herbert, 2005, 2006; Fitzsimons et al., 2013), but the effects of stress hormone may differ between GRs and mineralocorticoid receptors (Anacker et al., 2013). In addition, activation of GRs modulates gene expression (Anacker et al., 2013), which could have profound effects on adult neurogenesis. In addition to glucocorticoid signaling, stress could elicit other signaling pathways such as cytokines (Johnson et al., 2005; Goshen et al., 2008) and morphogens (Matrisciano et al., 2011).

Strikingly, adult neurogenesis is required for some of the beneficial effects of antidepressants acting through serotonin, BDNF, and BMP signaling in animal models (Malberg et al., 2000; Santarelli et al., 2003; Li et al., 2008; Bessa et al., 2009; David et al., 2009; Surget et al., 2011; Brooker et al., 2017). This may also be true in some cases of human patients with major depression disorder (Campbell et al., 2004; Perera et al., 2007; Boldrini et al., 2009, 2012, 2013; Lucassen et al., 2010), suggesting that adult hippocampal neurogenesis could be a key target for the treatment of mental illness (see further discussion in section 9.8.2). Recent studies have proposed different functionality between the dorsal and ventral hippocampus. Neural activity in the ventral hippocampus is associated with social memory and anxiety (Kheirbek et al., 2013; Danielson et al., 2016; T Okuyama et al., 2016; Jimenez et al., 2018), and adult neurogenesis in the ventral hippocampus confers resilience to chronic stress by inhibiting the activity of ventral DGCs (Anacker et al., 2018), suggesting that distinct circuits along the dorsoventral axis of the hippocampus may mediate different hippocampal functions. Of note, the dorsal hippocampus could also regulate mood-related behavior through the amygdala (Ramirez et al., 2015). Further investigation will be needed to tease out how adult-born neurons along the dorsoventral axis differentially contribute to hippocampal function.

9.4.3 Interaction with other organ systems

In addition to the environmental niche within the SGZ of the DG, recent findings have revealed that interactions with other organs systems in the body, such as systemic factors circulating in the blood and the microbiome, can exert a significant impact on the regulation of adult hippocampal neurogenesis. Wyss-Coray and his colleagues employed a classical parabiosis approach, in which the blood from one organism is circulated through a second, to explore the roles of the systemic milieu in adult hippocampal neurogenesis and hippocampus-dependent cognitive ability. They found that the systemic milieu in old animals attenuates adult neurogenesis and synaptic plasticity and impairs cognitive function through changes in chemokine signaling (Villeda et al., 2011). They also found that systemic factors could increase hippocampal neurogenesis in young animals and hippocampal plasticity in aged mice (Villeda et al., 2014).

Follow-up studies identified β2-microglobulin, a component of the major histocompatibility complex class 1 molecule, as a systemic negative regulator of adult hippocampal neurogenesis (Smith et al., 2015). Thus, changes in chemokine and immune signaling during aging appears to mediate age-related changes in adult hippocampal neurogenesis. Wyss-Coray and colleagues demonstrated that tissue inhibitor of metalloproteinase (TIMP2) is enriched both in human umbilical cord and young mouse plasma, and that both TIMP2 and human umbilical cord plasma could improve synaptic plasticity and cognitive ability (Castellano et al., 2017). Further studies revealed that liver-derived Gpld1 and platelet-derived factors mediate an exercise-induced increase in adult hippocampal neurogenesis (Leiter et al., 2019; Horowitz et al., 2020). Together, these observations suggest that systemic changes, as well as environmental changes in the local niche of the SGZ, can affect the process of adult hippocampal neurogenesis during aging, and the impact of these changes can be partially reversed. However, it is still not entirely clear how these systemic changes affect adult neurogenesis and hippocampal function, or whether the systemic changes during aging affect cognitive abilities and adult hippocampal neurogenesis in humans. Future investigation may uncover the underlying mechanisms and may lead to novel clinical approaches.

Finally, evidence suggests that both the immune system and the microbiome of the gut may interact with the neurogenic niche to modulate neurogenesis. CD4-positive T-cells are required in adult neurogenesis (Wolf et al., 2009), but the infiltration of T-cells into the hippocampus in the aged brain may negatively regulate adult neurogenesis (Dulken et al., 2019), indicating an age-dependent role of T-cells in the regulation of adult neurogenesis. Recent experiments show that signals from the gut microbiome set the levels of adult hippocampal neurogenesis and morphological maturation in very early life (Ogbonnaya et al., 2015; Luczynski et al., 2016). Moreover, long-term treatment with antibiotics reduces adult neurogenesis and impairs cognitive function (Wolf et al., 2009; Mohle et al., 2016), and alteration of the gut microbiome in early life can lead to behavioral deficits (Foley et al., 2014). It has been suggested that disruption of the microbiome by an excess usage of antibiotics or changes in diet, may affect the developmental processes of the brain as well as the maintenance of brain functions, including adult neurogenesis. Additional work is necessary to translate these findings into specific dietary recommendations for improving health. A recent study reported the surprising finding that the microbiota modulates neuroinflammation and motor functions in Parkinson's disease through the activation of microglia (Sampson et al., 2016), which have been identified as important regulators of adult neurogenesis (Sierra et al., 2010; Matsuda et al., 2015; de Lucia et al., 2016). Further investigation is needed to better understand the complex interactions between the immune system, the microbiome, and the nervous system under both physiological and pathological conditions.

9.5 Approaches for measuring and manipulating adult neurogenesis

9.5.1 Pulse chase techniques: autoradiography, BrdU, and Mo-MLV

Throughout the history of adult neurogenesis research, important discoveries can be traced to key technological advances (section

9.2). This is evident beginning with the birth of the field, when in the early 1960s Joseph Altman adapted techniques for "high" resolution brain autoradiography using tritiated thymidine ([³H]-thymidine), developed by Messiet and colleagues a few years before (Leblond and Messier, 1958). Nucleosides and their analogues are actively transported across the blood-brain barrier (G Lee et al., 2001; Lovitt et al., 2016), allowing systemic administration of [³H]-thymidine and other thymidine analogues to be incorporated into the DNA of dividing cells in the brain during S-phase. While thymidine analogues are cleared within a couple of hours (less than the typical S-phase duration) in the blood, the half-life of tritium exceeds 12 years, effectively providing a permanent marker for cells that are dividing at the time of [³H]-thymidine injection. These pulse chase experiments allowed Altman and Das to demonstrate that adult-born cells are long-lived and could be observed 2 months or more after mitosis, and that their frequency exhibits steep age dependence. It was not until 30 years later that [³H]-thymidine autoradiography was combined with immunohistochemistry by Cameron et al. to demonstrate that [³H]-thymidine labels dividing cells in the adult DG that mature into neurons and co-stain with neuronspecific enolase (NSE) (Cameron, Wooley, McEwen, et al., 1993). However, emitted radioactive beta particles are short-lived and are detected only at the surface of the brain slice coated with a radiosensitive emulsion, resulting in poor detection from cells deeper within the tissue. Around the same time, the nonradioactive thymidine analog 5-bromo-2'-deoxyuridine (BrdU) along with antibodies against BrdU were developed, which together with the neuronal markers NSE and calretinin were used to identify dividing adult-born neurons in the subependymal zone using immunofluorescence (Corotto et al., 1993). This finding led to progressively more complex studies in this and other neurogenic regions, taking advantage of confocal imaging and colabeling with multiple immunofluorescent markers for NPCs and developing neurons (Kuhn et al., 1996; Steiner et al., 2006; Hodge and Hevner, 2011; Kempermann, 2012). Subsequently, additional thymidine analogues with nonoverlapping immunoreactivity with BrdU were developed, including 5-Chloro-2'-deoxyuridine (CldU) and 5-Iodo-2'-deoxyuridine (IdU), allowing for sequential labeling of distinct cohorts of adult-born cells (Llorens-Martín, 2011).

One feature that limits the efficacy of these halogenated thymidine analogues is that the tertiary structure of DNA can preclude the binding of their antibodies, requiring harsh denaturing conditions to expose their epitopes. This prolonged tissue treatment with acid or heat may interfere with the immunohistochemical detection of other markers. There is also evidence that thymidine analogues such as BrdU mark not only dividing cells but also those undergoing DNA repair (Kao et al., 2001; Cooper-Kuhn and Georg Kuhn, 2002; S Lee et al., 2012). Finally, multiple studies report BrdU toxicity, where thymidine analogues are thought to alter cell migration and various aspects of the cell cycle (Duque and Rakic, 2011; Lehner et al., 2011). Some of these unfavorable characteristics of halogenated thymidine analogues are avoided by using 5-Ethynyl-2'-deoxyuridine (EdU) (Zeng et al., 2010; Bordiuk et al., 2014) and its prodrugs (Lovitt et al., 2016), which are detected through copper-catalyzed azide-alkyne cycloaddition (CuAAC) "click" chemistry. This approach allows detection of EdU, containing an alkyne ($C \equiv C$) group, with a small molecule fluorescent azide ($N = N = N$) within intact DNA, precluding the need for DNA denaturing tissue treatments.

Unfortunately, techniques for identifying adult-born neurons by incorporating nucleotide analogues are typically limited to visualization within fixed tissue and only label the nucleus, precluding physiological and detailed anatomical studies of adult-born neurons and their processes. In 2002, van Praag et al. described the use of an engineered Moloney murine leukemia virus (Mo-MLV), a single-stranded RNA oncoretrovirus, to genetically target and label adult-born neurons in the DG (van Praag et al., 2002). These oncoretroviruses are well suited for targeting NPCs in the SGZ, as they can only access the nucleus during initiation of mitosis and infect only dividing cells (Tashiro et al., 2015). Like other retroviruses, Mo-MLV encodes a reverse transcriptase that converts viral RNA into double-stranded DNA, which permanently integrates into the host genome and exhibits long-term expression of transgenes in both mitotic cells and their progeny. The engineered Mo-MLV genome contains three components, which can be supplied in trans during viral production. The *gag* gene encodes the capsid, matrix, and nucleocapsid proteins, which are necessary for the synthesis of viral particles. Transcription of the *pol* gene supplies multiple enzymes needed for replication and integration of the viral genome, including reverse transcriptase and integrase. Finally, to increase the neuronal tropism of the Mo-MLV retrovirus, vesicular stomatitis virus glycoprotein (VSV-G) is used to pseudotype the viral capsid. By introducing the green fluorescent protein (GFP) driven by the ubiquitous CAG promoter, van Praag et al. were able to identify adult-born neurons and study the development of their dendritic and axonal processes, including dendritic spines. By preparing acute brain slices and performing whole-cell recordings from GFP⁺ neurons 4 weeks after viral injection, they demonstrated that adult-born neurons establish synaptic connections, including perforant path inputs. This was the first of numerous studies to use retroviral techniques to characterize the development of adult-born neurons and their functional integration into the network of the DG (C Zhao, 2006).

9.5.2 Transgenic mice for labeling adult-born neurons

While pulse chase techniques have been invaluable in dissecting the development of adult-born DGCs, only a modest number of NPCs are dividing during the time pulse chase agents like Mo-MLV retrovirus are active. As a result, multiple stereotactic injections over hours to days delivered in multiple locations within each DG bilaterally are required to target a sufficient number of cells for behavioral or imaging studies (Gu et al., 2012; Zhuo et al., 2016), which can be cumbersome or impractical. Also, because these approaches primarily label dividing Type II progenitors, other approaches are required to label rarely dividing (Type I) or nondividing (immature neuron) populations participating in adult-born DGC development. Crowther et al. demonstrated that recombinant adenosine-associated virus (AAV) serotype 4 preferentially labels quiescent Type I cells in the adult DG (Crowther et al., 2018). These experiments must be performed at low-titers of ~1E10 viral particles per milliliter (vp/mL) to achieve specific labeling and avoid killing NPCs and immature neurons, which are particularly sensitive to the AAV-induced toxicity (Johnston et al., 2021). These and other limitations have motivated the use of transgenic animals for studying adult neurogenesis (Imayoshi et al., 2011; Enikolopov et al., 2015; Semerci and Maletic-Savatic, 2016), with an impressive range of experiments from lineage tracing to behavior. This approach relies on promoter-driven expression with (variable) specificity for cells at different stages of adult-DGC development. Both Cre recombinase independent (e.g., Nestin-GFP) (Filippov et al., 2003) and dependent (e.g., Nestin-Cre-ER2) (Sun and Kawata, 2004) strategies are available to drive expression of fluorescent proteins and other genetically encoded tools (Semerci and Maletic-Savatic, 2016). In using these models, one must be cognizant of the fact that promoter-driven expression of fluorescent proteins (e.g., Nestin-GFP) can often be detected beyond the temporal window of expression of the native protein (e.g., Nestin). Regardless, due to the utility of these approaches, the number of available transgenic animals and associated promoters continues to expand and they have become a mainstay in the field of adult neurogenesis (see Semerci and Maletic-Savatic, 2016 for a comprehensive list of transgenic lines).

9.5.3 Pharmacological and nongenetic ablation and enhancement of adult neurogenesis

To establish the role of adult-born DGCs in learning and memory and disease, it is critical to perturb their function. This can be accomplished by diminishing or eliminating immature neurons or their precursors for a given time period and testing the effects of attenuating neurogenesis. Traditionally, this is achieved using chemotherapeutic agents, which preferentially target dividing cells. Thus, Type II transient amplifying cells in the SGZ are thought to be more susceptible to these manipulations than postmitotic immature DGCs or Type I quiescent neural stem cells. A number of chemotherapeutic drugs, including methotrexate, cytosine arabinoside, and methylazoxymethanol, have been used as experimental agents to attenuate adult neurogenesis. More recent work relies on temozolomide (TMZ), which has become a popular choice due to effective elimination (~80%) of immature dentate granule neurons and a preferable side-effect profile compared with other agents (Garthe et al., 2009). In principle, short-duration chemotherapy allows for temporary depletion of neural precursor cells and their progeny, followed by repopulation presumably through the action of Type I cells. While cognitive side effects are a common complaint in patients undergoing chemotherapy, it is unclear to what extent these deficits can be attributed to the attenuation of adult neurogenesis (Monje et al., 2007). Rodent studies confirm that animals treated with chemotherapeutic agents exhibit deficits in hippocampus-dependent learning (Seigers et al., 2008; Garthe et al., 2009; Seigers et al., 2009). Some experiments indicate that cognitive deficits and their recovery are associated with the loss and return of adult-born DGCs, respectively, and that these deficits do not appear to have a significant extrahippocampal contribution (Shors et al., 2001).

Like chemotherapeutic agents, delivery of X-ray and gamma radiation and ionizing particles preferentially eliminate dividing cells in the brain, including NPCs in the SGZ. However, these treatments can result in dose-dependent inflammation within the hippocampus and other brain regions (Monje et al., 2003), and loss of neurogenesis, with prolonged or no recovery (Tada et al., 2000; Monje et al., 2002). Delivery of radiation has been used to investigate the role of adult-born DGCs in hippocampus-dependent learning, revealing deficits in spatial learning tasks such as the MWM and in working memory tasks (Madsen et al., 2003; Snyder et al., 2005; Wojtowicz et al., 2008; Clelland et al., 2009; ben Abdallah et al., 2013). However, as with chemotherapeutic agents, ablation of adult-born cells with radiation can yield mixed results (Shors et al., 2002; Raber et al., 2004; Hernández-Rabaza et al., 2009) and unwanted side effects.

There are a modest number of pharmacological agents that enhance neurogenesis. Memantine is an NMDA receptor antagonist and a D2 receptor agonist approved for the treatment of cognitive symptoms in Alzheimer's disease. Jin et al. demonstrated that similar to other NMDA antagonists (MK-801, D-APV, CGP-4387), memantine augments proliferation of BrdU+ cells in the SGZ of the DG (Jin et al., 2006; Cameron et al., 1995; Cameron et al., 1997; Gould et al., 1997; Hirasawa et al., 2003; Nacher et al., 2003; N Okuyama et al., 2003). Maekawa et al. later confirmed these results, showing that a single administration of memantine (50 mg/kg) augmented proliferation and survival, resulting in an almost sevenfold increase in BrdU+ DGCs (labeled 3 days after memantine) 4 weeks later (Maekawa et al, 2009). Administration of memantine reproduces the behavioral effects of running, which also enhances proliferation during adult neurogenesis (Akers et al., 2014) (section 9.4.1). Because clinicians have almost two decades of experience using memantine and it is well tolerated by elderly patients, memantine is an intriguing experimental pharmacological agent for studying the effects of augmenting adult neurogenesis in both patients and healthy human research subjects in the future (Lucassen et al., 2010). Other FDA-approved drugs that promote neurogenesis in animal models include SSRIs such as fluoxetine (section 9.8.2), mood stabilizers such as lithium (but not valproic acid), and the diabetes drug metformin.

9.5.4 Genetic ablation and enhancement of adult neurogenesis

In an attempt to avoid the off-target effects of radiation and pharmacologic manipulation of neurogenesis, researchers have turned to transgenic animal models to ablate or enhance adult neurogenesis (Imayoshi et al., 2011). In 2004, Garcia et al. utilized GFAP-tk mice to demonstrate that nearly all adult-born neurons are generated from GFAP-expressing progenitors (Garcia et al., 2004). Here, transgenic mice express the herpes simplex virus thymidine kinase (HSV-tk) driven by the GFAP promoter. Administration of the antiviral drug ganciclovir, which is metabolized into nucleotide analogues by HSV-tk, perturbs DNA synthesis and induces cell death in proliferating cells expressing GFAP. This technique is effective at ablating dividing radial glia-like cells while sparing the majority of astrocytes, which exhibit minimal proliferation under physiological conditions (Snyder et al., 2011). Ablation of GFAP+ progenitors using this approach resulted in impairment of context-dependent fear conditioning (Saxe et al., 2006), which may be due to alterations in neurogenesis-dependent stress responses in this model (Snyder et al., 2011). To increase the specificity of HSV-tk induced ablation, Deng et al. (2009) and Singer et al. (2009) developed transgenic mice that express the herpes transgene in Nestin-expressing cells. These Nestin-tk mice have been used to study the role of adult neurogenesis in a number of hippocampus-dependent behaviors, affective disorders, and other disease states (Hamilton et al., 2015; Seo et al., 2015; Hollands et al., 2017). Limitations on the use of HSV-tk-expressing models include systemic toxicities associated with ganciclovir and the slow onset of ablation and recovery of neurogenesis, which limits the temporal resolution of this technique to weeks or longer. Other models that induce toxicity in genetically defined neural progenitor populations include the NSE-DTA mouse, which expresses the diphtheria toxin fragment A (DTA) in cells that express Cre (Imayoshi et al., 2008). By crossing NSE-DTA with Nestin-CreERT2 mouse, one can kill Nestin-expressing cells upon administration of tamoxifen.

As an alternative to delivery or expression of toxins, others have developed transgenic models that use conditional knockout of transcription factors expressed in adult animals exclusively by neural progenitors. Among these approaches, the one with perhaps the most specificity utilizes a conditional knockout of the Tbr2 transcription factor, which is expressed during a developmentally narrow window defined by Type II neural progenitors (Figure 9.2, section 9.3.2). Tsai et al. crossed Tbr2 floxed mice with GLAST-CreER mice expressing the tamoxifen-inducible Cre recombinase in GLAST+ radial glia-like cells (and astrocytes). In contrast to other transgenic approaches for manipulating adult neurogenesis, this results in ablation of adult neurogenesis, as measured by Tbr2 and DCX expression, only in the hippocampus (Tsai et al., 2015) and not in the *adult* subventricular zone, where Tbr2 is not expressed (Arnold et al., 2008). Finally, transgenic approaches are available for increasing the survival of immature neurons to examine the effects of augmenting adult neurogenesis on hippocampal physiology. Sahay and coworkers demonstrated that conditional deletion of the proapoptotic factor *Bax* in Nestin-expressing cells resulted in an approximately 2-fold increase in DCX+ cells and 3.6-fold increase in BrdU-labeled cells 8 weeks after tamoxifen administration (Sahay et al., 2011). Bax transgenic mice with genetically augmented adult neurogenesis exhibited enhanced behavioral pattern separation.

9.5.5 Modulation of adult-born DGC function using optogenetics and chemogenetics

Modulating the activity of adult-born DGCs using opto- or chemogenetics has proven to be a powerful tool for mapping the changing connectivity of these cells during their development (sections 9.3 and 9.4). Coupled with intracellular recordings, optogenetics allows one to probe synaptic connections between genetically and anatomically defined neuronal cell types where paired electrical recordings alone are low yield or impractical. Toni et al. were among the first to deliver channelrhodopsin-2 (ChR2) to adult-born DGCs using Mo-MLV retrovirus, establishing that mossy fibers from immature adult-born neurons form excitatory synaptic connections with CA3 pyramidal neurons, hilar interneurons, and mossy cells similar to their mature counterparts (Toni et al., 2008). Using a similar approach, Gu et al. were able to define the onset and maturation time course of adult-born DGC connections to CA3 pyramidal cells (Gu et al., 2012). Temparana et al. utilized Ascl1-CreERT2 mice crossed with mice expressing Cre-dependent Chr2 (CAG-floxStopChr2) to achieve inducible expression of ChR2 in adult-born DGCs. Experiments in these mice revealed that excitatory output from immature DGCs onto CA3 pyramidal cells are established before connections to hilar inhibitory neurons are made, delaying the formation of (surround) inhibitory feedback onto neighboring mature DGCs relative to feedforward excitation (Temprana et al., 2015). Later, the timing of adult-born DGC synaptic connections onto PV and SOM hilar interneurons was more precisely mapped using optogenetic techniques by Groisman et al. (2020). Using a combination of the transgenic strategy described above and excitatory DREADDs delivered by Mo-MLV retrovirus, Alvarez et al. demonstrated that enhanced activity in the mature DGCs, such as experienced during exposure to EEs, augments dendritic development of immature DGCs less than 2 weeks old via a disynaptic connection; mature DGC -> PV interneuron -> immature DGC (Alvarez et al., 2016) (Figure 9.3).

An ambitious use of opto- and chemogenetic techniques is the study of time-sensitive contributions of adult-born DGC activity to learning and memory (Aimone et al., 2006). Gu et al. used Mo-MLV to express the inhibitory opsin Arch to suppress activity of immature DGCs during probe trials of the MWM test (Gu et al., 2012). Suppression of 4-week-old, but not 2- or 8-week-old DGCs impaired memory retrieval during this task. They demonstrated that a similar temporal pattern of immature DGC-dependent impairment was also observed during the retrieval phase of context-, but not tone-dependent fear conditioning. Zhuo et al. (2016) used a similar approach to study the effect of suppressing immature and mature adult-born DGC activity during a touchscreen location discrimination task pioneered by Clelland et al. (2009). Here mice underwent training when Mo-MLV targeted cells were 1- to 5-weeks-old followed by testing of mice from weeks 5 to 10 and again at weeks 14 to 18. Inhibiting the cells during weeks 5 to 10, but not weeks 14 to 18, impaired fine (but not gross) spatial discrimination in these mice. The effect of silencing 5- to 10-week-old cells was not observed when the training phase occurred prior to the birth of the adult-born DGCs. More recently, Masachs et al. used Mo-MLV delivery of Arch to show that mouse DGCs born during adolescence (4 weeks of age) are required for memory retrieval during MWM, but not DGCs born during embryonic development or adulthood (2 months of age; Masachs et al., 2021). Clearly, additional studies are required to paint a comprehensive picture of the contribution of newborn DGCs to hippocampal function at different time points in both CNS and granule cell development. The reversibility and temporal resolution offered by opto- and chemogenetics makes them well suited for answering these questions.

9.6 The role of adult neurogenesis in circuit function and learning and memory

9.6.1 Age-dependent contribution of adult-born neurons to learning and memory

The nontrivial challenge of integrating new neurons into a mature adult brain has sparked considerable speculation as to why such a metabolically expensive process as generating, culling, and differentiating new neurons has been conserved in the hippocampus. What advantage do adult-born granule cells provide that evolution has judged important to the hippocampal circuit but dispensable in other areas of the mammalian brain? As described in section 9.3, adult-born neurons develop incoming and outgoing synaptic connections by 3 weeks of age. However, immature adult-born neurons remain physiologically distinct from their mature counterparts through at least 6 weeks of age. During the period between 4 and–6 weeks, they are hyperexcitable (Mongiat et al., 2009), have enhanced synaptic plasticity (Ge et al., 2007), and are more broadly responsive to perforant path inputs (Marin-Burgin et al., 2012) than mature granule cells. One key question has been whether adult-born neurons themselves convey a distinct signal during this critical period, or if they play a more supportive role in modulating the connectivity and excitability of neighboring mature granule cells (Piatti et al., 2011).

The role of newborn neurons must thus be understood within the context of the DG and hippocampus as a whole. As discussed in more detail in Chapters 13 and 14, the hippocampus is critical for the formation of episodic or declarative memories: memories of events that occur in a specific place and at a specific time. It has also been implicated in spatial learning more broadly. To begin to investigate adult-born neuron function, numerous studies have manipulated neurogenesis levels and examined the outcome on known hippocampus-dependent behaviors. In rodent models, the two most popular assays of hippocampus-dependent memory have been the MWM and CFC. Manipulating neurogenesis during MWM has produced rather mixed results. Most common implementations of the MWM task have two to three distinct phases. Mice must first learn the location of a hidden platform (acquisition). They are then tested for memory of the platform's location by removing it and tracking the animal's search path (probe test). Finally, they are optionally asked to learn a new, different platform location (reversal learning). Some reports have observed that ablating neurogenesis has no effect at all on MWM performance (Saxe et al., 2006), whereas others have observed a reduction in long-term retention of the hidden platform location (Deng et al., 2009), or a reduction in both acquisition and reversal learning (Garthe et al., 2009). The contrary manipulation of increasing neurogenesis has sometimes resulted in improved performance throughout acquisition, probe, and reversal (W Wang et al., 2014). Other studies have seen more limited effects, with a deficit apparent only when animals have learned at least one prior location and are probed for spatial memory of a new location (McAvoy et al., 2016), and still others have observed no impact (Sahay et al., 2011). CFC experiments have more convincingly implicated adult-born neurons in overall hippocampal function, but still not entirely consistently. Reducing neurogenesis has been reported to impair acquisition of CFC (Saxe et al., 2006; Kitamura et al., 2009; Denny et al., 2012), to leave acquisition intact but impair extinction (Deng et al., 2009), or to have an effect on acquisition only if 1 but not 3 shocks are used during training (Denny et al., 2014). Long-term retention of the fear memory has been reported to be either unaffected (Kitamura et al., 2009) or reduced (Zou et al., 2015) in the absence of neurogenesis.

While the above studies relied mainly on long-term manipulations such as irradiation or genetic ablation, more recent work has used techniques capable of manipulating adult-born neurons acutely. Some of the disparity in results could be due to differences in the magnitude of neurogenesis knockdown that was achieved or the precise age of the targeted cells. If the 4- to 6-week period reflects a particularly important developmental stage, targeting this population would be most informative for inferring function. Using optogenetics to specifically silence populations of different ages, it was observed that silencing 4-week-old, but not 2- or 8-week-old cells, impaired MWM probe performance (Gu et al., 2012). Using optogenetic (Danielson et al., 2016) or chemogenetic (Huckleberry et al., 2018) methods to silence immature cells also produces a deficit in CFC acquisition, and silencing of 4-week-old but not 8-week-old cells impairs retrieval (Gu et al., 2012). These studies suggest that the function of adult-born neurons does in fact change as those cells mature.

9.6.2 Pattern separation and cognitive flexibility

Mixed results from tasks of overall hippocampal function suggest that to reveal the functional relevance of adult-born neurons, a closer examination of the specific contribution of the DG is required. The anatomy of the hippocampal trisynaptic circuit has inspired substantial theoretical and computational work. Among the

results of this work has been a proposed division of labor that assigns complementary functions to the DG and CA3 (Marr, 1971; McNaughton and Morris, 1987; Rolls and Kesner, 2006; Aimone et al., 2009; Yassa and Stark, 2011). When the DG receives cortical input, the presence of several-fold more principal neurons in the DG than in the source population of entorhinal cortex has the effect of spreading out and sparsifying the signal. For two input patterns of neuronal activity with a given similarity from entorhinal cortex, the corresponding two output patterns from dentate are likely to be less similar. This process of orthogonalizing neuronal activity has been dubbed *pattern separation*. In contrast, CA3 pyramidal neurons have recurrent collaterals onto other CA3 neurons, and theorists have suggested that this type of connectivity is likely to create an autoassociative network. Instead of making two similar inputs more distinct, the CA3 circuitry is set up to take a small fraction of the original input and use that to recreate a fuller pattern. This process of recreating a pattern from incomplete or degraded input has been dubbed *pattern completion*.

To apply the concept of pattern separation to a measurable behavioral assay, different research groups have adapted a range of spatial and contextual learning tasks. Typically, the more similar two options are, the more they are considered to tax pattern separation. Clelland et al. ablated neurogenesis and then assessed performance on the radial arm maze (Clelland et al., 2009). Lack of neurogenesis impaired the ability to discriminate near but not distant separations on the maze. Similarly, lack of neurogenesis impaired discrimination of small but not large separations on a touchscreen-based location discrimination task (Clelland et al., 2009; see Swan et al., 2014, for a more limited separation-independent effect) and of small but not large separations during a spontaneous location recognition task (Bekinschtein et al., 2014). Neurogenesis knockdown also decreased the ability to differentiate between two similar contexts during CFC (Nakashiba et al., 2012; Tronel et al., 2012). Complementarily, boosting neurogenesis was observed to improve discrimination of similar contexts (Sahay et al., 2011; McAvoy et al., 2016) and small separations on a touchscreen-based task (Creer et al., 2010). In a correlational study, rats with higher neurogenesis levels were better at discriminating nearby locations on the radial arm maze. Strategy matters for this effect, however, with performance correlating with neurogenesis only in spatial rather than idiothetic strategy users (Yagi et al., 2016). Taking advantage of optogenetic or chemogenetic techniques, it is also becoming feasible to tease apart the role of adult-born neurons during different phases of learning. Silencing adult-born neurons under 6 weeks of age impaired contextual fear discrimination only when silencing was performed in the similar lure context, but not the original training context (Danielson et al., 2016). Silencing 5- to 10-week-old cells impaired touchscreen-based location discrimination learning, but only if the silencing was performed prior to reaching asymptotic performance (Zhuo et al., 2016).

Although the view that adult-born neurons are improving pattern separation is widespread, there are some interpretations that emphasize cognitive flexibility rather than discrimination ability. For example, Swan et al. (2014) observed a deficit in touchscreen-based location discrimination only after the side of the correct location was reversed. To the authors, this signaled a deficit in ability to change the contingencies associated with learned information, not a deficit in determining precise spatial locations per se. Indeed, ablation of neurogenesis impairs other forms of reversal learning. On an active place avoidance task, lack of neurogenesis had no impact on learning the initial site of the shock zone, but did impair learning when the location was switched (Burghardt et al., 2012; Park et al., 2015). These interpretations do share the conclusion that neurogenesis is particularly important when learned information conflicts, either due to similarity or due to a change in the contingencies of the environment. Without knowing what the incoming and outgoing neuronal activity patterns look like during a particular learning episode or task, it is impossible to know whether behavioral changes actually reflect changes in pattern separation at a circuit level within the hippocampus, or whether altered task conditions recruit other brain regions to make use of learned information in a different way. Other criticisms stem from direct experimental evidence inconsistent with the idea of adult-born neurons enhancing pattern separation. Huckleberry et al. (2018) observed that although silencing immature DGCs impaired both CFC acquisition and retrieval, generalization was also reduced, leading to a net increase in discrimination capacity. This result is contrary to the expected impact of silencing immature cells, which would be to reduce discrimination capacity. This is an area that requires additional study.

9.6.3 Network level effects of neurogenesis on sparse coding

If loss of adult-born neurons impairs aspects of hippocampus function, what are the mechanistic underpinnings of the impairment? Immature cells are capable of firing action potentials by 1–3 weeks (Schmidt-Hieber et al., 2004; Mongiat et al., 2009), of forming synaptic connections in CA3 between 2 and 4 weeks of age (Toni et al., 2008; Gu et al., 2012) and of expressing immediate early genes in response to stimulation within 3–4 weeks of age (Jessberger and Kempermann, 2003; Snyder et al., 2009; Veyrac et al., 2013). Adult-born neurons are incorporated into memory traces, as indicated by IEG expression, if they are available (Kee et al., 2007). Posttraining ablation of adult-born neurons disrupts memory, leading to reduced ability to discriminate fear conditioning contexts 1 week later (Arruda-Carvalho et al., 2011), but no impairment occurs if cells are instead ablated in the week leading up to training. However, these ablated cells, although generated in adulthood, were largely mature (several months of age) at the time of the behavioral training. Evidence for direct encoding of memories by engram-bearing (i.e., IEG-expressing) immature granule cells, such as has been shown for mature granule cells (X Liu et al., 2012; Ramirez et al., 2013) is limited. Perhaps this is a mere technical limitation associated with the challenge of identifying and then reactivating a very small population of immature cells. Alternatively, some of the effects attributed to adult-born neurons may be occurring indirectly, through broader network level effects.

The impact of a small population of hyperexcitable adult-born neurons may be to control the overall excitability of the surrounding DG network. Several studies suggest that highly active immature cells lead to less activity in surrounding mature cells. Ablating or silencing adult-born neurons leads to greater spread of excitation in hippocampal slices as detected by voltage-sensitive dyes (Ikrar et al., 2013), greater IEG activation in vivo (Anacker et al., 2018), and greater susceptibility to seizure-inducing compounds (Iyengar et al., 2015). Chemogenetic inhibition of adult-born neurons in the ventral dentate not only led to greater cfos activation of mature ventral granule cells but also to increased responses to perforant path stimulation and altered behavioral responsiveness to social defeat stress (Anacker et al., 2018). Complementarily, increasing neurogenesis reduced cfos activation in the ventral DG of mice exposed to repeated social defeat (Anacker et al., 2018). This suppression of activity was specific to behaviorally stimulated conditions and not present in untrained animals. In vivo calcium imaging revealed that increased neurogenesis specifically attenuated the increase in Ca^{2+} transients during the time period when the defeated mouse received attacks from the resident aggressor mouse (Anacker et al., 2018). Optogenetic stimulation of immature granule cells less than 7 weeks of age in another study also reduced the fraction of IEG+ mature granule cells, whereas stimulation of a comparably sized population of mature cells had no effect on total IEG expression (Drew et al., 2016). However, not all reports have unanimously argued that immature neurons reduce dentate excitability. Lacefield et al. (2012) found bidirectional effects, with a loss of immature neurons leading to a reduction of evoked responses from the perforant path, but an increase in spontaneous gamma frequency bursts. The effect of immature neurons also appears to depend on the precise source of inputs, with adult-born DGCs exerting an inhibitory effect on inputs from the lateral entorhinal cortex but an excitatory effect on inputs from the medial entorhinal cortex (Luna et al., 2019). According to Luna et al.'s model, lateral perforant path input tends to activate a small number of immature DGCs, triggering them to release a small amount of extrasynaptic glutamate, which preferentially binds group II metabotropic glutamate receptors to inhibit mature DGCs. In contrast, medial perforant path input is more effective in recruiting immature DGCs, triggering larger extrasynaptic glutamate release that in turn excites mature DGCs via NMDARs.

Overall, adult-born neurons may enhance an already-noteworthy feature of the DG: its sparsity. The precise mechanism by which this enhanced sparsity is achieved remains to be clarified. From ex vivo slice recordings, stimulation of immature adult-born neurons at 4 weeks of age is less effective in recruiting feedback inhibition onto the granule cell layer than stimulation of mature granule cells (Temprana et al., 2015). The authors concluded that mature, rather than immature, DGCs recruit the critical feedback inhibition that limits the size of the active DGC population. However, other findings suggest alternative means for immature neurons to exert some control over hippocampal activity. As discussed above, immature DGCs may inhibit mature DGCs via extrasynaptic transmission at metabotropic glutamate receptors (Luna et al., 2019). Immature DGCs also have functional contacts with CA3, including more filopodial contacts on GABAergic CA3 interneurons than mature cells (Restivo et al., 2015). One report also suggests that adult-born neurons may directly release GABA onto mature cells (Drew et al., 2016), a synaptic connection not present at maturity. Another study observed that SOM-expressing interneurons, rather than the PV-expressing interneurons studied by Temprana et. al, are more important for determining the size of the active DGC ensemble in vivo, but this group did not examine adult-born neurons (Stefanelli et al., 2016). Because slice preparations unavoidably sever some projections compared with the in vivo case, more direct investigation of in vivo physiology from DGCs spanning an age range from immature to mature will be necessary for understanding circuit-level mechanisms.

Another possible explanation is that immature DGCs at 4 weeks of age still have fewer synapses from the entorhinal cortex, leading immature cells to sample their inputs from a smaller fraction of incoming fibers (Dieni et al., 2016). A model of network activity suggested that such poorly connected but intrinsically hyperexcitable immature neurons would provide fewer correlated signals than mature cells, and their presence would allow the dentate to better separate patterns when entorhinal cortex activity is high (Dieni et al., 2016). A reduced number of synapses would also serve to counterbalance the high intrinsic excitability of adult-born neurons, preventing stimulation in vivo from being dominated by immature DGCs. Indeed, limited excitatory drive plays a greater role in restricting immature DGC spiking up to 4 weeks of age than it does in more mature DGCs (Mongiat et al., 2009; Dieni et al., 2013), and entorhinal cortex stimulation that was sufficient to trigger spiking in mature DGCs failed to do the same in immature cells (Dieni et al., 2016).

While the above results have demonstrated a link between adult neurogenesis and the sparsity of the DG, it seems unlikely that imposing sparsity on the network is the only role of adult-born granule cells. There is no overarching network design principle that would require neurogenesis to create a sparsely active network. Further, a DG with neurogenesis ablated is still considerably quieter than neighboring CA3 or CA1. Whether there are additional physiological impacts of immature DGCs remains an open question. Over an individual's lifetime, both memory specificity and flexibility are required, and it may be that immature DGCs contribute differently depending on whether they are present during the formation of a memory or only during its recall, as discussed in the next section.

9.6.4 Neurogenesis and forgetting: bug or feature?

Most studies have manipulated neurogenesis first and then looked at the effects of that manipulation on later learning. A consequence of the competition for synaptic input and circuit rewiring that accompanies neurogenesis (Toni et al., 2007; McAvoy et al., 2016; Adlaf et al., 2017) could, however, be that already-formed memories are either overwritten or rendered difficult to access. To test this prediction, Akers et al. (2014) trained mice on a CFC task and then provided running wheels to enhance neurogenesis. Compared with sedentary animals, those who ran after the fear conditioning experience showed reduced freezing upon context re-exposure 4–6 weeks later, suggesting that more neurogenesis led to a less robust memory of the training event. Increasing neurogenesis pharmacologically with memantine treatment or genetically with p53 knockout in NPCs produced a similar pattern of forgetting (Akers et al., 2014). This phenomenon was not specific to contextual fear memory but was also observed for memories of the hidden platform location in the MWM and of paired associates in an odor discrimination task (Epp et al., 2016; but see Kodali et al., 2016 for a counterexample in rats trained on the MWM then given running wheel access). Enhanced neurogenesis was most critical in stimulating forgetting in the first 2 weeks following the conditioning experience, with 2 weeks of running nearly as effective as 4 weeks (Gao et al., 2018), but a lack of enhanced forgetting with only a week of running. Forgetting was temporally graded, as expected based on the time-limited role of the hippocampus in memory. Delaying the running period for 2 weeks prevented significant forgetting (Gao et al., 2018). However, even at remote time points, prolonged reexposure to the training context may open a reconsolidation window. Although the hippocampus becomes less critical for retrieval of remote memories over time, prolonged reexposure followed by memantine treatment or running 2 months after the original training period enabled forgetting 1 month later (Ishikawa

et al., 2016). Opening a second forgetting window appeared to be hippocampus- and protein-synthesis-dependent, and only a long (10 min) re-exposure to the training context was sufficient to induce IEG activation in the hippocampus 1 month after training, suggesting hippocampus reactivation is a component of the destabilization process (Ishikawa et al., 2016). Such findings are a promising new avenue for treatment of traumatic memories, such as those associated with PTSD.

These results offer further support that the enhanced flexibility and pattern separation enabled by adult neurogenesis come with a trade-off in stability. Indeed, reversal learning is enhanced in mice whose memory of the original escape platform in the MWM has been weakened by running (Epp et al., 2016). Ablating neurogenesis in contrast slows down reversal learning. On a paired associates odor discrimination task, forgetting of the original odor-context pairs due to running was also accompanied by enhanced learning of new, conflicting information when the original pairings were reversed (Epp et al., 2016). Consistent with a role of neurogenesis in mitigating interference, no difference in performance was observed when the new pairings were entirely novel rather than a reassignment of existing pairings. Naturally occurring variations in the level of neurogenesis provide further evidence for this relationship. In infant mice, neurogenesis levels are substantially higher than in adults, and memories formed on postnatal day 17 are forgotten within 2–4 weeks, a retention interval that can be improved by ablating neurogenesis (Akers et al., 2014). Such infantile amnesia is lacking in species with little early postnatal neurogenesis such as degus and guinea pigs, although running or memantine treatment can also trigger infantile amnesia in these animals (Akers et al., 2014). However, not all evidence is consistent with an enhancement of new learning by more new neurons. In rats, the number of immature cells was correlated with learning speed for a reference memory version of the MWM, but not a working memory version, which would be expected to create more interference (Aasebo et al., 2018). Although the impact of adult neurogenesis on previously formed memories is a relatively new area of experimental research, evidence thus far suggests increased neurogenesis is beneficial for learning new, conflicting information at the expense of the stability of older memories.

9.7 Adult neurogenesis in healthy humans

9.7.1 Evidence for adult hippocampal neurogenesis in humans

Adult neurogenesis has been firmly established in rodents. Does the same hold true for humans? Very few studies have been able to provide direct and unquestionable evidence for or against the existence of adult neurogenesis in humans, but the key evidence to date has been in favor. A landmark study by Eriksson and colleagues (1998) examined cancer patients who had been administered BrdU, the same compound used regularly in studies of rodents, prior to death (section 9.5.1). Tissue samples from these patients were then examined postmortem, and the researchers found colocalization of BrdU with the neuronal markers NeuN, calbindin, and neuron-specific enolase. Colocalization of BrdU and neuron-specific markers was observed in the SGZ and granule cell layer of all 5 BrdU-treated patients, who had a maximum age of 72 years. This study provided compelling evidence for the existence of adult neurogenesis in humans and suggested it could continue even into advanced age (Eriksson et al., 1998). A second report using IdU also found colocalization of IdU and neuronal markers in the DG in individuals ranging from 20 to 71 years of age (Ernst et al., 2014).

Another critical study used known variations in radioactive 14C due to nuclear testing to birthdate cells in individuals without any drug administration (Spalding et al., 2013). This carbon-dating approach led to an estimate of 700 new neurons produced in the adult human hippocampus per day, or about 0.004% of the DGC population. Not all hippocampal neurons were predicted to be part of the renewable population, but the approximately one-third that turned over would correspond to the vast majority of DGCs. The half-life of adult-born cells was estimated at 7.7 years, and neurogenesis persisted into at least the fifth decade of life. Although turnover declined with age, the trajectory was mild in comparison with rodents, corresponding to an approximately fourfold decline during adult life.

Corroborating, albeit indirect evidence, has come from immunohistochemical studies of postmortem tissue. In general, results from immunohistochemistry have been more contradictory than the clear results from birthdating studies. These methods are unable to identify a cell birthdate, but they can provide additional support to the extent that rodents and humans share markers of immaturity during development and adult neurogenesis. A study of 54 individuals ranging in age from 0 to 100 years observed an age-related decline in DCX, but coexpression of DCX and multiple markers of cell proliferation continued through 30 to 40 years of age, with DCX and Mcm2 coexpression detectable until at least 65 years of age (Knoth et al., 2010). However, this study did not control for psychiatric history or drug use. Another study of individuals 0–59 years of age also noted a sharp decline in proliferating cells and immature DCX+ neurons in early childhood, suggesting most proliferating cells in the adult brain are microglia (Dennis et al., 2016). At the RNA level, a study of presumably neurologically typical human subjects 18–88 years of age reported decreased DCX with age, but stable expression of eomesodermin (Tbr2), which is expressed in intermediate progenitors (section 9.3.2) (K Mathews et al., 2017). In individuals without neuropsychiatric disease, neuropsychiatric medication, or cognitive impairment, there is a decline in the quiescent Sox2+ stem cell population in the anterior hippocampus with age, but a stable pool of proliferating progenitors (Sox2+ Nestin+ or Sox2-Nestin+) and immature DCX+ or DCX+ PSA-NCAM+ neurons from the teen years through the eighth decade of life (Boldrini et al., 2018). Angiogenesis declined with age, as did total PSA-NCAM+ cells, suggesting a decrease in neuroplasticity with age (Boldrini et al., 2018). In sum, these studies suggest that some level of neurogenesis persists in the human hippocampus despite a steep decline during childhood.

Neurodegenerative disease alters the neurogenic landscape relative to healthy aging. While DCX+ immature neurons have been identified postmortem in neurologically healthy subjects as old as 87 years, fewer immature cells are present in subjects with Alzheimer's disease (AD) (Moreno-Jiménez et al., 2019). Other neurodegenerative diseases have been observed to impact the course of neurogenesis at the level of cell maturation and development (Terreros-Roncal et al., 2021). Immature DGCs appear more prevalent in amyotrophic lateral sclerosis (ALS), Huntington's disease, and Parkinson's disease than in healthy aging, but these immature cells are accompanied by increased pyknotic cells within the DG.

Along with reduced microglial phagocytic capacity and astrogliosis, these results suggest a failure to remove dying or poorly integrating cells, disrupting the neurogenic niche in the disease state. This work is still a recent addition to the neurogenesis literature and would benefit from further study.

In addition to this immunohistochemical evidence, progenitor cells isolated from hippocampal tissue in adults as part of surgical resection have been successfully isolated and expanded in vitro, generating neurons from the endogenous progenitor cells (Roy et al., 2000; Palmer et al., 2001; Hermann et al., 2006). Progenitors have been isolated from DG tissue across a wide age range, including adults up to 63 years old (Roy et al., 2000). Surgical samples of course come with caveats as to their applicability to healthy individuals, as the majority of resected tissue samples were obtained from patients with epilepsy.

9.7.2 Generalizability of rodent studies to humans?

Findings of adult neurogenesis in humans have occasionally sparked controversy. Sorrells et al. (2018) observed a sharp decline in neurogenesis during childhood and concluded that almost no adult neurogenesis occurs in adult humans. Shortly afterward, two reports put forward a competing claim, observing sustained adult neurogenesis for many decades (Boldrini et al., 2018; Moreno-Jiménez et al., 2019). What accounts for the difference? Kempermann and colleagues (Kempermann et al., 2018) pointed to a number of differences between the two 2018 studies. Boldrini et al. used a postmortem interval of less than 26 hours in contrast to a longer window of less than 48 hours in the work of Sorrells et al. (2018). Some of the markers used to investigate neurogenesis become degraded within hours after death, most notably DCX (Boekhoorn et al., 2006; Terstege et al., 2022). Sorrells et al. (2018) also used tissue from individuals with less well-defined clinical histories, whereas the individuals in Boldrini et al's report were free of known neurological or psychiatric disease. Even with short postmortem collection intervals, histological markers are sensitive to fixation conditions (Lyck et al., 2008; Flor-Garcia et al., 2020). Thus, numerous factors combine to make definitive detection of protein markers difficult in human samples. A best practices protocol for human tissue is available from the same investigators, who successfully detected immature neurons in aged healthy subjects and saw a decline with AD (Flor-Garcia et al., 2020). Specific areas of concern highlighted by the authors include strict sample curation to avoid using samples with a long postmortem delay period or neuropathology, fixation in 4% paraformaldehyde for only 24 hours, use of pretreatment procedures such as antigen retrieval and $NaBH_4$ incubation to minimize autofluorescence, and validation of antibodies (Flor-Garcia et al., 2020).

Ultimately, some of the debate surrounding these papers may reflect differences in opinion over what constitutes "significant" vs. "minimal" neurogenesis. Sorrells et al. included samples from fetal brain and early childhood, whereas the youngest age in Boldrini et al's work was 14 years, and Moreno-Jimenez et. al studied adults at least 43 years old. The comparative decline in neurogenesis from early development to old age is unsurprisingly greater in the Sorrells et al. (2018) study. If the estimate by Spalding et al. (2013) of 0.004% turnover per day holds, the question for further research becomes whether this number of cells is relevant and can provide the same unique processing capabilities attributed to neurogenesis in rodents.

Additional fodder for this debate has come from a report that single-nucleus transcriptomes from the hippocampus reveal a clear neurogenic trajectory in mice, pigs, and macaques, but not in human samples (Franjic et al., 2022). After sequencing transcriptomes in nearly 140,000 human DG cells, the authors reported only 1 convincing neural progenitor and 1 convincing neuroblast among 6 human subjects. These results suggest dramatically lower numbers of immature neurons in humans than estimates made via immunohistochemistry, questioning the relevance of adult neurogenesis in humans. This study raises important questions about how to interpret cross-species comparisons not just of immunohistochemistry but also of more recent and rapidly advancing sequencing methods. Again, the difficulty of obtaining high-quality human postmortem tissue may be a confounding factor. In this study, the authors did attempt to demonstrate an ability to detect progenitors and neuroblasts in pig samples over an extended post mortem interval of 7 hours at room temperature. However, these pig samples were very young in comparison to the humans studied (weanlings at 3 months of age compared with humans averaging slightly over 50 years), and still had a shorter postmortem time than the human samples (average 15 hours predominantly under refrigeration). Some cell types are also likely to be more sensitive and difficult to capture after nuclei isolation, though it is unclear why this process would specifically affect progenitors from human samples and not other organisms. It will be critical for future efforts to attempt to process human and nonhuman samples as similarly as possible to rule out interactions of age, postmortem time, and sample handling to reconcile the significant differences observed in levels of adult neurogenesis among human studies (Terstege et al., 2022).

Another explanation may be that analysis of hippocampal transcriptomes requires different approaches in humans compared with other species. Most recently, Zhou et al. (2022) reported detecting immature DGCs across the human lifespan using single-nuclei RNA-seq in samples spanning infancy to 92 years of age. In contrast to data from mouse models, immature DGCs in humans did not readily segregate into their own cluster using unbiased clustering algorithms. Instead, the authors were able to detect these cells via a supervised machine learning approach that compared the transcriptome of individual nuclei to "prototype" DCX+ PROX1+ CALBINDIN- immature hippocampal DGCs from subjects aged 0–2 as well as prototypes of mature nonneuronal cell types. Although immature DGCs were more common during infancy and early childhood, the authors estimated that immature DGCs represented ~3.1%–7.5% of DGCs detected in samples from ages 40–92. As in prior immunohistochemical work, samples from individuals with AD had lower percentages of immature DGCs than healthy aged controls. Because supporting immunohistochemistry experiments yielded low numbers of actively dividing Ki67+ or Tbr2+ progenitors even in samples from healthy individuals, the authors interpreted their results as supportive of a human neurogenic niche that generates low numbers of new cells but provides a prolonged maturation period.

In support of some conserved features of hippocampal neurogenesis through evolution are a number of studies showing adult neurogenesis in nonhuman primates. Injection of thymidine analogues into Old World monkeys (macaques) revealed proliferation in adulthood and coexpression of BrdU with neuronal markers such as NeuN, Tuj1, and calbindin in the DG (Gould et al., 1999; Kornack and Rakic, 1999; Koketsu et al., 2006), with a decline in older animals (Gould et al., 1999). Age-related declines in BrdU incorporation are also observed in the common marmoset. As reported between childhood and old age in humans, markers of immature neurons also decline dramatically with age in macaques (Sorrells et al., 2018) and marmosets. Some of the same environmental factors that influence neurogenesis levels in rodents are also shared with nonhuman primates. Newborn cells detected in the DG after BrdU injection in New World monkeys (marmosets) showed decreased proliferation with acute stress (Gould et al., 1998). Chronic stressors such as repeated social isolation have also been observed to decrease hippocampal neurogenesis in bonnet macaques (Perera et al., 2011). Conversely, antidepressant electroconvulsive shock treatment increased proliferation in the SGZ of adult bonnet macaques (Perera et al., 2007).

Other aspects of neurogenesis show greater cross-species variability. For example, markers of immature cells such as calretinin show pronounced differences between mouse and rat DG, with many more calretinin + immature DGCs in mouse (Liu et al., 1996; Brandt et al., 2003). There may be additional markers of neuronal development or plasticity that are present in humans but not in other species. Further, it has not been possible to determine how the maturation period of adult-born neurons compares in humans and other animals. It is possible that humans, whose average lifespan greatly exceeds that of rodents, face specific challenges in maintaining plasticity over decades, and neurons may take longer to mature. Based on the lack of mature neuronal marker expression and continued dendritic tree development, it has been suggested that the maturation process is prolonged in nonhuman primates relative to rodents, extending for at least 6 months in macaques (Kohler et al., 2011), although other studies have found substantial colocalization of BrdU-labeled cells with NeuN at 8 weeks (Perera et al., 2011), or even at 4 weeks (Koketsu et al., 2006; Perera et al., 2007).

Finally, although the hippocampal neurogenic niche may be conserved between rodents and humans, other neurogenic niches are not. The human SVZ does contain a population of proliferating cells (Johansson et al., 1999; Sanai et al., 2004; C Wang et al., 2011), as in rodents. However, these proliferating cells do not generate any significant number of new neurons in the olfactory bulb (Sanai et al., 2011; C Wang et al., 2011; Bergmann et al., 2012). What is the fate of cells derived from neural progenitors in the SVZ? In humans, these cells may migrate to the striatum instead. Carbon-dating evidence demonstrates turnover of a population of striatal interneurons during adulthood (Ernst et al., 2014). The renewable population is more restricted than in the case of the DG, with only 25% of neurons subject to turnover, but within this population 2.7% were expected to turn over annually. As in the study from Eriksson et al. (1998), samples were also obtained from cancer patients receiving a thymidine analogue (in this case, IdU). Postmortem examination of the striatum from these patients revealed IdU+ cells in both the caudate and putamen that coexpressed neuronal markers NeuN, MAP2, or calretinin. The reasons for such species differences in the ultimate destination of adult-born neurons are unknown, and uncovering those reasons may inform new hypotheses about the role of adult neurogenesis in humans specifically.

9.8 The implications of adult neurogenesis for psychiatric and neurological disease

9.8.1 Epilepsy

The sparse activity of DGCs is thought to be important not only for proper memory formation and recall (section 9.6.3) but also for controlling the spread of activity throughout the rest of the hippocampus. This ability of the DG to regulate and gate hippocampal excitability is severely altered in mesial temporal lobe epilepsy (mTLE) (Collins et al., 1983; Stringer et al., 1989; Heinemann et al., 1992; Krook-Magnuson et al., 2015), the most common form of epilepsy in adults (see Chapter 18, on epilepsy). Multiple cell types within the DG and hilus, including immature DGCs, contribute to setting the excitatory tone of the DG under both physiological and pathological settings. Under most conditions (see Lacefield et al., 2012, and Luna et al., 2019, for exceptions), immature DGCs appear to quiet the DG and facilitate the sparse activity observed in mature DGCs in part by recruiting inhibitory feedback onto these cells (section 9.6.3). However, in mTLE both the number of adult-born DGCs and their physiology are significantly altered. Compounding the effects of loss of interneurons observed in mTLE, changes in adult neurogenesis are thought to impact the excitability of the DG and downstream networks within the hippocampal formation and to play an important role in epileptogenesis.

9.8.1.1 Seizures augment proliferation and maturation of adult-born neurons

Enhanced proliferation of adult-born DGCs after seizure was first described by Parent et al. (1997) who demonstrated an approximately 10-fold increase in the number of BrdU+ and PCNA+ newborn DGCs starting 3 days following pharmacologically induced status epilepticus (SE) in rats. Similar findings of seizure-induced proliferation were reported by Bengzon et al. (1997) around the same time, and they have since been reproduced in numerous studies (Gray and Sundstrom, 1998; Scott et al., 1998; Huttmann et al., 2003; Jessberger et al., 2005; Lugert et al., 2010). However, there is some disagreement regarding the source of additional proliferating cells. Huttmann et al. found that seizures preferentially activate proliferation of GFAP+ Type I radial glia-like cells 72 hours after kainic acid administration in GFAP-GFP expressing transgenic mice (Huttmann et al., 2003). However, this increase in GFP+ and GFP+ BrdU+ radial glia-like cells accounted for a minority of the respective increase in GFP+ and GFP+ BrdU+ total cells of all morphologies in their experimental system. Moreover, the increase in BrdU+ GFP+ cells accounted for less than half of the increase in total BrdU+ cells, indicating that the majority of BrdU+ proliferating cells do not express GFAP, despite being exposed to BrdU only 2 hours prior to fixation. Using immunohistochemistry, Jessberger and colleagues did not observe an increase in the number of GFAP+ Type I radial glia-like cells under similar conditions, albeit at later time points after SE (Jessberger et al., 2005). Their experiments point toward Type III DCX+ neuroblasts as being the primary source for enhanced proliferation following seizure. In contrast, under physiological conditions proliferation of Type II cells is observed in response to running (sections 9.3 and 9.4, Figure 9.3). However, it should be noted that expression of the DCX marker is temporally quite broad, and experiments addressing the source of proliferating cells after seizure using the Tbr2 marker, whose

expression is highly specific for Type II cells, are lacking. Despite potential differences in the population of proliferating cells, many of the same factors are thought to regulate activity-dependent proliferation under these different conditions. These include (1) sensing of extrasynaptic GABA, which increases in response to PV cell recruitment and is sensed by NPCs; (2) changes in Shh, Notch, and Wnt signaling (Banerjee et al., 2005; Sibbe et al., 2012; Jang et al., 2013); and (3) enhanced expression of neurotrophic factors such as BDNF (Isackson et al., 1991; Gall, 1993; Newton et al., 2003) and VEGF (Jessberger and Parent, 2015). Finally, there is evidence indicating that the increased proliferation of NPCs after SE may not be long-lived in rodents, with return to basal levels of proliferation approximately 1 month later (Parent et al., 1997; Bonde et al., 2006). In fact, late in epileptogenesis the regenerative capacity of the SGZ niche is thought to be depleted compared with control animals (Hattiangady et al., 2004; Kralic et al., 2005).

Similar to proliferation, the functional and morphological maturation of NPCs is also enhanced by EE and running and is altered by seizures (Jessberger et al., 2007; Alvarez et al., 2016). However, unlike EE and running (Gonçalves, Schafer, et al., 2016), seizures appear to disrupt the normal homeostatic mechanisms that control dendritic tree development and maturation (Overstreet-Wadiche, 2006b). Overstreet et al. showed that 2 weeks after pilocarpine-induced seizures the total dendritic length of immature adult-born neurons labeled with POMC-GFP increased by almost 60% and extended beyond the inner molecular layer that was observed in control animals, reaching the middle and outer molecular layers. In pilocarpine-treated animals, excitatory postsynaptic currents (EPSCs) could be evoked in almost half of the GFP+ immature neurons via stimulation of the medial perforant path, compared with no observed responses in labeled cells from control animals. Together, the effects of enhanced proliferation and maturation of adult-born DGCs can have a long-term impact on the function of the DG, as increased numbers of neurons, including those with augmented dendritic arbors, survive and persist for at least weeks to months after SE (Jessberger et al., 2005; Overstreet-Wadiche, 2006b).

9.8.1.2 Aberrant development of adult-born neurons in epilepsy

Perhaps the most dramatic rewiring of adult-born DGCs observed in the setting of epilepsy is the abnormal projection of their axons, termed mossy fibers, onto the dendrites of local DGCs, termed "mossy fiber sprouting" (Zimmer, 1973; Victor Nadler et al., 1980; Tauck and Nadler, 1985; Represa et al., 1989; Sutula et al., 1989; Houser et al., 1990; Parent and Lowenstein, 1997). Mossy fibers are rich in zinc, allowing mossy fiber sprouting to be visualized via Timm's sulfide-silver-staining technique (Parent and Lowenstein, 1997). Using this staining approach, mossy fiber sprouting manifests as a dark band containing aberrant mossy fibers and terminals in the inner molecular layer of hippocampal slices from epileptic animals and humans. Studies show that immature DGCs born 1 to 4 weeks prior to SE (Jessberger et al., 2007; Kron et al., 2010), and not mature cells or DGCs born after SE (Parent et al., 1999), contribute to mossy fiber sprouting observed 4 weeks later. However, immature adult-born neurons born after SE continue to contribute to mossy fiber sprouting at later time points after SE (Kron et al., 2010). This aberrant rewiring of adult-born DGCs axons onto mature DGCs forms an excitatory positive feedback loop that is hypothesized to contribute to the hyperexcitability of the DG observed in mTLE (see dentate gate hypothesis Chapter 18). However, the causal role of mossy fiber sprouting in epileptogenesis is still a matter of debate as mossy fiber sprouting alone does not appear to be sufficient to produce seizures in mTLE (Hunt et al., 2012).

Normally, Type III neuroblasts migrate from the SGZ into the granule cell layer. In both human mTLE and rodent models of mTLE, an increased proportion of adult-born neurons exhibit ectopic migration, terminating in the hilus or the molecular layer. In contrast to mossy fiber sprouting, only adult-born cells born after SE exhibited aberrant migration into the hilus in rodents (Walter et al., 2007; Kron et al., 2010), consistent with the idea that seizure activity cannot alter the migration of cells that have completed migration. Hilar ectopic DGCs exhibit abnormal excitation (Scharfman et al., 2000), and their prevalence predicts seizure frequency after pilocarpine-SE in rodents. Interestingly, transgenic mice carrying loss-of-function mutations in genes encoding proteins with a variety of functions, including Reelin and PTEN, also exhibit ectopic migration of DGCs and have been implicated in epilepsy (Gong et al., 2007; Pun et al., 2012; Teixeira et al., 2012; Myers et al., 2013; Jiang et al., 2016). Whether these heterogeneous pathways reflect the diversity of insults that can lead to aberrant neurogenesis and epilepsy, or whether they belong to a common pathway is not known. Finally, similar to mossy fiber sprouting, it is not clear to what extent ectopic DGCs contribute to epileptogenesis or are simply a consequence of seizures. In an attempt to address this question, Lybrand et al. used retrovirally delivered hM3Dq to chemogenetically activate adult-born DGCs during their 1st or 2nd postmitotic week (Lybrand et al., 2021). This stimulation not only resulted in an increased number of these cell migrating to the hilus compared with DGCs without activation but also increased the incidence of spontaneous seizures in mice approximately 2 months later.

With rare exceptions, mature DGCs in rodents do not display basilar dendrites that extend into the hilus (Gonçalves, Schafer, et al., 2016). However, 5% of total DGCs exhibit hilar basal dendrites in pilocarpine treated epileptic rats (Ribak et al., 2000). Between one-third and one-half of immature DGCs in epileptic animals exhibit this morphological change (Walter et al., 2007; Kron et al., 2010). Ninety-three percent of the synaptic inputs received on these dendrites are excitatory (Thind et al., 2008), often with mossy appearance indicative of DGC innervation (Spigelman et al., 1998; Buckmaster and Dudek, 1999). Like other forms of seizure-induced aberrant neurogenesis, the contribution of hilar basal dendrites to network hyperexcitability and epileptogenesis are unknown. In fact, approximately 20% to 50% of DGCs in humans exhibit hilar basal dendrites, which appears to be a normal finding in both healthy adult humans and nonhuman primates (Seress and Mrzljak, 1987; Al-Hussain and Al-Ali, 1995; Lim et al., 1997; Lauer et al., 2003; Austin and Buckmaster, 2004). However, DGCs with basal dendrites are more prevalent in humans with epilepsy and other diseases that exhibit neuronal hyperexcitability such as schizophrenia, which suggests that the recurrent excitation recruited by these cells may contribute to pathology (Lauer et al., 2003; see below).

9.8.1.3 Effect of manipulating adult neurogenesis in epilepsy

A number of studies have attempted to test the hypothesis that aberrant adult-born DGCs contribute to epileptogenesis and that attenuating adult neurogenesis can reduce seizures in mTLE. Early studies used pharmacologic treatments, typically antimitotic agents, to examine the effect of ablation of adult neurogenesis on epileptogenesis. Jung et al. administered intraventricular cytosine-b-D-arabinofuranoside (Ara-C) starting 1 day prior to pilocarpine-induced SE and continuing for 14 days, which decreased the number of BrdU+ NeuN+ neurons in the hilus (Jung et al., 2004). This treatment also reduced the frequency and duration of seizures in these mice compared with controls. Similar effects were later observed by the same group using celecoxib, a selective COX-2 inhibitor, which in addition to decreasing inflammation in the brain, decreases the proliferation of cultured neural stem cells. Later, Cho et al. showed that genetic ablation of Nestin+ cells in Nestin-tk mice via ganciclovir administration for 4 weeks prior to pilocarpine-induced SE, resulted in a 40% reduction in seizure frequency (Cho et al., 2015). This effect persisted and was even more pronounced at 1 year, with a several-fold reduction in spontaneous seizures at this time point. More recently, work by Lybrand et al. demonstrated that chemogenetic inhibition of adult-born neurons, born days prior to SE, for 2 weeks after SE decreased seizure frequency in these mice 2 months later (Lybrand et al., 2021). In addition, using a transgenic strategy in mice that relied on tamoxifen-inducible expression of Cre under the Nestin promoter, Hosford et al. induced expression of diphtheria toxin receptors in DGCs born starting 5 weeks prior to SE (Hosford et al., 2016). However, they delayed administration of diphtheria toxin, and thus ablation of these adult-born cells, until after SE. Administration of diphtheria toxin 3 days after SE resulted in a 50% reduction in spontaneous seizures at 2 months after SE. Remarkably, delaying ablation of adult-born DGCs expressing toxin receptor until 3–4 months after SE, prevented a 300% increase in seizure frequency that was observed in untreated epileptic mice. However, the treatment did not result in a reduction of seizures at this time point. Lastly, Varma et al. investigated whether ablation of adult-born DGCs born *after* SE could impact seizure frequency (Varma et al., 2019). Continuous ablation of neurogenesis for more than 5 weeks following SE reduced seizures by 65%. However, this reduction was only temporary and was not present 2 weeks later, despite continued ablation of neurogenesis during this time period. Thus, treatments targeting aberrant adult neurogenesis at clinically relevant time points, well into the disease, may have some efficacy in abrogating seizures.

9.8.2 Mood disorders and schizophrenia

9.8.2.1 Depression, antidepressants, and adult neurogenesis

The concept that depression and adult neurogenesis might be related began to emerge in the late 1990s, with stress being a strong modulator of both of these phenomena (section 9.4.2) (Cameron and Gould, 1994; Gould et al., 1998; Gould, 1999; Jacobs et al., 2000; Kempermann and Kronenberg, 2003). Not long after Parent et al. described enhanced proliferation of adult-born DGCs following pilocarpine-induced SE, Madsen et al. and Scott et al. demonstrated that rats experiencing electroconvulsive seizures, a model of electroconvulsive therapy for severe and treatment-resistant depression, exhibited similar augmentation of adult neurogenesis (Parent & Lowenstein, 1997; Madsen et al., 2000; Scott et al., 2000). Later the same year, Malberg et al. published work showing both electroconvulsive seizures and three classes of chemical antidepressants: monoamine oxidase inhibitor (tranylcypromine), serotonin-selective reuptake inhibitor (fluoxetine), and norepinephrine-selective reuptake inhibitor (reboxetine) all promote proliferation of adult-born DGCs (Malberg et al., 2000). Similar findings have since been reproduced for numerous antidepressants and mood stabilizers (Chen et al., 2002; Bai et al., 2003; Banasr et al., 2006; Encinas et al., 2006; Jaako-Movits et al., 2006; Jayatissa et al., 2006; Dekeyne et al., 2008; Surget et al., 2008; Boldrini et al., 2012) and in a number of species including non-human primates and humans (Perera et al., 2007; Perera et al., 2011). In particular, Boldrini et al. found increased numbers of Nestin+ NPCs in postmortem brain tissue of patients with MDD treated with SSRIs or TCAa compared with untreated patients and controls (Boldrini et al., 2009). Evidence for a causal link between neurogenesis and depression was provided by Santarelli et al., who used X-irradiation to ablate adult neurogenesis in mice experiencing chronic unpredictable stress, which results in a deterioration in grooming that responds to pharmacological treatment with antidepressants (Santarelli et al., 2003). They demonstrated that (1) the antidepressive effects of fluoxetine require intact neurogenesis and (2) serotonin agonists could reproduce the enhancement of neurogenesis induced by SSRIs. In addition, the time course of their findings supported the idea that the development and maturation of adult-born neurons over weeks underlie the delay in onset of symptomatic relief from ECT, SSRIs, and other pharmacological therapies for depression (Porsolt et al., 1978; Willner et al., 1987; Bodnoff et al., 1988; Duman, 1997; J Wang et al., 2008). This finding is in contrast to the rapid effect of these agents on neurotransmission. Finally, the efficacy of antidepressants in treating anxiety disorders and the overlap between the anxiolytic effects and the strong augmentation of adult neurogenesis by running have prompted speculation that adult neurogenesis might underlie the pathophysiology of some anxiety disorders, including PTSD (Revest et al., 2009; Besnard and Sahay, 2016; Ishikawa et al., 2019; Schoenfeld et al., 2019).

While there is substantial correlative evidence that many of the same environmental factors and agents that modulate adult neurogenesis also exacerbate or treat depression, experiments demonstrating a causal link between neurogenesis and depression are scant (Surget et al., 2011). Multiple studies indicate that there may be both neurogenesis-dependent and-independent mechanisms of action underlying the antidepressive effects of SSRIs in rodents (Holick et al., 2008; Surget et al., 2008; David et al., 2009). Interestingly, Holick et al. demonstrate that neurogenesis-mediated antidepressant effects are dependent on the experimental mouse strain. In contrast to the 129/Sv mice used by Santarelli et al., antidepressive effects of fluoxetine in BALB/cj mice are independent of both adult neurogenesis and serotonin signaling at 5-HT1A receptors. Also, experiments in postmortem brain tissue published by Reif et al. did not detect an increase in Ki67+ dividing cells in the SGZ in patients taking TCAs or SSRIs (Reif et al., 2006). However, this could be specific to Ki67+ cells, which in the study from Boldrini et al. (2009) only showed an increase in patients taking TCAs and not SSRIs. Finally, many of the same agents or exposures that are known to modulate neurogenesis do not induce or alleviate depression. For example, ablation of adult neurogenesis using radiation does not produce a depression-like phenotype in animals (Santarelli et al., 2003; Airan et al., 2007; Surget et al., 2008). Also, pharmacological agents such as memantine that substantially upregulate neurogenesis are not effective at treating depression (Kishi et al., 2017). Thus, more studies are required to dissect the complex relationship between depression, antidepressants, and adult neurogenesis.

9.8.2.2 Schizophrenia and adult neurogenesis

Schizophrenia is a chronic psychiatric illness that presents in late adolescence or early adulthood and is characterized by disorganized or abnormal thought including delusions and altered perception (hallucinations). Patients can also exhibit mood disturbances and social withdrawal or dysfunction. A number of studies, including twin studies, estimate a large genetic contribution (up to 80%) to schizophrenia (Hilker et al., 2018), with genome-wide studies implicating multiple genes active during neurodevelopment (Birnbaum and Weinberger, 2017). Impaired development resulting in abnormal structure and reduced size in a number of brain structures, including the hippocampus, have been observed in schizophrenia (Lawrie and Abukmeil, 1998; Nelson et al., 1998; Wright et al., 2000; Cachia et al., 2020). Consistent with this, decreased immunohistological markers of proliferation and NPCs have been observed in the SGZ of postmortem brains of patients with schizophrenia (Barbeau et al., 1995; Reif et al., 2006), whereas other studies show increased numbers of calretinin+ immature neurons (Walton et al., 2012). Whether abnormal neurogenesis independently contributes to impairment in the pathophysiology of schizophrenia or is simply a bystander that shares defective genetic programs with those mechanisms that actually drive pathology earlier in neural development, is not known.

To answer this and other questions, investigators have turned to rodent models. Among these is the rat neonatal ventral hippocampal lesion model that reproduces many of the hallmarks of schizophrenia including delayed onset during adolescence, abnormal dopaminergic signaling, and schizophrenic-like behaviors (Tseng et al., 2009; O'Donnell, 2012). However, given the strong inheritable component of the disease, genetic models have begun to play a larger role. Mice have been developed carrying mutations in a number of genes identified either from families with multiple individuals suffering from schizophrenia and other psychiatric disorders or population studies identifying genes that impart increased risk of developing schizophrenia. Among these is the Disrupted in Schizophrenia 1 (DISC1) gene, which was first identified as altered in members of a Scottish family with schizophrenia and bipolar disorder. DISC1 is expressed throughout the developing brain, but is largely constrained to the hippocampus during adulthood. Loss of DISC1 impairs nearly all aspects of development of adult-born neurons, from neural precursor proliferation, to migration, to dendritic outgrowth and excitability. This can likely be explained by the fact that DISC1 is a highly connected node at the intersection of several pathways that are critical for neural development including the GSK-3β/β-catenin, AKT/mTOR, and NDEL1/LIS1 pathways. Other commonly studied genes in schizophrenia include NPAS3, which was identified through genome-wide association studies. Mice with loss-of-function mutations in NPAS3 demonstrate impaired prepulse inhibition (PPI) of the startle response, hyperactivity, memory deficits, and anxiety-like behaviors. Analogous to findings in postmortem tissue from schizophrenic patients, loss of NPAS3 function leads to markedly reduced proliferation of Brdu + cells in the adult DG (Pieper et al., 2005). Finally, loss of a number of synaptic proteins implicated in schizophrenia impact adult neurogenesis in mice. These include the SNARE protein SNAP-25 and the neurexin family of synaptic cell-adhesion molecules (NRXNs). Knockout of these genes results in impaired maturation and decreased survival of adult-born DGCs, respectively. Collectively, the diversity of these genes and their function in adult neurogenesis and neuronal development highlight the complexity of the disease and its pathophysiology.

9.8.3 Neurodegenerative disorders

Alzheimer's disease (AD) is a rampant and progressive age-related dementia of unknown etiology characterized by synaptic and neuronal loss and brain atrophy. AD pathology demonstrates aggregation of amyloid beta (Aβ) plaques and neurofibrillary tangles (NFTs). As discussed in detail in Chapter 20, extracellular plaques are composed primarily of aggregated Aβ peptide, containing between 36 and 43 amino acids. Aβ and other peptide fragments are generated from the amyloid precursor protein (APP) through enzymatic cleavage by a number of proteases including α-, β-, and γ-secretase. Patients with inheritable or familial AD (FAD) carry mutations in genes that encode APP or one of the proteins within the secretase complexes, which favor Aβ formation. The other major component of AD pathology, NFTs, are found intracellularly and consist of hyperphosphorylated tau, a microtubule-associated protein. NFTs spread throughout the brain in a stereotypic fashion, first appearing in the entorhinal cortex, followed by CA1, and then in the other hippocampal subfields before there is extensive neocortical involvement (Braak and Braak, 1991). The triggers that induce formation of Aβ and pathological tau species and how this process leads to neuronal loss in AD are not fully understood. Moreover, deposits of aggregated Aβ and tau can be found in cognitively normal subjects (Lue et al., 1999; Riudavets et al., 2007; Iacono et al., 2008; Erten-Lyons et al., 2009; Kramer et al., 2011; Bjorklund et al., 2012) and multiple clinical trials testing treatments that substantially reduce the accumulation of Aβ and tau show no effect on the progression or symptoms of AD (Doody et al., 2014; Gauthier et al., 2016; Honig et al., 2018; Cummings et al., 2019). Thus, despite more than a century of investigation, the etiology of AD is currently unknown and there exist no disease modifying therapies for this devastating illness.

9.8.3.1 Adult neurogenesis is attenuated in Alzheimer's disease

Questions about the causative role of Aβ plaques and NFTs have motivated investigation of alternative risk factors for developing AD, including deficits in adult neurogenesis. Whether adult neurogenesis is present in the hippocampal DG of aged humans and could be affected in neurodegenerative diseases remains a matter of some debate (Kempermann et al., 2018; Sorrells et al., 2018; Snyder, 2019; section 9.7). Nonetheless, studies suggests that the severity and perhaps even the development of AD is related to the loss of adult neurogenesis (Mu and Gage, 2011; Choi et al., 2018; Choi and Tanzi, 2019; Moreno-Jiménez et al., 2019). Indeed, adult neurogenesis is markedly decreased in the postmortem brains of AD patients, even at Braak stage I before NFTs can be identified in the hippocampus (Moreno-Jiménez et al., 2019). In contrast, people without dementia demonstrate intact neurogenesis late into adulthood (Eriksson et al., 1998; Spalding et al., 2013; Boldrini et al., 2018; Moreno-Jiménez et al., 2019), including healthy subjects who are nondemented but exhibit AD neuropathology (NDAN) at autopsy (Briley et al., 2016). Consistent with this idea, memantine improves cognition in patients with AD and has been shown to

sharply enhance adult neurogenesis in animals (Akers et al., 2014). Whether newborn DGCs are sentinel neurons ("canaries in the coal mine") for degenerative changes in AD or whether there is a causal link between attenuation of neurogenesis and the development of AD is an open question.

Questions of causality can perhaps best be addressed in animal models of familial Alzheimer's disease (FAD) that contain one or more mutations in the genes encoding APP or the presenilin proteins. Attenuation of adult neurogenesis has been identified in a number of these transgenic mice (Zhang et al., 2007; Demars et al., 2010; Choi et al., 2018), but is not universal among murine models of FAD (Jin et al., 2004; López-Toledano and Shelanski, 2007; Gan et al., 2008; Kolecki et al., 2008; Mirochnic et al., 2009). Similar to humans with sporadic AD, some FAD mice demonstrate attenuated neurogenesis early in adulthood, prior to the onset of NFTs and perhaps Aβ pathology (Demars et al., 2010). Interestingly, Choi et al. showed that enhancing adult neurogenesis through exercise improves cognitive function in FAD mice, requiring both increased neurogenesis and BNDF expression in the adult hippocampus. Likewise, attenuating adult neurogenesis in FAD mice significantly impaired cognitive function compared with FAD mice with intact neurogenesis and wildtype control animals (Choi et al., 2018).

While the mechanism of impaired neurogenesis in AD is not known, there is growing evidence that APP and presenilins are expressed in NPCs and developing DGCs and participate in the regulation of neurogenesis in rodents (Jaworski et al., 2009; Gadadhar et al., 2011; Fuster-Matanzo et al., 2012; Demars et al., 2013; Bonds et al., 2015; Komuro et al., 2015; Joseph et al., 2017; Choi et al., 2018). For example, sAPPα, the intracellular product of the AAP protein cleaved by α-secretase, enhances proliferation of NPCs in the SGZ of the DG. In contrast, sAPPβ, the extracellular product of the competing β-secretase pathway implicated in AD pathology, exhibits an inhibitory effect on proliferating cells (Demars et al., 2013). In addition, knockdown of presenilin-1, part of the γ-secretase complex that processes APP, results in decreased proliferation of NPCs and increased differentiation of these cells into neurons and glia in the adult DG (Gadadhar et al., 2011). This presenilin-1 knockdown-induced impairment of neurogenesis is accompanied by behavioral deficits including impaired pattern separation and novel object recognition (Bonds et al., 2015). Collectively, these studies suggest that the attenuation of adult neurogenesis observed in AD may result from impairment of AAP processing.

In addition, numerous studies show that tau is also expressed in NPCs and developing neurons (Kosik et al., 1989; Sah et al., 1997; Tatebayashi et al., 1999; Hong et al., 2010; Llorens-Martin et al., 2012) and regulate neurogenesis during development and adulthood (Sennvik et al., 2007; Jaworski et al., 2009; Hong et al., 2010; Fuster-Matanzo et al., 2012; Komuro et al., 2015; Dioli et al., 2017; Joseph et al., 2017). Consistent with these observations, chromosomal abnormalities at 17q21.3, which contains the *mapt* gene encoding the tau protein, is associated with microcephaly (Kirchhoff et al., 2007; Adams et al., 2016). Tau transcripts undergo alternative splicing yielding at least six tau isoforms, with zero (0N), one (1N), or two (2) N-terminal exons and either three (3R) or four (4R) microtubule repeat binding domains. The 3R and 4R isomers express differently during development and adulthood. In mice, 3R tau is expressed predominantly during embryonic and early postnatal development. Whole brain western blot analysis demonstrates a dramatic decrease in 3R expression around postnatal day 24 (P24) in mice and is not detectable at P90 (McMillan et al., 2008). However, immunofluorescence shows significant expression throughout the cortex at P24, particularly in the outer layers where there is an abundance of axons. Notably, there is clear expression of 3R in the SGZ of the DG at P24 (McMillan et al., 2008). Expression of 4R tau is almost undetectable via whole brain western blot prior to approximately P3 and is first detected throughout cortex and hippocampus by immunofluorescence around P6 and continues into adulthood (Sennvik et al., 2007; McMillan et al., 2008).

Knockout of the *mapt* gene in mice results in enhanced neurogenesis in both the DG and subventricular zone at 14 months of age (Criado-Marrero et al., 2020). However, this effect was not observed in other studies using the same strain of transgenic mice at 6–7 months of age (Dioli et al., 2017). Sennvik et al. use a knockin/knockout (KI/KO) model, where endogenous mouse tau is knocked out and only the human tau4R/2N gene without introns (and thus no alternative splicing) is knocked in. Similar to mouse 4R/2N, the human 4R/2N tau begins expression around P12–P15 in mice (which is somewhat delayed compared with 4R/1N and total 4R, see above). Prior to this time point, tau expression is absent and results in increased neurogenesis in the DG and CA1 (born during embryonic day 14 (E14)–E17 to P2) and larger overall hippocampal size in these mice. The authors went on to show that loss of tau in these mice results in increased proliferation and delayed maturation of DGCs. In addition, expression of human tau with an antiaggregate mutation results in increased neurogenesis (proliferation) and a larger hippocampus with more neurons (Joseph et al., 2017). In contrast, expressing wild type human tau in a *mapt$^{-/-}$* knockout mouse results in expression of phosphorylated tau in DCX+ cells within the SGZ. In addition, these animals exhibited attenuated neurogenesis resulting from decreased proliferation as measured by BrdU. Finally, there is evidence that tau promotes survival of newborn DGCs in response to enrichment (Pallas-Bazarra et al., 2016) and mediates cell-death during stress (Pallas-Bazarra et al., 2016; Dioli et al., 2017). Collectively, these studies indicate that tau may play an important role in regulating adult-born neurons, providing another potential link between the empirical observations of altered adult neurogenesis and the pathophysiology of AD.

Fewer studies have been able to examine adult neurogenesis in the context of other neurodegenerative disorders, but a recent investigation shed light on variations in neurogenesis that accompany ALS, Huntington's disease, dementia with Lewy bodies, frontotemporal dementia, and Parkinson's disease (Terreros-Roncal et al., 2021). The authors detected commonalties within the DG neurogenic niche across several neurodegenerative diseases when compared with neurologically healthy controls. All diseases except dementia with Lewy bodies showed evidence of astrogliosis, and all except frontotemporal dementia showed evidence of reduced microglial phagocytic capacity. Dead, uncleared pyknotic cells were increased in all disease states. When examining histological markers of neurogenesis, the authors actually detected increased Type I cells, cellular proliferation, and numbers of immature neurons in ALS, Huntington's, and Parkinson's diseases, but these cells appeared to have altered morphological maturation. Together, these results suggest that changes in the neurogenic niche during neurodegenerative disease are associated with a reduced ability to clear dying or aberrantly connected cells, leaving behind immature cells that may not properly integrate into the DG circuit. The functional implications of these findings will require additional clarification.

Acknowledgements

We thank Sergei Rusakoff for his work on the graphic design and scientific illustrations, Jahfreen Alam for her help with collating the references, and Mary Lynn Gage for comments on the manuscript. This work was made possible by our funding sources: National Institutes of Health grants K08NS093130 and R01 MH114030, the McKnight Endowment Fund for Neuroscience, the Whitehall Foundation, the American Heart Association, and the Paul G. Allen Frontiers Group Grant #19PABHI34610000/TEAM LEADER: Fred H. Gage/2019, and the JPB Foundation.

REFERENCES

Aarum J, Sandberg K, Haeberlein SLB, Persson MAA (2003) Migration and differentiation of neural precursor cells can be directed by microglia. *Proceedings of the National Academy of Sciences* 100:15983–15988.

Aasebo IEJ, Kasture AS, Passeggeri M, Tashiro A (2018) A behavioral task with more opportunities for memory acquisition promotes the survival of new neurons in the adult dentate gyrus. *Scientific Reports* 8:7369.

Åberg MAI, Åberg ND, Hedbäcker H, Oscarsson J, Eriksson PS (2000) Peripheral infusion of IGF-I selectively induces neurogenesis in the adult rat hippocampus. *Journal of Neuroscience* 20:2896–2903.

Adams HH, Hibar DP, Chouraki V, Stein JL, Nyquist PA, Rentería ME, et al. (2016) Novel genetic loci underlying human intracranial volume identified through genome-wide association. *Nature Neuroscience* 19:1569–1582.

Adlaf EW, Vaden RJ, Niver AJ, Manuel AF, Onyilo VC, Araujo MT, Dieni CV, Vo HT, King GD, Wadiche JI, et al. (2017) Adult-born neurons modify excitatory synaptic transmission to existing neurons. *Elife* 30:6.

Aimone JB, Wiles J, Gage FH (2006) Potential role for adult neurogenesis in the encoding of time in new memories. *Nature Neuroscience* 9:723–727.

Aimone JB, Wiles J, Gage FH (2009) Computational influence of adult neurogenesis on memory encoding. *Neuron* 61:187–202.

Airan RD, Meltzer LA, Roy M, Gong Y, Chen H, Deisseroth K (2007) High-speed imaging reveals neurophysiological links to behavior in an animal model of depression. *Science* 317:819–823.

Aizawa K, Ageyama N, Yokoyama C, Hisatsune T (2009) Age-dependent alteration in hippocampal neurogenesis correlates with learning performance of Macaque monkeys. *Experimental Animals* 58:403–407.

Akers KG, Martinez-Canabal A, Restivo L, Yiu AP, de Cristofaro A, Hsiang H-L (Liz), Wheeler AL, Guskjolen A, Niibori Y, Shoji H, et al. (2014) Hippocampal neurogenesis regulates forgetting during adulthood and infancy. *Science* 344:598–602.

Al-Hussain S, Al-Ali S (1995) A golgi study of cell types in the dentate gyrus of the adult human brain. *Cellular and Molecular Neurobiology* 15:207–220.

Allen E (1912) The cessation of mitosis in the central nervous system of the albino rat. *Journal of Comparative Neurology* 19:547–568.

Altman J (1962) Are new neurons formed in the brains of adult mammals? *Science* 135:1127–1128

Altman J (1963) Autoradiographic investigation of cell proliferation in the brains of rats and cats. *Anatomical Record* 145:573–591.

Altman J, Das GD (1965) Autoradiographic and histological evidence of postnatal hippocampal neurogenesis in rats. *Journal of Comparative Neurology* 124:319–335.

Altman J, Das GD (1966) Autoradiographic and histological studies of postnatal neurogenesis: I. A longitudinal investigation of the kinetics, migration and transformation of cells incorporating tritiated thymidine in neonate rats, with special reference to postnatal neurogenesis in some brain regions. *Journal of Comparative Neurology* 126:337–389.

Alvarez DD, Giacomini D, Yang SM, Trinchero MF, Temprana SG, Buttner KA, Beltramone N, Schinder AF (2016) A disynaptic feedback network activated by experience promotes the integration of new granule cells. *Science* 354:459–465.

Ambrogini P, Cuppini R, Cuppini C, Ciaroni S, Cecchini T, Ferri P, Sartini S, del Grande P (2000) Spatial learning affects immature granule cell survival in adult rat dentate gyrus. *Neuroscience Letters* 286:21–24.

Ambrogini P, Orsini L, Mancini C, Ferri P, Ciaroni S, Cuppini R (2004) Learning may reduce neurogenesis in adult rat dentate gyrus. *Neuroscience Letters* 359:13–16.

Amrein I, Isler K, Lipp H-P (2011) Comparing adult hippocampal neurogenesis in mammalian species and orders: influence of chronological age and life history stage. *European Journal of Neuroscience* 34:978–987.

Anacker C, Cattaneo A, Luoni A, Musaelyan K, Zunszain PA, Milanesi E, Rybka J, Berry A, Cirulli F, Thuret S, et al. (2013) Glucocorticoid-related molecular signaling pathways regulating hippocampal neurogenesis. *Neuropsychopharmacology* 38:872–883.

Anacker C, Hen R (2017) Adult hippocampal neurogenesis and cognitive flexibility—linking memory and mood. *Nature Reviews Neuroscience* 18:335–346.

Anacker C, Luna VM, Stevens GS, Millette A, Shores R, Jimenez JC, Chen B, Hen R (2018) Hippocampal neurogenesis confers stress resilience by inhibiting the ventral dentate gyrus. *Nature* 559:98–102.

Anderson RW, Strowbridge BW (2014) Regulation of persistent activity in hippocampal mossy cells by inhibitory synaptic potentials. *Learning and Memory* 21:263–271.

Arnold SJ, Huang G-J, Cheung AFP, Era T, Nishikawa S-I, Bikoff EK, Molnár Z, Robertson EJ, Groszer M (2008) The T-box transcription factor Eomes/Tbr2 regulates neurogenesis in the cortical subventricular zone. *Genes and Development* 22:2479–2484.

Arruda-Carvalho M, Sakaguchi M, Akers KG, Josselyn SA, Frankland PW (2011) Posttraining ablation of adult-generated neurons degrades previously acquired memories. *Journal of Neuroscience* 31:15113–15127.

Artegiani B, Lyubimova A, Muraro M, van Es JH, van Oudenaarden A, Clevers H (2017) A single-cell RNA sequencing study reveals cellular and molecular dynamics of the hippocampal neurogenic niche. *Cell Reports* 21:3271–3284.

Austin JE, Buckmaster PS (2004) Recurrent excitation of granule cells with basal dendrites and low interneuron density and inhibitory postsynaptic current frequency in the dentate gyrus of macaque monkeys. *Journal of Comparative Neurology* 476:205–218.

Bachstetter AD, Morganti JM, Jernberg J, Schlunk A, Mitchell SH, Brewster KW, Hudson CE, Cole MJ, Harrison JK, Bickford PC, et al. (2011) Fractalkine and CX 3CR1 regulate hippocampal neurogenesis in adult and aged rats. *Neurobiology of Aging* 32:2030–2044.

Bai F, Bergeron M, Nelson DL (2003) Chronic AMPA receptor potentiator (LY451646) treatment increases cell proliferation in adult rat hippocampus. *Neuropharmacology* 44:1013–1021.

Banasr M, Soumier A, Hery M, Mocaër E, Daszuta A (2006) Agomelatine, a new antidepressant, induces regional changes in hippocampal neurogenesis. *Biological Psychiatry* 59:1087–1096.

Banerjee SB, Rajendran R, Dias BG, Ladiwala U, Tole S, Vaidya VA (2005) Recruitment of the Sonic hedgehog signalling cascade in electroconvulsive seizure-mediated regulation of adult rat hippocampal neurogenesis. *European Journal of Neuroscience* 22:1570–1580.

Bao H, Asrican B, Li W, Gu B, Wen Z, Lim SA, Haniff I, Ramakrishnan C, Deisseroth K, Philpot B, et al. (2017) Long-Range GABAergic inputs regulate neural stem cell quiescence and control adult hippocampal neurogenesis. *Cell Stem Cell* 21:604–617.

Barbeau D, Liang JJ, Robitalille Y, Quirion R, Srivastava LK (1995) Decreased expression of the embryonic form of the neural cell adhesion molecule in schizophrenic brains. *Proceedings of the National Academy of Sciences* 92:2785–2789.

Barkho BZ, Song H, Aimone JB, Smrt RD, Kuwabara T, Nakashima K, Gage FH, Zhao X (2006) Identification of astrocyte-expressed factors that modulate neural stem/progenitor cell differentiation. *Stem Cells and Development* 15:407–421.

Barnea A, Nottebohm F (1994) Seasonal recruitment of hippocampal neurons in adult free-ranging black-capped chickadees. *Proceedings of the National Academy of Sciences of the United States of America* 91:11217–11221.

Barnea A, Nottebohm F (1996) Recruitment and replacement of hippocampal neurons in young and adult chickadees: an addition to the theory of hippocampal learning. *Proceedings of the National Academy of Sciences of the United States of America* 93:714–718.

Bartoletti A, Medini P, Berardi N, Maffei L (2004) Environmental enrichment prevents effects of dark-rearing in the rat visual cortex. *Nature Neuroscience* 7:215–216.

Beckervordersandforth R, Ebert B, Schäffner I, Moss J, Fiebig C, Shin J, et al. (2017) Role of mitochondrial metabolism in the control of early lineage progression and aging phenotypes in adult hippocampal neurogenesis. *Neuron* 93:560–573.

Beckervordersandforth R, Zhang CL, Lie DC (2015) Transcription-factor-dependent control of adult hippocampal neurogenesis. *Cold Spring Harbor Perspectives in Biology* 7:1–21.

Bedrosian TA, Houtman J, Eguiguren JS, Ghassemzadeh S, Rund N, Novaresi NM, Hu L, Parylak SL, Denli AM, Randolph-Moore L, et al. (2021) Lamin B1 decline underlies age-related loss of adult hippocampal neurogenesis. *EMBO Journal* 1;40(3). https://www.embopress.org/doi/full/10.15252/embj.2020105819

Bekinschtein P, Kent BA, Oomen CA, Clemenson GD, Gage FH, Saksida LM, Bussey TJ (2014) Brain-derived neurotrophic factor interacts with adult-born immature cells in the dentate gyrus during consolidation of overlapping memories. *Hippocampus* 24:905–911.

ben Abdallah NM-B, Filipkowski RK, Pruschy M, Jaholkowski P, Winkler J, Kaczmarek L, Lipp H-P (2013) Impaired long-term memory retention: common denominator for acutely or genetically reduced hippocampal neurogenesis in adult mice. *Behavioural Brain Research* 252:275–286.

Bengzon J, Kokaia Z, Elmer E, Nanobashvili A, Kokaia M, Lindvall O (1997) Apoptosis and proliferation of dentate gyrus neurons after single and intermittent limbic seizures. *Proceedings of the National Academy of Sciences* 94:10432–10437.

Berdugo-Vega G, Arias-Gil G, Lopez-Fernandez A, Artegiani B, Wasielewska JM, Lee CC, Lippert MT, Kempermann G, Takagaki K, Calegari F (2020) Increasing neurogenesis refines hippocampal activity rejuvenating navigational learning strategies and contextual memory throughout life. *Nature Communications* 11:135.

Berg DA, Yoon K-J, Will B, Xiao AY, Kim N-S, Christian KM, Song H, Ming G (2015) Tbr2-expressing intermediate progenitor cells in the adult mouse hippocampus are unipotent neuronal precursors with limited amplification capacity under homeostasis. *Frontiers in Biology* 10:262–271.

Bergami M, Rimondini R, Santi S, Blum R, Gotz M, Canossa M (2008) Deletion of TrkB in adult progenitors alters newborn neuron integration into hippocampal circuits and increases anxiety-like behavior. *Proceedings of the National Academy of Sciences of the United States of America* **105**:15570–15575.

Bergmann O, Liebl J, Bernard S, Alkass K, Yeung MS, Steier P, Kutschera W, Johnson L, Landen M, Druid H, et al. (2012) The age of olfactory bulb neurons in humans. *Neuron* **74**:634–639.

Besnard A, Sahay A (2016) Adult hippocampal neurogenesis, fear generalization, and stress. *Neuropsychopharmacology* **41**:24–44.

Bessa JM, Ferreira D, Melo I, Marques F, Cerqueira JJ, Palha JA, Almeida OF, Sousa N (2009) The mood-improving actions of antidepressants do not depend on neurogenesis but are associated with neuronal remodeling. *Molecular Psychiatry* **14**:739, 764–773.

bin Imtiaz MK, Jaeger BN, Bottes S, Machado RAC, Vidmar M, Moore DL, Jessberger S (2021) Declining lamin B1 expression mediates age-dependent decreases of hippocampal stem cell activity. *Cell Stem Cell* **28**:967–977.

Birnbaum R, Weinberger DR (2017) Genetic insights into the neurodevelopmental origins of schizophrenia. *Nature Reviews Neuroscience* **18**:727–740.

Bjorklund NL, Reese LC, Sadagoparamanujam V-M, Ghirardi V, Woltjer RL, Taglialatela G (2012) Absence of amyloid β oligomers at the postsynapse and regulated synaptic Zn2+ in cognitively intact aged individuals with Alzheimer's disease neuropathology. *Molecular Neurodegeneration* **7**:23.

Bodnoff SR, Suranyi-Cadotte B, Aitken DH, Quirion R, Meaney MJ (1988) The effects of chronic antidepressant treatment in an animal model of anxiety. *Psychopharmacology* **95**(3):298–302.

Boekhoorn K, Joels M, Lucassen PJ (2006) Increased proliferation reflects glial and vascular-associated changes, but not neurogenesis in the presenile Alzheimer hippocampus. *Neurobiology of Disease* **24**:1–14.

Boldrini M, Fulmore CA, Tartt AN, Simeon LR, Pavlova I, Poposka V, Rosoklija GB, Stankov A, Arango V, Dwork AJ, et al. (2018) Human hippocampal neurogenesis persists throughout aging. *Cell Stem Cell* **22**:589–599.

Boldrini M, Hen R, Underwood MD, Rosoklija GB, Dwork AJ, Mann JJ, Arango V (2012) Hippocampal angiogenesis and progenitor cell proliferation are increased with antidepressant use in major depression. *Biological Psychiatry* **72**:562–571.

Boldrini M, Santiago AN, Hen R, Dwork AJ, Rosoklija GB, Tamir H, Arango V, John Mann J (2013) Hippocampal granule neuron number and dentate gyrus volume in antidepressant-treated and untreated major depression. *Neuropsychopharmacology* **38**:1068–1077.

Boldrini M, Underwood MD, Hen R, Rosoklija GB, Dwork AJ, John Mann J, Arango V (2009) Antidepressants increase neural progenitor cells in the human hippocampus. *Neuropsychopharmacology* **34**:2376–2389.

Bonaguidi MA, Wheeler MA, Shapiro JS, Stadel RP, Sun GJ, Ming GL, Song H (2011) In vivo clonal analysis reveals self-renewing and multipotent adult neural stem cell characteristics. *Cell* **145**:1142–1155.

Bonde S, Ekdahl CT, Lindvall O (2006) Long-term neuronal replacement in adult rat hippocampus after status epilepticus despite chronic inflammation. *European Journal of Neuroscience* **23**:965–974.

Bonds JA, Kuttner-Hirshler Y, Bartolotti N, Tobin MK, Pizzi M, Marr R, Lazarov O (2015) Presenilin-1 dependent neurogenesis regulates hippocampal learning and memory. *PLoS ONE* 22;**10**(6).

Bordiuk OL, Smith K, Morin PJ, Semënov MV (2014) Cell proliferation and neurogenesis in adult mouse brain. *PLoS ONE* **9**:1–17.

Bottes S, Jaeger BN, Pilz GA, Jorg DJ, Cole JD, Kruse M, Harris L, Korobeynyk VI, Mallona I, Helmchen F, Guillemot F, Simons BD, Jessberger S (2021) Long-term self-renewing stem cells in the adult mouse hippocampus identified by intravital imaging. *Nature Neuroscience* **24**:225–233.

Braak H, Braak E (1991) Neuropathological stageing of Alzheimer-related changes. *Acta Neuropathologica* **82**:239–259.

Brandt MD, Jessberger S, Steiner B, Kronenberg G, Reuter K, Bick-Sander A, Behrens W von der, Kempermann G (2003) Transient calretinin expression defines early postmitotic step of neuronal differentiation in adult hippocampal neurogenesis of mice. *Molecular and Cellular Neuroscience* **24**:603–613.

Briley D, Ghirardi V, Woltjer R, Renck A, Zolochevska O, Taglialatela G, Micci M-A (2016) Preserved neurogenesis in non-demented individuals with AD neuropathology. *Scientific Reports* **6**:27812.

Brooker SM, Bond AM, Peng C-Y, Kessler JA (2016) β1-integrin restricts astrocytic differentiation of adult hippocampal neural stem cells. *Glia* **64**:1235–1251.

Brooker SM, Gobeske KT, Chen J, Peng CY, Kessler JA (2017) Hippocampal bone morphogenetic protein signaling mediates behavioral effects of antidepressant treatment. *Molecular Psychiatry* **22**:910–919.

Brown JP, Couillard-Després S, Cooper-Kuhn CM, Winkler J, Aigner L, Kuhn HG (2003) Transient expression of doublecortin during adult neurogenesis. *Journal of Comparative Neurology* **467**:1–10.

Bryans WA (1959) Mitotic activity in the brain of the adult white rat. *Anatomical Record* **133**:65–71.

Buckmaster PS, Dudek FE (1999) In vivo intracellular analysis of granule cell axon reorganization in epileptic rats. *Journal of Neurophysiology* **81**:712–721.

Burd GD, Nottebohm F (1985) Ultrastructural characterization of synaptic terminals formed on newly generated neurons in a song control nucleus of the adult canary forebrain. *Journal of Comparative Neurology* **240**:143–152.

Burghardt NS, Park EH, Hen R, Fenton AA (2012) Adult-born hippocampal neurons promote cognitive flexibility in mice. *Hippocampus* **22**:1795–1808.

Cachia A, Cury C, Brunelin J, Plaze M, Delmaire C, Oppenheim C, Medjkane F, Thomas P, Jardri R (2020) Deviations in early hippocampus development contribute to visual hallucinations in schizophrenia. *Translational Psychiatry* **10**:102.

Cameron HA, Gould E (1994) Adult neurogenesis is regulated by adrenal steroids in the dentate gyrus. *Neuroscience* **61**:203–209.

Cameron HA, McEwen BS, Gould E (1995) Regulation of adult neurogenesis by excitatory input and NMDA receptor activation in the dentate gyrus. *Journal of Neuroscience* **15**:4687–4692.

Cameron HA, McKay RD (1999) Restoring production of hippocampal neurons in old age. *Nature Neuroscience* **2**:894–897.

Cameron HA, Tanapat P, Gould E (1997) Adrenal steroids and N-methyl-D-aspartate receptor activation regulate neurogenesis in the dentate gyrus of adult rats through a common pathway. *Neuroscience* **82**:349–354.

Cameron HA, Woolley CS, Gould E (1993) Adrenal steroid receptor immunoreactivity in cells born in the adult rat dentate gyrus. *Brain Research* **611**:342–346.

Cameron HA, Woolley CS, McEwen BS, Gould E (1993) Differentiation of newly born neurons and glia in the dentate gyrus of the adult rat. *Neuroscience* **56**:337–344.

Campbell S, Marriott M, Nahmias C, MacQueen GM (2004) Lower hippocampal volume in patients suffering from depression: a meta-analysis. *American Journal of Psychiatry* **161**:598–607.

Cao L, Jiao X, Zuzga DS, Liu Y, Fong DM, Young D, During MJ (2004) VEGF links hippocampal activity with neurogenesis, learning and memory. *Nature Genetics* **36**:827–835.;

Castellano JM, Mosher KI, Abbey RJ, McBride AA, James ML, Berdnik D, Shen JC, Zou B, Xie XS, Tingle M, et al. (2017) Human umbilical cord plasma proteins revitalize hippocampal function in aged mice. *Nature* 544:488–492.

Chen G, Rajkowska G, Du F, Seraji-Bozorgzad N, Manji HK (2002) Enhancement of hippocampal neurogenesis by lithium. *Journal of Neurochemistry* 75:1729–1734.

Choi KO, Lybrand ZR, Ito N, Brulet R, Tafacory F, Zhang L, Good L, Ure K, Kernie SG, Birnbaum SG, Scharfman HE, Eisch A, Hsieh J (2015) Aberrant hippocampal neurogenesis contributes to epilepsy and associated cognitive decline. *Nature Communications* 6(6606).

Choi SH, Bylykbashi E, Chatila ZK, Lee SW, Pulli B, Clemenson GD, et al. (2018) Combined adult neurogenesis and BDNF mimic exercise effects on cognition in an Alzheimer's mouse model. *Science* 7;361(6406).

Choi SH, Tanzi RE (2019) Is Alzheimer's disease a neurogenesis disorder? *Cell Stem Cell* 25:7–8.

Clelland CD, Choi M, Romberg C, Clemenson GD, Fragniere A, Tyers P, Jessberger S, Saksida LM, Barker RA, Gage FH, et al. (2009) A functional role for adult hippocampal neurogenesis in spatial pattern separation. *Science* 325:210–213.

Collins RC, Tearse RG, Lothman EW (1983) Functional anatomy of limbic seizures: focal discharges from medial entorhinal cortex in rat. *Brain Research* 280:25–40.

Cooper-Kuhn CM, Georg Kuhn H (2002) Is it all DNA repair? *Developmental Brain Research* 134:13–21.

Corenblum MJ, Ray S, Remley QW, Long M, Harder B, Zhang DD, Barnes CA, Madhavan L (2016) Reduced Nrf2 expression mediates the decline in neural stem cell function during a critical middle-age period. *Aging Cell* 15:725–736.

Corotto FS, Henegar JA, Maruniak JA (1993) Neurogenesis persists in the subependymal layer of the adult mouse brain. *Neuroscience Letters* 149:111–114.

Creer DJ, Romberg C, Saksida LM, van Praag H, Bussey TJ (2010) Running enhances spatial pattern separation in mice. *Proceedings of the National Academy of Sciences of the United States of America* 107:2367–2372.

Criado-Marrero M, Sabbagh JJ, Jones MR, Chaput D, Dickey CA, Blair LJ (2020) Hippocampal neurogenesis is enhanced in adult tau deficient mice. *Cells* 9:210.

Crowther AJ, Lim S-A, Asrican B, Albright BH, Wooten J, Yeh C-Y, Bao H, Cerri DH, Hu J, Ian Shih Y-Y, Asokan A, Song J (2018) An adeno-associated virus-based toolkit for preferential targeting and manipulating quiescent neural stem cells in the adult hippocampus. *Stem Cell Reports* 10:1146–1159.

Cummings J, Blennow K, Johnson K, Keeley M, Bateman RJ, Molinuevo JL, Touchon J, Aisen P, Vellas B (2019) Anti-tau trials for Alzheimer's disease: a report from the EU/US/CTAD task force. *Journal of Prevention of Alzheimer's Disease* 6:157–163.

Czeh B, Michaelis T, Watanabe T, Frahm J, de Biurrun G, van Kampen M, Bartolomucci A, Fuchs E (2001) Stress-induced changes in cerebral metabolites, hippocampal volume, and cell proliferation are prevented by antidepressant treatment with tianeptine. *Proceedings of the National Academy of Sciences of the United States of America* 98:12796–12801.

Danielson NB, Kaifosh P, Zaremba JD, Lovett-Barron M, Tsai J, Denny CA, Balough EM, Goldberg AR, Drew LJ, Hen R, et al. (2016) Distinct contribution of adult-born hippocampal granule cells to context encoding. *Neuron* 90:101–112.

David DJ, Samuels BA, Rainer Q, Wang J-W, Marsteller D, Mendez I, Drew M, Craig DA, Guiard BP, Guilloux J-P, et al. (2009) Neurogenesis-dependent and -independent effects of Fluoxetine in an animal model of anxiety/depression. *Neuron* 62:479–493.

DeCarolis NA, Mechanic M, Petrik D, Carlton A, Ables JL, Malhotra S, Bachoo R, Götz M, Lagace DC, Eisch AJ (2013) *In vivo* contribution of nestin- and GLAST-lineage cells to adult hippocampal neurogenesis. *Hippocampus* 23:708–719.

Dekeyne A, Mannoury la Cour C, Gobert A, Brocco M, Lejeune F, Serres F, Sharp T, Daszuta A, Soumier A, et al. (2008) S32006, a novel 5-HT2C receptor antagonist displaying broad-based antidepressant and anxiolytic properties in rodent models. *Psychopharmacology* 199:549–568.

de Lucia C, Rinchon A, Olmos-Alonso A, Riecken K, Fehse B, Boche D, Perry VH, Gomez-Nicola D (2016) Microglia regulate hippocampal neurogenesis during chronic neurodegeneration. *Brain, Behavior, and Immunity* 55:179–190.

Demars MP, Hollands C, Zhao KD (Tommy), Lazarov O (2013) Soluble amyloid precursor protein-α rescues age-linked decline in neural progenitor cell proliferation. *Neurobiology of Aging* 34:2431–2440.

Demars M, Hu Y-S, Gadadhar A, Lazarov O (2010) Impaired neurogenesis is an early event in the etiology of familial Alzheimer's disease in transgenic mice. *Journal of Neuroscience Research* 88:2103–2117.

Deng W, Saxe MD, Gallina IS, Gage FH (2009) Adult-born hippocampal dentate granule cells undergoing maturation modulate learning and memory in the brain. *Journal of Neuroscience* 29:13532–13542.

Dennis CV, Suh LS, Rodriguez ML, Kril JJ, Sutherland GT (2016) Human adult neurogenesis across the ages: an immunohistochemical study. *Neuropathology and Applied Neurobiology* 42:621–638.

Denny CA, Burghardt NS, Schachter DM, Hen R, Drew MR (2012) 4- to 6-week-old adult-born hippocampal neurons influence novelty-evoked exploration and contextual fear conditioning. *Hippocampus* 22:1188–1201.

Denny CA, Kheirbek MA, Alba EL, Tanaka KF, Brachman RA, Laughman KB, Tomm NK, Turi GF, Losonczy A, Hen R (2014) Hippocampal memory traces are differentially modulated by experience, time, and adult neurogenesis. *Neuron* 83:189–201.

Dieni CV, Nietz AK, Panichi R, Wadiche JI, Overstreet-Wadiche L (2013) Distinct determinants of sparse activation during granule cell maturation. *Journal of Neuroscience* 33:19131–19142.

Dieni CV, Panichi R, Aimone JB, Kuo CT, Wadiche JI, Overstreet-Wadiche L (2016) Low excitatory innervation balances high intrinsic excitability of immature dentate neurons. *Nature Communications* 7:11313.

Dioli C, Patrício P, Trindade R, Pinto LG, Silva JM, Morais M, Ferreiro E, Borges S, Mateus-Pinheiro A, Rodrigues AJ, et al. (2017) Tau-dependent suppression of adult neurogenesis in the stressed hippocampus. *Molecular Psychiatry* 22:1110–1118.

Dityatev A, Schachner M, Sonderegger P (2010) The dual role of the extracellular matrix in synaptic plasticity and homeostasis. *Nature Reviews Neuroscience* 11:735–746.

Doody RS, Thomas RG, Farlow M, Iwatsubo T, Vellas B, Joffe S, Kieburtz K, Raman R, Sun X, Aisen PS, et al. (2014) Phase 3 trials of Solanezumab for mild-to-moderate Alzheimer's disease. *New England Journal of Medicine* 370:311–321.

Drapeau E, Montaron M-F, Aguerre S, Abrous DN (2007) Learning-induced survival of new neurons depends on the cognitive status of aged rats. *Journal of Neuroscience* 27:6037–6044.

Drew LJ, Kheirbek MA, Luna VM, Denny CA, Cloidt MA, Wu MV, Jain S, Scharfman HE, Hen R (2016) Activation of local inhibitory circuits in the dentate gyrus by adult-born neurons. *Hippocampus* 26:763–778.

Dulken BW, Buckley MT, Navarro Negredo P, Saligrama N, Cayrol R, Leeman DS, George BM, Boutet SC, Hebestreit K, Pluvinage JV, et al. (2019) Single-cell analysis reveals T cell infiltration in old neurogenic niches. *Nature* **571**:205–210.

Dulken BW, Leeman DS, Boutet SC, Hebestreit K, Brunet A (2017) Single-cell transcriptomic analysis defines heterogeneity and transcriptional dynamics in the adult neural stem cell lineage. *Cell Reports* **18**:777–790.

Duman RS (1997) A molecular and cellular theory of depression. *Archives of General Psychiatry* **54**:597.

Dupret D, Fabre A, Döbrössy MD, Panatier A, Rodríguez JJ, Lamarque S, Lemaire V, Oliet SHR, Piazza P-V, Abrous DN (2007) Spatial learning depends on both the addition and removal of new hippocampal neurons. *PLoS Biology* **5**(8):1683–1694.

Duque A, Rakic P (2011) Different effects of Bromodeoxyuridine and [3H]Thymidine incorporation into DNA on cell proliferation, position, and fate. *Journal of Neuroscience* **31**:15205–15217.

Eckenhoff MF, Rakic P (1988) Nature and fate of proliferative cells in the hippocampal dentate gyrus during the life span of the rhesus monkey. *Journal of Neuroscience* **8**:2729–2747.

Encinas JM, Michurina T v, Peunova N, Park JH, Tordo J, Peterson DA, Fishell G, Koulakov A, Enikolopov G (2011) Division-coupled astrocytic differentiation and age-related depletion of neural stem cells in the adult hippocampus. *Cell Stem Cell* **8**:566–579.

Encinas JM, Vaahtokari A, Enikolopov G (2006) Fluoxetine targets early progenitor cells in the adult brain. *Proceedings of the National Academy of Sciences* **103**:8233–8238.

Enikolopov G, Overstreet-Wadiche L, Ge S (2015) Viral and transgenic reporters and genetic analysis of adult neurogenesis. *Cold Spring Harbor Perspectives in Biology* **7**(8).

Epp JR, Scott NA, Galea LAM (2011) Strain differences in neurogenesis and activation of new neurons in the dentate gyrus in response to spatial learning. *Neuroscience* **172**:342–354.

Epp JR, Silva Mera R, Kohler S, Josselyn SA, Frankland PW (2016) Neurogenesis-mediated forgetting minimizes proactive interference. *Nature Communications* **7**:10838.

Eriksson PS, Perfilieva E, Björk-Eriksson T, Alborn A-M, Nordborg C, Peterson DA, Gage FH (1998) Neurogenesis in the adult human hippocampus. *Nature Medicine* **4**:1313–1317.

Ernst A, Alkass K, Bernard S, Salehpour M, Perl S, Tisdale J, Possnert G, Druid H, Frisen J (2014) Neurogenesis in the striatum of the adult human brain. *Cell* **156**:1072–1083.

Erten-Lyons D, Woltjer RL, Dodge H, Nixon R, Vorobik R, Calvert JF, Leahy M, Montine T, Kaye J (2009) Factors associated with resistance to dementia despite high Alzheimer disease pathology. *Neurology* **72**:354–360.

Espósito MS, Piatti VC, Laplagne DA, Morgenstern NA, Ferrari CC, Pitossi FJ, Schinder AF (2005) Neuronal differentiation in the adult hippocampus recapitulates embryonic development. *Journal of Neuroscience: The Official Journal of the Society for Neuroscience* **25**:10074–10086.

Fabel K (2009) Additive effects of physical exercise and environmental enrichment on adult hippocampal neurogenesis in mice. *Frontiers in Neuroscience* **3**:50.

Fatemi SH (2001) Reelin mutations in mouse and man: from reeler mouse to schizophrenia, mood disorders, autism and lissencephaly. *Molecular Psychiatry* **6**:129–133.

Faulkner RL, Jang M-H, Liu X-B, Duan X, Sailor KA, Kim JY, Ge S, Jones EG, Ming G -l., Song H, Cheng H-J (2008) Development of hippocampal mossy fiber synaptic outputs by new neurons in the adult brain. *Proceedings of the National Academy of Sciences* **105**:14157–14162.

Fiala BA, Joyce JN, Greenough WT (1978) Environmental complexity modulates growth of granule cell dendrites in developing but not adult hippocampus of rats. *Experimental Neurology* **59**:372–383.

Filippov V, Kronenberg G, Pivneva T, Reuter K, Steiner B, Wang L-P, Yamaguchi M, Kettenmann H, Kempermann G (2003) Subpopulation of nestin-expressing progenitor cells in the adult murine hippocampus shows electrophysiological and morphological characteristics of astrocytes. *Molecular and Cellular Neuroscience* **23**:373–382.

Fitzsimons CP, van Hooijdonk LW, Schouten M, Zalachoras I, Brinks V, Zheng T, Schouten TG, Saaltink DJ, Dijkmans T, Steindler DA, et al. (2013) Knockdown of the glucocorticoid receptor alters functional integration of newborn neurons in the adult hippocampus and impairs fear-motivated behavior. *Molecular Psychiatry* **18**:993–100.

Flor-Garcia M, Terreros-Roncal J, Moreno-Jimenez EP, Avila J, Rabano A, Llorens-Martin M (2020) Unraveling human adult hippocampal neurogenesis. *Nature Protocols* **15**:668–69.

Foley KA, Ossenkopp KP, Kavaliers M, Macfabe DF (2014) Pre- and neonatal exposure to lipopolysaccharide or the enteric metabolite, propionic acid, alters development and behavior in adolescent rats in a sexually dimorphic manner. *PLoS ONE* **9**(1).

Franjic D, Skarica M, Ma S, Arellano JI, Tebbenkamp AT, Choi J, et al. (2022) Transcriptomic taxonomy and neurogenic trajectories of adult human, macaque, and pig hippocampal and entorhinal cells. *Neuron* **110**:452–469.

Frantz C, Stewart KM, Weaver VM (2010) The extracellular matrix at a glance. *Journal of Cell Science* **123**:4195–4200.

Fuchs E, Chen T (2013) A matter of life and death: self-renewal in stem cells. *EMBO Reports* **14**:39–48.

Fukuda S, Kato F, Tozuka Y, Yamaguchi M, Miyamoto Y, Hisatsune T (2003) Two distinct subpopulations of nestin-positive cells in adult mouse dentate gyrus. *Journal of Neuroscience* **23**:9357–9366.

Fuster-Matanzo A, Llorens-Martín M, Jurado-Arjona J, Avila J, Hernández F (2012) Tau protein and adult hippocampal neurogenesis. *Frontiers in Neuroscience* **6**:104.

Gadadhar A, Marr R, Lazarov O (2011) Presenilin-1 regulates neural progenitor cell differentiation in the adult brain. *Journal of Neuroscience* **31**:2615–2623.

Gall CM (1993) Seizure-induced changes in neurotrophin expression: implications for epilepsy. *Experimental Neurology* **124**:150–166.

Gan L, Qiao S, Lan X, Chi L, Luo C, Lien L, Yan Liu Q, Liu R (2008) Neurogenic responses to amyloid-beta plaques in the brain of Alzheimer's disease-like transgenic (pPDGF-APPSw,Ind) mice. *Neurobiology of Disease* **29**:71–80.

Gao A, Xia F, Guskjolen AJ, Ramsaran AI, Santoro A, Josselyn SA, Frankland PW (2018) Elevation of hippocampal neurogenesis induces a temporally graded pattern of forgetting of contextual fear memories. *Journal of Neuroscience* **38**:3190–3198.

Gao Z, Ure K, Ables JL, Lagace DC, Nave K-A, Goebbels S, Eisch AJ, Hsieh J (2009) Neurod1 is essential for the survival and maturation of adult-born neurons. *Nature Neuroscience* **12**:1090–1092.

Garcia A, Steiner B, Kronenberg G, Bick-Sander A, Kempermann G (2004) Age-dependent expression of glucocorticoid- and mineralocorticoid receptors on neural precursor cell populations in the adult murine hippocampus. *Aging Cell* **3**:363–371.

Garthe A, Behr J, Kempermann G (2009) Adult-generated hippocampal neurons allow the flexible use of spatially precise learning strategies. *PLoS ONE* **4**:e5464.

Gauthier S, Feldman HH, Schneider LS, Wilcock GK, Frisoni GB, Hardlund JH, Moebius HJ, Bentham P, Kook KA, Wischik DJ, et al. (2016) Efficacy and safety of tau-aggregation inhibitor therapy in patients with mild or moderate Alzheimer's disease: a randomised, controlled, double-blind, parallel-arm, phase 3 trial. *Lancet* 388:2873–2884.

Ge S, Goh EL, Sailor KA, Kitabatake Y, Ming GL, Song H (2006) GABA regulates synaptic integration of newly generated neurons in the adult brain. *Nature* 439:589–593.

Ge S, Yang CH, Hsu KS, Ming GL, Song H (2007) A critical period for enhanced synaptic plasticity in newly generated neurons of the adult brain. *Neuron* 54:559–566.

Gebara E, Bonaguidi MA, Beckervordersandforth R, Sultan S, Udry F, Gijs PJ, Lie DC, Ming GL, Song H, Toni N (2016) Heterogeneity of radial glia-like cells in the adult hippocampus. *Stem Cells* 34:997–1010.

Gemma C, Bachstetter AD (2013) The role of microglia in adult hippocampal neurogenesis. *Frontiers in Cellular Neuroscience* 7:1–5.

Goldman SA, Nottebohm F (1983) Neuronal production, migration, and differentiation in a vocal control nucleus of the adult female canary brain. *Proceedings of the National Academy of Sciences of the United States of America* 80:2390–2394.

Gonçalves JT, Bloyd CW, Shtrahman M, Johnston ST, Schafer ST, Parylak SL, Tran T, Chang T, Gage FH (2016) In vivo imaging of dendritic pruning in dentate granule cells. *Nature Neuroscience* 19:788–791.

Gonçalves JT, Schafer ST, Gage FH (2016) Adult neurogenesis in the hippocampus: from stem cells to behavior. *Cell* 167:897–914.

Gong C, Wang T-W, Huang HS, Parent JM (2007) Reelin regulates neuronal progenitor migration in intact and epileptic hippocampus. *Journal of Neuroscience* 27:1803–1811.

Goshen I, Kreisel T, Ben-Menachem-Zidon O, Licht T, Weidenfeld J, Ben-Hur T, Yirmiya R (2008) Brain interleukin-1 mediates chronic stress-induced depression in mice via adrenocortical activation and hippocampal neurogenesis suppression. *Molecular Psychiatry* 13:717–728.

Gould E (1999) Serotonin and hippocampal neurogenesis. *Neuropsychopharmacology* 21:46S–51S.

Gould E, Cameron HA, Daniels DC, Woolley CS, McEwen BS (1992) Adrenal hormones suppress cell division in the adult rat dentate gyrus. *Journal of Neuroscience* 12:3642–3650.

Gould E, McEwen BS, Tanapat P, Galea LA, Fuchs E (1997) Neurogenesis in the dentate gyrus of the adult tree shrew is regulated by psychosocial stress and NMDA receptor activation. *Journal of Neuroscience* 17:2492–2498.

Gould E, Reeves AJ, Fallah M, Tanapat P, Gross CG, Fuchs E (1999) Hippocampal neurogenesis in adult Old World primates. *Proceedings of the National Academy of Sciences of the United States of America* 96:5263–5267.

Gould E, Tanapat P, McEwen BS, Flugge G, Fuchs E (1998) Proliferation of granule cell precursors in the dentate gyrus of adult monkeys is diminished by stress. *Proceedings of the National Academy of Sciences of the United States of America* 95:3168–3171.

Gratzner HG (1982) Monoclonal antibody to 5-bromo- and 5-iododeoxyuridine: A new reagent for detection of DNA replication. *Science* 218:474–475.

Gray WP, Sundstrom LE (1998) Kainic acid increases the proliferation of granule cell progenitors in the dentate gyrus of the adult rat. *Brain Research* 790:52–59.

Groisman AI, Yang SM, Schinder AF (2020) Differential coupling of adult-born granule cells to parvalbumin and somatostatin interneurons. *Cell Reports* 30:202–214.

Gu Y, Arruda-Carvalho M, Wang J, Janoschka SR, Josselyn SA, Frankland PW, Ge S (2012) Optical controlling reveals time-dependent roles for adult-born dentate granule cells. *Nature Neuroscience* 15:1700–1706.

Hamilton A (1901) The division of differentiated cells in the central nervous system of the white rat. *Journal of Comparative Neurology* 11:297–320.

Hamilton GF, Majdak P, Miller DS, Bucko PJ, Merritt JR, Krebs CP, Rhodes JS (2015) Evaluation of a C57BL/6J x 129S1/SvImJ hybrid nestin-thymidine kinase transgenic mouse model for studying the functional significance of exercise-induced adult hippocampal neurogenesis. *Brain Plasticity* 1:83–95.

Han YG, Spassky N, Romaguera-Ros M, Garcia-Verdugo JM, Aguilar A, Schneider-Maunoury S, Alvarez-Buylla A (2008) Hedgehog signaling and primary cilia are required for the formation of adult neural stem cells. *Nature Neuroscience* 11:277–284.

Harris L, Rigo P, Stiehl T, Gaber ZB, Austin SHL, Masdeu MDM, Edwards A, Urban N, Marciniak-Czochra A, Guillemot F (2021) Coordinated changes in cellular behavior ensure the lifelong maintenance of the hippocampal stem cell population. *Cell Stem Cell* 28:863–876.

Hastings NB, Gould E (1999) Rapid extension of axons into the CA3 region by adult-generated granule cells. *Journal of Comparative Neurology* 413:146–154.

Hattiangady B, Rao M, Shetty A (2004) Chronic temporal lobe epilepsy is associated with severely declined dentate neurogenesis in the adult hippocampus. *Neurobiology of Disease* 17:473–490.

Heigele S, Sultan S, Toni N, Bischofberger J (2016) Bidirectional GABAergic control of action potential firing in newborn hippocampal granule cells. *Nature Neuroscience* 19:263–270.

Heinemann U, Beck H, Dreier JP, Ficker E, Stabel J, Zhang CL (1992) The dentate gyrus as a regulated gate for the propagation of epileptiform activity. *Epilepsy Research Supplement* 7:273–280.

Hermann A, Maisel M, Liebau S, Gerlach M, Kleger A, Schwarz J, Kim KS, Antoniadis G, Lerche H, Storch A (2006) Mesodermal cell types induce neurogenesis from adult human hippocampal progenitor cells. *Journal of Neurochemistry* 98:629–640.

Hernández-Rabaza V, Llorens-Martín M, Velázquez-Sánchez C, Ferragud A, Arcusa A, Gumus HG, Gómez-Pinedo U, Pérez-Villalba A, Roselló J, Trejo JL, et al. (2009) Inhibition of adult hippocampal neurogenesis disrupts contextual learning but spares spatial working memory, long-term conditional rule retention and spatial reversal. *Neuroscience* 159:59–68.

Hevner RF (2016) Evolution of the mammalian dentate gyrus. *Journal of Comparative Neurology* 524:578–594.

Hilker R, Helenius D, Fagerlund B, Skytthe A, Christensen K, Werge TM, Nordentoft M, Glenthøj B (2018) Heritability of schizophrenia and schizophrenia spectrum based on the nationwide Danish twin register. *Biological Psychiatry* 83:492–498.

Hill AS, Sahay A, Hen R (2015) Increasing adult hippocampal neurogenesis is sufficient to reduce anxiety and depression-like behaviors. *Neuropsychopharmacology* 40:2368–2378.

Hirasawa T, Wada H, Kohsaka S, Uchino S (2003) Inhibition of NMDA receptors induces delayed neuronal maturation and sustained proliferation of progenitor cells during neocortical development. *Journal of Neuroscience Research* 74:676–687.

His W (1904) Die Entwickelung des menschlichen Gehirns. Leipzig: Hirzel.

Hochgerner H, Zeisel A, Lonnerberg P, Linnarsson S (2018) Conserved properties of dentate gyrus neurogenesis across postnatal development revealed by single-cell RNA sequencing. *Nature Neuroscience* 21:290–299.

Hodge RD, Hevner RF (2011) Expression and actions of transcription factors in adult hippocampal neurogenesis. *Developmental Neurobiology* 71:680–689.

Hodge RD, Kowalczyk TD, Wolf SA, Encinas JM, Rippey C, Enikolopov G, Kempermann G, Hevner RF (2008) Intermediate progenitors in adult hippocampal neurogenesis: Tbr2 expression and coordinate regulation of neuronal output. *Journal of Neuroscience* 28:3707–3717.

Holick KA, Lee DC, Hen R, Dulawa SC (2008) Behavioral effects of chronic fluoxetine in BALB/cJ mice do not require adult hippocampal neurogenesis or the serotonin 1A receptor. *Neuropsychopharmacology* 33:406–417.

Hollands C, Tobin MK, Hsu M, Musaraca K, Yu T-S, Mishra R, Kernie SG, Lazarov O (2017) Depletion of adult neurogenesis exacerbates cognitive deficits in Alzheimer's disease by compromising hippocampal inhibition. *Molecular Neurodegeneration* 12:64.

Hong XP, Peng CX, Wei W, Tian Q, Liu YH, Yao XQ, Zhang Y, Cao FY, Wang Q, Wang JZ (2010) Essential role of tau phosphorylation in adult hippocampal neurogenesis. *Hippocampus* 20:1339–1349.

Honig LS, Vellas B, Woodward M, Boada M, Bullock R, Borrie M, et al. (2018) Trial of Solanezumab for mild dementia due to Alzheimer's disease. *New England Journal of Medicine* 378:321–330.

Horowitz AM, Fan X, Bieri G, Smith LK, Sanchez-Diaz CI, Schroer AB, Gontier G, Casaletto KB, Kramer JH, Williams KE, et al. (2020) Blood factors transfer beneficial effects of exercise on neurogenesis and cognition to the aged brain. *Science* 369:167–173.

Hosford BE, Liska JP, Danzer SC (2016) Ablation of newly generated hippocampal granule cells has disease-modifying effects in epilepsy. *Journal of Neuroscience* 36:11013–11023.

Houser C, Miyashiro J, Swartz B, Walsh G, Rich J, Delgado-Escueta A (1990) Altered patterns of dynorphin immunoreactivity suggest mossy fiber reorganization in human hippocampal epilepsy. *Journal of Neuroscience* 10:267–282.

Hsieh J, Zhao X (2016) Genetics and epigenetics in adult neurogenesis. *Cold Spring Harbor Perspectives in Biology* 8(6).

Huckleberry KA, Shue F, Copeland T, Chitwood RA, Yin W, Drew MR (2018) Dorsal and ventral hippocampal adult-born neurons contribute to context fear memory. *Neuropsychopharmacology* 43:2487–2496.

Hunt RF, Haselhorst LA, Schoch KM, Bach EC, Rios-Pilier J, Scheff SW, Saatman KE, Smith BN (2012) Posttraumatic mossy fiber sprouting is related to the degree of cortical damage in three mouse strains. *Epilepsy Research* 99:167–170.

Huttmann K, Sadgrove M, Wallraff A, Hinterkeuser S, Kirchhoff F, Steinhauser C, Gray WP (2003) Seizures preferentially stimulate proliferation of radial glia-like astrocytes in the adult dentate gyrus: functional and immunocytochemical analysis. *European Journal of Neuroscience* 18:2769–2778.

Iacono D, O'Brien R, Resnick SM, Zonderman AB, Pletnikova O, Rudow G, An Y, West MJ, Crain B, Troncoso JC (2008) Neuronal hypertrophy in asymptomatic Alzheimer disease. *Journal of Neuropathology and Experimental Neurology* 67:578–589.

Ibrayeva A, Bay M, Pu E, Jorg DJ, Peng L, Jun H, Zhang N, Aaron D, Lin C, Resler G, et al. (2021) Early stem cell aging in the mature brain. *Cell Stem Cell* 28:955–966.

Ikrar T, Guo N, He K, Besnard A, Levinson S, Hill A, Lee HK, Hen R, Xu X, Sahay A (2013) Adult neurogenesis modifies excitability of the dentate gyrus. *Frontiers in Neural Circuits* 7:204.

Imayoshi I, Sakamoto M, Kageyama R (2011) Genetic methods to identify and manipulate newly born neurons in the adult brain. *Frontiers in Neuroscience* 5:64.

Imayoshi I, Sakamoto M, Ohtsuka T, Takao K, Miyakawa T, Yamaguchi M, Mori K, Ikeda T, Itohara S, Kageyama R (2008) Roles of continuous neurogenesis in the structural and functional integrity of the adult forebrain. *Nature Neuroscience* 11:1153–1161.

Isackson PJ, Huntsman MM, Murray KD, Gall CM (1991) BDNF mRNA expression is increased in adult rat forebrain after limbic seizures: temporal patterns of induction distinct from NGF. *Neuron* 6:937–948.

Ishikawa R, Fukushima H, Frankland PW, Kida S (2016) Hippocampal neurogenesis enhancers promote forgetting of remote fear memory after hippocampal reactivation by retrieval. *Elife* 26:5.

Ishikawa R, Uchida C, Kitaoka S, Furuyashiki T, Kida S (2019) Improvement of PTSD-like behavior by the forgetting effect of hippocampal neurogenesis enhancer memantine in a social defeat stress paradigm. *Molecular Brain* 12:68.

Iyengar SS, LaFrancois JJ, Friedman D, Drew LJ, Denny CA, Burghardt NS, Wu MV, Hsieh J, Hen R, Scharfman HE (2015) Suppression of adult neurogenesis increases the acute effects of kainic acid. *Experimental Neurology* 264:135–149.

Jaako-Movits K, Zharkovsky T, Pedersen M, Zharkovsky A (2006) Decreased hippocampal neurogenesis following olfactory bulbectomy is reversed by repeated citalopram administration. *Cellular and Molecular Neurobiology* 26:1557–1568.

Jacobs BL, van Praag H, Gage FH (2000) Adult brain neurogenesis and psychiatry: a novel theory of depression. *Molecular Psychiatry* 5:262–269.

Jang MH, Bonaguidi MA, Kitabatake Y, Sun J, Song J, Kang E, Jun H, Zhong C, Su Y, Guo JU, et al. (2013) Secreted frizzled-related protein 3 regulates activity-dependent adult hippocampal neurogenesis. *Cell Stem Cell* 12:215–223.

Jaworski T, Dewachter I, Lechat B, Croes S, Termont A, Demedts D, Borghgraef P, Devijver H, Filipkowski RK, Kaczmarek L, et al. (2009) AAV-tau mediates pyramidal neurodegeneration by cell-cycle re-entry without neurofibrillary tangle formation in wild-type mice. *PLoS ONE* 4(10).

Jayatissa MN, Bisgaard C, Tingström A, Papp M, Wiborg O (2006) Hippocampal cytogenesis correlates to escitalopram-mediated recovery in a chronic mild stress rat model of depression. *Neuropsychopharmacology* 31:2395–2404.

Jessberger S, Kempermann G (2003) Adult-born hippocampal neurons mature into activity-dependent responsiveness. *European Journal of Neuroscience* 18:2707–2712.

Jessberger S, Parent JM (2015) Epilepsy and adult neurogenesis. *Cold Spring Harbor Perspectives in Biology* 7(12).

Jessberger S, Römer B, Babu H, Kempermann G (2005) Seizures induce proliferation and dispersion of doublecortin-positive hippocampal progenitor cells. *Experimental Neurology* 196:342–351.

Jessberger S, Zhao C, Toni N, Clemenson GD, Li Y, Gage FH (2007) Seizure-associated, aberrant neurogenesis in adult rats characterized with retrovirus-mediated cell labeling. *Journal of Neuroscience* 27:9400–9407.

Jhaveri DJ, O'Keeffe I, Robinson GJ, Zhao QY, Zhang ZH, Nink V, Narayanan RK, Osborne GW, Wray NR, Bartlett PF (2015) Purification of neural precursor cells reveals the presence of distinct, stimulus-specific subpopulations of quiescent precursors in the adult mouse hippocampus. *Journal of Neuroscience* 35:8132–8144.

Jiang Y, Gavrilovici C, Chansard M, Liu RH, Kiroski I, Parsons K, Park SK, Teskey GC, Rho JM, Nguyen MD (2016) Ndel1 and Reelin maintain postnatal CA1 hippocampus integrity. *Journal of Neuroscience* 36:6538–6552.

Jimenez JC, Su K, Goldberg AR, Luna VM, Biane JS, Ordek G, Zhou P, Ong SK, Wright MA, Zweifel L, et al. (2018) Anxiety cells in a hippocampal-hypothalamic circuit. *Neuron* 97:670–683.

Jin K, Peel AL, Mao XO, Xie L, Cottrell BA, Henshall DC, Greenberg DA (2004) Increased hippocampal neurogenesis in Alzheimer's disease. *Proceedings of the National Academy of Sciences* 101:343–347.

Jin K, Xie L, Mao XO, Greenberg DA (2006) Alzheimer's disease drugs promote neurogenesis. *Brain Research* 1085(1):183–188.

Jin K, Zhu Y, Sun Y, Mao XO, Xie L, Greenberg DA (2002) Vascular endothelial growth factor (VEGF) stimulates neurogenesis in vitro and in vivo. *Proceedings of the National Academy of Sciences* **99**:11946–11950.

Johansson CB, Svensson M, Wallstedt L, Janson AM, Frisen J (1999) Neural stem cells in the adult human brain. *Experimental Cell Research* **253**:733–736.

Johnson JD, Campisi J, Sharkey CM, Kennedy SL, Nickerson M, Greenwood BN, Fleshner M (2005) Catecholamines mediate stress-induced increases in peripheral and central inflammatory cytokines. *Neuroscience* **135**:1295–1307.

Johnston S, Parylak SL, Kim S, Mac N, Lim C, Gallina I, Bloyd C, Newberry A, Saavedra CD, Novak O, et al. (2021) AAV ablates neurogenesis in the adult murine hippocampus. *eLife* **14**:10.

Joseph M, Anglada-Huguet M, Paesler K, Mandelkow E, Mandelkow E-M (2017) Anti-aggregant tau mutant promotes neurogenesis. *Molecular Neurodegeneration* **12**:88.

Jung KH, Chu K, Kim M, Jeong S-W, Song Y-M, Lee S-T, Kim J-Y, Lee SK, Roh J-K, Eur JN (2004) Continuous cytosine-b-D-arabinofuranoside infusion reduces ectopic granule cells in adult rat hippocampus with attenuation of spontaneous recurrent seizures following pilocarpine-induced status epilepticus. *European Journal of Neuroscience* **19**:3219–3226.

Kao GD, McKenna WG, Yen TJ (2001) Detection of repair activity during the DNA damage-induced G2 delay in human cancer cells. *Oncogene* **20**:3486–3496.

Kaplan MS (1983) Proliferation of subependymal cells in the adult primate CNS: differential uptake of DNA labelled precursors. *J Hirnforsch* **24**:23–33.

Kaplan MS (1985) Formation and turnover of neurons in young and senescent animals: an electronmicroscopic and morphometric analysis. *Annals of the New York Academy of Sciences* **457**:173–192.

Kaplan MS, Bell DH (1984) Mitotic neuroblasts in the 9-day-old and 11-month-old rodent hippocampus. *Journal of Neuroscience* **4**:1429–1441.

Kaplan MS, Hinds JW (1977) Neurogenesis in the adult rat: electron microscopic analysis of light radioautographs. *Science* **197**:1092–1094.

Katsimpardi L, Litterman NK, Schein PA, Miller CM, Loffredo FS, Wojtkiewicz GR, Chen JW, Lee RT, Wagers AJ, Rubin LL (2014) Vascular and neurogenic rejuvenation of the aging mouse brain by young systemic factors. *Science* **344**:630–634.

Kee N, Teixeira CM, Wang AH, Frankland PW (2007) Preferential incorporation of adult-generated granule cells into spatial memory networks in the dentate gyrus. *Nature Neuroscience* **10**:355–362.

Kempermann G, Brandon EP, Gage FH (1998) Environmental stimulation of 129/SvJ mice causes increased cell proliferation and neurogenesis in the adult dentate gyrus. *Current Biology* **8**:939–942.

Kempermann G, Chesler EJ, Lu L, Williams RW, Gage FH (2006) Natural variation and genetic covariance in adult hippocampal neurogenesis. *Proceedings of the National Academy of Sciences of the United States of America* **103**:780–785.

Kempermann G, Gage FH, Aigner L, Song H, Curtis MA, Thuret S, Kuhn HG, Jessberger S, Frankland PW, Cameron HA, et al. (2018) Human adult neurogenesis: evidence and remaining questions. *Cell Stem Cell* **23**:25–30.

Kempermann G, Gast D, Gage FH (2002) Neuroplasticity in old age: sustained fivefold induction of hippocampal neurogenesis by long-term environmental enrichment. *Annals of Neurology* **52**:135–143.

Kempermann G, Jessberger S, Steiner B, Kronenberg G (2004) Milestones of neuronal development in the adult hippocampus. *Trends in Neurosciences* **27**:447–452.

Kempermann G, Kronenberg G (2003) Depressed new neurons?—Adult hippocampal neurogenesis and a cellular plasticity hypothesis of major depression. *Biological Psychiatry* **54**:499–503.

Kempermann G, Kuhn HG, Gage FH (1997a) Genetic influence on neurogenesis in the dentate gyrus of adult mice. *Proceedings of the National Academy of Sciences of the United States of America* **94**:10409–10414.

Kempermann G, Kuhn HG, Gage FH (1997b) More hippocampal neurons in adult mice living in an enriched environment. *Nature* **386**:493–495.

Kempermann G, Kuhn HG, Gage FH (1998) Experience-induced neurogenesis in the senescent dentate gyrus. *Journal of Neuroscience* **18**:3206–3212.

Kempermann MG (2012) Adult Neurogenesis 2. Oxford University Press.

Kheirbek MA, Drew LJ, Burghardt NS, Costantini DO, Tannenholz L, Ahmari SE, Zeng H, Fenton AA, Henl R (2013) Differential control of learning and anxiety along the dorsoventral axis of the dentate gyrus. *Neuron* **77**:955–968.

Kim J-E, O'Sullivan ML, Sanchez CA, Hwang M, Israel MA, Brennand K, Deerinck TJ, Goldstein LSB, Gage FH, Ellisman MH, et al. (2011) Investigating synapse formation and function using human pluripotent stem cell-derived neurons. *Proceedings of the National Academy of Sciences* **108**:3005–3010.

Kirby ED, Kuwahara AA, Messer RL, Wyss-Coray T (2015) Adult hippocampal neural stem and progenitor cells regulate the neurogenic niche by secreting VEGF. *Proceedings of the National Academy of Sciences* **112**:4128–4133.

Kirchhoff M, Bisgaard A-M, Duno M, Hansen FJ, Schwartz M (2007) A 17q21.31 microduplication, reciprocal to the newly described 17q21.31 microdeletion, in a girl with severe psychomotor developmental delay and dysmorphic craniofacial features. *European Journal of Medical Genetics* **50**:256–263.

Kirschen GW, Shen J, Tian M, Schroeder B, Wang J, Man G, Wu S, Ge S (2017) Active dentate granule cells encode experience to promote the addition of adult-born hippocampal neurons. *Journal of Neuroscience* **37**:4661–4678.

Kishi T, Matsunaga S, Iwata N (2017) A meta-analysis of memantine for depression. *Journal of Alzheimer's Disease* **57**:113–121.

Kitamura T, Mishina M, Sugiyama H (2003) Enhancement of neurogenesis by running wheel exercises is suppressed in mice lacking NMDA receptor epsilon 1 subunit. *Neuroscience Research* **47**:55–63.

Kitamura T, Saitoh Y, Takashima N, Murayama A, Niibori Y, Ageta H, Sekiguchi M, Sugiyama H, Inokuchi K (2009) Adult neurogenesis modulates the hippocampus-dependent period of associative fear memory. *Cell* **139**:814–827.

Knoth R, Singec I, Ditter M, Pantazis G, Capetian P, Meyer RP, Horvat V, Volk B, Kempermann G (2010) Murine features of neurogenesis in the human hippocampus across the lifespan from 0 to 100 years. *PLoS ONE* **5**(1).

Kobilo T, Liu QR, Gandhi K, Mughal M, Shaham Y, van Praag H (2011) Running is the neurogenic and neurotrophic stimulus in environmental enrichment. *Learning and Memory* **18**:605–609.

Kodali M, Megahed T, Mishra V, Shuai B, Hattiangady B, Shetty AK (2016) Voluntary running exercise-mediated enhanced neurogenesis does not obliterate retrograde spatial memory. *Journal of Neuroscience* **36**:8112–8122.

Koelliker A (1896) Handbuch der Gewebelehre des Menschen. Leipzig: Engelmann.

Kohler SJ, Williams NI, Stanton GB, Cameron JL, Greenough WT (2011) Maturation time of new granule cells in the dentate gyrus of adult macaque monkeys exceeds six months. *Proceedings of*

Mirochnic S, Wolf S, Staufenbiel M, Kempermann G (2009) Age effects on the regulation of adult hippocampal neurogenesis by physical activity and environmental enrichment in the APP23 mouse model of Alzheimer disease. *Hippocampus* 19:1008–1018.

Mohle L, Mattei D, Heimesaat MM, Bereswill S, Fischer A, Alutis M, French T, Hambardzumyan D, Matzinger P, Dunay IR, et al. (2016) Ly6C(hi) monocytes provide a link between antibiotic-induced changes in gut microbiota and adult hippocampal neurogenesis. *Cell Reports* 15:1945–1956.

Mongiat LA, Espósito MS, Lombardi G, Schinder AF (2009) Reliable activation of immature neurons in the adult hippocampus. *PLoS ONE* 4(4).

Monje ML, Mizumatsu S, Fike JR, Palmer TD (2002) Irradiation induces neural precursor-cell dysfunction. *Nature Medicine* 8:955–962.

Monje ML, Toda H, Palmer TD (2003) Inflammatory blockade restores adult hippocampal neurogenesis. *Science* 302:1760–1765.

Monje ML, Vogel H, Masek M, Ligon KL, Fisher PG, Palmer TD (2007) Impaired human hippocampal neurogenesis after treatment for central nervous system malignancies. *Annals of Neurology* 62:515–520.

Moore DL, Pilz GA, Arauzo-Bravo MJ, Barral Y, Jessberger S (2015) A mechanism for the segregation of age in mammalian neural stem cells. *Science* 349:1334–1338.

Moreno-Jiménez EP, Flor-García M, Terreros-Roncal J, Rábano A, Cafini F, Pallas-Bazarra N, Ávila J, Llorens-Martín M (2019) Adult hippocampal neurogenesis is abundant in neurologically healthy subjects and drops sharply in patients with Alzheimer's disease. *Nature Medicine* 25:554–560.

Morgan SC, Taylor DL, Pocock JM (2004) Microglia release activators of neuronal proliferation mediated by activation of mitogen-activated protein kinase, phosphatidylinositol-3-kinase/Akt and delta-Notch signaling cascades. *Journal of Neurochemistry* 90:89–101.

Mu Y, Gage FH (2011) Adult hippocampal neurogenesis and its role in Alzheimer's disease. *Molecular Neurodegeneration* 6:85.

Mullen RJ, Buck CR, Smith AM (1992) NeuN, a neuronal specific nuclear protein in vertebrates. *Development* 116:201–211.

Müller C, Remy S (2018) Septo–hippocampal interaction. *Cell and Tissue Research* 373:565–575.

Myers CE, Bermudez-Hernandez K, Scharfman HE (2013) The influence of ectopic migration of granule cells into the hilus on dentate gyrus-CA3 function. *PLoS ONE* 8(6).

Nacher J, Alonso-Llosa G, Rosell DR, McEwen BS (2003) NMDA receptor antagonist treatment increases the production of new neurons in the aged rat hippocampus. *Neurobiology of Aging* 24:273–284.

Nakajima K, Honda S, Tohyama Y, Imai Y, Kohsaka S, Kurihara T (2001) Neurotrophin secretion from cultured microglia. *Journal of Neuroscience Research* 65:322–331.

Nakashiba T, Cushman JD, Pelkey KA, Renaudineau S, Buhl DL, McHugh TJ, Rodriguez Barrera V, Chittajallu R, Iwamoto KS, McBain CJ, et al. (2012) Young dentate granule cells mediate pattern separation, whereas old granule cells facilitate pattern completion. *Cell* 149:188–201.

Neeper SA, Gomez-Pinilla F, Choi J, Cotman C (1995) Exercise and brain neurotrophins. *Nature* 373:109.

Nelson MD, Saykin AJ, Flashman LA, Riordan HJ (1998) Hippocampal volume reduction in schizophrenia as assessed by magnetic resonance imaging. *Archives of General Psychiatry* 55:433.

Newton SS, Collier EF, Hunsberger J, Adams D, Terwilliger R, Selvanayagam E, Duman RS (2003) Gene profile of electroconvulsive seizures: induction of neurotrophic and angiogenic factors. *Journal of Neuroscience* 23:10841–10851.

Nicola Z, Fabel K, Kempermann G (2015) Development of the adult neurogenic niche in the hippocampus of mice. *Frontiers in Neuroanatomy* 9:1–13.

Nowakowski RS, Lewin SB, Miller MW (1989) Bromodeoxyuridine immunohistochemical determination of the lengths of the cell cycle and the DNA-synthetic phase for an anatomically defined population. *Journal of Neurocytology* 18:311–318.

O'Donnell P (2012) Cortical disinhibition in the neonatal ventral hippocampus lesion model of schizophrenia: new vistas on possible therapeutic approaches. *Pharmacology and Therapeutics* 133:19–25.

Ogbonnaya ES, Clarke G, Shanahan F, Dinan TG, Cryan JF, O'Leary OF (2015) Adult hippocampal neurogenesis is regulated by the microbiome. *Biological Psychiatry* 78(4).

Okuyama N, Takagi N, Kawai T, Miyake-Takagi K, Takeo S (2003) Phosphorylation of extracellular-regulating kinase in NMDA receptor antagonist-induced newly generated neurons in the adult rat dentate gyrus. *Journal of Neurochemistry* 88:717–725.

Okuyama T, Kitamura T, Roy DS, Itohara S, Tonegawa S (2016) Ventral CA1 neurons store social memory. *Science* 353:1536–1541.

Overstreet-Wadiche LS (2006a) Delayed development of adult-generated granule cells in dentate gyrus. *Journal of Neuroscience* 26:2326–2334.

Overstreet-Wadiche LS (2006b) Seizures accelerate functional integration of adult-generated granule cells. *Journal of Neuroscience* 26:4095–4103.

Pallas-Bazarra N, Jurado-Arjona J, Navarrete M, Esteban JA, Hernández F, Ávila J, Llorens-Martín M (2016) Novel function of Tau in regulating the effects of external stimuli on adult hippocampal neurogenesis. *EMBO Journal* 35:1417–1436.

Palmer TD, Ray J, Gage FH (1995) FGF-2-responsive neuronal progenitors reside in proliferative and quiescent regions of the adult rodent brain. *Molecular and Cellular Neuroscience* 6:474–486.

Palmer TD, Schwartz PH, Taupin P, Kaspar B, Stein SA, Gage FH (2001) Cell culture: progenitor cells from human brain after death. *Nature* 411:42–43.

Palmer TD, Willhoite AR, Gage FH (2000) Vascular niche for adult hippocampal neurogenesis. *Journal of Comparative Neurology* 425:479–494.

Parent JM, Lowenstein DH (1997) Mossy fiber reorganization in the epileptic hippocampus. *Current Opinion in Neurology* 10:103–109.

Parent JM, Tada E, Fike JR, Lowenstein DH (1999) Inhibition of dentate granule cell neurogenesis with brain irradiation does not prevent seizure-induced mossy fiber synaptic reorganization in the rat. *Journal of Neuroscience* 19:4508–4519.

Parent JM, Yu TW, Leibowitz RT, Geschwind DH, Sloviter RS, Lowenstein DH (1997) Dentate granule cell neurogenesis is increased by seizures and contributes to aberrant network reorganization in the adult rat hippocampus. *Journal of Neuroscience* 17:3727–3738.

Park EH, Burghardt NS, Dvorak D, Hen R, Fenton AA (2015) Experience-dependent regulation of dentate gyrus excitability by adult-born granule cells. *Journal of Neuroscience* 35:11656–11666.

Paton JA, Nottebohm FN (1984) Neurons generated in the adult brain are recruited into functional circuits. *Science* 225:1046–1048.

Patzke N, Spocter MA, Karlsson KAE, Bertelsen MF, Haagensen M, Chawana R, Streicher S, Kaswera C, Gilissen E, Alagaili AN, et al. (2015) In contrast to many other mammals, cetaceans have relatively small hippocampi that appear to lack adult neurogenesis. *Brain Structure and Function* 220:361–383.

Perera TD, Coplan JD, Lisanby SH, Lipira CM, Arif M, Carpio C, Spitzer G, Santarelli L, Scharf B, Hen R, et al. (2007)

Antidepressant-induced neurogenesis in the hippocampus of adult nonhuman primates. *Journal of Neuroscience* 27:4894–4901.

Perera TD, Dwork AJ, Keegan KA, Thirumangalakudi L, Lipira CM, Joyce N, Lange C, Higley JD, Rosoklija G, Hen R, et al. (2011) Necessity of hippocampal neurogenesis for the therapeutic action of antidepressants in adult nonhuman primates. *PLoS ONE* 6(4).

Pham K, Nacher J, Hof PR, McEwen BS (2003) Repeated restraint stress suppresses neurogenesis and induces biphasic PSA-NCAM expression in the adult rat dentate gyrus. *European Journal of Neuroscience* 17:879–886.

Piatti VC, Davies-Sala MG, Esposito MS, Mongiat LA, Trinchero MF, Schinder AF (2011) The timing for neuronal maturation in the adult hippocampus is modulated by local network activity. *Journal of Neuroscience* 31:7715–7728.

Pieper AA, Wu X, Han TW, Estill SJ, Dang Q, Wu LC, Reece-Fincanon S, Dudley CA, Richardson JA, Brat DJ, et al. (2005) The neuronal PAS domain protein 3 transcription factor controls FGF-mediated adult hippocampal neurogenesis in mice. *Proceedings of the National Academy of Sciences* 102:14052–14057.

Pilz GA, Bottes S, Betizeau M, Jorg DJ, Carta S, Simons BD, Helmchen F, Jessberger S (2018) Live imaging of neurogenesis in the adult mouse hippocampus. *Science* 359:658–662.

Plümpe T, Ehninger D, Steiner B, Klempin F, Jessberger S, Brandt M, Römer B, Rodriguez GR, Kronenberg G, Kempermann G (2006) Variability of doublecortin-associated dendrite maturation in adult hippocampal neurogenesis is independent of the regulation of precursor cell proliferation. *BMC Neuroscience* 7:77.

Porcheri C, Suter U, Jessberger S (2014) Dissecting integrin-dependent regulation of neural stem cell proliferation in the adult brain. *Journal of Neuroscience* 34:5222–5232.

Porsolt RD, Anton G, Blavet N, Jalfre M (1978) Behavioural despair in rats: a new model sensitive to antidepressant treatments. *European Journal of Pharmacology* 47:379–391.

Pun RYK, Rolle IJ, LaSarge CL, Hosford BE, Rosen JM, Uhl JD, Schmeltzer SN, Faulkner C, Bronson SL, Murphy BL, et al. (2012) Excessive activation of mTOR in postnatally generated granule cells is sufficient to cause epilepsy. *Neuron* 75:1022–1034.

Raber J, Rola R, LeFevour A, Morhardt D, Curley J, Mizumatsu S, VandenBerg SR, Fike JR (2004) Radiation-induced cognitive impairments are associated with changes in indicators of hippocampal neurogenesis. *Radiation Research* 162:39–47.

Rakic P (1985a) Limits of neurogenesis in primates. *Science* 227:1054–1056.

Rakic P (1985b) DNA synthesis and cell division in the adult primate brain. *Annals of the New York Academy of Sciences* 457:193–211.

Ramirez S, Liu X, Lin PA, Suh J, Pignatelli M, Redondo RL, Ryan TJ, Tonegawa S (2013) Creating a false memory in the hippocampus. *Science* 341:387–391.

Ramirez S, Liu X, MacDonald CJ, Moffa A, Zhou J, Redondo RL, Tonegawa S (2015) Activating positive memory engrams suppresses depression-like behaviour. *Nature* 522:335–339.

Ramón y Cajal S (1928) Degeneration and Regeneration of the Nervous System. Oxford University Press.

Ramón y Cajal S (1999) Texture of the Nervous System of Man and the Vertebrates. Springer.

Rampon C, Jiang CH, Dong H, Tang YP, Lockhart DJ, Schultz PG, Tsien JZ, Hu Y (2000) Effects of environmental enrichment on gene expression in the brain. *Proceedings of the National Academy of Sciences of the United States of America* 97:12880–12884.

Ray J, Gage FH (1994) Spinal cord neuroblasts proliferate in response to basic fibroblast growth factor. *Journal of Neuroscience* 14:3548–3564.

Ray J, Peterson DA, Schinstine M, Gage FH (1993) Proliferation, differentiation, and long-term culture of primary hippocampal neurons. *Proceedings of the National Academy of Sciences of the United States of America* 90:3602–3606.

Reif A, Fritzen S, Finger M, Strobel A, Lauer M, Schmitt A, Lesch K-P (2006) Neural stem cell proliferation is decreased in schizophrenia, but not in depression. *Molecular Psychiatry* 11:514–522.

Represa A, Robain O, Tremblay E, Ben-Ari Y (1989) Hippocampal plasticity in childhood epilepsy. *Neuroscience Letters* 99:351–355.

Restivo L, Niibori Y, Mercaldo V, Josselyn SA, Frankland PW (2015) Development of adult-generated cell connectivity with excitatory and inhibitory cell populations in the hippocampus. *Journal of Neuroscience* 35:10600–10612.

Revest JM, Dupret D, Koehl M, Funk-Reiter C, Grosjean N, Piazza PV, Abrous DN (2009) Adult hippocampal neurogenesis is involved in anxiety-related behaviors. *Molecular Psychiatry* 14:959–967.

Reynolds BA, Weiss S (1992) Generation of neurons and astrocytes from isolated cells of the adult mammalian central nervous system. *Science* 255:1707–171.

Ribak CE, Tran PH, Spigelman I, Okazaki MM, Nadler JV (2000) Status epilepticus-induced hilar basal dendrites on rodent granule cells contribute to recurrent excitatory circuitry. *Journal of Comparative Neurology* 428:240–253.

Riudavets MA, Iacono D, Resnick SM, O'Brien R, Zonderman AB, Martin LJ, Rudow G, Pletnikova O, Troncoso JC (2007) Resistance to Alzheimer's pathology is associated with nuclear hypertrophy in neurons. *Neurobiology of Aging* 28:1484–1492.

Rogers GL, Martino AT, Aslanidi G v, Jayandharan GR, Srivastava A, Herzog RW (2011) Innate immune responses to AAV vectors. *Frontiers in Microbiology* 2:1–10.

Rolls ET, Kesner RP (2006) A computational theory of hippocampal function, and empirical tests of the theory. *Progress in Neurobiology* 79:1–48.

Rosenzweig MR, Krech D, Bennett EL, Diamond MC (1962) Effects of environmental complexity and training on brain chemistry and anatomy: a replication and extension. *Journal of Comparative and Physiological Psychology* 55:429–437.

Rossi C, Angelucci A, Costantin L, Braschi C, Mazzantini M, Babbini F, Fabbri ME, Tessarollo L, Maffei L, Berardi N, et al. (2006) Brain-derived neurotrophic factor (BDNF) is required for the enhancement of hippocampal neurogenesis following environmental enrichment. *European Journal of Neuroscience* 24:1850–1856.

Roy NS, Wang S, Jiang L, Kang J, Benraiss A, Harrison-Restelli C, Fraser RA, Couldwell WT, Kawaguchi A, Okano H, et al. (2000) In vitro neurogenesis by progenitor cells isolated from the adult human hippocampus. *Nature Medicine* 6:271–277.

Sah DWY, Ray J, Gage FH (1997) Regulation of voltage- and ligand-gated currents in rat hippocampal progenitor cells in vitro. *Journal of Neurobiology* 32:95–110.

Sahay A, Scobie KN, Hill AS, O'Carroll CM, Kheirbek MA, Burghardt NS, Fenton AA, Dranovsky A, Hen R (2011) Increasing adult hippocampal neurogenesis is sufficient to improve pattern separation. *Nature* 472:466–470.

Sampson TR, Debelius JW, Thron T, Janssen S, Shastri GG, Ilhan ZE, Challis C, Schretter CE, Rocha S, Gradinaru V, et al. (2016) Gut microbiota regulate motor deficits and neuroinflammation in a model of Parkinson's disease. *Cell* 167:1469–1480.

Sanai N, Nguyen T, Ihrie RA, Mirzadeh Z, Tsai HH, Wong M, Gupta N, Berger MS, Huang E, Garcia-Verdugo JM, et al. (2011) Corridors of migrating neurons in the human brain and their decline during infancy. *Nature* 478:382–386.

Sanai N, Tramontin AD, Quinones-Hinojosa A, Barbaro NM, Gupta N, Kunwar S, Lawton MT, McDermott MW, Parsa AT, Manuel-Garcia Verdugo J, et al. (2004) Unique astrocyte ribbon in adult human brain contains neural stem cells but lacks chain migration. *Nature* 427:740–744.

Santarelli L, Saxe M, Gross C, Surget A, Battaglia F, Dulawa S, Weisstaub N, Lee J, Duman R, Arancio O, et al. (2003) Requirement of hippocampal neurogenesis for the behavioral effects of antidepressants. *Science* 301:805–809.

Saxe MD, Battaglia F, Wang J-W, Malleret G, David DJ, Monckton JE, Garcia ADR, Sofroniew MV, Kandel ER, Santarelli L, et al. (2006) Ablation of hippocampal neurogenesis impairs contextual fear conditioning and synaptic plasticity in the dentate gyrus. *Proceedings of the National Academy of Sciences* 103:17501–17506.

Schänzer A, Wachs F-P, Wilhelm D, Acker T, Cooper-Kuhn C, Beck H, Winkler J, Aigner L, Plate KH, Kuhn HG (2006) Direct stimulation of adult neural stem cells in vitro and neurogenesis in vivo by vascular endothelial growth factor. *Brain Pathology* 14:237–248.

Scharfman HE, Goodman JH, Sollas AL (2000) Granule-like neurons at the hilar/CA3 border after status epilepticus and their synchrony with area CA3 pyramidal cells: functional implications of seizure-induced neurogenesis. *Journal of Neuroscience* 20:6144–6158.

Schmidt-Hieber C, Jonas P, Bischofberger J (2004) Enhanced synaptic plasticity in newly generated granule cells of the adult hippocampus. *Nature* 429:184–187.

Schoenfeld TJ, Rhee D, Martin L, Smith JA, Sonti AN, Padmanaban V, Cameron HA (2019) New neurons restore structural and behavioral abnormalities in a rat model of PTSD. *Hippocampus* 29:848–861.

Scott BW, Wang S, Burnham WM, de Boni U, Wojtowicz JM (1998) Kindling-induced neurogenesis in the dentate gyrus of the rat. *Neuroscience Letters* 248:73–76.

Scott BW, Wojtowicz JM, Burnham WM (2000) Neurogenesis in the dentate gyrus of the rat following electroconvulsive shock seizures. *Experimental Neurology* 165:231–236.

Seib DR, Corsini NS, Ellwanger K, Plaas C, Mateos A, Pitzer C, Niehrs C, Celikel T, Martin-Villalba A (2013) Loss of Dickkopf-1 restores neurogenesis in old age and counteracts cognitive decline. *Cell Stem Cell* 12:204–214.

Seigers R, Schagen S, Beerlings W, Boogerd W, Vantellingen O, Vandam F, Koolhaas J, Buwalda B (2008) Long-lasting suppression of hippocampal cell proliferation and impaired cognitive performance by methotrexate in the rat. *Behavioural Brain Research* 186:168–175.

Seigers R, Schagen SB, Coppens CM, van der Most PJ, van Dam FSAM, Koolhaas JM, Buwalda B (2009) Methotrexate decreases hippocampal cell proliferation and induces memory deficits in rats. *Behavioural Brain Research* 201:279–284.

Seki T, Arai Y (1993) Highly polysialylated neural cell adhesion molecule (NCAM-H) is expressed by newly generated granule cells in the dentate gyrus of the adult rat. *Journal of Neuroscience* 13:2351–2358.

Semerci F, Maletic-Savatic M (2016) Transgenic mouse models for studying adult neurogenesis. *Frontiers in Biology* 11:151–167.

Sennvik K, Boekhoorn K, Lasrado R, Terwel D, Verhaeghe S, Korr H, Schmitz C, Tomiyama T, Mori H, Krugers H, et al. (2007) Tau-4R suppresses proliferation and promotes neuronal differentiation in the hippocampus of tau knockin/knockout mice. *FASEB Journal* 21:2149–2161.

Seo D-o., Carillo MA, Chih-Hsiung Lim S, Tanaka KF, Drew MR (2015) Adult hippocampal neurogenesis modulates fear learning through associative and nonassociative mechanisms. *Journal of Neuroscience* 35:11330–11345.

Seress L, Mrzljak L (1987) Basal dendrites of granule cells are normal features of the fetal and adult dentate gyrus of both monkey and human hippocampal formations. *Brain Research* 405:169–174.

Shah S, Lubeck E, Zhou W, Cai L (2016) In situ transcription profiling of single cells reveals spatial organization of cells in the mouse hippocampus. *Neuron* 92:342–357.

Shapiro LA, Korn MJ, Shan Z, Ribak CE (2005) GFAP-expressing radial glia-like cell bodies are involved in a one-to-one relationship with doublecortin-immunolabeled newborn neurons in the adult dentate gyrus. *Brain Research* 1040:81–91.

Shihabuddin LS, Horner PJ, Ray J, Gage FH (2000) Adult spinal cord stem cells generate neurons after transplantation in the adult dentate gyrus. *Journal of Neuroscience* 20:8727–8735.

Shin J, Berg DA, Zhu Y, Shin JY, Song J, Bonaguidi MA, Enikolopov G, Nauen DW, Christian KM, Ming GL, et al. (2015) Single-cell RNA-seq with waterfall reveals molecular cascades underlying adult neurogenesis. *Cell Stem Cell* 17:360–372.

Shors TJ, Miesegaes G, Beylin A, Zhao M, Rydel T, Gould E (2001) Neurogenesis in the adult is involved in the formation of trace memories. *Nature* 410:372–376.

Shors TJ, Townsend DA, Zhao M, Kozorovitskiy Y, Gould E (2002) Neurogenesis may relate to some but not all types of hippocampal-dependent learning. *Hippocampus* 12:578–584.

Sibbe M, Häussler U, Dieni S, Althof D, Haas CA, Frotscher M (2012) Experimental epilepsy affects Notch1 signalling and the stem cell pool in the dentate gyrus. *European Journal of Neuroscience* 36:3643–3652.

Sibbe M, Kuner E, Althof D, Frotscher M (2015) Stem- and progenitor cell proliferation in the dentate gyrus of the Reeler mouse. *PLoS ONE* 10(3).

Sierra A, Encinas JM, Deudero JJ, Chancey JH, Enikolopov G, Overstreet-Wadiche LS, Tsirka SE, Maletic-Savatic M (2010) Microglia shape adult hippocampal neurogenesis through apoptosis-coupled phagocytosis. *Cell Stem Cell* 7:483–495.

Silva-Vargas V, Crouch EE, Doetsch F (2013) Adult neural stem cells and their niche: a dynamic duo during homeostasis, regeneration, and aging. *Current Opinion in Neurobiology* 23:935–942.

Singer BH, Jutkiewicz EM, Fuller CL, Lichtenwalner RJ, Zhang H, Velander AJ, Li X, Gnegy ME, Burant CF, et al. (2009) Conditional ablation and recovery of forebrain neurogenesis in the mouse. *Journal of Comparative Neurology* 514:567–582.

Smith LK, He Y, Park JS, Bieri G, Snethlage CE, Lin K, Gontier G, Wabl R, Plambeck KE, Udeochu J, et al. (2015) beta2-microglobulin is a systemic pro-aging factor that impairs cognitive function and neurogenesis. *Nature Medicine* 21:932–937.

Smith LK, White CW, Villeda SA (2018) The systemic environment: at the interface of aging and adult neurogenesis. *Cell and Tissue Research* 371:105–113.

Snyder JS (2019) Recalibrating the relevance of adult neurogenesis. *Trends in Neurosciences* 42:164–178.

Snyder JS, Hong NS, McDonald RJ, Wojtowicz JM (2005) A role for adult neurogenesis in spatial long-term memory. *Neuroscience* 130:843–852.

Snyder JS, Radik R, Wojtowicz JM, Cameron HA (2009) Anatomical gradients of adult neurogenesis and activity: young neurons in the ventral dentate gyrus are activated by water maze training. *Hippocampus* 19:360–370.

Snyder JS, Soumier A, Brewer M, Pickel J, Cameron HA (2011) Adult hippocampal neurogenesis buffers stress responses and depressive behaviour. *Nature* 476:458–461.

Song H, Stevens CF, Gage FH (2002) Astroglia induce neurogenesis from adult neural stem cells. *Nature* 417:39–44.

Song J, Sun J, Moss J, Wen Z, Sun GJ, Hsu D, Zhong C, Davoudi H, Christian KM, Toni N, et al. (2013) Parvalbumin interneurons mediate neuronal circuitry: neurogenesis coupling in the adult hippocampus. *Nature Neuroscience* 16:1728–1730.

Song J, Zhong C, Bonaguidi MA, Sun GJ, Hsu D, Gu Y, Meletis K, Huang ZJ, Ge S, Enikolopov G, et al. (2012) Neuronal circuitry mechanism regulating adult quiescent neural stem-cell fate decision. *Nature* 489:150–154.

Sorrells SF, Paredes MF, Cebrian-Silla A, Sandoval K, Qi D, Kelley KW, James D, Mayer S, Chang J, Auguste KI, et al. (2018) Human hippocampal neurogenesis drops sharply in children to undetectable levels in adults. *Nature* 555:377–381.

Spalding KL, Bergmann O, Alkass K, Bernard S, Salehpour M, Huttner HB, Boström E, Westerlund I, et al. (2013) Dynamics of hippocampal neurogenesis in adult humans. *Cell* 153:1219–1227.

Spigelman I, Yan X-X, Obenaus A, Lee EY-S, Wasterlain CG, Ribak CE (1998) Dentate granule cells form novel basal dendrites in a rat model of temporal lobe epilepsy. *Neuroscience* 86:109–120.

Stanfield BB, Trice JE (1988) Evidence that granule cells generated in the dentate gyrus of adult rats extend axonal projections. *Experimental Brain Research* 72:399–406.

Stefanelli T, Bertollini C, Luscher C, Muller D, Mendez P (2016) Hippocampal somatostatin interneurons control the size of neuronal memory ensembles. *Neuron* 89:1074–1085.

Steiner B, Klempin F, Wang L, Kott M, Kettenmann H, Kempermann G (2006) Type-2 cells as link between glial and neuronal lineage in adult hippocampal neurogenesis. *Glia* 54:805–814.

Steiner B, Zurborg S, Hörster H, Fabel K, Kempermann G (2008) Differential 24 h responsiveness of Prox1–expressing precursor cells in adult hippocampal neurogenesis to physical activity, environmental enrichment, and kainic acid–induced seizures. *Neuroscience* 154:521–529.

Stringer JL, Williamson JM, Lothman EW (1989) Induction of paroxysmal discharges in the dentate gyrus: frequency dependence and relationship to afterdischarge production. *Journal of Neurophysiology* 62:126–135.

Sugita N (1918) Comparative studies on the growth of the cerebral cortex. *Journal of Comparative Neurology* 29:61–117.

Suh H, Consiglio A, Ray J, Sawai T, D'Amour KA, Gage FH (2007) In vivo fate analysis reveals the multipotent and self-renewal capacities of Sox2+ neural stem cells in the adult hippocampus. *Cell Stem Cell* 1:515–528.

Suhonen JO, Peterson DA, Ray J, Gage FH (1996) Differentiation of adult hippocampus-derived progenitors into olfactory neurons in vivo. *Nature* 383:624–627.

Sun HB, Kawata S (2004) Two-photon photopolymerization and 3D lithographic microfabrication. *Advances in Polymer Science* 170:169–273.

Surget A, Saxe M, Leman S, Ibarguen-Vargas Y, Chalon S, Griebel G, Hen R, Belzung C (2008) Drug-dependent requirement of hippocampal neurogenesis in a model of depression and of antidepressant reversal. *Biological Psychiatry* 64:293–301.

Surget A, Tanti A, Leonardo ED, Laugeray A, Rainer Q, Touma C, Palme R, Griebel G, Ibarguen-Vargas Y, Hen R, Belzung C (2011) Antidepressants recruit new neurons to improve stress response regulation. *Molecular Psychiatry* 16:1177–1188.

Sutula T, Cascino G, Cavazos J, Parada I, Ramirez L (1989) Mossy fiber synaptic reorganization in the epileptic human temporal lobe. *Annals of Neurology* 26:321–330.

Swan AA, Clutton JE, Chary PK, Cook SG, Liu GG, Drew MR (2014) Characterization of the role of adult neurogenesis in touch-screen discrimination learning. *Hippocampus* 24:1581–1591.

Tada E, Parent JM, Lowenstein DH, Fike JR (2000) X-irradiation causes a prolonged reduction in cell proliferation in the dentate gyrus of adult rats. *Neuroscience* 99:33–41.

Tajerian M, Hung V, Nguyen H, Lee G, Joubert LM, Malkovskiy AV, Zou B, Xie S, Huang TT, Clark JD (2018) The hippocampal extracellular matrix regulates pain and memory after injury. *Molecular Psychiatry* 23:2302–2313.

Tashiro A, Makino H, Gage FH (2007) Experience-specific functional modification of the dentate gyrus through adult neurogenesis: a critical period during an immature stage. *Journal of Neuroscience* 27:3252–3259.

Tashiro A, Sandler VM, Toni N, Zhao C, Gage FH (2006) NMDA-receptor-mediated, cell-specific integration of new neurons in adult dentate gyrus. *Nature* 442:929–933.

Tashiro A, Zhao C, Suh H, Gage FH (2015) Preparation and use of retroviral vectors for labeling, imaging, and genetically manipulating cells. *Cold Spring Harbor Protocols* 2015:883–888.

Tatebayashi Y, Iqbal K, Grundke-Iqbal I (1999) Dynamic regulation of expression and phosphorylation of tau by fibroblast growth factor-2 in neural progenitor cells from adult rat hippocampus. *Journal of Neuroscience* 19:5245–5254.

Tauck D, Nadler J (1985) Evidence of functional mossy fiber sprouting in hippocampal formation of kainic acid-treated rats. *Journal of Neuroscience* 5:1016–1022.

Teitelbaum H, Lee JF, Johannessen JN (1975) Behaviorally evoked hippocampal theta waves: a cholinergic response. *Science* 188:1114–1116.

Teixeira CM, Kron MM, Masachs N, Zhang H, Lagace DC, Martinez A, Reillo I, Duan X, Bosch C, Pujadas L, et al. (2012) Cell-autonomous inactivation of the Reelin pathway impairs adult neurogenesis in the hippocampus. *Journal of Neuroscience* 32:12051–12065.

Temprana SG, Mongiat LA, Yang SM, Trinchero MF, Alvarez DD, Kropff E, Giacomini D, Beltramone N, Lanuza GM, Schinder AF (2015) Delayed coupling to feedback inhibition during a critical period for the integration of adult-born granule cells. *Neuron* 85:116–130.

Terreros-Roncal J, Moreno-Jiménez EP, Flor-García M, Rodríguez-Moreno CB, Trinchero MF, Cafini F, Rábano A, Llorens-Martín M (2021) Impact of neurodegenerative diseases on human adult hippocampal neurogenesis. *Science* 374:1106–1113.

Terstege DJ, Addo-Osafo K, Teskey GC, Epp JR (2022) New neurons in old brains: a cautionary tale for the analysis of neurogenesis in post-mortem tissue. *Molecular Brain* 15(38).

Thind KK, Ribak CE, Buckmaster PS (2008) Synaptic input to dentate granule cell basal dendrites in a rat model of temporal lobe epilepsy. *Journal of Comparative Neurology* 509:190–202.

Toda T, Parylak SL, Linker SB, Gage FH (2018) The role of adult hippocampal neurogenesis in brain health and disease. *Molecular Psychiatry* 24(1):67–87.

Toni N, Laplagne DA, Zhao C, Lombardi G, Ribak CE, Gage FH, Schinder AF (2008) Neurons born in the adult dentate gyrus form functional synapses with target cells. *Nature Neuroscience* 11:901–907.

Toni N, Schinder AF (2016) Maturation and functional integration of new granule cells into the adult hippocampus. *Cold Spring Harbor Perspectives in Biology* 8(1).

Toni N, Teng EM, Bushong EA, Aimone JB, Zhao C, Consiglio A, van Praag H, Martone ME, Ellisman MH, Gage FH (2007) Synapse formation on neurons born in the adult hippocampus. *Nature Neuroscience* 10:727–734

Tozuka Y, Fukuda S, Namba T, Seki T, Hisatsune T (2005) GABAergic excitation promotes neuronal differentiation in adult hippocampal progenitor cells. *Neuron* 47:803–815.

Trinchero MF, Koehl M, Bechakra M, Delage P, Charrier V, Grosjean N, Ladeveze E, Schinder AF, Abrous DN (2015) Effects of spaced learning in the water maze on development of dentate granule cells generated in adult mice. *Hippocampus* 25:1314–1326.

Tronel S, Belnoue L, Grosjean N, Revest JM, Piazza P v, Koehl M, Abrous DN (2012) Adult-born neurons are necessary for extended contextual discrimination. *Hippocampus* 22:292–298.

Tsai C-Y, Tsai C-Y, Arnold SJ, Huang G-J (2015) Ablation of hippocampal neurogenesis in mice impairs the response to stress during the dark cycle. *Nature Communications* 6:8373.

Tseng KY, Chambers RA, Lipska BK (2009) The neonatal ventral hippocampal lesion as a heuristic neurodevelopmental model of schizophrenia. *Behavioural Brain Research* 204:295–305.

van Praag H, Kempermann G, Gage FH (1999) Running increases cell proliferation and neurogenesis in the adult mouse dentate gyrus. *Nature Neuroscience* 2:266–270.

van Praag H, Schinder AF, Christie BR, Toni N, Palmer TD, Gage FH (2002) Functional neurogenesis in the adult hippocampus. *Nature* 415:1030–1034.

van Praag H, Shubert T, Zhao C, Gage FH (2005) Exercise enhances learning and hippocampal neurogenesis in aged mice. *Journal of Neuroscience* 25:8680–8685.

Vanderwolf CH (1969) Hippocampal electrical activity and voluntary movement in the rat. *Electroencephalography and Clinical Neurophysiology* 26:407–418.

Varma P, Brulet R, Zhang L, Hsieh J (2019) Targeting seizure-induced neurogenesis in a clinically relevant time period leads to transient but not persistent seizure reduction. *Journal of Neuroscience* 39:7019–7028.

Veyrac A, Gros A, Bruel-Jungerman E, Rochefort C, Kleine Borgmann FB, Jessberger S, Laroche S (2013) Zif268/egr1 gene controls the selection, maturation and functional integration of adult hippocampal newborn neurons by learning. *Proceedings of the National Academy of Sciences of the United States of America* 110:7062–7067.

Victor Nadler J, Perry BW, Cotman CW (1980) Selective reinnervation of hippocampal area CA1 and the fascia dentata after destruction of CA3-CA4 afferents with kainic acid. *Brain Research* 182:1–9.

Villeda SA, et al. (2011) The ageing systemic milieu negatively regulates neurogenesis and cognitive function. *Nature* 477:90–94.

Villeda SA, Plambeck KE, Middeldorp J, Castellano JM, Mosher KI, Luo J, Smith LK, Bieri G, Lin K, Berdnik D, et al. (2014) Young blood reverses age-related impairments in cognitive function and synaptic plasticity in mice. *Nature Medicine* 20:659–663.

Walter C, Murphy BL, Pun RYK, Spieles-Engemann AL, Danzer SC (2007) Pilocarpine-induced seizures cause selective time-dependent changes to adult-generated hippocampal dentate granule cells. *Journal of Neuroscience* 27:7541–7552.

Walton NM, Zhou Y, Kogan JH, Shin R, Webster M, Gross AK, Heusner CL, Chen Q, Miyake S, Tajinda K, et al. (2012) Detection of an immature dentate gyrus feature in human schizophrenia/bipolar patients. *Translational Psychiatry* 2(7).

Wang C, Liu F, Liu YY, Zhao CH, You Y, Wang L, Zhang J, Wei B, Ma T, Zhang Q, et al. (2011) Identification and characterization of neuroblasts in the subventricular zone and rostral migratory stream of the adult human brain. *Cell Research* 21:1534–1550.

Wang JW, David DJ, Monckton JE, Battaglia F, Hen R (2008) Chronic fluoxetine stimulates maturation and synaptic plasticity of adult-born hippocampal granule cells. *Journal of Neuroscience* 28:1374–1384.

Wang L, Chang X, She L, Xu D, Huang W, Poo MM (2015) Autocrine action of BDNF on dendrite development of adult-born hippocampal neurons. *Journal of Neuroscience* 35:8384–8393.

Wang W, Pan YW, Zou J, Li T, Abel GM, Palmiter RD, Storm DR, Xia Z (2014) Genetic activation of ERK5 MAP kinase enhances adult neurogenesis and extends hippocampus-dependent long-term memory. *Journal of Neuroscience* 34:2130–2147.

Wang X, Allen WE, Wright MA, Sylwestrak EL, Samusik N, Vesuna S, Evans K, Liu C, Ramakrishnan C, Liu J, et al. (2018) Three-dimensional intact-tissue sequencing of single-cell transcriptional states. *Science* 361(6400).

Wexler EM, Paucer A, Kornblum HI, Palmer TD, Geschwind DH (2009) Endogenous Wnt signaling maintains neural progenitor cell potency. *Stem Cells* 27:1130–1141.

Willner P, Towell A, Sampson D, Sophokleous S, Muscat R (1987) Reduction of sucrose preference by chronic unpredictable mild stress, and its restoration by a tricyclic antidepressant. *Psychopharmacology* 93:358–364.

Wojtowicz JM, Askew ML, Winocur G (2008) The effects of running and of inhibiting adult neurogenesis on learning and memory in rats. *European Journal of Neuroscience* 27:1494–1502.

Wolf SA, Steiner B, Akpinarli A, Kammertoens T, Nassenstein C, Braun A, Blankenstein T, Kempermann G (2009) CD4-positive T lymphocytes provide a neuroimmunological link in the control of adult hippocampal neurogenesis. *Journal of Immunology* 182:3979–3984.

Wong EY, Herbert J (2005) Roles of mineralocorticoid and glucocorticoid receptors in the regulation of progenitor proliferation in the adult hippocampus. *European Journal of Neuroscience* 22:785–792.

Wong EY, Herbert J (2006) Raised circulating corticosterone inhibits neuronal differentiation of progenitor cells in the adult hippocampus. *Neuroscience* 137:83–92.

Wright IC, Rabe-Hesketh S, Woodruff PWR, David AS, Murray RM, Bullmore ET (2000) Meta-analysis of regional brain volumes in schizophrenia. *American Journal of Psychiatry* 157:16–25.

Xu J-C, Xiao M-F, Jakovcevski I, Sivukhina E, Hargus G, Cui Y-F, Irintchev A, Schachner M, Bernreuther C (2014) The extracellular matrix glycoprotein tenascin-R regulates neurogenesis during development and in the adult dentate gyrus of mice. *Journal of Cell Science* 127:641–652.

Yagi S, Chow C, Lieblich SE, Galea LA (2016) Sex and strategy use matters for pattern separation, adult neurogenesis, and immediate early gene expression in the hippocampus. *Hippocampus* 26:87–101.

Yao B, Christian KM, He C, Jin P, Ming GL, Song H (2016) Epigenetic mechanisms in neurogenesis. *Nature Reviews Neuroscience* 17:537–549.

Yassa MA, Stark CE (2011) Pattern separation in the hippocampus. *Trends in Neurosciences* 34:515–525.

Yoder RM, Pang KC (2005) Involvement of GABAergic and cholinergic medial septal neurons in hippocampal theta rhythm. *Hippocampus* 15:381–392.

Yousef H, Morgenthaler A, Schlesinger C, Bugaj L, Conboy IM, Schaffer D v (2015) Age-associated increase in BMP signaling inhibits hippocampal neurogenesis. *Stem Cells* 33:1577–1588.

Yun S, Reynolds RP, Masiulis I, Eisch AJ (2016) Re-evaluating the link between neuropsychiatric disorders and dysregulated adult neurogenesis. *Nature Medicine* 22:1239–1247.

Zeng C, Pan F, Jones LA, Lim MM, Griffin EA, Sheline YI, Mintun MA, Holtzman DM, Mach RH (2010) Evaluation of 5-ethynyl-2'-deoxyuridine staining as a sensitive and reliable method for studying cell proliferation in the adult nervous system. *Brain Research* **1319**:21–32.

Zhang C, McNeil E, Dressler L, Siman R (2007) Long-lasting impairment in hippocampal neurogenesis associated with amyloid deposition in a knock-in mouse model of familial Alzheimer's disease. *Experimental Neurology* **204**:77–87.

Zhang H, Ryu D, Wu Y, Gariani K, Wang X, Luan P, D'Amico D, Ropelle ER, Lutolf MP, Aebersold R, et al. (2016) NAD(+) repletion improves mitochondrial and stem cell function and enhances life span in mice. *Science* **352**:1436–1443.

Zhao C (2006) Distinct morphological stages of dentate granule neuron maturation in the adult mouse hippocampus. *Journal of Neuroscience* **26**:3–11.

Zhao S, Chai X, Frotscher M (2007) Balance between neurogenesis and gliogenesis in the adult hippocampus: role for Reelin. *Developmental Neuroscience* **29**:84–90.

Zhou Y, Su Y, Li S, Kennedy BC, Zhang DY, Bond AM, et al. (2022) Molecular landscapes of human hippocampal immature neurons across lifespan. *Nature* **607**(7919):527–533.

Zhuo J-M, Tseng H, Desai M, Bucklin ME, Mohammed AI, Robinson NT, Boyden ES, Rangel LM, et al. (2016) Young adult born neurons enhance hippocampal dependent performance via influences on bilateral networks. *eLife* **3**:5.

Zimmer J (1973) Changes in the Timm sulfide silver staining pattern of the rat hippocampus and fascia dentata following early postnatal deafferentation. *Brain Research* **64**:313–326.

Ziv Y, Ron N, Butovsky O, Landa G, Sudai E, Greenberg N, Cohen H, Kipnis J, Schwartz M (2006) Immune cells contribute to the maintenance of neurogenesis and spatial learning abilities in adulthood. *Nature Neuroscience* **9**:268–275.

Ziv Y, Schwartz M (2008) Immune-based regulation of adult neurogenesis: Implications for learning and memory. *Brain, Behavior, and Immunity* **22**:167–176.

Zou J, Wang W, Pan YW, Abel GM, Storm DR, Xia Z (2015) Conditional inhibition of adult neurogenesis by inducible and targeted deletion of ERK5 MAP kinase is not associated with anxiety/depression-like behaviors. *eNeuro* **2**(2).

10

Synaptic Plasticity in the Hippocampus

Tim Bliss, Graham Collingridge, Sam Cooke, John Georgiou, and Richard Morris

10.1 Overview

10.1.1 Introduction

In the first edition of this book, published in 2007, we were able to give a reasonably comprehensive overview of the types of activity-dependent synaptic plasticity that had been identified in the hippocampus and of the mechanisms that generated and sustained them. In the intervening decade and a half, the number of papers on plasticity at hippocampal synapses has nearly tripled and it is no longer possible in the space available to aim for completeness. Our intention therefore is to cover the core elements of hippocampal synaptic plasticity with more detailed forays into selected branches of this endlessly fascinating phenomenon.

This initial section covers the basic properties of plasticity in the pathways that constitute the core hippocampal trisynaptic circuit: the perforant path input from medial entorhinal cortex (EC) to granule cells, the mossy fiber projection from granule cells to the proximal dendrites of CA3 pyramidal cells, and the mixed pathway containing Schaffer collateral axons from ipsilateral CA3 neurons and commissural axons from the contralateral CA3 neurons to the CA1 pyramidal cell field (Figure 10.1). The mixed pathway is collectively known as the Schaffer collateral/commissural (SCC) pathway. Other significant but less studied pathways are also introduced in the first section, including the projections from medial and lateral EC to the distal dendrites of principal cells in all hippocampal subfields, and projections from CA3 to CA2 pyramidal cells. Subsequent sections (10.2–10.7) take up selected aspects of the cell biology of hippocampal synaptic plasticity in greater detail, followed by a consideration of how plasticity contributes to hippocampus-dependent memory (10.8). The final section, 10.9, summarizes recent data supporting the growing realization that deficits in hippocampal synaptic plasticity are a common and perhaps causative feature in a substantial number of brain disorders.

10.1.2 Basic properties and mechanisms of LTP at hippocampal synapses

The early experiments on synaptic plasticity at perforant path synapses by Bliss and Lømo (1973) and Bliss and Gardner-Medwin (1973), described in Chapter 2, had suggested that long-term potentiation (LTP) was input-specific and that its induction required a threshold intensity of stimulation. Moreover, two components of LTP could be distinguished: first, potentiation of the field excitatory postsynaptic potential (fEPSP) and a corresponding increase in the population spike; second, an additional component of spike potentiation, which could not be accounted for by the degree of potentiation of the fEPSP, and which sometimes occurred in the absence of any synaptic potentiation. This component was termed EPSP-spike (E-S) potentiation by Andersen et al. (1980). Direct confirmation of the input specificity of LTP came from two-pathway experiments in hippocampal slices (Andersen et al., 1977; Dunwiddie and Lynch, 1978). Bliss and Gardner-Medwin (1973) had found that strong high-frequency trains were more effective at producing LTP in the freely moving rabbit than weak trains, and this property was confirmed by McNaughton et al. (1978) in the anesthetized rat, and termed "cooperativity." Another key feature of LTP was discovered independently by Goddard et al. (1978) and by Levy and Steward (1983) and named "associativity." If a weak input that, given alone, does not produce LTP is combined with a strong input that does, then both inputs are potentiated. The three properties of cooperativity, input specificity, and associativity were displayed in an experiment carried out for a review on LTP several years later (Figure 10.2A).

Ten years after the initial description of LTP, two papers appeared that laid the foundations for our current understanding of the mechanisms underlying the induction of LTP. Lynch et al. (1983) showed that the induction of LTP in pyramidal cells of CA1 could be blocked by the injection of a Ca^{2+} chelator EGTA (ethylene glycol-bis(β-aminoethyl ether)-N,N,N′,N′-tetraacetic acid) into the postsynaptic cell. In the same year Collingridge et al. (1983) reported that the specific N-methyl-D-aspartate (NMDA) receptor (NMDAR) blocker AP5 (also called APV: 2-amino-5-phosphonopentanoic acid), recently developed by Watkins et al. (1981), completely blocked the induction of LTP in CA1 pyramidal cells in vitro, while having no effect on synaptic responses evoked by single stimuli either before or after the induction of LTP (Figure 10.2B). It had already been shown that the NMDAR channel was blocked by Mg^{2+} ions in spinal cord neurons (Evans et al., 1977), and in cultured cortical neurons (MacDonald and Wojtowicz, 1980). Uniquely for ligand-gated receptors, the receptor exhibited a voltage-dependent conductance, the channel not fully opening until the membrane was substantially depolarized. Then, in 1984, two groups showed that these two observations were interlinked—the block by Mg^{2+} ions is voltage-dependent, and is progressively

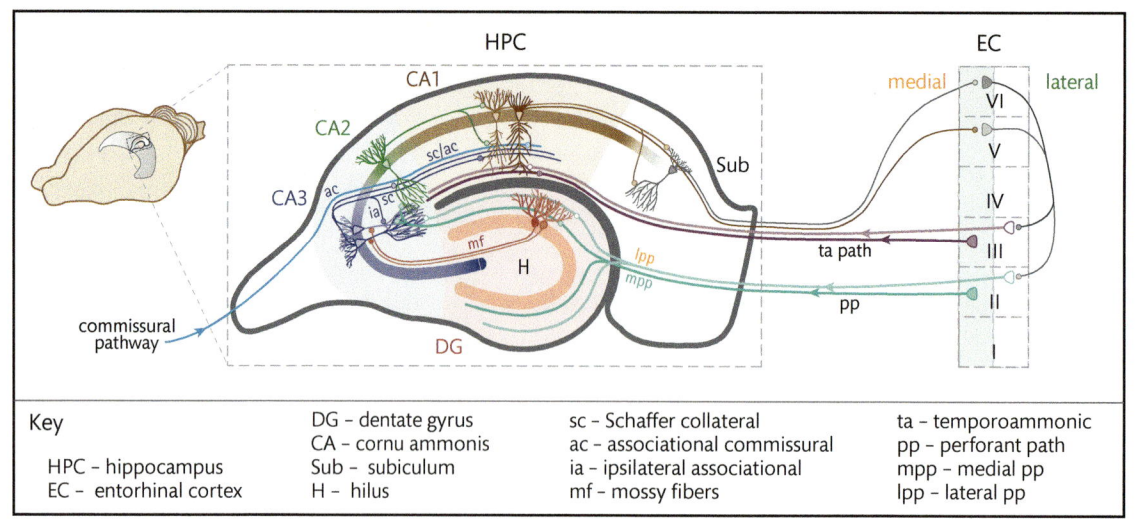

Figure 10.1 Hippocampal subregions. The diagram depicts a transverse section through the hippocampus, which is the orientation commonly used for in vitro experiments. The interconnectivity with the entorhinal cortex is also shown.

relieved as the membrane is depolarized (Mayer et al., 1984; Nowak et al., 1984). These characteristics of the NMDAR provide an elegant molecular explanation for the three properties that characterize the induction of LTP: input specificity, cooperativity, and associativity (Collingridge, 1985; Wigström and Gustafsson, 1985). Understanding of the voltage-dependent properties of the NMDAR allowed an induction rule for LTP to be formulated: *A synapse will be potentiated if, and only if, it is active at a time when its dendritic spine is sufficiently depolarized* (Figure 10.2C). This rule is based on the observation that activation of the NMDAR results in its ion-channel opening if and only if (1) synapses binding the glutamate ligand are embedded in a strongly depolarized section of dendrite (cooperativity), (2) synapses are active (input specificity), and (3) weakly active synapses can share the depolarization produced by strongly active synapses (associativity). The final clue to the role of the NMDAR in the induction of LTP was the demonstration that the channel is permeable to Ca^{2+} ions (MacDermott et al., 1986; Jahr and Stevens, 1993). The events that lead to NMDAR-dependent LTP (often referred to as NMDAR-LTP) can now be summarized: release of glutamate from a synapse, or a group of coactivated synapses, in sufficient quantities to produce strong postsynaptic depolarization allows the entry of Ca^{2+} into the spine and the triggering of Ca^{2+}-sensitive processes that lead to potentiation of transmission at that synapse (Figure 10.2D).

The importance of neuromodulatory influences on the induction of LTP has been known since the early 1980s (Bliss, Goddard, et al., 1983; Dingledine et al., 1986). An early example was the observation that blocking the actions of the inhibitory neurotransmitter gamma-aminobutyric acid (GABA), facilitates the induction of LTP by enhancing the synaptic activation of NMDARs (Wigström and Gustafsson, 1983; Herron et al., 1985). This occurs because the hyperpolarizing action of GABAergic inhibition ordinarily intensifies the Mg^{2+} block of NMDARs (Collingridge et al., 1988). A mechanistically distinct form of neuromodulation is the phosphorylation of NMDARs by the tyrosine kinase c-Src (cellular Src; derived from "sarcoma" owing to the original identification of the related viral v-Src oncogene in Rous sarcoma virus), which directly facilitates permeation through the NMDAR (YM Lu et al., 1998; Y-Q Huang et al.,

2001; H Li et al., 2024). A third, mechanistically distinct example of neuromodulation is the action of dopamine in facilitating signaling processes downstream of the NMDAR (U Frey et al., 1991), via the enhanced activation of protein kinase A (PKA). Neuromodulation is an important feature of synaptic plasticity and is considered in more detail in sections 10.2.1 and 10.5.

Expression mechanisms are considered in greater detail later in the chapter. In brief, while most attention has been paid to LTP-associated changes in postsynaptic glutamate receptor trafficking (Herring and Nicoll, 2016), there is also substantial evidence for presynaptic contributions to the maintenance of LTP in the SCC projection to CA1 (Bliss and Collingridge, 2013). In area CA1 in vitro, where the site of expression has been most extensively investigated, the locus and mechanisms of expression are strongly influenced by the induction protocol (Bliss and Collingridge, 2013; Padamsey and Emptage, 2014).

The induction of LTP at the giant synapses made by the mossy fiber axons of granule cells on the proximal dendrites of CA3 pyramidal cells is not NMDAR-dependent, and its expression is entirely presynaptic (see section 10.2.3). Synapses linking CA3 to CA2 pyramidal cells do not respond to conventional LTP-inducing stimulation (Carstens and Dudek, 2019), as their capacity to do so is gated by the Group III type of metabotropic glutamate receptors (mGluRs, Dasgupta et al., 2020). The SCC projection from CA3 to CA1 contains both ipsilateral projection axons (Schaffer collaterals) and commissural axons originating from contralateral CA3 neurons. The ease with which LTP can be obtained in this pathway in vitro (in contrast to the dentate gyrus, DG, where the bath application of a $GABA_A$ receptor antagonist is required to elicit LTP) has made the SCC projection the default pathway for the study of NMDAR-LTP in the hippocampus.

10.1.2.1 Signaling pathways in hippocampal plasticity

The question of what links activation of the NMDAR to the expression mechanisms of LTP, for example, an increase in the probability of release p(r), changes in α-amino-3-hydroxy-5-methyl-4-isoxazolepropionic acid receptor (AMPAR) properties, and/or structural alterations, has its origins in the late 1970s

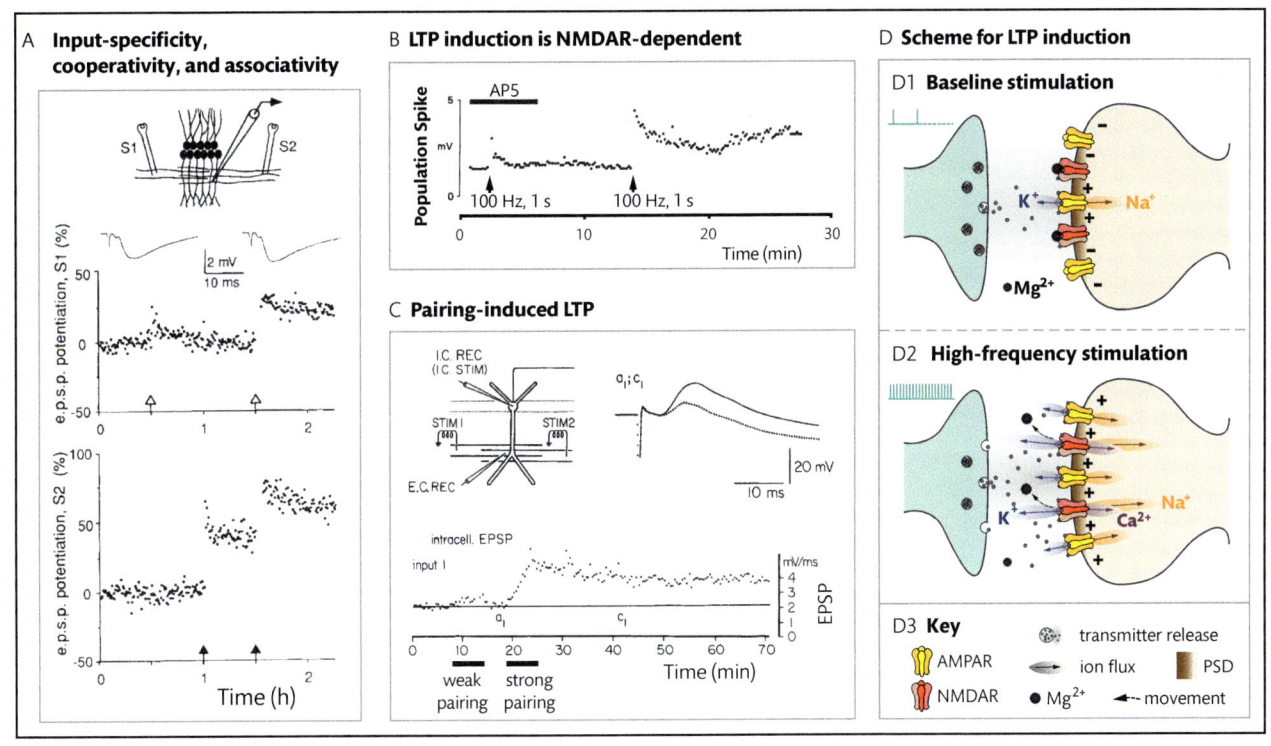

Figure 10.2 Properties and induction of NMDAR-LTP. (A) Three basic properties of LTP: A two-pathway in vivo experiment showing the properties of input specificity, cooperativity, and associativity that characterize LTP at the majority of hippocampal excitatory pathways, in this case the SCC pathway from CA3 to CA1 pyramidal cells. Stimulating electrodes S1 and S2 are positioned either side of the recording electrode to excite two independent pathways, one orthodromically (S1) and the other antidromically (S2), converging on a population of cells whose subthreshold field EPSPs are detected by a single recording electrode positioned in the stratum radiatum of an anesthetized rat. The independence of the two pathways is established by the absence of paired-pulse facilitation when a pair of stimuli are given at a 10–15 ms interval to the two pathways (not shown). A weak stimulus train given to S1 fails to produce LTP (first open arrow, top graph). A strong stimulus train, S2 (filled arrow), given to the second pathway produces robust LTP. The dependence of LTP on stimulus strength is referred to as cooperativity. Note that the strong stimulus, S2, does not induce LTP in the pathway activated by the weak stimulus. This is the property of input specificity. However, when the weak and strong stimulus trains are given together, both pathways are potentiated, demonstrating the property of cooperativity (from Bliss and Collingridge, 1993b). (B) Induction of NMDAR-LTP. The specific NMDAR blocker AP5 suppresses the induction of LTP at SCC-CA1 synapses. AP5 was applied iontophoretically for the period indicated by the bar. After washout, a repetition of the tetanus (100 Hz for 1 s) produced robust potentiation of the field response (from Collingridge et al., 1983). (C) Pairing low-frequency stimulation and depolarization induces LTP. A two-pathway experiment with intracellular recording establishes that what is required for the induction of LTP at SCC-CA1 synapses is the coincidence of synaptic activity and strong depolarization. Each pathway is stimulated alternately at 1 Hz. For the duration of the bar marked "strong pairing" a brief depolarizing pulse is delivered through the electrode to coincide with the stimulus to input 1. LTP is induced in this pathway, while the other pathway (not illustrated here) is unaffected (adapted from Gustafsson et al., 1987). (D) The mechanism for the induction of NMDAR-LTP. This widely accepted scheme depicts an excitatory synapse in area CA1. (D1) During baseline stimulation, the neurotransmitter L-glutamate, binds AMPARs to mediate the fast synaptic response. It also binds to NMDARs, but these contribute little to the synaptic response since they are blocked by Mg^{2+}. (D2) During HFS there is a longer lasting depolarization of the postsynaptic membrane, due in part to the temporal summation of AMPAR EPSPs, and this alleviates the Mg^{2+} block of NMDARs. While they are binding L-glutamate, NMDARs provide additional depolarization (mainly due to Na^+ entry) and a highly localized Ca^{2+} signal. Key aspects of this scheme are the relatively slow activation and deactivation kinetics of NMDARs (compared with AMPARs) and the powerful hyperpolarizing influence of synaptic inhibition (not illustrated). The highly localized nature of the Ca^{2+} signal confers the property of *input specificity*. The need for sufficient depolarization that cannot typically be provided by a single input underlies the property of *cooperativity*. The ability of the depolarization to spread to other inputs enables a weak input, defined as one that by itself is below the cooperativity threshold, to induce LTP, via the property of *associativity*. This scheme, which requires the conjunction of presynaptic activity to release L-glutamate and postsynaptic depolarization to relieve the Mg^{2+} block of NMDARs, confers the synapse with 'Hebbian' characteristics. (D3) Key.

with the suggestion that phosphorylation may be involved (Lynch et al., 1979). Since that time, a relatively large number of kinases have been identified as mediators of LTP, including protein kinase C (PKC), Ca^{2+}/calmodulin (CaM)-dependent protein kinases (CaMKs) such as CaMKII, PKA, mitogen-activated protein kinase (MAPK), phosphoinositide 3-kinase (PI3K), and c-Src (see first edition, pp 369–374). At mossy fiber synapses, where LTP is typically NMDAR-independent, PKA is a primary kinase that links the presynaptic Ca^{2+} signal with alterations in the presynaptic release machinery (first edition, pp 401–403).

With the discovery of robust ways to produce synaptic long-term depression (LTD), it was found that NMDAR-dependent LTD (NMDAR-LTD) involves the activation of a Ser/Thr protein phosphatase cascade (Mulkey et al., 1993; and see first edition, pp 410–412). This led to the simple concept that LTP involves phosphorylation and LTD involves dephosphorylation of critical substrates, most notably AMPARs. However, more recent work has revealed far greater complexity, as described in section 10.2.2 below. The mGluR-dependent form of LTD (mGluR-LTD) involves the activation of both kinases and phosphatases that largely differ from the ones involved in NMDAR-LTD. For example, mGluR-LTD involves the activation of a tyrosine phosphatase cascade (see first edition, p 416). How these signaling pathways interact in a coordinated manner to effect synaptic change is considered in more detail below.

10.1.2.2 Noncanonical LTP at other hippocampal pathways

As we have seen, medial perforant path (MPP) projections from layer II cells of the medial EC to granule cells of the DG, and the SCC-CA1 pathway from ipsilateral and contralateral CA3 pyramidal cells to CA1 neurons display the canonical form of LTP, characterized by insertion of AMPARs into the postsynaptic membrane, with synaptic growth on both sides of the synapse, and the potential for increases in transmitter release. Another type of expression mechanism is encountered at mossy fiber giant synapses, connecting granule cells to CA3 pyramidal cells, where both the induction and the expression of LTP is presynaptic, resulting in a sustained increase in transmitter release (see section 10.2.3). The lateral perforant path, originating with layer II cells of the lateral EC and projecting to the distal dendrites of granule cells in the DG and pyramidal cells of CA3, displays a third kind of synaptic plasticity; the induction of LTP at these synapses is blocked by the opioid inhibitor naloxone and not by the NMDAR antagonist AP5 (Bramham et al., 1991; Do et al., 2002). A more recent analysis of LTP in this pathway suggests that it is induced postsynaptically but expressed presynaptically and relies on an endocannabinoid retrograde messenger to provide the transsynaptic potentiating signal (W Wang, Jia, et al., 2018). Intriguingly, the synapses made by axon collaterals projecting to distal CA3 apical dendrites have properties consistent with a postsynaptic expression mechanism, suggesting that the target cell controls the mode of expression (Quintanilla et al., 2024). LTP has also been documented at excitatory synapses on dendrites of inhibitory cells, and at inhibitory synapses on pyramidal neurons (see section 10.3.1).

Finally, the SCC input to CA2 pyramidal cells in adult rodents is reluctant to display either LTP or LTD (Zhao et al., 2007). Area CA2 occupies a small region between the CA3 and CA1 cell fields. Pyramidal cells in this field receive SCC inputs from contra- and ipsilateral CA1 neurons and direct perforant paths inputs to distal dendrites from layer II stellate cells in EC. In a reversal of the usual situation, the distal inputs exert a stronger influence on CA2 neurons than do SCC axons (Chevaleyre and Siegelbaum, 2010). The SCC input to CA2 pyramidal cells while not exhibiting tetanus-induced LTP can be potentiated in vitro by prior injection of the live animal with domestically-relevant doses of the adenosine receptor antagonist, caffeine (Simons et al., 2011). A potential clue to the lack of activity-induced LTP at SCC-CA2 synapses is the perineural net (PNN), which surrounds CA2 neurons—LTP is more pronounced in young animals before the PNN has developed (Carstens and Dudek, 2019). Area CA2 plays an important role in social behavior and social memory (Hitti and Siegelbaum, 2014).

10.1.3 Temporal components of LTP: STP, LTP1, LTP2, and LTP3

In the first edition of this book, we described three well-recognized temporal components of LTP, referred to as STP, E-LTP, and L-LTP, acronyms for short-term potentiation, and early and late LTP respectively. They were defined, in reverse order, by the following characteristics: L-LTP is produced by strong tetanic stimulation, lasts for at least several hours, but if induced in the presence of a protein synthesis inhibitor, typically decays back to baseline within 1–3 h. The potentiation that remains, termed E-LTP, is itself sensitive to broad-spectrum protein kinase inhibitors, in the presence of which a brief potentiation, STP, survives, lasting typically 30–40 min. In a recent review (Bliss et al., 2018), we have advocated an alternative designation for the temporal components of LTP. This revised terminology (see also Raymond, 2007), recognizes four components of increasing persistence: STP, LTP1, LTP2, and LTP3. We consider the characteristics of these four components in more detail in section 10.2.1. In brief, while usually short-lived, the duration of STP is use-dependent—the less frequent the test stimulation, the longer the duration of STP. In contrast, the three components of LTP do not exhibit this exquisite sensitivity to use-dependent decay, and their time course is defined by the underlying cell biological processes that determine their expression or by the drugs that block them. LTP1 is blocked by kinase inhibitors, LTP2 by translation inhibitors, and LTP3 by transcription inhibitors. Which component is induced, and how long it lasts, can also be affected by the pattern of stimulation used to induce potentiation. There is likely to be a substantial temporal overlap between STP and LTP1–3, and further work in the freely moving animal is required to determine the temporal characteristics of each component.

10.1.4 Transition from LTP1 to LTP2, 3: the synaptic tagging and capture (STC) hypothesis

Although LTP2, unlike LTP1, is blocked by protein synthesis inhibitors, it can be induced in isolated CA1 dendrites (Cracco et al., 2005; Vickers et al., 2005), indicating that the protein synthesis required occurs locally. For LTP3, signals must pass from the synapse to the nucleus to initiate gene transcription, and newly expressed transcripts must then be transported to the appropriate synapses, either as proteins newly translated in the nucleus or as messenger ribonucleic acid (mRNA) destined for translation into protein by synthesizing machinery available at the base of the synapse. How is this achieved? The problem was addressed by U. Frey and Morris (1997) in area CA1 of the hippocampal slice. U. Frey and Morris found it hard to imagine that newly synthesized plasticity factors (i.e., PRPs, plasticity-related products including mRNA or proteins) in the nucleus could somehow acquire the dendritic "address" of recently active synapses. It seemed more likely that a mass mailing of newly synthesized somatic proteins or transcripts is dispatched to dendrites indiscriminately and these are captured by molecular tags established at activated synapses (Takeuchi et al., 2014). U. Frey and Morris proposed that both early and late forms of LTP set a synaptic tag, but that only strong tetanization led to the somatic transcription and translation of plasticity factors necessary for sustained synaptic potentiation—possibly because strong tetanization coactivates neuromodulatory inputs. In the synaptic tagging and capture (STC) hypothesis, one neuromodulatory influence that appears to be particularly important for promoting the conversion of LTP1 to LTP2 is the dopaminergic system, operating via dopamine 1 (D1) and D5 receptors (U Frey et al., 1990; O'Carroll and Morris, 2004). U. Frey and Morris (1997) showed that a weak protocol, which given alone produced only transient LTP, could produce persistent LTP if it were paired within about 90 min before or after a strong protocol to a neighboring pathway. The theory that plasticity factors, either dendritically targeted mRNA or somatically translated proteins, seek out active areas of the dendritic tree received some support from the finding that after prolonged (but not brief) tetanization of the MPP, mRNA for the immediate early gene *Arc/Arg3.1* (activity-regulated cytoskeleton-associated) becomes concentrated in the middle of the dendritic tree, where MPP fibers terminate (Steward et al., 1998). However, the identity of the synaptic tag has not been definitively established (Farris et al., 2014; see also section 10.6.2).

10.1.5 Other forms of long-term synaptic plasticity in the hippocampus: E-S potentiation, metaplasticity, LTD, STDP, and homeostatic plasticity

As mentioned above, two components of potentiation commonly result from high-frequency stimulation (HFS) of hippocampal excitatory pathways: first, the potentiation of the synaptic response together with the corresponding increase in the spike component of the evoked response, normally referred to simply as LTP; and second, an additional component of spike potentiation that cannot be accounted for by the increase in synaptic drive. This relatively little studied but potentially significant component of potentiation, referred to as EPSP-spike or E-S potentiation, is discussed further in section 10.4.

Metaplasticity, or the "plasticity of plasticity," has a long history. Saturation, an extreme form of metaplasticity, was evident in the early experiments of Lømo, Bliss, and Gardner-Medwin, in which repeated episodes of tetanic stimulation led to LTP reaching a maximal value, after which the tetanus that had initially produced potentiation no longer did so. The term "metaplasticity" was introduced by Abraham and colleagues to describe ways in which the magnitude and direction of activity-dependent changes in synaptic weight could be modified by prior activity (Abraham and Bear, 1996; Abraham and Tate, 1997). For example, in area CA1 in vitro, low-intensity priming trains, which do not themselves affect the response to test pulse stimulation, can suppress the subsequent induction of LTP (Y-Y Huang et al., 1992). We will revisit metaplasticity below in the context of homeostasis (see section 10.6).

Concerns about runaway excitation in a brain without a brake on LTP appeared early in the LTP literature (Stent, 1973; Sejnowski, 1977). But although there was evidence for heterosynaptic depression (Lynch et al., 1977; Abraham and Goddard, 1983; Stanton and Sejnowski, 1989), and LTP was known to be susceptible to homosynaptic depotentiation (DP) for a few minutes after induction (Staubli and Lynch, 1990), it was not until 1992 that the first protocol for obtaining de novo homosynaptic LTD appeared. Dudek and Bear (1992) reported that long, low-frequency trains (typically 1 Hz for 15 min) produced a persistent NMDAR-LTD of synaptic transmission in SCC synapses of young rats in vitro. LTD is much easier to elicit in vitro in young than in mature animals, and its induction is markedly facilitated by stress (L Xu et al., 1997). In awake mice LTD elicited by low-frequency trains rarely lasts longer than 60 min (Goh and Manahan-Vaughan, 2013). At SCC synapses an mGluR-dependent form of LTD can be induced either by bath application of the mGluR agonist dihydroxyphenylglycine (DHPG) or, in vivo, by a modified form of low-frequency stimulation using pairs of pulses (reviewed by Lüscher and Huber, 2010). Despite the relative difficulty of inducing LTD, its expression mechanisms are broadly understood (see section 10.2.2) and it is now as much an accepted feature of the landscape of synaptic plasticity as LTP.

A more recent development has been an interest in the precise timing criteria for Hebbian plasticity. Clearly, a Hebbian rule for potentiation requires cell A to fire before cell B if it is to take part in firing it; but what are the consequences of cell B firing before cell A? The discovery of local and propagated dendritic spikes (Stuart and Sakmann, 1994) made it possible to design experiments in which the interval between presynaptic and postsynaptic spikes could be precisely timed, yielding spike-timing-dependent plasticity (STDP). In general, LTP occurs when presynaptic spiking precedes postsynaptic spiking by a few milliseconds, and depression occurs when post- precedes pre-, with a rapid reversal through coincidence. The same induction and expression mechanisms hold for STDP as for LTP and LTD.

Homeostatic plasticity refers to the idea that there exists a mechanism for the overall control of the excitability of a network of cells, so that while there may be a potentiation of synaptic strength within a subset of neurons, this will be counterbalanced by a general reduction in synaptic strength and/or excitability of other cells so that the mean synaptic strength of the network remains within set limits (Turrigiano, 2017). We consider this topic in more detail in section 10.6.2.

10.1.6 Synaptic plasticity in the primate hippocampus

What is the evidence for synaptic plasticity in the nonhuman primate and human hippocampus? Both NMDAR-dependent and NMDAR-independent forms of LTP can be induced in area CA3 of hippocampal slices from *Macaca fascicularis* (cynomolgus monkeys; see Urban et al., 1996). In humans, plasticity has been examined in hippocampal tissue removed from patients suffering from intractable epilepsy. Beck and colleagues (2000) found that NMDAR-LTP could readily be elicited by HFS of the perforant path input to the DG. Transcranial magnetic stimulation (TMS) is a noninvasive technique that has yielded convincing evidence for activity-dependent plasticity in the human neocortex (reviewed by Bliss and Cooke, 2011). The hippocampus was thought to lie too deep in the brain for this technique to be useful, but a recent study targeting the hippocampus with brief volleys of TMS delivered in theta-burst mode revealed an increased functional magnetic resonance imaging (fMRI) blood-oxygen-level-dependent (BOLD) signal on the targeted side during a scene-encoding task, leading to enhanced subsequent recollection (Hermiller et al., 2020).

10.1.7 The role of hippocampal synaptic plasticity in learning and memory

A key question about synaptic plasticity concerns its function. Bliss and Lømo's (1973) article anticipated interest in this question in their concluding sentence: "Whether or not the intact animal makes use in real life of a property which has been revealed by synchronous, repetitive volleys to a population of fibers the normal rate and pattern of activity along which are unknown, is another matter." Their "other matter" soon became a topic of wide interest, with research on the possibility of a role in learning and memory triggered by Barnes's observation of a correlation between the decay of LTP in vivo and forgetting of spatial memory (Barnes, 1979). Diverse later studies have examined the impact of blocking the induction of LTP with appropriate antagonists on hippocampus-dependent learning. More recently, the use of genetic manipulations targeting neurons activated during hippocampus-dependent learning in a region-specific and time-dependent manner has emphasized the importance of hippocampal synaptic plasticity in learning. LTP-like phenomena in other regions of the brain have also been linked to forms of memory that are not hippocampus-dependent, such as auditory fear conditioning. Section 10.8 documents the evidence for an essential functional role for hippocampal synaptic plasticity in hippocampus-dependent learning and memory.

10.1.8 Hippocampal synaptic plasticity and brain disorders

A movement to characterize how synaptic plasticity is compromised in, and contributes to, disorders of learning and memory has been gathering momentum in recent years. Prominent among disorders involving the hippocampus is Alzheimer's disease (AD), the pathology of which originates in the hippocampus and associated medial temporal lobe structures, and whose primary symptom is memory loss. AD is a highly prevalent condition with growing incidence. Strong hypotheses have been developed concerning the root causes of the pathology, including the dominant amyloid hypothesis, which holds that amyloid beta (Aβ) fragments cleaved from the amyloid precursor protein (APP) are the originating pathological entities (Selkoe and Hardy, 2016). Additionally, there has been a focus on dysregulation of TAU (encoded by *MAPT*, the microtubule-associated protein tau gene) as a key endpoint to the pathology of AD and other dementias collectively known as tauopathies (Goedert, 2018). The pathology of the disorder includes significant cell death, progressing from the medial temporal lobe to the rest of the brain with increasingly severe symptomatology. Early investigations took two approaches, either applying Aβ fragments, particularly the highly hydrophobic and pathogenic Aβ 1-42 (Aβ42) fragments (Pike et al., 1995) to rat hippocampal slices, or studying synaptic plasticity in genetically defined mouse models that expressed mutations responsible for familial AD (Rowan et al., 2003). Experiments in rodent models were key to revealing that synaptic pathology may start long before neurons die and have been critical in developing the idea that the disorder is primarily synaptic in origin (Selkoe and Hardy, 2016). Moreover, deficits in synaptic plasticity and accompanying mild cognitive impairment may be present decades before AD is diagnosed, potentially providing a time window prior to major cell death in which candidate therapies may be maximally effective (Selkoe and Hardy, 2016). The role played by synaptic plasticity in AD, and in animal models of neurodevelopmental disorders, is discussed more fully in section 10.9.

10.2 Mechanisms of synaptic plasticity

Synaptic plasticity is a widespread phenomenon exhibited to a greater or lesser extent by most synapses in the brain, whether excitatory or inhibitory. Mechanistically, several different forms of synaptic plasticity can be distinguished (see Box 10.1). The most obvious distinction is whether synapses are potentiated (STP and LTP) or depressed (DP and LTD). Another important factor is whether the modification is homosynaptic (restricted to the pathway in which plasticity is induced) or heterosynaptic (affecting independent pathways converging on the same target cells). A third defining feature is the nature of the induction trigger—in most cases this is activation of the NMDAR, but there are examples of NMDAR-independent synaptic plasticity such as mossy fiber LTP (mf-LTP) and mGluR-LTD. Synaptic plasticity thus defined may comprise several mechanistically distinct components: Notably, at

SCC synapses, activity-dependent potentiation can be divided into four distinct NMDAR-dependent components:

- STP decays at a rate that is use-dependent.
- LTP1 is typically more sustained than STP and does not depend on protein synthesis.
- LTP2 often persists for longer than LTP1 and requires de novo protein synthesis.
- LTP3 requires transcription and is potentially the most persistent form of synaptic plasticity.

10.2.1 NMDAR-dependent synaptic potentiation

Many pathways in the central nervous system (CNS) express NMDAR-synaptic plasticity. In this section we describe primarily CA3 to CA1 plasticity, since the underlying mechanisms are best understood at these synapses.

10.2.1.1 Short-term potentiation (STP)

STP is induced rapidly in response to HFS and decays in an activity-dependent manner—in the absence of stimulation the potentiation can be stored without decrement for several hours (Volianskis et al., 2015). The extent to which STP contributes to synaptic potentiation varies according to the induction protocols employed. It is most pronounced after a brief period of continuous HFS or theta-burst stimulation (TBS), but is absent when a continuous low-frequency train (as used for pairing-induced LTP) is delivered. Since CA3 neurons fire in high-frequency synchronized bursts during the theta rhythm, STP is likely to be a widely occurring form of NMDAR-dependent synaptic plasticity in the behaving animal.

STP is readily distinguishable from LTP in that it is generally resistant to the kinase inhibitors that block the induction of all forms of LTP. Unlike LTP, its expression is associated with a decrease in paired-pulse facilitation that is most likely due to an increase in p(r) at individual synapses (Figure 10.3). STP can be further subdivided into two kinetically distinct components. In the absence of stimulation, both are stored without decrement for, at least, many hours, but STP1 decays more rapidly than STP2 when basal stimulation is delivered. STP1 and STP2 can also be distinguished by the NMDAR subunit (GluN) composition involved in their induction. STP1 involves GluN2A and GluN2B subunits, principally in the form of a heterotrimer, and STP2 involves GluN2B and GluN2D subunits, probably also in the form of a heterotrimer (Volianskis, Bannister, et al., 2013). Note, the latter receptor combination has a low sensitivity to the commonly used NMDAR antagonist, D-AP5, and so STP2 may falsely appear to be NMDAR-independent (Pradier et al., 2018). In recent work, it has been suggested that GluN2A- and GluN2B-containing NMDARs form distinct receptor subtypes that differentially regulate neurotransmitter release via the regulation of presynaptic SK (small conductance calcium-activated potassium) channels (Schmidt et al., 2024). The roles of these two receptor subtypes that are presumably heterodimers, in STP, is unclear. Clearly more work is required to understand the full complement of presynaptic NMDARs and their respective roles in the various forms of synaptic plasticity at hippocampal synapses.

It has been proposed that STP1 and STP2 converge on the same presynaptic expression mechanism and that the relative contributions of STP1 and STP2 vary according to the nature of the stimuli used to induce STP (Eapen et al., 2021). One possibility is that STP1 engages mainly high p(r) synapses and is triggered

Box 10.1 Presynaptic and postsynaptic changes contribute to the expression of LTP and LTD at Schaffer collateral/commissural (SCC) synapses

The central role of postsynaptic NMDARs in the induction of LTP has been accepted for nearly 40 years. The locus of expression of LTP remains controversial. While there is abundant evidence for changes in the number and distribution of postsynaptic AMPARs following the induction of LTP and LTD, there is also compelling evidence that in some experimental situations LTP can be sustained solely by an increase in release probability, p(r), without a change in synaptic potency (Enoki et al., 2009). Interestingly, as noted in Box 10.2, the size of the pre- and postsynaptic densities at hippocampal synapses are invariably well matched, suggesting that mechanisms are in place to keep the pre- and postsynaptic sides of the synapse in lockstep. In this box we summarize the current state of play in this long-running debate.

The molecular machinery of the dendritic spine comprises a system for on-demand delivery of additional AMPARs to the PSD, by exocytosis from delivery organelles to the plasma membrane and thence by lateral diffusion to the perisynaptic membrane (reviewed by (Herring and Nicoll, 2016). This mechanism has been visualized by single-molecule imaging using quantum dot technology (Penn et al., 2017; Choquet, 2018). Conversely, NMDAR-dependent LTD in the SCC pathway is associated with a reduction in surface delivery of AMPARs to the synapse (Collingridge et al., 2010). Moreover, AMPAR trafficking has been linked to learning; a buildup of synaptic AMPARs occurs in neurons of the lateral amygdala following cued fear conditioning (CFC) (Rumpel et al., 2005), and restricting the lateral diffusion of AMPARs in hippocampal neurons impairs CFC (Penn et al., 2017). Thus, there is compelling evidence that AMPARs are inserted into the perisynaptic membrane in LTP, and further evidence that this increase occurs during, and is necessary for, learning. Note however, that direct evidence that this translates to an increase in potency at individual synapses is lacking.

On the presynaptic side, evidence supports a change in p(r) during STP, which has the capacity to last several hours (see section 10.2.1). Is there evidence that LTP1 and LTP2 are associated with changes in the presynaptic parameters of synaptic transmission, p(r), or quantal content, n, the number of quanta released per release event? Convincing data at hippocampal synapses has been hard to obtain by purely electrophysiological means. The situation changed with the availability of Ca^{2+}-sensitive fluorescent dyes and the additional optical resolution offered by two-photon microscopy. This allowed optical quantal analysis to be carried out on LTP and LTD at SCC synapses. In this approach, a CA1 pyramidal cell is loaded with a Ca^{2+}-sensitive dye through a sharp recording electrode, a stimulating electrode is positioned nearby to activate afferent SCC fibers, test stimuli are delivered, a responding spine is located, and an estimate made of p(r) for that single connection. LTP is then induced by HFS and at later times further estimates are made of p(r). This approach has provided direct evidence for an increase in p(r) following the induction of LTP at single, visualized SCC synapses (Emptage et al., 2003; Enoki et al., 2009). An increase in q, the quantal amplitude or potency, estimated by subtracting the compound EPSPs associated with a success at the imaged spine from those associated with a failure, was not seen, as would be expected if there were an increase in the number of AMPARs in the subsynaptic zone (Enoki et al., 2009). There is corresponding evidence for an increase in the population of release-ready vesicles in LTP (Rey et al., 2020). Do similar presynaptic changes occur in learning? Evidence here relies on the assumption, well documented in vitro, that a decrease in PPF in hippocampal field responses reflects an increase in p(r) (McNaughton, 1982). Decreases in PPF in hippocampus-dependent tasks have been reported following trace eyeblink conditioning (Madronal et al., 2009) and inhibitory avoidance learning (Paw Min Thein et al., 2020).

How is what we may term this *pre-posterous* debate to be resolved? The question has been asked with varying degrees of perplexity (by Lisman, 2009; Bliss and Collingridge, 2013; MacDougall and Fine, 2014, 2019; and Padamsey and Emptage, 2014). Whatever the reason, the fact that both pre- and postsynaptic changes occur after learning suggests that animals can exploit the ability to modify either component of synaptic transmission at SCC synapses to sustain the changes in synaptic efficacy needed for learning.

Emptage and colleagues reexamined the role of the postsynaptic cell in presynaptic plasticity at SCC synapses using optical quantal analysis (Padamsey et al., 2017). They find that potentiation of p(r) occurs when a presynaptic action potential is paired with the postsynaptic release of the retrograde signaling molecule nitric oxide. The latter event requires strong membrane depolarization to activate VGCCs in the perisynaptic membrane, enabling the activation of postsynaptic NO synthase. The necessary depolarization may be provided by a backpropagating action potential or dendritic spike. The sequence of presynaptic action potential followed within a few ms by the transsynaptic release of NO activates an unidentified coincidence detector in the presynaptic terminal, leading to an increase in p(r). Interestingly, this mechanism for the persistent modulation of p(r) is not dependent on the release of glutamate. Padamsey (2017) also provide evidence for a population of presynaptic NMDARs that are negatively coupled to the release machinery, with the consequence that the release of glutamate leads to a reduction in p(r). A follow-up theoretical study (Tong et al., 2020) considered how this combination of pre- and postsynaptic control over synaptic efficacy might work together to control synaptic function. Postsynaptic changes, for instance an increase in the number of synaptic AMPARs, act as a gain control that applies equally to all successful release events. In contrast, a change in p(r) affects the fate of trains of action potentials, since a release event reduces the readily releasable pool of vesicles and so reduces p(r) for later action potentials in the train (Markram and Tsodyks, 1996; Dobrunz and Stevens, 1997). Thus, presynaptic plasticity events act as a low-pass filter to modulate the flow of neural traffic across the synapse.

The introduction of the glutamate-sensitive fluorescent reporter, GluSnFR ("glutamate sniffer"), offers a promising real-time approach for measuring glutamate release following the induction of LTP. In two studies (Kopach et al., 2020; Ucar et al., 2021), LTP was linked to an increase in the concentration of extracellular glutamate, though in the absence of glutamate-uptake inhibitors it was not possible to distinguish between an increase in glutamate release and a decrease in uptake, potentially linked to the withdrawal of perisynaptic astroglia that follows the induction of LTP (Henneberger et al., 2020).

How will this debate play out? Three decades of research have produced incontrovertible evidence for postsynaptic changes in LTP and LTD, though evidence linking these changes to potentiation at individual synapses is still lacking. In contrast, the findings from optical quantal analysis provide direct evidence for presynaptic changes at potentiated synapses 30–60 min after induction of LTP in vitro, without change in postsynaptic potency. A reconciliation of these two views remains elusive. One synapse back along the trisynaptic pathway, the site of LTP at mossy fiber synapses on CA3 cells, is incontrovertibly presynaptic in both its induction and expression. There is also evidence for glial involvement in the regulation of synaptic plasticity at SCC synapses on CA1 pyramidal neurons, both through release from astroglia of D-serine, a coagonist at NMDARs (Henneberger et al., 2010), and via control of the half-width distribution of p(r) at SCC terminals (Chipman et al., 2021). Synaptic strength may thus fall under the jurisdiction of a tripartite alliance, with presynaptic, postsynaptic, and glial participation.

by the activation of postsynaptic NMDARs that signal to the presynaptic terminals via K^+ efflux, potentially directly through the open channels of postsynaptic NMDARs. In contrast, STP2 engages low p(r) synapses via presynaptic NMDARs. Evidence for K^+ serving as a retrograde messenger in LTP (Shih et al., 2013) and for the existence of presynaptic GluN2B-containing NMDARs at the SCC terminals (McGuinness et al., 2010) are consistent with this hypothesis.

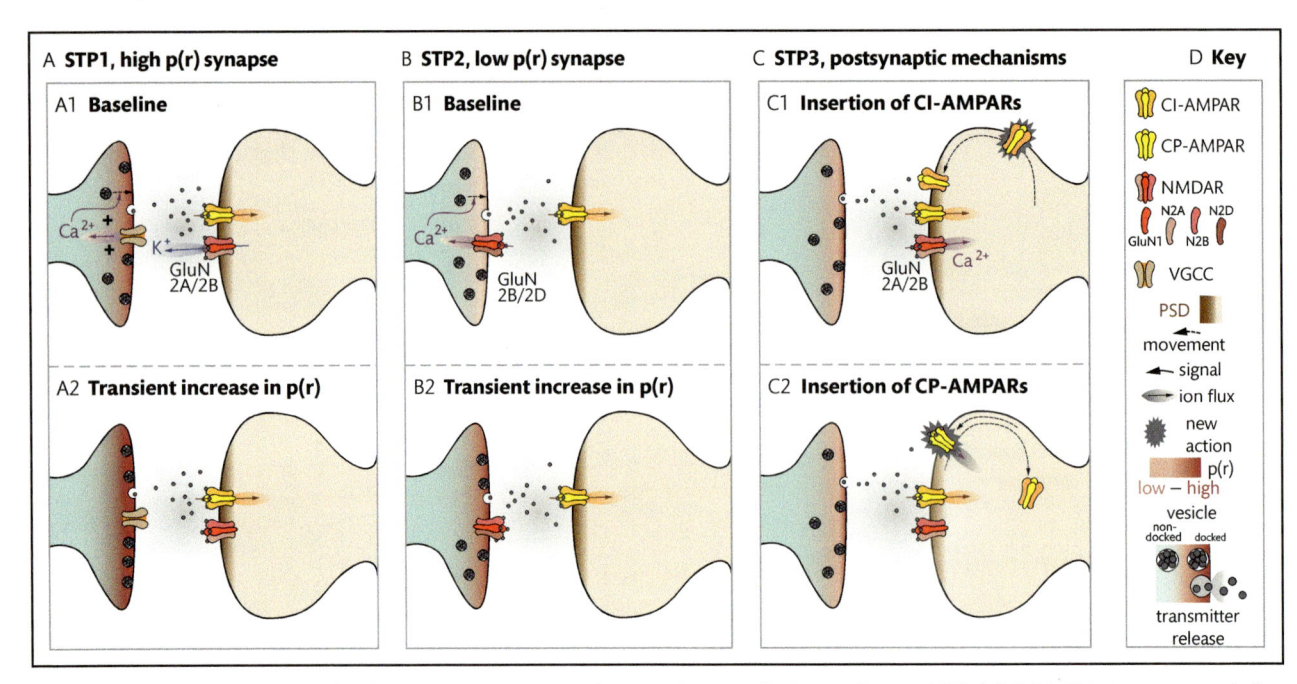

Figure 10.3 Short-term potentiation (STP). The schematic depicts three mechanistically distinct forms of STP. (A) STP1. This is a presynaptic form of STP that is expressed by an increase in p(r) and requires activation of GluN2A- and GluN2B-containing NMDARs (potentially a heterotrimer). This form of STP may be preferentially expressed at high p(r) synapses and involves signaling of postsynaptic NMDAR activation via K⁺ efflux, leading to a depolarization of presynaptic terminals and associated local Ca²⁺ influx (see text). (B) STP2. This is also a presynaptic form of STP that is expressed as an increase in p(r) and requires activation of GluN2B- and GluN2D-containing NMDARs (potentially a heterotrimer). This form of STP may be preferentially expressed at low p(r) synapses and involves signaling via presynaptic NMDARs generating a local Ca²⁺ influx. In both cases it is likely that the Ca²⁺ transient leads to an increase in docked vesicles, such that the next action potential is associated with a higher p(r). (C) STP3. This constitutes a family of possible postsynaptic mechanisms. (C1) Depicted here is STP reflecting a transient increase in synaptic AMPARs resulting from the transient insertion of CI-AMPARs, via the action of a CaMK. (C2) Another possibility is the transient homoexchange of CP-AMPARs for CI-AMPARs. (D) Key of major components.

What triggers the increase in p(r) and how is this process reversed by activity? A strong hint comes from a study of posttetanic potentiation (PTP) at mossy fiber synapses where the tetanus leads to a buildup of the readily releasable pool (RRP) of vesicles. The enlarged RRP acts as a resource that remains undepleted until used and supports an increase in p(r) until continuing stimulation depletes the RRP back to resting levels (Vandael et al., 2020). A resource-based mechanism of this sort is likely to support STP. A key question pertains to the functions of STP. Because STP affects p(r), it alters the dynamics within a burst discharge, whereas LTP, in cases where its expression is purely postsynaptic, scales all responses equally (Volianskis, Collingridge, et al., 2013; and see Box 10.1). The balance between these two modes of expression will affect the transmission of information through networks. Because STP does not decay until afferent activity occurs, it has the potential to store memories of the kind that are needed to hold information for a variable but indefinite time, and which can then, after recall, be safely deleted—for example, where I parked my car when I arrived at work this morning. This type of working memory is arguably accessed more often than the lifelong memories that LTP has the potential to deliver.

In addition to the presynaptic forms of STP, there is also evidence that a postsynaptic mechanism involving AMPARs can underlie some types of STP. For example, the transient movement of Ca²⁺-impermeable AMPARs (CI-AMPARs) into and out of the synapse could result in an enhanced response. The rapid movement of AMPARs between synaptic and perisynaptic sites can affect the amplitude of synaptic currents by enabling a rapid exchange of AMPARs that are in the desensitized and nondesensitized states. Such an effect limits the activity-dependent depression of AMPAR-mediated EPSCs during high-frequency trains (Heine et al., 2008; Constals et al., 2015). However, this desensitization-based mechanism is unlikely to impact STP at SCC-CA1 synapses, where both the rate of baseline stimulation and the average p(r) are low. Another potential postsynaptic mechanism for STP is the transient synaptic insertion of Ca²⁺-permeable AMPARs (CP-AMPARs); indeed, a homo-exchange with CI-AMPARs followed by a reverse homo-exchange would result in a transient synaptic enhancement due to the larger single-channel conductance of CP-AMPARs (Park, Georgiou, et al., 2021). Here, we refer to transient postsynaptic changes as STP3. By virtue of the likely equal scaling of all synaptic responses, STP3 will not alter the dynamics within a burst in the same manner as STP1 and STP2.

In conclusion, the relative contributions of STP1, STP2, and STP3 to the total STP will depend on the induction protocols and will affect the temporal dynamics of potentiation differently.

10.2.1.2 Long-term potentiation (LTP)

The role of the NMDAR

The biophysical properties of the NMDAR provide the hallmark features of this form of LTP: input specificity, cooperativity, and associativity. It also underpins the Hebbian nature of LTP, requiring the conjunction of presynaptic and postsynaptic activity for its activation (see first edition, pp 357–358). NMDARs comprise multiple subtypes, and recent work has identified a heterotrimeric subtype comprising GluN1, GluN2A. and GluN2B subunits as the major subtype involved in the induction of LTP in both adult (Volianskis, Bannister, et al., 2013) and juvenile postnatal day 14 (P14) rats (France et al., 2017).

Induction protocols

LTP can be readily induced by a small number of appropriately timed stimuli—the optimal timing being brief high-frequency bursts with an interburst interval within the theta range. Typically, 5–10 stimuli are used to trigger a weak LTP. These parameters require stimulating multiple fibers to exceed the cooperativity threshold (the minimum stimulus strength required to elicit LTP) and to mimic the synchronized firing that is seen in the freely exploring animal. If a single neuron is recorded from, then a single input may be sufficient to induce LTP, if the cooperativity requirement is met by depolarizing the neuron artificially. Also, in the latter case, HFS is no longer required to provide the depolarization to alleviate the Mg^{2+} block of NMDARs and some components of LTP can be induced by pairing artificial depolarization with basal frequency stimulation (see Box 10.1). NMDARs can also be triggered by appropriately timed pre- and postsynaptic action potentials that similarly reduce the Mg^{2+} block as NMDARs are being activated (for more details, see Bliss et al., 2018).

An important early discovery by the Magdeburg group (Frey et al., 1988) showed that multiple spaced induction protocols can induce a stronger LTP than a single period of induction (see Bliss et al., 2018). It is now established that the critical factor is the timing between the episodes and that the optimal timing is in the order of minutes. When the episodes are delivered close together (compressed), or when a continuous train is used, the resulting LTP is usually independent of protein synthesis (LTP1). In contrast, when spacing in the order of minutes is employed (10–20 min is optimal) there is an additional component that requires de novo protein synthesis (LTP2; see Figure 10.4). The third component, LTP3, defined by its dependence on transcription, likely involves the same induction protocols as LTP2.

The role of GABAergic inhibition

A key regulator in the induction of LTP is the potentially powerful suppression exerted by GABA-mediated synaptic inhibition. This is partly due to the increase in conductance, which will act to limit the local depolarization produced by an excitatory postsynaptic current EPSC, but the predominant factor is the hyperpolarizing influence that will intensify the voltage-dependent Mg^{2+} block. GABA is often blocked pharmacologically in experiments, and indeed in some cases, such as LTP at the MPP in vitro, this is a requisite for the efficient induction of LTP. Regulation by GABA-mediated synaptic inhibition plays a crucial physiological role in LTP, as discussed in the first edition (pp 361–363).

The role of tyrosine phosphorylation

The induction of LTP is strongly influenced by the tyrosine phosphorylation of NMDARs (YM Lu et al., 1998; Y-Q Huang et al., 2001; Rajani et al., 2021). In brief, c-Src potentiates NMDAR currents and thereby regulates the induction of LTP. This nonreceptor tyrosine kinase is anchored within the NMDAR complex by ND2 (NADH dehydrogenase subunit 2), a mitochondrial-encoded protein that is part of the NADH ubiquinone oxidoreductase complex I, which binds to both the GluN1 subunit and c-Src. Note that c-Src also binds to postsynaptic density 95 (PSD-95), which regulates its catalytic activity. Another member of the Src-family kinases (SFKs), Fyn, also potentiates NMDAR currents via an action on GluN2 subunits. Fyn is held in proximity to GluN2 subunits, since these proteins bind to different PDZ (PSD-95/Disc large/Zonula occludens-1) domains on PSD-95.

A variety of intracellular modulators of c-Src activity, which include CAKβ/Pyk2, C-terminal Src Kinase (CSK), H-Ras, and PTPα, can regulate LTP. Particularly notable is STEP (striatal-enriched protein tyrosine phosphatase), which regulates the activity of SFKs. A variety of transmembrane receptors can also modulate c-Src and/or Fyn activity and thereby regulate the induction of LTP. For example, stimulation of insulin receptors (IRs), by insulin, can potentiate NMDARs via activation of c-Src, whereas stimulation of EphB4 receptors, by neuroligin 1, can inhibit NMDARs via inhibition of c-Src. Other important regulators of synaptic plasticity affect NMDAR function via regulation of Fyn, such as BDNF acting on TrkB receptors.

Additionally, G-protein-coupled receptors (GPCRs) regulate NMDAR function using SFKs via several mechanisms. For example, activation of group II mGluRs in the hippocampus potentiates NMDARs via c-Src-mediated phosphorylation of GluN2A, and activation of dopamine D1 receptors in the hippocampus potentiates NMDARs via Fyn-mediated phosphorylation of GluN2B. These forms of regulation seem to involve CSK. Additionally, other forms of positive regulation of NMDARs by, for example, M1 muscarinic acetylcholine receptors and group I mGluRs operate via CAKβ/Pyk2 regulation of c-Src.

Any regulation of NMDAR function would be predicted to affect the induction of LTP in the hippocampus. Indeed, in several situations, manipulation of SFK signaling has been observed to regulate synaptic plasticity and metaplasticity. For example, activation of pituitary adenylate cyclase-activating polypeptide type I receptor (PACAP-R1/PAC1R) and dopamine D1 receptor had differential effects on the crossover frequency between LTP and LTD (K Yang et al., 2012). Adding further diversity to the regulation of NMDARs, the GluN1 subunit has multiple splice variants which can influence the induction of LTP. Notably, alternative splicing of *Grin1* exon 5 affects the magnitude of LTP and its regulation by c-Src-dependent phosphorylation (Li et al., 2024).

The role of Ca²⁺-permeable AMPARs (CP-AMPARs)

In a pivotal study, the Roder lab constitutively deleted the GluA2 subunit of AMPARs, rendering the receptor Ca^{2+}-permeable and demonstrated an NMDAR-independent form of LTP that is additive with NMDAR-LTP (see Gugustea and Jia, 2021). Subsequently, a role for CP-AMPARs in LTP in wild-type rodents was observed, but it initially proved controversial (for references see P Park et al., 2018). Some clarity was provided with the demonstration that CP-AMPARs are required for the induction of LTP2 but not LTP1 (P Park et al., 2016; P Park et al., 2018). Based on earlier studies using GluA2 knockout (KO) mice, it seems likely that CP-AMPARs trigger LTP2, via activation of PI3K and the MAPK cascade (Asrar, Zhou, et al., 2009). In wild-type animals CP-AMPARs work in concert with NMDARs via a multistep induction mechanism (see Figure 10.4 for details). It should also be noted that the role of CP-AMPARs in LTP is subject to developmental regulation. At around

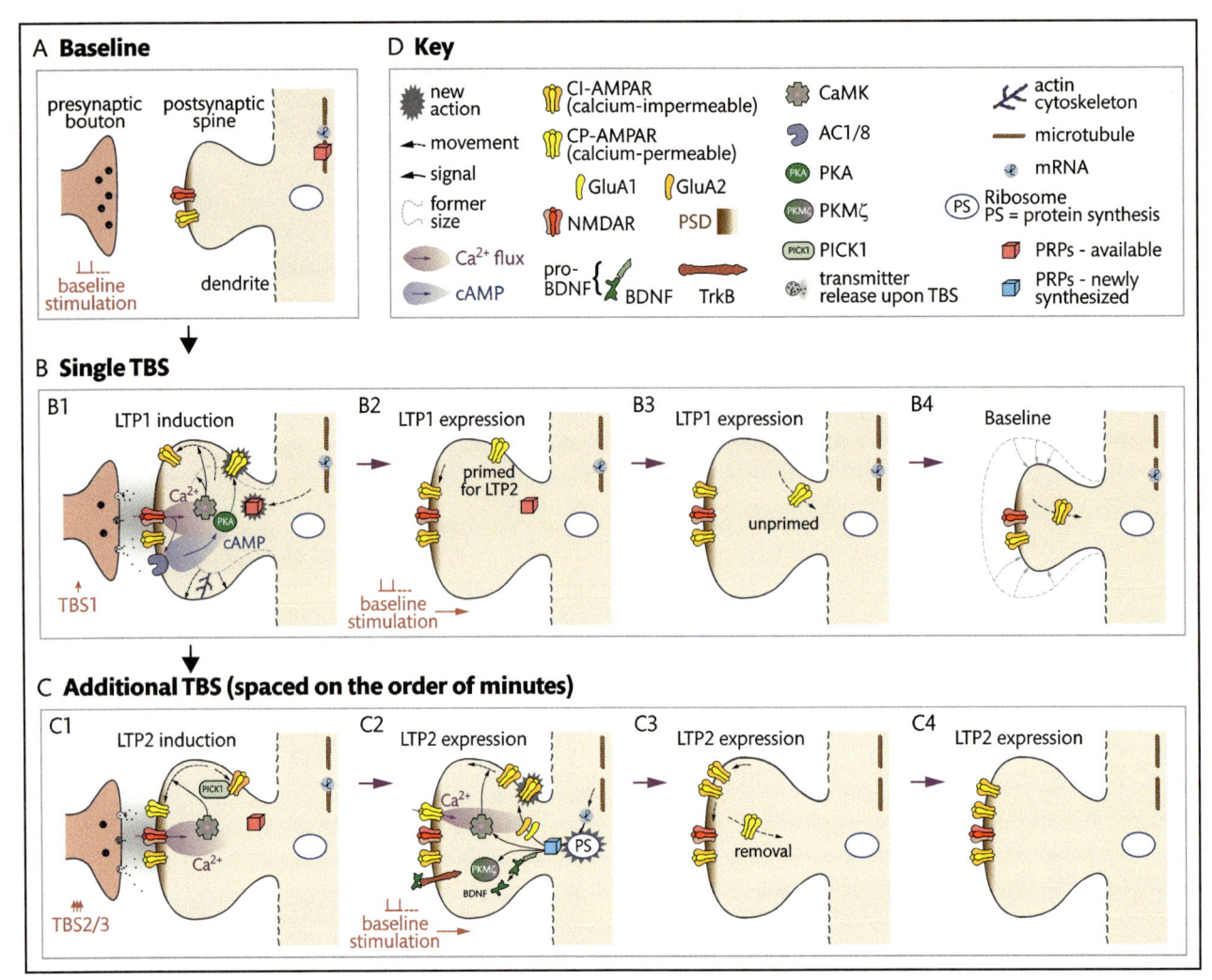

Figure 10.4 Long-term potentiation (LTP). The schematic depicts two mechanistically distinct forms of LTP (LTP1 and LTP2). (A) A schematic of a synapse comprising a presynaptic bouton and a postsynaptic spine that contains NMDARs and AMPARs, one of each is shown here. (B) LTP1. (B1) The induction stimulus (here shown as a single TBS) activates NMDARs. Ca^{2+} flux through these receptors triggers a CaMK, here CaMKII, which drives AMPARs into the synapse to enhance the synaptic response, via exocytosis and lateral diffusion. The increase in these GluA2-containing, and hence Ca^{2+}-impermeable (CI) AMPARs, may be associated with spine growth, presumably utilizing stored components. The NMDAR-associated Ca^{2+} flux also activates AC (1 and/or 8), which generates cAMP to activate PKA. PKA drives Ca^{2+}-permeable (CP) AMPARs into a perisynaptic site. (B2) LTP1 is expressed by the greater number of CI-AMPARs. The CP-AMPARs reside at the perisynaptic site, too far away to be activated by transmitter release (not shown) and so cannot contribute to the synaptic response. Rather, they *prime* the synapse for LTP2. B3. After time (tens of minutes) the CI-AMPARs are removed from the perisynaptic region, so that the synapse is no longer *primed*. (B4) After a variable period of time (that can last min or h) the synaptic response returns to baseline. (C) LTP2. (C1) If one or more TBS are delivered while the synapse is *primed*, then the perisynaptic CP-AMPARs are driven by a CaMK into the synapses, where they increase the size of the synaptic response. A one-to-one homoexchange, involving the coordinated actions of a CaMK and PICK1, increases the synaptic response due to the greater single channel conductance of CP-AMPARs. (C2) Continued activation of CP-AMPARs, during baseline stimulation, generates a Ca^{2+} signal that triggers protein synthesis. Among the many rapidly translated proteins, additional AMPAR subunits, signaling components such as BDNF, CaMKII, and PKMζ, and structural components are likely generated and required for LTP2 expression. (C3) The synaptic insertion of CP-AMPARs is only transient, and these are replaced with CI-AMPARs (with a greater number to maintain the potentiation). (C4) The enhanced spine size and additional AMPARs can persist for a long time, though transcription and additional rounds of protein synthesis are likely required (i.e., LTP3). Note that LTP also involves presynaptic changes (see Box 10.1). (D) Key of major components.

P14, a protocol that would be expected to induce LTP1 in adult animals generates an LTP that requires the activation of CP-AMPARs (J Sanderson et al., 2016).

The expression of LTP

The locus and mechanisms of expression of LTP were discussed in depth in the first edition (pp 376–383), and here we present an update (see Box 10.1). Importantly, many of the earlier controversies have been explained on the basis of multiple forms of LTP that are differentially engaged according to the protocols used (Bliss and Collingridge, 2013).

LTP1

A vast body of evidence suggests that LTP1 is triggered by the NMDAR-associated Ca^{2+} flux that activates CaMKs, notably CaMKII, which in turn triggers exocytosis of AMPARs. The insertion of AMPARs into the plasma membrane probably occurs at sites near, but outside, the postsynaptic density (PSD) and is rapidly

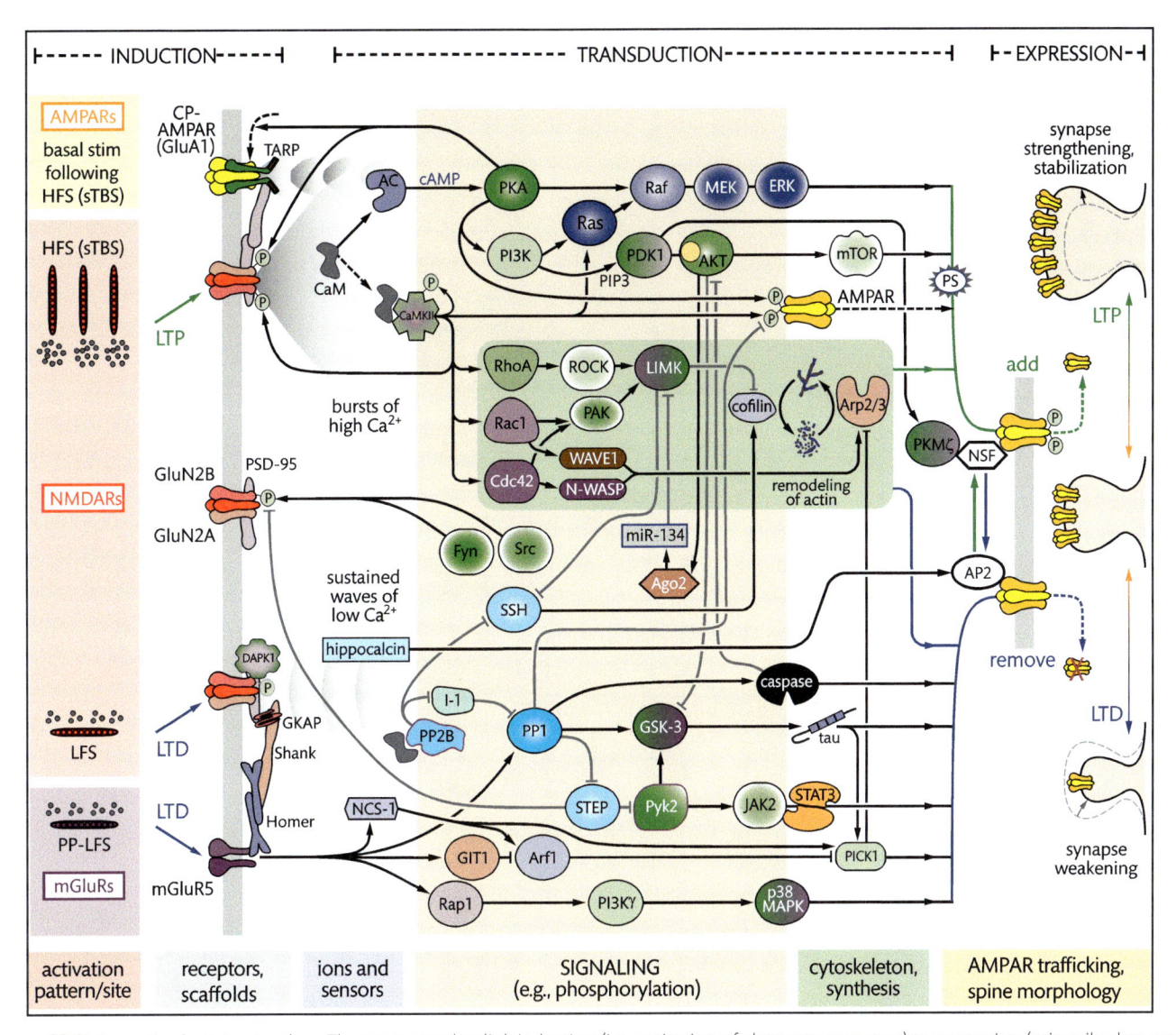

Figure 10.5 Synaptic plasticity signaling. The processes that link induction (i.e., activation of glutamate receptors) to expression (primarily changes in AMPAR number and associated alterations in spine volume) are extremely complex. This figure shows a subset of the molecules and pathways that are known to be involved.

followed by the lateral diffusion of AMPARs from these perisynaptic sites into the PSD, where they become anchored to scaffolding proteins, in particular PSD-95 (see first edition, pp 377–381). A variety of other proteins including SAP97 (synapse-associated protein 97), AKAP79/150 (A-kinase anchoring protein 79/150), certain TARPs (transmembrane AMPAR regulatory proteins), γ2 and γ8 (J Watson et al., 2021), cornichon family homologues (Zhang et al., 2021), and regulatory processes, such as palmitoylation, are involved in the trafficking and anchoring of AMPARs (see Hansen et al., 2021; Matt et al., 2019; Sumi and Harada, 2020; Nowacka et al., 2024). Intracellular trafficking involves vesicular transport along microtubules and actin filaments followed by regulated exocytosis, via a soluble-NSF-attachment protein receptor (SNARE)-dependent mechanism (Jurado et al., 2013; Bin et al., 2018) that utilizes synaptotagmin 1 and 7 as the Ca²⁺ sensor (Sumi and Harada, 2020). Simplified schematics of some of the trafficking steps involved in LTP are presented in Figures 10.5 and 10.6.

One area of recent debate has been the role of specific AMPAR subunits in LTP. Early work identified proteins that interact with GluA1 as crucial for LTP and implicated the direct phosphorylation of GluA1 at Ser831 on the C-terminal tail as a key regulatory step (see first edition, pp 381–382). Subsequently, it was shown that LTP can be generated in a manner that is independent of the AMPAR subtype and indeed can be induced in the absence of AMPARs altogether (Granger et al., 2013), the notion being that CaMKII activity drives vesicle fusion independent of the cargo, although this would ordinarily be AMPARs. This controversy was directly addressed using mice in which the C-terminal tails of GluA1 and GluA2 had been interchanged. This latter study reinforced the view that the C-terminal tail of the GluA1 subunit is important for LTP (Zhou et al., 2018), although it is possible to induce LTP under certain circumstances in the absence of the GluA1 C-terminal tail (Liu et al., 2020). These studies further attest to the complexity and adaptability of LTP. A reasonable conclusion is that while subunit-dependent mechanisms are generally involved in LTP, these processes can be bypassed under certain experimental conditions. Whether such conditions are physiological or not is unknown. More recently, detailed structural information using cryogenic

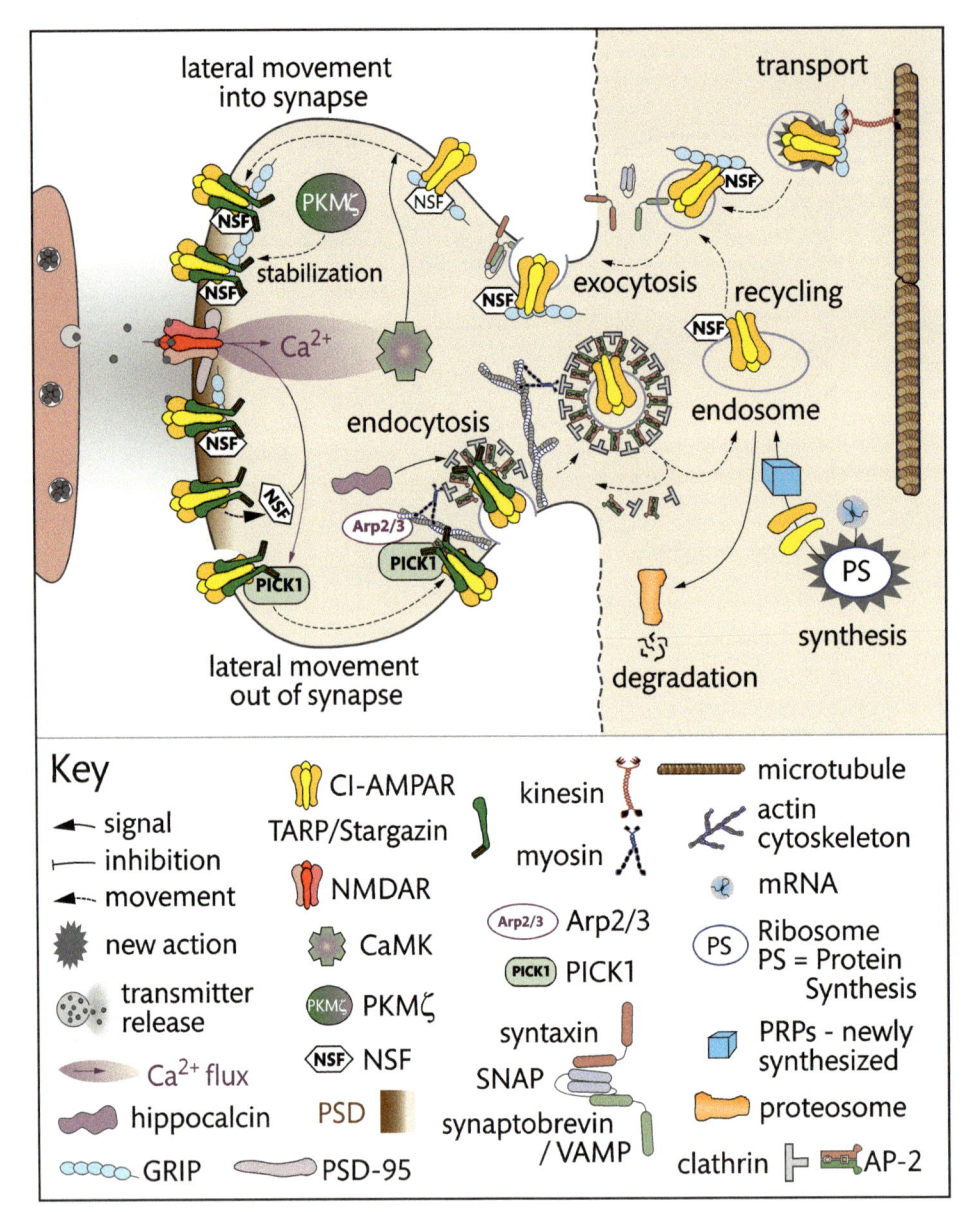

Figure 10.6 Postsynaptic expression mechanisms. A simplified scheme of AMPAR trafficking in NMDAR-LTP and -LTD. During LTP, the NMDAR-mediated Ca^{2+} signal drives exocytosis of AMPARs, via a SNARE-dependent mechanism. AMPARs are then stabilized at the synapse by the binding of NSF to the GluA2 subunit, a reaction promoted by PKMζ. During LTD, AP-2 displaces NSF to drive clathrin-dependent endocytosis of AMPARs. LTP and LTD are regulated by different Ca^{2+} sensors: synaptobrevin/VAMP and hippocalcin, respectively. Another Ca^{2+} sensor, PICK1 helps coordinate endocytosis and cytoskeletal adjustments. Once internalized, AMPARs can either be recycled or degraded.

electron microscopy (cryo-EM) is starting to explain in precise molecular terms how the different AMPAR subunits confer the distinct physiological properties of AMPARs that may underlie their roles in synaptic plasticity (Zhang et al., 2023).

The importance of AMPAR mobility and stabilization at the synapse followed the discovery that NSF (N-ethylmaleimide sensitive fusion protein) binds directly to the C-terminal tail of the GluA2 subunit: preventing this interaction leads to a rapid reduction in synaptic transmission over a time course of minutes. The inhibition is partial (~50%), implying that there are both mobile and anchored pools of AMPARs at the synapse. Although the mobile fraction of AMPARs is normally stabilized by the binding of NSF to the GluA2 subunit, this interaction can be inhibited to allow adaptor protein 2 (AP2) to bind and trigger endocytosis. This process is regulated by Ca^{2+} sensors, such as hippocalcin (see the first edition for details).

More recently direct evidence has been provided that the surface diffusion of AMPARs is necessary for LTP (Getz et al., 2022). It should be noted that regulated AMPAR trafficking could apply to both LTP1 and, as discussed below, LTP2. The extent to which LTP1 and LTP2 engage the same molecular mechanism of AMPAR trafficking has not been elucidated.

There is also evidence for an involvement of presynaptic expression of LTP1. Notably, an optical quantal analysis applied to acute hippocampal slices identified synapses where the LTP, measured 30–60 min after induction, could largely, and in some cases entirely, be explained by an increase in p(r) (see Enoki et al., 2009). Determining the factors that reflect distinct pre- vs. postsynaptic mechanisms of expression of LTP1 remains a challenge.

Finally, a rapid increase in spine size has been observed in the presence of blockers of de novo protein synthesis (Tanaka et al.,

2008), suggesting that LTP1 may, at least under certain conditions, be associated with structural changes. Hypothetically, preassembled PRPs may enable a rapid increase in the size of both boutons and spines to provide space for more docked vesicles and AMPARs, respectively. However, this increased size may not be stable over time as LTP1 decays to baseline.

LTP2

The locus of expression of LTP2 has been less intensively studied. However, current evidence points to a stable increase in the size of synapses (see Box 10.2 on structural plasticity) and accordingly most likely corresponds to functional changes on both side of the synapse (see Bliss and Collingridge, 2013). As described above, its defining feature is the requirement for de novo protein synthesis. This is accompanied by an increase in protein degradation (Fonseca et al., 2006), resulting in a rapid increase in protein turnover.

In terms of postsynaptic alterations, it has been shown that LTP2, but not LTP1, is associated with a transient increase in single-channel conductance reflecting the insertion of CP-AMPARs (Park, Georgiou, et al., 2021). It is likely that these replace existing synaptic CI-AMPARs via a 1:1 exchange and that this is driven by a process dependent on protein interacting with C kinase 1 (PICK1; see Terashima et al., 2008; Y Yang et al., 2010). The increase in synaptic conductance that CP-AMPARs confer can contribute to the initial expression of short-term potentiation (STP), but the inserted CP-AMPARs are rapidly replaced by CI-AMPARs. Moreover, a 1:1 exchange would result in a decrease in response size, which is generally not seen. It is likely therefore that the removal of CP-AMPARs is associated with the insertion of a greater number of CI-AMPARs. As LTP is probably associated with a rapid increase in spine size (Y Yang et al., 2010) it seems plausible that this growth creates more space to accommodate the increased number of CI-AMPARs.

The insertion of CP-AMPARs is probably a two-step process, along the following lines. In response to the first episode of a spaced-induction protocol, CP-AMPARs are inserted into a perisynaptic site driven by the phosphorylation of Ser845 by PKA. In response to subsequent episodes, these CP-AMPARs are driven into the synapse via an additional phosphorylation step that probably involves CaMKs, such as CaMKII or CaMKK/CaMKI (Guire et al., 2008). Both PKA and CaMKII are necessary for LTP2 and in combination are sufficient for LTP2 (P Park, Georgiou, et al., 2021). The dwell time of the CP-AMPARs at perisynaptic sites, which is on the order of minutes, probably explains the timing requirements of the spaced-induction protocol.

In this scenario, the first episode of HFS can be considered a priming stimulus or tag for LTP2. NMDARs activate CaMKII to trigger LTP1 and also activate PKA, via adenylyl cyclase 1 and/or 8 (AC1/8) and cAMP (cyclic adenosine monophosphate), to prime for LTP2. With subsequent episodes NMDARs further activate CaMK to drive the perisynaptic CP-AMPARs into the synapse. Once inserted into the synapse, CP-AMPARs need to be activated, typically via basal stimulation. Consequently, if stimulation is paused during this time, LTP2 is not produced and only the residual LTP1, which is not sensitive to lack of stimulation, remains. The stimulation of CP-AMPARs is required to provide a Ca^{2+} flux into the synapse (Morita et al., 2014). Why then the need for two Ca^{2+} sources—NMDARs and CP-AMPARs? The most likely explanation is that these receptors provide highly localized Ca^{2+} signals and that within these nanodomains different enzymes are activated. In the

case of NMDARs this includes CaM, which activates Ca^{2+}-sensitive AC isoforms (AC1 and/or AC8) and CaMKs, such as CaMKII. NMDARs, via these enzymes, control AMPAR insertion, and, additionally, contribute to initiating the alterations in translation and, for LTP3, transcription. CP-AMPARs in contrast may trigger protein synthesis by activating PI3K and MAPK (Asrar, Zhou, et al., 2009). So why has this seemingly convoluted mechanism evolved when LTP1 is generated much more simply? The likely answer is that CP-AMPARs are exploited by the neuron to encode the effects of spaced-induction protocols that trigger translation and transcription. Significantly, it is well established that spaced learning is more effective than massed (i.e., compressed) learning (Cepeda et al., 2006). Additionally, CP-AMPARs may also be part of the mechanism by which heterosynaptic LTP is triggered, thereby further increasing the strength or duration of the potentiation (Park, Kang, et al., 2019).

A growth in spines to accommodate more AMPARs is sufficient to explain the postsynaptic component of LTP2, provided that the AMPARs remain anchored. AMPARs are highly mobile in the plasma membrane unless anchored to PSD proteins (Nowacka et al., 2024). Anchoring is regulated by a number of mechanisms. Notably, as mentioned above, accessory subunits of the AMPAR, such as γ2 and γ8, bind tightly to PSD-95 and may regulate their diffusion and trafficking within the postsynaptic density. The accessory subunits are themselves regulated by phosphorylation by CaMKII and other kinases.

Interestingly, around the time of the first edition (see p 393), Todd Sacktor and colleagues demonstrated that protein kinase M ζ (PKMζ) activity is necessary to maintain LTP by using a peptide inhibitor, zeta inhibitory peptide (ZIP), that reversed established LTP. During LTP2, PKMζ is rapidly translated from dendritically located mRNA and, because it lacks a regulatory domain, is persistently active in regulating synaptic AMPAR function until it is degraded. Regulation involves the stabilization of the GluA2-NSF interaction by PKMζ (Yao et al., 2008). A seeming controversy arose when it was found that LTP could still be induced in mice lacking PKMζ and that ZIP remained effective at reversing preestablished LTP, indicating a nonspecific action of this inhibitor (Volk et al., 2013). However, it was then demonstrated that in PKMζ knockout (KO) mice there is compensation by the closely related PKMι/λ and that in wild-type mice the actions of ZIP are specific to PKMζ (Tsokas et al., 2016).

Another kinase that has also been extensively investigated in the context of a "memory molecule" is CaMKII, which can autophosphorylate to maintain a persistent active state (Lisman, 2017). CaMKII can regulate synaptic plasticity by virtue of its enzymatic activity and through its role as a structural molecule in the synapse, a role described in more detail in section 10.2.4. The relative roles of these two actions remains controversial (Tullis et al., 2023; Claiborne et al., 2024; see review by Nicoll and Schulman, 2023), though it may depend on the type of LTP under investigation.

A detailed discussion on the relative merits of CaMKII and PKMζ as memory molecules is presented elsewhere (Bear et al., 2018). Suffice it to say that both kinases seem to be important cogs in the wheel that drive AMPARs into the synapse and help keep them there. Since constitutively active PKMζ is a key component of this process, it provides a potential way to mark potentiated synapses (Hsieh et al., 2021). In summary, rather than searching for a memory molecule, more insight is likely to be gained by thinking

Box 10.2 Structural plasticity

In this box we consider activity-dependent structural changes associated with LTP and LTD (often referred to as sLTP and sLTD) in those two remarkable biological micromachines, the presynaptic bouton and the postsynaptic dendritic spine. Excitatory synapses in the hippocampus are found almost exclusively on dendritic spines, complex microstructures with a narrow stalk (maximum length less than 2 μm) and a bulbous head (maximum volume of less than 0.05 μm³ (Kashiwagi et al., 2019), with a specialized area, the postsynaptic density (PSD), facing the presynaptic bouton. The PSD is a dense protein mat that floats on the lipid bilayer enclosing the interior of the spine head (Zeng et al., 2018) and supports a population of many hundreds of different proteins, including glutamate receptors and the auxiliary proteins that anchor receptors to scaffolding proteins in the spine head (Broadhead et al., 2016; R Frank et al., 2016). The complex molecular machinery enclosed within the spine head (Murakoshi and Yasuda, 2012) is responsible for transducing the chemical signal received from the presynaptic terminal into the excitatory current that is injected through the spine shaft to influence the moment-to-moment excitability of the parent neuron.

Structural changes in dendritic spines and synaptic boutons associated with LTP and LTD

A question that was raised early in the study of synaptic plasticity was whether LTP is accompanied by an increase in the size of potentiated synapses. Early ultrastructural studies revealed that spines on distal dendrites of granule cells in animals in which the perforant path had been tetanized were larger than in control animals at time points up to 24 h after tetanization; no changes were seen in spines on nontetanized proximal dendrites (Van Harreveld and Fifkova, 1975; Desmond and Levy, 1983). A study of Golgi-stained material from control and potentiated tissue suggested that LTP is accompanied by new spines rather than bigger spines (Trommald et al., 1996). The issue was revisited in a serial-section EM study by Bourne and Harris (2011), who compared spines in potentiated and control tissue and found an increase in the number of large spines, and a decrease in the number of small spines on CA1 pyramidal cells 2 h after the induction of LTP. A follow-up study reported a corresponding reduction in the number of small synaptic boutons in potentiated tissue (Bourne et al., 2013). This set of results is consistent with a shift toward larger spines following the induction of LTP, without a change in the number of spines. Engert and Bonhoeffer (1999) examined changes in the size and number of a visualized population of spines in organotypic cultures before and after the induction of LTP. The experimental design restricted synaptic transmission to a small region of dendrite on a dye-filled CA1 neuron. Pairing-induced LTP was followed, usually after a delay of a few minutes, by the appearance of one or more new spines, which remained in place for the duration of the experiment, in some cases several hours. This was the first direct evidence that plasticity might involve not only the Hebbian enhancement of the efficacy of existing synapses but also the generation of new synapses. The same laboratory later showed that LTD at SCC-CA1 synapses was associated with the retraction of spines (Nägerl et al., 2004) and a delayed reduction in the number of SCC bouton-spine pairs on CA1 pyramidal cells (Becker et al., 2008).

The introduction of 4-methoxy-7-nitroindolinyl (MNI)-caged glutamate (MNI-Glu), from which glutamate can be released by a laser pulse of the appropriate frequency, made it possible to induce localized "gluLTP" by releasing glutamate over a single spine on a CA1 pyramidal cell filled with the fluorescent dye eGFP to allow the dimension of the spine to be monitored. At the same time the amplitude of the electrical response in the soma to the release of a single pulse of glutamate at the spine of interest was monitored (Matsuzaki et al., 2004). This technical tour de force established that glu-LTP of the electrical response in CA1 pyramidal cells was accompanied by a rapid enlargement of the spine. The effect was transient in larger spines, but long-lasting in smaller spines. Both spine enlargement and the enhanced electrical response in the soma declined over a few minutes to a smaller, maintained increase. These results were confirmed and extended by C. Harvey et al. (2008) in hippocampal pyramidal cells in organotypic culture. Changes to the presynaptic bouton could not be assessed with this approach, and the artificial nature of the

stimulus, in which the presynaptic bouton is not invaded by an action potential, makes it difficult to assess its physiological relevance. The first problem was addressed in a combined uncaging and EM study by Meyer et al. (2014), who reported that when uncaged glutamate was used to enhance spine size, the presynaptic bouton was also enlarged in those cases where there was a permanent change in spine size. A persistent expansion in spine size, confined to the zone of potentiation, was also noted in experiments in which TBS was used to induce LTP (X Wang et al., 2008; Y Yang et al., 2008). Further work is required to resolve the nature of the link between LTP and spine enlargement, particularly in adult animals. The bulk of evidence suggests that LTP goes hand in hand with an increase in the size of spines, only a proportion of which show a persistent increase, accompanied in the latter case by a corresponding enlargement of the presynaptic bouton (Meyer et al., 2014) and, in the late phase of LTP, by an increase in vesicle numbers (Y Sun et al., 2021). An increase in multi-innervated spines has also been noted in LTP (Giese et al., 2015; McLeod et al., 2020). Insights into how the shape and release apparatus of the presynaptic bouton is influenced by active expansion of the postsynaptic spine has come from Ucar et al. (2021). This study revealed that the expansion of the spine head following localized uncaging of glutamate leads to a mechanical interaction with the expanded presynaptic bouton resulting in an increase in actin polymerization and assembly of SNARE proteins at the terminal, and an increase in presynaptic glutamate release that could be sustained for at least 20 min. Given that the growth of spines following glutamate uncaging is often temporary, a mechanical linkage may be required to keep pre- and postsynaptic sides of the synapse in correspondence, provided perhaps by adhesion or other molecules that bridge the synaptic divide. Perhaps this linkage remains when the physical specializations of bouton and spine disappear, accounting for the apparent loss and gain of synapses that has been observed by many during sLTP and sLTD and that seems so counterintuitive from a Hebbian perspective.

Two groups have used correlated light and electron microscopy to examine LTP-associated formation of new spines and boutons on CA1 pyramidal cells in organotypic hippocampal cultures. Nägerl et al. (2007) found that new spines are formed following the induction of LTP. These rapidly (within an hour) make contact with existing presynaptic boutons, but do not develop into mature synapses for several more hours. These structural changes cannot explain changes in synaptic efficacy occurring immediately or shortly after induction. In contrast, Y. Sun et al. (2021) found that the induction of LTP led to a rapid and maintained increase in the structural complexity of the PSD on existing spines, an increase in the length of the apposition between spine and bouton, and a delayed increase in vesicle number. A combination of rapid structural changes on existing spines followed by a slower reorganization involving new spines and rewiring of boutons could accommodate both sets of findings, although perforation of existing spines would be the only way to modify connectivity within an Hebbian framework.

Mechanisms underlying changes in spine size

As with the induction and/or expression of LTP, changes in spine size are NMDAR-dependent (Matsuzaki et al., 2004), and require PKA activation (Y Yang et al., 2008), CaMKII (K Kim et al., 2015), and protein synthesis (Govindarajan et al., 2011; Heumüller et al., 2019). Moreover, the cytoskeletal changes underlying the persistent increase in spine volume that can follow the induction of LTP are beginning to be identified (see reviews by Bosch et al., 2014; Nakahata and Yasuda, 2018). The basic structure of the spine is determined by its network of actin filaments. In a stable spine, the network is in a state of dynamic equilibrium in which molecules of globular G-actin are removed from the tail of a filament of F-actin at the same rate at which they are added to its head, a process known as treadmilling. Accessory actin-binding proteins, including cofilin, further stabilize the network. Following the induction of LTP, cofilin dissociates from F-actin, and the equilibrium established by treadmilling is broken, with G-actin added only at the head of the F-actin filaments, which tend to be oriented toward the periphery. This leads to a peripheral extension of the F-actin network and a consequent increase in spine volume (see Nakahata and Yasuda, 2018).

Box 10.2 Continued

A novel pathway for regulating sLTP involving release of Ca^{2+} from dendritic lysosomes by backpropagating dendritic action potentials has been described by Padamsey et al. (2017). Release of Ca^{2+} leads to fusion of the lysosome with the dendritic membrane and release of Cathepsin B into the extracellular space, stimulating matrix metalloproteinase 9 and extracellular matrix remodeling. Inhibition of this process suppresses activity-related spine growth.

Evidence that sLTP is necessary for hippocampus-dependent learning has been supplied by Hayashi and colleagues, who developed a genetically encoded, light-sensitive method for dismantling cofilactin, the macromolecule formed when cofilin binds with actin during spine enlargement (Goto et al., 2021). Mice were engineered to express a fusion protein, CFL-SN, consisting of cofilin fused to a light-sensitive protein, SuperNova, which when illuminated with yellow light generates reactive oxygen species that inactivate the protein to which it fused. In vitro experiments confirmed that LTP in mutant mice was abolished by exposure of the slice to light, without affecting the ability to generate LTP in the same pathway subsequently. sLTP, induced by uncaging MNI-glutamate, was reversed by activation of CFL-SN. There was no effect of uncaging before or, surprisingly, more than ~30 min after the induction of LTP, suggesting that sLTP underpins only the initial phase of LTP (see also Matsuzaki et al., 2004). Performance in a hippocampus-dependent inhibitory-avoidance learning task was impaired by light-activation of CFL-SN in the dorsal hippocampus, when the light was given up to 20 min after one-trial learning, but not before or at longer intervals.

Spine dynamics in behaving animals

Evidence that learning can lead to changes in spine number is best documented in motor cortex, where it is easier to monitor the growth and shrinkage of spines in dye-filled cells for long periods in behaving animals (T Xu et al., 2009; G Yang et al., 2009; Ma et al., 2015). Even here, little is known about the growth of axons or axon collaterals that would be required to form functioning synapses on new spines. Less attention has been given to the structural correlates of LTD, but reductions in spine size have been reported following the induction of both LTD (Okamoto et al., 2004; Zhou et al., 2004) and DP (Y Yang et al., 2008).

While it has not so far been possible to follow the fate of individual spines in the hippocampus in the behaving animal, there is evidence from between-animal experiments that the size and density of spines on hippocampal engram cells can change following hippocampus-dependent learning. Several studies from the Tonegawa group have documented an increase in spine density in engram cells in the DG (i.e., granule cells expressing an immediate early gene after CFC, see Ryan et al., 2015; Roy et al., 2017). Using an ingenious modification of the GRASP technique, which allows synapses to be visualized by fusing two halves of the GFP protein to pre- and postsynaptically expressed proteins, Kaang and colleagues documented changes in the number and size of engram and non-engram CA3-CA1 synapses after CFC (J Choi et al., 2018; see also D Choi et al., 2021). CFC leads both to larger synapses, and to an increase in the number of synapses between engram CA3 and CA1 cells. Finally, as we have seen, it is likely that changes induced on one side of the synapse will be mirrored by corresponding changes on the other. There is thus good evidence that learning can lead to changes not only in the size but also the number of spines on engram neurons. What is less clear is how this relates to changes in connectivity. LTP-associated spinogenesis tends to occur in clusters (De Roo et al., 2008), and one possibility is that the new spines make multispine synapses with existing boutons, so that initially no new wiring is involved.

---

about a molecular memory process—a major part of which is regulated AMPAR trafficking (Figure 10.6).

LTP2 is characterized by its dependence on de novo protein synthesis, a process which is capable of producing proteins within a few minutes of induction. Many (>100) new protein products are rapidly translated from preexisting mRNAs (see Chapter 8), but the timing of their requirements is largely a matter of speculation. One scenario is as follows: preassembled CP-AMPARs are inserted into the membrane and their activation, along with NMDARs, is required to trigger de novo protein synthesis. Brain-derived neurotrophic factor (BDNF; see section 10.5.6) is rapidly synthesized and prevents the breakdown of PKMζ. This stabilizes the preexisting CI-AMPARs by favoring their interaction with NSF. Newly synthesized structural components, such as filamentous actin (F-actin), enable spine growth, and newly synthesized AMPAR subunits provide more CI-AMPARs for incorporation into these larger spines. Newly synthesized CaMKII drives the newly made AMPARs into the synapse and newly synthesized PKMζ helps keep them there (Panja and Bramham, 2014). BDNF may also signal to the presynaptic bouton to enable coordinated pre- and postsynaptic protein synthesis. Many other proteins are also newly synthesized to build and regulate the larger synapse, which may contain both more AMPARs and docked presynaptic vesicles, to increase p(r).

LTP3

LTP3, the most persistent form of LTP, is defined by its sensitivity to transcriptional inhibitors. Quite possibly, it is the continuation of LTP2, for which gene transcription is required to provide the necessary protein synthesis beyond that which occurs locally to generate LTP2. It has long been known that LTP is associated with the transcription of immediate early genes (IEGs), such as *Zif268* (zinc finger-containing transcription factor 268; also known as *Egr1*, early growth response protein 1, which encodes EGR-1) and *Arc/Arg3.1*, and that these IEGs are involved in LTP and LTD, though many aspects remain controversial (see Kyrke-Smith et al., 2021). It is also notable that engram cells are experimentally identified by the expression of IEGs and so it is LTP3, the least studied form of LTP, that may relate most closely to these memory modules. We included a detailed discussion of synapse to soma to synapse signaling in the first edition of this book (pp 388–393) and here provide only a brief summary and update.

One area of investigation has been to identify the factors that signal the induction of synaptic plasticity to the nucleus. There are several general categories of molecules that may serve this function. Activation of NMDARs generates a depolarization that will help activate somatic voltage-gated calcium channels (VGCCs) to trigger gene expression. Another candidate is cAMP, which is also required for LTP2 and is able to diffuse along dendrites. In principle, cAMP could initiate somatic signaling via EPAC and/or PKA to trigger gene expression, via activation of, for example, CREB. In addition to these features, cAMP is a likely candidate because the modulatory processes that promote learning and memory, such as dopamine and noradrenaline receptor-mediated signaling, activate this second messenger. Other mechanisms that have been suggested to invoke LTP3 include the translocation of signaling molecules, such as CaM and ERK, from synapse to nucleus.

The next step in the process of inducing LTP3 is the triggering of transcription factors, the first identified and best characterized of which is CREB, followed by inducible transcription factors, such as Zif268. Since these initial studies, a growing number of transcription factors have been associated with hippocampal LTP and related processes. These include c-fos, CRTC1 (CREB-regulated transcriptional coactivator 1), FOXP1 (forkhead box protein P1), junB, Mef2 (myocyte enhancer factor-2), NF-κB (nuclear factor kappa-light-chain-enhancer of activated B cells), c-Rel, Npas4 (neuronal PAS domain protein 4), Nr4a1/2/3 (nuclear receptor subfamily 4 group A member), SRF (serum response factor), and XBP1, X-box binding protein 1 (Abraham et al., 2019; Hegde and Smith, 2019).

These factors regulate transcription that leads to the translation of mRNAs that sustain the potentiated state. In principle, somatically synthesized proteins could then be targeted to appropriate synapses, that have been tagged as activated. Another possibility is that mRNAs are transported to tagged synapses to enable local protein synthesis. In both cases, the "synaptic tag" alerting the PRP that it has arrived at the correct location may be structural (e.g., spine enlargement) and/or metabolic (e.g., CP-AMPAR insertion) as described in Boxes 10.2 and 10.3. Another possibility is that appropriate synapses are tagged by the local depletion of mRNAs.

The involvement of transcription opens up many additional levels of regulation and modulation of synaptic plasticity. An important level of control is via transcriptional repressors, which may act to negatively impact synaptic plasticity. One example is cAMP-dependent transcription factor ATF4 (also known as CREB2), which acts as a CREB repressor. To enable transcription to proceed, ATF4 inhibition is removed, most likely by targeted degradation via the ubiquitin-proteosome pathway (Dong et al., 2008). Plasticity-related transcription is also subject to epigenetic regulation via both DNA methylation and histone modification (Abraham et al., 2019; Hegde and Smith, 2019). With respect to histone modifications, acetylation of histones on lysine residues facilitates transcription, whereas deacetylation blocks transcription. Methylation of histones can also regulate transcription. A variety of different histone modifications have been observed following LTP, several of which lead to activation of the *Zif268* promoter (Hegde and Smith, 2019).

Other sources of regulation include noncoding RNAs (ncRNAs). The best-studied ncRNAs in this context are the microRNAs (miRNAs), which bind to complementary sequences on mRNA to suppress their translation or cause their degradation (Mohammadi et al., 2022). For example, miR-26a and miR-384-5p are downregulated during NMDAR-LTP and this removes the suppression on the translation of a translational regulator of the ribosomal S6 kinase (S6K) family (RSK3, see Gu et al., 2015). Another example is miR-134, which inhibits the translation of LIMK during NMDAR-LTD (Rajgor et al., 2018). The miRNAs are themselves subject to regulation by transcription factors, such as CREB, and transcriptional regulators, such as Satb2 (Jaitner et al., 2016).

10.2.2 NMDAR-dependent synaptic depression

Depotentiation (DP) and de novo LTD are mechanisms by which synaptic efficacy is decreased for periods of time. In the former case, this is a reversal of LTP to (or toward) the basal state, whereas in the latter case it is the depression of synaptic transmission from baseline to below the basal state. These two forms of LTD have both overlapping and distinct mechanisms and are likely to serve differing functions in the brain. It is therefore important to make a clear distinction between de novo LTD (which is often referred to simply as LTD) and DP; see first edition, pp 407–419, for more detail on these two forms of LTD.

10.2.2.1 Depotentiation (DP)

The reversal of LTP by low-frequency trains is generally assumed to reset recently enhanced synaptic strength. It may enable forgetting (Moreno, 2021), or may be part of the process of memory reconsolidation, and can also reset synaptic tags (Sajikumar and Frey, 2004). There are both NMDAR-dependent and NMDAR-independent (principally mGluR-dependent) forms of DP, and the efficiency of DP depends on the underlying form of synaptic potentiation (P Park, Sanderson, et al., 2019). DP may also vary according to the animal's age. For example, in contrast to LTD, DP is more readily induced in the DG of adult than juvenile animals; an effect attributable to a switch from GluN2B- to GluN2A-containing NMDARs (Ge et al., 2019).

10.2.2.2 De novo long-term depression (LTD)

De novo NMDAR-LTD is particularly pronounced early in development. In adult tissues it is more difficult to induce NMDAR-LTD physiologically, but the process can be facilitated by chronic stress and other pathological conditions (see Collingridge et al., 2010).

10.2.2.3 The role of NMDARs in the induction of LTD

Early studies suggested that LTP and LTD involve different subtypes of NMDARs, but this remains highly controversial (see Collingridge et al., 2010). In terms of LTD, there is evidence for GluN2B-containing NMDARs (France et al., 2017) and GluN2D-containing NMDARs (Bartlett et al., 2007), possibly in the form of a heterotrimeric complex (Amici et al., 2021).

An interesting development was the finding that during the induction of LTD, NMDARs can function in a metabotropic manner (Nabavi et al., 2013). Thus, blocking NMDAR function with a glycine site antagonist or channel blocker did not prevent NMDARs from eliciting LTD, leading to the conclusion that binding of L-glutamate to the NMDAR was able to signal to the neuron without flux through the receptor. The mechanism seems to involve a conformational change in the C-terminal region of the NMDAR (Dore et al., 2015). However, this result is not obtained uniformly, with examples of NMDAR-LTD fully blocked by antagonists that are not competitive in nature (e.g., Babiec et al., 2014; Volianskis et al., 2015). One likely explanation for these disparate findings is that NMDARs can trigger LTD via both ionotropic and metabotropic mechanisms, the extent to which varies according to a number of factors, such as the developmental stage of the animal (Dore and Malinow, 2021).

How do NMDARs trigger either LTP or LTD?

The classical interpretation is that a brief high-frequency train, as typically used for inducing LTP, provides a higher Ca^{2+} concentration than a prolonged low-frequency train, which typically induces LTD. It then follows that the Ca^{2+} levels influence the relative induction of LTP and LTD by activating kinases and phosphatases, which have differing Ca^{2+} sensitivities. Although there is good evidence that Ca^{2+} levels play an important role, the situation is more complex because the activation of different NMDAR subtypes leads to different outcomes; thus, activation of GluN2A/B heterotrimers leads to LTP, while LTD is more likely to result from activation of GluN2B heterodimers or GluN2B/D heterotrimers (Volianskis, Bannister, et al., 2013). Different NMDAR subtypes not only have differing locations (classically, LTP-producing subtypes are more centrally located at the synapse) but also different molecules bound to their C-terminal tails. The notion that local Ca²⁺ nanodomains activate a different subset of signaling molecules depending on the activated NMDAR subtype is an appealing one. This would suggest that the direction of synaptic change is determined by different induction protocols favoring activation of the different subtypes. For classical induction protocols, using trains of stimuli, this can be explained by brief high-frequency stimuli producing a glutamate transient that is largely restricted to the PSD region while a continuous low-frequency stimulation produces a Ca²⁺ transient that spreads to extrasynaptic sites by overwhelming the uptake mechanisms that normally restrict its spread. But for STDP, where the number of pre- and postsynaptic stimuli is usually the same, but the order reversed, this is a less likely explanation. Here the determining factor may come down to how the timing determines the level of NMDAR activation and hence the local Ca²⁺ concentration within the same nanodomain.

Irrespective of how NMDARs are activated during LTP vs. LTD, the differing NMDAR subtype preferences for the two forms of plasticity probably reflect Ca²⁺ nanodomains engaging different subsets of signaling molecules, which are directly or indirectly associated with their C-terminal tails. This leads to the key question of the identity of these molecules. The answer is likely to be complex, with each subunit subject to multiple regulation, by Ser/Thr and Tyr phosphorylation, palmitoylation, and ubiquitination, with considerable overlap between their interacting partners (Gardoni and Di Luca, 2021; Ishchenko et al., 2021).

One molecule that seems to play a central role is CaMKII. Both α and β isoforms typically form a holoenzyme comprising 12 subunits, and this is important for its function, in particular, the autophosphorylation of Thr286, which triggers CaMKII binding to the GluN2B subunit where it maintains a partially autonomous state (Buonarati et al., 2021). Originally thought of as a molecule specific to LTP, it was subsequently found that it could trigger LTD when phosphorylated on Thr286 and that Thr305/306 residues are critical for determining the direction of synaptic change (Pi et al., 2010). The mechanism may involve CaMKII either promoting LTP via phosphorylation of GluA1-Ser831, or LTD, via phosphorylation of GluA1-Ser567, depending on its phosphorylation status (Coultrap et al., 2014). In addition, the death-associated protein kinase 1 (DAPK1) plays a critical role (Goodell et al., 2017). The idea is that the Ca²⁺ flux associated with LTD favors activation of DAPK1, via CaM-dependent dephosphorylation of Ser308, and this results in DAPK1 phosphorylation of GluN2B, at Ser1303. These alterations in phosphorylation enhance DAPK1/GluN2B interactions at the expense of the CaMKII/GluN2B interaction thereby inhibiting LTP. However, the Ca²⁺ flux associated with LTP favors CaM-mediated activation of CaMKII by inhibiting the competition of DAPK1.

Other important factors are the mechanisms that localize NMDARs either to the synapse, where they more readily induce LTP, or to peri/extrasynaptic sites, where they are likely to induce LTD. The interaction between the GluN2B subunit and PSD-95 is important for the synaptic localization of NMDARs (Gardoni et al., 2009). Casein kinase 2 phosphorylation of GluN2B at Ser1480, within the PDZ domain, disrupts this interaction and enables the

lateral diffusion of NMDARs to extrasynaptic sites, where they are endocytozed (Sanz-Clemente et al., 2010); this action is promoted by CaMKII (Sanz-Clemente et al., 2013). At extrasynaptic sites, NMDARs bind protein phosphatase 1 (PP1) and require PP1-dependent dephosphorylation of Ser1480 to enable reinsertion into the PSD (Chiu et al., 2019).

The role of CP-AMPARs in the induction of LTD

Just as CP-AMPARs are involved in the induction of some forms of LTP, they are also involved in the induction of NMDAR-LTD. Thus, during LTD induction, CP-AMPARs are recruited to the synapse, from which they are then rapidly removed (J Sanderson et al., 2016). This process is orchestrated by AKAP150, which anchors PKA and calcineurin at the correct locations within the synapse for this regulated process to occur. These findings build on the earlier discovery that AKAP150-bound PKA activity is required during the induction of NMDAR-LTD for the effect to be fully realized (Lu et al., 2008). It is intriguing that PKA and CP-AMPARs are both involved in the induction of certain forms of both NMDAR-LTP and NMDAR-LTD, emphasizing further the complexity of these induction processes (Hell, 2016).

Signaling mechanisms in LTD

There is strong evidence that de novo LTD is triggered by a protein phosphatase cascade, comprising CaM, calcineurin (PP2B), inhibitor-1 (I-1), and PP1, with one function of PP1 being to dephosphorylate AMPARs to regulate their trafficking. There is also good evidence that LTD-inducing stimulation promotes clathrin-dependent endocytosis of AMPARs at extrasynaptic sites by promoting the exchange of AP2 for NSF, which is ordinarily bound to the GluA2 subunit to stabilize AMPARs at the synapse. In addition to CaM, it has been suggested that Ca²⁺ activates the high-affinity neuronal Ca²⁺ sensor, hippocalcin, to initiate the AP2/NSF exchange and to activate PICK1 with the consequence of dissociating AMPARs from their tethering to GRIP (glutamate receptor interacting protein) as described in the first edition (see pp 412–414). Progress since 2006 has been extensive. Space constraints prevent a comprehensive coverage here, and instead we will focus on a subset of new discoveries—primarily those that uncover new principles.

GSK-3 regulates NMDAR-LTD

The simple concept that kinases regulate NMDAR-LTP and phosphatases regulate NMDAR-LTD (see first edition, Chapter 10) was dispelled with the discovery that the Ser/Thr kinase GSK-3 is required for NMDAR-LTD (Peineau et al., 2007). Conversely, the overexpression of GSK-3β inhibits the induction of LTP (Hooper et al., 2007). Collectively, these studies demonstrate that GSK-3 controls the balance between LTP and LTD. LTD is associated with the activation of both GSK-3β (Peineau et al., 2007) and GSK-3α (Draffin et al., 2021), and both paralogs have been implicated in the regulation of NMDAR-dependent synaptic plasticity (McCamphill et al., 2020; Draffin et al., 2021; Ebrahim Amini et al., 2022). However, the relative roles of GSK-3α and GSK-3β in synaptic plasticity remain to be fully established.

GSK-3 can phosphorylate many targets and has the potential to orchestrate the direction and extent of synaptic plasticity by integrating many different types of input signals and regulating a diverse array of effector mechanisms (Bradley et al., 2012). In the context of NMDAR-dependent LTD, GSK-3 is probably activated by dephosphorylation of Ser9/Ser21 via the well-established LTD phosphatase cascade (PP2B/I-1/PP1) (Peineau et al., 2009). Significantly, GSK-3 is phosphorylated on these residues by Akt/PKB (AK strain transforming (thymoma)/protein kinase B), resulting in its inhibition. Indeed, LTP directly inhibits LTD via activation of the PI3K-Akt pathway (Peineau et al., 2007). This allows a direct molecular crosstalk to occur, in which the level of LTP directly influences the ability of synapses to undergo LTD. Conceivably, other signaling systems that activate PI3K, for example insulin and growth factors, could also regulate LTD via this pathway. Another way in which GSK-3 may be regulated is via proteolytic cleavage of Akt, which removes the inhibitory brake on LTD. Significantly, during LTD, cytochrome C released from mitochondria activates a caspase cascade culminating in caspase-3-mediated cleavage of Akt (Z Li et al., 2010).

Although several GSK-3 substrates have been found to play a role in synaptic plasticity, it is likely that many more remain to be identified. The GSK-3 substrates that may regulate postsynaptic changes in synaptic plasticity include kinesin light chain 2 (KLC2) (Bourne and Harris, 2011), PSD-95 (Nelson et al., 2013), TAU (Kimura et al., 2014), PICK1 (Yagishita et al., 2015), and PI4KIIα (phosphatidylinositol 4-kinase IIα) (Robinson et al.,

2014; Amici et al., 2021). GSK-3 may also regulate presynaptic function. For example, GSK-3-mediated phosphorylation of dynamin 1, following priming by cyclin-dependent 5, regulates activity-dependent bulk endocytosis, and so may serve to increase the availability of presynaptic vesicles to boost transmitter release (Clayton et al., 2010).

Because of its many potential substrates, it is likely that GSK-3 signaling is highly compartmentalized. In particular, some neuronal GSK-3β is bound to Axin, where it forms a complex with adenomatous polyposis coli (APC) and β-catenin and is involved in wingless-integrated (Wnt) signaling. Wnt signaling is implicated both in developmental plasticity and synaptic plasticity more generally. For example, the induction of LTP is associated with an increase in Wnt7a/b levels, and acute blockade of endogenous Wnts, or loss of Frizzled-7 receptors, impairs LTP via an effect on AMPAR trafficking involving regulation by PKA and CaMKII (McLeod et al., 2018). A proposal for how GSK-3 may serve as the master regulator for synaptic plasticity is presented in Figure 10.7.

JAK2/STAT3

In addition to GSK-3, another kinase that is involved in NMDAR-LTD is JAK2, a tyrosine kinase that signals via STAT3 (Nicolas

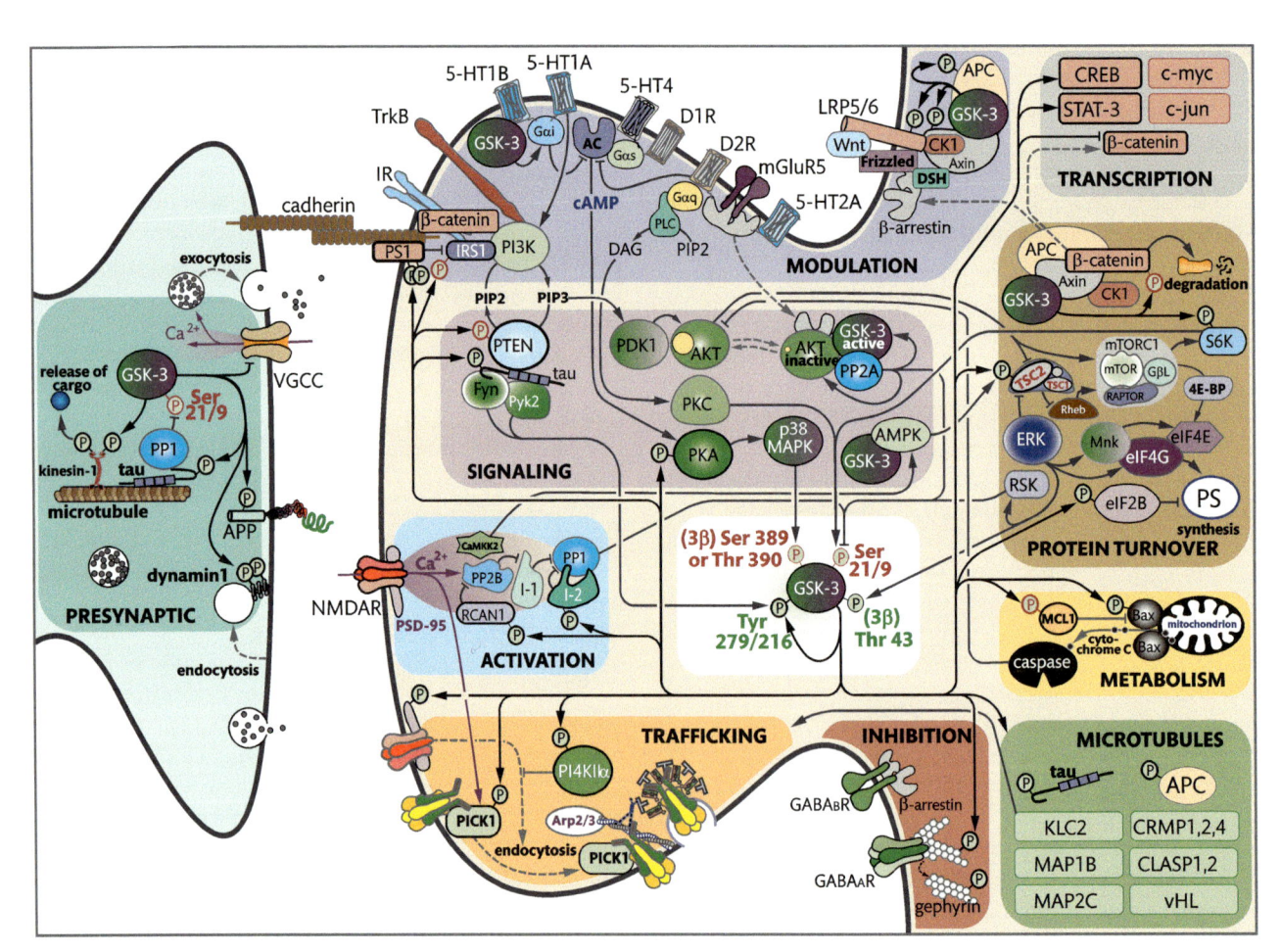

Figure 10.7 GSK-3 as a master regulator of NMDAR-mediated synaptic plasticity. GSK-3 phosphorylates numerous proteins involved in synaptic plasticity, many of which are likely still to be identified. Key substrates are clustered according to the processes they are involved in. In this diagram no distinction is made between the two paralogs (GSK-3α and GSK-3β) since little is known about which enzyme phosphorylates which substrates. Although the proteins shown are likely involved in synaptic plasticity and are bona fide GSK-3 substrates, in many cases the direct involvement of GSK-3 phosphorylation of the substrate has not been demonstrated during synaptic plasticity.

et al., 2012). At least initially, JAK-STAT's actions are confined to the cytoplasm, though it is reasonable to suppose that they may trigger transcriptional changes that impact LTD at later time points. A likely upstream regulator/downstream effector of JAK2 is proline-rich tyrosine kinase 2 (Pyk2), the activation of which is required for NMDAR-LTD (Hsin et al., 2010). The downstream targets of the JAK2/STAT3 pathway at synapses are largely unknown. A role for JAK/STAT in NMDAR-LTD has also been described at the entorhinal (temporoammonic) input to area CA1 of adult rats. Here the actions of the JAK/STAT pathway involves the classical regulation of gene transcription (McGregor et al., 2017). Interestingly, leptin can also induce LTD at this pathway via the activation of JAK2 (McGregor et al., 2018).

10.2.3 NMDAR-independent synaptic plasticity

10.2.3.1 Mossy fiber LTP (mf-LTP)

The first identified, and most extensively studied, form of NMDAR-independent LTP is at the mossy fiber pathway connecting dentate granule cells to CA3 pyramidal neurons (mf-LTP). The characterization of this form of LTP and insights into underlying mechanisms are described in detail in the first edition (pp 398–403). Here we provide an update.

The role of kainate receptors in the induction of mf-LTP

An unresolved issue is the role of kainate receptors (KARs) in the induction of mf-LTP and in the pronounced frequency facilitation seen at these synapses (Valbuena and Lerma, 2021). Most, but not all (Kwon and Castillo, 2008), evidence points to a critical role for presynaptic KARs as the triggers for both processes, consistent with the high levels of KARs and low levels of NMDARs at the mossy fiber pathway. However, there is still uncertainty regarding the subunit composition of these receptors (Pinheiro et al., 2007; Jane et al., 2009; Pinheiro et al., 2013). An important point to note is that the mossy fiber pathway is heterogeneous, with a comparatively small number of giant mossy boutons that innervate CA3 pyramidal neurons and numerous filipodia, which synapse onto GABAergic interneurons (Pelkey and McBain, 2008). The sensitivity of mf-LTP to KAR antagonists in vitro depends, surprisingly, on the orientation of hippocampal slices, suggesting the existence of two anatomically and functionally distinct synaptic components to the mossy fiber pathway running at different angles with respect to the long axis of the hippocampus (Sherwood et al., 2012). Importantly, brief high-frequency activation of individual granule cells elicits Ca^{2+} transients in individual mossy fiber boutons, the facilitation of which is sensitive to KAR antagonists (Scott et al., 2008; Dargan et al., 2009). These data suggest that GluK1- or GluK2/5-containing KARs are present at mossy fiber giant boutons, where they regulate frequency facilitation and the induction of mf-LTP.

There are synergistic actions of KARs and mGluRs in mf-LTP. Thus, a GluK1-selective agonist (ATPA; 2-Amino-3-[3-hydroxy-5-tert-butylisoxazol-4-yl]propanoic acid) can induce mf-LTP, provided either mGluR1 or mGluR5 is coactivated. This effect involved activation of PKA, the release of Ca^{2+} from stores, the facilitation of bouton Ca^{2+} transients, evoked by an action potential in a single granule cell, and an increase in resting Ca^{2+} in individual giant mossy fiber boutons (Nisticò et al., 2011). An interaction between mGluRs and KARs is also observed in vivo (Wallis et al., 2015). As described previously, HFS within the DG elicits a slowly developing, NMDAR-independent LTP devoid of frequency facilitation or STP.

This form of LTP was prevented by KAR antagonists, provided that group I mGluRs (both mGluR1 and mGluR5) were simultaneously blocked. These observations suggest that in vivo group I mGluRs and KARs cooperate in the induction of mf-LTP. In summary, current evidence suggests that activation of both KARs and mGluRs are necessary, and together sufficient, to regulate Ca^{2+} signaling in giant mossy fiber boutons and to generate LTP in vitro and in vivo.

Multiple forms of mf-LTP

In addition to the classic NMDAR-independent presynaptic LTP at mossy fiber synapses, there is also a postsynaptic form of LTP that is expressed as an increase in NMDAR-mediated synaptic responses (Kwon and Castillo, 2008; Rebola et al., 2008). This process is induced by coactivation of NMDARs and mGluR5s and involves a postsynaptic Ca^{2+} and PKC-dependent delivery of NMDARs via a SNARE-dependent process (Kwon and Castillo, 2008). It also involves activation of c-Src and adenosine A_{2A} receptors (A2AR, see Rebola et al., 2008) and has a lower threshold of induction than the classic presynaptic form of mf-LTP. Possible functions of mf-LTP of NMDAR-mediated synaptic transmission is to permit subsequent classical NMDAR-LTP of AMPAR-mediated synaptic transmission at mf synapses (Rebola et al., 2011) and to engage in associative LTP at associational/commissural inputs (Hunt et al., 2013).

Another well-established function of KARs is to mediate a relatively slow EPSP in CA3 pyramidal neurons. The depolarization that this provides may facilitate NMDAR-LTP at associational/commissural inputs, and thereby enable an associative form of LTP involving two functionally distinct inputs onto the same neurons (Sachidhanandam et al., 2009). Indeed, an EPSP evoked by subthreshold mossy fiber stimulation, which will contain both AMPAR and KAR components, is highly effective at enabling LTP at CA3-recurrent synapses (Brandalise and Gerber, 2014). Another study revealed the importance of NMDAR activation for STDP (both LTP and LTD) at the mossy fiber pathway (Astori et al., 2010). These findings illustrate how distinct forms of LTP at CA3 neurons may interact, the relative involvement of which may be subject to regulatory mechanisms, for example by synaptically released Zn^{2+} (Pan et al., 2011).

Recent evidence also suggests that mossy fibers contain presynaptic NMDARs that facilitate frequency facilitation and the associated giant bouton Ca^{2+} signaling during brief periods of HFS (Lituma et al., 2021), functions that are reminiscent of that provided by KARs. What determines the relative roles of NMDAR and KARs in this process remains to be determined. But why do mossy fibers exhibit such pronounced frequency facilitation? One function maybe to enable the EPSP evoked by the discharge of a single granule cell to facilitate sufficiently to discharge the CA3 pyramidal neurons it innervates (Vyleta et al., 2016).

Mechanisms of expression of mf-LTP

It is well established that presynaptic mf-LTP involves a PKA-dependent phosphorylation of RIM1α (Rab3-interacting molecule 1α) to increase p(r) via a mechanism also involving Rab3a. Additional PKA substrates that have been identified in mf-LTP include Munc13-1 (Yang and Calakos, 2011) and synaptotagmin-12 (Kaeser-Woo et al., 2013). In terms of the mechanism that promotes the increase in p(r), it has been shown that cAMP within the mossy fiber bouton probably increases the coupling between Ca^{2+} channels and the RRP of vesicles that are docked and primed ready to discharge their contents (Midorikawa and Sakaba, 2017). Recent evidence has suggested that PTP at mf synapses is due to an expansion in the RRP of synaptic vesicles and that these are depleted by synaptic activity (Vandael et al., 2020). Therefore, the duration of PTP can be prolonged by the absence of stimulation, a property also displayed by STP at CA1 synapses (see section 10.2.1).

Mechanisms of mf-LTD

Mossy fibers also exhibit LTD. Notably, a reduction in cAMP signaling opposes the PKA-dependent mechanism that underlies NMDAR-independent LTP at these synapses (Shahoha et al., 2022). A prominent, but not the only, mechanism by which LTD is induced at these synapses is via the activation of group II mGluRs (Lyon et al., 2011), which lowers cAMP levels. Further work is needed to understand the functional significance of LTD at mossy fiber synapses.

10.2.3.2 mGluR-LTD

LTD can also be induced by the activation of mGluRs, typically mGlu1 or mGlu5, as described in the first edition (pp 414–417). mGluR-LTD can be readily induced, in both adult and juvenile animals, by paired-pulse low-frequency stimulation (PP-LFS) or by pharmacological activation, typically by brief exposure to the group I mGluR selective compound, DHPG (DHPG-LTD). Induction of mGluR-LTD by DHPG and by PP-LFS may utilize overlapping but not necessarily identical mechanisms. Interestingly, mGluR-LTD involves different signaling mechanisms from NMDAR-LTD. In particular, whereas NMDAR-LTD involves Ser/Thr phosphatases, mGluR-LTD involves Tyr phosphatases, such as striatal-enriched protein tyrosine phosphatase (STEP; see Zhang et al., 2008).

Multiple forms of mGluR-LTD can be distinguished based on several criteria: the requirement for coactivation of NMDARs, the signaling mechanisms involved (such as the type of MAPK), the requirement for de novo protein synthesis, and the locus of expression (see Sanderson et al., 2016). In one form of mGluR-LTD, triggered by the activation of mGluR5, tyrosine dephosphorylation works in concert with p38MAPK phosphorylation, with both processes being necessary and together sufficient to induce a protein synthesis-insensitive form of LTD (Moult et al., 2008). This form of mGluR-LTD can be induced synaptically in the presence of a glycine site NMDAR antagonist and engages similar mechanisms to the more recently described metabotropic NMDAR form of LTD. A somewhat surprising observation is that a postsynaptic form of mGluR-LTD is influenced by p(r); activation of mGluR1 can lead to greater internalization of AMPARs at low-p(r) synapses than at high-p(r) synapses (T Sanderson et al., 2018). This is due to the activity-dependent internalization of mGluR1 and provides a mechanism to stabilize strong synapses at the expense of weak ones.

10.2.4 Cellular substrates of synaptic structure and structural plasticity

10.2.4.1 The nanostructure of synapses

There have been major advances since the first edition of this book in the identification of the nanoarchitecture of the synapse, driven largely by technological advancement in imaging techniques such as superresolution microscopy. Here we highlight principles that are directly relevant to synaptic plasticity.

At the presynapse, detailed serial EM has revealed how presynaptic vesicles relate to stages of synaptic plasticity (Harris

et al., 2024). There are three distinct classes of pre- to postsynaptic arrangements—strong active zones with tightly docked vesicles, weak active zones with loose or nondocked vesicles, and nascent zones with presynaptic vesicles but no PSD. During LTP, vesicles are recruited to nascent zones and converted to active zones and active zones are enlarged. These effects take time to develop, are associated with smooth endoplasmic reticulum (SER), and presumably relate to LTP2. A key feature of this process is the existence of "sentinel spines" that contain the SER and around which small spines cluster.

At the postsynapse, glutamate receptors form synaptic clusters (Nowacka et al., 2024). Typically, there is a single NMDAR cluster near the center of the PSD and one or a few AMPAR clusters that surround the NMDAR cluster. Each AMPAR cluster contains ~20–25 densely packed AMPARs. Since AMPARs have a relatively low affinity for L-glutamate, the position of these clusters in relationship to release sites is a critical factor. The positioning of AMPAR clusters directly opposed to release sites is controlled by scaffolding molecules, to form nanocolumns (A Tang et al., 2016). Interestingly, the position of the AMPAR clusters in relationship to presynaptic release sites depends on AMPAR subunit composition (Hruska et al., 2022).

A number of molecules have been proposed to orchestrate this transsynaptic alignment: These include cell adhesion molecules (CAMs), notably the neurexins and neuroligins, that may form a transsynaptic bridge. SynCAM1 and N-cadherin are other candidates that may mark the postsynaptic edge (Perez de Arce et al., 2015). Interestingly, N-cadherin binds to the N-terminus of GluA2 and regulates synaptic plasticity (Saglietti et al., 2007; Z Zhou et al., 2011). Neuroplastin-65 is another CAM that binds the N-terminus of GluA1 and is important for LTP (C Jiang et al., 2021). β3-integrin also binds GluA2, via a C-terminus interaction, and may mediate cell-cell adhesion (Pozo et al., 2012). LRRTM2 is a CAM that can align AMPARs opposite to release sites (Ramsey et al., 2021). Other candidate molecules include liprin-α that binds to RIM and LAR family tyrosine phosphatases, the latter of which can bind several synaptic proteins. Indeed, liprin-α interactions with GRIP are required for LTD induced by activation of muscarinic receptors but not mGluRs (Dickinson et al., 2009). Additionally, SynCAM1 and EphB2 have distinct synaptic localizations (Perez de Arce et al., 2015). Matrix proteins, such as the neuronal pentraxin receptors (SJ Lee et al., 2017) and Noelin-1 (Pandya et al., 2018), bind to AMPARs and may also play a role in transsynaptic alignment and synaptic plasticity. Presumably, these, and other organizers of synaptic nanoarchitecture still to be identified, have distinct roles to play in LTP, LTD, and other synaptic functions.

10.2.4.2 The cytoskeleton

Alterations in the cytoskeleton are crucial for bidirectional synaptic plasticity. They may be temporary or more lasting, but they provide the foundation stones for alterations in, for example, the expression of AMPARs in the PSD. These changes are critical for LTP2 and LTP3, but may also be involved in LTP1. Although the importance of the cytoskeleton was acknowledged in the first edition (pp 397–398), the underlying molecular mechanisms had hardly been explored at that time. Since then, a bewildering array of cytoskeletal molecules have been identified as playing a role in synaptic plasticity (see Borovac et al., 2018), as briefly outlined in Figure 10.5. The regulation of cytoskeletal elements is important for postsynaptic glutamate receptor trafficking, both to and from the synapse, and for insertion and removal of receptors at the plasma membrane. They are also the critical drivers of the changes in spine morphology and the formation and loss of spines that in many cases accompany and define long-term changes in synaptic function (see Box 10.2). A comprehensive account of the complex mechanisms involved in these processes is beyond the scope of this chapter, where we focus on the few molecules known to be involved in the regulation of the postsynaptic spine to highlight key principles. It is pertinent to point out, however, that the presynaptic cytoskeleton also plays a crucial role in transmitter release and synaptic plasticity. Unraveling the pre- and postsynaptic mechanisms of structural change is important not only for understanding the physiology of synaptic plasticity but also because errors in these processes are likely to contribute to hippocampal dysfunction (see section 10.9).

The actin cytoskeleton

A central player in the regulation of the actin cytoskeleton in dendritic spines is actin depolymerization factor (ADF)/cofilin (see Ben Zablah et al., 2020). Interestingly, N-cofilin regulates spine F-actin content to affect AMPAR trafficking, spine morphology, and spine density (Rust et al., 2010). Cofilin is inhibited via phosphorylation on Ser3 by LIM (Lin-11, Isl-1, and MEC-3) domain kinases (LIMKs, primarily LIMK1) and is activated by dephosphorylation of Ser3 by slingshot phosphatases. In turn, LIMK1 is activated through its phosphorylation by a variety of kinases, including Rho-associated protein kinases (ROCKs) (Z Zhou et al., 2009) and p21-activated kinases (PAKs) (Asrar, Meng, et al., 2009). These kinases are activated by the Rho family of small guanosine triphosphatases (GTPases) and constitute the central mediators of actin reorganization in response to a diverse array of external signals. One intriguing mechanism underlying mGluR-LTD involves an extracellular interaction between the GluA2 subunit of AMPARs and N-cadherin. These regulate cofilin via Rho-GTPase Rac1 (Ras-related C3 botulinum toxin substrate 1; see Z Zhou et al., 2011). Although cofilin is a key regulator of actin polymerization, its involvement is synaptic plasticity may be developmentally regulated. This is suggested by the observation that peptide inhibitors and activators of cofilin affect metabotropic LTD in mature but not juvenile mice (Cao et al., 2017), possibly because other regulators of the actin cytoskeleton are more important early on.

LIMK1 is also subject to different forms of regulation, in addition to its phosphorylation status. For example, during LTD, NMDAR activation leads to Akt-dependent phosphorylation of protein argonaute-2 (Ago2), which results in a reduction in the translation of LIMK1 via the miRNA miR-134 (Rajgor et al., 2018). Knockdown of Ago2 results in block of the induction of NMDAR-LTD, demonstrating the importance of RISC-mediated suppression of miRNAs, such as miR-191 and miR-135 (Z Hu et al., 2014), in this form of synaptic plasticity. However, while phosphoregulation of Ago2 (at Ser387) is required for translational suppression of LIMK1 and spine shrinkage, it is not required for AMPAR endocytosis or LTD. Thus, partially divergent pathways regulate functional and morphological plasticity.

Another central molecule in the regulation of the actin cytoskeleton is the actin-related 2/3 (Arp2/3) complex, which catalyzes the formation of branched actin networks to regulate cell geometry. A role of the Arp2/3 complex in synaptic plasticity was suggested by the finding that PICK1 binds to Arp2/3 to inhibit actin assembly and AMPAR trafficking (Rocca et al., 2008). This interaction is important

for the induction of NMDAR-LTD (Nakamura et al., 2011) via a pathway involving the small GTPase Arf1 (ADP-ribosylation factor 1; see Rocca et al., 2013). During NMDAR-LTD, an Arf GAP (GTPase-activating protein), GIT1 (G-protein-coupled receptor kinase-interactor 1), deactivates Arf1, which allows for the PICK1-mediated inhibition of Arp2/3 to promote AMPAR internalization and spine shrinkage.

The development of sophisticated imaging approaches has allowed for molecular interactions and structural changes to be studied at the single synapse in real time. Initial work focused on the organization and dynamics of F-actin within spines (Honkura et al., 2008) and the role of established LTP molecules, such as Ras (Harvey et al., 2008), CaMKII (SJ Lee et al., 2009), and Arp2/3 (I Kim et al., 2013), to study their spatiotemporal properties in structural LTP, induced by the uncaging of L-glutamate. Whereas CaMKII is highly localized to the active spine, Ras diffuses to neighboring spines along the same dendritic branch.

Investigations of structural LTP showed that the reorganization of the spine actin cytoskeleton occurs in a number of stages (Bosch et al., 2014). In the first few minutes after the induction of LTP, there is a large increase in the formation of F-actin and associated regulatory proteins, notably cofilin, Arp2/3 and Aip1 (actin-interacting protein 1), that are involved in modifying F-actin via severing, branching, and capping, respectively. This generates a labile state where cofilin and Arp2/3 may cooperate to form new branched filaments to initiate the structural growth of spines. Over the next ~1 h, the newly remodeled actin cytoskeleton is stabilized at a new level that determines the geometry of the enlarged spine. Finally, during a subsequent third phase, there is a remodeling of the PSD. An important trigger to initiate spine remodeling during LTP is CaMKII (Kim et al., 2015). Inactive CaMKII binds to and stabilizes F-actin; but when activated, CaMKII dissociates and permits remodeling of F-actin. CaMKII does this via activation of the RhoA (Ras homolog family member A)-ROCK pathway to initiate the initial spine growth and via activation of Cdc42 (cell division control protein 42 homolog) and PAK for maintenance of the structural plasticity (Murakoshi et al., 2011; I Kim et al., 2014). Interestingly, the different spatiotemporal characteristics of three small GTPases, Rho, Rac1, and Cdc42, may help determine some key properties of LTP: Cdc42 is localized to active spines, where it may orchestrate input-specificity, whereas Rho and Rac1 can diffuse to neighboring spines, where they act in a coordinated manner to enable heterosynaptic plasticity (Hedrick et al., 2016). A distinction between the roles of these two GTPases in heterosynaptic LTP is the requirement for both BDNF-TrkB (tyrosine kinase receptor B/tropomyosin receptor kinase B) (Hedrick et al., 2016) and PKC alpha (Tu et al., 2020) with respect to the actions of Rac1 but not of Rho. To sustain structural plasticity, Rac1 activation is prolonged via CaMKII-mediated phosphorylation of Tiam1 (T-cell lymphoma invasion and metastasis-inducing protein 1), a Rac GEF (guanine nucleotide exchange factor; see Saneyoshi et al., 2019).

Microtubules

Microtubules also play an important role in synaptic plasticity in providing the scaffold along which cargo is transported to and from the synapse. Microtubules are highly dynamic and can transiently enter and leave spines (Mitsuyama et al., 2008; Jaworski et al., 2009; Kapitein et al., 2011; Saneyoshi et al., 2019). It seems probable, therefore, that interactions between the actin cytoskeleton and microtubules are crucial for the delivery and removal of glutamate receptors and other key components of synaptic plasticity. One possibility is that actin polymerization in the spine neck provides a point of access for microtubules (Korobova and Svitkina, 2010), and that the actin cytoskeleton serves as a substrate along which the microtubules polymerize. The dynamics of microtubules is controlled by NMDAR-mediated Ca²⁺ flux (Jaworski et al., 2009; Kapitein et al., 2011) and involves interactions between the +TIP protein, the end-binding protein 3 (EB3), and the actin-associated protein debrin and a variety of signaling components, including CaMKII (Merriam et al., 2011; McVicker et al., 2015; McVicker et al., 2016). The frequency of microtubule polymerization into spines is increased during LTP (Merriam et al., 2011) and decreased during LTD (Kapitein et al., 2011).

Microtubules within dendrites are of mixed polarity and so +end- or –end-directed motor proteins could theoretically bring cargo to or from the synapse. However, since microtubules polymerize into spines via their +end leading edge, it is likely that kinesin motor proteins will convey cargo into spines while dynein will convey cargo out of spines. An example of a cargo that is brought into spines via microtubules is a member of the synaptotagmin family, syt4, which engages the kinesin motor protein KIF1A (Kinesin Family Member 1A; see McVicker et al., 2016).

The direction of microtubule transport is regulated by a number of different microtubule-associated proteins (MAPs), including MAP2 and TAU (Monroy et al., 2020). For example, TAU inhibits the kinesin motors, kinesin-1 and kinesin-3. TAU is a particularly important MAP, since mutations in or dysregulation of this protein underlies tauopathies, including frontotemporal dementia and AD (see section 10.9). The physiological function of TAU is suggested by its concentration in axons, where it stabilizes microtubules, and its presence in dendritic spines (see Ittner and Ittner, 2018). With respect to its dendritic function, knockout (KO) of TAU in mice impairs NMDAR-LTD without affecting LTP (Kimura et al., 2014). TAU is phosphorylated by GSK-3 (Kimura et al., 2014) at residue Ser396 (Regan et al., 2015). This suggests that NMDAR-mediated activation of GSK-3, via its dephosphorylation, will result in phosphorylation of TAU, an integral part of the LTD process. It is unclear what TAU then does, though one possibility is that it inhibits kinesin motors from importing cargo into spines, thus shifting the balance toward cargo export. In addition to LTD induced via synaptic activation, LTD induced by transient application of insulin is also absent in the TAU KO (Marciniak et al., 2017). However, in another study using a TAU KO there was inhibition of LTP but not LTD (Ahmed et al., 2014). The reason for this is currently unclear, but the discrepancy suggests that other factors contribute to the involvement of TAU in synaptic plasticity. Given the central role of TAU in numerous major brain disorders, it is clearly important to fully understand its role in synaptic physiology.

10.3 Synaptic plasticity at inhibitory pathways

We have so far considered synapses where both pre- and postsynaptic neurons are excitatory (E-E synapses). We turn now to a consideration of plasticity at synapses where one or both of the neurons is inhibitory. It is convenient to label these three classes as E-I (excitatory-inhibitory), I-E (inhibitory-excitatory), and I-I (inhibitory-inhibitory) synapses. Inhibitory interneurons make up 15%–30% of the neuronal count in the hippocampus (Sukenik et al.,

2021; and see Chapter 7). Approximately 6% of synapses on pyramidal cells are inhibitory (Megías et al., 2001). On interneurons, the proportion of inhibitory synapses varies between 6% for parvalbumin (PV)-expressing cells to 29% for calbindin-expressing cells (Gulyás et al., 1999). Thus, a sizable minority of synapses are inhibitory, and plasticity at inhibitory synapses on excitatory neurons (I-E plasticity; sometimes referred to as iLTP and iLTD), is of potential significance for cell and circuit behavior. In this section, we discuss synaptic plasticity both at I-E synapses and at E-I synapses in the hippocampus. (For reviews on plasticity at inhibitory pathways, see Kullmann et al., 2012; Moreau and Kullmann, 2013; Chevaleyre and Piskorowski, 2014; Artinian and Lacaille, 2018.)

10.3.1 LTP and LTD at glutamatergic synapses on hippocampal interneurons (E-I plasticity)

The subunit composition of AMPARs and NMDARs on interneurons differs from that on pyramidal cells. The dominant NMDAR subunit is GluN2B, the presence of which prolongs NMDAR-mediated currents (McBain et al., 1999). The AMPAR subunit GluA2, which in its edited form limits the Ca²⁺ permeability of the AMPAR ion channel, is generally in low abundance at synapses on inhibitory interneurons, and AMPAR-mediated Ca²⁺ fluxes are correspondingly higher (Lawrence and McBain, 2003). The distinct assemblage of glutamate receptor subtypes at interneuron synaptic membranes is reflected in the types of plasticity observed; high-frequency trains can, depending on the protocol or cell type, induce either LTP or LTD (Maccaferri and McBain, 1996; Perez et al., 2001; Lapointe et al., 2003; McMahon and Kauer, 1997). Induction of LTP in interneurons in the stratum oriens is mGluR1-dependent and requires postsynaptic Ca²⁺ entry (Lapointe et al., 2003).

There are no reports that prolonged low-frequency trains produce LTD at E-I synapses as they do at E-E synapses. However, LTD at feedforward excitatory synapses on CA1 interneurons can be induced by HFS (McMahon and Kauer, 1997). Functional suppression, via LTD, of excitatory feedforward synapses onto interneurons in the stratum radiatum provides a potential mechanism for the phenomenon of E-S potentiation (see section 10.4).

10.3.1.1 DG

Fast-spiking perisomatic interneurons such as basket cells, receive feedforward inputs from the perforant path, and feedback excitatory inputs from granule cell axons. Feedforward synapses lack CP-AMPARs and do not exhibit LTP, while feedback synapses support LTP via CP-AMPARs (Sambandan et al., 2010). However, NMDAR-LTD has been described at feedforward E-I synapses made by perforant path fibers onto dendrite-targeting interneurons with cell bodies lying at the border of the hilus and granule cell layer (Harney and Anwyl, 2012). NMDAR- and mGluR1-dependent LTP can also be induced at E-I mossy fiber synapses on somatostatin-expressing interneurons in the hilus (Grigoryan et al., 2023).

10.3.1.2 CA3

McBain and colleagues have described an intriguing example of bimodal feedforward E-I plasticity at synapses made by mossy fibers on SLINs (stratum lucidum inhibitory neurons). Mossy fiber collaterals to these interneurons express mGluR7 on their presynaptic terminals. HFS leads to presynaptically expressed LTD, with a consequent decrease in the inhibitory input to CA3 pyramidal cells, and, in addition, to the internalization of the population of presynaptic mGluR7s. A subsequent episode of HFS now produces LTP, also presynaptically expressed. Thus, mGluR7s act as a synapse-specific homeostatic molecular switch to regulate the level of inhibitory tone to pyramidal cells of area CA3 (Pelkey et al., 2005).

Plasticity at feedforward and feedback excitatory inputs to aspiny CA3 interneurons in stratum radiatum and stratum lacunosum-moleculare has also been described (Galvan et al., 2015). At recurrent collateral connections, the induction of LTP by HFS requires the coactivation of NMDARs and CP-AMPARs, and its expression is CaMKII-dependent. LTP can also be induced at feedforward (mossy fiber) inputs to these interneurons, but here LTP expression is CaMKII-independent (see Galvan et al., 2011, for review).

The efficacy of feedforward inhibition provided by the SLIN network onto CA3 pyramidal cells affects the specificity of DG engrams. The strength of mossy fiber synapses on SLINs is regulated by a presynaptic cytoskeletal actin-binding LIM protein, abLIM3. Following contextual fear conditioning (CFC), abLIM3 levels decline, leading to an increase in feedforward inhibition onto CA3 cells. The depressed linkage between the DG and CA3 networks contributes to the context specificity of fear conditioning (Guo et al., 2018).

10.3.1.3 CA1

Plasticity occurs at both feedforward and feedback excitatory connections to CA1 inhibitory neurons with cell bodies lying in stratum radiatum and stratum lacunosum-moleculare. Kullmann and colleagues were the first to examine LTP at feedforward SCC inputs to interneurons in stratum radiatum of area CA1 (Lamsa et al., 2005). In about half the cells, pathway-specific LTP occurred following a pairing induction protocol. The resulting enhancement of inhibition was necessary for the accurate timing of CA1 cell firing following the induction of LTP at SCC synapses on CA1 cells.

An unconventional "anti-Hebbian" form of LTP has been described by Lamsa et al. (2007) at feedback synapses made by axon collaterals of CA1 pyramidal cells synapsing on oriens–lacunosum-moleculare (OLM) interneurons, whose cell bodies and dendrites lie in stratum oriens. LTP at these synapses requires the pairing of presynaptic activity with hyperpolarization of the postsynaptic cell. Anti-Hebbian LTP occurs at synapses where CP-AMPARs lacking the GluA2 subunit are expressed on the postsynaptic membrane; Ca^{2+} entry though activated CP-AMPARs is enhanced by the Ca^{2+} concentration gradient at hyperpolarizing potentials and blocked at depolarizing potentials by cytoplasmic polyamines. LTP at recurrent collateral synapses between CA1 and somatostatin-expressing OLM interneurons is also dependent on the activation of group I mGluRs (Perez et al., 2001; Vasuta et al., 2015) and T-type Ca^{2+} channels (Nicholson and Kullmann, 2017). A consequence of the TBS stimulation of somatostatin-expressing OLM interneurons is an enhancement of NMDAR-LTP at the SCC projection to CA1 neurons (Vasuta et al., 2015), presumably as the result of increased transmission between OLM interneurons and interneurons in stratum radiatum, with a consequent disinhibition of CA1 apical dendrites—if so, a rare example of I-I potentiation.

Most interneurons lack spines, but about 20% of interneurons in stratum lacunosum-moleculare and stratum radiatum exhibit spines displaying CP-AMPARs and NMDARs. A proportion of such spines show morphological plasticity in response to repetitive glutamate uncaging (Scheuss and Bonhoeffer, 2014).

Another study of plasticity at E-I synapses found that LTP was induced in PV-expressing basket cells innervating the soma of CA1 pyramidal cells while LTD was expressed in PV-expressing bistratified cells innervating their dendrites (Nissen et al., 2010). The induction of both LTP and LTD was blocked by CP-AMPAR antagonists but not by NMDAR antagonists, supporting the conclusion that the induction of plasticity at E-I synapses is in general CP-AMPAR-dependent. Not all inhibitory interneurons displayed plasticity, among them basket cells expressing cannabinoid receptor 1 (CB1R).

The great majority of experiments on plasticity at E-I synapses have been performed in vitro. A study in the anesthetized rat documented LTP and LTD in PV-expressing basket cells in area CA1 in response to TBS of commissural inputs (Lau et al., 2017).

Research into plasticity at connections to and from inhibitory neurons is at an early stage, but it is already clear that plasticity at E-I synapses has the potential to influence the sculpting of hippocampal engrams (N Guo et al., 2018; Lamsa and Lau, 2019; He et al., 2021).

10.3.2 LTP and LTD at GABAergic synapses on excitatory neurons (I-E plasticity)

The first studies of plasticity at inhibitory synapses in the hippocampus were performed by Ben-Ari and colleagues on inhibitory inputs to pyramidal cells in neonatal hippocampal slices (McLean et al., 1996). In the presence of CNQX (6-cyano-7-nitroquinoxaline-2,3-dione) to block AMPAR-mediated responses, HFS produced LTD of inhibitory responses. However, if AP5 was present, HFS led to LTP of IPSPs. The authors concluded that plasticity of IPSPs was sustained by presynaptic mechanisms, though postsynaptic NMDARs controlled the direction of plasticity. Subsequent work by Marsden et al. (2007) showed that application of NMDA to hippocampal cultures leads to exocytosis of GABA receptors and internalization of AMPARs. This form of chemical I-E LTD also requires the scaffolding protein gephyrin (Petrini et al., 2014). Plasticity at I-E synapses can display different signatures at different synapses—for instance, in mouse medial prefrontal cortex, application of NMDA in vitro produces potentiation of IPSPs at SST-expressing interneurons, but not at PV- or VIP (vasoactive intestinal polypeptide)-expressing interneurons (Chiu et al., 2019).

An intriguing form of heterosynaptic plasticity called depolarization-induced suppression of inhibition (DSI) was discovered by Chevaleyre and Castillo (2003) at GABAergic synapses on CA1 pyramidal cells. Under ionotropic glutamate receptor blockade, HFS of SCC fibers in stratum radiatum results in a persistent reduction of evoked IPSPs. The effect is mediated by activation of mGluRs on pyramidal cell dendrites, leading to the retrograde release of the endocannabinoid 2-arachidonoylglycerol (2-AG), which binds to 2-AG receptors located on local inhibitory terminals, resulting in a sustained reduction of GABA release (reviewed by Min et al., 2010). The effect has been confirmed in mice navigating a linear track (Dudok et al., 2024). Endocannabinoids also mediate the induction of synaptic LTD and of a sustained decrease in intrinsic excitability in OLM interneurons in stratum oriens of area CA1 following HFS of the SCC pathway through an upregulation of the voltage-gated K^+ channel 7 (Kv7) (Incontro et al., 2021). A striking example of the targeted nature of endocannabinoid-mediated inhibition has been provided by Jensen et al. (2021). In the DG, granule cells and excitatory mossy cells are connected in a positive feedback loop. Mossy cells express constitutively active cannabinoid receptors on axon terminals synapsing on granule cells but not on interneurons, increasing the net inhibitory drive on granule cells and thus preserving the sparse firing pattern of granule cells required for pattern separation.

An intriguing observation that emphasizes the complexity of plasticity in inhibitory signaling was reported by Yap et al. (2021) in experiments revealing how spatial exploration drives changes in perisomatic inhibition at cFos-expressing CA1 cells. These are the cells that constitute the engram for an explored environment, and in those engram cells there is a characteristic alteration in the balance of perisomatic inhibition: that from PV interneurons is enhanced while inhibition from CCK-expressing interneurons is diminished.

10.3.3 Plasticity at inhibitory connections to interneurons (I-I plasticity)

Little work has been done on I-I plasticity, though a possible example of I-I potentiation was noted in section 10.3.1. An intriguing example of the ability of an inhibitory input to an inhibitory neuron to produce a long-lasting heterosynaptic change has been observed in area CA2, where the activity of pyramidal cells is strongly suppressed by PV-expressing interneurons. Trains of stimuli to SCC fibers projecting to area CA2 result in LTD of the inhibitory input from PV-expressing interneurons to CA2 pyramidal cells, leading to substantial disinhibition of the latter, and a consequent increase in the flow of excitatory traffic through CA2 (Piskorowski and Chevaleyre, 2013). This effect is achieved by the activated Schaffer-commissural fibers stimulating the release of enkephalin from VIP-containing interneurons. Enkephalin then binds to delta-opioid receptors on PV-expressing interneurons, resulting in suppression of their activity, and a consequent disinhibition of CA2 neurons (Leroy et al., 2022).

10.3.4 The role of persistent disinhibition in controlling the activity of principal cells in the hippocampus

There is increasing evidence that VIP-expressing interneurons acting on PV- or somatostatin (SST)-expressing interneurons to produce disinhibition of principal hippocampal neurons can play a significant role in sculpting the synaptic engram supporting spatial learning in the hippocampus (Donato et al., 2013; Letzkus et al., 2015; Artinian and Lacaille, 2018; Turi et al., 2019). Udakis et al. (2020) examined plasticity at monosynaptic connections made by PV-expressing interneurons onto CA1 pyramidal cell somata, and at synapses made by SST-expressing cells onto distal apical dendrites, using separate optogenetic mouse lines, expressing channelrhodopsin either in PV-expressing interneurons or in SST-expressing interneurons. TBS with blue light produced LTD at synapses made by PV interneurons, with a consequent disinhibition of pyramidal cells. In contrast, TBS of SST-expressing interneurons led to LTP of inhibitory synapses on distal dendrites of pyramidal cells. Modeling studies predicted that the consequence of these two opposing effects would be to stabilize place cell firing while maximizing the number of independent place fields that the hippocampal network could represent.

10.3.5 Homeostatic modulation of synaptic efficacy at I-E and E-I synapses

In addition to the examples of synaptic plasticity at I-E and E-I synapses discussed above, an increase in the firing rate of CA1 pyramidal cells, or of excitatory synaptic input to pyramidal cells, can cause compensatory homeostatic adjustment of the strength of inhibitory inputs at I-E synapses. This can happen in one of two ways. First, an increase in pyramidal cell firing leads to a compensatory increase in perisomatic inhibition from PV interneurons via a pathway that involves voltage-gated Na^+ channels (Na_Vs), L-type Ca^{2+} channels and neuroregulin 2. Second, an increase in activity at excitatory inputs on distal dendritic spines results in an increase in the strength of synapses of SST-expressing interneurons terminating on the same or neighboring spines or dendrites, through a mechanism involving the transsynaptic membrane signaling proteins neuroligin-2 and neuroligin-3 (Horn and Nicoll, 2018).

10.4 E-S potentiation

The relationship between the slope of the field EPSP and the amplitude of the population spike can be assessed by varying the strength of stimulation. The E-S curve obtained in this way after the induction of LTP is often shifted to the left relative to the preinduction E-S curve, indicating the recruitment of an additional component of spike potentiation over and above that due to EPSP potentiation (Bliss and Lømo, 1973). This persistent increase in excitability, referred to as E-S potentiation, is seen at the single cell level as an increase in the probability of spike discharge for a given EPSP slope (Chavez-Noriega et al., 1989). E-S potentiation in the DG has been followed for up to 4 hours in the anesthetized rat (Truchet et al., 2012).

The balance of evidence at the time of the first edition suggested that E-S potentiation is due to persistent disinhibition, perhaps caused by LTD in inhibitory inputs to principal excitatory neurons. Madison and colleagues reported that Aβ42 peptide caused a reduction in E-S potentiation at SCC synapses in vitro by depressing endocannabinoid-induced disinhibition (Orr et al., 2014), but a more recent report from the same laboratory attributes the effect to an increase in coupling between the somatic EPSP and the generation of the spike (Clark and Madison, 2020). A curious and unexplained feature of E-S potentiation is its apparent input specificity (Abraham et al., 1987), which runs counter to the idea that it reflects a general increase in neuronal excitability.

Evidence suggesting that E-S potentiation is important in facilitating the projection of activity from the hippocampus to extrahippocampal regions has come from a pioneering fMRI study of LTP in anesthetized rats (Canals et al., 2009). In naive animals, stimulation of the perforant path, irrespective of stimulus strength produced a BOLD signal that was always confined to the hippocampus. However, following the induction of LTP at perforant path–granule cell synapses, the BOLD signal spread to a number of extrahippocampal regions, notably the prefrontal cortex. These results suggest that an increase in synaptic strength alone is insufficient to allow mnemonic information to reach extrahippocampal targets; an additional boost is required, potentially supplied by E-S potentiation. Subsequent work by the same group indicates that the spread of the BOLD signal depends on disinhibition at recurrent basket cell–granule cell synapses (Caramés et al., 2020). Changes in the excitability of neural ensembles without change in synaptic coupling, an extreme form of E-S potentiation, has been generated in visual cortex by Yuste and his colleagues (Alejandre-García et al., 2022). An increase in the excitability of a network of neurons also feeds into the notion that excitable neurons are more likely to be allocated to information-storing networks (Rogerson et al., 2014).

10.5 Neuromodulation

In the first edition of *The Hippocampus Book* (pp 403–406), we described the actions of some of the key neuromodulators, including ACh, dopamine, BDNF, IL-1β (interleukin-1β), TNFα (tumor necrosis factor α), corticosterone, and estrogen. Since space precludes a comprehensive account of all neuromodulatory influences, here we describe a few exemplars to highlight key principles of neuromodulation. Neuromodulation generally has a similar impact on synaptic plasticity induced by conventional induction protocols and by STDP protocols. Here we will focus on traditional stimulus paradigms. The reader is referred to Brzosko et al. (2019) for a comprehensive account of neuromodulation of STDP. The present section is best read in conjunction with the first edition (Chapter 10, pp 403–406).

10.5.1 Acetylcholine (ACh)

Cholinergic systems of the brain are important for learning and memory, and the loss of cholinergic inputs is associated with dementia (see section 10.9). Cholinergic inputs to the hippocampus arise from the medial septum and diagonal band of Broca, are activated by arousal, and may be particularly important for reinforcing synaptic plasticity at times of uncertainty. ACh activates ionotropic receptors (principally the nicotinic α4β2, α3β4, and α7 receptors) and metabotropic receptors (muscarinic M1–M4) in the hippocampus.

Cholinergic modulation of synaptic plasticity operates predominantly through the facilitation of NMDAR-LTP and NMDAR-LTD, via a variety of distinct mechanisms (Palacios-Filardo and Mellor, 2019). Activation of muscarinic receptors facilitates the activation of NMDARs in multiple ways: (1) it directly boosts the NMDAR conductance via a membrane delineated process; (2) it triggers intracellular signaling cascades that regulate the NMDAR conductance directly (via phosphorylation) or indirectly via membrane depolarization (e.g., Buchanan et al., 2010); (3) it regulates the activity of GABAergic neurons, which in turn directly influences the synaptic activation of NMDARs via regulation of the membrane potential and hence the level of Mg^{2+} block; (4) it engages signaling mechanisms downstream of NMDAR activation to directly influence the level of expression of synaptic plasticity (e.g., Jo et al., 2010). Activation of nicotinic receptors also regulates the induction of synaptic plasticity via multiple mechanisms, including an action on astrocytes to release D-serine to enhance NMDAR activation (Papouin et al., 2017).

10.5.2 Dopamine

Of the monoamine neurotransmitters, the one most studied in the context of LTP is dopamine. Dopamine is associated with reward, prediction errors, novelty, and salience in distinct neural networks. Dopaminergic afferents to the hippocampus may influence the magnitude or persistence of synaptic plasticity during various emotional and behavioral states. Dopamine modulation is complex, since it acts via D1-like (D1 and D5) receptors, which elevate cAMP levels, and D2-like (D2, D3, and D4) receptors, which lower cAMP levels, and may also form heterodimeric assemblies with other G-protein-coupled subunits. One well-established role of dopamine, acting via D1-like receptors, is to engage the PKA-dependent signaling pathway to promote de novo protein synthesis, and hence transform LTP1 into LTP2 (Reymann and Frey, 2007). Dopamine

also regulates synaptic plasticity by influencing the synaptic activation of NMDARs in complex ways (Hammad and Wagner, 2006; Varela et al., 2009).

Much of our understanding of the actions of dopamine on synaptic plasticity has been derived from pharmacological experiments. However, the use of optogenetics to activate dopamine inputs selectively has highlighted some possible differences between physiological and pharmacological activation (Rosen et al., 2015). Intriguingly, optogenetic experiments have also shown that the dopamine that modulates LTP in the hippocampus may originate largely from the locus coeruleus rather than from the ventral tegmental area (Takeuchi et al., 2016). It will be important to determine how synaptic plasticity is modulated by different physiological patterns of activity in the various dopaminergic afferent populations.

10.5.3 Noradrenaline (norepinephrine)

Noradrenaline, sometimes referred to as norepinephrine, has long been implicated in memory function and accordingly, there has been widespread interest in how it is involved in hippocampal LTP (see first edition, pp 403–404). Noradrenaline released from the locus coeruleus signals attention and other cognitive processes that enhance learning and memory. Within the hippocampus, noradrenaline principally affects β-adrenergic receptors (both $β_1$ and $β_2$) to promote LTP2, via the activation of cAMP-driven mechanisms and triggering of protein synthesis. Interestingly, this signaling involves EPAC 1 (exchange protein directly activated by cAMP; also known as RAPGEF3, Rap guanine nucleotide exchange factor 3) as opposed to PKA (Maity et al., 2020). The combination of a tetanus, to activate NMDARs, and noradrenaline converts LTP1 not just to LTP2 but also to LTP3. The full potentiating action of noradrenaline is prevented by transcription inhibitors and involves epigenetic modifications, including DNA methylation (Maity et al., 2016).

10.5.4 5-Hydroxytryptamine (5-HT)

5-HT (serotonin) also has important modulatory effects on synaptic plasticity in the hippocampus. In mammals, 5-HT activates 14 subtypes of receptors, which are grouped into 7 distinct families (5-HT_{1-7}). With the exception of 5-HT_3, which is a ligand-gated ion channel, these receptors couple to G proteins (5-HT_1 and 5-HT_5 to G_i/G_o, 5-HT_2 to G_q/G_{11} and 5-HT_4, 5-HT_6 and 5-HT_7 to G_s). A major question is precisely how 5-HT modulates synaptic plasticity when there are many 5-HT receptors capable of inducing a variety of different, and sometimes opposing, effects. In part, their activation may be determined by the levels of 5-HT released. In the hippocampus, activation of 5-HT_{1A} is dominant and this inhibits the activation of GSK-3, which will limit the generation of NMDAR-LTD. Conversely, a reduction in 5-HT levels will tend to promote LTD, an effect that could contribute to major depressive disorder (MDD; see section 10.9) and be reversible by treatment with a selective serotonin-reuptake inhibitor (SSRI; Beurel et al., 2015). Clearly more work is required to understand the complexity of 5-HT receptor regulation of synaptic plasticity in the hippocampus.

10.5.5 Corticosteroids

Stress has profound effects on synaptic plasticity in the hippocampus. Early findings were touched on in the first edition (pp 405–406) and are covered in more detail in Chapter 17 of this edition. It is well established that stress can modulate hippocampal NMDAR-LTP in a bidirectional manner, with mild stress promoting and chronic stress inhibiting the process, and that inhibition of hippocampal LTP is associated with augmentation of LTD. Thus, mild stress provides a mechanism to enhance synaptic plasticity, and hence learning and memory, during everyday life, and is therefore an important adaptive process. However, excessive stress becomes maladaptive. Here we summarize how stress imparts its rapid, physiological action of enhancing the level of hippocampal LTP.

A number of rapid, nongenomic actions of corticosterone have been described in rodents, including a presynaptic effect, that involves extracellular signal-regulated kinase 1/2 (ERK1/2) signaling, and a postsynaptic action on A-type K current (I_A) currents (Olijslagers et al., 2008; Pasricha et al., 2011). One major target of corticosteroid is at the level of AMPAR trafficking. For example, the hormone increases the mobility and surface expression of AMPARs (Groc et al., 2008). This effect is itself dependent on regulation of the trafficking of GluN2B-containing NMDARs (Mikasova et al., 2017). A potential mechanism to account for the role of AMPARs in acute stress was suggested by the finding that corticosteroid treatment or brief restraint stress led, via activation of glucocorticoid receptors and PKA activity, to an enhanced LTP at dorsal SCC-CA1 synapses (Whitehead et al., 2013). In short, brief stress enables a stimulus that would typically only induce LTP1 to trigger LTP2 in addition.

10.5.6 BDNF

BDNF is the most highly expressed neurotrophin in the brain, and its role in hippocampal synaptic plasticity has been intensively studied. However, many unresolved issues remain (see Panja and Bramham, 2014; De Vincenti et al., 2019). BDNF is located in, and released from, both presynaptic and postsynaptic compartments of hippocampal pyramidal cells, as well as from a variety of other cell types (Edelmann et al., 2014). It seems likely, therefore, that BDNF contributes to regulation of pre- and postsynaptic protein synthesis that is required for coordinated structural alterations at both synaptic loci (see Chapter 8). One interesting idea is that BDNF released from the presynaptic terminal helps trigger the induction of LTP postsynaptically, via an anterograde signaling mechanism, while BDNF released postsynaptically maintains LTP via actions that are both pre- and postsynaptic (Lin et al., 2018).

In contrast, endogenous release of the immature precursor protein pro-BDNF, opposes the action of BDNF via facilitation of LTD (Yang et al., 2014). This effect is mediated via the low-affinity, pan neurotrophin receptor p75 (p75^{NTR}). The propeptide, generated when pro-BDNF is cleaved to liberate BDNF, facilitates LTD by regulating the surface distribution of GluN2B-containing NMDARs and promoting the endocytosis of AMPARs (Mizui et al., 2015). It is well established that a common human variant (Val66Met) affects memory function (Bath and Lee, 2006). Interestingly, propeptides that contain the Val version facilitate LTD whereas those that contain Met block LTD (Mizui et al., 2015). A likely mechanism for the effect of the mutation on synaptic plasticity involves the disruption of the binding of BDNF to the glycoprotein sortilin within secretary granules, and consequently to an impairment of BDNF release.

An important regulator of BDNF- and pro-BDNF-induced synaptic plasticity is SorCS2 (sortilin-related Vps10p domain containing receptor 2). SorCS2 binds both p75^{NTR} and TrkB to regulate LTD and LTP, respectively (Glerup et al., 2016). The effects of both BDNF and pro-BDNF are thus mediated via the regulation of complex signaling pathways. For BDNF this includes the PI3K/Akt pathway, the PLC (phospholipase C)/PKC/CaMKII pathway and the Raf/MEK/ERK (rapidly accelerated fibrosarcoma kinase/mitogen-activated protein kinase/ERK) pathway, with the latter resulting in activation of mitogen- and stress-activated kinase 1 (MSK1) to regulate protein synthesis (Cooper and Frenguelli, 2021).

10.5.7 Insulin and related substances

Several hormones and peptides involved in glucose homeostasis, including insulin, insulin-like growth factor 1 (IGF-1), ghrelin (growth hormone-releasing peptide), and glucagon-like peptide-1 (GLP-1), are important modulators of synaptic plasticity (Mainardi et al., 2015). Here, we focus on insulin, a hormone that can affect hippocampal synaptic plasticity in several ways (Kamal et al., 2012; Gralle, 2017; Ferrario and Reagan, 2018; F Zhao et al., 2019). Classically, insulin signals via the family of insulin receptor substrates (IRS) to regulate PI3K/Akt and MAPK cascades, both of which affect synaptic function. Also, activation of the brain-specific insulin receptor substrate of 53 kD (IRSp53) affects the level of NMDARs and LTP at SCC synapses (Kim et al., 2009; Sawallisch et al., 2009). IRS2 is also critically involved in LTP at SCC synapses, potentially via regulation of fyn, Akt, and MAPK pathways (Martín et al., 2012), and influences spine density and memory formation (Irvine et al., 2011). Understanding how insulin regulates these synaptic processes is important, since disruption of insulin signaling may contribute to cognitive decline in AD. One possibility, by analogy to its role in glycogen metabolism, is that a critical synaptic role of insulin is to activate the PI3K/Akt pathway to inhibit GSK-3 and thereby suppress LTD—in which case, insulin resistance or insulin depletion (Gabbouj et al., 2019; Imamura et al., 2020) could facilitate the induction of LTD, leading to the potential elimination of synapses.

10.6 Metaplasticity and homeostasis

10.6.1 Metaplasticity

Metaplasticity refers to the plasticity of plasticity; it is the process whereby a plasticity-inducing stimulus affects subsequent synaptic plasticity in the same or a different pathway. Metaplasticity comes in many guises.

10.6.1.1 Saturation

The first example of metaplasticity to be discovered was the saturation of LTP. When repeated HFS is delivered, the degree of LTP induced gets less each time and a point is reached where no further LTP can be induced (Bliss and Lømo, 1973). The ceiling effect may reflect the point at which no further AMPARs can be accommodated at the PSD and/or there is no further space for docked vesicles.

10.6.1.2 Depotentiation (DP)

DP (see also section 10.2.1) is a form of synaptic depression that is only observed following the induction of LTP. In other words, the induction of LTP has altered the sensitivity of the affected synapses to synaptic depression. As such, it constitutes a form of metaplasticity. Importantly, in healthy adult tissue, DP is much more readily induced than de novo LTD. It is therefore likely to be the dominant form of synaptic depression contributing to normal cognitive processes in the adult animal.

10.6.1.3 Homosynaptic priming

This takes many forms. For example, a weak HFS that does not induce LTP may enhance the magnitude, and alter the pharmacological properties, of the LTP induced by a subsequent HFS. A priming stimulus enables a subsequent stimulus, that would ordinarily trigger just LTP1, to induce both LTP1 and LTP2 (reviewed by Collingridge and Abraham, 2022). This process, which

led to the coining of the term "metaplasticity" by Cliff Abraham, is probably achieved by the priming stimulus activating mGluR5 to trigger de novo protein synthesis (see Figure 10.8). Priming requires extremely modest activation of mGluR5 (threshold ~5 stimuli at ~3 Hz; Bortolotto et al., 2008) and is exquisitely sensitive to neuromodulation. Notably, transient prior activation of β-adrenergic receptors enables a stimulus that would ordinarily trigger

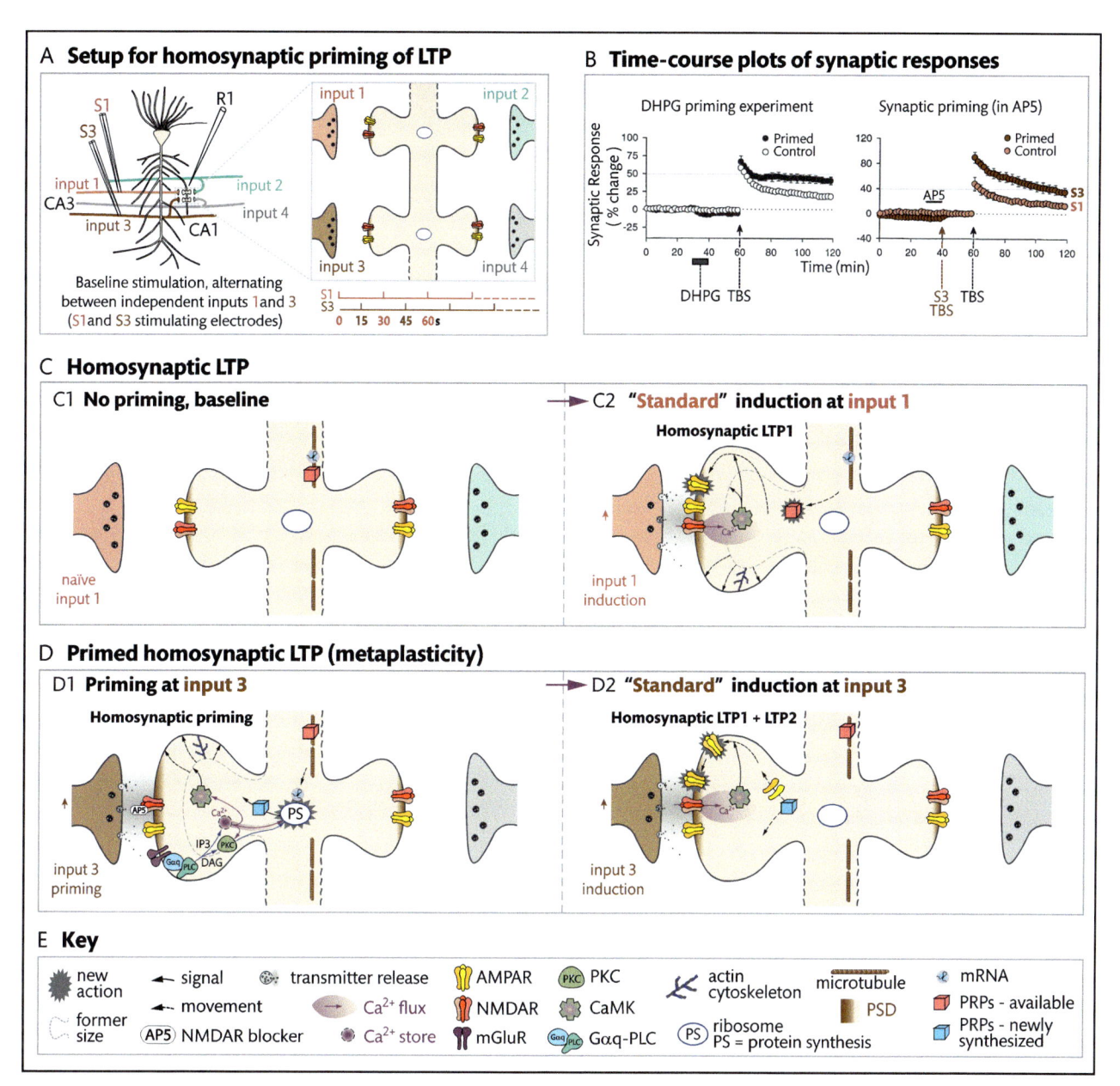

Figure 10.8 Homosynaptic priming of LTP. (A) A schematic of a typical priming experiment. This is based on the schematic described in Box 10.3. The brown input 3 is *primed*, whereas the pink input 1 is not, prior to the induction of LTP. The green and gray inputs 3 and 4 only receive test-pulse stimulation and are unaffected throughout. (B) Typical priming experiment. Left-hand graph: Following 1 h of baseline, an induction stimulus was applied (arrow pointing up), which induced LTP1 (open symbol). In interleaved experiments, slices were *primed* by brief application of the group I mGluR agonist, DHPG (20 μM, 10 min). The subsequent LTP was larger in magnitude (LTP1 + LTP2). Right-hand graph: Equivalent experiments where the priming was performed using a tetanus in the presence of an NMDAR antagonist, D-AP5 (modified from Raymond et al., 2000). (C) A schematic to illustrate LTP1 in the *nonprimed* input. The induction stimulus (tetanus or TBS) induces LTP1, via activation of NMDARs (as described in Figure 10.4). (D) Schematic to illustrate LTP1 + LTP2 in the *primed* input. (D1) The priming stimulus activates mGluR5 that initiates a cascade involving Ca^{2+} release from stores, CaMKII, PKC, and de novo protein synthesis. The protein synthesis is required for the priming but not for the subsequent induction of LTP2. It is assumed that this provides the components required to enable the induction of LTP2, including spine growth to accommodate the additional AMPARs. However, it is not known whether there is spine growth associated with priming (as depicted here). (D2) The subsequent LTP induction stimulus (tetanus or TBS) induces LTP1 + LTP2 at the same input, via activation of NMDARs (as described in Figure 10.4). (E) Key of major components.

LTP1 to trigger LTP2 (Tenorio et al., 2010). Considered together, these observations suggest that mGluR-dependent homosynaptic metaplasticity may be a common occurrence in vivo.

10.6.1.4 Heterosynaptic priming

Heterosynaptic priming constitutes a family of distinct mechanisms that allow the conditioning of one input to affect subsequent synaptic plasticity at a separate input. The best-known example of localized heterosynaptic priming is the STC process, introduced in section 10.1.4, whereby a strong HFS (defined as one that triggers LTP2) to one input enables a weak HFS (that would ordinarily only induce LTP1) to induce both LTP1 and LTP2 on an independent input (see Box 10.3). The extensive literature includes several authoritative reviews (e.g., Redondo and Morris, 2011; Bin Ibrahim et al., 2021; Okuda et al., 2021; Bin Ibrahim et al., 2024). In Box 10.3 we build on these foundations and incorporate the notion that CP-AMPARs may serve as the synaptic tag and also help trigger the formation of PRPs (P Park et al., 2018; P Park, Kang, et al., 2021).

Metaplastic interactions may also involve long-range interactions between synapses spread across dendritic compartments (Hulme et al., 2014). The mechanism of long-range heterosynaptic metaplasticity is complex and involves hydrolysis of ATP, acting via A2 adenosine receptors, gap junctions, and TNFα (Jones et al., 2013; Singh et al., 2022).

10.6.2 Homeostasis

The simple yet powerful Hebbian synaptic plasticity rule, that existing synaptic connections increase in strength when pre- and postsynaptic neurons are coactive (Hebb, 1949), lacks one essential element: a homeostatic mechanism to prevent runaway synaptic potentiation. The original version of Hebbian synaptic plasticity exhibits the property of positive feedback: the more a synapse is potentiated, the greater will be the depolarization its activation produces in the postsynaptic cell, leading to further potentiation and the prospect of runaway excitation in the neural network. The consequence would be an inevitable introduction of spurious noise into the hippocampal network, severely degrading memory storage, in addition to the potential for pathological hyperexcitability, including epilepsy. Indeed, failures of synaptic homeostasis have been invoked as causes of epilepsy (Staley, 2015).

10.6.2.1 Heterosynaptic LTD

Initially, the reverse synaptic process of input-specific synaptic depression (LTD), which had not been included in Hebb's original thesis, was proposed as a likely homeostatic mechanism under the rationale that "what goes up must come down" (Morris and Willshaw, 1989; Dayan and Willshaw, 1991). A protocol was eventually identified that could produce reliable long-lasting homosynaptic LTD at SCC-CA1 pyramidal cell synapses in young animals (Dudek and Bear, 1992; Mulkey and Malenka, 1992). Homosynaptic LTD, which was described in more detail in section 10.2.2, is commonly induced with LFS (1 Hz) over 15 min; similar effects can be induced under appropriate spike-timing protocols, with the postsynaptic cell firing immediately prior to the presynaptic cell (Levy and Steward, 1983; Bi and Poo, 1998). This form of plasticity is potentially relevant to forgetting (Tsumoto, 1993), memory extinction or reversal (Nabavi et al., 2014), or de novo learning (Kemp and Manahan-Vaughan,

2007; S Griffiths et al., 2008), but it is also theoretically attractive as a candidate homeostatic mechanism.

In isolation, LTD also suffers from a similar "runaway" propensity, although in the opposite direction to LTP; as synapses weaken, the conditions for further weakening are enhanced, since the likelihood that the synapse contributes to postsynaptic activation is reduced, leading eventually to a silencing of the network. One solution could be that LTP and LTD are distributed across a synaptic network, serving not only to maintain balanced levels of excitation but also to increase signal-to-noise in the network (Dayan and Willshaw, 1991). This is most clearly demonstrated at perforant path–granule cell synapses (Bear and Abraham, 1996), where heterosynaptic LTD occurs in a nontetanized pathway while LTP is induced in tetanized synapses. A similar phenomenon has been observed at SCC-CA1 synapses, but the authors argue that this LTD, though manifest heterosynaptically, is in fact a homosynaptic phenomenon that occurs due to uncorrelated pre- and postsynaptic activity (Stanton and Sejnowski, 1989). More recent work (Okuno et al., 2012) has shown that a very localized version of LTD at inactive synapses directly neighboring a potentiated synapse is supported by the protein product of the immediate early gene *Arc/Arg3.1*, a known LTD effector that facilitates clathrin-mediated AMPAR endocytosis (Chowdhury et al., 2006). Related work in neocortex reveals that Arc/Arg3.1-dependent heterosynaptic depression accompanies homosynaptic potentiation resulting from STDP (El-Boustani et al., 2018). Indeed, the process of heterosynaptic LTD may capture core aspects of STDP (Levy and Steward, 1983; Debanne et al., 1994).

When spike timing is investigated at hippocampal synapses (Bi and Poo, 1998), it is consistently observed that synapses potentiate when presynaptic neurons fire shortly before postsynaptic neurons (see section 10.2.5). The time window of pairing within which this synaptic potentiation occurs (~30 ms) reflects the likely period of integration for synaptic inputs that summate to cause a postsynaptic action potential, as Hebb predicted (Hebb, 1949). Reversal of this timing, so that the postsynaptic neuron fires before the presynaptic neuron, results in LTD, which is commonly invoked as a mechanism that weakens all active synapses that did not contribute to causing a postsynaptic action potential (Markram et al., 2012). The time window for t-LTD is longer than for t-LTP (Bi and Poo, 1998), which is likely a factor in the striking finding that net synaptic weakening results from randomized stimulation (Feldman, 2012). It is intriguing to consider that the default state for hippocampal and neocortical networks may be gradual synaptic weakening. A default state in which synaptic activity drives gradual synaptic weakening could serve as a natural safety valve for excessive Hebbian potentiation but, as we will see later in the chapter, it may also be a contributory factor in dementia processes (Sheng et al., 2012).

Examples such as those described above provide encouraging experimental evidence that mechanisms exist in the hippocampus to maintain network stability as Hebbian synaptic plasticity occurs during learning, and there are models of stable neural networks that invoke no more than a hard ceiling on synaptic strength (which surely exists due to physical limits if nothing else and is manifest as saturation, as described above) and the bidirectional forces of Hebbian STDP (Song et al., 2000). Nevertheless, most theoretical approaches have favored the inclusion of additional homeostatic factors to further extend memory storage capacity (Bienenstock et al., 1982; Oja, 1982).

10.6.2.2 Metaplasticity as a homeostatic mechanism

One theoretical solution to the homeostasis problem starts with the concept of a variable threshold in the frequency of postsynaptic activity, known as a modification threshold (θ_m), above which LTP occurs and below which LTD occurs (Cooper et al., 1979). That such a threshold exists in the hippocampus and elsewhere is now clearly established and can be defined by stimulus frequency (Dudek and Bear, 1993), spike timing (Bi and Poo, 1998), or postsynaptic Ca^{2+} concentration (Cummings et al., 1996; S Yang et al., 1999). A critical conceptual insight in relation to homeostasis is the notion that this threshold can vary or "slide" depending on the recent history of activity at that synapse. Following prolonged firing, θ_m shifts to the right, so that continued activity is more likely to lead to depression. This form of synaptic metaplasticity is embodied in the Bienenstock-Cooper-Munro (BCM) model of network stability (Bienenstock et al., 1982); also see Box 10.2, p 366 in the first edition of this book), which has often focused on the response of visual neocortex to sensory deprivation and experience as a primary exemplar (Cooper and Bear, 2012). Here, deprivation of various kinds serves to alter the average firing rates of neurons for long enough to evoke a homeostatic shift (Hengen et al., 2013), but it has been more challenging to come up with an appropriate environmental treatment that can produce a BCM-like shift in the hippocampus. Nevertheless, artificially altering average postsynaptic firing by delivering a priming burst of HFS is sufficient to cause a shift in θ_m (Abraham et al., 2001; Hulme et al., 2014).

Within the context of the BCM model, changes in Ca^{2+} conductance or Ca^{2+}-dependent signaling at the synapse are the likeliest biophysical mechanisms to shift θ_m (Yeung et al., 2004). Given the evidence that activation of the NMDAR serves as the primary induction mechanism for canonical forms of LTP and LTD (Dudek and Bear, 1992; Bliss and Collingridge, 1993a) and that the concentration of postsynaptic Ca^{2+} produced by influx through this receptor determines the direction of synaptic change (Lisman, 1989; Mulkey and Malenka, 1992), the most direct way of shifting θ_m would be to modify the subunit composition of the heterotetrameric NMDAR to alter its Ca^{2+} conductivity. The ratio of GluN2A/GluN2B subunits is most relevant in this regard as the GluN2A/2B composition governs Ca^{2+} conductance of the receptor (Cull-Candy and Leszkiewicz, 2004) and the polarity of plasticity resulting from patterned stimulation (Barria and Malinow, 2005; Morishita et al., 2007). Thus, a dynamically regulated GluN2A/2B ratio presents itself as an ideal molecular mechanism for synaptic metaplasticity. It is well known that the GluN2A/2B ratio is increased through development, coinciding with a change in the direction and magnitude of synaptic plasticity (Monyer et al., 1994; Sheng et al., 1994), but the ratio can also be influenced by experience and deprivation (Quinlan, Olstein, et al., 1999; Quinlan, Philpot, et al., 1999; Philpot et al., 2001). Evidence that this is a mechanism of sliding θ_m based on the prior history of synaptic activity is now strong in neocortex (L Cooper and Bear, 2012). Although the methods of constraining activity levels to drive metaplasticity in the hippocampus have so far not been as naturalistic as those applied in the visual system, there is evidence that synaptic activity levels can quickly alter the GluN2A/2B ratio and influence the direction of subsequent plasticity, both in vitro (Bellone and Nicoll, 2007; MC Lee et al., 2010) and in vivo (Abraham et al., 2001). There is particularly compelling evidence that uncaging glutamate at individual CA1 spines, using a protocol that induces Hebbian LTP of AMPA currents, also reduces the Ca^{2+} conductivity of NMDAR due to GluN2B subunit modification (Sobczyk and Svoboda 2007), a kind of LTD of NMDAR that could

---

Box 10.3 Synaptic tagging and capture (STC) mechanisms

STC is the term used to describe a cellular phenomenon whereby a "strong" input (defined as one sufficient to induce LTP2) enables a "weak" input (defined as one that only induces LTP1) to generate LTP2 on the weak pathway (see section 10.1.4). STC often alters the magnitude at the synaptic population level and significantly increases the retention of LTP induced by the weak input. Classically, the underlying mechanism involves (1) the setting of a local "synaptic tag" at the time of LTP (whether induced by weak or strong stimulation) and (2) the upregulation of de novo protein synthesis with the products of this process "captured" by the synaptic tag to stabilize local LTP. STC has been extensively studied, shown to be important for memory consolidation and associative learning (Moncada and Viola, 2007; S Wang et al., 2010), and its mechanisms and function are the subject of many reviews (e.g., Redondo and Morris, 2011; Pinho et al., 2020; Bin Ibrahim et al., 2021; Okuda et al., 2021; Bin Ibrahim et al., 2024) and two dedicated books (Sajikumar, 2015; Sajikumar and Abel, 2024), which may be consulted for additional details including the historical background.

One key element of the STC process is the setting of the synaptic tag. This is known to be posttranslational in that its setting is unaffected by anisomycin (U Frey and Morris, 1997), to last between 1 and 2 h, but capable of being reset by low-frequency activity (Sajikumar and Frey, 2004b). Various molecular candidates have been considered, with a consensus emerging that the tag may be more complex than a single molecule (or its phosphorylation) and may include also the transient destabilization of the actin cytoskeleton; this is permissive for the insertion of additional AMPARs to the PSD. The second key element is the concept of the role of plasticity-related products (PRPs) that include mRNAs and newly synthesized proteins. These can be triggered by the "strong" glutamatergic input and/or by neuromodulatory inputs, such as those that release dopamine. These inputs induce signal transduction pathway activation that triggers the synthesis of PRPs. Once PRPs are "captured" by the tag, the conjunction serves to stabilize the synaptic potentiation that had earlier been induced. Interestingly, PRPs induced in association with LTP2 can stabilize LTD, and vice versa (Sajikumar and Frey, 2004a). In a striking demonstration of the phenomenon of STC at work at the single synapse level, confocal microscopy was used to show the stabilization of changes to the size and shape of individual dendritic spines when the combination of release of caged MNI-glutamate is coupled to forskolin activation of neighboring regions of the dendrite (Govindarajan et al., 2011). Normally, the interaction of synaptic tags and PRPs is synergistic, i.e., LTP lasts longer, but in circumstances of limited PRP availability, it can be competitive (Govindarajan et al., 2011). A phenomenon called "inverse tagging" has also been described in which Arc protein produced as a result of strong synaptic stimulation is targeted to weak synapses to weaken them further by removal of surface GluA1-containing AMPARs (Okuno et al., 2012).

The STC process functions when, within a critical time window, the weak (W) input either precedes or follows the strong (S) input (W → S and S → W, respectively). The accompanying figure outlines the key molecular steps in STC, including the idea that CP-AMPARs may serve as the synaptic tag and trigger the formation of PRPs (P Park, Kang, et al., 2019; P Park, Kang, et al., 2021). We follow the sequence of figure panels A - G.

Box 10.3 Continued

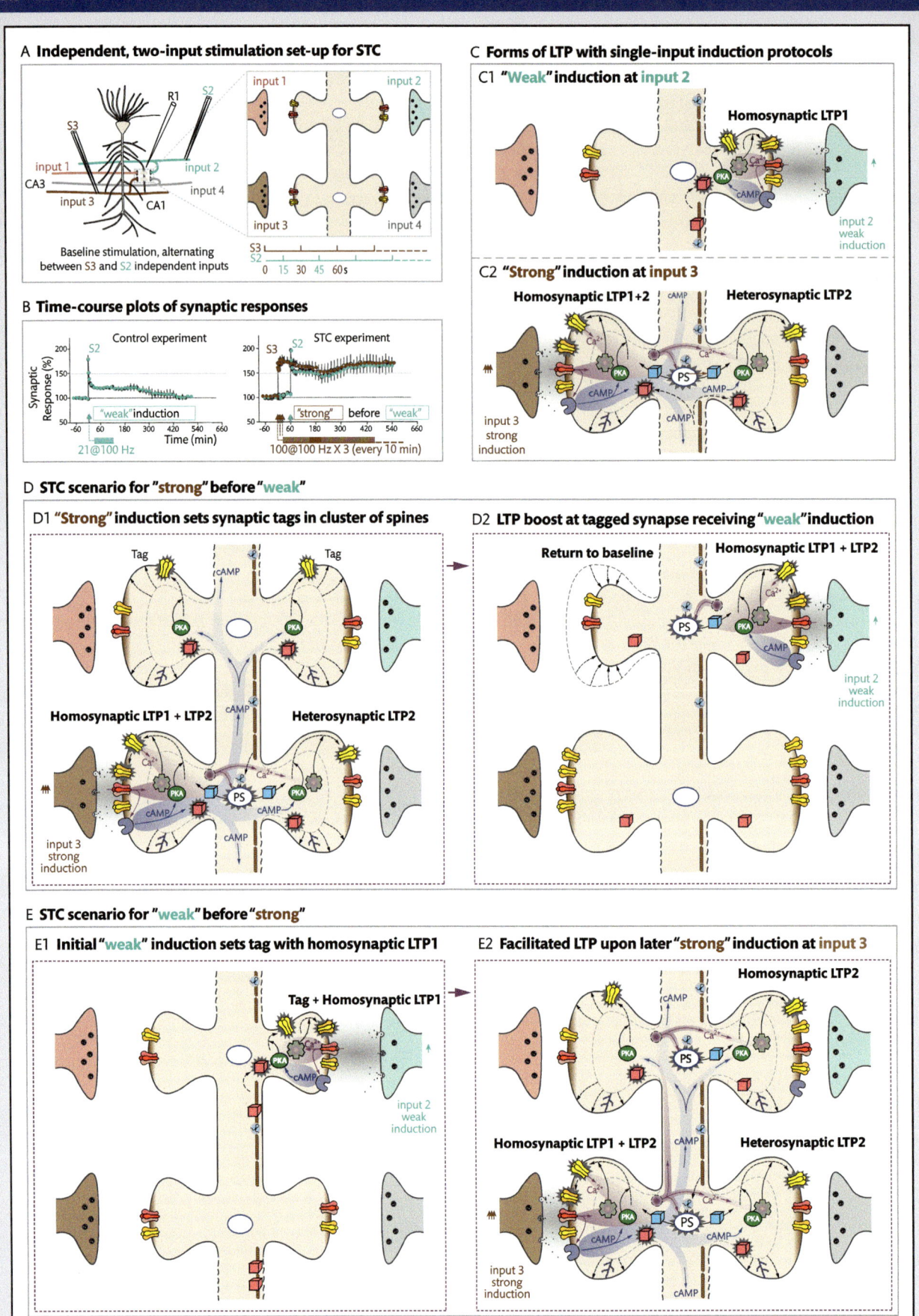

A Independent, two-input stimulation set-up for STC

R1 S2
S3
input 1   input 2
CA3   input 4
input 3   CA1

input 1   input 2
input 3   input 4

Baseline stimulation, alternating
between S3 and S2 independent inputs

S3
S2
0 15 30 45 60s

B Time-course plots of synaptic responses

Control experiment

Synaptic Response (%)
200
150
100
50
S2

"weak" induction
-60 60 180 300 420 540 660
Time (min)
21@100 Hz

STC experiment
200
150
100
50
S3 S2

"strong" before "weak"
-60 60 180 300 420 540 660
100@100 Hz X 3 (every 10 min)

C Forms of LTP with single-input induction protocols

C1 "Weak" induction at input 2

Homosynaptic LTP1

input 2
weak
induction

C2 "Strong" induction at input 3

Homosynaptic LTP1+2   cAMP   Heterosynaptic LTP2

input 3
strong
induction

D STC scenario for "strong" before "weak"

D1 "Strong" induction sets synaptic tags in cluster of spines

Tag   Tag
cAMP
PKA   PKA

Homosynaptic LTP1 + LTP2   Heterosynaptic LTP2
cAMP
PKA   PKA
cAMP
input 3
strong
induction
cAMP

D2 LTP boost at tagged synapse receiving "weak" induction

Return to baseline   Homosynaptic LTP1 + LTP2
PS
PKA
cAMP
input 2
weak
induction

E STC scenario for "weak" before "strong"

E1 Initial "weak" induction sets tag with homosynaptic LTP1

Tag + Homosynaptic LTP1
PKA
cAMP
input 2
weak
induction

E2 Facilitated LTP upon later "strong" induction at input 3

Homosynaptic LTP2
cAMP
PS

Homosynaptic LTP1 + LTP2   cAMP   Heterosynaptic LTP2
PS
PKA   PKA
cAMP   cAMP
input 3
strong
induction
cAMP

Box 10.3 Continued

A. Schematic of a typical STC experiment

Typically, multiple axons are activated (usually one set orthodromically and one set antidromically), with stimulating electrodes set either side of the recording electrode in the SCC terminal field in stratum radiatum. The field EPSP is generated by multiple neurons, only one of which is shown for clarity. The independence of the inputs is defined by the absence of heterosynaptic paired-pulse facilitation. Two inputs are stimulated alternately to evoke single responses that monitor synaptic strength. In this example of S → W, a period of high-frequency stimulation, in the form of repeated tetani or TBS, is delivered via stimulation of S3 to activate input 3 (brown) and subsequently a period of high-frequency stimulation, typically a single tetanus or TBS episode, is delivered via S2 to activate input 2 (blue). Inset: A zoomed-in view of four synapses. Each synapse contains multiple NMDARs (red) and AMPARs (yellow), only one of which per synapse are shown for clarity. Ribosomes (white ovals) are available to rapidly synthesize new proteins from existing mRNAs.

B. A typical STC experiment

Left-hand graph: Following 1 h of baseline, a weak tetanus is delivered to input 2 (blue arrow, S2) to induce LTP1, which in this example decayed to baseline within a few hours. Right-hand graph: In contrast, when preceded by a strong tetanus delivered 1 h earlier to input 3 (S3), the same weak tetanus applied to input 2 (S2) now induced LTP2, a larger LTP that persisted throughout the recording period (9 h). (Modified from U Frey and Morris, 1997.)

C. The key components of LTP1 and LTP2

A schematic to illustrate the key elements involved in triggering LTP1 (at input 2) and LTP1 + LTP2 (at input 3). See Figure 10.4 for temporal details. (C1) At input 2, the weak stimulus induces just LTP1; Ca^{2+} permeating through NMDARs activates CaMKII to drive additional CI-AMPARs into the synapse. The increase in the number of CI-AMPARs may be associated with spine growth (not illustrated) using a reserve of previously synthesized components (pink box). Concurrent activation of Ca^{2+}-sensitive AC1 and/ or AC8, generates cAMP to activate PKA and drive CP-AMPARs into perisynaptic sites, where they reside but do not contribute to the synaptic response. The LTP is homosynaptic since the neighboring spines, which are not activated by the weak stimulus, are not potentiated. (C2) At input 3, the strong stimulus induces both LTP1 (as described above) and LTP2; the latter also requires the activation of CaMKII (or a related kinase) to drive CP-AMPARs from perisynaptic sites to the PSD. Subsequent activation of these CP-AMPARs, typically via basal stimulation, provides a Ca^{2+} signal that drives local de novo protein synthesis (PS), resulting in the formation of additional AMPARs and the products required to make larger spines (blue boxes). Strong induction commonly leads to LTP2 at heterosynaptic sites that receive independent inputs. This may be due to spillover of the Ca^{2+}, potentially via calcium-induced calcium release (CICR; see Koek et al., 2024); and/or cAMP signals to neighboring spines; and/or due to the local protein synthesis affecting neighboring spines to trigger the synaptic insertion of CP-AMPARs. In this example, LTP2 is associated with an increase in spine size (i.e., structural LTP) at both the homo- and heterosynaptic sites. The critical activation of PKA for the generation of LTP2 may require and/or be augmented by neuromodulatory systems, such as dopaminergic inputs (not illustrated).

D. An outline of the STC process, where strong precedes weak induction

(D1) The lower two spines depict homo- and heterosynaptic LTP induced by the "strong" stimulus (as shown in C2). The strong stimulus not only induces LTP2 at the activated and some neighboring synapses but also tags other synapses that are within proximity of the potentiated ones. The upper spines are marked with both a metabolic tag (in this case, CP-AMPARs) and a structural tag (depicted as spine growth and which might involve newly synthesized cytoskeletal components). Regarding the metabolic tag, in this hypothetical scheme, cAMP spreads to neighboring synapses, where it activates local PKA, which in turn phosphorylates GluA1(Ser845) to drive CP-AMPARs into the perisynaptic plasma membrane, where they dwell for minutes to hours. (D2) Depiction of

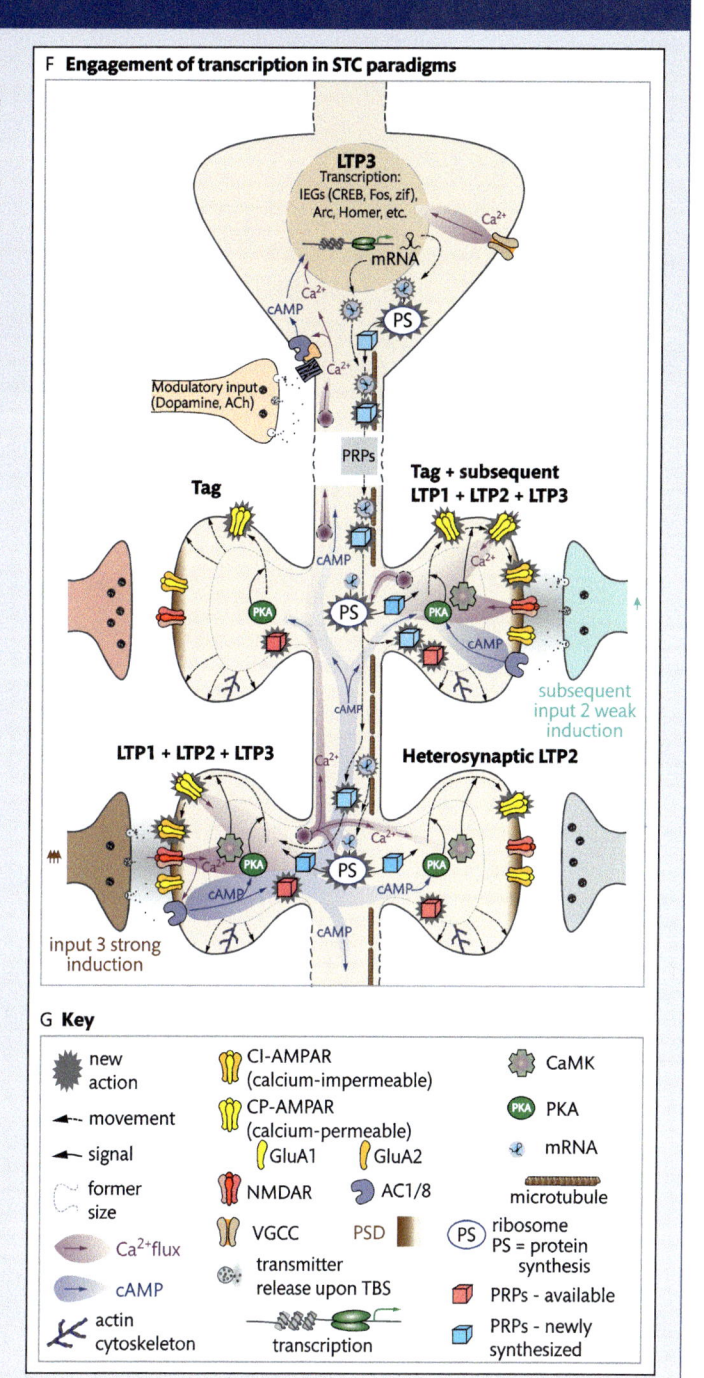

F Engagement of transcription in STC paradigms

LTP3
Transcription:
IEGs (CREB, Fos, zif),
Arc, Homer, etc.
mRNA

cAMP

Modulatory input
(Dopamine, ACh)

PRPs

Tag

Tag + subsequent
LTP1 + LTP2 + LTP3

cAMP

PKA   PKA

PS   cAMP

cAMP

subsequent
input 2 weak
induction

LTP1 + LTP2 + LTP3

Heterosynaptic LTP2

PKA   PKA

cAMP   PS   cAMP

input 3 strong
induction

cAMP

G Key

new action	CI-AMPAR (calcium-impermeable)	CaMK
movement	CP-AMPAR (calcium-permeable)	PKA
signal	GluA1 GluA2	mRNA
former size	NMDAR AC1/8	microtubule
Ca^{2+} flux	VGCC PSD	PS = ribosome PS = protein synthesis
cAMP	transmitter release upon TBS	PRPs - available
actin cytoskeleton	transcription	PRPs - newly synthesized

the consequence of delivering a weak stimulus at the independent input 2 within a limited time after the strong trigger at input 3. In the lower spines, LTP is maintained by the increase in the number of CI-AMPARs. In the tagged upper spines, the weak trigger, delivered to input 2, is now able to engage the protein-synthesis machinery to generate both LTP1 and LTP2 rather than just LTP1. Regarding the metabolic tag, the weak trigger stimulates NMDARs to activate CaMKII (or a related kinase) and drive CP-AMPARs into the synapse, from where they are able to trigger additional local protein synthesis to generate LTP2. Synapses that are tagged but not subject to an induction stimulus either return to baseline (as shown here, upper left spine), remain tagged, or become subject to heterosynaptic LTP2. In this model CP-AMPARs serve as (1) the synaptic tag, (2) the trigger for the generation of PRPs, and (3) one of the PRPs. Other PRPs may include GluA2 subunits to make additional CI-AMPARs

Box 10.3 Continued

that replace the CP-AMPARs, PKMζ to stabilize these new AMPARs at the synapses, CaMKII, pro-BDNF, and the structural components required to make larger synapses. Central to this mechanism is the perisynaptic insertion of CP-AMPARs into synapses, which do not necessarily themselves receive a weak or strong stimulus. Consistent with this model, structural LTP induced by local uncaging of MNI-glutamate leads to activation of PKA at surrounding synapses (Yang and Yasuda, 2017). This is most likely due to the diffusion of cAMP between spines within a dendritic compartment. Because cAMP signaling is central to STC, the process is geared for modulation by agents that regulate the levels of this second messenger, such as dopamine.

A question that remains is what determines whether the effect at neighboring spines is heterosynaptic potentiation (i.e., heterosynaptic LTP2) or heterosynaptic metaplasticity (i.e., STC as originally defined). One possibility, alluded to in panel D1, is that the heterosynaptic surround is defined by the diffusion of cAMP and the heterosynaptic potentiation within this surround is defined by the spread of Ca^{2+}, beyond the synapses receiving the strong input. This could occur via CICR that enables Ca^{2+} waves to propagate within neurons and for which some evidence exists (Sajikumar et al., 2009; Koek et al., 2024).

E. An outline of the STC process, when "weak" precedes "strong"

(E1) In a different scenario where the weak stimulus (at input 2) occurs first, LTP1 is generated, and the synapse is tagged. This LTP1 might be associated with spine growth (not illustrated). Here, CP-AMPARs are likely to be inserted into the perisynaptic membrane but not the synapse, where they could serve as a tag. (E2) The subsequent strong stimulus (to input 3) generates homosynaptic LTP1 + LTP2 at this input

and heterosynaptic LTP2 at input 4 (as depicted in C2) and additionally induces LTP2 at input 2. This might be due to activation of a CaMK (such as CaMKII) at input 2 by a propagated Ca^{2+} signal initiated in input 3.

F. An outline of the STC process involving transcription

In addition to local protein synthesis, transcription and somatic protein synthesis are also required at some point. Of relevance, the induction of LTP is associated with the upregulation of IEGs (e.g., *Zif268*, *CREB*, *Arc*, *c-Fos*) and there is evidence that LTP involves transcription (defined in this chapter as LTP3). One possibility is that tag specificity (defined here as inputs tagged for conversion from LTP1 to LTP2) is determined by the local events and somatically derived proteins/mRNAs are used to top up locally depleted resources. The other is that a classical STC operates, where the somatically derived PRPs are captured by tagged synapses. A potential candidate for such a process is Homer1a (Okada et al., 2009). Here, neuromodulation may be more of a cell-wide phenomenon, to facilitate the communication with the nucleus and to engage somatic protein synthesis. Increases in cell excitability, possibly involving E-S potentiation, may help to trigger somatic protein synthesis, via the activation of VGCCs.

Note also that, while this scheme focuses on some of the postsynaptic modifications, it is likely that an STC process operates presynaptically to coordinate the structural and functional alterations at both sides of the synapse. Indeed, there is evidence that PKA also plays a central role in this presynaptic process (A Park et al., 2014).

G. Key

---

be considered as homeostatic metaplasticity. Other candidate molecular mechanisms for sliding θ_m include Ca^{2+}-responsive signaling pathways, such as those initiated by CaMKII (Mayford et al., 1995; Yeung et al., 2004), or changes in dendritic excitability, such as those mediated by I_h, the HCN cation current (Narayanan and Johnston, 2010). A key missing link remains the feedback mechanism that detects changes in neuronal firing or internal Ca^{2+} to trigger the compensatory shift in θ_m (Hulme et al., 2012). A major advantage of BCM-like metaplasticity is that it is a closed-loop system that harnesses Hebbian plasticity itself to achieve homeostasis. However, a disadvantage is that at the heart of this homeostatic mechanism is the tendency to reverse synaptic changes induced by learning, posing a clear challenge to memory maintenance. For this reason, we now consider other solutions, invoking entirely distinct forms of plasticity that counteract Hebbian plasticity through synaptic normalization that nevertheless retain distributions of synaptic weights.

10.6.2.3 Synaptic normalization

Within a memory system such as the hippocampus, it may be highly beneficial to achieve homeostasis while also maintaining the relative strengths of synapses distributed across a neuron through a normalization process. Thus, if memories are stored as a distributed synaptic engram (S Martin and Morris, 2002; Govindarajan et al., 2006), that engram maintained in the relative distribution of synaptic strengths, even if the overall output of neurons is altered. The first major version of the normalization process was the Oja rule (Oja, 1982), which added the critical concept of a "forgetting" constant to Hebb's plasticity rule to counteract the issue of boundless synaptic growth through positive feedback. Importantly, this "forgetting" constant differs from standard LTD, because not only is it applied equally to all synapses on a neuron but also it is proportional to the overall output of the neuron. Subtractive normalization is, however, a highly

competitive process that punishes weaker synapses more than strong synapses and can lead to their elimination (Dayan and Abbott, 2001). Exact maintenance of the relative contributions of each synapse within a synaptic engram could only be achieved if the normalization process is multiplicative/divisive, or "scaled" (Turrigiano et al., 1998). Thus, the last two decades have seen a ramping up of interest in a homeostatic process that is now universally described as synaptic scaling (Turrigiano, 2017).

Synaptic scaling is a cell-autonomous property in which persistent changes in the level of cell firing multiplies or divides the strength of all synapses by the same factor on that cell to constrain its mean firing level within circumscribed limits. In early experiments, Gina Turrigiano and colleagues reported that suppressing action potentials with TTX in cortical neuronal cultures resulted in an increase in mean conductance at glutamatergic synapses, which scaled multiplicatively to the control condition (Turrigiano et al., 1998; Turrigiano, 2017). This process was described as synaptic upscaling, but the reverse process of synaptic downscaling of AMPAR conductance could also be produced through prolonged application of the $GABA_A$ receptor blockers picrotoxin or bicuculline to induce neuronal hyperactivity, this time in hippocampal cultures (Lissin et al., 1998). Most treatments that result in scaling are extreme both in terms of the degree of manipulation of neural activity and the length of time required for scaling to become manifest (Turrigiano et al., 1998; Turrigiano, 2017). As with BCM metaplasticity, much research has therefore focused on demonstrating that naturalistic interventions can produce scaling in the living animal. Again, primary sensory neocortex has provided the favored preparation due to the easy implementation of sensory enhancement or deprivation. In the visual cortex, homeostasis is clearly apparent as a rebounding of neural firing after binocular deprivation (Hengen et al., 2013), but the nature of that homeostasis remains to be fully understood and this lack of understanding is particularly acute in the hippocampus. Gaining a deeper appreciation of the divergent molecular mechanisms supporting each candidate form of synaptic homeostasis will enable targeted interventions in vivo to establish the consequences of each being lost.

AMPAR trafficking is a form of expression that is common within not only Hebbian plasticity but also scaling. A major focus of investigation on scaling has been a search for the mechanisms that differentiate it from Hebbian LTP. Initially, the most striking difference between hippocampal scaling and LTP was in the induction mechanism, as most forms of LTP are NMDAR-dependent whereas upscaling appears to be NMDAR-independent (O'Brien et al., 1998; Turrigiano et al., 1998). Other studies, however, have indicated that upscaling is prevented by genetic knockdown of NMDAR expression (Pawlak et al., 2005; Rodriguez et al., 2019), and there is currently no clear consensus. Another difference that has been emphasized is that glial release of the cytokine TNFα (Stellwagen and Malenka, 2006; Steinmetz and Turrigiano, 2010), is both necessary and sufficient to cause upscaling (Beattie et al., 2002; Stellwagen and Malenka, 2006), whereas Hebbian LTP, at least in young animals, is unaffected by genetic ablation of TNFα (Kaneko et al., 2008), though BCM-like metaplasticity may be affected (Singh et al., 2022). However, this too remains contentious as there is evidence that synaptic transmission can be enhanced by exogenous TNFα application in the hippocampus (Tancredi et al., 1992) and at high doses this effect may occlude the subsequent induction of LTP (Butler et al., 2004). Another feature that may differentiate scaling from Hebbian plasticity is a reliance on the GluA2 subunit for expression (Gainey et al., 2009; Ancona Esselmann et al., 2017). GluA2 is also likely to be the critical subunit for synaptic downscaling (Fiore et al., 2014). In contrast, the expression of most forms of LTP require upregulation of the GluA1 rather than the GluA2 subunit of the AMPAR (Malenka and Bear, 2004). There is also a divergence of opinion regarding the involvement of PSD-95 in LTP and scaling. Whereas PSD-95 overexpression induces a potentiation that occludes further induction of LTP in the hippocampus (Ehrlich and Malinow, 2004; Ehrlich et al., 2007), it does not produce a similar effect by occluding upscaling (Sun and Turrigiano, 2011). Complications exist here too, though, as genetic knockdown of PSD-95 impairs upscaling but enhances LTP in the hippocampus (Carlisle et al., 2008; Q Sun and Turrigiano, 2011). The reverse process of downscaling is left intact by loss of the GluA2 binding protein PICK1 (Anggono et al., 2011), which is required for canonical LTD in the hippocampus (Terashima et al., 2008; Volk et al., 2010).

As for the all-important feedback mechanism itself, which determines when activity is aberrant and homeostasis is required, evidence currently favors the level of free Ca^{2+} in the nucleus as the molecular monitor of overall neural activity, and that, accordingly, drives expression of GluA2 (Turrigiano, 2008). The details of the central signaling pathway have not yet been fully elucidated, but up- or downscaling of excitatory synaptic transmission, as well as homeostasis of intrinsic excitability, is regulated by CaMKIV (Ibata et al., 2008; Goold and Nicoll, 2010; Joseph and Turrigiano, 2017). A still murky picture is emerging of divergent induction and expression mechanisms for Hebbian plasticity and scaling that may be targeted to investigate synaptic homeostasis in living animals. Thus far, attempts to observe homeostatic plasticity in vivo have yielded mixed insights, as delayed increases in cortical responses after sensory deprivation require NMDAR activation and sensory experience (Cooper and Bear, 2012), contrary to expectations for scaling.

However, scaling is dependent on TNFα (Kaneko et al., 2008), at least in young animals (Ranson et al., 2012), which is consistent with the occurrence of scaling rather than Hebbian plasticity following a θ_m shift (though see Singh et al., 2022).

One important final consideration, however, is that there is little evidence of downscaling during in vivo hippocampal LTP experiments. Because these studies in unanesthetized rodents measure synaptic strength of both tetanized and control pathways over months, they seem the ideal situation within which to study hippocampal synaptic homeostasis. Control pathways, however, do not reveal evidence of reduced strength as saturated LTP is maintained over many weeks in the tetanized pathway (Abraham et al., 2002). Further work, therefore, will be required to confirm whether Hebbian or scaling mechanisms support in vivo homeostasis in the brain and, in particular, in the hippocampus.

10.7 Physiological engagement

In this section we discuss aspects of LTP that relate to the intersection of synaptic plasticity with the physiology of the organism. We begin with a brief overview of a type of plasticity that depends on the precise timing of the firing of pre- and postsynaptic hippocampal neurons.

10.7.1 Spike timing-dependent plasticity (STDP) and input timing-dependent plasticity (ITDP)

The importance of the temporal order of presynaptic and postsynaptic firing in establishing the polarity of changes in synaptic strength was first established at local excitatory connections between cortical pyramidal cells (Markram et al., 1997). Initially given the name STDP, its two components are often referred to as t-LTP and t-LTD. The familiar biphasic curve (see first edition, Figure 10.9C,D, p 413) in which potentiation occurs after multiple pairings in which the EPSP precedes the dendritic spike, and depression when the spike precedes the EPSP was first reported in the hippocampus by Bi and Poo (1998), working with dissociated cultures. Typically, LTP results when the EPSP precedes the spike by less than 20–40 ms, the magnitude increasing as the E-S interval decreases. LTP is replaced by LTD when the EPSP precedes the spike, the effect again being maximal at short intervals, and decaying to zero after a few tens of milliseconds. The effect is NMDAR-dependent (Andrade-Talavera et al., 2016). At SCC-CA1 synapses, STDP can be elicited by as few as six pairings of single pre- and postsynaptic spikes (Cepeda-Prado et al., 2022). There is evidence for both presynaptic (Cepeda-Prado et al., 2022) and postsynaptic (Andrade-Talavera et al., 2016) expression at SCC-CA1 synapses. The modest number of pairings required for STDP suggest that it may be of physiological relevance. However, while STDP has been widely adopted as a synaptic plasticity rule in the field of neural computation, its physiological relevance has been questioned (Lisman and Spruston, 2010), in part because of the artificial nature of the depolarization-induced postsynaptic spike. Moreover, the amplitude and polarity of STDP are highly dependent on the concentration of extracellular Ca^{2+}, which in in vitro studies is often maintained at unphysiological levels. When extracellular Ca^{2+} is lowered to more normal levels, pairing single pre- and postsynaptic spikes is without effect at any interval, and as Ca^{2+} levels are raised LTD occurs at both pre-before-post and post-before-pre intervals (Inglebert et al., 2020). Because of these and other reservations (see Lisman and Spruston, 2010), the role that STDP plays in hippocampal physiology is difficult to assess and will remain so until more is known about the spike-timing rules that govern synaptic plasticity in the behaving animal.

Another form of timing-dependent plasticity, called ITDP (input timing-dependent plasticity) has been described by Siegelbaum and colleagues. When monosynaptic inputs from EC layer II stellate cells to CA1 are stimulated 20 ms before stimulation of SCC inputs to CA1, the result is a persistent potentiation of the SCC input to pyramidal cells, generated largely by LTD of the Schaffer projection to local cholecystokinin-expressing inhibitory neurons (Basu et al., 2013). A similar phenomenon is seen in area CA2, where ITDP is linked to SCC-induced LTD of PV-expressing interneurons projecting to CA2 cells and is associated with enhanced social memory (Leroy et al., 2017).

10.7.2 Sleep and LTP

How is LTP affected by the circadian rhythms of sleep and wakefulness? In an early examination of this question in the intact rat, Leonard et al. (1987) found that, relative to the awake state, LTP in the DG was depressed during slow-wave sleep. Can the often-fleeting nature of memory for dreams be linked to a similar loss of synaptic plasticity during REM (rapid eye movement) sleep? Apparently not, since the magnitude of LTP in the DG is similar during REM sleep and in the awake animal (Bramham and Srebro, 1989). In rat hippocampal slices prepared at different phases of the diurnal light-dark cycle, Harris and Tyler (1983) found that LTP in the DG was greater in slices cut when the animal was behaviorally active, consistent with the result of Leonard et al. (1987); however, the reverse was the case in area CA1, where LTP in vitro was greater in slices cut during the light half of the cycle, when the animal was less active.

There is general agreement that sleep deprivation is associated with reversible deficits in LTP (Campbell et al., 2002; Ravassard et al., 2009; Prince et al., 2014). Interest in the interactions between synaptic plasticity and sleep has been stimulated by the sleep and synaptic homeostasis hypothesis (SHY) proposed by Tononi and Cirelli (2003), which addresses directly the perennial mystery of why animals sleep. During wake (the woke word used by the sleep community to describe the state of being awake), an event to be remembered is encoded as changes in synaptic strength, predominantly LTP, at synapses activated by the event. Thus, during wake, there is a net increase in synaptic efficacy. If unchecked, this will eventually lead to saturation and the failure of the network as a memory storage device (see section 10.5). According to SHY, sleep allows this synaptic apocalypse to be avoided by enabling a general downregulation of synaptic strength, particularly during slow-wave sleep. In short, "sleep is the price the brain pays for plasticity" (Tononi and Cirelli, 2014). While there is evidence that sleep is accompanied by changes that are consistent with the hypothesis—for instance, sleep is associated with a downregulation of cortical AMPARs and of the synaptic scaffolding Homer protein homolog 1 (Homer1, see Diering et al., 2017), and by a reduction in spine numbers (de Vivo et al., 2017), there is also evidence that downregulation is not universal (Frank, 2012; Puentes-Mestril and Aton, 2017). For example, visual cortical neurons increase rather than decrease their firing rates in slow-wave sleep and in REM sleep (Durkin and Aton, 2016), and large-scale monitoring of cortical

neuron firing rates suggest that sleep is associated with a tightening of variance rather than a homeostatic downscaling (Watson et al., 2016). An alternative proposal, reviewed by Rasch and Born (2013), posits that synapses strengthened during sleep enable the encoding of recent memories to be consolidated. Thus, while SHY has generated great interest as a theory that seeks to explain why animals sleep, the evidence that sleep leads to a universal downregulation of synaptic strength during slow-wave sleep is far from established. As Timofeev and Chauvette (2018) point out, a definitive resolution will depend on the ability to identify the engram cells for a particular memory, and access to labeling techniques that allow synaptic strength to be monitored and compared in a population of engram and non-engram synapses before, during and after learning—and again during sleep. Moreover, sleep is unlikely to have evolved with the primary function of consolidating plasticity, given that most analyses indicate that the strongest correlates of the amount of sleep from species to species are with metabolic factors such as size or diet rather than cognitive capacity; mice sleep considerably more than humans, and gerbils sleep more than elephants (Siegel, 2005). Any role for sleep in memory is likely to be a secondary adaptation (Siegel, 2001).

10.7.3 Sex differences in LTP and hippocampus-dependent learning

Differences in the properties of LTP between male and female rodents have emerged in a number of recent studies (reviewed by Baudry et al., 2013; Koss and Frick, 2017; Gall et al., 2021; Gall et al., 2024). The major circulating estrogen, estradiol, is found in the hippocampus of both male and female rats, where it binds to a variety of membrane-bound estrogen receptors including estrogen receptor α (ERα), ERβ and G-protein-coupled ER 1 (GPER1). Estradiol is also synthesized in principal hippocampal neurons of both sexes (Kretz et al., 2004), but is required for LTP only in female rats (Vierk et al., 2012). The concentration of circulating estradiol varies during the 4-day estrus cycle, reaching its maximum during proestrus. Interestingly, 17β-estradiol (E2), acting via the membrane estrogen receptor ERα, differentially regulates NMDAR-LTP at CA1 synapses in male and female rats (W Wang, Le, et al., 2018). This regulation, affecting key LTP-related signaling processes such as c-Src regulation and ERK1/2 signaling, may be responsible for sex-dependent differences in learning and memory. Another study revealed that PKA signaling was mandatory for LTP elicited by application of E2 in vitro in female but not in male rats (Jain et al., 2019). The significant differences in the ways that circulating estrogens affect LTP in the hippocampus of male and female rodents emphasizes the importance of taking sex differences into consideration when investigating hippocampal synaptic plasticity and hippocampus-dependent behavior. For example, female rats perform markedly better during proestrus in a hippocampus-dependent task measuring memory for object location (W Wang, Le, et al., 2018).

In an intriguing study of how puberty differentially affects male and female rats, Lynch, Gall, and colleagues found that while both LTP and spatial learning are stronger in female than male rats before puberty, this situation is reversed at puberty (Le et al., 2022). The mechanism in female rats centered on the level of expression of the $\alpha5$-GABA$_A$ receptor, which was relatively low in the hippocampus of prepubertal female rats, but after puberty switched to a more elevated level. This caused a shunting of synaptic current during LTP-inducing trains, leading to a reduced level of LTP, accompanied by impaired performance in two hippocampus-dependent tasks. The opposite changes occurred in males, via an unknown mechanism. Prepubertal male rats were unable to learn the tasks that prepubertal females mastered, but males exceeded the performance of females following puberty. The improvement in male rats was not due to changes in the expression of α5-GABA$_A$ receptors, which remained low both before and after puberty, and the mechanism behind the postpubertal improvements in LTP and learning of spatial tasks in males is unknown.

10.7.4 Changes in spine density, synaptic plasticity, and hippocampus-dependent learning during the estrus cycle

During proestrus in female rats, when levels of estrogens reach a peak, the number of spines on CA1 pyramidal cells is as much as 30% higher than during estrus (Woolley et al., 1990; see Chapter 9). These striking results have been confirmed several times (reviewed by Kato et al., 2013; Frick et al., 2015). In ovariectomized rats, replacement of E2/progesterone leads to an increase in spine density in area CA1 within hours (Gould et al., 1990; MacLusky et al., 2005).

The most direct evidence for the effect of E2 on spine density comes from studies of CA1 pyramidal cells in hippocampal organotypic cultures from both male and female mice (Mendez et al., 2011). Estradiol increases the rate of spinogenesis while removal of estradiol leads to the preferential retraction of the new spines.

There are subfield variations in the effects of E2 on spine density (see Sheppard et al., 2019, for review). Most studies have concentrated on area CA1, where the effects of E2 are most pronounced. E2 drives spinogenesis in CA1 in both sexes but has little effect on spine density in CA3 pyramidal neurons in male or female rodents, nor does CA3 spine density vary across the estrus cycle (Woolley et al., 1990). Intriguingly, in a study on acute slices in male rats, application of E2 led to a decrease in the density of thorny excrescences, the postsynaptic components of mossy fiber giant synapses (Tsurugizawa et al., 2005). In male rats, both E2 and testosterone rapidly enhance spine density on CA1 pyramidal cells (Jacome et al., 2016).

The variation in spine density during the estrus cycle raises some intriguing questions. Does performance in hippocampus-dependent tasks vary during the cycle, and is there a similar cyclical variation in synaptic plasticity? In 1995, Warren et al. (1995) found no difference in LTP across the estrus cycle. However, applied E2 increases LTP in vitro in males (Warren et al., 1995) and ovariectomized females (Cordoba Montoya and Carrer, 1997), possibly mediated by an increase in the recruitment of NMDARs at synaptic sites (Snyder et al., 2011). The behavioral literature is inconsistent. Warren and Juraska (1997) reported a surprising enhancement in watermaze performance during proestrus, when estradiol levels are at their lowest. However, Berry et al. (1997) found no difference in learning or retrieval in the watermaze across the phases of the estrus cycle. Other studies have found that in another hippocampus-dependent task, object place recognition, the higher the level of estrogen the better the performance (Frick et al., 2015; Wang, Le, et al., 2018).

How hippocampus-dependent memory remains constant (if indeed it does) in the face of the substantial cycling of spine numbers remains an intriguing question. Is it possible that spines retain their

presynaptic partners as they retreat into the dendrite, to form asymmetric dendritic shaft synapses on CA1 pyramidal cell dendrites? While this may happen during hibernation (Popov et al., 2007), it seems unlikely that it occurs to any great extent during the estrus cycle. Asymmetric synapses on CA1 pyramidal cell dendrites have a very low and constant density at all stages of estrus (Woolley and McEwen, 1992), and, in an EM study, asymmetric synapses were found only on dendrites in stratum lacunosum-moleculare (Megías et al., 2001).

10.7.5 Left-right asymmetries in receptor distribution and in intrahippocampal projections

Left-right differences in the distribution of glutamate receptor subunits in the hippocampus was first described by Kawakami et al. (2003), who found that the distribution of GluN2B receptors on CA1 neurons was not symmetrical. In the left hemisphere of adult mice, GluN2B-containing receptors were predominantly expressed at synapses made by ipsilateral CA3 cells onto apical dendrites of CA1 cells, while in the right hemisphere, GluN2B-containing receptors were concentrated at ipsilateral CA3 inputs onto basal CA1 dendrites. A converse pattern was found at synapses made by commissural inputs from CA3 to CA1 pyramidal cells. Left-right asymmetry of glutamate subunit expression was further emphasized in a study, also in mice, by Shinohara et al. (2008), who found that synapses made on CA1 cells by axons originating from CA3 cells in the right hemisphere were larger and had twice the level of GluA1 subunits as those originating from CA3 cells in the left hemisphere (reviewed in Shinohara and Hirase, 2009). An opposite result was reached in experiments using optogenetic methods to restrict activation to fibers from one or other hemisphere of the mouse hippocampus: only CA3 projections from the left hemisphere exhibited LTP (Kohl et al., 2011), a conclusion supported by subsequent behavioral studies (Shipton et al., 2014). But there may be a species differences in these left-right asymmetries, since in an earlier study in anesthetized rats, using kainic acid to destroy CA3 cells unilaterally in the left hippocampus, leaving fibers of passage unaffected, robust LTP was reported in ipsilateral and contralateral projections from the CA3 population in the surviving right hemisphere (Bliss, Lancaster, et al., 1983). Similarly, Martin et al. (2019) found no difference in the magnitude of LTP in the CA3 projection to contralateral CA1 originating in left or right hemispheres in the anesthetized rat.

10.7.6 Circadian variations in synaptic transmission and LTP in hippocampal pathways

It has long been known that the amplitude of field EPSPs in the DG of the unanesthetized rat varies over the 24 h light-dark cycle, reaching its maximum amplitude in the dark phase (Barnes et al., 1977). This may reflect changes in synaptic strength, but could also be caused by changes in brain temperature, which are known to affect the amplitude of field responses (Moser et al., 1993) as animals move from rest to activity (Barnes, personal communication). Are there circadian variations in any of the parameters of synaptic plasticity? Bowden and colleagues (2012) examined the magnitude and duration of LTP at MPP synapses, and the accompanying heterosynaptic LTD in the lateral perforant path, in unanesthetized rats. They found that LTP of the field EPSP induced by HFS of the medial pathway, as well as E-S potentiation, was maximal during the dark phase. For area CA1, data are only available from slices taken from mice at different phases of the light-dark cycle. Nakatsuka and Natsume (2014) found no diurnal variation in the magnitude of LTP in the SCC projection to CA1, though E-S potentiation was maximal in the dark phase, as was spike potentiation itself (Chaudhury et al., 2005). McCauley (2020) noted a diurnal variation in the fEPSP slope in mouse slices of either sex, with a peak in the middle of the light phase; LTP was also greater during the light phase. It is difficult to draw general conclusions from this rather disparate set of results; but it is clear, particularly from the in vivo data in the DG, that circadian variations exist, both in the strength of synaptic connections and in the capacity for synaptic plasticity.

10.7.7 Reward-based learning and behavioral time scale plasticity (BTSP)

It has long been recognized that in the case of reward-based learning, where the reward may occur a substantial time—seconds or even minutes—after the event that led to the reward, a Hebbian mechanism, with its emphasis on near-simultaneous pre- and postsynaptic events, cannot alone provide a synaptic explanation for the learned response (Crow, 1968). In reward learning what is needed is a mechanism that allows synapses that are engaged during a particular behavior, that may or may not be rewarded, to be marked or tagged in a way that does not immediately affect their strength (the so-called eligibility trace). Reward signals, such as dopamine, can then act specifically on tagged synapses to enhance (or possibly diminish) their strength. Direct evidence for this kind of plasticity was provided by Brzosko et al. (2015), who showed in hippocampal slices that t-LTD in the Schaffer projection to CA1 pyramidal cells could be converted to LTP by dopamine applied 10 min after pairing.

Bittner et al. (2017) studied the formation of place fields in head-fixed mice running on a linear maze and showed that place fields were induced in CA1 pyramidal cells when spontaneous or induced dendritic calcium transients were paired with stimulated input from area CA3 arriving seconds before or after the dendritic event. They named this non-Hebbian type of plasticity, with seconds-long intervals between pre- and postsynaptic induction events, behavioral timescale plasticity or BTSP. The results were broadly confirmed in an all-optical study, in which membrane potential of CA1 cells was measured using a voltage-sensitive indicator, and control of cell firing in CA1 and CA3 cells was under separate optogenetic control (Fan et al., 2023). Inhibition of CaMKII blocks BTSP (Xiao et al., 2023), and in a study of BTSP at single spines Jain et al. (2023) have shown that the activation of CaMKII is delayed and distributed widely within the dendrite that harbors the potentiated synapse. The study of BTSP is at an early stage but given the behavioral significance of reward-based learning, research into the properties and cellular and molecular basis of BTSP is likely to assume increasing prominence.

10.8 Synaptic plasticity in the hippocampus mediates memory encoding and storage

Beguiling analogies between LTP and learning have long been noted: (1) *persistence*—both LTP and memory long outlast the brief patterns of neural stimulation that trigger their induction and expression; (2) *specificity*—the input-specificity of LTP and the stimulus-specificity of memory are clearly analogous, and likely respect the complexities of distributed representations and sparse coding; and (3) *associativity and cooperativity*—both LTP-induction and learning are fundamentally associative and depend, in part, on stimulus strength with respect to an LTP induction threshold reflecting the activation of sufficient synaptic afferents (McNaughton et al., 1978; Lynch and Baudry, 1984; Morris, 1990b; Barnes, 1995; Jeffery, 1997; Takeuchi et al., 2014; Abraham et al., 2019; Humeau and Choquet, 2019).

With respect to the mammalian brain, a reasonable debating position at the time of the first edition of this book was to argue that LTP and LTD are fascinating laboratory phenomena, but ones whose function was still under debate (Shors and Matzel, 1997). The situation has moved on since, with numerous studies showing that synaptic potentiation and/or synaptic depression are induced in behaving animals during learning and that interventions which compromise their induction or expression have predictably deleterious effects on memory encoding or retrieval. Successful occlusion studies have also been conducted to establish some commonality of underlying mechanism between LTP and learning. Older techniques are now complemented by state-of-the-art biochemical and imaging studies that offer insights into the underlying neural mechanisms of learning-associated potentiation or depression.

Advanced neural network modeling has also greatly expanded our understanding of the properties of distributed associative memory systems and the dynamics of information processing in the hippocampus (see Chapter 16). This work includes functions such as the need for sparsity in neural representations, for pattern separation and pattern completion, dendritic computation, the contribution of inhibitory neurons, and the impact of neuromodulation by neurotransmitters such as catecholamines. Figure 10.9 illustrates a central idea about this modeling. First, in a linear sensory-motor reflex pathway with embedded synaptic plasticity, the strength of the output given a fixed input can be modulated upward or downward by synaptic potentiation and depression (Figure 10.9A). Given that LTP and LTD do precisely that, it is tempting to suppose that their role in brain circuits is primarily to make things "stronger" or "weaker." However, an important insight from models of distributed associative memory systems is that LTP and LTD can have very different functions. Specifically, they allow a neural pattern corresponding to an input (i.e., cue 1) to be associated with a neural pattern corresponding to different input (cue 2, see Figure 10.9B, and Morris, 1990a). In both cases, synaptic plasticity is the underlying mechanism of association when embedded in specific anatomical architecture. Neural network models emphasize the role of sparse coding of sensory inputs with respect to distinct anatomical architectures (as in DG) or re-entrant circuitry (CA3) to model associative representations (McNaughton and Morris, 1987).

In keeping with the second theme of this book (see Chapter 1), important lessons have also been learned from studies of the hippocampus that are relevant to new studies of the functional role of synaptic plasticity in other brain areas—such as the amygdala and motor cortex. One lesson is that the emphasis of the SPM (synaptic plasticity and memory) hypothesis on strictly synaptic storage mechanisms is at risk of ignoring a role for altered neuronal excitability in memory formation. Excitability plays a key role in allocating memory traces. First discovered in the lateral amygdala (Han et al., 2007; Silva et al., 2009), the allocation concept has now been extended to include situations in which memory traces formed at

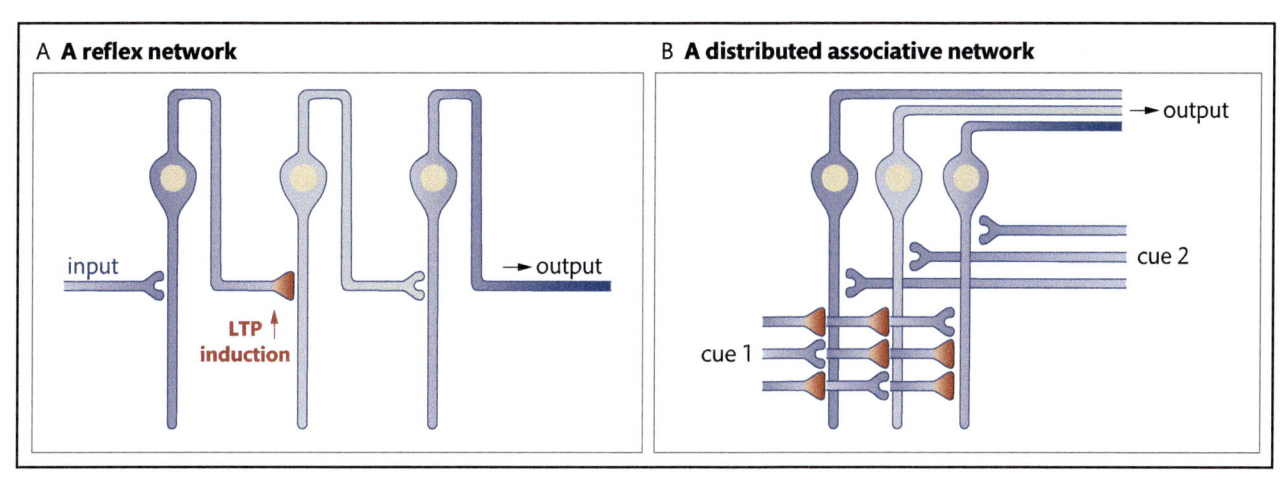

Figure 10.9 Anatomy meets plasticity. Synaptic plasticity embedded into a "reflex" pathway compared with its presence in a distributed associative network. Both use plasticity to fine-tune existing hardwired connections but the reflex network (A) permits, primarily, only increases or decreases in output to a given input stimulus; whereas the distributed network (B) is a fusion of a specific type of anatomical circuit with synaptic plasticity to enable associations to be formed such that one cue can evoke the memory of another.

different but closely related times are assigned to common neurons provided they occur in a common spatiotemporal context (Cai et al., 2016). Timing considerations were largely ignored in early studies of the relevance of LTP to memory, but they are central to understanding the speed with which dendritic spine enlargement might occur and thus be able to represent experience (Kasai et al., 2010). At a more cellular level, neuronal oscillations, sharp-wave ripples, and plateau potentials in the absence of cell-spiking could all play key roles in effective memory processing, including the formation of place fields, associative binding, the representation of sequences, and memory consolidation (Buzsáki, 2009; Hasselmo, 2011; Bittner et al., 2017). Work ranging from studies of perceptual learning (Cooke and Bear, 2010) to experiential aspects of social dominance (Zhou et al., 2017) also support a causal role for neocortical synaptic potentiation in learning and memory. The neocortex was, after all, Hebb's own focus (Hebb, 1949).

10.8.1 Experimental tests of the synaptic plasticity and memory (SPM) hypothesis

Working in Canada, and inspired by the ideas of Donald Hebb, Barnes and McNaughton observed in studies of aging that the persistence of LTP in the DG over days was statistically correlated with the degree of retention of spatial memory in a circular arena task (now called the Barnes maze, see Chapters 14 and 15, and Barnes and McNaughton, 1985; Barnes, 1988). Older animals lost synaptic enhancement and showed forgetting over the same time course. These pioneering experimental studies implicating LTP in memory were correlational, but they were a key step toward testing the generic SPM hypothesis later summarized by S. Martin, Grimwood, and Morris (2000) as follows: "Activity-dependent synaptic plasticity is induced at appropriate synapses during memory formation, and is both necessary and sufficient for the information storage underlying the type of memory mediated by the brain area in which that plasticity is observed" (Martin et al., 2000). They proposed four criteria for a rigorous test of the SPM hypothesis: detectability, anterograde interference, retrograde interference, and mimicry. Broadly speaking, they correspond to correlation, necessity (the two interference strategies), and sufficiency.

The first of three of these criteria, *detectability*, refers to the idea that, in association with the formation of memory lasting any length of time, LTP- or LTD-like changes should occur at certain synapses in one or more brain areas and should be detectable. The second, *anterograde interference*, asserts that blocking (or enhancing) the mechanisms that induce or express changes in synaptic weights should have the anterograde effect of impairing (or perhaps enhancing) new learning. Interventions are achieved in various ways: physiologically, pharmacologically, or through molecular-genetic manipulations including optogenetic stimulation. The third, *retrograde interference*, asserts that altering the pattern of synaptic weights *after* learning has taken place will affect an animal's ability to recall a memory. Altering the spatial distribution of synaptic weights within a distributed associative matrix should cause interference and so alter the ability to retrieve learned associations from such a network. Targeted manipulations specific to potentiated synapses should also cause forgetting. There is now strong evidence that each of these three formal criteria have been met in experimental studies, notably in those in which memory formation and memory recall are carefully distinguished.

The fourth criterion—the engineering challenge—is proving more difficult. The *mimicry* criterion states that if changes in synaptic weight are the neural basis of trace storage, the artificial induction of a specific spatial pattern of weights may give rise to an apparent memory for an event that did not actually occur. This is sometimes informally referred to as the "Marilyn Monroe/Cary Grant" criterion—the idea being that mimicry would allow a person to have a fictitious memory of a meeting with one of these movie stars. Although realizing this false memory criterion may seem experimentally fanciful, it has been a subject of study as described below.

10.8.2 Memory formation is associated with the induction of detectable synaptic potentiation

The prediction of the detectability criterion is that persistent changes in synaptic efficacy should occur at network-appropriate synapses in association with certain types of memory. This idea has been tested in the hippocampal formation and other brain areas.

Marr's notion that the hippocampus is involved in the "automatic-encoding" of facets of ongoing episodic experience using a conjunctive Hebb-like learning rule (Marr, 1971; Morris and Frey, 1997) implies that, during a typical day, many hundreds of memory traces may be created with most decaying relatively soon thereafter. This state-of-affairs is a necessary property of automatic encoding within the available storage capacity of the hippocampus. Consequently, there are challenges to detecting such synaptic potentiation. First, it will occur only at the activated subset of synapses distributed across one or more Hebbian cell-assemblies, possibly with concomitant heterosynaptic LTD at other synapses (Figure 10.10A). Traditional extracellular field-potential recording might *not* detect such a pattern, pointing to the need for more exacting optical approaches (Humeau and Choquet, 2019). Even with such techniques, finding the relevant subset of potentiated synapses would be akin to finding a needle in a haystack due to sparse coding (Willshaw and Dayan, 1990).

The detectability prediction has nonetheless been upheld. A classic demonstration is trace eyeblink conditioning in mice (Gruart et al., 2006). In this well-established hippocampus-dependent task, a small but steady increase in the size of hippocampal field potentials was seen as associative conditioning proceeded (Figure 10.10B). Moreover, both trace-conditioning and the synaptic potentiation were blocked by an NMDAR antagonist, and the synaptic potentials declined over the course of extinction.

A problem is that global changes in fEPSPs in behaving animals may not necessarily reflect synaptic potentiation. The discovery of what appeared to be striking short-term modulation of perforant-path evoked EPSPs in the DG during spatial exploration (Sharp et al., 1985) turned out to be due to changes in brain temperature (Moser et al., 1993). The clue was that exploratory activity caused simultaneously an *increase* in the fEPSP but a *decrease* of the population spike, this pattern being somewhat alarmingly confirmed by gentle heating of the animal with a hair-dryer (Moser et al., 1993). Once calibration functions relating brain temperature to fEPSP magnitude had been worked out, a small temperature-independent component of the increase in fEPSP was nonetheless observed during novelty exploration (Moser et al., 1994). This increased rapidly at the start of exploration but declined to baseline over 15 min. Exploratory behavior is also associated with the rapid activation of IEGs such as *c-fos* (Gall et al., 1998) and *Arc/Arg3.1* (Guzowski et al., 1999). The spatial overlap in Arc-expressing cells in area CA1 activated by exposure to a novel context and the population activated by exploration of a second enclosure is a function of the spatial similarity of the two enclosures in which testing takes place. IEG markers such as these are generally cell-wide rather than synapse-specific, and have much lower temporal resolution than electrophysiology, but are now also proving valuable in studies of engram cells (section 10.8.5 below).

In a different approach to overcoming the sparse coding problem, Whitlock et al. (2006) used multiple electrode arrays to target the apical dendrites of CA1 in behaving animals. Potentiation was observed on some electrodes but not others, pointing to the sensible possibility of a heterogeneous synaptic potentiation in some but not all recording locations (Figure 10.10C). An occlusion experiment revealed no further LTP at those electrodes which had shown learning-associated potentiation, but successful LTP induction at those electrodes which had not. Biochemical assays revealed

evidence of phosphorylation of GluA1 at Ser831 and a transient incorporation of additional GluA receptor components. This study generated much excitement because it overcame the previous concerns of temperature-related effects and provided the added dimension of occlusion of LTP by learning-induced synaptic change.

Similar work in other brain areas has been conducted. For example, amygdala-dependent fear conditioning is associated with lasting rather than transient changes in GluA expression. As discussed in the first edition, Rogan (1997) monitored evoked potentials elicited by an auditory conditional stimulus (CS) in the lateral amygdala in vivo before and after auditory fear conditioning. Paired presentations of the auditory CS and foot shock resulted in increased freezing behavior and a concomitant potentiation of the CS-evoked potential. Likewise, using the rectification of AMPAR-mediated transmission as an index of mutated GluA1 subunit incorporation (Rumpel et al., 2005), tone-fear conditioning was shown to be linked to an increase in EPSCs associated with AMPAR trafficking in the pathway from the auditory thalamus to the amygdala in vitro (Figure 10.10D). The change was greater when paired conditioning trials were used in which the tone preceded the fear-evoking shock by an optimum CS–US interval but much weaker after unpaired conditioning. Use of a "plasticity-block" vector to interfere with AMPAR trafficking (Malinow and Malenka, 2002) prevented learning-associated rectification of AMPA-mediated transmission and learning itself. Intriguingly, plasticity needed to be disturbed (or blocked) in only a small percentage of neurons (approximately 27%), raising the possibility that combinatorial effects may be responsible for the learning of different CS–US (conditioned stimulus–unconditioned stimulus) pairings.

In the primary motor cortex, a phenomenon resembling LTP also occurs in association with the acquisition of a motor skill in rats (Rioult-Pedotti et al., 1998; Monfils and Teskey, 2004; Roth et al., 2020). Of these studies, Roth et al. (2020) used imaging techniques to look at the dynamics of AMPAR trafficking via visualization of fluorescent AMPARs that were incorporated into existing spines resulting in apparent changes in receptor number. The focus of this work was on postsynaptic changes, and, using a pHluorin fluorescent marker for GluA1, they present striking evidence of a training-associated redistribution of spine GluA1 (Figure 10.10E). Training was associated with greater increases in this marker at individual spines than decreases (although, interestingly, some showed a decrease), whereas a control condition showed the opposite pattern (mainly decreases, but again, not exclusively). In keeping with the concept of clustered plasticity at specific regions of the dendritic arbor, there was a highly significant tendency for neighboring regions to go up or to go down, but this correlation was not absolute. The issue of whether the dendritic spine changes seen in motor cortex are *necessary* for the associated motor learning will be considered later (section 10.8.4, below) in relation to a further feature of a study by Hayashi-Tagaki et al. (2015).

An interesting extension of the relevance of synaptic plasticity to learning beyond the hippocampus is with respect to social learning. F. Wang et al. (2011) observed that social dominance status is statistically correlated with EPSC frequency in the medial prefrontal cortex of rats and, in a follow-up, T. Zhou and colleagues (2017) found that both behaviorally and optogenetically induced changes in social dominance rank were associated with altered connection strengths between the thalamus and prefrontal cortex.

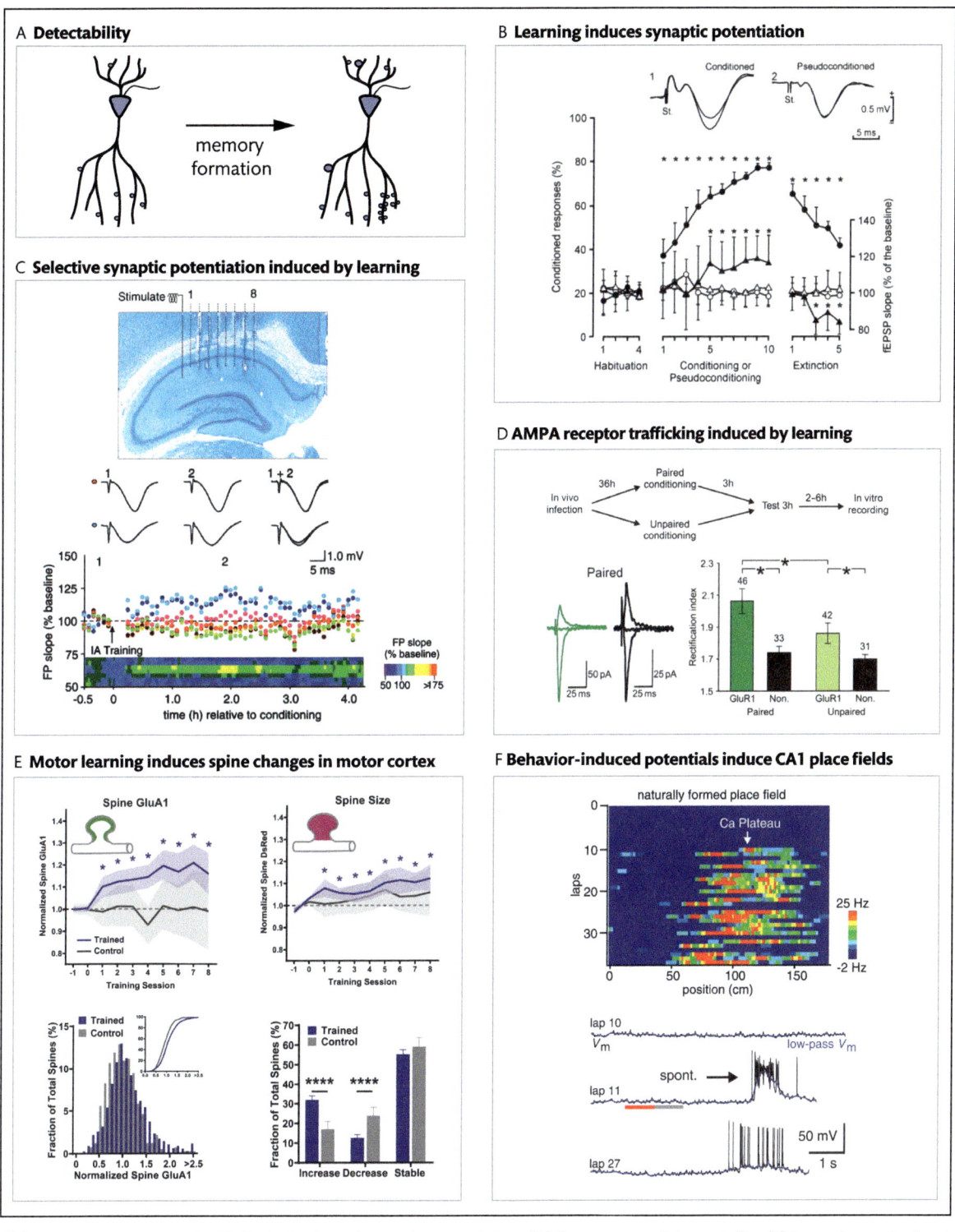

Figure 10.10 Learning is associated with the induction of synaptic potentiation. (A) The concept of detectability. (B) Exemplar study showing how the learning (filled circles) of a hippocampus-dependent task, trace eyeblink conditioning, is associated with a detectable increase in the fEPSP in hippocampus (filled triangles) relative to control conditions (after Gruart et al., 2006). (C) The placement of multiple extracellular electrodes in the hippocampus revealed learning-associated potentiation at some sites (blue symbols) but not others (inhibitory avoidance learning). This makes sense with respect to a distributed-associative memory system (from Whitlock et al., 2006). (D) Physiological evidence (rectification ratio) that AMPAR insertion made by auditory afferents to the amygdala is higher after paired rather than nonpaired auditory fear conditioning (after Rumpel et al., 2005). (E) Motor learning is associated with changes in mean GluA1 in dendritic spines and an associated change in spine size. Most spines stay stable, but learning is associated with more spines that are increased in size whereas control conditions show the reverse (Roth et al, 2020). (F) Somatic firing may not be necessary for learning-associated potentiation. In this example, a Ca^{2+} plateau potential in hippocampus occurred on lap 11 of an animal running around an initially unfamiliar track, and this was associated with the creation of a subsequently stable place field (Bittner et al., 2017).

A potential challenge to the Hebbian perspective that cell connections which are strengthened are between cells that regularly "take part in firing together" has now emerged in studies of dendritic computation in which the receptive-field properties of CA1 cells, such as place cells, occur in association with an unusual form of synaptic potentiation. Using intracellular recording in awake animals, Bittner et al. (2017) reported that plateau potentials may develop in the dendrites as cells started to exhibit a place field. For example, when running on a treadmill affording multiple "laps" of a virtual maze, little happened over the first few laps, a plateau potential then emerged, and this was soon associated with place-cell firing at this virtual location (Figure 10.10F). These and other findings point to a form of "behavioral time-scale" potentiation, which has some properties in common with classical LTP, but the timing considerations with respect to induction are strikingly different.

What about the presynaptically expressed component of LTP? It is now established that both pre- and postsynaptic changes can accompany learning in vivo (Richter-Levin et al., 1997; J Choi et al., 2018). Does the presence of presynaptic changes have any implications for the relationship between activity-dependent synaptic plasticity and memory? Padamsey and Emptage (2014) note that "discrepancies in the literature have raised doubts over a presynaptic locus of LTP" but argue that there are in fact two mechanistically distinct forms of LTP: one mechanism being postsynaptic (NMDAR-LTP) and the other expressed presynaptically (induced following postsynaptic Ca^{2+} influx through postsynaptic L-type VGCCs leading to the generation of a retrograde messenger, most likely nitric oxide). Interestingly, many computational models are agnostic about the locus of expression—all that matters is that the synapse is stronger. However, there are several ways in which it might matter. For example, the level of presynaptic potentiation at the mossy fiber terminals in CA3 could be important—the greater it is, the more likely will be the associative conjunction of pre- and postsynaptic activity at the terminals of the perforant path from EC in the outer dendritic layers of CA3. Given that mossy fiber potentiation is presynaptic, this could be an instance where its presence augments the memory encoding of timed sequences of events at synapses in the outer layers of CA3 reflecting the sequential events of an episode. However, even in this case, a computational model might only require a mathematical parameter reflecting the "strength" of mossy fiber synaptic terminals without regard to whether it is expressed pre- or postsynaptically (Tong et al., 2020).

10.8.3 Blocking the induction or expression of synaptic plasticity at the time of learning impairs memory formation

The SPM hypothesis predicts that interventions that block the induction or expression of synaptic plasticity in the hippocampus should have corresponding effects on hippocampus-dependent learning (Figure 10.11A). Addressing this test was a popular early approach, with results showing that, by and large, interference with hippocampal LTP prevents effective hippocampus-dependent learning.

However, there is devil in the experimental detail because, if a blocking intervention is applied *before* or *at the time of learning*, the encoding of a new memory trace and its later expression in behavior should both be impaired; applied *after* learning, only treatments that affect expression and maintenance would be expected to have an effect (S Martin et al., 2000). A second point is that certain

hippocampus-dependent tasks may result eventually in information storage outside of hippocampus in cortex, such that predictions of the SPM hypothesis must take on board wider systems consolidation considerations (McNaughton and Morris, 1987). A third detail relates to differential predictions arising from learning being mediated by the underlying mechanisms of LTP1, LTP2, or LTP3. Recent studies have expanded the scope of earlier studies with respect to blocking or enhancing LTP1 or LTP2—such as interventions that leave decaying LTP1 unaffected but enhance the availability of PRPs necessary for LTP2 that otherwise may not be expressed fully. This should and can enhance memory retention while leaving initial encoding and storage unaffected (Moncada and Viola, 2007). Humeau and Choquet (2019) consider the possibility of bringing contemporary imaging techniques at the level of the single spine or PSD into the picture to investigate, for example, the functional consequences of altering AMPAR exo- and endocytosis.

10.8.3.1 Physiological occlusion of LTP impairs learning

Saturation of LTP prior to behavioral training should *prevent* new learning. A key discovery was confirmation of this prediction in the context of spatial learning (Castro et al., 1989; Figure 10.11B). This observation was later confirmed using a very different hippocampus-dependent task—trace eyeblink conditioning (Gruart et al., 2006).

An impasse developed, however, following the failure of other groups to replicate the originally observed impairment of spatial learning (Cain et al., 1993; Jeffery and Morris, 1993; Korol et al., 1993; Sutherland et al., 1993). One creditable aspect of these four papers is that one of them—Korol et al. (1993)—was coauthored by McNaughton. Science works by self-correction and, while these failures were rightly published, no one could quite believe that this would be the end of the story. Bliss (1993) suggested that: (1) cumulative LTP of perforant path terminals may not have reached a true state of saturation; (2) perforant path terminals may have been sufficiently saturated, but not those on other hippocampal pathways (e.g., CA3-CA1 and EC-CA1 inputs); (3) saturation of the full septotemporal axis of the hippocampus may sometimes be necessary but would likely not have been achieved with electrical stimulation at a single site in the angular bundle. Evidence consistent with this third idea was presented by Barnes (1994), who found that upregulation of the immediate early gene *Zif268* was restricted to the dorsal hippocampus after stimulation at a single site in the angular bundle.

With these three caveats in mind, Moser (1998) designed a study that (1) used an array of cross-bundle stimulation electrodes to maximally activate the perforant path, with the cathode and anode switched frequently between active electrodes (Figure 10.11C); (2) employed a separate "probe" stimulating electrode to test whether the asymptotic LTP induced by the electrode array was a true saturation of LTP rather than some change in excitability at the stimulating electrode; and (3) made use of animals with large unilateral hippocampal lesions to reduce the amount of tissue to be potentiated. They confirmed the original findings of Castro et al. (1989), but with an interesting twist. When all animals were subsequently tested for induction of LTP from the probe site in the perforant path, some animals showed occlusion while others did not. Pleasingly, it turned out that only the subgroup in which LTP was successfully saturated failed to learn the watermaze, whereas those in which some LTP could still be induced did learn. Moreover, Brun et al. (2001) later observed that if the NMDAR antagonist CPP [(±)-3-(2-carboxypiperazin-4-yl)propyl-1-phosphonic acid], was

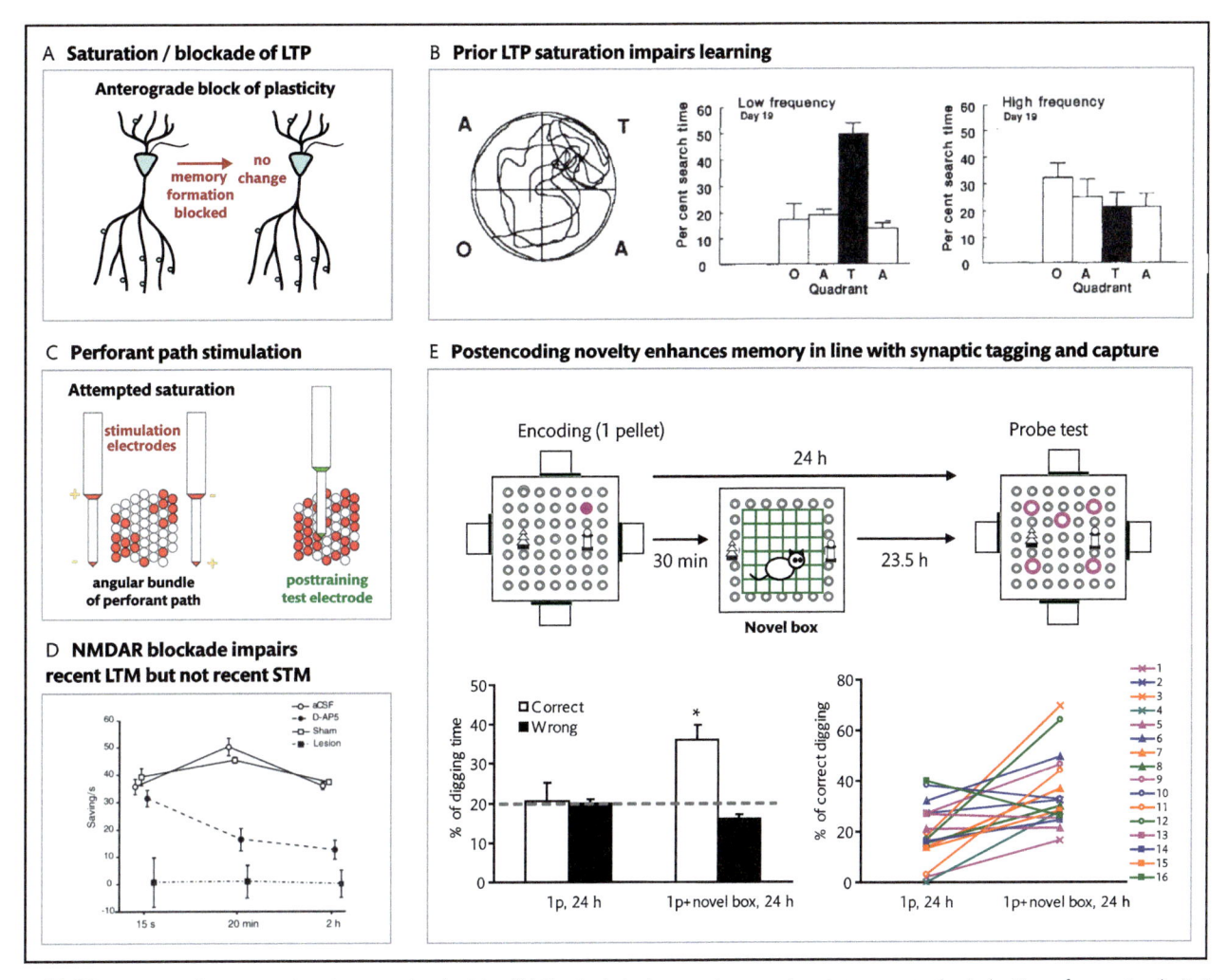

Figure 10.11 Anterograde interventions in synaptic plasticity. (A) The logic is that any intervention that prevents the induction of synaptic plasticity at the time of memory formation should block new learning. (B) Saturation of LTP prior to learning a water maze task caused impaired memory (after Castro et al., 1989). (C) Later replication using an enhanced arrangement of stimulating electrodes resolved a long-standing debate about this prediction in support of the original study (after Moser et al., 1998). (D) Task specificity is important, as pharmacological blockade of NMDARs has no effect in an everyday recency memory task when the memory interval is short (15 s) but causes a clear impairment at 2 h (from Steele and Morris, 1999). (E) The experience of something novel or surprising soon after learning does not change the neural representation of what has been learned but can strikingly enhance the retention of such information over time. Anterograde manipulations of neuromodulatory inputs can change memory persistence (after Wang et al., 2010).

locally infused into the hippocampus at the time of tetanization, which blocked intrahippocampal LTP induction but would have allowed any side-effects of this tetanization on other brain structures, there was no impairment of spatial learning. These newer findings vindicate both Castro et al.'s (1989) original observations and Barnes et al.'s (1994) timely concern about task variables.

LTP saturation might be achieved in other ways than angular bundle stimulation, such as bilateral stimulation of the ventral hippocampal commissure to potentiate the SCC pathway in CA3 and CA1. Indeed, as noted above, even a single LTP-inducing tetanus delivered to the SCC can impair trace eyeblink conditioning (Gruart et al., 2006). A pharmacological, rather than an electro-physiological, approach to saturation should also be considered, using, for example, BDNF (Bramham and Messaoudi, 2005), activators of AC, PKA, MAPK, or other signal-transduction cascades to induce asymptotic, slow-onset synaptic potentiation that, were it to saturate the capacity for further LTP induction, should impair learning.

10.8.3.2 Pharmacological blockade of the NMDAR impairs learning

A different approach is to block LTP induction at the time of learning directly using drugs. Morris et al. (1986) showed that chronic intraventricular infusion of the NMDAR antagonist D,L-AP5 blocked spatial but not visual discrimination learning in a watermaze (see first edition). Later work established that this effect was due to the active D-isomer of AP5 with a dose-response profile comparable to that established in studies on hippocampal LTP in vitro and in vivo (S Davis et al., 1992) and was seen also with acute intrahippocampal infusions of D-AP5 (Morris, 1989). When D-AP5 or the noncompetitive antagonist MK-801 ((5R,10S)-(+)-5-methyl-10,11-dihydro-5H-dibenzo[a,d] cyclohepten-5,10-imine) was applied after learning, however, there was no impairment of memory retrieval (Morris, 1989; Staubli et al., 1989; Shapiro and O'Connor, 1992) consistent with a role for NMDARs in the induction of LTP/memory but not their expression.

Using single-unit recording in conjunction with CPP, Kentros et al. (1998) showed that previously established hippocampal place fields were unchanged, but new place fields acquired under CPP in a new environment were unstable. A theoretical review of many further studies of the role of NMDAR activation on place- and grid-cell firing fields identified studies showing that sequence learning relies specifically on synaptic plasticity (Mehta, 2015). That is, learning a spatial sequence in which an animal moves from place A to place B, then from B to C to D, and so on, would sequentially activate a succession of overlapping place fields leading to the possibility that the sequence becomes encoded. This raises the fascinating question of whether spatial maps can be plastic. If so, how does such firing field plasticity contribute to sequence learning? Mehta (2015) summarizes a number of computational and experimental studies which indicate that NMDAR-mediated plasticity and the theta rhythm have specific effects on the experiential modification of spatial maps to facilitate predictive coding.

There is a pleasing generality to the involvement of NMDAR-dependent plasticity in learning. Numerous studies have found that competitive NMDAR antagonists impair diverse forms of learning. Learning paradigms used include spatial learning, T-maze alternation, certain types of olfactory learning, CFC, social transmission of food preference, flavor-place paired associate learning, differential reinforcement of low rates (DRL), and a number of operant tasks (for reviews, see Danysz et al., 1995; Lynch, 2004; Mehta, 2015). A similar involvement of the NMDAR is found for emotional learning tasks for which the underlying circuitry is focused on synaptic connectivity to and between distinct subregions of the amygdala (Davis et al., 1993; LeDoux, 2000). Indeed, the biophysical properties of the NMDAR make it ideal as a "coincidence detector" in many brain regions.

These data support the SPM hypothesis, but some ambiguities have been raised. One is that NMDAR blockade also affects LTD and so the pharmacological blockade approach cannot distinguish between a deleterious effect on learning mediated by blocking LTP or LTD or both. A second is that the use of NMDAR antagonists can cause a diverse array of sensorimotor disturbances. This is not surprising, as studies with the earliest glutamate antagonists in the early 1980s revealed the involvement of NMDAR-mediated currents in suprasegmental reflexes (Watkins and Jane, 2006) and NMDAR involvement in swimming by tadpoles (Dale and Roberts, 1985) and the lamprey (Grillner, 2006). In the watermaze, following intraperitoneal or intraventricular administration, these disturbances can include animals sometimes falling off the escape platform during a "wet-dog" shake, thigmotaxis, or even difficulties in climbing onto the platform early in training (S Davis et al., 1992; Saucier et al., 1996). Peter Cain therefore raised the possibility that, rather than NMDAR antagonists having a direct effect on memory encoding, these drug-induced "side-effects" might be the real cause of what he judged to be a spurious association between LTP blockade and memory. This is an important argument, but it was not supported in follow-up studies. Morris et al.'s (1986) original study used ventricular infusion, but in studies using acute infusion restricted to the hippocampus, sensorimotor deficits are not seen although the spatial learning impairment remains (Morris, 1989; Bast et al., 2005). The same dissociative pattern is seen with local infusions of D-AP5 into the prefrontal cortex in schema tasks—no

motor abnormalities, but clear learning/assimilation difficulties (Tse et al., 2011). The sensorimotor impairment hypothesis also wrongly predicts that memory retrieval would be abnormal under the influence of an NMDAR antagonist, as described earlier, because the motor problems would remain. A further puzzle that took some time to work out is that various forms of pretraining in behavioral tasks, with massed or spaced training in the same or different environments, alter the expression of drug-induced sensorimotor abnormalities and the impact of NMDAR antagonists on learning (Morris, 1989; Bannerman et al., 1995; Uekita and Okaichi, 2009; Inglis et al., 2013). Bye and McDonald (2019) provide a fascinating insight into this puzzle with a series of analytically powerful studies. Paradoxically, it seems that the causal impact of the drug-associated side-effects may be partially in the opposite direction from that envisaged by Cain—a deficit in learning in the watermaze caused by an NMDAR antagonist can exacerbate what would otherwise be minor sensorimotor abnormalities.

10.8.3.3 Task-specificity: differential impact on reference and recency memory

The induction/expression distinction in LTP is important in recognizing that two tasks classified as hippocampus-dependent may differ with respect to their daily involvement in two processes—making a memory and its long-term expression. A so-called reference memory task requires hippocampal synaptic plasticity at the outset, but little or none in experienced animals once a stable memory trace has been created; in contrast, substantial NMDAR-dependent plasticity remains essential for "everyday memory tasks" that entail regular one-trial encoding and a daily judgement of associative recency (see Chapter 14). In an everyday memory task in the watermaze, originally called "delayed matching-to-place" (DMP; see Steele and Morris, 1999), the animals cannot merely access a trace in long-term memory (LTM) and express this; they must access the most recent memory of where the escape platform is located and update this in an episodic-like manner.

Steele (1999) used this still poorly known modification of the watermaze protocol in which the hidden escape platform moves location from session to session. The animals' task was not just "to learn the watermaze" (in lab jargon), but to remember only where the escape platform was located most recently in an already well-learned spatial environment. Intrahippocampal D-AP5 caused a delay-dependent memory deficit that was seen day after day (Figure 10.11D). At short memory intervals (15 s), there was no memory deficit; at longer time intervals akin to those which would require an LTP-like process to induce a lasting memory trace (2 h), NMDAR blockade caused a major impairment in memory formation in every session irrespective of the extent of earlier training. When the dopamine D1/D5 receptor antagonist SCH23390 (7-chloro-3-methyl-1-phenyl-1,2,4,5-tetrahydro-3-benzazepin-8-ol) was infused into the hippocampus, likely affecting LTP2 but not LTP1, the deleterious impact on memory was seen only at the longer time period (2 h) but not at shorter ones (O'Carroll and Morris, 2004; O'Carroll et al., 2006).

Extensive training on a reference memory task in a watermaze can also eventually result in good spatial memory in animals treated with intrahippocampal D-AP5 (Bannerman et al., 1995). Learning is slower but not abolished. The gradual improvement even happens with hippocampal lesions (Morris et al., 1990) in which the cortex has to learn alone, albeit in an inflexible way (Eichenbaum et al., 1990). These findings are consistent with there being parallel memory encoding in hippocampus and neocortex that can be effective for stable unchanging long-term memory, with the cortex gradually able to overcome limitations arising from the compromise of the rapid space/time memory encoding in hippocampus caused by NMDAR blockade. This distinction between remembering something that is *always the case* and something that *happened most recently* is important (see Chapters 13 and 14).

10.8.3.4 Treatments that enhance LTP can also enhance memory and its persistence over time

The circuit-level consequences of enhancing synaptic plasticity through an anterograde intervention may be far from straightforward. Synaptic plasticity might normally be optimally tuned for the efficient encoding of information, such that any disturbance—even an enhancement—could have a paradoxically disruptive effect on hippocampal physiology. Nonetheless, considerable effort has been made to design experiments to test whether enhancing LTP would also enhance memory (Y Tang et al., 1999; Lynch, 2006). Well-known examples include "ampakines"—putative cognitive enhancers—which decrease the rate of AMPAR desensitization and slow the deactivation of receptor currents after agonist application (Arai et al., 1996), facilitate the induction of hippocampal LTP (Staubli et al., 1994), and can enhance the encoding of memory in a variety of tasks (Lynch and Gall, 2013). A number of other compounds, including phosphodiesterase inhibitors and drugs targeting the α7 nicotinic ACh receptors, have also been reported to enhance both learning and the induction, expression, or maintenance of hippocampal LTP (Cooke and Bliss, 2005; Peters et al., 2015). The successful development of such drugs, if without side-effects, would be an invaluable translational benefit of this area of research.

A separate focus of "enhancement" efforts has been on the differential effects of interventions affecting LTP2 rather than LTP1. As discussed in section 10.2.1, LTP2 is a form of potentiation that requires synthesis of new proteins and lasts longer than 4 h, unlike LTP1 which normally decays to baseline within 1–2 h. Importantly, however, the events triggering protein synthesis do not have to occur at *exactly* the same time as the stimulation that induces synaptic potentiation. They can be shortly before or after (up to approximately 1.5 h). The evidence for this is that tetanization in the presence of a protein synthesis inhibitor (such as anisomycin or emetine) still results in LTP2 if a strong tetanus is applied to a separate pathway up to 1.5 h previously (Frey and Morris, 1997). Together with other findings, this observation led to the notion that tetanization sets local "synaptic tags" that capture plasticity proteins as they become available—the so-called STC hypothesis (see Box 10.3, and U Frey and Morris, 1998a). Key support for this idea came from an early study establishing a temporal symmetry of the two processes of tagging and the availability of PRPs (Frey and Morris, 1998b), and from a heroic study involving the simultaneous use of laser-evoked glutamate uncaging in the presence of forskolin and 2-photon imaging of dendritic spines which showed STC at the single-spine level (Govindarajan et al., 2011).

The same flexibility with respect to timing may also be true of memory formation. In the phenomenon of "flashbulb memory," we not only remember certain very emotionally significant events for an inordinately long period of time (such as the birth of a child),

but we may also remember certain trivial facets happening around the same time. Such memories are annealed into our frameworks of semantic knowledge with a loss of spatiotemporal context information, but may also remain as event memories that can be brought to mind years later. The same happens with very surprising events. Activation of neuromodulatory systems by novelty, reward, or punishment (S Frey et al., 2001; Richter-Levin and Akirav, 2003; Lisman and Grace, 2005) may cause neuron-wide upregulation of gene expression and protein synthesis in the intrahippocampal target regions via activation of cAMP-, PKA-, and CREB-dependent pathways. This would enhance the somatic synthesis of PRPs and so enhance their capture by synapses that have recently been potentiated and tagged, as outlined in the original STC hypothesis (Frey and Morris, 1998a). The original somatically focused hypothesis now needs modification as an additional likely site of the synthesis of PRPs is dendritic (see Chapter 8).

Following pioneering work by Moncada et al. (2007) and their introduction of the concept of "behavioral tagging," S. Wang et al. (2010) went on to investigate this idea in a behavioral task in which rats were trained on the everyday memory spatial recency task in an event-arena in which they had to find and dig up food reward from sandwells (Figure 10.11E). Memory that was ordinarily forgotten rapidly was retained by short periods of task-independent novelty exploration scheduled 30 min *after* initial spatial memory encoding. Bilateral infusion of the D1/D5 antagonist SCH23390 or anisomycin into the dorsal hippocampus, in association with the novel experience (but after initial memory encoding), blocked the retention of memory. These and other findings of the study were interpreted in terms of STC, pointing to the possibility of catecholaminergic modulation of memory maintenance via control of protein synthesis.

In a follow-up study, Takeuchi et al. (2016) have investigated the impact of optogenetic activation of the ventral tegmental area (VTA) or locus coeruleus (LC) in *Th (tyrosine hydroxylase)*-cre mice to see if this could substitute for novelty exploration. The reason for using *Th*-cre mice was to explore the consequences of novelty-associated activation of TH+ (tyrosine hydroxylase-expressing) neurons in line with ideas developed by Lisman and Grace (2005). The findings showed, surprisingly, that what had been intended to be the control condition with only LC activation actually resulted in enhanced 24 h memory, whereas the VTA activation condition did not. Paradoxically, the light-evoked activation of LC caused modulation in hippocampus that was blocked by the D1/D5 receptor antagonist SCH23390 but not by the noradrenaline receptor antagonist propranolol. Parallel in vitro electrophysiology studies confirmed this puzzling dissociation. The possibility that, under some circumstances, LC innervation of hippocampus can lead to concomitant dopamine release as well as that of noradrenaline (Kempadoo et al., 2016) needs to be followed up. Interestingly, the effectiveness of unrelated novelty in enhancing memory retention by school children has also been explored and confirmed in exciting work by Viola's group in Buenos Aires (Viola et al., 2014).

10.8.4 Induction of synaptic potentiation after learning and interference with its expression both disrupt memory retrieval

If memory is mediated by reactivation of stable dendritic patterns of synaptic weights, firing of the correct ensemble of neurons in a learned cell-assembly is essential. The disruption of such patterns or ensembles should cause retrieval failure. This would be a *retrograde manipulation*—a test of the SPM hypothesis that differs from those discussed in the immediately preceding section because it is carried out *after* learning has taken place (Figure 10.12A).

One approach has been to induce or saturate LTP physiologically after learning with a view to "scrambling" the spatial pattern of synaptic weights. A second approach, again after learning, is to apply pharmacological or other brain-region-specific treatments to erase recent LTP expression. Again, correct recall should be disrupted. Both are "loss-of-function" approaches. However, a complementary prediction is that if the usual decay of memory over time seen with only modest training were to be prevented by a treatment that *enhanced* the retention of LTP, memory should last longer. This "gain-of-function" prediction has been explored using peptides targeting the dynamics of AMPAR endo- and exocytosis. A distinct approach to inducing forgetting is to disrupt the learned cell-assembly through a manipulation that induces adult neurogenesis. Whereas this does not affect synaptic weights, it could have a similar effect in altering the ensemble of active cells at the time of recall.

Retrograde manipulations cut across the logically separate issues of induction, expression, and maintenance of LTP/LTD. In the first approach above, new LTP is *induced* at additional synapses such that the spatial pattern of cell firing during retrieval should differ from the pattern expected from the initially stored memory trace. A manipulation affecting neurogenesis in the DG should have much the same effect, as the neurons participating in memory recall would overlap with but differ from those of learning. In the second approach, LTP *expression* is selectively blocked with a view to seeing whether a commensurate change in memory persistence occurs. In the third approach, the focus is on *selectivity*—interfering with some but not other memory traces that may overlap spatially in a population of cells. That is, one memory trace may be expressed and maintained largely by potentiated synapses that are selectively tagged for the purposes of the experiment, whereas another and possibly overlapping memory trace would be at synapses that are untagged. Neural mechanisms of pattern completion should generally enable the correct memory to be recalled even in the presence of some degradation through interference, but there will be a threshold beyond which it fails to help.

One computational complication to such experiments is that the pattern of firing of cells in a distributed associative memory system (such as CA3) will include those that fire *and* those that don't. A development of this argument is that, even if the induction of synaptic potentiation is necessary for memory formation, it does not mean that synaptic transmission at connections unaffected during learning, or the firing of cells whose connections were unchanged, may not also be involved in memory expression. Whereas the detectability and anterograde interventions discussed so far do not address this point, the postlearning induction and/or saturation of LTP would be an intervention that is indiscriminant between (1) potentiated connections; (2) unchanged connections on cells subject to synaptic potentiation; or (3) cells that fire during memory retrieval but have been unchanged during memory encoding. That is, this postlearning manipulation is aimed only at "scrambling" the spatial pattern of potentiated *and* baseline synapses across many cells.

McNaughton (1986) was the first to show that spatial memory retrieval could be disrupted by postlearning LTP induction. Brun et al. (2001) followed up this finding by training rats in a spatial reference memory task in the watermaze for several sessions before then inducing NMDAR-LTP via, again, an array of stimulating electrodes that straddled the angular bundle of the perforant path. Rats that had been subjected to HFS were unable to recall the platform location in a subsequent probe trial (Figure 10.12B). In an independent study of this same type, postlearning induction of LTP at CA3–CA1 synapses prevented the successful recall of trace eyeblink conditioning in mice (Gruart et al., 2006).

The SPM hypothesis predicts that scrambling the spatial pattern of synaptic weights in various subregions of the hippocampal formation by tetanic activation of the angular bundle should cause true forgetting, but can this manipulation be done more selectively in specific subregions of hippocampal circuitry? Madronal et al. (2016) devised one method of selectively inhibiting the granule cells of the DG without affecting other parts of the hippocampus, pointing out that "a major limitation of resolving the mechanisms of hippocampal function has been the lack of tools that allow for rapid, transient, efficient and specific inhibition of hippocampal cell-types." The technique deployed was systemic administration of the 5-HT$_{1A}$ receptor agonist, 8-OH-DPAT (7-(Dipropylamino)-5,6,7,8-tetrahydronaphthalen-1-ol) to transgenic mice expressing this receptor exclusively on DG granule cells. This inhibited field-potentials recorded in CA3 (one synapse downstream), and thus communication through the DG-CA3 component of hippocampal circuitry, but it had no effect on the direct input to CA1 from the EC that bypasses DG and CA3. Using a hippocampus-dependent trace eyeblink paradigm, this form of DG inhibition caused a loss of conditioned responding. This was apparently "true forgetting," because the transient inhibition induced by 8-OH-DPAT resulted in long-lasting loss of conditioned responding over several days, outlasting the transient inhibition of the DG (Figure 10.12C). Madronal et al. (2016) proposed a model suggesting that CA1 synaptic efficacy may be held in balance through interaction of the trisynaptic and the temporoammonic pathway inputs.

The experimental induction of adult neurogenesis constitutes another approach to scrambling the pattern of cell firing after learning. Akers (2014) trained rats in a hippocampus-dependent CFC task and measured the extent of freezing many days afterward (42 days). Rats required to run extensively (in a running wheel) soon after training were found, at this extended period later, to freeze less than the control group (Figure 10.12D). Histochemical data showed that the experience of running triggered augmented adult neurogenesis in the DG, with 42 days being enough time for these cells to make functional connections. This would likely have affected pattern separation in a manner that would have disrupted the cell-assembly encoding the context memory.

Specificity is increasingly the name of the game in contemporary neuroscience, with optogenetic techniques now being one exciting route to achieve this in causal studies. Using the behavioral technique of conditioned suppression in which fear causes a decrease in appetitively motivated lever-press responding for reward in an operant chamber, Nabavi (2014) examined associative fear conditioning mediated by specific connections in a small enough region of the amygdala to be sufficiently activated by focal light stimulation (i.e., the viral-spread, light-spread concerns were minimal). Rats were conditioned to associate a foot-shock with an auditory

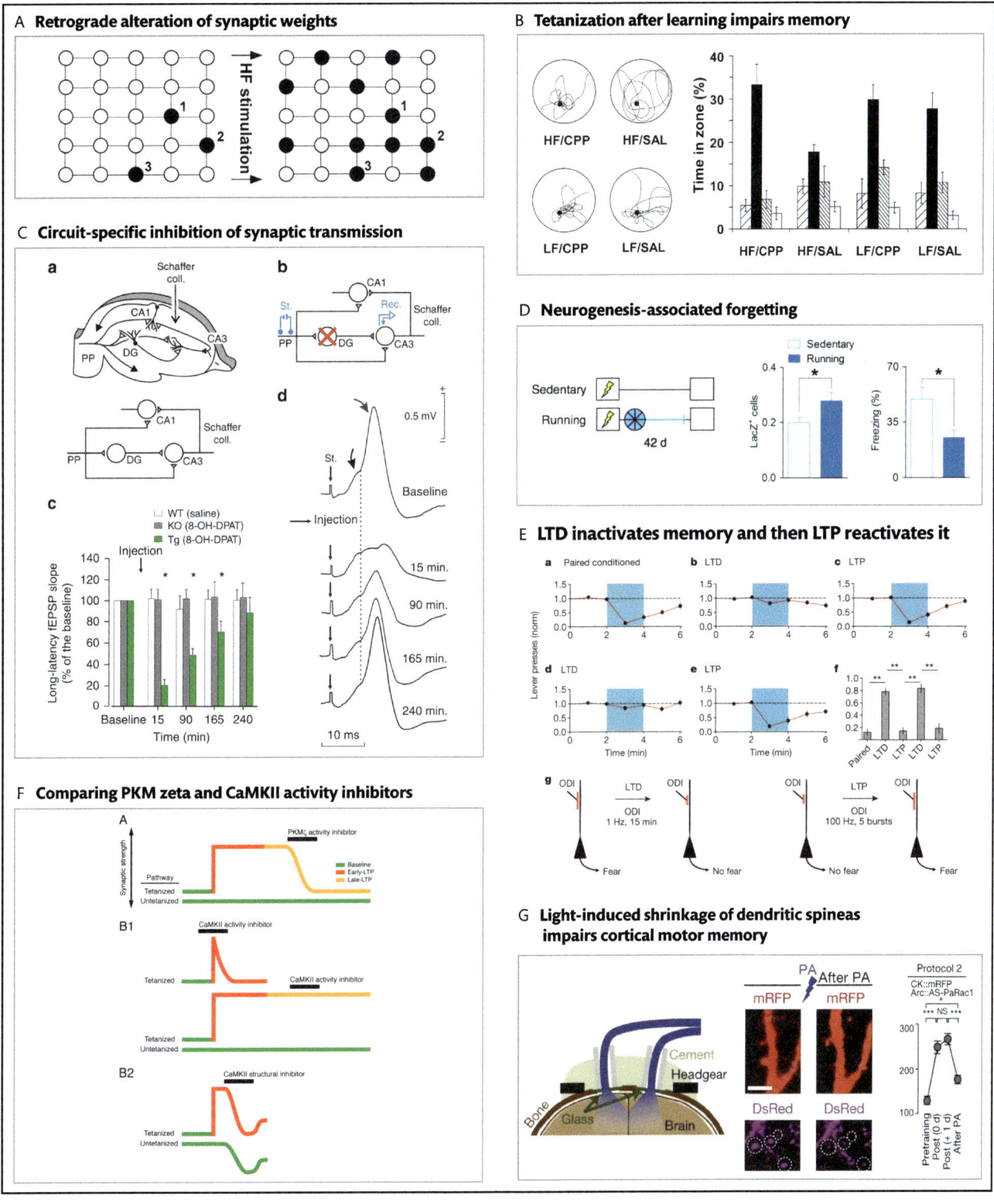

Figure 10.12 Retrograde manipulations affect memory. (A) The general concept is that induction of LTP after learning will change the spatial pattern of potentiated synapses, affecting the ability to correctly recall a learned task. (B) Posttraining tetanization of the perforant path blocks spatial memory unless the NMDAR antagonist CPP is present (after Brun et al., 2001). (C) Local circuit-specific inhibition of synaptic transmission in the dentate gyrus affects the balance of inputs to CA1 from the trisynaptic and temporoammonic pathways (after Madronal et al., 2016). (D) Postlearning exercise triggers neurogenesis that, weeks later, impairs memory (from Akers et al., 2014). (E) When animals express an amygdala-dependent fear memory that diminishes the incentive for appetitive behavior in an operant task, the induction of LTD rescues and the subsequent induction of LTP reinstates the memory (after Nabavi et al., 2014). (F) Inhibitors of PKMζ and CaMKII (activity and structure) have distinctive impacts on hippocampal synaptic potentiation (after Sacktor and Fenton, 2018). (G) A genetic construct that tags recently active synaptic inputs can in response to diffuse intracranial light cause shrinkage of tagged dendritic spines and a selective loss of a specific learned motor-skill (from Hayashi-Takagi et al., 2015).

tone and later to maintain the memory using optogenetic stimulation of the auditory inputs to the amygdala that the tone would have activated. Optogenetic induction of LTD of these same auditory inputs inactivated the memory, while subsequent optogenetic induction of LTP on the same auditory input had the "yo-yo" effect of reactivating memory (Figure 10.12E)—a "now-you-see-it-now-you-don't" sequence that could be readily repeated. The authors suggested that their findings support a causal link between LTP/LTD and memory as they had engineered both inactivation and reactivation of memory. The study did nonetheless find that optogenetic fear conditioning on its own, prior to tone fear conditioning, was insufficient to induce learning. Thus, optogenetic LTD and LTP can modulate the strength of synapses on a pathway in which successful fear conditioning has already occurred.

The second conceptual approach to retrograde manipulation aims to induce or block "synaptic forgetting" pharmacologically. This approach has a long history, much of it focused on second-messenger events downstream of NMDAR activation that may be mediating AMPAR mobilization, which the late James Schwartz aptly called "cognitive kinases" (Schwartz, 1993). A prominent example has been the idea that the autophosphorylated state of CaMKII could be maintaining synaptic potentiation and thus memory traces (Lisman, 1985). Whereas CaMKII phosphorylation is normally triggered by Ca^{2+}/CaM, the structure of this protein is such that, once activated, it can maintain this phosphorylated state autonomously (S Miller and Kennedy, 1986). Lisman (2017) elegantly summarized criteria for identifying the molecular basis of memory traces with respect to LTP induction, expression, and erasure tests, arguing that the key test is the latter. He describes experiments in which, after LTP induction, application of a specific peptide that interrupts autophosphorylation (TatCN21) reversed LTP expression back to baseline. Complementary behavioral studies using the transient Herpes simplex viral expression of a dominant-negative CaMKIIα (Lys42Met) in the hippocampus induced a persistent erasure of a conditioned place avoidance task (Rossetti et al., 2017). Honoring John Lisman's contributions to neuroscience, Bear and colleagues outlined the ingenuity but also certain caveats of Lisman's erasure approach (Bear et al., 2018).

An analogous but molecularly distinct theory has focused on an atypical protein kinase also proposed to be at the heart of the molecular mechanism of LTM–PKMζ. This idea, developed by Sacktor (2011) is that persistent memory may be caused by the persistent increase of an unusual isoform of protein kinase C. Some key evidence in support of this notion is that PKMζ is synthesized by stimulus protocols that lead to synaptic plasticity, can also be autonomously active like CaMKII, and demonstrably enhances synaptic transmission. Moreover, specific inhibitors and dominant negative mutations of PKMζ reverse LTP2 back to a baseline nonmemory state, with commensurate forgetting seen in relevant memory tasks in behaving animals. One key experimental study was the observation that ZIP could both reverse established LTP and cause forgetting of a hippocampus-dependent place avoidance task (Pastalkova et al., 2006). Figure 10.12F outlines the logic that differentiates experiments testing the distinct CaMKII and PKMζ hypotheses of memory maintenance. Whereas the CaMKII hypothesis appears to have focused on early LTP induction and structural stability, PKMζ is held to mediate late-LTP more selectively.

The PKMζ hypothesis was undermined by the publication in 2013 of two papers showing normal LTP and normal LTM in PKMζ knockout mice (A Lee et al., 2013; Volk et al., 2013) including mice with a regionally specific deletion of PKMζ in hippocampus. Moreover, whereas ZIP—an ostensibly specific pharmacological inhibitor of PKMζ—successfully abolished memory, it also did so in the PKMζ knockout mice. However, there is the possibility of genetic compensation. Tsokas (2016) describe one example of compensation by another atypical kinase—PKCι/λ—that is only upregulated in the absence of PKMζ and may take over some of its functions. They confirmed the earlier and problematic 2013 observation that ZIP successfully reduces late-LTP in PKMζ null mice, but also showed that ZIP inhibits the parallel self-sustaining function of PKCι/λ. In contrast, a different antisense molecule targeting the translation start site of PKMζ, successfully abolished late-LTP in wild-type, but not in PKMζ-null mice. Whereas PKCι/λ only increases transiently after LTP induction in wild-type mice (in which PKMζ is ostensibly doing the work of sustaining memory), the level of PKCι/λ was seen to be increased in PKMζ-null mice for the full duration of the study. Symmetrically, a different molecule called ICAP (4-(5-amino-4-carbamoylimidazol-1-yl)-2,3-dihydroxycyclopentyl] methyl dihydrogen) that affects PKCι/λ selectively reversed late-LTP in PKMζ-null but not in wild-type mice. Thus, PKMζ appears to be the first-team player, but PKCι/λ is an able substitute. In parallel behavioral studies using place-avoidance, PKMζ-antisense successfully disrupted LTM in wild-type but not in PKMζ-null mice, whereas ICAP worked in PKMζ-null mice.

A conceptual concern with respect to the autoregulation idea is whether it is likely that memory is maintained by a single molecule, as Lisman and Sacktor surmise (Rossetti et al., 2017; Sacktor and Fenton, 2018). In an insightful commentary, Kennedy is skeptical that a molecule implicated in memory retention really does need to be sustained throughout the lifetime of the memory trace (see Bear et al., 2018). By analogy with a classic problem in physics, it used to be thought long ago that mysterious "movers" were required to sustain the dynamics of the celestial spheres. But the Newtonian revolution did away with this necessity through the linked concepts of force, mass, and acceleration. Adopting this metaphor, an alternative possibility is that "cognitive kinases" may be key elements of the cascade of signal-transduction events *triggering* structural change but, like "acceleration," once they have done their job, a new stable structural state-of-affairs becomes passively responsible for lasting LTP expression (LTP2 and LTP3) in the manner of Newton's concept of a "uniform motion." It is, of course, not really "passive," because structural changes will be dynamically recycled during protein turnover, faithfully recreating the stable state and unaware, so to speak, that their recycling is sustaining a memory (Humeau and Choquet, 2019). This state of blissful ignorance would have first involved a transition from one maintained state to a new, no less dynamic, but distinct and structurally stable state—the transition reflecting the induction of memory. Sacktor has considered this issue in an implicit retreat to a position in which "the persistent action of PKMζ could function to launch or to sustain for a period the structural changes such as new synaptic connections which once established become independent of PKMζ" (Tsokas et al., 2016). Tests of the successful degradation of memory by ZIP have been successfully done up to 3 months after initial learning, but future studies should not only examine consolidated memories for which the long-term trace may be in cortex and not hippocampus. Studies are also required to address whether structural changes in spine stability in the hippocampus are sufficient to mediate lasting memory and spine stability once the involvement of PKMζ has passed (Attardo et al., 2018).

Finally, postlearning "gain-of-function" approaches have considered how to enable more lasting memory from an already formed LTM trace. For example, Migues et al. (2016) note that in certain learning tasks, the strength of LTM correlates positively with the level of GluA2-containing AMPARs at postsynaptic sites, and that active removal of these receptors from postsynaptic sites causes forgetting. Their study, using a novelty exploration task called object-place recognition memory (see Chapter 14), revealed that interfering with the removal of postsynaptic GluA2-containing AMPARs would prevent forgetting over time. Parallel electrophysiological studies implicated the process of synaptic depotentiation as a likely contributor to forgetting, just as Madronal et al. (2016) had also suggested with a different approach and a different task. Blocking depotentiation should therefore enhance memory. For example, in a study anticipating contemporary approaches conducted some while ago, L. Xu (1998) reported that after recent induction of LTP, exposing freely moving animals to a novel but nonstressful recording chamber can reverse the LTP without affecting the baseline on a control pathway. They speculated that exposure to novelty may sometimes erase hitherto consolidated information by an LTD-like mechanism, possibility related to "theta" activity (see also Manahan-Vaughan and Braunewell, 1999). Note in passing that the postencoding novelty that has the opposite effect in functional studies of synaptic tagging and capture is not typically given until 30 min after memory encoding, at a time when depotentiation can no longer be induced.

A further causal approach has explored whether synaptic potentiation of specific subsets of synapses located on dendritic spines in motor cortex is indispensable for learning (Kasai et al., 2010). Hayashi-Takagi (2015) showed that targeted removal of spines tagged during motor learning resulted in a selective loss of the very motor-skill that triggered the tagging, but not of another motor skill that did not, even though it utilized an overlapping population of neurons (Figure 10.12G). The new technical contribution was the development of a novel synaptic optoprobe, AS-PaRac1 (activated synapse targeting photoactivatable Rac1), which was designed to reflect and restrict labeling to recently potentiated spines without affecting nearby spines that might, in a different and much earlier training session, have participated in the learning of a different motor skill. Measurements were made on approximately 4,000+ neurons and 400,000+ spines. The optoprobe was calibrated using LTP-like protocols in which Hayashi-Takagi et al. (2015) observed that a protein synthesis-dependent potentiation protocol for single spine LTP involving both (1) glutamate uncaging, and (2) the AC activator forskolin, which selectively induced the accumulation of AS-PaRac1 in the stimulated spines (see Govindarajan et al., 2011). Glutamate uncaging alone, which induces only short-term changes in spine size, did not cause spine tagging.

Taken together, these results demonstrate that both exercise and a newly acquired motor skill depends on the formation of a task-specific "synaptic ensemble." Commenting on these results, Lu (2015) made the following interesting point which is worthy of extended quotation:

> Methods for labelling, imaging, activating and silencing neurons in animals have enabled researchers to map the ensemble of neurons that correlates with a particular learning task, to manipulate their activities, and even to generate artificial memory traces. However, a single neuron may participate in the processing and storage of more than one distinct piece of information. Therefore, the engram of a particular memory involves not only the identity of the constituent neurons, but also the entire set of synaptic connections between these neurons. How memory is allocated at this synaptic level remains unclear. (J Lu and Zuo, 2015, p 324)

These comments need to be borne in mind as we consider a very different "gain-of-function" approach to memory research based on the call rather than the synapse; this is the "engram cells and circuits" approach, to which we now turn, along with the last criterion—mimicry.

10.8.5 Cellular change, synaptic change or both: engram cells, engram circuits, and memory

The final criterion for testing the SPM hypothesis is mimicry—making an apparent memory from constituent bits and pieces—a kind of "Lego" of memory. Artificial engineering of spatiotemporal patterns of synaptic potentiation and depression should create, when reactivated, the experience of remembering something that never happened. Memory would then have been "mimicked." Recalling time spent with Marilyn Monroe or Cary Grant is one fantasy version of this hypothesis, being attacked by an octopus when sailing might be another (Figure 10.13A). A prominent feature of this field of research is the use of gain-of-function experimental designs in which a cellular optical construct enables memory traces to be reactivated by light.

10.8.5.1 The mimicry problem

Neves et al. (2008) sketched out the issue with two *gedanken* experiments (Figure 10.13B). One involved monitoring memory formation between areas CA3 and CA1 using very high-density electrode arrays to map connectivity between the subset of pairs of CA3 and CA1 cells. A recently formed synaptic memory, encoded as a sparse pattern of potentiated CA3–CA1 connections, might be erased by means of either a low-frequency DP or STDP to suppress LTP specifically between potentiated CA3–CA1 pairs. The memory would then be reinstated using STDP of these same pairs. The other thought experiment involved the "use of an imaginary but not wholly implausible molecular device" in an "ideal transgenic mouse." They imagined a transgenically forgetful mouse which had just learned and then soon after forgotten something. With suitable molecular ingenuity, this mouse would have its memory restored. Prophetically, they suggested that: "An immediate-early gene promoter can be used to drive transcription of a molecular LTP device in recently activated synapses," adding that, "In the current state of knowledge this is not feasible, and it is unlikely to become so any time soon."

However, only a few years later, a new engineering approach emerged using IEGs and transgenic mice—the technology that underpins an approach to memory called "engram cells" (Tonegawa, Pignatelli, et al., 2015; Josselyn and Tonegawa, 2020). It both differs from and is a challenge to the SPM hypothesis because it focuses on *cells* rather than *synapses* (Figure 10.13C). Both hypotheses link back to Hebb's ideas about the physical basis of memory reflecting activity in "cell-assemblies" (Hebb, 1949). The SPM hypothesis supposes that a memory trace is the specific distribution of synaptic potentiation (and depression) across multiple neurons, while the new engram-cell idea puts its emphasis on neuronal activity representations. The wider relevance of engram cells to hippocampal memory is considered in Chapter 14 (section 14.8).

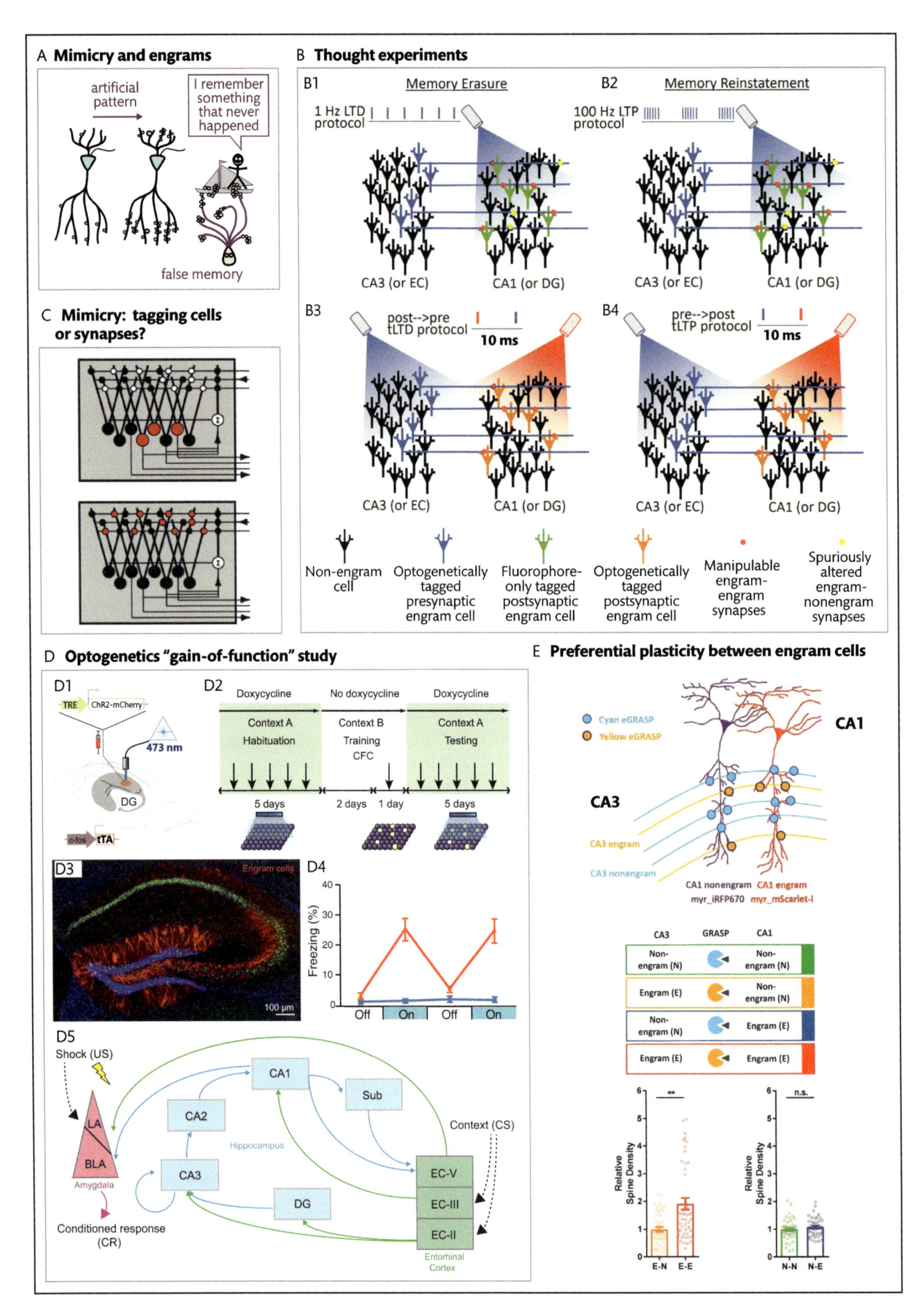

Figure 10.13 Mimicry and engram circuits. (A) The general concept is to test "sufficiency" by inducing an artificial pattern of potentiated synapses on a large number of cells (only one is shown) and thus cause the person to remember something that never happened, such as being attacked by an octopus while sailing. (B) In these thought experiments, the strength of connections between engram cells encoding a memory (for example, in the

Consider first the perspective of the SPM hypothesis. The challenge of mimicry is to find a way to create synaptic potentiation or depression *selectively* within a subset of the large number of synapses distributed across an even larger number of cells. Selectivity is critical, and it is no coincidence that an efficient pattern separation device (DG) serves as an entry point for hippocampal processing to help ensure sparse coding. The necessity for sparse coding (see Chapter 16) arises because, of the approximately 30,000 spines at each CA1 cell, spread across three main afferent pathways (strata oriens, radiatum, and lacunosum-moleculare), and a total of 300,000+ CA1 cells (in the rat, see Megías et al., 2001), storage capacity considerations require that only a relatively small number of these connections should have their synaptic weights changed for any one event memory (McNaughton and Morris, 1987; Treves and Rolls, 1994; Rolls and Treves, 2011). However, for a viable experiment, it is not immediately clear how to potentiate (say) 100 connections on one cell, still less to do so in a pattern, or to do so across a subset of cells. The Neves et al. (2008) proposal is a partial solution to the mimicry problem based on first forming, then suppressing, and then re-expressing a memory mediated by a subset of identifiable connections between connected CA3 and CA1 cells which are involved a specific memory. The yo-yo processes of depotentiating and then repotentiating to inhibit and then re-create memory will likely be experimentally challenging even with the optogenetic approach sketched out in Figure 10.13B. The silver lining to this cloud is that a distributed memory might work better if it got most of its synaptic weights down to baseline before it started on the daily task of keeping track of new experience. This might happen if the most widely expressed form of LTP is merely LTP1, which decays to baseline in 2–4 h, helping to ensure that the "slate is clean" as each new day unfolds (an assumption taken on board in the STC framework). Given that systems consolidation of memory happens largely during NREM slow-wave sleep (Diekelmann and Born, 2010), perhaps this process operates only on the information encoded via LTP2, which lasts sufficiently long to still be above baseline during sleep. The potentiated strength of synapses subject to LTP2 should therefore be long enough to allow successful hippocampal–neocortical interconnectivity to replay information encoded by selective potentiation into permanent neocortical sites of storage.

It needs to be stressed that a distributed memory trace is the entire set of synaptic weights including those that have not changed during learning. If CA3 and CA1 store a large number of distinct memories in a distributed associative manner, activity in CA3 will be changing from moment-to-moment and converging on *both* the subset of synaptic connections that comprise the putative engineered memory *and* on many other synapses in CA1 that were unchanged during memory formation. Thus, the probability of firing of the appropriate subset of CA1 cells to retrieve a memory cannot be solely determined by the engineered pattern of synaptic potentiation in CA1, but rather by the conjunction of two patterns—(1) the relatively static pattern of synaptic potentiation/depression and synaptic stability in CA1 on the one hand, and (2) the continuously changing afferent activity of CA3 cells on the other (not forgetting the stratum lacunosum-moleculare input from EC layer III also). Synaptic plasticity as a memory mechanism (SPM) only makes theoretical sense in the context of both the anatomical architecture in which it is embedded and the dynamic physiological patterns of activity.

Even if this could be done, how would the experimenter know or be able to test what the animal was remembering? The usual way forward is, of course, to simplify. In the search for tractability, neuroscientists of memory turn to simple behavioral tasks that require the animal to do one thing or another—to GO or to NO-GO, to turn LEFT or to turn RIGHT, to FREEZE or NOT-TO-FREEZE, and so on. Having a memory, even having a false memory, is then expressing A or B of these binary alternatives as an expression of memory read-out. This is not quite the same as

---

Figure 10.13 Continued

entorhinal cortex to granule cell projection, or the projection from CA3 to CA1) are manipulated by low- or high-frequency light stimulation (B1, B2), or by spike-timing-dependent plasticity (STDP) protocols (B3, B4), leading in each case to memory erasure or reinstatement. (B1) Engram synapses (red), connecting pre- and postsynaptic engram cells, are depotentiated by 1 Hz stimulation, leading to erasure of the memory. Note that some noise will be introduced in this approach by potential LTD at synapses (yellow) between presynaptic engram cells and non-engram postsynaptic cells. (B2) Reinstatement of the memory can be achieved by reinducing LTP at engram synapses by stimulating blue axons at 100 Hz. (B3, B4) An STDP protocol allows a more precise targeting of engram synapses. (B3) A post-before-pre protocol will cause memory erasure by inducing depotentiation only at engram synapses. (B4) Memory reinstatement can be achieved by reinducing LTP only at engram synapses with a pre-before-post protocol (after Neves et al., 2008). (C) A cross-section of cells in the dentate gyrus might be tagged at the cellular level (red cells) following, for example, *c-fos* activation (as in the Tonegawa experiments); alternatively, specific synapses onto DG granule cells might be tagged in some way, such as according to a Hebbian principle of synapses that were activated presynaptically at the time of postsynaptic cell activation. (D) At the heart of the Tonegawa approach is the use of tTA (tet transactivator), a bacterial protein that activates the tet promoter. In the Tonegawa strategy, a transgenic animal is produced in which a construct consisting of the promoter for the cFos protein drives expression of tTA. Expression of tTA will occur in any cell in which the cFos promoter happens to be activated. In animals that are fed doxycycline in their diet, the tTA so produced binds to doxycycline in the cytosol (D1). A further inducible step allows tTA to control local expression of a transgene expressing the light-gated cation channel channelrhodopsin. A viral construct containing the tet promoter linked to the gene encoding channelrhodopsin is injected locally into the hippocampus. Expression of channelrhodopsin will only occur in those hippocampal cells in which some significant event (e.g., a shock) has activated the cFos promoter, driving expression of the tet transactivator tTA, which, when and only when doxycycline (dox) is removed, binds to and activates the tet promoter, leading to expression of channelrhodopsin in the population of engram cells (D2). Subsequently it is possible to activate channelrhodopsin-expressing engram cells by exposing them to blue light (D3), leading to memory reactivation across repeated sessions (D4). Panel D5 outlines the concept of an engram-circuit consisting of different regions representing the context of experience (entorhinal cortex to dentate gyrus), its association with a fearful experience (basolateral amygdala, CA1 to BLA) and then the expression of the conditional response in the outputs of the basolateral amygdala (from Josselyn and Tonegawa, 2020). (E) An investigation into the interaction between CA3 and CA1 engram cells. Is the memory in the cells or in their connections? Using a novel two-color technique called dual-eGRASP, the Kaang laboratory examined the relative density of labeled connections between engram (E) and non-engram (N) cells, finding a higher density for E–E pairs than any other combination (after Choi et al., 2018).

remembering the "smell of grandma's apple pie," but we have to start somewhere.

10.8.5.2 Engram cells and circuits

These conceptual considerations set the stage for recognizing the value (and limitations) of a radically different approach, involving what are commonly called "engram cells" (Tonegawa, Liu, et al., 2015). Tonegawa defines an engram as the constellation of cells whose patterns of activity change during learning. Engram cells are part of a wider "engram circuit," in which different facets of experience are represented at different points. Read-out of memory is (generally) a straightforward matter of reactivating these (and only these) cells with the behavioral outcome being an A vs. B type of response.

The technology for making all this possible is truly awesome (Figure 10.13D). Typically, it involves specific transgenic lines of animals (usually mice) in which immediate-early gene activation triggers the cell-specific expression of Cre only during transient experimenter-defined time-windows controlled by removing access to doxycycline (usually available in the drinking water). Separate viral microinfusion of a Cre-dependent optogenetic construct, such as an AAV (adeno-associated virus)-mediated expression of channelrhodopsin-2 (ChR2), is made into a specific area of the brain. The tagging of neurons is then thought to occur largely during specific learning experiences in a behavioral task. After learning, light is shone onto a region of brain containing the very cells that have been tagged with ChR2 to see whether memory retrieval occurs. Such mice, with what one can only describe as a somewhat aristocratic pedigree, have to date been largely tested in CFC, one component of which is hippocampus-dependent. More sophisticated behavioral approaches involving operant or multichoice outputs will also prove valuable in the future.

X. Liu et al. (2012) used *cfos*-tTA (tetracycline transactivator) mice, generated by Reijmers et al. (2009), whose drinking water contained doxycycline (dox). The experimenters then removed it from the water, opening up a "tagging-window," during which memory encoding could take place. The animals had much earlier been given bilateral surgical infusion of an AAV-expressed ChR2-EYFP marker into the DG, together with implantation of miniature light guides aimed at the cells of DG. In that way, the light did not shine everywhere in the darkness, but just on the DG. With "dox" removed, the animals explored a novel box (context A) for several minutes (Figure 10.13D). A subset of DG neurons would have fired during this period, causing a cumulative tagging with ChR2 of all the DG neurons that fired during exploration of this space, together with the accumulation of any neurons tagged in the home-cage during the off-dox period. Given the pattern-separating functions of the DG, different subsets of DG neurons would be active in different contexts and thus a different subset of DG neurons would have been tagged with ChR2 in different environments (also in the off-dox state). Soon after initial context exposure, the animals were subject to Pavlovian fear conditioning (using electric shock) in a separate brain area—the basolateral amygdala—the site at which "neutral" information about the context relayed from the hippocampus and a neural representation of the painful stimulation would be associated. On the next day, these conditioned animals were placed in a very different context that did not induce fear (context B). They showed no behavior indicative of fear and no electric shocks were delivered. However, when blue light was shone through

the light guides onto DG neurons while the animals were in context B, a freezing response was observed. Freezing decreased soon after the light went off and intensified when the light came on, in an experimentally controllable up-down-up fashion. X. Liu et al. (2012) was the first of an impressive series of studies from the Tonegawa group. Other groups have confirmed the efficacy of the approach including, for example, an early study focused on the cingulate cortex rather than the DG (Cowansage et al., 2014).

X. Liu et al.'s 's (2012) pioneering gain-of function study was followed up by numerous other studies that are described in detail in Chapter 14. However, the approach raises the question, "where" and "what" is the memory trace itself? Is it synaptic or cellular? (see Box 10.4). An important challenge to the SPM hypothesis emerged in two further experiments from the MIT group. Ryan (2015) examined memory consolidation and queried whether protein synthesis-dependent memory consolidation exclusively reflects an underlying protein synthesis-dependent mechanism regulating the persistence of memory traces in hippocampus (i.e., LTP2). The key finding was that, even when the protein synthesis inhibitor anisomycin was injected into mice immediately after context fear conditioning causing the usual overnight forgetting of the fearful nature of the context where conditioning took place, it was still possible to evoke a learned fear response (freezing) by selectively activating the DG neurons that had been actively tagged during the task. That is, memory could be evoked even though the synapses ostensibly holding the memory had been bypassed. The message was that memory could be "recovered" under amnesia. It appears to follow that a synaptic mechanism cannot be the exclusive site of a memory trace or engram. In fact, the Ryan et al. (2015) study, titled "Memory: Engram Cells Retain Memory under Retrograde Amnesia," was presented as a major challenge to the SPM hypothesis at the time.

We query this interpretation because the study needs to be seen from two distinct perspectives. From an engram-cell point of view, the synaptic potentiation that would have mediated initial learning had demonstrably and measurably declined to baseline—but the memory could still be reactivated. This is an unavoidable fact. However, the introduction of *c-fos*-driven *cre*-dependent labeling with ChR2 is an engineering trick, not something that would ordinarily happen in daily life, and one that bypasses the usual physiological process of memory formation, expression, and decay. Once labeled with a virus, the ChR2 expression remains and does not decay according to a timescale comparable to the decay time course of potentiation or memory. Unlike synapses whose strength can wax and wane in response to experience, the dynamics of ChR2 expression is presumably quite stable and quite unlike the normal dynamics of physiology. Accordingly, from the perspective of the SPM hypothesis, this tagging trick could arguably be seen as "the exception that proves the rule."

There are also some other puzzles, of which one is that the anisomycin, which caused the failure to transform LTP1 into LTP2 at perforant path synapses of the DG in the Ryan et al. (2015) study, should *also* have had the same effect at the synapses in the basolateral amygdala receiving hippocampal input. One possibility is that the hippocampal-amygdala pathway displays a long-lasting form of protein synthesis-independent LTP2 mediated by CP-AMPARs (P Park, Kang, et al., 2019; P Park, Kang, et al., 2021). However, even this is not quite enough, as there is also the curious matter that c-fos protein itself was synthesized by the expression of its IEG. Anisomycin may not have inhibited this process, as the drug was given after the shock and thus after the amygdala component of the learning.

A further challenging study, but this time of mice harboring genetic mutations observed in AD, presents a similar conundrum associated with memory reactivation after forgetting. It is not always clear whether forgetfulness observed in AD is due to problems at the time of learning (e.g., a failure of encoding), or at the time of recall despite effective earlier storage (e.g., retrieval failure). One way to distinguish these in an animal model is to conduct recall tests very soon after encoding (e.g., 1 h) and after a longer delay (24 h–7 days) and look for accelerated decay of memory. Roy (2016) did this in an APP/PS1 (presenilin-1) murine model of AD, at an optimum age of 7 months, which was prior to their age-dependent amyloid plaque deposition (Saura et al., 2004). Their learning paradigms included CFC, but also inhibitory avoidance learning and novel object recognition memory. In each case, the "AD mouse" showed accelerated forgetting over time after apparently normal memory at the 1 h interval). Roy et al.'s analysis included looking at measures of dendritic spine density in DG at perforant pathway terminals from EC. A 25% reduction in spine density was observed in the AD mice—pointing to a possible compromise in the ability of neural activity in EC to activate the pattern separating machinery of DG. This was followed by the heroic step of putting different engram-labeling "virus cocktails" into the afferent EC neurons (including a rapidly activating form of channelrhodopsin, called oCHIEF). These cocktails enabled high-frequency optogenetic LTP-inducing stimulation of *only* those afferents from engram cells in EC that projected to engram cells in DG (i.e., across brain area neurons participating in the full "engram circuit" in the manner of a Hebbian cell-assembly, and presumably then with the basolateral amygdala [BLA] neurons further downstream). With LTP induced, not only was there a restoration of dendritic spine density in the AD mice but also indications of natural context evoked freezing in the CFC task (up from around 20% freezing to >40% freezing). Interestingly, it was essential that *only* the engram cells of both EC and DG were allowed to participate in this selective restoration of memory because, in an important control, a global induction of LTP in DG afferents had the opposite effect of impairing memory (as in the LTP saturation studies discussed earlier).

Roy et al. (2016) concluded that the AD-associated deficits were in memory retrieval. The memory traces cannot have been lost because—their critical piece of evidence—they could restore memory using a selective LTP induction protocol on the pathway between the engram cells of EC and hippocampus, a tagging status ostensibly unaffected by the degenerative processes of AD. However, once again, we query whether this is the only possible interpretation of the data. A true "retrieval deficit" occurs when memory traces *really are there* but for some reason cannot be accessed. So-called "tip-of-the-tongue" phenomena are a case in point, as are instances of metamemory, in which you have the dissociative mental experience of knowing that you know something but cannot, at that moment, recall what you know you know. Roy et al.'s (2016) fascinating experiment describes a situation that appears to be a retrieval deficit of this kind, because both the deficit in memory and its later restoration is only measured at retrieval. The alternative, as we have argued in the case of Ryan et al. (2015), is that the memory trace is a distributed array of synaptic weights in a circuit that, in this case, includes the pathway from EC to the pattern separation machinery of the DG and thence via CA3 and CA1 to the amygdala. Over 24 h,

the array of synaptic weights on the EC to DG part of this pathway may indeed have decayed to baseline due to AD-associated degenerative mechanisms. On this view, the memory trace *really was lost* (true "storage failure"). However, the optogenetic viral cocktails would have enabled the two subsets of relevant cells in EC and DG to be tagged in a manner that they, *and only they*, could be subject to synaptic potentiation. Accordingly, although the memory trace really was lost, it rose from the dead by reactivating the relevant two subsets of "engram" cells. As with the work of a skilled picture restorer, the damaged neural portrait is repaired without paint being splashed all over the canvas. To call the deficit in the Roy et al. (2016) study one of retrieval because it is seen at the time of retrieval is, on this view, misleading.

The difference between the SPM and engram-circuit view may be more a matter of emphasis than of substance. The power of the cell focused, gain-of-function, engram-cell approach is summarized beautifully by Josselyn and Tonegawa (2020), but we reassert that both theories see a central place for synaptic plasticity. It is fitting to end with a study that presents data indicating that the site-specific substrate of engram cell connectivity likely involves synaptic plasticity (J Choi et al., 2018). The Kaang Lab has developed an enhanced form of a technique called GRASP (GFP Reconstitution Across Synaptic Partners) which labels both pre- and postsynaptic partners. Connections from presynaptic engram- or non-engram cells to postsynaptic engram- or non-engram cells could be distinguished by distinct fluorescent markers. Using a *cFos*-rtTA (reverse rTA) system to allow cell marking only in the presence of dox (rather than its absence, as above), and a variety of control conditions, they observed that the connectivity between defined cells in CA3 and CA1 in association with context fear conditioning was highest between engram cells (Figure 10.13E). Moreover, when the conditions of training were modified to allow either weak or strong training, a correlation was observed between connectivity and memory strength and, finally, that the enhanced synaptic strength between engram cells was associated with a reduction in the ability to induce new LTP (occlusion).

Clearly there is much more to be done to understand memory mechanisms in detail, but the idea that strength of connectivity between memory-related cells is the substrate of memory, an idea dating back to Cajal, Hebb, Kandel, Bliss and Lømo, and many others since, appears to capture a fundamental mechanism in the brain. Not for the first time, study of the hippocampus has helped to reveal the brain's secrets.

10.9 Disordered hippocampal synaptic plasticity

10.9.1 Introduction to synaptopathies

We here consider the evidence for aberrant hippocampal plasticity in three broad categories of cognitive disorder: neurodevelopmental disorders, neurodegenerative disorders, and psychiatric disorders. The degree to which hippocampal plasticity phenotypes contribute to these cognitive deficits is open to debate. However, there can be no doubt that studying hippocampal plasticity has provided valuable insights into the underlying synaptic and cellular dysfunctions.

Collectively, these disorders account for an astonishingly large healthcare burden across the world and their incidence is growing: dementia is on the rise because age is the primary risk

Box 10.4 The engram: synaptic or cellular? Evidence from neocortex and hippocampus

Is the engram cellular or synaptic? Is memory encoded by a group of interconnected cells rendered more excitable as the result of learning so that, independent of synaptic changes, their firing as an ensemble is facilitated, as suggested by studies in both the hippocampus (Ryan et al., 2015) and cortex (Alejandre-García et al., 2022)? Or is memory more accurately captured by a traditional Hebbian model in which information is encoded as changes in synaptic strength, specifically at synapses that have been active during the laying down of the memory?

Problems with the synaptic engram: the spine population varies over time

The classical Hebb synapse has provided the dominant model for the neural basis of memory since the Hebbian properties of LTP were uncovered in the 1980s. But cracks in the Hebbian facade have appeared in the last decade. First, the realization that not all spines are permanent structures has raised the obvious question: if spines are not permanent, how can a Hebbian engram encode a memory for a lifetime? Mongillo et al. (2017) proposed a number of potential solutions to this quandary. First, as we discuss below, while some spines are transient structures, others are permanent, and it could be these that support lifelong memories. Second, if neurons in the ensemble representing the conditioned stimulus, for instance, CA1 neurons in CFC, make multiple synapses with each of their target neurons in the BLA, then the loss of individual spines in the BLA neurons would have a reduced and perhaps insignificant impact. And finally, the target ensemble may form a self-repairing attractor state in which loss of individual connections is compensated for by activity, leading to Hebbian restoration of the attractor state.

Long-term in vivo imaging of dye-filled neurons in neocortex has revealed that the majority of thicker spines are permanent structures, with the proportion of stable spines increasing with age (Holtmaat et al., 2005; Steffens et al., 2021). Nevertheless, both the growth and shrinkage of spines as well as the elimination of spines and the formation of stable new spines have been detected in motor cortex following motor learning (T Xu et al., 2009; G Yang et al., 2009). That spines are necessary for the maintenance of motor memory has been demonstrated by Kasai and his colleagues, who developed a method of targeting and shrinking a population of spines in motor cortex that are activated during the acquisition of a motor task (Hayashi-Takagi et al., 2015), with a consequent reduction in performance in the motor task. In this study, transgenic mice bearing a cassette containing the dendritic targeting element (DTE) of the *Arc/Arg3.1* gene was used to drive expression of a photo-activatable version of the small GTPase Rac1 into spines that were active during acquisition of a motor learning task. Active Rac1 is known to shrink spines, and to the extent that the Arc DTE drives Rac1 specifically into potentiated spines, this result offers causal evidence that the motor engram is synaptic. However, while *Arc/Arg3.1* mRNA accumulates locally following prolonged (but not brief) stimulation of a restricted dendritic region (Steward and Worley, 2001), Arc/Arg3.1 protein becomes concentrated, in a process known as inverse-tagging, in neighboring rather than potentiated spines, where, in a CaMKIIβ-dependent process, it directs the internalization of AMPARs (Okuno et al., 2012; Okuno et al., 2018). Thus, it is not clear that the Arc/Arg3.1 DTE directs transcripts exclusively to spines of potentiated synapses, and further refinement of this approach is needed to allow the conclusion that an acquired motor memory can be abolished by specific destruction of a synaptic engram.

In contrast to the stability of larger spines on pyramidal cells in the neocortex, spines on hippocampal neurons are essentially transient structures, with the majority turning over within 2–3 weeks (Attardo et al., 2015) or less. Memories whose formation requires the hippocampus can become independent of the hippocampus after 3–4 weeks, and are then supported by the neocortex alone, a process referred to as systems consolidation (JJ Kim and Fanselow, 1992; Frankland and Bontempi, 2005; Goshen et al., 2011). The rapid turnover of spines in the hippocampus is therefore not necessarily incompatible with the concept of a synaptic engram. The Kaang laboratory has documented LTP at existing synapses between engram CA3 and CA1 cells and a learning-induced increase in the size and/or number of synapses between CA3 and CA1 engram cells

in mice, following CFC (J Choi et al., 2018). These findings point to a synaptic rather than a cellular basis for the engram. A similar learning-induced increase in both the strength of existing synapses connecting two ensembles and an apparent increase in the number of spines on target cells occurred in a study of conditioned place preference, in which a rat's choice of two adjacent contexts is biased toward the context in which it had previously received an injection of cocaine (Y Zhou et al., 2019). The context-driven behavior was underpinned by an ensemble of CA1 pyramidal cells in the ventral hippocampus that projected to an ensemble of D1 medium spiny cells in the core of the nucleus accumbens. Synapses connecting the two cell ensembles were potentiated, and there was an increase in the number of mushroom spines on the D1 medium spiny neurons that were incorporated in the postsynaptic ensemble (Y Zhou et al., 2019). These two studies suggest that learning is associated either with the enlargement of spines or with the formation of new spines—the latter possibility may or may not be consistent with a strictly Hebbian mechanism, depending on whether or not the new spines contact active boutons to form multispine synapses.

Other observations raise difficulties for both synaptic and cellular theories of the engram. There is evidence that the group of cells, and the synapses that drive them, which together encode a particular memory—for instance memory of receiving a shock in a particular place in CFC—is not constant over time, but may "drift" across the neuronal space of area CA1 (reviewed by D Han et al., 2021). How this could be consistent with a simple Hebbian model is unclear, but a distinction is made between the role of place cells encoding context, and engram cells, with the former outnumbering the latter.

Evidence favoring a synaptic engram

Convincing evidence that information is stored at the synaptic rather than the cellular level comes from studies of a hippocampus-independent task, cued auditory fear conditioning in the rodent. Axons from cells in auditory cortex conveying specific frequency information converge on cells in the BLA, which mediate the unconditioned freezing response to electric shock. Following conditioning to a specific tone, low-frequency stimulation of auditory cells or axons encoding the conditioned frequency leads to a depotentiation of the conditioned response, while low-frequency stimulation of axons encoding a different tone and projecting to the same individual BLA neurons has no effect (W Kim and Cho, 2017; Abdou et al., 2018). Another study (D Choi et al., 2021) examined changes in the size of "engram spines" on BLA neurons after auditory conditioning and extinction. Engram spines are here defined as spines on engram BLA neurons, which are contacted by axons from engram neurons in the auditory cortex (in both cases, an engram neuron is one in which an immediate-early gene was activated during auditory fear conditioning). These synapses can be identified using the GRASP technique (Feinberg et al., 2008). By splitting a fluorescent molecule into two parts, one expressed presynaptically and the other postsynaptically, fluorescence is restricted to the synaptic contact (if any) between the two neurons. Using this technique, together with dye labeling of the postsynaptic neuron to allow clear visualization of the spine, D Choi et al. (2021) found that the mean size of engram spines increased following auditory fear conditioning and decreased following extinction. Clearly, in this case the information that drives the conditioned response is held at the synaptic rather than the cellular level.

Evidence favoring a nonsynaptic engram

Synaptic plasticity in the form of LTP and LTD has long seemed the obvious candidate to support a synaptic engram, and several decades of research has overwhelmingly supported this view, as documented in this chapter. However, there remain findings that cannot easily be explained in terms of synaptic potentiation, notably the fact that a cell assembly of light-activatable CA1 neurons formed during one-trial CFC can continue to elicit a fear response after conditioning in the presence of the protein synthesis-inhibitor anisomycin, which blocks long-lasting LTP (Ryan et al., 2015), indicating that long-lasting synaptic change is not required for memory storage. Interestingly, a randomly selected set of pyramidal cells in ventral CA1 rendered activatable by light can, when paired with shock,

Box 10.4 Continued

form a persistent cellular engram (W Kim and Cho, 2020; see also Vetere et al., 2019). Whether or not the persistence of these arbitrarily constructed cellular engrams, or of those reported in motor cortex (Alejandre-García et al., 2022), are also resistant to anisomycin is not known. An analogous phenomenon in the LTP literature to persistent excitability changes is E-S potentiation (see section 10.4), but again the sensitivity of this component of LTP to anisomycin, or whether it outlasts synaptic change, has not been investigated. Finally, there is intriguing evidence that hippocampus-dependent memories are associated with a set of neurons, distinct from engram cells, in which an inflammatory response to DNA damage, marked by the expression of the protein TLR9, can persist for several days after learning. Disruption of this process blocked retrieval of a fear memory (Jovasevic et al., 2024). The relation between these inflammatory memory cells and engram cells remains to be established.

The engram: synaptic or cellular? Or both?

In any discussion of the synaptic engram, the presynaptic side of the equation also needs to be considered. While a cell's population of spines can be readily catalogued by light microscopy, the cells of origin of its presynaptic terminals are much less easy to visualize. Nevertheless, as previously emphasized, EM studies show a good match between the dimensions of pre- and postsynaptic specializations in the hippocampus (Bourne et al., 2013; Meyer et al., 2014; Harris, 2020). Moreover, since EM surveys reveal a very low incidence of orphan spines, it can be assumed that the appearance of a new spine is accompanied by the budding of a matching presynaptic terminal from a passing axon. What is not obvious is how this process could lead to the creation of new synaptic or cellular engrams in response to experience rather than having the counterproductive effect of introducing noise. Finally, an important aspect of the cellular engram is the notion that a subset of neurons, by virtue of their increased intrinsic excitability, have privileged access to the process of forming a cellular engram, a process termed "allocation." There is good evidence, for example, that neurons with high expression levels of the transcription factor CREB are more likely to be selected for memory allocation (J Choi et al., 2018; Josselyn and Tonegawa, 2020; de Sousa et al., 2021; D Han et al., 2021). This is clearly a cellular rather than a synaptic phenomenon and suggests that there are both cellular and synaptic elements to the formation of an engram.

---

factor and humans are, on average, living longer (Wimo et al., 2017, also see Chapter 20). Similarly, for many neurodevelopmental disorders, the incidence is also rising, in part due to improved diagnosis (Elsabbagh et al., 2012). Several environmental factors, including increased urbanicity, recreational drug use, and social media, may be contributing to a rise in psychiatric disorders (Schmitt et al., 2014). While the human tragedy is impossible to overstate, we must also acknowledge the economic burden that they impose, which dwarfs current investment made in funding the development of treatments (Luengo-Fernandez et al., 2012). To put this in perspective, the global annual cost of dementia in 2017 was estimated to be approaching the trillion-dollar threshold (J Xu et al., 2017). Despite lower incidence, the impact of neurodevelopmental and psychiatric disorders is often comparable as they emerge much earlier in life and last a lifetime.

Study of the contribution of deficits in hippocampal synaptic plasticity to the symptoms of these brain disorders is hampered by the difficulties in measuring synaptic plasticity in the brains of living humans. Electrophysiology has been performed in the medial temporal lobes, including the hippocampus, of awake human subjects undergoing surgical resection for treatment of epilepsy, which is itself a neurodevelopmental disorder (Quiroga et al., 2005). Excised tissue has also been used to demonstrate that the adult human hippocampus displays LTP with the properties already described for rodent models (Beck et al., 2000). However, it is fair to say that this approach, while unique in the insight it can provide about basic function (Beck et al., 2000; Quiroga et al., 2005) and pathology (Lie et al., 1998), is hampered by the impossibility of harvesting from healthy controls. For this reason, much of the current mechanistic insight into the role of hippocampal synaptic plasticity in neural disorders has arisen from animal models that, alongside suitable controls, attempt to replicate a particular human disorder by imposing a known genetic or environmental factor that substantially contributes to either the cause or pathology of the disorder. Disorders that arise from a highly penetrant alteration of a single, known gene are far easier to model in a mouse or rat than diseases that arise either from known multifactorial causes or have unknown origins (Nestler and Hyman, 2010).

A growing, complementary avenue of research to work on human subjects is becoming available by taking advantage of the remarkable induced pluripotent stem cell (iPSC) technology that has been developed in recent years (Li et al., 2018). This allows reprogramming of easily harvested cells, such as hairs, into neurons. These can, in turn, be grown into neural networks in a dish. The parallel development of CRISPR-Cas9 genome-editing technology (Doudna and Charpentier, 2014) has made it possible to rescue potential genetic causes within these cultures and create congenic control lines, which will prove critical in demonstrating a specific genetic contribution to the disorder. The degree to which iPSC-derived preparations replicate the hippocampus is open to question, so a further major step of humanizing animal models by inserting these iPSC-derived neurons into intact hippocampal networks may allow them to be studied more readily in the intact, living animal (Espuny-Camacho et al., 2017). Overall, this approach provides great promise for studying idiopathic conditions, in which the underlying cause of pathology is not understood. Another approach that has been used for conditions in which the genetic etiology is hard to model, such as schizophrenia, exposes animals to specific environmental factors that contribute to the human condition, including drug use (Javitt et al., 2012) and maternal immune response during pregnancy (Knuesel et al., 2014).

Within this chapter there will be some bias toward those conditions that are familial or syndromic and are therefore currently easier to model in animals, as that has been the dominant approach, but future work will likely attend to the more prevalent yet more challenging idiopathic conditions.

10.9.2 Neurodevelopmental disorders

Neurodevelopmental disorders are a set of conditions that specifically arise from disruptions of neural development, even if the symptoms do not always emerge until adolescence or early adulthood (Marin, 2016). Neurodevelopmental disorders include, in rough order of prevalence: epilepsy, attention-deficit hyperactivity disorder (ADHD), autism spectrum disorder (ASD), and intellectual disability (ID) (defined by an intelligence quotient under 70). There is major overlap across the conditions such that several of them—for example epilepsy, ASD, and ID, frequently occur together in individuals (Tuchman et al., 2010).

A wealth of evidence now implicates synaptic dysfunction as a primary feature of most neurodevelopmental disorders (see Figure 10.14). Genome-wide association studies (GWAS) show that genetic risk converges on synaptic proteins (Gilbert and Man, 2017), and synapses commonly exhibit aberrant morphology (Martinez-Cerdeno, 2017) and function (Zoghbi and Bear, 2012) in these conditions. A picture is now emerging in which multiple known risk factors for neurodevelopmental disorders influence synaptic signaling through a number of convergent routes (see Figure 10.15). Cognitive symptoms characterize all neurodevelopmental disorders (Renner et al., 2000; Ranganath et al., 2008; Fabio et al., 2020). Hippocampal pathology and aberrant plasticity are strongly implicated in most cases (Li et al., 2019). In addition, the study of aberrant synaptic plasticity in the hippocampus may provide insight into far-reaching cellular deficits such as altered protein synthesis, excitatory/inhibitory (E/I) balance (Rubenstein and Merzenich, 2003), disrupted homeostasis (Mullins et al., 2016),

or dysregulated epigenetic/transcriptional mechanisms (see Chapter 8). For reasons already stated, we will focus primarily on a few exemplar conditions that are defined by a known genetic cause, with the hope that this will provide insight into the more common idiopathic conditions.

10.9.2.1 Fragile X syndrome—exemplary insight from hippocampal synaptic plasticity

Fragile X syndrome (FXS) is a genetically determined form of ID that exhibits features of epilepsy, ASD, and ADHD (Farzin et al., 2006). It is among the most common form of ID arising from a highly penetrant, inherited dysfunction of a single known gene, affecting ~1:4000 boys and ~1:8000 girls (Crawford et al., 2001). This sex linkage results from miscoding in the *Fragile X messenger ribonucleoprotein 1* (*FMR1*) gene and dysregulation of the encoded protein (FMRP), which is housed on the X chromosome, giving rise to the disorder's name. FMRP is a negative regulator of protein translation, which binds to mRNA and is located at polyribosomes (Brown et al., 1998). Loss of FMRP function therefore leads to excessive protein translation and, given that protein translation

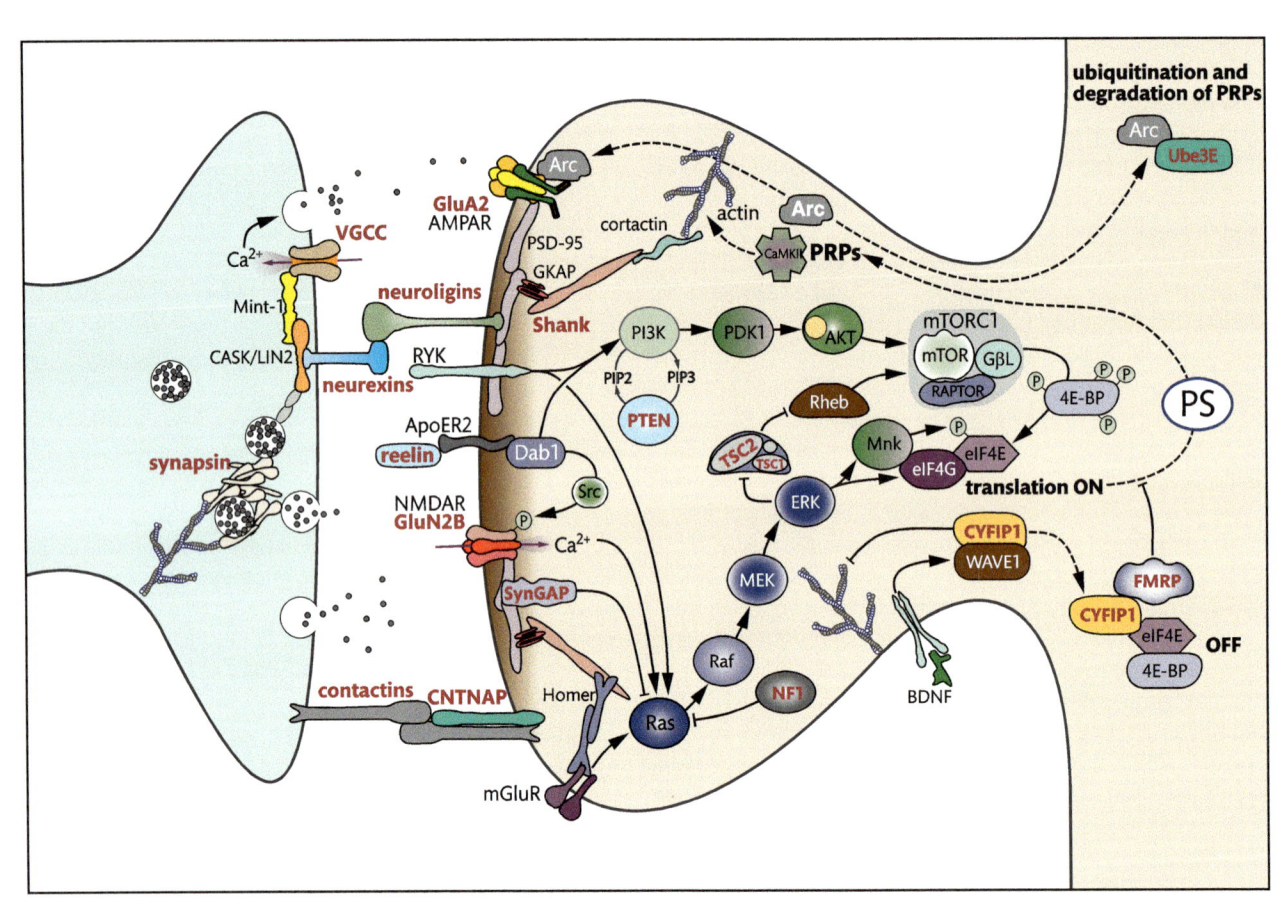

Figure 10.14 Synaptopathy underlying neurodevelopmental disorders. A simplified schematic describing some of the strongest genetic contributors to neurodevelopmental disorders and their role in hippocampal synaptic signaling. Risk factors are labeled in red: These include voltage-gated calcium channels (VGCC), neurexins, neuroligins, synapsin, contactins, contactin-associated proteins (CNTNAPs), reelin, some AMPAR subunits (GluA2), some NMDAR subunits (GluN2B), Synaptic GTPase-activating protein (SynGAP), Shank, Phosphatase and Tensin homolog (PTEN), neurofibromatosis type 1 (NF1), Tuberous Sclerosis Complex 1 and 2 (TSC1 and TSC2), FMRP (protein encoded by *FMR1*, *Fragile X messenger ribonucleoprotein 1*, Cytoplasmic FMR1 Interacting Protein 1 (CYFIP1), and Ubiquitin Protein ligase E3A (Ube3a). We have only addressed a subset of these risk factors directly in the chapter, but the schematic is designed to illustrate the convergence of many highly penetrant risk factors on the synapse and on signaling functions that relate to synaptic plasticity. Other binding partners and relevant signaling cascades are included in part and shown in black or white text within their respective schematic shapes. Solid arrow lines indicate direct activation. Dashed lines with arrows indicate indirect activation. Flat ended lines indicate inhibition. PS: protein synthesis. PRPs: plasticity-related proteins.

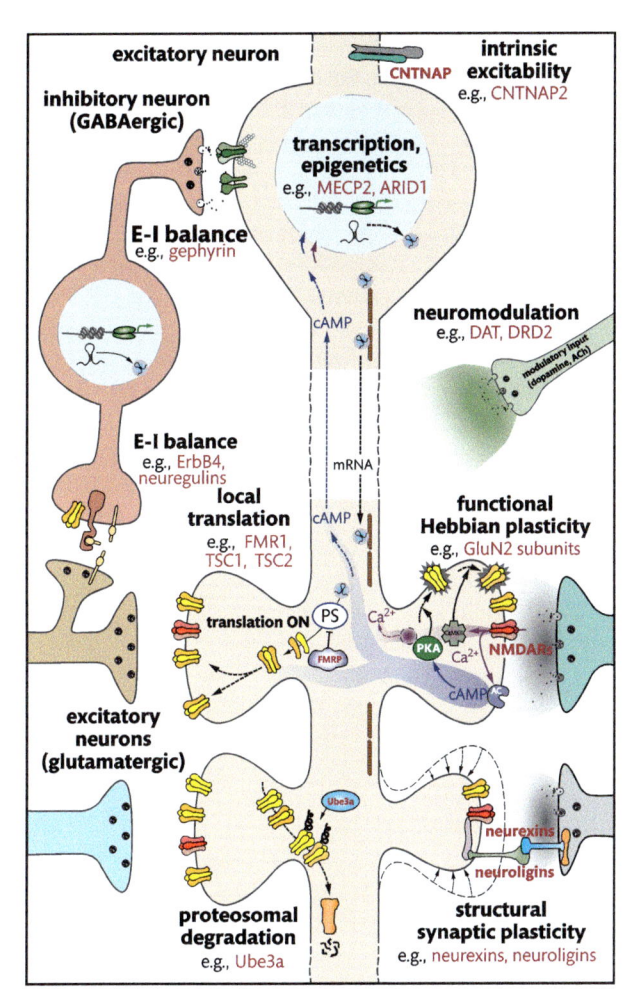

Figure 10.15 Neuronal functions affected in neurodevelopmental disorders that may influence synaptic plasticity. A schematic depicting neuronal functions that are affected by genetic risk factors for neurodevelopmental disorders, including excitatory/inhibitory (E-I) balance, intrinsic excitability, transcription and epigenetics, neuromodulation, local translation of proteins, functional Hebbian plasticity at the synapse, proteosomal degradation, and structural synaptic plasticity. Risk factors are again depicted in red, including contactin-associated protein 2 (CNTNAP2), methyl CpG binding protein 2 (MECP2), ATP-rich interactive domain-containing protein 1 (ARID1), gephyrin, dopamine transporter (DAT), dopamine 2 receptor (DRD2), Erb-B2 receptor tyrosine kinase 4 (ErbB4), neuregulins, Fragile X messenger ribonucleoprotein 1 (FMR1), Tuberous Sclerosis Complex 1 and 2 (TSC1 and TSC2), GluN2 NMDAR subunits, ubiquitin protein ligase E3A (Ube3a), neurexins, and neuroligins. AMPARs are depicted in yellow, NMDARs in red, and GABA receptors in green. PS: protein synthesis.

is required for several forms of hippocampal synaptic plasticity, it is not surprising that some forms of hippocampal synaptic plasticity are dysregulated in mouse models of FXS (Bear et al., 2004). Research on a mouse model in which *Fmr1* is genetically ablated (now complemented by studies in rats, see Asiminas et al., 2019), has been integral to our understanding of this underlying pathophysiology. This mouse model exhibits a wide variety of phenotypes, including altered dendritic spine density, protein synthesis, sensory-induced seizures, synaptic plasticity, and learning (Dolen et al., 2007), and has inspired several potential routes of treatment for ID and ASD within FXS. At the time of writing, none has

successfully passed through clinical trials in human patients, but clear promise exists.

A leading theory on the etiology of FXS holds that exaggerated protein synthesis linked to group I mGluR activation results in changes in synaptic structure and function (Bear et al., 2004). Group I mGluRs, which comprise mGluR1 and mGluR5, are widespread and potent regulators of local synaptic protein translation. Signaling through group I mGluRs plays a central role in the induction of a form of LTD at SCC-CA1 synapses (Palmer et al., 1997). This form of mGluR-LTD, can be induced by delivering PP of LFS, or by direct application of a group I, mGluR-specific agonist, such as DHPG. It is important to note that DHPG induces two mechanistically distinct forms of LTD, one of which requires coactivation of NMDARs (Palmer et al., 1997), and recent evidence suggests that the two forms may have different loci of expression (T Sanderson et al., 2022) (see sections 10.2.2 and 10.2.3 above on LTD mechanisms). Since there is a direct functional interaction between NMDARs and group I mGluRs (J Harvey et al., 1996), mGluR-LTD is often studied under conditions where NMDAR function is under complete block with AP5 (Huber et al., 2000). At SCC-CA1 synapses, the mGluR form of hippocampal LTD may require rapid protein synthesis, while the form induced exclusively via activation of NMDARs (i.e., NMDAR-LTD) typically does not (Huber et al., 2000). It should be noted that mGluR-LTD does not invariably require protein synthesis (e.g., Nosyreva and Huber, 2005; Moult et al., 2008; Toft et al., 2016). Potentially, this can be explained by the coexistence of an NMDAR-dependent, protein synthesis-independent presynaptic form and an NMDAR-independent, protein synthesis-dependent postsynaptic form of mGluR-LTD.

Importantly, mGluR-LTD is exaggerated in FXS model mice while NMDAR-LTD remains normal (Huber et al., 2002). In contrast to wild-type littermate control mice, the exaggerated mGluR-LTD in the FXS model mouse is not sensitive to blockade with protein translation inhibitors, indicating that exuberant ongoing protein synthesis in the absence of *Fmr1* has already synthesized enough proteins to support mGluR-LTD (Huber et al., 2002). An unexplored possibility is that the absence of *Fmr1* enables the protein synthesis-independent form of mGluR-LTD to be observed without the normal requirement of coactivation of NMDARs. Whatever the explanation, mGluR-LTD can provide a simple readout of aberrant activity-dependent protein translation in FXS model mice (Lüscher and Huber, 2010). Surprisingly, other forms of protein synthesis-dependent synaptic plasticity, such as LTP2 in the hippocampus, do not appear to be affected in FXS mice (Connor et al., 2011).

A genetic strategy to rescue the FXS phenotype involved reduced mGluR5 expression by 50% in the *Fmr1* knockout (KO) mice, restoring all aberrant phenotypes to normal levels, including protein synthesis-dependent SCC-CA1 mGluR-LTD, and hippocampus-dependent learning (Dolen et al., 2007). More recent work has indicated that many of these dysfunctions, starting with exaggerated, anisomycin-insensitive hippocampal mGluR-LTD, can be reversed by a month-long application of negative allosteric modulation of mGluR5 in young animals (Michalon et al., 2012). This is a particularly striking result as it indicates that a so-called neurodevelopmental effect can be reversed in the almost fully developed brain, motivating clinical trials that progressed all the way to phase III. Unfortunately, the trials eventually failed to meet their specified outcomes, which may support alternative views of the mechanistic underpinnings of FXS or reflect limitations of the current clinical trial process (Berry-Kravis et al., 2018).

A prominent competing approach to treatment strategies for FXS has focused on another well-studied signaling pathway that plays a critical role in protein synthesis, known as the mammalian target of rapamycin (mTOR) signaling pathway. Given the key role that the protein kinase mTOR plays in cell growth as a core component of the mTOR complex 1, and its major role in regulating protein synthesis at the synapse (S Tang and Schuman, 2002), it is perhaps unsurprising that mTOR inhibition should prevent mGluR-LTD (Hou and Klann, 2004). In the FXS model mouse, mTOR activity and downstream signaling, such as activation of S6 kinase (S6K) and the formation of eukaryotic initiation factor complex 4F (eiF4F, a critical step in local protein translation), are all elevated (Sharma et al., 2010). Inhibition of mTOR with the selective inhibitor rapamycin, which normally blocks mGluR-LTD by suppressing synaptic protein synthesis, has no effect on mGluR-LTD in FXS mice, presumably due to a profusion of protein synthesis (Sharma et al., 2010). Genetic knockdown of S6K, a key intermediary in this alternative signaling pathway that is elevated in the FXS mouse, rescues hippocampal mGluR-LTD to normal levels and sensitivities, and recovers cognition in FXS mice, just as was observed using the mGluR5 knockdown strategy.

Thus, it appears there are multiple routes to normalizing synaptic protein synthesis in FXS. To date there have been at least nine different genetic targets that have been reduced in expression to rescue hippocampal plasticity and recover cognitive function in FXS model mice (Richter et al., 2015). It therefore remains a strong possibility that the protein synthesis theory of FXS does capture the core dysfunction of the disorder and that the failure of clinical trials can be accounted for by three key practical limitations:

1. a failure to effectively stratify patients into likely responders and those that could be adversely affected,
2. the occurrence of unwanted side effects, and
3. the development of tolerance to the drug treatment.

To overcome the latter two factors, alternative approaches have focused on reducing activity in intracellular signaling pathways that trigger protein translation. One promising candidate, lovastatin, subtly reduces the activation of the ERK1/2 signaling pathway by the GTPase RAS (derived from "Rat sarcoma virus"). This cascade triggers protein translation not only because of mGluR5 activation but also due to other extracellular signals. Once again, SCC-CA1 mGluR-LTD has been used as a bedrock assay to establish the efficacy of lovastatin (Osterweil et al., 2013), as this form of plasticity is normalized by lovastatin in the FXS mouse. On further investigation, lovastatin application also reduced sensory-induced seizure (Osterweil et al., 2013) and improved specific hippocampus-dependent cognitive deficits (Asiminas et al., 2019) in FXS animal models, and clinical trials using this drug to treat FXS are currently ongoing (Thurman et al., 2020). Lovastatin is already widely used without major side effects in children and adults to manage high cholesterol and, as we will see later, the drug has been used with some success in another neurodevelopmental disorder, neurofibromatosis type 1 (NF1, Bearden et al., 2016), suggesting a potential clustering of neurodevelopmental disorders around aberrant RAS signaling. The use of lovastatin reflects the growing approach of drug repurposing that bypasses the lengthy and often unsuccessful attempt to bring new compounds to market.

Given the long-established importance of NMDARs in cognition, it is surprising that the possibility of direct impairment of NMDAR-dependent synaptic plasticity is only now coming to the fore in FXS research. A reduction in NMDAR-LTP at SCC-CA1 synapses was found using a weak TBS in an FXS animal model, a deficit that could be reversed by treatment with BDNF (Lauterborn et al., 2007). No deficit was observed with a stronger TBS, and in another study published around the same time, LTP was enhanced when induced by a pairing protocol (Pilpel et al., 2009). Interestingly, the impaired LTP, observed with a weak TBS protocol, can be restored by either the selective pharmacological inhibition or genetic elimination of the GluN2A subunit (Lundbye et al., 2018). In the DG, deficits in both NMDAR-LTP and NMDAR-LTD have been described in FXS mice (Yun and Trommer, 2011; Eadie et al., 2012). Interestingly, in adult FXS mice, the LTP deficit is extremely prominent in the dentate and LTP can be restored using a NMDAR glycine site agonist, suggesting that potentiating NMDAR function could be a useful therapeutic strategy in FXS (Bostrom et al., 2015). For example, a deficit in NMDAR-LTP and NMDAR-LTD in the DG that can be reversed by treatment with glycine site agonists, is observed in adult female FXS mice (Yau et al., 2016). The ability of minocycline, which is used to treat some FXS symptoms, to potentiate NMDAR function in the DG is also consistent with an NMDAR-mediated rescue strategy (Yau et al., 2016).

We have dwelled at some length on FXS because the work discussed provides instructive and cautionary insight into the development of viable treatments. The mGluR hypothesis has often been misinterpreted to indicate that mGluR-LTD is the core dysfunction in FXS (Mullins et al., 2016). In reality, SCC-CA1 mGluR-LTD is used as a window onto a much broader cellular process—activity-dependent protein translation—that is likely dysregulated throughout the brain in FXS. Whether meaningful therapy arises from this work or not, it provides a strong example of how basic mechanistic understanding of fundamental biological phenomena, in this case a form of synaptic plasticity in the hippocampus, can provide both deep and broad insight into disorders of the brain.

10.9.2.2 Neurofibromatosis 1—a window onto RASopathies

Neurofibromin is a protein that serves to restrain the GTPase RAS and thereby influence RAS/MAPK signaling. Thus, reduced neurofibromin function, which can result from one of several mutations in the encoding gene, results in a classic RASopathy, known as neurofibromatosis 1 (NF1). This disorder has an incidence of ~1:3500 (Cutting and Levine, 2010), making it a relatively common single-gene cause of neurodevelopmental disorder. Around 90% of individuals with NF1 show cognitive deficits (such as impaired working memory, executive function, and attention), although these are not often severe enough to be classed as ID (incidence of ~8%). More specific cognitive manifestations include ASD (~40%) and ADHD (~40%), in addition to other consistent symptoms such as epilepsy and noncancerous tumors along nerves (R Costa and Silva, 2002). A strikingly consistent cognitive phenotype is disrupted spatial cognition, implicating hippocampal dysfunction (Diggs-Andrews and Gutmann, 2013), and it is the study of hippocampus-dependent learning and related synaptic plasticity that has once again provided insights into the molecular origins of the symptoms, and potential treatments (Schwetye and Gutmann, 2014).

A mouse model which is heterozygous for NF1 has provided useful insight into hippocampal dysfunction. These mice exhibit deficient hippocampus-dependent learning and impaired induction of SCC-CA1 LTP1 using a TBS protocol (Silva et al., 1997). Both the LTP and learning deficits could be rescued using a genetic strategy in which NF1 heterozygous mice were crossed either with *K-Ras* or *N-Ras* heterozygous mice, to diminish the respective expression of two of three *Ras* genes (R Costa et al., 2002). To complicate matters, excitatory synaptic transmission was reduced overall in NF1 heterozygous mice, while inhibition was enhanced, and both were normalized by the genetic cross with the Ras heterozygous mice. Further investigation, using several cell-type conditional NF1 KOs, revealed that the primary RASopathy arises in inhibitory neurons and not forebrain excitatory neurons (Cui et al., 2008), indicating that the LTP deficit likely arises from increased feedforward inhibition that reduces postsynaptic activation during the inducing stimulus. This interpretation is confirmed by the fact that application of picrotoxin to block GABA$_A$ receptors restored SCC-CA1 LTP to control levels (R Costa et al., 2002). Thus, in this case LTP deficits do not arise directly from deficits in excitatory transmission, but rather reflect other permissive factors (Ehninger et al., 2008).

Pharmaceutical routes to normalizing signaling in NF1 model mice have been tested using the MEK inhibitor U0126, which reduces phospho-ERK, phospho-CREB, and LTP to normal levels (Guilding et al., 2007). The possibility of functional recovery through drug treatment in adult mice is encouraging, and lovastatin, which blocks farnesylation of Ras and reduces its activity, is again a most promising avenue for treatment as it is already widely used for other conditions. This drug restores normal SCC-CA1 LTP and spatial learning in NF1 model mice (W Li et al., 2005) and the closely related drug simvastatin shows efficacy in treating the cognitive symptoms of NF1 in children (Krab et al., 2008). A further group of syndromes that feature dysregulated RAS signaling are described as RASopathies. Along with NF1, they include Noonan syndrome, LEOPARD syndrome, cardiofaciocutaneous syndrome, capillary malformation-arteriovenous malformation syndrome, Legius syndrome, and Costello syndrome (Rauen, 2013; see Figure 10.16). All arise from mutations in genes encoding proteins that regulate RAS/MAPK signaling, but, other than a few cases of Noonan and cardiofaciocutaneous syndrome, only Costello syndrome results directly from a mutation in a RAS gene, in this case *H-RAS*, which causes H-RAS to be constitutively active (Aoki et al., 2005). All these disorders feature cognitive deficits, which are sometimes recapitulated in mouse models along with SCC-CA1 LTP deficits (Denayer et al., 2008), and the insight provided by the work on hippocampal synaptic plasticity in NF1 mice holds promise for each condition that shares dysregulation of RAS-MAPK signaling, pointing once again to a significant clustering of dysfunctions in signaling that may also be present in many idiopathic forms of epilepsy, ID, ASD,

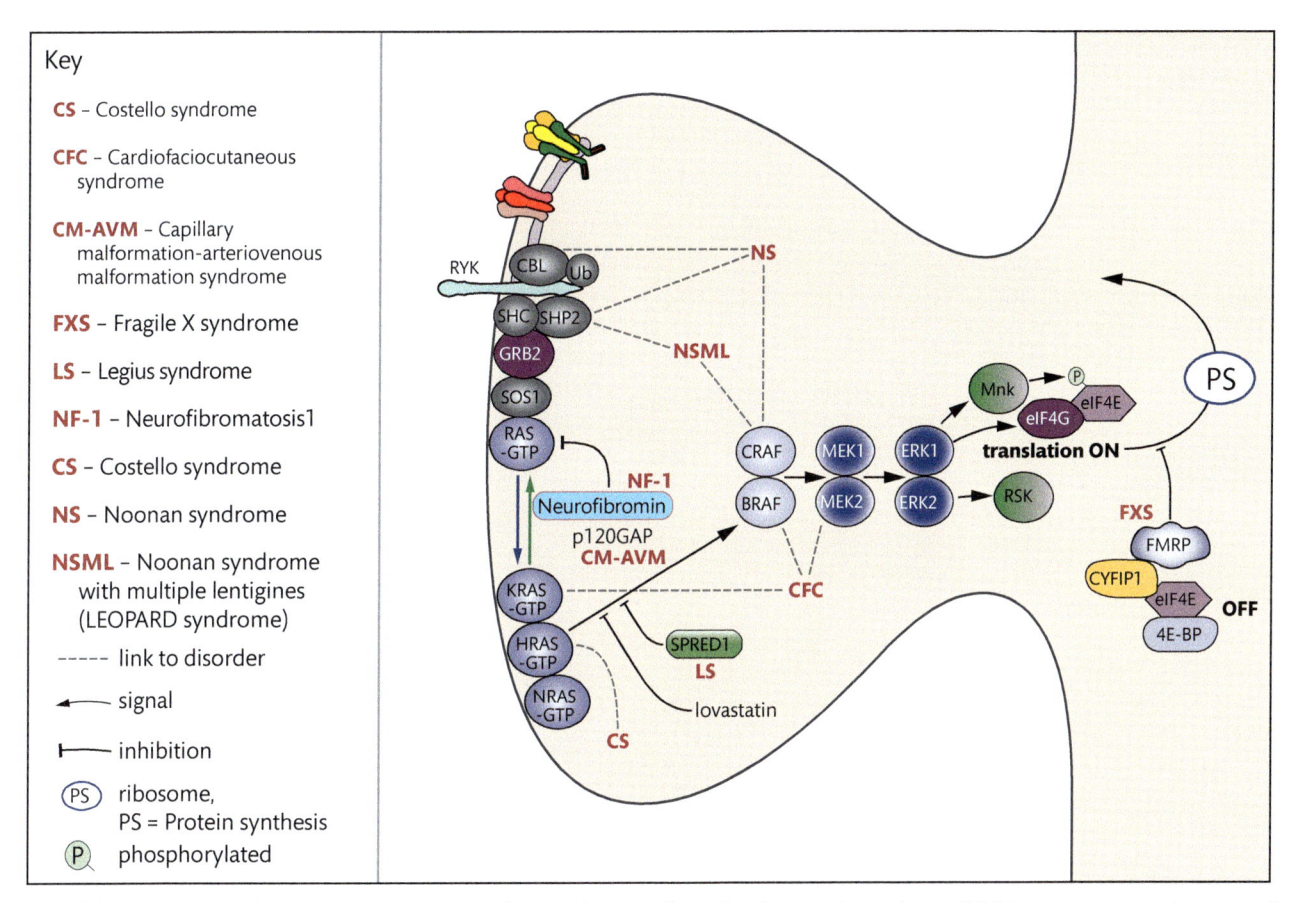

Figure 10.16 Rasopathies—when is a rasopathy a rasopathy? A schematic illustrating the protein products of highly penetrant genetic causes of canonical rasopathies embedded within the rat sarcoma virus GTPase (Ras)-extracellular signal-regulated kinase (ERK) signaling pathway at a synapse. Although not all rasopathies are addressed in this chapter, the figure illustrates the variety of impacts these risk factors have on the Ras-ERK pathway and is designed to convey the concept of clusters of risk factors for neurodevelopmental disorders that converge on a common endpoint. The rasopathy syndromes are listed in red with a key included in the figure, along with another neurodevelopmental disorder, FXS, that converges on the same endpoint. The dashed lines indicate the protein products that are modified in each syndrome while arrows indicate direct activation by one protein on another. Flat ended lines indicate inhibition. PS: protein synthesis.

or ADHD. The seeming success of treating many of the symptoms of FXS with lovastatin to normalize ERK signaling (Osterweil et al., 2013) indicates that FXS may fall under an extended RASopathy umbrella, although the broader the definition of a RASopathy, the less useful that concept may become. This also opens a key question as to whether treatments that are described as rescuing a signaling deficit instead reflect a compensation through an entirely separate signaling pathway with a common endpoint, such as protein translation or E/I imbalance.

10.9.2.3 Rett syndrome—disorder of development or maintenance?

Several genetically defined, syndromic forms of ID arise from dysregulated transcription. Best characterized among these and relatively high in prevalence is Rett syndrome (RTT), which is a monogenic disorder that manifests as ID, ASD, epilepsy, and motor dysfunction, typically observed in girls (with an incidence of ~1:10,000, see Hagberg et al., 1983). It emerges within the first year or so of life after an early relatively normal developmental trajectory, swiftly leading to catastrophic decline. Most cases arise from a loss of function in Methyl CpG binding protein 2 (MeCP2, see Amir et al., 1999), which detects methylation of genes and acts as a repressor of expression (Nan et al., 1998). Mutations in another protein, the cyclin-dependent kinase-like 5 (CDKL5), also cause RTT symptoms, and it is thought that these symptoms result from a failure of MeCP2 phosphorylation by CDKL5 (Grosso et al., 2007).

In mouse models of RTT that either do not express *Mecp2* within the brain or carry mutations that truncate MeCP2 to mimic RTT, not only are there significant RTT-like motor phenotypes, but deficits in hippocampus-dependent learning are apparent (Moretti et al., 2006), consistent with observations in RTT. Notably, only once these behaviorally manifest cognitive deficits arise, there are clear hippocampal synaptic plasticity phenotypes (Moretti et al., 2006; Asgarihafsheiani et al., 2024). Paired pulse facilitation (PPF) is drastically impaired at short intervals, there is less LTP1, and the longevity of LTP2 is reduced, with responses returning to baseline after an hour. Interestingly, hippocampal learning deficits are also apparent in mice in which there is overexpression of MeCP2, although these may result from a perseverative memory rather than a learning deficit (Na et al., 2012). Overexpression of MeCP2 can also cause severe learning deficits, in a syndrome simply described as *MECP2* duplication syndrome (Van Esch, 2012). This synaptic plasticity phenotype appears to be the reverse of that observed in *MeCP2*-null mice, as PPF is enhanced and LTP1 is also increased in magnitude (Collins et al., 2004). Interestingly, however, if the *MeCP2* duplication is modeled in postmitotic neurons only, hippocampal LTP1 shows a deficiency that is comparable to null mice (Na et al., 2012), perhaps implying that MeCP2 plays different roles in hippocampal synaptic function in the developing and adult animal.

One major way in which MeCP2 dysfunction could influence bidirectional hippocampal synaptic plasticity is through its role in the expression of the key growth factor BDNF. Neuronal activity leads to phosphorylation of MeCP2, which derepresses BDNF and enables CREB-mediated expression of BDNF. While MeCP2 is generally regarded as occupying this transcriptional repressor role, many genes are downregulated when *Mecp2* expression is reduced, as in the RTT model mice, showing that MeCP2 has a more complex role in the regulation of transcription (Li and Pozzo-Miller, 2014). One such paradoxically reduced gene product is BDNF, which shows normal expression levels presymptomatically, but is then greatly reduced as behavioral symptoms emerge in RTT model mice (Chang et al., 2006). While the reason for this reduction in expression is not fully understood, it is a strong candidate for the mechanism that has gone awry in hippocampal synaptic plasticity, given that conditional deletion of BDNF in postnatal forebrain neurons of mice results in phenotypes reminiscent of *Mecp2*-null RTT model mice (Chang et al., 2006). RTT patients also exhibit reduced BDNF expression (YE Sun and Wu, 2006), and BDNF application can be used to rescue some synaptic (Kline et al., 2010) and hippocampal phenotypes in RTT model mice (Larimore et al., 2009). It has long been known that *Bdnf* KO (knockout) mice have severely deficient hippocampal LTP, which can be rescued in adult mice through BDNF application (Patterson et al., 1996). Both LTP1 and LTP2 are potently modulated by the availability of BDNF (see section 10.5.4). The induction of LTP1 is enhanced by BDNF upregulating release mechanisms presynaptically (Jovanovic et al., 2000). Expression of LTP1 may also be enhanced by BDNF interactions with cytoskeletal machinery necessary for AMPAR trafficking (Rex et al., 2007). The importance of BDNF in the long-lasting nature of LTP2 is emphasized by the fact that prevention of sustained LTP2 by application of general protein synthesis inhibitors during induction can be prevented if exogenous BDNF is also applied, casting BDNF as one of the keys to the expression of LTP2 (Pang and Lu, 2004). While there is much to be understood mechanistically, BDNF expression deficits remain the likeliest cause of hippocampal synaptic plasticity deficits in RTT.

Strikingly, it has been possible to rescue almost all the deleterious symptoms in a *Mecp2*-null mouse model of RTT, including the hippocampal synaptic plasticity deficits, simply by re-expressing MECP2 in neurons even in early adulthood (Guy et al., 2007). Conversely, suppression of MeCP2 in normal adult mice leads to the swift development of RTT-like symptoms (McGraw et al., 2011; Nguyen et al., 2012). The capacity for cell type-specific knockdown or rescue by re-expression has also made it possible to assess the contribution of different neuronal subtypes to the RTT phenotype. Importantly, it has been found that loss of *Mecp2* expression selectively in inhibitory neurons recapitulates most RTT-like symptoms observed in the pan neuronal *Mecp2*-null mice, including deficits in hippocampus-dependent learning and hippocampal LTP (Chao et al., 2010). This finding is complemented beautifully by a substantial rescue of the pan-neuronal *Mecp2* knockdown mutant mouse with an inhibitory neuron-specific rescue of *Mecp2* expression (Ure et al., 2016), indicating that GABAergic neuronal dysfunction may be the originating site of RTT symptoms. As with the NF1 work described above, these findings indicate that aberrant inhibition may contribute to deficient plasticity in glutamatergic hippocampal neurons through its permissive role in activity-dependent Hebbian plasticity.

That many aspects of a disorder as severe as RTT should be rescuable in adulthood implies not only that it is not an irreversible disruption of development that causes RTT but also that there has been no neurodegeneration. A bigger question arises, therefore, as to whether a larger group of so-called neurodevelopmental disorders may, in fact, result from failures of neural maintenance. This possibility is likely to be a focus of work in the coming years for, not only does it provide hope of treating RTT after early development, when challenging treatment may be better tolerated, but it also provides promise for idiopathic disorders that are unlikely to be diagnosed until major symptoms start to emerge, making prophylactic treatment unfeasible. As we have already seen, evidence from FXS suggests that RTT may not be the only disorder that fits this profile.

There are a large number of syndromic forms of ID/ASD caused by highly penetrant mutations in a single or few known genes that are now being modeled in mice, including tuberous sclerosis complex (TSC), Angelman's syndrome, SynGAP1 (Synaptic Ras GTPase-activating protein 1) syndrome, and Neurexin1-deletion syndrome, among others. We do not have space to discuss these individually, but the hope is that in the coming decade or so, commonalities in the underlying dysfunction in these disorders with some of those that we have already discussed may not only inspire new treatments but also have implications for related idiopathic conditions, which affect a much larger number of individuals. Before completing this section, we will consider the most common genetically determined form of ID, which is Down syndrome.

10.9.2.4 Down syndrome–crossover between neurodevelopment and neurodegeneration

Down syndrome (DS) has the highest incidence among genetic forms of ID, occurring in ~1:850 births (Dierssen, 2012). DS is a well-known syndrome characterized by cardiac defects, craniofacial differences, and cognitive impairments often crossing the threshold for ID. It arises from a triplicate expression of chromosome 21, leading to overexpression of more than 200 genes (Lejeune et al., 1959). As well as a wide range of nonneural symptoms, cognitive symptoms likely arise from several different genetic sources, and cognitive tests indicate that hippocampal function is disproportionately affected (Pennington et al., 2003). One striking observation has been that AD arises in DS with an early onset in almost all cases, an observation that proved instrumental in the emergence of the amyloid hypothesis of AD, as the gene encoding *APP* is present on chromosome 21 and is therefore overexpressed in DS (Selkoe and Hardy, 2016). However, this is not the sole source of deficits in synaptic plasticity and cognition, as other overexpressed genes have a profound influence on these processes, particularly in the hippocampus (Dierssen, 2012). Several mouse models have been generated to study these deficits, including *Tc(has21)1TybEmcf* (transchromosomal, human 21, line 1, Victor Tybulewicz and Elizabeth M C Fisher), known as Tc1, in which the majority of human chromosome 21 is overexpressed (O'Doherty et al., 2005) and alternative strategies that overexpress the regions of mouse genome syntenic to human chromosome 21 (Davisson et al., 1993), of which the most used is *Ts(17^{16})65Dn* (trisomy, Chr 16 translocation to Chr 17; Davisson), known as Ts65Dn. The latter model has become favored as it does not produce the genetic mosaic expression, in which only a subset of neurons is triplicate for genes on chromosome 21, as in the Tc1 model. Although genetic mosaicism is present in a small subset of cases of DS, it produces an atypical, milder cognitive phenotype (Richards, 1969). It is important to note that the Ts65Dn model does not overexpress all mouse homologues of genes on human chromosome 21, and there are several mouse genes that are overexpressed which are not on human chromosome 21. Nevertheless, the findings from these different mouse models are largely complementary and they enable investigation of the molecular underpinnings of hippocampal learning deficits.

Both models show reduced DG LTP1 (Kleschevnikov et al., 2004; O'Doherty et al., 2005) in addition to deficits in a wide range of hippocampus-dependent memory tests. Interestingly, the Tc1 mouse, in which LTP was studied in vivo, does not show the same deficiency in lasting LTP, presumably LTP2 and 3. Although LTP in awake, freely moving mice is impaired within the first hour, when recorded 24 h later it is comparable to controls, suggesting an effect on LTP1 but not LTP2/3 (Morice et al., 2008). This finding is particularly striking given that hippocampus-dependent short-term memory deficits are present while LTM appears intact, consistent with the view that these are separable, parallel processes and not, as was previously the dominant view, one serial process (McGaugh, 2000). In the Ts65Dn model, SCC-CA1 LTP1 is also deficient when evoked with TBS (A Costa and Grybko, 2005), but, most intriguingly, NMDAR-LTD is exaggerated in magnitude (Siarey et al., 1999), indicating that some shift in the normal modification threshold for LTP/LTD may have occurred. Altered NMDAR properties can produce just such a shift in the modification threshold (Philpot et al., 2003). Consistent with this interpretation is the observation that acute application of the noncompetitive NMDAR antagonist memantine in Ts65Dn mice recovers TBS-induced SCC-CA1 LTP to control levels (Scott-McKean et al., 2018) while also reducing enhanced LTD and recovering hippocampus-dependent memory (Rueda et al., 2010; Lockrow et al., 2011; Scott-McKean and Costa, 2011). Memantine has for some time been one of the only approved compounds/drugs for treating symptoms in severe AD (Melnikova, 2007), suggesting that the overexpression of APP in the mouse model of DS may account for the hippocampal synaptic plasticity phenotype. Indeed, knockdown of overexpressed Aβ rescues deficits in hippocampus-dependent cognition even in young Ts65Dn mice (Netzer et al., 2010). However, much work indicates that several other overexpressed genes make major contributions to the cognitive deficits of DS.

Among several other strong candidate overexpressed genes, *DYRK1A* has been a focus of work on altered inhibition contributing to modified hippocampal plasticity. This gene encodes the kinase dual-specificity tyrosine phosphorylation-regulated kinase 1A (DYRK1A), which is implicated in cell proliferation and the development of the nervous system (Hammerle et al., 2011). Mutations in *DYRK1A* that lead to loss of function are the cause of a rare form of neurodevelopmental disorder that causes ID and ASD known simply as DYRK1A-syndrome (Blackburn et al., 2019). However, the gene's overexpression in DS contributes to altered synaptic plasticity within the hippocampus as overexpression of *Dyrk1a* mimics the diminished LTP and hippocampus-dependent cognitive deficits (Garcia-Cerro et al., 2014) and specific knockdown of *Dyrk1a* within the Ts65Dn mouse model recovers the hippocampal LTP deficit (Altafaj et al., 2013). Critically, a greater number of inhibitory neurons in the hippocampus and reduced susceptibility to drug-induced seizure arise from overexpression of *Dyrk1a* (Souchet et al., 2014). Direct assessment of inhibitory currents in the Ts65Dn DS model reveals increased inhibition in the dendrites of hippocampal pyramidal cells (Kleschevnikov et al., 2004; Schulz et al., 2019). Synaptic plasticity can be rescued in these mice by applying the GABA$_A$ receptor blocker picrotoxin (Kleschevnikov et al., 2004). Drugs that can be applied systemically to reduce inhibition, particularly safer negative allosteric modulators, do produce improvements in hippocampus-dependent learning and memory in DS model mice (Braudeau et al., 2011; Martinez-Cue et al., 2013). The most striking therapeutic development for DS has been the impact of the green tea extract epigallocatechin-3-gallate (EGCG), which is a noncompetitive inhibitor of DYRK1A. Prenatal treatment with EGCG reduces hippocampal inhibition and recovers hippocampus-dependent learning (Souchet et al., 2014), as well as normalizing hippocampal plasticity (Xie et al., 2008). Amazingly, it also reduces craniofacial dysmorphology in both the Ts65Dn mouse model and in children administered with EGCG from prior to birth (Starbuck et al., 2021). Consistent with EGCG exerting its effect specifically by mitigating the impact of *Dyrk1a* overexpression, similar cognitive-enhancing effects of EGCG are found in Dyrk1a overexpressing mice (Thomazeau et al., 2014). Given that green tea is freely available and does not need to pass through clinical trials, this is a very exciting outcome, and its use has been adopted by many DS individuals.

Overall, modeling DS provides an example of how the difficulties in pinpointing the biological mechanism at play are more challenging the larger the genetic alteration that produces the human condition. Nevertheless, very substantial progress has been made and, moreover, as discussed above and in the following section, the study of plasticity deficits in DS has provided the origins for the amyloid hypothesis, which is the leading candidate explanation for the etiology of AD (Selkoe and Hardy, 2016).

10.9.2.5 Autism spectrum disorder (ASD)

Although the focus of this section has been on neurodevelopmental disorders, including those with an identified genetic cause, such as FXS, there is good reason to believe that alterations in synaptic plasticity are central to ASD more generally. However, establishing the underlying causes has been very challenging. The Simons Foundation lists well over 1,000 genes that have been linked to ASD in humans (https://gene.sfari.org/) and also includes data from mouse models. Among the high confidence gene products are numerous synaptic proteins, many of which are involved in synaptic plasticity. These include glutamate receptor subunits (GluA1, GluA2, GluN1, GluN2A, GluN2B), neuroligins, neurexins, and scaffolding proteins (SHANK2 and SHANK3). Each genetic mutation has a small effect, and the overall effect will depend on the influence of many genes (both positive and negative), epigenetics, and environmental factors. Experimentally, identifying the influence of a defined genetic mutation is also complex. For example, two different mutations in two different exons of the Shank2 scaffolding protein can result either in enhanced NMDAR-LTP (Schmeisser et al., 2012) or inhibition of NMDAR-LTP (Won et al., 2012). Teasing out the relevance to ASD is further complicated by the fact that animal ASD models often have comorbidities, such as ID.

Mouse models of ASD have been used to examine the effects of lifestyle changes, such as ketogenic diet and supplements. For example, increasing dietary zinc can reduce ASD-like behaviors in *Shank2* and *Shank3* KO mice, although there are some differences depending on the SHANK isoform studied (K Lee et al., 2024).

10.9.3 Dementia

Age is the greatest risk factor for dementia (Hebert et al., 2010) and the incidence is consequently on the rise with ever improving healthcare. As full-time care is required at advanced stages of dementia, massive welfare costs are now being accrued (Wittenberg et al., 2019), which should make research on dementia a high priority. The most common disease that manifests as dementia is AD (~65% of cases), followed in prevalence by vascular dementia (VD,

~20%), Lewy body dementias (LBD, ~10%) and frontotemporal dementia (FTD, ~5%). Finding effective treatments to slow or reverse these dementias is a major strategic priority and many of the relevant issues are discussed in Chapter 20.

Notwithstanding a diversity of approaches, studying hippocampal synaptic plasticity is likely to provide key insight because, in all these prevalent forms of dementia, the hippocampus and related temporal lobe structures are among the most severely and, in some cases, the earliest affected regions in the brain (Armstrong and Cairns, 2015). Moreover, while focus on characteristic anatomical hallmarks of dementia pathology, such as amyloid plaques, neurofibrillary tangles, and Lewy bodies (Lovestone and McLoughlin, 2002) had long supported the idea that cell death accounts for the cognitive symptoms of dementia, there is now a growing consensus that deficits in synaptic function, and plasticity in particular, occur earlier and lead to synapse loss in living cells long before cell death (Selkoe and Hardy, 2016). If this is correct, one might expect a significant prodromal period during which mild cognitive symptoms emerge, in which cells remain alive, offering hope for an opportunity to completely reverse pathology (Selkoe and Hardy, 2016). Indeed, although recent clinical trials for rationally designed treatments of dementias have failed to meet their predesignated outcomes, post hoc analysis has revealed that patients with very mild cognitive deficits, indicating early stages of disorder, did show beneficial effects of treatment, while those with moderate or severe cognitive deficits did not (McDade, 2019). Studying the causes of early hippocampal synaptic plasticity deficits in dementia and finding ways to prevent these deficits is therefore of paramount importance. In this chapter we will focus our discussion of dementia on AD, as this is not only the commonest form of dementia but also the one that is most clearly associated with hippocampal dysfunction.

10.9.3.1 Alzheimer's disease (AD)

As discussed in detail in Chapter 20, three major hypotheses concerning AD etiology have focused on: (1) accumulation of peptide fragments cleaved from the transmembrane protein APP, which leads to the characteristic amyloid plaques (Selkoe and Hardy, 2016); (2) pathological intracellular buildup of hyperphosphorylated TAU, a microtubule-associated peptide, which leads to the formation of another pathological hallmark of the disease, the neurofibrillary tangles (NFT; see Goedert, 2018); (3) dysfunction of cholinergic inputs to the hippocampus, which consistently exhibit pathology in AD (P Davies and Maloney, 1976). Original versions of these hypotheses focused on degenerative processes of cell death, but contemporary versions posit an earlier deleterious effect on hippocampal synaptic plasticity. An additional hypothesis, which has received considerable attention recently, is that AD involves an alteration in insulin signaling in the brain (and as such is sometimes referred to as Type III diabetes). Space precludes a detailed consideration of this potential factor, but the role of insulin in synaptic plasticity is discussed in section 10.5.7. It is important to note that synaptic dysfunction is again central to this idea. Though one hypothesis may capture the true origin of the disorder better than the others, they may collectively reflect separate stages of a cascade of events that all contribute to dysfunctional hippocampal plasticity. It should also be noted that AD is a highly heterogenous disorder and so the relative contributions of these various factors may vary considerably from patient to patient.

The dominant theory for AD origins has been the amyloid hypothesis (Selkoe and Hardy, 2016), which holds that the disease is caused by increased production or reduced clearance of soluble forms of Aβ, including Aβ42, which is the main component of the amyloid plaques. Mutations that promote the occurrence of this accumulation may occur in *APP* itself, but also in other key contributors to this process, such as presenilin 1 and 2 (*PSEN1* and *2*), which encode gamma secretases that cleave APP into peptide fragments, or apolipoprotein E (APOE), which is a lipid-binding protein that can clear excessive Aβ42. It had initially been imagined that the accumulation of Aβ42 in extracellular plaques provided the major pathological entity, but multiple lines of evidence now indicate that Aβ42 can have deleterious effects on synaptic function prior to or without ever forming plaques (Tomiyama et al., 2008). In addition to DS, other highly penetrant genetic causes of AD run in families. Autosomal dominant forms of AD predominantly arise from increased Aβ42 production due to mutations either in *APP* or the genes that encode *PSEN1* and *2* (Campion et al., 1999; Kurt et al., 2001; Saura et al., 2004). Sporadic forms of AD often have a major genetic contribution, the best known of which is carrying the E4 allele of *APOE*, which makes APOE considerably less effective at clearing Aβ42 (Safieh et al., 2019). Mutations of the gene that encodes TAU (*MAPT*) are not in themselves risk factors for AD. Consistent with the idea that TAU pathology is a major factor in synaptic/cellular dysfunction, this pathology may arise from other causes, likely including amyloidosis (Strang et al., 2019). Thus, while hyperphosphorylation of TAU is a good correlate of cognitive dysfunction, mutations in TAU do not cause AD. Still, the wide range of mouse models that have been used to understand the hippocampal synaptopathy underlying cognitive deficits in AD have recapitulated one or a combination of mutations that cause familial or sporadic AD, sometimes in addition to mutations in TAU that mimic hyperphosphorylation (Klonarakis et al., 2022).

Disrupted LTP/LTD balance in AD

It has proved challenging to arrive at a clear understanding of how AD affects plasticity at hippocampal synapses, given the variety of rodent models and the ages at which they have been assessed. Even when equivalent models are compared under similar conditions marked differences are reported. For example, at SCC-CA1 synapses studies are divided as to whether basal synaptic transmission is unaffected or reduced. There are rarely reports of any striking effects on short-term plasticity as assessed with PP interactions (for review, see Marchetti and Marie, 2011; Mango et al., 2019). For long-term plasticity, when the amyloid hypothesis is being explicitly tested using transgenic mice expressing an AD-associated mutation in *APP*, such as the Swedish mutation (Hsiao et al., 1996), or in *PSEN1* (Q Guo et al., 1999), or a combination of these two mutations, then MPP-DG LTP1 is reduced in magnitude in most cases (Chapman et al., 1999). There is less consistency in findings relating to LTP at SCC-CA1 synapses, where LTP1 appears either normal (Fitzjohn et al., 2001; Volianskis et al., 2010) or deficient (Chapman et al., 1999; Jacobsen et al., 2006), suggesting that these synapses could be more resilient to the loss of plasticity imposed by Aβ42 dysregulation. When a triple transgenic model is used in which a mutation in *MAPT* (P301L) is also introduced, then the loss of LTP at both MPP-DG and SCC-CA1 synapses is apparent by around 6 months of age (Oddo et al., 2003). In this formative study on this mouse model, there is a very useful comparison between these triple

mutants and littermates expressing only the *PSEN1* knockin mutation or double transgenics also expressing the APP Swedish mutation. Interestingly, SCC-CA1 LTP appears near normal in these other two genotypes, indicating that the most profound impact on synaptic plasticity may arise from the *MAPT* mutation (Oddo et al., 2003). As we have already stated, however, mutations in *MAPT* are not themselves risk factors for AD but instead have been identified in FTD, casting some doubt on the validity of the model. Thus, tauopathy arising in AD, which is clearly a critical factor given that reversal can return synaptic function to normality (Shipton et al., 2011; Sydow et al., 2011), is likely a consequence of earlier pathology arising from a different source.

There is also a substantial body of work initiated by the Dublin group of Roger Anwyl and Michael Rowan (Cullen et al., 1997) that showed how soluble Aβ fragments, which are either secreted from cultured neurons, artificially synthesized, or harvested from tissue of AD patients, rapidly disrupt synaptic plasticity in the hippocampus (e.g., Walsh et al., 2002; Shankar et al., 2008; Jo et al., 2011). At first glance, one may question how a chronic disease that takes years to develop can be realistically modeled by an acute application of Aβ. There is a growing body of thought, however, that AD may, in at least some cases, result from acute synaptic exposure to Aβ and that the very slow progression of the disease is due to the extremely slow buildup of toxic levels. Indeed, it has been suggested that plaques may be a compensatory attempt by the brain to sequester toxic oligomeric species of Aβ and that only when these and other defense mechanisms break down does toxicity kick in. The use of acute Aβ application has led to several major advances in the AD field. It has been shown, for example, that application of soluble Aβ extracted from the brains of AD patients suppresses SCC-CA1 LTP1 in mouse hippocampal slices without altering basal synaptic transmission. Importantly, this suppressing effect on LTP is neutralized by application of an antiserum against Aβ and is not observed when extracts from brains of patients with either FTD or LBD are applied (Shankar et al., 2008). These observations strongly support the validity of the acute Aβ application models for understanding the etiology of the disease proper.

More generally, major insights into possible mechanisms of synaptic dysfunction, the likely initiating factor in AD, have been made using these acute models. Indeed, the Dublin group provided the first evidence for critical roles for mGluR5 as well as a complex array of signaling molecules including c-Jun N-terminal kinase, cyclin-dependent kinase 5 and p38 MAPK (Q Wang, Walsh, et al., 2004). They also identified a role for microglia, as well as NO and superoxide (Q Wang, Rowan, et al., 2004) long before the genetic associations of microglial specific genes and AD. Numerous studies by many groups have since added to the list of molecules involved in Aβ-induced effects on synaptic function, painting a picture of a complex cascade of serial and parallel components that maintain the integrity of synaptic plasticity.

In another study, it was shown that intracellularly applied Aβ was able to alter synaptic properties within a few minutes, corresponding roughly to the time it would take for the peptide to diffuse from the soma to the dendrites (Whitcomb et al., 2015). This observation suggests that Aβ exerts its toxicity almost immediately as it reaches its site of action and that this site is within the synaptic spine, leading to the question as to how Aβ, which is cleaved extracellularly, is able to enter neurons to initiate synaptopathy. An interesting candidate is mGluR5, which Aβ binds to in a manner that requires the cellular prion protein (PrPc) (Um et al., 2013) and could be carried into the cell when the receptor complex is endocytozed. Alternatively, or additionally, Aβ binding might trigger aberrant mGluR5 signaling which may lead to excessive mGluR-LTD. Interestingly, a complex involving mGluR5 and PrPc is required for the Aβ-induced inhibition of NMDAR-LTP and facilitation of NMDAR-LTD (N Hu et al., 2014), making mGluR5 an interesting therapeutic target for the treatment of AD (Abd-Elrahman et al., 2020).

The rate at which Aβ fragments are cleared is substantially determined by the protease neprilysin, and the activity of this enzyme is reduced with both age and, more extremely, in dementia (Yasojima et al., 2001). Loss of neprilysin expression in KO mice produces a mild impairment in perforant path-DG and SCC-CA1 LTP, a deficiency which is profoundly exacerbated and accompanied by a pronounced deficit in hippocampus-dependent learning if the neprilysin KO is crossed with APP overexpressing transgenic mice (S Huang et al., 2006), indicating that neprilysin dysregulation may contribute to synaptopathy. Hippocampal overexpression of neprilysin improves synaptic plasticity and cognitive function in APP mouse models (Iwata et al., 2004; Iwata et al., 2013) and therefore presents itself as an interesting therapeutic target in AD (M Park et al., 2013).

While LTP is impaired in APP-related rodent models of AD, most studies indicate that there is an enhancement of LTD at SCC-CA1 synapses in these AD model mice by 4 months of age (JH Kim et al., 2001; D'Amelio et al., 2011; Lante et al., 2015), much like observations at younger ages in DS model mice (Scott-McKean and Costa, 2011). Moreover, loss of synaptic spines is also observed, consistent with the idea that persistent LTD eventually leads to synaptic loss (Bastrikova et al., 2008). In hippocampal slices, acute treatment with exogenous soluble Aβ fragments produces an enhancement of both NMDAR- and mGluR-LTD (Mango et al., 2019) and 300 pulses of 1 Hz stimulation, not normally sufficient to induce lasting LTD, does so at SCC-CA1 synapses in slices of rat hippocampus treated with Aβ extracts of brain tissue from AD patients (Shankar et al., 2008). Interestingly, this enhanced LTD induction was found to depend on mGluRs but not NMDARs, while the accompanying loss of spines showed the opposite dependency, indicating that they may be parallel rather than sequential effects (Shankar et al., 2008). Thus, though the current view is confused, we can build a working hypothesis that, due to an increase in Aβ42, a wider range of activity patterns will lead to synaptic weakening, manifested in the laboratory as LTD, while LTP becomes harder to induce. Thus, spontaneous activity may lead to a net weakening and eventual loss of hippocampal synapses, and progressively reduced levels of evoked activity in neurons, potentially contributing to the cellular pathology that then develops (Nisticò et al., 2012).

GSK-3

At the heart of AD and likely many other brain disorders are the two paralogs GSK-3α and GSK-3β (collectively referred to here as GSK-3, Beurel et al., 2015). As described in more detail in section 10.2.2, GSK-3 directly regulates the balance between LTP and LTD. In many cell types it has been shown that GSK-3 acts as master regulator of cellular function by integrating a wide variety of external signals and controlling many effector mechanisms. Although the picture is far from complete, it seems extremely likely that GSK-3 plays a similar role in synaptic plasticity (see Figure 10.7). Here, we focus on the relevance of GSK-3 for AD, though it is likely that similar considerations apply in varying degrees to most, if not all, neurodegenerative disorders. GSK-3 is one of the key kinases responsible for the hyperphosphorylation of TAU. Therefore, the finding that activation of GSK-3 is required for NMDAR-LTD (Peineau et al., 2007) provides, in molecular terms, a direct connection between AD and LTD, giving support to the emerging hypothesis that AD involves dysregulated LTD. It is probably extremely significant that the process of LTP inhibits LTD by suppressing the activity of this kinase, via the activation of the PI3K and Akt pathway. Thus, when LTP is triggered, GSK-3 is inhibited, and this prevents LTD. Consequently, factors that promote LTP can limit LTD whereas factors that limit LTP can enhance LTD, excessively weakening synapses and eventually causing synaptic loss. Accordingly, AD may be triggered by an imbalance of synaptic plasticity through dysregulation of LTP and/or LTD mechanisms such that LTP is reduced and LTD is enhanced. GSK-3 phosphorylation of the tubulin-binding protein TAU is well established in AD, so the finding that GSK-3 also phosphorylates TAU during LTD (Kimura et al., 2014) adds considerable weight to the idea that AD is caused by LTD gone awry. In other words, phosphorylation of TAU by GSK-3 is a normal physiological process involved in synaptic weakening and elimination of synapses can result from exuberant LTD, triggering the early stages of AD.

Direct evidence that toxic Aβ products may promote synaptic loss was provided by the observation that the inhibition of LTP by the oligomeric species of Aβ(1-42) can be completely prevented by inhibition of GSK-3 (Jo et al., 2011). Furthermore, this pathway activates caspase-3, leading to cleavage of Akt and hence dysregulation of GSK-3. Not only does this provide direct experimental support for the dysregulation of synaptic plasticity hypothesis of AD but also it provides a possible link for another feature of the disease, which is apoptosis. In this scenario, LTD involves localized synaptic apoptosis for the reversible elimination of synapses, but excessive LTD due to overactivation of GSK-3 may result in a more widespread apoptosis, culminating in the death of affected neurons.

A bridge from insoluble Aβ fragments to increased activity of GSK-3 is provided by the Wnt/β-Catenin signaling pathway, via interactions with Frizzled receptors (Palomer et al., 2019); direct interventions to mimic each stage of this pathological cascade reduces hippocampal LTP and enhances LTD (Jo et al., 2011; also see Figure 10.17; Marzo et al., 2016; McLeod et al., 2018).

TAU

Although mutations in TAU are not themselves causes of AD, the normal association of TAU with axonal microtubules is altered through hyperphosphorylation so that it becomes distributed into dendrites and eventually forms neurofibrillary tangles (Kowall and Kosik, 1987). This process is triggered by overabundance of insoluble Aβ fragments. Indeed, the impairment of hippocampal LTP caused by exogenous Aβ fragments is prevented in the *Mapt* KO mouse (Shipton et al., 2011). Tauopathy is a hallmark of AD, and modeling this TAU aggregation in mice by transgenic overexpression of human aggregating TAU for several months leads to reduced hippocampal LTP and memory loss (Sydow et al., 2011). Surprisingly, the effect on synaptic plasticity can be reversed by preventing expression of the human transgene for several weeks, despite the persistence of already formed aggregates, indicating that TAU itself may have an acute effect at synapses, rather than the aggregates leading to irreversible synaptic pathology (Sydow et al.,

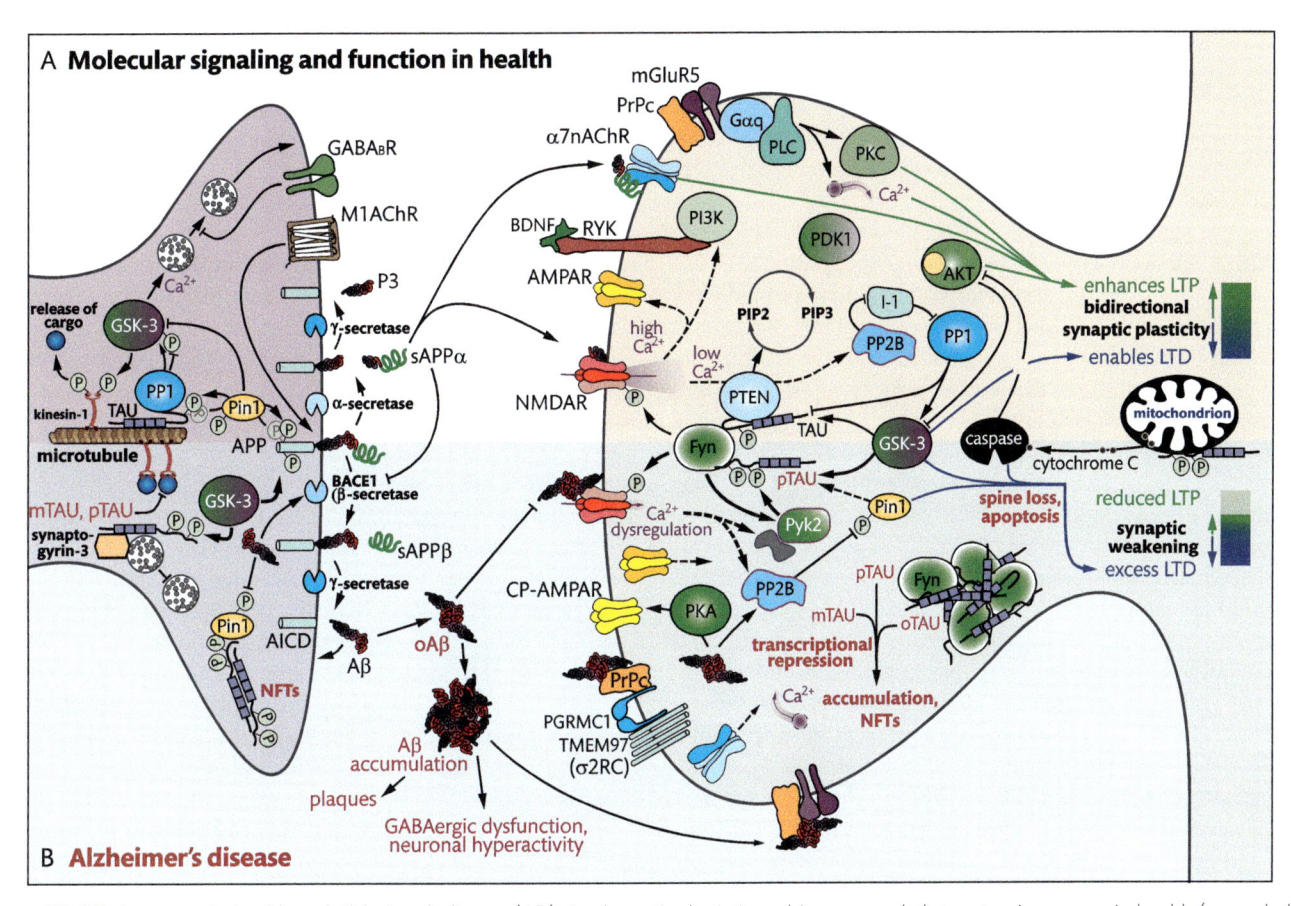

Figure 10.17 A synapse in health and Alzheimer's disease (AD). A schematic depicting a hippocampal glutamatergic synapse in health (upper half, white background) and AD, lower half, blue background). The schematic is designed to convey the concept of balanced Hebbian LTP and LTD in health (upper half), compared with the early stages of AD, in which the synapse is predisposed to excess LTD and reduced LTP. Progressive weakening of the synapse eventually leads to degeneration. In red are shown some of the key pathological effects that result from the synaptic balance being tipped toward an early AD state. The cascade of synaptic pathology may start with altered amyloid precursor protein (APP) cleavage, resulting in accumulation of Aβ fragments, eventually leading to extracellular plaque formation. Altered phosphorylation of TAU, which is a common endpoint for degenerative conditions called tauopathies, leads to a variety of pathological outcomes, several of which are depicted here, including the formation of intracellular neurofibrillary tangles.

2011). Although TAU is considered an axonal protein under normal circumstances, there is now good evidence that it is expressed at low levels in the postsynaptic compartment of healthy animals (Kimura et al., 2014). Also, as discussed above, TAU itself is required for hippocampal LTD, as LTD is absent in *Mapt* KO mice and in wild-type mice in which TAU is knocked down with short hairpin RNA (shRNA, see Kimura et al., 2014; Regan et al., 2015). Thus, the increased presence of TAU at the synapse in the progression of AD likely promotes LTD. As stated above, it is believed that this process occurs through GSK-3, which is a principal contributor to TAU hyperphosphorylation (Hooper et al., 2008) and to LTD (Peineau et al., 2007). Interestingly, as with tauopathy (Sydow et al., 2011), many of these aberrant signaling effects can be reversed to recover normal synaptic function and cognition (Marzo et al., 2016), presenting yet further therapeutic targets should we be able to identify AD at an early enough stage in its progression.

There is an increasing interest in the synergistic toxic actions of TAU and Aβ. For example, it has been shown that either recombinant human TAU or patient-derived TAU rapidly and persistently inhibits LTP, and that the threshold for TAU's action is lowered in APP transgenic rats (Ondrejcak et al., 2024). The effects of TAU on LTP could be rapidly reversed by anti-TAU monoclonal antibodies,

which may be highly relevant to the potential therapeutic strategies that target TAU.

Other LTD signaling molecules

It is important to note that other core hippocampal LTD signaling mechanisms are also known to be affected in AD. The phosphatase PP2B has long been implicated in the induction of LTD by dephosphorylating AMPARs to reduce their conductivity (Baumgartel and Mansuy, 2012). Like GSK-3, PP2B is overactive in the brains of AD patients (Lian et al., 2001; F Liu et al., 2005; Wu et al., 2010) and AD mouse models (Reese et al., 2008), and inhibition of this phosphatase normalizes LTD (Cavallucci et al., 2013) and accompanying spine loss (Rozkalne et al., 2011) in AD mouse models. A potential explanation for this observation is that PP2B is part of the pathway that activates GSK-3. Collectively, the data points to a causal, rather than simply a correlative, relationship between exaggerated LTD and spine loss and eventual neurodegeneration and that GSK-3 is at the heart of the matter.

Acetylcholine (ACh)

The third major hypothesis about the etiology of AD, which has in recent years fallen somewhat out of favor, is that a reduction in cholinergic tone in the hippocampus reduces the magnitude and longevity of synaptic plasticity (Bartus et al., 1982; Coyle et al., 1983). ACh has been established as a critical neuromodulator subserving processes that are important for the formation of long-lasting hippocampus-dependent memory (Decker et al., 2020). Current theories of learning and memory posit a key role for high hippocampal cholinergic tone in learning and low cholinergic tone during memory retrieval (Hasselmo, 2006), positioning this neurotransmitter in a critical role for both learning and memory. The theory is based on two intertwined concepts: First, that cholinergic action through nicotinic receptors increases the feedforward glutamatergic transmission that carries sensory information into the hippocampus (Gray et al., 1996; Giocomo and Hasselmo, 2005), thereby enhancing the likelihood of hippocampal LTP (Fujii et al., 2000; Ji et al., 2001; Welsby et al., 2006), particularly by converting STP into LTP (S Ge and Dani, 2005), and, in turn, promoting hippocampus-dependent learning (Bernal et al., 1999; J Davis et al., 2007). Second, ACh suppresses feedback excitation within CA3 that is required for memory retrieval (Hasselmo et al., 1995) through muscarinic receptor action on presynaptic terminals (Kremin et al., 2006). Within this compelling framework, phases of high cholinergic tone are required to improve encoding by amplifying sensory inputs and suppressing competing feedback from memory stores, while low cholinergic tone facilitates memory retrieval by enhancing feedback excitation required for pattern completion and suppressing new learning by quashing competing sensory inputs. These brain states may roughly equate to modes of active exploration, when ACh-induced theta oscillations are apparent in hippocampal local field potentials (O'Keefe, 1993), and quiet wakefulness, when sharp wave ripples emerge, and off-line memory consolidation processes occur (Buzsaki, 2015). Dysregulation of such a dynamic system would have crippling effects on learning and memory (Hasselmo, 2006).

More specifically, the cholinergic hypothesis arose from the observations that there is significant loss in AD of cholinergic basal forebrain neurons that project to the hippocampus (P Davies and Maloney, 1976; Whitehouse et al., 1982). This loss of cholinergic input is a consequence of tauopathy (Mesulam et al., 2004) and depleted cholinergic synthesis in the cerebral cortex/hippocampus in brains of AD patients which correlates with AD severity (Francis et al., 1985; Mesulam et al., 2004). Drugs that reduce the breakdown of ACh by inhibiting cholinesterase showed some promise in treating the memory deficits in AD (Summers et al., 1986). These drugs, such as the now widely used donepezil, were the first to be approved for treatment in AD and remain one of the few approved treatments for the condition. However, their efficacy is modest, possibly reflecting the fact that a drug that simply increases cholinergic tone is not likely to respect the distinction between high tone for laying down memories and low tone for consolidation. Of cholinergic receptors, nicotinic receptors, but not muscarinic receptors, are strikingly reduced by Aβ overexpression (Guan et al., 2001). Agonists of nicotinic AChRs, particularly those containing the alpha7 subunit, enhance LTP and can counteract deficits in LTP arising in the presence of Aβ (Ondrejcak et al., 2012).

Other considerations

Given the evidence for a shift toward reduced synaptic potentiation and increased synaptic weakening during the progression of AD, the reliable observation that hippocampal and neocortical activity is increased across the same period is counterintuitive. Hippocampal activity, as measured with fMRI, is increased in human subjects who carry mutations that produce familial AD (Mondadori et al., 2006; Filippini et al., 2009; Kunz et al., 2015). Temporal lobe epilepsy is often observed during the progression to mild cognitive impairment in patients before they develop full-blown AD (Vossel et al., 2013; Cretin et al., 2016), the occurrence of which predicts a faster decline of cognition (Vossel et al., 2016), and cognition can be improved using epilepsy treatments that reduce network activity, such as Levetiracetam (Bakker et al., 2012). Highly penetrant mutations that lead to familial AD also produce epileptiform activity (Lozsadi and Larner, 2006), and mouse models based on familial AD mutations exhibit hyperexcitable hippocampal networks and epileptiform activity (Palop et al., 2007; Busche et al., 2008; Minkeviciene et al., 2009; Sanchez et al., 2012), providing preclinical systems to investigate the origins of this network excitability. There is a developing view that a failure of homeostatic plasticity is the key factor that leads to this increased excitability (see section 10.6.2 for a more in-depth discussion of homeostatic plasticity).

A major remaining mystery is the basic function of APP. APP is highly conserved throughout the animal kingdom and clearly has a fundamentally important yet ill-defined role in synaptic/neuronal function. Mice in which *App* is knocked out show a deficit in LTP in later life, as well as accompanying learning and memory deficits (Ring et al., 2007), but remain viable due to compensation by the very closely related-proteins amyloid-like protein 1 and 2 (APLP1 and APLP2), and when all are knocked out, mice die soon after birth due to neuromuscular dysfunction (P Wang et al., 2005). A conditional knockdown of all family members after birth allows for progression to adulthood but with a severe neurodevelopmental phenotype resembling ASD (Steubler et al., 2021), whereas conditional knockdown only in the forebrain produces a far more subtle phenotype that nevertheless features clear hippocampal plasticity and learning deficits (SH Lee et al., 2020). Thus, APP and other family members that can compensate for its loss clearly play key roles in synaptic function. At the heart of the neuroprotective functions of APP is the cleavage of APP by α-secretase, producing the secreted, soluble APP (sAPP) fragment known as sAPPα, and it seems likely that this is the product that mediates the key role of APP in healthy synaptic function, given its ability to rescue synaptic plasticity and learning in the hippocampus of *App* KO mice (Ring et al., 2007, also see Figure 10.17). Reduced production of sAPPα, by inhibiting α-secretase, or direct blockade of sAPPα through antibody application, impairs MPP-DG LTP (Taylor et al., 2008), and application of this seemingly beneficial product of APP also shifts synaptic modification thresholds to reduce the likelihood of LTD and promote LTP (Ishida et al., 1997), thereby counteracting an early stage of synaptic dysfunction in aging (Xiong et al., 2017). There is now much interest in exactly how sAPPα has this effect, with evidence that it binds to key targets to affect the likelihood of LTP, including a direct facilitation of NMDAR currents (Taylor et al., 2008) and binding to GABA$_B$ receptors to diminish spontaneous release but enhance short-term synaptic plasticity in the hippocampus (Rice et al., 2019). It also interacts with K$^+$ channels to reduce neuronal excitability, which may be an additional protective effect (Furukawa et al., 1996). Perhaps most importantly, sAPPα suppresses BACE1 (β-site APP-cleaving enzyme 1; β-secretase) which is the enzyme that further cleaves APP into sAPPβ. This event, in turn, enables cleavage into the pathological product of Aβ oligomers. Thus, the balance of sAPPα and other APP cleavage products may serve as a kind of bistable switch between a healthy synapse that has great capacity for potentiation and a pathologically destabilized synapse that is committed to progressive weakening (Figure 10.17). Thus, there is huge potential for developing therapeutic strategies that aim to elevate sAPPα at hippocampal synapses.

In summary, there have been a bewildering number of molecules whose dysregulation has been implicated in AD. To conclude this section, we provide a hypothesis that may provide a framework for understanding this complexity and which builds on the work of many groups in the field.

We propose that the core concept is the balance between LTP and LTD; normal physiological function requires reversible synaptic strengthening and reversible synaptic weakening. Any factor (genetic, epigenetic, or environmental) that tips the balance in favor of LTD promotes AD whereas any factor that promotes LTP helps ward off AD. Since both processes involve highly complex signaling machinery, there are many potential causes of this dysregulation, all of which can potentially be reversed by the appropriate correction of the LTP/LTD imbalance. From a clinical perspective, cholinesterase inhibitors can theoretically do this by promoting LTP, while cholinergic systems remain intact, memantine may do this by restoring aberrant NMDAR signaling, and antibody treatment may be effective where the driver of the imbalance is accessible to manipulation. Indeed, there are numerous potential ways to restore the LTP/LTD imbalance. This could involve pharmacological approaches aimed at facilitating LTP or suppressing LTD, antibody approaches that target a driver of the imbalance (such as monoclonal antibodies against Aβ), genetic therapy where the underlying genetic cause is known and lifestyle choices that promote LTP (cognitive training) or in other ways impact LTP pathways (e.g., exercise to increase hippocampal BDNF). However, all potential treatments will likely need to be applied much earlier than is currently typical, which will require a major improvement in our ability to predict those who will eventually be diagnosed with AD without one or more of these interventions.

10.9.4 Psychiatric conditions

10.9.4.1 Schizophrenia

Schizophrenia is a complex psychiatric condition that affects around 1% of the population, typically arising in later teenage years or the early 20s. It is characterized not only by the so-called positive symptoms, which include delusions and hallucinations, and negative symptoms, which include anhedonia and social withdrawal, but also less well studied cognitive symptoms, notably including deficits in learning and memory, which are the major contributors to poor outcomes and failure of employability and are often the earliest symptoms to emerge (McGurk, 2000). The role of the hippocampus in schizophrenia is further discussed in Chapter 19.

Currently available treatments for schizophrenia are poor in efficacy and produce serious side effects (Dibonaventura et al., 2012). These treatments have been motivated by the "dopamine" hypothesis, which posits that dysregulations of striatal dopamine give rise to the symptoms of schizophrenia (Howes and Kapur, 2009) and while they exhibit moderate efficacy in treating the positive symptoms of the disorder, they produce little impact on the negative and cognitive symptoms (Coyle, 2006). Though the evidence is

strong for a key role of dopamine dysregulation in the etiology of schizophrenia, this is likely to be a secondary effect of a wider dysregulation of synaptic function, which accounts also for the cognitive symptoms and perhaps contributes to the negative symptoms. Hippocampal dysfunction is heavily implicated as an underlying cause of many symptoms of schizophrenia across all domains (Lodge and Grace, 2007; Lisman, 2012; Brugger and Howes, 2017). A now influential "glutamate" hypothesis for the originating dysfunction in schizophrenia (Coyle, 2006; Moghaddam and Javitt, 2012), posits that disruptions to NMDAR function at glutamatergic synapses are a cause of the cognitive symptoms, as well as producing knock-on effects that impair dopaminergic function and produce positive symptoms (Maatz et al., 2015). Clearly, then, there would be an expectation of deficient hippocampal synaptic plasticity in schizophrenia.

One of the major challenges to studying hippocampal plasticity in this disorder has been in modeling the condition for investigation of hippocampal synaptic function. While it has long been known that there is a major genetic contribution to schizophrenia (Kallmann, 1946), it has become clear that there is no one highly penetrant genetic contributor to the etiology of the disorder, and a polygenic risk score has therefore been adopted as the best assessment of susceptibility to schizophrenia (Gejman et al., 2011). Nevertheless, there is growing evidence for a convergence of genetic risk factors on synaptic plasticity hubs such as the NMDAR, the immediate early gene *Arc/Arg3.1*, and FMRP (Fromer et al., 2014). Despite this insight, it has been a challenge to develop genetically defined mouse models of schizophrenia and more emphasis has been placed on environmental factors, such as stress, maternal immune activation, and drug abuse, which are also known contributors to the disorder (Howes et al., 2004), or two-hit models in which a genetic risk factor is combined with an environmental factor (Guerrin et al., 2021). Even if we take the approach of using mouse models in which a genetic risk factor for schizophrenia has been modified to understand the disorder, we are left with the twin issues of trying to create a model based on a genetic risk factor that is highly unlikely to precipitate schizophrenia in humans, while studying behavioral manifestations that are also highly unlikely in any substantial way to capture the human condition. Thus, it may be important to search for more highly penetrant factors, which need not necessarily be genetic, and move away from claiming psychiatric validity for behavioral effects in animal models (Nestler and Hyman, 2010). At least this approach may provide insight into aberrant hippocampal physiology in schizophrenia.

Psychotomimetics and schizophrenia

One of the most striking, and some would argue, convincing models of schizophrenia is the administration of a group of substances that are described as psychotomimetic because they reliably recapitulate many of the symptoms of schizophrenia in humans. These drugs have a diverse range of effects on hippocampal synaptic plasticity. Probably those substances that will immediately spring to mind are classical psychedelic drugs like LSD and psilocybin, which is the active hallucinogenic ingredient in magic mushrooms. Acutely, these substances can produce hallucinations, and the actions of both are attributed to partial agonism of the G-protein-coupled 5-HT$_{2A}$ receptors (Nichols, 2016). Strikingly, the action of these substances on 5-HT$_{2A}$ receptors at very low doses shows promise as an antidepressant treatment, and this is a very active area of research, which we discuss below in the context of depression (R Griffiths et al., 2016; Palhano-Fontes et al., 2019).

An interesting possible route of influence of these substances is via synaptic plasticity and elevated BDNF levels (Lepack et al., 2016). However, the effects of these psychedelics only superficially resemble the positive symptoms of schizophrenia and do not convincingly recapitulate any of the other symptoms of the disorder. Among the more dramatic psychotomimetics are methamphetamine and cocaine, which prevent reuptake of dopamine and noradrenaline and produce in humans many of the positive symptoms of schizophrenia, particularly after repeated doses (Bramness et al., 2012). Indeed, it was this observation that partially fueled the original "dopamine" hypothesis. These recreational drugs, and related substances, elicit a pronounced enhancement of both the magnitude and longevity of hippocampal LTP and learning (Gold et al., 1984; Preston et al., 2019), likely because they increase cAMP levels postsynaptically and drive protein synthesis (U Frey et al., 1993). However, even in human subjects, while these substances produce positive symptoms, they do not recapitulate any cognitive or negative symptoms of schizophrenia, so cannot be classed as fully psychotomimetic.

Another group of substances frequently used as recreational drugs, which includes ketamine and phencyclidine (PCP), are not only psychotomimetic at high but subanesthetic doses, but also recapitulate the cognitive symptoms of the disorder, even to the extent that psychiatrists may diagnose an abuser as schizophrenic (Krystal et al., 1994; K Xu et al., 2015). Moreover, their effect is faster and more striking in schizophrenic subjects (Lahti et al., 2001). It was this evidence that first led to the foundation of the "glutamate" hypothesis, given that ketamine and PCP are both noncompetitive, use-dependent blockers of NMDAR, among many other actions (Lodge and Mercier, 2015). Of course, application of these substances, or related noncompetitive NMDAR blockers such as MK-801, completely prevent the induction of most forms of LTP in the hippocampus and related learning and memory (Ribeiro et al., 2014), thereby producing a strikingly opposing effect on synaptic plasticity to the delivery of methamphetamine or cocaine, and perhaps accounting for the uniquely emergent mimicry of the cognitive symptoms of schizophrenia. There are, however, other NMDAR-dependent hippocampal processes that could be affected to produce these symptoms. For instance, preferential action on NMDARs expressed by fast-spiking GABAergic inhibitory neurons, which are more prone to blockade by use-dependent antagonists because the channel of this voltage-gated receptor is more often open, leads to elevated, but noisy neural activity, thereby disrupting hippocampus-dependent cognition and increasing activity in other brain structures that are efferent to the hippocampus (Homayoun and Moghaddam, 2007). Selective genetic knockdown of NMDAR from parvalbumin-expressing, fast-spiking inhibitory neurons produces striking hippocampus-dependent cognitive deficits and disrupts gamma frequency oscillations (Korotkova et al., 2010), suggesting that the effects of ketamine/PCP on hippocampal function could largely be explained through this route. The idea that the impact on NMDAR that causes schizophrenia is primarily through inhibitory neurons is consistent with the observation that hippocampal activity is elevated in the condition and the dominant model posits a key role for increased hippocampal output in driving dopaminergic dysfunction in the striatum (Lodge and Grace, 2007). The possibility remains that much of the effect of these drugs is exerted through

non-NMDAR targets, given that many other such targets exist for these relatively promiscuous substances (Lodge and Mercier, 2015). However, many of the psychotomimetic effects that are present in mice when appropriate doses of these drugs are delivered do not manifest in NMDAR hypomorphs (Carlen et al., 2012).

Contributions of the immune response to schizophrenia

Perhaps the most fascinating recent finding to bolster the "glutamate" hypothesis of schizophrenia is the observation that NMDAR encephalitis often produces a mimicry of the full range of symptoms of the disorder in humans (Guasp and Dalmau, 2018). This is a condition in which inflammation usually results from an infection and autoantibodies against key targets are produced as a result (Bseikri et al., 2012). In this case, the antibodies target NMDARs and cause them to be internalized (Guasp and Dalmau, 2018), thereby producing NMDAR knockdown that produces the full range of symptoms of schizophrenia. Even more strikingly, given the lack of other highly penetrant causes of schizophrenia that can be used to model the disorder, antibodies against the NMDAR are found in ~5% of cases of first episode psychosis, with very few cases observed in control subjects (Gable et al., 2012). Preclinical mouse models of this condition can be produced either by infusion of serum derived from NMDAR encephalitis patients (Planaguma et al., 2015) or production of antibodies against NMDARs in mice, by injecting the stabilized NMDARs themselves (B Jones et al., 2019). In both cases, NMDAR currents are reduced in the hippocampus and cognitive deficits arise consistent with hippocampal dysfunction. Unfortunately, the interpretation of the origins of this pathology is complicated by the additional cell death that arises from inflammation in the hippocampus. However, not only is this observation consistent with the psychotomimetic effects of ketamine/PCP resulting from NMDAR blockade but also it implies that the positive symptoms of schizophrenia that result from dopamine dysregulation may be a consequence of NMDAR dysregulation and that the brain of any individual has the capacity to produce the full range of psychosis, even without a genetic or perinatal predisposition to schizophrenia. Whether the NMDAR function that is most consequential is hippocampal plasticity remains to be seen, but treatments that facilitate NMDAR, such as novel positive allosteric modulators, are a strong line of investigation, with hippocampal plasticity likely being at least a very useful readout of efficacy during the discovery phase of research. It is interesting to note that atypical antipsychotic substances, such as clozapine, do not specifically target dopamine dysregulation, and unlike dopamine 2 (D2) receptor antagonists that serve as typical antipsychotics, produce some beneficial effect on the cognitive symptoms of schizophrenia (MA Lee et al., 1999). There is some indication that clozapine, which can be effective in treating some of the symptoms of NMDAR encephalitis, may act to facilitate NMDAR function by binding to the glycine modulatory site (P Yang et al., 2019).

While NMDAR encephalitis is an acute cause of psychosis that arises from an immune response, it is also believed that immune events that cause inflammation may contribute to schizophrenia in other ways. Perhaps the best studied example of this is maternal immune activation (MIA), in which a mother's immune response to viral infection, or other pathogen, during pregnancy also produces an inflammatory immune response in the unborn fetus, in turn causing a range of neurodevelopmental disorders after birth, including schizophrenia (Canetta and Brown, 2012). This likely contributory factor in schizophrenia can be modeled in rodents by timed viral infection, or mimicking viral infection, in pregnant mothers (Estes and McAllister, 2016), and the insult can result in clear alterations of hippocampal plasticity. The results have been predictably variable given the likely complexity of this effect in progeny of mother rats in which immune activation occurred during pregnancy, with some studies finding reductions in DG or CA1 LTP (Oh-Nishi et al., 2010) and others unusual persistence of LTP (Savanthrapadian et al., 2013). Notably, disruptions to both short-term presynaptic plasticity (Oh-Nishi et al., 2010), in the form of PPF, and increases in neuronal excitability, likely due to altered inhibition, have also been described (Savanthrapadian et al., 2013). Overall, the most consistent observation is one of altered hippocampal E/I balance as a result of MIA (Z Zhang and van Praag, 2015; Patrich et al., 2016), which is again a consistent theme in neurodevelopmental disorders overall, and especially schizophrenia (Lisman, 2012). Much further work will be required to understand how MIA contributes to the causes of schizophrenia and related psychiatric disorders, but it is a rare known environmental factor that can be manipulated to model the disorder. In the future, combination of MIA with genetic models or other environmental factors such as drugs, in a so-called two-hit model, could prove not only the most reliable way to produce disorder in the hippocampus but also perhaps the most relevant to the actual etiology of the schizophrenia (Feigenson et al., 2014).

10.9.4.2 Depression

The effective treatment of major depressive disorder (MDD) has proved incredibly challenging but remains an important target for medical science given the over 100 million sufferers globally (Reddy, 2010). This burden primarily reflects substantial human suffering, but also leads to debilitation of the workforce and a requirement for major healthcare and welfare provisions, so the development of new cognitive or pharmaceutical therapeutics would amount to a major breakthrough in psychiatry.

The case for studying hippocampal dysfunction in this disorder is persuasive given that the most consistent observation in the brains of depressive patients is reduced hippocampal volume (Roddy et al., 2019). Moreover, it is a strong hypothesis that depression is a disorder of synaptic plasticity because there is a general reduction in the expression of synaptic proteins in depression as well as a convergence of a range of effective antidepressants on core mechanisms of long-lasting synaptic plasticity, including NMDAR, CREB, and GSK-3β (Pittenger and Duman, 2008). As with other psychiatric conditions such as schizophrenia, compelling preclinical models for MDD have been hard to come by. While there are genetic risk factors for MDD (Lohoff, 2010), they are of similarly low penetrance to those found in schizophrenia and, again, attempts to model the behavioral manifestation of depression in animals is challenging (Nestler and Hyman, 2010). Environmental factors that lead to depression in humans provide some hope for modeling the condition to study underlying etiology. These factors include learned helplessness (Castagne et al., 2010), aberrant light (LeGates et al., 2012), and chronic stress (JJ Kim and Diamond, 2002; see also Chapter 17), all of which cause reduced hippocampal LTP but with mixed effects on LTD. Given that aberrant light arising from jet lag, shift work, and computer/phone use is likely to become an increasingly prevalent element of modern life, the impact on plasticity is poised to become a major area of research in the coming years.

The most exciting breakthrough in psychiatry for decades has been the emergence of a range of relatively fast-acting and efficacious antidepressant substances that seem likely to produce their effect by restoring aberrant synaptic plasticity. As we discussed in the section on schizophrenia, there are several substances that are often described as psychotomimetic when delivered at high but subanesthetic doses, because they recapitulate all or some of the key behavioral symptoms of schizophrenia. Among these substances are ketamine, which has its own dedicated section in Box 10.5, and the psychedelics psilocybin and ayahuasca (a psychedelic that is brewed or smoked by the indigenous people of the Amazon basin in spiritual rituals). Recent, exciting developments demonstrate that lower doses of all these substances act with a striking efficacy in treating the psychiatric condition of MDD in patients resistant to other available treatments, without producing those psychotomimetic effects (Zarate et al., 2006; R Griffiths et al., 2016; Palhano-Fontes et al., 2019).

As with so many drugs approved for use in psychiatry, the mechanism of action of these substances remains poorly understood, just as the pathophysiology underlying the disorder is equally poorly understood. Consequently, animal and cell culture experiments are required not necessarily to model the disorder but rather to pick apart the potential mechanisms of action. This process of reverse translation is likely to become a dominant theme in brain science over the coming decades. While drugs can enter the clinic without deep understanding of mechanism of action, once proven safe, gaining a deeper understanding of the mode of action of effective therapeutics is likely to reveal key aspects of the etiology of the disorder, as well as opening the door to discovering more effective treatments. For example, while the improvements in mood produced by hallucinogens and psychedelics are pronounced, they are not always long-lasting (Zarate et al., 2006). One strong hypothesis for their effect in depression, given their relatively fast action of a day or less (Zarate et al., 2006; R Griffiths et al., 2016; Palhano-Fontes et al., 2019), is that they induce pronounced synaptic potentiation, reinvigorating the reduced functional connectivity in the brain that had given rise to the depression itself. This interpretation would explain why the effects of a single dose last for a week or two afterward, long after the drug is no longer in the brain. Indeed, synaptic number is greatly reduced in the hippocampus and prefrontal cortex of individuals suffering from depression (Duman and Li, 2012). Furthermore, the reinstatement of functional synaptic connectivity is consistent with the effect of deep brain stimulation, which produces striatocortical LTP (Creed et al., 2015) and is an invasive treatment that has been used as an effective therapy for depression that is resistant to other forms of treatment (Mayberg et al., 2005). Although noninvasive versions of LTP-inducing deep brain stimulation have been developed (reviewed by Bliss and Cooke, 2011), they do not appear to be as effective, making drugs that will achieve equivalent results highly attractive.

The pharmacology of psychedelic drugs is complex. Psilocybin and ayahuasca overlap in their composition and are somewhat related to LSD in that they are considered to exert their primary effect through partial agonism of 5-HT$_{2A}$, but their action is by no means restricted to this receptor (Carhart-Harris et al., 2017). Ayahuasca is particularly complex and has several active ingredients, including dimethyltryptamine (DMT), which is an analogue of psilocybin. The potential mechanistic action of these agents on the serotonergic system aligns them with the mode of action of other approved treatments for depression such as SSRIs. However, SSRIs are much slower (their effects taking weeks to emerge), and are ineffective in many individuals, with some claims that they have no greater effect than placebo (Kirsch et al., 2008). The overlap between psilocybin/ayahuasca and ketamine antidepressant actions remains unclear. While there may be some ill-defined common mechanism, it is important to entertain the perspective that there is no proximal point of convergence. Ketamine receives further discussion in Box 10.5.

It will be fascinating to establish which effect, or combination of effects, is required for the antidepressant action of these substances, given their pharmacological complexity. To answer this question, it will be necessary to conduct preclinical studies in mice in which individual targets are genetically ablated and clinical trials in humans in which drugs that are more restricted in their action are applied. Other possible core effects remain that do not relate to synaptic plasticity, such as increasing intrinsic excitability of neurons, but reinforcement of synaptic potentiation remains a strong hypothetical mechanism underlying the success of these substances in alleviating depressive symptoms, and this area of research promises to be a major focus for treatment of severe depression in the future.

Box 10.5 Ketamine

The notion that ketamine might exert its central actions via an effect on synaptic plasticity can be traced back to 1983, long before its rapid and relatively persistent antidepressant action was described at the turn of the millennium (Berman et al., 2000, also see Krystal et al., 2019). Three papers, which at the time seemed unrelated, showed that (1) ketamine blocks the induction of LTP (Stringer and Guyenet, 1983), (2) NMDARs are a trigger for the induction of LTP (Collingridge et al., 1983), and (3) ketamine is an NMDAR antagonist (Anis et al., 1983). In retrospect, it may therefore be postulated that ketamine's antidepressant action is via an effect on NMDAR-dependent synaptic plasticity in various regions of the CNS, including the hippocampus. Such a mechanism could account for the rapid onset and relatively persistent action, since NMDAR-mediated plasticity in the brain can manifest quickly and can also account for why the effects last much longer than the time the drug is present in the system. However, although considered an attractive possibility by many, the evidence in support of this hypothesis is still controversial (see Y Jiang et al., 2024, for a thorough discussion of the evidence).

There are a number of issues to consider. Foremost, are the antidepressant effects of ketamine due to its well-described actions on NMDARs or via effects at other sites where it is known to interact? This includes alpha7 subunit containing nicotinic ACh receptors, opioid receptors, HCN1 pacemaker channels, and 5-HT$_3$ receptors (Zanos et al., 2018). Indeed, its effects could be a result of a polypharmacology that involves multiple sites of action that may, or may not, involve the NMDAR. However, a careful pharmacological analysis strongly points to the NMDAR as the primary site of action of ketamine when used at therapeutic doses (Lodge and Mercier, 2015).

An action that is independent of NMDARs might still involve a regulation of NMDAR-dependent synaptic plasticity, via a modulatory influence mediated by one or more of its other targets. Indeed, one recent idea, which has received prominent attention, is that ketamine affects NMDAR-LTP by acting downstream of NMDARs (Zanos et al., 2016). The suggestion is that ketamine triggers the same increase in AMPAR function that is the basis of the expression of NMDAR-LTP, although the mechanism by which it does this is unclear. It was further suggested that this NMDAR-independent action is due to metabolites of ketamine, notably (2R,6R)-hydroxynorketamine (HNK), rather than ketamine itself (Zanos et al., 2016, see Highland et al., 2021). However, (2R,6R)-HNK has been found to inhibit NMDARs (Suzuki et al., 2017) and to prevent the induction of NMDAR-LTP (Kang et al., 2020).

Most researchers continue to favor the NMDAR as the principal target for the rapid antidepressant actions of ketamine. But if so, how is this manifest? One suggestion is that ketamine normalizes NMDAR-mediated synaptic transmission, via an action in a brain region involved in mood regulation such as the lateral habenula (Y Yang et al., 2018). Although an effect on NMDAR-mediated transmission can explain its rapid onset of action, it cannot alone explain a persistent effect unless the alteration in transmission itself leads to plasticity. This seems plausible, given the close association of NMDAR-mediated synaptic transmission and plasticity.

On the assumption that the ultimate target is NMDAR-mediated synaptic plasticity then how is the antidepressant effect achieved? One popular idea is that ketamine preferentially blocks NMDARs that are involved in the excitation of inhibitory interneurons and thereby reduces inhibitory drive. A reduction in synaptic inhibition is well known to facilitate the induction of NMDAR-LTP in principal neurons, by enabling synaptic excitation to more effectively remove the Mg^{2+} block of the NMDAR. So, a preferential reduction in NMDARs on GABAergic interneurons would boost NMDAR-LTP. But why are NMDARs on GABAergic interneurons more susceptible to the actions of ketamine? There are at least two, nonexclusive possibilities. First, inhibitory interneurons tend to be more depolarized and active, conditions that could favor use- and/or voltage-dependent compounds such as ketamine to block NMDARs (Honey et al., 1985; S Davies et al., 1988). Second, the subunit composition of NMDARs involved in the excitation of interneurons and principal neurons is likely different; with both GluN2B and GluN2D subunits (probably in the form of heterotrimers) being prominent in the excitation of interneurons. This is highly relevant since GluN2B-containing NMDARs have been implicated in the rapid antidepressant effects of ketamine (O Miller et al., 2014). However, ketamine has been shown to preferentially inhibit GluN2C- and GluN2D-containing NMDARs in the presence of physiological concentrations of Mg^{2+} (Kotermanski and Johnson, 2009). Therefore, the rapid antidepressant effect of ketamine may be mediated, at least in part, by a GluN2B/2D heterotrimer. Another target for ketamine could be STP2, a form of synaptic plasticity that involves GluN2B- and 2D-containing NMDARs and is extremely sensitive to the actions of ketamine (Ingram et al., 2018).

Irrespective of whether the persistent effects of ketamine are initiated via inhibition of NMDARs or not, an important question pertains to the underlying signaling mechanisms that are triggered by ketamine. In this context, there is evidence that ketamine engages de novo protein synthesis, via eIF4E (Aguilar-Valles et al., 2021), which is a component of the initiation factor complex that is required for the generation of LTP2 (Hoeffer et al., 2013).

The augmentation of LTP in structures such as the hippocampus could promote the reversal of synaptic loss that it associated with major depressive disorder (MDD) and result in an elevated mood. Alternatively (or additionally) a reduction in LTD could achieve the same effect. Indeed, chronic stress can lead to MDD and augments NMDAR-LTD, suggesting that there may be a causal link between LTD and MDD. The net result is that a shift in the LTP/LTD balance toward LTD may promote MDD; accordingly, ketamine may act to normalize this balance by promoting LTP and/or inhibiting LTD.

Another point to note is that many memories involve consolidation followed by extinction or reconsolidation, at which point the memory can be modified. The processes of extinction and reconsolidation have as their synaptic correlates NMDAR-dependent DP, and repotentiation (LTP), respectively. Ketamine could theoretically act on these forms of synaptic plasticity. In this scenario, depression might persist due to NMDAR-dependent consolidation of a negative mood state, which could be counteracted by the actions of ketamine on NMDAR-dependent synaptic plasticity.

10.10 Synaptic plasticity and hippocampal function: future perspectives

We end this chapter with a summary of some of the major unresolved questions relating to synaptic plasticity and its relationship to the neural basis of learning and memory. Given the dizzying rate of progress in memory research, it seems likely that answers to many of these questions will be found in the next decade or two.

1. How do the various components of synaptic plasticity interact with intrinsic plasticity to preserve hippocampus-dependent memory?

The SPM hypothesis supposes that changes in synaptic weight are the locus of memory storage, a proposal that has the advantage of affording greater fidelity for separating patterns and greater storage capacity. However, there may be circumstances in which alterations in cell excitability, typified by E-S potentiation, either together with, or in the absence of synaptic potentiation, could be an integral component of a Hebbian "cell-assembly." Such alterations could mediate memory allocation during encoding and foster more effective recall. An unresolved question is whether such persistent changes in cell excitability are also exploited for information storage.

2. How important is metaplasticity (in particular homosynaptic priming and STC) in hippocampal memory formation?

Metaplasticity, the plasticity of synaptic plasticity, comes in several guises, the relationship between which is not fully understood. Most prominent are "priming," which is typically homosynaptic, and STC, which involves cross-talk between synapses. The molecular mechanisms of STC are still under intense investigation, but the "synaptic tag" is now generally thought to involve actin destabilization leading to a temporary change in spine structure, with PRPs likely mediating the stabilization of such changes. A number of candidate molecules have been identified in both protocols (see Box 10.3 for a discussion of CP-AMPARs as a candidate tag in the "strong before weak" protocol), but the exact molecular mechanisms remain to be determined.

3. Is there a role for synaptogenesis in memory storage in the hippocampus?

Imaging studies of dendritic spines on dye-filled neurons in the neocortex of behaving animals have shown that motor training is associated with the extrusion and absorption of dendritic spines; fewer observations have been made in deep structures such as the hippocampus, where average spine lifetime is estimated at around 3 weeks. How in the face of such synaptic flux can a memory system based on changes in synaptic strength be maintained? The answer to this question is far from clear.

4. How do inhibitory neurons impact mnemonic function?

Most work on activity-dependent synaptic potentiation has focused on excitatory synapses but, in hippocampus and cortex, numerous different classes of inhibitory neurons are differentially activated to enable neural processing in distinct dendritic domains (somatic, proximal, distal, etc). How this process supports mnemonic function remains largely unknown.

5. How do homeostatic plasticity and synaptic plasticity interact in the hippocampus?

Synaptic homeostasis has become an extremely active topic since the previous edition of this book. General questions include how it is implemented (scaling or metaplasticity?) and, also given the reliance on reduced preparations, what the true biological boundary conditions might be for the phenomenon (i.e., how far must hippocampal networks be pushed from the normal range before homeostatic mechanisms are triggered?). It is interesting to note that many in vivo LTP experiments have been conducted in which large numbers of hippocampal synapses are potentiated for days or more, but data on counteracting homeostatic plasticity is lacking. Various issues arising from the concept of homeostasis are likely to continue to present challenges for future research.

6. How do neuromodulatory factors, individually and in combination, regulate synaptic plasticity to impact learning and memory?

Since the importance of monoamines for the induction of LTP was described some 40 years ago, a huge and diverse number of regulators of synaptic plasticity have been described. This includes neurotransmitters, neuropeptides, cytokines, growth factors, and hormones. These modulators provide the means for intrinsic and environmental factors to impact synaptic plasticity. A major challenge is to understand how these diverse signals are integrated at the synaptic level to influence plasticity in health and disease.

7. How do circulating and locally released sex hormones impact synaptic plasticity to influence learning and memory?

Growing evidence suggests that there are significant sex-differences in hippocampus-dependent synaptic plasticity and that both puberty and the estrus cycle impact these processes. Although a key role of estrogen receptors in LTP has been established, there are likely to be many other sex-related processes that are involved. Neuroendocrinological mechanisms are important to understand not only from a fundamental perspective but also because evidence is emerging that some potential therapeutic approaches for the treatment of cognitive decline may be sex-dependent.

8. What is the role of synaptic plasticity in neurodevelopmental disorders?

There is now a convergence of evidence that many neurodevelopmental disorders arise from synaptopathy. However, a disproportionate amount of research on neurodevelopmental disorders has focused specifically on synaptic plasticity in the hippocampus. This is in part due to the clear cognitive disturbances that are apparent in these disorders but, probably also reflects the ease with which synaptic plasticity can be measured in the hippocampus. Whether there is a particular prevalence of hippocampal disturbances in neurodevelopmental disorders compared to other regions of the brain remains to be seen.

9. What is the role of synaptic plasticity in neuropsychiatric disorders?

Hippocampal synaptic plasticity deficits are commonly observed in animal models of major depressive disorder. As discussed in this chapter, the efficacy of a new group of substances, including

NMDAR blockers such as ketamine, in the treatment of depression, implicate synaptic plasticity. However, it remains unconfirmed whether these drugs exert their antidepressant actions through the NMDAR or via some other target (of which there are many for these substances). Moreover, even if blockade of NMDARs is a key event, why should this promote plasticity or relieve depression? These key questions remain to be addressed.

10. What is the role of synaptic plasticity in neurodegenerative diseases?

As discussed above, a dominant hypothesis proposes that the earliest stages of AD, and potentially other tauopathies, emerge from altered synaptic function in medial temporal lobe structures such as the hippocampus, predisposing these synapses to weakening through a Hebbian LTD-like process that eventually cascades into synapse loss. Many treatment candidates exist based on this hypothesis, but because we cannot currently predict the individuals in which the disorder will arise, it has so far been challenging to test the efficacy of these treatments, and thus to assess the value of the hypothesis. It is therefore imperative to identify affordable, noninvasive measures of hippocampal synaptic plasticity in humans to screen for the earliest emergence of these synaptic phenotypes. Such a biomarker would have a huge range of potential applications.

Acknowledgments

The authors thank current and former lab members for their numerous valuable contributions. We are grateful for the financial support of granting agencies and donors over many years.

REFERENCES

Abd-Elrahman KS, Albaker A, de Souza JM, Ribeiro FM, Schlossmacher MG, Tiberi M, Hamilton A, Ferguson SSG (2020) Aβ oligomers induce pathophysiological mGluR5 signaling in Alzheimer's disease model mice in a sex-selective manner. *Sci Signal* 13:eabd2494. doi:10.1126/scisignal.abd2494

Abdou K, Shehata M, Choko K, Nishizono H, Matsuo M, Muramatsu SI, Inokuchi K (2018) Synapse-specific representation of the identity of overlapping memory engrams. *Science* 360:1227–1231.

Abraham WC, Bear MF (1996) Metaplasticity: the plasticity of synaptic plasticity. *Trends Neurosci* 19:126–130.

Abraham WC, Goddard GV (1983) Asymmetric relationships between homosynaptic long-term potentiation and heterosynaptic long-term depression. *Nature* 305:717–719.

Abraham WC, Gustafsson B, Wigström H (1987) Long-term potentiation involves enhanced synaptic excitation relative to synaptic inhibition in guinea pig hippocampus. *J Physiol* 394:367–380.

Abraham WC, Jones OD, Glanzman DL (2019) Is plasticity of synapses the mechanism of long-term memory storage? *NPJ Sci Learn* 4:9.

Abraham WC, Logan B, Greenwood JM, Dragunow M (2002) Induction and experience-dependent consolidation of stable long-term potentiation lasting months in the hippocampus. *J Neurosci* 22:9626–9634.

Abraham WC, Mason-Parker SE, Bear MF, Webb S, Tate WP (2001) Heterosynaptic metaplasticity in the hippocampus in vivo: a BCM-like modifiable threshold for LTP. *Proc Natl Acad Sci U S A* 98:10924–10929.

Abraham WC, Tate WP (1997) Metaplasticity: a new vista across the field of synaptic plasticity. *Prog Neurobiol* 52:303–323.

Aguilar-Valles A, De Gregorio D, Matta-Camacho E, Eslamizade MJ, Khlaifia A, Skaleka A, Lopez-Canul M, Torres-Berrio A, Bermudez S, Rurak GM, et al. (2021) Antidepressant actions of ketamine engage cell-specific translation via eIF4E. *Nature* 590:315–319.

Ahmed T, Van der Jeugd A, Blum D, Galas MC, D'Hooge R, Buee L, Balschun D (2014) Cognition and hippocampal synaptic plasticity in mice with a homozygous tau deletion. *Neurobiol Aging* 35:2474–2478.

Akers KG, Martinez-Canabal A, Restivo L, Yiu AP, De Cristofaro A, Hsiang HL, Wheeler AL, Guskjolen A, Niibori Y, Shoji H, et al. (2014) Hippocampal neurogenesis regulates forgetting during adulthood and infancy. *Science* 344:598–602.

Alejandre-García T, Kim S, Pérez-Ortega J, Yuste R (2022) Intrinsic excitability mechanisms of neuronal ensemble formation. *Elife* 11:e77470.

Altafaj X, Martin ED, Ortiz-Abalia J, Valderrama A, Lao-Peregrin C, Dierssen M, Fillat C (2013) Normalization of Dyrk1A expression by AAV2/1-shDyrk1A attenuates hippocampal-dependent defects in the Ts65Dn mouse model of Down syndrome. *Neurobiol Dis* 52:117–127.

Amici M, Lee Y, Pope RJP, Bradley CA, Cole A, Collingridge GL (2021) GSK-3β regulates the synaptic expression of NMDA receptors via phosphorylation of phosphatidylinositol 4 kinase type IIα. *Eur J Neurosci* 54:6815–6825.

Amir RE, Van den Veyver IB, Wan M, Tran CQ, Francke U, Zoghbi HY (1999) Rett syndrome is caused by mutations in X-linked MECP2, encoding methyl-CpG-binding protein 2. *Nat Genet* 23:185–188.

Ancona Esselmann SG, Diaz-Alonso J, Levy JM, Bemben MA, Nicoll RA (2017) Synaptic homeostasis requires the membrane-proximal carboxy tail of GluA2. *Proc Natl Acad Sci U S A* 114:13266–13271.

Andersen P, Sundberg SH, Sveen O, Swann JW, Wigström H (1980) Possible mechanisms for long-lasting potentiation of synaptic transmission in hippocampal slices from guinea-pigs. *J Physiol* 302:463–482.

Andersen P, Sundberg SH, Sveen O, Wigström H (1977) Specific long-lasting potentiation of synaptic transmission in hippocampal slices. *Nature* 266:736–737.

Andrade-Talavera Y, Duque-Feria P, Paulsen O, Rodriguez-Moreno A (2016) Presynaptic spike timing-dependent long-term depression in the mouse hippocampus. *Cereb Cortex* 26:3637–3654.

Anggono V, Clem RL, Huganir RL (2011) PICK1 loss of function occludes homeostatic synaptic scaling. *J Neurosci* 31:2188–2196.

Anis NA, Berry SC, Burton NR, Lodge D (1983) The dissociative anaesthetics, ketamine and phencyclidine, selectively reduce excitation of central mammalian neurones by N-methyl-aspartate. *Br J Pharmacol* 79:565–575.

Aoki Y, Niihori T, Kawame H, Kurosawa K, Ohashi H, Tanaka Y, Filocamo M, Kato K, Suzuki Y, Kure S, et al. (2005) Germline mutations in HRAS proto-oncogene cause Costello syndrome. *Nat Genet* 37:1038–1040.

Arai A, Kessler M, Ambros-Ingerson J, Quan A, Yigiter E, Rogers G, Lynch G (1996) Effects of a centrally active benzoylpyrrolidine drug on AMPA receptor kinetics. *Neuroscience* 75:573–585.

Armstrong RA, Cairns NJ (2015) Comparative quantitative study of "signature" pathological lesions in the hippocampus and adjacent gyri of 12 neurodegenerative disorders. *J Neural Transm (Vienna)* 122:1355–1367.

Artinian J, Lacaille JC (2018) Disinhibition in learning and memory circuits: new vistas for somatostatin interneurons and long-term synaptic plasticity. *Brain Res Bull* 141:20–26.

Asgarihafshejani A, Raveendran VA, Pressey JC, Woodin MA (2024) LTP is absent in the CA1 region of the hippocampus of male and female Rett Syndrome mouse models. *Neuroscience* 537:189–204.

Asiminas A, Jackson AD, Louros SR, Till SM, Spano T, Dando O, Bear MF, Chattarji S, Hardingham GE, Osterweil EK, et al. (2019) Sustained correction of associative learning deficits after brief, early treatment in a rat model of Fragile X Syndrome. *Sci Transl Med* 11(494):eaao0498.

Asrar S, Meng Y, Zhou Z, Todorovski Z, Huang WW, Jia Z (2009) Regulation of hippocampal long-term potentiation by p21-activated protein kinase 1 (PAK1). *Neuropharmacology* 56:73–80.

Asrar S, Zhou Z, Ren W, Jia Z (2009) Ca^{2+} permeable AMPA receptor induced long-term potentiation requires PI3/MAP kinases but not Ca/CaM-dependent kinase II. *PLoS One* 4:e4339.

Astori S, Pawlak V, Kohr G (2010) Spike-timing-dependent plasticity in hippocampal CA3 neurons. *J Physiol* 588:4475–4488.

Attardo A, Fitzgerald JE, Schnitzer MJ (2015) Impermanence of dendritic spines in live adult CA1 hippocampus. *Nature* 523:592–596.

Attardo A, Lu J, Kawashima T, Okuno H, Fitzgerald JE, Bito H, Schnitzer MJ (2018) Long-term consolidation of ensemble neural plasticity patterns in hippocampal area CA1. *Cell Rep* 25:640–650, e642.

Babiec WE, Guglietta R, Jami SA, Morishita W, Malenka RC, O'Dell TJ (2014) Ionotropic NMDA receptor signaling is required for the induction of long-term depression in the mouse hippocampal CA1 region. *J Neurosci* 34:5285–5290.

Bakker A, Krauss GL, Albert MS, Speck CL, Jones LR, Stark CE, Yassa MA, Bassett SS, Shelton AL, Gallagher M (2012) Reduction of hippocampal hyperactivity improves cognition in amnestic mild cognitive impairment. *Neuron* 74:467–474.

Bannerman DM, Good MA, Butcher SP, Ramsay MF, Morris RG (1995) Distinct components of spatial learning revealed by prior training and NMDA receptor blockade. *Nature* 378:182–186.

Barnes CA (1979) Memory deficits associated with senescence: a neurophysiological and behavioral study in the rat. *J Comp Physiol Psych* 93:74–104.

Barnes CA (1988) Spatial learning and memory processes: the search for their neurobiological mechanisms in the rat. *Trends Neurosci* 11:163–169.

Barnes CA (1995) Involvement of LTP in memory: are we "searching under the street light." *Neuron* 15:751–754.

Barnes CA, Jung MW, McNaughton BL, Korol DL, Andreasson K, Worley PF (1994) LTP saturation and spatial learning disruption: effects of task variables and saturation levels. *J Neurosci* 14:5793–5806.

Barnes CA, McNaughton BL (1985) An age comparison of the rates of acquisition and forgetting of spatial information in relation to long-term enhancement of hippocampal synapses. *Behav Neurosci* 99:1040–1048.

Barnes CA, McNaughton BL, Goddard GV, Douglas RM, Adamec R (1977) Circadian rhythm of synaptic excitability in rat and monkey central nervous system. *Science* 197:91–92.

Barria A, Malinow R (2005) NMDA receptor subunit composition controls synaptic plasticity by regulating binding to CaMKII. *Neuron* 48:289–301.

Bartlett TE, Bannister NJ, Collett VJ, Dargan SL, Massey PV, Bortolotto ZA, Fitzjohn SM, Bashir ZI, Collingridge GL, Lodge D (2007) Differential roles of NR2A and NR2B-containing NMDA receptors in LTP and LTD in the CA1 region of two-week old rat hippocampus. *Neuropharmacology* 52:60–70.

Bartus RT, Dean RL, 3rd, Beer B, Lippa AS (1982) The cholinergic hypothesis of geriatric memory dysfunction. *Science* 217:408–414.

Bast T, da Silva BM, Morris RGM (2005) Distinct contributions of hippocampal NMDA and AMPA receptors to encoding and retrieval of one-trial place memory. *J Neurosci* 25:5845–5856.

Bastrikova N, Gardner GA, Reece JM, Jeromin A, Dudek SM (2008) Synapse elimination accompanies functional plasticity in hippocampal neurons. *Proc Natl Acad Sci U S A* 105:3123–3127.

Basu J, Srinivas KV, Cheung SK, Taniguchi H, Huang ZJ, Siegelbaum SA (2013) A cortico-hippocampal learning rule shapes inhibitory microcircuit activity to enhance hippocampal information flow. *Neuron* 79:1208–1221.

Bath KG, Lee FS (2006) Variant BDNF (Val66Met) impact on brain structure and function. *Cogn Affect Behav Neurosci* 6:79–85.

Baudry M, Bi X, Aguirre C (2013) Progesterone-estrogen interactions in synaptic plasticity and neuroprotection. *Neuroscience* 239:280–294.

Baumgartel K, Mansuy IM (2012) Neural functions of calcineurin in synaptic plasticity and memory. *Learn Mem* 19:375–384.

Bear MF, Abraham WC (1996) Long-term depression in hippocampus. *Annu Rev Neurosci* 19:437–462.

Bear MF, Cooke SF, Giese KP, Kaang BK, Kennedy MB, Kim JI, Morris RGM, Park P (2018) In memoriam: John Lisman—commentaries on CaMKII as a memory molecule. *Mol Brain* 11:76.

Bear MF, Huber KM, Warren ST (2004) The mGluR theory of fragile X mental retardation. *Trends Neurosci* 27:370–377.

Bearden CE, Hellemann GS, Rosser T, Montojo C, Jonas R, Enrique N, Pacheco L, Hussain SA, Wu JY, Ho JS, et al. (2016) A randomized placebo-controlled lovastatin trial for neurobehavioral function in neurofibromatosis I. *Ann Clin Transl Neurol* 3:266–279.

Beattie EC, Stellwagen D, Morishita W, Bresnahan JC, Ha BK, Von Zastrow M, Beattie MS, Malenka RC (2002) Control of synaptic strength by glial TNFalpha. *Science* 295:2282–2285.

Beck H, Goussakov IV, Lie A, Helmstaedter C, Elger CE (2000) Synaptic plasticity in the human dentate gyrus. *J Neurosci* 20:7080–7086.

Becker N, Wierenga CJ, Fonseca R, Bonhoeffer T, Nägerl UV (2008) LTD induction causes morphological changes of presynaptic boutons and reduces their contacts with spines. *Neuron* 60:590–597.

Bellone C, Nicoll RA (2007) Rapid bidirectional switching of synaptic NMDA receptors. *Neuron* 55:779–785.

Ben Zablah Y, Merovitch N, Jia Z (2020) The role of ADF/Cofilin in synaptic physiology and Alzheimer's disease. *Front Cell Dev Biol* 8:594998.

Berman RM, Cappiello A, Anand A, Oren DA, Heninger GR, Charney DS, Krystal JH (2000) Antidepressant effects of ketamine in depressed patients. *Biol Psychiatry* 47:351–354.

Bernal MC, Vicens P, Carrasco MC, Redolat R (1999) Effects of nicotine on spatial learning in C57BL mice. *Behav Pharmacol* 10:333–336.

Berry B, McMahan R, Gallagher M (1997) Spatial learning and memory at defined points of the estrous cycle: effects on performance of a hippocampal-dependent task. *Behav Neurosci* 111:267–274.

Berry-Kravis EM, Lindemann L, Jonch AE, Apostol G, Bear MF, Carpenter RL, Crawley JN, Curie A, Des Portes V, Hossain F, et al. (2018) Drug development for neurodevelopmental disorders: lessons learned from fragile X syndrome. *Nat Rev Drug Discov* 17:280–299.

Beurel E, Grieco SF, Jope RS (2015) Glycogen synthase kinase-3 (GSK3): regulation, actions, and diseases. *Pharmacol Ther* 148:114–131.

Bi GQ, Poo MM (1998) Synaptic modifications in cultured hippocampal neurons: dependence on spike timing, synaptic strength, and postsynaptic cell type. *J Neurosci* 18:10464–10472.

Bienenstock EL, Cooper LN, Munro PW (1982) Theory for the development of neuron selectivity: orientation specificity and binocular interaction in visual cortex. *J Neurosci* 2:32–48.

Bin NR, Ma K, Harada H, Tien CW, Bergin F, Sugita K, Luyben TT, Narimatsu M, Jia Z, Wrana JL, et al. (2018) Crucial role of postsynaptic syntaxin 4 in mediating basal neurotransmission and synaptic plasticity in hippocampal CA1 neurons. *Cell Rep* 23:2955–2966.

Bin Ibrahim MZ, Benoy A, Sajikumar S (2021) Long-term plasticity in the hippocampus: maintaining within and "tagging" between synapses. *FEBS J* 289:2176–2201.

Bin Ibrahim MZ, Wang Z, Sajikumar S (2024) Synapses tagged, memories kept: synaptic tagging and capture hypothesis in brain health and disease. *Philos Trans R Soc Lond B* 379(1906):20230237.

Bittner KC, Milstein AD, Grienberger C, Romani S, Magee JC (2017) Behavioral time scale synaptic plasticity underlies CA1 place fields. *Science* 357:1033–1036.

Blackburn ATM, Bekheirnia N, Uma VC, Corkins ME, Xu Y, Rosenfeld JA, Bainbridge MN, Yang Y, Liu P, Madan-Khetarpal S, et al. (2019) DYRK1A-related intellectual disability: a syndrome associated with congenital anomalies of the kidney and urinary tract. *Genet Med* 21:2755–2764.

Bliss TVP, Collingridge GL (1993) A synaptic model of memory: long-term potentiation in the hippocampus. *Nature* 361:31–39.

Bliss TVP, Collingridge GL (1993b) A synaptic model of memory: long-term potentiation in the hippocampus. *Nature* 361:31–39.

Bliss TV, Collingridge GL (2013) Expression of NMDA receptor-dependent LTP in the hippocampus: bridging the divide. *Mol Brain* 6:5.

Bliss TVP, Collingridge GL, Morris RGM, Reymann KG (2018) Long-term potentiation in the hippocampus: discovery, mechanisms and function. *Neuroforum* 24:A103–A120.

Bliss TV, Cooke SF (2011) Long-term potentiation and long-term depression: a clinical perspective. *Clinics (Sao Paulo)* 66(Suppl 1):3–17.

Bliss TVP, Gardner-Medwin AR (1973) Long-lasting potentiation of synaptic transmission in the dentate area of the unanaesthetized rabbit following stimulation of the perforant path. *J Physiol (Lond)* 232:357–374.

Bliss TVP, Goddard GV, Riives M (1983) Reduction of long-term potentiation in the dentate gyrus of the rat following selective depletion of monoamines. *J Physiol* 334:475–491.

Bliss TVP, Lancaster B, Wheal HV (1983) Long-term potentiation in commissural and Schaffer projections to hippocampal CA1 cells: an in vivo study in the rat. *J Physiol (Lond)* 341:617–626.

Bliss TV, Lømo T (1973) Long-lasting potentiation of synaptic transmission in the dentate area of the anaesthetized rabbit following stimulation of the perforant path. *J Physiol (Lond)* 232:331–356.

Borovac J, Bosch M, Okamoto K (2018) Regulation of actin dynamics during structural plasticity of dendritic spines: signaling messengers and actin-binding proteins. *Mol Cell Neurosci* 91:122–130.

Bortolotto ZA, Collett VJ, Conquet F, Jia Z and Collingridge GL (2008) An analysis of the stimulus requirements for setting the molecular switch reveals a lower threshold for metaplasticity than synaptic plasticity. *Neuropharmacology* 55:454–458.

Bosch M, Castro J, Saneyoshi T, Matsuno H, Sur M, Hayashi Y (2014) Structural and molecular remodeling of dendritic spine substructures during long-term potentiation. *Neuron* 82:444–459.

Bostrom CA, Majaess NM, Morch K, White E, Eadie BD, Christie BR (2015) Rescue of NMDAR-dependent synaptic plasticity in Fmr1 knock-out mice. *Cereb Cortex* 25:271–279.

Bourne JN, Chirillo MA, Harris KM (2013) Presynaptic ultrastructural plasticity along CA3→CA1 axons during long-term potentiation in mature hippocampus. *J Comp Neurol* 521:3898–3912.

Bourne JN, Harris KM (2011) Coordination of size and number of excitatory and inhibitory synapses results in a balanced structural plasticity along mature hippocampal CA1 dendrites during LTP. *Hippocampus* 21:354–373.

Bowden JB, Abraham WC, Harris KM (2012) Differential effects of strain, circadian cycle, and stimulation pattern on LTP and concurrent LTD in the dentate gyrus of freely moving rats. *Hippocampus* 22:1363–1370.

Bradley CA, Peineau S, Taghibiglou C, Nicolas CS, Whitcomb DJ, Bortolotto ZA, Kaang BK, Cho K, Wang YT, Collingridge GL (2012) A pivotal role of GSK-3 in synaptic plasticity. *Front Mol Neurosci* 5:13.

Bramham CR, Messaoudi E (2005) BDNF function in adult synaptic plasticity: the synaptic consolidation hypothesis. *Prog Neurobiol* 76:99–125.

Bramham CR, Milgram NW, Srebro B (1991) Activation of AP5-sensitive NMDA receptors is not required to induce LTP of synaptic transmission in the lateral perforant path. *Eur J Neurosci* 3:1300–1308.

Bramham CR, Srebro B (1989) Synaptic plasticity in the hippocampus is modulated by behavioral state. *Brain Res* 493:74–86.

Bramness JG, Gundersen OH, Guterstam J, Rognli EB, Konstenius M, Loberg EM, Medhus S, Tanum L, Franck J (2012) Amphetamine-induced psychosis—a separate diagnostic entity or primary psychosis triggered in the vulnerable? *BMC Psychiatry* 12:221.

Brandalise F, Gerber U (2014) Mossy fiber-evoked subthreshold responses induce timing-dependent plasticity at hippocampal CA3 recurrent synapses. *Proc Natl Acad Sci U S A* 111:4303–4308.

Braudeau J, Delatour B, Duchon A, Pereira PL, Dauphinot L, de Chaumont F, Olivo-Marin JC, Dodd RH, Herault Y, Potier MC (2011) Specific targeting of the GABA-A receptor alpha5 subtype by a selective inverse agonist restores cognitive deficits in Down syndrome mice. *J Psychopharmacol* 25:1030–1042.

Broadhead MJ, Horrocks MH, Zhu F, Muresan L, Benavides-Piccione R, DeFelipe J, Fricker D, Kopanitsa MV, Duncan RR, Klenerman D, et al. (2016) PSD95 nanoclusters are postsynaptic building blocks in hippocampus circuits. *Sci Rep* 6:24626.

Brown V, Small K, Lakkis L, Feng Y, Gunter C, Wilkinson KD, Warren ST (1998) Purified recombinant Fmrp exhibits selective RNA binding as an intrinsic property of the fragile X mental retardation protein. *J Biol Chem* 273:15521–15527.

Brugger SP, Howes OD (2017) Heterogeneity and homogeneity of regional brain structure in schizophrenia: a meta-analysis. *JAMA Psychiatry* 74:1104–1111.

Brun VH, Ytterbo K, Morris RGM, Moser MB, Moser EI (2001) Retrograde amnesia for spatial memory induced by NMDA receptor-mediated long-term potentiation. *J Neurosci* 21:356–362.

Brzosko Z, Mierau SB, Paulsen O (2019) Neuromodulation of spike-timing-dependent plasticity: past, present, and future. *Neuron* 103:563–581.

Brzosko Z, Schultz W, Paulsen O (2015) Retroactive modulation of spike timing-dependent plasticity by dopamine. *Elife* 4:e09685.

Bseikri MR, Barton JR, Kulhanjian JA, Dalmau J, Cohen RA, Glaser CA, Roy-Burman A (2012) Anti-N-methyl D-aspartate receptor encephalitis mimics viral encephalitis. *Pediatr Infect Dis J* 31:202–204.

Buchanan KA, Petrovic MM, Chamberlain SE, Marrion NV, Mellor JR (2010) Facilitation of long-term potentiation by muscarinic M(1) receptors is mediated by inhibition of SK channels. *Neuron* 68:948–963.

Buonarati OR, Miller AP, Coultrap SJ, Bayer KU, Reichow SL (2021) Conserved and divergent features of neuronal CaMKII holoenzyme structure, function, and high-order assembly. *Cell Rep* 37:110168.

Busche MA, Eichhoff G, Adelsberger H, Abramowski D, Wiederhold KH, Haass C, Staufenbiel M, Konnerth A, Garaschuk O (2008) Clusters of hyperactive neurons near amyloid plaques in a mouse model of Alzheimer's disease. *Science* 321:1686–1689.

Butler MP, O'Connor JJ, Moynagh PN (2004) Dissection of tumor-necrosis factor-alpha inhibition of long-term potentiation (LTP) reveals a p38 mitogen-activated protein kinase-dependent mechanism which maps to early-but not late-phase LTP. *Neuroscience* 124:319–326.

Buzsáki G (2009) Rhythms of the Brain. Oxford: Oxford University Press.

Buzsaki G (2015) Hippocampal sharp wave-ripple: a cognitive biomarker for episodic memory and planning. *Hippocampus* 25:1073–1188.

Bye CM, McDonald RJ (2019) A specific role of hippocampal NMDA receptors and arc protein in rapid encoding of novel environmental representations and a more general long-term consolidation function. *Front Behav Neurosci* 13:8.

Cai DJ, Aharoni D, Shuman T, Shobe J, Biane J, Song W, Wei B, Veshkini M, La-Vu M, Lou J, et al. (2016) A shared neural ensemble links distinct contextual memories encoded close in time. *Nature* 534:115–118.

Cain DP, Hargreaves EL, Boon F, Dennison Z (1993) An examination of the relations between hippocampal long-term potentiation, kindling, afterdischarge, and place learning in the water maze. *Hippocampus* 3:153–163.

Campbell IG, Guinan MJ, Horowitz JM (2002) Sleep deprivation impairs long-term potentiation in rat hippocampal slices. *J Neurophysiol* 88:1073–1076.

Campion D, Dumanchin C, Hannequin D, Dubois B, Belliard S, Puel M, Thomas-Anterion C, Michon A, Martin C, Charbonnier F, et al. (1999) Early-onset autosomal dominant Alzheimer disease: prevalence, genetic heterogeneity, and mutation spectrum. *Am J Hum Genet* 65:664–670.

Canals S, Beyerlein M, Merkle H, Logothetis NK (2009) Functional MRI evidence for LTP-induced neural network reorganization. *Curr Biol* 19:398–403.

Canetta SE, Brown AS (2012) Prenatal infection, maternal immune activation, and risk for schizophrenia. *Transl Neurosci* 3:320–327.

Cao F, Zhou Z, Pan X, Leung C, Xie W, Collingridge G, Jia Z (2017) Developmental regulation of hippocampal long-term depression by cofilin-mediated actin reorganization. *Neuropharmacology* 112:66–75.

Caramés JM, Pérez-Montoyo E, Garcia-Hernandez R, Canals S (2020) Hippocampal dentate gyrus coordinates brain-wide communication and memory updating through an inhibitory gating. *bioRxiv* 2020. 07. 14.202218.

Carhart-Harris RL, Roseman L, Bolstridge M, Demetriou L, Pannekoek JN, Wall MB, Tanner M, Kaelen M, McGonigle J, Murphy K, et al. (2017) Psilocybin for treatment-resistant depression: fMRI-measured brain mechanisms. *Sci Rep* 7:13187.

Carlen M, Meletis K, Siegle JH, Cardin JA, Futai K, Vierling-Claassen D, Ruhlmann C, Jones SR, Deisseroth K, Sheng M, et al. (2012) A critical role for NMDA receptors in parvalbumin interneurons for gamma rhythm induction and behavior. *Mol Psychiatry* 17:537–548.

Carlisle HJ, Fink AE, Grant SG, O'Dell TJ (2008) Opposing effects of PSD-93 and PSD-95 on long-term potentiation and spike timing-dependent plasticity. *J Physiol* 586:5885–5900.

Carstens KE, Dudek SM (2019) Regulation of synaptic plasticity in hippocampal area CA2. *Curr Opin Neurobiol* 54:194–199.

Castagné V, Moser P, Roux S, Porsolt RD (2010) Rodent models of depression: forced swim and tail suspension behavioral despair tests in rats and mice. *Curr Protoc Pharmacol* Chapter 5: Unit 5.8. doi:10.1002/0471141755.ph0508s49

Castro CA, Silbert LH, McNaughton BL, Barnes CA (1989) Recovery of spatial learning deficits after decay of electrically induced synaptic enhancement in the hippocampus. *Nature* 342:545–548.

Cavallucci V, Berretta N, Nobili A, Nistico R, Mercuri NB, D'Amelio M (2013) Calcineurin inhibition rescues early synaptic plasticity deficits in a mouse model of Alzheimer's disease. *Neuromolecular Med* 15:541–548.

Cepeda NJ, Pashler H, Vul E, Wixted JT, Rohrer D (2006) Distributed practice in verbal recall tasks: a review and quantitative synthesis. *Psychol Bull* 132:354–380.

Cepeda-Prado EA, Khodaie B, Quiceno GD, Beythien S, Edelmann E, Lessmann V (2022) Calcium-permeable AMPA receptors mediate timing-dependent LTP elicited by low repeat coincident pre- and postsynaptic activity at Schaffer collateral-CA1 synapses. *Cereb Cortex* 32:1682–1703.

Chang Q, Khare G, Dani V, Nelson S, Jaenisch R (2006) The disease progression of Mecp2 mutant mice is affected by the level of BDNF expression. *Neuron* 49:341–348.

Chao HT, Chen H, Samaco RC, Xue M, Chahrour M, Yoo J, Neul JL, Gong S, Lu HC, Heintz N, et al. (2010) Dysfunction in GABA signalling mediates autism-like stereotypies and Rett syndrome phenotypes. *Nature* 468:263–269.

Chapman PF, White GL, Jones MW, Cooper-Blacketer D, Marshall VJ, Irizarry M, Younkin L, Good MA, Bliss TV, Hyman BT, et al. (1999) Impaired synaptic plasticity and learning in aged amyloid precursor protein transgenic mice. *Nat Neurosci* 2:271–276.

Chaudhury D, Wang LM, Colwell CS (2005) Circadian regulation of hippocampal long-term potentiation. *J Biol Rhythms* 20:225–236.

Chavez-Noriega LE, Bliss TVP, Halliwell JV (1989) The EPSP-spike (E-S) component of long-term potentiation in the rat hippocampal slice is modulated by GABAergic but not cholinergic mechanisms. *Neurosci Lett* 104:58–64.

Chevaleyre V, Castillo PE (2003) Heterosynaptic LTD of hippocampal GABAergic synapses: a novel role of endocannabinoids in regulating excitability. *Neuron* 38:461–472.

Chevaleyre V, Piskorowski R (2014) Modulating excitation through plasticity at inhibitory synapses. *Front Cell Neurosci* 8:93.

Chevaleyre V, Siegelbaum SA (2010) Strong CA2 pyramidal neuron synapses define a powerful disynaptic cortico-hippocampal loop. *Neuron* 66:560–572.

Chipman PH, Fung CCA, Pazo Fernandez A, Sawant A, Tedoldi A, Kawai A, Ghimire Gautam S, Kurosawa M, Abe M, Sakimura K, et al. (2021) Astrocyte GluN2C NMDA receptors control basal synaptic strengths of hippocampal CA1 pyramidal neurons in the stratum radiatum. *Elife* 10:e70818.

Chiu AM, Wang J, Fiske MP, Hubalkova P, Barse L, Gray JA, Sanz-Clemente A (2019) NMDAR-Activated PP1 dephosphorylates GluN2B to modulate NMDAR synaptic content. *Cell Rep* 28:332–341, e335.

Choi DI, Kim J, Lee H, Kim JI, Sung Y, Choi JE, Venkat SJ, Park P, Jung H, Kaang BK (2021) Synaptic correlates of associative fear memory in the lateral amygdala. *Neuron* 109:2717–2726, e2713.

Choi JH, Sim SE, Kim JI, Choi DI, Oh J, Ye S, Lee J, Kim T, Ko HG, Lim CS, et al. (2018) Interregional synaptic maps among engram cells underlie memory formation. *Science* 360:430–435.

Choquet D (2018) Linking nanoscale dynamics of AMPA receptor organization to plasticity of excitatory synapses and learning. *J Neurosci* **38**:9318–9329.

Chowdhury S, Shepherd JD, Okuno H, Lyford G, Petralia RS, Plath N, Kuhl D, Huganir RL, Worley PF (2006) Arc/Arg3.1 interacts with the endocytic machinery to regulate AMPA receptor trafficking. *Neuron* **52**:445–459.

Claiborne N, Anisimova M, Zito K (2024) Activity-dependent stabilization of nascent dendritic spines requires nonenzymatic CaMKIIα function. *J Neurosci* **44**:e1393222023.

Clark JK, Madison DV (2020) Control of E-S potentiation at two different sites in the dendro-somatic axis. *bioRxiv* 2020.02.21.960138.

Clayton EL, Sue N, Smillie KJ, O'Leary T, Bache N, Cheung G, Cole AR, Wyllie DJ, Sutherland C, Robinson PJ, et al. (2010) Dynamin I phosphorylation by GSK3 controls activity-dependent bulk endocytosis of synaptic vesicles. *Nat Neurosci* **13**:845–851.

Collingridge GL (1985) Long-term potentiation in the hippocampus— mechanisms of initiation and modulation by neurotransmitters. *Trends Pharmacol Sci* **6**:407–411.

Collingridge GL, Abraham WC (2022) Glutamate receptors and synaptic plasticity: the impact of Evans and Watkins. *Neuropharmacology* **206**:108922.

Collingridge GL, Herron C, Lester RAJ (1988) Synaptic activation of N-methyl-D-aspartate receptors in the Schaffer collateral-commissural pathway of rat hippocampus. *J Physiol* **399**:283–300.

Collingridge GL, Kehl SJ, McLennan H (1983) Excitatory amino acids in synaptic transmission in the Schaffer collateral-commissural pathway of the rat hippocampus. *J Physiol* **334**:33–46.

Collingridge GL, Peineau S, Howland JG, Wang YT (2010) Long-term depression in the CNS. *Nat Rev Neurosci* **11**:459–473.

Collins AL, Levenson JM, Vilaythong AP, Richman R, Armstrong DL, Noebels JL, David Sweatt J, Zoghbi HY (2004) Mild overexpression of MeCP2 causes a progressive neurological disorder in mice. *Hum Mol Genet* **13**:2679–2689.

Connor SA, Hoeffer CA, Klann E, Nguyen PV (2011) Fragile X mental retardation protein regulates heterosynaptic plasticity in the hippocampus. *Learn Mem* **18**:207–220.

Constals A, Penn AC, Compans B, Toulmé E, Phillipat A, Marais S, Retailleau N, Hafner AS, Coussen F, Hosy E, et al. (2015) Glutamate-induced AMPA receptor desensitization increases their mobility and modulates short-term plasticity through unbinding from Stargazin. *Neuron* **85**:787–803.

Cooke SF, Bear MF (2010) Visual experience induces long-term potentiation in the primary visual cortex. *J Neurosci* **30**:16304–16313.

Cooke SF, Bliss TV (2005) Long-term potentiation and cognitive drug discovery. *Curr Opin Investig Drugs* **6**:25–34.

Cooper DD, Frenguelli BG (2021) The influence of sensory experience on the glutamatergic synapse. *Neuropharmacology* **193**:108620.

Cooper LN, Bear MF (2012) The BCM theory of synapse modification at 30: interaction of theory with experiment. *Nat Rev Neurosci* **13**:798–810.

Cooper LN, Liberman F, Oja E (1979) A theory for the acquisition and loss of neuron specificity in visual cortex. *Biol Cybern* **33**:9–28.

Cordoba Montoya DA, Carrer HF (1997) Estrogen facilitates induction of long term potentiation in the hippocampus of awake rats. *Brain Res* **778**:430–438.

Costa AC, Grybko MJ (2005) Deficits in hippocampal CA1 LTP induced by TBS but not HFS in the Ts65Dn mouse: a model of Down syndrome. *Neurosci Lett* **382**:317–322.

Costa RM, Federov NB, Kogan JH, Murphy GG, Stern J, Ohno M, Kucherlapati R, Jacks T, Silva AJ (2002) Mechanism for the learning deficits in a mouse model of neurofibromatosis type 1. *Nature* **415**:526–530.

Costa RM, Silva AJ (2002) Molecular and cellular mechanisms underlying the cognitive deficits associated with neurofibromatosis 1. *J Child Neurol* **17**:622–626; discussion 627–629, 646–651.

Coultrap SJ, Freund RK, O'Leary H, Sanderson JL, Roche KW, Dell'Acqua ML, Bayer KU (2014) Autonomous CaMKII mediates both LTP and LTD using a mechanism for differential substrate site selection. *Cell Rep* **6**:431–437.

Cowansage KK, Shuman T, Dillingham BC, Chang A, Golshani P, Mayford M (2014) Direct reactivation of a coherent neocortical memory of context. *Neuron* **84**:432–441.

Coyle JT (2006) Glutamate and schizophrenia: beyond the dopamine hypothesis. *Cell Mol Neurobiol* **26**:365–384.

Coyle JT, Price DL, DeLong MR (1983) Alzheimer's disease: a disorder of cortical cholinergic innervation. *Science* **219**:1184–1190.

Cracco JB, Serrano P, Moskowitz SI, Bergold PJ, Sacktor TC (2005) Protein synthesis-dependent LTP in isolated dendrites of CA1 pyramidal cells. *Hippocampus* **15**:551–556.

Crawford DC, Acuna JM, Sherman SL (2001) FMR1 and the fragile X syndrome: human genome epidemiology review. *Genet Med* **3**:359–371.

Creed M, Pascoli VJ, Luscher C (2015) Addiction therapy: refining deep brain stimulation to emulate optogenetic treatment of synaptic pathology. *Science* **347**:659–664.

Cretin B, Sellal F, Philippi N, Bousiges O, Di Bitonto L, Martin-Hunyadi C, Blanc F (2016) Epileptic prodromal Alzheimer's disease, a retrospective study of 13 new cases: expanding the spectrum of Alzheimer's disease to an epileptic variant? *J Alzheimers Dis* **52**:1125–1133.

Crow TJ (1968) Cortical synapses and reinforcement: a hypothesis. *Nature* **219**:736–737.

Cui Y, Costa RM, Murphy GG, Elgersma Y, Zhu Y, Gutmann DH, Parada LF, Mody I, Silva AJ (2008) Neurofibromin regulation of ERK signaling modulates GABA release and learning. *Cell* **135**:549–560.

Cull-Candy SG, Leszkiewicz DN (2004) Role of distinct NMDA receptor subtypes at central synapses. *Sci STKE* **2004**:re16.

Cullen WK, Suh YH, Anwyl R, Rowan MJ (1997) Block of LTP in rat hippocampus in vivo by beta-amyloid precursor protein fragments. *Neuroreport* **8**:3213–3217.

Cummings JA, Mulkey RM, Nicoll RA, Malenka RC (1996) Ca^{2+} signaling requirements for long-term depression in the hippocampus. *Neuron* **16**:825–833.

Cutting LE, Levine TM (2010) Cognitive profile of children with neurofibromatosis and reading disabilities. *Child Neuropsychol* **16**:417–432.

Dale N, Roberts A (1985) Dual-component amino-acid-mediated synaptic potentials: excitatory drive for swimming in Xenopus embryos. *J Physiol* **363**:35–59.

D'Amelio M, Cavallucci V, Middei S, Marchetti C, Pacioni S, Ferri A, Diamantini A, De Zio D, Carrara P, Battistini L, et al. (2011) Caspase-3 triggers early synaptic dysfunction in a mouse model of Alzheimer's disease. *Nat Neurosci* **14**:69–76.

Danysz W, Zajaczkowski W, Parsons CG (1995) Modulation of learning processes by ionotropic glutamate receptor ligands. *Behav Pharmacol* **6**:455–474.

Dargan SL, Clarke VR, Alushin GM, Sherwood JL, Nisticò R, Bortolotto ZA, Ogden AM, Bleakman D, Doherty AJ, Lodge D, et al. (2009) ACET is a highly potent and specific kainate receptor antagonist: characterisation and effects on hippocampal mossy fibre function. *Neuropharmacology* **56**:121–130.

Dasgupta A, Lim YJ, Kumar K, Baby N, Pang KLK, Benoy A, Behnisch T, Sajikumar S (2020) Group III metabotropic glutamate receptors gate long-term potentiation and synaptic tagging/capture in rat hippocampal area CA2. *Elife* 9:e55344.

Davies P, Maloney AJ (1976) Selective loss of central cholinergic neurons in Alzheimer's disease. *Lancet* 2:1403.

Davies SN, Alford ST, Coan EJ, Lester RA, Collingridge GL (1988) Ketamine blocks an NMDA receptor-mediated component of synaptic transmission in rat hippocampus in a voltage-dependent manner. *Neurosci Lett* 92:213–217.

Davis JA, Kenney JW, Gould TJ (2007) Hippocampal alpha4beta2 nicotinic acetylcholine receptor involvement in the enhancing effect of acute nicotine on contextual fear conditioning. *J Neurosci* 27:10870–10877.

Davis M, Falls WA, Campeau S, Kim M (1993) Fear-potentiated startle: a neural and pharmacological analysis. *Behav Brain Res* 58:175–198.

Davis S, Butcher SP, Morris RG (1992) The NMDA receptor antagonist D-2-amino-5-phosphonopentanoate (D-AP5) impairs spatial learning and LTP in vivo at intracerebral concentrations comparable to those that block LTP in vitro. *J Neurosci* 12:21–34.

Davisson MT, Schmidt C, Reeves RH, Irving NG, Akeson EC, Harris BS, Bronson RT (1993) Segmental trisomy as a mouse model for Down syndrome. *Prog Clin Biol Res* 384:117–133.

Dayan P, Abbott LF (2001) Theoretical neuroscience: computational and mathematical modeling of neural systems. Cambridge, MA: Massachusetts Institute of Technology Press.

Dayan P, Willshaw DJ (1991) Optimising synaptic learning rules in linear associative memories. *Biol Cybern* 65:253–265.

Debanne D, Gahwiler BH, Thompson SM (1994) Asynchronous pre- and postsynaptic activity induces associative long-term depression in area CA1 of the rat hippocampus in vitro. *Proc Natl Acad Sci U S A* 91:1148–1152.

Decker A, Finn A, Duncan K (2020) Errors lead to transient impairments in memory formation. *Cognition* 204:104338.

Denayer E, Ahmed T, Brems H, Van Woerden G, Borgesius NZ, Callaerts-Vegh Z, Yoshimura A, Hartmann D, Elgersma Y, D'Hooge R, et al. (2008) Spred1 is required for synaptic plasticity and hippocampus-dependent learning. *J Neurosci* 28:14443–14449.

De Roo M, Klauser P, Muller D (2008) LTP promotes a selective long-term stabilization and clustering of dendritic spines. *PLoS Biol* 6:e219.

Desmond NL, Levy WB (1983) Synaptic correlates of associative potentiation/depression: an ultrastructural study in the hippocampus. *Brain Res* 265:21–30.

de Sousa AF, Chowdhury A, Silva AJ (2021) Dimensions and mechanisms of memory organization. *Neuron* 109:2649–2662.

De Vincenti AP, Ríos AS, Paratcha G, Ledda F (2019) Mechanisms that modulate and diversify BDNF functions: implications for hippocampal synaptic plasticity. *Front Cell Neurosci* 13:135.

de Vivo L, Bellesi M, Marshall W, Bushong EA, Ellisman MH, Tononi G, Cirelli C (2017) Ultrastructural evidence for synaptic scaling across the wake/sleep cycle. *Science* 355:507–510.

Dibonaventura M, Gabriel S, Dupclay L, Gupta S, Kim E (2012) A patient perspective of the impact of medication side effects on adherence: results of a cross-sectional nationwide survey of patients with schizophrenia. *BMC Psychiatry* 12:20.

Dickinson BA, Jo J, Seok H, Son GH, Whitcomb DJ, Davies CH, Sheng M, Collingridge GL, Cho K (2009) A novel mechanism of hippocampal LTD involving muscarinic receptor-triggered interactions between AMPARs, GRIP and liprin-alpha. *Mol Brain* 2:18.

Diekelmann S, Born J (2010) The memory function of sleep. *Nat Rev Neurosci* 11:114–126.

Diering GH, Nirujogi RS, Roth RH, Worley PF, Pandey A, Huganir RL (2017) Homer1a drives homeostatic scaling-down of excitatory synapses during sleep. *Science* 355:511–515.

Dierssen M (2012) Down syndrome: the brain in trisomic mode. *Nat Rev Neurosci* 13:844–858.

Diggs-Andrews KA, Gutmann DH (2013) Modeling cognitive dysfunction in neurofibromatosis-1. *Trends Neurosci* 36:237–247.

Dingledine R, Hynes MA, King GL (1986) Involvement of N-methyl-D-aspartate receptors in epileptiform bursting in the rat hippocampal slice. *J Physiol* 380:175–189.

Do VH, Martinez CO, Martinez JL, Jr, Derrick BE (2002) Long-term potentiation in direct perforant path projections to the hippocampal CA3 region in vivo. *J Neurophysiol* 87:669–678.

Dobrunz LE, Stevens CF (1997) Heterogeneity of release probability, facilitation, and depletion at central synapses. *Neuron* 18:995–1008.

Dolen G, Osterweil E, Rao BS, Smith GB, Auerbach BD, Chattarji S, Bear MF (2007) Correction of fragile X syndrome in mice. *Neuron* 56:955–962.

Donato F, Rompani SB, Caroni P (2013) Parvalbumin-expressing basket-cell network plasticity induced by experience regulates adult learning. *Nature* 504:272–276.

Dong C, Upadhya SC, Ding L, Smith TK, Hegde AN (2008) Proteasome inhibition enhances the induction and impairs the maintenance of late-phase long-term potentiation. *Learn Mem* 15:335–347.

Dore K, Aow J, Malinow R (2015) Agonist binding to the NMDA receptor drives movement of its cytoplasmic domain without ion flow. *Proc Natl Acad Sci U S A* 112:14705–14710.

Dore K, Malinow R (2021) Elevated PSD-95 blocks ion-flux independent LTD: a potential new role for PSD-95 in synaptic plasticity. *Neuroscience* 456:43–49.

Doudna JA, Charpentier E (2014) Genome editing: the new frontier of genome engineering with CRISPR-Cas9. *Science* 346:1258096.

Draffin JE, Sánchez-Castillo C, Fernández-Rodrigo A, Sánchez-Sáez X, Ávila J, Wagner FF, Esteban JA (2021) GSK3α, not GSK3β, drives hippocampal NMDAR-dependent LTD via tau-mediated spine anchoring. *Embo J* 40:e105513.

Dudek SM, Bear MF (1992) Homosynaptic long-term depression in area CA1 of hippocampus and effects of N-methyl-D-aspartate receptor blockade. *Proc Natl Acad Sci U S A* 89:4363–4367.

Dudek SM, Bear MF (1993) Bidirectional long-term modification of synaptic effectiveness in the adult and immature hippocampus. *J Neurosci* 13:2910–2918.

Dudok B, Fan LZ, Farrell JS, Malhotra S, Homidan J, Kim DK, Wenardy C, Ramakrishnan C, Li Y, Deisseroth K, et al. (2024) Retrograde endocannabinoid signaling at inhibitory synapses in vivo. *Science* 383:967–970.

Duman RS, Li N (2012) A neurotrophic hypothesis of depression: role of synaptogenesis in the actions of NMDA receptor antagonists. *Philos Trans R Soc Lond B Biol Sci* 367:2475–2484.

Dunwiddie T, Lynch G (1978) Long-term potentiation and depression of synaptic responses in the rat hippocampus: localization and frequency dependency. *J Physiol (Lond)* 276:353–367.

Durkin J, Aton SJ (2016) Sleep-dependent potentiation in the visual system is at odds with the synaptic homeostasis hypothesis. *Sleep* 39:155–159.

Eadie BD, Cushman J, Kannangara TS, Fanselow MS, Christie BR (2012) NMDA receptor hypofunction in the dentate gyrus and impaired context discrimination in adult Fmr1 knockout mice. *Hippocampus* 22:241–254.

Eapen AV, Fernández-Fernández D, Georgiou J, Bortolotto ZA, Lightman S, Jane DE, Volianskis A, Collingridge GL (2021) Multiple roles of GluN2D-containing NMDA receptors in short-term potentiation and long-term potentiation in mouse hippocampal slices. *Neuropharmacology* 201:108833.

Ebrahim Amini A, Miyata T, Lei G, Jin F, Rubie E, Bradley CA, Woodgett JR, Collingridge GL, Georgiou J (2022) Specific role for GSK3α in limiting long-term potentiation in CA1 pyramidal neurons of adult mouse hippocampus. *Front Mol Neurosci* 15:852171.

Edelmann E, Lessmann V, Brigadski T (2014) Pre- and postsynaptic twists in BDNF secretion and action in synaptic plasticity. *Neuropharmacology* 76(Pt C):610–627.

Ehninger D, Li W, Fox K, Stryker MP, Silva AJ (2008) Reversing neurodevelopmental disorders in adults. *Neuron* 60:950–960.

Ehrlich I, Klein M, Rumpel S, Malinow R (2007) PSD-95 is required for activity-driven synapse stabilization. *Proc Natl Acad Sci U S A* 104:4176–4181.

Ehrlich I, Malinow R (2004) Postsynaptic density 95 controls AMPA receptor incorporation during long-term potentiation and experience-driven synaptic plasticity. *J Neurosci* 24:916–927.

Eichenbaum H, Stewart C, Morris RGM (1990) Hippocampal representation in place learning. *J Neurosci* 10:3531–3542.

El-Boustani S, Ip JPK, Breton-Provencher V, Knott GW, Okuno H, Bito H, Sur M (2018) Locally coordinated synaptic plasticity of visual cortex neurons in vivo. *Science* 360:1349–1354.

Elsabbagh M, Divan G, Koh YJ, Kim YS, Kauchali S, Marcin C, Montiel-Nava C, Patel V, Paula CS, Wang C, et al. (2012) Global prevalence of autism and other pervasive developmental disorders. *Autism Res* 5:160–179.

Emptage NJ, Fine A, Bliss TVP (2003) Optical quantal analysis reveals a presynaptic component of LTP at hippocampal Schaffer-associational synapses. Neuron 38:797–804.

Engert F, Bonhoeffer T (1999) Dendritic spine changes associated with hippocampal long-term synaptic plasticity. *Nature* 399:66–70.

Enoki R, Hu YL, Hamilton D, Fine A (2009) Expression of long-term plasticity at individual synapses in hippocampus is graded, bidirectional, and mainly presynaptic: optical quantal analysis. *Neuron* 62:242–253.

Espuny-Camacho I, Arranz AM, Fiers M, Snellinx A, Ando K, Munck S, Bonnefont J, Lambot L, Corthout N, Omodho L, et al. (2017) Hallmarks of Alzheimer's disease in stem-cell-derived human neurons transplanted into mouse brain. *Neuron* 93:1066–1081, e1068.

Estes ML, McAllister AK (2016) Maternal immune activation: implications for neuropsychiatric disorders. *Science* 353:772–777.

Evans RH, Francis WW, Watkins JC (1977) Selective antagonism by Mg2+ of amino acid-induced depolarization of spinal neurones. *Experientia* 15:489–491.

Fabio RA, Bianco M, Capri T, Marino F, Ruta L, Vagni D, Pioggia G (2020) Working memory and decision making in children with ADHD: an analysis of delay discounting with the use of the dual-task paradigm. *BMC Psychiatry* 20:272.

Fan LZ, Kim DK, Jennings JH, Tian H, Wang PY, Ramakrishnan C, Randles S, Sun Y, Thadhani E, Kim YS, et al. (2023) All-optical physiology resolves a synaptic basis for behavioral timescale plasticity. *Cell* 186:543–559, e19.

Farris S, Lewandowski G, Cox CD, Steward O (2014) Selective localization of arc mRNA in dendrites involves activity- and translation-dependent mRNA degradation. *J Neurosci* 34:4481–4493.

Farzin F, Perry H, Hessl D, Loesch D, Cohen J, Bacalman S, Gane L, Tassone F, Hagerman P, Hagerman R (2006) Autism spectrum disorders and attention-deficit/hyperactivity disorder in boys with the fragile X premutation. *J Dev Behav Pediatr* 27:S137–144.

Feigenson KA, Kusnecov AW, Silverstein SM (2014) Inflammation and the two-hit hypothesis of schizophrenia. *Neurosci Biobehav Rev* 38:72–93.

Feinberg EH, Vanhoven MK, Bendesky A, Wang G, Fetter RD, Shen K, Bargmann CI (2008) GFP Reconstitution Across Synaptic Partners (GRASP) defines cell contacts and synapses in living nervous systems. *Neuron* 57:353–363.

Feldman DE (2012) The spike-timing dependence of plasticity. *Neuron* 75:556–571.

Ferrario CR, Reagan LP (2018) Insulin-mediated synaptic plasticity in the CNS: anatomical, functional and temporal contexts. *Neuropharmacology* 136:182–191.

Filippini N, MacIntosh BJ, Hough MG, Goodwin GM, Frisoni GB, Smith SM, Matthews PM, Beckmann CF, Mackay CE (2009) Distinct patterns of brain activity in young carriers of the APOE-epsilon4 allele. *Proc Natl Acad Sci U S A* 106:7209–7214.

Fiore R, Rajman M, Schwale C, Bicker S, Antoniou A, Bruehl C, Draguhn A, Schratt G (2014) MiR-134-dependent regulation of Pumilio-2 is necessary for homeostatic synaptic depression. *EMBO J* 33:2231–2246.

Fitzjohn SM, Morton RA, Kuenzi F, Rosahl TW, Shearman M, Lewis H, Smith D, Reynolds DS, Davies CH, Collingridge GL, et al. (2001) Age-related impairment of synaptic transmission but normal long-term potentiation in transgenic mice that overexpress the human APP695SWE mutant form of amyloid precursor protein. *J Neurosci* 21:4691–4698.

Fonseca R, Vabulas RM, Hartl FU, Bonhoeffer T, Nägerl UV (2006) A balance of protein synthesis and proteasome-dependent degradation determines the maintenance of LTP. *Neuron* 52:239–245.

France G, Fernández-Fernández D, Burnell ES, Irvine MW, Monaghan DT, Jane DE, Bortolotto ZA, Collingridge GL, Volianskis A (2017) Multiple roles of GluN2B-containing NMDA receptors in synaptic plasticity in juvenile hippocampus. *Neuropharmacology* 112:76–83.

Francis PT, Palmer AM, Sims NR, Bowen DM, Davison AN, Esiri MM, Neary D, Snowden JS, Wilcock GK (1985) Neurochemical studies of early-onset Alzheimer's disease: possible influence on treatment. *N Engl J Med* 313:7–11.

Frank MG (2012) Erasing synapses in sleep: is it time to be SHY? *Neural Plast* 2012:264378.

Frank RA, Komiyama NH, Ryan TJ, Zhu F, O'Dell TJ, Grant SG (2016) NMDA receptors are selectively partitioned into complexes and supercomplexes during synapse maturation. *Nat Commun* 7:11264.

Frankland PW, Bontempi B (2005) The organization of recent and remote memories. *Nat Rev Neurosci* 6:119–130.

Frey S, Bergado-Rosado J, Seidenbecher T, Pape HC, Frey JU (2001) Reinforcement of early long-term potentiation (early-LTP) in dentate gyrus by stimulation of the basolateral amygdala: heterosynaptic induction mechanisms of late-LTP. *J Neurosci* 21:3697–3703.

Frey U, Huang YY, Kandel ER (1993) Effects of cAMP simulate a late stage of LTP in hippocampal CA1 neurons. *Science* 260:1661–1664.

Frey U, Krug M, Reymann KG, Matthies H (1988) Anisomycin, an inhibitor of protein synthesis, blocks late phases of LTP phenomena in the hippocampal CA1 region in vitro. *Brain Res* 452:57–65.

Frey U, Matthies H, Reymann KG (1991) The effect of dopaminergic D1 receptor blockade during tetanization on the expression of long-term potentiation in the rat CA1 region in vitro. *Neurosci Lett* 129:111–114.

Frey U, Morris RG (1997) Synaptic tagging and long-term potentiation. *Nature* 385:533–536.

Frey U, Morris RGM (1998a) Synaptic tagging: implications for late maintenance of hippocampal long-term potentiation. *Trends Neurosci* 21:181–188.

Frey U, Morris RGM (1998b) Weak before strong: dissociating synaptic tagging and plasticity-factor accounts of late-LTP. *Neuropharmacology* 37:545–552.

Frey U, Schroeder H, Matthies H (1990) Dopaminergic antagonists prevent long-term maintenance of posttetanic LTP in the CA1 region of rat hippocampal slices. *Brain Res* 522:69–75.

Frick KM, Kim J, Tuscher JJ, Fortress AM (2015) Sex steroid hormones matter for learning and memory: estrogenic regulation of hippocampal function in male and female rodents. *Learn Mem* 22:472–493.

Fromer M, Pocklington AJ, Kavanagh DH, Williams HJ, Dwyer S, Gormley P, Georgieva L, Rees E, Palta P, Ruderfer DM, et al. (2014) De novo mutations in schizophrenia implicate synaptic networks. *Nature* 506:179–184.

Fujii S, Jia Y, Yang A, Sumikawa K (2000) Nicotine reverses GABAergic inhibition of long-term potentiation induction in the hippocampal CA1 region. *Brain Res* 863:259–265.

Furukawa K, Barger SW, Blalock EM, Mattson MP (1996) Activation of K+ channels and suppression of neuronal activity by secreted beta-amyloid-precursor protein. *Nature* 379:74–78.

Gabbouj S, Ryhänen S, Marttinen M, Wittrahm R, Takalo M, Kemppainen S, Martiskainen H, Tanila H, Haapasalo A, Hiltunen M, et al. (2019) Altered insulin signaling in Alzheimer's disease brain—special emphasis on PI3K-Akt pathway. *Front Neurosci* 13:629.

Gable MS, Sheriff H, Dalmau J, Tilley DH, Glaser CA (2012) The frequency of autoimmune N-methyl-D-aspartate receptor encephalitis surpasses that of individual viral etiologies in young individuals enrolled in the California Encephalitis Project. *Clin Infect Dis* 54:899–904.

Gainey MA, Hurvitz-Wolff JR, Lambo ME, Turrigiano GG (2009) Synaptic scaling requires the GluR2 subunit of the AMPA receptor. *J Neurosci* 29:6479–6489.

Gall CM, Hess US, Lynch G (1998) Mapping brain networks engaged by, and changed by, learning. *Neurobiol Learn Mem* 70:14–36.

Gall CM, Le AA, Lynch G (2021) Sex differences in synaptic plasticity underlying learning. *J Neurosci Res* 101:764–782.

Gall CM, Le AA, Lynch G (2024) Contributions of site- and sex-specific LTPs to everyday memory. *Philos Trans R Soc Lond B Biol Sci* 379:20230223 https://doi.org/10.1098/rstb.2023.0223.

Galvan EJ, Cosgrove KE, Barrionuevo G (2011) Multiple forms of long-term synaptic plasticity at hippocampal mossy fiber synapses on interneurons. *Neuropharmacology* 60:740–747.

Galvan EJ, Perez-Rosello T, Gomez-Lira G, Lara E, Gutierrez R, Barrionuevo G (2015) Synapse-specific compartmentalization of signaling cascades for LTP induction in CA3 interneurons. *Neuroscience* 290:332–345.

Garcia-Cerro S, Martinez P, Vidal V, Corrales A, Florez J, Vidal R, Rueda N, Arbones ML, Martinez-Cue C (2014) Overexpression of Dyrk1A is implicated in several cognitive, electrophysiological and neuromorphological alterations found in a mouse model of Down syndrome. *PLoS One* 9:e106572.

Gardoni F, Di Luca M (2021) Protein-protein interactions at the NMDA receptor complex: from synaptic retention to synaptonuclear protein messengers. *Neuropharmacology* 190:108551.

Gardoni F, Mauceri D, Malinverno M, Polli F, Costa C, Tozzi A, Siliquini S, Picconi B, Cattabeni F, Calabresi P, et al. (2009) Decreased NR2B subunit synaptic levels cause impaired long-term potentiation but not long-term depression. *J Neurosci* 29:669–677.

Ge M, Song H, Li H, Li R, Tao X, Zhan X, Yu N, Sun N, Lu Y, Mu Y (2019) Memory susceptibility to retroactive interference is developmentally regulated by NMDA receptors. *Cell Rep* 26:2052–2063, e2054.

Ge S, Dani JA (2005) Nicotinic acetylcholine receptors at glutamate synapses facilitate long-term depression or potentiation. *J Neurosci* 25:6084–6091.

Gejman PV, Sanders AR, Kendler KS (2011) Genetics of schizophrenia: new findings and challenges. *Annu Rev Genomics Hum Genet* 12:121–144.

Getz AM, Ducros M, Breillat C, Lampin-Saint-Amaux A, Daburon S, François U, Nowacka A, Fernández-Monreal M, Hosy E, Lanore F, et al. (2022) High-resolution imaging and manipulation of endogenous AMPA receptor surface mobility during synaptic plasticity and learning. *Sci Adv* 8:eabm5298.

Giese KP, Aziz W, Kraev I, Stewart MG (2015) Generation of multi-innervated dendritic spines as a novel mechanism of long-term memory formation. *Neurobiol Learn Mem* 124:48–51.

Gilbert J, Man HY (2017) Fundamental elements in autism: from neurogenesis and neurite growth to synaptic plasticity. *Front Cell Neurosci* 11:359.

Giocomo LM, Hasselmo ME (2005) Nicotinic modulation of glutamatergic synaptic transmission in region CA3 of the hippocampus. *Eur J Neurosci* 22:1349–1356.

Glerup S, Bolcho U, Mølgaard S, Bøggild S, Vaegter CB, Smith AH, Nieto-Gonzalez JL, Ovesen PL, Pedersen LF, Fjorback AN, et al. (2016) SorCS2 is required for BDNF-dependent plasticity in the hippocampus. *Mol Psychiatry* 21:1740–1751.

Goddard GV, McNaughton BL, Douglas RM, Barnes CA (1978) Synaptic change in the limbic system; evidence from studies using electrical stimulation with and without seizure activity. In: Limbic Mechanisms (Livingston KE Hornykiewicz O, eds), pp 355–368. Boston, MA: Springer. https://doi.org/10.1007/978-1-4757-0716-8_14.

Goedert M (2018) Tau filaments in neurodegenerative diseases. *FEBS Lett* 592:2383–2391.

Goh JJ, Manahan-Vaughan D (2013) Synaptic depression in the CA1 region of freely behaving mice is highly dependent on afferent stimulation parameters. *Front Integr Neurosci* 7:1.

Gold PE, Delanoy RL, Merrin J (1984) Modulation of long-term potentiation by peripherally administered amphetamine and epinephrine. *Brain Res* 305:103–107.

Goodell DJ, Zaegel V, Coultrap SJ, Hell JW, Bayer KU (2017) DAPK1 mediates LTD by making CaMKII/GluN2B binding LTP specific. *Cell Rep* 19:2231–2243.

Goold CP, Nicoll RA (2010) Single-cell optogenetic excitation drives homeostatic synaptic depression. *Neuron* 68:512–528.

Goshen I, Brodsky M, Prakash R, Wallace J, Gradinaru V, Ramakrishnan C, Deisseroth K (2011) Dynamics of retrieval strategies for remote memories. *Cell* 147:678–689.

Goto A, Bota A, Miya K, Wang J, Tsukamoto S, Jiang X, Hirai D, Murayama M, Matsuda T, McHugh TJ, et al. (2021) Stepwise synaptic plasticity events drive the early phase of memory consolidation. *Science* 374:857–863.

Gould E, Wooley CS, Frandkfurt M, McEwen BS (1990) Gonadal-steroids regulate dendritic spine density in hippocampal pyramidal cells in adulthood. *J Neurosci* 10:1286–1291.

Govindarajan A, Israely I, Huang SY, Tonegawa S (2011) The dendritic branch is the preferred integrative unit for protein synthesis-dependent LTP. *Neuron* 69:132–146.

Govindarajan A, Kelleher RJ, Tonegawa S (2006) A clustered plasticity model of long-term memory engrams. *Nat Rev Neurosci* 7:575–583.

Gralle M (2017) The neuronal insulin receptor in its environment. *J Neurochem* 140:359–367.

Granger AJ, Shi Y, Lu W, Cerpas M, Nicoll RA (2013) LTP requires a reserve pool of glutamate receptors independent of subunit type. *Nature* 493:495–500.

Gray R, Rajan AS, Radcliffe KA, Yakehiro M, Dani JA (1996) Hippocampal synaptic transmission enhanced by low concentrations of nicotine. *Nature* 383:713–716.

Griffiths RR, Johnson MW, Carducci MA, Umbricht A, Richards WA, Richards BD, Cosimano MP, Klinedinst MA (2016) Psilocybin produces substantial and sustained decreases in depression and anxiety in patients with life-threatening cancer: a randomized double-blind trial. *J Psychopharmacol* 30:1181–1197.

Griffiths S, Scott H, Glover C, Bienemann A, Ghorbel MT, Uney J, Brown MW, Warburton EC, Bashir ZI (2008) Expression of long-term depression underlies visual recognition memory. *Neuron* 58:186–194.

Grigoryan G, Harada H, Knobloch-Bollmann HS, Kilias A, Kaufhold D, Kulik A, Eyre MD, Bartos M (2023) Synaptic plasticity at the dentate gyrus granule cell to somatostatin-expressing interneuron synapses supports object location memory. *Proc Natl Acad Sci U S A* 120:e2312752120.

Grillner S (2006) Biological pattern generation: the cellular and computational logic of networks in motion. *Neuron* 52:751–766.

Groc L, Choquet D, Chaouloff F (2008) The stress hormone corticosterone conditions AMPAR surface trafficking and synaptic potentiation. *Nat Neurosci* 11:868–870.

Grosso S, Brogna A, Bazzotti S, Renieri A, Morgese G, Balestri P (2007) Seizures and electroencephalographic findings in CDKL5 mutations: case report and review. *Brain Dev* 29:239–242.

Gruart A, Munoz MD, Delgado-Garcia JM (2006) Involvement of the CA3-CA1 synapse in the acquisition of associative learning in behaving mice. *J Neurosci* 26:1077–1087.

Gu QH, Yu D, Hu Z, Liu X, Yang Y, Luo Y, Zhu J, Li Z (2015) miR-26a and miR-384-5p are required for LTP maintenance and spine enlargement. *Nat Commun* 6:6789.

Guan ZZ, Miao H, Tian JY, Unger C, Nordberg A, Zhang X (2001) Suppressed expression of nicotinic acetylcholine receptors by nanomolar beta-amyloid peptides in PC12 cells. *J Neural Transm (Vienna)* 108:1417–1433.

Guasp M, Dalmau J (2018) Encephalitis associated with antibodies against the NMDA receptor. *Med Clin (Barc)* 151:71–79.

Guerrin CGJ, Doorduin J, Sommer IE, de Vries EFJ (2021) The dual hit hypothesis of schizophrenia: evidence from animal models. *Neurosci Biobehav Rev* 131:1150–1168.

Gugustea R, Jia Z (2021) Genetic manipulations of AMPA glutamate receptors in hippocampal synaptic plasticity. *Neuropharmacology* 194:108630.

Guilding C, McNair K, Stone TW, Morris BJ (2007) Restored plasticity in a mouse model of neurofibromatosis type 1 via inhibition of hyperactive ERK and CREB. *Eur J Neurosci* 25:99–105.

Guire ES, Oh MC, Soderling TR, Derkach VA (2008) Recruitment of calcium-permeable AMPA receptors during synaptic potentiation is regulated by CaM-kinase I. *J Neurosci* 28:6000–6009.

Gulyás AI, Megías M, Emri Z, Freund TF (1999) Total number and ratio of excitatory and inhibitory synapses converging onto single interneurons of different types in the CA1 area of the rat hippocampus. *J Neurosci* 19:10082–10097.

Guo N, Soden ME, Herber C, Kim MT, Besnard A, Lin P, Ma X, Cepko CL, Zweifel LS, Sahay A (2018) Dentate granule cell recruitment of feedforward inhibition governs engram maintenance and remote memory generalization. *Nat Med* 24:438–449.

Guo Q, Fu W, Sopher BL, Miller MW, Ware CB, Martin GM, Mattson MP (1999) Increased vulnerability of hippocampal neurons to excitotoxic necrosis in presenilin-1 mutant knock-in mice. *Nat Med* 5:101–106.

Gustafsson B, Wigstrom H, Abraham WC, Huang YY (1987) Long-term potentiation in the hippocampus using depolarizing current pulses as the conditioning stimulus to single volley synaptic potentials. *J Neurosci* 7:774–780.

Guy J, Gan J, Selfridge J, Cobb S, Bird A (2007) Reversal of neurological defects in a mouse model of Rett syndrome. *Science* 315:1143–1147.

Guzowski JF, McNaughton BL, Barnes CA, Worley PF (1999) Environment-specific expression of the immediate-early gene Arc in hippocampal neuronal ensembles. *Nat Neurosci* 2:1120–1124.

Hagberg B, Aicardi J, Dias K, Ramos O (1983) A progressive syndrome of autism, dementia, ataxia, and loss of purposeful hand use in girls: Rett's syndrome: report of 35 cases. *Ann Neurol* 14:471–479.

Hammad H, Wagner JJ (2006) Dopamine-mediated disinhibition in the CA1 region of rat hippocampus via D3 receptor activation. *J Pharmacol Exp Ther* 316:113–120.

Hammerle B, Ulin E, Guimera J, Becker W, Guillemot F, Tejedor FJ (2011) Transient expression of Mnb/Dyrk1a couples cell cycle exit and differentiation of neuronal precursors by inducing p27KIP1 expression and suppressing NOTCH signaling. *Development* 138:2543–2554.

Han DH, Park P, Choi DI, Bliss TVP, Kaang BK (2021) The essence of the engram: cellular or synaptic? *Semin Cell Dev Biol* 125:122–135.

Han JH, Kushner SA, Yiu AP, Cole CJ, Matynia A, Brown RA, Neve RL, Guzowski JF, Silva AJ, Josselyn SA (2007) Neuronal competition and selection during memory formation. *Science* 316:457–460.

Hansen KB, Wollmuth LP, Bowie D, Furukawa H, Menniti FS, Sobolevsky AI, Swanson GT, Swanger SA, Greger IH, Nakagawa T, et al. (2021) Structure, function, and pharmacology of glutamate receptor ion channels. *Pharmacol Rev* 73:298–487.

Harney SC, Anwyl R (2012) Plasticity of NMDA receptor-mediated excitatory postsynaptic currents at perforant path inputs to dendrite-targeting interneurons. *J Physiol* 590:3771–3786.

Harris KM (2020) Structural LTP: from synaptogenesis to regulated synapse enlargement and clustering. *Curr Opin Neurobiol* 63:189–197.

Harris KM, Teyler TJ (1983) Age differences on a circadian influence on hippocampal LTP. *Brain Res* 261:69–73.

Harris KM, Kuwajima M, Flores JC, Zito K (2024) Synapse-specific structural plasticity that protects and refines local circuits during LTP and LTD. *Philos Trans R Soc Lond B Biol Sci* 379(1906):20230224.

Harvey CD, Yasuda R, Zhong H, Svoboda K (2008) The spread of Ras activity triggered by activation of a single dendritic spine. *Science* 321:136–140.

Harvey J, Palmer MJ, Irving AJ, Clarke VR, Collingridge GL (1996) NMDA receptor dependence of mGlu-mediated depression of synaptic transmission in the CA1 region of the rat hippocampus. *Br J Pharmacol* 119:1239–1247.

Hasselmo ME (2006) The role of acetylcholine in learning and memory. *Curr Opin Neurobiol* 16:710–715.

Hasselmo ME (2011) How We Remember. Cambridge, MA: MIT Press.

Hasselmo ME, Schnell E, Barkai E (1995) Dynamics of learning and recall at excitatory recurrent synapses and cholinergic modulation in rat hippocampal region CA3. *J Neurosci* 15:5249–5262.

Hayashi-Takagi A, Yagishita S, Nakamura M, Shirai F, Wu YI, Loshbaugh AL, Kuhlman B, Hahn KM, Kasai H (2015) Labelling and optical erasure of synaptic memory traces in the motor cortex. *Nature* 525:333–338.

He X, Li J, Zhou G, Yang J, McKenzie S, Li Y, Li W, Yu J, Wang Y, Qu J, et al. (2021) Gating of hippocampal rhythms and memory by synaptic plasticity in inhibitory interneurons. *Neuron* 109:1013–1028, e1019.

Hebb DO (1949) The Organization of Behavior; a Neuropsychological Theory. New York: Wiley.

Hebert LE, Bienias JL, Aggarwal NT, Wilson RS, Bennett DA, Shah RC, Evans DA (2010) Change in risk of Alzheimer disease over time. *Neurology* 75:786–791.

Hedrick NG, Harward SC, Hall CE, Murakoshi H, McNamara JO, Yasuda R (2016) Rho GTPase complementation underlies BDNF-dependent homo- and heterosynaptic plasticity. *Nature* 538:104–108.

Hegde AN, Smith SG (2019) Recent developments in transcriptional and translational regulation underlying long-term synaptic plasticity and memory. *Learn Mem* 26:307–317.

Heine M, Groc L, Frischknecht R, Béïque JC, Lounis B, Rumbaugh G, Huganir RL, Cognet L, Choquet D (2008) Surface mobility of postsynaptic AMPARs tunes synaptic transmission. *Science* 320:201–205.

Hell JW (2016) How Ca2+-permeable AMPA receptors, the kinase PKA, and the phosphatase PP2B are intertwined in synaptic LTP and LTD. *Sci Signal* 9:e2.

Hengen KB, Lambo ME, Van Hooser SD, Katz DB, Turrigiano GG (2013) Firing rate homeostasis in visual cortex of freely behaving rodents. *Neuron* 80:335–342.

Henneberger C, Bard L, Panatier A, Reynolds JP, Kopach O, Medvedev NI, Minge D, Herde MK, Anders S, Kraev I, et al. (2020) LTP induction boosts glutamate spillover by driving withdrawal of perisynaptic astroglia. *Neuron* 108:919–936, e911.

Henneberger C, Papouin T, Oliet SH, Rusakov DA (2010) Long-term potentiation depends on release of D-serine from astrocytes. *Nature* 463:232–236.

Hermiller MS, Chen YF, Parrish TB, Voss JL (2020) Evidence for immediate enhancement of hippocampal memory encoding by network-targeted theta-burst stimulation during concurrent fMRI. *J Neurosci* 40:7155–7168.

Herring BE, Nicoll RA (2016) Long-term potentiation: from CaMKII to AMPA receptor trafficking. *Annu Rev Physiol* 78:351–365.

Herron CE, Williamson R, Collingridge GL (1985) A selective N-methyl-D-aspartate antagonist depresses epileptiform activity in rat hippocampal slices. *Neurosci Lett* 61:255–260.

Heumüller M, Glock C, Rangaraju V, Biever A, Schuman EM (2019) A genetically encodable cell-type-specific protein synthesis inhibitor. *Nat Methods* 16:699–702.

Highland JN, Zanos P, Riggs LM, Georgiou P, Clark SM, Morris PJ, Moaddel R, Thomas CJ, Zarate CA, Jr, Pereira EFR et al. (2021) Hydroxynorketamines: pharmacology and potential therapeutic applications. *Pharmacol Rev* 73:763–791.

Hitti FL, Siegelbaum SA (2014) The hippocampal CA2 region is essential for social memory. *Nature* 508:88–92.

Hoeffer CA, Santini E, Ma T, Arnold EC, Whelan AM, Wong H, Pierre P, Pelletier J, Klann E (2013) Multiple components of eIF4F are required for protein synthesis-dependent hippocampal long-term potentiation. *J Neurophysiol* 109:68–76.

Holtmaat AJ, Trachtenberg JT, Wilbrecht L, Shepherd GM, Zhang X, Knott GW, Svoboda K (2005) Transient and persistent dendritic spines in the neocortex in vivo. *Neuron* 45:279–291.

Homayoun H, Moghaddam B (2007) NMDA receptor hypofunction produces opposite effects on prefrontal cortex interneurons and pyramidal neurons. *J Neurosci* 27:11496–11500.

Honey CR, Miljkovic Z, MacDonald JF (1985) Ketamine and phencyclidine cause a voltage-dependent block of responses to L-aspartic acid. *Neurosci Lett* 61:135–139.

Honkura N, Matsuzaki M, Noguchi J, Ellis-Davies GC, Kasai H (2008) The subspine organization of actin fibers regulates the structure and plasticity of dendritic spines. *Neuron* 57:719–729.

Hooper C, Killick R, Lovestone S (2008) The GSK3 hypothesis of Alzheimer's disease. *J Neurochem* 104:1433–1439.

Hooper C, Markevich V, Plattner F, Killick R, Schofield E, Engel T, Hernandez F, Anderton B, Rosenblum K, Bliss T, et al. (2007) Glycogen synthase kinase-3 inhibition is integral to long-term potentiation. *Eur J Neurosci* 25:81–86.

Horn ME, Nicoll RA (2018) Somatostatin and parvalbumin inhibitory synapses onto hippocampal pyramidal neurons are regulated by distinct mechanisms. *Proc Natl Acad Sci U S A* 115:589–594.

Hou L, Klann E (2004) Activation of the phosphoinositide 3-kinase-Akt-mammalian target of rapamycin signaling pathway is required for metabotropic glutamate receptor-dependent long-term depression. *J Neurosci* 24:6352–6361.

Howes OD, Kapur S (2009) The dopamine hypothesis of schizophrenia: version III—the final common pathway. *Schizophr Bull* 35:549–562.

Howes OD, McDonald C, Cannon M, Arseneault L, Boydell J, Murray RM (2004) Pathways to schizophrenia: the impact of environmental factors. *Int J Neuropsychopharmacol* 7(Suppl 1):S7–S13.

Hruska M, Cain RE, Dalva MB (2022) Nanoscale rules governing the organization of glutamate receptors in spine synapses are subunit specific. *Nat Commun* 13:920.

Hsiao K, Chapman P, Nilsen S, Eckman C, Harigaya Y, Younkin S, Yang F, Cole G (1996) Correlative memory deficits, Abeta elevation, and amyloid plaques in transgenic mice. *Science* 274:99–102.

Hsieh C, Tsokas P, Grau-Perales A, Lesburguères E, Bukai J, Khanna K, Chorny J, Chung A, Jou C, Burghardt NS, et al. (2021) Persistent increases of PKMζ in memory-activated neurons trace LTP maintenance during spatial long-term memory storage. *Eur J Neurosci* 54:6795–6814.

Hsin H, Kim MJ, Wang CF, Sheng M (2010) Proline-rich tyrosine kinase 2 regulates hippocampal long-term depression. *J Neurosci* 30:11983–11993.

Hu NW, Nicoll AJ, Zhang D, Mably AJ, O'Malley T, Purro SA, Terry C, Collinge J, Walsh DM, Rowan MJ (2014) mGlu5 receptors and cellular prion protein mediate amyloid-β-facilitated synaptic long-term depression in vivo. *Nat Commun* 5:3374.

Hu Z, Yu D, Gu QH, Yang Y, Tu K, Zhu J, Li Z (2014) miR-191 and miR-135 are required for long-lasting spine remodelling associated with synaptic long-term depression. *Nat Commun* 5:3263.

Huang SM, Mouri A, Kokubo H, Nakajima R, Suemoto T, Higuchi M, Staufenbiel M, Noda Y, Yamaguchi H, Nabeshima T, et al. (2006) Neprilysin-sensitive synapse-associated amyloid-beta peptide oligomers impair neuronal plasticity and cognitive function. *J Biol Chem* 281:17941–17951.

Huang Y-Q, Lu W-Y, Ali DW, Pelkey KA, Pitcher GM, Lu YM, Aoto H, Roder JC, Sasaki T, Salter MW, et al. (2001) CAKbeta/Pyk2 kinase is a signaling link for induction of long-term potentiation in CA1 hippocampus. *Neuron* 29:485–496.

Huang Y-Y, Colino A, Selig DK, Malenka RC (1992) The influence of prior synaptic activity on the induction of long-term potentiation. *Science* 255:730–733.

Huber KM, Gallagher SM, Warren ST, Bear MF (2002) Altered synaptic plasticity in a mouse model of fragile X mental retardation. *Proc Natl Acad Sci U S A* 99:7746–7750.

Huber KM, Kayser MS, Bear MF (2000) Role for rapid dendritic protein synthesis in hippocampal mGluR-dependent long-term depression. *Science* **288**:1254–1257.

Hulme SR, Jones OD, Ireland DR, Abraham WC (2012) Calcium-dependent but action potential-independent BCM-like metaplasticity in the hippocampus. *J Neurosci* **32**:6785–6794.

Hulme SR, Jones OD, Raymond CR, Sah P, Abraham WC (2014) Mechanisms of heterosynaptic metaplasticity. *Philos Trans R Soc Lond B Biol Sci* **369**:20130148.

Humeau Y, Choquet D (2019) The next generation of approaches to investigate the link between synaptic plasticity and learning. *Nat Neurosci* **22**:1536–1543.

Hunt DL, Puente N, Grandes P, Castillo PE (2013) Bidirectional NMDA receptor plasticity controls CA3 output and heterosynaptic metaplasticity. *Nat Neurosci* **16**:1049–1059.

Ibata K, Sun Q, Turrigiano GG (2008) Rapid synaptic scaling induced by changes in postsynaptic firing. *Neuron* **57**:819–826.

Imamura T, Yanagihara YT, Ohyagi Y, Nakamura N, Iinuma KM, Yamasaki R, Asai H, Maeda M, Murakami K, Irie K, et al. (2020) Insulin deficiency promotes formation of toxic amyloid-β42 conformer co-aggregating with hyper-phosphorylated tau oligomer in an Alzheimer's disease model. *Neurobiol Dis* **137**:104739.

Incontro S, Sammari M, Azzaz F, Inglebert Y, Ankri N, Russier M, Fantini J, Debanne D (2021) Endocannabinoids tune intrinsic excitability in O-LM interneurons by direct modulation of postsynaptic Kv7 channels. *J Neurosci* **41**:9521–9538.

Inglebert Y, Aljadeff J, Brunel N, Debanne D (2020) Synaptic plasticity rules with physiological calcium levels. *Proc Natl Acad Sci U S A* **117**:33639–33648.

Inglis J, Martin SJ, Morris RGM (2013) Upstairs-downstairs revisited: spatial pretraining-induced rescue of normal spatial learning during selective blockade of hippocampal N-methyl-D-aspartate receptors. *Eur J Neurosci* **37**:718–727.

Ingram R, Kang H, Lightman S, Jane DE, Bortolotto ZA, Collingridge GL, Lodge D, Volianskis A (2018) Some distorted thoughts about ketamine as a psychedelic and a novel hypothesis based on NMDA receptor-mediated synaptic plasticity. *Neuropharmacology* **142**:30–40.

Irvine EE, Drinkwater L, Radwanska K, Al-Qassab H, Smith MA, O'Brien M, Kielar C, Choudhury AI, Krauss S, Cooper JD, et al. (2011) Insulin receptor substrate 2 is a negative regulator of memory formation. *Learn Mem* **18**:375–383.

Ishchenko Y, Carrizales MG, Koleske AJ (2021) Regulation of the NMDA receptor by its cytoplasmic domains: (how) is the tail wagging the dog? *Neuropharmacology* **195**:108634.

Ishida A, Furukawa K, Keller JN, Mattson MP (1997) Secreted form of beta-amyloid precursor protein shifts the frequency dependency for induction of LTD, and enhances LTP in hippocampal slices. *Neuroreport* **8**:2133–2137.

Ittner A, Ittner LM (2018) Dendritic tau in Alzheimer's disease. *Neuron* **99**:13–27.

Iwata N, Mizukami H, Shirotani K, Takaki Y, Muramatsu S, Lu B, Gerard NP, Gerard C, Ozawa K, Saido TC (2004) Presynaptic localization of neprilysin contributes to efficient clearance of amyloid-beta peptide in mouse brain. *J Neurosci* **24**:991–998.

Iwata N, Sekiguchi M, Hattori Y, Takahashi A, Asai M, Ji B, Higuchi M, Staufenbiel M, Muramatsu S, Saido TC (2013) Global brain delivery of neprilysin gene by intravascular administration of AAV vector in mice. *Sci Rep* **3**:1472.

Jacobsen JS, Wu CC, Redwine JM, Comery TA, Arias R, Bowlby M, Martone R, Morrison JH, Pangalos MN, Reinhart PH, et al. (2006) Early-onset behavioral and synaptic deficits in a mouse model of Alzheimer's disease. *Proc Natl Acad Sci U S A* **103**:5161–5166.

Jacome LF, Barateli K, Buitrago D, Lema F, Frankfurt M, Luine VN (2016) Gonadal hormones rapidly enhance spatial memory and increase hippocampal spine density in male rats. *Endocrinology* **157**:1357–1362.

Jahr CE, Stevens CF (1993) Calcium permeability of the N-methyl-D-aspartate receptor-channel in hippocampal neurons in culture. *Proc Natl Acad Sci U S A* **90**:11573–11577.

Jain A, Huang GZ, Woolley CS (2019) Latent sex differences in molecular signaling that underlies excitatory synaptic potentiation in the hippocampus. *J Neurosci* **39**:1552–1565.

Jain A, Nakahata Y, Watabe T, Rusina P, South K, Adachi K, Yan L, Simorowski N, Furukawa H, Yasuda R (2023) Dendritic, delayed, and stochastic CaMKII activation underlies behavioral time scale plasticity in CA1 synapses. *bioRxiv* 2023.08.01.549180.

Jaitner C, Reddy C, Abentung A, Whittle N, Rieder D, Delekate A, Korte M, Jain G, Fischer A, Sananbenesi F, et al. (2016) Satb2 determines miRNA expression and long-term memory in the adult central nervous system. *Elife* **5**:e17361.

Jane DE, Lodge D, Collingridge GL (2009) Kainate receptors: pharmacology, function and therapeutic potential. *Neuropharmacology* **56**:90–113.

Javitt DC, Zukin SR, Heresco-Levy U, Umbricht D (2012) Has an angel shown the way? Etiological and therapeutic implications of the PCP/NMDA model of schizophrenia. *Schizophr Bull* **38**:958–966.

Jaworski J, Kapitein LC, Gouveia SM, Dortland BR, Wulf PS, Grigoriev I, Camera P, Spangler SA, Di Stefano P, Demmers J, et al. (2009) Dynamic microtubules regulate dendritic spine morphology and synaptic plasticity. *Neuron* **61**:85–100.

Jeffery KJ (1997) LTP and spatial learning—where to next? *Hippocampus* **7**:95–110.

Jeffery KJ, Morris RGM (1993) Cumulative long-term potentiation in the rat dentate gyrus correlates with, but does not modify, performance in the water maze. *Hippocampus* **3**:133–140.

Jensen KR, Berthoux C, Nasrallah K, Castillo PE (2021) Multiple cannabinoid signaling cascades powerfully suppress recurrent excitation in the hippocampus. *Proc Natl Acad Sci U S A* **118**(4):e2017590118.

Ji D, Lape R, Dani JA (2001) Timing and location of nicotinic activity enhances or depresses hippocampal synaptic plasticity. *Neuron* **31**:131–141.

Jiang CH, Wei M, Zhang C, Shi YS (2021) The amino-terminal domain of GluA1 mediates LTP maintenance via interaction with neuroplastin-65. *Proc Natl Acad Sci U S A* **118**:e2019194118.

Jiang Y, Dong Y, Hu H (2024) The NMDAR hypothesis of ketamine's antidepressant action: evidence and controversies. *Philos Trans R Soc Lond B Biol Sci* **379**:20230225.

Jo J, Son GH, Winters BL, Kim MJ, Whitcomb DJ, Dickinson BA, Lee YB, Futai K, Amici M, Sheng M, et al. (2010) Muscarinic receptors induce LTD of NMDAR EPSCs via a mechanism involving hippocalcin, AP2 and PSD-95. *Nat Neurosci* **13**:1216–1224.

Jo J, Whitcomb DJ, Olsen KM, Kerrigan TL, Lo SC, Bru-Mercier G, Dickinson B, Scullion S, Sheng M, Collingridge G, et al. (2011) Abeta(1–42) inhibition of LTP is mediated by a signaling pathway involving caspase-3, Akt1 and GSK-3beta. *Nat Neurosci* **14**:545–547.

Jones BE, Tovar KR, Goehring A, Jalali-Yazdi F, Okada NJ, Gouaux E, Westbrook GL (2019) Autoimmune receptor encephalitis in mice induced by active immunization with conformationally stabilized holoreceptors. *Sci Transl Med* **11**:eaaw0044.

Jones OD, Hulme SR, Abraham WC (2013) Purinergic receptor- and gap junction-mediated intercellular signalling as a mechanism of heterosynaptic metaplasticity. *Neurobiol Learn Mem* **105**:31–39.

Joseph A, Turrigiano GG (2017) All for one but not one for all: excitatory synaptic scaling and intrinsic excitability are coregulated by CaMKIV, whereas inhibitory synaptic scaling is under independent control. *J Neurosci* 37:6778–6785.

Josselyn SA, Tonegawa S (2020) Memory engrams: recalling the past and imagining the future. *Science* 367(6473):eaaw4325.

Jovanovic JN, Czernik AJ, Fienberg AA, Greengard P, Sihra TS (2000) Synapsins as mediators of BDNF-enhanced neurotransmitter release. *Nat Neurosci* 3:323–329.

Jovasevic V, Wood EM, Cicvaric A, Zhang H, Petrovic Z, Carboncino A, Parker KK, Bassett TE, Moltesen M, Yamawaki N, et al. (2024) Formation of memory assemblies through the DNA-sensing TLR9 pathway. *Nature* 628:145–153.

Jurado S, Goswami D, Zhang Y, Molina AJ, Südhof TC, Malenka RC (2013) LTP requires a unique postsynaptic SNARE fusion machinery. *Neuron* 77:542–558.

Kaeser-Woo YJ, Younts TJ, Yang X, Zhou P, Wu D, Castillo PE, Sudhof TC (2013) Synaptotagmin-12 phosphorylation by cAMP-dependent protein kinase is essential for hippocampal mossy fiber LTP. *J Neurosci* 33:9769–9780.

Kallmann FJ (1946) The genetic theory of schizophrenia; an analysis of 691 schizophrenic twin index families. *Am J Psychiatry* 103:309–322.

Kamal A, Ramakers GM, Gispen WH, Biessels GJ (2012) Effect of chronic intracerebroventricular insulin administration in rats on the peripheral glucose metabolism and synaptic plasticity of CA1 hippocampal neurons. *Brain Res* 1435:99–104.

Kaneko M, Stellwagen D, Malenka RC, Stryker MP (2008) Tumor necrosis factor-alpha mediates one component of competitive, experience-dependent plasticity in developing visual cortex. *Neuron* 58:673–680.

Kang H, Park P, Han M, Tidball P, Georgiou J, Bortolotto ZA, Lodge D, Kaang BK, Collingridge GL (2020) (2S,6S)- and (2R,6R)-hydroxynorketamine inhibit the induction of NMDA receptor-dependent LTP at hippocampal CA1 synapses in mice. *Brain Neurosci Adv* 4:2398212820957847.

Kapitein LC, Yau KW, Gouveia SM, van der Zwan WA, Wulf PS, Keijzer N, Demmers J, Jaworski J, Akhmanova A, Hoogenraad CC (2011) NMDA receptor activation suppresses microtubule growth and spine entry. *J Neurosci* 31:8194–8209.

Kasai H, Fukuda M, Watanabe S, Hayashi-Takagi A, Noguchi J (2010) Structural dynamics of dendritic spines in memory and cognition. *Trends Neurosci* 33:121–129.

Kashiwagi Y, Higashi T, Obashi K, Sato Y, Komiyama NH, Grant SGN, Okabe S (2019) Computational geometry analysis of dendritic spines by structured illumination microscopy. *Nat Commun* 10:1285.

Kato A, Hojo Y, Higo S, Komatsuzaki Y, Murakami G, Yoshino H, Uebayashi M, Kawato S (2013) Female hippocampal estrogens have a significant correlation with cyclic fluctuation of hippocampal spines. *Front Neural Circuits* 7:149.

Kawakami R, Shinohara Y, Kato Y, Sugiyama H, Shigemoto R, Ito I (2003) Asymmetrical allocation of NMDA receptor epsilon2 subunits in hippocampal circuitry. *Science* 300:990–994.

Kemp A, Manahan-Vaughan D (2007) Hippocampal long-term depression: master or minion in declarative memory processes? *Trends Neurosci* 30:111–118.

Kempadoo KA, Mosharov EV, Choi SJ, Sulzer D, Kandel ER (2016) Dopamine release from the locus coeruleus to the dorsal hippocampus promotes spatial learning and memory. *Proc Natl Acad Sci U S A* 113:14835–14840.

Kentros C, Hargreaves E, Hawkins RD, Kandel ER, Shapiro M, Muller RV (1998) Abolition of long-term stability of new hippocampal place cell maps by NMDA receptor blockade. *Science* 280:2121–2126.

Kim IH, Racz B, Wang H, Burianek L, Weinberg R, Yasuda R, Wetsel WC, Soderling SH (2013) Disruption of Arp2/3 results in asymmetric structural plasticity of dendritic spines and progressive synaptic and behavioral abnormalities. *J Neurosci* 33:6081–6092.

Kim IH, Wang H, Soderling SH, Yasuda R (2014) Loss of Cdc42 leads to defects in synaptic plasticity and remote memory recall. *Elife* 3:e02839.

Kim JH, Anwyl R, Suh YH, Djamgoz MB, Rowan MJ (2001) Use-dependent effects of amyloidogenic fragments of (beta)-amyloid precursor protein on synaptic plasticity in rat hippocampus in vivo. *J Neurosci* 21:1327–1333.

Kim JJ, Diamond DM (2002) The stressed hippocampus, synaptic plasticity and lost memories. *Nat Rev Neurosci* 3:453–462.

Kim JJ, Fanselow MS (1992) Modality-specific retrograde amnesia of fear. *Science* 256:675–677.

Kim K, Lakhanpal G, Lu HE, Khan M, Suzuki A, Hayashi MK, Narayanan R, Luyben TT, Matsuda T, Nagai T, et al. (2015) A temporary gating of actin remodeling during synaptic plasticity consists of the interplay between the kinase and structural functions of CaMKII. *Neuron* 87:813–826.

Kim MH, Choi J, Yang J, Chung W, Kim JH, Paik SK, Kim K, Han S, Won H, Bae YS, et al. (2009) Enhanced NMDA receptor-mediated synaptic transmission, enhanced long-term potentiation, and impaired learning and memory in mice lacking IRSp53. *J Neurosci* 29:1586–1595.

Kim WB, Cho JH (2017) Encoding of discriminative fear memory by input-specific LTP in the amygdala. *Neuron* 95:1129–1146, e1125.

Kim WB, Cho JH (2020) Encoding of contextual fear memory in hippocampal-amygdala circuit. *Nat Commun* 11:1382.

Kimura T, Whitcomb DJ, Jo J, Regan P, Piers T, Heo S, Brown C, Hashikawa T, Murayama M, Seok H, et al. (2014) Microtubule-associated protein tau is essential for long-term depression in the hippocampus. *Philos Trans R Soc Lond B Biol Sci* 369:20130144.

Kirsch I, Deacon BJ, Huedo-Medina TB, Scoboria A, Moore TJ, Johnson BT (2008) Initial severity and antidepressant benefits: a meta-analysis of data submitted to the Food and Drug Administration. *PLoS Med* 5:e45.

Kleschevnikov AM, Belichenko PV, Villar AJ, Epstein CJ, Malenka RC, Mobley WC (2004) Hippocampal long-term potentiation suppressed by increased inhibition in the Ts65Dn mouse, a genetic model of Down syndrome. *J Neurosci* 24:8153–8160.

Kline DD, Ogier M, Kunze DL, Katz DM (2010) Exogenous brain-derived neurotrophic factor rescues synaptic dysfunction in Mecp2-null mice. *J Neurosci* 30:5303–5310.

Klonarakis M, De Vos M, Woo EK, Ralph LT, Thacker JS, Gil-Mohapel J (2022) The three sisters of fate: genetics, pathophysiology and outcomes of animal models of neurodegenerative diseases. *Neurosci Biobehav Rev* 135:104541.

Knuesel I, Chicha L, Britschgi M, Schobel SA, Bodmer M, Hellings JA, Toovey S, Prinssen EP (2014) Maternal immune activation and abnormal brain development across CNS disorders. *Nat Rev Neurol* 10:643–660.

Koek L, Sanderson T, Georgiou J, Collingridge GL (2024) The role of calcium stores in long-term potentiation and synaptic tagging and capture in mouse hippocampus. *Philos Trans R Soc Lond B Biol Sci* 379:20230241.

Kohl MM, Shipton OA, Deacon RM, Rawlins JN, Deisseroth K, Paulsen O (2011) Hemisphere-specific optogenetic stimulation reveals left-right asymmetry of hippocampal plasticity. *Nat Neurosci* 14:1413–1415.

Kopach O, Zheng K, Rusakov DA (2020) Optical monitoring of glutamate release at multiple synapses in situ detects changes following LTP induction. *Mol Brain* **13**:39.

Korobova F, Svitkina T (2010) Molecular architecture of synaptic actin cytoskeleton in hippocampal neurons reveals a mechanism of dendritic spine morphogenesis. *Mol Biol Cell* **21**:165–176.

Korol DL, Abel TW, Church LT, Barnes CA, McNaughton BL (1993) Hippocampal synaptic enhancement and spatial learning in the Morris swim task. *Hippocampus* **3**:127–132.

Korotkova T, Fuchs EC, Ponomarenko A, von Engelhardt J, Monyer H (2010) NMDA receptor ablation on parvalbumin-positive interneurons impairs hippocampal synchrony, spatial representations, and working memory. *Neuron* **68**:557–569.

Koss WA, Frick KM (2017) Sex differences in hippocampal function. *J Neurosci Res* **95**:539–562.

Kotermanski SE, Johnson JW (2009) Mg^{2+} imparts NMDA receptor subtype selectivity to the Alzheimer's drug memantine. *J Neurosci* **29**:2774–2779.

Kowall NW, Kosik KS (1987) Axonal disruption and aberrant localization of tau protein characterize the neuropil pathology of Alzheimer's disease. *Ann Neurol* **22**:639–643.

Krab LC, de Goede-Bolder A, Aarsen FK, Pluijm SM, Bouman MJ, van der Geest JN, Lequin M, Catsman CE, Arts WF, Kushner SA, et al. (2008) Effect of simvastatin on cognitive functioning in children with neurofibromatosis type 1: a randomized controlled trial. *JAMA* **300**:287–294.

Kremin T, Gerber D, Giocomo LM, Huang SY, Tonegawa S, Hasselmo ME (2006) Muscarinic suppression in stratum radiatum of CA1 shows dependence on presynaptic M1 receptors and is not dependent on effects at GABA(B) receptors. *Neurobiol Learn Mem* **85**:153–163.

Kretz O, Fester L, Wehrenberg U, Zhou L, Brauckmann S, Zhao S, Prange-Kiel J, Naumann T, Jarry H, Frotscher M, et al. (2004) Hippocampal synapses depend on hippocampal estrogen synthesis. *J Neurosci* **24**:5913–5921.

Krystal JH, Abdallah CG, Sanacora G, Charney DS and Duman RS (2019) Ketamine: a paradigm shift for depression research and treatment. *Neuron* **101**:774–778.

Krystal JH, Karper LP, Seibyl JP, Freeman GK, Delaney R, Bremner JD, Heninger GR, Bowers MB, Jr, Charney DS (1994) Subanesthetic effects of the noncompetitive NMDA antagonist, ketamine, in humans: psychotomimetic, perceptual, cognitive, and neuroendocrine responses. *Arch Gen Psychiatry* **51**:199–214.

Kullmann DM, Moreau AW, Bakiri Y, Nicholson E (2012) Plasticity of inhibition. *Neuron* **75**:951–962.

Kunz L, Schroder TN, Lee H, Montag C, Lachmann B, Sariyska R, Reuter M, Stirnberg R, Stocker T, Messing-Floeter PC, et al. (2015) Reduced grid-cell-like representations in adults at genetic risk for Alzheimer's disease. *Science* **350**:430–433.

Kurt MA, Davies DC, Kidd M, Duff K, Rolph SC, Jennings KH, Howlett DR (2001) Neurodegenerative changes associated with beta-amyloid deposition in the brains of mice carrying mutant amyloid precursor protein and mutant presenilin-1 transgenes. *Exp Neurol* **171**:59–71.

Kwon HB, Castillo PE (2008) Role of glutamate autoreceptors at hippocampal mossy fiber synapses. *Neuron* **60**:1082–1094.

Kyrke-Smith M, Volk LJ, Cooke SF, Bear MF, Huganir RL, Shepherd JD (2021) The immediate early gene arc is not required for hippocampal long-term potentiation. *J Neurosci* **41**:4202–4211.

Lahti AC, Weiler MA, Tamara Michaelidis BA, Parwani A, Tamminga CA (2001) Effects of ketamine in normal and schizophrenic volunteers. *Neuropsychopharmacology* **25**:455–467.

Lamsa K, Heeroma JH, Kullmann DM (2005) Hebbian LTP in feedforward inhibitory interneurons and the temporal fidelity of input discrimination. *Nat Neurosci* **8**:916–924.

Lamsa KP, Heeroma JH, Somogyi P, Rusakov DA, Kullmann DM (2007) Anti-Hebbian long-term potentiation in the hippocampal feedback inhibitory circuit. *Science* **315**:1262–1266.

Lamsa K, Lau P (2019) Long-term plasticity of hippocampal interneurons during in vivo memory processes. *Curr Opin Neurobiol* **54**:20–27.

Lante F, Chafai M, Raymond EF, Pereira AR, Mouska X, Kootar S, Barik J, Bethus I, Marie H (2015) Subchronic glucocorticoid receptor inhibition rescues early episodic memory and synaptic plasticity deficits in a mouse model of Alzheimer's disease. *Neuropsychopharmacology* **40**:1772–1781.

Lapointe V, Morin F, Ratte S, Croce A, Conquet F, Lacaille JC (2003) Synapse-specific mGluR1-dependent long-term potentiation in interneurons regulates mouse hippocampal inhibition. *J Physiol (Lond)* **555**:125–135.

Larimore JL, Chapleau CA, Kudo S, Theibert A, Percy AK, Pozzo-Miller L (2009) Bdnf overexpression in hippocampal neurons prevents dendritic atrophy caused by Rett-associated MECP2 mutations. *Neurobiol Dis* **34**:199–211.

Lau PY, Katona L, Saghy P, Newton K, Somogyi P, Lamsa KP (2017) Long-term plasticity in identified hippocampal GABAergic interneurons in the CA1 area in vivo. *Brain Struct Funct* **222**:1809–1827.

Lauterborn JC, Rex CS, Kramár E, Chen LY, Pandyarajan V, Lynch G, Gall CM (2007) Brain-derived neurotrophic factor rescues synaptic plasticity in a mouse model of fragile X syndrome. *J Neurosci* **27**:10685–10694.

Lawrence JJ, McBain CJ (2003) Containing the detonation—feedforward inhibition in the CA3 hippocampus. *Trends Neurosci* **26**:631–640.

Le AA, Lauterborn JC, Jia Y, Wang W, Cox CD, Gall CM, Lynch G (2022) Prepubescent female rodents have enhanced hippocampal LTP and learning relative to males, reversing in adulthood as inhibition increases. *Nat Neurosci* **25**:180–190.

LeDoux JE (2000) Emotion circuits in the brain. *Ann Rev Neurosci* **23**:155–184.

Lee AM, Kanter BR, Wang D, Lim JP, Zou ME, Qiu C, McMahon T, Dadgar J, Fischbach-Weiss SC, Messing RO (2013) Prkcz null mice show normal learning and memory. *Nature* **493**:416–419.

Lee K, Jung Y, Vyas Y, Mills L, Monfgomery JM (2024) Differential effectiveness of dietary zinc supplementation with autism-related behaviour. *Philos Trans R Soc Lond B Biol* **379**(1906):20230230. https://doi.org/10.1098/rstb.2023.0230

Lee MA, Jayathilake K, Meltzer HY (1999) A comparison of the effect of clozapine with typical neuroleptics on cognitive function in neuroleptic-responsive schizophrenia. *Schizophr Res* **37**:1–11.

Lee MC, Yasuda R, Ehlers MD (2010) Metaplasticity at single glutamatergic synapses. *Neuron* **66**:859–870.

Lee SH, Kang J, Ho A, Watanabe H, Bolshakov VY, Shen J (2020) APP family regulates neuronal excitability and synaptic plasticity but not neuronal survival. *Neuron* **108**:676–690, e678.

Lee SJ, Escobedo-Lozoya Y, Szatmari EM, Yasuda R (2009) Activation of CaMKII in single dendritic spines during long-term potentiation. *Nature* **458**:299–304.

Lee SJ, Wei M, Zhang C, Maxeiner S, Pak C, Calado Botelho S, Trotter J, Sterky FH, Südhof TC (2017) Presynaptic neuronal pentraxin receptor organizes excitatory and inhibitory synapses. *J Neurosci* **37**:1062–1080.

LeGates TA, Altimus CM, Wang H, Lee HK, Yang S, Zhao H, Kirkwood A, Weber ET, Hattar S (2012) Aberrant light directly impairs mood and learning through melanopsin-expressing neurons. *Nature* 491:594–598.

Lejeune J, Turpin R, Gautier M (1959) [Mongolism; a chromosomal disease (trisomy)]. *Bull Acad Natl Med* 143:256–265.

Leonard BJ, McNaughton BL, Barnes CA (1987) Suppression of hippocampal synaptic plasticity during slow-wave sleep. *Brain Res* 425:174–177.

Lepack AE, Bang E, Lee B, Dwyer JM, Duman RS (2016) Fast-acting antidepressants rapidly stimulate ERK signaling and BDNF release in primary neuronal cultures. *Neuropharmacology* 111:242–252.

Leroy F, Brann DH, Meira T, Siegelbaum SA (2017) Input-timing-dependent plasticity in the hippocampal CA2 region and its potential role in social memory. *Neuron* 95:1089–1102, e1085.

Leroy F, de Solis CA, Boyle LM, Bock T, Lofaro OM, Buss EW, Asok A, Kandel ER, Siegelbaum SA (2022) Enkephalin release from VIP interneurons in the hippocampal CA2/3a region mediates heterosynaptic plasticity and social memory. *Mol Psychiatry* 27:2879–2900.

Letzkus JJ, Wolff SB, Lüthi A (2015) Disinhibition, a circuit mechanism for associative learning and memory. *Neuron* 88:264–276.

Levy WB, Steward O (1983) Temporal contiguity requirements for long-term associative potentiation/depression in the hippocampus. *Neuroscience* 8:791–797.

Li H, Rajani V, Sengar AS, Salter MW (2024) Src dependency of the regulation of LTP by alternative splicing of *GRIN1* exon 5. *Philos Trans R Soc Lond B Biol Sci* 379. https://doi.org/10.1098/rstb.2023.0236.

Li L, Chao J, Shi Y (2018) Modeling neurological diseases using iPSC-derived neural cells: iPSC modeling of neurological diseases. *Cell Tissue Res* 371:143–151.

Li W, Cui Y, Kushner SA, Brown RA, Jentsch JD, Frankland PW, Cannon TD, Silva AJ (2005) The HMG-CoA reductase inhibitor lovastatin reverses the learning and attention deficits in a mouse model of neurofibromatosis type 1. *Curr Biol* 15:1961–1967.

Li W, Pozzo-Miller L (2014) BDNF deregulation in Rett syndrome. *Neuropharmacology* 76(Pt C):737–746.

Li Y, Shen M, Stockton ME, Zhao X (2019) Hippocampal deficits in neurodevelopmental disorders. *Neurobiol Learn Mem* 165:106945.

Li Z, Jo J, Jia JM, Lo SC, Whitcomb DJ, Jiao S, Cho K, Sheng M (2010) Caspase-3 activation via mitochondria is required for long-term depression and AMPA receptor internalization. *Cell* 141:859–871.

Lian Q, Ladner CJ, Magnuson D, Lee JM (2001) Selective changes of calcineurin (protein phosphatase 2B) activity in Alzheimer's disease cerebral cortex. *Exp Neurol* 167:158–165.

Lie AA, Blumcke I, Beck H, Schramm J, Wiestler OD, Elger CE (1998) Altered patterns of Ca2+/calmodulin-dependent protein kinase II and calcineurin immunoreactivity in the hippocampus of patients with temporal lobe epilepsy. *J Neuropathol Exp Neurol* 57:1078–1088.

Lin PY, Kavalali ET, Monteggia LM (2018) Genetic dissection of pre-synaptic and postsynaptic BDNF-TrkB signaling in synaptic efficacy of CA3-CA1 synapses. *Cell Rep* 24:1550–1561.

Lisman JE (1985) A mechanism for memory storage insensitive to molecular turnover: a bistable autophosphorylating kinase. *Proc Natl Acad Sci U S A* 82:3055–3057.

Lisman J (1989) A mechanism for the Hebb and the anti-Hebb processes underlying learning and memory. *Proc Natl Acad Sci U S A* 86:9574–9578.

Lisman JE (2009) The pre/post LTP debate. *Neuron* 63:281–284.

Lisman J (2012) Excitation, inhibition, local oscillations, or large-scale loops: what causes the symptoms of schizophrenia? *Curr Opin Neurobiol* 22:537–544.

Lisman J (2017) Criteria for identifying the molecular basis of the engram (CaMKII, PKMzeta). *Mol Brain* 10:55.

Lisman JE, Grace AA (2005) The hippocampal-VTA loop: controlling the entry of information into long-term memory. *Neuron* 46:703–713.

Lisman J, Spruston N (2010) Questions about STDP as a general model of synaptic plasticity. *Front Synaptic Neurosci* 2:140.

Lissin DV, Gomperts SN, Carroll RC, Christine CW, Kalman D, Kitamura M, Hardy S, Nicoll RA, Malenka RC, von Zastrow M (1998) Activity differentially regulates the surface expression of synaptic AMPA and NMDA glutamate receptors. *Proc Natl Acad Sci U S A* 95:7097–7102.

Lituma PJ, Kwon HB, Alviña K, Luján R, Castillo PE (2021) Presynaptic NMDA receptors facilitate short-term plasticity and BDNF release at hippocampal mossy fiber synapses. *Elife* 10:e66612. doi:10.7554/eLife.66612.

Liu A, Ji H, Ren Q, Meng Y, Zhang H, Collingride G, Xie W, Jia Z (2020) The requirement of the C-terminal domain of GluA1 in different forms of long-term potentiation in the hippocampus is age-dependent. *Front Synaptic Neurosci* 12:588785.

Liu F, Grundke-Iqbal I, Iqbal K, Oda Y, Tomizawa K, Gong CX (2005) Truncation and activation of calcineurin A by calpain I in Alzheimer disease brain. *J Biol Chem* 280:37755–37762.

Liu X, Ramirez S, Pang PT, Puryear CB, Govindarajan A, Deisseroth K, Tonegawa S (2012) Optogenetic stimulation of a hippocampal engram activates fear memory recall. *Nature* 484:381–385.

Lockrow J, Boger H, Bimonte-Nelson H, Granholm AC (2011) Effects of long-term memantine on memory and neuropathology in Ts65Dn mice, a model for Down syndrome. *Behav Brain Res* 221:610–622.

Lodge D, Mercier MS (2015) Ketamine and phencyclidine: the good, the bad and the unexpected. *Br J Pharmacol* 172:4254–4276.

Lodge DJ, Grace AA (2007) Aberrant hippocampal activity underlies the dopamine dysregulation in an animal model of schizophrenia. *J Neurosci* 27:11424–11430.

Lohoff FW (2010) Overview of the genetics of major depressive disorder. *Curr Psychiatry Rep* 12:539–546.

Lovestone S, McLoughlin DM (2002) Protein aggregates and dementia: is there a common toxicity? *J Neurol Neurosurg Psychiatry* 72:152–161.

Lozsadi DA, Larner AJ (2006) Prevalence and causes of seizures at the time of diagnosis of probable Alzheimer's disease. *Dement Geriatr Cogn Disord* 22:121–124.

Lu J, Zuo Y (2015) Neuroscience: forgetfulness illuminated. *Nature* 525:324–325.

Lu Y, Zhang M, Lim IA, Hall DD, Allen M, Medvedeva Y, McKnight GS, Usachev YM, Hell JW (2008) AKAP150-anchored PKA activity is important for LTD during its induction phase. *J Physiol* 586:4155–4164.

Lu YM, Roder JC, Davidow J, Salter MW (1998) Src activation in the induction of long-term potentiation in CA1 hippocampal neurons. *Science* 279:1363–1367.

Luengo-Fernandez R, Leal J, Gray AM (2012) UK research expenditure on dementia, heart disease, stroke and cancer: are levels of spending related to disease burden? *Eur J Neurol* 19:149–154.

Lundbye CJ, Toft AKH, Banke TG (2018) Inhibition of GluN2A NMDA receptors ameliorates synaptic plasticity deficits in the Fmr1(-/y) mouse model. *J Physiol* 596(20):5017–5031.

Lüscher C, Huber KM (2010) Group 1 mGluR-dependent synaptic long-term depression: mechanisms and implications for circuitry and disease. *Neuron* 65:445–459.

Lynch G (2004) AMPA receptor modulators as cognitive enhancers. *Curr Opin Pharmacol* 4:4–11.

Lynch G (2006) Glutamate-based therapeutic approaches: ampakines. *Curr Opin Pharmacol* 6:82–88.

Lynch G, Baudry M (1984) The biochemistry of memory: a new and specific hypothesis. *Science* 224:1057–1063.

Lynch G, Browning M, Bennett WF (1979) Biochemical and physiological studies of long-term synaptic plasticity. *Fed Proc* 38:2117–2122.

Lynch GS, Dunwiddie T, Gribkoff V (1977) Heterosynaptic depression: a postsynaptic correlate of long-term potentiation. *Nature* 266:737–739.

Lynch G, Gall CM (2013) Mechanism based approaches for rescuing and enhancing cognition. *Front Neurosci* 7:143.

Lynch G, Larson J, Kelso S, Barrionuevo G, Schottler F (1983) Intracellular injections of EGTA block induction of hippocampal long-term potentiation. *Nature* 305:719–721.

Lyon L, Borel M, Carrión M, Kew JN, Corti C, Harrison PJ, Burnet PW, Paulsen O, Rodríguez-Moreno A (2011) Hippocampal mossy fiber long-term depression in Grm2/3 double knockout mice. *Synapse* 65:945–954.

Ma L, Qiao Q, Tsai JW, Yang G, Li W, Gan WB (2015) Experience-dependent plasticity of dendritic spines of layer 2/3 pyramidal neurons in the mouse cortex. *Dev Neurobiol* 76:277–286.

Maatz A, Hoff P, Angst J (2015) Eugen Bleuler's schizophrenia—a modern perspective. *Dialogues Clin Neurosci* 17:43–49.

Maccaferri G, McBain CJ (1996) Long-term potentiation in distinct subtypes of hippocampal nonpyramidal neurons. *J Neurosci* 16:5334–5343.

MacDermott AB, Mayer ML, Westbrook GL, Smith SJ, Barker JL (1986) NMDA-receptor activation increases cytoplasmic calcium concentration in cultured spinal cord neurones [published erratum appears in Nature 1986 Jun 26-Jul 2;321(6073):888]. *Nature* 321:519–522.

MacDonald JF, Wojtowicz JM (1980) Two conductance mechanisms activated by applications of L-glutamic, L-aspartic, DL-homocysteic, N-methyl-D-aspartic, and DL-kainic acids to cultured mammalian central neurones. *Can J Physiol Pharmacol* 58:1393–1397.

MacDougall MJ, Fine A (2014) The expression of long-term potentiation: reconciling the priests and the positivists. *Philos Trans R Soc Lond B Biol Sci* 369:20130135.

MacDougall MJ, Fine A (2019) Optical quantal analysis. *Front Synaptic Neurosci* 11:8.

MacLusky NJ, Luine VN, Hajszan T, Leranth C (2005) The 17alpha and 17beta isomers of estradiol both induce rapid spine synapse formation in the CA1 hippocampal subfield of ovariectomized female rats. *Endocrinology* 146:287–293.

Madronal N, Delgado-Garcia JM, Fernandez-Guizan A, Chatterjee J, Kohn M, Mattucci C, Jain A, Tsetsenis T, Illarionova A, Grinevich V, et al. (2016) Rapid erasure of hippocampal memory following inhibition of dentate gyrus granule cells. *Nat Commun* 7:10923.

Madronal N, Gruart A, Delgado-Garcia JM (2009) Differing presynaptic contributions to LTP and associative learning in behaving mice. *Front Behav Neurosci* 3:7.

Mainardi M, Fusco S, Grassi C (2015) Modulation of hippocampal neural plasticity by glucose-related signaling. *Neural Plast* 2015:657928.

Maity S, Chandanathil M, Millis RM, Connor SA (2020) Norepinephrine stabilizes translation-dependent, homosynaptic long-term potentiation through mechanisms requiring the cAMP sensor Epac, mTOR and MAPK. *Eur J Neurosci* 52:3679–3688.

Maity S, Jarome TJ, Blair J, Lubin FD, Nguyen PV (2016) Noradrenaline goes nuclear: epigenetic modifications during long-lasting synaptic potentiation triggered by activation of β-adrenergic receptors. *J Physiol* 594:863–881.

Malenka RC, Bear MF (2004) LTP and LTD: an embarrassment of riches. *Neuron* 44:5–21.

Malinow R, Malenka RC (2002) AMPA receptor trafficking and synaptic plasticity. *Ann Rev Neurosci* 25:103–126.

Manahan-Vaughan D, Braunewell KH (1999) Novelty acquisition is associated with induction of hippocampal long-term depression. *Proc Natl Acad Sci U S A* 96:8739–8744.

Mango D, Saidi A, Cisale GY, Feligioni M, Corbo M, Nistico R (2019) Targeting synaptic plasticity in experimental models of Alzheimer's disease. *Front Pharmacol* 10:778.

Marchetti C, Marie H (2011) Hippocampal synaptic plasticity in Alzheimer's disease: what have we learned so far from transgenic models? *Rev Neurosci* 22:373–402.

Marciniak E, Leboucher A, Caron E, Ahmed T, Tailleux A, Dumont J, Issad T, Gerhardt E, Pagesy P, Vileno M, et al. (2017) Tau deletion promotes brain insulin resistance. *J Exp Med* 214:2257–2269.

Marin O (2016) Developmental timing and critical windows for the treatment of psychiatric disorders. *Nat Med* 22:1229–1238.

Markram H, Gerstner W, Sjostrom PJ (2012) Spike-timing-dependent plasticity: a comprehensive overview. *Front Synaptic Neurosci* 4:2.

Markram H, Lubke J, Frotscher M, Sakmann B (1997) Regulation of synaptic efficacy by coincidence of postsynaptic APs and EPSPs. *Science* 275:213–215.

Markram H, Tsodyks M (1996) Redistribution of synaptic efficacy between neocortical pyramidal cells. *Nature* 382:807–810.

Marr D (1971) Simple memory: a theory for archicortex. *Phil Trans Roy Soc Lond B*:262:23–81.

Marsden KC, Beattie JB, Friedenthal J, Carroll RC (2007) NMDA receptor activation potentiates inhibitory transmission through GABA receptor-associated protein-dependent exocytosis of GABA(A) receptors. *J Neurosci* 27:14326–14337.

Martín ED, Sánchez-Perez A, Trejo JL, Martin-Aldana JA, Cano Jaimez M, Pons S, Acosta Umanzor C, Menes L, White MF, Burks DJ (2012) IRS-2 Deficiency impairs NMDA receptor-dependent long-term potentiation. *Cereb Cortex* 22:1717–1727.

Martin SJ, Grimwood PD, Morris RGM (2000) Synaptic plasticity and memory: an evaluation of the hypothesis. *Annu Rev Neurosci* 23:649–711.

Martin SJ, Morris RG (2002) New life in an old idea: the synaptic plasticity and memory hypothesis revisited. *Hippocampus* 12:609–636.

Martin SJ, Shires KL, da Silva BM (2019) Hippocampal lateralization and synaptic plasticity in the intact rat: no left-right asymmetry in electrically induced CA3-CA1 long-term potentiation. *Neuroscience* 397:147–158.

Martinez-Cerdeno V (2017) Dendrite and spine modifications in autism and related neurodevelopmental disorders in patients and animal models. *Dev Neurobiol* 77:393–404.

Martinez-Cue C, Martinez P, Rueda N, Vidal R, Garcia S, Vidal V, Corrales A, Montero JA, Pazos A, Florez J, et al. (2013) Reducing GABAA alpha5 receptor-mediated inhibition rescues functional and neuromorphological deficits in a mouse model of down syndrome. *J Neurosci* 33:3953–3966.

Marzo A, Galli S, Lopes D, McLeod F, Podpolny M, Segovia-Roldan M, Ciani L, Purro S, Cacucci F, Gibb A, et al. (2016) Reversal of synapse degeneration by restoring wnt signaling in the adult hippocampus. *Curr Biol* 26:2551–2561.

Matsuzaki M, Honkura N, Ellis-Davies GCR, Kasai H (2004) Structural basis of long-term potentiation in single dendritic spines. *Nature* 429:761–766.

Matt L, Kim K, Chowdhury D, Hell JW (2019) Role of palmitoylation of postsynaptic proteins in promoting synaptic plasticity. *Front Mol Neurosci* 12:8.

Mayberg HS, Lozano AM, Voon V, McNeely HE, Seminowicz D, Hamani C, Schwalb JM, Kennedy SH (2005) Deep brain stimulation for treatment-resistant depression. *Neuron* 45:651–660.

Mayer ML, Westbrook GL, Guthrie PB (1984) Voltage-dependent block by Mg2+ of NMDA responses in spinal cord neurones. *Nature* 309:261–263.

Mayford M, Wang J, Kandel ER, O'Dell TJ (1995) CaMKII regulates the frequency-response function of hippocampal synapses for the production of both LTD and LTP. *Cell* 81:891–904.

McBain CJ, Freund TF, Mody I (1999) Glutamatergic synapses onto hippocampal interneurons: precision timing without lasting plasticity. *Trends Neurosci* 22:228–235.

McCamphill PK, Stoppel LJ, Senter RK, Lewis MC, Heynen AJ, Stoppel DC, Sridhar V, Collins KA, Shi X, Pan JQ, et al. (2020) Selective inhibition of glycogen synthase kinase 3α corrects pathophysiology in a mouse model of fragile X syndrome. *Sci Transl Med* 12(544):eaam8572. doi:10.1126/scitranslmed.aam8572

McCauley JP, Petroccione MA, D'Brant LY, Todd GC, Affinnih N, Wisnoski JJ, Zahid S, Shree S, Sousa AA, De Guzman RM, et al. (2020) Circadian modulation of neurons and astrocytes controls synaptic plasticity in hippocampal area CA1. *Cell Rep* 33:108255.

McDade E (2019) Why amyloid is still a target for Alzheimer disease clinical trials. *J Am Geriatr Soc* 67:845–847.

McGaugh JL (2000) Memory—a century of consolidation. *Science* 287:248–251.

McGraw CM, Samaco RC, Zoghbi HY (2011) Adult neural function requires MeCP2. *Science* 333:186.

McGregor G, Clements L, Farah A, Irving AJ, Harvey J (2018) Age-dependent regulation of excitatory synaptic transmission at hippocampal temporoammonic-CA1 synapses by leptin. *Neurobiol Aging* 69:76–93.

McGregor G, Irving AJ, Harvey J (2017) Canonical JAK-STAT signaling is pivotal for long-term depression at adult hippocampal temporoammonic-CA1 synapses. *Faseb J* 31:3449–3466.

McGuinness L, Taylor C, Taylor RD, Yau C, Langenhan T, Hart ML, Christian H, Tynan PW, Donnelly P, Emptage NJ (2010) Presynaptic NMDARs in the hippocampus facilitate transmitter release at theta frequency. *Neuron* 68:1109–1127.

McGurk SR (2000) Neurocognition as a determinant of employment status in schizophrenia. *J Psychiatr Pract* 6:190–196.

McLean HA, Caillard O, Ben-Ari Y, Gaiarsa JL (1996) Bidirectional plasticity expressed by GABAergic synapses in the neonatal rat hippocampus. *J Physiol (Lond)* 496:471–477.

McLeod F, Bossio A, Marzo A, Ciani L, Sibilla S, Hannan S, Wilson GA, Palomer E, Smart TG, Gibb A, et al. (2018) Wnt signaling mediates LTP-dependent spine plasticity and AMPAR localization through frizzled-7 receptors. *Cell Rep* 23:1060–1071.

McLeod F, Boyle K, Marzo A, Martin-Flores N, Moe TZ, Palomer E, Gibb AJ, Salinas PC (2020) Wnt signaling through nitric oxide synthase promotes the formation of multi-innervated spines. *Front Synaptic Neurosci* 12:575863.

McMahon LL, Kauer JA (1997) Hippocampal interneurons express a novel form of synaptic plasticity. *Neuron* 18:295–305.

McNaughton BL (1982) Long-term synaptic enhancement and short-term potentiation in rat fascia dentata act through different mechanisms. *J Physiol* 324:249–262.

McNaughton BL, Barnes CA (1986) Long-term enhancement of hippocampal synaptic transmission and the acquisition of spatial information. *J Neurosci* 6:563–571.

McNaughton BL, Douglas RM, Goddard GV (1978) Synaptic enhancement in fascia dentata: cooperativity among coactive afferents. *Brain Res* 157:277–293.

McNaughton BL, Morris RGM (1987) Hippocampal synaptic enhancement and information storage within a distributed memory system. *TINS* 10:408–415.

McVicker DP, Awe AM, Richters KE, Wilson RL, Cowdrey DA, Hu X, Chapman ER, Dent EW (2016) Transport of a kinesin-cargo pair along microtubules into dendritic spines undergoing synaptic plasticity. *Nat Commun* 7:12741.

McVicker DP, Millette MM, Dent EW (2015) Signaling to the microtubule cytoskeleton: an unconventional role for CaMKII. *Dev Neurobiol* 75:423–434.

Megías M, Emri Z, Freund TF, Gulyás AI (2001) Total number and distribution of inhibitory and excitatory synapses on hippocampal CA1 pyramidal cells. *Neuroscience* 102:527–540.

Mehta MR (2015) From synaptic plasticity to spatial maps and sequence learning. *Hippocampus* 25:756–762.

Melnikova I (2007) Therapies for Alzheimer's disease. *Nat Rev Drug Discov* 6:341–342.

Mendez P, Garcia-Segura LM, Muller D (2011) Estradiol promotes spine growth and synapse formation without affecting pre-established networks. *Hippocampus* 21:1263–1267.

Merriam EB, Lumbard DC, Viesselmann C, Ballweg J, Stevenson M, Pietila L, Hu X, Dent EW (2011) Dynamic microtubules promote synaptic NMDA receptor-dependent spine enlargement. *PLoS One* 6:e27688.

Mesulam M, Shaw P, Mash D, Weintraub S (2004) Cholinergic nucleus basalis tauopathy emerges early in the aging-MCI-AD continuum. *Ann Neurol* 55:815–828.

Meyer D, Bonhoeffer T, Scheuss V (2014) Balance and stability of synaptic structures during synaptic plasticity. *Neuron* 82:430–443.

Michalon A, Sidorov M, Ballard TM, Ozmen L, Spooren W, Wettstein JG, Jaeschke G, Bear MF, Lindemann L (2012) Chronic pharmacological mGlu5 inhibition corrects fragile X in adult mice. *Neuron* 74:49–56.

Midorikawa M, Sakaba T (2017) Kinetics of releasable synaptic vesicles and their plastic changes at hippocampal mossy fiber synapses. *Neuron* 96:1033–1040, e1033.

Migues PV, Liu L, Archbold GE, Einarsson EO, Wong J, Bonasia K, Ko SH, Wang YT, Hardt O (2016) Blocking synaptic removal of GluA2-containing AMPA receptors prevents the natural forgetting of long-term memories. *J Neurosci* 36:3481–3494.

Mikasova L, Xiong H, Kerkhofs A, Bouchet D, Krugers HJ, Groc L (2017) Stress hormone rapidly tunes synaptic NMDA receptor through membrane dynamics and mineralocorticoid signalling. *Sci Rep* 7:8053.

Miller OH, Yang L, Wang CC, Hargroder EA, Zhang Y, Delpire E, Hall BJ (2014) GluN2B-containing NMDA receptors regulate depression-like behavior and are critical for the rapid antidepressant actions of ketamine. *Elife* 3:e03581.

Miller SG, Kennedy MB (1986) Regulation of brain type II Ca2+/calmodulin-dependent protein kinase by autophosphorylation: a Ca2+-triggered molecular switch. *Cell* 44:861–870.

Min R, Di Marzo V, Mansvelder HD (2010) DAG lipase involvement in depolarization-induced suppression of inhibition: does endocannabinoid biosynthesis always meet the demand? *Neuroscientist* 16:608–613.

Minkeviciene R, Rheims S, Dobszay MB, Zilberter M, Hartikainen J, Fulop L, Penke B, Zilberter Y, Harkany T, Pitkanen A, et al. (2009) Amyloid beta-induced neuronal hyperexcitability triggers progressive epilepsy. *J Neurosci* 29:3453–3462.

Mitsuyama F, Niimi G, Kato K, Hirosawa K, Mikoshiba K, Okuya M, Karagiozov K, Kato Y, Kanno T, Sanoe H, et al. (2008) Redistribution of microtubules in dendrites of hippocampal CA1 neurons after tetanic stimulation during long-term potentiation. *Ital J Anat Embryol* 113:17–27.

Mizui T, Ishikawa Y, Kumanogoh H, Lume M, Matsumoto T, Hara T, Yamawaki S, Takahashi M, Shiosaka S, Itami C, et al. (2015) BDNF pro-peptide actions facilitate hippocampal LTD and are altered by the common BDNF polymorphism Val66Met. *Proc Natl Acad Sci U S A* 112:E3067–3074.

Moghaddam B, Javitt D (2012) From revolution to evolution: the glutamate hypothesis of schizophrenia and its implication for treatment. *Neuropsychopharmacology* 37:4–15.

Mohammadi AH, Seyedmoalemi S, Moghanlou M, Akhlagh SA, Talaei Zavareh SA, Hamblin MR, Jafari A, Mirzaei H (2022) MicroRNAs and synaptic plasticity: from their molecular roles to response to therapy. *Mol Neurobiol* 59:5084–5102.

Moncada D, Viola H (2007) Induction of long-term memory by exposure to novelty requires protein synthesis: evidence for a behavioral tagging. *J Neurosci* 27:7476–7481.

Mondadori CR, Buchmann A, Mustovic H, Schmidt CF, Boesiger P, Nitsch RM, Hock C, Streffer J, Henke K (2006) Enhanced brain activity may precede the diagnosis of Alzheimer's disease by 30 years. *Brain* 129:2908–2922.

Monfils MH, Teskey GC (2004) Skilled-learning-induced potentiation in rat sensorimotor cortex: a transient form of behavioural long-term potentiation. *Neuroscience* 125:329–336.

Mongillo G, Rumpel S, Loewenstein Y (2017) Intrinsic volatility of synaptic connections—a challenge to the synaptic trace theory of memory. *Curr Opin Neurobiol* 46:7–13.

Monroy BY, Tan TC, Oclaman JM, Han JS, Simó S, Niwa S, Nowakowski DW, McKenney RJ, Ori-McKenney KM (2020) A combinatorial MAP code dictates polarized microtubule transport. *Dev Cell* 53:60–72, e64.

Monyer H, Burnashev N, Laurie DJ, Sakmann B, Seeburg PH (1994) Developmental and regional expression in the rat brain and functional properties of four NMDA receptors. *Neuron* 12:529–540.

Moreau AW, Kullmann DM (2013) NMDA receptor-dependent function and plasticity in inhibitory circuits. *Neuropharmacology* 74:23–31.

Moreno A (2021) Molecular mechanisms of forgetting. *Eur J Neurosci* 54:6912–6932.

Moretti P, Levenson JM, Battaglia F, Atkinson R, Teague R, Antalffy B, Armstrong D, Arancio O, Sweatt JD, Zoghbi HY (2006) Learning and memory and synaptic plasticity are impaired in a mouse model of Rett syndrome. *J Neurosci* 26:319–327.

Morice E, Andreae LC, Cooke SF, Vanes L, Fisher EM, Tybulewicz VL, Bliss TV (2008) Preservation of long-term memory and synaptic plasticity despite short-term impairments in the Tc1 mouse model of Down syndrome. *Learn Mem* 15:492–500.

Morishita W, Lu W, Smith GB, Nicoll RA, Bear MF, Malenka RC (2007) Activation of NR2B-containing NMDA receptors is not required for NMDA receptor-dependent long-term depression. *Neuropharmacology* 52:71–76.

Morita D, Rah JC, Isaac JT (2014) Incorporation of inwardly rectifying AMPA receptors at silent synapses during hippocampal long-term potentiation. *Philos Trans R Soc Lond B Biol Sci* 369:20130156.

Morris RG, Willshaw DJ (1989) Memory: must what goes up come down? *Nature* 339:175–176.

Morris RGM (1989) Synaptic plasticity and learning: selective impairment of learning rats and blockade of long-term potentiation in vivo by the N-methyl-D- aspartate receptor antagonist AP5. *J Neurosci* 9:3040–3057.

Morris RGM (1990a) Synaptic plasticity, neural architecture, and forms of memory. In: Brain Organization and Memory: Cells,

Systems and Circuits (McGaugh JL, Weinberger NM, Lynch G, eds), pp 52–77. New York: Oxford University Press.

Morris RGM (1990b) Toward a representational hypothesis of the role of hippocampal synaptic plasticity in spatial and other forms of learning. *Cold Spring Harb Symp Quant Biol* 55:161–173.

Morris RGM, Anderson E, Lynch GS, Baudry M (1986) Selective impairment of learning and blockade of long-term potentiation by an N-methyl-D-aspartate receptor antagonist, AP5. *Nature* 319:774–776.

Morris RGM, Frey U (1997) Hippocampal synaptic plasticity: role in spatial learning or the automatic recording of attended experience? *Philos Trans R Soc Lond B Biol Sci* 352:1489–1503.

Morris RGM, Schenk F, Tweedie F, Jarrard LE (1990) Ibotenate lesions of hippocampus and/or subiculum: dissociating components of allocentric spatial learning. *Eur J Neurosci* 2:1016–1028.

Moser EI, Krobert KA, Moser MB, Morris RGM (1998) Impaired spatial learning after saturation of long-term potentiation. *Science* 281:2038–2042.

Moser E, Mathiesen I, Andersen P (1993) Association between brain temperature and dentate field potentials in exploring and swimming rats. *Science* 259:1324–1326.

Moser EI, Moser MB, Andersen P (1994) Potentiation of dentate synapses iniated by exploratory learning in rats: dissociation from brain temperature, motor activity and arousal. *Learn Mem* 1:55–73.

Moult PR, Corrêa SA, Collingridge GL, Fitzjohn SM, Bashir ZI (2008) Co-activation of p38 mitogen-activated protein kinase and protein tyrosine phosphatase underlies metabotropic glutamate receptor-dependent long-term depression. *J Physiol* 586:2499–2510.

Mulkey RM, Herron CE, Malenka RC (1993) An essential role for protein phosphatases in hippocampal long-term depression. *Science* 261:1051–1055.

Mulkey RM, Malenka RC (1992) Mechanisms underlying induction of homosynaptic long-term depression in area CA1 of the hippocampus. *Neuron* 9:967–975.

Mullins C, Fishell G, Tsien RW (2016) Unifying views of autism spectrum disorders: a consideration of autoregulatory feedback loops. *Neuron* 89:1131–1156.

Murakoshi H, Wang H, Yasuda R (2011) Local, persistent activation of Rho GTPases during plasticity of single dendritic spines. *Nature* 472:100–104.

Murakoshi H, Yasuda R (2012) Postsynaptic signaling during plasticity of dendritic spines. *Trends Neurosci* 35:135–143.

Na ES, Nelson ED, Adachi M, Autry AE, Mahgoub MA, Kavalali ET, Monteggia LM (2012) A mouse model for MeCP2 duplication syndrome: MeCP2 overexpression impairs learning and memory and synaptic transmission. *J Neurosci* 32:3109–3117.

Nabavi S, Fox R, Proulx CD, Lin JY, Tsien RY, Malinow R (2014) Engineering a memory with LTD and LTP. *Nature* 511:348–352.

Nabavi S, Kessels HW, Alfonso S, Aow J, Fox R, Malinow R (2013) Metabotropic NMDA receptor function is required for NMDA receptor-dependent long-term depression. *Proc Natl Acad Sci U S A* 110:4027–4032.

Nägerl UV, Eberhorn N, Cambridge SB, Bonhoeffer T (2004) Bidirectional activity-dependent morphological plasticity in hippocampal neurons. *Neuron* 44:759–767.

Nägerl UV, Köstinger G, Anderson JC, Martin KA, Bonhoeffer T (2007) Protracted synaptogenesis after activity-dependent sporogenesis in hippocampal neurons. *J Neurosci* 27:8149–8156.

Nakahata Y, Yasuda R (2018) Plasticity of spine structure: local signaling, translation and cytoskeletal reorganization. *Front Synaptic Neurosci* 10:29.

Nakamura Y, Wood CL, Patton AP, Jafari N, Henley JM, Mellor JR, Hanley JG (2011) PICK1 inhibition of the Arp2/3 complex controls dendritic spine size and synaptic plasticity. *Embo J* 30:719–730.

Nakatsuka H, Natsume K (2014) Circadian rhythm modulates long-term potentiation induced at CA1 in rat hippocampal slices. *Neurosci Res* 80:1–9.

Nan X, Ng HH, Johnson CA, Laherty CD, Turner BM, Eisenman RN, Bird A (1998) Transcriptional repression by the methyl-CpG-binding protein MeCP2 involves a histone deacetylase complex. *Nature* 393:386–389.

Narayanan R, Johnston D (2010) The h current is a candidate mechanism for regulating the sliding modification threshold in a BCM-like synaptic learning rule. *J Neurophysiol* 104:1020–1033.

Nelson CD, Kim MJ, Hsin H, Chen Y, Sheng M (2013) Phosphorylation of threonine-19 of PSD-95 by GSK-3β is required for PSD-95 mobilization and long-term depression. *J Neurosci* 33:12122–12135.

Nestler EJ, Hyman SE (2010) Animal models of neuropsychiatric disorders. *Nat Neurosci* 13:1161–1169.

Netzer WJ, Powell C, Nong Y, Blundell J, Wong L, Duff K, Flajolet M, Greengard P (2010) Lowering beta-amyloid levels rescues learning and memory in a Down syndrome mouse model. *PLoS One* 5:e10943.

Neves G, Cooke SF, Bliss TVP (2008) Synaptic plasticity, memory and the hippocampus: a neural network approach to causality. *Nat Rev Neurosci* 9:65–75.

Nguyen MV, Du F, Felice CA, Shan X, Nigam A, Mandel G, Robinson JK, Ballas N (2012) MeCP2 is critical for maintaining mature neuronal networks and global brain anatomy during late stages of postnatal brain development and in the mature adult brain. *J Neurosci* 32:10021–10034.

Nichols DE (2016) Psychedelics. *Pharmacol Rev* 68:264–355.

Nicholson E, Kullmann DM (2017) T-type calcium channels contribute to NMDA receptor independent synaptic plasticity in hippocampal regular-spiking oriens-alveus interneurons. *J Physiol* 595:3449–3458.

Nicolas CS, Peineau S, Amici M, Csaba Z, Fafouri A, Javalet C, Collett VJ, Hildebrandt L, Seaton G, Choi SL, et al. (2012) The Jak/STAT pathway is involved in synaptic plasticity. *Neuron* 73:374–390.

Nicoll RA, Schulman H (2023) Synaptic memory and CaMKII. *Physiol Rev* 103:2877–2925.

Nissen W, Szabo A, Somogyi J, Somogyi P, Lamsa KP (2010) Cell type-specific long-term plasticity at glutamatergic synapses onto hippocampal interneurons expressing either parvalbumin or CB1 cannabinoid receptor. *J Neurosci* 30:1337–1347.

Nisticò R, Dargan SL, Amici M, Collingridge GL, Bortolotto ZA (2011) Synergistic interactions between kainate and mGlu receptors regulate bouton Ca signalling and mossy fibre LTP. *Sci Rep* 1:103.

Nisticò R, Pignatelli M, Piccinin S, Mercuri NB, Collingridge G (2012) Targeting synaptic dysfunction in Alzheimer's disease therapy. *Mol Neurobiol* 46:572–587.

Nosyreva ED, Huber KM (2005) Developmental switch in synaptic mechanisms of hippocampal metabotropic glutamate receptor-dependent long-term depression. *J Neurosci* 25:2992–3001.

Nowacka A, Getz AM, Bessa-Neto D, Choquet D (2024) Activity dependent diffusion-trapping of AMPA receptors as a key step for expression of early LTP. *Philos Trans R Soc Lond B Biol Sci* 379:20230220. doi.org/10.1098/rstb.2023.0220

Nowak L, Bregestovski P, Ascher P, Herbet A, Prochiantz A (1984) Magnesium gates glutamate-activated channels in mouse central neurones. *Nature* 307:462–465.

O'Brien RJ, Kamboj S, Ehlers MD, Rosen KR, Fischbach GD, Huganir RL (1998) Activity-dependent modulation of synaptic AMPA receptor accumulation. *Neuron* 21:1067–1078.

O'Carroll CM, Martin SJ, Sandin J, Frenguelli B, Morris RG (2006) Dopaminergic modulation of the persistence of one-trial hippocampus-dependent memory. *Learn Mem* 13:760–769.

O'Carroll CM, Morris RG (2004) Heterosynaptic co-activation of glutamatergic and dopaminergic afferents is required to induce persistent long-term potentiation. *Neuropharmacology* 47:324–332.

Oddo S, Caccamo A, Shepherd JD, Murphy MP, Golde TE, Kayed R, Metherate R, Mattson MP, Akbari Y, LaFerla FM (2003) Triple-transgenic model of Alzheimer's disease with plaques and tangles: intracellular Abeta and synaptic dysfunction. *Neuron* 39:409–421.

O'Doherty A, Ruf S, Mulligan C, Hildreth V, Errington ML, Cooke S, Sesay A, Modino S, Vanes L, Hernandez D, et al. (2005) An aneuploid mouse strain carrying human chromosome 21 with Down syndrome phenotypes. *Science* 309:2033–2037.

Oh-Nishi A, Obayashi S, Sugihara I, Minamimoto T, Suhara T (2010) Maternal immune activation by polyriboinosinic-polyribocytidilic acid injection produces synaptic dysfunction but not neuronal loss in the hippocampus of juvenile rat offspring. *Brain Res* 1363:170–179.

Oja E (1982) A simplified neuron model as a principal component analyzer. *J Math Biol* 15:267–273.

Okada D, Ozawa F, Inokuchi K (2009) Input-specific spine entry of soma-derived Vesl-1S protein conforms to synaptic tagging. *Science* 324:904–909.

Okamoto K-I, Nagai T, Miyawaki A, Hayashi Y (2004) Rapid and persistent modulation of actin dynamics regulates postsynaptic reorganisation underlying bidirectional plasticity. *Nature Neuroscience* 7:1104–1112.

O'Keefe J (1993) Hippocampus, theta, and spatial memory. *Curr Opin Neurobiol* 3:917–924.

Okuda K, Højgaard K, Privitera L, Bayraktar G, Takeuchi T (2021) Initial memory consolidation and the synaptic tagging and capture hypothesis. *Eur J Neurosci* 54:6826–6849.

Okuno H, Akashi K, Ishii Y, Yagishita-Kyo N, Suzuki K, Nonaka M, Kawashima T, Fujii H, Takemoto-Kimura S, Abe M, et al. (2012) Inverse synaptic tagging of inactive synapses via dynamic interaction of Arc/Arg3.1 with CaMKIIbeta. *Cell* 149:886–898.

Okuno H, Minatohara K, Bito H (2018) Inverse synaptic tagging: an inactive synapse-specific mechanism to capture activity-induced Arc/arg3.1 and to locally regulate spatial distribution of synaptic weights. *Semin Cell Dev Biol* 77:43–50.

Olijslagers JE, de Kloet ER, Elgersma Y, van Woerden GM, Joëls M, Karst H (2008) Rapid changes in hippocampal CA1 pyramidal cell function via pre- as well as postsynaptic membrane mineralocorticoid receptors. *Eur J Neurosci* 27:2542–2550.

Ondrejcak T, Kylubin I, Hu NW, Yang Y, Zhang Q, Rodriguez BJ, Rowan MJ (2024) Rapidly reversible persistent LTP inhibition by patient-derived brain tau and amyloid ß proteins. *Philos Trans R Soc Lond B Biol Sci* 379(1906):20230234. doi.org/10.1098/rstb.2023.0234.

Ondrejcak T, Wang Q, Kew JN, Virley DJ, Upton N, Anwyl R, Rowan MJ (2012) Activation of alpha7 nicotinic acetylcholine receptors persistently enhances hippocampal synaptic transmission and prevents Ass-mediated inhibition of LTP in the rat hippocampus. *Eur J Pharmacol* 677:63–70.

Orr AL, Hanson JE, Li D, Klotz A, Wright S, Schenk D, Seubert P, Madison DV (2014) beta-Amyloid inhibits E-S potentiation through suppression of cannabinoid receptor 1-dependent synaptic disinhibition. *Neuron* 82:1334–1345.

Osterweil EK, Chuang SC, Chubykin AA, Sidorov M, Bianchi R, Wong RK, Bear MF (2013) Lovastatin corrects excess protein synthesis and prevents epileptogenesis in a mouse model of fragile X syndrome. *Neuron* 77:243–250.

Padamsey Z, Emptage N (2014) Two sides to long-term potentiation: a view towards reconciliation. *Philos Trans R Soc Lond B Biol Sci* 369:20130154.

Padamsey Z, Tong R, Emptage N (2017) Glutamate is required for depression but not potentiation of long-term presynaptic function. *Elife* 6:e29688.

Palacios-Filardo J, Mellor JR (2019) Neuromodulation of hippocampal long-term synaptic plasticity. *Curr Opin Neurobiol* 54:37–43.

Palhano-Fontes F, Barreto D, Onias H, Andrade KC, Novaes MM, Pessoa JA, Mota-Rolim SA, Osorio FL, Sanches R, Dos Santos RG, et al. (2019) Rapid antidepressant effects of the psychedelic ayahuasca in treatment-resistant depression: a randomized placebo-controlled trial. *Psychol Med* 49:655–663.

Palmer MJ, Irving AJ, Seabrook GR, Jane DE, Collingridge GL (1997) The group I mGlu receptor agonist DHPG induces a novel form of LTD in the CA1 region of the hippocampus. *Neuropharmacology* 36:1517–1532.

Palomer E, Buechler J, Salinas PC (2019) Wnt signaling deregulation in the aging and Alzheimer's brain. *Front Cell Neurosci* 13:227.

Palop JJ, Chin J, Roberson ED, Wang J, Thwin MT, Bien-Ly N, Yoo J, Ho KO, Yu GQ, Kreitzer A, et al. (2007) Aberrant excitatory neuronal activity and compensatory remodeling of inhibitory hippocampal circuits in mouse models of Alzheimer's disease. *Neuron* 55:697–711.

Pan E, Zhang XA, Huang Z, Krezel A, Zhao M, Tinberg CE, Lippard SJ, McNamara JO (2011) Vesicular zinc promotes presynaptic and inhibits postsynaptic long-term potentiation of mossy fiber-CA3 synapse. *Neuron* 71:1116–1126.

Pandya NJ, Seeger C, Babai N, Gonzalez-Lozano MA, Mack V, Lodder JC, Gouwenberg Y, Mansvelder HD, Danielson UH, Li KW, et al. (2018) Noelin1 affects lateral mobility of synaptic AMPA receptors. *Cell Rep* 24:1218–1230.

Pang PT, Lu B (2004) Regulation of late-phase LTP and long-term memory in normal and aging hippocampus: role of secreted proteins tPA and BDNF. *Ageing Res Rev* 3:407–430.

Panja D, Bramham CR (2014) BDNF mechanisms in late LTP formation: a synthesis and breakdown. *Neuropharmacology* 76(Pt C):664–676.

Papouin T, Dunphy J, Tolman M, Foley JC, Haydon PG (2017) Astrocytic control of synaptic function. *Philos Trans R Soc Lond B Biol Sci* 372(1715):20160154. https://doi.org/10.1098/rstb.2016.0154

Park AJ, Havekes R, Choi JH, Luczak V, Nie T, Huang T, Abel T (2014) A presynaptic role for PKA in synaptic tagging and memory. *Neurobiol Learn Mem* 114:101–112.

Park MH, Lee JK, Choi S, Ahn J, Jin HK, Park JS, Bae JS (2013) Recombinant soluble neprilysin reduces amyloid-beta accumulation and improves memory impairment in Alzheimer's disease mice. *Brain Res* 1529:113–124.

Park P, Georgiou J, Sanderson TM, Ko KH, Kang H, Kim JI, Bradley CA, Bortolotto ZA, Zhuo M, Kaang BK, et al. (2021) PKA drives an increase in AMPA receptor unitary conductance during LTP in the hippocampus. *Nat Commun* 12:413.

Park P, Kang H, Georgiou J, Zhuo M, Kaang BK, Collingridge GL (2021) Further evidence that CP-AMPARs are critically involved in synaptic tag and capture at hippocampal CA1 synapses. *Mol Brain* 14:26.

Park P, Kang H, Sanderson TM, Bortolotto ZA, Georgiou J, Zhuo M, Kaang BK, Collingridge GL (2018) The role of calcium-permeable AMPARs in long-term potentiation at principal neurons in the rodent hippocampus. *Front Synaptic Neurosci* 10:42.

Park P, Kang H, Sanderson TM, Bortolotto ZA, Georgiou J, Zhuo M, Kaang BK, Collingridge GL (2019) On the role of calcium-permeable AMPARs in long-term potentiation and synaptic tagging in the rodent hippocampus. *Front Synaptic Neurosci* 11:4.

Park P, Sanderson TM, Amici M, Choi SL, Bortolotto ZA, Zhuo M, Kaang BK, Collingridge GL (2016) Calcium-permeable AMPA receptors mediate the induction of the protein kinase A-dependent component of long-term potentiation in the hippocampus. *J Neurosci* 36:622–631.

Park P, Sanderson TM, Bortolotto ZA, Georgiou J, Zhuo M, Kaang BK, Collingridge GL (2019) Differential sensitivity of three forms of hippocampal synaptic potentiation to depotentiation. *Mol Brain* 12:30.

Pasricha N, Joëls M, Karst H (2011) Rapid effects of corticosterone in the mouse dentate gyrus via a nongenomic pathway. *J Neuroendocrinol* 23:143–147.

Pastalkova E, Serrano P, Pinkhasova D, Wallace E, Fenton AA, Sacktor TC (2006) Storage of spatial information by the maintenance mechanism of LTP. *Science* 313:1141–1144.

Patrich E, Piontkewitz Y, Peretz A, Weiner I, Attali B (2016) Maternal immune activation produces neonatal excitability defects in offspring hippocampal neurons from pregnant rats treated with poly I:C. *Sci Rep* 6:19106.

Patterson SL, Abel T, Deuel TA, Martin KC, Rose JC, Kandel ER (1996) Recombinant BDNF rescues deficits in basal synaptic transmission and hippocampal LTP in BDNF knockout mice. *Neuron* 16:1137–1145.

Paw Min Thein O, Sakimoto Y, Kida H, Mitsushima D (2020) Proximodistal heterogeneity in learning-promoted pathway-specific plasticity at dorsal CA1 synapses. *Neuroscience* 437:184–195.

Pawlak V, Schupp BJ, Single FN, Seeburg PH, Kohr G (2005) Impaired synaptic scaling in mouse hippocampal neurones expressing NMDA receptors with reduced calcium permeability. *J Physiol* 562:771–783.

Peineau S, Nicolas CS, Bortolotto ZA, Bhat RV, Ryves WJ, Harwood AJ, Dournaud P, Fitzjohn SM, Collingridge GL (2009) A systematic investigation of the protein kinases involved in NMDA receptor-dependent LTD: evidence for a role of GSK-3 but not other serine/threonine kinases. *Mol Brain* 2:22.

Peineau S, Taghibiglou C, Bradley C, Wong TP, Liu L, Lu J, Lo E, Wu D, Saule E, Bouchet T, et al. (2007) LTP inhibits LTD in the hippocampus via regulation of GSK3beta. *Neuron* 53:703–717.

Pelkey KA, Lavezzari G, Racca C, Roche KW, McBain CJ (2005) mGluR7 is a metaplastic switch controlling bidirectional plasticity of feedforward inhibition. *Neuron* 46:89–102.

Pelkey KA, McBain CJ (2008) Target-cell-dependent plasticity within the mossy fibre-CA3 circuit reveals compartmentalized regulation of presynaptic function at divergent release sites. *J Physiol* 586:1495–1502.

Penn AC, Zhang CL, Georges F, Royer L, Breillat C, Hosy E, Petersen JD, Humeau Y, Choquet D (2017) Hippocampal LTP and contextual learning require surface diffusion of AMPA receptors. *Nature* 549:384–388.

Pennington BF, Moon J, Edgin J, Stedron J, Nadel L (2003) The neuropsychology of Down syndrome: evidence for hippocampal dysfunction. *Child Dev* 74:75–93.

Perez Y, Morin F, Lacaille JC (2001) A Hebbian form of long-term potentiation dependent on mGluR1a in hippocampal inhibitory interneurons. *Proc Natl Acad Sci U S A* 98:9401–9406.

Perez de Arce K, Schrod N, Metzbower SWR, Allgeyer E, Kong GK, Tang AH, Krupp AJ, Stein V, Liu X, Bewersdorf J, et al. (2015) Topographic mapping of the synaptic cleft into adhesive nanodomains. *Neuron* 88:1165–1172.

Peters M, Munoz-Lopez M, Morris RGM (2015) Spatial memory and hippocampal enhancement. *Curr Opin Behav Sci* 4:81–91.

Petrini EM, Ravasenga T, Hausrat TJ, Iurilli G, Olcese U, Racine V, Sibarita JB, Jacob TC, Moss SJ, Benfenati F, et al. (2014) Synaptic recruitment of gephyrin regulates surface GABAA receptor dynamics for the expression of inhibitory LTP. *Nat Commun* 5:3921.

Philpot BD, Espinosa JS, Bear MF (2003) Evidence for altered NMDA receptor function as a basis for metaplasticity in visual cortex. *J Neurosci* 23:5583–5588.

Philpot BD, Sekhar AK, Shouval HZ, Bear MF (2001) Visual experience and deprivation bidirectionally modify the composition and function of NMDA receptors in visual cortex. *Neuron* 29:157–169.

Pi HJ, Otmakhov N, Lemelin D, De Koninck P, Lisman J (2010) Autonomous CaMKII can promote either long-term potentiation or long-term depression, depending on the state of T305/T306 phosphorylation. *J Neurosci* 30:8704–8709.

Pike CJ, Walencewicz-Wasserman AJ, Kosmoski J, Cribbs DH, Glabe CG, Cotman CW (1995) Structure-activity analyses of beta-amyloid peptides: contributions of the beta 25–35 region to aggregation and neurotoxicity. *J Neurochem* 64:253–265.

Pilpel Y, Kolleker A, Berberich S, Ginger M, Frick A, Mientjes E, Oostra BA, Seeburg PH (2009) Synaptic ionotropic glutamate receptors and plasticity are developmentally altered in the CA1 field of Fmr1 knockout mice. *J Physiol* 587:787–804.

Pinheiro PS, Lanore F, Veran J, Artinian J, Blanchet C, Crépel V, Perrais D, Mulle C (2013) Selective block of postsynaptic kainate receptors reveals their function at hippocampal mossy fiber synapses. *Cereb Cortex* 23:323–331.

Pinheiro PS, Perrais D, Coussen F, Barhanin J, Bettler B, Mann JR, Malva JO, Heinemann SF, Mulle C (2007) GluR7 is an essential subunit of presynaptic kainate autoreceptors at hippocampal mossy fiber synapses. *Proc Natl Acad Sci U S A* 104:12181–12186.

Pinho J, Marcut C, Fonseca R (2020) Actin remodeling, the synaptic tag and the maintenance of synaptic plasticity. *IUBMB Life* 72:577–589.

Piskorowski RA, Chevaleyre V (2013) Delta-opioid receptors mediate unique plasticity onto parvalbumin-expressing interneurons in area CA2 of the hippocampus. *J Neurosci* 33:14567–14578.

Pittenger C, Duman RS (2008) Stress, depression, and neuroplasticity: a convergence of mechanisms. *Neuropsychopharmacology* 33:88–109.

Planaguma J, Leypoldt F, Mannara F, Gutierrez-Cuesta J, Martin-Garcia E, Aguilar E, Titulaer MJ, Petit-Pedrol M, Jain A, Balice-Gordon R, et al. (2015) Human N-methyl D-aspartate receptor antibodies alter memory and behaviour in mice. *Brain* 138:94–109.

Popov VI, Medvedev NI, Patrushev IV, Ignat'ev DA, Morenkov ED, Stewart MG (2007) Reversible reduction in dendritic spines in CA1 of rat and ground squirrel subjected to hypothermia-normothermia in vivo: a three-dimensional electron microscope study. *Neuroscience* 149:549–560.

Pozo K, Cingolani LA, Bassani S, Laurent F, Passafaro M, Goda Y (2012) β3 integrin interacts directly with GluA2 AMPA receptor subunit and regulates AMPA receptor expression in hippocampal neurons. *Proc Natl Acad Sci U S A* 109:1323–1328.

Pradier B, Lanning K, Taljan KT, Feuille CJ, Nagy MA, Kauer JA (2018) Persistent but labile synaptic plasticity at excitatory synapses. *J Neurosci* 38:5750–5758.

Preston CJ, Brown KA, Wagner JJ (2019) Cocaine conditioning induces persisting changes in ventral hippocampus synaptic transmission, long-term potentiation, and radial arm maze performance in the mouse. *Neuropharmacology* 150:27–37.

Prince TM, Wimmer M, Choi J, Havekes R, Aton S, Abel T (2014) Sleep deprivation during a specific 3-hour time window post-training impairs hippocampal synaptic plasticity and memory. *Neurobiol Learn Mem* 109:122–130.

Puentes-Mestril C, Aton SJ (2017) Linking network activity to synaptic plasticity during sleep: hypotheses and recent data. *Front Neural Circuits* 11:61.

Quinlan EM, Olstein DH, Bear MF (1999) Bidirectional, experience-dependent regulation of N-methyl-D-aspartate receptor subunit composition in the rat visual cortex during postnatal development. *Proc Natl Acad Sci U S A* 96:12876–12880.

Quinlan EM, Philpot BD, Huganir RL, Bear MF (1999) Rapid, experience-dependent expression of synaptic NMDA receptors in visual cortex in vivo. *Nat Neurosci* 2:352–357.

Quintanilla J, Jia Y, Pruess BS, Chavez J, Gall CM, Lynch G, Gunn BG (2024) Pre- versus post-synaptic forms of LTP in two branches of the same hippocampal afferent. *J Neurosci* 44:e1449232024.

Quiroga RQ, Reddy L, Kreiman G, Koch C, Fried I (2005) Invariant visual representation by single neurons in the human brain. *Nature* 435:1102–1107.

Rajani V, Sengar AS, Salter MW (2021) Src and Fyn regulation of NMDA receptors in health and disease. *Neuropharmacology* 193:108615.

Rajgor D, Sanderson TM, Amici M, Collingridge GL, Hanley JG (2018) NMDAR-dependent Argonaute 2 phosphorylation regulates miRNA activity and dendritic spine plasticity. *Embo J* 37:e97943.

Ramsey AM, Tang AH, LeGates TA, Gou XZ, Carbone BE, Thompson SM, Biederer T, Blanpied TA (2021) Subsynaptic positioning of AMPARs by LRRTM2 controls synaptic strength. *Sci Adv* 7:eabf3126.

Ranganath C, Minzenberg MJ, Ragland JD (2008) The cognitive neuroscience of memory function and dysfunction in schizophrenia. *Biol Psychiatry* 64:18–25.

Ranson A, Cheetham CE, Fox K, Sengpiel F (2012) Homeostatic plasticity mechanisms are required for juvenile, but not adult, ocular dominance plasticity. *Proc Natl Acad Sci U S A* 109:1311–1316.

Rasch B, Born J (2013) About sleep's role in memory. *Physiol Rev* 93:681–766.

Rauen KA (2013) The RASopathies. *Annu Rev Genomics Hum Genet* 14:355–369.

Ravassard P, Pachoud B, Comte JC, Mejia-Perez C, Scote-Blachon C, Gay N, Claustrat B, Touret M, Luppi PH, Salin PA (2009) Paradoxical (REM) sleep deprivation causes a large and rapidly reversible decrease in long-term potentiation, synaptic transmission, glutamate receptor protein levels, and ERK/MAPK activation in the dorsal hippocampus. *Sleep* 32:227–240.

Raymond CR (2007) LTP forms 1, 2 and 3: different mechanisms for the "long" in long-term potentiation. *Trends Neurosci* 30:167–175.

Raymond CR, Thompson VL, Tate WP, Abraham WC (2000) Metabotropic glutamate receptors trigger homosynaptic protein synthesis to prolong long-term potentiation. *J Neurosci* 20:969–976.

Rebola N, Carta M, Lanore F, Blanchet C, Mulle C (2011) NMDA receptor-dependent metaplasticity at hippocampal mossy fiber synapses. *Nat Neurosci* 14:691–693.

Rebola N, Lujan R, Cunha RA, Mulle C (2008) Adenosine A2A receptors are essential for long-term potentiation of NMDA-EPSCs at hippocampal mossy fiber synapses. *Neuron* 57:121–134.

Reddy MS (2010) Depression: the disorder and the burden. *Indian J Psychol Med* 32:1–2.

Redondo RL, Morris RG (2011) Making memories last: the synaptic tagging and capture hypothesis. *Nat Rev Neurosci* 12:17–30.

Reese LC, Zhang W, Dineley KT, Kayed R, Taglialatela G (2008) Selective induction of calcineurin activity and signaling by oligomeric amyloid beta. *Aging Cell* 7:824–835.

Regan P, Piers T, Yi JH, Kim DH, Huh S, Park SJ, Ryu JH, Whitcomb DJ, Cho K (2015) Tau phosphorylation at serine 396 residue is required for hippocampal LTD. *J Neurosci* 35:4804–4812.

Reijmers L, Mayford M (2009) Genetic control of active neural circuits. *Front Mol Neurosci* 2:27.

Renner P, Klinger LG, Klinger MR (2000) Implicit and explicit memory in autism: is autism an amnesic disorder? *J Autism Dev Disord* 30:3–14.

Rex CS, Lin CY, Kramar EA, Chen LY, Gall CM, Lynch G (2007) Brain-derived neurotrophic factor promotes long-term potentiation-related cytoskeletal changes in adult hippocampus. *J Neurosci* 27:3017–3029.

Rey S, Marra V, Smith C, Staras K (2020) Nanoscale remodeling of functional synaptic vesicle pools in Hebbian plasticity. *Cell Rep* 30:2006–2017, e2003.

Reymann KG, Frey JU (2007) The late maintenance of hippocampal LTP: requirements, phases, "synaptic tagging," "late-associativity" and implications. *Neuropharmacology* 52:24–40.

Ribeiro PO, Tome AR, Silva HB, Cunha RA, Antunes LM (2014) Clinically relevant concentrations of ketamine mainly affect long-term potentiation rather than basal excitatory synaptic transmission and do not change paired-pulse facilitation in mouse hippocampal slices. *Brain Res* 1560:10–17.

Rice HC, de Malmazet D, Schreurs A, Frere S, Van Molle I, Volkov AN, Creemers E, Vertkin I, Nys J, Ranaivoson FM, et al. (2019) Secreted amyloid-beta precursor protein functions as a GABABR1a ligand to modulate synaptic transmission. *Science* 363(6423):eaa04827. doi:10.1126/science.aao4827

Richards BW (1969) Mosaic mongolism. *J Ment Defic Res* 13:66–83.

Richter JD, Bassell GJ, Klann, E (2015) Dysregulation and restoration of translational homeostasis in fragile X syndrome. *Nature Rev Neurosci* 16:595–605.

Richter-Levin G, Akirav I (2003) Emotional tagging of memory formation—in the search for neural mechanisms. *Brain Res Brain Res Rev* 43:247–256.

Richter-Levin G, Canevari L, Bliss TVP (1997) Spatial training and high-frequency stimulation engage a common pathway to enhance glutamate release in the hippocampus. *Learn Mem* 4:445–450.

Ring S, Weyer SW, Kilian SB, Waldron E, Pietrzik CU, Filippov MA, Herms J, Buchholz C, Eckman CB, Korte M, et al. (2007) The secreted beta-amyloid precursor protein ectodomain APPs alpha is sufficient to rescue the anatomical, behavioral, and electrophysiological abnormalities of APP-deficient mice. *J Neurosci* 27:7817–7826.

Rioult-Pedotti MS, Friedman D, Hess G, Donoghue JP (1998) Strengthening of horizontal cortical connections following skill learning. *Nat Neurosci* 1:230–234.

Robinson JW, Leshchyns'ka I, Farghaian H, Hughes WE, Sytnyk V, Neely GG, Cole AR (2014) PI4KIIα phosphorylation by GSK3 directs vesicular trafficking to lysosomes. *Biochem J* 464:145–156.

Rocca DL, Amici M, Antoniou A, Blanco Suarez E, Halemani N, Murk K, McGarvey J, Jafari N, Mellor JR, Collingridge GL, et al. (2013) The small GTPase Arf1 modulates Arp2/3-mediated actin polymerization via PICK1 to regulate synaptic plasticity. *Neuron* 79:293–307.

Rocca DL, Martin S, Jenkins EL, Hanley JG (2008) Inhibition of Arp2/3-mediated actin polymerization by PICK1 regulates neuronal morphology and AMPA receptor endocytosis. *Nat Cell Biol* 10:259–271.

Roddy DW, Farrell C, Doolin K, Roman E, Tozzi L, Frodl T, O'Keane V, O'Hanlon E (2019) The hippocampus in depression: more than the sum of its parts? Advanced hippocampal substructure segmentation in depression. *Biol Psychiatry* 85:487–497.

Rodriguez G, Mesik L, Gao M, Parkins S, Saha R, Lee HK (2019) Disruption of NMDAR function prevents normal experience-dependent homeostatic synaptic plasticity in mouse primary visual cortex. *J Neurosci* 39:7664–7673.

Rogan MT, Staubli UV, LeDoux JE (1997) Fear conditioning induces associative long-term potentiation in the amygdala. *Nature* 390:604–607.

Rogerson T, Cai DJ, Frank A, Sano Y, Shobe J, Lopez-Aranda MF, Silva AJ (2014) Synaptic tagging during memory allocation. *Nat Rev Neurosci* 15:157–169.

Rolls ET, Treves A (2011) The neuronal encoding of information in the brain. *Prog Neurobiol* 95:448–490.

Rosen ZB, Cheung S, Siegelbaum SA (2015) Midbrain dopamine neurons bidirectionally regulate CA3-CA1 synaptic drive. *Nat Neurosci* 18:1763–1771.

Rossetti T, Banerjee S, Kim C, Leubner M, Lamar C, Gupta P, Lee B, Neve R, Lisman J (2017) memory erasure experiments indicate a critical role of CaMKII in memory storage. *Neuron* 96:207–216, e202.

Roth RH, Cudmore RH, Tan HL, Hong I, Zhang Y, Huganir RL (2020) Cortical synaptic AMPA receptor plasticity during motor learning. *Neuron* 105:895–908, e895.

Rowan MJ, Klyubin I, Cullen WK, Anwyl R (2003) Synaptic plasticity in animal models of early Alzheimer's disease. *Philos Trans R Soc Lond B Biol Sci* 358:821–828.

Roy DS, Arons A, Mitchell TI, Pignatelli M, Ryan TJ, Tonegawa S (2016) Memory retrieval by activating engram cells in mouse models of early Alzheimer's disease. *Nature* 531:508–512.

Roy DS, Muralidhar S, Smith LM, Tonegawa S (2017) Silent memory engrams as the basis for retrograde amnesia. *Proc Natl Acad Sci U S A* 114:e9972–e9979.

Rozkalne A, Hyman BT, Spires-Jones TL (2011) Calcineurin inhibition with FK506 ameliorates dendritic spine density deficits in plaque-bearing Alzheimer model mice. *Neurobiol Dis* 41:650–654.

Rubenstein JL, Merzenich MM (2003) Model of autism: increased ratio of excitation/inhibition in key neural systems. *Genes Brain Behav* 2:255–267.

Rueda N, Llorens-Martin M, Florez J, Valdizan E, Banerjee P, Trejo JL, Martinez-Cue C (2010) Memantine normalizes several phenotypic features in the Ts65Dn mouse model of Down syndrome. *J Alzheimers Dis* 21:277–290.

Rumpel S, LeDoux J, Zador A, Malinow R (2005) Postsynaptic receptor trafficking underlying a form of associative learning. *Science* 308:83–88.

Rust MB, Gurniak CB, Renner M, Vara H, Morando L, Görlich A, Sassoè-Pognetto M, Banchaabouchi MA, Giustetto M, Triller A, et al. (2010) Learning, AMPA receptor mobility and synaptic plasticity depend on n-cofilin-mediated actin dynamics. *Embo J* 29:1889–1902.

Ryan TJ, Roy DS, Pignatelli M, Arons A, Tonegawa S (2015) Memory: engram cells retain memory under retrograde amnesia. *Science* 348:1007–1013.

Sachidhanandam S, Blanchet C, Jeantet Y, Cho YH, Mulle C (2009) Kainate receptors act as conditional amplifiers of spike transmission at hippocampal mossy fiber synapses. *J Neurosci* 29:5000–5008.

Sacktor TC (2011) How does PKMzeta maintain long-term memory? *Nat Rev Neurosci* 12:9–15.

Sacktor TC, Fenton AA (2018) What does LTP tell us about the roles of CaMKII and PKMzeta in memory? *Mol Brain* 11:77.

Safieh M, Korczyn AD, Michaelson DM (2019) ApoE4: an emerging therapeutic target for Alzheimer's disease. *BMC Med* 17:64.

Saglietti L, Dequidt C, Kamieniarz K, Rousset MC, Valnegri P, Thoumine O, Beretta F, Fagni L, Choquet D, Sala C, et al. (2007) Extracellular interactions between GluR2 and N-cadherin in spine regulation. *Neuron* 54:461–477.

Sajikumar S (ed) (2015) Synaptic Tagging and Capture: From Synapses to Behavior. New York: Springer.

Sajikumar S, Abel T (eds) (2024) Synaptic Tagging and Capture: From Synapses to Behavior. New York: Springer.

Sajikumar S, Frey JU (2004a) Late-associativity, synaptic tagging, and the role of dopamine during LTP and LTD. *Neurobiol Learn Mem* 82:12–25.

Sajikumar S, Frey JU (2004b) Resetting of "synaptic tags" is time- and activity-dependent in rat hippocampal CA1 in vitro. *Neuroscience* 129:503–507.

Sajikumar S, Li Q, Abraham WC, Xiao ZC (2009) Priming of short-term potentiation and synaptic tagging/capture mechanisms by ryanodine receptor activation in rat hippocampal CA1. *Learn Mem* 16:178–186.

Sambandan S, Sauer JF, Vida I, Bartos M (2010) Associative plasticity at excitatory synapses facilitates recruitment of fast-spiking interneurons in the dentate gyrus. *J Neurosci* 30:11826–11837.

Sanchez PE, Zhu L, Verret L, Vossel KA, Orr AG, Cirrito JR, Devidze N, Ho K, Yu GQ, Palop JJ, et al. (2012) Levetiracetam suppresses neuronal network dysfunction and reverses synaptic and cognitive deficits in an Alzheimer's disease model. *Proc Natl Acad Sci U S A* 109:E2895–2903.

Sanderson JL, Gorski JA, Dell'Acqua ML (2016) NMDA receptor-dependent LTD requires transient synaptic incorporation of Ca^{2+}-permeable AMPARs mediated by AKAP150-anchored PKA and calcineurin. *Neuron* 89:1000–1015.

Sanderson TM, Bradley CA, Georgiou J, Hong YH, Ng AN, Lee Y, Kim HD, Kim D, Amici M, Son GH, et al. (2018) The probability of neurotransmitter release governs AMPA receptor trafficking via activity-dependent regulation of mGluR1 surface expression. *Cell Rep* 25:3631–3646, e3633.

Sanderson TM, Hogg EL, Collingridge GL, Corrêa SA (2016) Hippocampal metabotropic glutamate receptor long-term depression in health and disease: focus on mitogen-activated protein kinase pathways. *J Neurochem* 139(Suppl 2):200–214.

Sanderson TM, Ralph LT, Amici M, Ng AN, Kaang BK, Zhuo M, Kim SJ, Georgiou J, Collingridge GL (2022) Selective recruitment of presynaptic and postsynaptic forms of mGluR-LTD. *Front Synaptic Neurosci* 14:857675.

Saneyoshi T, Matsuno H, Suzuki A, Murakoshi H, Hedrick NG, Agnello E, O'Connell R, Stratton MM, Yasuda R, Hayashi Y (2019) Reciprocal activation within a kinase-effector complex underlying persistence of structural LTP. *Neuron* 102:1199–1210, e1196.

Sanz-Clemente A, Gray JA, Ogilvie KA, Nicoll RA, Roche KW (2013) Activated CaMKII couples GluN2B and casein kinase 2 to control synaptic NMDA receptors. *Cell Rep* 3:607–614.

Sanz-Clemente A, Matta JA, Isaac JT, Roche KW (2010) Casein kinase 2 regulates the NR2 subunit composition of synaptic NMDA receptors. *Neuron* 67:984–996.

Saucier D, Hargreaves EL, Boon F, Vanderwolf CH, Cain DP (1996) Detailed behavioral analysis of water maze acquisition under systemic NMDA or muscarinic antagonism: nonspatial pretraining eliminates spatial learning deficits. *Behav Neurosci* 110:103–116.

Saura CA, Choi SY, Beglopoulos V, Malkani S, Zhang D, Shankaranarayana Rao BS, Chattarji S, Kelleher RJ, 3rd, Kandel ER, Duff K, et al. (2004) Loss of presenilin function causes impairments of memory and synaptic plasticity followed by age-dependent neurodegeneration. *Neuron* 42:23–36.

Savanthrapadian S, Wolff AR, Logan BJ, Eckert MJ, Bilkey DK, Abraham WC (2013) Enhanced hippocampal neuronal excitability and LTP persistence associated with reduced behavioral flexibility in the maternal immune activation model of schizophrenia. *Hippocampus* 23:1395–1409.

Sawallisch C, Berhörster K, Disanza A, Mantoani S, Kintscher M, Stoenica L, Dityatev A, Sieber S, Kindler S, Morellini F, et al. (2009) The insulin receptor substrate of 53 kDa (IRSp53) limits hippocampal synaptic plasticity. *J Biol Chem* 284:9225–9236.

Scheuss V, Bonhoeffer T (2014) Function of dendritic spines on hippocampal inhibitory neurons. *Cereb Cortex* 24:3142–3153.

Schmeisser MJ, Ey E, Wegener S, Bockmann J, Stempel AV, Kuebler A, Janssen AL, Udvardi PT, Shiban E, Spilker C, et al. (2012) Autistic-like behaviours and hyperactivity in mice lacking ProSAP1/Shank2. *Nature* 486:256–260.

Schmidt CC, Tong R, Emptage NJ (2024) GluN2A- and GluN2B-containing pre-synaptic *N*-methyl-d-aspartate receptors differentially regulate action potential evoked Ca^{2+} influx via modulation of SK channels. *Philos Trans R Soc Lond B Biol Sci* 379. doi.org/10.1098/rstb.2023.0222

Schmitt A, Malchow B, Hasan A, Falkai P (2014) The impact of environmental factors in severe psychiatric disorders. *Front Neurosci* 8:19.

Schulz JM, Knoflach F, Hernandez MC, Bischofberger J (2019) Enhanced dendritic inhibition and impaired NMDAR activation in a mouse model of Down syndrome. *J Neurosci* 39:5210–5221.

Schwartz J (1993) Cognitive kinases. *Proc Natl Acad Sci U S A* 90:8310–8313.

Schwetye KE, Gutmann DH (2014) Cognitive and behavioral problems in children with neurofibromatosis type 1: challenges and future directions. *Expert Rev Neurother* 14:1139–1152.

Scott R, Lalic T, Kullmann DM, Capogna M, Rusakov DA (2008) Target-cell specificity of kainate autoreceptor and Ca2+-store-dependent short-term plasticity at hippocampal mossy fiber synapses. *J Neurosci* 28:13139–13149.

Scott-McKean JJ, Costa AC (2011) Exaggerated NMDA mediated LTD in a mouse model of Down syndrome and pharmacological rescuing by memantine. *Learn Mem* 18:774–778.

Scott-McKean JJ, Roque AL, Surewicz K, Johnson MW, Surewicz WK, Costa ACS (2018) Pharmacological modulation of three modalities of CA1 hippocampal long-term potentiation in the Ts65Dn mouse model of Down syndrome. *Neural Plast* 2018:9235796.

Sejnowski TJ (1977) Storing covariance with nonlinearly interacting neurons. *J Math Biol* 4:303–321.

Selkoe DJ, Hardy J (2016) The amyloid hypothesis of Alzheimer's disease at 25 years. *EMBO Mol Med* 8:595–608.

Shahoha M, Cohen R, Ben-Simon Y, Ashery U (2022) cAMP-dependent synaptic plasticity at the hippocampal mossy fiber terminal. *Front Synaptic Neurosci* 14:861215.

Shankar GM, Li S, Mehta TH, Garcia-Munoz A, Shepardson NE, Smith I, Brett FM, Farrell MA, Rowan MJ, Lemere CA, et al. (2008) Amyloid-beta protein dimers isolated directly from Alzheimer's brains impair synaptic plasticity and memory. *Nat Med* 14:837–842.

Shapiro ML, O'Connor C (1992) N-methyl-D-aspartate receptor antagonist MK-801 and spatial memory representation: working memory is impaired in an unfamiliar environment but not in a familiar environment. *Behav Neurosci* 106:604–612.

Sharma A, Hoeffer CA, Takayasu Y, Miyawaki T, McBride SM, Klann E, Zukin RS (2010) Dysregulation of mTOR signaling in fragile X syndrome. *J Neurosci* 30:694–702.

Sharp PE, McNaughton BL, Barnes CA (1985) Enhancement of hippocampal field potentials in rats exposed to a novel, complex environment. *Brain Res* 339:361–365.

Sheng M, Cummings J, Roldan LA, Jan YN, Jan LY (1994) Changing subunit composition of heteromeric NMDA receptors during development of rat cortex. *Nature* 368:144–147.

Sheng M, Sabatini BL, Sudhof TC (2012) Synapses and Alzheimer's disease. *Cold Spring Harb Perspect Biol* 4:a005777.

Sheppard PAS, Choleris E, Galea L (2019) Structural plasticity of the hippocampus in response to estrogens in female rodents. *Mol Brain* 12:22. doi:10.1186/s13041-019-0442-7.

Sherwood JL, Amici M, Dargan SL, Culley GR, Fitzjohn SM, Jane DE, Collingridge GL, Lodge D, Bortolotto ZA (2012) Differences in kainate receptor involvement in hippocampal mossy fibre long-term potentiation depending on slice orientation. *Neurochem Int* 61:482–489.

Shih PY, Savtchenko LP, Kamasawa N, Dembitskaya Y, McHugh TJ, Rusakov DA, Shigemoto R, Semyanov A (2013) Retrograde synaptic signaling mediated by K+ efflux through postsynaptic NMDA receptors. *Cell Rep* 5:941–951.

Shinohara Y, Hirase H (2009) Size and receptor density of glutamatergic synapses: a viewpoint from left-right asymmetry of CA3-CA1 connections. *Front Neuroanat* 3:10.

Shinohara Y, Hirase H, Watanabe M, Itakura M, Takahashi M, Shigemoto R (2008) Left-right asymmetry of the hippocampal synapses with differential subunit allocation of glutamate receptors. *Proc Natl Acad Sci U S A* 105:19498–19503.

Shipton OA, El-Gaby M, Apergis-Schoute J, Deisseroth K, Bannerman DM, Paulsen O, Kohl MM (2014) Left-right dissociation of hippocampal memory processes in mice. *Proc Natl Acad Sci U S A* 111:15238–15243.

Shipton OA, Leitz JR, Dworzak J, Acton CE, Tunbridge EM, Denk F, Dawson HN, Vitek MP, Wade-Martins R, Paulsen O, et al. (2011) Tau protein is required for amyloid {beta}-induced impairment of hippocampal long-term potentiation. *J Neurosci* 31:1688–1692.

Shors TJ, Matzel LD (1997) Long-term potentiation: what's learning got to do with it? *Behav Brain Sci* 20:597–614; discussion 614–655.

Siarey RJ, Carlson EJ, Epstein CJ, Balbo A, Rapoport SI, Galdzicki Z (1999) Increased synaptic depression in the Ts65Dn mouse, a model for mental retardation in Down syndrome. *Neuropharmacology* 38:1917–1920.

Siegel JM (2001) The REM sleep-memory consolidation hypothesis. *Science* 294:1058–1063.

Siegel JM (2005) Clues to the functions of mammalian sleep. *Nature* 437:1264–1271.

Silva AJ, Frankland PW, Marowitz Z, Friedman E, Laszlo GS, Cioffi D, Jacks T, Bourtchuladze R (1997) A mouse model for the learning and memory deficits associated with neurofibromatosis type I. *Nat Genet* 15:281–284.

Silva AJ, Zhou Y, Rogerson T, Shobe J, Balaji J (2009) Molecular and cellular approaches to memory allocation in neural circuits. *Science* 326:391–395.

Simons SB, Caruana DA, Zhao M, Dudek SM (2011) Caffeine-induced synaptic potentiation in hippocampal CA2 neurons. *Nat Neurosci* 15:23–25.

Singh A, Sateesh S, Jones OD, Abraham WC (2022) Pathway-specific TNF-mediated metaplasticity in hippocampal area CA1. *Sci Rep* 12:1746.

Snyder MA, Cooke BM, Woolley CS (2011) Estradiol potentiation of NR2B-dependent EPSCs is not due to changes in NR2B protein expression or phosphorylation. *Hippocampus* 21:398–408.

Sobczyk A, Svoboda K (2007) Activity-dependent plasticity of the NMDA-receptor fractional Ca2+ current. *Neuron* 53:17–24.

Song S, Miller KD, Abbott LF (2000) Competitive Hebbian learning through spike-timing-dependent synaptic plasticity. *Nat Neurosci* 3:919–926.

Souchet B, Guedj F, Sahun I, Duchon A, Daubigney F, Badel A, Yanagawa Y, Barallobre MJ, Dierssen M, Yu E, et al. (2014) Excitation/inhibition balance and learning are modified by Dyrk1a gene dosage. *Neurobiol Dis* 69:65–75.

Staley K (2015) Molecular mechanisms of epilepsy. *Nat Neurosci* 18:367–372.

Stanton PK, Sejnowski TJ (1989) Associative long-term depression in the hippocampus induced by Hebbian covariance. *Nature* 339:215–218.

Starbuck JM, Llambrich S, Gonzalez R, Albaiges J, Sarle A, Wouters J, Gonzalez A, Sevillano X, Sharpe J, De La Torre R, et al. (2021) Green tea extracts containing epigallocatechin-3-gallate modulate facial development in Down syndrome. *Sci Rep* 11:4715.

Staubli U, Lynch G (1990) Stable depression of potentiated synaptic responses in the hippocampus with 1–5Hz stimulation. *Brain Res* 513:113–118.

Staubli U, Perez Y, Xu FB, Rogers G, Ingvar M, Stone-Elander S, Lynch G (1994) Centrally active modulators of glutamate receptors facilitate the induction of long-term potentiation in vivo. *Proc Natl Acad Sci U S A* 91:11158–11162.

Staubli U, Thibault O, DiLorenzo M, Lynch G (1989) Antagonism of NMDA receptors impairs acquisition but not retention of olfactory memory. *Behav Neurosci* 103:54–60.

Steele RJ, Morris RGM (1999) Delay-dependent impairment of a matching-to-place task with chronic and intrahippocampal infusion of the NMDA-antagonist D-AP5. *Hippocampus* 9:118–136.

Steffens H, Mott AC, Li S, Wegner W, Švehla P, Kan VWY, Wolf F, Liebscher S, Willig KI (2021) Stable but not rigid: chronic in vivo STED nanoscopy reveals extensive remodeling of spines, indicating multiple drivers of plasticity. *Sci Adv* 7. doi:10.1126/sciadv.abf2806

Steinmetz CC, Turrigiano GG (2010) Tumor necrosis factor-alpha signaling maintains the ability of cortical synapses to express synaptic scaling. *J Neurosci* 30:14685–14690.

Stellwagen D, Malenka RC (2006) Synaptic scaling mediated by glial TNF-alpha. *Nature* 440:1054–1059.

Stent GS (1973) A physiological mechanism for Hebb's postulate of learning. *Proc Natl Acad Sci USA* 70:997–1001.

Steubler V, Erdinger S, Back MK, Ludewig S, Fassler D, Richter M, Han K, Slomianka L, Amrein I, von Engelhardt J, et al. (2021) Loss of all three APP family members during development impairs synaptic function and plasticity, disrupts learning, and causes an autism-like phenotype. *EMBO J* 40:e107471.

Steward O, Wallace CS, Lyford GL, Worley PF (1998) Synaptic activation causes the mRNA for the IEG Arc to localize selectively near activated postsynaptic sites on dendrites. *Neuron* 21:741–751.

Steward O, Worley P (2001) Selective targeting of newly synthesised *Arc* mRNA to active synapses requires NMDA receptor activation. *Neuron* 30:227–240.

Strang KH, Golde TE, Giasson BI (2019) MAPT mutations, tauopathy, and mechanisms of neurodegeneration. *Lab Invest* 99:912–928.

Stringer JL, Guyenet PG (1983) Elimination of long-term potentiation in the hippocampus by phencyclidine and ketamine. *Brain Res* 258:159–164.

Stuart GJ, Sakmann B (1994) Active propagation of somatic action potentials into neocortical pyramidal cell dendrites. *Nature* 367:69–72.

Sukenik N, Vinogradov O, Weinreb E, Segal M, Levina A, Moses E (2021) Neuronal circuits overcome imbalance in excitation and inhibition by adjusting connection numbers. *Proc Natl Acad Sci U S A* 118. doi.10.1073/pnas.2018459118

Sumi T, Harada K (2020) Mechanism underlying hippocampal long-term potentiation and depression based on competition between endocytosis and exocytosis of AMPA receptors. *Sci Rep* 10:14711.

Summers WK, Majovski LV, Marsh GM, Tachiki K, Kling A (1986) Oral tetrahydroaminoacridine in long-term treatment of senile dementia, Alzheimer type. *N Engl J Med* 315:1241–1245.

Sun Q, Turrigiano GG (2011) PSD-95 and PSD-93 play critical but distinct roles in synaptic scaling up and down. *J Neurosci* **31**:6800–6808.

Sun Y, Smirnov M, Kamasawa N, Yasuda R (2021) Rapid ultrastructural changes in the PSD and surrounding membrane after induction of structural LTP in single dendritic spines. *J Neurosci* **41**:7003–7014.

Sun YE, Wu H (2006) The ups and downs of BDNF in Rett syndrome. *Neuron* **49**:321–323.

Sutherland RJ, Dringenberg HC, Hoesing JM (1993) Induction of long-term potentiation at perforant path dentate synapses does not affect place learning or memory. *Hippocampus* **3**:141–147.

Suzuki K, Nosyreva E, Hunt KW, Kavalali ET, Monteggia LM (2017) Effects of a ketamine metabolite on synaptic NMDAR function. *Nature* **546**:E1–e3.

Sydow A, Van der Jeugd A, Zheng F, Ahmed T, Balschun D, Petrova O, Drexler D, Zhou L, Rune G, Mandelkow E, et al. (2011) Tau-induced defects in synaptic plasticity, learning, and memory are reversible in transgenic mice after switching off the toxic Tau mutant. *J Neurosci* **31**:2511–2525.

Takeuchi T, Duszkiewicz AJ, Morris RG (2014) The synaptic plasticity and memory hypothesis: encoding, storage and persistence. *Philos Trans R Soc Lond B Biol Sci* **369**:20130288.

Takeuchi T, Duszkiewicz AJ, Sonneborn A, Spooner PA, Yamasaki M, Watanabe M, Smith CC, Fernández G, Deisseroth K, Greene RW, et al. (2016) Locus coeruleus and dopaminergic consolidation of everyday memory. *Nature* **537**:357–362.

Tanaka J, Horiike Y, Matsuzaki M, Miyazaki T, Ellis-Davies GC, Kasai H (2008) Protein synthesis and neurotrophin-dependent structural plasticity of single dendritic spines. *Science* **319**:1683–1687.

Tancredi V, D'Arcangelo G, Grassi F, Tarroni P, Palmieri G, Santoni A, Eusebi F (1992) Tumor necrosis factor alters synaptic transmission in rat hippocampal slices. *Neurosci Lett* **146**:176–178.

Tang AH, Chen H, Li TP, Metzbower SR, MacGillavry HD, Blanpied TA (2016) A trans-synaptic nanocolumn aligns neurotransmitter release to receptors. *Nature* **536**:210–214.

Tang SJ, Schuman EM (2002) Protein synthesis in the dendrite. *Philos Trans R Soc Lond B Biol Sci* **357**:521–529.

Tang YP, Shimizu E, Dube GR, Rampon C, Kerchner GA, Zhuo M, Liu G, Tsien JZ (1999) Genetic enhancement of learning and memory in mice. *Nature* **401**:63–69.

Taylor CJ, Ireland DR, Ballagh I, Bourne K, Marechal NM, Turner PR, Bilkey DK, Tate WP, Abraham WC (2008) Endogenous secreted amyloid precursor protein-alpha regulates hippocampal NMDA receptor function, long-term potentiation and spatial memory. *Neurobiol Dis* **31**:250–260.

Tenorio G, Connor SA, Guévremont D, Abraham WC, Williams J, O'Dell TJ, Nguyen PV (2010) "Silent" priming of translation-dependent LTP by ß-adrenergic receptors involves phosphorylation and recruitment of AMPA receptors. *Learn Mem* **17**:627–638.

Terashima A, Pelkey KA, Rah JC, Suh YH, Roche KW, Collingridge GL, McBain CJ, Isaac JT (2008) An essential role for PICK1 in NMDA receptor-dependent bidirectional synaptic plasticity. *Neuron* **57**:872–882.

Thomazeau A, Lassalle O, Iafrati J, Souchet B, Guedj F, Janel N, Chavis P, Delabar J, Manzoni OJ (2014) Prefrontal deficits in a murine model overexpressing the down syndrome candidate gene dyrk1a. *J Neurosci* **34**:1138–1147.

Thurman AJ, Potter LA, Kim K, Tassone F, Banasik A, Potter SN, Bullard L, Nguyen V, McDuffie A, Hagerman R, et al. (2020) Controlled trial of lovastatin combined with an open-label treatment of a parent-implemented language intervention in youth with fragile X syndrome. *J Neurodev Disord* **12**:12.

Timofeev I, Chauvette S (2018) Sleep, anesthesia, and plasticity. *Neuron* **97**:1200–1202.

Toft AK, Lundbye CJ, Banke TG (2016) Dysregulated NMDA-receptor signaling inhibits long-term depression in a mouse model of fragile X syndrome. *J Neurosci* **36**:9817–9827.

Tomiyama T, Nagata T, Shimada H, Teraoka R, Fukushima A, Kanemitsu H, Takuma H, Kuwano R, Imagawa M, Ataka S, et al. (2008) A new amyloid beta variant favoring oligomerization in Alzheimer's-type dementia. *Ann Neurol* **63**:377–387.

Tonegawa S, Liu X, Ramirez S, Redondo R (2015) Memory engram cells have come of age. *Neuron* **87**:918–931.

Tonegawa S, Pignatelli M, Roy DS, Ryan TJ (2015) Memory engram storage and retrieval. *Curr Opin Neurobiol* **35**:101–109.

Tong R, Emptage NJ, Padamsey Z (2020) A two-compartment model of synaptic computation and plasticity. *Mol Brain* **13**:79.

Tononi G, Cirelli C (2003) Sleep and synaptic homeostasis: a hypothesis. *Brain Res Bull* **62**:143–150.

Tononi G, Cirelli C (2014) Sleep and the price of plasticity: from synaptic and cellular homeostasis to memory consolidation and integration. *Neuron* **81**:12–34.

Treves A, Rolls ET (1994) Computational analysis of the role of the hippocampus in memory. *Hippocampus* **4**:374–391.

Trommald M, Hulleberg G, Andersen P (1996) Long-term potentiation is associated with new excitatory spine synapses on rat dentate granule cells. *Learn Mem* **3**:218–228.

Truchet B, Manrique C, Sreng L, Chaillan FA, Roman FS, Mourre C (2012) Kv4 potassium channels modulate hippocampal EPSP-spike potentiation and spatial memory in rats. *Learn Mem* **19**:282–293.

Tse D, Takeuchi T, Kakeyama M, Kajii Y, Okuno H, Tohyama C, Bito H, Morris RG (2011) Schema-dependent gene activation and memory encoding in neocortex. *Science* **333**:891–895.

Tsokas P, Hsieh C, Yao Y, Lesburgueres E, Wallace EJ, Tcherepanov A, Jothianandan D, Hartley BR, Pan L, Rivard B, et al. (2016) Compensation for PKMzeta in long-term potentiation and spatial long-term memory in mutant mice. *Elife* **5**. doi:10.7554/eLife.14846.

Tsumoto T (1993) Long-term depression in cerebral cortex: a possible substrate of "forgetting" that should not be forgotten. *Neurosci Res* **16**:263–270.

Tsurugizawa T, Mukai H, Tanabe N, Murakami G, Hojo Y, Kominami S, Mitsuhashi K, Komatsuzaki Y, Morrison JH, Janssen WG, et al. (2005) Estrogen induces rapid decrease in dendritic thorns of CA3 pyramidal neurons in adult male rat hippocampus. *Biochem Biophys Res Commun* **337**:1345–1352.

Tu X, Yasuda R, Colgan LA (2020) Rac1 is a downstream effector of PKCα in structural synaptic plasticity. *Sci Rep* **10**:1777.

Tuchman R, Alessandri M, Cuccaro M (2010) Autism spectrum disorders and epilepsy: moving towards a comprehensive approach to treatment. *Brain Dev* **32**:719–730.

Tullis JE, Larsen ME, Rumian NL, Freund RK, Boxer EE, Brown CN, Coultrap SJ, Schulman H, Aoto J, Dell'Acqua ML, et al. (2023) LTP induction by structural rather than enzymatic functions of CaMKII. *Nature* **621**:146–153.

Turi GF, Li WK, Chavlis S, Pandi I, O'Hare J, Priestley JB, Grosmark AD, Liao Z, Ladow M, Zhang JF, et al. (2019) Vasoactive intestinal polypeptide-expressing interneurons in the hippocampus support goal-oriented spatial learning. *Neuron* **101**:1150–1165, e1158.

Turrigiano GG (2008) The self-tuning neuron: synaptic scaling of excitatory synapses. *Cell* **135**:422–435.

Turrigiano GG (2017) The dialectic of Hebb and homeostasis. *Philos Trans R Soc Lond B Biol Sci* **372**. doi: 10.1098/rstb.2016.0258.

Turrigiano GG, Leslie KR, Desai NS, Rutherford LC, Nelson SB (1998) Activity-dependent scaling of quantal amplitude in neocortical neurons. *Nature* **391**:892–896.

Ucar H, Watanabe S, Noguchi J, Morimoto Y, Iino Y, Yagishita S, Takahashi N, Kasai H (2021) Mechanical actions of dendritic-spine enlargement on presynaptic exocytosis. *Nature* **600**:686–689.

Udakis M, Pedrosa V, Chamberlain SEL, Clopath C, Mellor JR (2020) Interneuron-specific plasticity at parvalbumin and somatostatin inhibitory synapses onto CA1 pyramidal neurons shapes hippocampal output. *Nat Commun* **11**:4395.

Uekita T, Okaichi H (2009) Pretraining does not ameliorate spatial learning deficits induced by intrahippocampal infusion of AP5. *Behav Neurosci* **123**:520–526.

Um JW, Kaufman AC, Kostylev M, Heiss JK, Stagi M, Takahashi H, Kerrisk ME, Vortmeyer A, Wisniewski T, Koleske AJ, et al. (2013) Metabotropic glutamate receptor 5 is a coreceptor for Alzheimer aβ oligomer bound to cellular prion protein. *Neuron* **79**:887–902.

Urban NN, Henze DA, Lewis DA, Barrionuevo G (1996) Properties of LTP induction in the CA3 region of the primate hippocampus. *Learn Mem* **3**:86–95.

Ure K, Lu H, Wang W, Ito-Ishida A, Wu Z, He LJ, Sztainberg Y, Chen W, Tang J, Zoghbi HY (2016) Restoration of Mecp2 expression in GABAergic neurons is sufficient to rescue multiple disease features in a mouse model of Rett syndrome. *Elife* **5**:e14198. doi:10.7554/eLife.14198

Valbuena S, Lerma J (2021) Kainate receptors, homeostatic gatekeepers of synaptic plasticity. *Neuroscience* **456**:17–26.

Vandael D, Borges-Merjane C, Zhang X, Jonas P (2020) Short-term plasticity at hippocampal mossy fiber synapses is induced by natural activity patterns and associated with vesicle pool engram formation. *Neuron* **107**:509–521, e507.

Van Esch H (2012) MECP2 Duplication syndrome. *Mol Syndromol* **2**:128–136.

Van Harreveld A, Fifkova E (1975) Swelling of dendritic spines in the fascia dentata after stimulation of the perforant fibers as a mechanism of post-tetanic potentiation. *Exp Neurol* **49**:736–749.

Varela JA, Hirsch SJ, Chapman D, Leverich LS, Greene RW (2009) D1/D5 modulation of synaptic NMDA receptor currents. *J Neurosci* **29**:3109–3119.

Vasuta C, Artinian J, Laplante I, Hebert-Seropian S, Elayoubi K, Lacaille JC (2015) Metaplastic regulation of CA1 Schaffer collateral pathway plasticity by Hebbian MGluR1a-mediated plasticity at excitatory synapses onto somatostatin-expressing interneurons. *eNeuro* **2**. doi:10.1523/ENEURO.0051-15.2015

Vetere G, Tran LM, Moberg S, Steadman PE, Restivo L, Morrison FG, Ressler KJ, Josselyn SA, Frankland PW (2019) Memory formation in the absence of experience. *Nat Neurosci* **22**:933–940.

Vickers CA, Dickson KS, Wyllie DJ (2005) Induction and maintenance of late-phase long-term potentiation in isolated dendrites of rat hippocampal CA1 pyramidal neurones. *J Physiol (Lond)* **568**:803–813.

Vierk R, Glassmeier G, Zhou L, Brandt N, Fester L, Dudzinski D, Wilkars W, Bender RA, Lewerenz M, Gloger S, et al. (2012) Aromatase inhibition abolishes LTP generation in female but not in male mice. *J Neurosci* **32**:8116–8126.

Viola H, Ballarini F, Martinez MC, Moncada D (2014) The tagging and capture hypothesis from synapse to memory. *Prog Mol Biol Transl Sci* **122**:391–423.

Volianskis A, Bannister N, Collett VJ, Irvine MW, Monaghan DT, Fitzjohn SM, Jensen MS, Jane DE, Collingridge GL (2013) Different NMDA receptor subtypes mediate induction of long-term potentiation and two forms of short-term potentiation at CA1 synapses in rat hippocampus in vitro. *J Physiol* **591**:955–972.

Volianskis A, Collingridge GL, Jensen MS (2013) The roles of STP and LTP in synaptic encoding. *Peer J* **1**:e3.

Volianskis A, France G, Jensen MS, Bortolotto ZA, Jane DE, Collingridge GL (2015) Long-term potentiation and the role of N-methyl-D-aspartate receptors. *Brain Res* **1621**:5–16.

Volianskis A, Kostner R, Molgaard M, Hass S, Jensen MS (2010) Episodic memory deficits are not related to altered glutamatergic synaptic transmission and plasticity in the CA1 hippocampus of the APPswe/PS1deltaE9-deleted transgenic mice model of ss-amyloidosis. *Neurobiol Aging* **31**:1173–1187.

Volk LJ, Bachman JL, Johnson R, Yu Y, Huganir RL (2013) PKM-ζ is not required for hippocampal synaptic plasticity, learning and memory. *Nature* **493**:420–423.

Volk L, Kim CH, Takamiya K, Yu Y, Huganir RL (2010) Developmental regulation of protein interacting with C kinase 1 (PICK1) function in hippocampal synaptic plasticity and learning. *Proc Natl Acad Sci U S A* **107**:21784–21789.

Vossel KA, Beagle AJ, Rabinovici GD, Shu H, Lee SE, Naasan G, Hegde M, Cornes SB, Henry ML, Nelson AB, et al. (2013) Seizures and epileptiform activity in the early stages of Alzheimer disease. *JAMA Neurol* **70**:1158–1166.

Vossel KA, Ranasinghe KG, Beagle AJ, Mizuiri D, Honma SM, Dowling AF, Darwish SM, Van Berlo V, Barnes DE, Mantle M, et al. (2016) Incidence and impact of subclinical epileptiform activity in Alzheimer's disease. *Ann Neurol* **80**:858–870.

Vyleta NP, Borges-Merjane C, Jonas P (2016) Plasticity-dependent, full detonation at hippocampal mossy fiber-CA3 pyramidal neuron synapses. *Elife* **5**:e17977.

Wallis JL, Irvine MW, Jane DE, Lodge D, Collingridge GL, Bortolotto ZA (2015) An interchangeable role for kainate and metabotropic glutamate receptors in the induction of rat hippocampal mossy fiber long-term potentiation in vivo. *Hippocampus* **25**:1407–1417.

Walsh DM, Klyubin I, Fadeeva JV, Cullen WK, Anwyl R, Wolfe MS, Rowan MJ, Selkoe DJ (2002) Naturally secreted oligomers of amyloid beta protein potently inhibit hippocampal long-term potentiation in vivo. *Nature* **416**:535–539.

Wang F, Zhu J, Zhu H, Zhang Q, Lin Z, Hu H (2011) Bidirectional control of social hierarchy by synaptic efficacy in medial prefrontal cortex. *Science* **334**:693–697.

Wang P, Yang G, Mosier DR, Chang P, Zaidi T, Gong YD, Zhao NM, Dominguez B, Lee KF, Gan WB, et al. (2005) Defective neuromuscular synapses in mice lacking amyloid precursor protein (APP) and APP-Like protein 2. *J Neurosci* **25**:1219–1225.

Wang Q, Rowan MJ, Anwyl R (2004) Beta-amyloid-mediated inhibition of NMDA receptor-dependent long-term potentiation induction involves activation of microglia and stimulation of inducible nitric oxide synthase and superoxide. *J Neurosci* **24**:6049–6056.

Wang Q, Walsh DM, Rowan MJ, Selkoe DJ, Anwyl R (2004) Block of long-term potentiation by naturally secreted and synthetic amyloid beta-peptide in hippocampal slices is mediated via activation of the kinases c-Jun N-terminal kinase, cyclin-dependent kinase 5, and p38 mitogen-activated protein kinase as well as metabotropic glutamate receptor type 5. *J Neurosci* **24**:3370–3378.

Wang SH, Redondo RL, Morris RGM (2010) Relevance of synaptic tagging and capture to the persistence of long-term potentiation and everyday spatial memory. *Proc Natl Acad Sci U S A* **107**:19537–19542.

Wang W, Jia Y, Pham DT, Palmer LC, Jung KM, Cox CD, Rumbaugh G, Piomelli D, Gall CM, Lynch G (2018) Atypical endocannabinoid signaling initiates a new form of memory-related plasticity at a cortical input to hippocampus. *Cereb Cortex* **28**:2253–2266.

Wang W, Le AA, Hou B, Lauterborn JC, Cox CD, Levin ER, Lynch G, Gall CM (2018) Memory-related synaptic plasticity is sexually dimorphic in rodent hippocampus. *J Neurosci* 38:7935–7951.

Wang XB, Bozdagi O, Nikitczuk JS, Zhai ZW, Zhou Q, Huntley GW (2008) Extracellular proteolysis by matrix metalloproteinase-9 drives dendritic spine enlargement and long-term potentiation coordinately. *Proc Natl Acad Sci U S A* 105:19520–19525.

Warren SG, Humphreys AG, Juraska JM, Greenough WT (1995) LTP varies across the estrous cycle: enhanced synaptic plasticity in proestrus rats. *Brain Res* 703:26–30.

Warren SG, Juraska JM (1997) Spatial and nonspatial learning across the rat estrous cycle. *Behav Neurosci* 111:259–266.

Watkins JC, Davies J, Evans RH, Francis AA, Jones AW (1981) Pharmacology of receptors for excitatory amino acids. *Adv Biochem Psychopharmacol* 27:263–273.

Watkins JC, Jane DE (2006) The glutamate story. *Br J Pharmacol* 147(Suppl 1):S100–108.

Watson BO, Levenstein D, Greene JP, Gelinas JN, Buzsaki G (2016) Network homeostasis and state dynamics of neocortical sleep. *Neuron* 90:839–852.

Watson JF, Pinggera A, Ho H, Greger IH (2021) AMPA receptor anchoring at CA1 synapses is determined by N-terminal domain and TARP γ8 interactions. *Nat Commun* 12:5083.

Welsby P, Rowan M, Anwyl R (2006) Nicotinic receptor-mediated enhancement of long-term potentiation involves activation of metabotropic glutamate receptors and ryanodine-sensitive calcium stores in the dentate gyrus. *Eur J Neurosci* 24:3109–3118.

Whitcomb DJ, Hogg EL, Regan P, Piers T, Narayan P, Whitehead G, Winters BL, Kim DH, Kim E, St George-Hyslop P, et al. (2015) Intracellular oligomeric amyloid-beta rapidly regulates GluA1 subunit of AMPA receptor in the hippocampus. *Sci Rep* 5:10934.

Whitehead G, Jo J, Hogg EL, Piers T, Kim DH, Seaton G, Seok H, Bru-Mercier G, Son GH, Regan P, et al. (2013) Acute stress causes rapid synaptic insertion of Ca2+ -permeable AMPA receptors to facilitate long-term potentiation in the hippocampus. *Brain* 136:3753–3765.

Whitehouse PJ, Price DL, Struble RG, Clark AW, Coyle JT, Delon MR (1982) Alzheimer's disease and senile dementia: loss of neurons in the basal forebrain. *Science* 215:1237–1239.

Whitlock JR, Heynen AJ, Shuler MG, Bear MF (2006) Learning induces long-term potentiation in the hippocampus. *Science* 313:1093–1097.

Wigstrom H, Gustafsson B (1983) Facilitated induction of hippocampal long-lasting potentiation during blockade of inhibition. *Nature* 301:603–604.

Wigström H, Gustafsson B (1985) On long lasting potentiation in the hippocampus: a proposed mechanism for its dependence on coincident pre- and postsynaptic activity. *Acta Physiol Scand* 123:519–522.

Willshaw D, Dayan P (1990) Optimal plasticity from matrix memories: what goes up must come down. *Neural Computation* 2:85–93.

Wimo A, Guerchet M, Ali GC, Wu YT, Prina AM, Winblad B, Jonsson L, Liu Z, Prince M (2017) The worldwide costs of dementia 2015 and comparisons with 2010. *Alzheimers Dement* 13:1–7.

Wittenberg R, Knapp M, Hu B, Comas-Herrera A, King D, Rehill A, Shi C, Banerjee S, Patel A, Jagger C, et al. (2019) The costs of dementia in England. *Int J Geriatr Psychiatry* 34:1095–1103.

Won H, Lee HR, Gee HY, Mah W, Kim JI, Lee J, Ha S, Chung C, Jung ES, Cho YS, et al. (2012) Autistic-like social behaviour in Shank2-mutant mice improved by restoring NMDA receptor function. *Nature* 486:261–265.

Woolley CS, McEwen BS (1992) Estradiol mediates fluctuation in hippocampal synapse density during the estrous cycle in the adult rat. *J Neurosci* 12:2549–2554.

Woolley DE, Gould E, Frankfurt M, McEwen BS (1990) Naturally occurring fluctuations in dendritic spine density on adult hippocampal pyramidal neurons. *J Neurosci* 10:4035–4039.

Wu HY, Hudry E, Hashimoto T, Kuchibhotla K, Rozkalne A, Fan Z, Spires-Jones T, Xie H, Arbel-Ornath M, Grosskreutz CL, et al. (2010) Amyloid beta induces the morphological neurodegenerative triad of spine loss, dendritic simplification, and neuritic dystrophies through calcineurin activation. *J Neurosci* 30:2636–2649.

Xiao K, Li Y, Chitwood RA, Magee JC (2023) A critical role for CaMKII in behavioral timescale synaptic plasticity in hippocampal CA1 pyramidal neurons. *Sci Adv* 9:eadi3088.

Xie W, Ramakrishna N, Wieraszko A, Hwang YW (2008) Promotion of neuronal plasticity by (-)-epigallocatechin-3-gallate. *Neurochem Res* 33:776–783.

Xiong M, Jones OD, Peppercorn K, Ohline SM, Tate WP, Abraham WC (2017) Secreted amyloid precursor protein-alpha can restore novel object location memory and hippocampal LTP in aged rats. *Neurobiol Learn Mem* 138:291–299.

Xu J, Wang J, Wimo A, Fratiglioni L, Qiu C (2017) The economic burden of dementia in China, 1990–2030: implications for health policy. *Bull World Health Organ* 95:18–26.

Xu K, Krystal JH, Ning Y, Chen DC, He H, Wang D, Ke X, Zhang X, Ding Y, Liu Y, et al. (2015) Preliminary analysis of positive and negative syndrome scale in ketamine-associated psychosis in comparison with schizophrenia. *J Psychiatr Res* 61:64–72.

Xu L, Anwyl R, Rowan MJ (1997) Behavioural stress facilitates the induction of long-term depression in the hippocampus. *Nature* 387:497–500.

Xu L, Anwyl R, Rowan MJ (1998) Spatial exploration induces a persistent reversal of long-term potentiation in rat hippocampus. *Nature* 394:891–894.

Xu T, Yu X, Perlik AJ, Tobin WF, Zweig JA, Tennant K, Jones T, Zuo Y (2009) Rapid formation and selective stabilization of synapses for enduring motor memories. *Nature* 462:915–919.

Yagishita S, Murayama M, Ebihara T, Maruyama K, Takashima A (2015) Glycogen synthase kinase 3β-mediated phosphorylation in the most C-terminal region of protein interacting with C kinase 1 (PICK1) regulates the binding of PICK1 to glutamate receptor subunit GluA2. *J Biol Chem* 290:29438–29448.

Yang G, Pan F, Gan WB (2009) Stably maintained dendritic spines are associated with lifelong memories. *Nature* 462:920–924.

Yang J, Harte-Hargrove LC, Siao CJ, Marinic T, Clarke R, Ma Q, Jing D, Lafrancois JJ, Bath KG, Mark W, et al. (2014) proBDNF negatively regulates neuronal remodeling, synaptic transmission, and synaptic plasticity in hippocampus. *Cell Rep* 7:796–806.

Yang K, Trepanier C, Sidhu B, Xie YF, Li H, Lei G, Salter MW, Orser BA, Nakazawa T, Yamamoto T, et al. (2012) Metaplasticity gated through differential regulation of GluN2A versus GluN2B receptors by Src family kinases. *Embo J* 31:805–816.

Yang P, Li L, Xia S, Zhou B, Zhu Y, Zhou G, Tu E, Huang T, Huang H, Li F (2019) Effect of Clozapine on anti-N-methyl-D-aspartate receptor encephalitis with psychiatric symptoms: a series of three cases. *Front Neurosci* 13:315.

Yang SN, Tang YG, Zucker RS (1999) Selective induction of LTP and LTD by postsynaptic [Ca2+]i elevation. *J Neurophysiol* 81:781–787.

Yang Y, Calakos N (2011) Munc13–1 is required for presynaptic long-term potentiation. *J Neurosci* 31:12053–12057.

Yang Y, Cui Y, Sang K, Dong Y, Ni Z, Ma S, Hu H (2018) Ketamine blocks bursting in the lateral habenula to rapidly relieve depression. *Nature* 554:317–322.

Yang S, Yasuda R (2017) Imaging ERK and PKA activation in single dendritic spines during structural plasticity. Neuron 22:1315-1324

Yang Y, Wang XB, Frerking M, Zhou Q (2008) Spine expansion and stabilization associated with long-term potentiation. *J Neurosci* 28:5740–5751.

Yang Y, Wang XB, Zhou Q (2010) Perisynaptic GluR2-lacking AMPA receptors control the reversibility of synaptic and spines modifications. *Proc Natl Acad Sci U S A* 107:11999–12004.

Yao Y, Kelly MT, Sajikumar S, Serrano P, Tian D, Bergold PJ, Frey JU, Sacktor TC (2008) PKM zeta maintains late long-term potentiation by N-ethylmaleimide-sensitive factor/GluR2-dependent trafficking of postsynaptic AMPA receptors. *J Neurosci* 28:7820–7827.

Yap EL, Pettit NL, Davis CP, Nagy MA, Harmin DA, Golden E, Dagliyan O, Lin C, Rudolph S, Sharma N, et al. (2021) Bidirectional perisomatic inhibitory plasticity of a Fos neuronal network. *Nature* 590:115–121.

Yasojima K, Akiyama H, McGeer EG, McGeer PL (2001) Reduced neprilysin in high plaque areas of Alzheimer brain: a possible relationship to deficient degradation of beta-amyloid peptide. *Neurosci Lett* 297:97–100.

Yau SY, Bostrom CA, Chiu J, Fontaine CJ, Sawchuk S, Meconi A, Wortman RC, Truesdell E, Truesdell A, Chiu C, et al. (2016) Impaired bidirectional NMDA receptor dependent synaptic plasticity in the dentate gyrus of adult female Fmr1 heterozygous knockout mice. *Neurobiol Dis* 96:261–270.

Yeung LC, Shouval HZ, Blais BS, Cooper LN (2004) Synaptic homeostasis and input selectivity follow from a calcium-dependent plasticity model. *Proc Natl Acad Sci U S A* 101:14943–14948.

Yun SH, Trommer BL (2011) Fragile X mice: reduced long-term potentiation and N-Methyl-D-Aspartate receptor-mediated neurotransmission in dentate gyrus. *J Neurosci Res* 89:176–182.

Zanos P, Moaddel R, Morris PJ, Georgiou P, Fischell J, Elmer GI, Alkondon M, Yuan P, Pribut HJ, Singh NS, et al. (2016) NMDAR inhibition-independent antidepressant actions of ketamine metabolites. *Nature* 533:481–486.

Zanos P, Moaddel R, Morris PJ, Riggs LM, Highland JN, Georgiou P, Pereira EFR, Albuquerque EX, Thomas CJ, Zarate CA, Jr, et al. (2018) Ketamine and ketamine metabolite pharmacology: insights into therapeutic mechanisms. *Pharmacol Rev* 70:621–660.

Zarate CA, Jr, Singh JB, Carlson PJ, Brutsche NE, Ameli R, Luckenbaugh DA, Charney DS, Manji HK (2006) A randomized trial of an N-methyl-D-aspartate antagonist in treatment-resistant major depression. *Arch Gen Psychiatry* 63:856–864.

Zeng M, Chen X, Guan D, Xu J, Wu H, Tong P, Zhang M (2018) Reconstituted postsynaptic density as a molecular platform for understanding synapse formation and plasticity. *Cell* 174:1172–1187, e1116.

Zhang D, Ivica J, Krieger JM, Ho H, Yamashita K, Stockwell I, Baradaran R, Cais O, Greger IH (2023) Structural mobility tunes signalling of the GluA1 AMPA glutamate receptor. *Nature* 621:877–882.

Zhang D, Watson JF, Matthews PM, Cais O, Greger IH (2021) Gating and modulation of a hetero-octameric AMPA glutamate receptor. *Nature* 594:454–458.

Zhang Y, Venkitaramani DV, Gladding CM, Zhang Y, Kurup P, Molnar E, Collingridge GL, Lombroso PJ (2008) The tyrosine phosphatase STEP mediates AMPA receptor endocytosis after metabotropic glutamate receptor stimulation. *J Neurosci* 28:10561–10566.

Zhang Z, van Praag H (2015) Maternal immune activation differentially impacts mature and adult-born hippocampal neurons in male mice. *Brain Behav Immun* 45:60–70.

Zhao F, Siu JJ, Huang W, Askwith C, Cao L (2019) Insulin modulates excitatory synaptic transmission and synaptic plasticity in the mouse hippocampus. *Neuroscience* 411:237–254.

Zhao M, Choi YS, Obrietan K, Dudek SM (2007) Synaptic plasticity (and the lack thereof) in hippocampal CA2 neurons. *J Neurosci* 27:12025–12032.

Zhou Q, Homma KJ, Poo MM (2004) Shrinkage of dendritic spines associated with long-term depression of hippocampal synapses. *Neuron* 44:749–757.

Zhou T, Zhu H, Fan Z, Wang F, Chen Y, Liang H, Yang Z, Zhang L, Lin L, Zhan Y, et al. (2017) History of winning remodels thalamo-PFC circuit to reinforce social dominance. *Science* 357:162–168.

Zhou Y, Zhu H, Liu Z, Chen X, Su X, Ma C, Tian Z, Huang B, Yan E, Liu X, et al. (2019) A ventral CA1 to nucleus accumbens core engram circuit mediates conditioned place preference for cocaine. *Nat Neurosci* 22:1986–1999.

Zhou Z, Hu J, Passafaro M, Xie W, Jia Z (2011) GluA2 (GluR2) regulates metabotropic glutamate receptor-dependent long-term depression through N-cadherin-dependent and cofilin-mediated actin reorganization. *J Neurosci* 31:819–833.

Zhou Z, Liu A, Xia S, Leung C, Qi J, Meng Y, Xie W, Park P, Collingridge GL, Jia Z (2018) The C-terminal tails of endogenous GluA1 and GluA2 differentially contribute to hippocampal synaptic plasticity and learning. *Nat Neurosci* 21:50–62.

Zhou Z, Meng Y, Asrar S, Todorovski Z, Jia Z (2009) A critical role of Rho-kinase ROCK2 in the regulation of spine and synaptic function. *Neuropharmacology* 56:81–89.

Zoghbi HY, Bear MF (2012) Synaptic dysfunction in neurodevelopmental disorders associated with autism and intellectual disabilities. *Cold Spring Harb Perspect Biol* 4:a009886.

11

Hippocampal Physiology in the Behaving Animal

Julija Krupic and John O'Keefe

11.1 Introduction

In this chapter we will summarize what is known about the electrophysiological activity of the hippocampus in the behaving animal. We begin in section 11.2 with work on the hippocampal local field potential (LFP) and its role in organizing hippocampal cellular activity. The LFP represents the state of the hippocampus as it shifts from an active theta mode in which the hippocampus controls the behavior of the animal to a more passive state with large amplitude irregular activity (LIA) and sharp wave ripples (SWRs), which have more to do with internal housekeeping and communication with other parts of the brain, for example, during consolidation of memories. We will focus on hippocampal theta activity, which dominates the LFP when the animal is actively attending to and moving around the environment. We will discuss how theta occurs not only when animals move around in space but also during other types of nonspatial coding, for example, when pyramidal cells are coding for aspects of time. It appears to reflect activity at the cellular level, which has multiple functions, each related to a different septohippocampal neurotransmitter system. For example, theta dependent on glutamatergic input from the medial septum provides information about the speed of translation in an environment, while cholinergic theta is related to rotations in the environment. In addition, cholinergic theta also provides information about the presence of arousing or attention-grabbing stimuli, perhaps as a way of incorporating these into the hippocampal representation of the environment. In addition, the oscillatory theta system provides a clock function for temporal as well as rate coding of pyramidal cell activity and different phases of the theta control memory functions.

In section 11.3 we discuss the functional correlates of the different cell types in the hippocampal formation. Single-unit recording has revealed different classes of principal cell in the hippocampal formation, many with a spatial correlate: place cells in the hippocampus proper, head-direction cells in pre- and para-subiculum and entorhinal cortex, and grid cells in entorhinal cortex. In addition to the principal cells, theta cells, almost all of which are interneurons, show less dramatic spatial coding and are characterized by rate changes associated with hippocampal LFP theta. Many display strong phase relations to the hippocampal LFP theta, with different classes of interneuron preferring to fire at different phases. Since different classes of inhibitory interneurons target different parts of the pyramidal cell dendrites, one important function of the theta interneuronal mechanism may be to control access to these dendritic compartments at different phases of theta.

In section 11.4, we will examine some of the properties of spatial cells, and in the next section (11.5) will ask whether hippocampal pyramidal cells are influenced by nonspatial information either independently of the animal's location or in conjunction with it. We and others have previously argued that hippocampal pyramidal cells have space as their primary correlate and that many of the studies making claims for other correlates could be shown to be misinterpreted. This is a crucial question, since primary correlates other than space have been taken as support for other theories of hippocampal function—for example, the relational theory of Eichenbaum—and would necessitate a broadening of the function of the cognitive map theory beyond space. In addition to looking at sensory inputs to the pyramidal cells, we will ask whether their activity is influenced by goals and rewards and, importantly, whether they also signal the temporal aspects of events as well as their spatial ones. We will argue that many if not all these nonspatial correlates are secondary to the spatial ones, but at this stage this is still an open question. We will also ask whether place cells can be found in parts of the brain other than the hippocampal formation (11.6), and in section 11.7 will take an in-depth look at the relationship between the hippocampus and the entorhinal cortex, with which it is strongly connected. Section 11.8 asks whether place cells exist in species other than rats, including nonhuman primates and humans. In the subsequent sections, we tackle such questions as how place cells are created (11.9), and whether they relate to the animal's current position or to past or future locations (11.10).

An important role of the hippocampus is in the formation of spatial representations, which subserve spatial navigation. We will report recent work on this question in section 11.11 and show how during two-dimensional navigation place cells become directionally polarized and provide information about the direction of the goal from any location, which could be used by the brain to support flexible navigation. The hippocampus has long been recognized as having an important role to play in memory.

While evidence for lateralization in the human hippocampus is strong, it is less so in other animals such as the rodent. In section 11.12 we will deal with the question of hippocampal lateralization.

Other types of spatial cells, most notably head-direction cells and grid cells, contribute to the formation of spatial representations in the hippocampal formation. In addition, other types of spatial cells have been identified in the hippocampal formation: object-in-place cells, boundary vector cells, object vector cells, and speed cells, and their properties and roles in the formation of spatial representations will be discussed in Chapters 13 and 15.

11.2 The hippocampal local field potential

The hippocampal local field potential (LFP) reflects the synchronized activity of large numbers of neural elements. Since the function of the hippocampus depends on the differential activity of neighboring neurons, the LFP is best thought of as providing information about the different states of the hippocampus. This section is primarily about the two major types of hippocampal LFP, what we know about their generation, and, most importantly, what they tell us about the function of the hippocampus. The two states of the hippocampus reflected in the LFP are the theta (6–12 Hz)/gamma (30–100 Hz) state and the large amplitude irregular activity (LIA)/SWR state. The latter is characterized by a broad spectrum of frequencies intermittently punctuated by sharp waves of about 100 ms duration, on which higher frequency ripples (SWR, 100–200 Hz) ride. Figure 11.1 shows examples of each. Some patterns can co-occur (e.g., LIA with ripples, theta with gamma), while others appear to be mutually exclusive (e.g., theta and LIA). These latter waveforms appear to correspond to mutually exclusive states of hippocampal functioning. Theta/gamma occurs during movements

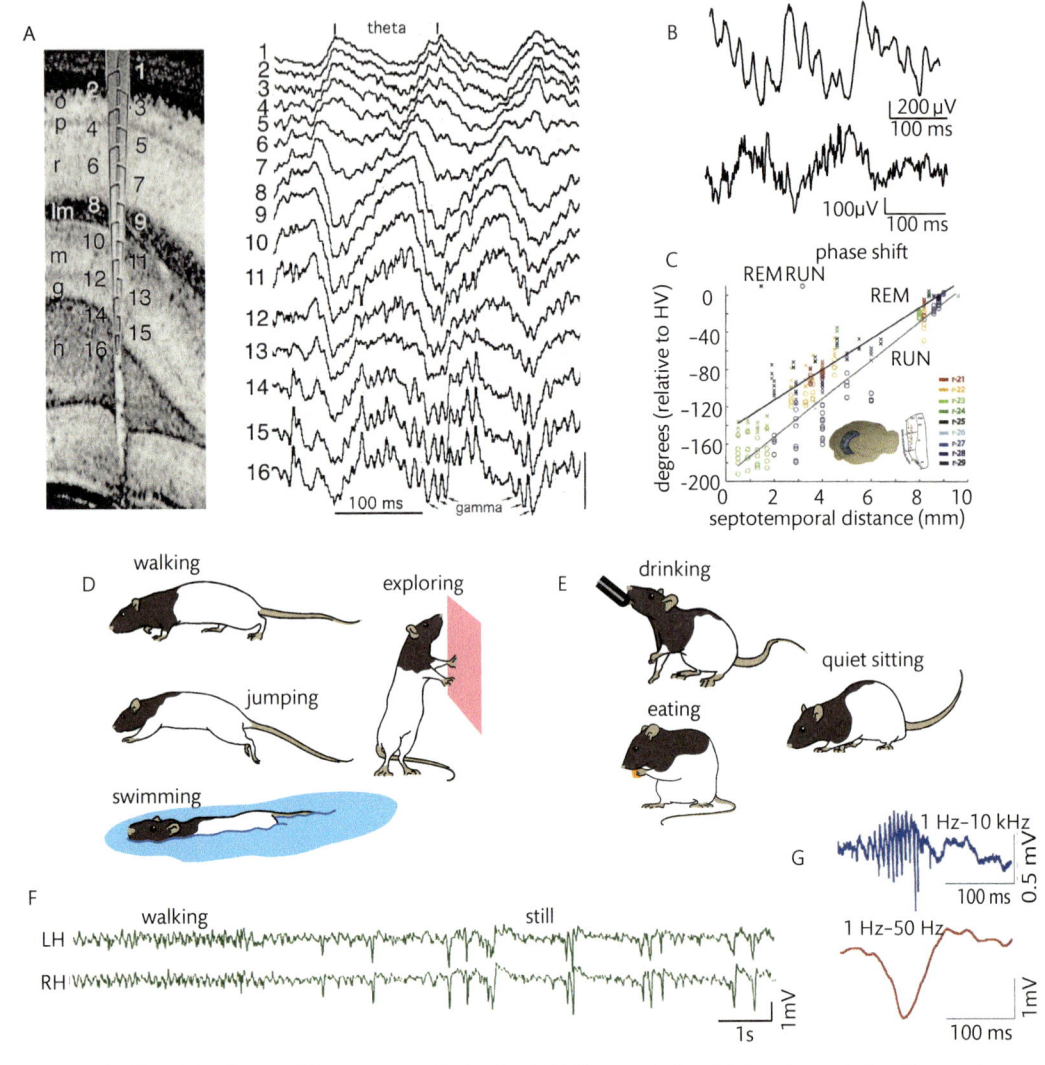

Figure 11.1 Hippocampal LFP activity during different types of behavior. (A) LFP recorded at 16 sites through the different layers of the hippocampus with a silicon probe (left) during walking. Note regular theta oscillations with gradual shift of theta phase from str. oriens (o) to str. lacunosum-moleculare (lm). Gamma waves superimposed on theta oscillations become more prominent on the lower recording sites (arrows). Numbers indicate recording sites (100 μm spacing). o, str. oriens; p, pyramidal layer; r, str. radiatum; lm, str. lacunosum-moleculare; g, granule cell layer; h, hilus. (B) Slow (above) and fast (below) gamma waves riding on hippocampal waves. (C) Theta waves shift phase along the longitudinal extent of the hippocampus (inset), theta during movement and REM sleep shown separately. (D) During behaviors such as walking, exploring, jumping, and swimming, theta dominates the hippocampal LFP. (E) During behaviors such as drinking, eating, and quiet sitting, LIA with sharp wave ripples dominates. (F) Bilateral hippocampal LFP with theta on the left and LIA/sharp wave ripples on the right. (G) Sharp wave ripples (blue) recorded from CA1 pyramidal cell layer and concurrent SPW in str. radiatum (red). (Reproduced with permission from Buzsaki et al., 1992, and Colgin et al., 2009.)

which changed the animal's location in an environment such as walking, exploring, swimming, and jumping (Figure 11.1D), and also during attention and arousal. The LIA/SWR state occurs when the animal is not actively attending to the environment including during quiet sitting, eating, and drinking (Figure 11.1E,F,G). In some animals the SWRs can be blocked by arousing stimuli, while in others it cannot. During sleep, the REM dreaming phase is associated with theta and the nondreaming sleep with LIA. In this section we will summarize work on these LFP patterns and provide some insight into their generation and functional significance.

11.2.1 Theta LFP

Theta waves are the macroscopic signature of the oscillatory properties of the hippocampal system and, in particular, the pyramidal cells. The waves themselves vary in phase and amplitude along all three axes of the hippocampus, forming a 3D traveling wave (Bragin, Jando, et al., 1995; Lubenov and Siapas, 2009; Patel, Fujisawa, et al., 2012; Buzsaki, Stark, et al., 2015). As shown in Figure 11.1A, they travel in depth from the stratum lacunosum-moleculare toward the stratum oriens and (C) longitudinally from the septal to the temporal poles of the hippocampus, changing phase by 180° in each direction.

The mechanisms underlying theta oscillations are complex, involving both single-cell and network processes. Single pyramidal cells contain the channels and intracellular feedback loops which cause them to oscillate under the right conditions. Strong dendritic depolarization by current injection leads to large amplitude, self-sustained oscillation in the theta frequency range (Kamondi, Acsady, et al., 1998). Distal dendritic depolarization of the pyramidal cell by the entorhinal input during theta usually overlaps in time with somatic hyperpolarization. As a result, most pyramidal cells are normally below the firing threshold, either silent or discharging with single spikes on the negative portion of local field theta (i.e., when the somatic region is least polarized). These individual oscillators are organized into a synchronous network by the operation of the inhibitory interneurons. Minimal intrahippocampal circuitry is necessary to produce theta as shown in isolated hippocampal slices bathed in a cholinergic agonist (Konopacki, MacIver, et al., 1987). These theta oscillations are part of the cholinergic theta system (see below) since they are blocked by atropine. The isolated hippocampus in the absence of the septal or entorhinal inputs is also capable of producing theta (Goutagny, Jackson, and Williams, 2009). Extracellular recordings from CA1 pyramidal cells in rats running in open fields or on linear tracks show that the cells are silent outside of the restricted region of the place field (see section 11.3 for description of place cells and place fields). In the place field, the cells began to fire in bursts with a frequency slightly higher than the field LFP, resulting in the phase precession effect (Figure 11.2B). Intracellular recordings from pyramidal cell soma of mice running in virtual reality environments show theta frequency oscillations in the membrane potential below the firing rate threshold outside of the place field in synchrony with the extracellular theta LFP (Harvey, Collman, et al., 2009), suggesting that the extracellular theta waves reflect the summed intracellular oscillations of large numbers of silent pyramidal cells outside of their place fields. In the place field, synaptic inputs drive the frequency of oscillations of individual pyramidal cells higher than those of the network oscillations, allowing them to escape from the blanket inhibition of the inhibitory networks and to fire the cells.

These network inhibitory theta potential oscillations in turn reflect and are synchronized by the activity of different groups of hippocampal interneurons (Figure 11.2A). These are connected together in feedback networks with time constants that reinforce the oscillations. These networks in turn can be driven by forcing inputs from the medial septum.

Different classes of hippocampal inhibitory interneurons can be distinguished by their location in different hippocampal strata, differential expression of molecular markers, responsiveness to distinct synaptic transmitters, and axonal targeting of different regions of the pyramidal cell dendrites. Importantly, they also have different phase relationships to different phases of the hippocampal theta (Klausberger and Somogyi, 2008), suggesting that different parts of the dendrites are inaccessible to synaptic inputs during different parts of the theta cycle. Figure 11.2A summarizes some of the distinct types of hippocampal interneuron (see Chapters 5 and 7 for more details). To take one example, the OLM cells that have their cell bodies in the stratum oriens synapse on the tips of the apical dendrites in the stratum lacunosum-moleculare, where they are in a good position to inhibit the inputs from the entorhinal cortex. O'Keefe and Nadel (1978, 1979, pp. 228–9) originally suggested that one of the functions of the interneuron network underlying theta was to act as a gate that opens and closes access to different parts of the dendrites during different phases of theta (see also McKenzie, 2018, for a good recent discussion of this idea). As we shall see, the activity of different classes of interneurons targeting different segments of the dendrites is controlled by different medial septal inputs presumably reflecting the operation of arousal/attentional processes and mechanisms for conveying the animal's rotational and translational movements in the environment.

Vanderwolf (1969) originally proposed that hippocampal theta activity was comprised of two components, which could be distinguished on the basis of behavioral correlates (active voluntary vs. quiescent involuntary states) and pharmacology (a cholinergic component sensitive to atropine and a noncholinergic component). We now know that there are at least three components to theta, each identifiable with a different pharmacological input from the medial septum (Figure 11.2A). *First* is sensory theta, which depends on the ACh input from the medial septum and has two functions: an arousal/attentional component that reflects the role of the hippocampus in processing exteroceptive sensory inputs such as strong aversive stimuli or ethologically arousing stimuli (Sainsbury, Heynen, and Montoya, 1987) and a behavioral component that reflects rotationally driven inputs from the vestibular system that signals the animal's rotation in space (Tai, Ma, et al., 2012). It occurs in isolation in the rat during freezing in the face of predator threats and other arousing stimuli, and in the 1–2 seconds before the start of translational movements. It is much more common in rabbits, guinea pigs, ferrets, and cats, where it often occurs in the absence of any movement. It is unclear how much of this theta response to arousing stimuli is related to preparation for movement. An important study supporting this interpretation (Balleine and Curthoys, 1991) found that pretraining animals on an inescapable shock paradigm resulted in the absence of theta to a subsequent single shock in contrast to the immobility theta found in animals without that pretraining or with training that allowed for escape.

Sensory theta may also be related to the synchronization that occurs between rhythmical myostatial sniffing movements involving

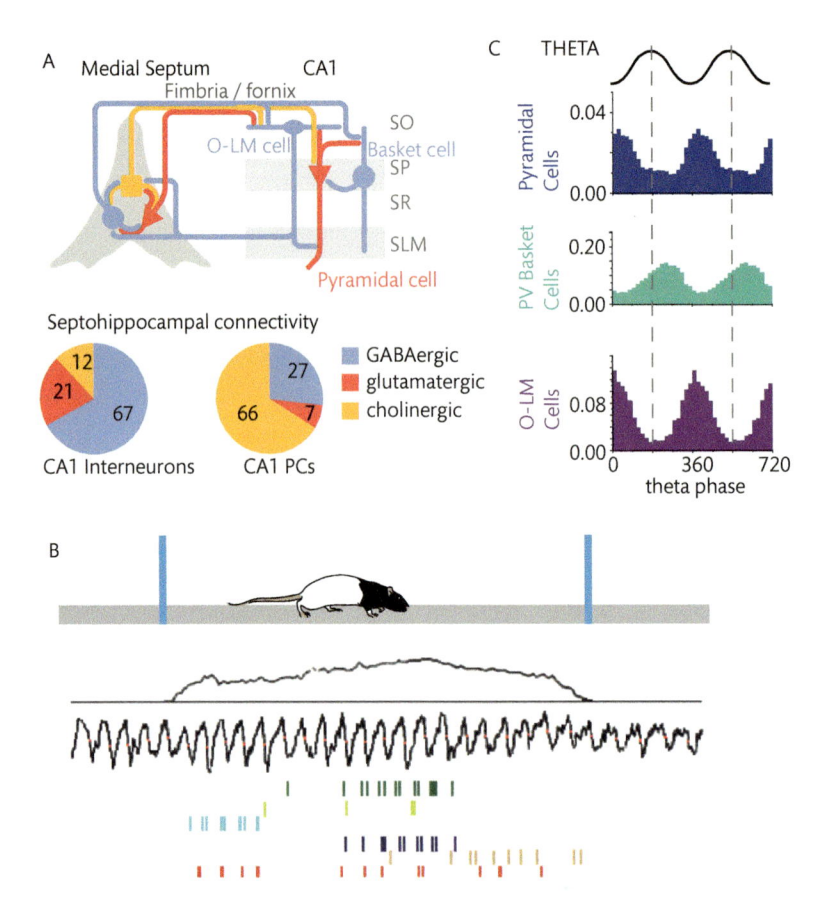

Figure 11.2 Simplified schema of medial septal circuitry and septohippocampal connections. (A) Anatomical arrangement within the medial septum (left) and simplified connectivity scheme focusing on medial septal connections to hippocampal CA1 pyramidal cells and interneurons. Septal cells shown in color: GABAergic (blue); glutamatergic (red); cholinergic (orange). Hippocampal cells: pyramidal cells (in red), together with PV-expressing basket cells and O-LM interneurons (in blue), which target different sections of the pyramidal cell soma and dendrites. Below, proportions of GABAergic, glutamatergic, and cholinergic projections terminating on CA1 interneurons and CA1 pyramidal neurons. (B) Hippocampal cells are velocity-tuned oscillators. When an animal runs on a linear track to obtain food at each end (top), hippocampal LFP shows rhythmical theta of 8–10 Hz. Pyramidal cells (top 5) fire at different locations on the track and oscillate at slightly higher frequencies than the theta frequency, showing phase precession. Interneurons (bottom, red) also fire along the track and usually do not depart from the LFP theta frequency and therefore do not show phase precession. Red ticks on the hippocampal LFP theta identify the + to - 0 crossing point of each wave for comparison to the spike times (O'Keefe, unpublished). (C) Oscillatory properties of different types of hippocampal cells. The firing probability histograms show that interneurons innervating different parts of the soma and dendrites of pyramidal cells fire with distinct temporal patterns during theta. PVC basket cells, which target the perisomatic region of the cell, fire earlier in the theta cycle than the pyramidal cells, while the O-LM cells, which target the apical dendrites, fire at approximately the same phase as the pyramidal cells. (Adapted with permission from Klausberger and Somogyi, 2008; Sun et al., 2014; and Muller and Remy, 2017.)

coupled whisker movements and sniffing (Welker, 1964). Kleinfeld (Kleinfeld, Deschenes, and Ulanovsky, 2016) has proposed that these active sniffing/head movements are controlled by the medial septum, tracing a pathway from the pontine rhythm generators to the nucleus. The MS/DB receives ascending projections from cholinergic neurons in the laterodorsal and pedunculopontine-tegmental nuclei (pontine respiratory group) (Fibiger, 1982; Woolf and Butcher, 1989). The same pontine nuclei send descending inputs to the dorsal and ventral respiratory groups (Jones, 1990; Semba and Fibiger, 1992) that generate the respiratory rhythm (Smith, Ellenberger, et al., 1991; Onimaru and Homma, 2003). Studies have shown that active sniffing movements and hippocampal theta briefly synchronize during the 1 second surrounding active olfactory/tactile discriminations (Macrides et al., 1982; Tsanov, Chah, et al.,

2014; Grion, Akrami, et al., 2016). However, injection of muscimol into the medial septum reduced the frequency of sniffing and theta (from 8.5 Hz to 7.5 Hz) but did not change the phase-locking, suggesting that the septal input is only one of several synchronizing theta with sensory inputs (Tsanov, Chah, et al., 2014). Overall, these results suggest that one function of hippocampal theta is to organize some of the sensory, and in particular, the olfactory and whisker, inputs to the hippocampus.

The *second* component, translational theta, is based on the glutamatergic/GABAergic septal input and reflects the exteroceptive and interoceptive inputs signaling translational movements in the environment (Fuhrmann, Justus, et al., 2015). In addition to its dependency on the medial septal in the rat, this component of theta (but not the ACh theta) is also dependent on the entorhinal cortex

(Vanderwolf, Leung, and Cooley, 1985). By way of contrast, both types of theta were affected by entorhinal lesions in the guinea pig (Montoya and Sainsbury, 1985). The frequency of glutamatergic theta is related to the speed of movement signaled by optic flow or stepping frequency.

Much is known about the role of theta in organizing spiking activity in the hippocampus. A *third* function for theta is to synchronize cellular activity across large regions of the hippocampus. In doing so it provides a neural clock against which the timing of place (and grid) cells can be measured to provide a basis for temporal as well as rate coding of location (Figure 11.2B). Temporal information provided by this phase precession phenomenon improves localization of the animal's position by 43% over that obtained using firing rates alone (Jensen and Lisman, 2000). As part of the temporal control of neuronal timing, theta exerts control over LTP induction. Inputs arriving at the +ve phase of CA1 theta will be more likely to result in synaptic potentiation while those arriving at the -ve phase will be more likely to result in depotentiation or depression (Huerta and Lisman, 1995).

The *fourth* function of theta is to signal novelty, either due to exposure to a novel environment or to changes to a familiar environment by the introduction of a novel object or the movement of a familiar object to another location. The novelty is signaled by a decrease in the frequency of theta related to a particular speed of movement. It should be noted that there is a methodological concern here, since novelty calls out exploratory behavior, which often consists of exploratory myostatial sniffing not usually seen in normal behavior. Therefore, it is inherently difficult to control for behavior between the novel and familiar situations. Despite this caveat, there is good evidence that novel situations are correlated with lower frequency theta compared with familiar ones, given the same general behaviors in terms of speed of movement, etc., or after controls for any changes in running speed (Jeewajee, Lever, et al., 2008) (Figure 11.3A). One component of novelty theta arises in the supramammillary nucleus, which projects directly to the hippocampus as well as via the medial septum and is responsible in part for the hippocampal response to social and environmental novelty (Chen, He, et al., 2020). We will discuss this in greater detail shortly.

The *fifth* function of theta is one we have already touched on, which is to control access of inputs to CA1 pyramidal cell dendrites, allowing different inputs access at different phases of the theta wave. This is implemented by the different interneuronal types that target different parts of the dendritic field and are maximally active at different parts of the theta wave.

The *final* function of theta is to control the reading in and out of information from individual pyramidal cells. This model (Hasselmo, Bodelon, and Wyble, 2002) is based on the fact that inputs to CA1 pyramidal cells from the medial entorhinal cortex target the tips of the apical dendrites and those from the CA3 field make contact closer to the soma, and that these two inputs arrive at different phases of the theta cycle. On this view, new associations are set up on the phase of the theta cycle during which synaptic input from entorhinal cortex onto the apical dendrites is strong but synaptic currents arising from CA3 input are weak (to prevent interference from prior learned associations). Conversely, retrieval of old associations occurs at the phase when the entorhinal input is weak and synaptic input from region CA3 is strong.

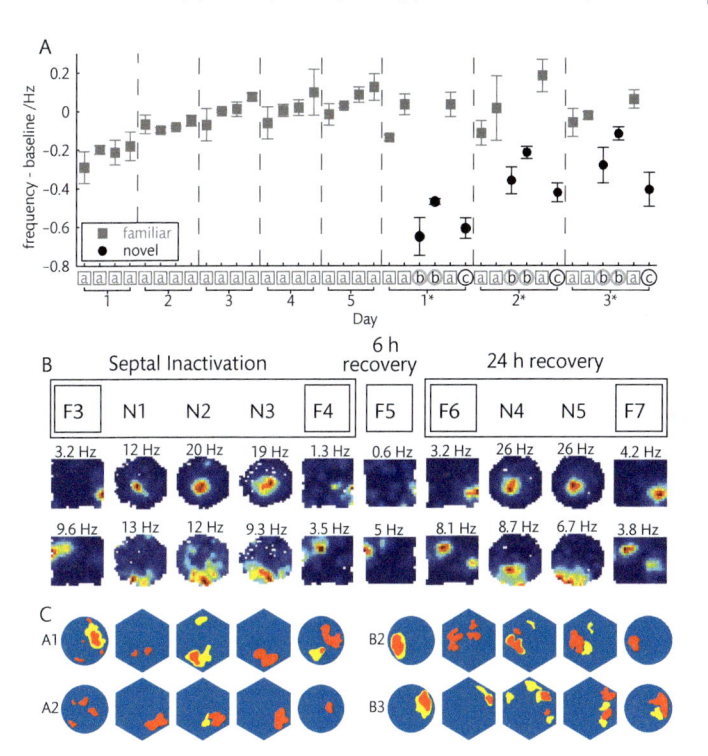

Figure 11.3 Effect of environmental novelty and septal inactivation on hippocampal LFP theta and place cells. (A) exposure to a novel environment decreases theta frequency. Animals were habituated to a square-shaped environment (A) for 5 days, resulting in stable theta frequency. On the next days (1*–3*), the 3rd, 4th, and 6th trials took place in novel environments, resulting in a reduced theta frequency, which slowly recovered over time as the environments became familiar. (After Jeewajee et al., 2008, with permission.) (B) During medial septal inactivation with muscimol, a GABAA-receptor agonist, hippocampal place cells (preinactivation, F3) form new place fields in a novel environment (N1–N3), which are maintained after recovery 24 hours later. Place cells in the original environment (F3–F7) are retained intact throughout the procedure. (After Brandon et al., 2014, with permission.) (C) Effect of the loss of medial septal cholinergic input to the hippocampus on place-cell stability during remapping. Cholinergic septal cells were lost following injection of IgG-saporin neurotoxic lesions. Animals were recorded on three trials in a novel octagon bracketed by two trials in a familiar circle. Two cells from control animals (left, A1, A2) showed stable remapping over several trials in the novel hexagonal environment while two cells from lesioned animals (right, B2, B3) originally remapped in the hexagon but over trials regressed to the original circular representation. (After Ikonen et al., 2002, with permission.)

11.2.2 Role of the medial septal/diagonal band of Broca pacemaker in the generation of hippocampal LFPs

The gross anatomical connections underlying theta activity are as follows. Increases in activity of ascending cholinergic and glutamatergic afferents from brainstem and hypothalamus to the medial septum drive oscillatory rhythms there. In turn, this oscillatory activity drives the hippocampal circuitry into theta mode. In addition to their interconnectedness within the medial septum, all three types of septal cells also project to the hippocampus through the fornix (Figure 11.2A). These three components can be separated on the basis of their pharmacology: cholinergic (Frotscher and Leranth, 1985), GABAergic (Kohler, Chan-Palay, and Wu, 1984; Freund and Antal, 1988), and glutamatergic (Colom, Castaneda, et al., 2005) (Figure 11.2A. Each has its own individual set of hippocampal formation targets in the hippocampus, which comprise primarily interneurons but also nonpyramidal principal cells such as the hilar cells (Leranth and Frotscher, 1987). These same septal afferents also project to EC (Manns, Mainville, and Jones, 2001), although this will not be addressed in detail in this chapter.

Medial septal cells are interconnected such that they form oscillators. Figure 11.2A shows some of the interconnections within the medial septum between the three types of septal projection cells. Cholinergic neurons provide a slow excitatory drive onto glutamatergic and GABAergic neurons, while glutamatergic neurons in turn provide strong fast excitatory drives onto the other two cell types with reciprocal projections forming recurrent connections. GABAergic neurons inhibit the others, synchronizing the septal network and pacing the rhythm of the theta oscillations. Some of these cells continuously oscillate at slightly different frequencies within the theta frequency range even in the absence of hippocampal theta (Kocsis, Martínez-Bellver, et al., 2021). During hippocampal theta, these different pacemaker neurons, identified as parvalbumin-expressing GABAergic neurons, synchronize their frequencies and increase firing rates, coming into phase alignment in a manner suggestive of the synchronization of Huygens clocks (Kocsis, Martínez-Bellver, et al., 2021).

The evidence suggests that the GABAergic cells directly drive the theta rhythms via their projections to inhibitory hippocampal interneurons, while glutamatergic inputs provide both rhythmical and nonrhythmical excitatory drive to both CA3 pyramidal cells and their associated interneurons, which in turn inhibit the pyramidal cells (Huh, Goutagny, and Williams, 2010). Direct cholinergic inputs only depolarize the pyramids and do not directly provide oscillatory input. They may, however, activate the intrinsic hippocampal oscillatory circuits indirectly instead.

In addition to their role in participating in hippocampal oscillations, some of the hippocampal inhibitory interneurons also project back to the medial and lateral septi, where it is thought they contribute to the synchronization of the septal/hippocampal oscillations, although these oscillations are not primarily dependent on this hippocamposeptal projection.

11.2.3 The role of theta in controlling hippocampal neuronal activity

The two major cell types in the hippocampus are the excitatory pyramidal cells and the inhibitory interneurons. Two major behavioral correlates of pyramidal cell activity are the animal's location (O'Keefe and Dostrovsky, 1971; O'Keefe, 1976) and the processing of sensory inputs (Bland and Oddie, 2001). The inhibitory interneurons are mostly theta cells. The name "theta cell" (Ranck, 1973) refers to the fact that they usually fire phase-locked to the local LFP. They have also been called "displace cells" (O'Keefe, 1976) to reflect the fact that one of their primary behavioral correlates in the rat is movement of a type that changes the animal's location in the environment. In addition, like the LFP theta itself, they also increase their firing under situations of high arousal or attention to sensory inputs. As pointed out in the LFP theta section above, this mode of theta occurs more frequently in animals such as rabbits and guinea pigs than in rodents. We will use these behavioral correlates of neural firing to elucidate some of the ways in which the theta system controls hippocampal activity. The spatial correlate of hippocampal pyramidal cells is immediately obvious as an animal engages in open field foraging. Here each cell

is typically silent as the rat moves around the foraging arena until it enters a small patch of the environment when the cell begins to fire (its place field). Within the place field, these cells also fire in a rhythmical bursting pattern during the LFP theta state. Unlike the theta cells, however, the frequency of bursting in the place cells is slightly higher than LFP theta, causing each successive burst to precess to successively earlier phases of the theta cycle as the animal moves through the place field (Figure 11.2B). This temporal code works together with the overall rate code to continuously update the animal's location. Phase precession is also seen during some aspects of sensory processing and during stationary running in place on a treadmill (e.g., Pastalkova, Itskov, et al., 2008).

At first glance, it might seem strange for a brain structure primarily involved in cognitive processing and memory to code explicitly for movements. As an example of how this might work, we turn to the role of movement in cognitive map theory. This theory postulates that there are two ways in which place cells can be activated. In the first, direct sensory inputs from the environment are used to uniquely identify the animal's location in a familiar environment. In the second, once its current location has been identified in the current map, it can subsequently be updated as the animal moves around the environment through the operation of internal hippocampal circuitry activated by information about translations and rotations resulting from those movements, a type of updating called "path integration" (O'Keefe, 1976; O'Keefe and Nadel, 1978; McNaughton, Chen et al. 1991). As we shall see, representations of translation and rotation movements are intimately connected with different aspects of theta activity.

11.2.4 GABAergic septal cells

The function of the GABAergic septal cells is to create rhythmical theta oscillatory firing, which is then transmitted to the hippocampal formation. GABAergic PV/HCN inputs drive the basic HPC theta oscillations via inhibitory inputs to HPC inhibitory interneurons (Freund and Antal, 1988; Hangya, 2009) and to EC interneurons (Gonzalez-Sulser, 2014). These inputs primarily target the perisomatic PV inhibitory interneurons, including the GABAergic basket cells (Figure 11.2A). Optogenetic driving of this pathway at frequencies above the normal theta range supersedes the spontaneously occurring theta frequency and drives theta oscillations in both hippocampal interneurons and place cells at slightly higher than the imposed frequency. The amplitude of LFP theta is still responsive to the animal's running speed, suggesting it is controlled independently by either another septal input or the entorhinal cortical input (Zutshi, Brandon, et al., 2018). Blocking this GABAergic septal input by injecting muscimol (a GABAa agonist) into the medial septum markedly attenuates hippocampal theta in much the same way as anesthetizing the medial septum. This suggests that the direct glutamatergic and cholinergic septal hippocampal projections must act in concert with GABAergic circuits and projections, and may have little independent influence on theta on their own.

GABAergic projections to HPC perisomatic inhibitory interneurons convey information about both the animal's translational running behavior, perhaps in conjunction with the glutamatergic projections (Joshi, Salib, et al., 2017) (see below), and about stimuli in different sensory modalities including noxious (aversive airpuffs to the face), auditory (10 KHz tones) and visual (light flashes) ones (Kaifosh, Lovett-Barron, et al., 2013). Rabies-tracing studies show that brainstem areas that project to the septal GABAergic cells and are presumed to convey these two types of information include posterior hypothalamic areas, supramammillary nucleus, interpeduncular nucleus, raphe nuclei, locus coeruleus, and the nucleus incertus (Lu, Ren, et al., 2020). It has long been recognized that posterior hypothalamic/supramammillary inputs to the medial septum are part of the circuitry that generates the translational hippocampal theta rhythm: electrical stimulation of these structures produces running or jumping, with the speed of the movement increasing as a function of stimulation intensity (Bland and Vanderwolf, 1972). The locus coeruleus has been implicated in the reorganization of goal information in the hippocampus (Kaufman, Geiller, and Losonczy, 2020) and in the consolidation of new spatial learning (Takeuchi, Duszkiewicz, et al., 2016), although whether this memory-related function involves the theta mechanism is not clear. See below for more information on the supramammillary contributions to the theta system.

Blocking the activity of cells in the medial septum using anesthetics or the GABA agonist muscimol has marked effects on hippocampal place-cell activity and different aspects of spatial recognition, memory, and navigation. Some studies report complete loss of CA3 and CA1 place fields (Bolding, Ferbinteanu, et al., 2020), while others report reductions in CA1 fields with partial sparing in CA3 (Mizumori, Barnes, and McNaughton, 1989; Koenig, Linder, et al., 2011). In an important study, Brandon (Brandon, Koenig, et al., 2014) used muscimol injections into the medial septum to completely block hippocampal theta and looked at the effect on place fields (Figure 11.3B). Surprisingly, new fields emerged immediately and remained stable during the septal inactivation and persisted when theta oscillations had recovered. This indicates that at least some place fields survive septal blockade and the creation of new place fields can take place independently of GABAergic inputs. Furthermore some aspects of the temporal dynamics of hippocampal cells including theta rhythmicity were abolished during muscimol. A similar study by Wang and colleagues (Wang, Romani, et al., 2015) supports the idea that these effects might be explained by the existence of two routes to place-field creation, as outlined at the beginning of this section. One route relies on the ability of exteroceptive sensory cues to create and maintain fields in the absence of septal inputs; the other updates place fields on the basis of the animal's own path integration inputs and is dependent on medial septal inputs. This latter study also showed that unlike some place-cell activity, "time cells" found in the running wheel component of a spatial memory task (see section 11.5) were solely dependent on septal integrity.

11.2.5 Glutamatergic septal cells

Glutamatergic septal cells participate in the circuitry that sets the running speed of the animal in the forward direction and concomitantly the frequency of theta oscillations. They provide excitatory inputs to a majority of local GABAergic and a minority of septal cholinergic neurons (J Robinson, Manseau, et al., 2016). Importantly, they also drive translational running and couple it to hippocampal theta frequency (Fuhrmann, Justus, et al., 2015). An early discovery relating hippocampal theta to running was the observation that electrical stimulation of the posterior hypothalamus causes the animal to run and greater amounts of stimulation power cause the animal to run faster (Bland and Vanderwolf, 1972). Concomitantly there is an increase in theta frequency. Stimulation during jumping

causes the animal to jump higher and the hippocampal theta to increase in frequency (Bland and Vanderwolf, 1972). These effects are probably mediated by the glutamatergic septal system. There is a good correlation between the firing rate of glutamatergic cells, the animal's speed, and the hippocampal theta frequency (Fuhrmann, Justus, et al., 2015). Pharmacological block of the medial septum abolishes these effects. Blocking glutamatergic transmission within the septum itself does not affect running speed but does uncouple speed from theta frequency. This suggests that the glutamatergic cells may control the activity of the theta-generating GABAergic cells via synaptic connections in the septum. Increased firing of glutamatergic cells takes place several hundred milliseconds before the animal begins to run. Conversely optogenetic stimulation of these cells causes the animal to run and the latency of onset depends on the strength of the stimulation (Fuhrmann, Justus, et al., 2015). They not only link theta to speed but also independently control speed via their projections to hypothalamus and brainstem. We can conclude that running speed can sometimes be controlled by the septum but sometimes not.

11.2.6 Cholinergic septal cells

Muscarinic cholinergic septal cells underlie the theta that accompanies arousal/attention and rotational movements. This theta occurs during nonmovement in response to sensory inputs including vestibular ones. These ACh septal cells provide excitation to other septal cells and to hippocampal pyramidal cells as well as to hippocampal interneurons (Figure 11.2A). Unlike GABAergic and glutamatergic septal cells, cholinergic cells do not have HCN channels or other resonant membrane properties, nor do they exhibit a theta rhythm, but increase their firing rates during sensory-related theta, increasing the cholinergic tone of hippocampal networks. Their firing rates are generally high during exploratory behaviors, leading to increased Ach tone, depolarizing hippocampal cell membrane potential, and increasing excitability in hippocampal pyramidal cells (see C Muller and Remy, 2018). Different levels of acetylcholine release may selectively recruit subsets of hippocampal interneurons and, in that way, control signal processing within the hippocampus. Hippocampal interneurons activated by muscarinic receptors respond more slowly than those activated by nicotinic receptors, which, in addition to being faster, are also more transient.

The effects of Ach on the gating of inputs to CA1 cells are complex. To take one example, ACh causes presynaptic inhibition of glutamatergic synaptic transmission from longitudinal association fibers and Schaffer collaterals in stratum radiatum of region CA1 but has little influence on the glutamatergic synaptic transmission from the entorhinal cortex in stratum lacunosum-moleculare of CA3 or CA1 (Dannenberg, Hinman, and Hasselmo, 2016). In contrast, OLM interneurons are activated by fast nicotinergic ACh excitation (Lovett-Barron, Kaifosh, et al., 2014) and these OLM axons inhibit the tufts of the apical dendrites where the entorhinal input synapses, controlling the effectiveness of that input. As can be seen in Figure 11.2C, the OLM cells fire preferentially on the negative trough of the extracellular LFP, at approximately the same time as the pyramidal cells. Therefore, increasing cholinergic activity might be expected to change the relative balance of control of the pyramidal cells between intrahippocampal signals and EC inputs in a complex way. One consequence might be that loss of cholinergic inputs might affect the ability of the hippocampal spatial representations to update maps of an environment in response to changes in sensory input.

Lovett Baron (Lovett-Barron, Kaifosh, et al., 2014) found that, in head-fixed mice, EC inputs drove the dendrites during the learning of a novel context, but following an aversive stimulus the somatostatin OLM cells inhibited this input, supporting (hippocampal-independent) fear conditioning.

The septal-to-hippocampal cholinergic inputs have been associated with several different functions, many but not all of them related to exteroceptive and interoceptive sensory inputs to the hippocampus. The first function is associated with theta that occurs in response to arousing/attention-grabbing sensory inputs, which include odors, loud noises, restraint, predators, and other signs of danger. As we saw earlier, this type of theta may be related to the subthreshold activation of avoidance motor systems. It may also be associated with the role of theta in signaling mismatches in the hippocampal representation of an environment. An example of this latter role would be object-in-place recognition tasks, in which objects change their location from one place to another. An interoceptive sensory input associated with cholinergic theta is the vestibular input resulting from rotational behavior, where the theta is related to angular velocity analogous to the relationship between glutamatergic theta and translational movements. Information about behavioral translation and rotation may relate to the role of the hippocampus in spatial tasks that require the use of path integration. An example would be the Olton radial arm maze with reduced extramaze cues, which can be solved on the basis of remembered body turns, but not the Morris watermaze, which forces the animal to use environmental cues.

11.2.7 ACh effects on hippocampal cells

Some properties of hippocampal pyramidal cells are dependent on the cholinergic inputs, while others are not. Removal of cholinergic inputs either through the injection of the ACh antagonist scopolamine into the ventricles or immunolesions of the cholinergic septal cells using the selective toxin IgG-saporin does not affect the basic firing fields of place cells but reduces the firing rate in the place field and changes the oscillatory properties of the cells including loss of phase precession. Another effect seems to be to reduce or abolish the control of place fields by proximal sensory inputs, causing them to rely to a greater extent than usual on distal cues or path-integration inputs. Brazhnik and colleagues (Brazhnik, Borgnis, et al., 2004) injected scopolamine into the lateral ventricles overlying the hippocampus and found that place fields remained intact but had smaller firing fields and lower firing rates. Ikonen (Ikonen, McMahan, et al., 2002) studied the effects of IgG-saporin neurotoxic lesions of the medial septum on the ability of place cells to represent two different environments. In line with the Brazhnik et al. (2004) results, CA1 cells in the lesioned animals were as capable of representing a familiar environment as those of controls (Figure 11.3C; compare cells A1,2 with B2,3, left-most circles). Moreover, when both lesioned and control animals were transferred to a novel octagonal environment, they both originally showed evidence of remapping, creating a new hippocampal representation (Figure 11.3C, column 2 octagons). However, on the second and subsequent exposures to the new environment, place cells in the control animals maintained their new representations but those of the lesioned animals reverted to a representation similar to the one in the original environment (Figure 11.3C, columns 3 and 4, octagons). As expected, these authors also found a loss of immobility-related theta during light restraint (Ikonen, McMahan, et al., 2002).

It is possible that the difference in the tasks that are selectively affected by cholinergic lesions may have something to do with the need to identify the sensory cues that distinguish between two environments and to use these to create two independent maps. Evidence in favor of this interpretation comes from a study in which animals were asked to choose one of eight central food wells in octagon and square environments with different cues on the walls. Lesioned animals could do so if trained first on one task and then the other, but not when trained together at the same time (Janisiewicz, Jackson, et al., 2004). Flexible switching back and forth between two cognitive maps seems to depend on the cholinergic system.

Lesions of the cholinergic component of the MS hippocampal projection also affect the use of the path-integration component of cognitive maps. This is clearly shown by the difference in their effects on navigation tasks such as the Morris watermaze and the Olton 8-arm maze tasks. In the first, the animal is required to swim directly to an escape location in a swimming pool regardless of where it is placed into the water; the use of multiple start locations forces the animal to use environmental cues to locate itself and navigate to the goal. The use of the path-integration system is precluded. In the Olton radial arm maze, on the other hand, the animal is required to visit each of eight arms radiating from a central platform without returning to one of the previously visited arms. The task can be learned using either an environmental cue or a path-integration strategy, depending on the availability of extramaze cues. Using a path-integration strategy, the animal has to keep track of its own behavior to update its location. Destruction of the entire medial septum by ibotenic acid usually results in large deficits in both tasks (e.g., Hagan, Salamone, et al., 1988), whereas use of the selective cholinergic toxin 192 IgG saporin leads to normal, or only mildly deficient, acquisition of the Morris watermaze (Berger-Sweeney, Heckers, et al., 1994; Baxter, Bucci, et al., 1996; Frielingsdorf, Thal, and Pizzo, 2006; and references in Frielingsdorf, Thal, and Pizzo, 2006). In contrast, some studies using this cholinergic toxin find deficits in radial arm maze tasks, whereas others do not. The former studies may limit access to external cues or in other ways bias a solution toward path integration strategies.

Strong evidence for the role of the cholinergic projection in path integration comes from studies of food hoarding in rats with IgG-saporin lesions of the medial septum (Martin, Horn, et al., 2007). Animals were trained to fetch nuts placed at different locations in an open area and take them back to their nest to hoard them. In the lights-on condition with both distal visual and path-integration cues available, both normals and lesioned animals performed normally. However, when required to return to the location of the nest using path-integration cues, either in the dark or with the nest box moved, the lesioned animals made large heading errors. This dissociation implied that the controls could use either extramaze visual cues or internal path-integration cues whereas the lesioned animals were confined to the use of the latter. No deficits in the Morris watermaze, which forces the use of distal cues, were found in the same study. Interestingly a subsequent study from the same group found similar deficits in path-integration-based hoarding following selective lesions of the septohippocampal GABAergic projection, suggesting that this is also involved in path integration functions, as suggested by the Joshi study (Joshi, Salib, et al., 2017) mentioned above. Presumably both inputs need to be working (as well as the glutamatergic input?) for the path-integration system to be intact. Atropine-sensitive cholinergic theta is produced during passive rotation in either the light or dark, presumably through vestibular activation (Gavrilov, Wiener, and Berthoz, 1995; Gavrilov, Wiener, and Berthoz, 1996; Shin, 2010) and is probably mediated by the cholinergic neurons of the medial septum (Tai and Leung, 2012; Tai, Ma, et al., 2012) since the effect is not found in septal cholinergic saporin-lesioned animals. Vestibular lesions decrease the power and the frequency of theta (Russell, Horii, et al., 2006; Neo, Carter, et al., 2012; Tai, Ma, et al., 2012). However, medial septum stimulation, which restores theta in rats with lesions of the vestibular system, is not sufficient to restore the spatial deficit induced by these lesions (Neo, Carter, et al., 2012), probably because it failed to restore cholinergic theta (Neo, Carter, et al., 2012).

Following saporin cholinergic lesions, a deleterious effect on object location recognition memory but not simple object recognition memory is often found. For example, Cai et al. (Cai, Gibbs, and Johnson, 2012) found a deficit in object location recognition but no significant effect on novel object recognition in the same animals. This is to be expected from the dependence of the former but not the latter on the spatial functions of the hippocampus (O'Keefe and Krupic, 2021), see the section on object recognition memory in this chapter (section 11.5). One interesting result at odds with this simple interpretation was found in a study by Easton, Fitchett, et al. (2011). They showed that neurotoxic saporin cholinergic lesions of the septum did not affect the ability of the rats to identify which object was in which place in which box, but did affect their ability to know that there had been an object (identity not specified) at a particular place. We now know that one cell type in the entorhinal cortex, the object-vector cell (Hoydal, Skytoen, et al., 2019), is not specific for a particular object but fires at a certain distance in a specific direction from any object in the environment and we might speculate that this cell's function remains intact following the lesion.

11.2.8 Role of the supramammillary nucleus in hippocampal theta

Not all hippocampal theta is dependent on the medial septum. The supramammillary nucleus contributes to hippocampal theta via direct projections to DG and CA2 as well as through indirect projections via the medial septum/diagonal band of Broca. Its main role seems to be to activate the component of theta that modulates inputs to these areas in support of hippocampal response to novelty. Like the septal projections, the SuM appears to exert its influence primarily via its inputs to the interneurons in the hippocampus, although it projects weakly to dentate granule cells as well. It is one of the two different circuits for control of speed signals in the hippocampus and entorhinal cortex. One circuit goes via the midbrain locomotion region (MLR) (AM Lee, Hoy, et al., 2014), which directly projects to the basal forebrain and controls motor stepping activity and is probably involved in flight behavior and other motivated behaviors. The other goes through the supramammillary nucleus (SuM), which projects directly to the hippocampus as well as via the septum and may control responses to novelty.

Supramammillary-cell firing rates correlate with the animal's speed and are predictive: the relation is best seen between SuM cell activity and the animal's speed 1.2 seconds later. Correlation with speed is better than with acceleration (Farrell, Lovett-Barron, et al., 2021). There are two kinds of SuM cells, those that express substance P (tac1+) and those that do not (tac1-), instead releasing GABA and glutamate. The two types of cells have slightly different projection patterns to the hippocampus (Hashimotodani, Karube, et al., 2018) and have different effects on it. The tac 1+ cells are involved in activation of the motor systems and particularly those driving exploration, whereas the tac1- cells are more related to control of activity within the hippocampus. Cells that receive tac1+ projections are related to midbrain PAG neurons, which in turn project to the midbrain locomotion region (MLR). MLR is a source of speed information to the EC speed cells via its projection to the DBB. Optogenetic activation of tac1+ cells drove a slow exploratory type of movement but did not entrain hippocampal LFP, whereas tac1- cells entrained hippocampal LFP (overriding the ongoing spontaneous theta LFP) at 8 and 12 Hz stimulation but only had very weak control over locomotion (Farrell, Lovett-Barron, et al., 2021). Tac1- cells also activate hippocampal speed cells but at a different phase from the spontaneous theta. Some putative tac1- cells (Farrell, Lovett-Barron, et al., 2021) might be involved in the detection and responses to novelty (S Chen, He, et al., 2020). Those projecting to the DG are activated by contextual novelty (placing animals in a new environment), those projecting to CA2 are activated by social novelty (such as a new juvenile mouse), and finally some are activated by both types of novelty.

11.2.9 LIA and sharp wave ripples

Large amplitude irregular activity (LIA) is characterized by a sharp wave of about 100 ms duration, which occurs at random with an average interval of about 1 second. Associated with these are high-frequency ripple oscillations of 100–200 Hz. Together these are called sharp wave ripples (SWRs) (Figure 11.1F right, G). Here we will briefly summarize their behavioral correlates and possible functions. (See Buzsaki, 2015, for a comprehensive review of sharp wave ripples.) SWRs have been suggested to signify a hippocampus that is disengaged from active place learning and navigation, occurring during behaviors that do not change an animal's location, such as sitting quietly, eating, drinking, grooming, and slow wave sleep (O'Keefe and Nadel, 1978; Buzsaki, 2015). They originate in the CA3 field and project to the CA1 fields via the Schaffer collaterals (Buzsaki, 2015). One view is that SWRs represent an inactive state of the hippocampus providing information to the rest of the brain about the strength and duration of previous theta states of the hippocampus, including the amount of recent translational and rotational behaviors. Some evidence for this more general metabolic function comes from a recent study showing an inverse correlation between SWRs and interstitial glucose concentrations (Tingley, McClain, et al., 2021). SWRs might also be involved in the homeostatic renormalization of recently activated synapses. Optogenetical stimulation of the cholinergic cells in the medial septum produce a loss of SWRs (Vandecasteele, Varga, et al., 2014), suggesting that they are a sign of reduced medial septal input. (For an extensive discussion of this idea, see Buzsaki, 2015.) Another possibility is that they represent a type of future thinking, trying out courses of action that an animal might take as it navigates through the environment. Finally, they have also been suggested to represent a neural correlate of memory consolidation.

On the consolidation view of LIA, the uncoupling of the hippocampus from the septum during SWRs is a necessary condition for hippocampal consolidation to occur, involving either transfer of information from hippocampus to neocortex or another type of hippocampus–neocortex interaction. The primary evidence for this view is twofold. During SWRs the temporal pattern of firing of place cells reproduces their recent activation on linear tracks on

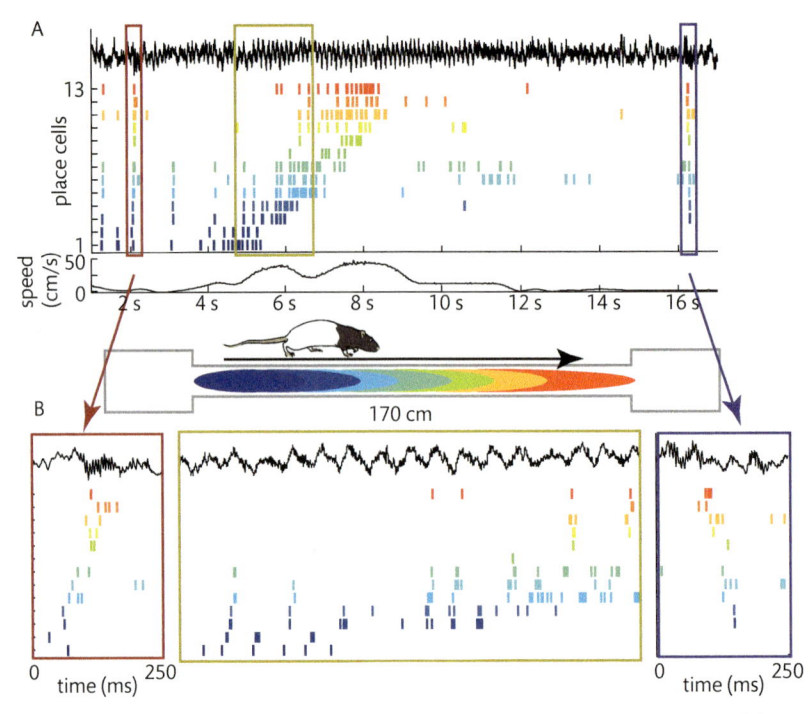

Figure 11.4 Place-cell replay occurs in both forward and reverse direction during awake sharp wave ripples. (A) Hippocampal LFP (top) showing sharp wave ripples (SWRs) at the beginning and end of a run during which hippocampal theta is prominent. During the run (middle rat cartoon), place cells fire in sequence as the animal enters and exits each place field. (B) SWRs prior to the run show forward replay reproducing the sequence in which the cells will fire; SWRs following the run show reverse replay firing in the opposite sequence to that seen in the run. (Adapted from Diba and Buzsaki, 2007.)

a compressed timescale. As an animal runs in a one-dimensional environment, place cells consistently fire at different locations along the track, although there is no relationship between the order of their firing and the anatomical location of the cells relative to each other in the hippocampus. In the original experiments it was shown that cells with overlapping fields tended to fire more often together during SWR than would be expected by chance (Wilson and McNaughton, 1994). Subsequent studies showed that, if enough cells are recorded simultaneously, one can reconstruct the awake firing pattern and hence the trajectory along the track from the firing pattern of the cells. During SWRs, firing of the same cells tends to replicate the temporal order of firing in a pattern, which is said to replay the recent experience (Nadasdy, Hirase, et al., 1999; AK Lee and Wilson, 2002). The pattern is compressed by an order of 20-fold so that it all fits within the 100–200 ms of the SWR (see Figure 11.4, left-hand side). While the original discovery of replay found a reflected or backward ordering of the cell firings (Figure 11.4, right-hand side), more recent work has found forward replays as well, where the cells fire in the same order is as during the real-world experience (Figure 11.4, left-hand side). Both of these observations have been taken as evidence that replay might be a means of rehearsing the original experience, perhaps leading to the consolidation of the memory of the experience or, at the systems level, to transferring information from the hippocampus to neocortical regions. Experiments that disrupted SWRs after each behavioral experience reported that learning was inferior to that seen in animals without such disruptions (Girardeau, Benchenane, et al., 2009; Ego-Stengel and Wilson, 2010).

Although replay was originally discovered during sleep, as shown above it can also occur during short movement pauses in the behaving animal. Notably, it can also occur in a different environment from that in which the original experience occurred, showing that it is not due to progressive activations of place cells from the animal's current position but more likely to be reactivation of recent experiences (Karlsson and Frank, 2009).

It has been suggested that the forward type of replay represents a type of planning in which the hippocampus is predicting the activation of place cells in a two-dimensional environment in the order in which they would be experienced as the animal runs to a goal from the animal's current location (Pfeiffer and Foster, 2013). Important variations on this are preplay experiences that take shortcuts between the animal's start and goal locations along right-angled routes, traversing paths that the animal could not in fact take or experience (Olafsdottir, Barry, et al., 2015).

The original idea that replay was a simple demonstration of the learned ordering of place-cell activations has been called into question by the finding that potential orderings of place cells exist prior to the animal's entering an environment and therefore may not be a reflection of past experience but rather a prediction of the possibility of that experience (Dragoi and Tonegawa, 2011). This suggests that at least part of the replay phenomenon might be due to preexisting connections between hippocampal pyramidal cells, which are then played out during exploration of a novel environment.

11.2.10 Gamma waves

Gamma oscillations span the frequency range 25–140 Hz. They co-occur with LFP theta, and their amplitude waxes and wanes as a function of theta phase. Two gamma generators have been identified, one in the dentate gyrus and another in the CA3–CA1 regions. Both pyramidal cells and interneurons are phase-locked to gamma waves (Csicsvari, Jamieson, et al., 2003). In CA1, they can roughly be divided into slow (~25–50 Hz) and fast (~65–140 Hz) gamma (Figure 11.1B, top and bottom, respectively) (Colgin, Denninger, et al., 2009). Simultaneous recordings in the CA1 and CA3 fields and the upper layers of the medial entorhinal cortex showed that the fast gamma couples CA1 to inputs from the medial entorhinal cortex, while the slow-frequency gamma provides access to inputs from CA3 on separate theta cycles. Importantly, fast and slow gamma occurred at different phases of the CA1 theta rhythm. These results suggest that gamma acts as a gate allowing information from different inputs to the CA1 field access to the pyramidal cells at different points in the theta cycle. Fast gamma occurred at the point in the theta cycle when place-cell firing was maximal, suggesting that the input from the entorhinal cortex was effective in firing the cells at this phase. A significantly lower percentage of place cells were phase-locked to slow gamma than to fast gamma. This gamma segregation of inputs to the CA1 field clearly relates to Hasselmo's idea that different parts of the theta cycle select for the current input to the CA1 fields whereas others select for the stored memory for that environment. In this model (Hasselmo, Bodelon, and Wyble, 2002), new associations are set up in the phase of the theta cycle during which synaptic input from entorhinal cortex is strong but synaptic currents arising from region CA3 input are weak (to prevent interference from prior learned associations). In contrast, retrieval of old associations occurs on the phase when entorhinal input is weak and input from region CA3 is strong. An alternative explanation is that the CA1 inputs are constantly flipping back and forth between the two inputs, entorhinal inputs being more related to the path integration support for navigation and the CA3 inputs more related to the environmental cue-control of location. CA1 is probably where these two inputs are compared, leading to exploration if there is a mismatch (O'Keefe and Nadel, 1978). As we saw on the section on theta (above, 11.2.1), CA1 is clearly involved in detecting changes in a familiar environment, whether it be the inclusion of a novel object in a familiar place or movement of a familiar object to a new place. Recall that O'Keefe (1976) and, more recently, Larkin and colleagues (Larkin, Lykken, et al., 2014) reported increased firing in CA1 place cells when the animal explored a novel object or a familiar object in a novel location. Surprisingly in the Larkin study, the increased firing rate occurred not only in cells with place fields containing the novel object but also in all place fields in that environment, suggesting that CA1 broadcasts a general novelty signal and does not provide information to direct behavior toward the experienced novelty. Sharp wave ripples recorded during and after a novel exploration reflected increased firing and coupling between coactive cells. The specific aspects of novelty might be detected in lateral entorhinal cortex, where cells responding to novel objects in specific contexts have also been detected (Deshmukh and Knierim, 2011).

11.3 Place cells

Single-unit recordings in freely behaving animals have revealed different classes of principal cell in the hippocampal formation that display spatial correlates: place cells in the hippocampus proper, head-direction cells in pre- and para-subiculum and entorhinal cortex, and grid cells in entorhinal cortex. In addition, there are interneuronal theta cells that show less dramatic spatial coding and

are characterized by rate changes associated with hippocampal LFP theta. They fire with a constant phase relation to the hippocampal LFP under most circumstances, with different classes of interneuron preferring to fire at different phases (see section 11.2.1 above).

Hippocampal place cells signal the animal's location in an environment. They are usually silent over most of the environment, but rates increase dramatically in one or, less frequently, two locations in small (circa 1–2 m dia.) environments (place field). Different cells have different place fields, and there does not seem to be any correspondence between the anatomical location of the neurons within the hippocampus and the location of their fields in the environment. Cells recorded next to each other in the CA1 field can have place field next to each other or distant from each other, and vice versa. In addition, variations in firing rate within the place field can signal aspects of behavior that occur there or the presence (or absence) of objects encountered there. The same cells will often fire in different environments, but the preferred locations are unrelated if the environments are sufficiently dissimilar to each other. One notable feature of place cells is that in unconstrained open field environments, in which the animal is free to move in all directions, the cells fire in the place field irrespective of the direction in which the animal is facing. In environments that constrain the animal's behavior to move toward a reward location, for example, when behavior is restricted to specific routes, as when an animal runs back and forth on a linear track or between two points in an open field, the cells become directionally sensitive and may be said to represent the successive locations along a path. During navigation to a single goal in a two-dimensional environment, place cells show both allocentric locational firing and egocentric directional firing oriented toward a specific location in the environment (see section 11.11 on place cells and navigation for more details). In many experiments in which nonspatial stimuli are always delivered in the same place, the response of hippocampal pyramidal cells is taken as evidence of nonspatial functions of the hippocampus. We shall see in section 11.5 that whenever the locational gating of these simple feature responses is tested by presenting the same stimuli in more than one place, they are almost invariably found to be location-dependent, activating the cells in one location but not in others.

The frame of reference of place fields can be provided by proximal or distal spatial cues, as shown by cue-rotation experiments. An experiment in two-dimensional rectilinear boxes showed that some place fields were controlled in the x dimension by intramaze cues and in the y dimension by extramaze cues, showing that the idea of a strict separation into two different sets of cues is unnecessary (O'Keefe and Burgess, 1996). In addition to this control by exteroceptive sensory cues, place fields can also be controlled by idiothetic cues. The proportion of pyramidal cells that are place cells depends on how many environments are tested. When the same cells are recorded in enough different environments, many have a field in at least one. In an experiment in which CA3 pyramidal cells were tested in 11 rooms, 210 of 342 (61%) were active in at least one environment (Alme, Miao, et al., 2014).

Are there other correlates than just space? It can be argued that hippocampal pyramidal cells have space as their primary correlate and that many of the studies making claims for other correlates can be shown to be misinterpreted. This is a crucial question, since primary correlates other than space might necessitate a broadening of the function of the cognitive map theory beyond space. There is now extensive evidence on this issue, which we will discuss later in section 11.5. Another important question is whether place-cell activity is influenced by goals, rewards, and other nonspatial cues, and we will examine this question in section 11.5 as well. There is good evidence for temporal as well as rate coding in hippocampal place-cell activity. When animals run through the place field of a hippocampal pyramidal cell, the cell fires a series of bursts at a slightly higher frequency than the ongoing theta, and the best correlate of the phase of firing is the animal's location within the place field. This *phase precession* phenomenon remains the best example of temporal coding in the nervous system to date. We now know that phase precession occurs in grid cells as well.

11.4 Place cells within the hippocampal formation

Place cells were first reported in the hippocampal CA1 region (O'Keefe and Dostrovsky, 1971), followed by CA3 (O'Keefe and Nadel, 1978; McNaughton, Barnes, and O'Keefe, 1983) and dentate gyrus (DG) (Jung and McNaughton, 1993). They were proposed to represent the main building blocks of the hippocampal cognitive map (O'Keefe and Nadel, 1978) where they combine multiple types of sensory and self-motion information (Figure 11.5A). In most cases no single external or internal input ("a feature") can completely determine a place-field location, although a single "feature" may significantly change place-cell firing rate and the place cell effectively becomes a feature-in-place cell (see section 11.5). Additionally, some place cells respond to the absence of a familiar cue and were originally termed mis-place cells (O'Keefe, 1976). Place cells can remain stable even in the absence of any external visual cues as long as the animal can predict where it should be based on previously received information, including its use of the path-integration system

to update its position within the map (O'Keefe, 1976; Quirk, Muller, and Kubie, 1990; G Chen, King, et al., 2013). Hence, place cells are the substructure of a coherent spatial internal map, with only sparse external inputs, which can be used to flexibly navigate between arbitrary "starting" and "goal" locations taking previously unvisited routes (Morris, Garrud, et al., 1982; R Wood, Bauza, et al., 2018). While there are many similarities (such as their spatial specificity) between place cells found in different hippocampal subregions, there are a number of important differences related to their stability and cue encoding properties.

In small environments typically used in laboratory experiments (e.g., 1 m dia circles), CA1 and CA3 place cells tend to have a single field (Park, Dvorak, and Fenton, 2011; Rich, Liaw, and Lee, 2014), while DG place cells often exhibit multiple fields (Leutgeb, Leutgeb, et al., 2007) (Figure 11.5B,C). The number of fields per place cell tends to increase with the size of the enclosure (Park, Dvorak, and Fenton, 2011; Rich, Liaw, and Lee, 2014), and the number of neurons with fields scales logarithmically with track length on a long linear track (Rich, Liaw, and Lee, 2014). The field sizes of CA1 place cells tend to be slightly larger than CA3 (Mizuseki, Royer, et al., 2012), while DG place cells tend to be smaller than either of the CA regions (Jung and McNaughton, 1993; Park, Dvorak, and Fenton, 2011). Interestingly, in larger environments CA1 place fields scale more with the size of the environment compared with CA3 or DG place fields, which show similar resizing (Park, Dvorak, and Fenton, 2011). Both CA1 and CA3 place cells can encode temporal information of ongoing experience (Pastalkova, Itskov, et al., 2008; Kraus, Robinson, et al., 2013; Salz, Tiganj, et al., 2016). On the other hand, it has been demonstrated that CA3 neurons show more coordinated responses to environmental cue manipulations compared with CA1 neurons (Lee, Yoganarasimha, et al., 2004). To demonstrate this, Lee and colleagues recorded from CA1 and CA3 neurons on a circular

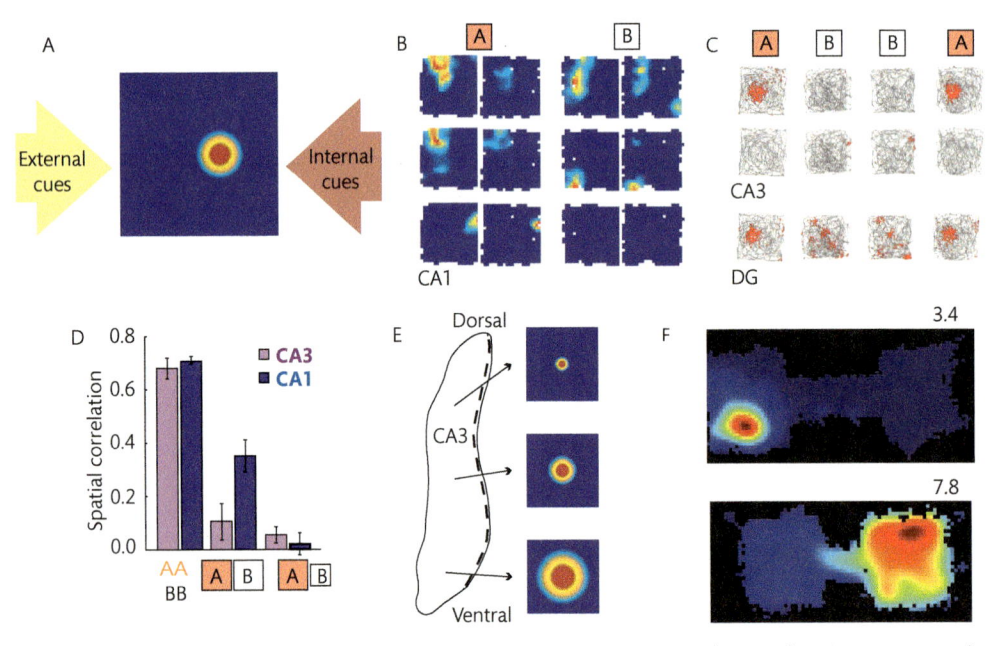

Figure 11.5 (A) Schemas illustrating that place cells receive two major inputs from exteroceptive (external) and interoceptive (internal) cues. (B) CA1 place cells show a wide range of responses in two different geometrically identical enclosures, with some cells approximately maintaining their positions (top), some becoming active at a different (middle) location, and others ceasing their activity altogether. (C) CA3 and DG place cells in two different enclosures. (Left: Adapted from Leutgeb et al., 2004, with permission. Right: Adapted from Leutgeb et al., 2007, with permission.) (D) The correlation between CA1 place cells is higher compared with CA3 cells. (E) Place fields increase in size along the dorsoventral hippocampal axis. (F) Ventral hippocampal place cells. (Adapted from Komorowski et al., 2013, with permission.)

linear track, where they rotated proximal and distal environmental cues to put them in conflict. The majority of CA3 place fields (~ 60%) rotated on the track with local cues (although they showed responses to distal cues as well), preserving their topological relation. By contrast, only a third of CA1 place fields responded similarly, most of the time showing some form of unpredictable remapping or compromised stability, especially with larger mismatches between proximal and distal cues. In addition, when the shape of the enclosure is changed, CA3 responses remain more stable compared with CA1 (Leutgeb, Leutgeb, et al., 2005) (Figure 11.5B–D). Taken together, these findings suggest that CA1 and CA3 place cells may encode distal and local cues differently. Moreover, CA1 cells may coexpress several "frames of references" (i.e., multiple autonomous maps of the environment; Fenton, Wesierska, et al., 1998) at the same time, a finding confirmed by multiple other studies as well (Zinyuk, Kubik, et al., 2000; Anderson and Jeffery, 2003), whereas CA3 cells carry a much more coherent representation, potentially defined by the most stable environmental cues and/or an animal's anticipation of being in a particular location (I Lee, Yoganarasimha, et al., 2004). It has also been shown that CA3 place cells tend to be more stable compared with CA1 (and CA2) place cells within the same enclosure across multiple days of recordings (Mankin, Sparks, et al., 2012; Mankin, Diehl, et al., 2015). Thus, CA3 cells appear to be more stable than those of CA1 in the same environment across time.

However, when the animal is transferred to a new enclosure in a new room, CA3 cells tend to remap more robustly than CA1 place cells (Leutgeb, Leutgeb, et al., 2005). DG place cells show even higher sensitivity to even small changes to the geometry of the enclosure (Leutgeb, Leutgeb, et al., 2007) (Figure 11.5B–D). Based on these overall findings, it has been suggested that DG and CA3 place cells play a key role in pattern separation and pattern completion, respectively, which is necessary for robust discrimination of different environments when sparse potentially overlapping information is available, while CA1 place cells convey multiple autonomous maps relevant for different actions the animal may need to undertake as it is comparing/reconciling the memory and expectations of the environment that it receives from CA3 region with ongoing inputs related to its current experience coming from the entorhinal cortex.

The finely tuned place cells described above are found in the dorsal part of CA1, CA3, and DG regions. Place cells in the ventral part of the hippocampus tend to be fewer in number, have much larger fields, and respond to the overall context of the environment (Jung and McNaughton, 1993; Kjelstrup, Solstad, et al., 2008; Komorowski, Garcia, et al., 2013). Currently, much less is known about the type of external and internal cues driving the responses in different parts of the ventral hippocampus. However, lesion studies (Moser et al., 1995) indicate that the dorsal and ventral parts of the hippocampus encode different types of information whereby the former represents a fine-grained cognitive map of the environment while the latter has been proposed to encode "internal states" such as hunger associated with this map (Davidson and Jarrard, 1993; Hock and Bunsey, 1998).

Different types of stable location-specific activity were also reported in the subiculum (Sharp, 1999a; Lever, Burton, et al., 2009) and in multiple areas of parahippocampal formation, e.g., the medial entorhinal cortex and pre- and parasubiculum (Quirk, Muller, et al., 1992; Taube, 1995a,b; Cacucci, Lever, et al., 2004;

Fyhn, Molden, et al., 2004; Hafting, Fyhn, et al., 2005; Hargreaves, Rao, et al., 2005; Solstad, Boccara, et al., 2008; Boccara, Sargolini, et al., 2010; Krupic, Burgess, and O'Keefe, 2012; Diehl, Hon, et al., 2017) (examples of these and other cells with place-like cell activity can be seen in section 11.6, Figure 11.15). Initially these subicular cells were thought to represent more sensory-driven, place-like activity, since they exhibited much more invariant location-specific response properties when the animal was transferred from one environment to the other (Quirk, Muller, et al., 1992; Sharp, 1999b). However, further examination revealed that location-specific neurons in the subiculum respond to the boundaries of the enclosure (Lever, Burton, et al., 2009) while spatial cells in the medial entorhinal cortex (and some other parahippocampal areas including pre- and parasubiculum; Boccara, Sargolini, et al., 2010) responded to both borders of the environment (Solstad, Boccara, et al., 2008) and exhibited symmetrical grid-like spatially periodic properties (Hafting, Fyhn, et al., 2005; Krupic, Burgess, and O'Keefe, 2012) proposed to be generated by path integration (McNaughton, Battaglia, et al., 2006). Other spatially modulated nongrid and nonborder cells (Diehl, Hon, et al., 2017) may be driven by specific visual landmarks (Casali, Shipley, et al., 2018; Kinkhabwala, Gu, et al., 2020) and possibly other types of sensory cues. Currently, the relation between all these hippocampal formation location-specific cells is poorly understood. After the discovery of grid cells (Hafting, Fyhn, et al., 2005), it was suggested that the combined input from multiple grid cells of different biologically plausible scales and orientations may produce a stable bump of activity, i.e., a place field (O'Keefe and Burgess, 2005; Solstad, Moser, and Einevoll, 2006). This idea can only be partially true, since it has become clear that the input from grid cells and more generally medial entorhinal cells is not necessary for CA1 place-field formation (Brandon et al., 2014; Brandon et al., 2011; Hales et al., 2014; Koenig et al., 2011; Langston et al., 2010; Wills et al., 2010). At best they can be only one of at least two routes by which place cells are formed, the second being through the use of environmental cues alone. Further evidence for this view is that bilateral medial entorhinal lesions only partially disrupt hippocampal place-cell activity and hippocampus-dependent memory (Hales, Schlesiger, et al., 2014). On the other hand, inactivation of the medial septum by muscimol or lidocaine obliterates the pattern of grid cell firing while other spatial cells, including head-direction, border, and place cells, remain intact (Brandon, Bogaard, et al., 2011; Koenig, Linder, et al., 2011) and can even be formed de novo in novel environments (Brandon, Koenig, et al., 2014). Indeed, using a viral approach combined with optogenetic stimulation, it has been shown that the whole range of different mEC cell types project to CA1 region (Zhang, Ye, et al., 2013). Moreover, in developing animals place cells emerge ~5 days before stable grid cells are found (Langston, Ainge, et al., 2010; Wills, Cacucci, et al., 2010). On the other hand, hippocampal inactivation with muscimol significantly impairs grid-like activity in the medial entorhinal cortex (Bonnevie, Dunn, et al., 2013). Currently it is not clear to what extent this inactivation affects other spatial cells in the parahippocampal formation. These results suggest that parahippocampal spatial maps may provide an internal metric, boundaries, and polarization (i.e., directionality in respect to local and global cues) of space, while the hippocampal neurons shape, update, and read out these entorhinal spatial inputs into specific cognitive map-like representations. In the absence of the entorhinal inputs, other environmentally generated inputs can still generate and subsequently activate the place of representation. We discuss the relation of the hippocampal place cells and the grid cells of the entorhinal cortex in greater detail in section 11.7

11.5 Conjunctive spatial representations in hippocampal pyramidal cells

The existence of nonspatial inputs has been taken to suggest the hippocampus has a broader function than spatial, see Chapter 14; alternatively, these nonspatial responses might actually be signaling a feature-in-place where the spatial nature of the response has been missed by the narrowness of the experimental design where the target features were only presented in one location or one environment. We look first at responses to simple stimuli such as olfactory and taste stimuli, then to other modalities, followed by higher-order features such as conspecifics, time, and rewards. As we discuss these results, we will point out where sensory responses have been shown to be dependent on the animal's location and where this question has been left unanswered.

11.5.1 Odor and taste responses in hippocampal pyramidal cells

There is considerable evidence of responses of single units in the hippocampal formation to simple sensory inputs. We look first at responses to olfactory and taste cues. A series of experiments on normal and hippocampal-lesioned animals have dissected the respective roles of the olfactory cues themselves and their spatial (and more recently temporal) context in successful performance on a variety of discrimination, inference, and memory tasks. In general, the hippocampus is not required for simple olfactory discriminations when both cues are present at the same time (Kaut and Bunsey, 2001; Kaut, Bunsey, and Riccio, 2003), nor for tasks involving a nonmatch to a previously presented sample (Mair, Burk, and Porter, 1998), nor for recognition paradigms where the animal has to respond to novel but not to recently experienced odors (Dudchenko, Wood, and Eichenbaum, 2000). To take one

illustrative example, rats were trained on an open platform to approach a small cup containing sand scented with one of up to 24 odors (Figure 11.6). On each trial, the cup was placed first in one location and then in another. If the second odor was different from the previous one (nonmatch), it contained food; if the odor was the same, there was no food (match). Performance was not disrupted by selective hippocampal damage; in fact, the lesioned animals were able to remember up to 24 previously experienced odors, a number comparable to controls (Figure 11.6B). In contrast, the same animals scored at chance on a spatial forced-choice T-maze alternation task (Figure 11.6C). While the hippocampus is clearly not involved in simple olfactory memory, simultaneous olfactory discrimination is affected by lesions of the perirhinal cortex (Otto and Garruto, 1997) and somewhat surprisingly, go/no-go discrimination (Otto, Schottler, et al., 1991) is significantly *improved* by lesions of the entorhinal cortex.

Where the hippocampus does become important is in learning about the temporal order of *sequences* of odors. Fortin and colleagues (Fortin, Agster, and Eichenbaum, 2002) presented rats with a sequence of 5 odors in the same place drawn at random from a library of 20 and asked them subsequently to identify which of a pair of the 5 was experienced earlier. Animals with hippocampal damage were severely impaired but could recognize the individual odors if each was paired with an odor that had not been experienced before. They could remember they had experienced the odor before but not its order in the sequence in which it had appeared. Although not obvious at first sight, a different study provided some evidence that odor-sequence memory may be dependent on place memory (Ergorul and Eichenbaum, 2004). Normal animals were trained on an odor-sequence task where each different odor was presented in a different location and subsequently memory for spatial location and for odor were tested independently. During probe experiments the pots containing the odors were presented in new locations, or in their old locations without the odors. The animals adopted a two-stage strategy of first going to the location of the correct pot, followed secondly by identifying whether it contained the correct odor. They approached the correct location 69% of the time

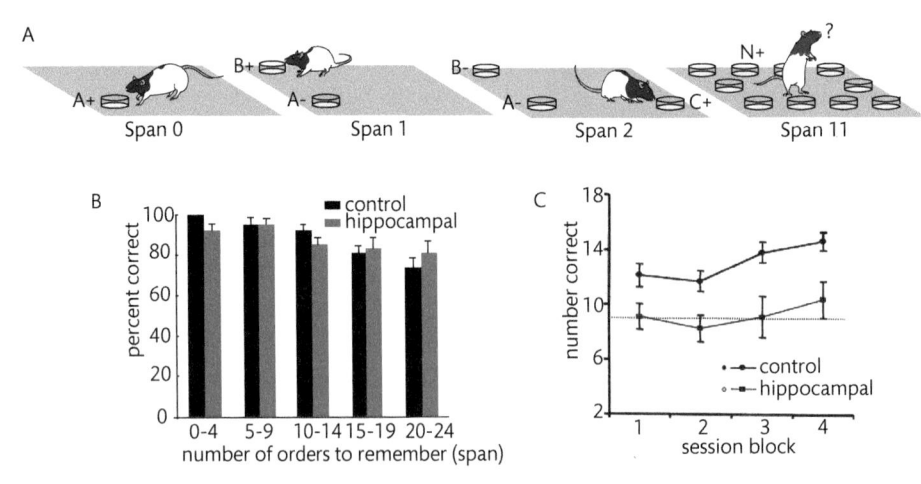

Figure 11.6 Olfaction and the hippocampus. (A) Schema of the olfactory memory span test. On the first part of the trial, the animal is allowed to sniff at a particular odor (A+); subsequently the animal is asked to choose a novel odor when paired with the previously experienced odor (Span 1, B+ vs A-) or odors (Span 2, C+ vs A-, B-), or up to 11 previously experienced odors (Span 11, N+). (B) Percentage of correct responses for the control and hippocampal groups in the 25-odor span probe session. Spans (number of odors to be remembered) are shown in blocks of five. There are no deficits in animals with hippocampal lesions on this type of recognition olfactory task. (C) Performance of the same animals on a spatial memory task showing profound deficits in the hippocampal group. (Adapted from Dudchenko et al., 2000, with permission.)

but switched to the other pot if this did not contain the correct odor, resulting in an overall performance of 76% correct. In further tests, location by itself proved incapable of supporting correct choice whereas odors by themselves when presented in new locations resulted in performance equal to that during the standard odor-in-place task. Animals with hippocampal lesions failed completely on the standard odor-in-place sequence task, showed normal performance on the odor-alone sequence probe, and showed significantly below chance performance on the location-alone sequence probe. These results show several things: despite the fact that hippocampal-lesioned animals can discriminate the odors and know which one was experienced earlier, they do not use this information by itself to solve the what-when task but rather rely on the hippocampal system representation of the temporal ordering of the odor-in-place experiences and this knowledge, when available, takes preference over the simpler odor-strength system. As we shall see subsequently, a similar strategy applies to object recognition memory.

Several studies have shown that hippocampal units respond selectively to the sequence of odors. Allen and colleagues (Allen, Salz, et al., 2016) reported that 11% of hippocampal cells respond differentially to correct and incorrect sequences of odors and this number correlated with task performance on a memory test (Figure 11.7A); of these, 40% showed selectivity for specific conjunctions of item and sequence position (Figure 11.7B). Rats first learned a sequence of five odors. On a probe trial, some of the odors were misplaced within the sequence and the rats were asked to hold the nosepoke response if an odor was presented in sequence or withdraw if presented out of sequence. Importantly, it is not possible to exclude that these were place-dependent responses, since all of the odors were presented in the same place. A study by Komorowski did include this control and provides good evidence for an odor-in-place role for hippocampal pyramidal cells (Komorowski, Manns, and Eichenbaum, 2009). The test was an odor/spatial context conditional discrimination task in which the animal had to use the box contextual cues to decide in which of two odor-scented pots to dig for food; in one context (left-side arena), one pot was correct and in the other (right-side arena), the other pot was correct (Figure 11.7C). The pots could occupy one of two locations (X or Y) in each arena to prevent the use of left/right egocentric spatial strategies. In total there were eight olfactory/location combinations. Only one of 52 neurons fired differentially to the 2 odors irrespective of location. By the end of the experiment, 31% of the cells responded to an odor in a place while pure place cells (which responded irrespective of the odor located there) represented another 47%. It is only by looking at the overall pattern of firing to both odors in both boxes that one can see that a cell is an odor-in-place cell. For comparison, the firing profile of a simple place cell that responded in a location irrespective of odors there is shown on the right-hand side of Figure 11.7D. Interestingly, the number of odor-in-place cells started at a low 6% of cells at the beginning of learning, and increased dramatically during the experiment to 31% at the end. The increase correlated with the learning of the task suggesting that this might be the signal used to make the discrimination. In contrast, the proportion of simple place cells did not change over the course of learning, going from 47% at the beginning to 38% at the end of learning, a change that was not significant. This change in percentage of different cell types was due to simple place cells developing odor-in-place responses and new simple place cells in turn developing from previously nonresponsive cells. No new

simple odor-only cells developed during the course of learning. We conclude that CA1/CA3 pyramidal cells have the potential to become place cells and can do that with increased familiarity of the environment even though the task the animal is engaged in does not rely on simple place cells and furthermore that many place cells have the potential to become odor-in-place cells or more generally feature-in-place cells and that this can occur under normal circumstances but may be accelerated during learning tasks that call attention to particular features in particular places. As we shall see later in this section, hippocampal feature-in-place cells occur in experimental paradigms where the animal is not rewarded for making the association (Herzog, Pascual, et al., 2019), or even when it is rewarded for paying attention to other aspects of the experiment (Manns and Eichenbaum, 2009). In contrast, if this study is representative, simple odor-cell responses independent of location do not appear to exist in the hippocampus before or after training on an odor/place association task.

Taking the animal's location into account is also crucial to the interpretation of hippocampal responses to taste stimuli. There is good behavioral evidence that the hippocampus is involved in regulating food intake and that this might be due to the inhibition of feeding after an animal has eaten food. The hippocampus is involved in the patterning of meals but not in the total amount of food ingested: animals with hippocampal lesions ate more often but took smaller meals than controls and consequently did not gain weight (Clifton, Vickers, and Somerville, 1998). In another study, animals with hippocampus lesions returned to eating following the last meal quicker than normal (Henderson, Smith, and Parent, 2013) perhaps because they forgot the last meal (Parent, Darling, and Henderson, 2014).

Herzog and colleagues (Herzog, Pascual, et al., 2019) studied the response to different-tasting fluids: sweet (saccharine), salty (sodium chloride), neutral (distilled water), and bitter (quinine) injected directly into the mouths of rats via an implanted cannula as they foraged in an open field (Figure 11.8A,B). They were not required to respond to the fluid or to location in any way. Despite this, 90% of CA1 pyramidal cells had place fields. Of these, 15% also responded to one or more injected fluids but only when the fluid was delivered in the cell's place field (Figure 11.8C). A much larger percentage of interneurons, 76%, also had taste responses. Place cells with taste responses had larger place fields; their spatial information content and the magnitude of the taste response were inversely correlated. Taking both place cells and interneurons together, cell firing provided information about the presence of a taste at short latencies (80%), the identity of the taste (37%), and its palatability (19%) at longer latencies, with some cells providing information about two or all three of these categories (Figure 11.8D).

11.5.2 Auditory, tactile, and visual responses

Hippocampal pyramidal cells have been shown to respond to auditory stimuli. Aronov and colleagues (Aronov, Nevers, and Tank, 2017) trained rats on a simple go/no-go auditory discrimination in which animals first had to hold down a lever to turn on a sound consisting of a frequency ramp ascending from 2 to 22 kHz, and then to release the lever when the frequency reached a window of 15 to 22 kHz to get a reward (Figure 11.9A). The speed of the frequency increase varied from trial to trial, ruling out the use of temporal coding. Forty percent of CA1 cells were engaged at different points in the task, with 5.5% responding at a particular point in the

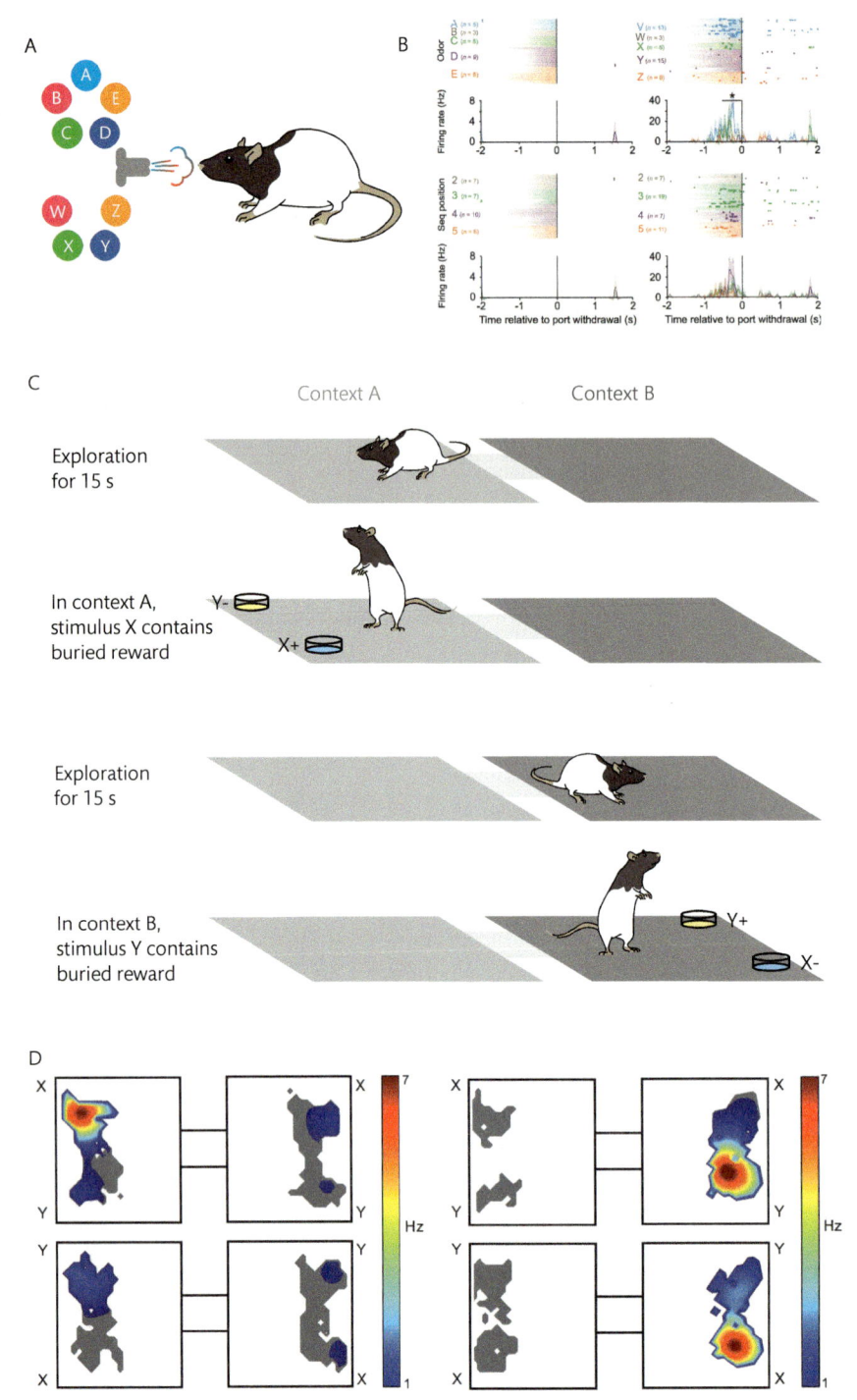

Figure 11.7 Olfactory responses of hippocampal pyramidal cells in an olfactory sequence spatial conditional discrimination. (A) Using an automated odor-delivery system, rats were presented with a sequence of five odors delivered in the same odor port. The same set of odors was presented multiple times with all items in sequence (e.g., ABCDE) or out of sequence (e.g., ABDDE). Each odor sequence presentation was initiated by a nosepoke, and rats were required to correctly identify the odor as either in sequence (by holding their nosepoke response until a signal at 1.2 s) or out of sequence (by withdrawing their nosepoke before the signal) to receive a water reward. (B) An example of a conjunctive sequence cell showing selectivity for a particular item (V) out of sequence (top) but not for which out-of-position it occupied (bottom). (After Allen, 2016, with permission.) (C) Schema of an olfactory context conditional learning task that consisted of two contexts connected by a corridor. Initially the animal was allowed to explore both contexts before the odor pots were introduced. The correct odor pot to dig in depended on the context in which the pots were placed. In context A, odor X was correct and odor Y incorrect; in context B, the opposite contingencies hold, Y was correct and X incorrect. (D) Left, Example of an odor-in-place cell recorded during the spatial conditional discrimination task. Place-field heat map shows that the cell fired when the animal sniffed at the X odor in the right-hand position in box A but not under any of the other conditions. (D) Right, Classic place cell responding to a location in box B irrespective of the odor there. In D, hotter colors represent higher rates. (After Komorowski et al., 2009, with permission.)

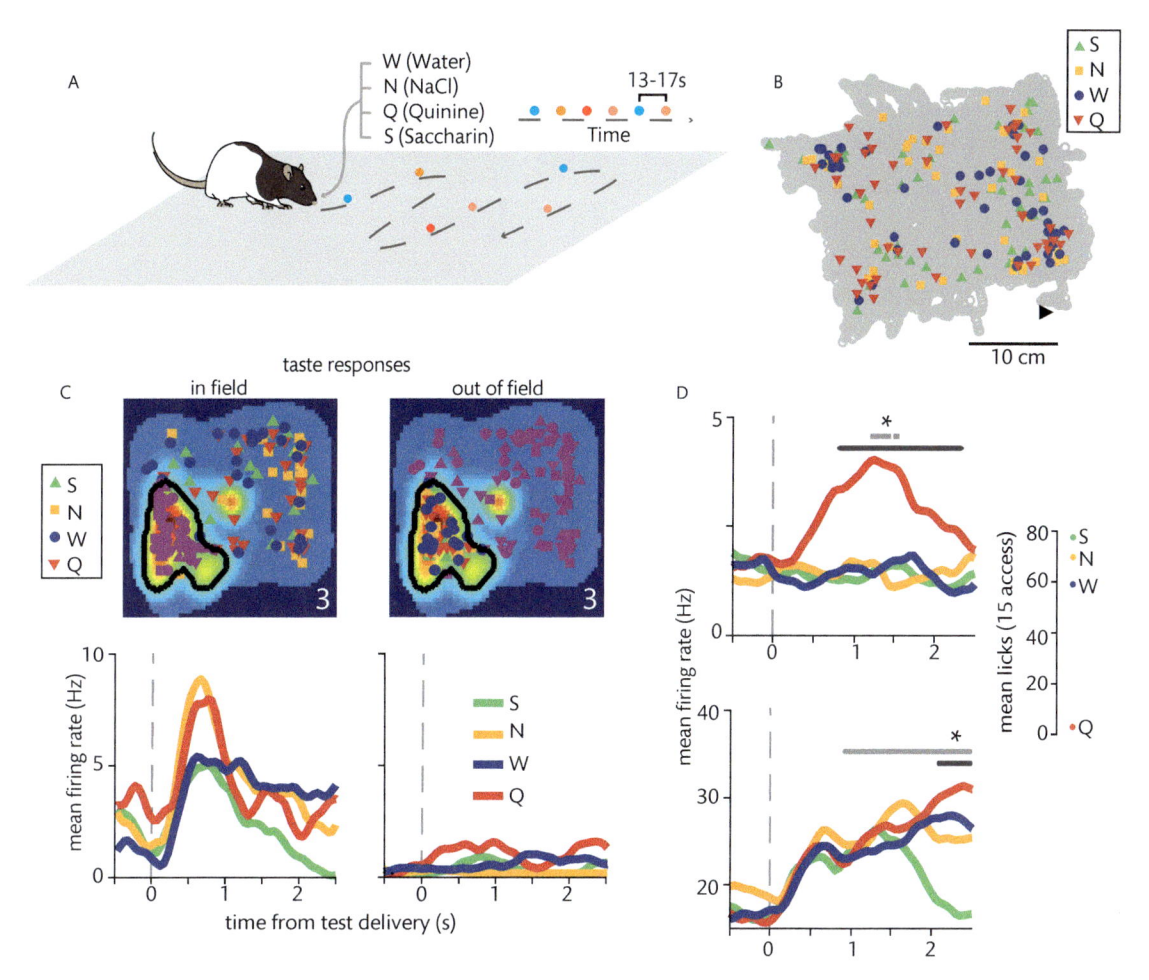

Figure 11.8 Hippocampal cell responses to fluids injected directly into the mouth via tubing while rats were foraging for food. (A) Schema of experiments showing four liquids, water, salt, quinine, or saccharin, injected at random locations as the rat searches for food randomly placed in the open-field environment. (B) Locations where different fluids were injected. (C) Typical place cell responded to injected fluids (purple) inside the place field (left) but not outside (right). The cell fired more to quinine (red) and saline (orange) than to water (blue) and saccharin (green). (D) Example pyramidal cell and interneuron responses to different tastes (in color) signaling the presence of the taste (light gray bar) and in addition the identity of the taste (dark gray bar) which correlated well with the palatability of the different tastes (far right) for these particular cells. (Adapted from Herzog et al., 2019, with permission.)

frequency ramp rather than more broadly or during behaviors before or after the ramp (Figure 11.9B). The comparable number for mEC cells was 9.4%. All frequencies were represented across both populations, despite the animals only being tasked with identifying frequencies within the target range. Hippocampal cells only responded if the animal was engaged in an appropriate task. For example, most did not respond during passive reproduction of the frequency ramp but did respond if the frequency ramp was automatically followed by a reward, although to a lesser extent than during the active lever-press task. There was some overlap between cells responding in this task and those with spatial fields tested in another environment. However, the authors did not record from the same tone-responsive cells in different parts of the same box or in different boxes and therefore we cannot rule out the possibility that these were in fact tone-in-place cells comparable to the odor-in-place cell responses just described.

Itskov and colleagues (Itskov, Vinnik, et al., 2012) did take into account the location dependency of auditory responses. They trained rats to discriminate between four auditory "vowels" or complex sounds while situated on two different platforms located in different parts of the same laboratory and facing in different directions

(Figure 11.9C). Two sounds required the animal to turn left on each platform to get reward; the other two, to turn right. Platforms were oriented at 180° to each other, so these two similar egocentric responses required turning in opposite allocentric directions. Twenty-one percent of hippocampal pyramids had significant responses to at least one of the sounds on at least one of the platforms (Figure 11.9D). Taking into account the location of a sound as well as its identity, they found that 87% of cells responded on only one of the four platform/response combinations, 13% on two, and none on more than two (Figure 11.9D,E). The authors concluded that this was what would be expected if a neuron's differentiation between two sound stimuli at one location did not predict whether it differentiated between the same sounds at a different location. The response to the sounds was context-dependent.

Hippocampal cells have also been shown to respond to an auditory CS in Pavlovian conditioning experiments, but the context-dependency of these responses is rarely tested. One experiment did study hippocampal cells during tone/eyeblink conditioning in rats running on a linear track for food reward (Shan, Lubenov, et al., 2016). The tone and eyelid-shock pairing occurred at random points on the track to test the importance of location. Sixty-three percent

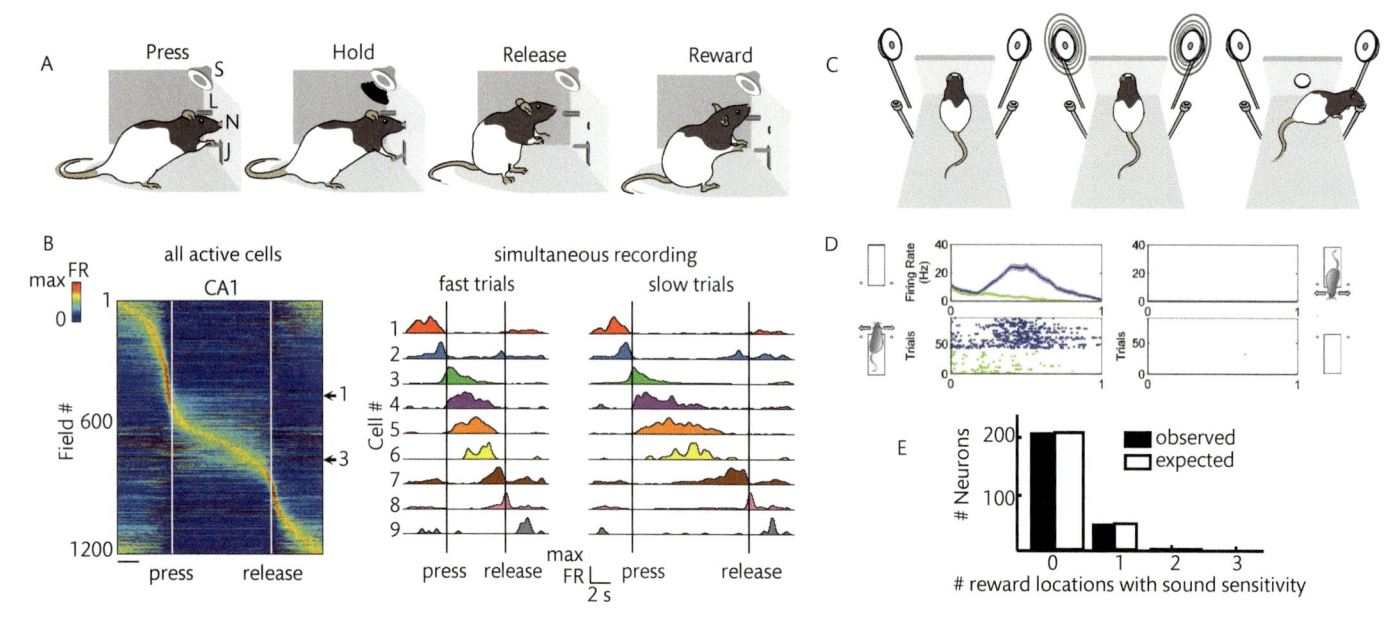

Figure 11.9 Acoustic responses in hippocampal neurons. (A) Schema of the auditory discrimination task: to get reward, the rat had to hold down a lever to turn on a sound stimulus consisting of a frequency ramp ascending from 2 to 22 kHz, and then release the lever when the frequency reached a window of 15–22 kHz. (B) Responses of all (left) and selected (right) cells during the auditory go/no-go frequency discrimination task. Some cells fire selectively to specific tones, and the entire frequency range was covered. (After Aranov, 2017, with permission.) (C) Schema of the context-dependent auditory discrimination task, in which the same auditory stimuli were presented on two platforms in different locations while the animal faced in different directions. One platform is shown. (D) Typical hippocampal cell, which only responded (in blue, average rate top, raster plots below) to specific auditory stimuli when the animal was on one platform (left) but not the other (right). (E) Observed and expected distribution of cell responses if cell responses to the auditory stimuli were completely independent on the two platforms, i.e., they were auditory stimulus-in-place responses. (After Itskov, et al 2012, with permission.)

of CA1 pyramids had place fields along the track or in the food boxes at each end of the track. In addition, some of these cells fired to the tone CS, but only when the animal was sitting quietly in the place field with sharp wave ripples (SWRs) in the hippocampal LFP (see section 11.2.9). The unit response was equivalent to the level of place-field activity observed when the animal ran through that part of the track in the absence of the tone. Unit activity outside the place field was inhibited by the CS. The authors concluded that the conditioned tone was arousing and the unit responses to the nonspatial auditory stimuli were due to an arousal-mediated resumption of place-specific firing. This explanation has the broader implication that place-field firing is partly dependent on the ongoing level of arousal and is suppressed during SWRs, a state of low arousal.

The Diamond group (Itskov, Vinnik, and Diamond, 2011) also used the same paradigm described above for testing hippocampal unit responses to auditory stimuli (4 different stimuli/2 responses in 2 different locations) to assess whether hippocampal neurons responded to texture stimuli and whether this tactile response was also independent of location. Similarly to the auditory results, 86% of neurons encoded texture on just one platform, failing to distinguish between the same textures when the rat was positioned on the opposite platform. Moreover, among 21 neurons that encoded a single texture pair on each platform, only 6 demonstrated consistent "texture tuning" independent of location; the remaining 15 either discriminated between the same texture pair on both platforms but switched preference within the pair, or else discriminated between different texture pairs on the two platforms. Texture was only represented in the hippocampal responses in conjunction with context.

There was no representation of the tactile stimulus independent of location.

The visual system provides a strong exteroceptive sensory input to the hippocampal place, grid, and head-direction cells, which controls their spatial firing and is used to locate the animal in a familiar environment. Rotating a single visual cue card on the wall of the testing enclosure rotates all of these spatial cells by a comparable amount (R Muller and Kubie, 1987; Knierim, Kudrimoti, and McNaughton, 1995). When pitted against other cues such as those of the path-integration system, visual cues strongly control the location of place fields (Jayakumar, Madhav, et al., 2019) as long as the reliability of these visual cues is not devalued by moving them in the animal's presence (Jeffery and O'Keefe, 1999) and the cues are not too small (e.g., ~350cm^2) (Scaplen, Gulati, et al., 2014). So, one might expect cells in the hippocampal formation to respond to visual cues, but do they do so independently of context? X. Zhao and colleagues recorded CA1 pyramidal cells intracellularly from mice running on an oval track in a virtual reality environment (Zhao, Wang, et al., 2020). They found that they could create place fields in silent pyramidal cells by intracellular depolarization sufficiently strong to produce plateau potentials and fire the cell at a particular location in the virtual environment, replicating previous work (see section 11.9 for a description of the role of plateau potentials in place-cell formation). The artificially created place cells followed the movement of local visual cues within the same environment but failed to respond to the same cues when the shape of the virtual reality environment was changed from an oval to a triangular track. Similar findings were found in naturally occurring extracellularly recorded CA3 cells, suggesting that the CA1 responses might have been inherited from there. Powerful visual stimuli that could be shown to drive place cells in one environment failed to do so in another. We can conclude that most or all of the responses of hippocampal cells to simple sensory stimuli are likely to be feature-in-place responses where the feature response is crucially dependent on the location of the animal. A potential route for visual information to access hippocampal pyramidal cells is by the visual cortex. Lesions of the striate cortex do not affect the basic statistics of place cells but reduce the ability of intramaze objects to control the orientation of place fields. Under normal circumstances, rotation of objects placed at the edge of the standard recording cylinder result in a comparable rotation of the orientation of place fields. Following visual cortex lesions this control is greatly diminished (Paz-Villagran, Lenck-Santini, et al., 2002) suggesting that although the animals can use other sensory modalities to control the angular location of fields in the cylinder, when visual stimuli are present they dominate. This influence is probably exerted via the head-direction system. The size and location of the visual stimulus is important (Scaplen, Gulati, et al., 2014). Rotation of large distal visual cues on the wall or floor of the environment resulted in concomitant rotation of approximately 52% and 44% of place fields, respectively. Rotation of smaller visual floor cues often resulted in remapping with only 2% of place fields following the rotated cues. The ability of visual stimuli to influence place cells depends on the size and location of these stimuli. Further insight into the properties of visual inputs to hippocampal pyramidal cells was gained in a VR experiment in which animals were first trained in a multistimulus visual world to navigate in a visually rich virtual maze where overhanging striped pillars indicated the location of the rewarded position (Purandare, Dhingra, et al., 2022). Subsequently the animal's position was fixed except for small head movements and a single vertical bar was moved either clockwise or counterclockwise around them. Thirty-nine percent of cells showed responses to the moving visual stimulus typically with a single preferred visual angle in either the clockwise or counterclockwise direction. Stimuli in front of the animal were preferred, but the entire visual field was represented. Approaching and receding stimuli were equally effective, but stimulus distance was better coded for approaching stimuli. Of the visually responsive cells, 79% were shown to be place cells in subsequent standard free-foraging experiments in a different environment. Since damage to the hippocampal system does not cause deficits in standard visual discrimination tests (O'Keefe and Nadel, 1978), it is reasonable to interpret these experiments as explorations of the visual inputs to the hippocampal pyramidal cells in the service of more abstract functions such as spatial or relational processing.

11.5.3 Hippocampal single units respond to combinations of simple sensory stimuli

It is clear from the studies described above that CA1 hippocampal pyramidal cells can respond to combinations of a sensory stimulus in a specific modality together with a location in the testing box or the room. Good examples of this are the Komorowski (Komorowski, Manns, and Eichenbaum, 2009) and Herzog (Herzog, Pascual, et al., 2019) studies described above. This leaves open the question as to whether single hippocampal cells can respond to multiple sensory cues in combination. Configural association theory (Rudy and Sutherland, 1989, 1995) suggested that

the hippocampus is necessary for discriminations that involve combining stimuli into a configuration in order to solve a problem that could not be solved by linear combinations of the individual stimuli by themselves. For example, an animal might be asked to respond positively to stimulus A+ or stimulus B+ but not respond to the combination of the two of them AB-. Another task in this domain is biconditional discrimination, in which the animal must respond positively to combinations AB+ and CD+ but not to combinations AC- and BD-. The theory met with mixed results, some studies finding deficits following hippocampal lesions and others not (summary in Rudy and Sutherland, 1995). An important lesion study (Albasser, Dumont, et al., 2013) showed that hippocampal-lesioned animals could learn bidirectional discriminations if the two stimuli to be configured were located in close approximation but not if one of them was a location in the environment determined by distal cues.

In a biconditional discrimination study by Terada and colleagues (Terada, Sakurai, et al., 2017) the two stimuli to be associated were an olfactory and an auditory cue presented one after another with partial overlap in time. CA1 hippocampal cells responded to either one or the other of the two stimuli individually or in some cells to the combination of the two. Interestingly, almost all cells were phase modulated relative to the theta LFP and the majority of pyramidal neurons demonstrated phase precession in at least one of the conditions in particular during the stimulus preferred by the cell or during the combination of stimuli.

There is some evidence that single cue information reaches the hippocampus from the anterior cingulate (AC) (Rajasethupathy, Sankaran, et al., 2015). In an experiment testing the role of the hippocampus in integrating multiple cues (Yadav, Noble, et al., 2022), three sets of cues from four different modalities (auditory, visual, tactile, and olfactory) were presented together, forming three different contexts in a virtual environment. Each set of cues was associated with either a positive, neutral, or aversive liquid stimulus. Animals learned to increase licking to the positive cue, inhibit licking to the aversive one, and ignore the neutral one. Each stimulus combination activated a set of hippocampal pyramidal cells, presumably because the animal thought they represented three different contexts each with a different valence. Following learning, different cells responded to different combinations of stimuli (e.g., olfactory plus tactile) but almost none (1% vs. 0.8% chance) to a single stimulus alone. Nearly all neurons that responded to a particular stimulus also showed significant and prominent responses to all other features of the same context group. In contrast to this multistimulus hippocampal response, neurons in the anterior cingulate, which projects to the hippocampus, responded to the single features of the compounds. Inhibition of the AC population silenced the hippocampal compound cells, suggesting that this is the source of the elemental feature input.

The results summarized in the previous sections make it clear that hippocampal pyramidal cells can respond to single sensory stimuli in different modalities and even to combinations of stimuli from different modalities such as olfactory, tactile, and auditory cues. Interesting questions that remain open are whether these responses are normally contextually dependent, as in the Yadav study, where the hippocampus is used as a framework to associate together stimuli that occur in specific places, or whether they are part of a more general relational response system capable of capturing the relationship between nonspatial as well as spatial information (N Cohen and Eichenbaum, 1993) (see Chapter 14 for further discussion).

11.5.4 Responses to objects in hippocampal pyramidal cells

Objects can be considered to be bundles of multimodal stimuli that maintain their coherence under spatial and temporal translation. Several studies have looked at the response of hippocampal cells to objects. This is usually done by presenting the animal with a novel object or moving the location of a familiar object. If the animal recognizes the novelty or change it should explore the object in preference to one that is not changed (Ennaceur and Delacoeur 1988). There is an extensive literature on object recognition and its neural substrates. Similar to odor recognition, there appear to be at least two brain mechanisms for responding to novel objects. In the first, the response is determined by the familiarity of the object, which depends ultimately on recency of experience with the object and decays reasonably rapidly as a function of time. This extrahippocampal brain region involved in novel-object recognition has been identified as the perirhinal cortex (Meunier, Bachevalier 1993; Mumby and Pinel, 1994), and therefore this type of familiarity-based object recognition should be intact in animals with damage to the hippocampus. The second system for detecting novel objects sits squarely in the hippocampal cognitive map and performs one of its core functions: the role of exploration of novelty for originally building and subsequently updating hippocampal representations of the environment. Here, exploration of novel objects is triggered by a mismatch between what the current representation within the hippocampus predicts will be found in a particular location and what is actually found there. This idea of a dual mechanism for detecting novelty has been espoused by several authors (e.g., O'Keefe and Nadel, 1978; Squire, 1992; Aggleton and Brown, 2006).

One widely used behavioral paradigm for testing novelty, the novel-object recognition (NOR) test, relies on exploratory behavior to assess whether a rodent remembers that it has recently experienced an object or that it has experienced one object more recently than another (Ennaceur and Delacoeur 1988). In the standard NOR experiment the animal is exposed to one or more objects in specific locations in a specific box (the context) and then subsequently their memory for this experience is tested by replacing one or more objects with new ones. One review of the effects of hippocampal lesions on NOR (S Cohen and Stackman, 2015) found that only between 28% and 33% of experiments found deficits, and this was independent of the method of lesioning. Presumably, the unaffected animals used one or more nonhippocampal structures, most probably the perirhinal cortex, to recognize the objects. In one interesting experiment (Gaskin, Tremblay, and Mumby, 2003), rats were impaired if the hippocampus was lesioned after initial exposure to familiar objects but were unimpaired when subsequently given a new test with novel objects. This suggests that extrahippocampal areas can support object recognition but only if the hippocampus does not participate in encoding the original encounter with the object. As with odor recognition, the simplest interpretation is that two memory systems underlie object recognition, a hippocampal one subserving long-term context-dependent object-in-place memory and a perirhinal one providing short-term context-independent familiarity-based object memory. Priority is normally given to the

hippocampal system, but if it is unavailable, the second system is brought into operation.

Hippocampal place cells respond to novel objects. O'Keefe (1976) and Larkin and colleagues (Larkin, Lykken, et al., 2014) reported increased firing in CA1 place cells when the animal explored a novel object or a familiar object in a novel location (see section 11.10 on place-field formation). Surprisingly, in the Larkin study, the increased firing rate occurred not only in cells with place fields containing the novel object but also in all place fields in that environment, suggesting that a general novelty signal is broadcast and may not provide specific information to direct behavior toward the experienced novelty. Sharp wave ripples recorded during and after a novel exploration also had increased firing and coupling between coactive cells. The specific aspects of novelty might be detected in lateral entorhinal cortex, where cells responding to novel objects in specific contexts have also been detected (Deshmukh and Knierim, 2011).

Single-unit recording experiments strongly support the dual center model. The standard object-recognition task needs to be modified for use in single-unit recording, since it is usually a one-shot event and would not provide enough cell data for statistical purposes. An experiment that successfully studied both object recognition and, independently, object-in-place recognition was carried out by Manns and Eichenbaum (2009) (Figure 11.10). Rats ran around an annular track for reward delivered once every circumnavigation and en route encountered a set of objects located at 12 different locations around the track of which a maximum of 10 were occupied on any given trial. A total of 40 different objects were used during the course of the experiment. After each group of three successive laps, new objects were added and old objects moved to new positions, allowing item memory to be dissociated from item-in-place memory (Figure 11.10A). Decreased exploration for repeated objects and repeated places reflected memory for each of these independently and showed that the animals recognized the objects and also the location in which each occurred. Sixty percent of cells responded to the location of the objects and, in addition, 17% signaled the identity of the objects (Figure 11.10C shows typical examples, location cells, top row; object cells, bottom). Importantly, a large component of the identification of objects was due to the identification of that object in a particular location. Similar to the behavioral recognition data, the single-unit population responses were slightly more similar when the same rather than a different object was re-experienced in the same place but decreased markedly when that object was moved to a new place (Figure 11.10B). It is clear from this experiment that the ability of hippocampal cells to distinguish objects from each other depends substantially on object-in-place recognition memory.

In other studies of dorsal hippocampal CA1 or CA2 unit responses to objects, a similar absence of specific responses to the object coupled with some evidence of modulation of the place response was found (Deshmukh and Knierim, 2011; von Heimendahl, Rao, and Brecht, 2012). For example, in the von Heimendahl, et al., study, 63% of cells were dependent on the animal's location, and no cells responded solely to objects or conspecifics independent of location. In other studies (Alexander, Farris, et al., 2016; Rao, von Heimendahl, et al., 2019), the dominant response was a remapping of the place field to a new location but no evidence of specific-object responses. Ventral hippocampal cells also did not show modulation by the presence of objects in contrast to the response of a small

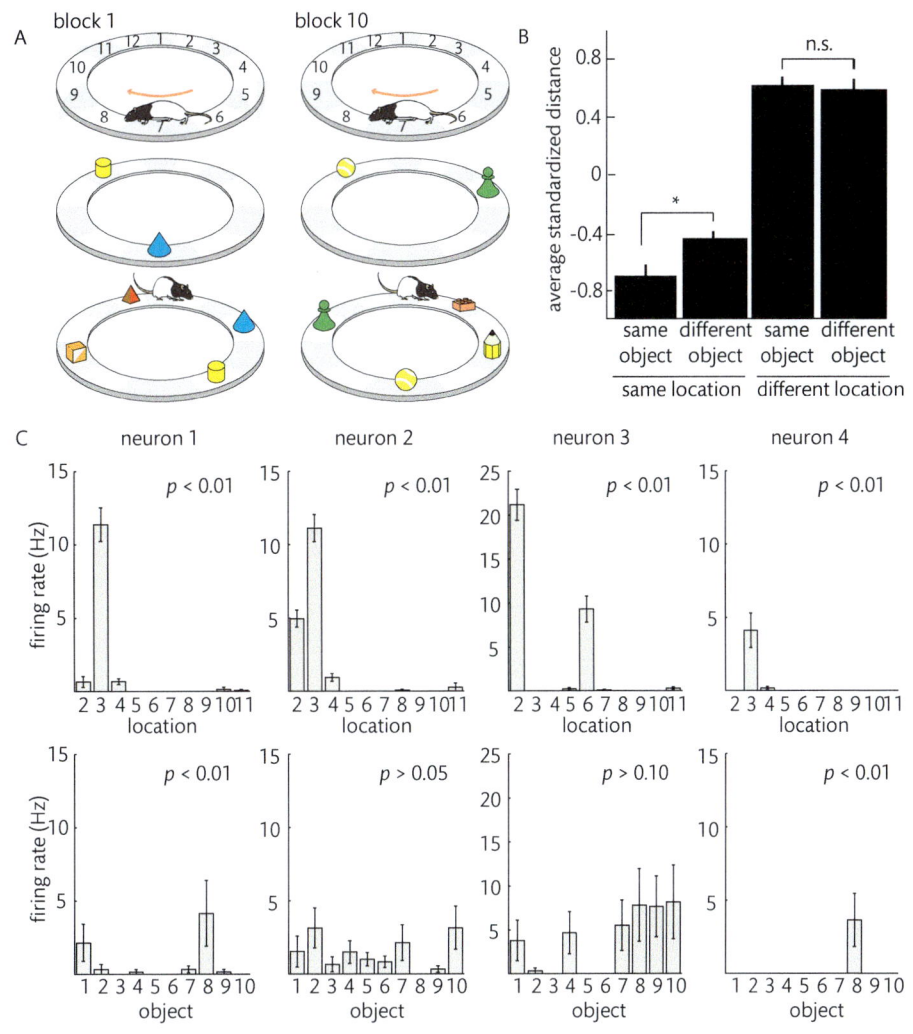

Figure 11.10 Object representation in the hippocampus is dependent on location. (A) Schema of the object and place recognition task: rats circumnavigated an annular track for food reward after each lap. Middle, items (e.g., plastic junk object) were originally placed in specific locations on the track for 3 laps and then (Bottom) moved to new locations and additional items (e.g., wooden toy) added in a new location for another 3 laps. During each block of 4 × 3 laps, 4 different objects were encountered in at least 2 different places. Right, after this block, a new set of items was used and the procedure repeated for a total of 10 blocks and 40 different items. (B) Hippocampal cells distinguish between different objects but only when these objects are encountered in the same location on the running track. When objects are presented in different locations (right 2 bars), hippocampal firing patterns do not distinguish between the same or different objects. When the objects are presented in the same location (left 2 bars), the firing patterns do distinguish between them. (C) Examples of 4 hippocampal pyramidal cells that coded for location (top, all 4 cells) and four different cells two of which coded for object identity (bottom, leftmost and rightmost cells). (After Manns and Eichenbaum, 2009, with permission.)

number to the presence of a conspecific (Rao, von Heimendahl, et al., 2019) (see below).

11.5.5 Responses to conspecifics in hippocampal pyramidal cells

Several studies have looked at whether hippocampal pyramidal cells respond to conspecifics using the response to objects as a control (see section 11.5.4 on object responses). Some of these suggest that dorsal CA2 and ventral hippocampal cells show such responses. Rao et al. (Rao, von Heimendahl, et al., 2019) used the same "gap paradigm" that they used to demonstrate the absence of responses to objects in dorsal CA1. It consists of two elevated platforms separated by a gap, with a rat on each platform spontaneously reaching out across the gap and performing facial interactions (see Figure 11.11A). Around 10% of ventral hippocampal cells showed strong firing modulation by the conspecific, especially in males, where

cells were highly selective for females. The same cells did not show such strong modulation by objects. Dorsal CA2 cells, the main hippocampal target for vasopressin (the neurohormone involved in social behavior) and oxytocin (Vaccari, Lolait, and Ostrowski, 1998), were also recorded in this study. These did not differentiate between the gender of the conspecific and never showed such a dramatic increase in activity as the ventral cells. Similar to ventral CA1–CA3 regions (Jung, Wiener, and McNaughton, 1994; Kjelstrup, Solstad, et al., 2008; Komorowski, Garcia, et al., 2013; Ciocchi, Passecker, et al., 2015), it has been reported that dorsal CA2 place cells have significantly larger fields compared with dorsal hippocampal CA1 place cells, which may signal the context the animal occupies rather than a location per se, with a large percentage of dorsal CA2 place fields remapping in response to the introduction of a novel or familiar conspecific but none representing conspecifics per se (N.B. the same effect was found upon the introduction of a novel

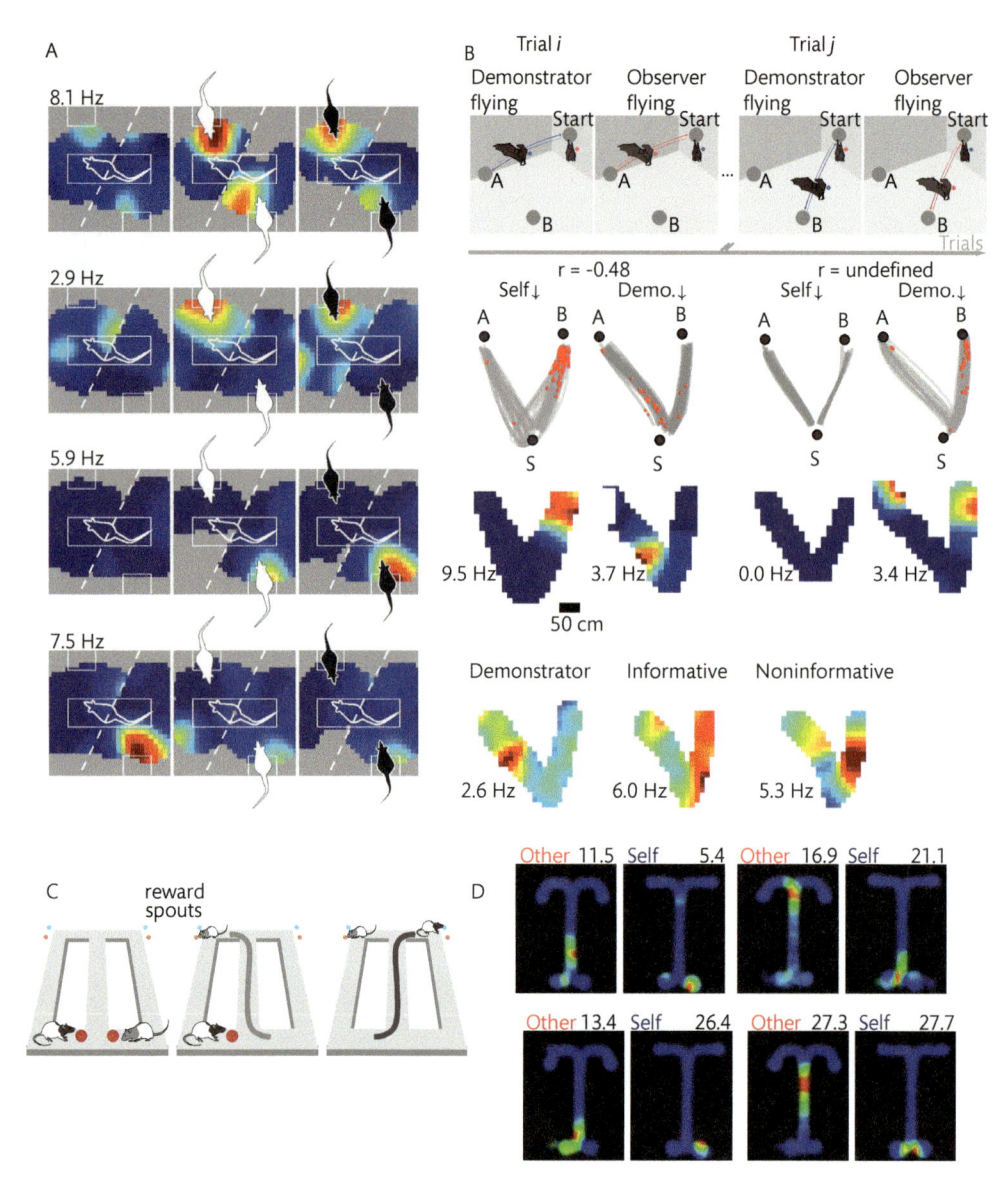

Figure 11.11 Place-cell responses to conspecifics. (A) Rat-modulated place cells. The recorded rat (in outline) sits on a central platform (either alone), or with a stimulus rat (black or white) presented on a platform on either side. Firing maps of 4 cells that had place fields modulated by the presence of a stimulus rat (deep red, maximal rate; deep blue, no firing). Top, Firing map of a weak place cell with fields on top and bottom, which increase firing in the presence of a rat. Middle 2 panels show place cells whose fields only appear when the stimulus rat is located in the field but not elsewhere. There is some evidence of preference for the black rat in the lower of the two middle panels. Bottom panel shows place cell whose field firing is strongly reduced during presence of a stimulus rat. (Adapted from Heimendahl et al., 2012.) (B) Hippocampal responses to conspecifics in bats. Top, schema of the bat conspecific location task: the subject bat flew itself or observed a conspecific demonstrator flying to and from 1 of 2 goals, A and B, from a common Start position. Below, 3 hippocampal cells that had social place fields as the observer bat either flew the route or watched another bat do so (cells and demonstration flight patterns shown in the second row). The left cell in the third row down fired in specific locations, both when the observer bat flew itself (left) or watched the flight of the demonstrator (right). The right cell only fired to the flight of the demonstrator and not to the observer bat's own flight. Another example cell (bottom row) fired to objects moved along the usual trajectories as well as to self flight (left), whether the observer bat was required to match the flight of the object (middle) or not (right). Cells responding to objects were often bidirectional, firing in both flight directions, whereas conspecific cells were usually unidirectional. (After Omer et al., 2018, with permission.) (C) Schema of the rat conspecific location task: the subject rat had to observe a conspecific running on a T maze and choose the arm not selected by the latter to obtain the reward. (D) Examples of 4 place cells whose firing was modulated by the location of the other rat (other) in addition to the subject rat's own location (Self). (After Danjo et al., 2018, with permission.)

object) (Wintzer, Boehringer, et al., 2014; Alexander, Farris, et al., 2016). The Siegelbaum lab has suggested that selective damage to dorsal CA2 pyramidal cells does result in alterations in social functions, perhaps via this remapping effect (Hitti and Siegelbaum, 2014).

There is little support for the idea that there are pure rat-specific cells in the dorsal hippocampus independent of the

animal's location. Instead it has been shown that the firing rate of hippocampal place fields is modulated by the presence of another rat: while Danjo and colleagues (Danjo, Toyoizumi, and Fujisawa, 2018) reported as many as 85% (Figure 11.11D), Von Heimendahl et al. (von Heimendahl, Rao, and Brecht, 2012) only found 7% (not significant) of such CA1 place cells (Figure 11.11A). The striking difference may be due to the attentional and behavioral demands of the tasks. In the former study the subject rats had to observe the conspecific and to follow its route in a stereotyped way to solve the T-maze task (Figure 11.11C), so there is the possibility that it had moved to slightly different positions as it moved to follow the other animal and these correlated with the position of the observed animal. In the Von Heimendahl experiment rats were simply interacting without any task. When objects were substituted for the conspecifics (von Heimendahl, Rao, and Brecht, 2012), if anything, there was a slightly stronger object-in-place response. A similar finding was reported by Zynyuk and colleagues (Zynyuk, Huxter, et al., 2012).

In the bat CA1, Omer et al. (Omer, Maimon, et al., 2018) reported that 18% of pyramidal cells responded to the positions of a demonstrator conspecific on an airborne version of a Y-maze task (Figure 11.11B). Similar to Danjo et al. (Danjo, Toyoizumi, and Fujisawa, 2018), the subject had to observe the conspecific to be able to subsequently choose the correct arm on the Y maze. Fifty-seven percent of these cells also had self-place fields during navigation (Figure 11.11B).

However, although the bats were clearly immobile during the observations, the authors did not vary the location of the sessile observer bat during the other-bat observation phase task, making it impossible to know whether the cells truly represented the position of a conspecific or, similarly to previous studies in rats, they were conjunctive place cells representing the subject bat's current location modulated by another conspecific's position on the Y-maze. Also, in line with previous studies, many of the place cells (65%) that responded to conspecifics also responded to moving inanimate objects (Figure 11.11B), although there were some differences: e.g., the responses were bidirectional for moving objects but not for conspecifics (however, note that the objects but not the bats looked similar during both moving directions).

11.5.6 Responses to rewards in hippocampal pyramidal cells

If the hippocampus is involved in learning, one might expect cellular activity there to reflect information about rewards and punishments. Except for one study (Gauthier and Tank, 2018; see below), there is no indication that hippocampal pyramidal cells signal reward independently of location. With a few exceptions, experiments have involved presenting rewards in goal locations. One important exception is the one on taste responses in hippocampal neurons by Herzog and colleagues (Herzog, Pascual, et al., 2019), discussed above. Recall that they injected solutions into the animal's mouth as it foraged in an open field and showed that almost all responses to the injected liquid were taste-in-place cell responses, i.e., they depended on the animal's location. Importantly they also showed that while a large majority of the cells identified the presence of the taste with short latency responses, another third identified the specific identity of the taste and a further fifth its palatability. The palatability information only appeared around 1,800 ms after taste delivery. It might be argued that some of these palatability-in-place responses and in particular those to the highly desirable sucrose could be used by downstream structures as a signal that reward had occurred in particular locations. The authors conclude, "the hippocampus does not contribute to an animal's decision to consume or expel a given taste. Rather, it responds to the hedonic value of tastes consumed within a particular context, forming associations between place and reward that may be relayed downstream via hippocampal projections to the ventral tegmental area and other neural reward centers.... This could serve as a means of relating place to taste in terms of its inherent reward value, allowing animals to use past experience to locate food sources" (p. 3067).

In most studies rewards are concentrated at goal locations, in some cases consistently so, in others variably so, and in still others they move from one location to another or alternate between locations. There are four different possible ways in which goals might be represented in hippocampal pyramidal cells: (1) overrepresentation of the goal location via fields moving toward the goal or new fields emerging; (2) the modulation of out-of-goal-location place-cell firing depending on whether the animal is heading toward the goal or not; (3) dedicated goal cells; or (4) goal-direction and -distance cells. In addition to reward location, the value of the reward as well as time spent in the goal may be reflected in the activity of hippocampal cells. We deal with each possibility in turn. Importantly, it must be noted that introduction of a goal often significantly changes an animal's behavior, resulting in strong directional, locational, and velocity sampling biases that can make experimental design and data interpretation challenging. In a subsequent section on the role of the place cells in navigation (11.11), we shall present a more complex picture of the role of reward in restructuring the firing of large numbers of cells in the CA1 field than is within the compass of this section.

Place fields have generally been found to cluster closer to or fire more action potentials near the goal/reward location, but there have been exceptions. Several studies show goals overrepresented in the number of place fields found there, but this usually differed for different goals. Dupret and colleagues (Dupret, O'Neill, et al., 2010) found that CA1 (but not CA3) place cells shifted their location toward the goal during rewarded navigation and this reorganization was NMDAR-dependent (Figure 11.12A). A subsequent study suggested that this movement was greater in deep CA1 pyramids than in superficial ones (Danielson, Zaremba, et al., 2016).

In contrast, Kobayashi et al. (Kobayashi, Nishijo, et al., 1997) used lateral hypothalamic stimulation as a reward in three tasks (Figure 11.13A) (random foraging where randomly chosen locations are rewarded; shuttling between two goals for reward in each; and a goal-directed task where repeated visits to a designated goal location were rewarded) and showed that the majority of place cells (92%) had significant reward correlates only inside the place fields, and that reward and place correlates of the neurons did not change between the random foraging and two goal-navigation tasks (Figure 11.13B,C). Only on the third, more complex, task, where the animal had to shuttle between two places but was only rewarded at one (Figure 11.13D), did a subset (19%) of place cells shift place fields.

I. Lee et al. (I Lee, Griffin, et al., 2006) found that during the course of running an automated T-maze alternation task in which a return path led the animal back to the start after each trial, 70% of place cells fired differently in the stem depending on the animal's previous and subsequent choice (Figure 11.12B), the "splitter effect". These cells progressively moved along the T toward the goal with experience while approximately one-third of did not change over time. Despite this movement toward the goal, simultaneously recorded cells maintained their relative topological position. Running the animal on one half of the T configuration without alternation of choices did not result in the forward shift effect (see section 11.10

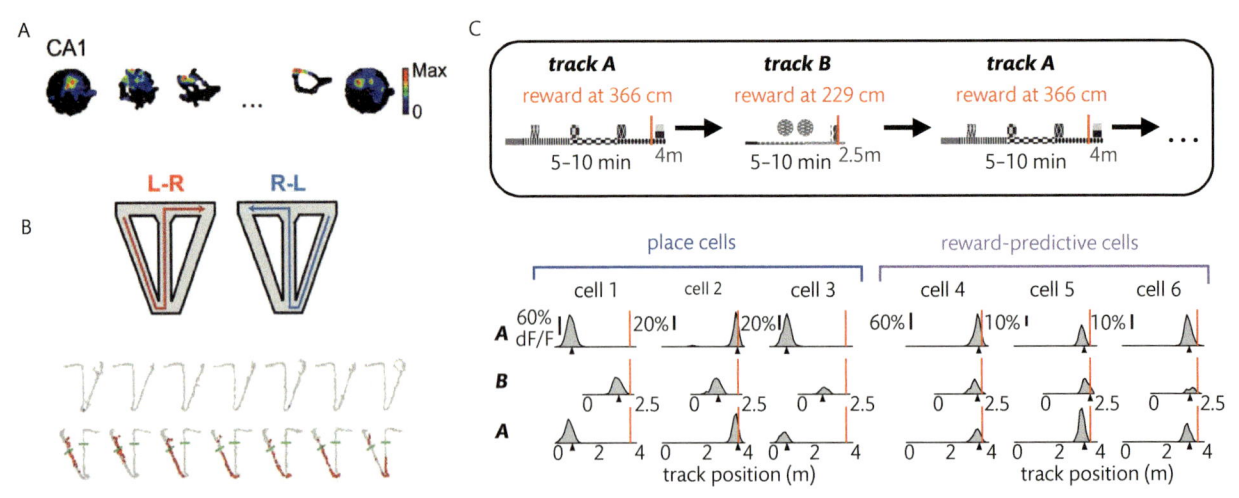

Figure 11.12 Place-cell responses to reward location I. (A) Example of place-field reorganization in an open-field whole-board task where the animal was required to find rewards in 3 different locations (small white dots). The field originally fired toward the middle of the environment, but after successive training trials (middle three pictures) moved to end up close to one of the goal locations. (After Dupret, 2010, with permission.) (B) Schema of continuous T-maze alternation task. Left: path on return from previous left goal and run on stem prior to right goal choice (L-R, in red). Right: path on return from previous right goal and run on stem prior to left goal choice (R-L, in blue). Below: an example of place cell that only fired on L-R red trials (bottom) showing firing field shifting toward the reward location from early (left) to late (right) trials. (C) Dedicated population of hippocampal place cells coding for reward location. Top: schema of 2 virtual reality tracks A and B of different lengths and cues with reward (red sticks) presented toward the end of the track in each. Bottom: examples of 3 classic place cells (cells 1–3, bottom left), which remap between environments and are not affected by reward location (shown by red line), and 3 reward-predictive cells (cells 4–6, bottom right), which always maintain their relative position to the reward in each environment. (From Gauthier and Tank, 2018.)

for further discussion of splitter cells in the context of predictive coding. In a candelabra maze task (Ainge, Tamosiunaite, et al., 2007) with one start arm and multiple goals visited on different trials, many cells (84%) had multiple fields involving one or more goals. Of these, 61% fired in only one goal, 39% fired in either two or three goals, but no cells fired in all four goals and nowhere else; thus there was no evidence that place cells represented goal locations per se. Instead, many cells also fired in the start arm as well as in the goal, and, similar to I. Lee et al., 46% of all place fields had different firing rates reflecting the destination on that trial while the rest ignored the destination and represented the animal's actual location in the start arm on all trials. A similar predilection for the start location shows up in other studies as well (Ainge, Tamosiunaite, et al., 2012; Grieves, Wood, and Dudchenko, 2016). This has been interpreted as activation of the intended route in the start arm before it is actually run or as conveying information about downstream locations. In general, studies that reported goal-related firing and that also required the animal to visit more than one goal, found evidence that the different goals were represented differently.

Only one study (Gauthier and Tank, 2018) reported a small number of cells that fired exclusively at the goal, either when it was shifted to a different location in the same virtual environment or to a totally different virtual environment (Figure 11.12C). These "reward-associated cells" made up 4.2% of cells with place fields in both conditions (or a tiny 0.8% of all recorded cells). They might form a small population of place cells with direct inputs from reward circuitry, which then inform other hippocampal cells of reward locations.

Several studies asked whether the value of the goal was represented in place-cell firing: if reward in the goal is varied, does place-cell firing in the goal or elsewhere on the maze represent the change in value (H Lee, Ghim, et al., 2012; S Lee, Huh, et al., 2017; Tryon,

Penner, et al., 2017; Duvelle, Grieves, et al., 2019)? H. Lee et al. (Lee, Ghim, et al., 2012) using an automated T-maze with varying probabilities of reward in the two arms over blocks of trials (signaled by different tones), found that both CA1 (15%) and subicular (11%) cells reflected the animal's goal choice and its outcome in the current as well as previous trials. In another study (Duvelle, Grieves, et al., 2019), two goal locations were used, each of which had a different reward value. The rat was required to go to a goal location and remain there for 2 seconds to earn a reward delivered elsewhere in the arena. The study failed to find place-field clustering at goals, but did find increased out-of-field population spiking at the goals occurring when the rat was paused or moving very slowly and only developing after ~1 second spent at the goal, as had previously been found in one-goal versions of the continuous navigation task (Hok, Lenck-Santini, Roux, et al., 2007; Hok, Lenck-Santini, Save, et al., 2007, Hok, Chah, et al., 2013; Hayashi, Sawa, and Hikida, 2016). This increased out-of-field firing may be related in some studies to SWR firing, which has been suggested to be involved in the replay of the previous locations and in the consolidation of the memory of the path to the goal (Lee and Wilson, 2002). However, it has not been seen in tasks in which animals did not have to wait at the goal (Zinyuk, Kubik, et al., 2000; Anderson, Killing, et al., 2006), or waited there for a shorter delay (Siegel, Neunuebel, and Knierim, 2008), suggesting that it is this slowing down and waiting in the goal zone that may be the cause of the slight increase in firing and not anything specific about goal location. In general, the amount of waiting time seems to be an important factor, with studies asking the animal to wait 1-second not showing firing and those requiring a 2-second wait showing it. McKenzie and colleagues (McKenzie, Robinson, et al., 2013) required a 5-second wait and noted that cells started firing on arrival at a goal but decayed in rate thereafter. Forty percent of cells only fired at one location, but another 25% fire at

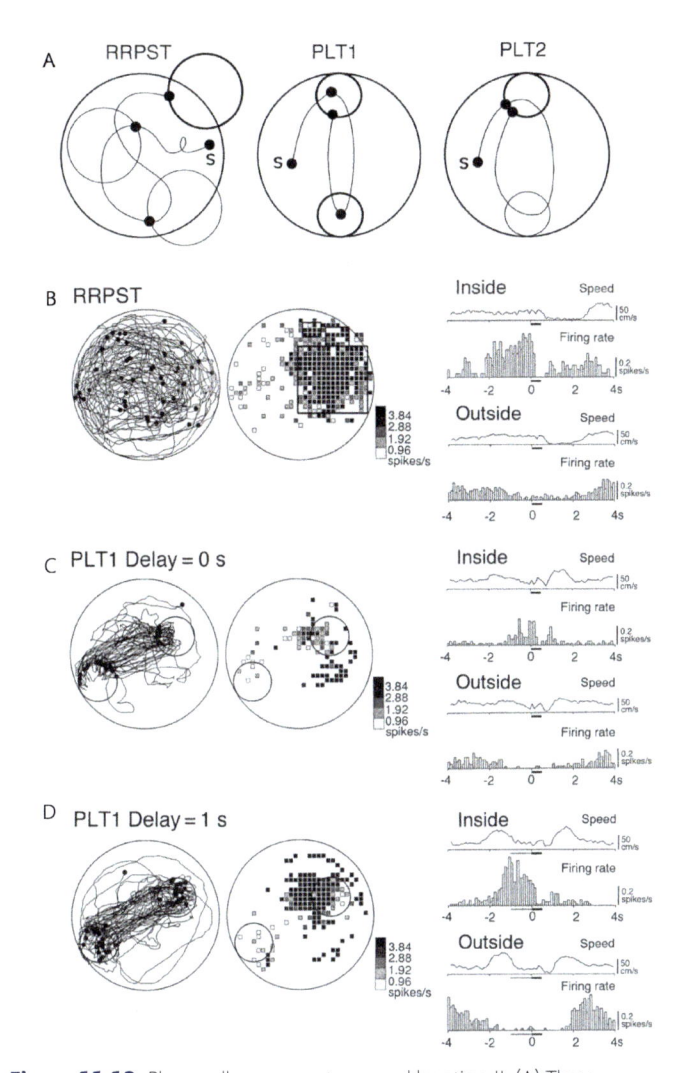

Figure 11.13 Place-cell responses to reward location II. (A) Three different behavior patterns were rewarded by the delivery of hypothalamic stimulation to animals in an open field: random foraging (left, random reward RRPST), reward for visiting each of 2 locations alternately without delays (middle, PLT1-0s), reward for alternating visits to 2 locations with 1 s delay and only one location rewarded (right, PLT1-1s). The rewarded zones were identified by an invisible circular location (small thick-line circle in the figures) at some randomly selected coordinate. The rat was rewarded with intracranial self-stimulation when it entered the reward site, which was then made inactive (changed to thin-line circle). After a 5 s interval, the reward site was moved to a different location and reactivated. Examples of behavior and place field under random reward condition (B), in Place-learning with no delay (C), and in Place-learning with 1 s delay (D). Note that the field does not change between the three different reinforcement schedules. Large dots, locations of reward delivery. (Adapted from Kobayashi et al., 2003, with permission.)

more than one, and overall, "It is important to note that cells never fired at all goal locations during WAIT events despite identical behavioral demands" (p. 10249). The amount of time spent at the reward location cannot be the whole story.

11.5.7 Representation of time in hippocampal pyramidal cells

The coding of time as a feature can take several different forms. At its simplest, the temporal signal can consist of a representation of the temporal ordering of events or features and their relative recency, such as whether the experience of a particular smell or sound

occurred before or after another. More complex temporal analyses involve the inclusion of metric information such as the duration of an event, or the length of time between events.

Lesion studies as well as single-unit recordings suggest that the hippocampus is important for some aspect of the processing of temporal information. However, it still remains unclear to what extent this merely reflects temporal information as a feature generated by other brain regions and embedded in hippocampal locations and contexts (similar to the way other features are so embedded as described above), or as a distinct encoding of a fourth dimension within the hippocampus that is independent of its three-dimensional coding of space (O'Keefe, 1996).

Let us look first at behavioral evidence that animals can use the time since the last visit to a location to control their behavior at that location. Clayton and Dickinson (1998) showed that Scrub jays could recognize the location and identity of self-cached foods. They trained birds that objects which they preferred such as worms decayed over time and lost their attractiveness while initially less preferred objects such as peanuts maintained their palatability over time. They then asked whether the birds could use the passage of time to decide which foods they had previously buried to retrieve. The optimal strategy would be to retrieve worms in preference to nuts after short periods since burial, and to retrieve nuts after longer periods, and this is what the birds did. Importantly they also showed that the birds dug in the correct location even if they only learned that worms were perishable after they had finished the burying phase of the experiment.

Babb and Crystal (Babb, 2005; Babb and Crystal, 2006b) designed a broadly similar task for rats and showed that they also could measure and compare relative time intervals between events, and associate them with different actions. Rats were trained on an eight-arm radial maze where the daily testing was divided into two phases. During the first phase, they were given access to only four randomly selected arms, three of which were baited with regular food pellets and the fourth with a more desirable chocolate pellet. After either 0.5 or 4 hours delay, they took part in the "free-choice" phase, where all arms were accessible, and the four previously unvisited ones were baited with regular food. In addition, the chocolate arm was replenished, but only after the longer interphase period. The animals revisited the chocolate arm significantly more often after longer interphase intervals, and this tendency could be reversed if, offline, chocolate was devalued by being associated with an unpleasant event such as the sickness resulting from lithium chloride poisoning. This would appear to be good evidence that the rats remembered the taste and valence of the chocolate as well as its location (Babb and Crystal, 2005). Even more convincingly, training with two flavors in two different arms followed by the devaluation of one by poisoning resulted in only that one being subsequently left unchosen (Babb and Crystal, 2006b). The choice of arms to visit after a delay did not rely on input from a circadian clock, since the choice could still be made if both choices took place at the same circadian time of day, after intervals of 1 hour or 25 hours (Babb and Crystal, 2006a). It should be noted that at least one alternative interpretation of these results may be that the rats were able to encode the recency of the events rather than the relative time intervals per se to solve the task. Importantly these results were not repeatable when unique movable objects placed at the ends of the radial maze arms were the predictors of reward instead of the locations themselves (Babb and Crystal, 2003). In a different set of experiments, the animals *could be trained* to use their circadian clocks to time-stamp experiences as occurring in the morning or the afternoon, and this did not depend on the interval between the feeding experience and subsequent testing (Zhou and Crystal, 2009). Overall, these findings suggest that, similar to Scrub jays, rats were able to form episodic-like associations of what-where-when at least within the time frame of a few hours to days.

Another approach to studying the role of time in a spatial context in rodents is to use a modified NOR paradigm (see NOR in section 11.5.4 on object recognition) where object familiarity is negatively correlated with the relative amount of time since an object was last encountered: higher familiarity leads to less time spent exploring an object (see above section 11.5.4 on object-in-place responses). A typical modification of the NOR paradigm (e.g., Dere, Huston, and De Souza Silva, 2005; Kart-Teke, De Souza Silva, et al., 2006) involves three consecutive exposures to four objects in the same open field box. In the first exposure four copies of the same object A are placed in four different locations; in the second exposure sometime later, there are four copies of a new object B, some of them in the same locations the As had occupied and some in novel locations. During the third (test) phase the animal was faced with one copy of A and B in old locations ("stationary") and one copy of each in different locations ("displaced"). The results showed that the animals explored old stationary objects (A) to a greater extent in comparison with more recent stationary objects (B), indicating that animals had a knowledge of the relative recency of A and B. The displacement of a familiar object itself is known to result in increased exploration, presumably triggering a novelty signal associated with mismatch of an animal's expectation to find a particular object in a particular place. Interestingly, object displacement reversed the recency-related trend of an animal's exploratory behavior: now the displaced objects experienced more recently (B) were explored for longer compared with displaced old objects (A). This indicates that the temporal recency and spatial object-mismatch are not simply added together to encode the amount of novelty generated by objects in new locations and their relative recency.

In another set of experiments, Chiba and colleagues (Chiba, Kesner, and Reynolds, 1994) showed that rodents can tell which of several locations was visited earlier. On each day, animals were forced to enter all of the arms on an eight-arm maze in a random sequence and then in a subsequent test session were asked to choose the earlier of two arms visited. The two choice arms could have been separated in the prior learning phase by a number of intervening arms ranging from 0 (i.e., sequential) to 6. Control animals performed excellently, showing a gradual improvement in choice accuracy with larger separation intervals. Only for choices experienced sequentially was the performance at chance level. Hippocampal-lesioned animals were severely impaired on this task, being at chance on all pairs except for those experienced successively, where performance was significantly improved. In the case of the latter, it is reasonable to assume that a different brain region was used to solve the task (perhaps using relative familiarity of sensory cues in each arm analogous to NOR task performance described above).

These behavioral experiments still do not address some major questions about temporal coding: do rodents measure the relative recency of various events using relative familiarity: A is more familiar than B and B more familiar than C; or, alternatively, can animals genuinely measure intervals between events, and if so, what are the time ranges available to them? On a behavioral level, our major source of information about animals' ability to make such "precise" time judgments mostly stems from operant experiments implementing differential reinforcement learning (DRL) or peak-timing schedules. In these tasks, after each operant response (e.g., a lever press) the animal is required to withhold responding for a predetermined period of time (usually of the order 10 to 20 seconds) before responding again. Premature responses reset the clock. Animals with hippocampal damage find this schedule particularly difficult, tending to respond again before the interval is up. In another test of timing ability, the peak procedure, a food pellet is delivered for the first lever press after 20 seconds of the onset of a stimulus, often auditory, on a fixed interval 20-second schedule. In 40-second nonrewarded probe trials designed to see how accurately the animal judge the 20-second interval, normal animals typically increase their lever presses to peak at the 20-second time point and then decrease them, demonstrating good duration timing. Both controls and rats with fimbria-fornix (FFx) lesions (which disconnect the hippocampus from septal and other subcortical regions) could perform this task, suggesting that the lesions caused no general impairment of the ability to perceive time intervals (although the time interval might be perceived to be slightly shorter). The same FFx lesions resulted in profound spatial memory deficits, comparable to hippocampal lesions. However, differences between the groups showed up when a short 5-second gap was introduced halfway through the 20-second stimulus. Whereas the controls quickly learned to adapt to the gap by increasing their estimate of the total length of time by 5 seconds, the FFx animals did not accommodate but instead acted as though the delay period reset after the gap interval, suggesting that the hippocampus is important for a correct selection of the onset and resetting of the timing mechanism (Meck, Church, and Olton, 1984). To our knowledge, the role of spatial context in this timing task has not been studied by, for example, training animals in one box and testing them in a different one.

Overall, then, the experimental findings suggest that the hippocampus is important for placing features encountered in a particular spatial context in their temporal order (sequence) and using this information to inform an animal's future actions. It is also important in setting and resetting animals' internal clocks to measure time lapsed in seconds, minutes, hours, and possibly even days (although more work is required to tell how precise the temporal resolution can be). However, the clocks themselves are likely to be located in different, possibly multiple, brain regions outside the hippocampus (Meck, Church, and Matell, 2013; Tsao, Sugar, et al., 2018). In general, it is difficult to unambiguously interpret the cause of impairments observed in hippocampal animals unless we know more about hippocampal cell activity or until behavioral readouts with a finer indication of an animal's perception of space and time during the task are developed. An impairment may have arisen due to an animal's inability to use the information about the temporal order of the events, but equally there might not have been a recollection of the events themselves (i.e., spatial maps of various features and the animal's actions associated with them), hence their temporal order becomes unavailable as well, as a secondary consequence.

We turn now to the single-unit data. There are several ways in which hippocampal pyramidal cells might code for temporal as well as spatial variables. In the simplest, their activity might reflect the amount of time elapsed since an event. That is, they might have time fields analogous to place fields and fire after, e.g., 4 seconds since a specific "starting" event. More complexly, time might be represented by a systematic change in place-cell firing, e.g., by a deviation with the passage of time from the initial coding for a place or an object-in-a-place either at the level of a single cell or of the population. Comparison of this deviated code with the original would act as a measure of time passed. As we shall see, there is evidence for both types of signal in the hippocampus (see Issa, Tocker, et al., 2020, for a recent review).

Eichenbaum and colleagues have reported that hippocampal pyramidal cells signal time within a short series of events as well as the location of those events. In an olfactory recency discrimination, they (Komorowski, Manns, and Eichenbaum, 2009, Manns, Howard, and Eichenbaum, 2007) found evidence of temporal coding based on systematic alterations in the hippocampal population code representing the sequence of five odor-sniffing events. Odor pots changed location across the sequence, permitting detection of firing-rate correlates to the odor pot itself, to its temporal sequence in the trial, and to the interaction of these with location. The population of cells showed an average change in absolute firing rates (some increasing and some decreasing) across the session, mostly due to rate changes in place cells and less so to the temporal ordering of the sniffing experiences. These changes were correlated with the animal's ability to perform the task, suggesting that success was due to the association of each odor with the changing place-cell activity across the trial and only slightly, if at all, to the temporal sequence in which the odor was experienced.

Another study (Macdonald, Lepage, et al., 2011) trained animals on an object/odor go/no-go short-term memory task. Each trial began with the animal sampling one of two objects at the beginning of the stem of a T-maze for a few seconds and then being held in the middle compartment of the stem for 10 seconds before being released to sniff at one of two odor pots toward the end of the stem. Each of the objects was matched with an odor pot, and digging at the odor pot of a matching pair yielded a reward; withholding digging to a mismatched pair also yielded reward farther down the maze. Many cells had place fields in the delay compartment whose field firing was modulated with time passed, forming a spatiotemporal code. For example, a cell might fire during the first few seconds after the animal reached the middle of the compartment while another might fire in the field during the last few seconds. Interestingly, when the length of the delay period was increased, 37% of cells continued to display peak firing during the same time from the start of the delay while 63% shifted their time correlate to maintain a fixed proportion of the delay. Other cells responded selectively to one of the objects or odors, as might be expected if these were object-in-place or odor-in-place cells.

Most of the remaining studies on short-term time coding relied on the technique of forcing the animal to run in position on a wheel or treadmill to look at the firing of pyramidal cells independently of changes in location. In their pioneering study, Czurko and colleagues (Czurko, Hirase, et al., 1999) recorded while animals explored a small square box or ran on a wheel attached to one side of the box for water reward. In addition to the usual place cells in the stationary box, a small percentage of cells became active as the animal ran on the wheel and continued to fire as long as the animal continued to run. The authors concluded that these were place cells with fields at the location of the wheel in the room, because rotating the box by 90° either abolished or reduced their wheel firing.

Presumably, the wheel had been moved out of the place fields or the preferred direction of the cells relative to the room cues. In a follow-up study, Pastalkova and colleagues (Pastalkova, Itskov, et al., 2008) incorporated the wheel into the starting stem of a figure-8 maze in which the animal was required to alternate choices between runs for reward. Each run began with the rat entering the running wheel and running for a short fixed period before being allowed to run down the central stem of the maze and choose left or right. Hippocampal pyramidal cells fired in the wheel as well as on the maze with different cells active during different times in the wheel-running period. The firing patterns of individual "wheel" cells differed between upcoming left and right choice trials and, in some animals, were predictive of the animal's choice on that trial. Thus, on each trial there was a specific sequence of pyramidal-cell firing from the beginning of wheel running through maze choice and on to the reward. Wheel cells had many properties in common with place cells, including showing phase precession. Control recordings were taken when the animals ran in a wheel box similar to that used by Czurko et al. (1999; see above) and also on a wheel in the animal's home cage. As in the Czurko et al. study, cells fired in these wheels but not in such delineated time periods and not in regular repeatable patterns correlated to the time of running in the wheel. Also similar to the Czurko et al. study, a different firing pattern was observed when the animals ran in the opposite direction in the wheel, implicating a substantial role for distal room or head-direction cues. Since the animals always ran in the same direction in the alternation figure-8 memory study, a role for room cues can be excluded as a source of variation in the temporal patterns found there. Clearly hippocampal pyramidal cells can generate sequences of activity during running on wheels independently of the current location in the environment. Something similar was shown in a virtual reality study (G Chen, King, et al., 2013) where place cells could be appropriately activated on a linear track following the brief presentation of visual cues at the start of the run which were then removed. In the appropriate experimental conditions, place cells can use some aspect of the animal's running to update the location of the place-cell representation.

Salz and colleagues (Salz, Tiganj, et al., 2016) repeated many of these findings in a slightly different paradigm. They recorded while animals were performing an alternation task on a similar figure-8 maze with a shared central stem containing a treadmill (Figure 11.14A). Twenty-seven percent of CA3 cells and 30% of CA1 cells increased their activity on the treadmill with peak firing ranging from the beginning of running until the end (Figure 11.14B). Interestingly, the time period during which the cells fired lengthened with increasing time during the run, resulting in decreased temporal resolution later in the period. Roughly the same percentage of "time" cells were recorded when the working-memory component of the task was removed by using only one-half of the figure-8 structure. In an important dissociation study, Kraus et al. (Kraus, Robinson, et al., 2013) forced the animal to run at different speeds on the figure-8 treadmill allowing dissociation of distance run from time spent running. Most neurons were influenced to varying extents by both variables, but there were cells at the extreme ends of the distribution that were influenced entirely by one or the other of these variables (Figure 11.14C).

A similar finding was reported by Villette, Malvache, et al. (2015) and Haimerl, Angulo-Garcia, et al. (2019), who imaged CA1 pyramidal cells as mice ran or stood still on a nonmotorized treadmill

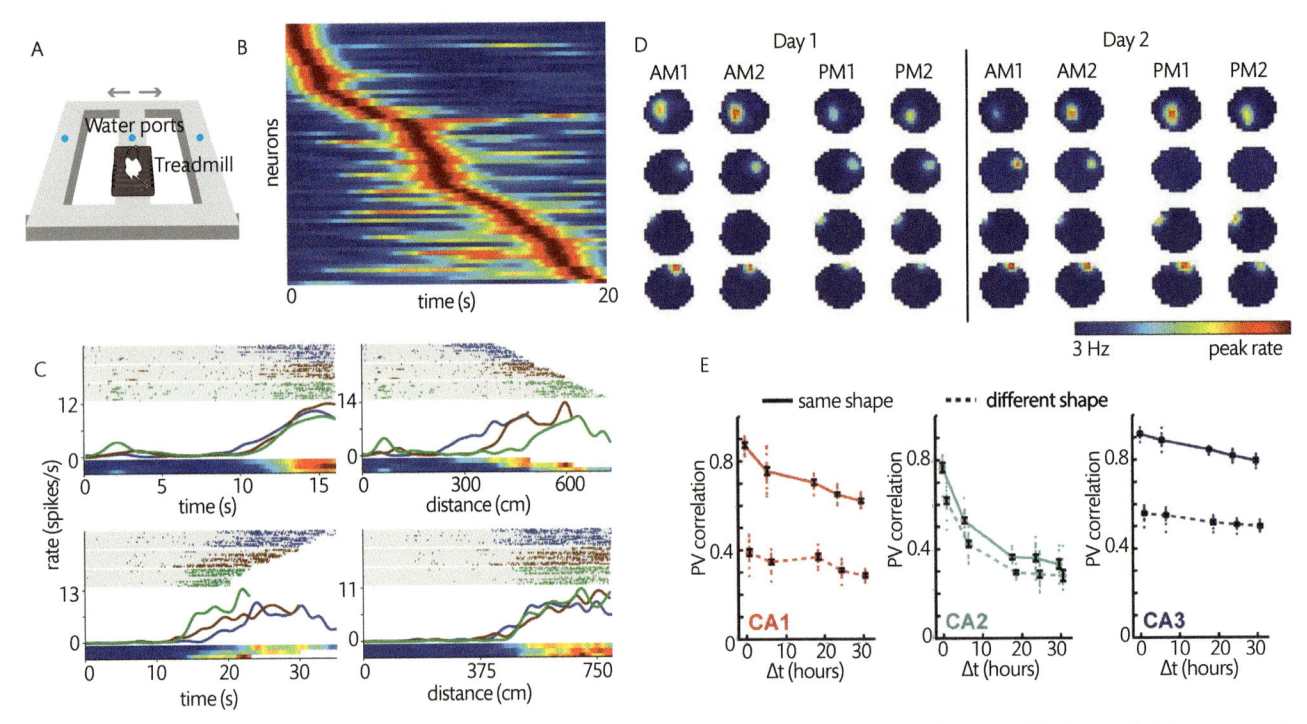

Figure 11.14 Hippocampal representation of time. (A) Schema of spatial alternation task with treadmill in stem. (B) Time-cell-firing patterns in CA3 as a function of time since treadmill start during treadmill running sessions. (After Salz, 2016, with permission.) (C) Two hippocampal cells on treadmill, one responding more to time (top) and the other to distance run since the start (bottom). Left: firing rate plotted as a function of time (at 3 different speeds) since beginning of run. Right: distance run. (After Kraus, 2013, with permission.) (D) Changes in firing rates of four CA1 place cells recorded in the same circular environment on eight sessions spread over 2 days. Note the field location remains the same but there is large variability in rates over time. (After Mankin et al. (2012), with permission.) (E) Change in population vector correlations with time in the same and different environments in the three CA fields. Note the larger slope in CA1 vs. that in CA3 in the same boxes, which might be used as a time signal. Note also the more rapid decay in CA2. (After Mankin, 2012, 2015, with permission.)

in a featureless environment in the dark. During spontaneous running, they observed spontaneous bursts of firing in populations of 5% of the cells ("sequences of neural activation"), which represented either the distance run (50% of sessions, 14/28), the duration of running (11%, 3/28), or a mixture of both (39%, 11/28); overall, the majority represented distance significantly stronger than time (Villette, Malvache, et al., 2015; Haimerl, Angulo-Garcia, et al., 2019). Animals tended to spontaneously run in bursts of distance lengths that were multiples of the neural activation sequence lengths, prompting Villette and colleagues to suggest that each population sequence encoded distance traveled in discrete "distance units" (Villette, Malvache, et al., 2015). It should be noted that sequences of neural activations were only present when the animal was running and not when it was standing still, suggesting that they may be important for integrating speed rather than measuring time intervals. This view was strengthened by the observation that short pauses in running during a sequence did not disrupt the sequence progression, suggesting that it was more related to distance than time. Importantly the bursts of activity in the same cells recorded on two consecutive days could switch from one mode of representation to the other, showing that the same circuits could provide either spatial or temporal information. Modeling the dynamics of the hippocampal circuitry and examining the variables that produced the switch suggested that a generalized input such as an increase in the power in the theta band could switch the network from the duration to the distance mode (Haimerl, Angulo-Garcia, et al.,

2019). One interpretation of these findings is that a decrease in the running speed information provided by the septally-generated theta signal removes the input necessary for the hippocampal network to calculate distances traveled by taking running speed into account. This idea that it is the sequential behavior of hippocampal pyramidal cells, whether representing temporal or spatial variables or both, that is important echoes a position advocated by Buzsaki (Buzsaki and Tingley, 2018). Before we accept the simple interpretation that there are "time" cells that have as their primary or sole correlate the time after an event, we might want to see what these same cells do on running wheels located in different parts of the maze or in different locations in the room, to see whether the time cells are actually time-in-place cells analogous to the feature-in-place cells described elsewhere in this chapter. To our knowledge, this experiment has not yet been carried out.

Another way in which a time code might be instantiated is by rate remapping of place cells across time. That is, place fields could stay in the same location over time but firing rates slowly diverge from the original in a probabilistic way, giving rise to a temporal signal at the population level. Several studies suggest this possibility. One line of support for this long-term temporal code in CA1 comes from a study that recorded calcium transients from large numbers of hippocampal pyramidal cells for up to 45 days (Ziv, Burns, et al., 2013). Place fields were stable but disappeared and reappeared or changed firing rates on a random basis, causing the cell population pattern to deviate from the original, similarly to the Mankin, et al., experiment (Mankin, Sparks, et al., 2012) described above. The deviation from the original pattern continued for as long as 30 days, reaching quite high levels, despite which there was enough similarity between any two patterns to enable a decoder to use the pattern recorded on the first occasion to identify the animal's position on the second. This means that in addition to providing a temporal code for the linear passage of time as the place-cell patterns deviate from each other, there is still enough stability in their firing to reliably reidentify the animal's position across considerable periods of time. We can expect this spatial code to be much more reproducible in CA3 if the pattern shown in the Mankin et al. experiment continues for the longer periods used in the Ziv et al. experiment. In a subsequent study, Rubin and colleagues trained mice in two distinct runways located in different parts of the same laboratory (Rubin, Geva, et al., 2015). Both population codes drifted away from the originals at roughly the same rates, and temporal decoders trained on one set of pyramidal cells could predict elapsed time on the other maze with a significant accuracy of 65% (compared with 98% within tracks). In a subsequent experiment (Geva, Deitch, et al., 2023), representational drift in the firing rates was similar in markedly different virtual reality environments sampled at different intervals, suggesting that hippocampal place cells signaled the same elapsed time in both environments. In contrast, the amount of experience with each environment was signaled by place-field location drift, where the exact location of the fields shifted with accumulated experience rather than time. These findings can be taken as some evidence for a cross-environment temporal code. It will be interesting to see whether these systematic changes in the place-cell firing patterns can be used to inform the animal's performance in behavioral experiments.

Another example of hippocampal encoding of the temporal sequence of events within a single overall experience was reported by Sun and colleagues (Sun, Yang, et al., 2020). The authors used one-photon microscopy to image calcium transients in a large number of CA1 pyramidal cells from mice running in a square-shaped linear track. A single running session comprised four laps, and animals were food-rewarded in the same corner of the track at the beginning of each session. The animals completed 15–20 sessions in succession. While 72% of the CA1 pyramidal cells had place fields, they also noted that for 31% of these cells (called event-specific rate-remapping [ESR] cells), the firing level within the place field varied with the number of laps after reward, for example, firing on the second, but not other, laps. Most of ESR cells fired on the first lap (~50%), but other laps were also represented (~16% of ESR cells for each subsequent lap). Importantly, they showed that these ESR responses could be dissociated from the location of the place fields. Switching to a circular maze caused the place fields to remap, but 38% of the cells with strong event-related responses continued to mark the same lap. Conversely, they were able to change the preferred lap by increasing the number of laps run before reward or by blocking the inputs from the MEC. This latter caused the preferred lap to shift but left the place field unaltered. Alterations of time elapsed or distance run after the reward did not affect the preferred lap. The effect increased with experience, and, conversely, rewarding the animal on each lap greatly reduced the effect (to 9% of cells; and in this case every lap was equally well represented), showing the importance of the lap-polarizing rewarding event. It is unfortunate that they did not alter the amount of reward or try

a different polarizing event, such as interrupting the animal's progress every fourth lap to demonstrate the generality of the effect. This experiment would seem to demonstrate that some aspect of the number of laps subsequent or prior to the feeding experience was being encoded in the pyramidal cells independent of the place code. However, it must be noted that on average only ~4.6% of place cells per animal (8 out of 179 of corecorded place cells) represented the order of each lap beyond the first lap (i.e., on the second, third, and fourth laps). Taken together with the observation that, in the majority of examples, these lap responses were not confined to just a single lap (i.e., they were nonbinary and often present on other laps only being strongest on a particular lap on average), this warrants more careful investigation whether ESR cells are really used to encode the order of the "events" beyond the first lap. The differential firing during the rewarded event (i.e., the first lap) may represent the presence of the reward rather than any temporal order per se. In the absence of evidence that animals can use these codes to guide their behavior, we should be cautious of overinterpreting them as evidence for temporal coding. An alternative possibility is that the ongoing changes of place-cell responses during different visits reflect the flexibility of the hippocampal code to adopt to constantly changing experience (each visit is different, even if it occurs in the same environment). Hence it may allow the animal to distinguish between different events in the same spatial context, but whether the animal can actually use the information to assess temporal relations between these events remains to be seen. As described above, Manns et al. (Manns, Howard, and Eichenbaum, 2007) found evidence of temporal coding based on systematic alterations in the locational population code representing the sequence of five odor-sniffing events and that these were correlated with the animal's ability to perform the task, suggesting that this form of spatiotemporal code could be useful in solving temporal sequence problems.

At this point, it is clear that the hippocampus incorporates a representation of time of different durations. Whether this is independent of the spatial mapping function is not clear, since in general the relevant experiments have not been done. In only a few experiments (Rubin, Geva, et al., 2015; Sun, Yang, et al., 2020, Geva, Deitch, et al., 2023) is there evidence that time can be represented independently and not as a variable within the spatial framework comparable to other features. To what extent hippocampal temporal coding is independent from spatial coding is an important question that needs more carefully controlled behavioral physiological experiments.

11.6 Place cells outside the hippocampal formation

Place-cell-like activity has been reported in a number of other extrahippocampal regions that have been associated with spatial learning and memory, such as retrosplenial, postrhinal, and posterior parietal cortices as well as rostral thalamus, claustrum, and primary cortical motor (M1 and PMd) and somatosensory (S1) cortices (Sutherland, Whishaw, and Kolb, 1988; Aggleton and Vann, 2004; Harker and Whishaw, 2004; Vann and Aggleton, 2005; Vann, Aggleton, and Maguire, 2009) (Figure 11.15F–M). We refer to these cells as "place-like" because although superficially like hippocampal place cells, they often exhibit fundamentally different properties.

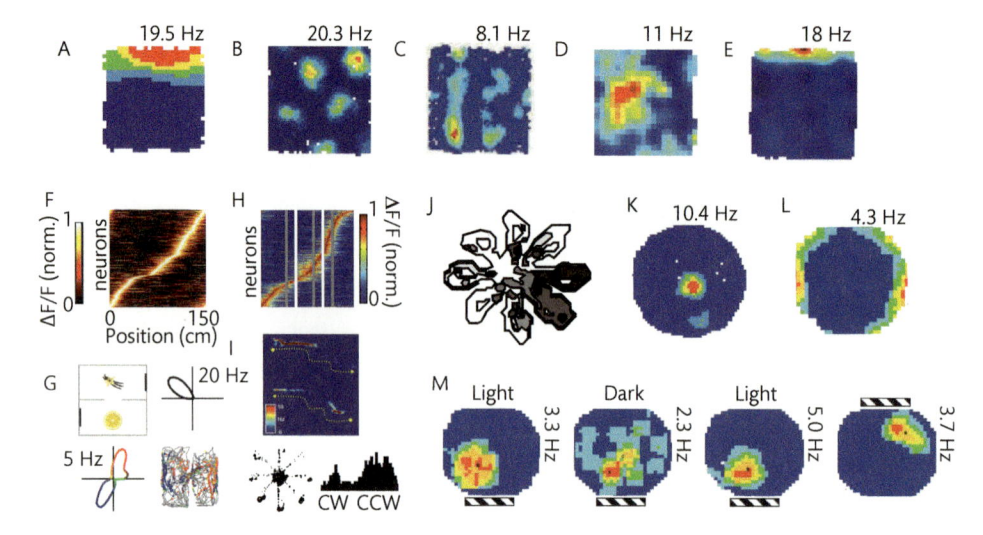

Figure 11.15 Spatial responses in different brain regions. (A) Subicular boundary cell. (Adapted from Lever et al., 2009, with permission.) (B) Grid cell. (C) mEC spatially periodic nongrid cells. (Adapted from Krupic et al., 2012, with permission.) (D) mEC spatially modulated cell. (Adapted from Diehl et al., 2017, with permission.) (E) mEC border cell. (Adapted from Solstad et al., 2008, with permission.) (F) Retrosplenial cells show place-like responses on a virtual linear track. Individual neurons represent discrete positions along the track and taken together represent the entire path. (Adapted from Mao et al., 2018, with permission.) (G) In real enclosures, retrosplenial cells show directional responses to cues (bottom). Head-direction cells (top right) recorded in ADT and parahippocampus maintain their directional tuning in a multiple compartment with a single visual cue but differing odor cues, vanilla above, lemon below (top left), while retrosplenial cue cells change their directional properties to follow the cues (bottom left). Raw data shows the color-coded red and blue directional firing in each box (bottom right). (Adapted from Jacob et al., 2017, with permission.) (H) Place-like choice-related PPC neurons. Individual neurons represent discrete positions in a virtual visual conditional T-maze where the choice of arm is dependent on the visual stimulus at the beginning. Taken together, the activity of the population represents the animal's path. Vertical gray lines divide the trajectory into cue section at the beginning, the run section and the goal choice section. (Adapted from Harvey et al., 2013, with permission.) (I) PPC cells respond to animals' trajectories in 2D enclosures. Top, cell firing on the left-to-right trajectory on a winding linear track (above) also fires at the beginning of the right-to-left trajectory (below). (Adapted from Nitz, 2006, with permission.) Bottom, a different PPC cell response to clockwise rotations at the ends of an eight-arm maze and in the center (McNaughton, 1994, with permission.) (J) Spatial responses in the lateral septum recorded on an eight-arm radial maze. Darker colors represent higher firing rates. (Adapted from Leutgeb and Mizumori, 2002, with permission.) (K) Place-cell responses in anterior thalamic nuclei. (Adapted from Jankowski et al., 2015, with permission.) (L) Boundary response in anterior claustrum. (M) Spatial cells in anterior claustrum are strongly modulated by the visual cues. Spatial field deteriorates in the dark and rotates with the visual cue. (Adapted from Jankowski et al., 2015, with permission.)

These relate to their spatial specificity, preferred response stimuli, stability, or other important features. Given that they have markedly different anatomical properties as well as neural network architecture, they are also likely to have distinct functional roles, which have yet to be uncovered. As we review these experiments, we will keep in mind that localized field firing can be generated by many different cues especially under constrained circumstances in which, for example, the animal only moves in one direction relative to the cues.

In retrosplenial cortex (RSC), place-like responses were observed in head-restrained mice navigating on a one-dimensional tactile-stimuli-based virtual reality (VR) linear track (Mao, Kandler, et al., 2017; Mao, Neumann, et al., 2018) (Figure 11.15F). Most of the place-like activity was found in the superficial (granular and agranular) layers (15%–60% of all cells vs. <5% in deep layers). RSC place-like cells showed similar field sizes and distributions compared with CA1 place cells recorded on the same task (Mao, Kandler, et al., 2017). During the task, a head-restrained mouse navigated on a linear 1.5 m belt with multiple tactile cues distributed along the belt. The proportion of RSC place-like cells, as well as their spatial specificity, increased with learning (Mao, Neumann, et al., 2018), growing from ~30% to 60% over 7 days of repeated exposures to the environment. This is in contrast to CA1 place cells, which rapidly reach high spatial specificity shortly after the first exposure to a new

environment (Wilson and McNaughton, 1993; Frank, Stanley, and Brown, 2004; Komorowski, Manns, and Eichenbaum, 2009) and remain relatively stable across many days (Mankin, Sparks, et al., 2012; Ziv, Burns, et al., 2013). Interestingly, although location-specific responses of CA1 place cells show rapid onset and remain stable, they often gradually develop a response to specific nonspatial features located in their place fields (e.g., smells, sounds, objects; see section 11.5), reminiscent of the gradual increase in spatial specificity with learning observed in the RSC. For example, Komorowski and colleagues (Komorowski, Manns, and Eichenbaum, 2009) reported that the percentage of CA1 place cells that showed a strong modulation by "item" (which in their case was a distinct smell) in addition to location increased from ~6% in the first 30 trial block to ~31% at the end of the learning session. At the same time the percentage of "pure" place cells (i.e., cells that were sensitive solely to an animal's location) decreased from ~48% to ~35% (n.s.). On close examination a significant portion of the original place cells became strongly modulated by item-in-place with learning and were replaced by newly developed place cells.

In contrast to this modulation of rate by item seen in the hippocampus, the slow emergence of location-specificity in the RSC suggests that it is might be provided by another brain region— for example the hippocampus, the medial entorhinal cortex, or presubiculum/postsubiculum—that has strong reciprocal connections with the retrosplenial cortex (Wyss and Van Groen, 1992; Van Groen and Wyss, 2003). Indeed, RSC place-like responses significantly deteriorated after bilateral hippocampal lesions (Mao, Neumann, et al., 2018), suggesting that they are likely receiving their spatial tuning from the hippocampal formation or possibly indirectly via inputs from grid cells, which were also shown to degrade after hippocampal inactivation (Bonnevie, Dunn, et al., 2013). After bilateral hippocampal inactivation, fewer RSC neurons develop location selectivity, their day-to-day stability deteriorated, and positional decoding errors became significantly larger. The lesion also significantly disrupted spatial learning in RSC cells, further suggesting that hippocampus (directly or indirectly) may be a key source for location-specific representations in the RSC (Mao, Neumann, et al., 2018). On the other hand, temporary bilateral RSC inactivation using tetracaine injection does not significantly affect basic properties of place-cell firing such as spatial specificity and firing rates (Cooper and Mizumori, 2001). It does, however, significantly compromise place-cell stability, causing fields to remap. The place fields return to their baseline positions after the tetracaine is metabolized (~20 min after the injection). These findings are in line with one of the prevailing hypotheses that RSC may play a key role in landmark processing (Mitchell, Czajkowski, et al., 2018): place cells may have remapped because they lost the input about their initial visual anchoring landmarks and instead had to use other types of cues.

In general, in one-dimensional tactile-stimuli-based VR environment, RSC place-like cells remain stable across multiple trials, although the stability and spatial specificity is markedly reduced by removing all the tactile cues from the track (Mao, Neumann, et al., 2018). By contrast, in the same experiments, CA1 place cells did not show a significant decrease in stability, suggesting that they can use path-integration signals to effectively update their position with respect to the reward position (which is presumably the only reliable fixed reference point on the virtual track after the tactile cues have been removed). This also suggests that the existence of stable spatial representations in the hippocampus is alone insufficient to provide equally stable representations in the RSC. Instead, stable external cues seem to be necessary to associate location representations with them. Somewhat surprisingly, despite strong connectivity with visual areas (Mitchell, Czajkowski, et al., 2018), RSC place-like cells showed largely stable responses in the dark (with tactile cues present) and when the reward was moved to another location.

Unlike hippocampal place cells, RSC cells show little location specificity in two-dimensional environments (L Chen, Lin, Barnes, et al., 1994; Cho and Sharp, 2001). Neural responses recorded in the RSC in two-dimensional environments include head-directional cells (Chen, Lin, Barnes, et al., 1994; Cho and Sharp, 2001; Jacob, Casali, et al., 2017; Keshavarzi, Bracey, et al., 2022) and various conjunctive cells, which incorporate signals for speed, angular head velocity, allocentric and egocentric directions, specific movements, and location. Interestingly, the location-specific responses were different in their nature compared with CA1 place cells: overall, cells were active across the entire environment, but with different conjunctive directional preferences in different parts of the environment (Cho and Sharp, 2001). Unlike head-direction cells found in anterior dorsal thalamus and parahippocampal areas (e.g., presubiculum, medial entorhinal cortex, etc.), many retrosplenial directional cells are responsive to specific environmental cues.

Jacob and colleagues used an enclosure consisting of two identical compartments with one strong identical polarizing cue available but placed on the opposite walls of each compartment (Figure 11.15G, top left). Cue-specific RSC head-direction cells rotated their preferred direction by 180° in different compartments (Figure 11.15G, bottom), whereas ADT and parahippocampal head-direction cells maintained their preferred direction in both compartments (Jacob, Casali, et al., 2017) (Figure 11.15G, top right). This suggests that place-like activity reported in the RSC combines different types of information about an animal's direction anchored to different types of stable sensory cues (visual, tactile, and other cues available), location, and running speed to maintain stable spatial maps. This observation is also in line with the findings in human subjects showing that although patients with selective damage to RSC were able to recognize neighborhood landmarks, they failed to navigate effectively in familiar environments, indicating that they are unable to derive directional information from landmark cues (Vann, Aggleton, and Maguire, 2009). In contrast, patients with selective hippocampal damage were able to maintain a sense of direction relative to the external landmarks even though they are significantly impaired at navigating in both novel and familiar environments (Maguire, Nannery, and Spiers, 2006). An important role for the RSC in integrating these different stimuli becomes apparent especially when animals are required to shift spatial strategies or "frames of reference," which may include shifting between external vs. internal (self-motion) cue navigation or between frames of references anchored to different external cues (Vann, Aggleton, and Maguire, 2009). This suggests that RSC may play a key role in selecting among multiple autonomous maps observed in CA1 (Fenton, Wesierska, et al., 1998; Zinyuk, Kubik, et al., 2000; Anderson and Jeffery, 2003). Indeed, Burgess and colleagues (Burgess, Becker, et al., 2001) proposed that RSC may play a key role in translating self-motion egocentric representations, possibly processed in the parietal cortex, into allocentric hippocampal-parahippocampal spatial representations as well as translating the latter representations into egocentric ones to guide and inform an animal's actions.

The posterior parietal cortex (PPC) has also been suggested to contain spatial cells. One-dimensional place-like responses were found there in head-fixed mice navigating in visually based virtual environments (Harvey, Coen, and Tank, 2012) (Figure 11.15H). PPC is reciprocally connected with all the primary sensory cortical regions, higher multimodal associative areas (e.g., prefrontal, temporal, and limbic association cortex), motor and premotor areas, RSC (Kolb and Walkey, 1987), and the dorsal part of the medial entorhinal cortex (Burwell and Amaral, 1998; Furtak, Wei, et al., 2007). It does not have direct connections with the hippocampal formation. It has been suggested that PPC mediates the egocentric spatial relationship between the body and external targets and is essential for computing coherent representations of movement trajectories across multiple bodycentric domains (e.g., eye, or limb movements) (McNaughton, Mizumori, et al., 1994; Nitz, 2006; Whitlock, Sutherland, et al., 2008; Calton and Taube, 2009). For example, PPC cells showed different responses depending on the type of movement (a reach vs. saccade) that an animal executed toward the same allocentric target (Cui and Andersen, 2007). More broadly, studies in primates indicate that PPC is essential for spatial perception, for correct real-time execution of visually guided motor actions, for sustaining and controlling attention over time, and for detecting salient events embedded in a sequence of events

(Husain and Nachev, 2007). PPC lesion studies in rats suggest that PPC together with MEC plays a key role in path integration (Parron and Save, 2004), possibly via converting an animal's movement in an egocentric frame of reference into an allocentric frame of reference, as observed in MEC neural responses (Whitlock, Sutherland, et al., 2008).

Harvey and colleagues showed that PPC is necessary for the correct execution of planned actions during a visual conditional discrimination in a virtual T-maze (Harvey, Coen, and Tank, 2012). In this experiment, head-fixed mice navigated in a virtual T-maze with a stem consisting of three parts: cue segment, delay segment, and choice segment. The delay and choice segments had the same visual landmarks independent of the choice to be made, whereas the cue segment had different visual cues indicating what choice the animal had to make at the choice segment in order to receive the reward. In this cue-conditional task, PPC cells (~73% of the highly active cells) formed a sequence of location-specific neuronal activations covering the entire track: i.e., the majority of PPC neurons were active in small portions of the T-maze (with only a small number of neurons having broad tuning curves). In the majority of cases, different neural sequences were active on left vs. right trials with only a third of neurons active on both. A similar activation sequence was observed in all three parts of the virtual T-maze. In another study, Nakamura (1999) recorded from PPC in head-restrained rats performing a directional delayed nonmatching-to-sample task where an auditory cue was presented from one of the six speakers positioned around the animal. The animal had to lick if a sample cue and an identical probe cue (which were separated by 2 seconds) came from different locations and withhold the licking if they came from the same locations. Nakamura found that PPC neurons showed auditory-cue-specific responses as well as broadly tuned directional responses and mnemonic responses (i.e., cells that were active during the delay period). When animals were rotated by 180° or when new auditory cues were presented, the majority of the cells maintained their directional responses, suggesting that they encoded directions in an allocentric frame of reference.

The findings observed in head-fixed animals are in contrast with experiments in freely moving rats, which showed little or no spatial location specificity in PPC neural responses (McNaughton, Mizumori, et al., 1994; Nitz, 2006). In freely moving rats navigating in mazes, PPC cells represented body trajectories such as inward and outward movements, turns, forward running, and absence of motion in one study (McNaughton, Mizumori, et al., 1994), and allocentric direction, external visual cues, and illuminance in another (L Chen, Lin, Barnes, et al., 1994) (Figure 11.15I). McNaughton and colleagues (McNaughton, Mizumori, et al., 1994) showed one cell with a high location specificity, which turned out to be responding to an illuminated spot rather than the more abstract place-field responses found in hippocampal maps. Indeed, when Nitz (2006) systematically investigated the response correlates of PPC cells in complex mazes, he found that, unlike CA1 place cells recorded in the same task, PPC cells showed little directional or location specificity. Instead, they had highly consistent response patterns related to the sequence of the rat's movements in line with observations that PPC neurons encode information about turns, speed, and other movement-related behavior.

Similar to observations related to the retrosplenial cortex, it is possible that any spatial modulations observed in PPC during head-fixed navigation task may be inherited from the medial entorhinal or indeed RSC, which has direct reciprocal connections with PPC (Mitchell, Czajkowski, et al., 2018). Currently, there are no reports of single-unit recordings in the PPC in animals with lesions in the hippocampus, medial entorhinal cortex, or RSC. However, it is clear that PPC is not essential for forming location-specific activity in CA1 place cells; instead it plays a key role in integrating local proximal cues into the hippocampal cognitive map (Save and Poucet, 2000). Save and colleagues showed that PPC lesions did not affect the formation or stability of CA1 place cells, although place cells in PPC animals tended to have significantly larger place fields (Save, Paz-Villagran, et al., 2005). However, after PPC lesions the control of proximal cues over place-cell firing was significantly reduced: the proportion of place fields that completely rotated with the proximal cues was significantly lower (64% in PPC lesioned vs. 93% in control animals). Moreover, even in cases where CA1 place fields in the lesioned animals did rotate with the cues, they tended to revert back to their initial locations after all the proximal cues were removed, whereas place fields in control animals tended to maintain their newly rotated positions (63% of place fields reverted to their initial prerotation field positions in PPC-lesioned rats, while 79% of place fields maintained their rotated positions in control rats). One possibility is that in the absence of the parietal cortex, proximal cues can still control location of hippocampal place fields but those fields are not integrated into the control by the stable background cues. An alternative possibility is that the parietal cortex mediates the control of place fields by path-integration cues that are maintaining the location of the fields after proximal cue removal.

Neurons with activity modulated by location have also been reported in postrhinal cortex (LaChance, Todd, and Taube, 2019). However, unlike the location-specific cells described above, these cells are strongly modulated by head-direction in an allocentric frame of reference, by distance to the center of the environment, and by the center-bearing angle (i.e., the angle between an animal's head axis and the line connecting the center of the environment and the animal's head). This can be interpreted as postrhinal cells encoding an animal's position in a spherical coordinate system with its center positioned at the center of the enclosure. This is in contrast to the hippocampal and mEC cells, which encode location in a Cartesian coordinate system.

A third of lateral septal neurons have been reported to show location specificity (Zhou, Tamura, et al., 1999; S Leutgeb and Mizumori, 2002) when rats were exploring two-dimensional enclosures or eight-arm mazes (Figure 11.15J). The hippocampus has two major efferent projections: one forms a part of a strong bidirectional pathway with the medial entorhinal cortex and the other consists of a unidirectional projection to the lateral septum. The activity of lateral septal cells might be expected to reflect this place-cell input. Interestingly, all of the lateral septal location cells had low firing rates (peak firing rate <7 Hz), whereas normally septal firing rates range from 0 to 125 Hz). Unlike cells located in the hippocampus, all the responses of the lateral septal cells are inhibitory and the fields are broader compared with hippocampal place cells (S Leutgeb and Mizumori, 2002). Currently it is unknown what stimuli drive these spatial responses. S. Leutgeb and Mizumori (2002) recorded simultaneously from LS and CA1 neurons in identical eight-arm mazes located in different enclosures with distinct distal visual cues. As expected, CA1 place cells immediately differentiated between the rooms by remapping in the novel room while maintaining a highly similar representation in the familiar room.

LS cells also showed a decrease in correlation between the familiar and novel room on the first day in the novel environment. However, unlike hippocampal place cells, which show higher decorrelation between two similar environments with experience (Lever, Wills, et al., 2002), LS showed higher similarity between two environments with increased number of re-exposures. The increased similarity may reflect more similar behavior exhibited by the animal in these highly similar environments (e.g., speed profile, body turns at particular space, and other). More systematic studies will have to be conducted in order to determine what drives location responses in the lateral septum. However, based on its strong anatomical connections with the hippocampal formation, it is likely that hippocampal place cells may be shaping LS spatial responses.

A small proportion of neurons in rostral thalamus also exhibit high and stable locational firing in two-dimensional environments (Jankowski, Passecker, et al., 2015). Jankowski and colleagues recorded from freely moving rats exploring a two-dimensional curtained circular enclosure with only one external cue present. They showed responses coding for place (Figure 11.15K), head-direction, and distance to the boundary (boundary cells) in parataenial nucleus (PT), anteromedial nucleus (AM), and nucleus reuniens (NRe) similar to those seen in the hippocampal-parahippocampal formation. The overall percentage of place-like cells in rostral thalamus was significantly smaller (29% in PT, but note that this estimation may be unreliable due to the very low total number of recorded cells: ~24 cells in 3 rats; 6.2% in AM, 329 cells recorded in 7 rats; and 2% in NRe, 550 cells recorded in 6 rats) compared with place-cell number reported in CA1 region (usually ~30%). The number of boundary cells was even lower (~2% vs. ~10% reported in the parahippocampal regions (Boccara, Sargolini, et al., 2010). Place-like cells in PT and AM tended to have smaller well-defined fields (often more than one field per cell) compared with NRe cells. They also did not exhibit any location clustering. Other spatial cell types found in all three nuclei of rostral thalamus include boundary cells and head-direction cells. The ranges of boundary cells were larger than the 90° degrees usually observed in mEC but often did not span the 360° observed in the claustrum (see below). Head-direction cells had a narrow tuning range comparable to cells found in the anterior dorsal thalamus and postsubiculum (Taube, Muller, and Ranck, 1990; Taube 1995a). Unfortunately, the authors did not conduct any environmental manipulations to examine what cues (internal and/or external) control the firing of these cells. Surprisingly, location-specific cells were also found in the rat's anterior claustrum of rats navigating in a circular or square enclosure (Jankowski and O'Mara, 2015) (Figure 11.15L). A small percentage of cells (4.3%) showed place-like activity similar to hippocampal CA1 cells; for example, their fields rotated in response to a rotation of a single external visual cue. Interestingly, they also showed significant clustering around that visual cue, unlike place cells, which exhibit uniform coverage of the enclosure in similar experiments. These cells showed poorer spatial specificity in the dark (the change was not significant although, as noted by the authors, visual inspection of the data clearly suggests otherwise) (Figure 11.15M). Finally, when recorded in a square environment, the spatial cells did not show the global remapping usually observed in CA1 place cells, instead preserving their position in close proximity to the visual cue. Other claustral cell types included boundary cells (2.6%) and object cells (5.5%). The claustrum has a diverse connectivity with a range of neocortical and subcortical regions including the medial septum, amygdala, subiculum, RSC, and medial and lateral entorhinal cortex (Wilhite, Teyler, and Hendricks, 1986; X Zhang, Hannesson, et al., 2001; Park, Dvorak, and Fenton, 2011; Zingg, Hintiryan, et al., 2014). As yet, too few single-unit recordings have been made in the claustrum to allow one to infer with any certainty the functional role of its location specificity. It appears likely that claustral cells may inherit their spatial specificity from medial entorhinal cells, which contain all the cell types described above (i.e., place-like cells, object-like cells, and boundary-like cells). However, some important differences are apparent: mEC border cells in a circular environment usually span ~90° range, whereas in claustrum they always covered an entire 360° perimeter. Also, no anatomical clustering was reported in the entorhinal spatial cells. Perhaps this is mediated by the RSC or is something computed within the claustrum to bind an animal's location to specific external cues. More experiments should be carried out to address this, including adding multiple external (distal) cues in the environment.

Location-specific cells have also been found in other cortical structures in nonhuman primates. Nicolelis and colleagues (Tseng, Rajangam, et al., 2018; Yin, Tseng, et al., 2018) reported location- and direction-specific neural responses in primary cortical motor (M1 and PMd) and somatosensory (S1) cortex during monkey whole-body navigation. The monkeys navigated to a grape dispenser reward located in a large real environment using a motorized wheelchair. On average ~40% of neurons encoded the location of the wheelchair within the allocentric room frame of reference. Many also showed directional modulation. These location specific cells had large spatial fields (often >2 m^2) and were stable across multiple days (Yin, Tseng, et al., 2018). The fields tended to cluster around the reward location and around the boundaries located in close proximity to the reward. Some of the fields could be rotated by rotating environmental cues (including a reward cue and a stationary conspecific) (Tseng, Rajangam, et al., 2018). Future experiments will explore the relation between these cortical cells and hippocampal place cells and how they are used for navigation and spatial learning and memory. For example, it will be important to determine how much they are determined by the task at hand: e.g., how sensory-motor neurons respond in the absence of a goal. It could be that the spatial responses will disappear similar to the way in which feature-driven responses in hippocampal place cells are not observed if no attention to them is required during the task (Pastalkova, Itskov, et al., 2008; Itskov, Vinnik, et al., 2012; Aronov, Nevers, and Tank, 2017; Danjo, Toyoizumi, and Fujisawa, 2018).

An outstanding issue is the development of place fields during infancy and immediately thereafter. The existing findings show that CA1 and CA3 regions develop place-cell representations as soon as the animal leaves the nest without any prior experience being required for their emergence (Langston, Ainge, et al., 2010; Wills, Cacucci, et al., 2010). This firing provides the building blocks for the hippocampal cognitive map. Border cells are also basic building blocks of the map and are also present as soon as an animal leaves the nest (Bjerknes, Moser, and Moser, 2014). Indeed, it has been suggested that inputs from border cells, which show higher stability, spatial specificity, and clustering close to the borders, may be important for early place-cell formation (Muessig, Hauser, et al., 2015). In line with this view, grid cells in adult mice are more stable at the borders, suggesting that border inputs may act as an error-correction signal (Hardcastle, Ganguli, and Giocomo, 2015); but see Nagele, Herz, and Stemmler (2020), who reported no increase in field firing variability with the distance to the wall. Grid cells may represent a universal metric for space and provide the neural basis for path integration (McNaughton, Battaglia, et al., 2006; Moser and Moser, 2008). Indeed, there is some experimental evidence showing that path integration is impaired in animals with degraded grid-cell representations (Gil, Ancau, et al., 2018) or after blocking the output from mEC layer II cells, which provide one of the main inputs to the hippocampal region (Tennant, Fischer, et al., 2018). However, multiple experiments have demonstrated that place cells can form place fields in the absence of grid cells (Langston, Ainge, et al., 2010; Wills, Cacucci, et al., 2010; Brandon, Koenig, et al., 2014; Hales, Schlesiger, et al., 2014). It is yet to be shown whether place cells can be formed in the absence of grid cells when only path-integration cues are available. Perhaps there are several independent pathways providing self-motion signals, including postrhinal and PPC signals. Similar to mEC grid cells, location selectivity in RSC also becomes impaired following hippocampal damage (Mao, Neumann, et al., 2018). It remains to be seen how hippocampal inactivation affects place-like cells in other regions including PPC, lateral septum, rostral thalamus, claustrum, and sensory-motor regions. Based on the current evidence, we may expect that inactivation of any of these regions will not result in significant degradation of place cells, whereas the opposite may be true. That is, extrahippocampal location-specificity in cell firing may be inherited from the hippocampus or another brain region. For example, with experience, the activity of V1 neurons can become modulated by stimulus location and this anticipatory response is mediated by anterior cingulate cortex (Fiser, Mahringer, et al., 2016), which receives direct inputs from the ventral hippocampus and appears to play a role in remote contextual and spatial memory (Frankland, Bontempi, et al., 2004; Maviel, Durkin, et al., 2004). Importantly, when the effect of learning was addressed by recording cells over prolonged periods of time in novel environments, the number and location selectivity of extrahippocampal place-like cells gradually increase with learning, unlike hippocampal place cells. In contrast, hippocampal place cells emerge rapidly and only gradually develop other nonspatial feature-in-place properties. One can speculate that other extrahippocampal place-like cells may have their primary correlate, such as a direction-modulated response to external cues in retrosplenial cortex or movement-related information in PPC, and then gradually map location modulation on top of these, for a more effective execution of optimal actions in particular spatial contexts (e.g., if you are in location A, run to the northeast to escape the predator vs. if you are in location B walk slowly until you hit the hidden food location). By working together, these systems provide the basis for learning and storing new environments, actions/goals associated with these environments, and movement motives, enabling effective execution of these actions.

11.7 Hippocampal–entorhinal cortex interactions

One of the major excitatory inputs to the hippocampus comes from the entorhinal cortex (mEC) (Witter, Doan, et al., 2017). Reciprocally, the hippocampus projects back to the entorhinal cortex (see Chapter 2). In this section, we will explore the relationship between these two areas. There have been multiple attempts to determine to what extent the spatial representations found in the hippocampus are already present in the entorhinal

cortex (Quirk, Muller, et al., 1992; Cacucci, Lever, et al., 2004; Fyhn, Molden, et al., 2004) or are built up from entorhinal inputs. Later in the section, we will also ask the reverse question: how dependent are entorhinal cell properties and in particular, grid cells, on hippocampal inputs? Grid cells represent one of the major cell types in the medial entorhinal cortex (mEC) (Hafting, Fyhn, et al., 2005; Sargolini, Fyhn, et al., 2006; Boccara, Sargolini, et al., 2010). Other functional cell types also found there include head-direction cells (Sargolini, Fyhn, et al., 2006; Boccara, Sargolini, et al., 2010), border cells (Solstad, Boccara, et al., 2008; Boccara, Sargolini, et al., 2010), speed cells (Kropff, Carmichael, et al., 2015), and theta cells (Boccara, Sargolini, et al., 2010; Deshmukh, Yoganarasimha, et al., 2010). Grid cells are predominantly located in mEC layers II and III (Hafting, Fyhn, et al., 2005; Sargolini, Fyhn, et al., 2006; Boccara, Sargolini, et al., 2010) and hence, based on anatomical connections of these layers to the hippocampal CA fields (Witter, Doan, et al., 2017), were thought to provide the major input to place cells. Shortly after grid cells were discovered, it was suggested that the summation of multiple grid cells of different scales and orientations could generate spatial representations in place cells (O'Keefe and Burgess, 2005; Solstad, Moser, and Einevoll, 2006; Monaco and Abbott, 2011). However, optogenetic (S Zhang, Ye, et al., 2013), lesion (Bonnevie, Dunn, et al., 2013; Hales, Schlesiger, et al., 2014), and pharmacological studies (Brandon et al., 2014; Brandon et al., 2011; Koenig et al., 2011; Wang et al., 2015; Brandon, Bogaard, et al., 2011; Brandon, Koenig, et al., 2014) as well as experiments in young animals (Langston, Ainge, et al., 2010; Wills, Cacucci, et al., 2010; Bjerknes, Moser, and Moser, 2014; Bjerknes, Langston, et al., 2015; Tan, Bassett, et al., 2015) pointed to a more complex relationship between place cells, grid cells, and other spatial cells in the hippocampal-mEC regions. For example, following mEC lesions, CA1 cells still exhibited location-selective firing (place fields), but typically in fewer numbers and with significantly reduced stability, ranging from 10 seconds to a few minutes (Hales, Schlesiger, et al., 2014; Schlesiger, Cannova, et al., 2015; Sabariego, Schonwald, et al., 2019). CA1 place cells showed impaired stability between recordings separated by a short interval. With longer intervals, there were even larger changes: the correlation coefficient between recordings in a square environment decreased from 0.6 after a 2-minute break to 0.4 after a 20-minute break, compared with a correlation coefficient of 0.8 in controls (Hales, Schlesiger, et al., 2014). Increasing the interval further to 6 and 24 hours only slightly affected stability in lesioned animals, with spatial correlation dropping to ~0.35 while it steadily decreased in control animals to 0.6 after 24 hours. In addition, CA1 place cells lacking mEC inputs also showed larger and less spatially tuned place fields (Hales, Schlesiger, et al., 2014). Unlike CA1 place cells, CA3 place cells did not show an increase in field size, and showed a much smaller decrease in spatial information and stability following mEC lesions (Sabariego, Schonwald, et al., 2019). These physiological changes were mirrored in behavioral deficits on a spatial working-memory task in a figure-8 maze. In this task, rats had to alternate between left and right arms of the figure-8 configuration to get reward with 0 s, 10 s, and 60 s delay periods in the stem arm between choices (Sabariego, Schonwald, et al., 2019). Notably, mEC lesions resulted in an impairment on the 60 s delay working-memory task but not in the continuous version of the task (i.e., with 0 s delay). However, even on the longer delays, performance significantly improved after 15–20 days of learning, reaching significantly above chance levels. This improvement with experience did not take place in animals with combined lesions of the mEC and the hippocampus. The unimpaired performance at 0 s delays may have been due to the use of a simple alternating-body-turn strategy, which was disrupted by the delays in the stem. MEC lesions also caused severe impairments on the Morris watermaze comparable with the ones observed in animals with selective hippocampal lesions, but milder than combined hippocampal-mEC lesions (Hales, Schlesiger, et al., 2014), indicating that place-cell stability may be crucial for executing this task. Importantly, the standard Morris watermaze task can eventually be learned by animals with selective mEC or hippocampal lesions (or both), but the training takes significantly longer compared with controls (5 and 9 days to reach control performance levels for time spent in the target quadrant and for time spent in a small circle around the platform location, respectively). Strikingly, animals with mEC lesions never exceeded chance performance for the probes involving time spent in a small circle around the platform location and were only slightly above chance levels for those involving time spent in the target quadrant even after 10 days of training on a goal relocation version of the Morris watermaze (i.e., when the platform was shifted to a different location). Instead, mEC rats kept on looking in the old platform location (reminiscent of observations made in patients with selective hippocampal damage [Schacter, Moscovitch, et al., 1986] who kept on looking for an object in its first hidden location even after the object was moved to a new position in front of the patient 15 minutes prior to the task). Surprisingly, there was no impairment observed in mEC rats in other well-established hippocampal-dependent tasks such as object-in-place recognition and contextual fear conditioning, or on a perirhinal and lEC-dependent task such as novel object recognition (Hales, Schlesiger, et al., 2014). CA3 place cells may be able to support these tasks. Importantly, such deficits were only present if learning occurred prior to lesions, but not if the task was presented postlesion (Hales, Schlesiger, et al., 2014), suggesting that the animals may be using a different mEC-independent strategy to solve the task if mEC is unavailable during the initial acquisition of the task. As we have seen in section 11.5, this seems to be a general rule with the hippocampal involvement in novel object recognition tasks.

Grid cells, as well as place cells, may be important for providing the "time" signal to the hippocampal place cells (Pastalkova, Itskov, et al., 2008; Kraus, Robinson, et al., 2013; Kraus, Brandon, et al., 2015) and thus possibly contributing to hippocampal-dependent spatial/episodic working memory (section 11.5). Recall that in these types of experiments, the animals are usually running on a stationary wheel or treadmill positioned in a stem arm of maze such as a figure-8 maze. The animal is allowed to run for 10–20 s ("a delay period") before turning left or right on the maze to get the reward. The animal has to alternate between the sides to get the reward. Hence, the correct execution of the task requires the memory of the previous choice to be maintained during the delay period. It has been suggested that hippocampal "time cells," cells firing sequentially in time on a stationary wheel or track may support such working memory, since distinct choices were correlated with distinct firing sequences of hippocampal time cells (Pastalkova, Itskov, et al., 2008). Pharmacological inactivation of the medial septum (MS) disrupts the sequential temporal hippocampal firing (i.e., time cells) while preserving place-cell firing on the maze (Wang, Romani, et al., 2015). Importantly MS pharmacological inactivation selectively impairs gird-cell firing patterns but spares other mEC spatial

cells (Koenig, Linder, et al., 2011; Brandon, Koenig, et al., 2014) as well as place cells, even in novel environments. Similar to the effect seen with mEC lesions, place cells become less stable and less selective (Koenig, Linder, et al., 2011; Brandon, Koenig, et al., 2014). It is important to note that MS inactivation also causes a significant reduction in theta modulation in neural firing as well as LFP oscillations in both mEC and hippocampal regions (see section 11.2). Thus, such loss of temporal sequences may be caused by reduced theta activity rather than the lack of inputs from grid cells, since mEC lesions do not have a similar effect (Sabariego, Schonwald, et al., 2019). Instead, removal of mEC significantly diminished CA1 place-cell phase precession (section 11.2), the coupling between the place cells with overlapping fields, and replay events during the resting states within a trial (Schlesiger, Cannova, et al., 2015; Chenani, Sabariego, et al., 2019). Hence, mEC inputs are important for coordinating place-cell activity on a population level as well as with respect to LFP theta oscillations. The deficit following mEC removal may reflect the reduced inputs from speed-modulated cells, which are abundant in the mEC (Kropff, Carmichael, et al., 2015). A different type of mEC manipulation was tested on a different spatial-memory task (N Robinson, Priestley, et al., 2017). Here the animals were presented with one of two objects before running on a stationary track for 10 seconds. They received reward by either digging in a well on the right or proceeding to the left arm at the end of the corridor. The performance on this task was significantly impaired after only 2 seconds of transient mEC optogenetic inactivation, which was delivered 2 s after the beginning of the 10 s run on the treadmill. On the other hand, behavioral performance was not affected by comparable inactivation delivered while the animal was running on the maze after turning right or when it was near the object. The decrease in performance was accompanied by a decrease in time-cell stability during the inactivation period. In contrast, place-cell firing remained stable on the maze as well as near the object after inactivation.

Inputs from mEC and more specifically from grid cells may drive place-cell remapping (Fyhn, Hafting, et al., 2007; Monaco and Abbott, 2011; Latuske, Kornienko, et al., 2017).When an animal is placed into a different familiar environment, grid cells change their offsets and rotate, while place cells exhibit "global remapping" by assuming new positions that cannot be predicted from their old arrangement measured in the first familiar environment (R Muller and Kubie, 1987; Leutgeb, Leutgeb, et al., 2005; Fyhn, Hafting, et al., 2007). Intermittent partial inactivation as well as activation of mEC caused global remapping in hippocampal place cells accompanied by behavioral deficits on spatial memory tasks (Miao, Cao, et al., 2015; Rueckemann, DiMauro, et al., 2016; R Zhao, Grunke, et al., 2016; Kanter, Lykken, et al., 2017).Transient optogenetic inactivation of dorsal mEC cells caused global remapping in one-third of CA1 place cells, while the rest did not change their position (Rueckemann, DiMauro, et al., 2016). Such partial global remapping may reflect incomplete inactivation of mEC cells due to light reaching only a fraction of the cells. In line with this assumption, similar inactivation using optogenetic or chemogenetic techniques induced even more substantial remapping in CA3 place cells (Miao, Cao, et al., 2015). Selective optogenetic inactivation of mEC-DG inputs in the hippocampal formation resulted in a similar remapping, suggesting that the global place-cell remapping resulted from direct mEC inputs rather than indirectly from other brain areas affected by mEC manipulation (Miao, Cao, et al., 2015). Inactivation restricted to dorsal mEC had a significantly larger effect compared with that restricted to the ventral mEC.

Interestingly, CA1 place cells maintained their newly acquired firing fields even after mEC inactivation was terminated (Brandon, Koenig, et al., 2014; Miao, Cao, et al., 2015; Rueckemann, DiMauro, et al., 2016); mEC manipulation may lead to a "switch" to a new place-cell ensemble: once engaged, its properties may be sustained via internal hippocampal network dynamics. Importantly, when chemogenetic manipulation was restricted primarily to the dorsoventral extent of layer II mEC, depolarization but not hyperpolarization using hM3 and hM4 DREADD mice, respectively, resulted in global place-cell remapping in a familiar enclosure (Kanter, Lykken, et al., 2017). The hM3 manipulation (intraperitoneal injection of the designer ligand clozapine N-oxide [CNO]) also caused a significant increase in firing rate and field size, which vanished >12 hours after the manipulation, presumably when CNO had been metabolized. Place cells resumed their initial place fields, and stability came back to its initial high levels (~0.8; comparable to controls) which is in contrast to previous pharmacological or optogenetic manipulations, after which place cells retained their newly formed fields. This discrepancy may be due to the specificity of chemogenetic manipulations compared with other types of manipulations: first, in the case of the former, the manipulation was restricted to layer II mEC cells; second, chemogenetic manipulation induced global CA1 place-cell remapping only when mEC cells were depolarized, whereas other less-specific mEC manipulations induced global inhibition of large mEC areas spanning all cell layers. Place-cell remapping after chemogenetic depolarization of layer II mEC cells was accompanied by behavioral deficits on the Morris watermaze (Kanter, Lykken, et al., 2017). In these experiments, hM3, hM4 and control mice were trained to swim to the escape platform and all mice showed comparable high levels of performance after 9 days. During the retraining phase on day 9 the mice were injected with CNO, after which only hM3 mice were impaired on the task, presumably due to the artificially induced global place-cell remapping. Importantly, grid cells showed only partial remapping during both types of manipulations, whereby individual grid fields changed their firing rates but not their positions. Other mEC spatial cells, including head-direction cells, also showed partial remapping. However, this was less pronounced compared with grid cells in the case of hM3 manipulation. Even though mEC manipulation (both activation as well as inactivation) can clearly drive CA1 (but less so CA3) place-cell remapping, CA1 place cells can also form and undergo global remapping even in the complete absence of mEC inputs. The similarity between rate maps in two distinct enclosures after complete mEC lesions were at a chance level for both mEC and control animal (Schlesiger, Boublil, et al., 2018). Place-field stability after mEC lesions can be improved by adding external cues such as objects, smells, and visual landmarks, and is especially degraded when the animal has to mostly rely on the information about self-motion (Jacob, Van Cauter, et al., 2020).

Although place cells can be formed in the absence of grid cells and even in the absence of the entire mEC, the opposite is not the case: grid cells require input from the hippocampus for their existence. Pharmacological inactivation of the hippocampal region using muscimol injection results in severe grid-cell pattern degeneration (Bonnevie, Dunn, et al., 2013). Other spatial cells appear to be unaffected. Interestingly, during the hippocampal inactivation grid cells began to be modulated by the animal's head direction in

an allocentric frame of reference similarly to mEC head-directional cells, despite their being omnidirectional during control trials prior to inactivation. Moreover, experiments in young animals demonstrated that place cells develop before grid cells: the former appears as soon as the animal leaves the nest at P16, while it takes another 5 days for the first grid-like representations to appear (Langston, Ainge, et al., 2010; Wills, Cacucci, et al., 2010). Both cell types continue to develop their firing properties, such as increasing stability and spatial tuning, until reaching P28, when they become adult-like. This also coincides with the development of the hippocampal-parahippocampal inhibitory network (Langston, Ainge, et al., 2010). On the other hand, head-direction cells as well as border cells appear even earlier than place cells (Bjerknes, Moser, and Moser, 2014; Bjerknes, Langston, et al., 2015; Tan, Bassett, et al., 2015). Border cells may significantly contribute to place-cell formation around the boundary of an environment during the early stages of an animal development (Muessig, Hauser, et al., 2015).

Much less is known about how lateral entorhinal cortex (lEC), another major excitatory input to the hippocampus, contributes to place-cell activity. lEC cells display only weak place specificity (Hargreaves, Rao, et al., 2005). Instead lEC neurons respond to behaviorally relevant stimuli such as an animal's location relative to objects (Suzuki, Miller, and Desimone, 1997; Deshmukh and Knierim, 2011; Tsao, Moser, and Moser, 2013) as well as memory for object location (Tsao, Moser, and Moser, 2013), odors (Young, Otto, et al., 1997; Petrulis, Alvarez, and Eichenbaum, 2005; Xu and Wilson, 2012), and time signals (Tsao, Sugar, et al., 2018). Lesions to lEC impair rate remapping (change in firing rates without change in place-field location) in CA3 place cells (Lu, Leutgeb, et al., 2013). Interestingly, lEC cells themselves are not sensitive to changes in the environment associated with partial remapping (e.g., changes in color of the walls), hence, currently it is not known how they might be influencing rate remapping in place cells.

In summary, mEC inputs are necessary for place-field stability and spatial specificity, but not for place-field formation. Perturbation of mEC input, either by removing it via lesion experiments or by inducing intermittent pharmacological, chemogenetic, or optogenetic inactivation as well as more specific chemogenetic activation of its layer II neurons, results in impaired CA1 (but not CA3) place-cell stability, lower location specificity, and impaired performance on navigational and spatial working-memory tests such as the Morris watermaze and the figure-8 maze. Chemogenetic manipulation of mEC layer II cells revealed that while activating layer II cells induced artificial global remapping in CA1 place cells, stimulated mEC grid cells did not change their offsets but instead changed the firing rates of their individual fields. Interestingly, mEC chemogenetic inactivation induced rate remapping in individual grid fields but not global remapping in place cells. Other mEC cell types showed significantly smaller responses to such manipulations. Specific chemogenetic perturbation of mEC led to reinstatement of initial CA1 place-field position 24 hours later, when the effect of the manipulation wore off. On the other hand, larger inactivations of mEC affecting all layers, whether by chemogenetic, optogenetic, or pharmacological approaches, resulted in permanent global place-cell remapping (i.e., place cells retained their newly acquired fields even 24 hours after the manipulation). This suggests that changes across all mEC layers may be necessary for long-term "rewiring" of hippocampal representations. All in all, it can be concluded that mEC plays a key role in global or partial CA1 place-cell remapping and this in turn underpins behavioral performance. However, it is not the sole initiator and contributor to hippocampal remapping, since global remapping can occur even in the complete absence of mEC. In this case, the newly formed maps are less specific and less stable, leading to severe behavioral impairments. The other major inputs underlying this second type of remapping are currently unknown but one candidate is the anterior cingulum (Rajasethupathy, Sankaran, et al., 2015, see section 11.5.3). They are unlikely to come from lEC, since its permanent removal induces only rate remapping in CA3 place cells. Medial septum may play an important role in hippocampal place-cell formation, although as in the case of mEC, pharmacological activation of GABAergic MS cells does not prevent place-field formation even though it completely abolishes grid-cell firing patterns, leaving other mEC spatial cells intact. Perhaps other non-GABAergic MS inputs can rescue location specificity and responses to novelty by global remapping in place cells. On the other hand, activation of MS GABAergic signal significantly disrupts hippocampal time signaling, leaving location specificity relatively intact. In delayed spatial working-memory tasks, disruption of time signaling in either the hippocampus or entorhinal grid cells during the delay period leads to significant impairments. Complete mEC lesions do not disrupt the hippocampal time signal, suggesting that time representation is either independent in these two regions or the EC time signal is inherited from the hippocampus. Importantly, mEC lesions significantly impair CA1 place-cell precession as well as the coupling between the place cells with overlapping fields. The mEC clearly has an important role in coordinating place-cell temporal firing properties, possibly with respect to the LFP.

11.8 Place cells in other species: mice, bats, monkeys, humans

Place cells were discovered in rats (O'Keefe and Dostrovsky, 1971), and since then have also been found in mice (Rotenberg, Mayford, et al., 1996), bats (Ulanovsky and Moss, 2007), primates (Ludvig, Tang, et al., 2004; Hori, Nishio, et al., 2005; Courellis, Nummela, et al., 2019; Mao, Avila, et al., 2021), and humans (Ekstrom et al., 2003). There are many similarities between place cells recorded in different species: cells are active in restricted locations of the environment and are modulated by different sensory stimuli, e.g., the presence of objects. It has been suggested that place cells in rats and mice are qualitatively similar (Figure 11.16A,B). When place cells were compared in rats and mice exploring identical novel linear tracks, they showed similar well-defined place fields, phase precession, and burst firing associated with SWR events (Mou, Cheng, et al., 2018). On average, mice tended to have more place fields per cell (1.2 vs. 0.9 in mice vs. rats, respectively), which were also significantly smaller (33 cm vs. 40 cm in mice vs. rats, respectively) and had lower peak firing rates. Mice also tended to have fewer SWR events, at a significantly lower frequency (154 Hz in mice vs. 190 Hz in rats).

Nevertheless, despite these quantitative differences, place cells and their major temporal and spatial characteristics are comparable in rats and mice and, when used for position decoding, provide broadly similar precision. Place cells in bats (Figure 11.16C) also show similar properties (Ulanovsky and Moss, 2007) in two-dimensional environments: around 31% of hippocampal cells exhibited high spatial selectivity (which is comparable to the numbers

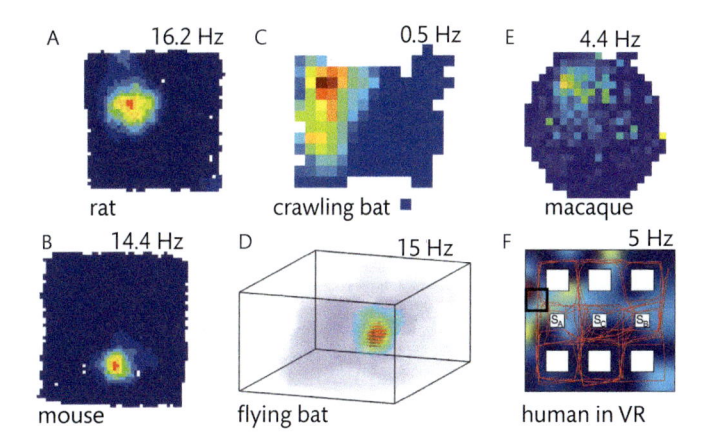

Figure 11.16 Place cells in different species. (A) Place cells in rats. (Adapted from Lever et al., 2002, with permission.) (B) Place cells in mice. (Adapted from Krupic lab with permission.) (C–D) Place cells in crawling (C) and flying (D) bats. (Adapted from Ulanovsky and Moss, 2007, and Yartsev and Ulanovsky, 2013, with permission.) (E) Place cells in macaques. (Adapted from Mao et al., 2021, with permission.) (F) Place cells in humans. (Adapted from Ekstrom et al., 2003, with permission.)

in rats, e.g., 34% reported in Wilson and McNaughton, 1993) and were stable across trials even when they potentially used different sensory modalities to navigate (echolocation in the dark vs. echolocation and visual inputs in lights-on conditions; see Quirk, Muller, and Kubie, 1990) for rats. Bats exhibit sphere-like fields in three-dimensional environments (Yartsev and Ulanovsky, 2013) (Figure 11.16D), as do rats (Grieves, Jedidi-Ayoub, et al., 2020).

However, one pronounced difference in place-cell firing between rodents and bats relates to the oscillatory activity in both single-unit activity and LFP. In bats high frequency (~123 Hz) oscillatory activity associated with bursts of neural activity appear in short bouts similar to SWRs observed in rodents (see section 11.2.9, "LIA and sharp wave ripples") albeit at lower average frequency. By contrast, bats, unlike rodents, do not show strong continuous LFP oscillations at 8–10 Hz theta frequency. Instead, prominent theta oscillations appear in 1–2 s bouts on average twice per minute. Unlike theta oscillations in rodents, which increase with running speed (both in terms of power and frequency), theta bouts in bats are associated with an increase in echolocation and a decrease in speed of movement. These findings are reminiscent of observations in cats, where theta power increases in immobile animals engaged in active visual behavior such as visually tracking prey, observing movement outside the window, etc., in addition to mobile behaviors (T Robinson, 1980). In marmosets, theta also occurs in short bursts and the relation between theta and locomotion is much less obvious if it exists at all (e.g., Courellis, Nummela, et al., 2019). Theta occurs in short 0.5 sec bouts in humans locomoting in real or virtual environments (Bohbot, Copara, et al., 2017), and there are more bouts during rapid movement (Aghajan, Schuette, et al., 2017).

Place cells have also been observed in primates (Matsumura, Nishijo, et al., 1999; Ludvig, Tang, et al., 2004), as have spatial view cells, which encode facing toward an environmental location (Rolls and O'Mara, 1995; Rolls, 1999) (Figure 11.16E). In these experiments, the animals were either freely moving in a large arena or were passively transported in a moveable chair controlled by an experimenter or the animal itself. Interestingly, in humans the majority of hippocampal cells encode the subject's location (Figure 11.16F), while the majority of "view cells" are located in the parahippocampal region (Ekstrom, Kahana, et al., 2003), whereas in monkeys there were more than two times as many view cells as place cells in the hippocampus (16% vs. 7%, respectively; Mao, Avila, et al., 2021). However, on the whole, the majority of view cells are found outside the hippocampus in the entorhinal cortex and subiculum (25% and 31%, respectively; Mao, Avila, et al., 2021). In general, place cells in primates show lower spatial specificity compared with rodents and bats. This is likely due to the fields being larger with more out-of-field background firing (Ekstrom, Kahana, et al., 2003). As in the case of rodents and bats, primate place cells are often modulated by other types of stimuli such as facing location (Ekstrom, Kahana, et al., 2003; Mao, Avila, et al., 2021), egocentric boundaries (Mao, Avila, et al., 2021), and goals (Ekstrom, Kahana, et al., 2003; Watrous, Miller, et al., 2018). It has been suggested that the dominance of view cells over place cells observed in nonhuman primates is due to their much more acute visual system than in rodents, leading them to rely more on visual landmarks to estimate their position (Ekstrom, 2015). In view of this, surprisingly, by tracking the monkey's head and eyes at the same time, it has been shown that the cells encoded a view toward which the head was pointing rather than the view of the animal's gaze (Mao, Avila, et al., 2021; but see Rolls, 1999). Also, it is not clear why there are place cells than view cells in the human hippocampal region (Ekstrom, Kahana, et al., 2003). Perhaps the recently discovered place ConSink cells in rats which have increased firing when the animal faces a place in the environment (Ormond and O'Keefe 2022, see section 11.11) will provide a resolution of these differences.

Similar to rodent place cells, which exhibit a phase precession as an animal traverses a place field (O'Keefe and Recce, 1993), and theta cells, which fire action potentials at theta (8–10 Hz) frequency (Ranck, 1973), human hippocampal cells also show phase-locking to LFP oscillations in the theta (4–8 Hz) band (Jacobs, Kahana, et al., 2007). However, the strongest phase-locking occurs in the delta (1–4 Hz) and gamma (30–90 Hz) frequency ranges (Jacobs, Kahana, et al., 2007) and firing mostly occurs at or just after the trough of the oscillation (Watrous, Miller, et al., 2018). Hippocampal neurons may exhibit different phase preferences to encode different goal locations (Watrous, Miller, et al., 2018): i.e., a neuron fires at a different phase (in delta or theta frequency range) depending on which goal location the patient is visiting. Importantly, the majority of these phase-coding cells (~80%) do not exhibit rate coding, meaning that the firing rate of the neurons does not distinguish between different goal locations while including information about their phases does. However, in some of the remaining examples both rate- and phase-coding were used to encode different goal locations. This indicates that hippocampal phase- and rate- coding present two different neural coding mechanisms similar to previously reported findings in rodents (Huxter, Burgess, and O'Keefe, 2003). Goal encoding by hippocampal neurons correlated with both the planning stage (when the subject was planning a route to the next goal location) and the goal approach stage.

Importantly, it has been shown that in humans the same place cells become activated during the recall of the event that happened in that location as well as the direct experience of the location (J Miller, Neufang, et al., 2013). Participants were asked to deliver different objects to different shops in a virtual reality town. The town had been explored beforehand, so the participants were familiar with its layout. After delivery of 12 different objects to 12 different shops, the participants were asked to recall what objects they had delivered. Strikingly, during free recall of item retrieval, the hippocampal neural activity highly correlated with locations associated with these items during the virtual navigation task, so that the closer the corresponding place cells were to the item/shop the higher the correlation observed during the free recall. The authors suggested that reinstating the spatial context provided the basis for item recall, hence reconciling the role of the hippocampal cells in episodic and spatial memory, and navigation.

Interestingly, in humans, as in rodents (see section 11.6 for details), single-unit place-like representations were also observed in other regions outside the hippocampus such as parahippocampal cortex, entorhinal cortex, amygdala, anterior medial temporal lobe, and prefrontal regions (J Miller, Neufang, et al., 2013; Ekstrom, 2015; Kornblith, Quian Quiroga, et al., 2017), with the highest percentage of such representations located in the parahippocampal cortex: 25% compared with the 17% in EC, 15% in the hippocampus, and 14% in the amygdala (Kornblith, Quian Quiroga, et al., 2017). Of course, these percentages can only be taken as rough estimates, given the inherent difficulties of placement and tracking of electrode locations in human patients. Future studies will be needed to identify the major differences and similarities between these representations. For example, it has been suggested that RSC may play a key role in visual landmark processing and representation (Wolbers and Buchel, 2005; Vann, Aggleton, and Maguire, 2009, Ekstrom, 2015) and hence may be important for generating view cells (for a more detailed discussion of extrahippocampal representations, see section 11.6).

Human hippocampal neurons also encode nonspatial abstract representations such as faces, objects, and visual scenes (Fried, MacDonald, and Wilson, 1997; Quiroga, Reddy, et al., 2005; Quian Quiroga, Kraskov, et al., 2009). In one set of experiments, patients with pharmacologically intractable epilepsy were implanted with depth electrodes to localize the focus of seizure onset. Single-unit activity was usually recorded in the hippocampus, parahippocampal region, entorhinal cortex, and amygdala while the patients were presented with a set of novel and familiar pictures of faces, objects, and/or buildings. A number of cells in these regions selectively responded only to a single or a small number of visual stimuli. For example, a hippocampal neuron became significantly more active when different pictures of Jennifer Aniston were presented but not to other images of celebrities or other individuals (Quiroga, Reddy, et al., 2005). Interestingly, in this particular example, the cell was not active when the image of Jennifer Aniston was presented together with Brad Pitt, implying that their conjunctive representation did not drive the cell firing. In general, the hippocampal responses often displayed conjunctive firing properties whereby the neurons were modulated not only by faces vs. objects but also by facial expression, gender, and other properties (Fried, MacDonald, and Wilson, 1997). Moreover, a neuron could often respond to several similar expressions such as anger and disgust, rather than unrelated or opposite ones such as joy and sadness. In general, as in the case of human place cells, the responses to nonspatial abstract stimuli showed poorer stimulus-tuning compared with rodent place cells. It is likely that similarly to rodent work, any given stimulus is represented by the population of neurons because a single cell often responded to more than one stimulus and because such specific responses were detected using just a handful of visual stimuli during the experiment (a range of stimuli: 71–114).

These hippocampal nonspatial neurons were active during the stimulus representation and often continued firing for a second or longer after removal of the stimulus, suggesting that they do not simply respond to the sensory features of the stimuli. The responses were present during the encoding phase when the stimulus was presented for the first time as well as during the recall phase when the already familiar stimulus was reintroduced. The responses to visual stimuli often significantly increased 300–600 ms after stimulus onset (Quiroga, Reddy, et al., 2005; Kornblith, Quian Quiroga, et al., 2017) and maintained sustained firing activity during the dark intertrial intervals (ITIs). In the experiments of Kornblith, Quian Quiroga, et al. (2017), the patients were briefly (200 ms) presented with eight or nine images of famous or familiar people, animals, and scenes with variable ITIs between the images (0 ms, 200 ms, 500 ms, and 800 ms). This was followed by a long delay period (~2.5 s), after which the patients were presented with two different images: a new one and a familiar image from the previous sequence. The patient had to indicate by pressing the left or right cursor which image was part of the last sequence. Increasing the ITI from 0 to 200 ms or 500 ms increased the duration of persistent firing. There was no significant difference in firing with a 500 ms vs. 800 ms ITI. A part of the firing variability in response to nonpreferred stimuli could be explained by the appearance of the preferred image in the sequence. Finally, sustained firing during the delay phase was strongest after sequences with preferred images. Importantly, the strength and duration of sustained firing activity also correlated with the behavioral performance levels. When patients were presented with a target image (e.g., a face of Bill Clinton) followed by five other images of the same person ("lure image") and a new face ("foil image") visually selective neurons had increased firing to the target image compared with a lure image and did not show increased responses to a foil image (Suthana, Parikshak, et al., 2015). The increase in response to the target image also correlated with performance. Importantly, such correlation with performance was only observed in hippocampal neurons (DG/CA3 and subiculum) and not in other regions in the medial temporal lobe such as entorhinal cortex, parahippocampal region, and amygdala (Suthana, Parikshak, et al., 2015).

Altogether, this strongly indicates that hippocampal neurons play a key role in image discrimination via increased firing to the target stimulus, which is maintained during a working memory task even in the absence of the stimulus. As with human place cells, at the moment, it is not clear how stable the stimulus response is during different re-exposures due to the difficulty of recording from the same cells over long periods of time.

Finally, in addition to responses to visual stimuli such as the face of Jennifer Aniston, nonspatial neurons could also be activated (8 out of 132 responsive units, 6.1%) when only a written or spoken name of the visual stimulus was presented (e.g., "Jennifer Aniston" but not to other names), pointing to the highly abstract conceptual nature of these neural responses (Quiroga, Reddy, et al., 2005; Quian Quiroga, Kraskov, et al., 2009). Interestingly, no example was found of cells responding to spoken names alone (Quian Quiroga, Kraskov, et al., 2009).

11.9 Place-field formation

The manner in which place fields are initially formed and subsequently maintained is still not settled. In the original experiments in which a small number of environmental cues were controlled by rotating them as a constellation from trial to trial, two types of cell were revealed by removal of some or all of these controlled cues (O'Keefe and Conway, 1978). The first class became silent when the cues were removed, while the second class increased their firing under these circumstances. When all the controlled cues were removed, these "lacuna" place units actually doubled the number of spikes on the maze, firing in previously silent areas. The place fields of this second class of place cell appeared to be the residual excitatory patches that escaped inhibitory influences presumably from neighboring active place cells. The original suggestion was that place fields could be activated directly by combinations of environmental cues or indirectly by a combination of the place fields representing the current location together with path integration based on the distance and direction of movement to the new location (O'Keefe, 1976; O'Keefe and Nadel, 1978). Mismatches between these two sources of information either by the introduction of new cues or removal of expected ones, including food, would result in exploration designed to identify the source of the mismatch. As we shall see it is still not clear how these two sources of information are integrated or compared in practice.

Around 30%–70% of CA1 place cells have at least one field in any given environment, while the remainder are silent (Thompson and Best, 1989; Wilson and McNaughton, 1993; Gothard, Skaggs, et al., 1996). Even the cells with active fields show a considerable variability in their activity; they often emerge later in the recording session, show intermittent cessation of activity, or altogether disappear. This variability has been linked to an animal's experience of the environment as novel or familiar (Hill, 1978; Frank, Stanley, and Brown, 2004), to attention and task performance (Markus, Qin, et al., 1995; Zinyuk, Kubik, et al., 2000; Kentros, Agnihotri, et al., 2004; Fenton, Lytton, et al., 2010), and to future goals and past destinations (Ferbinteanu and Shapiro, 2003; Jackson and Redish, 2007; Catanese, Viggiano, et al., 2014). The number of fields and the field properties (e.g., firing rate, size, shape, dispersion, etc.) largely depend on an animal's experience (Frank, Stanley, and Brown, 2004; Barry, Ginzberg, et al., 2012) as well as the size of the enclosure (Fenton, Kao, et al., 2008; Rich, Liaw, and Lee, 2014) and other external and internal cues (e.g., presence or absence of objects, smells, sounds, reward associated with that place) important in forming a cognitive map. Multiple studies have demonstrated that an animal's location is encoded by the coordinated activity of an ensemble of cells rather than through the activity of a single cell (Wilson and McNaughton, 1993). These cell ensembles may be constructed for each environment or they might be selected from prefigured ensembles. It has been suggested that these preconfigured ensembles may be based on "path-integration reference frames" potentially implemented via distinct connectivity patterns imposed during development (McNaughton, Barnes, et al., 1996). The idea is that these distinct preconfigured ensembles of place cells will become active during exploration of novel environments and the surrounding external stimuli and other types of information relevant to an animal's behavior in these environments will become uniquely associated with these "reference frames" (Figure 11.17A). Some evidence in support of the existence of preconfigured place-cell ensembles come from both neurodevelopmental and neurophysiological studies. Deguchi and colleagues (Deguchi, Donato, et al., 2011) described the existence of preferentially interconnected microcircuits of principal CA1, CA3, and DG neurons where their selective connectivity is likely achieved via partially overlapping developmental time

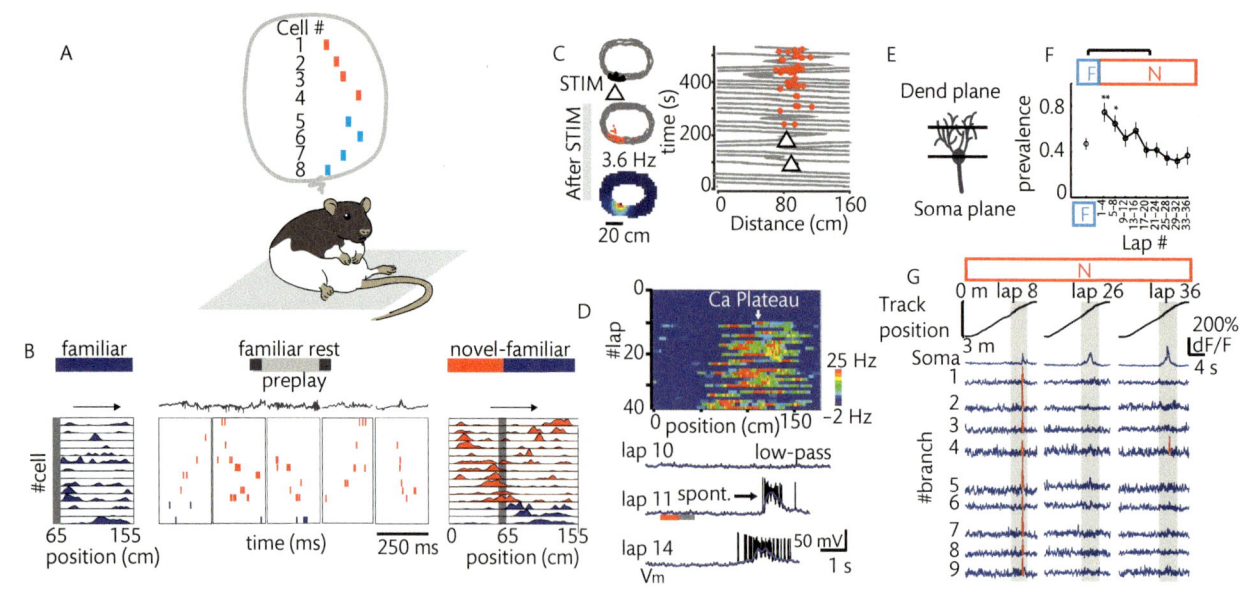

Figure 11.17 Place-cell formation. (A) Schema of prearranged place-cell sequences recorded in CA1 before a rat experiences a novel enclosure. As the animal rests between runs on the linear track, during SWRs, cells 1–4 predict the sequence which the animal will experience on the novel track, while cells 5 –8 replay the sequence previously experienced on the familiar track. (B) The preplay sequences were uncorrelated with the replay sequences of a recently visited familiar enclosure. First, the rat ran on a familiar linear track (65–155 cm, left) before experiencing a novel segment on the same track (0–65 cm, right). During the resting period prior to exposure to the novel segment of the track (central panel), some place cells (red) fired in the order subsequently observed on the novel track, in a phenomenon called preplay, while the activity of other place cells (blue) was arranged in the order observed on the familiar track (the phenomenon called replay). (Adapted from Dragoi and Tonegawa, 2011, with permission.) (C) Place-cell formation by current injection in a freely moving mouse. Juxtacellular electrical stimulation was applied to normally silent pyramidal cells at a specific point on a circular track. Upper left, point of stimulation, lower left, place fields created and maintained after stimulation. Right sequence of runs starting at bottom showing no firing prior to stimulation (triangles) and firing in the same location and subsequently. (Adapted from Diamantaki et al., 2018.) (D) Plateau potentials create place fields in silent cells. Intracellularly recorded CA1 place-cell responses in a head-fixed mouse running on a virtual linear track across 40 laps. Naturally occurring plateau potential on lap 11 produced a ramp-like depolarization of membrane potential (Vm) that drove place-field firing on subsequent trials, 12 onward (top). The induced Vm ramps extend back in time (bottom). Vm (black) and low-pass filtered Vm (blue) for laps preceding (lap 10), during (lap 11), and after plateau (lap 14). (Adapted from Bittner et al., 2017, with permission.) (E) Schema showing simultaneous two-photon imaging planes of a CA1 place-cell soma and basal dendrites. (F, G) Branch spikes are more prevalent during novel exposures to the place field then subsequently. (G) Simultaneous imaging of soma and nine dendritic branches during multiple laps. During the first 8 laps basal dendrites tended to show significant Ca2+ transients coinciding with somatic activity Ca2+ traces (top) from the soma and 9 dendritic branches during three place-field traversals (gray columns, mean place field over session). Red traces indicate significant Ca2+ transients, which are prevalent on all branches on the first run but reduced to branch 4 by the 3rd run. (F) On average the majority of dendritic branches are active during the eight initial traversal of a virtual linear track, after which their proportion gradually decreases to baseline levels measured on the familiar linear track. (Adapted from Sheffield et al., 2017, with permission.)

windows. They used two sparse Thy1 reporter lines (Lsi1 and Lsi2) to show that Lsi1 (Lsi2) neurons are more likely to be connected with other Lsi1 (Lsi2) neurons and that they matured and established synapses at different times from each other and from other principal neurons. However, one has to be careful in attributing any functional significance to such observed preferential connectivity. Some evidence in favor of hippocampal cell assemblies also comes from experiments on preplay. They show that connectivity between cells exists before an animal encounters an environment (McNaughton, Barnes, et al., 1996; Deguchi, Donato, et al., 2011; Dragoi and Tonegawa, 2011; D Lee, Lin, and Lee, 2012; Dragoi and Tonegawa, 2013). Such organization of future hippocampal cell assemblies is revealed via the coordinated activation of place cells while the animal is in a quiescent state or asleep *prior* to entering a novel environment (Dragoi and Tonegawa, 2011) (Figure 11.17B). It has been suggested that preplay may serve to depolarize the relevant cells bringing them closer to firing threshold. However, there is some skepticism about the existence of such predetermined states (see Bendor and Spiers, 2016, who point out that their number is close to not being statistically significant). It is still unclear how

these preexisting cell assemblies would be selected for any given environment. An experiment in which the cell assemblies originally activated in a novel environment were prevented from consolidation by the subsequent use of an NMDA blocker, found that re-exposure to the same environment resulted in a new set of place fields, raising problems for the idea of preexisting cell assemblies for any particular environment (Kentros, Hargreaves, et al., 1998). This supports the possibility is that the cell assembly is originally chosen at random and its association to that environment learned and consolidated by an NMDA-dependent process.

Hill (1978) was the first to address the question of whether experience was necessary for place-cell firing. He concluded that little, if any, experience was required. Ten of 12 cells studied showed firing as robust on the first visit to their place fields as on subsequent visits. The other two cases seemed to develop fields over the first 10 min. Wilson and McNaughton (1993), using parallel recording methods that enabled simultaneous study of more than 100 cells, provided evidence that place fields are less robust during the first 10 min of exploration of a novel 60 cm² arena than following this initial period of exploration. They suggested that place fields might develop, at least partially, as a result of rapid learning. A slightly different interpretation of these data, however, is that the fundamental, idiothetic relationships among the place fields were preconfigured. Under this interpretation, the initially lower precision of the place fields in the novel arena was due to the fact that they were initially driven entirely by path-integration mechanisms and hence subject to greater drift error. Over about 10 min, however, there would have been gradual associative binding of local-view information to place cells, which would have enabled a more-or-less continual correction for the cumulative error that is an unavoidable component in all path-integration systems. Hill's experiments were performed in a more geometrically restricted apparatus, where such cumulative error might have been attenuated because of the limitation of possible trajectories. Moreover, the position-tracking method available to Hill was not very precise, and it is likely that such subtle effects would have been missed. In the Wilson and McNaughton (1993) study, the apparatus consisted of two square arenas separated by a partition into familiar and novel halves. In a followup to this experiment, we repeated the partition removal procedure over several days until the rat was well familiarized with both halves of the apparatus. We then conducted a trial in which the second box, together with its associated visual cues, was removed altogether. When the partition was removed, the rat was free to explore an open tabletop in the region where the second box had stood. Consistent with the cue-removal experiments of O'Keefe and Speakman (1987), there were no pronounced changes in the distribution of place fields, even though, in this case, there was a rich array of distal cues. One interpretation of this observation is that the animal's idiothetically based sense of location relative to the stable, familiar arena exerted a more powerful control over the place fields than the proximal visual stimuli. An alternative possibility is that the fields were maintained by the remaining distal cues. Evidence that place cells are influenced by both proximal cues inside the testing box or environment and the distal room cues comes from many studies (O'Keefe and Speakman, 1987; O'Keefe and Burgess, 1996).

Strong support for the idiothetic basis of place-specific firing comes from a study by Quirk and colleagues (Quirk, Muller, and Kubie, 1990) in which rats were introduced into a cylindrical environment in total darkness. Although the animals had experienced the same environment previously under illumination, the condition of darkness resulted, in many cases, in the establishment of new place fields that persisted in subsequent light. These new fields ultimately came under the control of visual input in that they rotated when the single polarizing stimulus (a white cue card) was rotated. Thus, place fields can arise independently of the visual landmarks that eventually develop control over their expression. We cannot of course rule out the possibility that these dark fields were originally established on the basis of nonvisual cues, which then transferred control to the visual cues when they appeared.

Indirect support for a preconfiguration of place fields can also be derived from observations of the statistical interactions among populations of simultaneously recorded place cells while the animal is either asleep or in quiet wakefulness prior to exposure to a novel spatial situation. Contrary to an initial report based on a small number of experiments (Wilson and McNaughton, 1994), the extent to which two cells will have overlapping place fields in a novel environment can be predicted, to a small degree at least, by the strength of their activity correlation (i.e., the correlation of their firing rates over sequential 100 ms epochs) during sleep prior to the

experience (Kudrimoti, Barnes, and McNaughton, 1999). In agreement with the initial report, however, only those cells that actually end up having overlapping fields in a given environment exhibit enhanced correlations in subsequent sleep. It seems that the activation of specific groups of cells in a given environment results in some priming effect on these cells, possibly, but not necessarily, as a result of synaptic modification during exploration. This priming results in their increased likelihood of co-activation for periods of 30–60 min after the experience.

In recent experiments in our laboratory, we observed an even more dramatic metastable effect. The purpose of this experiment was to observe the effects of an extensive episode of exploration of novel spaces on the distribution of place fields in the familiar environment. The procedure involved an initial recording session in the familiar environment, followed by a 1 h period in which the rats were permitted 10 min of exploration, each in a different room in the laboratory facility. The animals were then returned to the familiar environment for further recording. The animals repeatedly ran around an elevated track (either triangular or rectangular) for food reinforcement. The animals were adapted to the particular task and environment for more than a week prior to the recording sessions. In many cases, the distribution of place fields (up to 80 simultaneously recorded) was completely rearranged following the intervening period of exploration. This effect was not a result of recording instability.

The stable states could be determined by patterns of connection strengths established through some developmental process. The usual conclusion is that the number of unique stable states is vast if each state involves activity of only a small fraction (about 0.01) of the total population of cells and each cell is involved in many different states. This is known as sparse, distributed coding. Suppose that, rather than forming through the storage of arbitrary events, the synaptic weight matrix was preconfigured in a manner that implicitly defined a large set of two-dimensional surfaces. These surfaces can be considered as "path-integration reference frames," and they can be envisioned as consisting of a random subset of the total population of place cells in CA3 in which the synaptic connections define metrical, two-dimensional neighborhood relationships. It has been shown (Shen and McNaughton, 1996), for example, that such a preconfigured system of spatial reference frames will spontaneously reactivate representations of locations within a given frame in the presence of random noise input. Moreover, representations associated with recently experienced locations can be preferentially reactivated either by increasing the excitability of recently active neurons or by superimposing a transient increase in the connection weight among coactive neurons with overlapping place fields. Such a model proposes that landmark and event information becomes secondarily bound to these preconfigured representations by Hebbian learning.

Place cells can be formed even in the complete absence of inputs from the medial entorhinal cortex (Hales, Schlesiger, et al., 2014). They are less abundant and less stable, and display inferior spatial tuning. Interestingly, further studies indicated that partial optogenetic inactivation of mEC did not affect the number of active place cells or their spatial tuning, but rather induced a global remapping with newly formed representations remaining stable even after mEC activity was reinstated (Rueckemann, DiMauro, et al., 2016; N Robinson, Priestley, et al., 2017). This type of manipulation mostly affected place-cell firing sequences.

In addition to neural network mechanisms, it has been shown that place cells themselves may play an active role in place-field formation through regenerative dendritic events, which are thought to be essential for inducing synaptic plasticity when paired with presynaptic input (Magee and Johnston, 1997; Schiller, Schiller, and Clapham, 1998; Golding, Staff, and Spruston, 2002). CA1 dendrites are able to generate and maintain nonlinear dendritic spike activity via voltage-gated Ca^{2+}-permeable NMDA receptors and/or backpropagating action potentials. Sheffield and colleagues (Sheffield and Dombeck, 2015; Sheffield, Adoff, and Dombeck, 2017) used two-photon imaging to record simultaneous activity in CA1 pyramidal cell soma and in basal and apical dendrites while a head-restrained mouse was navigating in novel and familiar enclosures. They showed that the emergence of a place field was strongly coupled to coordinated dendritic spiking detected across multiple dendritic branches. In some cases where the place field only appeared after an animal ran a few laps on a linear virtual track, the dendritic branch spikes preceded the somatic spikes and were more clustered around the future somatic place field. Interestingly, these preceding excitatory postsynaptic calcium transients were highly restricted to a single branch and only rarely were widely spread across the majority of branches.

These transients were considered nonregenerative depolarizations, generated by the excitatory inputs to a single spine, or regenerative ones (called "branch spikes") caused by backpropagating action potentials and/or dendritically generated spikes such as Na^+ and calcium spikes. It has been observed that the location where dendritic spikes occurred closely coincided with the respective somatic place fields. In extremely rare cases dendritic branch spiking was observed in the absence of somatic spiking (6 spikes in total inside or near the somatic place field and 2 outside the place field or in nonplace cells out of more than a thousand observed transients). In general, spatial heterogeneity of branch dendritic spikes was accompanied by temporal variability: i.e., different subsets of dendritic branches could become active on different place-field traversals. It has been shown that long-term stability and spatial tuning of a place cell significantly correlated with the dendritic branch-spike prevalence (BSP), a measure showing the percentage of branches with detectable branch spikes during each place-field traversal. Interestingly, place cells with multiple fields showed different BSP values for different fields, suggesting that the field properties are not solely determined by global cell properties such as cell excitability but also may be synaptic-input specific.

Place-field formation has been linked to the appearance/generation of somatically recorded plateau potentials, called dendritic plateau potentials (e.g., Takahashi and Magee, 2009; Bittner, Grienberger, et al., 2015) mediated by dendritic branch spiking events. It is possible to artificially induce a field by manipulating the excitability and/or activity of both silent CA1 neurons and active CA1 place cells. Such field induction can be achieved via direct manipulation of a neuron (Bittner, Grienberger, et al., 2015; Diamantaki, Frey, et al., 2016; Rueckemann, DiMauro, et al., 2016; Bittner, Milstein, et al., 2017; Kanter, Lykken, et al., 2017) and local place-cell activity (Schoenenberger, 2016, Diamantaki, Coletta, et al., 2018) or through bulk manipulation of its upstream entorhinal inputs (Miao et al., 2015) (Figure 11.17C). However the success rate of field induction by extracellular stimulation is relatively low (32%). The fields emerge after induction with an average latency of 55.6 ± 53 s. This procedure is effective for both silent cells and place cells.

Importantly, an artificially induced new field significantly weakens the firing properties of the old fields (Diamantaki, Coletta, et al., 2018). Surprisingly, extracellular optogenetic activation of about 10–50 pyramidal cells affects not only cells directly stimulated by the light but also more distant cells (McKenzie, Huszar, et al., 2021). Novel place fields emerged and existing fields disappeared both within and outside the stimulation zone. Furthermore, for CA1 neurons that remapped, the locations of the new place fields were not clustered around the stimulation zone. The 12% of directly stimulated cells in the stimulation zone that remapped did so immediately, while the roughly comparable number (10%) outside the stimulation zone that remapped took longer to do so, suggesting a second-order reorganization effect. Interneurons were synaptically driven by the stimulation and were probably responsible for this reorganization. Cells that developed place fields appeared to be the ones that were weakly active prior to the stimulation. The authors interpret the results as further evidence for preconfigured cell assemblies.

Surprisingly, neither the entorhinal nor septal inputs are necessary for the maintenance of hippocampal place cells. In an early work, V. Miller and Best (1980) showed that even with bilateral EC lesions, place cells were still present in hippocampus but the fields were more tuned to intramaze than extramaze cues. Thus, place cells may be formed in the absence of inputs from mEC. Furthermore, population coding of position is comparable between place cells with or without mEC inputs (Rueckemann, DiMauro, et al., 2016). As we saw in the section on theta, place cells can also be maintained and indeed established following medial septal lesions (e.g., Brandon, Koenig, et al., 2014).

11.10 Predictive coding in the hippocampal formation

During behavioral trajectories, spatial coding in the hippocampus often better reflects the future or past positions of an animal than it does the present ones. This phenomenon of coding for locations other than the current one can broadly be divided into two categories. The first is associated with very short (50–200 ms) time intervals, whereas the second operates at much longer timescales and is linked to trajectories the animal is going to take in the future. How these two types of nonpresent positional encodings are related is not clear.

Let us start with short-range coding. It was first described by R. Muller and Kubie (1989), who noticed that shifting spikes forward by ~120 ms along a rat's path of movement significantly improved the spatial tuning properties of hippocampal CA1 and CA3 place cells. The positive shifts resulted in smaller place fields and decreased patchiness (i.e., "tighter" and "cleaner" fields) as well as higher place-field coherence (Figure 11.18A). Subsequently, future (prospective) coding was found in both the subiculum (Sharp, 1999), the brain region that receives strong projections from CA1 region, and in the medial entorhinal cortex (De Almeida, Idiart, et al., 2012; Kropff, Carmichael, et al., 2015; Chaudhuri, Rule, et al. 2023)), which has bidirectional projections with CA1. Predictive coding was also reported in mammillary bodies (Cho and Sharp, 2001), anterior dorsal thalamic nucleus (Blair and Sharp, 1995; Blair, Lipscomb, and Sharp, 1997), and RSC (Cho and Sharp, 2001). While cells exhibiting future coding in the hippocampus (CA1/CA3 and subiculum) and

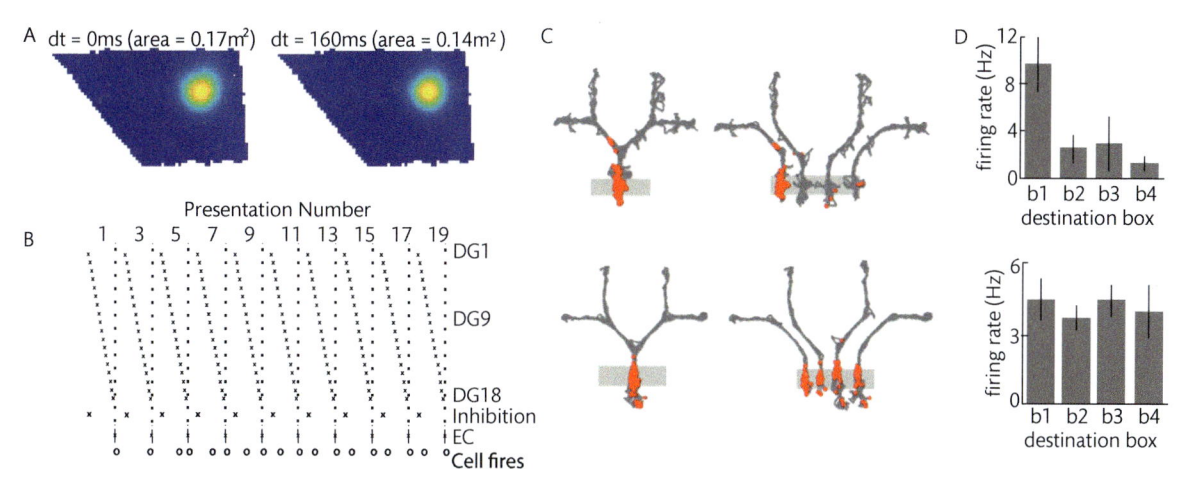

Figure 11.18 Predictive coding in place cells (A) An example of a place cell that better reflects an animal's location 160 ms ahead of the animal. Note the smaller area of the place field following timeshifting of the firing pattern relative to the animal's location. (Courtesy of Krupic lab.) (B) Potential mechanism for predictive learning in the hippocampus. (Adapted from Denham and McCabe, 1998, with permission.) (C) An example of splitter cell (top) and place cell (bottom). The firing of the splitter cell depends on the animal's future choice only active before left turns, whereas that of the place cell does not, always firing on every trial regardless of subsequent choice. (Adapted from Ainge et al., 2007, with permission.) (D) Firing rate of the cells shown in C in the start arm as a function of destination. (Adapted from Ainge et al., 2007, with permission.)

the medial entorhinal cortex can be identified as location-encoding cells such as place cells and grid cells, respectively, cells with predictive coding in the mammillary bodies, anterior dorsal thalamic nucleus, and RSC correspond to head-direction cells. Interestingly, head-direction cells in the postsubiculum (dorsal presubiculum), which is located at the top node of the classic head-direction cell hierarchy (Taube, 2007), do not show anticipatory coding and best encode an animal's current head direction (Blair and Sharp, 1995). In addition to prospective coding in spatial cells, speed cells in the medial entorhinal cortex also exhibit prospective coding, with time shifts equal to the ones observed in the corecorded grid cells (Kropff, Carmichael, et al., 2015), suggesting that they may be directly causing the temporal biases observed in the latter.

In general, within each anatomical region, time shifts showed broad distributions spanning tens of milliseconds. Different regions tended to exhibit different average time shifts even when recorded simultaneously (Sharp, 1999a; Kropff, Carmichael, et al., 2015; Chaudhuri, Rule, et al. 2023). Place cells tended to show the largest forward time shifts of around ~120ms (R Muller and Kubie, 1989; Battaglia, Sutherland, and McNaughton, 2004; Chaudhuri, Rule, et al. 2023) compared with other regions (but see Sharp, 1999a, Kropff, Carmichael, et al., 2015). Medial entorhinal grid cells and speed cells displayed ~50–80 ms forward shifts (Kropff, Carmichael, et al., 2015; Chaudhuri, Rule, et al. 2023) similar to what was reported in the subiculum (50–70 ms; Sharp 1999a). Head-directional cells had generally lower forward time shifts: ~25 ms in RSC (Cho and Sharp, 2001), ~23 ms in the anterior dorsal thalamus (ADT) (Blair and Sharp, 1995; Taube and Muller, 1998), ~67 ms in mammillary bodies (Blair, Cho, and Sharp, 1998; Stackman and Taube, 1998) and -6 ms (Taube and Muller, 1998) or 2 ms (Blair and Sharp, 1995) in the dorsal presubiculum, also known as the postsubiculum. However, it must be noted that in CA1 and CA3 regions others also reported much smaller 40 ms forward shifts (Sharp, 1999) or even no temporal shifts at all (Kropff, Carmichael, et al., 2015).

One of the possible explanations for such time shifts assumes that the "ego" or "self" of the animal is shifted slightly ~5 cm ahead of the animal. Alternatively, they may be of a purely methodological

nature, e.g., artifacts resulting from LEDs being slightly misplaced relative to the center of an animal's head (Huxter, Senior, 2008). The strongest argument against these simple explanations is that in some experiments different cell types were corecorded (Sharp, 1999a; Kropff, Carmichael, et al., 2015), in which case it is reasonable to expect that the time shifts should be similar in these cells, but they were not.

An alternative hypothesis assumes that inputs related to the animal's movement may be responsible for creating the time shifts (McNaughton, Chen, and Markus, 1991; Blair, Lipscomb, and Sharp, 1997; Taube and Muller, 1998; Kropff, Carmichael, et al., 2015). Currently, the source of these anticipatory motor commands is unclear, but it has been suggested that they may represent a motor efference copy (e.g., an angular head velocity in case of head-direction cells). For example, it has been demonstrated that motor cortical cells discharge about 100–120 ms prior to an animal's movement (Thach, 1978). Indeed, the possibility of active movement is important for place cells (Foster, Castro, and McNaughton, 1989) and ADT head-direction cells (Knierim, Kudrimoti, and McNaughton, 1995; Taube, 1995a), as they significantly reduce their firing rates or cease activity altogether if the animal is restrained. Notably, such effect of restraint was not observed in presubicular head-direction cells (Taube, Muller, and Ranck, 1990). Moreover, head-direction cells modulated by the animal's turns were reported in the presubiculum and the lateral mammillary nucleus, which provide the direct input to ADT cells (Blair, Lipscomb, and Sharp, 1997), while cells modulated by the animal's speed were reported in the medial entorhinal cortex (Kropff, Carmichael, et al., 2015). Both of these cell types also exhibit time biases possibly driven by the motor efference copy, as previously discussed.

This alternative hypothesis further suggests that anticipatory signals may combine sensory input from the recent past with motor information to predict future sensory input, thereby updating the spatial representation (McNaughton, Chen, and Markus, 1991; Taube and Muller, 1998). Interestingly, lesion of the dorsal presubiculum, which has been reported to contain head-direction cells with zero or small negative lag, does significantly increase anticipatory timing in the ADT cells (Goodridge and Taube, 1997). One strong prediction of this hypothesis is that in case of passive movements the anticipatory bias should be attenuated or abolished. In one experiment, ADT or presubicular head-direction neurons were recorded while the animal's ability to control its directional headings via its own movement was manipulated by either placing it in a cart moved by the experimenter or gently restraining its head and body and orienting it back and forward by 180 degrees (Bassett, Zugaro, et al., 2005). In both cases the animal could move its head, but the movement resulted in a different orientation than without interference, limiting the animal's predictive powers about its own movements. In this case, the authors showed that instead of reducing the anticipatory time shifts in ADT cells, the time shifts were actually increased (Bassett, Zugaro, et al., 2005). The anticipatory shifts were near zero under both experimental conditions in PreS cells, suggesting that they may be generated independently. Although this manipulation provides some evidence that observed time bias in ADT head-direction cells cannot be accounted for solely by a motor corollary discharge, the experiment does not completely rule out such a possibility, as the animal was actively moving.

The third proposed hypothesis relates to the underlying mechanism of how information may be stored and retrieved. Namely, the observed differences in optimal time shifts may be a necessary consequence of "separating" the signal into several parts encoding different communication modes, one of which corresponds to encoding the current and anticipatory information while the other corresponds to comparing the current and past information for novelty detection. The timing of these modes may be controlled by the inhibitory neural network, which on the population level is defined/described by the LFP oscillations (Hasselmo, Bodelon, and Wyble, 2002). The 100 ms ranges may simply reflect this division. Mechanistically it may be implemented through LTP facilitation mechanisms, which preferentially strengthens the connections between the pre- and postsynaptic cell if the latter fires 10–100 ms ahead of the former (Denham 1998) (Figure 11.18B). The suggestion is that it may be implemented through LTP facilitation mechanisms that preferentially strengthen the connections between the pre- and postsynaptic cell if the former fires 10–100 ms ahead of the latter (Markram et al., 1997). The synapses between cells with the reversed firing order (i.e., where a postsynaptic cell fires before a presynaptic cell) or simultaneously firing cells become weakened (Markram et al., 1997).

In principle, the second and the third hypotheses are not mutually exclusive, and indeed there is good evidence that temporal biases observed in different regions seem to be independent (Goodridge and Taube, 1997; Kropff, Carmichael, et al., 2015; Chaudhuri, Rule, et al. 2023). Indeed, it may be that in some regions (e.g., mEC and ADT) the anticipatory signal arises from motor command-related inputs, while in other regions (e.g., hippocampus and presubiculum) they may result as a consequence of splitting the signal processing into two different stages separated in time within individual theta cycles. Different time shifts in both the hippocampus and mEC tend to occur at different hippocampal theta phases. (Chaudhuri, Rule, et al. 2023).

Another type of future (or past) encoding encompasses significantly larger time shifts and is related to trajectories animals have taken or are going to take after decision points in goal-directed tasks. These types of activity have been studied on "search tree" mazes, where the animal has to make one or more turns to reach the "goal"

location. On such tasks the hippocampal place cells often show different firing properties depending on which turn the animal has taken or is going to take (Dudchenko and Wood, 2014). Place cells showing trajectory-dependent differential activity are also known as "splitter cells" (Dudchenko and Wood, 2014). Early evidence for this type of longer-range trajectory-dependent coding was reported by E. Wood and colleagues, who studied CA1 place-cell responses as rats were engaged in a continuous spatial-alternation task on a modified T-maze with return arms from the goals back to the start of the maze (E Wood, Dudchenko, et al., 2000). The authors showed that the firing rates of the majority of place cells (71%, 22/31 cells) were significantly modulated by the type of trajectory (left or right turn at the choice point) the animal was going to take even after any differences in other behavioral variables (e.g., speed and head direction) were taken into account. The differences in firing rates were often higher than 10-fold. The design of the study did not permit disambiguation between the influence of future or past trajectories, since, on successful trials, a future left turn was always preceded by a past right turn and vice versa. Using another modified continuous-alternation task on a W-shaped track where the animal ran continuously from a stem arm to the left, back to the stem arm, and to the right, and so on (Frank, Brown, and Wilson, 2000), it was shown that the majority of cell firing represented retrospective coding, i.e., where the animal had just come from (81%, 13/16 cells). Interestingly, in this study, in addition to CA1 place-cell recordings, the authors also recorded from the superficial and deep layers of the medial entorhinal cortex (mEC). The result suggested that, similar to CA1 place cells, spatial cells in the superficial layers of mEC also displayed retrospective coding (71%, 5/7 cells), whereas those in deep layers seemed to contain more cells displaying prospective coding (40%, 12/30 cells). However, it should be noted that the number of recorded cells was generally quite small, making it difficult to arrive at a strong conclusion.

While the first studies on splitter cells generally agree with each other (Frank, Brown, and Wilson, 2000; E Wood, Dudchenko, et al., 2000; Ferbinteanu and Shapiro, 2003), subsequent work called into question the significance and interpretation of the general phenomenon. First, a follow-up study in the lab that made the original discovery showed that the continuous-alternation task described by E. Wood and colleagues was not hippocampal-dependent (Ainge, van der Meer, et al., 2007). In this experiment, the authors slightly modified the T-maze to add a small waiting area in the beginning of the stem corridor in order to introduce a short 2 s or 10 s delay between the choices in addition to the uninterrupted continuous-alternation task previously used by E. Wood and colleagues (E Wood, Dudchenko, et al., 2000). This study showed that the continuous task is not hippocampal-dependent. However, introduction of even short delays significantly impaired the performance in the hippocampal-lesioned animals. Importantly, in the alternation tasks with delays, hardly any splitter cells were observed in the stem corridor (1/27). Instead, the trajectory-dependent activity was only present in the waiting area (7/22), and was exclusively of anticipatory nature. Moreover, two earlier studies that used other versions of T-maze like tasks could not find any significant modulation by the animal's future or past trajectories in CA1 place-cell firing: none was reported by Lenck-Santini and colleagues (Lenck-Santini, Save, and Poucet, 2001), and only 4/45 cells were reported by Hölscher and colleagues (Holscher, Jacob, and Mallot, 2004). Lenck-Santini and colleagues concluded that the differences in exact animal trajectories may have fully accounted for any observed trajectory-dependent differences in CA1 place-cell firing; Hölscher and colleagues proposed that the animals may have used a different strategy to solve superficially similar tasks depending on the differences in animal training, the exact details of the experimental setup, etc. For example, in the initial E. Wood et al. study (E Wood, Dudchenko, et al., 2000) the animals were trained by blocking the incorrect arm choice during the training stage, while Hölscher and colleagues allowed the animals to make incorrect choices at the training stage and discouraged the wrong choices by gently pushing the animals from the incorrectly chosen arm rather than blocking it altogether. The authors suggested that if no choice is given, animals might be encouraged to learn a routine motor program and "splitter cells" (called "turn cells" by the authors) emerge. However, by giving an animal a choice, the acquisition of a stereotypic motor program may have been prevented.

Another version of delayed-alternation task conducted by Pastalkova and colleagues (Pastalkova, Itskov, et al., 2008) showed qualitatively similar results during the waiting phase. In this version of the task, the delay period was introduced at the turning point into the stem. Instead of a small waiting compartment, the animal was confined to a stationary running wheel. The authors reported that CA1 place-cell activity was modulated by time lapsed on the running wheel (time cells encoding 0–20 s time intervals, see section on hippocampal cells and time, 11.5, for fuller description) and, in some cases, the activity of these cells could reliably predict the future trajectory of the animal. Because running on the stationary wheel appeared to be highly stereotypical and did not obviously differ between an animal's future trajectories, the authors argued that the differences observed in cell firing related to the animal's future choices could not be simply explained by the differences in motor activity. On the contrary, the behavioral activity in the standard waiting compartment may have exhibited substantial differences and hence would not be able to conclusively rule out this possibility (Ainge, van der Meer, et al., 2007). It must be noted however, that no detailed analysis of an animal's behavior on the wheel was reported by Pastalkova and colleagues.

Multiple studies also showed that journeys (defined as going between a specific start and goal location independent of the exact trajectory taken) influenced place fields more than either spatial trajectory, a combination of views and body turns, on the one hand, or the correctness of the choice, on the other (Ferbinteanu and Shapiro, 2003; Griffin, Eichenbaum, and Hasselmo, 2007; Pastalkova, Itskov, et al., 2008). For example, on a modified T-maze task implemented on the plus maze, the activity of 49% (27/55) of place fields were consistent with the origin of the journey despite varied detours and trajectories. These fields were dependent on the starting location even in the presence of the same goal. However, the exact trajectory of the animal, or whether it was correct or not, was not important. Notably, the activity is tied to the trajectory the animal takes rather than to the goal it is heading to (Grieves, Wood, and Dudchenko, 2016). In this experiment, the animals ran on a multiple-arm maze where the overlapping combination of the maze arms led to different goals; or conversely, the same goal could be reached by multiple different routes with some nonoverlapping parts. The place-cell activity only depended on what trajectory the animal took rather than the goal it was trying to reach.

The importance of the exact route taken was emphasized by another experiment, showing that when the same stem corridor leads to four different choices, the cell activity differentiates between the routes to all four different choices rather than two most proximal ones (Ainge, Tamosiunaite, et al., 2007) (Figure 11.18C,D). The difference in activity could be observed already at the beginning of the first stem corridor, which was multiple "turns and segments" away from the goal locations, demonstrating a possible long-range (in time and/or space) anticipatory encoding in splitter cells.

Several studies also investigated how quickly the splitter cells develop, reasoning that this may provide important clues on their potential functional role. In the study by I. Lee and colleagues (I Lee, Griffin, et al., 2006) it was reported that the differential place-cell activity was formed instantaneously on the first exposure to the continuous-alternation T-maze task, thus questioning the "motor-strategy hypothesis," as it has been previously shown that motor learning takes place over many trials (Packard and Knowlton, 2002). However, in this study the animals were pretrained to run unidirectional laps on one side of the T-maze by blocking the opposite arm; and on the first day of the alternation task they ran two blocks of unidirectional laps. Hence, it is possible that the conjunctive place-motor representations developed prior to the spatial-alternation task. Some evidence in support of this argument comes from Dudchenko and Wood (2014), who showed that when no prior exposure to the T-maze alternation task occurred prior to recordings only 10% of cells showed differential modulation by the animal's trajectory. The percentage of cells increased to 45% over the several days of training (reaching 50% peak after 3 days), which positively correlated with the animal's performance on the task (the performance increased from chance levels to 80% over 2 days of training). Curiously, similar increase in the proportion of odor-in-place cells with learning the spatial-odor-discrimination task was reported by Komorowski and colleagues (Komorowski et al., 2009; see section 11.5 for details), further suggesting that there may be communalities between the two, i.e., that both represent distinct types of feature-in-place cells.

In addition to encoding differential activity that depended on the animal's trajectories, Griffin and colleagues (Griffin, Eichenbaum, and Hasselmo, 2007) reported that CA1 place cells showed differential activity that depended on the phase of the trial, i.e., whether it represented a sample vs. a probe trial. In this experiment, the authors used a discrete-trial delayed-nonmatch-to-place (DNMP) paradigm, which required continuous switching between cue-based encoding and memory-dependent retrieval phases of each trial. Previously it has been shown that this task is hippocampal-dependent (Dudchenko, Wood, and Eichenbaum, 2000). They reported that the majority of place cells were sensitive to the phase of the task (45.5%) and only a minority displayed strong modulation by the animal's future trajectory (3.9%; 0% in the stem of the maze). The authors concluded that the former may be sensitive to the memory demands of the task, with some neurons participating in encoding on the sample phase and some neurons participating in retrieval on the choice phase.

In summary, hippocampal place cells and mEC spatial cells can represent both short-range (20–500 ms) as well as longer-range (seconds or more) prospective and retrospective coding, whereby a cell more precisely represents future or past location of an animal than its current location. How these different types of representations of the future or the past are related is currently unknown. The functional significance of these phenomena also remains to be established, with some theories arguing that such representations are used to predict and possibly plan future "states" of the animal (Stachenfeld, Botvinick, and Gershman, 2017) and update the information about the past. The demonstration that CA1 pyramidal cell firing is not homogeneous in goal-directed behavior but instead generates vector fields oriented toward the goal from any location in the environment may explain some of this splitter phenomena (Ormond and O'Keefe, 2022). We will describe these results in greater detail in section 11.11.

Other theories offer more mechanistic explanations, suggesting that it may result as a necessary outcome of LTP implementation and its relation to LFP theta activity and may provide a way to separate the information flow between different parts within the hippocampus proper and the medial entorhinal cortex into different processing stages such as memory retrieval, encoding of the present, and comparisons between past and present for the novelty detection (Hasselmo, Bodelon, and Wyble, 2002). The latter more mechanistic hypothesis primarily relates to the shorter time ranges. Yet the third possible explanation related to the longer-range representations suggests that the differences may reflect the variations related to motor or other behavioral or "context-related" activity, as different trajectories may result in substantially different motor execution, which was shown to be used by rodents to successfully solve cognitively demanding tasks (Kawai, Markman, et al., 2015). As a result of these differences, feature-in-place cells develop with learning (O'Keefe and Krupic, 2021).

11.11 Hippocampal place cells support navigation

It is widely accepted that the hippocampal formation supports flexible navigation to a goal or away from a dangerous location in a familiar environment, for example, in the Morris watermaze and Bures's place-avoidance task, respectively. How it does so is less clear, and this has been a significant deficiency in the cognitive map theory since its inception.

Put simply, what is needed for efficient flexible navigation to a goal location in two-dimensional environments is either a signal that tells the animal the direction to move at each point in the environment or a signal providing the information about the probability of getting to the goal as a function of each movement at any particular location in the environment. One clue as to how this might be accomplished in the hippocampus comes from the observation that although hippocampal place fields are nondirectional in open-field foraging tasks (R Muller, Kubie, and Ranck, 1987) they become directional once a goal (or goals) is introduced, as for example on the Olton radial arm maze (McNaughton, Barnes, and O'Keefe, 1983) or linear track (O'Keefe 1993). Could this directionality be part of the mechanism for supporting navigation to a goal?

Several experiments have shown that the fields of place cells move toward a new goal (Dupret, O'Neill, et al., 2010) (Figure 11.13A) and continue to move closer to the goal arms of a T-maze with continued training (I Lee, Griffin, et al., 2006) (Figure 11.13B). Furthermore, there are studies reporting the existence of goal-direction and distance cells, which point in the direction of the goal from various different locations, or fire as a function of distance to the goal, respectively. Evidence for CA1 nonplace goal-direction and goal-distance cells was reported in bats (Sarel, Finkelstein, et al., 2017) These cells were tuned to directions in a polar coordinate framework centered on the goal, some of which pointed to the goal,

and goal-distance cells tuned to specific distances to the goal. Work on rats found weak evidence for goal-direction cells (Aoki, Igata, et al., 2019) and stronger evidence for goal-distance cells (Spiers, Olafsdottir, and Lever, 2018). The population activity of these latter cells was directly correlated with the distance from the goal, i.e., cells fired more the farther away the animal was from the goal. Together these two cell types could provide information to create a vector to the goal, guiding the animal's behavior in that direction.

One of the technical problems with studying navigation is that once the animal has learned that there is a constant goal location in an environment, it heads toward that location when placed into the environment, so that the sampling of place cells is restricted to these paths to the goal. Changing the goal location regularly to increase the variety of paths does not solve the problem, since there is no reason to believe that cellular activity as an animal navigates to one goal is the same or similar to that toward a different goal and unless goal changes are done within a session it is hard to be sure that one is recording from the same cells across sessions or days when goals are switched between days.

Perhaps more important, the nature of the situation makes it difficult to explore the properties of place cells at points along the path. For example, although we know that the place cells become directional when there is a single or small number of goals in an environment, it is not clear what this means, since directionality in any given point on a given trajectory is undersampled. Even on a one-dimensional linear track we do not know what the cell response would be in the opposite or other directions during each trajectory.

One solution to this problem is to break the two-dimensional environment up into a large number of sections where the animal can be confined to any one section along its path to the goal. Navigation on a new maze called the "honeycomb maze" accomplishes this parcellation and makes it possible to obtain information about place-cell directional preferences at all points on the maze on all trajectories. The maze consists of a series of hexagonal platforms that can be raised or lowered independently so that the animal can be trapped on any one of them as it makes its way to the goal (R Wood, Bauza, et al., 2018) (Figure 11.19A–C). At each point along its trajectory to the goal, the animal is offered a choice of two adjacent platforms and is expected to pick the platform that has the best heading direction to the goal (Figure 11.19C,D). Because the experimenter is in control of the choices offered to the animal on different routes to the same goal, an animal can be asked to approach the goal by way of a different path on each trial, ruling out the use of simple sequential strategies. Looking at the effect of variations in the angle and distance of the choice platforms to the goal shows that several factors are important in determining response performance. Normal animals make more mistakes as the angle between the choice platforms decreases (F), the distance from the goal increases (G), and most importantly as the angle of the best choice platform with the goal direction increases (H). Hippocampal lesions impair the animal's ability to learn this task (Figure 11.19E). Importantly, this lesion selectively impairs all three aspects of normal performance, which offer an insight into how the task is solved. The results suggest that the hippocampus generates both the direct vector to the goal and some measure of deviation from this goal vector.

CA1 place-cell recordings during navigation on the honeycomb maze provide evidence as to how the hippocampus provides the information necessary to support flexible navigation (Ormond and O'Keefe, 2022). As expected, many cells have circumscribed place fields on the maze (example in Figure 11.20A). Importantly, CA1

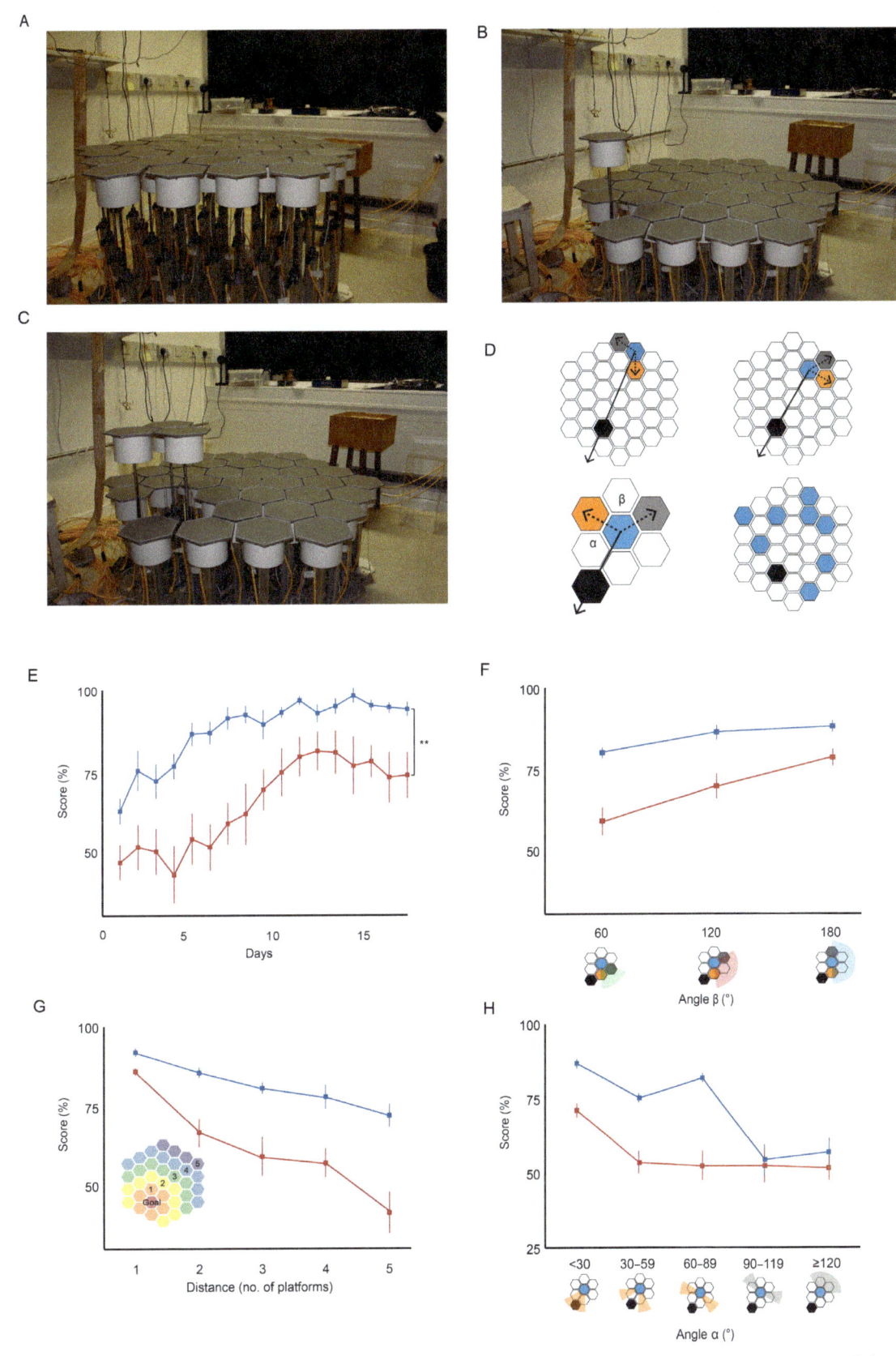

Figure 11.19 Honeycomb Maze reveals hippocampal contribution to navigation. Pictures of the maze with all platforms raised (A), one platform raised (B), and three platforms raised (C). (D) Schematic of the navigation paradigm: *Upper left*, at any given location (e.g., blue start platform) two choices are offered, correct (orange) having a smaller heading direction toward the goal (black) than the other (gray). *Upper right*, after the animal makes its choice, the platform chosen becomes the new "occupied" platform (blue), and two more choice platforms are raised. This pattern continues until the animal reaches the goal. *Lower left*, each choice is described by two angles: α between the correct choice and the goal-heading direction, and β between correct and incorrect choices. *Lower right*, eight different start platforms (blue). (E) Performance of control animals (blue) and animals with hippocampal lesions (red) in learning the maze. Six trials per day. Error bars equal SEMs. (F) Control performance increased with increasing separation of the choice platforms and the hippocampal animals were differentially affected by this measure. (G) Performance in controls decreased with the distance of the animal from the goal, and this affected the hippocampal animals to a greater extent. (H) Performance decreased as the angle of the best- choice platform with the heading direction to the maze increased, and this also affected the hippocampal animals to a greater extent.

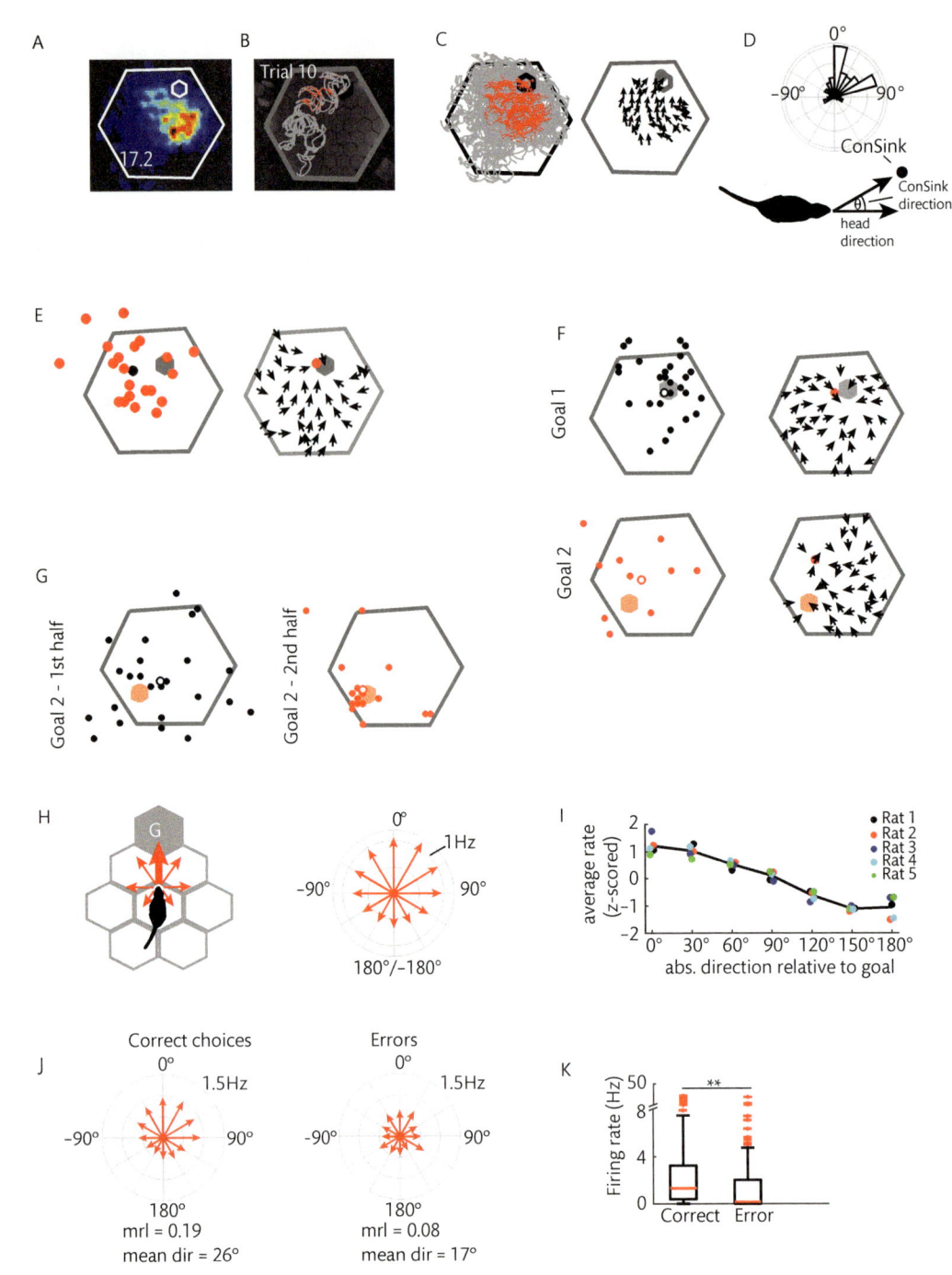

Figure 11.20. Place-cell firing during navigation on the honeycomb maze. (A) Typical place field on the honeycomb maze as the animal navigates to the goal platform (white hexagon). (B) Cell firing (red dots)is not omnidirectional but consists of arcs of spikes oriented in a particular direction. (C) Firing across a set of trials (left) can be characterized as a set of vectors on each platform oriented around a location somewhere on the maze (right). In this example this organizing location (gray spot)is close to the goal (gray hexagon). (D) Animal needs to keep this organizing location (called ConSink) at a constant angle (θ) relative to its egocentric axis. For the cell shown, that angle is between zero and 90°. (E) Example ConSinks (in red) from one rat. ConSinks for the population of cells recorded in each animal are scattered around the maze but centered on a location (black spot) close to the goal (left). The population vectors summed across all these cells point to a location (red spot) near the goal (right). (F) When the goal location is changed, the ConSinks and the vector fields reorganize toward the new goal. Goal 1 (above), original goal; goal 2 (below), new goal. (G) With experience, the ConSinks move closer to the goal location. Left side, ConSinks on the first half of trials with the new goal; right side, second half. (H) For flexible navigation, when the choice of heading directly toward the goal is not available, the brain needs to know the next best alternatives (vectors of decreasing size with angle to the goal direction) (left side). Firing pattern of the population of place cells provides this information in the form of vectors of decreasing amplitudes as a function of the angle to the goal direction (Fantail, right side). (I) Each vectorial component of the Fantail in each of 5 rats is formed by the firing rate of the place-cell population as the animal points in different directions relative to the goal direction. (J) Fantails on correct trials are better organized, with an average mean vector length (mrl) of 0.19 (left), than fantails on error trials that are less well organized and have a mean length of 0.08 (right). (K) Firing rate on correct trials is significantly higher than on error trials.

place cells that are normally nondirectional in open field environments become directional during navigation on the honeycomb maze (Figure 11.20B). This directionality of cell firing on each platform can be characterized by a vector and taken together the vector field formed across the entire place field is best organized when the animal has a specific egocentric orientation relative to a location somewhere on or occasionally off the maze (Figure 11.20C). These orientation locations or convergence sinks (ConSinks) are sometimes in front of the animal, but quite often are off to one side of the animal's heading, forming an angle as shown in Figure 11.20D.

Early in the learning of the navigation task, these convergence sinks are scattered around the environment but are clustered closer to the goal than expected by chance and have their centroid near to it (Figure 11.20E left). Importantly for the claim that these vector fields support navigation, when averaged across all of the CA1 place cells recorded from each animal, they point to a location close to the goal, providing a signal for navigation when there is an unencumbered route to the goal (Figure 11.20E right). If the vector field and ConSink organization are identifying the direction to the goal, then changing the goal location should result in a reorganization of the ConSink population around the new goal and redirection of the population vector field toward it. And this is exactly what happens (Figure 11.20F). Interestingly most of the CA1 place cells that contribute to the new ConSink/vector field representation are different from the ones involved in the original goal. The representation of the goal direction can only be seen at the cell population level. As learning progresses, many ConSinks move closer toward the goal as does their average location (Figure 11.20G).

Equally interesting, hippocampal activity also provides the information for solving indirect trajectories to the goal, the hallmark of flexible navigation. At many points along paths to a goal the choice of directly approaching the goal may not be available, but the animal is forced to choose between two non-goal-directed alternatives. A representation of the sort shown in Figure 11.20H (left) would be one way of providing information to support the choice between less-than-optimal directions. On the honeycomb maze, while the animal is confined to one of the platforms waiting for the choice platforms to be offered, it often rotates through 360°, allowing a hippocampus-dependent evaluation of the different possible directions it might be asked to choose amongst when the two platforms are raised. And this is exactly what is found in the hippocampal pyramidal cell-firing patterns (Figure 11.20H, right-hand side). The lengths of the arrows represent the rate of pyramidal cell firing as the animal points in the different directions. It is important to note that these *fantail* firing patterns provide a representation of the local environment before the animal has any idea of the choice it will be asked to make. The results show peak firing rates in the direction of the goal but then a monotonic decrease in rate with increasing angle from the goal direction (Figure 11.20I). When faced with two platforms neither of which points in the direction of the goal, the solution to the navigation problem is to choose the one in the direction of the highest firing rate. Importantly the fantails before an incorrect choice are less well organized, and do not point toward the goal direction (Figure 11.20J), and the firing rates on average are lower (Figure 11.20K).

The global population firing patterns of CA1 place cells provide sufficient information to guide navigation to a goal under conditions where the animal is not allowed to move directly toward the goal. It will be interesting to see whether modification of these vector fields/fantail structures modify the animal's choices during navigation.

These findings raise a number of questions about how the different components of the representation, the ConSinks, vector fields, and fantails are constructed, and what are the learning mechanisms underlying the movement of the ConSinks toward the goal. Further issues concern whether the fantails carry additional information, such as areas on the maze to be avoided, and more generally what is the downstream mechanism that compares the two arms of the fantail and selects the best direction (best branch of the fantail) when the animal is actually offered a choice between two platforms. Finally, it is not lost on us that a number of puzzling features exhibited by place cells in experiments with more than one goal, such as their unidirectionality on linear tracks, the splitter cell phenomenon, and the gradual movement of place fields to the goal in both T-mazes and open fields, may be explicable by the ConSink phenomenon.

11.12 Lateralization of function in human and animal hippocampus

Growing molecular, morphological, neurophysiological and behavioral evidence points to lateralization in the dorsal hippocampus in humans and other mammals, including rodents. For example, when human subjects navigated in large virtual spaces, only the activity of the right hippocampus significantly correlated with navigational accuracy (i.e., the ability to take the most direct path to the goal) (Maguire, Burgess, et al., 1998). Moreover, patients with selective damage to the right temporal lobe displayed impairments in remembering object's locations (O'Keefe, Burgess, et al., 1998). It has been suggested that the left hippocampus in humans may be storing spatial information about locations of "important" landmarks, e.g., goal locations (O'Keefe, Burgess, et al., 1998; Jordan, 2020), or it may be necessary for processing episodic (O'Keefe, Burgess, et al., 1998) or linguistic memory (O'Keefe 1996). To investigate differences between the left and right hemispheres, the majority of studies concentrated on using fMRI in humans partially due to the lack of commissural CA3–CA1 and CA3–CA3 connections. These connections exist in other nonprimate mammals, including rodents, that have strong commissural connections (Amaral and Lavenex, 2007). Otherwise, the hippocampal formation is largely preserved across all mammals (Amaral and Lavenex, 2007). More recent studies in rodents point to clear differences in processing hippocampal-dependent long-term (left hippocampus) vs. short-term (right hippocampus) memory, possibly mediated by differences in LTP properties.

Some of the first evidence for hippocampal lateralization in rodents came from a seminal study in hippocampal mouse slices showing different distribution of NMDA NR2B receptor subunits (also known as GluN2B and ε2) in the left and right hippocampi (Kawakami, Shinohara, et al., 2003). The relative amount of NR2B with respect to other NMDA receptor subunits (e.g., NR2A) is thought to play an important role in regulation of synaptic plasticity (Shi, Hayashi, et al., 1999; Morishita, Lu, et al., 2007) and may be critical for allowing calcium influx into synapses in order to modify synapse efficacy (Shinohara and Hirase, 2009; El-Gaby, Shipton, and Paulsen, 2015). Ipsilateral (via Schaffer fibers) CA3–CA1 pyramidal cell synapses in the stratum radiatum in the left CA1 were shown to be ~50% more sensitive to NR2B-subunit-specific antagonist compared with those in the right CA1(Kawakami, Shinohara, et al., 2003). The contralateral (via commissural fibers) CA3–CA1 pyramidal synapses had the opposite asymmetry. Thus, CA3–CA1 pyramidal cell synapses in the stratum radiatum of CA1 region displayed significantly higher density of NR2B receptor subunits in the synapses connected to axons from the left CA3 compared with the right CA3, independent of whether those connections were ipsi- or contralateral (Shinohara, Hirase, et al., 2008; Shinohara and Hirase, 2009; El-Gaby, Shipton, and Paulsen, 2015; Jordan, 2020). Studies using an anterograde viral tracing technique combined with fluorescent and electron microscopy to differentiate between ipsilateral and contralateral CA3–CA1 inputs showed that the CA1 stratum radiatum spines connected with right CA3 pyramidal neurons had ~70% larger head volume (0.278 μm^3 vs. 0.166 μm^3), were more likely to display "mushroom-type" morphology (35% vs. 20% of all synapses), and had ~40% larger postsynaptic density area compared with the ones in contact with the left CA3 pyramidal neurons (Shinohara, Hirase, et al., 2008). Synaptic area had a significant positive correlation with synaptic GluR1 density and negative correlation with NR2B density (Shinohara et al., 2008), suggesting that right CA3 axons preferentially connect to the spines with higher GluR1 density while left CA3 axons connect to spines with a higher density of NR2B. It has been previously demonstrated that increase in GluR1-containing AMPA receptors in postsynaptic sites is also associated with LTP induction and enlargement of spines (Kopec, Real, et al., 2007). Thus at least in principle, both right and left, ipsilateral and contralateral CA3–CA1 connections, have distinct molecular and morphological patterns that may potentially support different aspects of hippocampal-dependent learning, spatial memory, and navigation. It has been suggested that the increased spine volume as well as postsynaptic areas with high concentration of GluR1 receptor subunits may provide "a close-to-saturation state" of synapses receiving inputs from the right CA3, leading to reduced capacity for LTP induction (El-Gaby, Shipton, and Paulsen, 2015; Jordan, 2020). On the other hand, synapses with a high density of NR2B subunits receiving inputs from the left CA3 region may be perfectly suited for effective LTP, allowing associative learning. Indeed, using optogenetic stimulation of ipsilateral and contralateral CA3–CA1 inputs in mouse hippocampal slices, it has been shown that the selective stimulation of left (but not right) CA3–CA1 inputs induced robust LTP responses (Kohl, Shipton, et al., 2011). Moreover, application of an NR2B antagonist reversed LTP induction, thus pointing at a causal link between increased concentration of NR2B receptors subunits in postsynaptic densities between left CA3 axons and CA1 spines, and LTP. Metabotropic glutamate receptor 5 (mGluR5), associated with long-term depression (LTD), shows a similar asymmetrical expression pattern to NR2B (Shinohara and Hirase, 2009; Jordan, 2020) while other NMDA receptors do not show significant differences between the left and right hippocampi (Kawakami, Shinohara, et al., 2003; Shinohara and Hirase, 2009). There is also no difference between any of these measures in left and right CA1 pyramidal neurons. Thus laterality in mice is solely determined by the differences between left and right CA3 inputs (Shinohara, Hirase, et al., 2008).

Behavioral studies using lesions, pharmacological or optogenetic inactivation, and early gene imaging also point to a different role of left vs. right hippocampus, especially in processing long- vs. short-term memory as well as possible different involvement in specific spatial tasks. It has been demonstrated that unilateral hippocampal lesions (the differences between sides were not reported) induce long-term (rats tested 30 days after the training) but not short- (1 day after the training) or medium-term (7 days after training) memory deficits on a fear-conditioning task (H Zhou, Zhou, and Xu, 2016). In all the cases lesions were induced prior to training. Rats with bilateral hippocampal lesions were significantly deficient on all pretest trial durations.

It has been suggested that, similar to findings in humans, the right rodent hippocampus may be more heavily involved in real-time-processing of external and internal cues during navigation. In one study examining distinct functions of the left and right hippocampi, mice underwent transection of ventral hippocampal commissure (VHC; VHC transection disrupts connectivity between the left and the right sides of both ventral and dorsal hippocampi) and corpus callosum (CC) with right or left eye permanently closed (Shinohara, Hosoya, et al., 2012). Since most of the connections from the retina are contralateral, such visual deprivation resulted in visual processing confined mostly to right hippocampus when the right eye was closed (ΔR) and left hippocampus when the left eye was closed (ΔL). Mice, released from random starting locations with a number of distal landmarks available to them, had to navigate to a goal location on the Barnes maze (Barnes, 1979). While both ΔR and ΔL could learn the task as well as controls, ΔR mice showed significantly more accurate (i.e., direct) trajectories to the goal location compared with ΔL mice, suggesting that the right hippocampus may be more involved in real-time processing distal landmarks or coordinating an animal's movements/trajectories toward the goal in relation to the visual landmarks. The right hippocampus also shows differential gene expression compared with the left hippocampus after rats undergo training in the Morris watermaze: 623 genes, mostly associated with metabolism, synaptic plasticity, memory, and other neurophysiological function, were differentially expressed in the right hippocampus (299 genes were induced, 324 were repressed), compared with 74 in the left hippocampus (Klur, Muller, et al., 2009).

In line with the hypothesis that real-time spatial information processing during navigation may be more heavily weighted on the right hippocampus, it has been suggested that the right hippocampus may also be more important for processing short-term spatial memory, possibly acting as a "memory buffer" or alternatively by providing preconfigured place-cell ensembles (Dragoi and Tonegawa, 2011), which could act as a "scaffold" on which other features associated with a particular place may be stored (El-Gaby, Shipton, and Paulsen, 2015; Jordan, 2020). There is some evidence indicating that unilateral lesions in the right hippocampus (but not left) significantly affect short-term working memory tested on a spontaneous-alternation task in a T-maze, a well-established hippocampal-dependent working-memory task, and novel-arm exploration in a Y-maze, whereas unilateral left-hippocampal lesions (but not right) resulted in severe impairments in an object-in-place recognition task. In the latter task, the animal was presented with two identical objects in two corners of the environments for 10 min of free exploration. After 24 hours the rat was allowed to explore the two objects, one identical novel object placed in another corner, and one previously encountered object in its former position, for another 3 min. Rats with left unilateral hippocampal lesion discriminated significantly worse between the familiar and the displaced object compared with controls (Sakaguchi and Sakurai, 2020).

Further support for distinct roles in short- and long-term memory comes from selective in vivo optogenetic inactivation of either left or right CA3 to CA1 inputs. Silencing of the right CA3 to CA1 inputs resulted in significantly larger reduction of performance on a spontaneous alternation task in a T-maze compared with silencing left CA3 to CA1 inputs (Shipton, El-Gaby, et al., 2014). Such inactivation also disrupted performance on a spatial novelty preference task in a Y-maze. On the other hand, long-term memory behavioral tests using a modified Y-maze with three fixed external cues present, revealed that inactivation of left (but not right) CA3 to CA1connections resulted in impaired learning of a reward location using distal cues, suggesting that left CA3 to CA1 connections may have a special role in processing hippocampal-dependent learning and long-term memory (Shipton, El-Gaby, et al., 2014). During this task, mice were trained in a Y-maze to navigate to the reward location with a fixed relation to available distal cues that was kept constant for each mouse throughout the entire duration of the experiment. The starting location was randomly chosen between trials and the Y-maze was rotated before each trial to ensure that proximal cues could not be used. While inactivation of right CA3 neurons had no effect on behavioral performance, inactivation of left CA3 neurons significantly reduced performance levels, which did not reach the level of the controls even after 11 consecutive days of training. Similarly, temporary pharmacological inactivation of left (but not right) hippocampus (both CA1, CA3, and DG areas, and likely some other areas in the vicinity of the injection site) via infusion of lidocaine during the acquisition stage (i.e., during the 6 days of training) on the Morris watermaze spatial-memory task resulted in an inferior ability to locate the hidden platform 24 hours after the training (retention trial with no prior lidocaine infusion) (Klur, Muller, et al., 2009).On the contrary, only the injection to the right hippocampus (and not the left) during the retention trial resulted in spatial memory deficits on the Morris watermaze.

Some studies also suggest that left hippocampus may be more important in processing novel objects. Using expressions of Immediate Early Gene (IEG) c-Fos as a marker for neural activity during the behavioral tasks showed that left dentate gyrus exhibited an increased neural activation compared with the right dentate gyrus when the animal was presented with a new object (Jordan, Shanley, and Pytte, 2019). No asymmetry in activity levels was observed when the animal was running on the stationary wheel, even though, as expected, the activity was highly upregulated during this behavior in both left and right DG compared with the neural activity measured in a control home cage.

Left-right hippocampal asymmetry appears to be determined by both genetic and epigenetic factors. For example, it has been shown that hippocampal left-right symmetry can be abolished by mutating the gene encoding the motor protein, left-right dynein (Lrd) crucial for driving left-right axis determination process necessary for normal asymmetric arrangements of organs (Nonaka, Tanaka, et al., 1998; Kawakami, Dobi, et al., 2008). These mutants exhibited "right-hippocampus" isomorphism of NMDA NR2B receptor subunits independent of presence of abnormal arrangements of organs (Kawakami, Dobi, et al., 2008).

On the other hand, a "right-shift" in hippocampal asymmetry may be induced by epigenetic factors such as novelty or stress (Tang, Zou, et al., 2008). In these experiments young pups were daily taken for 3 min outside their home environments during the 3 initial weeks of their life. Unilateral stimulation of right but not left

hippocampus induced stronger LTP at 7 months of age compared with their control littermates, which did not undergo such displacement procedure as pups. This epigenetic manipulation has also been associated with enhanced LTP (Tang and Zou, 2002), increase in the right hippocampal volume (Verstynen, Tierney, et al., 2001), enhanced social behavior (Tang and Reeb, 2004), and hippocampal-dependent spatial memory (Tang, 2001), such as Morris watermaze with a moving platform (Whishaw, 1985), during adulthood.

In summary, there is growing evidence pointing to different roles of left and right hippocampi, with the latter being more involved in real-time cognitive map generation during navigation and short-term spatial memory while the former appears to be more important in processing long-term episodic-like memory and long-term encoding of salient environmental cues. These differences are likely to be mediated by different molecular signatures underpinning the connections between the left and right CA3–CA1 area with the former being rich in NMDA NR2B receptor subunits crucial for LTP induction, while the latter appears to be in a "close-to-saturation state" with much lower degree of rapid modification available. Finally, this lateralization is largely predetermined by genetic factors such as the motor protein left-right dynein (Lrd) crucial for driving left-right axis determination process. However, environmental factors such as novelty and stress also play an important role in modifying asymmetry properties.

11.13 Conclusions

In this final section, we will summarize and draw conclusions from some of the major findings of the previous sections.

Hippocampal pyramidal cells clearly represent important features of the environment and, in common with cortical representations in general, these representations are created by the combination of exteroceptive and interoceptive inputs. In the case of the hippocampus, pyramidal cells represent many features of the present, past, and future, but most or all of these are organized around the animal's location. In addition to telling the animal where it is in environment and what it is currently experiencing there, the cells also provide information about what has been experienced in the past and what will be experienced in the future under certain conditions or if certain actions are taken. They also provide information about desirable places such as goals and how to navigate to them and undesirable places to be avoided.

The second major type of cell in the hippocampus are the interneurons, which set up the environmental representations, control movement from one representation to the next, help to structure the type of information that comes into the hippocampus from different brain regions, and maintain overall neural activity within manageable levels, for example, by preventing large-scale synchronous activity from developing into epileptiform discharges.

Hippocampus receives its main inputs from entorhinal cortex and medial septum. Together these bring information about the sensory environment and also about the animal's movements. Both can independently provide information about the animal's location in the environment. A major clue to the functions of the medial septum comes from the correlates of the hippocampal LFP activity, in particular, the theta waves, which reflect the synchronized intracellular voltages of the pyramidal cells controlled primarily by the hippocampal interneurons. In section 11.2 we showed that the synchronization of the activity of large parts of the hippocampus allows it to act as an integrated system rather than as a simple collection of independent neurons. Importantly, we now know that one of the major functions of the medial septal inputs to the hippocampus is to provide path-integration information in a form that allows the hippocampus to predict the outcome of present movements in terms of changes in the animal's location in the environment. To this end, the cholinergic septal input provides information about the animal's rotations in space based partly on vestibular inputs, while the glutamatergic inputs provide information about the rate of linear forward translation on the basis of inputs from the midbrain locomotion region to the entorhinal speed cells. The combination of these two inputs together with representations of the current location should be sufficient to update the animal's location in the absence of further inputs from the environment, e.g., in the dark. It is likely that some of the effect of these spatial translocation inputs is mediated via the medial entorhinal cortex and to some extent the hippocampal interneuronal networks. As we saw in section 11.2, different classes of hippocampal interneurons target different parts of the pyramidal cell dendrites as well as the soma, and, although it is not clear how these gating inputs control movements within the spatial representational network, this would seem to be one of their functions. As we saw in section 11.7, some of the updating of the hippocampal locational representations is dependent on the entorhinal cortical input, in particular the grid cells, one of whose functions appears to be to provide metric information to the place cells about distance traveled in particular directions. As we also saw in section 11.7, the grid cells appear to be more dependent on the place cells than vice versa, and one suggestion is that the grid structure might be a way of organizing the anatomically disorganized spatial relationships among the place fields representing an environment and to allow them to relate to the more organized neocortical representations of the environment.

11.13.1 What do place cells represent?

The CA1 pyramidal cells probably have the most extensive representational capacities of any cells in the brain. The evidence presented in sections 11.3 to 11.7 strongly support the idea that the fundamental thing represented by these cells is the animal's location in the environment and it was this discovery that originally suggested the hippocampal cognitive map theory in the, 1970 s. But they clearly can represent many other aspects of the environment as well, as predicted by that theory. As detailed in section 11.5, they can represent the animal's current, past, and future locations, objects, and features to be found in those locations including those from every sensory modality, as well as higher-order entities such as conspecifics and rewards. They also represent time that has passed in a particular location since it was last visited and provide the higher-order information about features to be found in the environment, including the order in which they were experienced. Information from different sensory modalities may be more easy to bind together if they occur in the same location. In addition, place-cell firing patterns are influenced by distant goals and places to be avoided. Crucially, they provide important information supporting navigation to those distant goals and, although there is little evidence on this point, we assume to avoid dangerous places as well. When an animal is navigating to a distant goal, the vector-field representations of the place cells provide information about the direction and distance of that goal and in addition evaluate all other possible directions in terms of their relative usefulness in reaching the goal if the direct path to the goal is not available (section 11.11). The hippocampus seems to operate in several different states: when there is no clear goal in an environment, firing in the place fields is omnidirectional. Introduction of a single or small number of goals causes a switch into a different mode in which the firing of the place cells is organized around the goal location. This information is not available at the single cell level but is carried by the neuronal population in the form of vector fields that point to a location close to the goal. Switching the goal location alters the hippocampal vector-field representation, which primarily involves changing the place cells participating in the representation. Errors are reflected in this representation, suggesting that it might be used to guide the animal's decisions during navigation.

Although it is postulated that the hippocampal pyramidal cells act together as elements of multiple different networks, there is relatively little empirical evidence to support this. Some indirect evidence points to the fact that in any environment, the place fields tend to distribute themselves somewhat evenly across the environment so as to fill up the representation and not leave any unrepresented spatial scotoma. This suggests that there is some inhibitory interaction between the place cells where something like a first-past-the-post network sort out the distribution of fields. Further evidence for network interactions comes from experiments attempting to alter a small number of place fields through direct electrical or optogenetic stimulation. In these experiments, it is typically found that place-field remapping is not confined to the stimulated cells but involves cells outside the stimulated population, suggesting that there is an integrated network within which each cell finds its place and alterations occur at the network rather than the single-cell level. Further evidence for network interactions comes from the preplay phenomenon, in which there is evidence of preordained connections between groups of cells prior to experiencing an environment, which may determine the pattern of activity in that environment. Finally, recordings during navigation on the honeycomb maze show that the representation of the goal, the direct path to the goal, and the utility of possible alternative directions are all based on population activity and not on the behavior of any individual neuron.

11.13.2 Hippocampal learning rules

Learning clearly modifies many aspects of hippocampal representation. The combination of inputs necessary to fire a pyramidal cell in the place field may not be dependent on learning originally but the maintenance and strengthening of these input patterns is clearly dependent on plasticity processes, since newly development place fields in a novel environment are only maintained during a postevent consolidation and can be blocked by the use of NMDA blockers during that postevent period. The place cells of these animals treat the previously experienced environment as a novel one and set up an entirely new and different representation in the hippocampus.

One can also assume that the association of particular objects or features with particular places should be dependent on the LTP processes outlined in Chapter 10. However, there is also evidence from the Magee lab for much more complicated learning mechanisms involving much longer time courses. Something similar might be occurring during navigation as studied on the honeycomb maze. The changes in vector fields and associated ConSink locations as part of learning the navigation task suggests a learning mechanism more complicated than simple scalar strengthening of synapses and might involve something more akin to the comparison and modification of groups of vectors. This learning will probably be found to be taking place at the population level and might not be understandable at the single cell or synaptic level.

There are still many more aspects of hippocampal function that are not well understood and remain to be explored. While the basic functions of the hippocampus probably remain unchanged across different species, it is clear that there are differences between rodent and human hippocampal function, and future work will be needed to explore how much these involve specifically human capacities such as language and self-consciousness.

REFERENCES

Aggleton JP, MW Brown (2006) Interleaving brain systems for episodic and recognition memory 55. *Trends Cogn Sci* **10**(10):455–463.

Aggleton JP, SD Vann (2004) Testing the importance of the retrosplenial navigation system: lesion size but not strain matters: a reply to Harker and Whishaw 67. *Neurosci Biobehav Rev* **28**(5):525–531.

Aghajan M, P Schuette, TA Fields, ME Tran, SM Siddiqui, NR Hasulak, TK Tcheng, D Eliashiv, EA Mankin, J Stern, I Fried, N Suthana (2017) Theta oscillations in the human medial temporal lobe during real-world ambulatory movement. *Curr Biol* **27**(24):3743–3751, e3743.

Ainge JA, M Tamosiunaite, F Woergoetter, PA Dudchenko (2007) Hippocampal CA1 place cells encode intended destination on a maze with multiple choice points. *J Neurosci* **27**(36):9769–9779.

Ainge JA, M Tamosiunaite, F Woergoetter, PA Dudchenko (2012) Hippocampal place cells encode intended destination, and not a discriminative stimulus, in a conditional T-maze task. *Hippocampus* **22**(3):534–543.

Ainge JA, MA van der Meer, RF Langston, ER Wood (2007) Exploring the role of context-dependent hippocampal activity in spatial alternation behavior. *Hippocampus* **17**(10):988–1002.

Albasser MM, JR Dumont, E Amin, JD Holmes, MR Horne, JM Pearce, JP Aggleton (2013) Association rules for rat spatial learning: the importance of the hippocampus for binding item identity with item location. *Hippocampus* **23**(12):1162–1178.

Alexander GM, S Farris, JR Pirone, C Zheng, LL Colgin, SM Dudek (2016) Social and novel contexts modify hippocampal CA2 representations of space. *Nat Commun* **7**:10300.

Allen TA, DM Salz, S McKenzie, NJ Fortin (2016) Nonspatial sequence coding in CA1 neurons. *J Neurosci* **36**(5):1547–1563.

Alme CB, C Miao, K Jezek, A Treves, EI Moser, MB Moser (2014) Place cells in the hippocampus: eleven maps for eleven rooms. *Proc Natl Acad Sci U S A* **111**(52):18428–18435.

Amaral D, P Lavenex (2007) Hippocampal neuroanatomy. In: The Hippocampus Book (Anderson P, Morris RGM, Amaral DG, Bliss TVP, O'Keefe J, eds), pp 37–114. New York: Oxford University Press.

Anderson MI, KJ Jeffery (2003) Heterogeneous modulation of place cell firing by changes in context. *J Neurosci* **23**(26):8827–8835.

Anderson MI, S Killing, C Morris, A O'Donoghue, D Onyiagha, R Stevenson, M Verriotis, KJ Jeffery (2006) Behavioral correlates of the distributed coding of spatial context. *Hippocampus* **16**(9):730–742.

Aoki Y, H Igata, Y Ikegaya, T Sasaki (2019) The integration of goal-directed signals onto spatial maps of hippocampal place cells. *Cell Rep* **27**(5):1516–1527, e1515.

Aronov D, R Nevers, DW Tank (2017) Mapping of a non-spatial dimension by the hippocampal-entorhinal circuit. *Nature* **543**(7647):719–722.

Babb SJ, JD Crystal (2003) Spatial navigation on the radial maze with trial-unique intramaze cues and restricted extramaze cues. *Behav Processes* **64**(1):103–111.

Babb SJ, JD Crystal (2005) Discrimination of what, when, and where: implications for episodic-like memory in rat. *Learning and Motivation* **36**:177–189.

Babb SJ, JD Crystal (2006a) Discrimination of what, when, and where is not based on time of day. *Learn Behav* **34**(2):124–130.

Babb SJ, JD Crystal (2006b) Episodic-like memory in the rat. *Curr Biol* **16**(13):1317–1321.

Balleine BW, IS Curthoys (1991) Differential effects of escapable and inescapable footshock on hippocampal theta activity. *Behav Neurosci* **105**(1):202–209.

Barnes CA (1979) Memory deficits associated with senescence: a neurophysiological and behavioral study in the rat. *J Comp Physiol Psychol* **93**(1):74–104.

Barry C, LL Ginzberg, J. O'Keefe, N Burgess (2012) Grid cell firing patterns signal environmental novelty by expansion. *Proc Natl Acad Sci U S A* **109**(43):17687–17692.

Bassett JP, MB Zugaro, GM Muir, EJ Golob, RU Muller, JS Taube (2005) Passive movements of the head do not abolish anticipatory firing properties of head direction cells. *J Neurophysiol* **93**(3):1304–1316.

Battaglia FP, GR Sutherland, BL McNaughton (2004) Local sensory cues and place cell directionality: additional evidence of prospective coding in the hippocampus. *J Neurosci* **24**(19):4541–4550.

Baxter MG, DJ Bucci, TJ Sobel, MJ Williams, LK Gorman, M Gallagher (1996) Intact spatial learning following lesions of basal forebrain cholinergic neurons. *Neuroreport* **7**(8):1417–1420.

Bendor D, HJ Spiers (2016) Does the Hippocampus map out the future? *Trends Cogn Sci* **20**(3):167–169.

Berger-Sweeney, J, S Heckers, MM Mesulam, RG Wiley, DA Lappi, M Sharma (1994) Differential effects on spatial navigation of immunotoxin-induced cholinergic lesions of the medial septal area and nucleus basalis magnocellularis. *J Neurosci* **14**(7):4507–4519.

Bittner KC, C Grienberger, SP Vaidya, AD Milstein, JJ Macklin, J Suh, S Tonegawa, JC Magee (2015) Conjunctive input processing drives feature selectivity in hippocampal CA1 neurons. *Nat Neurosci* **18**(8):1133–1142.

Bittner KC, AD Milstein, C Grienberger, S Romani, JC Magee (2017) Behavioral time scale synaptic plasticity underlies CA1 place fields. *Science* **357**(6355):1033–1036.

Bjerknes TL, RF Langston, IU Kruge, EI Moser, MB Moser (2015) Coherence among head direction cells before eye opening in rat pups. *Curr Biol* **25**(1):103–108.

Bjerknes TL, EI Moser, MB Moser (2014) Representation of geometric borders in the developing rat. *Neuron* **82**(1):71–78.

Blair HT, J Cho, PE Sharp (1998) Role of the lateral mammillary nucleus in the rat head direction circuit: a combined single unit recording and lesion study. *Neuron* **21**(6):1387–1397.

Blair HT, BW Lipscomb, PE Sharp (1997) Anticipatory time intervals of head-direction cells in the anterior thalamus of the rat: implications for path integration in the head-direction circuit. *J Neurophysiol* **78**(1):145–159.

Blair HT, PE Sharp (1995) Anticipatory head direction signals in anterior thalamus: evidence for a thalamocortical circuit that integrates angular head motion to compute head direction. *J Neurosci* **15**(9):6260–6270.

Bland BH, SD Oddie (2001) Theta band oscillation and synchrony in the hippocampal formation and associated structures: the case for its role in sensorimotor integration. *Behav Brain Res* **127**(1–2):119–136.

Bland BH, CH Vanderwolf (1972) Diencephalic and hippocampal mechanisms of motor activity in the rat: effects of posterior hypothalamic stimulation on behavior and hippocampal slow wave activity. *Brain Res* 43(1):67–88.

Boccara CN, F Sargolini, VH Thoresen, T Solstad, MP Witter, EI Moser, MB Moser (2010) Grid cells in pre- and parasubiculum. *Nat Neurosci* 13(8):987–994.

Bohbot VD, MS Copara, J Gotman, AD Ekstrom (2017) Low-frequency theta oscillations in the human hippocampus during real-world and virtual navigation. *Nat Commun* 8:14415.

Bolding KA, J Ferbinteanu, SE Fox, RU Muller (2020) Place cell firing cannot support navigation without intact septal circuits. *Hippocampus* 30(3):175–191.

Bonnevie T, B Dunn, M Fyhn, T Hafting, D Derdikman, JL Kubie, Y Roudi, EI Moser, MB Moser (2013) Grid cells require excitatory drive from the hippocampus. *Nat Neurosci* 16(3):309–317.

Bragin A, G Jando, Z Nadasdy, J Hetke, K Wise, G Buzsaki (1995) Gamma (40–100 Hz) oscillation in the hippocampus of the behaving rat. *J Neurosci* 15(1 Pt 1):47–60.

Brandon MP, AR Bogaard, CP Libby, MA Connerney, K Gupta, ME Hasselmo (2011) Reduction of theta rhythm dissociates grid cell spatial periodicity from directional tuning. *Science* 332(6029):595–599.

Brandon MP, J Koenig, JK Leutgeb, S Leutgeb (2014) New and distinct hippocampal place codes are generated in a new environment during septal inactivation. *Neuron* 82(4):789–796.

Brazhnik E, R Borgnis, RU Muller, SE Fox (2004) The effects on place cells of local scopolamine dialysis are mimicked by a mixture of two specific muscarinic antagonists. *J Neurosci* 24(42):9313–9323.

Burgess N, S Becker, JA King, J O'Keefe (2001) Memory for events and their spatial context: models and experiments. *Philos Trans R Soc Lond B Biol Sci.* 356(1413):1493–1503.

Burwell RD, DG Amaral (1998) Cortical afferents of the perirhinal, postrhinal, and entorhinal cortices of the rat. *J Comp Neurol* 398(2):179–205.

Buzsaki G (2015) Hippocampal sharp wave-ripple: a cognitive biomarker for episodic memory and planning. *Hippocampus* 25(10):1073–1188.

Buzsaki G, E Stark, A Berenyi, D Khodagholy, DR Kipke, E Yoon, KD Wise (2015) Tools for probing local circuits: high-density silicon probes combined with optogenetics. *Neuron* 86(1):92–105.

Buzsaki G, D Tingley (2018) Space and time: the hippocampus as a sequence generator. *Trends Cogn Sci* 22(10):853–869.

Cacucci F, C Lever, TJ Wills, N Burgess, J O'Keefe (2004) Theta-modulated place-by-direction cells in the hippocampal formation in the rat. *J Neurosci* 24(38):8265–8277.

Cai L, RB Gibbs, DA Johnson (2012) Recognition of novel objects and their location in rats with selective cholinergic lesion of the medial septum. *Neurosci Lett* 506(2):261–265.

Calton JL, JS Taube (2009) Where am I and how will I get there from here? a role for posterior parietal cortex in the integration of spatial information and route planning. *Neurobiol Learn Mem* 91(2):186–196.

Casali G, S Shipley, C Dowell, R Hayman, C Barry (2018) Entorhinal neurons exhibit cue locking in rodent VR. *Front Cell Neurosci* 12:512.

Catanese J, A Viggiano, E Cerasti, MB Zugaro, SI Wiener (2014) Retrospectively and prospectively modulated hippocampal place responses are differentially distributed along a common path in a continuous T-maze. *J Neurosci* 34(39):13163–13169.

Chaudhuri-Vayalambrone P, ME Rule, M Bauza, M Krstulovic, P Kerekes, S Burton, T O'Leary, J Krupic (2023) Simultaneous representation of multiple time horizons by entorhinal grid cells and CA1 place cells. Cell Reports 42:112716.

Chen G, JA King, N Burgess, J O'Keefe (2013) How vision and movement combine in the hippocampal place code. *Proc Natl Acad Sci U S A* 110(1):378–383.

Chen LL, LH Lin, CA Barnes, BL McNaughton (1994) Head-direction cells in the rat posterior cortex: II. Contributions of visual and ideothetic information to the directional firing. *Exp Brain Res* 101(1):24–34.

Chen LL, LH Lin, EJ Green, CA Barnes, BL McNaughton (1994) Head-direction cells in the rat posterior cortex: I. Anatomical distribution and behavioral modulation. *Exp Brain Res* 101(1):8–23.

Chen S, L He, AJY Huang, R Boehringer, V Robert, ME Wintzer, D Polygalov, AZ Weitemier, Y Tao, M Gu, et al. (2020) A hypothalamic novelty signal modulates hippocampal memory. *Nature* 586(7828):270–274.

Chenani A, M Sabariego, MI Schlesiger, JK Leutgeb, S Leutgeb, C Leibold (2019) Hippocampal CA1 replay becomes less prominent but more rigid without inputs from medial entorhinal cortex. *Nat Commun* 10(1):1341.

Chiba AA, RP Kesner, AM Reynolds (1994) Memory for spatial location as a function of temporal lag in rats: role of hippocampus and medial prefrontal cortex. *Behav Neural Biol* 61(2):123–131.

Cho J, PE Sharp (2001) Head direction, place, and movement correlates for cells in the rat retrosplenial cortex. *Behav Neurosci* 115(1):3–25.

Ciocchi S, J Passecker, H Malagon-Vina, N Mikus, T Klausberger (2015) Brain computation: selective information routing by ventral hippocampal CA1 projection neurons. *Science* 348(6234):560–563.

Clayton NS, A Dickinson (1998) Episodic-like memory during cache recovery by scrub jays [see comments]. *Nature* 395(6699):272–274.

Clifton PG, SP Vickers, EM Somerville (1998) Little and often: ingestive behavior patterns following hippocampal lesions in rats. *Behav Neurosci* 112(3):502–511.

Cohen NJ, H Eichenbaum (1993) Memory, Amnesia, the Hippocampal System. Cambridge, MA: MIT Press.

Cohen SJ, RW Stackman, Jr (2015) Assessing rodent hippocampal involvement in the novel object recognition task: a review. *Behav Brain Res* 285:105–117.

Colgin LL, T Denninger, M Fyhn, T Hafting, T Bonnevie, O Jensen, MB Moser, EI Moser (2009) Frequency of gamma oscillations routes flow of information in the hippocampus. *Nature* 462(7271):353–357.

Colom LV, MT Castaneda, T Reyna, S Hernandez, E Garrido-Sanabria (2005) Characterization of medial septal glutamatergic neurons and their projection to the hippocampus. *Synapse* 58(3):151–164.

Cooper BG, SJ Mizumori (2001) Temporary inactivation of the retrosplenial cortex causes a transient reorganization of spatial coding in the hippocampus. *J Neurosci* 21(11):3986–4001.

Courellis HS, SU Nummela, M Metke, GW Diehl, R Bussell, G Cauwenberghs, CT Miller (2019) Spatial encoding in primate hippocampus during free navigation. *PLoS Biol* 17(12):e3000546.

Csicsvari J, B Jamieson, KD Wise, G Buzsaki (2003) Mechanisms of gamma oscillations in the hippocampus of the behaving rat. *Neuron* 37(2):311–322.

Cui H, RA Andersen (2007) Posterior parietal cortex encodes autonomously selected motor plans. *Neuron* 56(3):552–559.

Czurko A, H Hirase, J Csicsvari, G Buzsaki (1999) Sustained activation of hippocampal pyramidal cells by "space clamping" in a running wheel. *Eur J Neurosci* 11(1):344–352.

Danielson NB, JD Zaremba, P Kaifosh, J Bowler, M Ladow, A Losonczy (2016) Sublayer-specific coding dynamics during spatial navigation and learning in hippocampal area CA1. *Neuron* 91(3):652–665.

Danjo T, T Toyoizumi, S Fujisawa (2018) Spatial representations of self and other in the hippocampus. *Science* 359(6372):213–218.

Dannenberg H, JR Hinman, ME Hasselmo (2016) Potential roles of cholinergic modulation in the neural coding of location and movement speed. *J Physiol Paris* 110(1–2):52–64.

Davidson TL, LE Jarrard (1993) A role for hippocampus in the utilization of hunger signals. *Behav Neural Biol* 59(2):167–171.

De Almeida, L, M Idiart, A Villavicencio, J Lisman (2012) Alternating predictive and short-term memory modes of entorhinal grid cells. *Hippocampus* 22(8):1647–1651.

Deguchi Y, F Donato, I Galimberti, E Cabuy, P Caroni (2011) Temporally matched subpopulations of selectively interconnected principal neurons in the hippocampus. *Nat Neurosci* 14(4):495–504.

Denham MJ, SL McCabe (1998) A model of predictive learning in the rat Hippocampal principal cells during spatial activity. *IEEE International Joint Conference on Neural Networks Proceedings. IEEE World Congress on Computational Intelligence* 1547–1552.

Dere E, JP Huston, MA De Souza Silva (2005) Integrated memory for objects, places, and temporal order: evidence for episodic-like memory in mice. *Neurobiol Learn Mem* 84(3):214–221.

Deshmukh SS, JJ Knierim (2011) Representation of non-spatial and spatial information in the lateral entorhinal cortex. *Front Behav Neurosci* 5:69.

Deshmukh SS, D Yoganarasimha, H Voicu, JJ Knierim (2010) Theta modulation in the medial and the lateral entorhinal cortices 10. *J Neurophysiol* 104(2):994–1006.

Diamantaki M, S Coletta, K Nasr, R Zeraati, S Laturnus, P Berens, P Preston-Ferrer, A Burgalossi (2018) Manipulating hippocampal place cell activity by single-cell stimulation in freely moving mice. *Cell Rep* 23(1):32–38.

Diamantaki M, M Frey, P Preston-Ferrer, A Burgalossi (2016) Priming spatial activity by single-cell stimulation in the dentate gyrus of freely moving rats. *Curr Biol* 26(4):536–541.

Diba K, G Buzsaki (2007) Forward and reverse hippocampal place-cell sequences during ripples. *Nat Neurosci* 10(10):1241–1242.

Diehl GW, OJ Hon, S Leutgeb, JK Leutgeb (2017) Grid and nongrid cells in medial entorhinal cortex represent spatial location and environmental features with complementary coding schemes. *Neuron* 94(1):83–92, e86.

Dragoi G, S Tonegawa (2011) Preplay of future place cell sequences by hippocampal cellular assemblies. *Nature* 469(7330):397–401.

Dragoi G, S Tonegawa (2013) Distinct preplay of multiple novel spatial experiences in the rat. *Proc Natl Acad Sci U S A* 110(22):9100–9105.

Dudchenko PA, ER Wood (2014) Splitter cells: hippocampal place cells whose firing is modulated by where the animal is going or where it has been. In: Space, Time, Memory in the Hippocampal Formation (Derdikman D, Knierim JJ, eds), pp 253–272. Vienna: Springer.

Dudchenko PA, ER Wood, H Eichenbaum (2000) Neurotoxic hippocampal lesions have no effect on odor span and little effect on odor recognition memory but produce significant impairments on spatial span, recognition, and alternation [in process citation]. *J Neurosci* 20(8):2964–2977.

Dupret D, J O'Neill, B Pleydell-Bouverie, J Csicsvari (2010) The reorganization and reactivation of hippocampal maps predict spatial memory performance. *Nat Neurosci* 13(8):995–1002.

Duvelle E, RM Grieves, V Hok, B Poucet, A Arleo, KJ Jeffery, E Save (2019) Insensitivity of place cells to the value of spatial goals in a two-choice flexible navigation task. *J Neurosci* 39(13):2522–2541.

Easton A, AE Fitchett, MJ Eacott, MG Baxter (2011) Medial septal cholinergic neurons are necessary for context-place memory but not episodic-like memory. *Hippocampus* 21(9):1021–1027.

Ego-Stengel V, MA Wilson (2010) Disruption of ripple-associated hippocampal activity during rest impairs spatial learning in the rat 4. *Hippocampus* 20(1):1–10.

Ekstrom AD (2015) Why vision is important to how we navigate. *Hippocampus* 25(6):731–735.

Ekstrom AD, MJ Kahana, JB Caplan, TA Fields, EA Isham, EL Newman, I Fried (2003) Cellular networks underlying human spatial navigation. *Nature* 425(6954):184–188.

El-Gaby, M, OA Shipton, O Paulsen (2015) Synaptic plasticity and memory: new insights from hippocampal left-right asymmetries. *Neuroscientist* 21(5):490–502.

Ennaceur A, J Delacour (1988) A new one-trial test for neurobiological studies of memory in rats. 1: Behavioral data. *Behav Brain Res* 31(1):47–59.

Ergorul C, H Eichenbaum (2004) The hippocampus and memory for what, where, and when. *Learn Mem* 11(4):397–405.

Farrell JS, M Lovett-Barron, PM Klein, FT Sparks, T Gschwind, AL Ortiz, B Ahanonu, S Bradbury, S Terada, M Oijala, et al. (2021) Supramammillary regulation of locomotion and hippocampal activity. *Science* 374(6574):1492–1496.

Fenton AA, HY Kao, SA Neymotin, A Olypher, Y Vayntrub, WW Lytton, N Ludvig (2008) Unmasking the CA1 ensemble place code by exposures to small and large environments: more place cells and multiple, irregularly arranged, and expanded place fields in the larger space. *J Neurosci* 28(44):11250–11262.

Fenton AA, WW Lytton, JM Barry, PP Lenck-Santini, LE Zinyuk, S Kubik, J Bures, B Poucet, RU Muller, AV Olypher (2010) Attention-like modulation of hippocampus place cell discharge. *J Neurosci* 30(13):4613–4625.

Fenton AA, M Wesierska, Y Kaminsky, J Bures (1998) Both here and there: simultaneous expression of autonomous spatial memories in rats. *Proc Natl Acad Sci U S A* 95(19):11493–11498.

Ferbinteanu J, ML Shapiro (2003) Prospective and retrospective memory coding in the hippocampus. *Neuron* 40(6):1227–1239.

Fibiger HC (1982) The organization and some projections of cholinergic neurons of the mammalian forebrain. *Brain Res* 257(3):327–388.

Fiser A, D Mahringer, HK Oyibo, AV Petersen, M Leinweber, GB Keller (2016) Experience-dependent spatial expectations in mouse visual cortex. *Nat Neurosci* 19(12):1658–1664.

Fortin NJ, KL Agster, HB Eichenbaum (2002) Critical role of the hippocampus in memory for sequences of events. *Nat Neurosci* 5(5):458–462.

Foster TC, CA Castro, BL McNaughton (1989) Spatial selectivity of rat hippocampal neurons: dependence on preparedness for movement. *Science* 244(4912):1580–1582.

Frank LM, EN Brown, M Wilson (2000) Trajectory encoding in the hippocampus and entorhinal cortex. *Neuron* 27(1):169–178.

Frank LM, GB Stanley, EN Brown (2004) Hippocampal plasticity across multiple days of exposure to novel environments. *J Neurosci* 24(35):7681–7689.

Frankland PW, B Bontempi, LE Talton, L Kaczmarek, AJ Silva (2004) The involvement of the anterior cingulate cortex in remote contextual fear memory. *Science* 304(5672):881–883.

Freund TF, M Antal (1988) GABA-containing neurons in the septum control inhibitory interneurons in the hippocampus. *Nature* 336(6195):170–173.

Fried I, KA MacDonald, CL Wilson (1997) Single neuron activity in human hippocampus and amygdala during recognition of faces and objects. *Neuron* 18(5):753–765.

Frielingsdorf H, LJ Thal, DP Pizzo (2006) The septohippocampal cholinergic system and spatial working memory in the Morris water maze. *Behav Brain Res* 168(1):37–46.

Frotscher M, C Leranth (1985) Cholinergic innervation of the rat hippocampus as revealed by choline acetyltransferase immunocytochemistry: a combined light and electron microscopic study. *J Comp Neurol* 239(2):237–246.

Fuhrmann F, D Justus, L Sosulina, H Kaneko, T Beutel, D Friedrichs, S Schoch, MK Schwarz, M Fuhrmann, S Remy (2015) Locomotion, theta oscillations, and the speed-correlated firing of hippocampal neurons are controlled by a medial septal glutamatergic circuit. *Neuron* 86(5):1253–1264.

Furtak SC, SM Wei, KL Agster, RD Burwell (2007) Functional neuroanatomy of the parahippocampal region in the rat: the perirhinal and postrhinal cortices. *Hippocampus* 17(9):709–722.

Fyhn M, T Hafting, A Treves, MB Moser, EI Moser (2007) Hippocampal remapping and grid realignment in entorhinal cortex. *Nature* 446(7132):190–194.

Fyhn M, S Molden, MP Witter, EI Moser, MB Moser (2004) Spatial representation in the entorhinal cortex. *Science* 305(5688):1258–1264.

Gaskin S, A Tremblay, DG Mumby (2003) Retrograde and anterograde object recognition in rats with hippocampal lesions. *Hippocampus* 13(8):962–969.

Gauthier JL, DW Tank (2018) A dedicated population for reward coding in the hippocampus. *Neuron* 99(1):179–193, e177.

Gavrilov VV, SI Wiener, A Berthoz (1995) Enhanced hippocampal theta EEG during whole body rotations in awake restrained rats. *Neurosci Lett* 197(3):239–241.

Gavrilov VV, SI Wiener, A Berthoz (1996) Whole-body rotations enhance hippocampal theta rhythmic slow activity in awake rats passively transported on a mobile robot. *Ann N Y Acad Sci* 781:385–398.

Geva N, D Deitch, A Rubin, Y Ziv (2023) Time and experience differentially affect distinct aspects of hippocampal representational drift. *Neuron* 111(15):2357–2366, e2355.

Gil M, M Ancau, MI Schlesiger, A Neitz, K Allen, RJ De Marco, H Monyer (2018) Impaired path integration in mice with disrupted grid cell firing. *Nat Neurosci* 21(1):81–91.

Girardeau G, K Benchenane, SI Wiener, G Buzsaki, MB Zugaro (2009) Selective suppression of hippocampal ripples impairs spatial memory. *Nat Neurosci* 12(10):1222–1223.

Golding NL, NP Staff, N Spruston (2002) Dendritic spikes as a mechanism for cooperative long-term potentiation. *Nature* 418(6895):326–331.

Gonzalez-Sulser A, D Parthier, A Candela, C McClure, H Pastoll, D Garden, G Surmeli, MF Nolan (2014) GABAergic projections from the medial septum selectively inhibit interneurons in the medial entorhinal cortex. *J Neurosci* 34(50):16739–16743.

Goodridge JP, JS Taube (1997) Interaction between the postsubiculum and anterior thalamus in the generation of head direction cell activity. *J Neurosci* 17(23):9315–9330.

Gothard KM, WE Skaggs, KM Moore, BL McNaughton (1996) Binding of hippocampal CA1 neural activity to multiple reference frames in a landmark-based navigation task. *J Neurosci* 16(2):823–835.

Goutagny R, J Jackson, S Williams (2009) Self-generated theta oscillations in the hippocampus. *Nat Neurosci* 12(12):1491–1493.

Grieves RM, S Jedidi-Ayoub, K Mishchanchuk, A Liu, S Renaudineau, KJ Jeffery (2020) The place-cell representation of volumetric space in rats. *Nat Commun* 11(1):789.

Grieves RM, ER Wood, PA Dudchenko (2016) Place cells on a maze encode routes rather than destinations. *Elife* 5(5):e15986.

Griffin AL, H Eichenbaum, ME Hasselmo (2007) Spatial representations of hippocampal CA1 neurons are modulated by behavioral context in a hippocampus-dependent memory task. *J Neurosci* 27(9):2416–2423.

Grion N, A Akrami, Y Zuo, F Stella, ME Diamond (2016) Coherence between rat sensorimotor system and hippocampus is enhanced during tactile discrimination. *PLoS Biol* 14(2):e1002384.

Hafting T, M Fyhn, S Molden, MB Moser, EI Moser (2005) Microstructure of a spatial map in the entorhinal cortex. *Nature* 436(7052):801–806.

Hagan JJ, JD Salamone, J Simpson, SD Iversen, RG Morris (1988) Place navigation in rats is impaired by lesions of medial septum and diagonal band but not nucleus basalis magnocellularis. *Behav Brain Res* 27(1):9–20.

Haimerl C, D Angulo-Garcia, V Villette, S Reichinnek, A Torcini, R Cossart, A Malvache (2019) Internal representation of hippocampal neuronal population spans a time-distance continuum. *Proc Natl Acad Sci U S A* 116(15):7477–7482.

Hales JB, MI Schlesiger, JK Leutgeb, LR Squire, S Leutgeb, RE Clark (2014) Medial entorhinal cortex lesions only partially disrupt hippocampal place cells and hippocampus-dependent place memory. *Cell Rep* 9(3):893–901.

Hardcastle K, S Ganguli, LM Giocomo (2015) Environmental boundaries as an error correction mechanism for grid cells. *Neuron* 86(3):827–839.

Hargreaves EL, G Rao, I Lee, JJ Knierim (2005) Major dissociation between medial and lateral entorhinal input to dorsal hippocampus. *Science* 308(5729):1792–1794.

Harker KT, IQ Whishaw (2004) Impaired place navigation in place and matching-to-place swimming pool tasks follows both retrosplenial cortex lesions and cingulum bundle lesions in rats. *Hippocampus* 14(2):224–231.

Harvey CD, P Coen, DW Tank (2012) Choice-specific sequences in parietal cortex during a virtual-navigation decision task. *Nature* 484(7392):62–68.

Harvey CD, F Collman, DA Dombeck, DW Tank (2009) Intracellular dynamics of hippocampal place cells during virtual navigation. *Nature* 461(7266):941–946.

Hashimotodani Y, F Karube, Y Yanagawa, F Fujiyama, M Kano (2018) Supramammillary nucleus afferents to the dentate gyrus co-release glutamate and GABA and potentiate granule cell output. *Cell Rep* 25(10):2704–2715, e2704.

Hasselmo ME, C Bodelon, BP Wyble (2002) A proposed function for hippocampal theta rhythm: separate phases of encoding and retrieval enhance reversal of prior learning. *Neural Comput* 14(4):793–817.

Hayashi Y, A Sawa, T Hikida (2016) Impaired hippocampal activity at the goal zone on the place preference task in a DISC1 mouse model. *Neurosci Res* 106:70–73.

Henderson YO, GP Smith, MB Parent (2013) Hippocampal neurons inhibit meal onset. *Hippocampus* 23(1):100–107.

Herzog LE, LM Pascual, SJ Scott, ER Mathieson, DB Katz, SP Jadhav (2019) Interaction of taste and place coding in the hippocampus. *J Neurosci* 39(16):3057–3069.

Hill AJ (1978) First occurrence of hippocampal spatial firing in a new environment. *Exp Neurol* 62(2):282–297.

Hitti FL, SA Siegelbaum (2014) The hippocampal CA2 region is essential for social memory. *Nature* 508(7494):88–92.

Hock BJ, Jr, MD Bunsey (1998) Differential effects of dorsal and ventral hippocampal lesions. *J Neurosci* 18(17):7027–7032.

Hok V, E Chah, E Save, B Poucet (2013) Prefrontal cortex focally modulates hippocampal place cell firing patterns. *J Neurosci* 33(8):3443–3451.

Hok V, PP Lenck-Santini, S Roux, E Save, RU Muller, B Poucet (2007) Goal-related activity in hippocampal place cells 8. *J Neurosci* 27(3):472–482.

Hok V, PP Lenck-Santini, E Save, P Gaussier, JP Banquet, B Poucet (2007) A test of the time estimation hypothesis of place cell goal-related activity. *J Integr Neurosci* 6(3):367–378.

Holscher C, W Jacob, HA Mallot (2004) Learned association of allocentric and egocentric information in the hippocampus. *Exp Brain Res* 158(2):233–240.

Hori E, Y Nishio, K Kazui, K Umeno, E Tabuchi, K Sasaki, S Endo, T Ono, H Nishijo (2005) Place-related neural responses in the monkey hippocampal formation in a virtual space. *Hippocampus* 15(8):991–996.

Hoydal OA, ER Skytoen, SO Andersson, MB Moser, EI Moser (2019) Object-vector coding in the medial entorhinal cortex. *Nature* 568(7752):400–404.

Huerta PT, JE Lisman (1995) Bidirectional synaptic plasticity induced by a single burst during cholinergic theta oscillation in CA1 in vitro. *Neuron* 15(5):1053–1063.

Huh CY, R Goutagny, S Williams (2010) Glutamatergic neurons of the mouse medial septum and diagonal band of Broca synaptically drive hippocampal pyramidal cells: relevance for hippocampal theta rhythm. *J Neurosci* 30(47):15951–15961.

Husain M, P Nachev (2007) Space and the parietal cortex. *Trends Cogn Sci* 11(1):30–36.

Huxter J, N Burgess, J O'Keefe (2003) Independent rate and temporal coding in hippocampal pyramidal cells. *Nature* 425(6960):828–832.

Huxter J, T Senior, K Allen, J Csicsvari (2008) Theta phase-specific codes for two-dimensional position, trajectory and heading in the hippocampus. *Nature Neuroscience* 11:587–594.

Ikonen S, R McMahan, M Gallagher, H Eichenbaum, H Tanila (2002) Cholinergic system regulation of spatial representation by the hippocampus. *Hippocampus* 12(3):386–397.

Issa JB, G Tocker, ME Hasselmo, JG Heys, DA Dombeck (2020) Navigating through time: a spatial navigation perspective on how the brain may encode time. *Annu Rev Neurosci* (43):73–93.

Itskov PM, E Vinnik, ME Diamond (2011) Hippocampal representation of touch-guided behavior in rats: persistent and independent traces of stimulus and reward location. *PLoS One* 6(1):e16462.

Itskov PM, E Vinnik, C Honey, J Schnupp, ME Diamond (2012) Sound sensitivity of neurons in rat hippocampus during performance of a sound-guided task. *J Neurophysiol* 107(7):1822–1834.

Jackson J, AD Redish (2007) Network dynamics of hippocampal cell-assemblies resemble multiple spatial maps within single tasks. *Hippocampus* 17(12):1209–1229.

Jacob PY, G Casali, L Spieser, H Page, D Overington, K Jeffery (2017) An independent, landmark-dominated head-direction signal in dysgranular retrosplenial cortex. *Nat Neurosci* 20(2):173–175.

Jacob PY, T Van Cauter, B Poucet, F Sargolini, E Save (2020) Medial entorhinal cortex lesions induce degradation of CA1 place cell firing stability when self-motion information is used. *Brain Neuroscience Advances* 4(10):1177/2398212820953004.

Jacobs J, MJ Kahana, AD Ekstrom, I Fried (2007) Brain oscillations control timing of single-neuron activity in humans. *J Neurosci* 27(14):3839–3844.

Janisiewicz AM, O Jackson, 3rd, EF Firoz, MG Baxter (2004) Environment-spatial conditional learning in rats with selective lesions of medial septal cholinergic neurons. *Hippocampus* 14(2):265–273.

Jankowski MM, SM O'Mara (2015) Dynamics of place, boundary and object encoding in rat anterior claustrum. *Front Behav Neurosci* 9:250.

Jankowski MM, J Passecker, MN Islam, S Vann, JT Erichsen, JP Aggleton, SM O'Mara (2015) Evidence for spatially-responsive neurons in the rostral thalamus. *Front Behav Neurosci* 9:256.

Jayakumar RP, MS Madhav, F Savelli, HT Blair, NJ Cowan, JJ Knierim (2019) Recalibration of path integration in hippocampal place cells. *Nature* 566(7745):533–537.

Jeewajee A, C Lever, S Burton, J O'Keefe, N Burgess (2008) Environmental novelty is signaled by reduction of the hippocampal theta frequency. *Hippocampus* 18(4):340–348.

Jeffery KJ, JM O'Keefe (1999) Learned interaction of visual and idiothetic cues in the control of place field orientation. *Exp Brain Res* 127(2):151–161.

Jensen O, JE Lisman (2000) Position reconstruction from an ensemble of hippocampal place cells: contribution of theta phase coding. *J Neurophysiol* 83(5):2602–2609.

Jones BE (1990) Immunohistochemical study of choline acetyltransferase-immunoreactive processes and cells innervating the pontomedullary reticular formation in the rat. *J Comp Neurol* 295(3):485–514.

Jordan JT (2020) The rodent hippocampus as a bilateral structure: a review of hemispheric lateralization. *Hippocampus* 30(3):278–292.

Jordan JT, MR Shanley, CL Pytte (2019) Behavioral state-dependent lateralization of dorsal dentate gyrus c-Fos expression in mice. *Neuronal Signal* 3(1):NS20180206.

Joshi A, M Salib, TJ Viney, D Dupret, P Somogyi (2017) Behavior-dependent activity and synaptic organization of septo-hippocampal GABAergic neurons selectively targeting the hippocampal CA3 area. *Neuron* 96(6):1342–1357, e1345.

Jung MW, BL McNaughton (1993) Spatial selectivity of unit activity in the hippocampal granular layer. *Hippocampus* 3(2):165–182.

Jung MW, SI Wiener, BL McNaughton (1994) Comparison of spatial firing characteristics of units in dorsal and ventral hippocampus of the rat. *J Neurosci* 14(12):7347–7356.

Kaifosh P, M Lovett-Barron, GF Turi, TR Reardon, A Losonczy (2013) Septo-hippocampal GABAergic signaling across multiple modalities in awake mice. *Nat Neurosci* 16(9):1182–1184.

Kamondi A, L Acsady, XJ Wang, G Buzsaki (1998) Theta oscillations in somata and dendrites of hippocampal pyramidal cells in vivo: activity-dependent phase-precession of action potentials. *Hippocampus* 8(3):244–261.

Kanter BR, CM Lykken, D Avesar, A Weible, J Dickinson, B Dunn, NZ Borgesius, Y Roudi, CG Kentros (2017) A novel mechanism for the grid-to-place cell transformation revealed by transgenic depolarization of medial entorhinal cortex layer II. *Neuron* 93(6):1480–1492, e1486.

Karlsson MP, LM Frank (2009) Awake replay of remote experiences in the hippocampus. *Nat Neurosci* 12(7):913–918.

Kart-Teke, E, MA De Souza Silva, JP Huston, E Dere (2006) Wistar rats show episodic-like memory for unique experiences. *Neurobiol Learn Mem* 85(2):173–182.

Kaufman AM, T Geiller, A Losonczy (2020) A role for the locus coeruleus in hippocampal CA1 place cell reorganization during spatial reward learning. *Neuron* 105(6):1018–1026, e1014.

Kaut KP, MD Bunsey (2001) The effects of lesions to the rat hippocampus or rhinal cortex on olfactory and spatial memory: retrograde and anterograde findings. *Cogn Affect Behav Neurosci* 1(3):270–286.

Kaut KP, MD Bunsey, DC Riccio (2003) Olfactory learning and memory impairments following lesions to the hippocampus and perirhinal-entorhinal cortex. *Behav Neurosci* 117(2):304–319.

Kawai R, T Markman, R Poddar, R Ko, AL Fantana, AK Dhawale, AR Kampff, BP Olveczky (2015) Motor cortex is required for learning but not for executing a motor skill. *Neuron* 86(3):800–812.

Kawakami R, A Dobi, R Shigemoto, I Ito (2008) Right isomerism of the brain in inversus viscerum mutant mice. *PLoS One* 3(4):e1945.

Kawakami R, Y Shinohara, Y Kato, H Sugiyama, R Shigemoto, I Ito (2003) Asymmetrical allocation of NMDA receptor epsilon2 subunits in hippocampal circuitry. *Science* 300(5621):990–994.

Kentros CG, NT Agnihotri, S Streater, RD Hawkins, ER Kandel (2004) Increased attention to spatial context increases both place field stability and spatial memory. *Neuron* 42(2):283–295.

Kentros C, E Hargreaves, RD Hawkins, ER Kandel, M Shapiro, RU Muller (1998) Abolition of long-term stability of new hippocampal place cell maps by NMDA receptor blockade. *Science* 280(5372):2121–2126.

Keshavarzi S, EF Bracey, RA Faville, D Campagner, AL Tyson, SC Lenzi, T Branco, TW Margrie (2022) Multisensory coding of angular head velocity in the retrosplenial cortex. *Neuron* 110(3):532–543, e539.

Kinkhabwala AA, Y Gu, D Aronov, DW Tank (2020) Visual cue-related activity of cells in the medial entorhinal cortex during navigation in virtual reality. *Elife* 9:e43140.

Kjelstrup KB, T Solstad, VH Brun, T Hafting, S Leutgeb, MP Witter, EI Moser, MB Moser (2008) Finite scale of spatial representation in the hippocampus. *Science* 321(5885):140–143.

Klausberger T, P Somogyi (2008) Neuronal diversity and temporal dynamics: the unity of hippocampal circuit operations. *Science* 321(5885):53–57.

Kleinfeld D, M Deschenes, N Ulanovsky (2016) Whisking, sniffing, and the hippocampal theta-rhythm: a tale of two oscillators. *PLoS Biol* 14(2):e1002385.

Klur S, C Muller, A Pereira de Vasconcelos, T Ballard, J Lopez, R Galani, U Certa, JC Cassel (2009) Hippocampal-dependent spatial memory functions might be lateralized in rats: an approach combining gene expression profiling and reversible inactivation. *Hippocampus* 19(9):800–816.

Knierim JJ, HS Kudrimoti, BL McNaughton (1995) Place cells, head direction cells, and the learning of landmark stability. *J Neurosci* 15(3 Pt 1):1648–1659.

Kobayashi T, H Nishijo, M Fukuda, J Bures, T Ono (1997) Task-dependent representations in rat hippocampal place neurons. *J Neurophysiol* 78(2):597–613.

Kocsis B, S Martínez-Bellver, R Fiáth, A Domonkos, K Sviatkó, P Barthó, TF Freund, I Ulbert, S Káli, V Varga, et al. (2022) Huygens synchronization of medial septal pacemaker neurons generates hippocampal theta oscillation. *Cell Rep* 40(5):111149.

Koenig J, AN Linder, JK Leutgeb, S Leutgeb (2011) The spatial periodicity of grid cells is not sustained during reduced theta oscillations. *Science* 332(6029):592–595.

Kohl MM, OA Shipton, RM Deacon, JN Rawlins, K Deisseroth, O Paulsen (2011) Hemisphere-specific optogenetic stimulation reveals left-right asymmetry of hippocampal plasticity 5. *Nat Neurosci* 14(11):1413–1415.

Kohler C, V Chan-Palay, JY Wu (1984) Septal neurons containing glutamic acid decarboxylase immunoreactivity project to the hippocampal region in the rat brain. *Anat Embryol (Berl)* 169(1):41–44.

Kolb B, J Walkey (1987) Behavioural and anatomical studies of the posterior parietal cortex in the rat. *Behav Brain Res* 23(2):127–145.

Komorowski RW, CG Garcia, A Wilson, S Hattori, MW Howard, H Eichenbaum (2013) Ventral hippocampal neurons are shaped by experience to represent behaviorally relevant contexts. *J Neurosci* 33(18):8079–8087.

Komorowski RW, JR Manns, H Eichenbaum (2009) Robust conjunctive item-place coding by hippocampal neurons parallels learning what happens where. *J Neurosci* 29(31):9918–9929.

Konopacki J, MB MacIver, BH Bland, SH Roth (1987) Carbachol-induced EEG "theta" activity in hippocampal brain slices. *Brain Res* 405(1):196–198.

Kopec CD, E Real, HW Kessels, R Malinow (2007) GluR1 links structural and functional plasticity at excitatory synapses. *J Neurosci* 27(50):13706–13718.

Kornblith S, R Quian Quiroga, C Koch, I Fried, F Mormann (2017) Persistent single-neuron activity during working memory in the human medial temporal lobe. *Curr Biol* 27(7):1026–1032.

Kraus BJ, MP Brandon, RJ Robinson, 2nd, MA Connerney, ME Hasselmo, H Eichenbaum (2015) During running in place, grid cells integrate elapsed time and distance run. *Neuron* 88(3):578–589.

Kraus BJ, RJ Robinson, 2nd, JA White, H Eichenbaum, ME Hasselmo (2013) Hippocampal time cells: time versus path integration. *Neuron* 78(6):1090–1101.

Kropff E, JE Carmichael, MB Moser, EI Moser (2015) Speed cells in the medial entorhinal cortex. *Nature* 523(7561):419–424.

Krupic J, N Burgess, J O'Keefe (2012) Neural representations of location composed of spatially periodic bands 1. *Science* 337(6096):853–857.

Kudrimoti HS, CA Barnes, BL McNaughton (1999) Reactivation of hippocampal cell assemblies: effects of behavioral state, experience, and EEG dynamics. *J Neurosci* 19(10):4090–4101.

LaChance PA, TP Todd, JS Taube (2019) A sense of space in postrhinal cortex. *Science* 365(6449):eaax4192.

Langston RF, JA Ainge, JJ Couey, CB Canto, TL Bjerknes, MP Witter, EI Moser, MB Moser (2010) Development of the spatial representation system in the rat. *Science* 328(5985):1576–1580.

Larkin MC, C Lykken, LD Tye, JG Wickelgren, LM Frank (2014) Hippocampal output area CA1 broadcasts a generalized novelty signal during an object-place recognition task. *Hippocampus* 24(7):773–783.

Latuske P, O Kornienko, L Kohler, K Allen (2017) Hippocampal remapping and its entorhinal origin. *Front Behav Neurosci* 11:253.

Lee AK, MA Wilson (2002) Memory of sequential experience in the hippocampus during slow wave sleep. *Neuron* 36(6):1183–1194.

Lee AM, JL Hoy, A Bonci, L Wilbrecht, MP Stryker, CM Niell (2014) Identification of a brainstem circuit regulating visual cortical state in parallel with locomotion. *Neuron* 83(2):455–466.

Lee D, BJ Lin, AK Lee (2012) Hippocampal place fields emerge upon single-cell manipulation of excitability during behavior. *Science* 337(6096):849–853.

Lee H, JW Ghim, H Kim, D Lee, M Jung (2012) Hippocampal neural correlates for values of experienced events. *J Neurosci* 32(43):15053–15065.

Lee I, AL Griffin, EA Zilli, H Eichenbaum, ME Hasselmo (2006) Gradual translocation of spatial correlates of neuronal firing in the hippocampus toward prospective reward locations. *Neuron* 51(5):639–650.

Lee I, D Yoganarasimha, G Rao, JJ Knierim (2004) Comparison of population coherence of place cells in hippocampal subfields CA1 and CA3. *Nature* 430(6998):456–459.

Lee SH, N Huh, JW Lee, JW Ghim, I Lee, MW Jung (2017) Neural signals related to outcome evaluation are stronger in CA1 than CA3. *Front Neural Circuits* 11:40.

Lenck-Santini PP, E Save, B Poucet (2001) Place-cell firing does not depend on the direction of turn in a Y-maze alternation task. *Eur J Neurosci* 13(5):1055–1058.

Leranth C, M Frotscher (1987) Cholinergic innervation of hippocampal GAD- and somatostatin-immunoreactive commissural neurons. *J Comp Neurol* 261(1):33–47.

Leutgeb JK, S Leutgeb, MB Moser, EI Moser (2007) Pattern separation in the dentate gyrus and CA3 of the hippocampus. *Science* 315(5814):961–966.

Leutgeb JK, S Leutgeb, A Treves, R Meyer, CA Barnes, BL McNaughton, MB Moser, EI Moser (2005) Progressive transformation of hippocampal neuronal representations in morphed environments. *Neuron* 48(2):345–358.

Leutgeb S, JK Leutgeb, A Treves, MB Moser, EI Moser (2004) Distinct ensemble codes in hippocampal areas CA3 and CA1. *Science* 305(5688):1295–1298.

Leutgeb S, JK Leutgeb, CA Barnes, EI Moser, BL McNaughton, MB Moser (2005) Independent codes for spatial and episodic memory in hippocampal neuronal ensembles. *Science* 309(5734):619–623.

Leutgeb S, SJ Mizumori (2002) Context-specific spatial representations by lateral septal cells. *Neuroscience* 112(3):655–663.

Lever C, S Burton, A Jeewajee, J O'Keefe, N Burgess (2009) Boundary vector cells in the subiculum of the hippocampal formation. *J Neurosci* 29(31):9771–9777.

Lever C, T Wills, F Cacucci, N Burgess, J O'Keefe (2002) Long-term plasticity in hippocampal place-cell representation of environmental geometry. *Nature* 416(6876):90–94.

Lovett-Barron, M, P Kaifosh, MA Kheirbek, N Danielson, JD Zaremba, TR Reardon, GF Turi, R Hen, BV Zemelman, A Losonczy (2014) Dendritic inhibition in the hippocampus supports fear learning. *Science* 343(6173):857–863.

Lu L, JK Leutgeb, A Tsao, EJ Henriksen, S Leutgeb, CA Barnes, MP Witter, MB Moser, EI Moser (2013) Impaired hippocampal rate coding after lesions of the lateral entorhinal cortex. *Nat Neurosci* 16(8):1085–1093.

Lu L, Y Ren, T Yu, Z Liu, S Wang, L Tan, J Zeng, Q Feng, R Lin, Y Liu, et al. (2020) Control of locomotor speed, arousal, and hippocampal theta rhythms by the nucleus incertus. *Nat Commun* 11(1):262.

Lubenov EV, AG Siapas (2009) Hippocampal theta oscillations are travelling waves. *Nature* 459(7246):534–539.

Ludvig N, HM Tang, BC Gohil, JM Botero (2004) Detecting location-specific neuronal firing rate increases in the hippocampus of freely-moving monkeys. *Brain Res* 1014(1–2):97–109.

Macdonald CJ, KQ Lepage, UT Eden, H Eichenbaum (2011) Hippocampal time cells bridge the gap in memory for discontiguous events 7. *Neuron* 71(4):737–749.

Macrides F, HB Eichenbaum, WB Forbes (1982) Temporal relationship between sniffing and the limbic theta rhythm during odor discrimination reversal learning. *J.Neurosci* 2(12):1705–1717.

Magee JC, D Johnston (1997) A synaptically controlled, associative signal for Hebbian plasticity in hippocampal neurons. *Science* 275(5297):209–213.

Maguire EA, N Burgess, JG Donnett, RS Frackowiak, CD Frith, J O'Keefe (1998) Knowing where and getting there: a human navigation network. *Science* 280(5365):921–924.

Maguire EA, R Nannery, HJ Spiers (2006) Navigation around London by a taxi driver with bilateral hippocampal lesions. *Brain* 129(Pt 11):2894–2907.

Mair RG, JA Burk, MC Porter (1998) Lesions of the frontal cortex, hippocampus, and intralaminar thalamic nuclei have distinct effects on remembering in rats. *Behav Neurosci* 112(4):772–792.

Mankin EA, GW Diehl, FT Sparks, S Leutgeb, JK Leutgeb (2015) Hippocampal CA2 activity patterns change over time to a larger extent than between spatial contexts. *Neuron* 85(1):190–201.

Mankin EA, FT Sparks, B Slayyeh, RJ Sutherland, S Leutgeb, JK Leutgeb (2012) Neuronal code for extended time in the hippocampus. *Proc Natl Acad Sci U S A* 109(47):19462–19467.

Manns ID, L Mainville, BE Jones (2001) Evidence for glutamate, in addition to acetylcholine and GABA, neurotransmitter synthesis in basal forebrain neurons projecting to the entorhinal cortex. *Neuroscience* 107(2):249–263.

Manns JR, H Eichenbaum (2009) A cognitive map for object memory in the hippocampus. *Learn Mem* 16(10):616–624.

Manns JR, MW Howard, H Eichenbaum (2007) Gradual changes in hippocampal activity support remembering the order of events. *Neuron* 56(3):530–540.

Markram H, J Lubke, M Frotscher, B Sakmann (1997) Regulation of synaptic efficacy by coincidence of postsynaptic APs and EPSPs. *Science* 275(5297):213–215.

Mao D, E Avila, B Caziot, J Laurens, JD Dickman, DE Angelaki (2021) Spatial modulation of hippocampal activity in freely moving macaques. *Neuron* 109(21):3521–3534, e3526.

Mao D, S Kandler, BL McNaughton, V Bonin (2017) Sparse orthogonal population representation of spatial context in the retrosplenial cortex. *Nat Commun* 8(1):243.

Mao D, AR Neumann, J Sun, V Bonin, MH Mohajerani, BL McNaughton (2018) Hippocampus-dependent emergence of spatial sequence coding in retrosplenial cortex. *Proc Natl Acad Sci U S A* 115(31):8015–8018.

Markus EJ, YL Qin, B Leonard, WE Skaggs, BL McNaughton, CA Barnes (1995) Interactions between location and task affect the spatial and directional firing of hippocampal neurons. *J Neurosci* 15(11):7079–7094.

Martin MM, KL Horn, KJ Kusman, DG Wallace (2007) Medial septum lesions disrupt exploratory trip organization: evidence for septohippocampal involvement in dead reckoning. *Physiol Behav* 90(2–3):412–424.

Matsumura N, H Nishijo, R Tamura, S Eifuku, S Endo, T Ono (1999) Spatial- and task-dependent neuronal responses during real and virtual translocation in the monkey hippocampal formation. *J Neurosci* 19(6):2381–2393.

Maviel T, TP Durkin, F Menzaghi, B Bontempi (2004) Sites of neocortical reorganization critical for remote spatial memory. *Science* 305(5680):96–99.

McKenzie S, R Huszar, DF English, K Kim, F Christensen, E Yoon, G Buzsaki (2021) Preexisting hippocampal network dynamics constrain optogenetically induced place fields. *Neuron* 109(6):1040–1054, e1047.

McKenzie S, NT Robinson, L Herrera, JC Churchill, H Eichenbaum (2013) Learning causes reorganization of neuronal firing patterns to represent related experiences within a hippocampal schema. *J Neurosci* 33(25):10243–10256.

McKenzie S (2018) Inhibition shapes the organization of hippocampal representations. *Hippocampus* 28(9):659–671.

McNaughton BL, CA Barnes, JL Gerrard, K Gothard, MW Jung, JJ Knierim, H Kudrimoti, Y Qin, WE Skaggs, M Suster, et al. (1996) Deciphering the hippocampal polyglot: the hippocampus as a path integration system. *J Exp Biol* 199 (Pt 1):173–185.

McNaughton BL, CA Barnes, J O'Keefe (1983) The contributions of position, direction, and velocity to single unit activity in the hippocampus of freely-moving rats. *Exp Brain Res* 52(1):41–49.

McNaughton BL, FP Battaglia, O Jensen, EI Moser, MB Moser (2006) Path integration and the neural basis of the "cognitive map." *Nat Rev Neurosci* 7(8):663–678.

McNaughton BL, LL Chen, EJ Markus (1991) Dead reckoning, landmark learning, and the sense of direction: a neurophysiological and computational hypothesis. *J Cogn Neurosci* 3(2):190–202.

McNaughton BL, SJ Mizumori, CA Barnes, BJ Leonard, M Marquis, EJ Green (1994) Cortical representation of motion during unrestrained spatial navigation in the rat. *Cereb Cortex* 4(1):27–39.

Meck WH, RM Church, MS Matell (2013) Hippocampus, time, and memory—a retrospective analysis. *Behav Neurosci* 127(5):642–654.

Meck WH, RM Church, DS Olton (1984) Hippocampus, time, and memory. *Behav Neurosci* 98(1):3–22.

Miao C, Q Cao, HT Ito, H Yamahachi, MP Witter, MB Moser, EI Moser (2015) Hippocampal remapping after partial inactivation of the medial entorhinal cortex. *Neuron* 88(3):590–603.

Miller JF, M Neufang, A Solway, A Brandt, M Trippel, I Mader, S Hefft, M Merkow, SM Polyn, J Jacobs, et al. (2013) Neural activity in human hippocampal formation reveals the spatial context of retrieved memories. *Science* 342(6162):1111–1114.

Miller VM, PJ Best (1980) Spatial correlates of hippocampal unit activity are altered by lesions of the fornix and endorhinal cortex. *Brain Res* 194(2):311–323.

Mitchell AS, R Czajkowski, N Zhang, K Jeffery, A. JD Nelson (2018) Retrosplenial cortex and its role in spatial cognition. *Brain Neurosci Adv* 2:2398212818757098.

Mizumori SJ, CA Barnes, BL McNaughton (1989) Reversible inactivation of the medial septum: selective effects on the spontaneous unit activity of different hippocampal cell types. *Brain Res* 500(1–2):99–106.

Mizuseki K, S Royer, K Diba, G Buzsaki (2012) Activity dynamics and behavioral correlates of CA3 and CA1 hippocampal pyramidal neurons 10. *Hippocampus* 22(8):1659–1680.

Monaco JD, LF Abbott (2011) Modular realignment of entorhinal grid cell activity as a basis for hippocampal remapping. *J Neurosci* 31(25):9414–9425.

Montoya CP, RS Sainsbury (1985) The effects of entorhinal cortex lesions on type 1 and type 2 theta. *Physiol Behav* 35(1):121–126.

Morishita W, W Lu, GB Smith, RA Nicoll, MF Bear, RC Malenka (2007) Activation of NR2B-containing NMDA receptors is not required for NMDA receptor-dependent long-term depression. *Neuropharmacology* 52(1):71–76.

Morris RG, P Garrud, JN Rawlins, J O'Keefe (1982) Place navigation impaired in rats with hippocampal lesions. *Nature* 297(5868):681–683.

Moser EI, MB Moser (2008) A metric for space. *Hippocampus* 18(12):1142–1156.

Moser MB, EI Moser, E Forrest, P Andersen, RG Morris (1995) Spatial learning with a minislab in the dorsal hippocampus. *Proc Natl Acad Sci U S A* 92(21):9697–9701.

Mou X, J Cheng, YSW Yu, SE Kee, D Ji (2018) Comparing mouse and rat hippocampal place cell activities and firing sequences in the same environments. *Front Cell Neurosci* 12:332.

Muessig L, J Hauser, TJ Wills, F Cacucci (2015) A developmental switch in place cell accuracy coincides with grid cell maturation. *Neuron* 86(5):1167–1173.

Muller C, S Remy (2018) Septo-hippocampal interaction. *Cell Tissue Res* 373(3):565–575.

Muller RU, JL Kubie (1987) The effects of changes in the environment on the spatial firing of hippocampal complex-spike cells. *J Neurosci* 7(7):1951–1968.

Muller RU, JL Kubie (1989) The firing of hippocampal place cells predicts the future position of freely moving rats. *J Neurosci* 9(12):4101–4110.

Muller RU, JL Kubie, JB Ranck, Jr (1987) Spatial firing patterns of hippocampal complex-spike cells in a fixed environment. *J Neurosci* 7(7):1935–1950.

Mumby DG, JP Pinel (1994) Rhinal cortex lesions and object recognition in rats. *Behav Neurosci* 108(1):11–18.

Nadasdy Z, H Hirase, A Czurko, J Csicsvari, G Buzsaki (1999) Replay and time compression of recurring spike sequences in the hippocampus. *J Neurosci* 19(21):9497–9507.

Nagele J, A VM Herz, MB Stemmler (2020) Untethered firing fields and intermittent silences: why grid-cell discharge is so variable. *Hippocampus* 30(4):367–383.

Nakamura K (1999) Auditory spatial discriminatory and mnemonic neurons in rat posterior parietal cortex. *J Neurophysiol* 82(5):2503–2517.

Neo P, D Carter, Y Zheng, P Smith, C Darlington, N McNaughton (2012) Septal elicitation of hippocampal theta rhythm did not repair cognitive and emotional deficits resulting from vestibular lesions. *Hippocampus* 22(5):1176–1187.

Nitz DA (2006) Tracking route progression in the posterior parietal cortex. *Neuron* 49(5):747–756.

Nonaka S, Y Tanaka, Y Okada, S Takeda, A Harada, Y Kanai, M Kido, N Hirokawa (1998) Randomization of left-right asymmetry due to loss of nodal cilia generating leftward flow of extraembryonic fluid in mice lacking KIF3B motor protein. *Cell* 95(6):829–837.

O'Keefe J (1976) Place units in the hippocampus of the freely moving rat. *Exp Neurol* 51(1):78–109.

O'Keefe J (1996) The spatial prepositions in English, vector grammar, the cognitive map theory. In: Language, Space (Bloom P, Peterson M, Nadel L, Garrett M, eds), pp 277–316. Cambridge, MA: MIT Press.

O'Keefe J, N Burgess (1996) Geometric determinants of the place fields of hippocampal neurons. *Nature* 381(6581):425–428.

O'Keefe J, N Burgess (2005) Dual phase and rate coding in hippocampal place cells: theoretical significance and relationship to entorhinal grid cells. *Hippocampus* 15(7):853–866.

O'Keefe J, N Burgess, JG Donnett, KJ Jeffery, EA Maguire (1998) Place cells, navigational accuracy, and the human hippocampus. *Philos Trans R Soc Lond B Biol Sci* 353(1373):1333–1340.

O'Keefe J, DH Conway (1978) Hippocampal place units in the freely moving rat: why they fire where they fire. *Exp Brain Res* 31(4):573–590.

O'Keefe J, J Dostrovsky (1971) The hippocampus as a spatial map: preliminary evidence from unit activity in the freely-moving rat. *Brain Res* 34(1):171–175.

O'Keefe J, J Krupic (2021) Do hippocampal pyramidal cells respond to nonspatial stimuli? *Physiol Rev* 101(3):1427–1456.

O'Keefe J, L Nadel (1978) The Hippocampus as a Cognitive Map. Oxford University Press, Oxford.

O'Keefe J, L Nadel (1979) Precis of O'Keefe and Nadel's *The Hippocampus as a Cognitive Map. The Behavioral and Brain Sciences* 2:487–533.

O'Keefe J, ML Recce (1993) Phase relationship between hippocampal place units and the EEG theta rhythm. *Hippocampus* 3(3):317–330.

O'Keefe J, A Speakman (1987) Single unit activity in the rat hippocampus during a spatial memory task. *Exp Brain Res* 68(1):1–27.

Olafsdottir HF, C Barry, AB Saleem, D Hassabis, HJ Spiers (2015) Hippocampal place cells construct reward related sequences through unexplored space. *Elife* 4:e06063.

Omer DB, SR Maimon, L Las, N Ulanovsky (2018) Social place-cells in the bat hippocampus. *Science* 359(6372):218–224.

Onimaru H, I Homma (2003) A novel functional neuron group for respiratory rhythm generation in the ventral medulla. *J Neurosci* 23(4):1478–1486.

Ormond J, J O'Keefe (2022) Hippocampal place cells have goal-oriented vector fields during navigation. *Nature* 607(7920):741–746.

Otto T, D Garruto (1997) Rhinal cortex lesions impair simultaneous olfactory discrimination learning in rats. *Behav Neurosci* 111(5):1146–1150.

Otto T, F Schottler, U Staubli, H Eichenbaum, G Lynch (1991) Hippocampus and olfactory discrimination learning: effects of entorhinal cortex lesions on olfactory learning and memory in a successive-cue, go-no-go task. *Behav Neurosci* 105(1):111–119.

Packard MG, BJ Knowlton (2002) Learning and memory functions of the basal ganglia. *Annu Rev Neurosci* 25:563–593.

Patel J, S Fujisawa, A Berenyi, S Royer, G Buzsaki (2012) Traveling theta waves along the entire septotemporal axis of the hippocampus 3. *Neuron* 75(3):410–417.

Parent MB, JN Darling, YO Henderson (2014) Remembering to eat: hippocampal regulation of meal onset. *Am J Physiol Regul Integr Comp Physiol* 306(10):R701–713.

Park E, D Dvorak, AA Fenton (2011) Ensemble place codes in hippocampus: CA1, CA3, and dentate gyrus place cells have multiple place fields in large environments 6. *PLoS ONE* **6**(7):e22349.

Parron C, E Save (2004) Evidence for entorhinal and parietal cortices involvement in path integration in the rat. *Exp Brain Res* **159**(3):349–359.

Pastalkova E, V Itskov, A Amarasingham, G Buzsaki (2008) Internally generated cell assembly sequences in the rat hippocampus. *Science* **321**(5894):1322–1327.

Patel J, S Fujisawa, A Berenyi, S Royer, G Buzsaki (2012) Traveling theta waves along the entire septotemporal axis of the hippocampus 3. *Neuron* **75**(3):410–417.

Paz-Villagran, V, PP Lenck-Santini, E Save, B Poucet (2002) Properties of place cell firing after damage to the visual cortex. *Eur J Neurosci* **16**(4):771–776.

Petrulis A, P Alvarez, H Eichenbaum (2005) Neural correlates of social odor recognition and the representation of individual distinctive social odors within entorhinal cortex and ventral subiculum. *Neuroscience* **130**(1):259–274.

Pfeiffer BE, DJ Foster (2013) Hippocampal place-cell sequences depict future paths to remembered goals. *Nature* **497**(7447):74–79.

Purandare CS, S Dhingra, R Rios, C Vuong, T To, A Hachisuka, K Choudhary, MR Mehta (2022) Moving bar of light evokes vectorial spatial selectivity in the immobile rat hippocampus. *Nature* **602**(7897):461–467.

Quian Quiroga R, A Kraskov, C Koch, I Fried (2009) Explicit encoding of multimodal percepts by single neurons in the human brain. *Curr Biol* **19**(15):1308–1313.

Quirk GJ, RU Muller, JL Kubie (1990) The firing of hippocampal place cells in the dark depends on the rat's recent experience. *J Neurosci* **10**(6):2008–2017.

Quirk GJ, RU Muller, JL Kubie, JB Ranck, Jr (1992) The positional firing properties of medial entorhinal neurons: description and comparison with hippocampal place cells. *J Neurosci* **12**(5):1945–1963.

Quiroga RQ, L Reddy, G Kreiman, C Koch, I Fried (2005) Invariant visual representation by single neurons in the human brain. *Nature* **435**(7045):1102–1107.

Rajasethupathy P, S Sankaran, JH Marshel, CK Kim, E Ferenczi, SY Lee, A Berndt, C Ramakrishnan, A Jaffe, M Lo, C Liston, K Deisseroth (2015) Projections from neocortex mediate top-down control of memory retrieval. *Nature* **526**(7575):653–659.

Ranck JB (1973) Studies on single neurons in dorsal hippocampal formation and septum in unrestrained rats: I. Behavioral correlates and firing repertoires. *Exp Neurol* **41**(2):461–531.

Rao RP, M von Heimendahl, V Bahr, M Brecht (2019) Neuronal responses to conspecifics in the ventral CA1. *Cell Rep* **27**(12):3460–3472, e3463.

Rich PD, HP Liaw, AK Lee (2014) Place cells: large environments reveal the statistical structure governing hippocampal representations. *Science* **345**(6198):814–817.

Robinson J, F Manseau, G Ducharme, B Amilhon, E Vigneault, S El Mestikawy, S Williams (2016) Optogenetic activation of septal glutamatergic neurons drive hippocampal theta rhythms. *J Neurosci* **36**(10):3016–3023.

Robinson NTM, JB Priestley, JW Rueckemann, AD Garcia, VA Smeglin, FA Marino, H Eichenbaum (2017) Medial entorhinal cortex selectively supports temporal coding by hippocampal neurons. *Neuron* **94**(3):677–688, e676.

Robinson TE (1980) Hippocampal rhythmic slow activity (RSA; theta): a critical analysis of selected studies and discussion of possible species-differences. *Brain Res* **203**(1):69–101.

Rolls ET (1999) Spatial view cells and the representation of place in the primate hippocampus. *Hippocampus* **9**(4):467–480.

Rolls ET, SM O'Mara (1995) View-responsive neurons in the primate hippocampal complex. *Hippocampus* **5**(5):409–424.

Rotenberg A, M Mayford, RD Hawkins, ER Kandel, RU Muller (1996) Mice expressing activated CaMKII lack low frequency LTP and do not form stable place cells in the CA1 region of the hippocampus. *Cell* **87**(7):1351–1361.

Rubin A, N Geva, L Sheintuch, Y Ziv (2015) Hippocampal ensemble dynamics timestamp events in long-term memory. *Elife* **4e:12247**.

Rudy JW, RJ Sutherland (1989) The hippocampal formation is necessary for rats to learn and remember configural discriminations. *Behav Brain Res* **34**(1–2):97–109.

Rudy JW, RJ Sutherland (1995) Configural association theory and the hippocampal formation: an appraisal and reconfiguration. *Hippocampus* **5**(5):375–389.

Rueckemann JW, AJ DiMauro, LM Rangel, X Han, ES Boyden, H Eichenbaum (2016) Transient optogenetic inactivation of the medial entorhinal cortex biases the active population of hippocampal neurons. *Hippocampus* **26**(2):246–260.

Russell NA, A Horii, PF Smith, CL Darlington, DK Bilkey (2006) Lesions of the vestibular system disrupt hippocampal theta rhythm in the rat. *J Neurophysiol* **96**(1):4–14.

Sabariego M, A Schonwald, BL Boublil, DT Zimmerman, S Ahmadi, N Gonzalez, C Leibold, RE Clark, JK Leutgeb, S Leutgeb (2019) Time cells in the hippocampus are neither dependent on medial entorhinal cortex inputs nor necessary for spatial working memory. *Neuron* **102**(6):1235–1248, e1235.

Sainsbury RS, A Heynen, CP Montoya (1987) Behavioral correlates of hippocampal type 2 theta in the rat. *Physiol Behav* **39**(4):513–519.

Sakaguchi Y, Y Sakurai (2020) Left-right functional difference of the rat dorsal hippocampus for short-term memory and long-term memory. *Behav Brain Res* **382**:112478.

Salz DM, Z Tiganj, S Khasnabish, A Kohley, D Sheehan, MW Howard, H Eichenbaum (2016) Time cells in hippocampal area CA3. *J Neurosci* **36**(28):7476–7484.

Sarel A, A Finkelstein, L Las, N Ulanovsky (2017) Vectorial representation of spatial goals in the hippocampus of bats. *Science* **355**(6321):176–180.

Sargolini F, M Fyhn, T Hafting, BL McNaughton, MP Witter, MB Moser, EI Moser (2006) Conjunctive representation of position, direction, and velocity in entorhinal cortex. *Science* **312**(5774):758–762.

Save E, V Paz-Villagran, T Alexinsky, B Poucet (2005) Functional interaction between the associative parietal cortex and hippocampal place cell firing in the rat. *Eur J Neurosci* **21**(2):522–530.

Save E, B Poucet (2000) Involvement of the hippocampus and associative parietal cortex in the use of proximal and distal landmarks for navigation. *Behav Brain Res* **109**(2):195–206.

Scaplen KM, AA Gulati, VL Heimer-McGinn, RD Burwell (2014) Objects and landmarks: hippocampal place cells respond differently to manipulations of visual cues depending on size, perspective, and experience. *Hippocampus* **24**(11):1287–1299.

Schacter DL, M Moscovitch, E Tulving, DR McLachlan, M Freedman (1986) Mnemonic precedence in amnesic patients: an analogue of the AB error in infants? *Child Dev* **57**(3):816–823.

Schiller J, Y Schiller, DE Clapham (1998) NMDA receptors amplify calcium influx into dendritic spines during associative pre- and postsynaptic activation. *Nat Neurosci* **1**(2):114–118.

Schlesiger MI, BL Boublil, JB Hales, JK Leutgeb, S Leutgeb (2018) Hippocampal global remapping can occur without input from the medial entorhinal cortex. *Cell Rep* **22**(12):3152–3159.

Schlesiger MI, CC Cannova, BL Boublil, JB Hales, EA Mankin, MP Brandon, JK Leutgeb, C Leibold, S Leutgeb (2015) The medial entorhinal cortex is necessary for temporal organization of hippocampal neuronal activity. *Nat Neurosci* **18**(8):1123–1132.

Schoenenberger P, J O'Neill, J Csicsvari (2016) Activity-dependent plasticity of hippocampal place maps. *Nat Commun* 7:11824.

Semba K, HC Fibiger (1992) Afferent connections of the laterodorsal and the pedunculopontine tegmental nuclei in the rat: a retro- and antero-grade transport and immunohistochemical study. *J Comp Neurol* 323(3):387–410.

Shan KQ, EV Lubenov, M Papadopoulou, AG Siapas (2016) Spatial tuning and brain state account for dorsal hippocampal CA1 activity in a non-spatial learning task. *Elife* 5:e14321.

Sharp PE (1999a) Comparison of the timing of hippocampal and subicular spatial signals: implications for path integration. *Hippocampus* 9(2):158–172.

Sharp PE (1999b) Complimentary roles for hippocampal versus subicular/entorhinal place cells in coding place, context, and events. *Hippocampus* 9(4):432–443.

Sheffield ME, DA Dombeck (2015) Calcium transient prevalence across the dendritic arbour predicts place field properties. *Nature* 517(7533):200–204.

Sheffield MEJ, MD Adoff, DA Dombeck (2017) Increased prevalence of calcium transients across the dendritic arbor during place field formation. *Neuron* 96(2):490–504, e495.

Shi SH, Y Hayashi, RS Petralia, SH Zaman, RJ Wenthold, K Svoboda, R Malinow (1999) Rapid spine delivery and redistribution of AMPA receptors after synaptic NMDA receptor activation. *Science* 284(5421):1811–1816.

Shin J (2010) Passive rotation-induced theta rhythm and orientation homeostasis response. *Synapse* 64(5):409–415.

Shinohara Y, H Hirase (2009) Size and receptor density of glutamatergic synapses: a viewpoint from left-right asymmetry of CA3-CA1 connections. *Front Neuroanat* 3:10.

Shinohara Y, H Hirase, M Watanabe, M Itakura, M Takahashi, R Shigemoto (2008) Left-right asymmetry of the hippocampal synapses with differential subunit allocation of glutamate receptors. *Proc Natl Acad Sci U S A* 105(49):19498–19503.

Shinohara Y, A Hosoya, N Yamasaki, H Ahmed, S Hattori, M Eguchi, S Yamaguchi, T Miyakawa, H Hirase, R Shigemoto (2012) Right-hemispheric dominance of spatial memory in split-brain mice. *Hippocampus* 22(2):117–121.

Shipton OA, M El-Gaby, J Apergis-Schoute, K Deisseroth, DM Bannerman, O Paulsen, MM Kohl (2014) Left-right dissociation of hippocampal memory processes in mice. *Proc Natl Acad Sci U S A* 111(42):15238–15243.

Siegel JJ, JP Neunuebel, JJ Knierim (2008) Dominance of the proximal coordinate frame in determining the locations of hippocampal place cell activity during navigation. *J Neurophysiol* 99(1):60–76.

Smith JC, HH Ellenberger, K Ballanyi, DW Richter, JL Feldman (1991) Pre-Botzinger complex: a brainstem region that may generate respiratory rhythm in mammals. *Science* 254(5032):726–729.

Solstad T, CN Boccara, E Kropff, MB Moser, EI Moser (2008) Representation of geometric borders in the entorhinal cortex. *Science* 322(5909):1865–1868.

Solstad T, EI Moser, GT Einevoll (2006) From grid cells to place cells: a mathematical model. *Hippocampus* 16(12):1026–1031.

Spiers HJ, HF Olafsdottir, C Lever (2018) Hippocampal CA1 activity correlated with the distance to the goal and navigation performance. *Hippocampus* 28(9):644–658.

Squire LR (1992) Memory and the hippocampus: a synthesis from findings with rats, monkeys, and humans [published erratum appears in Psychol Rev 1992 Jul;99(3):582]. *Psychol Rev* 99(2):195–231.

Stachenfeld KL, MM Botvinick, SJ Gershman (2017) The hippocampus as a predictive map. *Nat Neurosci* 20(11):1643–1653.

Stackman RW, JS Taube (1998) Firing properties of rat lateral mammillary single units: head direction, head pitch, and angular head velocity. *J Neurosci* 18(21):9020–9037.

Sun C, W Yang, J Martin, S Tonegawa (2020) Hippocampal neurons represent events as transferable units of experience. *Nat Neurosci* 23(5):651–663.

Suthana NA, NN Parikshak, AD Ekstrom, MJ Ison, BJ Knowlton, SY Bookheimer, I Fried (2015) Specific responses of human hippocampal neurons are associated with better memory. *Proc Natl Acad Sci U S A* 112(33):10503–10508.

Sutherland RJ, IQ Whishaw, B Kolb (1988) Contributions of cingulate cortex to two forms of spatial learning and memory. *J Neurosci* 8(6):1863–1872.

Suzuki WA, EK Miller, R Desimone (1997) Object and place memory in the macaque entorhinal cortex. *J Neurophysiol* 78(2):1062–1081.

Tai SK, LS Leung (2012) Vestibular stimulation enhances hippocampal long-term potentiation via activation of cholinergic septohippocampal cells. *Behav Brain Res* 232(1):174–182.

Tai SK, J Ma, KP Ossenkopp, LS Leung (2012) Activation of immobility-related hippocampal theta by cholinergic septohippocampal neurons during vestibular stimulation. *Hippocampus* 22(4):914–925.

Takahashi H, JC Magee (2009) Pathway interactions and synaptic plasticity in the dendritic tuft regions of CA1 pyramidal neurons. *Neuron* 62(1):102–111.

Takeuchi T, AJ Duszkiewicz, A Sonneborn, PA Spooner, M Yamasaki, M Watanabe, CC Smith, G Fernandez, K Deisseroth, RW Greene, et al. (2016) Locus coeruleus and dopaminergic consolidation of everyday memory. *Nature* 537(7620):357–362.

Tan HM, JP Bassett, J O'Keefe, F Cacucci, TJ Wills (2015) The development of the head direction system before eye opening in the rat. *Curr Biol* 25(4):479–483.

Tang AC (2001) Neonatal exposure to novel environment enhances hippocampal-dependent memory function during infancy and adulthood. *Learn Mem* 8(5):257–264.

Tang AC, BC Reeb (2004) Neonatal novelty exposure, dynamics of brain asymmetry, and social recognition memory. *Dev Psychobiol* 44(1):84–93.

Tang AC, B Zou (2002) Neonatal exposure to novelty enhances long-term potentiation in CA1 of the rat hippocampus. *Hippocampus* 12(3):398–404.

Tang AC, B Zou, BC Reeb, JA Connor (2008) An epigenetic induction of a right-shift in hippocampal asymmetry: selectivity for short- and long-term potentiation but not post-tetanic potentiation. *Hippocampus* 18(1):5–10.

Taube JS (1995a) Head direction cells recorded in the anterior thalamic nuclei of freely moving rats. *J Neurosci* 15(1 Pt 1):70–86.

Taube JS (1995b) Place cells recorded in the parasubiculum of freely moving rats. *Hippocampus* 5(6):569–583.

Taube JS (2007) The head direction signal: origins and sensory-motor integration 21. *Annu Rev Neurosci* 30:181–207.

Taube JS, RU Muller (1998) Comparisons of head direction cell activity in the postsubiculum and anterior thalamus of freely moving rats. *Hippocampus* 8(2):87–108.

Taube JS, RU Muller, JB Ranck, Jr (1990) Head-direction cells recorded from the postsubiculum in freely moving rats: II. Effects of environmental manipulations. *J Neurosci* 10(2):436–447.

Tennant SA, L Fischer, DLF Garden, KZ Gerlei, C Martinez-Gonzalez, C McClure, ER Wood, MF Nolan (2018) Stellate cells in the medial entorhinal cortex are required for spatial learning. *Cell Rep* 22(5):1313–1324.

Terada S, Y Sakurai, H Nakahara, S Fujisawa (2017) Temporal and rate coding for discrete event sequences in the hippocampus. *Neuron* 94(6):1248–1262, e1244.

Thach WT (1978) Correlation of neural discharge with pattern and force of muscular activity, joint position, and direction of intended next movement in motor cortex and cerebellum. *J Neurophysiol* 41(3):654–676.

Thompson LT, PJ Best (1989) Place cells and silent cells in the hippocampus of freely-behaving rats. *J Neurosci* 9(7):2382–2390.

Tingley D, K McClain, E Kaya, J Carpenter, G Buzsaki (2021) A metabolic function of the hippocampal sharp wave-ripple. *Nature* 597(7874):82–86.

Tryon VL, MR Penner, SW Heide, HO King, J Larkin, S. JY Mizumori (2017) Hippocampal neural activity reflects the economy of choices during goal-directed navigation. *Hippocampus* 27(7):743–758.

Tsanov M, E Chah, R Reilly, SM O'Mara (2014) Respiratory cycle entrainment of septal neurons mediates the fast coupling of sniffing rate and hippocampal theta rhythm. *Eur J Neurosci* 39(6):957–974.

Tsao A, MB Moser, EI Moser (2013) Traces of experience in the lateral entorhinal cortex. *Curr Biol* 23(5):399–405.

Tsao A, J Sugar, L Lu, C Wang, JJ Knierim, MB Moser, EI Moser (2018) Integrating time from experience in the lateral entorhinal cortex. *Nature* 561(7721):57–62.

Tseng PH, S Rajangam, G Lehew, MA Lebedev, M. AL Nicolelis (2018) Interbrain cortical synchronization encodes multiple aspects of social interactions in monkey pairs. *Sci Rep* 8(1):4699.

Ulanovsky N, CF Moss (2007) Hippocampal cellular and network activity in freely moving echolocating bats. *Nat Neurosci* 10(2):224–233.

Vaccari C, SJ Lolait, NL Ostrowski (1998) Comparative distribution of vasopressin V1b and oxytocin receptor messenger ribonucleic acids in brain. *Endocrinology* 139(12):5015–5033.

Van Groen, T, JM Wyss (2003) Connections of the retrosplenial granular b cortex in the rat. *J Comp Neurol* 463(3):249–263.

Vandecasteele M, V Varga, A Berenyi, E Papp, P Bartho, L Venance, TF Freund, G Buzsaki (2014) Optogenetic activation of septal cholinergic neurons suppresses sharp wave ripples and enhances theta oscillations in the hippocampus. *Proc Natl Acad Sci U S A* 111(37):13535–13540.

Vanderwolf CH (1969) Hippocampal electrical activity and voluntary movement in the rat. *Electroencephalogr Clin Neurophysiol* 26:407–418.

Vanderwolf CH, LW Leung, RK Cooley (1985) Pathways through cingulate, neo- and entorhinal cortices mediate atropine-resistant hippocampal rhythmical slow activity. *Brain Res* 347(1):58–73.

Vann SD, JP Aggleton (2005) Selective dysgranular retrosplenial cortex lesions in rats disrupt allocentric performance of the radial-arm maze task 59. *Behav Neurosci* 119(6):1682–1686.

Vann SD, JP Aggleton, EA Maguire (2009) What does the retrosplenial cortex do? 32. *Nat Rev Neurosci* 10(11):792–802.

Verstynen T, R Tierney, T Urbanski, A Tang (2001) Neonatal novelty exposure modulates hippocampal volumetric asymmetry in the rat. *Neuroreport* 12(14):3019–3022.

Villette V, A Malvache, T Tressard, N Dupuy, R Cossart (2015) Internally recurring hippocampal sequences as a population template of spatiotemporal information. *Neuron* 88(2):357–366.

von Heimendahl, M, RP Rao, M Brecht (2012) Weak and nondiscriminative responses to conspecifics in the rat hippocampus. *J Neurosci* 32(6):2129–2141.

Wang Y, S Romani, B Lustig, A Leonardo, E Pastalkova (2015) Theta sequences are essential for internally generated hippocampal firing fields. *Nat Neurosci* 18(2):282–288.

Watrous AJ, J Miller, SE Qasim, I Fried, J Jacobs (2018) Phase-tuned neuronal firing encodes human contextual representations for navigational goals. *Elife* 7:e32554.

Welker WI (1964) Analysis of sniffing of the albino rat. *Behaviour* 22(3/4):223–244.

Whishaw IQ (1985) Formation of a place learning-set by the rat: a new paradigm for neurobehavioral studies. *Physiol Behav* 35(1):139–143.

Whitlock JR, RJ Sutherland, MP Witter, MB Moser, EI Moser (2008) Navigating from hippocampus to parietal cortex. *Proc Natl Acad Sci U S A* 105(39):14755–14762.

Wilhite BL, TJ Teyler, C Hendricks (1986) Functional relations of the rodent claustral-entorhinal-hippocampal system. *Brain Res* 365(1):54–60.

Wills TJ, F Cacucci, N Burgess, J O'Keefe (2010) Development of the hippocampal cognitive map in preweanling rats. *Science* 328(5985):1573–1576.

Wilson MA, BL McNaughton (1993) Dynamics of the hippocampal ensemble code for space. *Science* 261(5124):1055–1058.

Wilson MA, BL McNaughton (1994) Reactivation of hippocampal ensemble memories during sleep. *Science* 265(5172):676–679.

Wintzer ME, R Boehringer, D Polygalov, TJ McHugh (2014) The hippocampal CA2 ensemble is sensitive to contextual change. *J Neurosci* 34(8):3056–3066.

Witter MP, TP Doan, B Jacobsen, ES Nilssen, S Ohara (2017) Architecture of the entorhinal cortex a review of entorhinal anatomy in rodents with some comparative notes. *Front Syst Neurosci* 11:46.

Wolbers T, C Buchel (2005) Dissociable retrosplenial and hippocampal contributions to successful formation of survey representations. *J Neurosci* 25(13):3333–3340.

Wood ER, PA Dudchenko, RJ Robitsek, H Eichenbaum (2000) Hippocampal neurons encode information about different types of memory episodes occurring in the same location. *Neuron* 27(3):623–633.

Wood RA, M Bauza, J Krupic, S Burton, A Delekate, D Chan, J O'Keefe (2018) The honeycomb maze provides a novel test to study hippocampal-dependent spatial navigation. *Nature* 554(7690):102–105.

Woolf NJ, LL Butcher (1989) Cholinergic systems in the rat brain: IV. Descending projections of the pontomesencephalic tegmentum. *Brain Res Bull* 23(6):519–540.

Wyss JM, T Van Groen (1992) Connections between the retrosplenial cortex and the hippocampal formation in the rat: a review. *Hippocampus* 2(1):1–11.

Xu W, DA Wilson (2012) Odor-evoked activity in the mouse lateral entorhinal cortex. *Neuroscience* 223:12–20.

Yadav N, C Noble, JE Niemeyer, A Terceros, J Victor, C Liston, P Rajasethupathy (2022) Prefrontal feature representations drive memory recall. *Nature* 608(7921):153–160.

Yartsev MM, N Ulanovsky (2013) Representation of three-dimensional space in the hippocampus of flying bats. *Science* 340(6130):367–372.

Yin A, PH Tseng, S Rajangam, MA Lebedev, MAL Nicolelis (2018) Place cell-like activity in the primary sensorimotor and premotor cortex during monkey whole-body navigation. *Sci Rep* 8(1):9184.

Young BJ, T Otto, GD Fox, H Eichenbaum (1997) Memory representation within the parahippocampal region. *J Neurosci* 17(13):5183–5195.

Zhang SJ, J Ye, C Miao, A Tsao, I Cerniauskas, D Ledergerber, MB Moser, EI Moser (2013) Optogenetic dissection of entorhinal-hippocampal functional connectivity. *Science* 340(6128):1232627.

Zhang X, DK Hannesson, DM Saucier, AE Wallace, J Howland, ME Corcoran (2001) Susceptibility to kindling and neuronal connections of the anterior claustrum. *J Neurosci* **21**(10):3674–3687.

Zhao R, SD Grunke, MM Keralapurath, MJ Yetman, A Lam, TC Lee, K Sousounis, Y Jiang, DA Swing, L Tessarollo, et al. (2016) Impaired recall of positional memory following chemogenetic disruption of place field stability. *Cell Rep* **16**(3):793–804.

Zhao X, Y Wang, N Spruston, JC Magee (2020) Membrane potential dynamics underlying context-dependent sensory responses in the hippocampus. *Nat Neurosci* **23**(7):881–891.

Zhou H, Q Zhou, L Xu (2016) Unilateral hippocampal inactivation or lesion selectively impairs remote contextual fear memory. *Psychopharmacology (Berl)* **233**(19–20):3639–3646.

Zhou TL, R Tamura, J Kuriwaki, T Ono (1999) Comparison of medial and lateral septal neuron activity during performance of spatial tasks in rats. *Hippocampus* **9**(3):220–234.

Zhou W, JD Crystal (2009) Evidence for remembering when events occurred in a rodent model of episodic memory. *Proc Natl Acad Sci U S A* **106**(23):9525–9529.

Zingg B, H Hintiryan, L Gou, MY Song, M Bay, MS Bienkowski, NN Foster, S Yamashita, I Bowman, AW Toga, et al. (2014) Neural networks of the mouse neocortex. *Cell* **156**(5):1096–1111.

Zinyuk L, S Kubik, Y Kaminsky, AA Fenton, J Bures (2000) Understanding hippocampal activity by using purposeful behavior: place navigation induces place cell discharge in both task-relevant and task- irrelevant spatial reference frames. *Proc Natl Acad Sci U S A* **97**(7):3771–3776.

Ziv Y, LD Burns, ED Cocker, EO Hamel, KK Ghosh, LJ Kitch, A El Gamal, MJ Schnitzer (2013) Long-term dynamics of CA1 hippocampal place codes. *Nat Neurosci* **16**(3):264–266.

Zutshi I, MP Brandon, ML Fu, ML Donegan, JK Leutgeb, S Leutgeb (2018) Hippocampal neural circuits respond to optogenetic pacing of theta frequencies by generating accelerated oscillation frequencies. *Curr Biol* **28**(8):1179–1188, e1173.

Zynyuk L, J Huxter, RU Muller, SE Fox (2012) The presence of a second rat has only subtle effects on the location-specific firing of hippocampal place cells. *Hippocampus* **22**(6):1405–1416.

12

The Entorhinal Cortex

Benjamin R. Kanter, Edvard I. Moser, and Menno P. Witter

12.1 Introduction

The entorhinal cortex (EC) is part of the multilayered cortical domain, directly adjacent to the archetypal three-layered hippocampal formation. EC shares several gross morphological features with the medially adjacent pre- and parasubiculum and all three are connectionally closely associated with the hippocampal formation and with each other. The laterally adjacent perirhinal cortex and the more caudally positioned parahippocampal (in primates) or postrhinal cortex (in nonprimates) form major cortical input and output structures of EC. These two areas share morphological features with adjacent neocortical areas and are generally considered to represent a kind of transition between pallial areas that originate the hippocampal formation and areas of the developing cortex from which the neocortex originates (see Chapter 4). Since these areas in the human brain are all part of, or directly adjacent to, the parahippocampal gyrus, they are often referred to together as the parahippocampal region (see also Chapter 3, sections 3.7.4 and 3.8).

Thanks to the early works of Ramón y Cajal, EC was considered an integral part of the hippocampal formation, mainly due to the strong connectivity between the two (see also Chapter 3). This concept was further strengthened by the seminal publications in the 1970s and 1980s showing that EC not only provides the main input pathway for cortical information to reach the hippocampal formation but also includes circuits to send hippocampally processed information back to the neocortex (Van Hoesen and Pandya, 1975; Steward, 1976; Steward and Scoville, 1976; Rosene and Van Hoesen, 1977). This notion provided strong support for the by now classical concept of hippocampal-neocortical interactions underlying episodic memory (Squire and Zola-Morgan, 1991; Buzsáki, 1996). Over time, EC became appreciated as a separate entity, contributing an additional and unique neural computational component to the circuits of the medial temporal lobe system. The discovery of the grid cell (Fyhn et al., 2004; Hafting et al., 2005) sparked a strong focus on EC, though mainly concerning the medial entorhinal cortex (MEC) and the spatially modulated neurons therein. This explosion of research on EC resulted in vast amounts of data and many new theoretical concepts on how the brain might represent higher order cognitive information.

Notions on the relevance of EC and how it contributes to the overall functions of the medial temporal lobe memory system have also changed dramatically since the times of Cajal and the first detailed anatomical and electrophysiological experiments on the system. In 1971, the place cell was first described in CA1 of the hippocampus (O'Keefe and Dostrovsky, 1971), and this observation was embedded in the then known canonical trisynaptic circuit, which has been extremely influential in the first decades of focused research on the hippocampal formation. Note that this circuit was not like what Cajal initially proposed, in which he emphasized the entorhinal to CA projections, but was based on contemporary connectivity studies in which EC to DG projections became the main point of entry for cortical information to enter the hippocampal formation (cf. Witter, Doan, et al., 2017) (Figure 12.1A). The trisynaptic circuit has been expanded and adjusted over the years, aiming to encompass a wealth of new data, pointing to complex connectional and functional diversities, but still maintained the concept of EC as being the start of a series of unidirectional connections, looping through HF with different points of entry, eventually returning to EC (Figure 12.1B). Further, EC was considered the structure holding reciprocal connections with the neocortex (see also Chapter 3). In our view, this connectional scheme (Figure 12.1) no longer adequately describes the current knowledge, and it does not facilitate an open exploration of the functional relevance of EC.

12.2 Definition of entorhinal cortex

12.2.1 Nomenclature, subdivisions, and macroscopic features

The name "the entorhinal cortex" refers to its position as a cortical area (partially) enclosed by the rhinal (olfactory) sulcus. Attention to this area was first raised by Ramón y Cajal, who described a particular part of the posterior temporal cortex, which he referred to as sphenoidal cortex/angular ganglion. He was impressed by the massive connection between this part of the cortex and the hippocampus by way of the temporoammonic tract, and this feature led him to propose a strong functional relationship between the two structures. It was Brodmann in 1909 who described EC based on cytoarchitectonic criteria, referring to it as area 28. Although Brodmann divided area 28 into two cytoarchitectonically different areas a and b, neither Ramón y Cajal nor his student Lorente de Nó saw reasons for such a subdivision. The latter author, however, related cytoarchitectonic differences to the hippocampal projections, so he distinguished lateral, intermediate, and medial subdivisions of

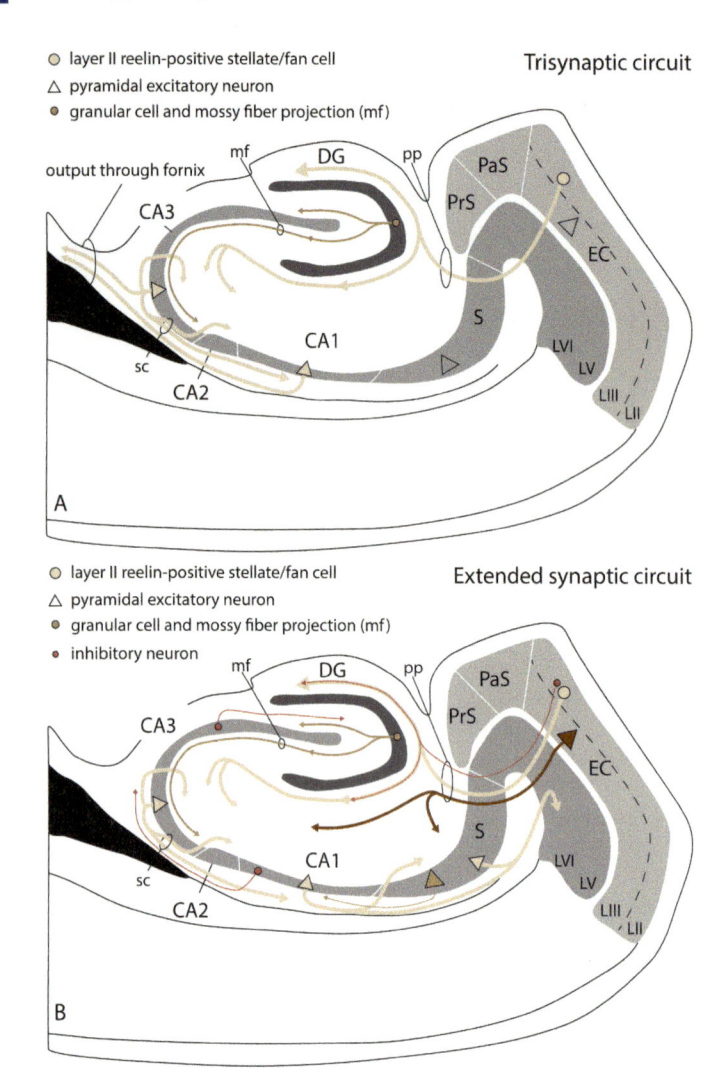

Trisynaptic circuit

○ layer II reelin-positive stellate/fan cell
△ pyramidal excitatory neuron
● granular cell and mossy fiber projection (mf)

Extended synaptic circuit

○ layer II reelin-positive stellate/fan cell
△ pyramidal excitatory neuron
● granular cell and mossy fiber projection (mf)
● inhibitory neuron

Figure 12.1 Schematic representation of entorhinal-hippocampal circuits. (A) The "standard" trisynaptic circuit. (B) The extended synaptic circuit.

EC. Combined cytoarchitectural and connectivity data still form a commonly accepted basis to define brain entities, although the addition of gene-expression profiles in adult and embryological brains has become a useful and often used additional criterion, supporting the view that EC, at least its lateral part, might be considered an entity separate from the hippocampal formation (Medina et al., 2017). Following the initial proposition of Ramón y Cajal, EC can be best defined based on its projections to the hippocampus. Since EC targets neurons in all main hippocampal subdivisions, and other parahippocampal divisions at least project to the CA field (especially CA1) and to the subiculum, it has become accepted to use projections to the dentate gyrus as the defining feature of EC. When knowledge of projections is not available, advancements in genetic profiling together with cyto- and chemoarchitectural criteria have enabled reliable delineation of EC.

In most rodents and insectivores, EC is situated in a ventroposterior part of the cortical mantle. In most carnivores, herbivores, bats, and lagomorphs, as well as in the guinea pig, EC occupies the posterior half to two-thirds of the so-called piriform lobe on the ventral surface of the brain. In rodents, lacking a well-developed ventrally positioned piriform lobe, EC is positioned ventrocaudally in the brain,

whereas in species with a less differentiated cortical mantle, as in both the erinaceous and tenrec hedgehog, EC is mainly found at the dorsocaudal surface of the hemisphere. In all these species, EC is surrounded by the rhinal sulcus. In primates, EC is positioned at the posterior part of the uncus of the medial temporal lobe, very close to the level of the optic chiasm and the hypothalamic area (Figure 12.2). In monkeys, EC is also associated with the rhinal sulcus along most of its anteroposterior extent, but in humans this sulcus is generally underdeveloped and only present anteriorly. Posteriorly, it is replaced by the collateral sulcus. In all mammalian species, as far as they have been studied, EC has several cortical areas as its neighbors, such as the piriform cortex anterolaterally, the periamygdaloid cortex anteromedially, and the parasubiculum medially. The lateral aspect of EC borders the perirhinal cortex anteriorly and the postrhinal/parahippocampal cortex at more posterior levels.

Histologically, in all species studied there is a part of EC characterized by a regular six-layered structure and a relatively homogeneous distribution of neurons in all layers. This subregion resembles Brodmann's area 28b and has now become known as the medial entorhinal cortex (MEC). The complementary anterolateral part has a comparable laminar structure, but the overall distribution of neurons and layers is less homogeneous. This resembles the cytoarchitecture of area 28a, which has now become known as the lateral entorhinal cortex (LEC). Note that there is generally an area in between these extremes and in various species this intermediate area has been subdivided differently. Moreover, the cytoarchitectonically based subdivision of this intermediate area is increasingly complex in primates, resulting in an increased number of subdivisions in nonhuman primates (Amaral et al., 1987) and even more in the human (Insausti et al., 1995).

In rodents, EC projections to the dentate gyrus (DG) has been taken as a strong argument supporting the main subdivision into two subareas (see Witter, 2007), and the projections to the other subdivisions may be organized in a comparable way. In the monkey, the terminal distribution of the entorhinal-to-dentate projection does not provide such a clear argument to subdivide EC and arguably supports the existence of a substantial intermediate area of EC (Witter and Amaral, 1991). In contrast, in all mammalian species studied thus far, the entorhinal projections to CA1 and subiculum show a strikingly similar organization (see section 12.3 for further details). It is of interest that recent gene expression data led to the suggestion that the two entorhinal subdivisions originate from two different pallial structures and should therefore be considered two different cortical domains, instead of subdivisions of one area (Medina et al., 2017). This proposition obviously needs further study. For the sake of simplicity, and in line with our voiced opinions (Doan et al., 2019; Nilssen et al., 2019; Witter and Amaral, 2020), here we will use the connotation that EC comprises two subdivisions, referred to as LEC and MEC or anterolateral and posteromedial entorhinal cortex in primates. The two notations will be used interchangeably when convenient.

12.2.2 Laminar structure of entorhinal cortex

EC is a cortical area characterized by a striking separation between a superficial and a deep sheet of neurons, separated by a cell-sparse zone, generally referred to as the lamina dissecans (the separating lamina; Figures 12.2 and 12.3). The lamina dissecans essentially lacks neuronal somata, and it is positioned where in the neocortex one would expect to find the granular cell layer populated by small,

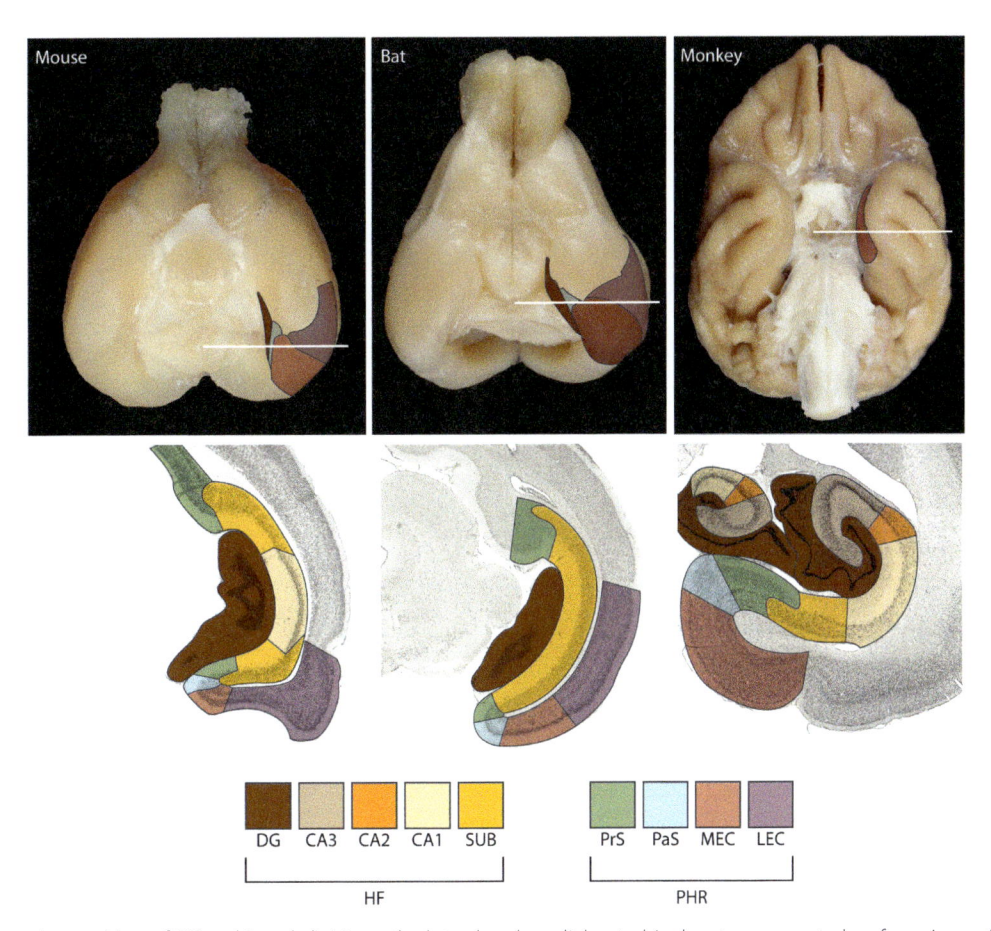

Figure 12.2 Comparative position of EC and its subdivisions, the lateral and medial entorhinal cortex, on ventral surface views of the brain (top row) and in a coronal section (bottom row), which includes subdivisions of the hippocampal formation and pre- and parasubiculum as well. The level of the coronal section is indicated by white lines in the top row images. Abbreviations: HF, hippocampal formation; PHR, parahippocampal region.

star-shaped neurons, i.e., the thalamic input layer of the neocortex. Superficial to it are layers I–III and deep to it are layers V and VI.[1] Layer I, the molecular layer, has only few neuronal somata, which are locally projecting interneurons. Layer II contains many large neurons, traditionally described as stellate-like neurons, and pyramidal neurons. Stellate-like neurons, in most species occupying layer IIa, express the protein reelin, which is absent in the layer II pyramidal neurons in layer IIb, the majority of which express the calcium-binding protein calbindin. Both the reelin-positive and the calbindin-positive neurons tend to cluster, and this differs across the extent of EC as well as between species (Tunon et al., 1992; Fujimaru and Kosaka, 1996; Solodkin and Vanhoesen, 1996; Varga et al., 2010; Kitamura et al., 2014; Naumann et al., 2016). Layer III is composed of pyramidal neurons with an apical dendrite extending up to the pial surface. Layer V is commonly subdivided into two or more sublayers, where the most superficial one is populated with relatively large pyramidal neurons that stain darkly with basic dye preparations. In rodents, these neurons express the transcription factor Evt1, and we will refer to this layer as Va. In the deep sublayer(s), which we will refer to as layer Vb, medium-sized

pyramidal neurons with long and short apical dendrites are common. These neurons express CTip2 and/or PCP4 (Ramsden et al., 2015; Surmeli et al., 2015; Ohara et al., 2018; Ohara, Yoshimo, et al., 2021). PCP4 seems specific for excitatory principal neurons, whereas CTip2 is present in both principal cells and interneurons (Ohara, Blankvoort, et al., 2021). Finally, in layer VI, one finds a mixture of pyramidal and multipolar neurons that give this layer a more heterogeneous cytoarchitectonic appearance (not indicated in Figure 12.3). All layers comprise a variety of smaller neurons of different morphologies associated with the various subtypes of interneurons (see section 12.4). Recently, single-cell analyses provided additional expression patterns that need further exploration (Ramsden et al., 2015; Grubman et al., 2019).

12.3 Main afferent and efferent connections of lateral and medial entorhinal cortex

12.3.1 Hippocampal connectivity

Both LEC and MEC contribute to what is the main cortical input to the hippocampus, and entorhinal axons target principal neurons and interneurons in all hippocampal subfields. Neurons in layer II that express the protein reelin are the main source of the entorhinal projections to the dentate gyrus and fields CA2 and CA3 (Witter, Doan, et al., 2017) and these projections likely originate as collaterals from

[1] Although there is consensus about the presence of a lamina dissecans in the entorhinal cortex, the numbers of the layers may vary. In this chapter, the lamina dissecans is considered to be layer IV, but in some accounts, layer IV is used to indicate the superficial part of layer V (Va). See also Chapter 3, section 3.9.5.

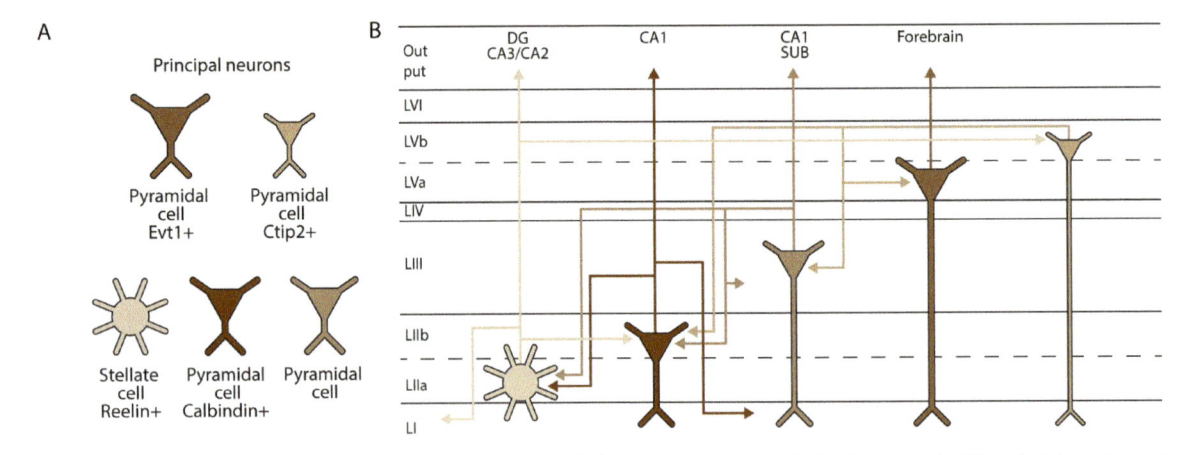

Figure 12.3 Schematic representation of laminar distribution of defined classes of excitatory principal neurons in EC and their main projections. Due to lack of details, neurons in layer VI are not represented, but this layer contributes to projections that reach the thalamus.

single neurons (Tamamaki and Nojyo, 1993).[2] The latter authors also reported axon collaterals that apparently terminate in the subiculum. Pyramidal neurons in layer III give rise to the entorhinal projections to CA1 and subiculum, and it has not been established whether these projections arise as collaterals from single layer III neurons.[3] In addition to these anatomically massive, superficially originating, entorhinal-hippocampal projections, it is well established in rodents, cats, and primates that neurons in layers V and VI project to hippocampal fields as well (van Groen et al., 1986; Witter and Amaral, 1991; Deller et al., 1996; Dugladze et al., 2001; van Groen et al., 2003).

12.3.1.1 Layer II projection

Reelin neurons in layer II of EC are the source of the projections to DG, CA2, and CA3, terminating in the molecular layer of the hippocampal subfields in a gradient along the proximodistal axis of the apical dendrites. This proximodistal terminal gradient corresponds to the anterolateral-to-posteromedial origin in EC. This organization appears quite discrete in rodents, such that axons originating in LEC terminate in the outer one-third and those from MEC in the middle one-third of the molecular layer/stratum lacunosum-moleculare of CA2/CA3 (Ino et al., 1998; Witter, 2007) (Figure 12.4). In contrast, in primates this projection shows a more gradient-like organization (Witter and Amaral, 1991; see also Chapter 3). In addition, there is a weaker projection originating from a small percentage of the layer II neurons that express the calcium-binding protein calbindin. This projection, which originates both in LEC and MEC calbindin-positive neurons, selectively distributes in stratum lacunosum of CA1 (see also section on cortical and subcortical connectivity; Kitamura et al., 2014; Ohara et al., 2019). Calbindin-positive neurons throughout EC contribute also to the commissural projections of EC (Fuchs et al.,

2016; Leitner et al., 2016; Ohara et al., 2019; see also next section on layer III).

12.3.1.2 Layer III projection

Pyramidal neurons in layer III give rise to projections to CA1 and subiculum, terminating in stratum lacunosum-moleculare in CA1 and in the superficial molecular layer of the subiculum. Comparable to the layer II projections, the layer III projections show a topographic organization related to the origin along the anterolateral-to-posteromedial gradient in EC. In rodents and primates, including humans, this origin is correlated with a distal-to-proximal termination along the transverse axis in CA1 and the opposite axis in case of the subiculum (Witter and Amaral, 1991; Ino et al., 1998; Naber et al., 2001; van Groen et al., 2003; Maass et al., 2015) (Figures 12.4 and 12.5). Moreover, there is evidence in rodents indicating that MEC inputs mainly target deep neurons in proximal CA1, whereas LEC inputs mainly target superficial neurons in distal CA1 (Masurkar et al., 2017).

In rodents, a substantial percentage of the layer III pyramidal cells contribute to the crossed projections that target the contralateral hippocampus and EC (Steward and Scoville, 1976). About 40% of the layer III hippocampal projecting cells in MEC send collaterals to the contralateral MEC (Tang et al., 2015). The axons of the commissural projecting cells in MEC apparently distribute mainly to layer III, thus contrasting with the commissural calbindin-positive neurons in layer II in both MEC and LEC, of which the axons preferentially distribute in layer I of the contralateral MEC or LEC, respectively (Fuchs et al., 2016; Leitner et al., 2016; Ohara et al., 2019). In primates, commissural projections are well developed in MEC, but are seemingly absent in LEC (Amaral et al., 1984).

The hippocampus sends projections back to EC, and these originate almost exclusively in CA1 and the subiculum. The origins of these projections and the terminal distributions show a topographic organization very similar to the layer III input system. The proximal CA1 and distal subiculum project to MEC, whereas distal CA1 and proximal subiculum project to LEC (Witter and Amaral, 2020).

The hippocampal projections distribute predominantly to layer V of EC, although weaker projections distribute to superficial layer III (Kloosterman et al., 2003; Cenquizca and Swanson, 2007), and in rodents and cats a specific projection from CA2 targeting layer II of MEC has been reported (Ino et al., 2001; Rowland et al., 2013). Regarding the projection to layer V in MEC of rodents, the terminal

---

[2] Due to space limitations, we only provide a limited bibliography. We opted not to include extensive citations of older literature, particularly on anatomy of the rat EC, that has been extensively summarized (Witter, Groenewegen, et al., 1989; Cappaert et al., 2015) A version of the chapter with a full bibliography will be available upon request to the last author: menno.witter@ntnu.no.

[3] The layer II to dentate projection is often erroneously referred to as the perforant pathway, contrasting with the layer III projection to CA1, which is referred to as the temporoammonic tract. This is confusing because layer II cells also project to the CA2 and CA3 fields and layer III neurons also project to the subiculum. We will therefore refer to layer II and layer III hippocampal projections (for a more detailed discussion, see Witter, Kleven, et al., 2017; see also Chapter 3, section 3.7.2).

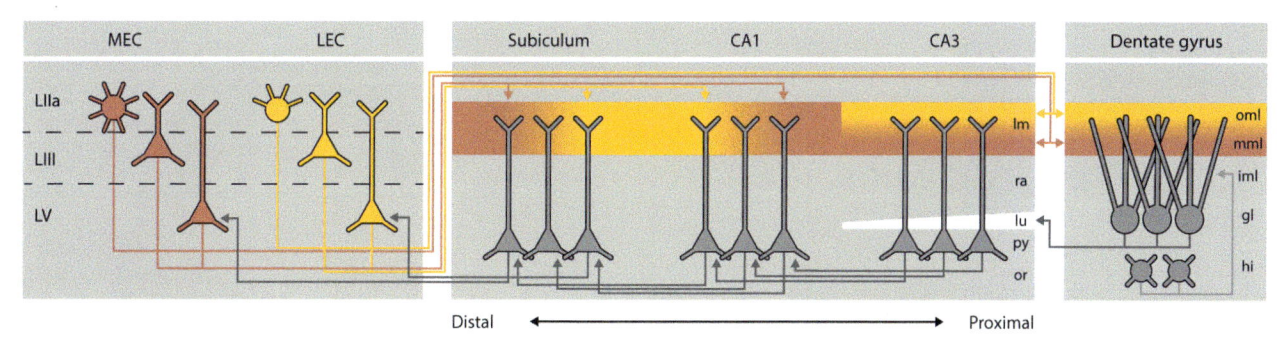

Figure 12.4 Schematic representation of the differential distribution of medial and lateral perforant path in most nonprimate species. The figure includes the main excitatory intrinsic hippocampal projections as well as those from CA1 and subiculum back to EC (gray arrows). MEC and LEC both send projections to all subdivisions of the hippocampal formation (yellow and purple arrows, respectively). Neurons in layer II project to DG and to CA3/CA2, where projections from LEC terminate in the outer one-third of the molecular layer (oml) and those from MEC terminate in the middle one-third (mml). Note that the inner one-third (iml) is the main terminal zone for intrinsic DG ipsilateral and contralateral association projections from DG mossy cells (see Chapter 3 for details). Neurons in layer III send a main projection to hippocampal fields CA1 and subiculum. MEC neurons target preferentially neurons in proximal CA1 and distal subiculum, whereas LEC layer III neurons target neurons in distal CA1 and the bordering proximal subiculum (see text for more details; see also Figure 12.5). Abbreviations: gl, stratum granulare; hi, hilus; iml, inner molecular layer; lm, stratum lacunosum-moleculare; lu, stratum lucidum; mml, middle molecular layer; oml, outer molecular layer; or, stratum oriens; py, stratum pyramidale; ra, stratum radiatum.

distribution seems to vary associated with the dorsoventral origin in CA1 and subiculum. Projections from dorsal hippocampus to dorsal MEC preferentially target layer Vb, whereas more ventral projections seem to project to both layers Va and Vb, or specifically to Va in dorsal MEC (Surmeli et al., 2015; Rozov et al., 2020; Ohara et al., 2023).

12.3.1.3 Longitudinal topography

There is a main topographical axis that pertains to the connectivity between EC and the hippocampal formation. This axis in EC runs from the rhinal/collateral sulcus toward the EC-hippocampal junction and is thus best described in terms of close to the sulcus versus more distant from the sulcus.[4] This axis in EC thus encompasses both LEC and MEC, and it relates to the long axis of the hippocampal formation. Areas of LEC and MEC that are close to the sulcus send projections to all subfields in the most dorsal (nonprimate) or caudodorsal (primate) hippocampal formation and receive projections from CA1 and subiculum in the same territory. In contrast, areas of EC progressively more distant from the sulcus map connectionally on to progressively more ventral (nonprimate) or rostroventral (primate) parts of the hippocampal formation (Witter and Groenewegen, 1984; van Groen et al., 1986; Witter, Van Hoesen, et al., 1989; Witter and Amaral, 1991, 2020; Dolorfo and Amaral, 1998; Kloosterman et al., 2003; van Groen et al., 2003) (Figure 12.5).

12.3.2 Cortical connectivity

Cortical input areas to EC include olfactory areas, medial prefrontal, orbitofrontal, insular, parietal, anterior cingulate, retrosplenial, visual, and temporal association cortex, as well as all parahippocampal areas. The latter include the perirhinal and postrhinal cortices[5] as well as the presubiculum[6] and parasubiculum (Figures 12.6D, 12.7D, and 12.8). Extensive retrograde tracing studies in rats have indicated that

the most substantial inputs to EC arise from olfactory domains, in particular the piriform cortex (44% of inputs to LEC originate from piriform cortex, followed by 24% from insular cortex, and 13% from frontal areas; for MEC these percentages are 34% from piriform cortex, 15% occipital cortex, and 13% cingulate (mainly retrosplenial) cortex (Kerr et al., 2007). Summarizing these analyses in a different way, in addition to the main piriform input to both, they receive high input levels from unimodal (40%) and polymodal (55% LEC; 43% MEC) association cortex, where input to MEC is strongly dominated by higher-order visual areas (Burwell and Amaral, 1998). Although knowledge derived from other species is less complete, the data corroborate the rodent-based conclusion of an anatomically dominant input from adjacent higher-order multisensory cortical domains (see below for details and references). Neurons in EC, specifically in layer Va, reciprocate most of these inputs (Surmeli et al., 2015; Ohara et al., 2018; Ohara, Blankvoort, et al., 2021), and the origin of these entorhinal efferents shows a pattern that is remarkably like the terminal distribution of cortical inputs. A beautiful and convincing representation of this rather strict reciprocity in rats is provided in the review of Kerr (Kerr et al., 2007; see also Witter, Groenewegen, et al., 1989; and, for monkeys, Suzuki and Amaral, 1994b).

In many contemporary accounts of EC, which are strongly influenced by work in rodents, emphasis has been on the distribution of cortical inputs to either one or both subdivisions, LEC and MEC. However, to allow for a more encompassing and comparative account, we describe input distributions related to the location of the rhinal/collateral sulcus as described above, although we have indicated a tentative border between LEC and MEC for both rodent and monkey data (see below; Figure 12.8; see also Figure 12.5) (cf. Witter, Groenewegen, et al., 1989). Relevant references in rats and monkeys on which the following descriptions and Figure 12.8 are based are listed in the legend of Figure 12.8. In the following text, we will only reference papers specific for

---

[4] This gradient has often been referred to as the lateral-to-medial axis of origin, but this has led to confusion. We therefore opt to change this (for details, see Kobro-Flatmoen and Witter, 2019).

[5] The postrhinal cortex in rodents has been proposed as the homologue of the parahippocampal cortex in primates (Burwell et al., 1995). In several rodent accounts, the postrhinal cortex is handled as the posterior part of the perirhinal cortex.

[6] According to some authors the presubiculum is considered to have a separate dorsal component referred to as the postsubiculum (van Groen and Wyss, 1990b). We consider this as part of the presubiculum in this chapter, in line with Chapters 2 and 3.

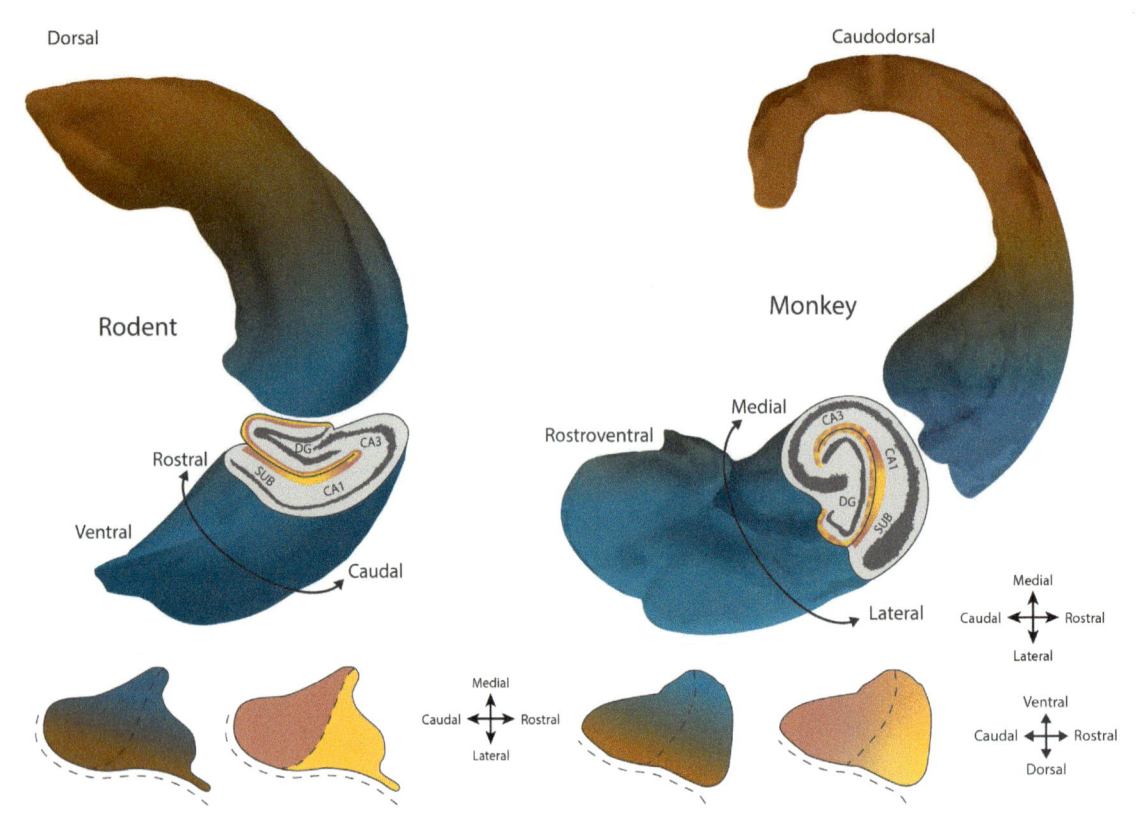

Figure 12.5 Longitudinal, transverse, and radial distributions of the entorhinal-hippocampal projections in the rodent and the primate. The longitudinal terminal distribution (cyan–orange gradient) is correlated to the left unfolded EC, and the transverse and radial distribution (purple–yellow gradient) is correlated to the right unfolded EC.

one connection or species other than rats and monkeys and that are not already included in Witter, Groenewegen, et al. (1989) or Cappaert et al. (2015).[7]

In rodents, as well as in animals with a marked piriform lobe, such as guinea pigs and cats, olfactory axons preferentially terminate laterally and centrally in LEC and in MEC, avoiding the most caudodorsal portion of MEC. In monkeys, olfactory inputs are much more restricted, only targeting a small anterior portion of EC. Reciprocal connections to the anterior olfactory nucleus and primary olfactory/piriform cortex have been reported, whereas the entorhinal projections to the olfactory bulb are sparse.

The infralimbic, prelimbic, anterior cingulate, and retrosplenial cortex all project to EC, although striking density gradients are apparent. Infralimbic and ventral prelimbic cortex innervate central parts of LEC, with weaker innervation of the central and medial parts of MEC. Dorsal prelimbic and directly adjacent anterior parts of anterior cingulate cortex innervate lateral and intermediate parts of EC, with projections to LEC being stronger than those to MEC, whereas the density of projections to MEC increases at the expense of those to LEC when the origin is more posterior in ACC (Vertes, 2004; B Jones and Witter, 2007). These connections look very similar in cats. In the monkey, projections from infralimbic and prelimbic cortex and dorsally adjacent anterior cingulate cortex

show comparable distributions (Arikuni et al., 1994; Chiba et al., 2001), and some studies support the general notion of reciprocity of these connections (Arikuni et al., 1994; Munoz and Insausti, 2005). The gradual change related to origin along the anteroposterior axis of the midline cortex continues such that projections from the retrosplenial cortex almost exclusively innervate caudodorsal parts of EC, close to the sulcus. In both primates and rodents, the more ventral parts of the retrosplenial cortex (area 29 in rodents, and areas 29 and 23v in primates) originate the densest projections (B Jones and Witter, 2007; Kobayashi and Amaral, 2007). The reciprocating efferent projections in EC originate from neurons predominantly coinciding with the areas receiving the corresponding afferent input (Morris et al., 1999; Kobayashi and Amaral, 2003; Kerr et al., 2007; Kobayashi and Amaral, 2007; Aggleton et al., 2012).

In all species studied, the most lateral parts of EC have reciprocal connections with the insular and orbitofrontal cortices. All of these connections are shared with adjacent parts of perirhinal cortex. In the rat, it has been reported that a restricted ventral part of the orbitofrontal cortex preferentially has reciprocal connections with MEC (Kerr et al., 2007; Price, 2007; Saleem et al., 2008; Hoover and Vertes, 2011; Kondo and Witter, 2014; Mathiasen et al., 2015). It remains to be determined whether this is true in primates. Similarly, in rodents, connections with areas of temporal cortex are restricted to the extreme lateral parts of EC, whereas in monkeys these projections have a substantially more widespread distribution. This distribution is likely associated with the increased functional diversity of temporal areas, including temporal polar cortex, higher-order auditory cortex/superior temporal gyrus, and area TE (Saleem and Tanaka, 1996). Projections from the posterior parietal

---

[7] It is important to point out that most of the rodent cortical connections have been detailed in the rat, though several have been corroborated by experiments made available in public mouse connectome data such as can be found at https://connectivity.brain-map.org/static/brainexplorer and www.brainarchitecture.org.

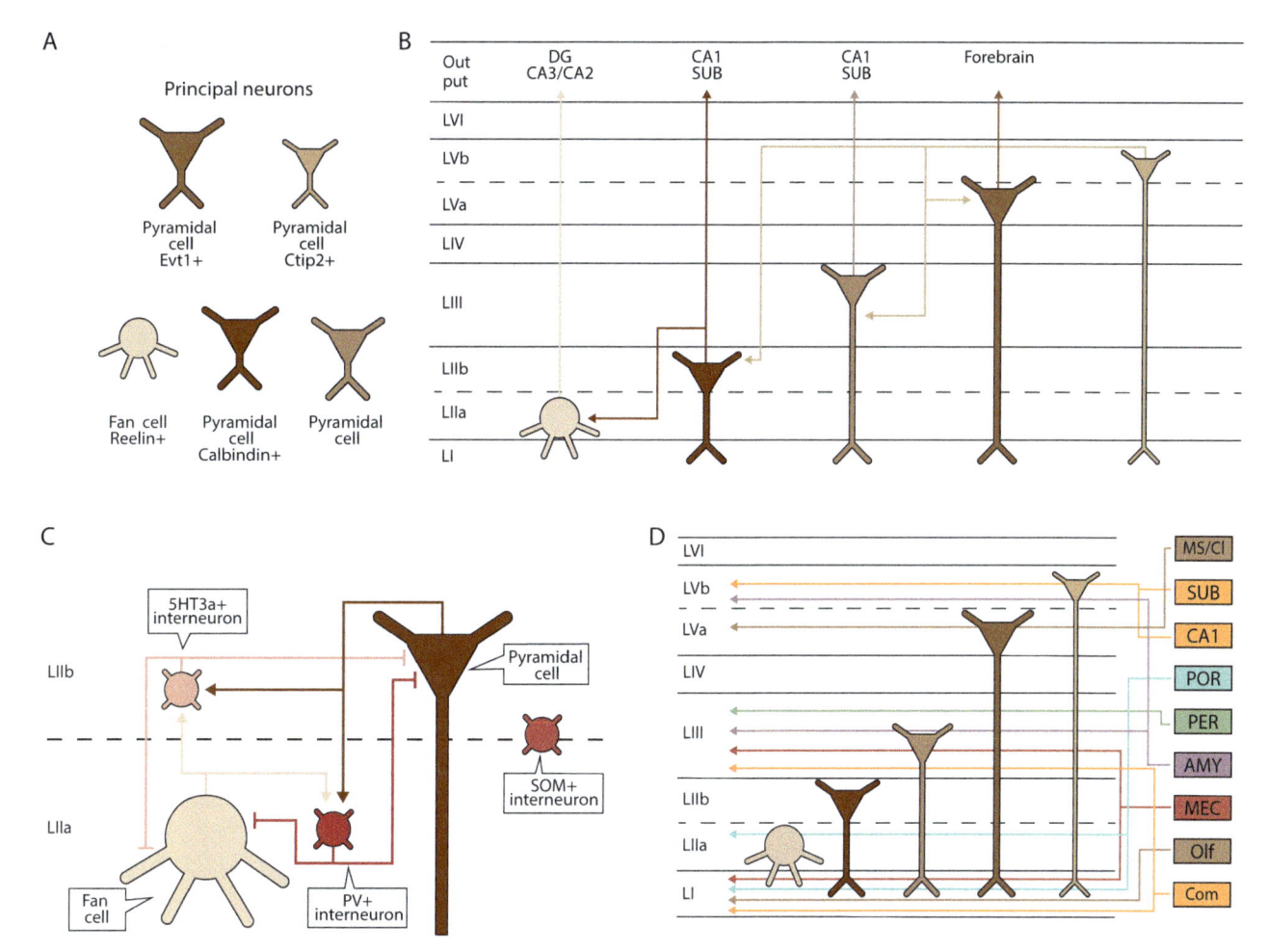

Figure 12.6 Connectivity summary for LEC. (A) Summary of main principal cell types. (B) Summary of laminar neuronal distribution, main outputs, and main interlaminar projections. (C) Details of intralaminar connectivity of layer II. (D) Summary of laminar distribution of main cortical and subcortical input. Abbreviations: AMY, amygdala; CA, cornu ammonis; Ctip2, chicken ovalbumin upstream promoter transcription factor interacting protein 2; EvT1, E twenty-six (ETS) variant 1; MEC, medial entorhinal cortex; Olf, olfactory areas; PER, perirhinal cortex; POR, postrhinal cortex; PV, parvalbumin; SOM, somatostatin; SUB, subiculum; 5HT3aR, serotonin 3a receptor.

cortex to EC are relatively weak and innervate an area close to the sulcus showing a density preference for LEC over MEC (Olsen et al., 2017). In the monkey, weak reciprocal connections of EC with posterior parietal area 7, which is likely homologous to posterior parietal cortex in the rodent, have been reported as well (Ding et al., 2000; Munoz and Insausti, 2005; Insausti and Amaral, 2008). Interestingly, connections with parietal area 5 seem to be absent. Note that both in rats and monkeys, connections of posterior parietal cortex are much stronger with other parahippocampal areas, in particular with postrhinal/parahippocampal area TF and the presubiculum, with less dense projections to the perirhinal cortex (Cavada and Goldman-Rakic, 1989; Suzuki and Amaral, 1994a; Lavenex et al., 2002; Munoz and Insausti, 2005; Olsen et al., 2017; see also Chapter 3).

Regarding EC connections with the other parahippocampal domains, some striking topographic features need to be emphasized. First, in nonprimate species, the projections from the presubiculum are confined to the caudal portions of EC, which strictly overlaps with the cytoarchitectonically defined MEC. Moreover, the presubiculum is the only parahippocampal area that projects bilaterally with almost equal densities (van Groen and Wyss, 1990a; Caballero-Bleda and Witter, 1993). In monkeys, inputs from the

presubiculum also distribute bilaterally to a restricted posterior portion of EC (Witter and Amaral, 2020), and this area may thus represent the homologue of MEC as defined in nonprimates. Note, however, that in monkeys the distribution of the presubicular inputs is not restricted to one or several cytoarchitectonically defined subdivisions but apparently stops approximately halfway through the caudorostral extent of the intermediate entorhinal area (Witter and Amaral, 2020). In contrast, projections from the parasubiculum, although densest to the area also receiving the presubicular input, extend more rostrally and laterally in all species studied.

Contemporary descriptions of the connectivity of EC with its direct lateral and posterior neighbors, the perirhinal and postrhinal/parahippocampal cortex, generally emphasize a preferred connectivity between the perirhinal cortex and LEC, and the postrhinal/parahippocampal cortex domain and MEC. A recent re-evaluation, however, led to a revised connectivity scheme. In the rat, postrhinal projections target the more anterior portions of EC more densely than the posterior parts, indicating that the densest projections target LEC and a small anterior part of MEC (Doan et al., 2019). In the monkey, sparse data indicate that both areas TF and TH have strong reciprocal connections with EC (Mohedano-Moriano et al., 2007; Insausti and Amaral, 2008) and

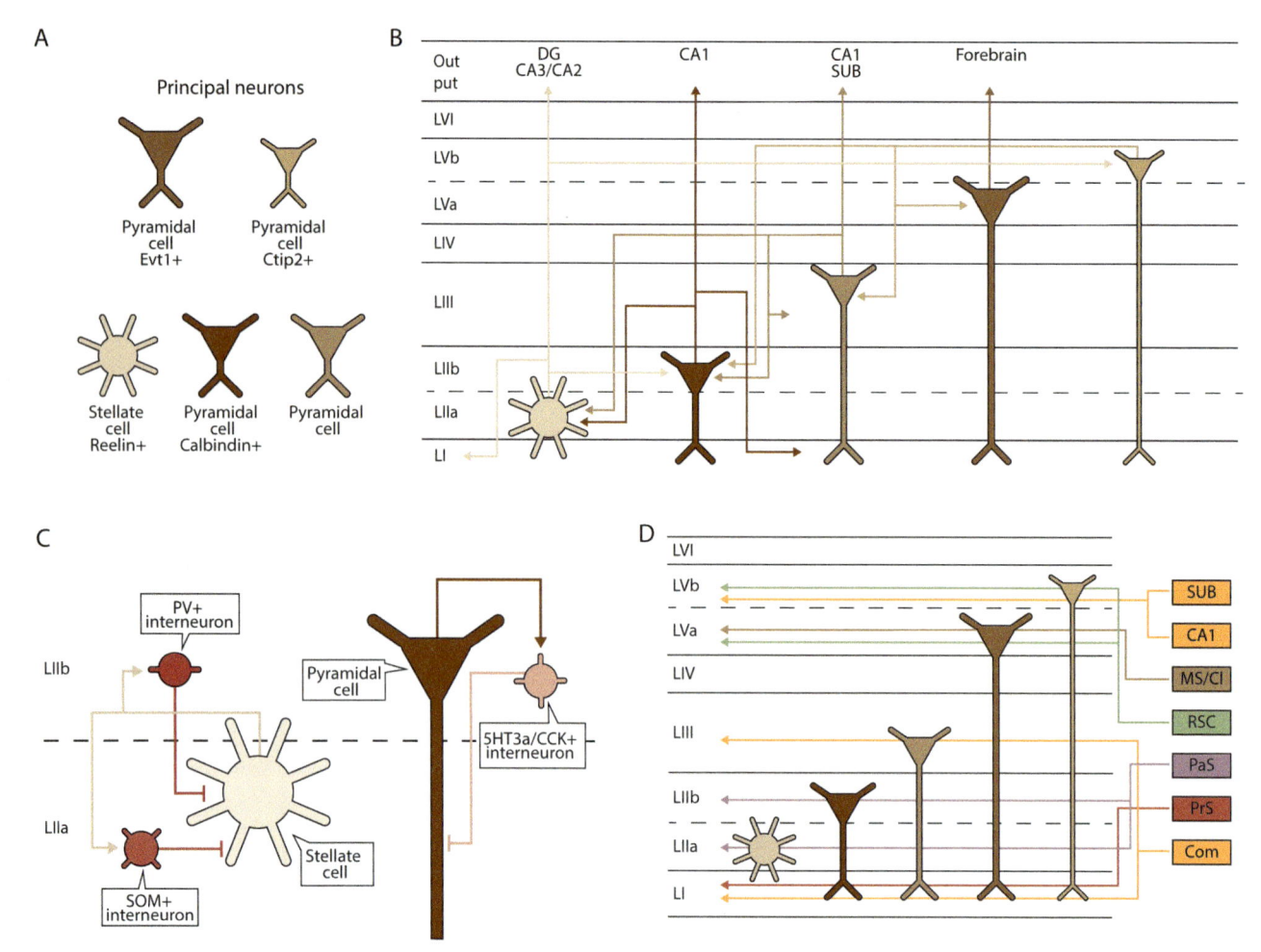

Figure 12.7 Connectivity summary for MEC. (A) Summary of main principal cell types. (B) Summary of laminar neuronal distribution, main outputs, and main interlaminar projections. (C) Details of intralaminar connectivity of layer II. (D) Summary of laminar distribution of main cortical and subcortical input. Abbreviations: AMY, amygdala; CA, cornu ammonis; CCK, cholecystokinin; Com, commissural; Ctip2, chicken ovalbumin upstream promoter transcription factor interacting protein 2; EvT1, E twenty-six (ETS) variant 1; MS/Cl, medial septum/claustrum; PaS, parasubiculum; PrS, presubiculum; PV, parvalbumin; RSC, retrosplenial cortex; SOM, somatostatin; SUB, subiculum; 5HT3aR, serotonin 3a receptor.

that there is an apparent difference between the two areas. Whereas area TH strongly projects to the more posteromedial part of EC, projections from TF cover a more extensive area, including antero-lateral parts of EC as well (Suzuki and Amaral, 1994b; Wellman and Rockland, 1997). Connectional MRI studies in humans have pointed to a comparable connectional bipartite system separating anterolateral from posteromedial EC, showing clear differences with respect to connectivity measures with perirhinal and parahippocampal cortex, although the parahippocampal areas TF and TH were not analysed separately (Maass et al., 2015; Navarro Schroder et al., 2015).

12.3.3 Subcortical connectivity

Subcortical connections of EC have been extensively studied across species and are remarkably conserved (for detailed overviews, see Witter, Groenewegen, et al., 1989; Kerr et al., 2007; Cappaert et al., 2015; Agster et al., 2016; Tomas Pereira et al., 2016). Retrograde tracing studies indicated that inputs originate from the medial septum/ diagonal band/nucleus basalis complex, the amygdala and bed nucleus of the stria terminalis, endopiriform nucleus, claustrum, and midline thalamus as well as several ascending modulatory inputs from the hypothalamic supramammillary and tuberomammillary

nuclei, and from brainstem structures such as the ventral tegmental area, raphe nuclei, and locus coeruleus (Insausti et al., 1987; Witter, Groenewegen, et al., 1989).

With the exception of inputs from the medial septum/diagonal band/nucleus basalis complex and those from the hypothalamic and brainstem domains, these connections are reciprocal in rats and cats. Regarding the septal complex, EC projects weakly to the medial domain but sends strong projections to lateral septal nuclei. In addition, entorhinal projections to the ventral striatum/nucleus accumbens and adjacent parts of the olfactory tubercle have been reported.

EC has very strong reciprocal connections with the endopiriform nucleus. These connections terminate in and originate from widespread domains, with some preference for lateral parts of both LEC and MEC in rodents. Equally strong connections exist with the amygdala, though these connections are more prominent in the most lateral parts of LEC in all species studied, but connections between the amygdala and MEC do exist. All of these connections are shared with adjacent parts of perirhinal cortex. Whereas in rodents the amygdaloid connections are mainly with the basal nucleus, in cats, there is a substantial connectivity with the lateral nucleus as well. In monkeys, the lateral and accessory basal nucleus are the

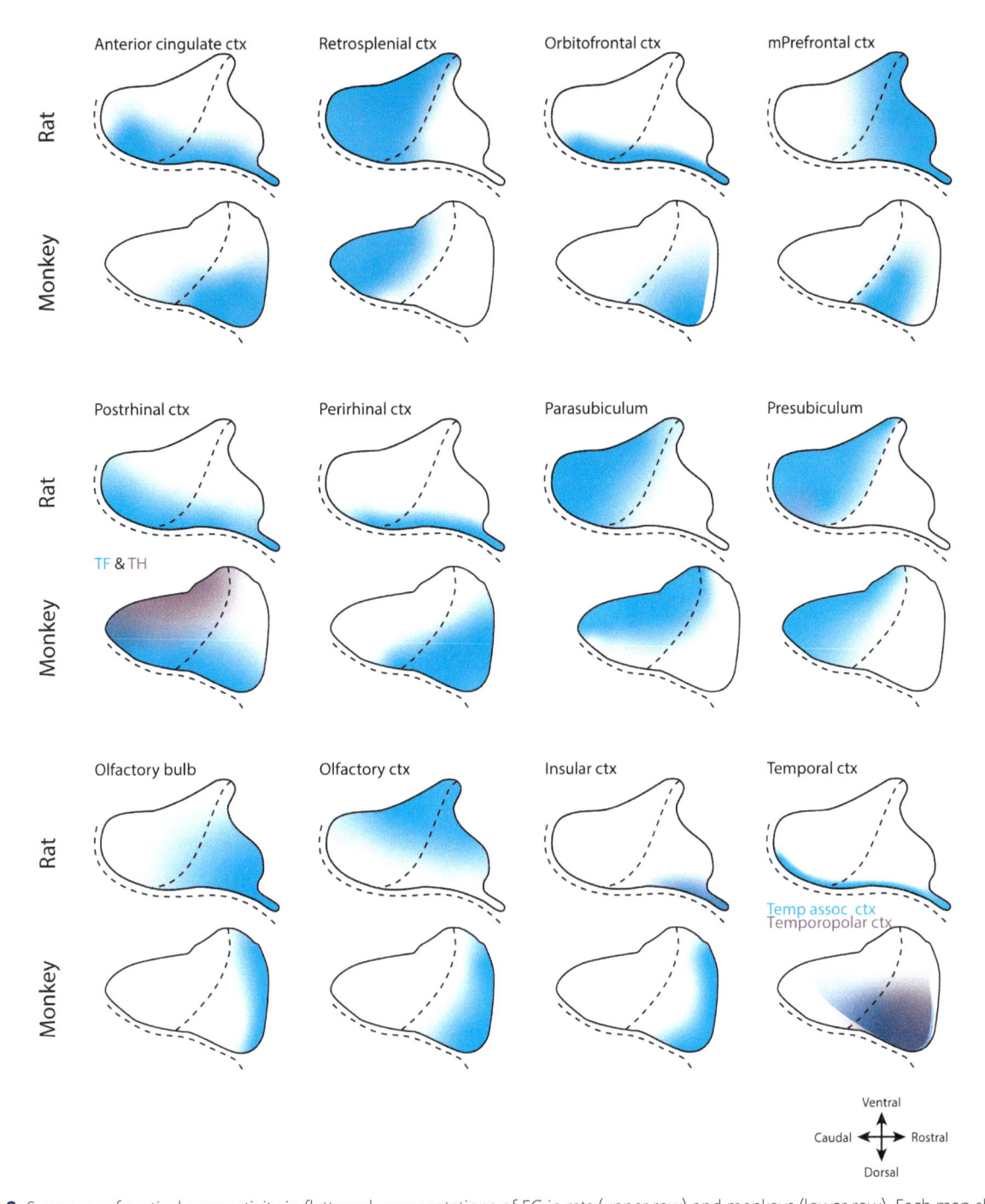

Figure 12.8 Summary of cortical connectivity in flattened representations of EC in rats (upper row) and monkeys (lower row). Each map shows a schematic surface distribution of cortical inputs, where the intensity of the color is proportional to the density of the input (high intensity = dense input). Each flatmap has an indication of the rhinal sulcus/collateral sulcus (dashed line below) and a tentative indication of the border between MEC and LEC (dashed line across the surface) based on the distribution of the input from the presubiculum. The surface distribution represents what is considered the main terminal distribution, irrespective of the layer it is in. (For the preferred laminar distribution of each input, see section 12.3.4, "Laminar profiles of termination and origin." The distributions are mainly based on the following references: Amaral et al., 1987; Insausti et al., 1987; Burwell and Amaral, 1998; Kerr et al., 2007; Mohedano-Moriano et al., 2007; Insausti and Amaral, 2008; Agster and Burwell, 2009; Cappaert et al., 2015, and the references provided in the text.) Abbreviations: ctx, cortex; Temp assoc, temporal association cortex; TF&TH, temporal fields F & H, likely homologue of postrhinal cortex.

main structures involved (Pitkanen et al., 2000; Kemppainen et al., 2002; Pitkanen et al., 2002; Majak and Pitkanen, 2003). EC further shows a strong reciprocal connectivity with ventral parts of the claustrum in all species studies (Pearson et al., 1982; Kitanishi and Matsuo, 2017).

With respect to the connectivity with the thalamus, studies in rodents have shown the strongest connections with the midline nucleus reuniens and to a lesser extent with other midline nuclei, such as the paraventricular, central, and rhomboid nuclei (van der Werf et al., 2002; Cassel et al., 2013). In monkeys, however, the strongest input to EC has been reported to originate in the central part of the central thalamic complex (Insausti et al., 1987; Moga et al., 1995).

Hypothalamic inputs have mainly been studied in some detail in rodents and preferentially target MEC, whereas brainstem inputs show a widespread and diffuse terminal distribution in EC. Inputs from the dopaminergic ventral tegmental area show a particularly dense patch-like terminal distribution in anterolateral parts of LEC, influencing both excitatory and inhibitory neurons (Cilz et al., 2014). Effects of dopamine on neurons in layers II and III in LEC include a concentration-dependent inhibition or excitation of input-driven responses as well as the blocking of persistent firing in LEC layer III (Caruana et al., 2006; Batallan-Burrowes and Chapman, 2018). A recent study in mice reported that inhibition of dopamine inputs disrupted the associative encoding of layer IIa fan cells in LEC and impaired learning performance (Lee et al., 2021). The raphe nucleus projects to EC, sending both serotonergic and nonserotonergic projections to EC, with the serotonergic projections showing a slight preference for LEC. The locus coeruleus provides a light, diffusely organized noradrenergic input to EC that exhibits a slightly denser termination in layer I. This projection originates from noradrenergic neurons expressing neuropeptide Y. Minor pontine projections arise from the parabrachial nucleus, the dorsal tegmental nucleus, and the nucleus subcoeruleus. An additional moderate input originates from the nucleus incertus.

Several of the subcortical connections of EC show a topographical organization that is similar to that of the cortical connectivity; they are thus also organized along the axis that starts from the rhinal/collateral sulcus running perpendicular to it (Figure 12.8) (Akil and Lewis, 1994; Kobro-Flatmoen and Witter, 2019). This axis corresponds roughly to a dorsomedial-to-ventrolateral axis in the septal complex (Kondo and Zaborszky, 2016), a lateromedial axis in both the amygdala and the ventral striatum, and a dorsoventral axis in the claustrum.

12.3.4 Laminar profiles of termination and origin

EC is a layered cortex, and many of its input terminal distributions and output origins show a certain level of laminar specificity, comparable to what has been described for other cortical areas in the brain. Below we aim to describe the laminar organization of EC in anatomical terms first. It is important to emphasize that in terms of inputs, the laminar organization may point to preferred synaptic interactions with neurons that have their somata or main dendritic tree in that particular layer, but many neuron types in EC have dendrites that extend across multiple layers, thus greatly enhancing the integrative complexity of the networks in EC (Figures 12.6 and 12.7).

Cortical inputs fall into two groups based on their preferred laminar terminal distributions: those that distribute preferentially to layers I–III, and those that preferentially target layer V (and VI). The inputs belonging to the superficial group include inputs from olfactory domains such as those from the olfactory bulb, the anterior olfactory nucleus, and the piriform cortex that all mainly distribute to layer I. An additional, almost exclusive, input to layer I is the commissural input originating from calbindin-positive layer II pyramidal neurons in EC (Fuchs et al., 2016; Leitner et al., 2016; Ohara et al., 2019). Additional inputs reaching layer I include those from presubiculum, perirhinal cortex, and postrhinal/parahippocampal cortex, as well as local intrinsic ipsilateral connections. These latter inputs have additional terminal fields in layer II, layer III, or both.

Projections from parasubiculum are mainly confined to layer II. Layer III in MEC is the main recipient of inputs from both ipsi- and contralateral presubiculum in rodents, cats, and monkeys (van Groen and Wyss, 1990a; Caballero-Bleda and Witter, 1993; Saunders et al., 2005; Witter and Amaral, 2020). Additional inputs originate from the parahippocampal/postrhinal cortex. Layer III of both LEC and MEC receives the commissural projections that originate in the contralateral layer III (Blackstad, 1956; Steward and Scoville, 1976; Ino et al., 2000; Ohara et al., 2019), although in monkeys the commissural projection seems limited to MEC, such that left and right LEC are apparently not connected (Amaral et al., 1984). In LEC, layer III receives additional inputs from insular cortex (Mesulam and Mufson, 1982; Price, 2007; Saleem et al., 2008; Mathiasen et al., 2015), perirhinal and postrhinal/parahippocampal cortex and adjacent temporal cortex (Vaudano et al., 1991; Saleem and Tanaka, 1996; Naber et al., 1997; Shi and Cassell, 1997; Naber et al., 1999; Pinto et al., 2006; Mohedano-Moriano et al., 2007; Insausti and Amaral, 2008; Koganezawa et al., 2015; Doan et al., 2019), orbitofrontal cortex (Insausti and Amaral, 2008; Hoover and Vertes, 2011; Kondo and Witter, 2014), and parietal cortex (Ding et al., 2000; Munoz and Insausti, 2005; Insausti and Amaral, 2008; Olsen et al., 2017). Several of the latter cortical inputs also have a weak distribution into layer V, except for those from the insular cortex, which prefer layer V. This layer is also the recipient of most of the inputs that originate from midline cortical areas, such as the medial prefrontal, infralimbic, and prelimbic areas, and from anterior cingulate and retrosplenial cortex (Arikuni et al., 1994; Chiba et al., 2001; Hoover and Vertes, 2007; B Jones and Witter, 2007; Kobayashi and Amaral, 2007).

EC, to a large extent, reciprocates the cortical inputs described above, and these projections originate mainly from neurons in layer V (Witter, Groenewegen, et al., 1989; Insausti et al., 1997; Munoz and Insausti, 2005; Cappaert et al., 2015). Neurons in layers II and III, however, contribute substantially to the projections to medial prefrontal and olfactory areas. As described above, layer V is generally subdivided into two or three sublayers, and recent data in rodents indicate that most, if not all, of the telencephalic layer V projections originate from neurons in layer Va (Surmeli et al., 2015; Ohara et al., 2018).

Subcortical inputs from the medial septum/diagonal band show a rather diffuse terminal distribution, though with a marked preference for layer Va, and the latter holds true for claustral inputs as well (Figures 12.6D and 12.7D) (Alonso and Kohler, 1984; Ohara et al., 2018). Since layer Va neurons originate the main forebrain outputs of EC, these two subcortical inputs are therefore in an optimal position to modulate this output pathway and/or modulate the substantial input from neurons in Vb (Ohara et al., 2018). Although little is known about the functional relevance of claustral inputs, the activity of cholinergic inputs seems to set the appropriate dynamics to facilitate or interfere with memory performance. These subcortical inputs also play an essential role in the oscillatory activity that is an elementary component of normal entorhinal function (Heys et al., 2012). Amygdala inputs have a preferred distribution in layer III, although this depends somewhat on the origin. Whereas other inputs, like hypothalamic, serotonergic, noradrenergic, and midline thalamic inputs are diffuse, dopaminergic inputs are strikingly selective in providing a patch-like innervation in superficial layers of lateral parts of LEC specifically, in addition to a more diffuse innervation throughout the remainder of EC (Herkenham, 1978; Swanson et al., 1987; Witter, Groenewegen, et al., 1989; Wouterlood et al., 1990; Akil and Lewis, 1993; Akil and Lewis, 1994; Dolleman-Van der Weel and Witter, 1996; Vertes et al., 2006; Vertes and Hoover, 2008; Cappaert et al., 2015; Lee et al., 2021)

12.4. Neurons and local circuits in lateral and medial entorhinal cortex

Most of the detailed information concerning neuron types and local circuits in EC has been obtained in rodents. With original studies mainly in rats, the recent decade has seen an enormous increase of data obtained in mice using genetic approaches. The following account is therefore mainly based on rat and mouse data with an occasional insertion of references to other species where relevant (Figures 12.6 and 12.7).

12.4.1 Neurons

12.4.1.1 Layer II

Principal cells in layer II of both subdivisions of EC come in two main morphological types, pyramidal cells and multipolar or stellate-like cells, although two intermediate subtypes have been described as well (Alonso and Klink, 1993; Klink and Alonso, 1997; Buckmaster et al., 2004; Tahvildari and Alonso, 2005; Canto and Witter, 2012a, 2012b; Fuchs et al., 2016; Leitner et al., 2016). Both cell types have the large part of their spiny dendrites confined to layers I and II. They also have a main axon that courses toward the underlying white matter, but the axon has many collaterals that mainly distribute within layers I–III, having a large extension in layers I and II, parallel to the pial plane (Quilichini et al., 2010). In both rodents and monkeys, only sparse collaterals seem to distribute in deep layers V and VI.

In MEC, stellate cells and intermediate stellate cells, which make up approximately 67% of principal cells in layer II (Gatome et al., 2010; Witter, Doan, et al., 2017), have multiple primary dendrites that radiate out from the soma. The pyramidal cells typically have a well-developed thick apical dendrite with a marked tuft in layer I. The two main subtypes in LEC are fan cells and pyramidal cells with two intermediate subtypes, as in MEC. Fan cells, originally referred to as stellate-like cells, were renamed since they lack a distinct basal dendritic tree and have extremely large dendritic trees with a diameter close to the pial surface of layer I that can reach up to 900 μm in rats (Tahvildari and Alonso, 2005; Leitner et al., 2016; Nilssen et al., 2018; Doan et al., 2019). The pyramidal cells are morphologically similar to those described in MEC. In MEC, the two main morphological cell types show electrophysiological and chemical differences. Stellate cells show subthreshold membrane oscillations in the theta range and a large depolarizing sag potential in response to hyperpolarizing voltage steps (Alonso and Llinas, 1989; Dickson et al., 2000; Canto and Witter, 2012b; Pastoll et al., 2012; Couey et al., 2013; Pastoll et al., 2013; Fuchs et al., 2016). Pyramidal cells show much smaller or no sag potentials (Alonso and Klink, 1993; Canto and Witter, 2012b; Winterer et al., 2017). In contrast, in LEC, the two main cell types do not show such striking differences in electrophysiological properties, though subtle differences between the two classes have been reported (Tahvildari and Alonso, 2005; Canto and Witter, 2012a; Leitner et al., 2016; Nilssen et al., 2018; Doan et al., 2019). Chemically, stellate-like

cells express the glycoprotein reelin, whereas the pyramidal-like cells express the calcium-binding protein calbindin and WFS-1. In MEC the expression patterns of these latter chemical markers match almost completely and adhere to the morphological classification, i.e., all pyramidal cells do express both calbindin and WFS-1. In contrast, in LEC the overlap is less precise, i.e., multipolar neurons are either reelin- or calbindin-expressing, a small proportion of pyramidal cells express reelin instead of calbindin, and there is not perfect overlap between calbindin and WFS-1 expression patterns (Kitamura et al., 2014; Fuchs et al., 2016; Leitner et al., 2016; Nilssen et al., 2018; Kobro-Flatmoen and Witter, 2019) (Figures 12.6A, 12.7A, and 12.9). It is likely, however, that all reelin-positive neurons in EC form the origin of the projections to DG, CA3, and CA2, whereas only a small proportion of calbindin-positive neurons project to the hippocampus, particularly sending terminating axons to stratum lacunosum of CA1 (Kitamura et al., 2014; Surmeli et al., 2015; Ohara et al., 2019).

In MEC, calbindin-positive cells and reelin-positive cells appear to be grouped in patches, whereas in LEC, the two cell types are confined to two separate sublayers, reelin cells in the superficial layer IIa and calbindin cells in the deeper layer IIb. The reported clustering of calbindin-positive neurons is particularly striking in limited parts of MEC (Naumann et al., 2016). Only in mice, the MEC calbindin-positive neurons are located superficial to the reelin positive neurons (Figure 12.9A; (Fujimaru and Kosaka, 1996; Kitamura et al., 2014; Fuchs et al., 2016; Leitner et al., 2016; Ohara et al., 2019). In monkeys, calbindin-positive clusters of neurons are localized deep to the typically large cell clusters assumed to originate the EC–DG projections (Suzuki and Porteros, 2002). EC in humans is known for its wart-like bumps or verrucae, as described in older human anatomical accounts by Retzius and Klinger (see Solodkin and Vanhoesen, 1996), which in the largest centrally located part of EC are composed of the large multipolar reelin-positive layer II cells. In our view, it is therefore confusing to refer to calbindin-positive cells in layer II as island cells embedded in an ocean of reelin-positive cells (Kitamura et al., 2014), since this organization likely only applies for a small part of EC.

12.4.1.2 Layer III

Compared with what is known about neurons and connectivity in layers II and V, layer III is still largely terra incognita. Layer III in both LEC and MEC comprises a homogeneous population of spiny excitatory pyramidal neurons (Gloveli, Schmitz, Empson, et al., 1997; Buckmaster et al., 2004; Tahvildari and Alonso, 2005; Canto and Witter, 2012a, 2012b; Tang et al., 2015) that project to CA1 and subiculum as well as to the contralateral homotopic part of EC (Steward and Scoville, 1976; Amaral et al., 1984; Witter and Amaral, 1991; Tang et al., 2015). In addition, layer III also contains a population of nonspiny pyramidal cells, sending axons toward the angular bundle. Collaterals originate from the main axon close to the cell body, and those traveling toward the superficial layers distribute over their own dendritic extent (Gloveli, Schmitz, Empson, et al., 1997). The third principal neuron type in layer III is formed by multipolar neurons. These contribute to the hippocampal projections. Currently, no correlations have been reported between morphology, connectional profile, and electrophysiological properties of neurons in layer III (Canto and Witter, 2012a, 2012b; Tang et al., 2015).

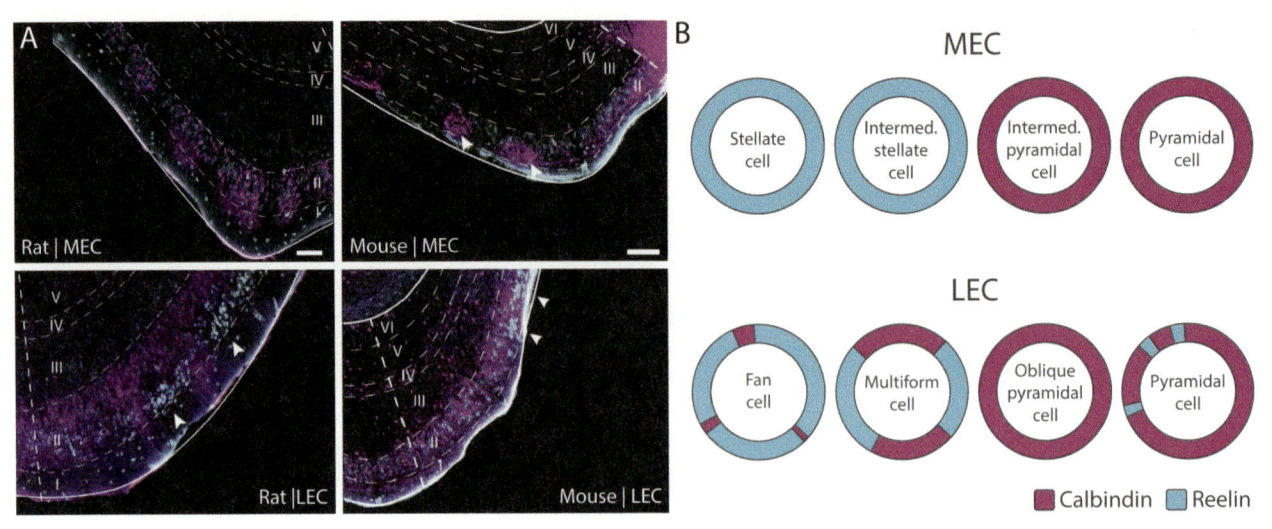

Figure 12.9 Summary of the chemical nature of morphologically defined principal neurons in rodent entorhinal cortex layer II. (Modified with permission from Witter et al., 2017a.) (A) Coronal sections of the entorhinal cortex (EC) of the rat (left) and mouse (right), stained for two main markers calbindin (magenta) and reelin (cyan). Note the different position of the two cell populations in the two species and the two subdivisions of EC. Scale bars equal 100 mm. (B) Schematic representation of the relationships of morphologically, electrophysiologically, and connectionally defined cell types, and their respective expression of calbindin (magenta) or reelin (cyan) in LEC and MEC. Width of circle segments indicate approximate percentages of the two markers. Abbreviations: Fan, fan cell; IMSC, intermediate stellate cell; IMPC, intermediate pyramidal cell; multi, multipolar cell; ObPC, oblique pyramidal cell; PC, pyramidal cell; SC, stellate cell.

12.4.1.3 Layer V

As described above, layer V is commonly subdivided into layers Va and Vb. The superficial layer Va, adjacent to layer IV (lamina dissecans), comprises mainly large pyramidal neurons that are unequally distributed along the extent of both MEC and LEC. Cells in layer Vb are smaller, more uniform in soma size, and more densely packed than their counterparts in layer Va (Amaral et al., 1987; Insausti et al., 1995; Insausti et al., 1997); see also (Hamam et al., 2000; Hamam et al., 2002; Canto and Witter, 2012a, 2012b). Layer Vb of both MEC and LEC also contains multipolar and tilted pyramidal neurons and a population of GABA-negative, calretinin-positive neurons (Miettinen et al., 1997), providing additional markers for principal cell types in the layer V network. All these studies seem to agree that neurons in layer V are morphologically and electrophysiologically not very different between LEC and MEC, and that clear correlations between morphology and electrophysiology are not apparent. With the emergence of tools to genetically differentiate between neuron types, it became clear that in rodents, the expression patterns of the transcription factors Etv1 and Ctip2/PCP4 provide for the differentiation between two molecularly distinct sublayers Va and Vb, respectively. This organization prevails across the whole mediolateral and dorsoventral extent of EC (Surmeli et al., 2015; Ohara et al., 2018; Ohara, Blankvoort, et al., 2021). Using neuron-specific tools, based on these and other markers (Ramsden et al., 2015), the connections of specific populations of neurons indicate that neurons in layer Va in both of EC subdivisions are indistinguishable. In contrast, neurons in layer Vb of MEC and LEC show striking differences in the morphology of the apical dendrite. Neurons in MEC-LVb have an apical dendrite that heads straight to the pia, such that distal branches reach all the way up into LI, whereas the apical dendrites of LEC-LVb neurons have a more complex branching pattern and they do not extend beyond LIII. These neurons further differ in their electrophysiological properties (Ohara, Blankvoort, et al., 2021). Finally, pyramidal cells in

layer V show regular spiking, strongly adapting physiological profiles, whereas multipolar neurons respond to a depolarization with delayed firing and show little adaptation. Both layer V cell types correlate with the persistent firing neurons, which can be found in EC when muscarinic acetylcholine receptors are activated (Egorov et al., 2002).

12.4.1.4 Layer VI

Data for neurons in layer VI are sparse but show that there are two main cell types: pyramidal and multipolar neurons. Data in monkeys and rats differ in that the pyramidal neurons in monkeys have a spiny apical dendrite reaching up to superficial layer II/III (Buckmaster et al., 2004), whereas all layer VI pyramidal cells in rats are tilted or have a main dendrite running more or less parallel to the cell layer (Canto and Witter, 2012a, 2012b). All neurons that have been described show an axon traveling into the white matter, some of which reach the subiculum (Dugladze et al., 2001), and giving off local collaterals that distribute superficially reaching up to layer III and interacting with neurons in all superficial levels.

12.4.1.5 Interneurons

Similar to what has been reported for neocortical areas, EC contains three main subgroups of interneurons: parvalbumin- (PV), somatostatin- (SOM), and 5-HT3a-receptor-expressing cells (Wouterlood, 2002; Fuchs et al., 2016; Leitner et al., 2016; Ferrante et al., 2017). In the neocortex, PV-positive and SOM-positive neurons derive from the medial ganglionic eminence, whereas 5-HT3aR-positive neurons have their embryonic origin in the caudal ganglionic eminence, and this likely holds true for interneurons in EC as well. PV-positive interneurons constitute approximately half of the interneuron population across EC, making them the largest subgroup of interneurons in the area. PV-positive cell bodies are present across all layers of EC (except layer I) but are more common in layers II and III. Layer I, however, does contain thick, radiating PV-positive dendrites that reach all the way to the pial surface. Layer II of MEC has many PV-positive neurons and heavy neuropil staining. Layer IIa of LEC has comparatively weak PV staining, with few neurons and light neuropil staining, with the exception of the area close to the rhinal/collateral sulcus in which the densities of neurons and neuropil are substantially higher (Wouterlood et al., 1995; Fujimaru and Kosaka, 1996; Leitner et al., 2016). A similar gradient is present in MEC (Beed et al., 2013; Kobro-Flatmoen and Witter, 2019). It appears that the lower number of PV-positive neurons in layer II of LEC is compensated for by a substantially higher number of the 5-HT3aR-positive cells (Leitner et al., 2016). Most PV-positive neurons belong to the class of basket cells, providing strong perisomatic inhibition onto reelin-positive principal cells in layer II and pyramidal neurons in layer III. Like PV-positive cells in other parts of the brain, they display a fast-spiking physiological profile (R Jones, 1994; Varga et al., 2010; Fuchs et al., 2016; Leitner et al., 2016; Ferrante et al., 2017).

The second PV-positive interneuron in layer II, also present in layer III, is the chandelier or axo-axonic cell. Chandelier cells are characterized by vertical aggregations of axonal boutons called cartridges, which mainly make synapses on the initial axon segments of principal cells. Both vertical and horizontal chandelier cells are present in MEC, but the horizontal subtype is dominant in LEC. The local axon branches of these neurons are largely confined to layers II and III (Soriano et al., 1993). The deeper layers V and VI do comprise PV-positive interneurons, but less is known about their specific pre- and postsynaptic contacts, their axon distribution onto the postsynaptic neurons, and their firing properties.

The proportion of SOM-positive interneurons in EC has not been properly quantified, but in other cortical regions SOM-positive cells typically account for approximately 30% of the interneuron population. SOM-positive interneurons are located across all layers of EC but are most numerous in layers V and VI (Köhler and Chan-Palay, 1983; Carboni et al., 1990), and there are no major differences between LEC and MEC in this respect. SOM-positive axonal fibers also run along superficial layer I, close to the pial surface. The axonal plexus in layer I of EC suggests that Martinotti cells make up a substantial portion of the SOM-positive interneurons in EC, as in other cortical regions. SOM-positive interneurons in rats often express calbindin as well. In MEC, SOM-positive interneurons selectively inhibit pyramidal neurons in layers III and V (Kecskés et al., 2020).

The third group of interneurons in EC, the 5-HT3aR-expressing neurons, comprise a large variety of yet poorly described cells, such as those expressing calretinin, VIP, and CCK. One subtype is formed by the CCK-expressing basket cell in layer II of MEC. Whereas CCK-positive basket cells preferentially target layer II calbindin-positive pyramidal cells, avoiding the reelin positive stellate neurons, single parvalbumin-positive basket cells do innervate both reelin- and calbindin-positive neurons (Varga et al., 2010; Armstrong et al., 2016). Similar CCK-positive basket cells are present in LEC (Köhler, 1986).

VIP-interneurons are a second class of 5-HT3aR-expressing neurons, and they are found in all layers of EC. As in the hippocampus and the neocortex, preliminary data indicate that EC VIP-positive neurons mainly have other inhibitory neurons as their main postsynaptic targets. Calretinin-expressing neurons in EC show a very tight overlap with VIP-positive interneurons, but do include excitatory neurons as well, similar to what has been reported for calbindin-positive neurons, though to a much lesser extent

(Miettinen et al., 1997; Wouterlood et al., 2000). There is very little data on either type of these neurons aside from their overall distribution patterns and morphology, as summarized recently (Kobro-Flatmoen and Witter, 2019).

There is a population of medium-to-small, round, or fusiform cells that express substance P in layers III and V in both LEC and MEC. These neurons give rise to a widespread and weak innervation across all layers, though they have a striking preference for layer Va in both the entorhinal subdivisions. Additionally, neurons expressing enkephalin, neuropeptide Y, and corticotropin releasing factor have been reported (for review, see Wouterlood, 2002). For an extensive comparative description of many chemically marked neurons and neuropil distribution, we refer the reader to the recent review paper of Kobro-Flatmoen and Witter (2019).

12.4.2 Intralaminar and interlaminar circuits and the specific involvement of interneurons and principal neurons

Since the 1980s, reports have addressed the organization of intrinsic connections in the entorhinal network. Initial studies were strongly guided by two main factors: the potential relevance of such networks in the generation of epileptic network activity (see also section 12.6.2) and, associated with the potential to generate rhythmic activity, how such cortical oscillations might impact information transfer within the entorhinal-hippocampal network, a process thought to be critical for learning and memory. Most of the data came from networks in layers II, III, and V, and data on layer VI are lacking. In what follows, we will therefore not include layer VI. In recent years, more data have become available on the differential wiring and functional contributions of the two main layer V sublayers (Va and Vb). These sublayer-specific insights are included below, but we note that the focus of these studies has been on MEC, thus this level of detail in LEC is somewhat lagging.

12.4.2.1 Intralaminar networks layer II

The local circuit of stellate cells has been probed in several studies using in vitro patch clamp recordings, and it is now well established that individual stellate cells form only very sparse monosynaptic connections with other stellate cells (reported percentages range from 0.2% to 2.5%) (Dhillon and Jones, 2000; Couey et al., 2013; Pastoll et al., 2013). Communication between stellate cells occurs through an intermediate inhibitory interneuron whereby activation of one or more stellate cells evokes disynaptic inhibitory currents in neighboring stellate cells. Paired recordings have revealed strong connectivity in both directions between stellate cells and PV-positive fast spiking cells (R Jones and Buhl, 1993; Couey et al., 2013; Pastoll et al., 2013) and, to a much lesser extent, between stellate cells and low-threshold spiking interneurons. In LEC, a rather similar network organization has been reported between fan cells, which are the principal cell counterparts to the MEC stellate cells (Tahvildari and Alonso, 2005), and fast-spiking interneurons (Nilssen et al., 2018) (Figures 12.6C and 12.7C).

The local network of layer II pyramidal cells has been explored using similar methods and, like the stellate and fan cell network, rather sparse monosynaptic connectivity was detected between pyramidal cells (in MEC, 1.6%; in LEC, 2.9%), with somewhat higher connectivity between other intermediate cell types (Fuchs et al., 2016; Winterer et al., 2017; Nilssen et al., 2018). These results suggest that the general principle of disynaptic inhibitory connectivity as described for the stellate cell network also applies to the layer II pyramidal cells but is less likely to apply to the other classes of principal neurons.

Contacts from layer II pyramidal cells with stellate and fan cells might be more frequent, and although authors do not agree on whether these are mediated by all pyramidal cells, or more specifically through intermediate pyramidal cells, the evidence in MEC points to a relatively strong calbindin-positive pyramidal cell-mediated input to stellate cells, which may go up to 13.5% (Fuchs et al., 2016; Winterer et al., 2017). Comparable connectivity percentages have been reported in LEC (Nilssen et al., 2018). This is in line with preliminary data that about 50% of calbindin-positive neurons in both MEC and LEC contribute to local connectivity (Ohara et al., 2019), and a recent in vivo study showing strong transient excitatory and inhibitory responses in layer II neurons, but not in layer III neurons, following optogenetic perturbations of calbindin-positive pyramidal cells (Zutshi et al., 2018). The connectional embedding of identified interneurons has been studied in substantial detail in MEC (Fuchs et al., 2016), though some information is available in LEC as well (Nilssen et al., 2018). Using the fast-spiking property of neurons as an indication for PV-positive interneurons, it is clear that they preferentially connect reciprocally with stellate and fan cells, as well as with the intermediate stellate and intermediate pyramidal cells in MEC, but they are not connected with pyramidal cells in MEC. In LEC, the situation differs in that both pyramidal and oblique pyramidal cells are reciprocally connected with fast-spiking interneurons. The firing pattern of SOM-positive interneurons in MEC layer II is characterized by low-threshold firing and the presence of a prominent sag potential (Fuchs et al., 2016; Ferrante et al., 2017), and since interneurons with the exact same properties have also been described in LEC layer II (Nilssen et al., 2018), we assume that these are likely SOM-positive neurons. These interneurons are reciprocally connected with stellate and intermediate pyramidal cells in MEC and with fan cells in LEC, although there are little connectional data from LEC. In MEC, pyramidal and intermediate stellate cells are not connected, although the latter class seems to synaptically contact SOM-positive neurons. In contrast, there are essentially no connections between the nonfan cell population and SOM-positive neurons in LEC.

The third class of 5-HT3aR-expressing interneurons have been characterized in the somatosensory cortex as being rather diverse electrophysiologically, but a substantial part can likely be clustered as non-fast-spiking neurons (Fuchs et al., 2016; Nilssen et al., 2018). In MEC, these neurons seem to be reciprocally connected to all types of principal cells, though with a preference for the intermediate pyramidal cells and pyramidal cells. In LEC, these interneurons show a preferential connectivity with fan cells and oblique pyramidal neurons, lesser connectivity with pyramidal neurons, and no connections with multipolar cells.

12.4.2.2 Intralaminar networks layer III

The microcircuits of layer III are only sparsely studied but seem to be markedly different from those seen in layer II, showing a much stronger monosynaptic principal-to-principal neuron connectivity, reported to be 5.7%–8.4%, at least in MEC (Dhillon and Jones, 2000; Tang et al., 2015; Winterer et al., 2017). This high interpyramidal connectivity in both LEC and MEC, together with specific channels/receptors (Jochems et al., 2013) present in these pyramidal neurons,

may be relevant for the strongly coordinated and persistent firing observed in layer III neurons. These features are likely also under the influence of combinatorial effects of certain inputs (Tahvildari et al., 2008; Beed et al., 2020). There are indications that different types of interneurons interact with principal cells. In vitro slice data in MEC show that layer III might have at least two electrophysiologically different local circuit neurons that seem to result in strong, long-lasting hyperpolarization of layer III hippocampal projecting neurons (Gloveli, Schmitz, Empson, et al., 1997; Gloveli, Schmitz, and Heinemann, 1997), and among these are likely SOM-positive interneurons (Kecskés et al., 2020).

12.4.2.3 Intralaminar networks layer V

Data on the intralaminar connectivity in layer V are extremely sparse. This sparsity becomes even more striking if we consider, as described above, that layer V seems to comprise at least two sublayers, one of which, layer Va, originates most of the cortical and subcortical forebrain projections. In contrast, neurons in layer Vb almost exclusively give rise to interlaminar projections to superficial layers (see section below). Paired recordings in dorsal MEC showed that functional connections between neurons in layer V is quite high, around 11% (Dhillon and Jones, 2000), but variable across sublayers (Rozov et al., 2020). The latter authors reported connectivity between LVa and LVb neurons being fairly low (~3% in both directions); cross-connectivity of neurons within LVb is 5.9%, but reciprocal connectivity between LVa neurons is rather high (15.6%). Principal neurons in both layers Va and Vb both contact fast-spiking interneurons, but that connectivity is much stronger in Va neurons (50%) compared to Vb neurons (5%). Principal neurons in MEC layer V seem to receive a strong inhibitory control of SOM-positive neurons (Kecskés et al., 2020). In MEC, layer V neurons show clear persistent firing that is likely generated intrinsically, in that it does not need, but is modulated by, extrinsic inputs (Egorov et al., 2002).

12.4.2.4 Interlaminar connections originating in layer II

Stellate and fan cells in layer II of MEC and LEC, respectively, originate elaborate local axon collaterals distributing densely in layer I and superficial layer II. The density tapers off rapidly in deep layer II and stays sparse in layers III and V (Tamamaki and Nojyo, 1993; Klink and Alonso, 1997; Buckmaster et al., 2004; Canto and Witter, 2012a, 2012b). Very little is known about the postsynaptic targets of these local superficial collaterals, aside from the already described strong innervation of PV-positive basket cells. Calbindin-positive layer II pyramidal cells and layer III pyramidal cells are apparently not among the main postsynaptic neurons (Fuchs et al., 2016; Winterer et al., 2017). The main axon, traveling to the hippocampal formation, emits sparse collaterals in layers III and V, likely targeting neurons (Surmeli et al., 2015). In contrast, calbindin-positive layer II neurons provide strong intrinsic projections (Ohara et al., 2019) that, at least in MEC, but likely also in LEC, distribute quite selectively in layers II and I. Perturbing this strong connectivity resulted in clear responses in grid cells, speed cells, and broadly tuned head direction cells in both layers II and III, but did not affect the sharply tuned head direction cells (Zutshi et al., 2018). In layer II, approximately one quarter of the neurons was inhibited, likely due to feedforward inhibition. In layer III, however, almost three-quarters of the neurons showed inhibitory responses.

12.4.2.5 Interlaminar connections originating in layer III

Data on interlaminar connections originating from layer III neurons are almost exclusively available in MEC. The neurons in layer III seem to exert a powerful control over neurons in both deeper and superficial layers. As referred to above, layer III pyramidal cells make direct synaptic contacts with layer II stellate cells (about 7% of the studied neuron pairs in in vitro slice recordings), which is potentially even a higher incidence than between layer III pyramidal cells. Even more surprising is the finding that the layer III-to-stellate cell connections are stronger than the pyramidal-to-pyramidal cell connections (Winterer et al., 2017). Similarly, layer III exerts a strong driving input to neurons in layer Vb, and up-down state activity generated in layer III is followed by neurons in layer Vb, but not in layer Va (Beed et al., 2020).

12.4.2.6 Interlaminar connections originating in layer V

Neurons in layer V originate strong projections to superficial layers in both LEC and MEC and include both excitatory and inhibitory projections. Older in vitro data indicated that superficial projections might preferentially originate from neurons in the deeper part of layer V (Hamam et al., 2000; Hamam et al., 2002; Buckmaster et al., 2004; Canto and Witter, 2012a, 2012b). This has been substantiated and detailed in a series of recent studies in rodents, convincingly showing that these superficially directed intrinsic projections arise mainly from neurons in layer Vb, and not from neurons in layer Va (Surmeli et al., 2015; Ohara et al., 2018; Ohara, Blankvoort, et al., 2021). In addition, these layer Vb projections show a marked preference for pyramidal neurons in layers III and II over the nonpyramidal stellate and fan neurons in layer II (Beed et al., 2010; Ohara, Blankvoort, et al., 2021). Quantitative data in MEC show that over 80% of inputs to stellate cells originate from superficial layers. For layer II pyramidal cells this percentage is approximately 70%, and the area of layer V originating inputs to a single stellate cell has a significantly smaller diameter than that projecting to the pyramidal cells in layers II and III (Beed et al., 2010). Moreover, postsynaptic responses following stimulation of layer Vb neurons in both LEC and MEC are significantly smaller in stellate and fan cells than in layer II or layer III pyramidal cells (Ohara, Blankvoort, et al., 2021).

12.4.3 Integrating local network features with extrinsic connectivity

We have thus far used the entorhinal layers as a major organizing dimension because cell types, intrinsic circuits, and many inputs and outputs show a striking laminar organization. It is important to emphasize, however, that a laminar preference does not necessarily imply a synaptic preference for neurons localized in that layer. This is mainly due to the fact that neurons with a soma in a particular layer may have dendrites extending into other layers, and the dendritic variation will thus add to the complexity of the network. For example, inputs confined to layer I will likely contact dendrites belonging to the sparse interneuron population present there, but will also contact dendrites belonging to neurons in the deeper layers II–V. Indeed, olfactory fibers in rats make synaptic contacts with apical dendrites of neurons in layers II and III (Wouterlood and Nederlof, 1983). Differences in dendritic branching may thus strongly influence the potential integrative properties of identified neurons. One example is that neurons in MEC layer Vb have an apical dendrite with distal branches in the tuft reaching into layer I, whereas the apical dendrites of LEC layer Vb neurons have a more complex proximal branching pattern and they do not extend beyond layer III. This indicates that LEC layer Vb neurons are unlikely to have synapses from the olfactory inputs mentioned above or the commissural projection from CB-positive neurons, and that such superficial inputs, including the commissural projection, will likely target the apical dendrite of MEC layer Vb neurons. Since no such striking morphological differences have been reported for layer Va and layer III neurons, here the integrative properties will likely be more similar. This complexity increases if inputs distribute over multiple layers, and perhaps the most striking example is the input from pre/parasubiculum to MEC, for which electrophysiological data clearly indicate that neurons in all layers are targeted by both types of inputs with a high likelihood (Canto et al., 2012). It goes without saying that all such functional inferences strongly depend on dendritic integration and local properties such as types and density of different receptors, as well as differences in biophysical properties of the neurons. We currently lack sufficient data to provide an integrated representation of such complex interactions, but it is evident they play a role in the last-mentioned paper, where it is apparent that neurons in different layers show rather striking differences in response properties to the same stimulated input. Similarly, although neurons in layers II and III of MEC share many inputs, a recent study indicated that the spatiotemporal firing properties of layer III neurons are remarkably different from those in layer II (Tang et al., 2015).

12.5 Function of entorhinal cortex

EC serves as a critical interface between sensory and associative cortical areas and the hippocampus. Given its anatomical position in the medial temporal lobe, it should intuitively play a functional role in declarative memory processes. Pioneering work starting in the 1970s explored this role by using lesions and electrode recordings during memory tasks. Lesions of EC in rats impaired both spatial memory (Olton et al., 1978) and olfactory memory (Staubli et al., 1986). In one of these memory tasks, a delayed (non)match-to-sample (DMS) procedure was used to test recognition memory by presenting two stimuli sequentially with a delay period between them. The subject was rewarded for correctly identifying whether the second stimulus matched the first. Lesions of EC in monkeys caused memory deficits in this task (Meunier et al., 1993), and these deficits became progressively worse with longer delay periods between the stimuli (Leonard et al., 1995). Young et al. (1997) and Suzuki et al. (1997) were the first to record single entorhinal units in this task, in rats and in monkeys, respectively. They found multiple features of entorhinal activity supporting the idea that this area is important for recognition memory: (1) many entorhinal neurons were selective for specific visual or olfactory stimuli, (2) these responses could persist during the delay period, and (3) many neurons were also match-selective, i.e., their firing rates were either enhanced or suppressed based on whether the second stimulus matched the first.

Although the DMS task and many other memory tests are performed while subjects are immobile, memories are formed as we move throughout the world and are thought to be associated with the specific spatiotemporal context at the moment of encoding. Learning to navigate an environment is therefore tightly linked with the formation of episodic memories. As an animal moves through space, it continuously updates an estimate of its position by monitoring its direction of movement and distance traveled. This use of self-motion information as a navigational strategy is called path integration and is used by a wide range of species from insects (von Frisch, 1947) to mammals (Darwin, 1873). While effective across short distances, path integration is prone to accumulating error over time. To reduce these errors, animals can use environmental cues (e.g., landmarks) to reset their positional estimate. Importantly, these sensory cues could become bound to the spatial map through associative learning to create an allocentric (world-centered) representation of the environment. This relational representation of all objects and locations in an environment is referred to as a cognitive map (Tolman, 1948).

One of the key elements of the cognitive map is the hippocampal place cell, a neuron that is most active when an animal is in a particular place in a given environment (i.e., its "place field"; O'Keefe and Dostrovsky, 1971). Most principal cells in the hippocampus are place cells. Each place cell with activity in the environment has its place field in a different location such that a population of place cells collectively maps the entire environment. The discovery of place cells led O'Keefe and Nadel to propose in their book from 1978 (O'Keefe and Nadel, 1978) that the hippocampus was the neural substrate for the cognitive map, a theory that has inspired an entire field of research. Another key element needed for a cognitive map is a mental compass telling the animal which direction it is heading. Head direction cells serve this critical function: each cell is highly active only when the animal's head is pointing in a particular allocentric direction (Ranck, 1984; Clark and Taube, 2012). The discovery of head direction cells (first recorded in the dorsal presubiculum of rats) was momentous because it lent strong support to the cognitive map theory, and because neural representations of position and heading can be used to perform path integration. There is, however, a problem with the use of place cells for this purpose, because for each distinct environment that the animal visits, place cells *remap* by shuffling their firing fields to seemingly random locations (Muller and Kubie, 1987). This would require a unique network architecture for each environment (Samsonovich and McNaughton, 1997). It was thought that there should exist a simpler mechanism with a context-invariant spatial map, and that perhaps this more generalized spatial signal was the source of spatial input to place cells.

It was assumed for some time that the spatial specificity of place cells in area CA1 was created within the hippocampus because recordings upstream in EC showed considerably less spatial modulation (Barnes et al., 1990). To test this idea, a series of experiments lesioned the dentate gyrus (McNaughton et al., 1989), inactivated CA3 (Mizumori et al., 1989), or cut the projections from CA3 to CA1 (Brun et al., 2002). The results were clear: CA1 place fields persisted after all three manipulations, and therefore they do not exclusively rely on CA3 for their spatial tuning; rather they likely rely on direct spatial input from EC. Critically, early recordings in EC were not performed in the area that receives the most visual-tactile information and that projects most densely to the dorsal hippocampus, where place fields are most sharply tuned. This realization prompted the recording of neurons in the dorsal MEC for the first time (Fyhn et al., 2004), leading to the discovery of new dedicated cell types for each fundamental element needed to build a cognitive map.

In subsequent sections, we describe (1) the building blocks of the cognitive map that are found in EC, (2) the emergence and organization of the grid cell network, (3) the contribution of EC to hippocampal mapping, (4) the functional differences between medial and lateral entorhinal cortices, (5) entorhinal function in primates, and (6) entorhinal coding beyond physical space.

12.5.1 Dedicated cell types for elements of the cognitive map

12.5.1.1 Grid cells

In search of the origin of the spatial signal in the hippocampus, a team of researchers at the Norwegian University of Science and Technology began recording in the dorsalmost extent of MEC, close to neighboring postrhinal cortex (Fyhn et al., 2004). Cells in this dorsal part of MEC had substantially stronger spatial tuning compared with cells in more ventral parts, consistent with earlier recordings showing weak spatial modulation in ventral MEC (Barnes et al., 1990). These dorsal cells had well-defined firing fields, similar to place cells, but instead of having only one field, they typically had multiple sharply tuned fields (Fyhn et al., 2004). In fact, the fields seemed to be evenly spaced apart, thus creating a regular pattern throughout the environment, though it was unclear at the time exactly what that pattern was.

To have enough firing fields to identify any regularities in the firing pattern, Hafting et al. (2005) began recording animals in a much larger environment than the ones used conventionally for place cell recordings in the hippocampus. These experiments made it clear that a substantial number of neurons in dorsal MEC have firing fields that repeat at regular intervals, spaced ~30–50 cm apart. These firing fields tile the entire environment in a symmetric hexagonal pattern (Figure 12.10). Each grid cell has a grid pattern with three major features: (1) the *spacing* of the grid defines its size, calculated as the center-to-center distance between firing fields; (2) the *orientation* of the grid defines its rotation, calculated as the angular offset relative to a reference axis; and (3) the spatial *phase* of the grid defines the location of its firing fields, calculated as a two-dimensional offset relative to a reference point. Analyzing these features made it clear that neurons found more ventrally in MEC are indeed spatially tuned, but ventral grid cells have a much larger spacing between their firing fields (~3 m), making them difficult to recognize in smaller environments. This spacing increases on average from dorsal to ventral MEC (Fyhn et al., 2004; Brun, Solstad, et al., 2008). Interestingly, although neighboring grid cells share the same spacing and orientation, they have largely random phases (Hafting et al., 2005). This means that at each anatomical position along the dorsoventral axis of MEC, only a few grid cells are needed to tile the entire environment and form a complete spatial map.

Grid cell activity is extremely stable despite constant changes in the speed and direction of the animal as it freely moves about the environment. This stability could result from path integration or from a reliance on stable sensory cues. To test whether grid cell firing is controlled by sensory cues, Hafting et al. (2005) rotated a large cue card between trials in an otherwise uniform environment. The grid pattern followed the cue card by rotating by the same amount. Grid cells also have stable patterns across repeated trials in the same environment (Hafting et al., 2005), suggesting that available cues become bound to the grid pattern during its initial formation and subsequently act as an anchor to align the pattern.

Sensory cues, however, may not be strictly necessary for the expression of the grid pattern. When grid cells were recorded as

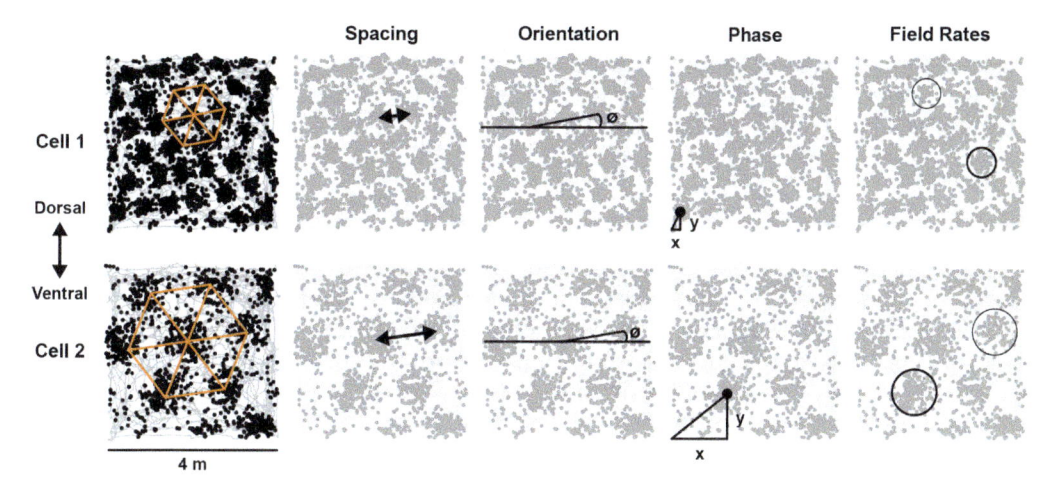

Figure 12.10 Grid cells in medial entorhinal cortex. Spike path plots for two grid cells, one cell per row. Gray lines indicate the trajectory of a rat as it foraged in a large open field environment (4 × 4 m). Black dots indicate locations of each spike. Spikes cluster into firing fields that repeat at regular intervals, covering the entire environment and creating a hexagonal grid pattern depicted in orange (first column). Grid cells are defined based on the existence of this grid pattern, but there are multiple features of the grid that vary between different grid cells. The spacing between firing fields varies from ~30 cm to >3 m, and this distance increases along the dorsoventral axis of medial entorhinal cortex (second column). The orientation of the grid relative to a horizontal reference axis also varies between cells (third column). Next, each grid cell has a particular spatial phase relative to a reference point (fourth column). Finally, grid cells exhibit highly variable firing field rates (fifth column). (Data collected by Valentin A. Normand in the Moser lab.)

rats ran in total darkness, the grid was intact (Hafting et al., 2005). Moreover, when animals were tested in a novel environment, the grid pattern was established almost instantaneously (Hafting et al., 2005). Place cells respond similarly to all of these manipulations: place fields follow a cue card that is rotated between trials (Muller and Kubie, 1987), they are stable over time (Thompson and Best, 1990), they persist during darkness (Quirk et al., 1990), and they are quickly expressed in novel environments (Hill, 1978). These commonalities between place cells and grid cells suggest that they both rely on path integration, because their spatial maps are instantly formed without any need for environmental cues. In contrast, self-motion information is necessary for normal spatial firing: passive transport in a car causes the grid pattern to disappear (Winter et al., 2015) and greatly reduces the spatial tuning of place cells (Terrazas et al., 2005). More recent work has demonstrated that the grid structure is even maintained during sleep (Gardner et al., 2019; Trettel et al., 2019), when sensory information is largely irrelevant. It is therefore likely that the grid structure is an intrinsic network property (see section 12.5.2) and that self-motion information provides smooth updating of the current position. Sensory cues, rather than creating the grid pattern, may be critical determinants of where in the environment a grid cell is active (e.g., setting its phase and orientation).

Perhaps the most salient aspect of any navigable space is its boundaries which restrict the animal's movement. So how do grid cells respond when the shape of the environment is changed? After rats are familiarized to a box of specific dimensions, grid cells will rescale their firing patterns to match a distorted version of that box, stretching or compressing to fill the available space (Barry et al., 2007). As above, this rescaling effect is consistent with the response of place cells (O'Keefe and Burgess, 1996) and indicates that the spatial map becomes linked to a set of stable cues in the environment. Moreover, if local and distal cues are put into conflict, the grid pattern is more strongly controlled by salient local cues (Savelli et al., 2017), presumably because they more directly impact

navigation. In more irregularly shaped environments, the grid pattern can become distorted (Krupic et al., 2015; T Stensola et al., 2015) or even break down completely (Krupic et al., 2015), regardless of past experience. In a trapezoid, the hexagonal symmetry of the firing fields is lost in the narrow portion of the environment (Krupic et al., 2015), presumably due to the nonparallel boundaries. These observations raised some discussion about whether grid cells can provide a useful spatial metric in these oddly shaped enclosures, but subsequent work has shown that position can be read out precisely from grid cell activity provided that cells respond coherently to distortions (Stemmler et al., 2015), which they appear to do (H Stensola et al., 2012; Wernle et al., 2017).

In addition to forming a link between the grid pattern and the environment, boundaries also prevent drift in the pattern over time. Hardcastle et al. (2015) showed that grid cell firing patterns continuously accumulate error as the animal explores an environment at a rate that would prevent an accurate representation of position after tens of minutes. When the animal encounters a boundary, however, the grid pattern is corrected in a direction-dependent manner (i.e., running north into a wall will correct the north–south estimate, but not the east–west estimate). While objects and other salient cues could play a similar role in more complex environments, boundaries likely play a critical role in anchoring and maintaining a regular grid pattern in geometrically simple environments.

The beautiful and striking regularity of the grid signal inspired many theoretical models attempting to explain the origin of the hexagonal pattern. While the details of some of the more influential models are described in section 12.5.2, here it is important to note how these early models motivated the search for other key components of the positioning system.

When grid cells were discovered, it was thought that the algorithms for updating position could be similar to those proposed for head direction cells and place cells. As described in section 12.4, the MEC microcircuit contains strong intrinsic connectivity (Witter, Doan, et al., 2017) which could enable a two-dimensional continuous attractor-based representation of the environment (McNaughton et al., 1996). Updating this representation could be accomplished using a path-integration based mechanism which requires that both direction and speed information are present in dorsal MEC. There was good reason to think that dorsal MEC cells would contain directional information due to inputs arising from dorsal presubiculum, although the source of a speed signal was less clear. Another critical component of this path integrator model is an intermediate layer of cells that conjunctively encodes position and head direction, which, together with speed information, enables movement of the activity bump. There were therefore explicit predictions from early computational models about the cell types that should exist in MEC if it were to perform path integration, and they would soon be discovered as well.

12.5.1.2 Head direction cells

If there is a path-integration-based spatial map in the MEC with grid cells representing the animal's position, where does the directional information come from? To test whether directional information was also encoded within the same local circuits, Sargolini et al. (2006) recorded neural activity from all principal layers of the MEC in rats. They found that while layer II mostly contained grid cells, layers III through V contained grid cells intermingled with many cells tuned to head direction. It was thought when grid cells were first discovered that directional information from upstream dorsal presubiculum was critical for updating position estimates. The finding that head direction cells exist within MEC and are situated near grid cells changed the anatomical constraints for path integration and suggested that hardwired local connectivity within MEC could be sufficient. In further support of the path integration model, many cells, particularly in deep layers of MEC, were conjunctive grid × head direction cells, meaning that they were only active when the animal passed through the grid fields in a specific allocentric direction (Sargolini et al., 2006). As mentioned above, this conjunctive coding is required to translate the activity bump in the appropriate direction.

While local head direction information within MEC simplifies the model structure for computing path integration, numerous brain areas encode head direction, and the relationships between these directional representations are important for understanding the transformation of spatial signals en route to the hippocampus. The origins of the head direction signal are found in the brainstem and mammillary bodies, where cells are tuned to angular head velocity, and these early areas are critical for forming the first pure allocentric head direction signal in the anterodorsal thalamic nucleus (Taube, 2007). This thalamic relay projects further to the retrosplenial cortex and the dorsal presubiculum, both of which have direct projections to MEC. In contrast to the pure allocentric head direction signal in the anterodorsal thalamic nucleus, head direction cells further downstream have more complex coding properties. Retrosplenial cells, for example, can have bidirectional tuning (i.e., equal preference for two distinct heading angles) and are heavily dependent on visual information (Jacob et al., 2017). Head direction cells in presubiculum (where the first such cells were reported; Taube et al., 1990), parasubiculum, and MEC can also exhibit conjunctive representations for head direction, grid, and/or theta phase (Sargolini et al., 2006). The head direction signal is therefore dominated by idiothetic information in the brainstem and mammillary bodies and becomes increasingly influenced by cognitive variables such as

visual landmarks (Jacob et al., 2017), and possibly even environmental geometry (Munn et al., 2020), as the information passes to the hippocampal formation and associated areas.

It is important to note here that path integration models rely on movement direction, not head direction. Movement direction denotes the direction of travel, whereas head direction denotes the orientation of the head. These two variables are often correlated, but are indeed distinct, and which brain areas encode movement direction is largely unknown (Raudies et al., 2015). In addition, movement direction and running speed must be multiplicatively integrated into a velocity signal, not simply summed.

12.5.1.3 Speed cells

For grid cells to perform path integration, they need to have access to information about moment-to-moment changes in the animal's running speed. While it was known that cells both in the hippocampus (McNaughton et al., 1983) and in subcortical areas that project to EC (King et al., 1998) are speed-responsive, it was unknown whether speed information was encoded locally within MEC. From the earliest studies of grid cells, it was already apparent that a subset of grid cells was weakly modulated by speed, particularly those grid cells in layers III and V (Sargolini et al., 2006). It was not until 2015, however, that Kropff et al. showed that a distinct subset of cells in MEC have strong linear relationships between firing rate and running speed (Kropff et al., 2015). Importantly, these speed cells have such reliable speed–rate relationships that the animal's speed can be decoded from the firing rate of only a handful of cells. Speed cells are mostly fast-spiking interneurons (Ye et al., 2018) and make up 15%–25% of cells in MEC across all layers. The density, distribution, and widespread projections of speed cells, together with their universal coding across contexts, lends further support to the notion that MEC forms a path-integration-based cognitive map.

While speed cells are an integral part of the local MEC network, they are also part of a brain-wide speed circuit. Hippocampal place cells encode running speed (McNaughton et al., 1983), and the hippocampus receives direct projections from the speed cells in MEC (Ye et al., 2018). The hippocampus and MEC both receive strong input from the medial septum, a region that exerts a powerful influence on spatial and temporal firing patterns in the hippocampal formation (Buzsáki and Moser, 2013) and contains speed modulated neurons as well (King et al., 1998). Carvalho et al. (2020) recently traced the origins of the entorhinal speed signal back to the pedunculopontine nuclei in the brainstem, a locomotor region with widespread projections throughout the brain. They found that the pedunculopontine nuclei send a running speed signal to MEC via the medial septum, where each area contains a substantial number of cells that linearly encode running speed. MEC thus has direct access to subcortical structures initiating locomotor programs, thereby enabling stable and regular spatial codes in the hippocampal formation.

12.5.1.4 Border cells

Shortly after the discovery of head direction cells in MEC, Solstad et al. (2008) and Savelli et al. (2008) independently found another key cell type for mapping an environment. Border cells are preferentially active along one or more specific boundaries, including walls of a box and edges of a platform (Figure 12.11A). Consistent with a universal map of space, border cells generalize across multiple walls of the same type. For example, a cell that fires along the right side of

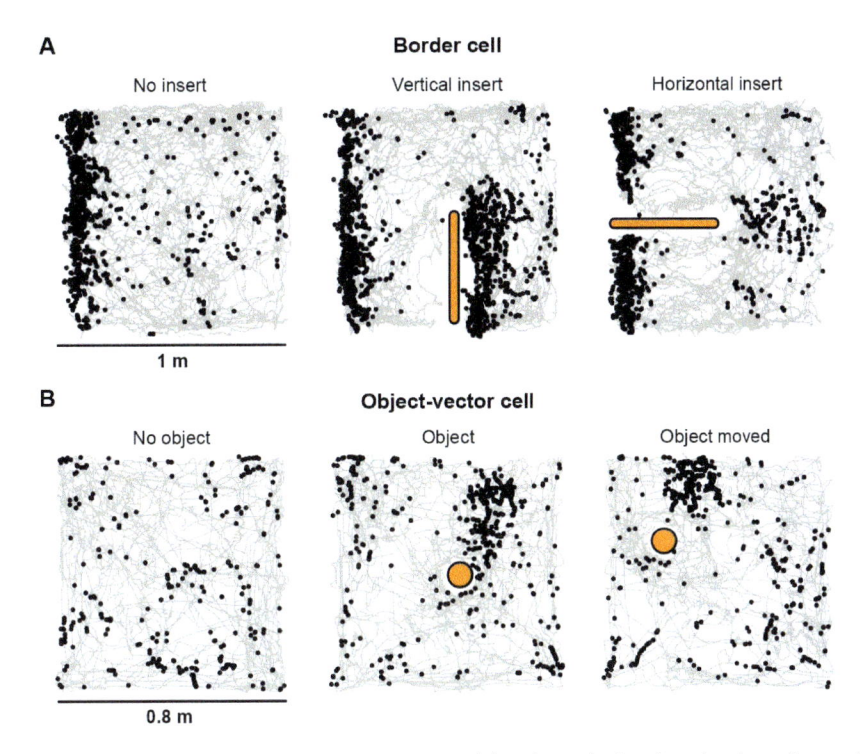

Figure 12.11 Border and object representations in medial entorhinal cortex. (A) Spike path plots for a border cell recorded in three different sessions (columns). Gray lines indicate the trajectory of the animal as it foraged in an open field environment (1 × 1 m). Black dots indicate locations of each spike. Spikes cluster into a firing field that spans the right side of the west wall of the environment (first column). When a vertical wall (thick orange line) is inserted, another firing field develops along the right side of this wall (second column), duplicating the pattern seen in the first session. When a horizontal wall is inserted, the original firing field is bisected, and a new firing field develops to the right of this wall (third column). This border cell thus encodes the right (east) edge of all walls. (Data from Solstad et al., 2008.) (B) Spike path plots for an object-vector cell recorded in three different sessions (columns). Same conventions as in (A). Very few spikes occur in the absence of objects (first column). After an object (orange circle) is introduced, spikes cluster into a firing field at a specific distance and allocentric direction from the object, here approximately 20 cm northeast (second column). When the object is moved to a new location, the firing field moves along with it, preserving the same distance and direction (third column). Note that object-vector cell responses are independent of head direction. (Data from Høydal et al., 2019.)

the west wall will also fire along the right side of a new wall inserted parallel to the first in the middle of the box. Border cells are found mostly in superficial layers II and III, nearby grid and head direction cells. Compared with grid cells and head direction cells, border cells are much sparser, comprising only 5%–10% of principal cells in MEC. This sparsity, however, does not rule out the possibility that they serve a critical role in anchoring the spatial map. Grid cells are strongly influenced by borders, as described above, and the entire grid pattern appears to be oriented with a specific angular offset relative to the walls (T Stensola et al., 2015). Border cells may be responsible for sharpening grid cell representations near walls and for resetting the path integrator, although a direct experimental link between the effects of boundaries on the cognitive map and the activity of border cells has not yet been made.

Border-selective cells are not restricted to MEC and are in fact even found within the hippocampus (Rivard et al., 2004) and the subiculum (Barry et al., 2006; Lever et al., 2009), thus raising the possibility that border representations are created in one area and inherited in downstream areas. Boundary-vector cells in the subiculum (Barry et al., 2006; Lever et al., 2009) are similar to MEC border cells, but instead of firing only along environmental borders, they fire in a distance-dependent manner from specific walls. This firing pattern yields band-like firing fields throughout the environment when considering a population of boundary-vector cells. The discovery of boundary-vector cells was an exciting confirmation of

theoretical predictions from O'Keefe and Burgess (1996) and later Hartley et al. (2000) that the building blocks of hippocampal place cell representations might encode specific distance–direction relationships to boundaries, a model discussed in section 12.5.3. The general direction of information flow suggested by the anatomy of the hippocampal formation, however, makes it more likely that border cells in MEC provide the dominant source of boundary-related input to the hippocampus.

12.5.1.5 Object-vector cells

The presence of grid cells, head direction cells, border cells, and speed cells in MEC enables a highly accurate representation of position which is easily updated as the animal explores its environment. Given the powerful influence of boundaries described above, it would make sense that prominent objects, especially those that impede the animal's movement and/or serve as landmarks, would also be incorporated into the spatial representation. In fact, McNaughton et al. (1995) predicted the existence of place fields that could be defined by vectorial relationships to landmarks in allocentric coordinates. Nearly all studies thus far of spatial cells in the hippocampal formation, however, had animals exploring empty environments. Høydal et al. (2019) recorded from MEC in mice exploring environments with one or more objects and found that a subset of cells encoded the allocentric distance and direction to objects, and thus named these cells object-vector cells (Figure 12.11B). The activity of object-vector cells is irrespective of both the number and the identity of the objects, and firing emerges during the first exposure to the object(s). Moreover, object-vector cells have the same firing patterns in distinct environments, consistent with a universal spatial map in MEC.

Much like other functional cell types in MEC, object-vector cells also resemble cells in other areas with the same general coding properties. The hippocampus contains so-called landmark vector cells (Deshmukh and Knierim, 2013), which fire at a specific distance and direction to objects but do not seem to generalize across all objects or immediately stabilize their firing patterns in novel environments. Similar findings of hippocampal cells firing in relation to landmarks were previously reported, although vectorial relationships were not examined (Gothard, Skaggs, Moore, et al., 1996). Boundary-vector cells in the subiculum, described above, also resemble object-vector cells due to their vectorial coding. Object-vector cells will continue to fire at the same distance and direction relative to an object even as it is stretched and transformed into a wall (Høydal et al., 2019). This is further indication that object-vector cell coding generalizes well, and boundary-vector cells may in fact be considered a subset of object-vector cells outside of MEC that only respond to elongated boundaries. Lastly, object-vector cells share some properties with border cells in MEC, especially when objects are stretched. An important distinction, however, is that border cells only respond to barriers that impede the animal's movement (Solstad et al., 2008), whereas object-vector cells also respond to objects suspended from the ceiling that the animal can run underneath (Høydal et al., 2019). Object-vector coding is therefore the most universal code for objects/boundaries in the hippocampal region and is tightly integrated with other MEC cell types.

12.5.1.6 Other cell types in medial entorhinal cortex

Other functional cell types within MEC are less well understood, such as aperiodic spatial cells (Zhang et al., 2013). With new entorhinal cell types described every few years, one wonders what the currently unclassified entorhinal cells may encode. Changing the experimental design may yield new insights, as it did for the discovery of object-vector cells (Høydal et al., 2019). Another possibility is that improved analysis methods will uncover new functional roles. Hardcastle et al. (2017), for example, used a generalized linear model (GLM) to classify cells, as opposed to using standard scores for each functional type, and found that nearly all MEC cells encoded some combination of position, speed, head direction, and theta phase, similar to the conjunction of grid and head direction patterns observed originally by Sargolini et al. (2006). The assessment of mixed selectivity in MEC will necessarily depend on the strictness of criteria for cell classification, but the findings so far suggest both that a large fraction of MEC cells respond to singular features of the environment (unlike cells in most other high-level cortical regions) and that conjunctive coding is present. Note that while some covariates such as speed may interact with many others, there are covariates that clearly do not overlap: grid cells and object-vector cells are distinct. Each cell type also retains its identity across different environments (i.e., grid cells are always grid cells). It will be important in future work to continue to develop theory regarding representations that are likely to exist in the network, and to carefully design experiments and statistical analyses that can reveal these representations.

12.5.1.7 Neighboring brain areas with coding similar to medial entorhinal cortex

As described above, many of the functional cell types in MEC have counterparts in nearby brain areas. Notably, grid cells are also found in presubiculum and parasubiculum (Boccara et al., 2010), two major inputs to MEC. These grid cells appear to be most like grid cells in the deep layers of MEC: their density is similar, they are intermixed with head direction and border cells, they often conjunctively encode head direction, and they exhibit less regular sixfold symmetry (Boccara et al., 2010). Due to differences in circuitry between MEC and pre/parasubiculum, the presence of grid cells in all regions constrains the possible mechanisms of grid formation, as discussed in the following section.

12.5.2 Emergence of the grid pattern and organization of the grid network

The striking regularity of grid cell receptive fields immediately raised questions about the mechanisms underlying the emergence of the grid. Is the sixfold symmetry determined by a single cell process or is it a consequence of intrinsic network connectivity? In addition, nearby grid cells seemed to have similar properties (spacing, orientation, etc.), suggesting that they could be grouped together into functional clusters. In this section, we describe recent progress toward understanding the origin and network structure of the grid signal.

12.5.2.1 Mechanisms of grid cell formation

Neural firing patterns within the positional system of EC are surprisingly resilient to perturbations, remaining intact in complete darkness and throughout continuous changes in the animal's running speed and direction. This stability of neural responses is a hallmark of self-sustained activity governed by recurrent connectivity within a neural network (Hebb, 1949; Amari, 1977). These so-called attractor networks have several advantageous computational properties. They have one or more stable points to which activity quickly converges. Once in a stable point, the network is highly resistant to noise and can remain in that state indefinitely, even in the absence of external input. While some networks exhibit one or more discrete attractors, other networks exhibit a continuum of attractor states. When neurons are strongly connected to their immediate neighbors and only weakly connected to neurons farther away, this leads to a stable "bump" of activity in a small group of nearby neurons (Amari, 1977; Ben-Yishai et al., 1995). The activity can smoothly transition around the network such that each active group of nearby neurons is a stable network state, thus creating a continuous attractor network (Figure 12.12).

Following the discovery of head direction cells in the dorsal presubiculum (Ranck, 1984), many researchers independently applied the ideas put forward by Hebb and Amari to explain the directional tuning of these cells (McNaughton et al., 1991; Skaggs et al., 1995). Neurons are arranged conceptually on a ring such that neighboring neurons have similar directional preferences (Figure 12.12A). Local excitatory and global inhibitory connectivity leads to a stable activity bump on the ring that moves in concert with the animal's heading, thus creating an allocentric neural network compass. The preserved angular relationships between head direction cells across conditions and environments implies a low-dimensional architecture, as expected if activity is driven around the ring by head

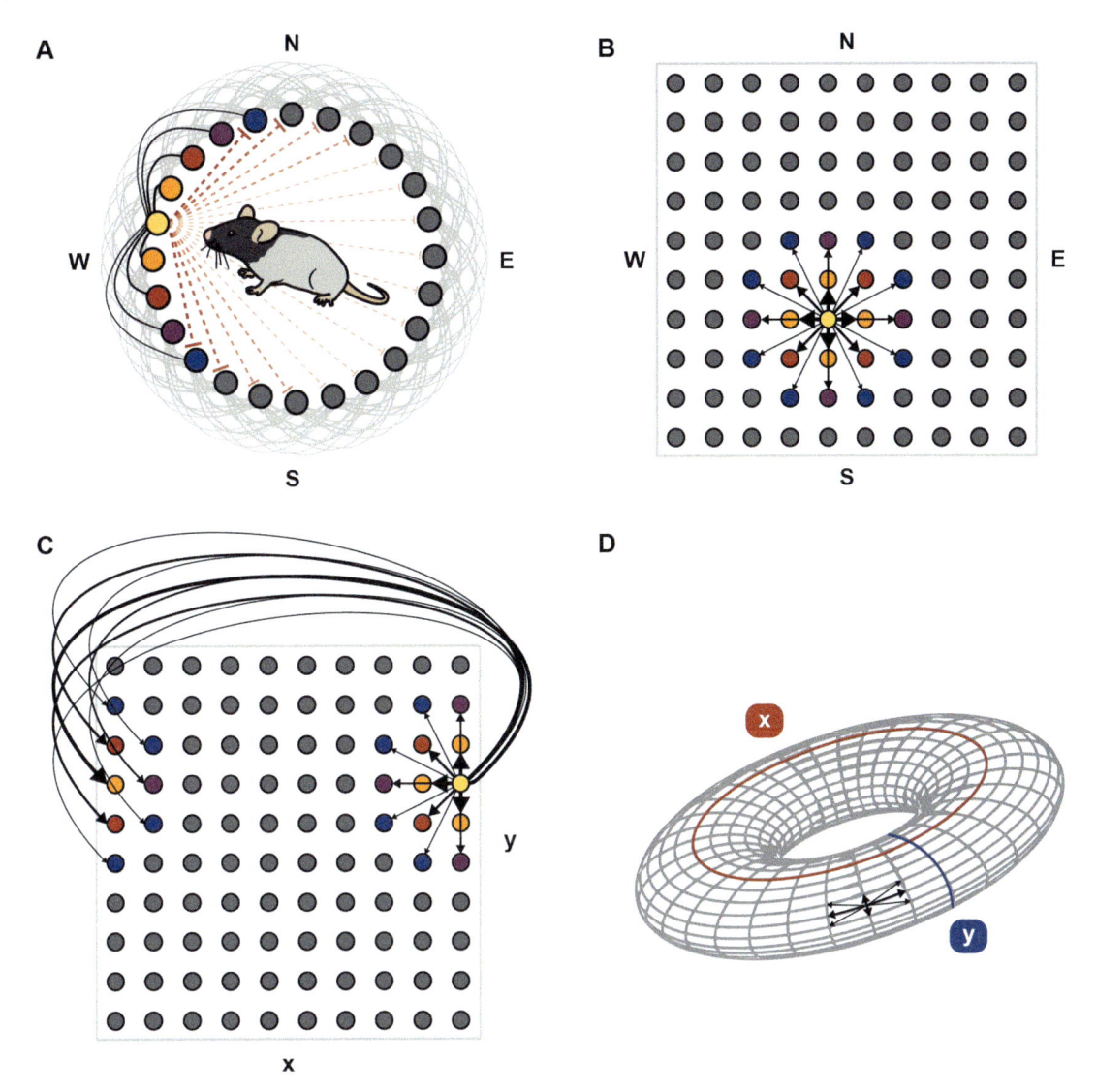

Figure 12.12 Continuous attractor networks in one and two dimensions. (A) One-dimensional continuous attractor network for head direction. Neurons (circles) are arranged around a ring corresponding to their preferred allocentric head direction. Each neuron sends strong excitatory connections to neighboring neurons with similar preferred directions (black lines), and the level of this excitation decreases with distance around the ring. Neurons with opposing preferred directions are inhibited (red dashed lines). At the snapshot in time depicted here, the rat is heading west. This results in high activity levels for the westward neurons (bright colors) and suppression of the remaining neurons (dark colors). The activity of this network of neurons thus codes for the heading direction of the rat. This stable activity bump on the west side of the ring will smoothly translate to other parts of the ring in concert with the heading of the animal and could stably remain at any of those positions, thus forming a continuum of stable states. (Rat modified from Tang, Wenbo, "Long-Evans Rat Still (Modified from Ethan Tyler's Drawing), " Zenodo, 2020, http://doi.org/ 10.5281/zenodo.3926042.) (B) Two-dimensional (2D) continuous attractor network for position. Neurons (circles) are arranged on a 2D neural sheet corresponding to their preferred firing location. As in (A), recurrent connectivity with local excitation (black arrows) and long-range inhibition (not shown) maintains a stable activity bump, which smoothly translates in concert with the position of the animal. At the snapshot in time depicted here, the rat is located slightly southwest of center in the environment. This results in high activity levels for the neurons preferring this location (bright colors) and suppression of the remaining neurons (dark colors). This stable activity bump has a 2D Gaussian shape and will smoothly translate to other parts of the environment as the animal changes location. As in (A), every position is a stable state. (C) Sharp boundaries at the edges of this two-dimensional neural sheet create a problem for mapping a continuous grid pattern. To resolve this issue, connections between neurons at the edges of the neural sheet wrap around to the other side in both the x and y directions. (D) The periodic boundary conditions imposed in (C) create a three-dimensional donut-shaped structure called a torus. (Figure inspired by McNaughton et al., 2006.)

velocity inputs. As mentioned above, a directional ring attractor likely resides in the brainstem and mammillary bodies (Clark and Taube, 2012). In recent years, exciting experiments have confirmed the major theoretical predictions of the ring attractor model in fruit flies, where is it possible to record from the whole network and the connectivity is known (Seelig and Jayaraman, 2015). Topological analyses in mammalian head direction circuits have also uncovered

a low-dimensional ring structure (Chaudhuri et al., 2019), which likely does not reflect physical topography as it does in the fruit fly.

It was quickly realized that the continuous attractor network model used in one dimension for head direction tuning could be extended to two dimensions for positional tuning (Tsodyks and Sejnowski, 1995). Rather than being arranged on a ring, neurons are arranged on a two-dimensional neural sheet based on their preferred location of firing (Figure 12.12B). Similar to the head direction model, recurrent connectivity with local excitation and global inhibition maintains a stable activity bump, and this bump moves across the network in concert with the animal's position. In place of conjunctive head direction × angular velocity cells, the two-dimensional model relies on conjunctive head direction × place cells for the smooth translation of activity. Interestingly, this model was first focused on CA3 place cells because of the known recurrent network architecture and because, at the time, they provided the clearest positional signal in the hippocampal formation. Due to the drastic reorganization of the active population of place cells in distinct environments, however, this continuous attractor model would require a distinct architecture for each environment (Samsonovich and McNaughton, 1997), a biologically implausible assumption.

After learning about the grid cell network in the next 10–20 years, it became clear that its properties were much more consistent with a universal path-integration-based positioning system (Fuhs and Touretzky, 2006; McNaughton et al., 2006; Guanella et al., 2007). In these models, grid cells with similar spatial phases typically have excitatory connections with each other. If each cell instead receives inhibition from neighboring neurons, however, this can also produce a hexagonal grid (Burak and Fiete, 2009), provided there is tonic global excitation. Both reelin-positive stellate cells and calbindin-positive pyramidal cells can be grid cells (Rowland et al., 2018), and each cell type communicates through its own class of inhibitory neurons: stellate cells connect to each other through parvalbumin cells and pyramidal cells connect to each other through 5-HT3a cells (Fuchs et al., 2016). To resolve the boundary problem of using a two-dimensional neural sheet for a periodic grid pattern, the connections of cells at the edges of the neural sheet wrap around (Figure 12.12C; Samsonovich and McNaughton, 1997; McNaughton et al., 2006). This periodic boundary condition converts the neural sheet into a torus (Figure 12.12D; Gardner et al., 2022). Grid cell activity therefore maps both onto physical space and onto a toroidal representation of that space.

A plausible alternative for the emergence of the grid pattern is that it arises from a single cell process, as opposed to arising through network interactions. Kropff and Treves (2008), for example, showed that any spatially organized input (including hippocampal place cells) to neurons that undergo adaptation results in grid-like firing patterns. As the animal explores an environment, spatial inputs drive an entorhinal unit and, if above a certain threshold, these connections are strengthened via Hebbian plasticity. After being highly active, the neuron is fatigued, and its firing rate will decrease. The neuron will exhibit multiple firing fields throughout the environment in this manner, and the triangular grid pattern appears to be a favored arrangement of the fields. Connections between neurons can be included in the model only to ensure that nearby neurons have the same grid spacing and orientation (Si et al., 2012). Importantly, firing patterns take a long time to develop in this adaptation model, so it may be most relevant early in an animal's development (Si et al., 2012). In the adult, attractor networks could take over, thus making it possible that both single-cell and network-level mechanisms are responsible for the grid pattern. Later work expanded on the foundation of Kropff and Treves (2008) by using spike-based models (D'Albis and Kempter, 2017) and deriving biologically plausible learning rules (Castro and Aguiar, 2014).

Another alternative model for grid formation was the oscillatory interference model (Burgess et al., 2007), which suggested that the firing fields arise due to temporal interference between sinusoidal waves with slightly different frequencies. The model was initially formulated to describe place fields (O'Keefe and Recce, 1993), where the field was produced due to interference between the global theta-frequency oscillation and a cell-specific velocity-controlled theta oscillation. After the discovery of grid cells, it was adapted to include not one cell-specific oscillator, but three different velocity-controlled oscillators with the velocity vectors separated by 60-degree intervals, each of which resided on separate dendrites. This mechanism creates band-like spatial firing patterns at each 60-degree orientation, and the combination of these bands creates a hexagonal grid.

While the oscillatory interference model had a tremendous impact on the study of grid cells, there now exists a large body of counterevidence. Perhaps most notably, Domnisoru et al. (2013) and Schmidt-Hieber and Häusser (2013) independently performed in vivo intracellular recordings from grid cells to test for the presence of a cell-specific theta oscillator and, as predicted by the attractor network models, a slow ramping depolarization. They found clear ramps of depolarization, no stable oscillations at a fixed theta frequency, and showed that ramps were the primary force driving firing field formation. In addition, grid patterns are expressed in crawling bats despite a lack of theta oscillations (Yartsev et al., 2011). The oscillatory interference model is therefore no longer considered a plausible mechanism for grid cell formation.

12.5.2.2 Grid cell network properties

Given the recurrent connectivity within the MEC and the strong explanatory power of attractor models for grid cell formation, it is important to consider the anatomical and functional organization of the grid cell network. As described above, grid cells initially appeared to cluster based on their field spacing and orientation, although each grid cell within a cluster had a random phase or spatial offset from one another (Hafting et al., 2005). Moreover, the grid spacing dramatically increases along the dorsoventral axis of MEC (Brun, Solstad, et al., 2008), much like the increase in place-field size along the dorsoventral axis of the hippocampus (Jung et al., 1994). This change in grid spacing could have proved problematic for attractor models, as they require each connected cell in the network to have the same spacing. Thus, the only way to have grid cells with different spacings governed by attractor dynamics is to have multiple discrete networks, each with their own gain control (i.e., slower movement of the activity bump for grid cells with larger spacing). Some years later, H. Stensola et al. (2012) were able to record enough grid cells in each animal to prove that the increase in grid spacing was not continuous but was in fact discrete (see also Barry et al., 2007). They found at least four of these grid modules, each with their own spacing, orientation, and asymmetry (Figure 12.13). It was subsequently shown that this modular organization is an extremely efficient way to represent space with a limited population of cells (Mathis et al., 2012a, 2012b).

Another prediction made by the attractor models is that all cells within the network should behave as a coherent group. In support of this prediction, grid cells within the same module maintain their spatial phase relationships across environments (Fyhn et al., 2007; Yoon et al., 2013). This is consistent with the notion that grid cell activity lies close to a two-dimensional manifold, meaning that the

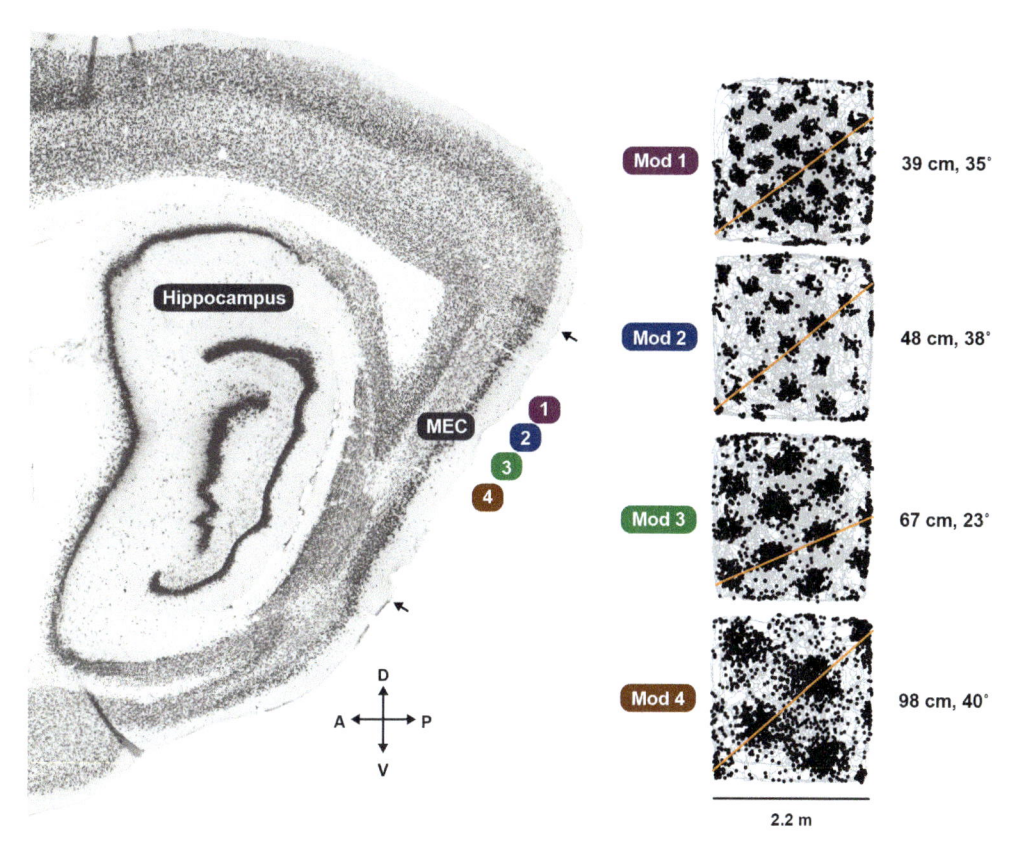

Figure 12.13 Grid modules with distinct spacing and orientation. (Left) Nissl-stained sagittal section of the rat brain. The hippocampus and medial entorhinal cortex (MEC) are indicated. The dorsoventral extent of MEC is indicated by two arrowheads. Numbers indicate approximate recording locations of each example grid cell shown on the right. (Right) The increase in grid spacing along the dorsoventral axis of MEC is divided into discrete modules. Within each module, all grid cells share the same spacing and orientation (values shown on the right, orientation also indicated by orange line.) Different modules have different spacings and orientations. At least four discrete modules have been found in the rat. Note that experiments thus far have focused on the dorsalmost portion of MEC so there likely exist larger modules more ventrally. (Data from Stensola et al., 2012.)

population activity of a grid cell module can be simply described by the animal's x-y position in space (Yoon et al., 2013). There is now abundant evidence of low-dimensional continuous attractor dynamics in grid cell networks: cell-to-cell spike relationships are expressed immediately in novel environments, remain stable over time, are not perturbed by manipulations of the environment (Yoon et al., 2013), are preserved across different sleep-wake states (Gardner et al., 2019; Trettel et al., 2019), and are even preserved when the grid pattern itself is compromised during inactivation of the hippocampus (Almog et al., 2019). Note that this universal relationship between cells within a grid module does not arise in the learning models of grid cell formation described above.

If the grid cell network is modular, and each module should comprise a unique attractor network, does each module function independently? Upon discovery of the modules, H. Stensola et al. (2012) compressed the recording environment by moving one wall inward to test how the modules would respond. They found that while all grid cells within the same module behaved coherently, different modules behaved differently. Some modules rescaled their grid pattern to accommodate the new shape of the environment, but others retained the same grid pattern, thus "losing" some firing fields beyond the compressed side of the environment. It was later shown that while grid cells within a module retain their spike time relationships during sleep, this relationship is not well preserved when comparing grid cell pairs from different modules (Gardner et al., 2019). These findings confirm grid modules can operate

independently, and ongoing theoretical work aims to address how, and under what conditions, the modules may coordinate with one another (Mosheiff and Burak, 2019).

One of the main difficulties in studying large networks of grid cells has been due to technical limitations. Most grid cell recordings have been made using tetrodes, which in rats can yield approximately 50–100 simultaneously recorded units at best (this number is typically much smaller in mice and bats). More recently, high channel count silicon probes (J Jun et al., 2017) and calcium imaging in animals expressing genetically encoded indicators (Ziv et al., 2013; C Stringer et al., 2019) has increased the yield to hundreds or thousands of simultaneously recorded units in behaving rodents. Silicon probes offer better temporal resolution compared with imaging slowly varying calcium dynamics, but the experimenter is blind to which cells are being recorded. Imaging enables visualization and targeting of specific cell populations, although high-resolution imaging has frequently relied on head-fixed behavior, which is known to differentially affect spatial firing patterns compared with freely moving behavior (Aronov and Tank, 2014; Aghajan et al., 2015). Due to recent advances, it is now possible to perform high-resolution (multiphoton) imaging under conditions where behavior is not constrained by the weight of the microscope or the flexibility of cable (Zong et al., 2022). We are thus amid a technical revolution enabling routine recordings of thousands of cells during natural behavior. These methods open the door for observing large-scale network dynamics and decoding latent variables from the population, likely revealing emergent properties that were hidden from view by focusing on single neuron responses and relationships between pairs of cells.

12.5.3 The contribution of the entorhinal cortex to hippocampal mapping

Given the critical role of the hippocampus in spatial navigation and memory, there is great interest in understanding the source of this spatial signal. As mentioned earlier in the chapter, attention shifted from intrinsic mechanisms within the hippocampus to EC in part because CA1 place cells persisted without any input from the dentate gyrus and CA3 (McNaughton et al., 1989; Mizumori et al., 1989; Brun et al., 2002). In this section, we discuss experimental evidence and theory exploring the contribution of EC to mapping (and remapping) in the hippocampus.

12.5.3.1 Experimental evidence

A straightforward way to test the necessity of EC in generating hippocampal place fields is to simply lesion it. Shortly after the discovery of place cells, it was shown that large lesions of EC (impinging on the surrounding subicular complex) did not prevent the existence of place fields (Miller and Best, 1980). In fact, place cells were still observed in all hippocampal subfields, though their firing fields were less spatially specific. Following the discovery of grid cells and the renewed interest in the spatial firing of EC, Van Cauter et al. (2008) performed bilateral entorhinal lesions, taking care to avoid damaging nearby areas, and found sharply tuned place cells in CA1. Similarly, lesioning layer III of MEC, which provides direct input to CA1, failed to abolish place fields there (Brun, Leutgeb, et al., 2008). Noting that the most dorsocaudal part of MEC, with the highest resolution spatial representations, had been spared in previous studies, Hales et al. (2014) repeated these experiments and lesioned the entirety of MEC. Yet again, CA1 place cells persisted (Hales et al., 2014; Schlesiger et al., 2015). These results consistently show that while EC may contribute to the spatial precision of place fields, the stability of place fields over time, and the temporal organization of place cell activity, it is clearly not absolutely necessary for the existence of place cells. In its absence, it remains possible that weak spatial input from other areas can be sharpened within the hippocampus.

A complementary approach to lesion studies, and one that avoids complicated issues of variability in lesion size and compensation by other brain areas, is to track the developmental time course of spatial representations in EC and hippocampus. If spatial activity of entorhinal units contributes to the formation of place fields, the entorhinal responses need to develop first. Place fields, however, are present during the first exploration after rat pups leave the nest, several days before the emergence of grid cell firing patterns (Langston et al., 2010; Wills et al., 2010). Consistent with the lesion literature, this suggests that the most spatially precise firing patterns in EC (those of grid cells) are not necessary for the expression of place fields, although they may contribute to their refinement as place cells become more sharply tuned over the next few weeks (Muessig et al., 2015). The responses of border cells, on the other hand, develop in tandem with those of place cells, and thus could contribute to initial place-field formation (Bjerknes et al., 2014). It is worth noting that head direction cells in the presubiculum and parasubiculum have adult-like directional tuning before pups have any substantial navigational experience (Langston et al., 2010; Wills et al., 2010). The

development of other functional cell types such as speed cells and object-vector cells remains to be determined. Together, these findings demonstrate that EC has weak spatial tuning and strong directional tuning at the time hippocampal place fields are first formed.

Place cell activity undergoes a drastic reorganization between distinct environments, both at the single-cell level, where place fields change location, and at the population level, where an independent subset of place cells becomes active. In parallel with this remapping, the entorhinal spatial representations should also change if they influence hippocampal maps. Soon after grid cells were discovered, Fyhn et al. (2007) found that the grid pattern shifts and/or rotates between distinct environments when place cells remap. Within one grid module, this realignment is coherent between all grid cells and is therefore a simple rigid transformation. If each module can change independently (Fyhn et al., 2007; Monaco and Abbott, 2011), however, this would elicit a large and complex change in the grid cell representation at the network level. Other entorhinal cell types, due to their apparent lack of functional modules, are unable to change in a nonlinear manner: border cells coherently rotate their activity such that their preferred activity is adjacent to a new boundary (Solstad et al., 2008), and head direction cells coherently rotate as well (Sargolini et al., 2006). Speed cells and object-vector cells seem to be insensitive to environmental context (Kropff et al., 2015; Høydal et al., 2019; but see Munn et al., 2020). Given their sharply tuned firing fields and sensitivity to contextual change, grid cells are thus uniquely positioned to influence hippocampal maps.

The fact that place cells persist after entorhinal lesions and are formed before grid cells during development does not preclude the possibility that grid cells strongly impact normal place cell functioning in adulthood. During inactivation of the medial septum, there is a drastic reduction in theta power in MEC and the hexagonal regularity of the grid pattern is lost (Brandon et al., 2011; Koenig et al., 2011). Surprisingly, although there is a large decrease in firing rate, CA1 place fields remain stable in a familiar environment (Koenig et al., 2011). Moreover, the same manipulation did not prevent place cell remapping in a novel environment; the fields developed normally, were stable over time, and persisted after theta power and grid cell activity returned to baseline levels (Brandon et al., 2014). These experiments raise important questions about how place cells remap and suggest that other spatial representations in EC can be used instead of purely relying on grid cells. While place cells are largely unaffected by the loss of the grid pattern, hippocampal activity is in fact critical for maintenance of the grid pattern. Bonnevie et al. (2013) found that inactivation of the hippocampus caused the grid to disintegrate, thus demonstrating a key role for excitatory drive to EC. Implications of this bidirectional communication between EC and hippocampus are discussed below.

With the advent of new tools for manipulating neural circuitry, it has become possible in recent years to probe spatial representations in the hippocampal formation in a more fine-grained manner. Multiple studies have now shown that place fields are altered to varying degrees following pharmacological (Ormond and McNaughton, 2015), chemogenetic (Miao et al., 2015), and optogenetic (Miao et al., 2015; Rueckemann et al., 2016) inactivation of MEC. These findings do not contradict earlier lesion and inactivation studies, but rather highlight the importance of local, short-term manipulations that reveal the contribution of MEC activity during normal brain function. Even these experiments, however, were incapable of targeting specific layers or cell types within

MEC due to the use of viruses or pharmacological agents infused as a diffuse bolus. Kanter et al. (2017) took advantage of a transgenic mouse line that enabled specific targeting of a subset of cells within a single layer of MEC (reelin-positive stellate cells in layer II), where grid cells are most abundant (Sargolini et al., 2006). Chemogenetic hyperpolarization of this highly specific population had negligible changes on CA1 place cells, but depolarization of the same subpopulation of cells caused strong remapping (Kanter et al., 2017). In fact, despite targeting a much more restricted population, the remapping was stronger than in the aforementioned studies and comparable to natural remapping between distinct environments. In addition, this approach is amenable to characterization of the affected local circuitry in MEC. It was shown that changes in individual grid field firing rates, but not their locations, were most likely responsible for the remapping in place cells (Kanter et al., 2017). This was the first study to identify a possible functional role for individual grid field rates (see Figure 12.10), and it was subsequently shown that they may also encode changes in environmental context (Diehl et al., 2017) and local positional information (Ismakov et al., 2017). Thus, with more precise perturbations comes a more nuanced understanding of the impact of the entorhinal representations on those of the hippocampus. While EC, and perhaps grid cells in particular, likely plays a critical role in shaping spatial representations in the hippocampus, the hippocampal circuit appears to have redundancies that render it resilient to insult.

12.5.3.2 Theory

Grid cells are the most abundant spatially modulated cell type in layer II of MEC (Sargolini et al., 2006), the major spatial input to the hippocampus. Moreover, grid cell firing patterns most resemble those of place cells. It is therefore not surprising that there has been a lot of emphasis placed on the notion of a grid- to place cell transformation. Here, we highlight two influential classes of models.

The first model of the grid- to place cell transformation implemented a simple weighted linear summation of grid cell inputs (Solstad et al., 2006). Integrating input from a small number of grid cells (10–50) was sufficient to produce single place fields in simulated hippocampal units. Importantly, place cells should receive input from grid cells with similar spatial phases, but diverse spacing and orientation, such that the firing in all but one field is cancelled out. This input pattern is consistent with the topographical organization of the hippocampal formation, where each dorsoventral level in EC projects to a fairly restricted region at a similar dorsoventral level in the hippocampus (Dolorfo and Amaral, 1998). Discrete grid modules would not be discovered until years later, but this does not change any major conclusions of the model. Later models paid increased attention to anatomical details and relied on competitive interactions between place cells, thus emphasizing that place-field creation is a network effect (de Almeida et al., 2009, 2012). Together, this class of models confirmed the intuitive idea that place cell responses can be generated through the simple integration of appropriate grid cell inputs (i.e., those with variable phase and orientation), and furthermore, they identified key constraints on the connectivity patterns.

A separate class of models achieved realistic simulated place cells by using Hebbian plasticity to learn the grid cell inputs. Rolls et al. (2006) used a feedforward network of grid cells and dentate gyrus place cells and, like de Almeida et al. (2009), implemented network-level inhibition to keep the active subset of hippocampal cells small.

Over the course of learning, dentate cells become associated with specific patterns of entorhinal activity and develop place fields. Savelli and Knierim (2010) later built on this work by showing that network competition is not strictly necessary for generating single place fields. Interestingly, they also found that place-field location was strongly influenced by the initial trajectory of the animal (or agent) such that, all else being equal, place fields would remap between each simulation. This raises an important point about the trade-off between stability and flexibility. It is still unknown how the hippocampal formation achieves the appropriate balance to have stable, unique maps for each distinct environment.

Despite the prominent role of grid cells, there is good reason (described above) to consider alternative mechanisms of place-field formation that do not rely purely on grid cells as the source of spatial input. Due to the focus of this chapter, we limit our discussion here to models deriving hippocampal spatial firing from the activity of their entorhinal inputs.

Based on findings that place fields are strongly controlled by the walls of an environment, O'Keefe and Burgess (1996) hypothesized that place cells receive input from neurons that are active at a specific distance from a particular wall. More specifically, place fields are formed by a thresholded sum of two or more of these distance-dependent, Gaussian-shaped receptive fields (Hartley et al., 2000; Barry et al., 2006). These input neurons were termed boundary-vector cells (Hartley et al., 2000), and cells with this firing pattern have been found in the subiculum (Barry et al., 2006; Lever et al., 2009), as described in section 12.5.1. Given the predominantly unidirectional flow through the hippocampal circuit, it is unlikely that boundary-vector cells in the subiculum give rise to place fields. There are, however, recent reports of direct connections from subiculum to CA1 (Sun et al., 2014; Sun et al., 2019), which leave that possibility open. If boundary-vector cells are not found in EC, a similar model could rely on entorhinal border cells (Savelli et al., 2008; Solstad et al., 2008), at least for creating place fields close to environmental boundaries.

More recently, models have begun to explore the recurrent nature of the hippocampal formation by using bidirectional connections between EC and the hippocampus. Rennó-Costa and Tort (2017) used recurrent connections both within the place- and grid cell populations, and between them. Place cells were additionally driven by nongrid cells (presumed to be other medial and lateral entorhinal neurons) while grid cells received velocity inputs. They found that place cells do not require grid cell input but are modulated by grid cell activity and may rely on grid cells to stabilize their place fields, consistent with experimental evidence described above. In addition, they showed for the first time that global remapping of place cells leads to grid cell realignment, as opposed to the commonly accepted notion of grid cell realignment causing remapping (Fyhn et al., 2007; Monaco and Abbott, 2011). Laptev and Burgess (2019) used a similar recurrent architecture with reciprocal interaction between place cells and grid cells but placed emphasis on the integration of environmental boundaries. Grid cells are still path integrating via a continuous attractor network, but place cells receive input from boundary-vector cells. This model recapitulates interesting experimental findings where self-motion information (grid cells) and sensory information (place cells) are put into conflict (Gothard, Skaggs, and McNaughton, 1996; Redish et al., 2000). Together, these models that incorporate projections from the hippocampus back to deep layers of MEC are not only more biologically realistic but are also powerful tools for explaining and predicting place cell responses. Similar models could explore the potential bidirectional communication between border cells in MEC and boundary-vector cells in subiculum.

12.5.4 Functional differences between medial and lateral entorhinal cortex

Our discussion of the function of EC thus far has focused almost exclusively on MEC. The reason for this bias is twofold. First, this is *The Hippocampus Book*. The hippocampus is widely known for its role in spatial navigation and spatial memory, and spatial information arrives to the hippocampus primarily via MEC. Second, neural correlates of LEC have proven more difficult to uncover. In this section, we discuss the differences in coding between MEC and LEC and emphasize what has recently been discovered regarding functional properties of the somewhat enigmatic LEC.

12.5.4.1 Allocentric spatial signals are significantly less prominent in lateral entorhinal cortex

Near the turn of the 21st century, functional heterogeneity along the dorsoventral axis of the hippocampus became increasingly apparent (Jung et al., 1994). This was followed shortly after by an analogous finding in MEC: there was a substantial decrease in sharp spatial tuning from dorsal to ventral MEC (Brun, Solstad, et al., 2008). At the same time, Hargreaves et al. (2005) tested whether there was a similar gradient along the orthogonal axis of EC. They found that MEC units exhibited multiple clear firing fields while LEC units generally lacked spatial firing. Moreover, MEC spatial firing patterns were twice as stable across consecutive sessions compared with those in LEC. In retrospect, many MEC units recorded in this study must have been grid cells. These findings and others (Yoganarasimha et al., 2011; Neunuebel et al., 2013) thus provide clear evidence of a functional dissociation between MEC and LEC, which is consistent with the idea of parallel input streams to the hippocampus: the MEC pathway carries spatial input and the LEC pathway carries nonspatial input (Witter, Groenewegen, et al., 1989; Burwell, 2000; but see Doan et al., 2019).

12.5.4.2 Lateral entorhinal cortex encodes objects and object history

While others had demonstrated that LEC neurons respond to individual items (Zhu et al., 1995), Deshmukh and Knierim (2011) were the first to directly compare MEC and LEC firing patterns during open field navigation in the presence of objects. LEC neurons were much more sensitive than MEC neurons to the presence of objects, the introduction of a novel object, and the movement of a familiar object. It was unknown, however, whether the object-related activity in LEC was due to low-level stimulus features or if it could be a higher-level code for the animal's experience. By performing a similar experiment where one or more objects were only present during specific trials, Tsao et al. (2013) revealed an additional class of LEC neurons that were only active at locations where objects had been in previous trials. By moving an object around on successive trials, one can observe these object-trace cells build up a spatial firing pattern over time, which could serve as a memory for past experience. The discovery of object and object-trace cells established LEC as a key component of the hippocampal circuit for object-place memory. This idea was recently validated by showing that silencing the activity of LEC layer II fan cells impairs

memory for objects in particular locations and contexts (Vandrey et al., 2020).

12.5.4.3 Lateral entorhinal cortex encodes episodic time

If the hippocampus constructs episodic memories using spatial ("where") input from the MEC and object ("what") input from the LEC, from where does it receive temporal ("when") input? Since LEC integrates input from an extremely diverse set of brain areas (Zingg et al., 2014; Bota et al., 2015) and contains object-memory traces (Tsao et al., 2013), as described in the previous section, it might be possible that LEC binds object information to a particular temporal context and that MEC helps place this memory into the appropriate spatial context. It was recently found that as rats explored black or white boxes in an alternating manner, a substantial fraction of LEC neurons encoded time within each individual trial or within the overall recording session (Tsao et al., 2018; See also Figure 12.14). At a population level, one could use LEC activity to accurately decode time across multiple scales from seconds to hours. Activity in MEC and CA3, on the other hand, was sensitive to box color and/or the animal's position, but not time. Importantly, a temporal code for episodic memory should be relative to the animal's experience, as opposed to metric time. When the task was changed from open field exploration to stereotyped trajectories in a figure-8 maze, the neural trajectories became stereotyped as well (Tsao et al., 2018). The temporal coding became relative to the start and end of each lap because the animal's experience was the same each time. These experiments therefore identified a temporal code in LEC that is distinct from timing mechanisms elsewhere in the brain and is well suited for the creation of episodic memories.

12.5.4.4 Both lateral and medial entorhinal cortex encode space, boundaries, objects, and time

Functional dissociations between brain areas are rarely absolute and the distinction between MEC and LEC is no exception. Based on the apparent segregation between spatial coding in MEC and contextual coding in LEC, Lisman (2007) proposed that the true distinction may instead be between coding motor/self information (i.e., position) vs. sensory/nonself information (i.e., objects). Representation of position by MEC is in an allocentric reference frame to give a sense of location within a fixed map of the world, but representation of objects by LEC should be in an egocentric reference frame because objects are experienced dynamically from a first-person perspective. While egocentric tuning during navigation had been explored in other brain areas such as posterior parietal cortex (Whitlock et al., 2012), only recently was it explored in LEC. As rats foraged in an empty box, some LEC neurons were preferentially active when the animal was facing in a specific egocentric direction relative to the nearest boundary (Wang et al., 2018). For example, a neuron may be active only when a nearby boundary is directly to the animal's left. This coding is in direct contrast to allocentric head direction tuning found in many MEC neurons. Egocentric tuning in LEC was also found for objects that were placed inside the box, and for a goal location that the animal navigated to for a food reward. This egocentric tuning is like object-vector cell representations in MEC (Høydal et al., 2019), except that the latter is in an allocentric reference frame and encodes a specific distance to the objects. The hippocampus may therefore receive a balanced representation of allocentric coding from MEC and egocentric coding

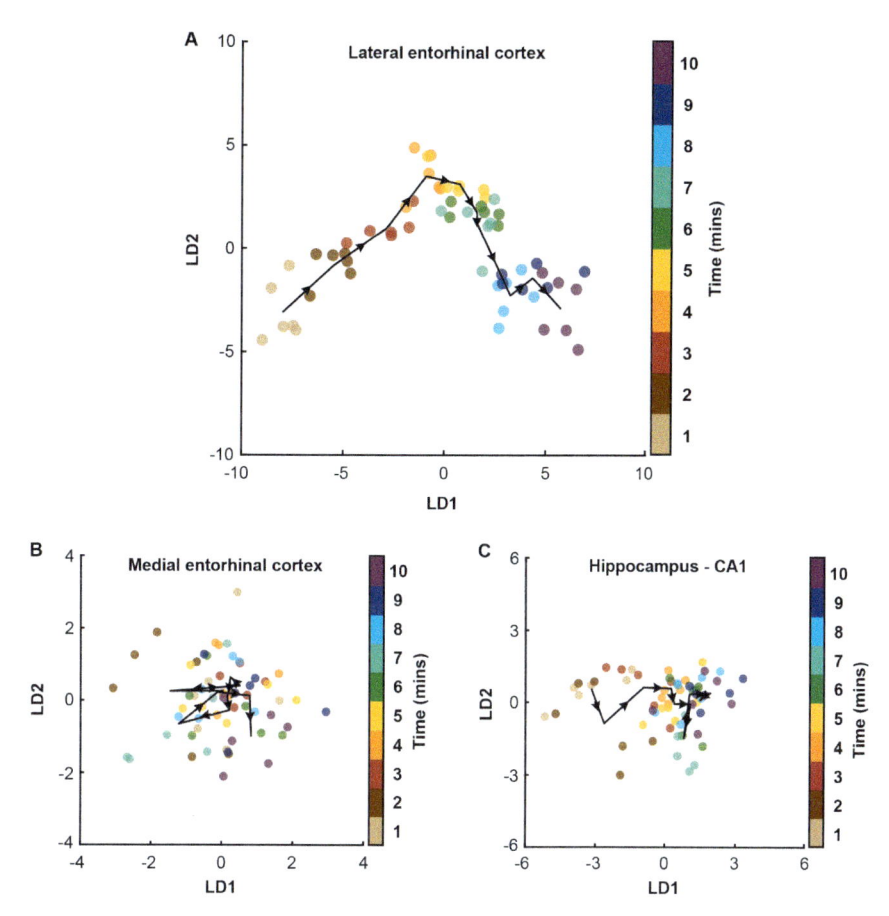

Figure 12.14 Lateral entorhinal cortex encodes episodic time. (A) 2D projection of the population activity of 164 simultaneously recorded neurons in LEC during open field foraging in a familiar environment. Each dot represents the population activity in a 10 s time bin. Each minute of the session is plotted in a different color from brown to purple, and the average activity of each minute is connected by a black trajectory to indicate movement within the state space over time. Note how the population activity travels smoothly throughout the space and does not revisit the same space twice. The continuous experience of time can therefore be easily decoded from the neural activity. The same analysis reveals a lack of temporal coding in size-matched populations from (B) MEC and (C) hippocampal area CA1 recorded simultaneously with the data from (A). Note how the population activity jumps randomly throughout the state space, as seen by the scrambled colors and overlapping trajectories. LD = linear discriminant. (Data collected by Benjamin R. Kanter and Christine M. Lykken in the Moser lab, consistent with findings from Tsao et al., 2018.)

from LEC, allowing it to place objects in their appropriate context. It is also interesting to note that following this report of egocentric representations in LEC (Wang et al., 2018), similar representations were quickly found in many interrelated areas including CA1 (see also Sarel et al., 2017; Jercog et al., 2019), postrhinal cortex (Gofman et al., 2019; LaChance et al., 2019), retrosplenial cortex (Alexander et al., 2020), and dorsal striatum (Hinman et al., 2019). Egocentric spatial representations may form a distributed network, much like allocentric head direction tuning, which funnels into the hippocampus via EC.

As described above, both LEC and MEC encode the presence of objects, albeit in separate spatial reference frames. In most of the studies described above, rodents navigate in an environment containing objects that have no significance to the animal. If the objects, their position, and the spatial context are made equally important to the animal such that their integration is critical for receiving a reward, a dissociation is seen at the neural population level (Keene et al., 2016). There is a hierarchical organization in which MEC is biased toward representing the animal's position over objects, and the opposite is true of LEC. Both regions are more sensitive to spatial context than either position or objects. It is therefore important to consider conjunctive and relational coding schemes when trying

to tease apart functional roles in higher-order cognitive areas such as EC. Interestingly, similar analysis of hippocampal representations in the same task revealed the same organization as in MEC (i.e., position > objects) (McKenzie et al., 2014). Thus, it seems that the hippocampus is strongly driven by the positional code in MEC, while object and temporal coding inherited from LEC may be secondary, at least during classic rodent behavioral tests.

Temporal coding is not exclusively found in LEC (Tsao et al., 2018), but is also prevalent in MEC, particularly in tasks with delay periods (Suh et al., 2011; Kitamura et al., 2014). As rats run in place on a treadmill, grid cells in MEC fire at specific times or distances relative to the onset of running (Kraus et al., 2015), as predicted by models of path integration in grid cells (McNaughton et al., 2006). When animals are sitting still during a delay period, however, it seems that a distinct population of cells in MEC encodes elapsed time, nonoverlapping with the grid cell population that is active during running (Heys and Dombeck, 2018). Importantly, these studies of temporal coding in MEC do not distinguish between metric time and episodic time (Tsao et al., 2018) by allowing variations in the animal's behavior. It may be that MEC and LEC provide metric and episodic temporal representations, respectively, to the hippocampus, where activity patterns similar to MEC are seen while running in place (Pastalkova et al., 2008) and sitting still (MacDonald et al., 2013).

12.5.5 Entorhinal function in primates

Recordings of neural activity in nonhuman primates and humans have revealed many of the same functional roles described above in rodents (see also Chapter 13), but they have also uncovered novel roles that may or may not be present in lower-order species.

12.5.5.1 Memory processing in the primate entorhinal cortex

Much of the rodent research on the role of EC in memory focuses on features of episodic memory because of the interplay between EC and the hippocampus. The content of episodic memory can be inferred using behavioral paradigms in rodents, but it can be more directly assessed in humans by asking participants to verbally describe their memories. It is therefore key to compare anatomical, electrophysiological, and behavioral data across species to understand episodic memory. Above we described the pioneering work of (Suzuki et al., 1997) showing that single units in monkey EC were active during a delayed (non)matching task, which indicated that they could support recognition memory. A few years later, it was found that individual neurons in the human EC were active while participants learned word pairs and that entorhinal activity during recall was correlated with success (Cameron et al., 2001). These early studies provided important evidence that individual entorhinal neurons are also important for memory in primates.

More recent work using functional neuroimaging has enabled greater functional parcellation of EC while humans perform behavioral tasks. To test whether a similar divide between spatial and nonspatial information processing was present in humans, as it is in rodents, Navarro Schroder et al. (2015) and Maass et al. (2015) used high-resolution fMRI to measure the functional connectivity between EC and the rest of the hippocampal formation (Maass et al., 2015) or broader cortical memory networks (Navarro Schroder et al., 2015). They found that the major axis of change within EC was in the anterior-posterior direction: posteromedial entorhinal cortex (pmEC) had stronger connectivity with parahippocampal cortex and anterolateral entorhinal cortex (alEC) had stronger connectivity with perirhinal cortex. In addition, pmEC was preferentially active when participants viewed pictures of scenes whereas alEC was more active when they viewed pictures of objects (Navarro Schroder et al., 2015). These studies thus demonstrated that pmEC and alEC might be considered homologues of rodent MEC and LEC, respectively.

In rodent studies, recent work has pointed to LEC as a site of integration where temporal information is encoded in addition to sensory stimuli (Doan et al., 2019). Human fMRI studies have also identified temporal signals in EC. Participants listened to a radio story and were later asked to judge the elapsed time between different segments of the story. The more that neural activity in EC drifted between the two clips, the longer the participants judged the elapsed time to be (Lositsky et al., 2016). In a follow-up study, participants watched a TV show and were later asked to report the exact time during the episode that a still-frame was taken from (Montchal et al., 2019). Activity in alEC was correlated with the precision of their judgments, but activity in pmEC was not. Finally, Bellmund et al. (2019) found that activity in alEC maps the temporal order in which objects are encountered along a route, but not the spatial location of those objects. There is therefore strong convergence between rodent and primate research indicating that EC is important for episodic memory, and that the posteromedial and anterolateral subdivisions have unique roles in spatial and nonspatial processing, respectively.

12.5.5.2 A grid-like signal in the primate entorhinal cortex

The discovery of grid cells in rodents was exciting due to their potential impact on navigation, hippocampal spatial maps, and memory, but do humans have grid cells as well? Finding grid cells in humans would not be easy because of the difficulty in recording human brain activity during movement. Doeller et al. (2010) therefore had human participants navigate in a virtual world while imaging the entorhinal activity using fMRI. They predicted that when participants move in the virtual world parallel to the axes of the grid pattern (i.e., passing through multiple grid fields), there should be stronger grid cell population activity than when they move along opposing axes. Because fMRI pools the activity of thousands of neurons into a single measurement, and because grid cells share a common orientation, this direction-specific activity modulation was expected to translate to a population-level activity bias observable with fMRI. Indeed, during virtual navigation it was possible to identify the predicted sixfold rotationally symmetric activity in the human EC, presumably reflecting a population of grid cells. Follow-up studies showed that this grid-like signal is also present when participants imagined the direction between two learned locations, suggesting that grid cells might be active even during mental navigation (Bellmund et al., 2016; Horner et al., 2016). It will be important for future work to address how the grid-like signal recorded by fMRI or other population recording techniques (Kunz et al., 2019) relates to grid cell activity, possibly using imaging in rodents.

Attempts to find allocentric spatial coding in monkeys resulted in the discovery of a novel type of cell, the spatial view cell (Rolls, 1999). These hippocampal neurons were like place cells, but rather than being active when the monkey visited a particular location, they were active when the monkey looked at a particular location in space. Following the logic that entorhinal neurons might similarly represent space independent of the monkey's position, Killian et al. (2012) recorded the activity of single entorhinal neurons while monkeys freely viewed natural images on a computer screen. They found a subset of entorhinal neurons that looked like rodent grid cells: the neurons were only active when the monkey looked at specific locations on the screen, and these locations formed a grid pattern tiling the whole visual display. Moreover, grid cells were modulated by the theta rhythm, showed an increase in grid spacing along EC, and were engaged during a recognition memory task (Killian et al., 2012). Similarly, recent work in humans has revealed a grid-like signal for gaze direction using fMRI. Two independent sets of studies found that when human participants either tracked a moving visual target (Nau, Julian, et al., 2018; Nau, Navarro Schröder, et al., 2018) or performed a visual search task (Julian et al., 2018), EC was preferentially active for movements in particular gaze directions with sixfold symmetry (see also Staudigl et al., 2018). Moreover, orientation of the grid pattern was anchored to the borders of the search display (Julian et al., 2018) and active (attentional) movements were required to drive grid-cell like activity (Nau, Navarro Schröder, et al., 2018), much like in rodents and nonhuman primates (Meister and Buffalo, 2018). Together, these results indicate that the primate EC represents locations in visual space in an analogous way to the mapping of physical space in the rodent EC (Nau, Julian, et al., 2018; Rolls and Wirth, 2018).

12.5.6 Entorhinal coding beyond physical space

There is now mounting evidence to suggest that the hippocampal region could be involved more generally in mapping task-relevant variables (Buzsáki and Moser, 2013). In rodents, a clever experimental design revealed that both place cells and grid cells can develop receptive fields for specific sound frequencies (Aronov et al., 2017). Rats were trained to navigate a continuous frequency space of tones using a joystick and were rewarded for releasing the joystick to stop at specific tones. A population of CA1 cells mapped the whole frequency space with each cell developing a "tone field." Similarly, a population of MEC cells were active for specific tones with regular spacing between them. These sound-modulated cells only partially overlapped with the true place cell and grid cell populations. In humans, EC likely also maps abstract space. Participants were trained to associate birds with various neck and leg lengths with Christmas symbols (Constantinescu et al., 2016). The participants were unaware that the Christmas symbols were in fact arranged on a two-dimensional map that corresponded to continuous changes in the bird's neck length (x-axis) and leg length (y-axis). They were then shown a bird morphing (i.e., neck and leg lengths changing) and were asked to imagine, "If it continues morphing in that direction, what Christmas symbol would the resulting bird be associated with?" fMRI activity in EC was higher when the participants imagined movement in particular directions with sixfold symmetry in this abstract space, despite them having never explicitly seen the underlying two-dimensional organization of that space.

Mapping physical space therefore may be a specific example of a broader role for EC and hippocampus in mapping cognitive spaces (Behrens et al., 2018; Bellmund et al., 2019). Grid cells and place cells could theoretically encode any continuous dimension of experience, where similar stimuli are close together in cognitive space and are encoded by overlapping neural population activity. In addition, the multiscale nature of grid cell and place cell populations bridges both general and specific representations. Because of the broad implications of this proposal, future work might aim to elucidate the mechanisms underlying the generation of this continuous neural code, probe the potential dimensionality of the space, and attempt to relate principles from the rodent grid cell code (e.g., modularity) to other cognitive spaces. While much less is known about the (antero)lateral EC, it will be similarly important to extend recent work on temporal coding to explore the neural correlates of the experience of time in humans.

12.6 Entorhinal cortex and brain disease

Neurons and networks in EC have intrigued neuroscientists for a long time, and one reason is the apparent association with a variety of brain diseases, including Alzheimer's disease, epilepsy, and schizophrenia. For some of these diseases, the emerging insight that many of the main characteristics of neurons and networks are relatively well conserved in many of the species resulted in relatively successful attempts to model some of the disease features in animals. The most successful attempts are those focusing on epilepsy, whereas models for Alzheimer's disease have been much less successful. It seems that many features of epilepsy can be mimicked in animals, whereas Alzheimer's disease seems a condition rather unique for the human brain. Attempts to model schizophrenia in animals have been rather limited and have not focused strongly on EC as a relevant factor. The association of specific EC pathology with a particular disease is strongest for Alzheimer's disease and temporal lobe epilepsy, and these have resulted in causal hypotheses. In contrast, the associations of alterations in EC with other diseases is less apparent and causal hypotheses have barely been formulated.

12.6.1 Alzheimer's disease

Alois Alzheimer described a striking case of dementia that was associated with two pathological hallmarks: intracellular neurofibrillary tangles (NFTs), now known to mainly consist of the aberrantly hyperphosphorylated microtubule associated protein tau, and extracellular amyloid-beta (Aβ) plaques, mainly consisting of Aβ aggregates. Soon after the initial report of this disease, which later came to be known as Alzheimer's disease (AD), it was found that EC was among the cortical areas that showed striking pathological alterations in postmortem brains of Alzheimer's patients (for a short historical account, see Van Hoesen, 2002). It not until the beginning of the 1980s, however, that a number of studies revealed that initial changes related to formation of NFTs occur in layer II of lateral parts of EC at the border with the perirhinal cortex (Hyman et al., 1984; Braak and Braak, 1991; see also Chapter 20, section 20.3.1.1). This has been confirmed by many more contemporary studies showing a massive neuronal loss in EC layer II already in early AD, a feature also evident in at least a subset of subjects with mild cognitive impairment, of which the majority are likely to convert to AD (Gomez-Isla et al., 1996; Kordower et al., 2001). Even more recent are the studies showing a significant volume reduction, likely due to thinning of EC, again corroborating the preferred initial involvement of anterolateral parts of EC and the adjacent part of the perirhinal cortex (Dickerson et al., 2001; Holbrook et al., 2020). Recently developed PET ligands for phosphorylated tau support these findings in patients, showing a preferred early binding in the domain of EC (Adams et al., 2019).

Several lines of evidence point to the population of reelin-positive neurons in EC as the neurons most likely to develop NFTs, and there is evidence in both animal models and postmortem brain tissue from patients that these neurons also selectively accumulate intracellular Aβ before showing signs of phosphorylated tau (Kobro-Flatmoen et al., 2016; Kobro-Flatmoen et al., 2021). As summarized in section 12.3, reelin-expressing neurons in EC layer II are likely the sole origin of the excitatory projection to DG (Witter, Doan, et al., 2017), and this projection shows severe loss of synaptic contacts during early-stage Alzheimer's disease (Scheff et al., 2006). The presence of reelin-positive principal neurons in superficial layers of the cortex, as seen in EC, is common in all species studied. This expression pattern is atypical, however, for cortex in general, where reelin is expressed primarily in a subset of principal cells of layer V (Pesold et al., 1998; Pérez-García et al., 2001; Martínez-Cerdeño and Clascá, 2002; Martínez-Cerdeño et al., 2003; Kobro-Flatmoen and Witter, 2019). The reason for this selective adult expression of reelin is currently unknown, but it is of interest that reelin is a modulatory protein involved in synaptic plasticity (Weeber et al., 2002; Qiu et al., 2006; Rogers et al., 2011).

The link between Alzheimer's disease and entorhinal pathology on the one hand and that of EC as part of the MTL on the other hand has triggered an interest to assess pathological changes in many other diseases that eventually cause dementia, such as argyrophilic grain disease, Pick's disease, idiopathic Parkinson's disease, Huntington's disease, and progressive nuclear palsy. Although many of these diseases are normally associated with specific pathological changes in other parts of the brain, they often also show changes in EC, and it has been argued that disruption of the MTL circuitry plays a role in this memory impairment. In this context, it is relevant to briefly mention that AD-associated changes induced in animals, such as the knockin of gene mutations associated with familial AD, result in functional defects as measured by behavioral and electrophysiological phenomena. These include deficits in spatial memory and a disruption of spatial coding in EC (H Jun et al., 2020). Interestingly, human carriers of the ε4 allele of the *APOE* gene, a strong risk factor for AD, show changes in activity in EC as measured by fMRI, and these changes are presumed to reflect altered grid-like activity in humans (Kunz et al., 2015). In view of the evidence that the earliest AD pathology is likely found in lateral parts of EC, behavioral deficits associated with this entorhinal area, likely LEC, might provide even more sensitive readouts associated with an early stage of AD.

12.6.2 Medial temporal lobe epilepsy

The hippocampal formation has always been at the core of research on the initiation and spread of seizures in the medial temporal lobe, although the relevance of the parahippocampal region has been considered significant as well (Chapter 18). EC has been a focus for two main reasons. First, it was reported that resected tissue from patients with pharmacologically intractable temporal lobe epilepsy showed profound and consistent loss of neurons in EC, specifically in layer III of the more posterior part (Du et al., 1993). The relevance of this entorhinal damage was corroborated in several neuroimaging studies, showing substantial volume loss in EC and in some cases not showing striking volume changes in the hippocampal formation (Bernasconi et al., 2001). Second, the productive modeling of epileptic phenomena in animals, using a variety of electrical and chemical induction approaches, all consistently replicated the finding that neurons in layer III of MEC are particularly vulnerable (Du et al., 1995). A crude though convincing argument for the relevance of EC in the induction of seizures came from studies showing that silencing or lesioning EC in animals prevents the development of seizure activity (J Stringer and Lothman, 1992). The specific relevance of MEC and of layer III was further corroborated by a series of elegant animal studies in which injections of neurotoxins in MEC resulted in the initiation of epileptic seizures, accompanied by specific death of the principle pyramidal neurons in layer III, though apparently sparing most of the interneurons (Du et al., 1995).

Interestingly, lesioning a main input to MEC layer III pyramidal neurons (see section 12.3) by selective lesions of the presubiculum and subsequent induction of status epilepticus blocked seizure induction and spared the pyramidal layer III neurons in MEC (Eid et al., 2001). There is now an extensive literature relating some of the specific neuron and network properties in layer III of MEC, as described in section 12.4, to this specific pathology seen in temporal lobe epilepsy (Vismer et al., 2015). It has further been shown that in animal models, temporal lobe epilepsy results in substantial connectivity rewiring including loss of hippocampal-to-MEC connections and rewiring of MEC-to-dentate projections. In contrast,

the local circuits of the two main types of basket cells in layer II, the PV-positive cells forming baskets with reelin-positive and calbindin-positive principal cells, and CCK-positive interneurons that preferentially target calbindin-positive neurons (section 12.4), remain unaltered. The question of why LEC is much less vulnerable to damage in temporal lobe epilepsy is relatively unexplored.

Synaptic reorganization in the MEC-hippocampal network produces robust changes in evoked and spontaneous activity in parts of the network that may impact the re-entrant activation in the network and will likely impact memory storage and recall processes that are mediated strongly, though not exclusively, by the layer III-CA1/SUB loops (Schwarcz and Witter, 2002). This is in line with reports that memory deficits in temporal lobe epilepsy do not seem to worsen over time when comparing deficits at the time of first diagnosis with a 5-year retest. This thus implies that the memory deficits are the result of the initial lesion associated with the onset. It remains to be established, however, whether the damage in layer III is a necessary and sufficient condition for temporal lobe epilepsy to emerge. Although there are convincing data supporting this concept, there are data supporting alternative views, for example, that temporal lobe epilepsy is due to an imbalance in the intricate and complex circuitry between EC and the hippocampal formation and structures that modulate these circuits. One of the latter structures implicated strongly by many authors is the midline thalamic nucleus reuniens, which interestingly has also been implicated in schizophrenia and Alzheimer's disease (for a recent review, see Dolleman-van der Weel and Witter, 2020). Another relevant network might include the primary olfactory or piriform cortex and the associated endopiriform nucleus (for a recent review, see Vismer et al., 2015).

Finally, it is worth mentioning that patients suffering from pharmacologically intractable temporal lobe epilepsy, or even more generalized epilepsy, are often evaluated for surgical interventions, aiming to localize a possible focus that can be surgically removed. This has resulted in a series of interesting electrophysiological studies in humans in which data have been obtained corroborating animal findings on functional correlates and functionally defined cell types in EC, such as grid cells, temporal coding, and neuronal properties underlying the more generalized cognitive map concept in hippocampus and parahippocampus (Mankin and Fried, 2020).

12.6.3 Schizophrenia

Schizophrenia is a severe brain disorder in which patients suffer from an abnormal interpretation of reality and that typically manifests in early adulthood. Although its specific causes remain unknown, there is a body of evidence that associates entorhinal pathology to the disease, likely resulting from developmental factors, including genetic and environmental influences. Though data are sparse and conflicting, there are 30–40 studies associating entorhinal disorganization and malfunctions with schizophrenia. Volume reductions of EC, as established in postmortem studies or using MRI analysis in patients, are commonly seen in schizophrenic patients, generally unilaterally, though reports on either left- or right-sided preferences are conflicting. The same is true for reports on possible sex differences. Such volume reductions are likely associated with structural anomalies in EC of schizophrenics that reportedly occur in up to half of the population of schizophrenics, although reports disagree on the exact percentages. Loss or displacement of neurons, or decreased volume have been repeatedly reported but also refuted (Talbot and Arnold, 2002). In more recent studies in which treatment-naive patients were involved, a slightly more stable picture emerges, although there are still inconsistencies regarding hemispheric preferences and sex differences. Cytoarchitectural changes, when observed, generally involve the large layer II neurons of EC (Arnold et al., 1991) in preferentially the anterolateral portion of EC (Falkai et al., 2000). Some studies assessed changes in number of GABAergic neurons and reported a reduction in schizophrenics, though animal model studies have not replicated these observations. One of the most striking additional changes is a substantial decrease in dopamine-positive innervation of anterolateral EC (Akil et al., 2000). In contrast, changes in expression levels and distribution of neurotensin receptors, although present in EC, do not seem to be specifically associated with schizophrenia (Hamid et al., 2002).

Whether or not EC is a key player in schizophrenia is still unclear (see also Chapter 19), and it remains to be determined what causes the changes in EC seen in schizophrenia. Although it is apparent that changes occur in the overall functional connectivity of the entorhinal network with a preference for layer II, studies should likely assess changes in adjacent parahippocampal areas as well.

Acknowledgments

We thank our colleagues Nathalie Cappaert, Alexei Egorov, Dietmar Schmitz, Matt Nolan, Niels van Strien, Benjamin Dunn, and Matthias Nau for their constructive comments on an earlier draft of this chapter. Bente Jacobsen receives our thanks, since she has been instrumental in the preparation of all anatomical illustrations, and Ingrid Riphagen for her help with the references. The preparation of this chapter was supported by a Synergy Grant from the European Research Council to E.I.M. ("KILONEURONS," Grant Agreement N° 951319), the Centre of Excellence Scheme of the Research Council of Norway—Centre for Neural Computation (Grant No. 223262) and the Kavli Foundation.

REFERENCES

Adams JN, Maass A, Harrison TM, Baker SL, Jagust WJ (2019) Cortical tau deposition follows patterns of entorhinal functional connectivity in aging. *eLife* 8:e49132.

Aggleton JP, Wright NF, Vann SD, Saunders RC (2012) Medial temporal lobe projections to the retrosplenial cortex of the macaque monkey. *Hippocampus* 22:1883–1900.

Aghajan ZM, Acharya L, Moore JJ, Cushman JD, Vuong C, Mehta MR (2015) Impaired spatial selectivity and intact phase precession in two-dimensional virtual reality. *Nat Neurosci* 18:121–128.

Agster KL, Burwell RD (2009) Cortical efferents of the perirhinal, postrhinal, and entorhinal cortices of the rat. *Hippocampus* 19:1159–1186.

Agster KL, Tomas Pereira I, Saddoris MP, Burwell RD (2016) Subcortical connections of the perirhinal, postrhinal, and entorhinal cortices of the rat: II. Efferents. *Hippocampus* 26:1213–1230.

Akil M, Edgar CL, Pierri JN, Casali S, Lewis DA (2000) Decreased density of tyrosine hydroxylase-immunoreactive axons in the entorhinal cortex of schizophrenic subjects. *Biol Psychiatry* 47:361–370.

Akil M, Lewis DA (1993) The dopaminergic innervation of monkey entorhinal cortex. *Cereb Cortex* 3:533–550.

Akil M, Lewis DA (1994) The distribution of tyrosine hydroxylase-immunoreactive fibers in the human entorhinal cortex. *Neuroscience* 60:857–874.

Alexander AS, Carstensen LC, Hinman JR, Raudies F, Chapman GW, Hasselmo ME (2020) Egocentric boundary vector tuning of the retrosplenial cortex. *Sci Adv* 6:eaaz2322.

Almog N, Tocker G, Bonnevie T, Moser EI, Moser M-B, Derdikman D (2019) During hippocampal inactivation, grid cells maintain synchrony, even when the grid pattern is lost. *eLife* 8:e47147.

Alonso A, Klink R (1993) Differential electroresponsiveness of stellate and pyramidal-like cells of medial entorhinal cortex layer II. *J Neurophysiol* 70:128–143.

Alonso A, Kohler C (1984) A study of the reciprocal connections between the septum and the entorhinal area using anterograde and retrograde axonal transport methods in the rat brain. *J Comp Neurol* 225:327–343.

Alonso A, Llinas RR (1989) Subthreshold Na+-dependent theta-like rhythmicity in stellate cells of entorhinal cortex layer II. *Nature* 342:175–177.

Amaral DG, Insausti R, Cowan WM (1984) The commissural connections of the monkey hippocampal formation. *J Comp Neurol* 224:307–336.

Amaral DG, Insausti R, Cowan WM (1987) The entorhinal cortex of the monkey: I. Cytoarchitectonic organization. *J Comp Neurol* 264:326–355.

Amari S-I (1977) Dynamics of pattern formation in lateral-inhibition type neural fields. *Biol Cybern* 27:77–87.

Arikuni T, Sako H, Murata A (1994) Ipsilateral connections of the anterior cingulate cortex with the frontal and medial temporal cortices in the macaque monkey. *Neurosci Res* 21:19–39.

Armstrong C, Wang J, Yeun Lee S, Broderick J, Bezaire MJ, Lee SH, Soltesz I (2016) Target-selectivity of parvalbumin-positive interneurons in layer II of medial entorhinal cortex in normal and epileptic animals. *Hippocampus* 26:779–793.

Arnold SE, Hyman BT, Van Hoesen GW, Damasio AR (1991) Some cytoarchitectural abnormalities of the entorhinal cortex in schizophrenia. *Arch Gen Psychiatry* 48:625–632.

Aronov D, Nevers R, Tank DW (2017) Mapping of a non-spatial dimension by the hippocampal-entorhinal circuit. *Nature* 543:719–722.

Aronov D, Tank DW (2014) Engagement of neural circuits underlying 2D spatial navigation in a rodent virtual reality system. *Neuron* 84:442–456.

Barnes CA, McNaughton BL, Mizumori SJ, Leonard BW, Lin LH (1990) Comparison of spatial and temporal characteristics of neuronal activity in sequential stages of hippocampal processing. *Prog Brain Res* 83:287–300.

Barry C, Hayman R, Burgess N, Jeffery KJ (2007) Experience-dependent rescaling of entorhinal grids. *Nat Neurosci* 10:682–684.

Barry C, Lever C, Hayman R, Hartley T, Burton S, O'Keefe J, Jeffery K, Burgess N (2006) The boundary vector cell model of place cell firing and spatial memory. *Rev Neurosci* 17:71–97.

Batallan-Burrowes AA, Chapman CA (2018) Dopamine suppresses persistent firing in layer III lateral entorhinal cortex neurons. *Neurosci Lett* 674:70–74.

Beed P, Bendels MH, Wiegand HF, Leibold C, Johenning FW, Schmitz D (2010) Analysis of excitatory microcircuitry in the medial entorhinal cortex reveals cell-type-specific differences. *Neuron* 68:1059–1066.

Beed P, de Filippo R, Holman C, Johenning FW, Leibold C, Caputi A, Monyer H, Schmitz D (2020) Layer 3 pyramidal cells in the medial entorhinal cortex orchestrate up-down states and entrain the deep layers differentially. *Cell Rep* 33:108470.

Beed P, Gundlfinger A, Schneiderbauer S, Song J, Böhm C, Burgalossi A, Brecht M, Vida I, Schmitz D (2013) Inhibitory gradient along the dorsoventral axis in the medial entorhinal cortex. *Neuron* 79:1197–1207.

Behrens TEJ, Muller TH, Whittington JCR, Mark S, Baram AB, Stachenfeld KL, Kurth-Nelson Z (2018) What is a cognitive map? Organizing knowledge for flexible behavior. *Neuron* 100:490–509.

Bellmund JL, Deuker L, Doeller CF (2019) Mapping sequence structure in the human lateral entorhinal cortex. *eLife* 8:e45333.

Bellmund JL, Deuker L, Navarro Schröder T, Doeller CF (2016) Grid-cell representations in mental simulation. *eLife* 5:e17089.

Ben-Yishai R, Bar-Or RL, Sompolinsky H (1995) Theory of orientation tuning in visual cortex. *Proc Natl Acad Sci* 92:3844–3848.

Bernasconi N, Bernasconi A, Caramanos Z, Dubeau F, Richardson J, Andermann F, Arnold DL (2001) Entorhinal cortex atrophy in epilepsy patients exhibiting normal hippocampal volumes. *Neurology* 56:1335–1339.

Bjerknes TL, Moser EI, Moser MB (2014) Representation of geometric borders in the developing rat. *Neuron* 82:71–78.

Blackstad TW (1956) Commissural connections of the hippocampal region in the rat, with special reference to their mode of termination. *J Comp Neurol* 105:417–537.

Boccara CN, Sargolini F, Thoresen V, Solstad T, Witter MP, Moser EI, Moser M-B (2010) Grid cells in pre- and parasubiculum. *Nat Neurosci* 13:987–994.

Bonnevie T, Dunn B, Fyhn M, Hafting T, Derdikman D, Kubie JL, Roudi Y, Moser EI, Moser M-B (2013) Grid cells require excitatory drive from the hippocampus. *Nat Neurosci* 16:309–317.

Bota M, Sporns O, Swanson LW (2015) Architecture of the cerebral cortical association connectome underlying cognition. *Proc Natl Acad Sci U S A* 112:E2093–2101.

Braak H, Braak E (1991) Neuropathological stageing of Alzheimer-related changes. *Acta Neuropathol* 82:239–259.

Brandon MP, Bogaard AR, Libby CP, Connerney MA, Gupta K, Hasselmo ME (2011) Reduction of theta rhythm dissociates grid cell spatial periodicity from directional tuning. *Science* 332:595–599.

Brandon MP, Koenig J, Leutgeb JK, Leutgeb S (2014) New and distinct hippocampal place codes are generated in a new environment during septal inactivation. *Neuron* 82:789–796.

Brun VH, Leutgeb S, Wu HQ, Schwarcz R, Witter MP, Moser EI, Moser MB (2008) Impaired spatial representation in CA1 after lesion of direct input from entorhinal cortex. *Neuron* 57:290–302.

Brun VH, Otnass MK, Molden S, Steffenach HA, Witter MP, Moser MB, Moser EI (2002) Place cells and place recognition maintained by direct entorhinal-hippocampal circuitry. *Science* 296:2243–2246.

Brun VH, Solstad T, Kjelstrup KB, Fyhn M, Witter MP, Moser EI, Moser MB (2008) Progressive increase in grid scale from dorsal to ventral medial entorhinal cortex. *Hippocampus* 18:1200–1212.

Buckmaster PS, Alonso A, Canfield DR, Amaral DG (2004) Dendritic morphology, local circuitry, and intrinsic electrophysiology of principal neurons in the entorhinal cortex of macaque monkeys. *J Comp Neurol* 470:317–329.

Burak Y, Fiete IR (2009) Accurate path integration in continuous attractor network models of grid cells. *PLoS Comput Biol* 5:e1000291.

Burgess N, Barry C, O'Keefe J (2007) An oscillatory interference model of grid cell firing. *Hippocampus* 17:801–812.

Burwell RD (2000) The parahippocampal region: corticocortical connectivity. *Ann N Y Acad Sci* 911:25–42.

Burwell RD, Amaral DG (1998) Cortical afferents of the perirhinal, postrhinal, and entorhinal cortices of the rat. *J Comp Neurol* 398:179–205.

Burwell RD, Witter MP, Amaral DG (1995) Perirhinal and postrhinal cortices of the rat: a review of the neuroanatomical literature and comparison with findings from the monkey brain. *Hippocampus* 5:390–408.

Buzsáki G (1996) The hippocampo-neocortical dialogue. *Cereb Cortex* 6:81–92.

Buzsáki G, Moser EI (2013) Memory, navigation and theta rhythm in the hippocampal-entorhinal system. *Nat Neurosci* 16:130–138.

Caballero-Bleda M, Witter MP (1993) Regional and laminar organization of projections from the presubiculum and parasubiculum to the entorhinal cortex: an anterograde tracing study in the rat. *J Comp Neurol* 328:115–129.

Cameron KA, Yashar S, Wilson CL, Fried I (2001) Human hippocampal neurons predict how well word pairs will be remembered. *Neuron* 30:289–298.

Canto CB, Koganezawa N, Beed P, Moser EI, Witter MP (2012) All layers of medial entorhinal cortex receive presubicular and parasubicular inputs. *J Neurosci* 32:17620–17631.

Canto CB, Witter MP (2012a) Cellular properties of principal neurons in the rat entorhinal cortex: I. The lateral entorhinal cortex. *Hippocampus* 22:1256–1276.

Canto CB, Witter MP (2012b) Cellular properties of principal neurons in the rat entorhinal cortex: II. The medial entorhinal cortex. *Hippocampus* 22:1277–1299.

Cappaert NLM, Van Strien NM, Witter MP (2015) Hippocampal formation. In: The Rat Nervous System (Paxinos G, ed), pp 511–574. San Diego, CA: Elsevier Academic Press.

Carboni AA, Lavelle WG, Barnes CL, Cipolloni PB (1990) Neurons of the lateral entorhinal cortex of the rhesus monkey: a Golgi, histochemical, and immunocytochemical characterization. *J Comp Neurol* 291:583–608.

Caruana DA, Sorge RE, Stewart J, Chapman CA (2006) Dopamine has bidirectional effects on synaptic responses to cortical inputs in layer II of the lateral entorhinal cortex. *J Neurophysiol* 96:3006–3015.

Carvalho MM, Tanke N, Kropff E, Witter MP, Moser MB, Moser EI (2020) A brainstem locomotor circuit drives the activity of speed cells in the medial entorhinal cortex. *Cell Rep* 32:108123.

Cassel JC, Pereira de Vasconcelos A, Loureiro M, Cholvin T, Dalrymple-Alford JC, Vertes RP (2013) The reuniens and rhomboid nuclei: neuroanatomy, electrophysiological characteristics and behavioral implications. *Prog Neurobiol* 111:34–52.

Castro L, Aguiar P (2014) A feedforward model for the formation of a grid field where spatial information is provided solely from place cells. *Biol Cybern* 108:133–143.

Cavada C, Goldman-Rakic PS (1989) Posterior parietal cortex in rhesus monkey: I. Parcellation of areas based on distinctive limbic and sensory corticocortical connections. *J Comp Neurol* 287:393–421.

Cenquizca LA, Swanson LW (2007) Spatial organization of direct hippocampal field CA1 axonal projections to the rest of the cerebral cortex. *Brain Res Rev* 56:1–26.

Chaudhuri R, Gercek B, Pandey B, Peyrache A, Fiete I (2019) The intrinsic attractor manifold and population dynamics of a canonical cognitive circuit across waking and sleep. *Nat Neurosci* 22:1512–1520.

Chiba T, Kayahara T, Nakano K (2001) Efferent projections of infralimbic and prelimbic areas of the medial prefrontal cortex in the Japanese monkey, Macaca fuscata. *Brain Res* 888:83–101.

Cilz NI, Kurada L, Hu B, Lei S (2014) Dopaminergic modulation of GABAergic transmission in the entorhinal cortex: concerted roles of $\alpha 1$ adrenoreceptors, inward rectifier K^+, and T-type Ca^{2+} channels. *Cereb Cortex* 24:3195–3208.

Clark B, Taube J (2012) Vestibular and attractor network basis of the head direction cell signal in subcortical circuits. *Front Neural Circuits* 6:7.

Constantinescu AO, O'Reilly JX, Behrens TEJ (2016) Organizing conceptual knowledge in humans with a gridlike code. *Science* 352:1464–1468.

Couey JJ, Witoelar A, Zhang SJ, Zheng K, Ye J, Dunn B, Czajkowski R, Moser MB, Moser EI, Roudi Y, et al. (2013) Recurrent inhibitory circuitry as a mechanism for grid formation. *Nat Neurosci* 16:318–324.

D'Albis T, Kempter R (2017) A single-cell spiking model for the origin of grid-cell patterns. *PLoS Comput Biol* 13:e1005782.

Darwin C (1873) Origin of certain instincts. *Nature* 7:417–418.

de Almeida L, Idiart M, Lisman JE (2009) The input-output transformation of the hippocampal granule cells: from grid cells to place fields. *J Neurosci* 29:7504–7512.

de Almeida L, Idiart M, Lisman JE (2012) The single place fields of CA3 cells: a two-stage transformation from grid cells. *Hippocampus* 22:200–208.

Deller T, Martinez A, Nitsch R, Frotscher M (1996) A novel entorhinal projection to the rat dentate gyrus: direct innervation of proximal dendrites and cell bodies of granule cells and GABAergic neurons. *J Neurosci* 16:3322–3333.

Deshmukh SS, Knierim JJ (2011) Representation of non-spatial and spatial information in the lateral entorhinal cortex. *Front Behav Neurosci* 5:69.

Deshmukh SS, Knierim JJ (2013) Influence of local objects on hippocampal representations: landmark vectors and memory. *Hippocampus* 23:253–267.

Dhillon A, Jones RS (2000) Laminar differences in recurrent excitatory transmission in the rat entorhinal cortex in vitro. *Neuroscience* 99:413–422.

Dickerson BC, Goncharova I, Sullivan MP, Forchetti C, Wilson RS, Bennett DA, Beckett LA, deToledo-Morrell L (2001) MRI-derived entorhinal and hippocampal atrophy in incipient and very mild Alzheimer's disease. *Neurobiol Aging* 22:747–754.

Dickson CT, Magistretti J, Shalinsky MH, Fransen E, Hasselmo ME, Alonso A (2000) Properties and role of I(h) in the pacing of subthreshold oscillations in entorhinal cortex layer II neurons. *J Neurophysiol* 83:2562–2579.

Diehl GW, Hon OJ, Leutgeb S, Leutgeb JK (2017) Grid and nongrid cells in medial entorhinal cortex represent spatial location and environmental features with complementary coding schemes. *Neuron* 94:83–92, e81–e86.

Ding SL, Van Hoesen G, Rockland KS (2000) Inferior parietal lobule projections to the presubiculum and neighboring ventromedial temporal cortical areas. *J Comp Neurol* 425:510–530.

Doan TP, Lagartos-Donate MJ, Nilssen ES, Ohara S, Witter MP (2019) Convergent projections from perirhinal and postrhinal cortices suggest a multisensory nature of lateral, but not medial, entorhinal cortex. *Cell Rep* 29:617–627, e617.

Doeller CF, Barry C, Burgess N (2010) Evidence for grid cells in a human memory network. *Nature* 463:657–661.

Dolleman-Van der Weel MJ, Witter MP (1996) Projections from the nucleus reuniens thalami to the entorhinal cortex, hippocampal field CA1, and the subiculum in the rat arise from different populations of neurons. *J Comp Neurol* 364:637–650.

Dolleman-van der Weel MJ, Witter MP (2020) The thalamic midline nucleus reuniens: potential relevance for schizophrenia and epilepsy. *Neurosci Biobehav Rev* 119:422–439.

Dolorfo CL, Amaral DG (1998) Entorhinal cortex of the rat: topographic organization of the cells of origin of the perforant path projection to the dentate gyrus. *J Comp Neurol* 398:25–48.

Domnisoru C, Kinkhabwala AA, Tank DW (2013) Membrane potential dynamics of grid cells. *Nature* 495:199–204.

Du F, Eid T, Lothman EW, Köhler C, Schwarcz R (1995) Preferential neuronal loss in layer III of the medial entorhinal cortex in rat models of temporal lobe epilepsy. *J Neurosci* 15:6301–6313.

Du F, Whetsell WO, Abou-Khalil B, Blumenkopf B, Lothman EW, Schwarcz R (1993) Preferential neuronal loss in layer III of the entorhinal cortex in patients with temporal lobe epilepsy. *Epilepsy Res* 16:223–233.

Dugladze T, Heinemann U, Gloveli T (2001) Entorhinal cortex projection cells to the hippocampal formation in vitro. *Brain Res* 905:224–231.

Egorov AV, Hamam BN, Fransen E, Hasselmo ME, Alonso AA (2002) Graded persistent activity in entorhinal cortex neurons. *Nature* 420:173–178.

Eid T, Du F, Schwarcz R (2001) Ibotenate injections into the pre- and parasubiculum provide partial protection against kainate-induced epileptic damage in layer III of rat entorhinal cortex. *Epilepsia* 42:817–824.

Falkai P, Schneider-Axmann T, Honer WG (2000) Entorhinal cortex pre-alpha cell clusters in schizophrenia: quantitative evidence of a developmental abnormality. *Biol Psychiatry* 47:937–943.

Ferrante M, Tahvildari B, Duque A, Hadzipasic M, Salkoff D, Zagha EW, Hasselmo ME, McCormick DA (2017) Distinct functional groups emerge from the intrinsic properties of molecularly identified entorhinal interneurons and principal cells. *Cereb Cortex* 27:3186–3207.

Fuchs EC, Neitz A, Pinna R, Melzer S, Caputi A, Monyer H (2016) Local and distant input controlling excitation in layer II of the medial entorhinal cortex. *Neuron* 89:194–208.

Fuhs MC, Touretzky DS (2006) A spin glass model of path integration in rat medial entorhinal cortex. *J Neurosci* 26:4266–4276.

Fujimaru Y, Kosaka T (1996) The distribution of two calcium binding proteins, calbindin D-28K and parvalbumin, in the entorhinal cortex of the adult mouse. *Neurosci Res* 24:329–343.

Fyhn M, Hafting T, Treves A, Moser MB, Moser EI (2007) Hippocampal remapping and grid realignment in entorhinal cortex. *Nature* 446:190–194.

Fyhn M, Molden S, Witter MP, Moser EI, Moser MB (2004) Spatial representation in the entorhinal cortex. *Science* 305:1258–1264.

Gardner RJ, Hermansen E, Patchitariu M, Burak Y, Baas NA, Dunn B, Moser M-B, Moser EI (2022) Toroidal topology of population activity in grid cells. *Nature* 602:123–128.

Gardner RJ, Lu L, Wernle T, Moser M-B, Moser EI (2019) Correlation structure of grid cells is preserved during sleep. *Nat Neurosci* 22:598–608.

Gatome CW, Slomianka L, Lipp HP, Amrein I (2010) Number estimates of neuronal phenotypes in layer II of the medial entorhinal cortex of rat and mouse. *Neuroscience* 170:156–165.

Gloveli T, Schmitz D, Empson RM, Dugladze T, Heinemann U (1997) Morphological and electrophysiological characterization of layer III cells of the medial entorhinal cortex of the rat. *Neuroscience* 77:629–648.

Gloveli T, Schmitz D, Heinemann U (1997) Prolonged inhibitory potentials in layer III projection cells of the rat medial entorhinal cortex induced by synaptic stimulation in vitro. *Neuroscience* 80:119–131.

Gofman X, Tocker G, Weiss S, Boccara CN, Lu L, Moser MB, Moser EI, Morris G, Derdikman D (2019) Dissociation between postrhinal cortex and downstream parahippocampal regions in the representation of egocentric boundaries. *Curr Biol* 29:2751–2757, e2754.

Gomez-Isla T, Price JL, McKeel DW, Morris JC, Growdon JH, Hyman BT (1996) Profound loss of layer II entorhinal cortex neurons occurs in very mild Alzheimer's disease. *J Neurosci* 16:4491–4500.

Gothard KM, Skaggs WE, McNaughton BL (1996) Dynamics of mismatch correction in the hippocampal ensemble code for space: interaction between path integration and environmental cues. *J Neurosci* **16**:8027–8040.

Gothard KM, Skaggs WE, Moore KM, McNaughton BL (1996) Binding of hippocampal CA1 neural activity to multiple reference frames in a landmark-based navigation task. *J Neurosci* **16**:823–835.

Grubman A, Chew G, Ouyang JF, Sun G, Choo XY, McLean C, Simmons RK, Buckberry S, Vargas-Landin DB, Poppe D, et al. (2019) A single-cell atlas of entorhinal cortex from individuals with Alzheimer's disease reveals cell-type-specific gene expression regulation. *Nat Neurosci* **22**:2087–2097.

Guanella A, Kiper D, Verschure P (2007) A model of grid cells based on a twisted torus topology. *Int J Neural Syst* **17**:231–240.

Hafting T, Fyhn M, Molden S, Moser MB, Moser EI (2005) Microstructure of a spatial map in the entorhinal cortex. *Nature* **436**:801–806.

Hales JB, Schlesiger MI, Leutgeb JK, Squire LR, Leutgeb S, Clark RE (2014) Medial entorhinal cortex lesions only partially disrupt hippocampal place cells and hippocampus-dependent place memory. *Cell Rep* **9**:893–901.

Hamam BN, Amaral DG, Alonso AA (2002) Morphological and electrophysiological characteristics of layer V neurons of the rat lateral entorhinal cortex. *J Comp Neurol* **451**:45–61.

Hamam BN, Kennedy TE, Alonso A, Amaral DG (2000) Morphological and electrophysiological characteristics of layer V neurons of the rat medial entorhinal cortex. *J Comp Neurol* **418**:457–472.

Hamid EH, Hyde TM, Egan MF, Wolf SS, Herman MM, Nemeroff CB, Kleinman JE (2002) Neurotensin receptor binding abnormalities in the entorhinal cortex in schizophrenia and affective disorders. *Biol Psychiatry* **51**:795–800.

Hardcastle K, Ganguli S, Giocomo LM (2015) Environmental boundaries as an error correction mechanism for grid cells. *Neuron* **86**:827–839.

Hardcastle K, Maheswaranathan N, Ganguli S, Giocomo LM (2017) A multiplexed, heterogeneous, and adaptive code for navigation in medial entorhinal cortex. *Neuron* **94**:375–387, e377.

Hargreaves EL, Rao G, Lee I, Knierim JJ (2005) Major dissociation between medial and lateral entorhinal input to dorsal hippocampus. *Science* **308**:1792–1794.

Hartley T, Burgess N, Lever C, Cacucci F, O'Keefe J (2000) Modeling place fields in terms of the cortical inputs to the hippocampus. *Hippocampus* **10**:369–379.

Hebb DO (1949) The Organization of Behavior: A Neuropsychological Theory. Oxford: Wiley.

Herkenham M (1978) The connections of the nucleus reuniens thalami: evidence for a direct thalamo-hippocampal pathway in the rat. *J Comp Neurol* **177**:589–610.

Heys JG, Dombeck DA (2018) Evidence for a subcircuit in medial entorhinal cortex representing elapsed time during immobility. *Nat Neurosci* **21**:1574–1582.

Heys JG, Schultheiss NW, Shay CF, Tsuno Y, Hasselmo ME (2012) Effects of acetylcholine on neuronal properties in entorhinal cortex. *Front Behav Neurosci* **6**:32.

Hill AJ (1978) First occurrence of hippocampal spatial firing in a new environment. *Exp Neurol* **62**:282–297.

Hinman JR, Chapman GW, Hasselmo ME (2019) Neuronal representation of environmental boundaries in egocentric coordinates. *Nat Commun*:**10**:2772.

Holbrook AJ, Tustison NJ, Marquez F, Roberts J, Yassa MA, Gillen DL (2020) Anterolateral entorhinal cortex thickness as a new biomarker for early detection of Alzheimer's disease. *Alzheimers Dement (Amst)* **12**:e12068.

Hoover WB, Vertes RP (2007) Anatomical analysis of afferent projections to the medial prefrontal cortex in the rat. *Brain Struct Funct* **212**:149–179.

Hoover WB, Vertes RP (2011) Projections of the medial orbital and ventral orbital cortex in the rat. *J Comp Neurol* **519**:3766–3801.

Horner AJ, Bisby JA, Zotow E, Bush D, Burgess N (2016) Grid-like processing of imagined navigation. *Curr Biol* **26**:842–847.

Hyman BT, Van Horsen GW, Damasio AR, Barnes CL (1984) Alzheimer's disease: cell-specific pathology isolates the hippocampal formation. *Science* **225**:1168–1170.

Høydal OA, Skytoen ER, Andersson SO, Moser MB, Moser EI (2019) Object-vector coding in the medial entorhinal cortex. *Nature* **568**:400–404.

Ino T, Kaneko T, Mizuno N (1998) Direct projections from the entorhinal cortical layers to the dentate gyrus, hippocampus, and subicular complex in the cat. *Neurosci Res* **32**:241–265.

Ino T, Kaneko T, Mizuno N (2000) Intrinsic and commissural connections within the entorhinal cortex: an anterograde and retrograde tract-tracing study in the cat. *Neurosci Res* **36**:45–60.

Ino T, Kaneko T, Mizuno N (2001) Projections from the hippocampal and parahippocampal regions to the entorhinal cortex: an anterograde and retrograde tract-tracing study in the cat. *Neurosci Res* **39**:51–69.

Insausti R, Amaral DG (2008) Entorhinal cortex of the monkey: IV. Topographical and laminar organization of cortical afferents. *J Comp Neurol* **509**:608–641.

Insausti R, Amaral DG, Cowan WM (1987) The entorhinal cortex of the monkey: III. Subcortical afferents. *J Comp Neurol* **264**:396–408.

Insausti R, Herrero MT, Witter MP (1997) Entorhinal cortex of the rat: cytoarchitectonic subdivisions and the origin and distribution of cortical efferents. *Hippocampus* **7**:146–183.

Insausti R, Tunon T, Sobreviela T, Insausti AM, Gonzalo LM (1995) The human entorhinal cortex: a cytoarchitectonic analysis. *J Comp Neurol* **355**:171–198.

Ismakov R, Barak O, Jeffery K, Derdikman D (2017) Grid cells encode local positional information. *Curr Biol* **27**:2337–2343.

Jacob P-Y, Casali G, Spieser L, Page H, Overington D, Jeffery K (2017) An independent, landmark-dominated head-direction signal in dysgranular retrosplenial cortex. *Nat Neurosci* **20**:173–175.

Jercog PE, Ahmadian Y, Woodruff C, Deb-Sen R, Abbott LF, Kandel ER (2019) Heading direction with respect to a reference point modulates place-cell activity. *Nat Commun*:**10**:2333.

Jochems A, Reboreda A, Hasselmo ME, Yoshida M (2013) Cholinergic receptor activation supports persistent firing in layer III neurons in the medial entorhinal cortex. *Behav Brain Res* **254**:108–115.

Jones BF, Witter MP (2007) Cingulate cortex projections to the parahippocampal region and hippocampal formation in the rat. *Hippocampus* **17**:957–976.

Jones RS (1994) Synaptic and intrinsic properties of neurons of origin of the perforant path in layer II of the rat entorhinal cortex in vitro. *Hippocampus* **4**:335–353.

Jones RS, Buhl EH (1993) Basket-like interneurones in layer II of the entorhinal cortex exhibit a powerful NMDA-mediated synaptic excitation. *Neurosci Lett* **149**:35–39.

Julian JB, Keinath AT, Frazzetta G, Epstein RA (2018) Human entorhinal cortex represents visual space using a boundary-anchored grid. *Nat Neurosci* **21**:191–194.

Jun H, Bramian A, Soma S, Saito T, Saido TC, Igarashi KM (2020) Disrupted place cell remapping and impaired grid cells in a knockin model of Alzheimer's disease. *Neuron* **107**:1095–1112.

Jun JJ, Steinmetz NA, Siegle JH, Denman DJ, Bauza M, Barbarits B, Lee AK, Anastassiou CA, Andrei A, Aydın Ç, et al. (2017) Fully integrated silicon probes for high-density recording of neural activity. *Nature* **551**:232–236.

Jung MW, Wiener SI, McNaughton BL (1994) Comparison of spatial firing characteristics of units in dorsal and ventral hippocampus of the rat. *J Neurosci* **14**:7347–7356.

Kanter BR, Lykken CM, Avesar D, Weible A, Dickinson J, Dunn B, Borgesius NZ, Roudi Y, Kentros CG (2017) A novel mechanism for the grid-to-place cell transformation revealed by transgenic depolarization of medial entorhinal cortex layer II. *Neuron* **93**:1480–1492, e1486.

Kecskés M, Henn-Mike N, Agócs-Laboda Á, Szőcs S, Petykó Z, Varga C (2020) Somatostatin expressing GABAergic interneurons in the medial entorhinal cortex preferentially inhibit layer(III-V) pyramidal cells. *Commun Biol* **3**:754.

Keene CS, Bladon J, McKenzie S, Liu CD, O'Keefe J, Eichenbaum H (2016) Complementary functional organization of neuronal activity patterns in the perirhinal, lateral entorhinal, and medial entorhinal cortices. *J Neurosci* **36**:3660–3675.

Kemppainen S, Jolkkonen E, Pitkanen A (2002) Projections from the posterior cortical nucleus of the amygdala to the hippocampal formation and parahippocampal region in rat. *Hippocampus* **12**:735–755.

Kerr KM, Agster KL, Furtak SC, Burwell RD (2007) Functional neuroanatomy of the parahippocampal region: the lateral and medial entorhinal areas. *Hippocampus* **17**:697–708.

Killian NJ, Jutras MJ, Buffalo EA (2012) A map of visual space in the primate entorhinal cortex. *Nature* **491**:761–764.

King C, Recce M, O'Keefe J (1998) The rhythmicity of cells of the medial septum/diagonal band of Broca in the awake freely moving rat: relationships with behaviour and hippocampal theta. *Eur J Neurosci* **10**:464–477.

Kitamura T, Pignatelli M, Suh J, Kohara K, Yoshiki A, Abe K, Tonegawa S (2014) Island cells control temporal association memory. *Science* **343**:896–901.

Kitanishi T, Matsuo N (2017) Organization of the claustrum-to-entorhinal cortical connection in mice. *J Neurosci* **37**:269–280.

Klink R, Alonso A (1997) Morphological characteristics of layer II projection neurons in the rat medial entorhinal cortex. *Hippocampus* **7**:571–583.

Kloosterman F, Witter MP, Van Haeften T (2003) Topographical and laminar organization of subicular projections to the parahippocampal region of the rat. *J Comp Neurol* **455**:156–171.

Kobayashi Y, Amaral DG (2003) Macaque monkey retrosplenial cortex: II. Cortical afferents. *J Comp Neurol* **466**:48–79.

Kobayashi Y, Amaral DG (2007) Macaque monkey retrosplenial cortex: III. Cortical efferents. *J Comp Neurol* **502**:810–833.

Kobro-Flatmoen A, Lagartos-Donate MJ, Aman Y, Edison P, Witter MP, Fang EF (2021) Re-emphasizing early Alzheimer's disease pathology starting in select entorhinal neurons, with a special focus on mitophagy. *Ageing Res Rev* **67**:101307.

Kobro-Flatmoen A, Nagelhus A, Witter MP (2016) Reelin-immunoreactive neurons in entorhinal cortex layer II selectively express intracellular amyloid in early Alzheimer's disease. *Neurobiol Dis* **93**:172–183.

Kobro-Flatmoen A, Witter MP (2019) Neuronal chemo-architecture of the entorhinal cortex: a comparative review. *Eur J Neurosci* **50**:3627–3662.

Koenig J, Linder AN, Leutgeb JK, Leutgeb S (2011) The spatial periodicity of grid cells is not sustained during reduced theta oscillations. *Science* **332**:592–595.

Koganezawa N, Gisetstad R, Husby E, Doan TP, Witter MP (2015) Excitatory postrhinal projections to principal cells in the medial entorhinal cortex. *J Neurosci* **35**:15860–15874.

Kondo H, Witter MP (2014) Topographic organization of orbitofrontal projections to the parahippocampal region in rats. *J Comp Neurol* **522**:772–793.

Kondo H, Zaborszky L (2016) Topographic organization of the basal forebrain projections to the perirhinal, postrhinal, and entorhinal cortex in rats. *J Comp Neurol* **524**:2503–2515.

Kordower JH, Chu Y, Stebbins GT, DeKosky ST, Cochran EJ, Bennett D, Mufson EJ (2001) Loss and atrophy of layer II entorhinal cortex neurons in elderly people with mild cognitive impairment. *Ann Neurol* **49**:202–213.

Kraus BJ, Brandon MP, Robinson RJ, Connerney MA, Hasselmo ME, Eichenbaum H (2015) During running in place, grid cells integrate elapsed time and distance run. *Neuron* **88**:578–589.

Kropff E, Carmichael JE, Moser MB, Moser EI (2015) Speed cells in the medial entorhinal cortex. *Nature* **523**:419–424.

Kropff E, Treves A (2008) The emergence of grid cells: intelligent design or just adaptation? *Hippocampus* **18**:1256–1269.

Krupic J, Bauza M, Burton S, Barry C, O'Keefe J (2015) Grid cell symmetry is shaped by environmental geometry. *Nature* **518**:232–235.

Kunz L, Maidenbaum S, Chen D, Wang L, Jacobs J, Axmacher N (2019) Mesoscopic neural representations in spatial navigation. *Trends Cogn Sci* **23**:615–630.

Kunz L, Schröder TN, Lee H, Montag C, Lachmann B, Sariyska R, Reuter M, Stirnberg R, Stöcker T, Messing-Floeter PC, et al. (2015) Reduced grid-cell-like representations in adults at genetic risk for Alzheimer's disease. *Science* **350**:430–433.

Köhler C (1986) Cytochemical architecture of the entorhinal area. *Adv Exp Med Biol* **203**:83–98.

Köhler C, Chan-Palay V (1983) Somatostatin and vasoactive intestinal polypeptide-like immunoreactive cells and terminals in the retrohippocampal region of the rat brain. *Anat Embryol (Berl)* **167**:151–172.

LaChance PA, Todd TP, Taube JS (2019) A sense of space in postrhinal cortex. *Science* **365**:eaax4192.

Langston RF, Ainge JA, Couey JJ, Canto CB, Bjerknes TL, Witter MP, Moser EI, Moser MB (2010) Development of the spatial representation system in the rat. *Science* **328**:1576–1580.

Laptev D, Burgess N (2019) Neural dynamics indicate parallel integration of environmental and self-motion information by place and grid cells. *Front Neural Circuits* **13**:59.

Lavenex P, Suzuki WA, Amaral DG (2002) Perirhinal and parahippocampal cortices of the macaque monkey: projections to the neocortex. *J Comp Neurol* **447**:394–420.

Lee JY, Jun H, Soma S, Nakazono T, Shiraiwa K, Dasgupta A, Nakagawa T, Xie JL, Chavez J, Romo R, et al. (2021) Dopamine facilitates associative memory encoding in the entorhinal cortex. *Nature* **598**:321–326.

Leitner FC, Melzer S, Lutcke H, Pinna R, Seeburg PH, Helmchen F, Monyer H (2016) Spatially segregated feedforward and feedback neurons support differential odor processing in the lateral entorhinal cortex. *Nat Neurosci* **19**:935–944.

Leonard BW, Amaral DG, Squire LR, Zola-Morgan S (1995) Transient memory impairment in monkeys with bilateral lesions of the entorhinal cortex. *J Neurosci* **15**:5637–5659.

Lever C, Burton S, Jeewajee A, O'Keefe J, Burgess N (2009) Boundary vector cells in the subiculum of the hippocampal formation. *J Neurosci* **29**:9771–9777.

Lisman JE (2007) Role of the dual entorhinal inputs to hippocampus: a hypothesis based on cue/action (non-self/self) couplets. *Prog Brain Res* **163**:615–625.

Lositsky O, Chen J, Toker D, Honey CJ, Shvartsman M, Poppenk JL, Hasson U, Norman KA (2016) Neural pattern change during encoding of a narrative predicts retrospective duration estimates. *eLife* **5**:e16070.

Maass A, Berron D, Libby LA, Ranganath C, Duzel E (2015) Functional subregions of the human entorhinal cortex. *eLife* **4**:e06426.

MacDonald CJ, Carrow S, Place R, Eichenbaum H (2013) Distinct hippocampal time cell sequences represent odor memories in immobilized rats. *J Neurosci* **33**:14607–14616.

Majak K, Pitkanen A (2003) Projections from the periamygdaloid cortex to the amygdaloid complex, the hippocampal formation, and the parahippocampal region: a PHA-L study in the rat. *Hippocampus* **13**:922–942.

Mankin EA, Fried I (2020) Modulation of human memory by deep brain stimulation of the entorhinal-hippocampal circuitry. *Neuron* **106**:218–235.

Martínez-Cerdeño V, Clascá F (2002) Reelin immunoreactivity in the adult neocortex: a comparative study in rodents, carnivores, and non-human primates. *Brain Res Bull* **57**:485–488.

Martínez-Cerdeño V, Galazo MJ, Clascá F (2003) Reelin-immunoreactive neurons, axons, and neuropil in the adult ferret brain: evidence for axonal secretion of reelin in long axonal pathways. *J Comp Neurol* **463**:92–116.

Masurkar AV, Srinivas KV, Brann DH, Warren R, Lowes DC, Siegelbaum SA (2017) Medial and lateral entorhinal cortex differentially excite deep versus superficial CA1 pyramidal neurons. *Cell Rep* **18**:148–160.

Mathiasen ML, Hansen L, Witter MP (2015) Insular projections to the parahippocampal region in the rat. *J Comp Neurol* **523**:1379–1398.

Mathis A, Herz AV, Stemmler M (2012a) Optimal population codes for space: grid cells outperform place cells. *Neural Comput* **24**:2280–2317.

Mathis A, Herz AV, Stemmler MB (2012b) Resolution of nested neuronal representations can be exponential in the number of neurons. *Phys Rev Lett* **109**:018103.

McKenzie S, Frank AJ, Kinsky NR, Porter B, Riviere PD, Eichenbaum H (2014) Hippocampal representation of related and opposing memories develop within distinct, hierarchically organized neural schemas. *Neuron* **83**:202–215.

McNaughton BL, Barnes CA, Gerrard JL, Gothard K, Jung MW, Knierim JJ, Kudrimoti H, Qin Y, Skaggs WE, Suster M, Weaver KL (1996) Deciphering the hippocampal polyglot: the hippocampus as a path integration system. *J Exp Biol* **199**:173–185.

McNaughton BL, Barnes CA, Meltzer J, Sutherland RJ (1989) Hippocampal granule cells are necessary for normal spatial learning but not for spatially-selective pyramidal cell discharge. *Exp Brain Res* **76**:485–496.

McNaughton BL, Barnes CA, O'Keefe J (1983) The contributions of position, direction, and velocity to single unit activity in the hippocampus of freely-moving rats. *Exp Brain Res* **52**:41–49.

McNaughton BL, Battaglia FP, Jensen O, Moser EI, Moser M-B (2006) Path integration and the neural basis of the "cognitive map." *Nat Rev Neurosci* **7**:663–678.

McNaughton BL, Chen LL, Markus EJ (1991) "Dead reckoning," landmark learning, and the sense of direction: a neurophysiological and computational hypothesis. *J Cogn Neurosci* **3**:190–202.

McNaughton BL, Knierim JJ, Wilson MA (1995) Vector encoding and the vestibular foundations of spatial cognition: neurophysiological and computational mechanisms. In: The Cognitive Neurosciences, pp 585–595. Cambridge, MA: MIT Press.

Medina L, Abellan A, Desfilis E (2017) Contribution of genoarchitecture to understanding hippocampal evolution and development. *Brain Behav Evol* **90**:25–40.

Meister MLR, Buffalo EA (2018) Neurons in primate entorhinal cortex represent gaze position in multiple spatial reference frames. *J Neurosci* **38**:2430–2441.

Mesulam MM, Mufson EJ (1982) Insula of the old world monkey: III: Efferent cortical output and comments on function. *J Comp Neurol* **212**:38–52.

Meunier M, Bachevalier J, Mishkin M, Murray EA (1993) Effects on visual recognition of combined and separate ablations of the entorhinal and perirhinal cortex in rhesus monkeys. *J Neurosci* **13**:5418–5432.

Miao C, Cao Q, Ito HT, Yamahachi H, Witter MP, Moser MB, Moser EI (2015) Hippocampal remapping after partial inactivation of the medial entorhinal cortex. *Neuron* **88**:590–603.

Miettinen M, Pitkanen A, Miettinen R (1997) Distribution of calretinin-immunoreactivity in the rat entorhinal cortex: coexistence with GABA. *J Comp Neurol* **378**:363–378.

Miller VM, Best PJ (1980) Spatial correlates of hippocampal unit activity are altered by lesions of the fornix and endorhinal cortex. *Brain Res* **194**:311–323.

Mizumori SJ, McNaughton BL, Barnes CA, Fox KB (1989) Preserved spatial coding in hippocampal CA1 pyramidal cells during reversible suppression of CA3c output: evidence for pattern completion in hippocampus. *J Neurosci* **9**:3915–3928.

Moga MM, Weis RP, Moore RY (1995) Efferent projections of the paraventricular thalamic nucleus in the rat. *J Comp Neurol* **359**:221–238.

Mohedano-Moriano A, Pro-Sistiaga P, Arroyo-Jimenez MM, Artacho-Perula E, Insausti AM, Marcos P, Cebada-Sanchez S, Martinez-Ruiz J, Munoz M, Blaizot X, et al. (2007) Topographical and laminar distribution of cortical input to the monkey entorhinal cortex. *J Anat* **211**:250–260.

Monaco JD, Abbott LF (2011) Modular realignment of entorhinal grid cell activity as a basis for hippocampal remapping. *J Neurosci* **31**:9414–9425.

Montchal ME, Reagh ZM, Yassa MA (2019) Precise temporal memories are supported by the lateral entorhinal cortex in humans. *Nat Neurosci* **22**:284–288.

Morris R, Petrides M, Pandya DN (1999) Architecture and connections of retrosplenial area 30 in the rhesus monkey (Macaca mulatta). *Eur J Neurosci* **11**:2506–2518.

Mosheiff N, Burak Y (2019) Velocity coupling of grid cell modules enables stable embedding of a low dimensional variable in a high dimensional neural attractor. *eLife* **8**:e48494.

Muessig L, Hauser J, Wills TJ, Cacucci F (2015) A developmental switch in place cell accuracy coincides with grid cell maturation. *Neuron* **86**:1167–1173.

Muller RU, Kubie JL (1987) The effects of changes in the environment on the spatial firing of hippocampal complex-spike cells. *J Neurosci* **7**:1951–1968.

Munn RGK, Mallory CS, Hardcastle K, Chetkovich DM, Giocomo LM (2020) Entorhinal velocity signals reflect environmental geometry. *Nat Neurosci* **23**:239–251.

Munoz M, Insausti R (2005) Cortical efferents of the entorhinal cortex and the adjacent parahippocampal region in the monkey (*Macaca fascicularis*). *Eur J Neurosci* **22**:1368–1388.

Naber PA, Caballero-Bleda M, Jorritsma-Byham B, Witter MP (1997) Parallel input to the hippocampal memory system through peri- and postrhinal cortices. *Neuroreport* **8**:2617–2621.

Naber PA, Lopes da Silva FH, Witter MP (2001) Reciprocal connections between the entorhinal cortex and hippocampal fields CA1 and the subiculum are in register with the projections from CA1 to the subiculum. *Hippocampus* **11**:99–104.

Naber PA, Witter MP, Lopez da Silva FH (1999) Perirhinal cortex input to the hippocampus in the rat: evidence for parallel pathways, both direct and indirect: a combined physiological and anatomical study. *Eur J Neurosci* **11**:4119–4133.

Nau M, Julian JB, Doeller CF (2018) How the brain's navigation system shapes our visual experience. *Trends Cogn Sci* **22**:810–825.

Nau M, Navarro Schröder T, Bellmund JLS, Doeller CF (2018) Hexadirectional coding of visual space in human entorhinal cortex. *Nat Neurosci* **21**:188–190.

Naumann RK, Ray S, Prokop S, Las L, Heppner FL, Brecht M (2016) Conserved size and periodicity of pyramidal patches in layer 2 of medial/caudal entorhinal cortex. *J Comp Neurol* **524**:783–806.

Navarro Schroder T, Haak KV, Zaragoza Jimenez NI, Beckmann CF, Doeller CF (2015) Functional topography of the human entorhinal cortex. *eLife* **4**:e06738.

Neunuebel JP, Yoganarasimha D, Rao G, Knierim JJ (2013) Conflicts between local and global spatial frameworks dissociate neural representations of the lateral and medial entorhinal cortex. *J Neurosci* **33**:9246–9258.

Nilssen ES, Doan TP, Nigro MJ, Ohara S, Witter MP (2019) Neurons and networks in the entorhinal cortex: a reappraisal of the lateral and medial entorhinal subdivisions mediating parallel cortical pathways. *Hippocampus* **29**:1238–1254.

Nilssen ES, Jacobsen B, Fjeld G, Nair RR, Blankvoort S, Kentros C, Witter MP (2018) Inhibitory connectivity dominates the fan cell network in layer II of lateral entorhinal cortex. *J Neurosci* **38**:9712–9727.

O'Keefe J, Burgess N (1996) Geometric determinants of the place fields of hippocampal neurons. *Nature* **381**:425–428.

O'Keefe J, Dostrovsky J (1971) The hippocampus as a spatial map: preliminary evidence from unit activity in the freely-moving rat. *Brain Res* **34**:171–175.

O'Keefe J, Nadel L (1978) The Hippocampus as a Cognitive Map, *Oxford University Press*. ISBN: 0-19-857206-9.

O'Keefe J, Recce ML (1993) Phase relationship between hippocampal place units and the EEG theta rhythm. *Hippocampus* **3**:317–330.

Ohara S, Blankvoort S, Nair RR, Nigro MJ, Nilssen ES, Kentros C, Witter MP (2021) Local projections of layer Vb-to-Va are more prominent in lateral than in medial entorhinal cortex. *eLife* **10**:e67262.

Ohara S, Gianatti M, Itou K, Berndtsson CH, Doan TP, Kitanishi T, Mizuseki K, Iijima T, Tsutsui KI, Witter MP (2019) Entorhinal layer II calbindin-expressing neurons originate widespread telencephalic and intrinsic projections. *Front Syst Neurosci* **13**:54.

Ohara S, Onodera M, Simonsen OW, Yoshino R, Hioki H, Iijima T, Tsutsui KI, Witter MP (2018) Intrinsic projections of layer Vb neurons to layers Va, III, and II in the lateral fixand medial entorhinal cortex of the rat. *Cell Rep* **24**:107–116.

Ohara S, Rannap M, Tsutsui K-I, Draguhn A, Egorov AV, Witter MP (2023) Hippocampal-medial entorhinal circuit is differently organized along the dorsoventral axis in rodents. *Cell Rep* **42**:112001.

Ohara S, Yoshino R, Kimura K, Kawamura T, Tanabe S, Zheng A, Nakamura S, Inoue K-I, Takada M, Tsutsui K-I, et al. (2021) Laminar organization of the entorhinal cortex in macaque monkeys based on cell-type-specific markers and connectivity. *Front Neural Circuits* **15**:790116.

Olsen GM, Ohara S, Iijima T, Witter MP (2017) Parahippocampal and retrosplenial connections of rat posterior parietal cortex. *Hippocampus* **27**:335–358.

Olton DS, Walker JA, Gage FH (1978) Hippocampal connections and spatial discrimination. *Brain Res* **139**:295–308.

Ormond J, McNaughton BL (2015) Place field expansion after focal MEC inactivations is consistent with loss of Fourier components and path integrator gain reduction. *Proc Natl Acad Sci U S A* **112**:4116–4121.

Pastalkova E, Itskov V, Amarasingham A, Buzsaki G (2008) Internally generated cell assembly sequences in the rat hippocampus. *Science* **321**:1322–1327.

Pastoll H, Ramsden HL, Nolan MF (2012) Intrinsic electrophysiological properties of entorhinal cortex stellate cells and their contribution to grid cell firing fields. *Front Neural Circuits* **6**:17.

Pastoll H, Solanka L, van Rossum MC, Nolan MF (2013) Feedback inhibition enables theta-nested gamma oscillations and grid firing fields. *Neuron* **77**:141–154.

Pearson RC, Brodal P, Gatter KC, Powell TP (1982) The organization of the connections between the cortex and the claustrum in the monkey. *Brain Res* **234**:435–441.

Pérez-García CG, González-Delgado FJ, Suárez-Solá ML, Castro-Fuentes R, Martín-Trujillo JM, Ferres-Torres R, Meyer G (2001) Reelin-immunoreactive neurons in the adult vertebrate pallium. *J Chem Neuroanat* **21**:41–51.

Pesold C, Pisu MG, Impagnatiello F, Uzunov DP, Caruncho HJ (1998) Simultaneous detection of glutamic acid decarboxylase and reelin mRNA in adult rat neurons using in situ hybridization and immunofluorescence. *Brain Res Brain Res Protoc* **3**:155–160.

Pinto A, Fuentes C, Pare D (2006) Feedforward inhibition regulates perirhinal transmission of neocortical inputs to the entorhinal cortex: ultrastructural study in guinea pigs. *J Comp Neurol* **495**:722–734.

Pitkanen A, Kelly JL, Amaral DG (2002) Projections from the lateral, basal, and accessory basal nuclei of the amygdala to the entorhinal cortex in the macaque monkey. *Hippocampus* **12**:186–205.

Pitkanen A, Pikkarainen M, Nurminen N, Ylinen A (2000) Reciprocal connections between the amygdala and the hippocampal formation, perirhinal cortex, and postrhinal cortex in rat: a review. *Ann N Y Acad Sci* **911**:369–391.

Price JL (2007) Definition of the orbital cortex in relation to specific connections with limbic and visceral structures and other cortical regions. *Ann N Y Acad Sci* **1121**:54–71.

Qiu S, Zhao LF, Korwek KM, Weeber EJ (2006) Differential reelin-induced enhancement of NMDA and AMPA receptor activity in the adult hippocampus. *J Neurosci* **26**:12943–12955.

Quilichini P, Sirota A, Buzsaki G (2010) Intrinsic circuit organization and theta-gamma oscillation dynamics in the entorhinal cortex of the rat. *J Neurosci* **30**:11128–11142.

Quirk GJ, Muller RU, Kubie JL (1990) The firing of hippocampal place cells in the dark depends on the rat's recent experience. *J Neurosci* **10**:2008–2017.

Ramsden HL, Surmeli G, McDonagh SG, Nolan MF (2015) Laminar and dorsoventral molecular organization of the medial entorhinal cortex revealed by large-scale anatomical analysis of gene expression. *PLoS Comput Biol* **11**:e1004032.

Ranck JB, Jr (1984) Head direction cells in the deep cell layer of dorsal presubiculum in freely moving rats. *Abstr Soc Neurosci* **10**.

Raudies F, Brandon MP, Chapman GW, Hasselmo ME (2015) Head direction is coded more strongly than movement direction in a population of entorhinal neurons. *Brain Res* **1621**:355–367.

Redish AD, Rosenzweig ES, Bohanick JD, McNaughton BL, Barnes CA (2000) Dynamics of hippocampal ensemble activity realignment: time versus space. *J Neurosci* **20**:9298–9309.

Rennó-Costa C, Tort ABL (2017) Place and grid cells in a loop: implications for memory function and spatial coding. *J Neurosci* **37**:8062–8076.

Rivard B, Li Y, Lenck-Santini PP, Poucet B, Muller RU (2004) Representation of objects in space by two classes of hippocampal pyramidal cells. *J Gen Physiol* **124**:9–25.

Rogers JT, Rusiana I, Trotter J, Zhao L, Donaldson E, Pak DT, Babus LW, Peters M, Banko JL, Chavis P, et al. (2011) Reelin supplementation enhances cognitive ability, synaptic plasticity, and dendritic spine density. *Learn Mem* **18**:558–564.

Rolls ET (1999) Spatial view cells and the representation of place in the primate hippocampus. *Hippocampus* 9:467–480.

Rolls ET, Stringer SM, Elliot T (2006) Entorhinal cortex grid cells can map to hippocampal place cells by competitive learning. *Network* 17:447–465.

Rolls ET, Wirth S (2018) Spatial representations in the primate hippocampus, and their functions in memory and navigation. *Prog Neurobiol* 171:90–113.

Rosene DL, Van Hoesen GW (1977) Hippocampal efferents reach widespread areas of cerebral cortex and amygdala in the rhesus monkey. *Science* 198:315–317.

Rowland DC, Obenhaus HA, Skytoen ER, Zhang Q, Kentros CG, Moser EI, Moser MB (2018) Functional properties of stellate cells in medial entorhinal cortex layer II. *eLife* 7:e36664.

Rowland DC, Weible AP, Wickersham IR, Wu H, Mayford M, Witter MP, Kentros CG (2013) Transgenically targeted rabies virus demonstrates a major monosynaptic projection from hippocampal area CA2 to medial entorhinal layer II neurons. *J Neurosci* 33:14889–14898.

Rozov A, Rannap M, Lorenz F, Nasretdinov A, Draguhn A, Egorov AV (2020) Processing of hippocampal network activity in the receiver network of the medial entorhinal cortex layer V. *J Neurosci* 40:8413–8425.

Rueckemann JW, DiMauro AJ, Rangel LM, Han X, Boyden ES, Eichenbaum H (2016) Transient optogenetic inactivation of the medial entorhinal cortex biases the active population of hippocampal neurons. *Hippocampus* 26:246–260.

Saleem KS, Kondo H, Price JL (2008) Complementary circuits connecting the orbital and medial prefrontal networks with the temporal, insular, and opercular cortex in the macaque monkey. *J Comp Neurol* 506:659–693.

Saleem KS, Tanaka K (1996) Divergent projections from the anterior inferotemporal area TE to the perirhinal and entorhinal cortices in the macaque monkey. *J Neurosci* 16:4757–4775.

Samsonovich A, McNaughton BL (1997) Path integration and cognitive mapping in a continuous attractor neural network model. *J Neurosci* 17:5900–5920.

Sarel A, Finkelstein A, Las L, Ulanovsky N (2017) Vectorial representation of spatial goals in the hippocampus of bats. *Science* 355:176–180.

Sargolini F, Fyhn M, Hafting T, McNaughton BL, Witter MP, Moser MB, Moser EI (2006) Conjunctive representation of position, direction, and velocity in entorhinal cortex. *Science* 312:758–762.

Saunders RC, Mishkin M, Aggleton JP (2005) Projections from the entorhinal cortex, perirhinal cortex, presubiculum, and parasubiculum to the medial thalamus in macaque monkeys: identifying different pathways using disconnection techniques. *Exp Brain Res* 167:1–16.

Savelli F, Knierim JJ (2010) Hebbian analysis of the transformation of medial entorhinal grid-cell inputs to hippocampal place fields. *J Neurophysiol* 103:3167–3183.

Savelli F, Luck JD, Knierim JJ (2017) Framing of grid cells within and beyond navigation boundaries. *eLife* 6:e21354.

Savelli F, Yoganarasimha D, Knierim JJ (2008) Influence of boundary removal on the spatial representations of the medial entorhinal cortex. *Hippocampus* 18:1270–1282.

Scheff SW, Price DA, Schmitt FA, Mufson EJ (2006) Hippocampal synaptic loss in early Alzheimer's disease and mild cognitive impairment. *Neurobiol Aging* 27:1372–1384.

Schlesiger MI, Cannova CC, Boublil BL, Hales JB, Mankin EA, Brandon MP, Leutgeb JK, Leibold C, Leutgeb S (2015) The medial entorhinal cortex is necessary for temporal organization of hippocampal neuronal activity. *Nat Neurosci* 18:1123–1132.

Schmidt-Hieber C, Häusser M (2013) Cellular mechanisms of spatial navigation in the medial entorhinal cortex. *Nat Neurosci* 16:325–331.

Schwarcz R, Witter MP (2002) Memory impairment in temporal lobe epilepsy: the role of entorhinal lesions. *Epilepsy Res* 50:161–177.

Seelig JD, Jayaraman V (2015) Neural dynamics for landmark orientation and angular path integration. *Nature* 521:186–191.

Shi CJ, Cassell MD (1997) Cortical, thalamic, and amygdaloid projections of rat temporal cortex. *J Comp Neurol* 382:153–175.

Si B, Kropff E, Treves A (2012) Grid alignment in entorhinal cortex. *Biol Cybern* 106:483–506.

Skaggs WE, Knierim JJ, Kudrimoti HS, McNaughton BL (1995) A model of the neural basis of the rat's sense of direction. *Adv Neural Inf Process Syst* 7:173–180.

Solodkin A, Vanhoesen GW (1996) Entorhinal cortex modules of the human brain. *J Comp Neurol* 365:610–627.

Solstad T, Boccara CN, Kropff E, Moser MB, Moser EI (2008) Representation of geometric borders in the entorhinal cortex. *Science* 322:1865–1868.

Solstad T, Moser EI, Einevoll GT (2006) From grid cells to place cells: a mathematical model. *Hippocampus* 16:1026–1031.

Soriano E, Martinez A, Farinas I, Frotscher M (1993) Chandelier cells in the hippocampal formation of the rat: the entorhinal area and subicular complex. *J Comp Neurol* 337:151–167.

Squire LR, Zola-Morgan SM (1991) The medial temporal lobe memory system. *Science* 253:1380–1386.

Staubli U, Fraser D, Kessler M, Lynch G (1986) Studies on retrograde and anterograde amnesia of olfactory memory after denervation of the hippocampus by entorhinal cortex lesions. *Behav Neural Biol* 46:432–444.

Staudigl T, Leszczynski M, Jacobs J, Sheth SA, Schroeder CE, Jensen O, Doeller CF (2018) Hexadirectional modulation of high-frequency electrophysiological activity in the human anterior medial temporal lobe maps visual space. *Curr Biol* 28:3325–3329, e3324.

Stemmler M, Mathis A, Herz AV (2015) Connecting multiple spatial scales to decode the population activity of grid cells. *Sci Adv* 1:e1500816.

Stensola H, Stensola T, Solstad T, Froland K, Moser MB, Moser EI (2012) The entorhinal grid map is discretized. *Nature* 492:72–78.

Stensola T, Stensola H, Moser MB, Moser EI (2015) Shearing-induced asymmetry in entorhinal grid cells. *Nature* 518:207–212.

Steward O (1976) Topographic organization of the projections from the entorhinal area to the hippocampal formation of the rat. *J Comp Neurol* 167:285–314.

Steward O, Scoville SA (1976) Cells of origin of entorhinal cortical afferents to the hippocampus and fascia dentata of the rat. *J Comp Neurol* 169:347–370.

Stringer C, Pachitariu M, Steinmetz N, Carandini M, Harris KD (2019) High-dimensional geometry of population responses in visual cortex. *Nature* 571:361–365.

Stringer JL, Lothman EW (1992) Reverberatory seizure discharges in hippocampal-parahippocampal circuits. *Exp Neurol* 116:198–203.

Suh J, Rivest AJ, Nakashiba T, Tominaga T, Tonegawa S (2011) Entorhinal cortex layer III input to the hippocampus is crucial for temporal association memory. *Science* 334:1415–1420.

Sun Y, Jin S, Lin X, Chen L, Qiao X, Jiang L, Zhou P, Johnston KG, Golshani P, Nie Q, et al. (2019) CA1-projecting subiculum neurons facilitate object–place learning. *Nat Neurosci* 22:1857–1870.

Sun Y, Nguyen AQ, Nguyen JP, Le L, Saur D, Choi J, Callaway EM, Xu X (2014) Cell-type-specific circuit connectivity of hippocampal CA1 revealed through Cre-dependent rabies tracing. *Cell Rep* 7:269–280.

Surmeli G, Marcu DC, McClure C, Garden DL, Pastoll H, Nolan MF (2015) Molecularly defined circuitry reveals input-output segregation in deep layers of the medial entorhinal cortex. *Neuron* **88**:1040–1053.

Suzuki WA, Amaral DG (1994a) Perirhinal and parahippocampal cortices of the macaque monkey: cortical afferents. *J Comp Neurol* **350**:497–533.

Suzuki WA, Amaral DG (1994b) Topographic organization of the reciprocal connections between the monkey entorhinal cortex and the perirhinal and parahippocampal cortices. *J Neurosci* **14**:1856–1877.

Suzuki WA, Miller EK, Desimone R (1997) Object and place memory in the macaque entorhinal cortex. *J Neurophysiol* **78**:1062–1081.

Suzuki WA, Porteros A (2002) Distribution of calbindin D-28k in the entorhinal, perirhinal, and parahippocampal cortices of the macaque monkey. *J Comp Neurol* **451**:392–412.

Swanson LW, Köhler C, Björklund A (1987) The limbic region, Part I. In: The Septohippocampal System Handbook of Chemical Neuroanatomy (Björklund A, Hökfelt T, Swanson LW, eds), vol 5, pp 125–227. Amsterdam: Elsevier.

Tahvildari B, Alonso A (2005) Morphological and electrophysiological properties of lateral entorhinal cortex layers II and III principal neurons. *J Comp Neurol* **491**:123–140.

Tahvildari B, Alonso AA, Bourque CW (2008) Ionic basis of ON and OFF persistent activity in layer III lateral entorhinal cortical principal neurons. *J Neurophysiol* **99**:2006–2011.

Talbot K, Arnold SE (2002) The parahippocampal region in schizophrenia. In: The Parahippocampal Region Organization and Role in Cognitive Function (Witter MP, Wouterlood FG, eds), pp 297–320. Oxford: Oxford University Press.

Tamamaki N, Nojyo Y (1993) Projection of the entorhinal layer II neurons in the rat as revealed by intracellular pressure-injection of neurobiotin. *Hippocampus* **3**:471–480.

Tang Q, Ebbesen CL, Sanguinetti-Scheck JI, Preston-Ferrer P, Gundlfinger A, Winterer J, Beed P, Ray S, Naumann R, Schmitz D, et al. (2015) Anatomical organization and spatiotemporal firing patterns of layer 3 neurons in the rat medial entorhinal cortex. *J Neurosci* **35**:12346–12354.

Taube JS (2007) The head direction signal: origins and sensory-motor integration. *Annu Rev Neurosci* **30**:181–207.

Taube JS, Muller RU, Ranck JB, Jr. (1990) Head-direction cells recorded from the postsubiculum in freely moving rats: I. Description and quantitative analysis. *J Neurosci* **10**:420–435.

Terrazas A, Krause M, Lipa P, Gothard KM, Barnes CA, McNaughton BL (2005) Self-motion and the hippocampal spatial metric. *J Neurosci* **25**:8085–8096.

Thompson LT, Best PJ (1990) Long-term stability of the place-field activity of single units recorded from the dorsal hippocampus of freely behaving rats. *Brain Res* **509**:299–308.

Tolman EC (1948) Cognitive maps in rats and men. *Psychol Rev* **55**:189–208.

Tomas Pereira I, Agster KL, Burwell RD (2016) Subcortical connections of the perirhinal, postrhinal, and entorhinal cortices of the rat: I. Afferents. *Hippocampus* **26**:1189–1212.

Trettel SG, Trimper JB, Hwaun E, Fiete IR, Colgin LL (2019) Grid cell co-activity patterns during sleep reflect spatial overlap of grid fields during active behaviors. *Nat Neurosci* **22**:609–617.

Tsao A, Moser MB, Moser EI (2013) Traces of experience in the lateral entorhinal cortex. *Curr Biol* **23**:399–405.

Tsao A, Sugar J, Lu L, Wang C, Knierim JJ, Moser M-B, Moser EI (2018) Integrating time from experience in the lateral entorhinal cortex. *Nature* **561**:57–62.

Tsodyks M, Sejnowski TJ (1995) Associative memory and hippocampal place cells. *Int J Neural Syst* **6**:91–86.

Tunon T, Insausti R, Ferrer I, Sobreviela T, Soriano E (1992) Parvalbumin and calbindin D-28K in the human entorhinal cortex. an immunohistochemical study. *Brain Res* **589**:24–32.

Van Cauter T, Poucet B, Save E (2008) Unstable CA1 place cell representation in rats with entorhinal cortex lesions. *Eur J Neurosci* **27**:1933–1946.

van der Werf YD, Witter MP, Groenewegen HJ (2002) The intralaminar and midline nuclei of the thalamus: anatomical and functional evidence for participation in processes of arousal and awareness. *Brain Res Brain Res Rev* **39**:107–140.

Vandrey B, Garden DLF, Ambrozova V, McClure C, Nolan MF, Ainge JA (2020) Fan cells in layer 2 of the lateral entorhinal cortex are critical for episodic-like memory. *Curr Biol* **30**:169–175, e165.

van Groen T, Miettinen P, Kadish I (2003) The entorhinal cortex of the mouse: organization of the projection to the hippocampal formation. *Hippocampus* **13**:133–149.

van Groen T, van Haren FJ, Witter MP, Groenewegen HJ (1986) The organization of the reciprocal connections between the subiculum and the entorhinal cortex in the cat: I. A neuroanatomical tracing study. *J Comp Neurol* **250**:485–497.

van Groen T, Wyss JM (1990a) The connections of presubiculum and parasubiculum in the rat. *Brain Res* **518**:227–243.

van Groen T, Wyss JM (1990b) The postsubicular cortex in the rat: characterization of the fourth region of the subicular cortex and its connections. *Brain Res* **529**:165–177.

Van Hoesen GW (2002) The human parahippocampal region in Alzheimer's disease, dementia, and ageing. In: The Parahippocampal Region Organization and Role in Cognitive Function (Witter MP, Wouterlood FG, eds), vol 1, pp 271–295. Oxford: Oxford University Press.

Van Hoesen GW, Pandya DN (1975) Some connections of the entorhinal (area 28) and perirhinal (area 35) cortices of the rhesus monkey: III. Efferent connections. *Brain Res* **95**:39–59.

Varga C, Lee SY, Soltesz I (2010) Target-selective GABAergic control of entorhinal cortex output. *Nat Neurosci* **13**:822–824.

Vaudano E, Legg CR, Glickstein M (1991) Afferent and efferent connections of temporal association cortex in the rat: a horseradish peroxidase study. *Eur J Neurosci* **3**:317–330.

Vertes RP (2004) Differential projections of the infralimbic and prelimbic cortex in the rat. *Synapse* **51**:32–58.

Vertes RP, Hoover WB (2008) Projections of the paraventricular and paratenial nuclei of the dorsal midline thalamus in the rat. *J Comp Neurol* **508**:212–237.

Vertes RP, Hoover WB, Do Valle AC, Sherman A, Rodriguez JJ (2006) Efferent projections of reuniens and rhomboid nuclei of the thalamus in the rat. *J Comp Neurol* **499**:768–796.

Vismer MS, Forcelli PA, Skopin MD, Gale K, Koubeissi MZ (2015) The piriform, perirhinal, and entorhinal cortex in seizure generation. *Front Neural Circuits* **9**:27.

von Frisch K (1947) The dance of the bees. *Bull Anim Behav* **5**:2–25.

Wang C, Chen X, Lee H, Deshmukh SS, Yoganarasimha D, Savelli F, Knierim JJ (2018) Egocentric coding of external items in the lateral entorhinal cortex. *Science* **362**:945.

Weeber EJ, Beffert U, Jones C, Christian JM, Forster E, Sweatt JD, Herz J (2002) Reelin and ApoE receptors cooperate to enhance hippocampal synaptic plasticity and learning. *J Biol Chem* **277**:39944–39952.

Wellman BJ, Rockland KS (1997) Divergent cortical connections to entorhinal cortex from area TF in the macaque. *J Comp Neurol* **389**:361–376.

Wernle T, Waaga T, Mørreaunet M, Treves A, Moser M-B, Moser EI (2017) Integration of grid maps in merged environments. *Nat Neurosci* 21:92–101.

Whitlock JR, Pfuhl G, Dagslott N, Moser MB, Moser EI (2012) Functional split between parietal and entorhinal cortices in the rat. *Neuron* 73:789–802.

Wills TJ, Cacucci F, Burgess N, O'Keefe J (2010) Development of the hippocampal cognitive map in preweanling rats. *Science* 328:1573–1576.

Winter SS, Mehlman ML, Clark BJ, Taube JS (2015) Passive transport disrupts grid signals in the parahippocampal cortex. *Curr Biol* 25:2493–2502.

Winterer J, Maier N, Wozny C, Beed P, Breustedt J, Evangelista R, Peng Y, D'Albis T, Kempter R, Schmitz D (2017) Excitatory microcircuits within superficial layers of the medial entorhinal cortex. *Cell Rep* 19:1110–1116.

Witter MP (2007) The perforant path: projections from the entorhinal cortex to the dentate gyrus. *Prog Brain Res* 163:43–61.

Witter MP, Amaral DG (1991) Entorhinal cortex of the monkey: V. Projections to the dentate gyrus, hippocampus, and subicular complex. *J Comp Neurol* 307:437–459.

Witter MP, Amaral DG (2020) The entorhinal cortex of the monkey: VI. Organization of projections from the hippocampus, subiculum, presubiculum, and parasubiculum. *J Comp Neurol* 529:828–852.

Witter MP, Doan TP, Jacobsen B, Nilssen ES, Ohara S (2017) Architecture of the entorhinal cortex: a review of entorhinal anatomy in rodents with some comparative notes. *Front Syst Neurosci* 11:46.

Witter MP, Groenewegen HJ (1984) Laminar origin and septotemporal distribution of entorhinal and perirhinal projections to the hippocampus in the cat. *J Comp Neurol* 224:371–385.

Witter MP, Groenewegen HJ, Lopes da Silva FH, Lohman AH (1989) Functional organization of the extrinsic and intrinsic circuitry of the parahippocampal region. *Prog Neurobiol* 33:161–253.

Witter MP, Kleven H, Kobro-Flatmoen A (2017) Comparative contemplations on the hippocampus. *Brain Behav Evol* 90:15–24.

Witter MP, Van Hoesen GW, Amaral DG (1989) Topographical organization of the entorhinal projection to the dentate gyrus of the monkey. *J Neurosci* 9:216–228.

Wouterlood FG (2002) Spotlight on the neurons (I): cell types, local connectivity, microcircuits, and distribution of markers. In: The Parahippocampal Region Organization and Role in Cognitive Function (Witter MP, Wouterlood FG, eds), pp 61–88. Oxford: Oxford University Press.

Wouterlood FG, Hartig W, Bruckner G, Witter MP (1995) Parvalbumin-immunoreactive neurons in the entorhinal cortex of the rat: localization, morphology, connectivity and ultrastructure. *J Neurocytol* 24:135–153.

Wouterlood FG, Nederlof J (1983) Terminations of olfactory afferents on layer II and III neurons in the entorhinal area: degeneration-Golgi-electron microscopic study in the rat. *Neurosci Lett* 36:105–110.

Wouterlood FG, Saldana E, Witter MP (1990) Projection from the nucleus reuniens thalami to the hippocampal region: light and electron microscopic tracing study in the rat with the anterograde tracer Phaseolus vulgaris-leucoagglutinin. *J Comp Neurol* 296:179–203.

Wouterlood FG, van Denderen JC, van Haeften T, Witter MP (2000) Calretinin in the entorhinal cortex of the rat: distribution, morphology, ultrastructure of neurons, and co-localization with gamma-aminobutyric acid and parvalbumin. *J Comp Neurol* 425:177–192.

Yartsev MM, Witter MP, Ulanovsky N (2011) Grid cells without theta oscillations in the entorhinal cortex of bats. *Nature* 479:103–107.

Ye J, Witter MP, Moser MB, Moser EI (2018) Entorhinal fast-spiking speed cells project to the hippocampus. *Proc Natl Acad Sci U S A* 115:E1627–E1636.

Yoganarasimha D, Rao G, Knierim JJ (2011) Lateral entorhinal neurons are not spatially selective in cue-rich environments. *Hippocampus* 21:1363–1374.

Yoon K, Buice MA, Barry C, Hayman R, Burgess N, Fiete IR (2013) Specific evidence of low-dimensional continuous attractor dynamics in grid cells. *Nat Neurosci* 16:1077–1084.

Young BJ, Otto T, Fox GD, Eichenbaum H (1997) Memory representation within the parahippocampal region. *J Neurosci* 17:5183–5195.

Zhang SJ, Ye J, Miao C, Tsao A, Cerniauskas I, Ledergerber D, Moser MB, Moser EI (2013) Optogenetic dissection of entorhinal-hippocampal functional connectivity. *Science* 340:1232627.

Zhu XO, Brown MW, Aggleton JP (1995) Neuronal signalling of information important to visual recognition memory in rat rhinal and neighbouring cortices. *Eur J Neurosci* 7:753–765.

Zingg B, Hintiryan H, Gou L, Song Monica Y, Bay M, Bienkowski Michael S, Foster Nicholas N, Yamashita S, Bowman I, Toga Arthur W, et al. (2014) Neural networks of the mouse neocortex. *Cell* 156:1096–1111.

Ziv Y, Burns LD, Cocker ED, Hamel EO, Ghosh KK, Kitch LJ, El Gamal A, Schnitzer MJ (2013) Long-term dynamics of CA1 hippocampal place codes. *Nat Neurosci* 16:264–266.

Zong W, Obenhaus HA, Skytøen ER, Eneqvist H, de Jong NL, Vale R, Jorge MR, Moser M-B, Moser EI (2022) Large-scale two-photon calcium imaging in freely moving mice. *Cell* 185(7):1240–1256.

Zutshi I, Fu ML, Lilascharoen V, Leutgeb JK, Lim BK, Leutgeb S (2018) Recurrent circuits within medial entorhinal cortex superficial layers support grid cell firing. *Nat Commun* 9:3701.

13

Functions of the Human Hippocampus

Daniel N. Barry and Eleanor A. Maguire

13.1 Overview

The last few decades have witnessed a considerable proliferation of research into the functions of the human hippocampus. This expanded understanding of hippocampal contributions to cognition has been derived from studies of diverse cohorts of people, with technological, analytical, and theoretical developments accelerating the pace of discovery. Perhaps the most striking and definitive evidence of hippocampal function can be observed in clinical cases involving surgical excision of the hippocampus (e.g., to reduce seizures; Scoville and Milner, 1957), or nonprogressive pathologies that result in more focal bilateral damage to this region. Neurodegenerative illnesses that affect the hippocampal formation in the context of wider brain pathology can also provide illumination, including assessing people who are genetically at risk of developing these disorders (Kunz et al., 2015; see Chapter 20). While patients with stable, focal hippocampal lesions are particularly useful to study, they are rare, and do not readily inform about the computations executed by an intact hippocampus. Much of our knowledge in this domain accrues from neuroimaging of healthy people during the performance of cognitive tasks. Further insights into hippocampal function in the healthy population are gained by examining relationships between cognitive performance and brain structure (e.g., gray matter volume) from early development through to healthy aging. Moreover, it can be informative to study changes in the hippocampi of individuals who have reached expert levels of knowledge in a particular domain over the course of time, or who demonstrate exceptionally high abilities.

An abundance of tools are used to study the different cohorts of humans mentioned above in order to characterize hippocampal structure and function from different perspectives (Figure 13.1). One such technique is magnetic resonance imaging (MRI), of which there are various types. Structural MRI (sMRI; reviewed in Symms et al., 2004) is typically employed to quantify the volume of gray matter, white matter, and other tissue microstructure properties in the hippocampus in healthy individuals, and to assess the nature and extent of hippocampal damage in patients. In particular, submillimeter high spatial resolution sMRI has transformed our ability to delineate the subfields of the human hippocampus (Dalton et al., 2017), enabling researchers to start interrogating intrahippocampal processing. Diffusion-weighted and diffusion tensor imaging (DWI/DTI; Le Bihan et al., 1986) permit a more detailed view of the microstructure of gray and white matter in the hippocampus. By contrast, functional MRI (fMRI), during cognitive task performance or while the brain is resting, measures changes in blood oxygenation levels as a proxy for increases or decreases in underlying neuronal activity (Ogawa et al., 1992). Magnetic resonance spectroscopy (MRS; Bottomley et al., 1985) complements this approach by offering a window into the biochemistry of the brain by detecting the in vivo concentration of specific metabolites. Other biomarkers in the hippocampus can be detected using positron emission tomography (PET), such as amyloid and tau burden (Brier et al., 2016). PET is also used to measure levels of energy consumption in the hippocampus during task performance (Squire et al., 1992); although it has in general been superseded by fMRI for this purpose due to its safety, ease of use and high degree of spatial precision. Increases in MRI scanner field strength, and optimization of scanning sequences, continues to allow for more sensitive and spatially precise detection of hippocampal structure and function. However, MRI and PET suffer from relatively poor temporal resolution (the hemodynamic delay during fMRI is ~4 seconds; West et al., 2019) and remain indirect measures of neuronal activity.

Other methods complement MRI by measuring human hippocampal electrophysiology directly and with millisecond precision. SQUID-based magnetoencephalography (MEG; Cohen, 1972) detects magnetic fields generated by neuronal activity in the hippocampus using sensors fixed in a cryogenically cooled dewar. More recently, optically pumped MEG (OP-MEG; Boto et al., 2018) has been developed that measures neural activity throughout the whole brain, including the hippocampus, but allows sensors to be placed flexibly, providing increased sensitivity and, crucially, permitting the people being scanned to move naturally, a limitation of all the aforementioned neuroimaging methods. The most direct measurement of human hippocampal neurophysiology is achieved through in vivo intracranial electrode recordings (intracranial electroencephalography, iEEG; Hayne et al., 1949; Reif et al., 2016) in patients who are being evaluated prior to epilepsy surgery, whereby local field potentials as well as the spiking of individual neurons can be recorded. While iEEG studies have been very informative, it should be borne in mind that such patients typically have uncontrolled, chronic epilepsy for many years, and so recordings are not being made from neurologically healthy brains.

These technological advances have been paralleled by increasingly sophisticated analysis methods that provide a better understanding of the nature and loci of hippocampal neural representations. For example, as noted above, more precise protocols for

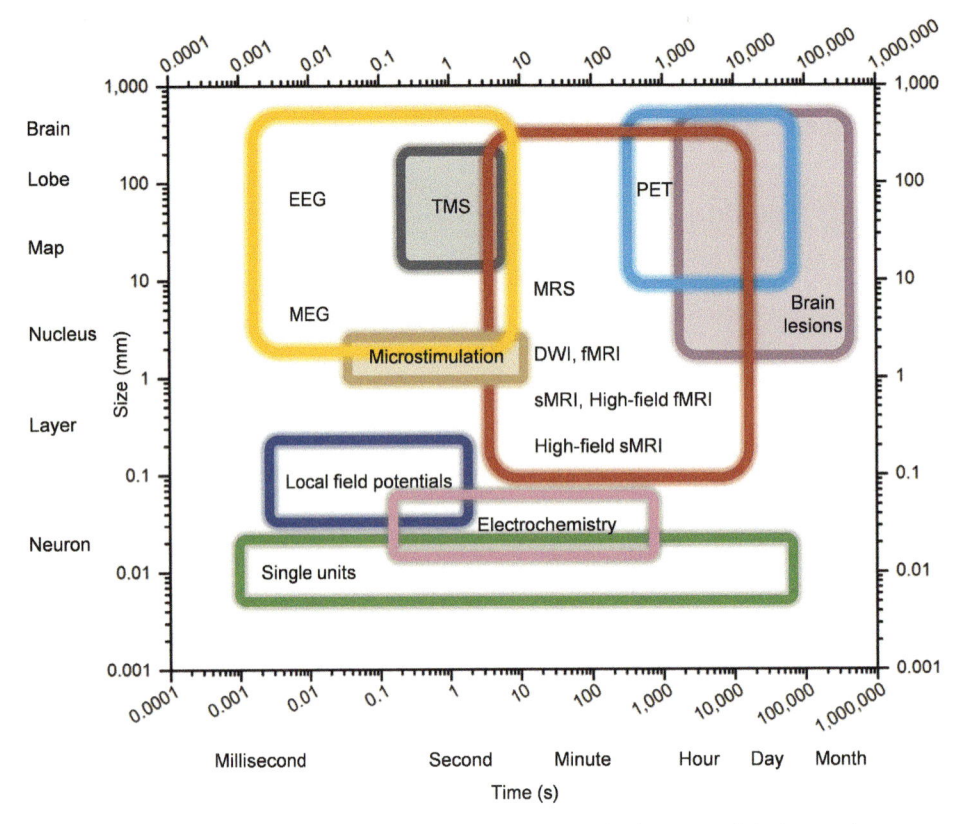

Figure 13.1 The spatiotemporal parameters of the methods commonly used to study the functions of the human hippocampus. Each colored region represents the spatial and temporal resolution of one method. Open regions depict measurement techniques, while filled regions indicate perturbations of function. EEG, electroencephalography; MEG, magnetoencephalography; TMS, transcranial magnetic stimulation; MRS, magnetic resonance spectroscopy; DWI, diffusion-weighted imaging; fMRI, functional magnetic resonance imaging; sMRI, structural magnetic resonance imaging; PET, positron emission tomography. (Adapted with permission from Sejnowski et al., 2014.)

segmenting human hippocampal subfields (Dalton et al., 2017) facilitates increased understanding of their differential contributions to cognitive processes. Multivoxel pattern analysis (Chadwick et al., 2012) and repetition suppression (Barron et al., 2016) approaches to fMRI data analysis allow for greater sensitivity in the detection of specific representations, while improved source localization techniques in MEG (Van Veen et al., 1997) have provided better detection of hippocampal signals. These methods are complemented by computational modeling, which can help to bridge the gap between observed hippocampal responses and cognitive task performance.

Of course, the wealth of data generated by these methods provides insights into hippocampal function mostly through the prism of behavior. Detailed neuropsychological investigation of hippocampal-damaged patients remains a powerful approach not only to understand hippocampal function but also to inform neuroimaging investigations in healthy people. Traditional laboratory-based tasks in this regard include the learning of controlled, simple stimuli in the form of words in a list, or the association between word pairs, more complex story narratives, or visuospatial memoranda such as faces or abstract images. Successful learning can be measured as either unprompted recollection from memory, recollection given an associated or helpful cue, or recognition of the stimuli on later exposure. Stimuli with greater ecological validity can also be leveraged, such as recollecting personal past experiences in the form of autobiographical memories (see Box 13.1 for more on memory definitions) or imagining life events, demonstrating factual knowledge

---

Box 13.1 Episodic and semantic memories

For many years, memories that are available to conscious awareness were known as declarative memories because they could be declared or described (Squire, 1992). These memories were held to be dependent on the hippocampus at least in the short term. However, declarative memories are heterogeneous, and another framework differentiated between the memory for past experiences or episodes that are specific to a particular time and place, referred to as episodic memories (Tulving, 1972), and conceptual knowledge including facts about the world, known as semantic memories. These latter memories are not associated with a specific spatiotemporal context, but instead the relevant information is thought to be extracted across many different experiences. It is now widely agreed that episodic memories are hippocampal-dependent, while semantic memories come to rely on neocortical areas such as the lateral temporal cortex.

Further nuances in terminology are also apparent in the literature. Episodic memories can cover a broad range of situations. For example, they can involve the event of learning a pair of words during a laboratory-based experiment, or a specific experience from the real world such as meeting someone for the first time, a graduation ceremony, or other life events. The personal relevance of these latter memories means they are often described as autobiographical memories. A further distinction is sometimes made between episodic autobiographical memories for past experiences that are specific in time and place, and semantic autobiographical memories (also called personal semantics) that concern facts about the self. As with the more general episodic-semantic distinction, only episodic autobiographical memories are thought to be hippocampal-dependent.

about the world, or being able to navigate through a spatial environment. In this chapter, the neuropsychological evidence that we consider concerns, for the most part, patients with nonprogressive damage that primarily involved the two hippocampi and little or no significant detectable damage elsewhere in the brain.

Methods to measure the success of memory recall, such as detailed scoring protocols (e.g., Levine et al., 2002), have also evolved to be more sensitive to hippocampal function. For example, during neuroimaging investigations, experimental stimuli are normally presented via computer, and this platform now allows for highly realistic virtual reality environments to be created to test hippocampus-dependent functions such as spatial navigation and to record and analyze naturalistic behaviors in these virtual worlds in great detail. Computer-based tasks are also useful in paradigms that require the presentation of stimuli to adapt to participants' individual performance. In addition, viewing naturalistic stimuli such as films during scanning can provide an avenue into understanding hippocampal function, because the exposure to perceptually rich narratives can be synchronized across participants. Eye-tracking technology also facilitates our understanding of the relationship between such viewing behaviors and hippocampal function. With "open science" being increasingly adopted across neuroscience, these rich stimuli, datasets and code are starting to be made publicly available and repurposed to address different questions about the hippocampus.

The wide range of human cohorts, rapidly evolving neuroimaging technologies, sophisticated analysis methods, and diversity of behavioral paradigms have substantially broadened the remit of the hippocampus to include functional domains with which it has traditionally not been associated. This chapter will reflect this expanded perspective on human hippocampal functions. We will not discuss research involving nonhumans in any detail, as this is amply covered elsewhere in the book; our focus is on the human hippocampus. We will primarily focus on the visual modality, as that embodies the vast majority of research into human hippocampal function, although we acknowledge fully the multimodal nature of hippocampal processing. The chapter's narrative will, in essence, consider the journey of signals once they enter the brain, and the roles played by the human hippocampus in their processing. We outline representative empirical findings at each staging post, and then toward the end of the chapter we consider traditional perspectives on hippocampal function, new frameworks that have emerged, whether these extant theories can account for the data, and where the gaps in our knowledge still remain.

The chapter begins with the hippocampal contribution to the online perceptual processing of the environment, and the maintenance of information in the hippocampus for a short period of time. Evidence that the hippocampus is sensitive to the presence of sequences and the boundaries between them will be presented. Finally, in this section, the hippocampal processes that support the committal of information to long-term memory will be outlined. We will then turn to the mechanisms underlying consolidation, in other words, the processing of recently encoded information in the hippocampus, including the replay, or reactivation, of recent experiences. We will discuss the functional significance of these processes, the kinds of memories that are processed, and how representations are transformed or lost over time. We will also consider in this section the time course of this process, and the long-term dependency of representations on the hippocampus. Following this, we will

Box 13.2 Laterality and human hippocampal function

It is rarely the case that one hippocampus is selectively damaged in humans because adjacent areas are often compromised also, for example, when surgery is performed to remove hippocampal and surrounding tissue for the relief of intractable epilepsy. In situations of unilateral temporal lobe damage that encroaches on the hippocampus, the most commonly reported dichotomy involves modality-specific deficits. Left-sided damage has been associated with verbal and right-sided damage with visuospatial impairments, particularly when simplified stimuli are used (Blakemore and Falconer, 1967; Milner, 1968; Hou et al., 2013; Jordan, 2020). Results are less clear-cut when paradigms are more complex, for instance, involving real-world behaviors such as navigation—while patients with right-sided damage have been found to be more impaired than those with left-sided lesions, the latter were still more impaired than healthy controls (e.g., Maguire et al., 1996; Spiers et al., 2001).

This lack of exclusivity in terms of lateralized hippocampal function has been amplified by neuroimaging studies especially those involving fMRI. While there is evidence for preferential involvement of the right hippocampus in spatial paradigms (Burgess et al., 2002) and left hippocampal engagement during autobiographical memory recall (Maguire, 2001), bilateral hippocampal activations are very commonly reported. With an increased focus on brain networks and connectivity between regions, it is fair to say that as the number of fMRI studies increased, the amount of attention paid to human hippocampal laterality has decreased over the last few decades.

Consequently, the significance of hippocampal functional asymmetry remains unclear, as does a potential basis for any left-right hippocampal differences. It has been suggested that the neuronal algorithms running in the two hippocampi are the same and it is merely the information being supplied to each hippocampus (i.e., more verbal or visuospatial inputs) that results in laterality differences (O'Keefe and Nadel, 1978; Burgess et al., 2002). However, another perspective holds that there may be underlying processing differences between the two hippocampi (Kennepohl et al., 2007). The tasks used to assess hippocampal function also need careful consideration. For example, many so-called verbal tests evoke visual imagery (Clark et al., 2018; 2020a), thus complicating the assessment of laterality effects further.

outline how the hippocampus reconstructs these representations during later retrieval and the nature of these reconstructions. This section will also discuss other flexible and adaptive applications of hippocampal representations, such as in planning for the future, imagining alternate scenarios, navigating through spatial and conceptual space, and decision-making. Finally, we will consider how prior consolidated experiences influence subsequent perception, attention, and memory. The structure of this chapter, therefore, reflects the contribution of the hippocampus to a continuous cycle of perceptual and constructive processes. Consideration of the historical (Chapter 2), developmental (Chapter 4), aging (Chapter 15), and dementia-related (Chapter 20) aspects of human hippocampal function, are presented elsewhere in this book, and a note on laterality is provided in Box 13.2.

13.2 The online hippocampus: from perception to memory

13.2.1 Sampling the environment

Perception is the gateway through which new neural representations are captured and processed by the hippocampus. It is perhaps unsurprising then that visual sampling of the environment is closely associated with hippocampal activity. Increased numbers of fixations to novel stimuli have been related to greater hippocampal activity in healthy people (Liu et al., 2017), suggesting cumulative sampling may help to assemble more complete representations. Aligning with this idea, the number of fixations a healthy person makes to a stimulus predicts whether or not they will later remember it, yet such a relationship between vision and memory is not present in patients with damaged hippocampi (Olsen et al., 2016; see also Munoz et al., 2010). However, it is not merely that the link between visual sampling and later recall is abolished; rather, viewing behavior is fundamentally changed following hippocampal damage. Relative to healthy control participants, the patients' viewing is more random in nature, and the extent of this disorganization is not related to subsequent memory (Lucas et al., 2019). The hippocampus, therefore, seems to assist with managing efficient visual exploration of the environment in order to actively build neural representations.

Direct neural recordings from the hippocampus provide an insight into how this process might take place. Low-frequency theta rhythms in the hippocampus align to the onset of a visual fixation to a new location in a scene, and persist for a short period afterward (Hoffman et al., 2013); however, this phenomenon is not observed during eye movements on a darkened screen. Therefore, the hippocampus appears to accumulate packets of information by synchronizing its activity with the sequential sampling of novel information in the environment. This visual input may be coordinated into a coherent structure in the entorhinal cortex, because during visual exploration in two-dimensional (2D) space, activity in this region is higher when eye movement direction aligns with a sixfold rotationally symmetric grid pattern (Nau et al., 2018).

Most studies investigating the association between visual sampling and hippocampal activity are restricted to paradigms where the person or the stimuli in question are static. However, during real-world exploration of an environment and memory formation, sampling is unrestricted, in that people physically move their bodies and head direction through space to collect more information. The deployment of virtual reality paradigms has enabled the monitoring of hippocampal activity while people navigate through virtual space. Intracranial recordings from the hippocampus have revealed increases in theta power during virtual navigation, albeit at a lower frequency and for shorter durations than that typically observed in rodent studies (Watrous et al., 2013). Advances in wireless technology have allowed patients undergoing intracranial recordings to physically move around their local environment, while immersed in a synchronized virtual environment, confirming this increase in theta power during ambulation (Aghajan et al., 2017; Figure 13.2). This increase was correlated with the speed of movement, suggesting greater information processing. However, given the aforementioned relationship between visual sampling and hippocampal activity, it is surprising that these effects were stronger in a congenitally blind patient (Aghajan et al., 2017). Therefore, the hippocampus likely integrates perceptual signals from multiple modalities during exploration. However, exploration in and of itself does not appear to be the main driving force behind hippocampal theta. Comparable increases in this frequency have been observed in patients whether they were ambulating toward a visible goal or exploring the environment for a hidden goal (Aghajan et al., 2019). Furthermore, in both tasks, modulation of theta in the entorhinal cortex and subiculum was observed when patients were moving in directions aligned to a hexagonal grid, similar to the grid-like neural patterns observed in visual space. The human hippocampus may therefore build rich, structured representations of the environment independent of sensory modality and the task at hand.

13.2.2 Making sense of sensory inputs

Given the hippocampus is engaged during perceptual exploration, how is this input transformed into a hippocampal representation? Across many perspectives on hippocampal function there is general agreement that the hippocampus constructs representations composed of numerous features (O'Keefe and Nadel, 1978; Cohen and Eichenbaum, 1993; Gaffan, 1994; Burgess et al., 2002; Lee et al., 2005; Hassabis and Maguire, 2007, 2009; Schacter and Addis, 2007; Yonelinas et al., 2019). Visual scenes have been deployed extensively to test hippocampal function, as they are paradigmatic multifeature stimuli. We define a scene as a naturalistic three-dimensional (3D)

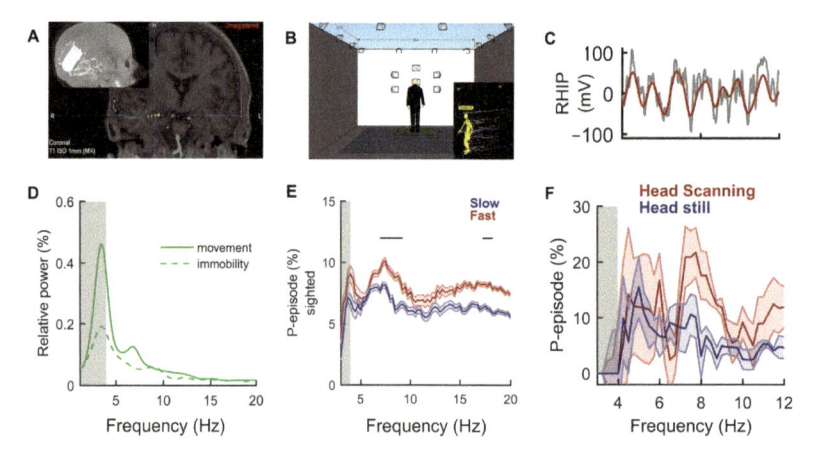

Figure 13.2 Hippocampal theta oscillations during exploration. (A) Postoperative CT scan of a participant with a wireless, chronically implanted electrode in the right hippocampus (inset) alongside a high-resolution structural MR image displaying electrode locations. (B) Schematic of cameras used for motion capture and real-time tracking of a participant (right inset). (C) Example raw iEEG trace from the hippocampus of one participant overlaid with filtered (3–12 Hz) theta oscillations. (D) Power spectra from the same participant showing higher theta power during movement periods when compared with immobility. (E) Fast movements were associated with more frequent occurrences of theta oscillations when compared with slow movements. (F) Theta oscillations were also more prevalent during head scanning behavior than when the head was kept still during locomotion. (Reproduced with permission from Aghajan et al., 2017.)

spatially coherent representation of the world typically populated by objects and viewed from an egocentric perspective (Dalton et al., 2018; Maguire and Mullally, 2013). Whether they are scenes from ongoing experience, or 2D representations (such as photographs) of 3D places, scenes are contexts that you could potentially step into (e.g., a forest) or operate within (e.g., a scene of the desk area in front of you) (Monk et al., 2021).

The hippocampus is more engaged during the perception of scenes compared with single objects (Hodgetts et al., 2016; Graham et al., 2010; Zeidman, Mullally, et al., 2015). Moreover, tasks that require participants to correctly identify the same scene from a different perspective—which taxes this constructive process because the scene representation has to be reconstructed to reflect the various views that can then be mentally compared—are associated with greater hippocampal activity (Barense et al., 2010). The hippocampus is also engaged during the viewing of spatially incoherent scenes that are not physically possible (e.g., Escher-type scenes), again indicating its role in constructing multiple scene representations for comparison, in this case between possible and impossible versions of a scene, which then facilitates violation detection (Douglas et al., 2017).

This perceptual processing appears to be limited to the spatial-constructive rather than the semantic domain, because patients with hippocampal damage are selectively impaired at identifying scenes that contain spatial-constructive abnormalities, whereas they readily detect semantic violations in scenes (McCormick et al., 2017). In a similar vein, patients are poor at noticing changes between scenes that are conjunctive in nature (i.e., the spatial relationship between components), but not those that are local and discrete, and these strength-based conjunctive judgments are correlated with hippocampal activity in healthy controls (Aly et al., 2013). The hippocampus, therefore, constructs multifeature representations from elements of perceived input. This is likely multimodal, but in humans has been examined extensively in the visual domain, and often using scene stimuli.

13.2.3 Holding items in working memory

The next question that arises is whether or not the hippocampus is involved in retaining the representations it has constructed prior to their consolidation into long-term memory. The capacity to temporarily maintain information in memory during the performance of a task is referred to as working memory (Miller et al., 1960; Baddeley, 2003, 2010). Patients with hippocampal damage perform similarly to healthy control participants in maintaining information in working memory over a short delay when the stimuli are simple, such as during a digit span task (Cave and Squire, 1992). However, when such patients are required to retain more complex stimuli in working memory, they demonstrate substantial impairment. For example, when presented with a scene, and then after a delay of just 2 seconds they are shown the same place from a different viewpoint, patients are unable to identify it as the same or a different place (Hartley et al., 2007). Further work has documented that patients with hippocampal damage can struggle to hold even simple stimuli in working memory if the task demands are increased. When rudimentary stimuli are obscured, scrambled, or fragmented, patients are significantly worse than healthy control participants at making comparative judgments or integrating information across samples, even when the time to hold such online representations is minimized by presenting stimuli simultaneously (Warren et al., 2012).

This rapid decay in online representations is further evidenced by patients' eye movements during performance on working memory tasks. For instance, when healthy controls search for a target stimulus among lures, fixation time varies as a function of similarity between the target and lures, but in the case of hippocampal damage, this effect is diminished during longer visual search paths (Warren et al., 2011). Therefore, high-fidelity information cannot be maintained without the hippocampus. Neuroimaging studies in healthy people have confirmed the involvement of the hippocampus in working memory. Hippocampal activity during a 7–13 second maintenance period of scene imagery predicts successful short-term retrieval from working memory (Bergmann et al., 2015; see Kumar et al., 2016, for an example of hippocampal involvement in auditory working memory). Furthermore, increasing the number of scene images that are held in working memory leads to a corresponding increase in posterior hippocampus activity (Barense et al., 2010). This association between hippocampal activity and working memory can be observed below the maximal amount that individuals can hold in memory (von Allmen et al., 2013), which then raises the question, what is the optimal working memory storage capacity of the hippocampus?

The hippocampus seems to be maximally recruited for the retrieval of items from what is termed "direct access," that is, a capacity of around four items that are just outside of the current perceptual input (Nee and Jonides, 2011). Intracranial recordings in patients provide some clues about how the hippocampus may hold such information in memory—low-frequency theta oscillations are coupled with high-frequency gamma during working memory. Memory performance is related to the precision of this coupling, and increases in working memory load are associated with lower frequency theta (Axmacher et al., 2010). This suggests that individual elements are activated in the hippocampus in the gamma frequency and groups of items are nested within theta cycles. This theta-gamma coupling is not observed during the maintenance of single items, but emerges when more items need to be maintained, and this load-dependent increase in coupling is associated with memory performance (Chaieb et al., 2015). The hippocampus, therefore, participates in the maintenance of multifeature stimuli, the performance of demanding working memory tasks, and its activity scales with working memory load.

13.2.4 Keeping track of time

While working memory capacity is critical for the online maintenance of multiple items, subsequent successful retrieval may further depend on preserving the temporal order in which items were experienced. This requirement appears to place a further load on the hippocampus, because maintaining the order of experienced stimuli in memory is associated with greater activation of the posterior hippocampus when compared with retaining just the stimuli in working memory (Roberts et al., 2018). More temporally resolved evidence that the hippocampus preserves such sequential order in working memory has been provided by MEG, whereby items learned early in a sequence result in increased high-frequency gamma at an early stage of the theta cycle, while items learned later show a similar increase but toward the end of the cycle (Heusser et al., 2016). In other words, items are repeatedly and rapidly activated in the correct sequence during online maintenance.

Whether or not the hippocampus is involved in the subsequent retrieval of the sequential aspect of an experience beyond the window of working memory has also been examined. Bilateral hippocampal damage leads to impaired recognition of the correct temporal order of verbal and visual stimuli following the performance of a distractor task, despite preserved recognition of the stimuli themselves (Mayes et al., 2001). This impairment in the recall of sequences also appears to extend to more naturalistic stimuli. For example, Dede et al. (2016) exposed hippocampal-damaged patients to a series of 11 staged autobiographical episodes over a period of 25 minutes and asked them to subsequently recall these experiences. In contrast to healthy controls, who recalled the events in the sequence in which they occurred, patients did not recall the episodes in any particular order. This suggests that the hippocampus may be necessary to preserve the integrity of such a sequence for subsequent memory retrieval.

Supporting evidence from fMRI studies involving healthy controls has demonstrated that hippocampal activation is higher during the learning of sequences that share an overlapping order with previously learned sequences, that is, where some stimuli occupy the same position in both sequences (Kumaran et al., 2006a). This observed increase in activation during sequence learning is also related to a participant's ability to recall the correct order of the sequence during a later memory test (Tubridy and Davachi, 2011). Another powerful approach to investigating the role of the hippocampus in the encoding of sequences is to transiently disrupt its activity during learning, which interferes with neural transmission. This is made possible by applying direct electrical stimulation via depth electrodes in patients undergoing neural recordings prior to epilepsy surgery. When this stimulation is applied during the learning of items, they are less likely to be recalled in the correct order in which they were learned, and they are less liable to be clustered with items that were temporally adjacent during learning (Goyal et al., 2018). Therefore, the hippocampus appears to encode sequential associations between items learned close together in time.

A different type of temporal information one can extract from ongoing experience is the perceived duration of an event itself. Patients with hippocampal damage perform similarly to healthy controls in estimating the duration of short naturalistic video clips that are less than 90 seconds long, but are impaired at durations of more than 4 minutes (Palombo et al., 2016). This pattern of results suggests different processes support duration estimation than those underlying sequence learning. A similar coarse measure of temporal estimation over a longer timescale can be obtained by asking a participant when a stimulus was presented over the course of an entire experiment. Hippocampal activity during initial learning, as measured by fMRI, predicts the subsequent accuracy of this temporal estimation (Jenkins and Ranganath, 2016). Moreover, further fMRI evidence suggests that hippocampal activity during retrieval is related to the precision of temporal estimation of scenes within a previously watched movie on a minute-level accuracy scale (Montchal et al., 2019).

However, when one considers the estimation of the temporal context of events on a much longer timescale, that encompassing the distant past and future, the hippocampus appears to be less involved. Patients with hippocampal damage do not have difficulty placing their autobiographical memories that have taken place over decades, on the correct position on a timeline (Tranel and Jones, 2006). Likewise, hippocampus-lesioned patients discount the value of proposed future rewards in accordance with increasing temporal distance in a similar way to healthy controls (Kwan et al., 2013).

This demonstrates a preserved understanding of the passage of long periods of time and an ability to project themselves forward. Therefore, while the hippocampus appears to encode unfolding sequences within events, and facilitate the estimation of event duration over the short term, this does not seem to apply over a longer timescale.

13.2.5 Setting boundaries

If the hippocampus represents sequences of information that take place over a short time period, how are such sequences packaged into self-contained events for later recall? One perspective on how this is achieved proposes that periods of perceptual stability are recognized as contiguous events, whereas significant changes in the environment are perceived as representing the boundaries of these events (Zacks et al., 2007). There is evidence that an individual's capacity to segment naturalistic event stimuli in this way is associated with their ability to remember an event later, suggesting it may play a role in determining successful memory encoding (Sargent et al., 2013). To investigate the role played by the hippocampus in this structuring of experience, Schapiro et al. (2016) exposed participants to a sequence of stimuli that shared an underlying community structure through their temporal proximity. That is, stimuli within the community would follow each other in sequence, comprising a single event, whereas each community of stimuli was connected via a single association, and this rare transition indicated an event boundary. Neural patterns of activity in the hippocampus were more similar within these communities, or contiguous events, than to others. Furthermore, the hippocampal BOLD response was lower during the transitions between these events. The hippocampus, therefore, clustered sequences of stimuli from different events together, even though participants were not explicitly informed about the underlying structure.

While hippocampal activity is, therefore, more similar within an event, does this change with increasing temporal distance from other events? Using more naturalistic stimuli in the form of movies, W. Liu et al. (2022) demonstrated that hippocampal neural patterns were most dissimilar for events that occurred close in time, suggesting that the hippocampus segments adjacent experience through encoding orthogonal patterns. The hippocampus shows a strong response at these event boundaries for naturalistic stimuli. For example, Ben-Yakov et al. (2018) asked participants to segment a movie into discrete events, and investigated whether these ratings of event transitions were associated with hippocampal activation in a separate group of participants watching the same movie. Hippocampal activity was consistently higher at these independently defined junctions, even when perceptual factors were taken into account, suggesting a parcelation of experience at these narrative boundaries. Using an approach driven by neural data rather than behavioral ratings, Baldassano et al. (2017) identified event boundaries within a movie from changing patterns of cortical activity. They discovered that these cortically defined event boundaries were reliably followed by a peak in hippocampal activity, indicating that the hippocampus may participate in integrating input from other regions to dissect experience.

While it is advantageous to segment experience into discrete events, there are circumstances where we may need to link information across multiple events. When participants attempt to learn a sequence across an event boundary, hippocampal activity predicts whether or not it will be subsequently recalled successfully

(DuBrow and Davachi, 2016). Therefore, piecing information together across changing contexts requires additional hippocampal processing. Similarly, one may wish to recall information across a previous event boundary, necessitating the reinstatement of a previous context. Swallow et al. (2011) asked participants to recall objects that appeared 5 seconds previously during the viewing of a film. Hippocampal activity was higher during object retrieval when an event boundary was present during that delay, indicating that the hippocampus is recruited to mentally traverse between segmented episodes. Overall, therefore, the online integration and segmentation of experience, identification of significant shifts in context, and the ability to both bridge and breach these boundaries appear to involve the hippocampus.

13.2.6 Committing information to memory

It is perhaps unsurprising then that, given the involvement of the hippocampus in maintaining recent information in working memory and its sensitivity to ongoing event structure, patients with bilateral hippocampal damage are unable to commit new everyday life experiences to long-term memory (Scoville and Milner, 1957). This mnemonic impairment is readily apparent during neuropsychological testing when a patient is asked to try and learn information that is presented to them in a standardized format. These stimuli can be visual in nature in the form of a picture, or verbal such as a list of words, or a narrated story. After a short delay, hippocampal-damaged patients are unable to recall most, if any, of this information (e.g., Scoville and Milner, 1957; Vargha-Khadem et al., 1997; Cipolotti et al., 2001; Zola-Morgan et al., 1986; reviewed in Spiers, Maguire, et al., 2001). One frequently employed task that involves the encoding of new information is paired associate learning, which requires a participant to form an arbitrary relationship between two different stimuli. Consistent with the role of the hippocampus in the integration of multimodal information, patients are particularly impaired at learning these associations when they span modalities, such as a combination of visual and verbal material (e.g., Mayes et al., 2004; Borders et al., 2017). This inability to commit new information to long-term memory is known as anterograde amnesia, and has devastating consequences for independent living.

High-resolution fMRI studies involving healthy people allow for inspection of hippocampal engagement during the learning of new information with a high degree of spatial specificity. Suthana et al. (2015) asked participants to learn associations between pairs of names and faces, or pairs of words and objects. They observed encoding-related increases in activity specifically in the CA2 and CA3 subfields of the hippocampus as well as in the subiculum. A subsequent fMRI investigation by Hrybouski et al. (2019) had participants learn abstract shapes, the locations in which they appeared, or both. These tasks recruited all subfields of the hippocampus, with the highest increase from baseline observed in the dentate gyrus (DG). Real-world events, however, take place over a more extended time period than many laboratory-based studies. Ben-Yakov and Dudai (2011) showed participants naturalistic movies and measured hippocampal signal change during and after viewing. They found a reliable hippocampal response to the offset of the movie clips, the magnitude of which correlated with subsequent memory of the event portrayed. Therefore, the integration and commitment to memory of real-world events may be delayed until an event boundary is recognized.

Solomon et al. (2019) used iEEG to examine the oscillations associated with encoding of word lists and found they were associated with decreases in low-frequency theta power in CA1, DG, and subiculum, and the magnitude of these decreases were predictive of later successful free recall. Despite this decrease in signal amplitude, successful encoding in the hippocampal formation was related to increased coupling, or synchronized activity, in the theta band between the entorhinal cortex and both the DG and CA1, followed by synchronization between the entorhinal cortex and the subiculum (Solomon et al., 2019). This timing of connectivity is suggestive of a flow of information through the hippocampal circuitry.

Successful encoding by the hippocampus is also associated with interactions across frequencies, specifically the amplitude of fast oscillations being modulated by the phase of slower rhythms, known as cross-frequency coupling. Increased theta-gamma phase-amplitude coupling in the human hippocampus during successful encoding takes place at the trough of the theta oscillation, when long-term potentiation is likely to occur (Lega et al., 2014). This may represent a critical mechanism for the encoding of new memories (Chapter 10). Another important electrophysiological feature that can affect the encoding of new memories is the prevalence of sharp wave ripples, brief bursts of high frequency (80–140 Hz) activity. The rate at which these ripples occur in the hippocampus during the initial (but not subsequent) presentation of pictures is associated with subsequent memory for these stimuli (Norman et al., 2019). Successful memory formation, therefore, is likely supported by a complex interaction between multiple frequencies in the hippocampus.

While these studies demonstrate a strong association between oscillations in the hippocampus and successful memory encoding, they do not provide a direct causal link. However, patients with electrodes implanted in the hippocampus provide researchers with an opportunity to apply direct electrical stimulation. This targeted intervention can be used to specifically disrupt neural activity in the hippocampus and reveal a more direct link with behavior. Jacobs et al. (2016) applied electrical stimulation at a frequency of 50 Hz to both the hippocampus and entorhinal cortex while patients learned either the location of an object in a virtual environment, or while they learned a list of 12 words. Stimulation impaired subsequent memory performance on both tasks. Stimulation protocols can also be adapted to enhance memory encoding. Titiz et al. (2017) applied brief bursts of stimulation to the entorhinal cortex in a periodical fashion to align with the theta frequency. The stimulation location was chosen to maximize input to the hippocampus and the protocol is known to induce long-term potentiation. When deployed just before learning of novel photographs of people, this stimulation enhanced subsequent recognition and also successful rejection of similar, but different, portraits indicating an improvement in the specificity of memory.

Transcranial magnetic stimulation (TMS) has been used to achieve noninvasive indirect modulation of hippocampal activity in healthy people. Hermiller et al. (2020) applied TMS at a scalp location chosen to affect hippocampal activity via stimulation of the wider brain memory network of which it is part, while participants performed an encoding task during an fMRI scan. Combining the two approaches reportedly allowed for an immediate measure of hippocampal activity in response to stimulation. TMS in the theta frequency increased hippocampal activity during the encoding of complex scenes, and was related to successful subsequent recollection of these scenes. Of note, stimulation in the beta frequency produced no significant effects. Therefore, theta power in the hippocampus appears to be essential to bind elements of experience together.

13.3 Consolidation: the restless state

13.3.1 Replay during wake and sleep

While the hippocampus captures ongoing experience, the processing of new information does not end there. Evidence is accumulating that the hippocampus reactivates recently learned representations for a period of time after encoding. For example, Tambini and Davachi (2013) asked participants to perform two different tasks, learning pairs of objects and faces, or scenes and faces, during an fMRI scan. They found the distinct patterns of hippocampal activation associated with each of these tasks persisted into a postlearning rest period of over 8 minutes. This enduring reactivation following learning has also been observed during fear conditioning, where participants associated a face with a mild electric shock (Hermans et al., 2017). In addition, replay during rest can be observed at the level of single items. Schapiro et al. (2018) tasked participants with learning an array of novel objects, each with distinctive features, and measured hippocampal activity during a rest period during an fMRI scan. Distinct patterns of activity across hippocampal voxels associated with each object were spontaneously reinstated during the rest period. Real-world memory, however, comprises sequences

of events, and there is evidence that replay adopts this sequential form. Schuck and Niv (2019) deployed a sequential decision-making task that was composed of 16 possible states. These states had a latent constrained structure that limited the range of possible transitions from one state to another. During a subsequent rest period in an MRI scanner, they assessed whether patterns of activity in the hippocampus associated with the different states occurred close together in time. They found that brief sequences (fewer than three steps in this structure) were most commonly observed to reactivate in succession during rest, suggesting the structure of experience is preserved during restful reactivation.

Reactivation of recent experience continues into periods of sleep. Schönauer et al. (2017) used electroencephalography (EEG) to measure patterns of activity during sleep after participants had performed a task where they learned pictures of either faces or houses. They successfully decoded which type of stimulus material participants had learned during the prior waking period, indicating that information is processed further during sleep. Analyses of intracranial recordings in patients during sleep reveals that such replay events have physiological correlates in the hippocampus. Zhang et al. (2018) discovered that during non–rapid eye movement sleep (NREM), replay events were triggered by spontaneous ripples (bursts of activity at a rate of 200 Hz). What followed was a pattern of hippocampal activity in the gamma frequency (30–90 Hz) that matched the specific patterns previously observed during the encoding of individual stimuli in the waking period (Figure 13.3).

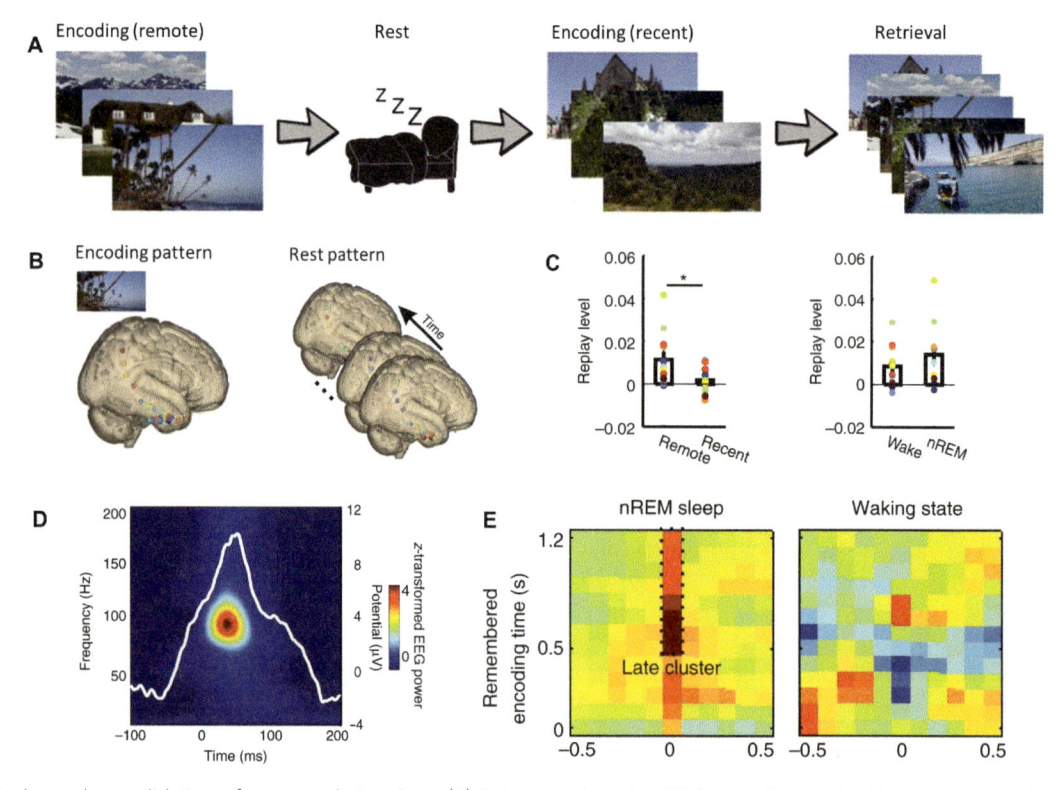

Figure 13.3 Replay and consolidation of memory during sleep. (A) Patients undergoing iEEG recordings in the hippocampus and multiple cortical sites learned a set of pictures (remote) and napped for 1 hour. Following this phase, they learned another set of pictures (recent). They were then administered a test to assess their memory for the pictures (retrieval). (B) Stimulus-specific patterns of neural activity were calculated for each image and were compared with patterns observed during the resting period. (C) Higher replay for pictures learned before the resting period was detected. Equivalent replay was observed during waking rest and sleep. (D) Average of high-frequency (80–100 Hz) ripples and ripple-triggered EEG traces in the hippocampus from all patients. (E) Ripple-triggered replay of neural representations during non-REM sleep from late in the encoding period (500–1200 ms) was associated with subsequent memory. (Reproduced with permission from Zhang et al., 2018.)

Therefore, individual stimuli are replayed and can be detected in the hippocampus during both wake and sleep.

13.3.2 The function and form of replay

What is the benefit of replaying stimuli or sequences in the hippocampus? At its most fundamental, replay is a proposed mechanism to preserve the memory of a recent experience by strengthening existing neural connections. There is evidence that replay serves this function. The level of reactivation in the hippocampus in the rest period after the learning of object-face or scene-face pairs predicts subsequent memory for these stimuli (Tambini and Davachi, 2013). The strength of reactivation of activity patterns in the hippocampus following fear conditioning also predicts subsequent spontaneous recovery of this memory 24 hours later (Hermans et al., 2017).

Consideration has also been given to how hippocampal replay strengthens such associations. The process, which is disrupted in patients with bilateral hippocampal damage (Spanò et al., 2020a), appears to involve spindles (12–16 Hz) in the neocortex during sleep, coupled with slower oscillations (<1.25 Hz), which are thought to trigger high-speed hippocampal ripples (80–120 Hz), which may then initiate information transfer from the hippocampus to neocortex (Helfrich et al., 2019). There is behavioral evidence that these oscillations facilitate learning in humans. Cowan et al. (2020) asked participants to encode a list of word–image pairs, and then recorded their brain activity during sleep. The next day participants restudied these words while undergoing an fMRI scan. They found that fast spindle density during sleep predicted subsequent increased functional connectivity between the hippocampus and ventromedial prefrontal cortex (vmPFC) during relearning of the list in the MRI scanner. This in turn was related to increased neural pattern similarity in the vmPFC between the two items in a remembered pair. This suggests the hippocampus helps to integrate learned associations in the neocortex during replay by transforming the neural representations of these hitherto unassociated stimuli to become more alike.

What kind of information is selected for replay in the hippocampus? There is evidence that specific items that are weakly learned, as measured by a memory test following training, are more likely to be replayed in the hippocampus during a subsequent rest period (Schapiro et al., 2018). This suggests that hippocampal replay may rescue items that are prone to forgetting. However, subsequent work has revealed a more complex picture. Sleep appears to benefit memory for successfully visualized items only, and within these items, the sleep-wake difference was found to be largest for more weakly encoded information (Denis et al., 2020). Therefore, vividness of visualization may be a key dimension along which items are pinpointed for subsequent replay. Another more nuanced issue is that replay is not always beneficial for memory retention. The effects of replay may depend on which segment of the encoding experience is replayed. Hippocampal reactivation during sleep of a stimulus from late in the encoding period (500–1,200 ms) benefits subsequent memory (Zhang, Fell, et al., 2018). However, reactivation from an earlier window of perceptual processing (100–500 ms) appears to be detrimental to memory stabilization, because it leads to forgetting of that stimulus. This temporal dissociation suggests that, as is the case with vividness, replay associated with a deeper processing of information determines the fate of memories.

Aside from tuning memory strength, hippocampal replay may serve a more adaptive function in humans, and that is to reorganize past experiences. Liu et al. (2019) trained participants to infer the correct order of scrambled sequences of stimuli based on prelearned rules. The experimenters then attempted to detect the replay of these stimuli during subsequent rest in an MEG scanner. Despite only experiencing the stimuli in their scrambled form during the experiment, participants replayed stimuli in the sequential order that would be dictated by the learned rules. A source-based analysis centered around the onset of these replay events revealed they were associated with high-frequency ripples in the hippocampus. Replay, therefore, does not just preserve the sequential nature of experience, it may dynamically restructure it in a way that is useful.

13.3.3 Further functions of consolidation

Consolidation, therefore, can assist in restructuring the temporal form of experience in the service of adaptive behavior. However, consolidation also serves to restructure other aspects of experience to the same end. One such hippocampus-dependent function is to extract common elements across multiple experiences. This form of learning helps us apply information learned in one context to another or, in other words, to generalize to a new situation. Kumaran et al. (2009) used a weather prediction task to encourage this form of learning. Participants could learn to predict weather conditions across multiple trials, based on either the copresentation of stimuli or their location on the screen. To test whether participants had extracted this knowledge across the experiment, a probe trial with partial information was administered, correct performance on which depended on having learned the rules over time. Hippocampal activity during learning predicted how well participants generalized this knowledge during the subsequent probe trial.

A key question is whether a prolonged period of consolidation further facilitates this kind of learning. Schapiro et al. (2017) investigated this issue by tasking participants with learning novel objects that belonged to one of three categories. This task was accomplished by extracting the overlapping features of these stimuli across trials. After one night of sleep, participants' memory for these shared features improved. Therefore, it is likely that offline replay during sleep enhances this kind of conceptual knowledge consolidation. Further evidence that this time-dependent consolidation is mediated by the hippocampus was provided by Sweegers et al. (2014). In this study, participants learned where faces would appear on a screen, and could work out a hidden rule to facilitate learning based on the features of the faces. Following 48 hours of consolidation, participants were asked to retrieve this knowledge, and connectivity between the hippocampus and prefrontal cortex was higher during retrieval of this rule-based knowledge, compared with retrieving arbitrary rule-free face-location associations. After an even longer consolidation period of several weeks after learning this task, participants' knowledge of these learned regularities was preserved, whereas arbitrary face-location pairings had been forgotten (Sweegers and Talamini, 2014).

Evidence from patients with hippocampal lesions suggests that conceptual knowledge is in fact continually extracted and updated throughout the life span. For example, this has been investigated by assessing patients' depth of vocabulary and the richness of their semantic associations where their original learning of these concepts occurred long before sustaining their hippocampal damage. When patients with hippocampal damage were given a word and asked to either identify words that were associated with it, list features that it brought to mind, or generate different interpretations of the word,

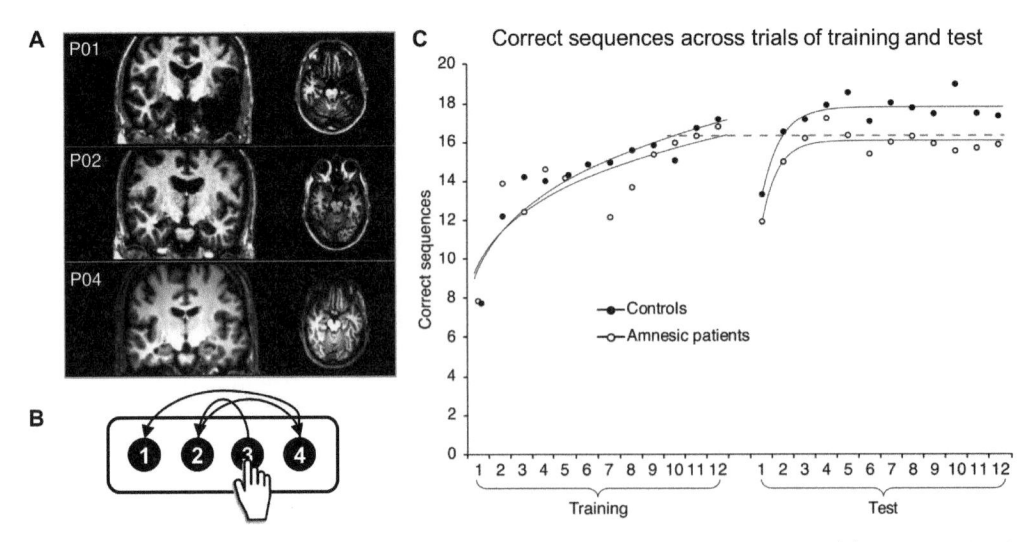

Figure 13.4 The hippocampus may be necessary for task consolidation without being required for learning. (A) Patients with selective (P02 and P04) and nonselective (P01) damage to the hippocampus performed a motor sequence task. (B) Patients and healthy controls learned to press a sequence of five digits on a four-button keypad. (C) Patients and controls reached the same level of performance at the end of training on the first day (dashed line). However, after a night of sleep, the healthy control participants improved during subsequent testing, benefiting from offline consolidation, whereas patients' performance remained the same. Curves fit to average performance are power functions for training and exponential functions for test. (Reproduced with permission from Schapiro et al., 2019.)

they were impaired on all three tasks (Klooster and Duff, 2015). These findings suggest that even remote conceptual knowledge is impoverished in such patients because the hippocampus may play a role in the maintenance and updating of knowledge beyond its initial acquisition. Overall, therefore, it seems that another function of consolidation is to extract conceptual knowledge over numerous, ongoing, episodic experiences.

However, while it can be useful to extract commonalities across numerous life experiences, it can be equally adaptive to forget information that is not beneficial to retain. This capacity to weaken or erase memories is another proposed function of consolidation. One way this has been investigated is through the deployment of a directed forgetting paradigm, in which participants are presented with a stimulus, but instructed not to remember it. This approach was used by Rauchs et al. (2011), who showed participants a list of words, followed by an instruction to either remember or forget each word. Memory performance was tested either after one night's sleep, or a period of sleep deprivation. Both groups successfully retrieved an equivalent number of the to-be-remembered words, but the sleep deprivation group remembered significantly more to-be-forgotten words. This suggests that sleep-dependent consolidation may erase memories that are not deemed significant. Moreover, hippocampal activity in the sleep group predicted subsequent memory, whereas no such association was found in the sleep-deprived group. These findings indicate that experiences may be tagged during encoding for subsequent weakening or strengthening during sleep.

One might assume, based on these discoveries, that the benefits of hippocampus-mediated consolidation are reserved for tasks that are hippocampus-dependent but, interestingly, this appears not to be the case. For example, Schapiro et al. (2019) had a group of patients with hippocampal damage and healthy controls to perform a motor task (Figure 13.4). This involved learning to press buttons in a defined sequence as quickly and accurately as possible. Patients showed remarkably similar learning trajectories to controls, indicating that the acquisition of this task does not depend on

hippocampal integrity. When tested after one night's sleep, however, the healthy controls displayed improved performance while the patients remained at the same level as the previous day. Therefore, hippocampus-dependent consolidation appears to provide an additional performance benefit for tasks that are not initially dependent on the hippocampus. This may be facilitated by the replay of the learning context during sleep, and demonstrates how hippocampal damage can result in impairments beyond functional domains traditionally associated with the hippocampus.

13.3.4 How long does consolidation take?

There is much evidence, therefore, that the hippocampus is recruited to learn new information, and is heavily involved in strengthening, restructuring, and updating this knowledge during offline periods. It may appear a reasonable assumption that the hippocampus retains a lifelong role in the subsequent instantiation of these experiences. However, despite the considerable accumulation of research on the mnemonic functions of the hippocampus, this remains a complex issue that awaits resolution. The seminal case of patient H.M. focused attention on the role of the hippocampus in memory retrieval (Scoville and Milner, 1957). After undergoing a bilateral excision of the medial temporal lobes, H.M. was observed to be incapable of remembering past, real-life experiences—episodic autobiographical memories—for a time period of 3 years prior to his operation. Under initial examination, his older memories appeared relatively unaffected, but later studies revealed them to be much more impaired (Corkin, 2002; Steinvorth et al., 2005). The apparent preservation of remote autobiographical memories, despite the loss of recent memories, is termed "temporally graded retrograde amnesia." Subsequent cases of hippocampal damage followed, presenting with a similar neuropsychological profile, and this motivated a perspective on the core function of the hippocampus in which its role in memory retrieval is time-limited (Squire, 1992; Squire and Alvarez, 1995). Known as standard consolidation theory (see more on this later in the chapter), this perspective proposes that the hippocampus stores memories initially, but they become strengthened in the neocortex over time, and eventually the hippocampus is not necessary for their retrieval.

One systematic method of assessing a person's ability to recall autobiographical memories from their recent and remote past is a test known as the Autobiographical Interview (AI; Levine et al., 2002). Participants are asked to provide memories from multiple life periods, and are then probed further to elicit as much specific information as possible about the events. This test can be administered to patients to assess the impact of hippocampal damage on their ability to retrieve past memories and, more specifically, whether or not their memory loss displays a temporal gradient. In support of standard consolidation theory, Kirwan et al. (2008) reported that three patients with selective hippocampal damage could recall an equivalent number of specific details from remote life periods when compared with healthy control participants, and were only impaired in the recollection of events from the year before testing.

However, this evidence is not conclusive, because other investigations have revealed strikingly different patterns of memory loss. For example, using the AI, Rosenbaum et al. (2008) found that hippocampal damage was associated with impairment in recalling memories across all life periods. This flat temporal gradient can be profound, with hippocampal damage often leading to a near total erasure of autobiographical memories regardless of memory age (Nadel and Moscovitch, 1997; Maguire et al., 2006; Cipolotti et al., 2001). There is further evidence that even when damage is confined to specific portions of the hippocampus, memory from all life periods can be compromised. Transient global amnesia is a condition characterized by the sudden onset of memory loss, but called "transient" as it lasts for only a limited period of time (Hodges and Warlow, 1990). Under fMRI investigation, it is associated with selective perturbations to CA1 of the hippocampus (Bartsch et al., 2006). This condition offers a unique time window within which to assess the effect of such interference with CA1 activity on remote memory recall. While the retrograde amnesia associated with this condition was found to have a temporal gradient, in that the ability to recall autobiographical events from early life periods was less affected, the recall of memories from all life periods was nevertheless impaired (Bartsch et al., 2011). Another condition that is uniquely illuminating due to the selective nature of its associated pathology, is LGI1-antibody-complex limbic encephalitis. This infection results in selective damage to CA3 (Miller et al., 2017). Despite such spatially confined lesions, a retrograde amnesia can span up to 50 years prior to the onset of the condition (Miller et al., 2020). As this represents an implausibly long time frame for the completion of systems-level consolidation, such findings cast doubt on the assertion that the retrieval of vivid, detailed autobiographical memories is a process that becomes entirely independent of the hippocampus.

While the existence of temporally graded retrograde amnesia for episodic autobiographical memories in cases of hippocampal damage remains disputed, its existence in the case of semantic memories is more generally accepted. One approach to assessing this kind of memory is to ask patients to recall public events, demonstrating factual knowledge about the world as opposed to the recollection of personal experiences. In one such study, Manns et al. (2003) required patients with hippocampal damage to recall news events from different periods of their lives. Patients were impaired up to around 11 years before the onset of amnesia, but their memory for news events from more remote periods was spared. Patients'

ability to recall semantic autobiographical information—facts about their personal life—is also preserved (Rosenbaum et al., 2008). Hence, there is a consensus that although following hippocampal damage semantic information is not updated, premorbidly acquired semantic memory can become independent of the hippocampus over time. However, whether or not hippocampal damage results in a lasting impairment in the recall of remote episodic autobiographical memories remains an open question that awaits further clarification.

An alternative approach to investigating hippocampal involvement in remote episodic autobiographical memory retrieval is the neuroimaging of healthy controls. If the hippocampus is engaged during the retrieval of autobiographical memories regardless of their age, then increased activity in this region should be observed. However, as is the case with neuropsychological studies, evidence from this domain is mixed. Piefke et al. (2003) asked participants to recall remote childhood memories alongside more recent events from the preceding 5 years while undergoing an fMRI scan. Consistent with standard consolidation theory and a gradual disengagement of the hippocampus over time, they observed greater activation for recent memories in the hippocampus when compared with earlier life periods. In contrast, Rekkas and Constable (2005) compared hippocampal activation during participants' recall of memories that were either a few days old, with that of more remote 8-year-old memories, and observed greater hippocampal engagement during the recall of more remote events.

Given that systems-level consolidation may take years, a more fine-grained analysis of hippocampal involvement is required to address this question. To this end, Viard et al. (2007) investigated hippocampal activation during the retrieval of memories across the entire life span in older adults, from time periods ranging from childhood to young and older adulthood. Despite this wide range in time periods, the hippocampus was equivalently active throughout. This challenges the notion that the retrieval of episodic autobiographical memories becomes hippocampus-independent over time. While one could argue that hippocampal activation in fMRI studies of remote memory is attributable to participants merely recollecting the period of memory harvesting just prior to scanning, this does not appear to be the case. Steinvorth et al. (2006) collected participants' autobiographical memories through long-unseen diary entries and from interviews with family and friends, and found equivalent hippocampal activation while participants recollected both recent and remote autobiographical memories during fMRI. Consistent with a dissociation between remote episodic and semantic memory, hippocampal activation was lower for the latter during a task that involved participants visualizing well-known objects.

A potential limitation of fMRI studies demonstrating increased hippocampal activation for remote memories is whether the observed activity represents the retrieval of specifically that experience rather than, for example, a more general process. Advanced fMRI analysis techniques, such as multivoxel pattern analysis (MVPA), are well suited to address this issue. Bonnici, Chadwick, Lutti, et al. (2012) asked participants to recall both recent (2-week-old) and remote (10-year-old) autobiographical memories while undergoing high-resolution fMRI scanning. An MVPA analysis demonstrated the patterns of activity observed in the hippocampus during memory recall were specific to individual memories. Furthermore, recent and remote memories could be decoded to a similar extent in the hippocampus. These findings provide additional evidence that the hippocampus supports episodic autobiographical memory recall regardless of remoteness.

Further evidence that the hippocampus is involved in the retrieval of remote memories has been observed with intracranial recordings from presurgical patients with epilepsy. During the presentation of an autobiographical memory cue that concerned an event at least 10 years old, there was increased high-frequency gamma activity in layers of the entorhinal cortex that project to the hippocampus (Steinvorth et al., 2010). During the subsequent retrieval of that memory, prolonged theta activity in layers of the entorhinal cortex that output to cortical areas was observed. This pattern is indicative of information flow in and out of the hippocampus during remote autobiographical memory recall, and these oscillatory signatures were less evident during the retrieval of semantic knowledge, whether personal or general in nature.

In summary, while the extant literature is not definitive, converging evidence from different investigative approaches suggests that the retrieval of detailed episodic autobiographical memories is likely to be dependent on hippocampal integrity over the long term. However, the precise nature of the hippocampal contribution to remote memory retrieval has itself been the subject of debate. The preponderance of data emphasizing a role for the hippocampus in remote memory retrieval motivated an alternative perspective to the standard consolidation theory.

Multiple trace theory posits that the hippocampus stores lasting traces of rich and vivid episodic autobiographical memories in perpetuity (Nadel et al., 2007; Moscovitch and Nadel, 2019; see more on this theory in a later section). This argument has been called into question (reviewed in Barry and Maguire, 2019a, 2019b), for example, by analyses of neurogenesis, the birth of new neurons throughout the adult life, in postmortem human hippocampal tissue samples. It has been estimated that continual neurogenesis in the DG contributes to a high turnover of hippocampal granule cells over the adult life span (Spalding et al., 2013). This structural instability permits the possibility that remote autobiographical memory retrieval by the hippocampus does not involve storage, but may instead represent a reconstructive process (Barry and Maguire, 2019a, 2019b). Therefore, while the duration of systems-level consolidation remains a critical issue, it may in fact be resolved by understanding how a memory is reconstructed once it has been consolidated. In the next section, we address in more detail the mechanisms underlying memory retrieval within the hippocampus.

13.4 The constructive use of hippocampal representations

13.4.1 Initiation of memory reconstruction

While the fate of memory traces in the hippocampus and neocortex remains a matter of dispute, there exists a consensus that the constituent elements of memories are stored in cortical regions in the longer term (as reviewed in Squire, 1992; Maguire, 2014; Squire et al., 2015; Moscovitch et al., 2016). The vmPFC is an area that is densely connected with the hippocampus, and there is considerable cross-species evidence that it plays an important role in the long-term consolidation of memories (van Kesteren et al., 2010; Nieuwenhuis and Takashima, 2011). In humans, Bonnici, Chadwick, Lutti, et al. (2012) applied MVPA to fMRI data and demonstrated that episodic autobiographical memories which had occurred at least one decade earlier were more detectable in vmPFC than those experienced in recent weeks. Follow-up work resolved this timescale even further by showing that autobiographical memory traces become stabilized in vmPFC in the first few months following their encoding (Barry et al., 2018), which indicates that the vmPFC may interact with the hippocampus during memory retrieval over this period.

Evidence from MEG studies suggests this is the case. Fuentemilla et al. (2017) asked participants to keep an audio diary of autobiographical memory episodes that were later used as cues during an MEG scan. Retrieval of these memories, which were between 2 and 7 months old, was associated with an increase in theta power in the left hippocampus and vmPFC, with both regions showing greater synchronization during recall of these episodes when compared with general semantic memories. In addition, the strength of this connectivity predicted more detailed visual imagery during retrieval. Therefore, the vmPFC seems to be recruited to support the hippocampus in reconstructing remote memories. In fact, the process of memory reconstruction appears to be initiated by the vmPFC. McCormick et al. (2020) asked participants to recall autobiographical memories while undergoing a MEG scan (Figure 13.5). These memories ranged in remoteness from less than 1 month old to 5 years of age. They found that the hippocampus and the vmPFC showed the greatest power changes across the whole brain during autobiographical memory retrieval. Notably, responses in the vmPFC preceded activity in the hippocampus during initiation of recall, except during retrieval of the most recent autobiographical memories. Moreover, an effective connectivity analysis revealed that the vmPFC drove hippocampal activity during recall initiation, and also as recollection unfolded over subsequent seconds, and this effect was evident regardless of memory age. These findings imply that memory retrieval in the hippocampus may be orchestrated by the vmPFC.

There is also evidence that the coordinated activity of the hippocampus and vmPFC is the strongest determinant of the vividness of recollected memories. Geib et al. (2017) tasked participants with encoding a series of scene images, and obtained vividness ratings for their memories of these scenes. They then assessed hippocampal functional connectivity while participants recalled the scenes, and compared vivid with dim retrieval trials. Of 90 brain regions analyzed, inferior frontal regions, including medial and orbital areas, displayed the largest increase in connectivity with the hippocampus for vivid memories. Therefore, the successful and vivid reconstruction of past events by the hippocampus seem to involve input from the vmPFC.

13.4.2 Reconstructing the past

Once recall is initiated, perhaps driven by the vmPFC, the hippocampus then appears to reconstruct the context of previously experienced events. "Context" is an often-used term that can mean simply a space or place in an environment, or a space and the elements within it (e.g., landmarks, objects, people), perhaps best exemplified in the notion of a scene, or it can have wider connotations in terms of the emotional and social milieu. We will elaborate further on this issue in later sections, but here consider some general points. For example, stronger hippocampal activation during fMRI was observed when participants recalled places in a virtual environment they had visited, compared with recalling individual objects they

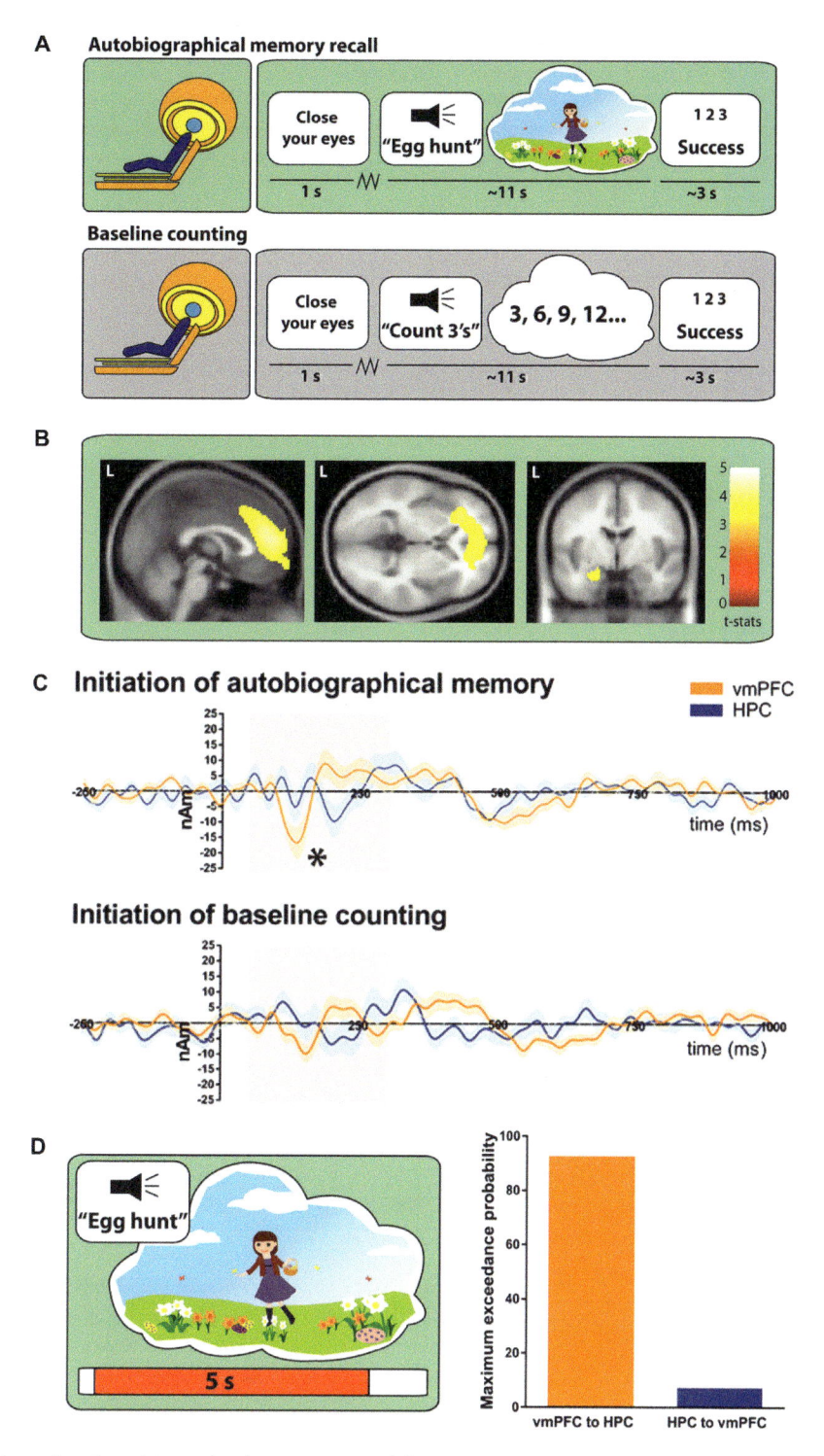

Figure 13.5 The temporal dynamics of autobiographical memory recall. (A) Participants recalled autobiographical memories while undergoing an MEG scan (upper panel). A baseline condition where participants mentally counted was also included (lower panel). (B) Power changes (1–30 Hz) during autobiographical memory retrieval showed engagement of the hippocampus and ventromedial prefrontal cortex (vmPFC). (C) Event-related signals during autobiographical memory retrieval revealed that activity in the hippocampus lagged behind that of the vmPFC (upper panel), an effect that was not evident during baseline counting (lower panel). (D) Dynamic causal modeling of neural interactions showed that the vmPFC drove hippocampal activity during the first 5 seconds of autobiographical memory retrieval (orange bar). (Reproduced with permission from McCormick et al., 2020).

received (Burgess et al., 2002). In a similar vein, Liang and Preston (2017) asked participants to visualize a place, person, or object in response to an adjective, while undergoing an fMRI scan. During a subsequent scan, they were shown the same adjectives and asked to recall which condition the word belonged to, and to visualize

their previous representation. When participants successfully recalled and visualized previous representations of places, patterns of neural activity observed during encoding were reinstated along the entire axis of the hippocampus during retrieval. This effect was not observed for the people or objects conditions, suggesting reinstatement of place information in the hippocampus is dominant during retrieval.

Direct hippocampal recordings from patients with intracranial electrodes has revealed more about the processes underlying the retrieval of context. Patients traversed a virtual reality environment, encountering objects in different rooms (Pacheco Estefan et al., 2019). During retrieval, objects were shown either in the original context or in a different room. The hippocampus reinstated time-frequency patterns of encoding activity during retrieval only when objects were shown in their original context, indicating that the hippocampus encodes and retrieves the association between an item and its context. As with encoding, reinstatement of electrophysiological patterns of activity was most prominent in the low-frequency theta and delta bands. Furthermore, as has been observed in the studies of human replay described in an earlier section, reinstatement was temporally compressed, in this case by a factor of three. Therefore, during recall, the hippocampus seems to rebuild the spatial and other event elements, and the associations between them, into a coherent representation. We will return to this issue further in a later section.

13.4.3 Separating and completing memory traces

One key function required by an effective memory system is the ability to retrieve one complete specific episode, while at the same time not confusing it with related events. Two hippocampal subregions that appear to be particularly important in memory recall and that support these complementary functions are the DG and CA3. There is evidence that the DG is recruited to disambiguate similar contexts, a process termed "pattern separation." For example, Berron et al. (2016) showed participants a sequence of stimuli that comprised two similar scenes, and asked them to identify when the first scene in a sequence was presented for the third time, while undergoing a high-resolution fMRI scanning. They compared activity in the hippocampus during repeated presentations of the target scene, with that present during the alternating lure. Activity in the DG was higher during lures than repeated presentations, consistent with a role for this region in pattern separation because of the requirement to disambiguate similar stimuli. Furthermore, using a neural pattern classification approach, Berron et al. (2016) could decode representations of lure stimuli in the DG, but not in any other hippocampal subregion or medial temporal lobe area, indicating that the DG may be specialized for this task.

The DG appears to accomplish this feat by orthogonalizing representations of similar stimuli (see Chapter 7). Lohnas et al. (2018) deployed a pattern separation task with patients undergoing intracranial recordings. The objects presented during retrieval were new, repeated, or highly similar to previous objects. Greater high-frequency (45–115 Hz) activity was observed in the hippocampus during the correct rejection of similar items, compared with those erroneously identified as old. This activity was present from 1 to 1.5 seconds after stimulus onset. Analysis of the spatiotemporal activity patterns across multiple hippocampal electrodes showed that the patterns for similar and new items were more dissimilar than the patterns for old and new items. The generation of orthogonal neural patterns therefore allows for more accurate discrimination. Of note, when patients performed the same task with the sole exception of having to classify similar items as new, these effects were not observed. Therefore, such mnemonic discrimination in the hippocampus appears to be deployed only when the task demands targeted attention toward the precise disambiguation of features.

The DG is thought to transfer these orthogonalized representations to CA3 (Rolls and Kesner, 2006), which then completes the representation of an event. This capacity to recall an entire episode given one or more associated elements is often termed "pattern completion." Horner et al. (2015) scrutinized the role of the hippocampus in this process using a learning paradigm consisting of "closed" or "open" loops. Stimuli from different categories (places, famous people, objects, animals) were associated with each other through pairwise presentation during learning where participants were required to imagine the two elements interacting in a meaningful way, typically in a scene, as vividly as possible. Open loops comprised a chain of four stimuli, where the first and last item were not connected. The closed loop stimuli represented a bound representation, where the cueing and retrieval of two of these items should result in an incidental activation, or pattern completion, of the third. Consistent with a role for the hippocampus in this process, incidental cortical reactivation of the third item in the closed loop correlated with hippocampal activity during retrieval. A subsequent high-resolution fMRI investigation using this task isolated this effect to area CA3 (Grande et al., 2019).

Another important capacity beyond linking different elements of a single memory together, is linking together different memories that share a common element. In contrast to the association of temporally contiguous events that we described in an earlier section, this may involve connecting memories that are far apart in time but share common features. Koster et al. (2018) investigated such integration across episodes by showing participants faces linked by either a scene or an object, through corresponding pairwise presentations. Subsequently, participants were shown one face, and had to identify the other, which involved linking the two through their common element. Using high-resolution fMRI, Koster et al. (2018) showed that during this retrieval process, activation of the linking scene or object was observed in both the deep and superficial layers of the entorhinal cortex. This indicates that the common elements were circulated out of the hippocampus and back in again, to help link the two faces together. In further support of this idea, connectivity between the deep and superficial layers of the entorhinal cortex predicted the strength of representation of the common elements. This connectivity also correlated with connectivity between the superficial layer of the entorhinal cortex and DG/CA3, and was associated with performance on the task. Hence, connecting different experiences through their overlapping components involves a loop of information flow in and out of the hippocampus that chains events together.

While it might be useful in some instances to integrate information across separate episodes, this may lead to impairments in memory when similar episodes become confused. Chadwick et al. (2014) investigated this potential problem by showing participants naturalistic video clips that contained overlapping elements (Figure 13.6). Participants subsequently recalled these events during high-resolution fMRI. Consistent with a role for CA3 in pattern completion, this hippocampal subregion contained partially overlapping memory traces of the individual events, as measured by voxel activity patterns. Furthermore, the degree of mnemonic confusion that participants reported during retrieval correlated with the extent to which the neural traces overlapped. Therefore, successful memory retrieval seems to rely on a delicate balance

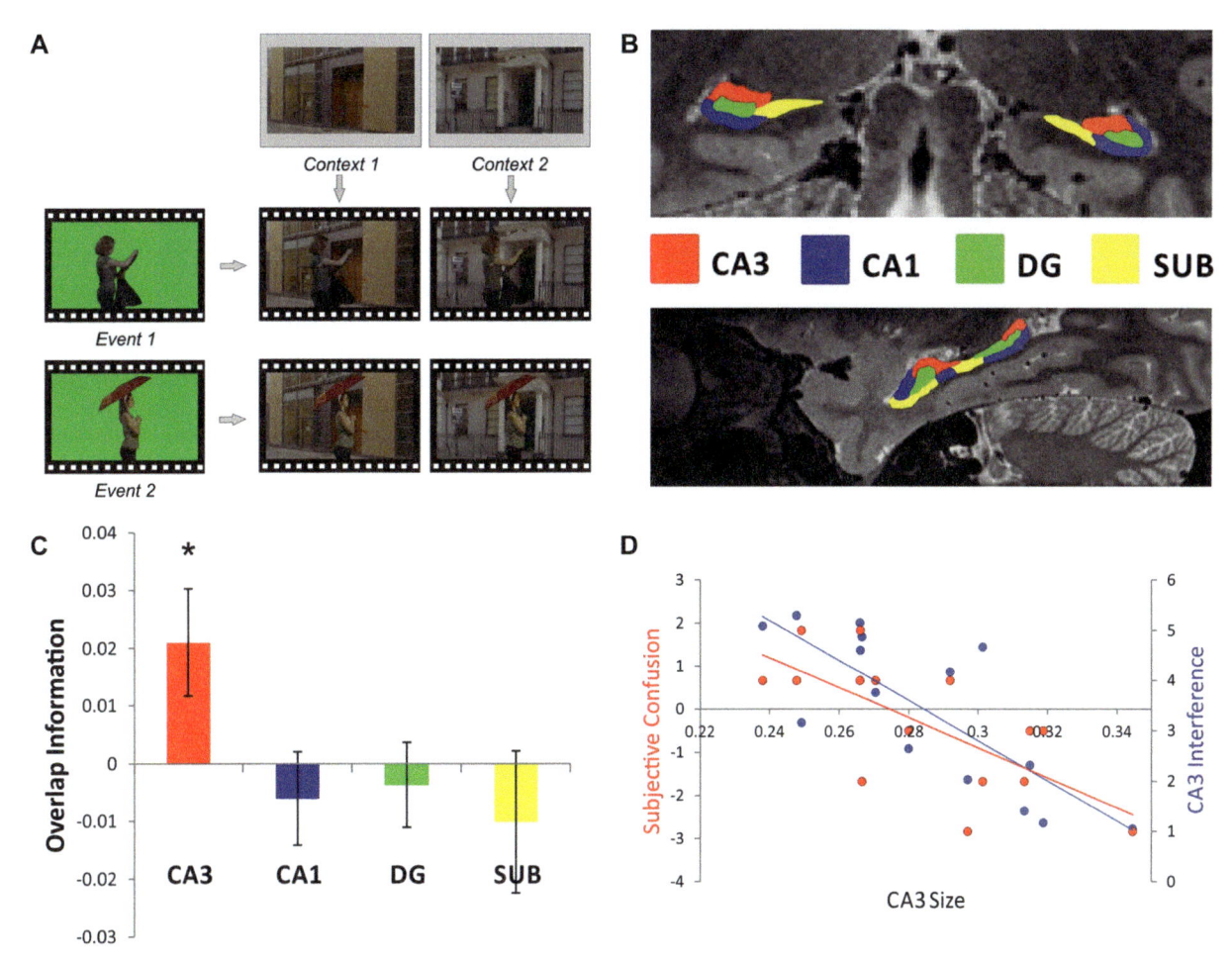

Figure 13.6 CA3 size predicts the precision of memory recall. (A) Participants viewed four unique events that contained overlapping people and contexts and then recalled them during fMRI scanning. (B) Delineation of an example participant's hippocampal subfields. (C) Only CA3 contained detectable evidence for informational overlap between memories. (D) A larger CA3 was associated with less interference in neural representations and less confusion between memories. (Reproduced with permission from Chadwick et al., 2014.)

between retrieving events in memory based on relevant learned associations, while successfully disambiguating these episodes from those that are irrelevant to the current task demands.

13.4.4 Recognition memory and familiarity

While it is clear that the hippocampus is involved in the detailed, vivid recollection of past experiences, we often do not remember an item or event until it is presented to us. This form of memory retrieval is termed "recognition memory," and is thought to involve two processes, the recollection itself, and a feeling of familiarity (Yonelinas, 2002). Some theories of memory do not draw any distinction between pure recollection and recognition memory in terms of the extent of hippocampal involvement (e.g., Squire, 1992). Other accounts propose that a sense of familiarity originates in regions outside of the hippocampus, such as the perirhinal cortex (Aggleton and Brown, 1999; Eichenbaum et al., 2007) and that, consequently, recognition memory may still be possible even in the case of hippocampal damage, as this component is preserved. There is evidence to support this latter view. For example, Aggleton et al. (2005) studied patient K.N., who had bilateral hippocampal damage while the rest of the medial temporal lobes appeared to be spared. He performed poorly on tests requiring the recall of people or shapes, but within normal levels

when recognizing doors and names. Further analyses of K.N.'s ratings of confidence during recognition memory revealed a different pattern to healthy controls in that he relied more on the familiarity of items, rather than recollection, and this was associated with lower confidence.

However, further research has suggested that the determinant of hippocampal involvement in recognition memory and familiarity may depend on the nature of the stimuli. For example, patients with hippocampal damage have been found to be more impaired at recognizing verbal stimuli than faces (Smith et al., 2014). Similarly, patient Jon, with bilateral hippocampal pathology and developmental amnesia, performed normally on a recognition memory test of faces, but was markedly impaired on an equivalent test of scene recognition (Bird et al., 2008). Only in other patients in whom brain damage extended to the neighboring perirhinal cortex did recognition memory for faces seem to be additionally compromised (Taylor et al., 2007). Furthermore, even familiarity-based recognition for spatial stimuli such as buildings or landscapes is affected by selective hippocampal damage (Cipolotti et al., 2006). Therefore, a sense of familiarity and the subsequent ability to recognize stimuli, may depend on the integrity of regions specialized for processing those kinds of stimuli. Accordingly, recognition memory in the scene or spatial domain, or in the case of verbal stimuli, which are facilitated by internally generated visual imagery during encoding and retrieval, may invariably involve the hippocampus.

13.4.5 Constructing the future

While research on the functions of the hippocampus has predominantly focused on the encoding and retrieval of prior experiences, over the years it has emerged that the temporal locus of hippocampal representations is not confined to the past (Tulving et al., 1988; Okuda et al., 2003; Rosenbaum et al., 2005). Hassabis et al. (2007a) examined this systematically by asking patients with hippocampal damage to project themselves forward into their personal future, and imagine plausible events such as meeting a friend, or an upcoming weekend activity. Compared with healthy controls, patients produced far fewer details. This deficit included a reduction in references to space and entities occupying it, the properties of these entities, and other aspects of the scenario, including their thoughts, emotions, or actions or those of others involved. A key feature of such an exercise is that its construction is not dependent on the recall of a specific personally experienced past event, presenting the possibility that the hippocampus may be involved in functions beyond recollection of the past.

Neuroimaging studies in healthy controls have provided further support for this idea. Addis et al. (2007) had participants remember past events or imagine episodes situated in the future, in response to cue phrases during fMRI. In either case an event could take place up to 20 years from the present moment. Future events were required to be plausible, but novel, avoiding memory retrieval processes. Both tasks recruited a similar network of brain regions, most notably the left hippocampus, suggesting similar processes may underlie both tasks. In fact, the right hippocampus was also strongly recruited for future events, which may indicate that future thinking taxes underlying processes more heavily.

One concern with comparing past and future events in such an unconstrained paradigm is that future events may be phenomenologically different from past events. To address this, in Weiler et al.'s (2010) fMRI experiment participants had to imagine multiple events that could theoretically take place during an upcoming seasonal holiday. After the holiday, participants returned to be scanned again, this time recalling actual events that had taken place. In this carefully controlled design, past and future events were closely matched in terms of their content and phenomenology. While hippocampal activity was similar across the two conditions during the early phase of event construction, the later elaboration stage during future imagining elicited more activity in the posterior hippocampus, again suggesting that future thinking may tax the hippocampus more than memory recall.

Another approach to investigating the extent to which the hippocampus is involved in these future projections, is to directly assess the relationship between the detail and phenomenology of constructed future events and hippocampal activity. Addis et al. (2011) had participants construct events that were temporally and contextually specific, occurring over a short time period such as a special dinner, or a more general, routine event. Hippocampal activity was higher when participants were constructing future compared with past experiences, but this only applied to specific events. There are other key features of imagined future experiences that modulate hippocampal activity. When participants plan their autobiographical future, the associated activity of the hippocampus is modulated by the amount of detail in these plans, the novelty of the imagined scenarios, and it even scales with the temporal distance of these future events (Spreng et al., 2015). Therefore, the hippocampus is not just involved in retrieving rich, vivid past experiences but also constructing future events, that are detailed, unique, and far ahead in time.

One might argue that such fictitious construction in a laboratory setting is not representative of, or relevant to, our daily mental lives, but this is not the case. In fact, much of our time when not attending to the external environment, or concentrating during a laboratory task, is spent engaging in past and future thinking. Karapanagiotidis et al. (2017) sampled the thoughts of participants at unpredictable moments during the performance of a simple laboratory task. Future and self-focused thoughts accounted for 29% of the variance in the recorded spontaneous thoughts, while past-focused social thoughts made up 19%. We, therefore, spend much of our time perceptually decoupled from the external environment, mentally traveling back and forth through experienced and potential future scenarios (Smallwood and Andrews-Hanna, 2013; Moneyham and Schooler, 2013). This study also revealed an association between the propensity to embark on such mental time travel and brain structure. Individuals who engaged in more mind-wandering had greater integrity of the temporolimbic tract, which is heavily connected to the hippocampus. In addition, an analysis of functional connectivity during rest as measured by fMRI revealed these individuals had higher connectivity between the hippocampus and the anterior cingulate cortex. Indeed, the consistently observed activity across a distributed set of brain areas, including the hippocampus, while the brain is at "rest," typically referred to as the "default mode network" (Buckner and Vincent, 2007; Raichle and Snyder, 2001), may well relate to mind-wandering during resting-state fMRI scans.

A more direct association between hippocampal activity and spontaneous thought was provided by Ellamil et al. (2016). Experienced mindfulness practitioners, who display heightened introspective abilities, were scanned while performing one of two tasks. The first was to monitor the emergence of their spontaneous thoughts and respond when one occurred. The second was to monitor their external environment for a word appearing on a screen. Just before the practitioners pressed a button to indicate spontaneous thought, bilateral activation of the hippocampus was observed, providing strong evidence for the hippocampus in mediating perceptually decoupled thoughts. Together, these results suggest that the interaction between the hippocampus and a wider network of brain regions underlies our capacity to mentally wander to the future and the past.

Studying these processes in patients with hippocampal damage provides a unique window into the contribution of the hippocampus to such mental time travel. McCormick et al. (2018) sampled patients' spontaneous thoughts and compared them to healthy controls. While patients spent an equivalent amount of time to controls perceptually decoupled from the external environment, the form and content of their thoughts were markedly different. Patients spent much less time pondering the past and future, instead remaining rooted to the present. In addition, while the mind-wandering of the healthy controls comprised mostly visual representations, which were predominantly scene-like, the patients' thoughts were verbal, abstract, and semantic in nature. Therefore, while healthy people are free to mentally escape to a rich past and future at any time, patients with hippocampal damage seem to remain captives of the present (Corkin, 2013).

The functional relevance of perceptual decoupling is particularly evident during the prolonged period of our night's sleep. For example, Wamsley and Stickgold (2019) tasked healthy participants with learning a maze in a virtual environment, and sampled their dream content from different sleep stages during the night. Incorporation of the maze task into dream content was observed in a proportion of participants across all phases of sleep, including onset, NREM, and rapid eye movement sleep (REM). Aligning with the reconstructive view of hippocampal functioning outlined earlier, the dream content differed from actual experience in almost every detail. Despite this, only the participants who incorporated such content during dreaming showed an improvement in maze performance the next day, highlighting the role of construction during dreaming in memory consolidation.

Further evidence that dreaming may be relevant for consolidation was revealed by Spanò et al. (2020b) by examining hippocampal-damaged patients with amnesia. Using a provoked awakening protocol, participants were woken up at various points throughout the night, including during NREM and REM sleep, and asked to report their thoughts in that moment. Despite being roused a similar number of times, dream frequency was significantly reduced in patients compared with healthy controls, and the few dreams the patients reported were less episodic-like in nature and lacked content. These findings suggest that healthy hippocampi are necessary for dreaming and perhaps, when dreaming is compromised, this contributes to amnesia.

Overall, therefore, re-experiencing the past and pre-experiencing the future, whether during wakefulness, idleness, or sleep, appears to critically depend on the hippocampus. Revealing the robust recruitment of the hippocampus in functions beyond memory in fact highlights the fundamental purpose of memory. We use memory to capture our experiences and accrue knowledge that we can deploy to shape our behavior in the future, thus promoting survival.

13.4.6 Constructing scenes

The hippocampus may support event construction, regardless of its temporal dimension, through a more fundamental process. There is converging evidence that one of its roles may be to construct imagery, and specifically imagery in a scene-like form. Hassabis et al. (2007a) asked patients with bilateral hippocampal damage to imagine and describe novel scenes. Despite these scenes being temporally agnostic, and not dependent on recalling past events, and even when they were cued with relevant elements from the scenes (such as objects, sounds, and smells), patients produced greatly impoverished scene descriptions compared with healthy controls. Closer inspection of patients' descriptions also revealed that their imagined scenes were spatially fragmented. The patients' imagination deficit seemed to be specific to scenes, because they could imagine single isolated objects with ease. Moreover, this scene imagination deficit, which has been since widely replicated (e.g., Irish et al., 2017; Wilson et al., 2020), cannot be attributed to problems with verbal output, fluency, or narrative construction (Race et al., 2011).

Aligning with the patient findings, constructing scenes in the imagination also recruits the hippocampus in healthy controls. When participants were asked to construct novel scenes while undergoing an fMRI scan, a network of regions was activated, including the hippocampus, when contrasted with imagining single objects in isolation (e.g., Hassabis et al., 2007b; Zeidman, Mullally, et al., 2015). Bonnici, Kumaran, et al. (2012) took this further and used multivoxel pattern analysis to demonstrate that viewed scenes of differing topology were uniquely identifiable in hippocampal activity patterns. Furthermore, and in line with the aforementioned role for the hippocampus in pattern separation, when participants were presented with images that were 50% morphs of two separate scenes, hippocampal activity patterns predicted the participants' decisions about which original scene it most resembled. This demonstrates that internally generated scene imagery can diverge from perceptual input, and this is especially evident in a phenomenon called "boundary extension" (Intraub and Richardson, 1989; Intraub, 2020). Specifically, when participants are shown the same scene twice in succession, even when separated by a short delay of just a few seconds, they often report the second presentation as a closer-up representation of the first (or in other words, remembering the initial presentation as more expansive than it was). This boundary extension effect suggests that people automatically and rapidly create an internal scene representation that extrapolates beyond the bounds of what has been seen. When this occurs, it is associated with increased activation of the hippocampus (Chadwick et al., 2013), whereas the boundary extension effect is significantly attenuated in hippocampal-damaged patients, in line with their impaired ability to imagine scenes (Mullally et al., 2012).

High-resolution fMRI also affords the opportunity to investigate whether the process of scene construction is associated with specific subfields of the hippocampus. Zeidman, Lutti, et al. (2015) reported increased activity of the anterior-medial pre- and parasubiculum during the construction of scene imagery compared with imagining single isolated objects. Dalton et al. (2018) took this further using a carefully controlled paradigm during fMRI (see Monk et al., 2021, for a similar MEG study), where in one condition participants gradually built scene imagery from three successive auditorily presented object descriptions and an imagined 3D space (Figure 13.7). This was contrasted with constructing mental images of nonscene arrays that were composed of three objects and an imagined 2D space. The scene and array stimuli were, therefore, highly matched in terms of content and the associative and constructive processes they evoked, but only one resulted in a scene representation. Mentally constructing scenes as opposed to arrays was specifically associated with activation of the pre- and parasubiculum. Of note, when the imagined 3D and 2D spaces alone (without objects) were examined, neither was associated with increased hippocampal activity. This echoed a previous finding where a 3D space did not provoke engagement of the hippocampus (Zeidman et al., 2012). Consequently, Dalton et al. (2018) concluded that it is specifically scene representations that consistently engage the hippocampus, and that the pre- and parasubiculum may be especially attuned to constructing these scene representations (Dalton and Maguire, 2017; see Chapter 3 for more on the anatomy of these regions).

Several lines of inquiry suggest that scene construction may be a process that underpins episodic memory and future thinking. First, the pre- and parasubiculum are also consistently activated in fMRI studies of autobiographical memory and imagination (reviewed in Zeidman and Maguire, 2016), and increased pre- and parasubiculum volume has been associated with the persistence of autobiographical memories over time (Barry et al., 2021). In addition, there is evidence that hippocampal activity during learning is related to imagery (Maguire and Mullally, 2013) rather than the formation of arbitrary associations between stimuli (Eichenbaum et al., 1992). For example, in an fMRI study, Clark et al. (2018) had participants encode pairs of words that described either scenes, or abstract concepts that were low on imageability. The anterior-medial hippocampus was engaged during processing of scene word pairs in comparison to abstract word pairs, despite binding occurring in both conditions. This was also the case when just subsequently remembered stimuli were considered.

In another study involving a large sample (n = 217) of healthy participants and multiple cognitive tests with a wide spread of individual differences in performance, Clark et al. (2019) performed a mediation analysis and found that the ability to construct scene imagery mediated the relationships between autobiographical memory, imagining the future and spatial navigation task performance. Put another way, these findings suggest that scene construction may be a significant cognitive process underlying the relationships between the different cognitive functions that are each associated with the hippocampus. The prominence of scene imagery was further emphasized in another study involving the same sample, where the explicit strategies used to perform autobiographical memory recall, future thinking, and spatial navigation tasks were assessed (Clark et al., 2020a). In each case, the use of scene imagery strategies was significantly higher than for all other types of strategies.

There are also strong parallels between the connectivity profiles of memory retrieval and the construction of scene imagery. As previously mentioned, the vmPFC has been found to drive hippocampal activity during autobiographical memory recall (McCormick et al., 2020), but this also seems to be the case during the construction of novel scene imagery. Barry et al. (2019) showed that during MEG,

scene construction was associated with theta power coherence between the anterior hippocampus and vmPFC, and that vmPFC activity also preceded and drove hippocampal activity during the generation of scene imagery. These neural dynamics have also been observed during MEG using an adaptation of the aforementioned paradigm (Dalton et al., 2018), where participants mentally constructed either a scene comprising three objects on a 3D background, or an array with three objects on a 2D background (Monk et al., 2021). Scene-related modulation of theta power in anterior hippocampus and vmPFC was observed during the early construction stage relative to array construction, again with hippocampal activity driven by the vmPFC (Figure 13.7).

In conclusion, hippocampal-damaged patients have wide-ranging impairments on tasks involving memory retrieval, future thinking, mind-wandering, dreaming, and the construction of scene imagery. Such findings, coupled with the comparable recruitment of the pre- and parasubiculum during autobiographical memory recall and the creation of novel scene imagery, and the observation of similar effective connectivity in both domains, suggest that a possible key contribution of the hippocampus to the generation of real or imagined events is the construction of spatially coherent scene imagery. Why might scene imagery be deployed so pervasively? The most obvious answer is that it mirrors how people experience and perceive the world. In pragmatic terms it makes sense that the neural hardware and software underpinning perception, including the hippocampus, would also be utilized during recall and for other mental representations where it would be advantageous. In

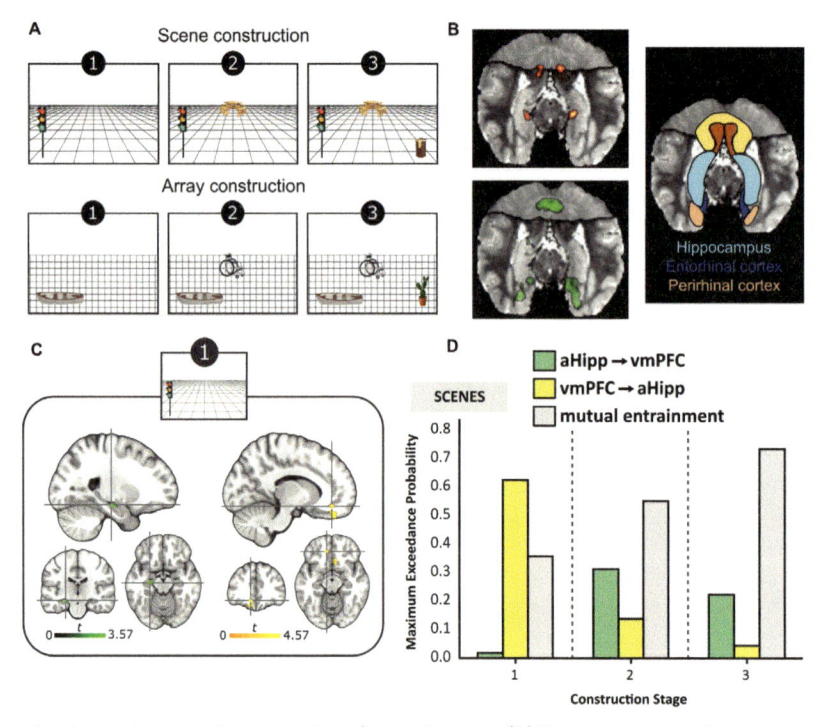

Figure 13.7 Hippocampal activity during the mental construction of scene imagery. (A) Participants mentally constructed scenes by sequentially imagining three objects on an imagined 3D grid while undergoing an fMRI or MEG scan (scene construction, upper panel). In a separate condition, participants imagined three objects against an imagined 2D background (array construction, lower panel). (B) fMRI analysis revealed that scene construction was associated with recruitment of the anterior medial hippocampus (upper panel), while array construction was associated with the activation of the entorhinal cortex and posterior hippocampus (lower panel). (C) Theta power changes in the hippocampus and ventromedial prefrontal cortex (vmPFC) were evident during the initial stage of scene construction compared with array construction. (D) Dynamic causal modeling of neural responses showed that the vmPFC drove the hippocampus during the initial stage of specifically scene construction. (Reproduced with permission from Dalton et al., 2018, and Monk et al., 2021.)

addition, scenes are a highly efficient means of packaging information. The apparent prevalence of scene imagery has even led some to suggest that it may be the currency of cognition (Maguire and Mullally, 2013). One such instance where the internal generation of scene imagery may be beneficial, is in navigating along routes from one location to another. In the next section we consider in more detail the contribution of the hippocampus to navigation, in both physical and abstract space.

13.4.7 Navigating in novel and familiar environments

The evidence assessed so far supports the idea that the hippocampus is involved in the encoding and retrieval of experiences, with an emergent view that it also supports the construction of imagined and future scenarios. Another essential behavior we must perform on a daily basis requires the successful integration of all of these functions, and that is the need to continuously navigate through space, planning and executing a route from one place to another (O'Keefe and Nadel, 1978). It is perhaps unsurprising, then, that given the impairments patients with bilateral hippocampal damage display on tasks assessing the aforementioned functions, that they also exhibit equivalently profound difficulties when trying to navigate an environment that has been experienced, even over a protracted period, following the onset of their lesions. One such patient, E.P., could not describe how to navigate to locations in his home neighborhood, despite having lived there for 6 years (Teng and Squire, 1999). Likewise, extensive attempts to teach patient K.C. how to navigate within a new building proved unsuccessful, nor could he display knowledge of the spatial layout of the library in which he had worked for 2 years (Rosenbaum et al., 2000).

These deficits appear to be related to the inability to learn new spatial information, rather than to navigate per se, because such patients seem to have a relatively preserved capacity to navigate around an environment that was learned long before hippocampal damage. Patient E.P. could describe how to navigate between his childhood home and other locations in the neighborhood. He could also plan a route between two locations in the area, even describing a detour when the main route was blocked. He could point in the direction of a specific landmark from the location of another landmark. Similarly, patient K.C. could also describe a route between two landmarks, including a detour via an alternative route. His performance in estimating the correct heading direction between two landmarks, or estimating the difference between them was also comparable to controls. These findings suggest that over time, the ability to navigate in a familiar environment becomes largely independent of the hippocampus, and that hippocampal damage does not preclude intact allocentric spatial processing. However, further investigations of remote spatial memory have revealed that it is not necessarily entirely spared following hippocampal damage.

Patient T.T., a licensed London taxi driver with bilateral hippocampal lesions, was tested on a virtual navigation task around London, a city with a complex layout that he had navigated for 40 years before his hippocampal damaged occurred (Maguire et al., 2006). While he could navigate successfully on well-practiced main routes, he became lost on minor roads, suggesting that detailed spatial knowledge was lost. More strikingly, despite having navigated certain routes perfectly, he could not visualize and describe such routes, indicative of an impairment in the construction of mental imagery related to the route, rather than the navigation of that route itself. Interestingly, the childhood neighborhoods of E.P. and K.C., about which they had apparently preserved information, were laid out in very simple, predictable grid patterns, unlike London, which may have masked the deficits that were detected in T.T. Taken together these neuropsychological findings suggest that allocentric spatial processing may be preserved in hippocampal-damaged patients, whereas egocentric representation of space may be more impaired in the context of hippocampal pathology, even in a highly familiar environment.

13.4.8 Navigation ability and hippocampal structure

The expertise of licensed London taxi drivers, therefore, allows for a more granular examination of the association between hippocampal integrity and the preservation of navigational ability. Taxi drivers in London train for many years to acquire "The Knowledge" of its 25,000 streets, their spatial layout, and associated landmarks. The slow and demanding acquisition of this knowledge also provides a unique opportunity to assess whether there is an association between navigational proficiency and hippocampal structure. Accordingly, it has been found that London taxi drivers have greater gray matter volume in their posterior hippocampus, but reduced gray matter in the anterior hippocampus, compared with healthy controls (Maguire et al., 2000), and even when compared with London bus drivers (Maguire et al., 2006b). The changes seem to be restricted to the spatial domain, as no such hippocampal changes were evident in the context of nonspatial expertise (Woollett et al., 2008). These structural differences are specifically related to the acquisition of The Knowledge, because a within-subjects longitudinal study involving trainee taxi drivers showed hippocampal volume changes after, but not before, training and successful qualification, compared with a control group (Woollett and Maguire, 2011). Therefore, the acquisition of spatial knowledge can show a striking relationship with the gray matter volume of the human hippocampus.

Attempts to demonstrate an association between navigation ability and hippocampal structure in non-taxi-driving healthy individuals have been mixed. Similar to the tasks performed by taxi drivers, Maguire et al. (2003) asked healthy controls to navigate to different locations by driving through a virtual environment. In these nonexperts, navigational accuracy was unrelated to hippocampal volume. This finding was subsequently confirmed in a larger sample of 90 healthy participants where participants learned two routes in a virtual environment, and their navigational ability was tested by asking them to point to particular landmarks elsewhere in the environment (Weisberg et al., 2019). An association between performance on this task and hippocampal volume was not observed. Definitive evidence to this end was provided by Clark et al. (2020b), who tested navigational ability in a large sample of 217 healthy controls. Participants watched a video of overlapping routes through an unfamiliar town, and were then tested on a range of spatial memory tasks. None of these measures correlated with hippocampal volume. Therefore, changes to hippocampal structure likely require extended and intensive spatial training in order to emerge.

13.4.9 Navigation as the crossroads of memory and imagination

Nevertheless, neuroimaging of both experts and healthy controls during navigation has revealed functional similarities in hippocampal activation. Spiers and Maguire (2006) tasked experienced taxi drivers with driving around a virtual recreation of London, simulating the delivery of passengers to particular locations, while being scanned with fMRI. Hippocampal activation was greatest during the initial planning of a route at the beginning of the journey. This observation suggests that the role of the hippocampus in navigation lies at the intersection of memory reconstruction and envisaging the future, and this prospective planning has also been decoded from hippocampal activity during navigation in healthy controls. Brown et al. (2016) had participants navigate from a start position to a goal that was on a path around a virtual circular arena. Along this route during the learning phase were distinct cues that could be decoded from patterns of hippocampal activation as measured by fMRI. During the initial phase of planning the best route to take, both the end-goal location and the intervening subgoal locations were more strongly represented in the hippocampus than alternative routes. Therefore, the hippocampus appears to rehearse the intended route before embarking on a journey.

In fact, the hippocampus may represent not just the most favored or intended route, but a number of potential avenues at the same time. Javadi et al. (2017) trained participants in situ to navigate around a spatially complex area of London, and subsequently asked them to make navigational decisions while watching movies of different routes through this environment during fMRI. As soon as participants entered a new street, the posterior hippocampus tracked the number of connected streets, or available routes to take. This effect was not observed in control participants who were untrained on the spatial layout, confirming that navigating participants were using prior experience to simulate a range of possible futures.

13.4.10 Hippocampal mechanisms underlying successful navigation

Studies of neural activity associated with spatial tasks during iEEG and MEG have revealed more about the mechanisms underlying successful human navigation. Bush et al. (2017) studied hippocampal activity in patients with implanted electrodes while they performed a spatial memory task. Patients navigated to the remembered location of an object within a virtual arena. Increases in low (2–5 Hz) and high (6–9 Hz) theta power in the hippocampus were associated with movement onset, and were sustained throughout long navigational paths, suggesting that theta power tracks self-motion throughout an environment. There is further evidence that hippocampal theta power contributes to successful navigation. Cornwell et al. (2008) used a human version of a virtual Morris watermaze task during MEG. Participants used cues to navigate to a hidden platform. Theta activity in the posterior hippocampus was negatively correlated with average path length, implicating this frequency in the efficient navigation of an environment.

While navigating in a virtual environment is different from moving through space in the real world, there is also evidence of theta power changes during real-world navigation. Aghajan et al. (2019) measured theta oscillations in the hippocampus of patients with intracranial electrodes, while they performed a navigation task in a real space that was augmented by virtual reality. Greater similarity between theta prevalence during encoding and retrieval was associated with superior navigation performance, suggesting theta power assists in the reinstatement of prior experience to aid

navigation. Further similar evidence, and echoing the fMRI findings that the hippocampus is involved in planning routes, was provided by Watrous et al. (2018). They observed that during the planning stage of navigation, the particular goal location of that trial could be decoded from neuronal activity during iEEG. More specifically, the firing of these neurons occurred at a specific phase of low-frequency 1–10 Hz oscillations. In other words, the hippocampus appears to represent prospective navigational goals through a unique neural code. It also appears that these unique codes are reactivated throughout the act of navigation. Kunz et al. (2019) trained patients with a range of intracranial electrodes to navigate through a virtual arena to the location of previously learned objects. Using a temporal similarity analysis, they found evidence for distinct representations of these objects throughout the brain. Each one of these goal objects was reactivated throughout the navigation process at distinct phases of the theta rhythm (3–4 Hz) in the hippocampus. In fact, the distinctiveness of these preferred phase reactivations was associated with better navigational performance in patients. The hippocampus, therefore, appears to help coordinate a detailed representation of the spatial environment during active navigation.

Of note, a similar pattern was also observed in the prefrontal cortex, where theta power tended to co-occur with that of the hippocampus. Large-scale reactivations of particular goal objects also occurred at distinct phases of the prefrontal theta rhythm, albeit within a faster oscillation (5–6 Hz). As was the case with the hippocampus, the distinctiveness of these preferred phase reactivations also predicted navigation performance. The co-occurrence of theta power in the hippocampus and prefrontal cortex has also been observed in healthy controls during a navigation task. Kaplan et al. (2014) reported increased theta phase coupling between the prefrontal cortex and the anterior medial temporal lobe during the planning phase prior to navigation toward a remembered goal. Therefore, as is the case with memory retrieval (McCormick et al., 2020) and imagination (Barry et al., 2019), the prefrontal cortex and hippocampus appear to cooperate in order to plan and execute a route through an environment.

While the available evidence supports a role for the hippocampus in simulating prospective routes, an obvious critical component of successful navigation is awareness of one's current position within an environment. There is evidence in humans that the hippocampus represents space in this manner. Ekstrom et al. (2003) had patients with implanted hippocampal electrodes play a virtual taxi driver game where they picked up passengers in one location and delivered them to another. Of the recorded cells in the hippocampus, 24% responded to the specific location of the patient in the virtual environment, suggesting this location information is continuously updated.

One feature of modern-day navigation, particularly in an urban environment, is that location is not exclusively restricted to a 2D plane, rather we are required to update our location within 3D space, such as the floor of a building. There is evidence in humans that the hippocampus also incorporates this additional dimension. Kim et al. (2017) immersed participants in a virtual environment during fMRI, where they moved through a 3D space on a rollercoaster-style vehicle. Multivoxel pattern analysis of fMRI activity in the hippocampus was deployed to determine if specific locations could be decoded. They observed the right anterior hippocampus was sensitive to changes in spatial location on the vertical as well as the horizontal plane.

13.4.11 Entorhinal cortex and the structure of physical space

The hippocampus therefore encodes a person's current position in multiple dimensions, and simulates future locations before travel, whereas there is evidence that the neighboring entorhinal cortex, which has strong bidirectional connections with the hippocampus (see Chapter 3), represents our surrounding space in a highly structured manner. Building on fMRI findings from Doeller et al. (2010), D. Chen et al. (2018) recorded directly from the entorhinal cortex in patients during iEEG, and asked them to perform a spatial navigation task in a virtual environment. Cells in this region increased their activity in a directional-dependent manner, firing at regularly spaced 60 degree angles. This sixfold rotational symmetry is taken as evidence that physical space is represented by the entorhinal cortex in a hexagonal grid that maps out the environment. As has been observed with other navigation tasks, this activity was confined to the theta frequency. The formation of these grid-like maps appears to take some time, emerging toward the end of training when the environment is more familiar. The effect was also observed to be stronger toward the edge of the arena, implicating a role for boundaries in the creation of these mental maps. Interestingly, Doeller et al. (2010) also found similar grid-like activity in medial prefrontal cortex, further emphasizing the close connection between this region and the medial temporal lobe.

Similar to the encoding of place in the hippocampus, these grid-like representations are not limited to navigation on a flat surface. Kim and Maguire (2019) trained participants in a 3D space during zero gravity in a virtual spaceship, and investigated the response of the entorhinal cortex to the direction that participants were facing as they moved throughout this space during fMRI. Entorhinal cortex signal was modulated based on the alignment to grid axes in three dimensions, suggesting volumetric space may also be mapped out in this way.

As is the case with the simulation of future routes by the hippocampus, grid-like activity in the entorhinal cortex is not limited to an actual position in (virtual) space, but can emerge during imagination. Horner et al. (2016) asked participants to learn six object locations in a virtual reality arena. Then, participants were required to either actually navigate between locations, or to imagine themselves doing so, while undergoing an fMRI scan. As expected, they observed sixfold rotational symmetry in the entorhinal cortex during actual movement. However, during imagined navigation, the same sensitivity to a grid-like structure in the environment emerged, with an offset of just 5.5 degrees from real navigation. Such grid-like modulation of entorhinal cortex activity was not observed during stationary periods, suggesting it is key to successful navigation, either real or imagined.

13.4.12 Mapping the structure of abstract knowledge

While the entorhinal cortex is involved in building a map-like representation of novel spatial environments to help us navigate through them, there is also evidence implicating this region in the application of a similar structure to acquired conceptual knowledge. Constantinescu et al. (2016) trained participants to navigate through a 2D conceptual space (Figure 13.8). The bird stimuli they employed could differ along two dimensions, the length of either their legs or neck. Participants imagined the birds morphing from one point in this feature space to another, akin to navigation in physical space. Using fMRI, they searched throughout the brain for a grid-like signal that would represent hexagonal symmetry within this 2D conceptual space; in other words, when participants imagined morphing birds along trajectories that differed by 60 degree increments. Similar to navigation in physical space, the entorhinal cortex signal was modulated by this sixfold symmetry. Moreover, a similar effect was found in the vmPFC, where the signal was aligned to the same angle, suggesting the two regions represent conceptual space in a structurally similar manner. Notably, participants who performed better at the task displayed stronger grid-like signals, highlighting the functional relevance of this organizing principle in supporting conceptual knowledge.

The entorhinal cortex also appears to arrange arbitrary stimuli into a map-like structure based on the sequence in which they are encountered. Garvert et al. (2017) presented participants with a series of object stimuli, ensuring participants' attention by simply asking them to identify whether a small gray patch was present on the stimulus in the previous trial. Unbeknownst to participants, the order of stimuli was not random, rather they were arranged in a latent map-like structure where there were a limited number of possible transitions from one stimulus to others. On a separate day, participants were shown stimuli from the same graph in a random order, representing small or large jumps through this map-like space. Repetition suppression, the attenuation of the fMRI blood-oxygen-level-dependent (BOLD) signal in response to stimuli presented adjacently, was used to test whether stimuli located closer together on this graph were represented more similarly in the brain. Despite participants being unaware of the hidden conceptual structure, signal in the entorhinal cortex was reduced for items that had fewer links to each other in the graph. This suggests that through the temporally proximal experience of previously unrelated stimuli, the entorhinal cortex automatically assembles this knowledge into a coherent structure that likely facilitates subsequent retrieval.

While much research on navigation through conceptual space has focused on traversing feature dimensions in the visual domain, the compiled structure of experience is not limited to this sensory modality. Bao et al. (2019) trained participants to mentally navigate through an odor space where the intensity of odors varied along two dimensions, banana and pine. During fMRI, navigation-related activity in the vmPFC was modulated by sixfold rotational symmetry in this 2D odor space. Multivoxel pattern analysis of the entorhinal cortex revealed that pattern similarity here was higher across trials that matched the preferred angle of the vmPFC, compared with trials offset by 30 degrees. Therefore, multisensory conceptual spaces appear to be constructed via a dialogue between the vmPFC and the hippocampal formation.

13.4.13 Computing the distance through conceptual space

While the entorhinal cortex helps to support a coherent map-like structure during learning, the hippocampus appears to be more involved in encoding distances through learned conceptual space. Theves et al. (2019) trained participants to associate object stimuli with specific abstract stimuli that varied along the dimensions of opacity and size. These abstract stimuli were therefore positioned in a 2D continuous space, and the participants learned to associate the particular object with this new location in this abstract feature space. After training, the objects were presented to participants during an fMRI scan to test whether objects that were

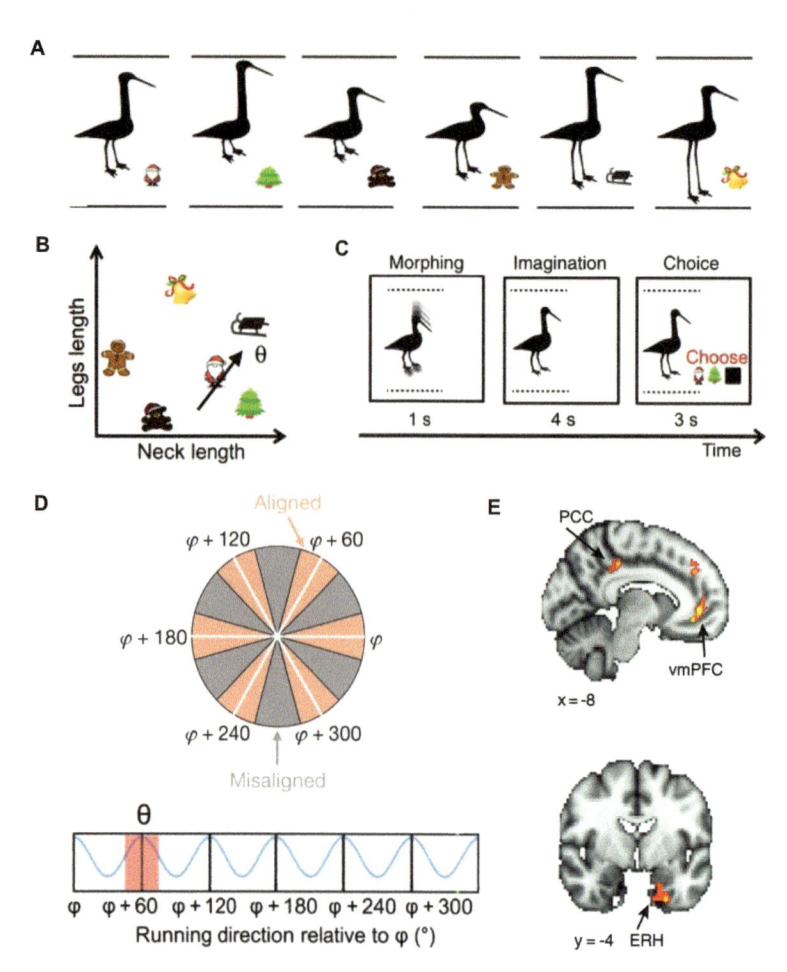

Figure 13.8 Grid-like coding of conceptual knowledge in humans. (A) Participants were trained to associate bird stimuli that had varying neck and leg lengths with symbols. (B) The symbols could be organized in 2D space with the associated neck and leg length on the two axes. The arrow indicates the potential trajectory when morphing one bird into another. (C) During an fMRI scan participants watched the leg and neck length begin to change and were asked to imagine the projected bird stimuli if the morphing continued, and to indicate if that projected stimulus led to a previously associated outcome. (D) Angles in 2D bird space could be aligned or misaligned with a hexagonal grid (upper panel). FMRI markers of grid cells showing hexagonal symmetry—the signal is bigger for trajectories aligned versus those misaligned with the grid (lower panel). (E) Hexagonal modulation of activity was observed in the medial entorhinal cortex (ERH) and the ventromedial prefrontal cortex (vmPFC). (Reproduced with permission from Constantinescu et al., 2016.)

trained to be close together in the associated abstract space were now represented more similarly in the brain than those further apart. In the anterior hippocampus, objects that were adjacent in feature space had more similar patterns of activation than those which were more distant, indicating the hippocampus is involved in restructuring existing knowledge to align with a learned conceptual space.

As with navigation through physical space, distance in conceptual space also seems to involve the theta rhythm. Solomon et al. (2019) had 189 patients learn series of word lists and recorded directly from the hippocampi during free recall following a delay. The conceptual distances between the stimuli in semantic space were calculated for each list using a method for creating vector representations of words based on regularities present in text corpuses. Just prior to the retrieval of each word, the magnitude of theta corresponded with the transition distance in this semantic space from the previous stimulus. In other words, the shorter the distance that had to be traveled in conceptual space from one word to another, the stronger the theta response. This effect, however, was only present along the primary dimension of that word list, representing

navigation through a one-dimensional semantic space. This suggests that when traveling through a conceptual environment, the hippocampus may favor a highly compressed representation of this space.

While it might be most efficient in some circumstances to navigate through a one-dimensional conceptual space, we may wish to switch our attention to different dimensions depending on the task at hand. Mack et al. (2016) investigated this issue by having participants allocate insects to particular categories that they could learn by attending to the morphology of insect features (Figure 13.9). However, the features that were useful for categorization in one task were not useful for another. Therefore, stimuli that were conceptually similar in one task due to sharing relevant features would become dissimilar in another task. Neural patterns in the anterior hippocampus indicated that conceptual space was reconfigured across the two tasks, such that attention was weighted toward different dimensions, despite the stimuli being the same. Furthermore, connectivity between the vmPFC and hippocampus was higher during early learning when compared with late learning, suggesting that the vmPFC may help to restructure

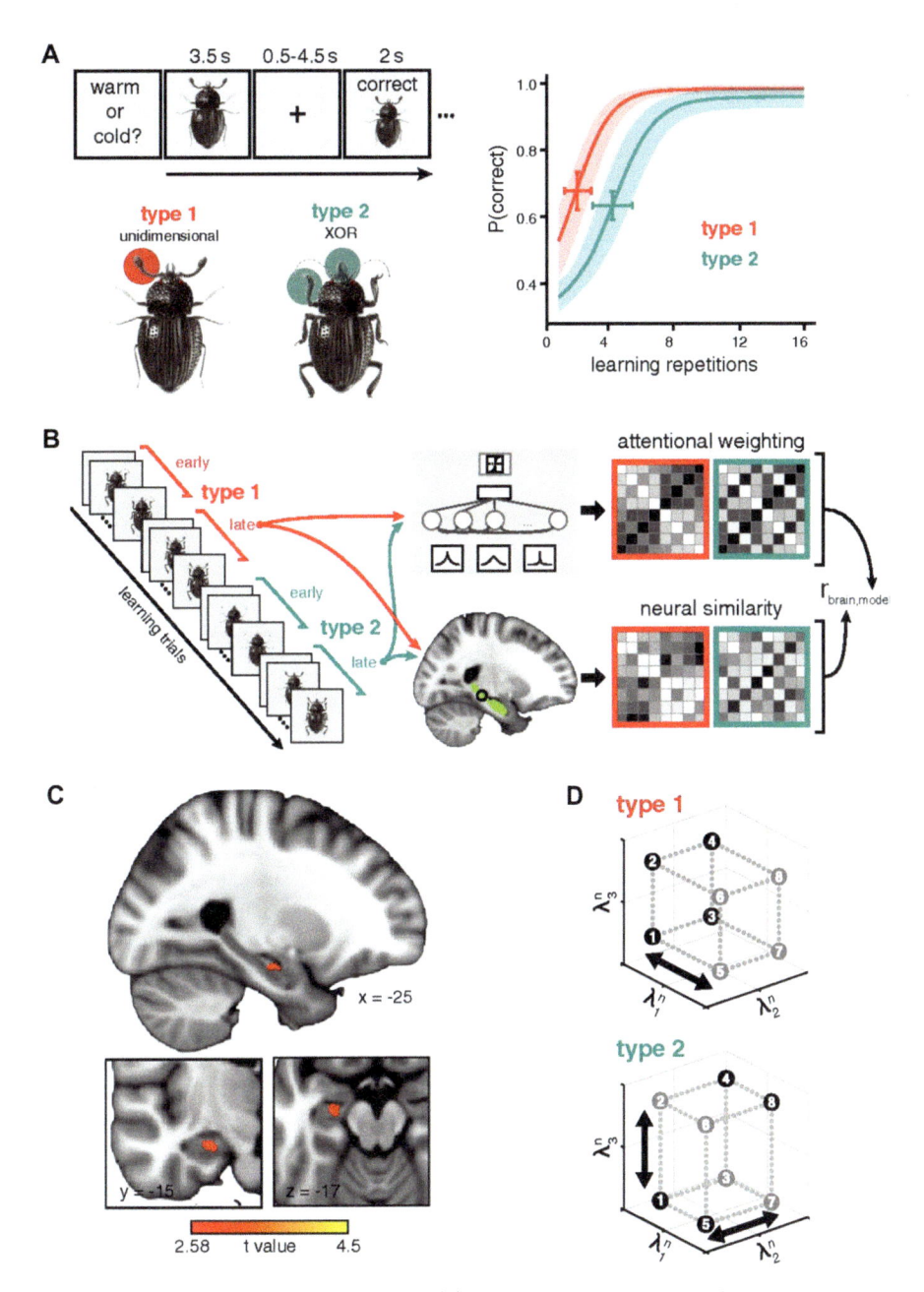

Figure 13.9 Updating of conceptual knowledge in the hippocampus. (A) Participants learned to classify insect images based on one feature, or a combination of two features. The two tasks were learned sequentially and required paying attention to different features of the same stimuli. (B) A model learned to classify the stimuli based on the task and was fitted to participants' behavior in order to generate representational similarity spaces. Neural similarity spaces were calculated by correlating the similarity of each stimulus in terms of hippocampal activity. Representational and neural similarity spaces were then correlated to assess where in the brain reflected the updating of conceptual knowledge. (C) Neural representations in the anterior hippocampus were consistent with model predictions of attention-weighted conceptual coding. (D) Neural representations from the hippocampus projected into feature space showed how stimulus space was reconfigured into task-relevant conceptual space. (Reproduced with permission from Mack et al., 2016.)

conceptual space when it is more useful to compare stimuli along different dimensions.

13.4.14 Navigating through social space

One important environment that we navigate on a daily basis is our social milieu. Kumaran and Maguire (2005) compared spatial and social navigation by asking participants to optimize routes either between their friends' London homes, so a spatial network, or between the same friends within their social network. The task in both cases was to get a virtual crate of wine from person A to person

B. On a trial tapping the spatial network, person A could live very close in physical space to person B, making the conveyance of wine easy between the two spatial locations. In contrast, on a trial tapping the social network, persons A and B may not be well acquainted with each other socially, and so to convey the wine between them may require passing it through other friends (nodes) in the social network. Spatial navigation within London was associated with increased activity in the hippocampus during fMRI compared with social navigation. More recent work, however, suggests a more nuanced story. Two important dimensions along which we can place others in our social network are affiliation and power, where affiliation reflects our desire to engage in personal communication with someone, and power the extent to which we would comply with their demands. Tavares et al. (2015) tasked participants with navigating through such a multidimensional social space by interacting with characters in a virtual environment. Novel characters would assume a neutral position in social space at the beginning, and the way in which participants chose to respond to these avatars in each interaction would shift that character along one of the two dimensions to a new location. This navigation through social space reflected the interaction between power and affiliation, and was tracked specifically by the left hippocampus.

One aspect of navigating a complex social landscape every day is that when we encounter new individuals and learn about their attributes and preferences, we often must compute how these relate to both our own and those of others who inhabit our social environment. Kaplan and Friston (2019) investigated such mental transformations by asking participants to rate their own preferences, those of close friends, and what they would consider the average preference, relative to the preferences of a new individual. Such a preference might involve eating a spicy food, for example. This task requires an existing knowledge of the distances between preferences for individuals and the self and, given a novel location in this social space (the new individual), to use these to navigate to a new relative position. The entorhinal cortex and subiculum displayed a strong relationship with participants' performance on this task, suggesting these regions assist in recalibrating distances in social space when we encounter new situations.

There is also evidence that 2D maps in social space can be constructed using limited information, and that subsequent navigation through this space can be supported by a grid-like code. Park et al. (2020) had participants learn the ranks of 16 "entrepreneurs" along two dimensions—popularity and competence. Participants learned these rankings through pairwise presentations of entrepreneurs' faces, and the two dimensions were learned on separate days. Participants were not informed that together the ratings on these two attributes formed a 2D social hierarchy, and each entrepreneur was located in a different part of this space. During fMRI participants had to choose the best business partner for a given entrepreneur given two possible choices. This decision would take into account the highest ranking on each dimension. Although participants were never exposed to the full 2D social hierarchy, the activity of hippocampal and entorhinal cortex voxels revealed that the closer entrepreneurs were located in this space, the more similar the neural representations. During the process of deciding the best partner for a given entrepreneur, participants had to navigate through the 2D space to the location of the partner, taking a route they had not experienced during training. As with navigation through physical 2D space, these trajectories could be represented in 60 degree angles in social space. Activity in the entorhinal cortex was modulated by this hexagonal symmetry, and the orientation of this grid aligned to a similar modulation in the medial prefrontal cortex. Therefore, grid-like modulation of physical, conceptual, and social space appears to be supported by similar representations in the hippocampal formation and the prefrontal cortex.

13.4.15 Decision-making

We have outlined how the hippocampus captures and updates representations of our environment, and how this knowledge can facilitate action, such as navigation toward a goal. In our daily lives, we are faced with continuous dilemmas, such as which route to take to get to our destination, or which food to order in a restaurant. To support such decision-making, we can draw on prior experience of encountering similar situations, and the rich representations of alternate scenarios that can be constructed by the hippocampus provide a possible mechanism to optimize this process.

There is evidence that the hippocampus facilitates deliberation prior to making decisions, as shown by Bakkour et al. (2019). Their study comprised two decision-making tasks. The first involved making a choice between two food items, where the preexisting value was known to participants. A second task required a perceptual choice about whether a display consisted of mostly blue or yellow dots. In both tasks, reaction times were longer when the decision was less obvious, indicating more extensive deliberation. For healthy participants who performed this paradigm during fMRI, activity in the hippocampus was more strongly correlated with reaction time for value-based rather than perceptual decisions. This suggests that the hippocampus draws more heavily on previous memory representations when they are useful for decision-making. Patients with hippocampal damage were also asked to perform the same tasks. While patients showed comparable performance to healthy controls on the perceptual task, a marked difference was observed on the value-based task. Patients took significantly longer to make these decisions, yet the increased deliberation did not boost their performance, and they were more stochastic in their responding. In other words, they were less sensitive to the differences in value that they had previously ascribed. Therefore, the hippocampus may be involved in the retrieval of prior experience to guide choice.

Additional evidence to support this thesis was provided by Mack and Preston (2016). Participants in their fMRI study learned to associate images of eight famous faces or places with a series of real-world objects. During a subsequent fMRI scan, they were presented with one of these objects and, following a 9-second delay, one of the items from the associated category. Participants had to indicate whether it was the correct place or face in the learned pair, or a lure item. During this delay period, the authors found evidence for item-specific reinstatement of places, but not faces, in the hippocampus. That is, the neural representations associated with the previously learned paired stimulus were reconstructed while participants were waiting for the probe stimulus to appear. The strength of the reinstatement of these neural patterns had a direct effect on subsequent decision-making. For example, in trials where the probe matched the learned place, stronger neural reinstatement of these stimuli in right CA1 facilitated rapid evidence accumulation and shorter response times. In contrast, weak reinstatement was associated with a need to gradually acquire more evidence to make a successful response. Therefore, successfully reconstructing previous experience in the hippocampus seems to facilitate effective decision-making.

In our daily lives, however, we can encounter choices that are novel, and in these circumstances drawing on direct prior experience is precluded. However, we are often able make these decisions with ease, and there is evidence that the hippocampus exploits the reinstatement of associations to facilitate this process. Wimmer and Shohamy (2012) trained participants to associate scene, face, or body part stimuli with colored fractals. Half of these fractals were subsequently paired with a reward. Then, in a decision-making task, participants were asked which of two stimuli they preferred from within the two sets. The tendency for participants to choose one of the face, scene or body part pictures that had been associated with a rewarded fractal was associated with increased activity in the posterior hippocampus. In other words, preferences "spread" to related memories through hippocampal mechanisms, offering one explanation as to why we can make confident decisions in novel scenarios.

Sometimes, in novel environments, the right option can be unclear, and it appears that the hippocampus helps to resolve such conflicts by attracting toward one option rather than another. This was examined by Steemers et al. (2016), who had participants learn the locations of four objects within two virtual environments. The same four objects were present in the two separate environments, but occupied different locations in each environment. Once the learning of these two environments was completed, participants were asked to place the objects in a series of four new environments that were linear morphs from the first learned environment to the second environment. Therefore, the participants performed the task in six virtual environments where the background landscapes gradually blended from one state, the first learned environment, via four morphed environments, into the second learned environment. However, participants did not replace the objects into locations that respected this linear transition of a gradual change from the first environment to the second environment. Rather, there was an abrupt shift in behavior between the two middle morphed environments, with participants tending to place objects closer to the initial locations in the original two learned environments on either side of this divide. Neural patterns of activity in the hippocampus reflected this sigmoid-like behavioral response, showing that representations in this region were attracted to one state or another where the choice between the two original learned environments was ambiguous. Participants who demonstrated the strongest sigmoid-like response in behavior also showed the strongest corresponding shift in hippocampal representations. Conversely, in the visual cortex, neural patterns respected the linear perceptual change in the environmental topography. Therefore, the human hippocampus displays attractor dynamics in memory when faced with ambiguous decisions.

While hippocampal reinstatement can help inform decisions, there is evidence of a two-way process, in that the act of decision-making itself can influence existing hippocampal representations. Luettgau et al. (2020) trained participants to associate originally neutral stimuli with different food items that were rated low, intermediate or high value. Following this Pavlovian learning, participants made choices between pairs of half of these conditioned stimuli. In a final decision-making task, participants chose between all pairs of stimuli. At this stage participants tended to prefer the items they had experienced choosing in the second phase of the experiment, indicating prior decisions, even without feedback, influence future behavior. The authors then investigated whether the act of choosing a stimulus more often also affected its underlying neural representations. Using repetition suppression, an fMRI approach where sequential presentation of associated stimuli can lead to a suppression of neural activity, they found that stronger associations emerged between the frequently chosen stimuli and their paired food items in the hippocampus, while the opposite pattern was present for the stimuli chosen less often, with a weakening of the original learned association. This effect was also present in the medial prefrontal cortex. Increased repetition suppression

following the additional choice valuation of stimuli also correlated with an individual participant's tendency to prefer the previously chosen stimuli.

Given the observed altering of memory representations in the hippocampus and medial prefrontal cortex in the aforementioned study, it is possible that a dialogue between the two regions facilitates decision-making. This was investigated in an fMRI study by Gluth et al. (2015), who trained participants to associate a food snack with a particular on-screen location. After a distractor task, they were shown highlighted locations and had to choose between the snacks that occupied these locations, a task drawing on prior memory representations. To manipulate memory strength during encoding, half of the snacks were exposed twice as opposed to once. Consistent with the idea that better-remembered stimuli are more likely to be chosen, participants showed a preference for the snacks presented more often during encoding, even if their value to the participant was the same. In a connectivity analysis, with the vmPFC used as a seed region, coupling with the hippocampus was higher when participants chose the better-remembered option, demonstrating that the medial prefrontal cortex and hippocampus interact to retrieve memories in the service of decision-making.

The mechanisms underlying this coupling were further revealed by Guitart-Masip et al. (2013) using MEG. In this study, participants were presented with three objects on each side of a screen. One of these groups contained a target object, and the participants had to select the group that contained it through a process of trial and error. The objects in each group were shuffled from trial to trial, and participants were deemed to have learned the rule after six consecutive correct responses. During this phase, where participants were performing better on the task, theta power was observed to increase in the anterior hippocampus and vmPFC. This theta power was negatively correlated with the number of decision errors, indicating its relevance for choice behavior. An analysis of theta phase synchrony with a seed located in the anterior hippocampus revealed increased coupling with the vmPFC. This coupling increased toward the end of the 2-second decision period, suggesting that the two regions interact to accumulate evidence from memory until a choice is made.

While the reconstruction of prior memory representations is useful for decision-making, there is considerable evidence that the hippocampus is necessary for constructing fictitious, future, and counterfactual scenarios. Often, we have to make decisions where the consequences have not been experienced before, and the potential outcomes must be imagined to help inform a rational decision. McCormick et al. (2016) investigated these processes with patients who had selective bilateral damage to their hippocampi. Deploying a moral decision-making task, they exposed patients to difficult scenarios designed to elicit high internal conflict. Such a scenario might involve (hypothetically) choosing whether or not to personally harm a single individual to save the lives of many people. While this is a difficult decision to make, it is also the more rational one. In contrast to healthy controls, patients with hippocampal damage were less likely to choose such a rational option, with their decisions guided instead by an aversive emotional response to harming anyone. Furthermore, control participants tended to visualize these scenarios in much greater detail than patients. These results suggest that an impairment in constructing detailed hypothetical scenarios, a known hippocampal function, has a detrimental effect on the ability to make rational decisions in morally ambiguous circumstances. Similar findings emerged in relation to counterfactual thinking, which involves reflecting on "what might have been." In two counterfactual thinking tasks, Mullally and Maguire (2014) found that patients with bilateral hippocampal damage performed comparably to matched controls in being able to determine plausible alternatives of complex episodes. A difference between the patients and control participants was evident, however, in the patients' subtle avoidance of counterfactual simulations that required the construction of an internal spatial representation.

In summary, in concert with the medial prefrontal cortex, the hippocampus has access to prior experience, and constructs scenarios that facilitate deliberation and decision-making across multiple domains, whether spatial, moral, or value-based.

13.5 Back to the future: predictive percepts

13.5.1 Memory-guided attention

At the beginning of this chapter we outlined how the hippocampus captures ongoing perceptual experience. Given that the hippocampus also helps to reconstruct the past, the two functions may combine to help focus attention toward relevant aspects of our environment, based on our previous experience.

Summerfield et al. (2006) investigated the influence of prior experience on attentional mechanisms. Participants were trained to locate an object within a range of scenes. Then, during a subsequent fMRI scan, participants were shown the same scene again, or a novel scene, and asked to detect when the previously encountered object appeared on screen. Participants were faster to detect the object when they had a prior memory of the scene on which it appeared. In addition, the hippocampus was more active during the memory-facilitated trials, and this activity correlated with the performance-enhancing attentional effect. Hence, reconstructed memories of scenes in the hippocampus boosted attention toward specific locations in the environment.

In the aforementioned study, participants were required to fixate in the center of the screen while attending toward objects in their peripheral vision. However, there is also evidence that memory reconstruction in the hippocampus guides visual exploration of the environment. Hannula et al. (2007) investigated this process first in healthy controls. The training task involved learning to pair faces with scenes. During a test phase, three faces were displayed with a single scene. When one of these faces had been shown with the displayed scene previously, participants spent significantly longer looking at it, highlighting an interaction between memory and visual sampling. This effect emerged naturally; regardless of whether participants were required to indicate they recognized the face. Furthermore, when participants were primed with the scene before the presentation of the faces, this behavioral effect was accelerated, indicating that the initial memory retrieval facilitated attention toward the associated face. The same task was then presented to patients with damage thought to be largely limited to the hippocampi. Patients did not display above-chance viewing of the correct matched face during the first 2,000 ms of presentation, and were also no better than chance at recognizing this face from the trio of faces. This suggests that the hippocampus is necessary for the successful retrieval of memory to guide viewing behavior.

Earlier in this chapter we also discussed subsequent memory effects in the hippocampus, that is, where activity in the hippocampus during the encoding of an event predicts whether the experience is subsequently remembered. Goldfarb et al. (2016) investigated whether hippocampal activity during encoding also predicted subsequent attentional effects. Participants performed a visual search task which involved looking for a rotated "T" in an array of distractors. As a specific search configuration was repeated throughout the experiment, participants became significantly faster at locating the target, indicating a facilitating effect of prior experienced context. The authors then analyzed the BOLD signal on a trial-by-trial basis, to determine whether the activity during one trial predicted attentional performance on a subsequent trial with the same configuration. In all hippocampal subregions, the BOLD signal on one trial predicted a boost in performance when that context was encountered again. Moreover, individual differences in the change in hippocampal signal throughout the experiment were correlated with the rate of learning across participants. Therefore, the state of hippocampal activity during learning predicts the extent to which attention is subsequently guided to the correct location.

The capacity of the hippocampus to facilitate memory-guided attention appears to also be determined by the state of neural representations during visual exploration. Aly and Turk-Browne (2016b) presented participants with images of a virtual art gallery during an fMRI scan. Each room contained a painting and a unique layout. Participants were shown a comparable sample image and asked to search throughout subsequent images for either a painting by the same artist, or a room with a similar layout. This task required the orienting of attention toward high-level features of novel stimuli. The same rooms were encountered in both tasks, therefore the task only differed in attentional demands. Patterns of neural activity in all hippocampal subfields were more similar within a task, than compared with a different task. Therefore, the hippocampus appeared to enter a state that facilitated attention toward particular dimensions of relevant stimuli, even if they had not been encountered before. This effect was greater when participants were searching for a similar room than a similar painting by the same artist. In addition, performance on the room task was associated with increased pattern similarity in subregions CA2/CA3/DG of the hippocampus. The stronger effect observed during the search for similar environmental topology emphasizes a role for the hippocampus in the processing of scene imagery.

These anticipatory representational states not only facilitate attentional performance but also "close the loop" in the sense of influencing whether the attended item is then subsequently remembered. After participants performed the virtual gallery task described above, they took part in a one-back task, and indicated whether the previous image contained a painting by the same artist or contained the same room layout (Aly and Turk-Browne, 2016a). Using the hippocampal attentional states from the first task as a template, they measured the extent to which hippocampal activity patterns matched that state for each item in the one-back task. This gave an indication of how strong the correct attentional state was in the hippocampus. Participants were given a surprise memory test afterward, and items that were subsequently remembered were associated with a stronger attentional state when the item was incidentally encoded. This effect was driven by patterns in CA2/CA3/DG. Taken together, these results indicate that prior experience can bias attentional states in the hippocampus, which in turn affects future memory and attentional performance in similar situations.

13.5.2 Generating predictive representations

Memory-guided attention is further facilitated by the capacity of the hippocampus to bias representations in other brain regions. For example, Hindy et al. (2016) trained participants to associate the same cue with different outcomes (stimulus A and B), depending on whether participants pressed a left or right key. Therefore, the same cue could elicit different expectations depending on the context of a participant's action. Using fMRI, they investigated neural activity in the hippocampus and visual cortex during this task. Neural patterns representing the full sequence of stimuli A and B were detectable in the hippocampus even if the second stimulus was never presented. This is consistent with a role for the hippocampus in pattern completion, and the effects were confined to areas CA2/CA3/DG and CA1. In contrast, there was stronger decoding of the outcome stimulus in areas V1 and V2. This suggests that the reconstruction of a sequence in the hippocampus biases the visual cortex to expect the next stimulus in that sequence. In support of this idea, more accurate decoding of the learned sequence in the hippocampus was associated with more reliable decoding of the expected stimulus in V1 and V2.

These predictions can also be cross-modal. For example, we may hear a sound that evokes a visual expectation, or vice versa. Kok and Turk-Browne (2018) presented participants with stimuli where certain shapes were more likely to be preceded by certain auditory cues. Therefore, an auditory cue would elicit an expectation of a specific shape even if it was not subsequently presented. Activity patterns in the hippocampus measured during fMRI revealed that the hippocampus represented the expected shape, rather than the presented shape, consistent with the idea that the hippocampus anticipates experience based on memory. These effects were observed in areas CA2/CA3/DG and the subiculum. The strength of these predicted representations in the hippocampus also correlated with a shift in decoding latency in the lateral occipital cortex between expected and unexpected shapes, providing further evidence for the facilitation of early visual processing by the hippocampus.

Given the role of the hippocampus in memory consolidation that we described earlier, one might expect that the relationship between predictive representations in the hippocampus and expectation effects in visual cortices strengthens with the passage of time. Hindy et al. (2019) investigated this by training participants to expect one of two stimuli to follow an initial cue depending on whether they pressed a left or right button, their actions, therefore, having a predictable outcome. In a nonpredictable control condition, pressing left or right in response to a different stimulus resulted in an equal probability of two cues. This task was performed twice, initially 3 days before an fMRI scan, and repeated with a new set of cues right before the scan. In the scanner, participants had to indicate the expected outcome for each cue by pressing left or right. After th3ree days, participants were significantly faster at responding to predictive cues, indicating offline consolidation of the task had taken place in the intervening period. In addition, connectivity between the hippocampus and visual cortex was higher during predictive actions compared with nonpredictive actions after 3 days of consolidation, but not immediately after learning. An analysis of the time course of the BOLD response also revealed that the visual cortex lagged behind the hippocampus during predictive trials from 3 days

previously, suggesting that the ability of the hippocampus to facilitate expectation in the visual cortex is further enhanced through offline consolidation.

While these studies suggest the hippocampus may be influencing early visual areas, it is also the case, as described throughout this chapter, that many functions of the human hippocampus, including memory, imagination, and decision-making, seem to depend on a dialogue between the hippocampus and vmPFC, with the latter often driving activity in the former. Consequently, we might expect the vmPFC to also display a similar preparatory attentional state. This was investigated by Günseli and Aly (2020) utilizing the same art gallery task as previously described (Aly and Turk-Browne, 2016a, 2016b). They searched for neural patterns associated with attending toward an artistic style compared with searching for a topographical layout of the environment. Both the hippocampus and vmPFC were biased toward the current task demands while in the process of attending toward different environmental features to search for a stimulus that matched the desired state. However, Günseli and Aly (2020) also investigated the preparatory period before each trial, where participants oriented themselves toward the task at hand. During this period, participants simply knew which type of trial was next, but did not yet know the artist or room type that they would be searching for. Both the hippocampus and vmPFC showed attentional effects for the upcoming trial, in that both regions were already biased toward the expected state. Therefore, both regions can enter a global attentional mode, which does not necessarily rely on the retrieval of a specific memory. Taken together, these results suggest that the hippocampus and vmPFC generate biased attentional states based on prior experience and current task demands that in turn activate and facilitate anticipatory representations in early visual areas to boost perceptual performance.

13.5.3 Detecting when prediction and perception deviate

The world, however, is not always predictable, and we often encounter surprising or novel information (van Kesteren et al., 2012; Fernandez and Morris, 2018). Recognizing when our environment deviates from the norm is an adaptive function, as new salient information may be important to notice. Just as the hippocampus is sensitive to expected information, it also seems to process these perceptual and contextual aberrations. The necessity of the hippocampus for this function was first demonstrated directly by Knight (1996), who asked patients with hippocampal damage to respond when they heard target computer-generated audio stimuli. On a random selection of trials, patients were also presented with unexpected stimuli, such as environmental noises. Unlike in healthy controls, where the presence of such deviant stimuli was associated with an evoked response in EEG, this novelty-related neural activity was dramatically attenuated in the patients. Subsequent fMRI investigations in healthy people have demonstrated that the hippocampus is sensitive to the mismatch between expected and unexpected information in a range of different contexts. For example, Strange and Dolan (2001) presented participants with a series of words in which there were embedded "oddball" stimuli. These could be perceptually different from the majority of stimuli because they were presented in a novel font, semantically deviant because they had a different meaning, or had an alternative emotional context because they were presented alongside aversive stimuli. fMRI scanning revealed that during the first exposure to the stimuli, the anterior hippocampus was sensitive to these deviant stimuli, and this response declined over subsequent fMRI sessions as participants began to expect the unexpected.

The aforementioned tasks demonstrate a hippocampal response to contextual novelty, where a stimulus appears out of place, however in our daily life we can also experience a different kind of surprise, when the expected order of events changes. Often, we associate the occurrence of one experience with the subsequent occurrence of another, with the hippocampus processing such learned sequences of events, as we have outlined previously. Kumaran and Maguire (2006b) investigated the hippocampal response to a change in an expected sequence. During fMRI, participants were presented with a series of objects superimposed on scenes. Participants were subsequently presented with the same objects, that could be repeated, completely rearranged, or the objects in the second half of the sequence switched places. In the latter task, the first half of the sequence set an expectation for the learned sequence to continue as it was originally experienced. When this expectation was not met, and participants encountered different objects than anticipated, greater activation of the left hippocampus was observed, indicating that it processes deviations of temporal order from experience. A subfield-specific investigation of associative novelty was conducted by Chen et al. (2011) and involved participants learning to associate faces and houses. During a later testing phase, participants were presented with one of these stimuli and had to imagine the associated stimulus from memory. Following this, they would either encounter the correct associate or a different one. Correct rejections of unexpected stimuli were associated with increased activity in CA1, suggesting such mismatch computations may be performed there.

A more fine-grained analysis of these computations was performed by Bein et al. (2020). Participants learned the layout of room images before an fMRI scan (Figure 13.10). During scanning, they were presented with an associated cue to help them recall the original room. They were subsequently shown a room layout that could be the original room, or contain up to four changes to the layout. Thus, participants were exposed to stimuli that differed from their original memory in a graded manner, from slightly unexpected to significantly so. Bein et al. (2020) compared neural patterns in CA1 during the cue presentation, when participants accessed the original memory, with the subsequent presentation of the altered room. An increase in the number of changes to the spatial layout in the room was associated with decreased pattern similarity between recall and perception, indicating that CA1 is sensitive to the degree of unexpected information. Therefore, such mismatch computations in the hippocampus may be a trigger to update prior representations, as generated predictions have not been realized in the environment and may no longer be useful.

As we have noted, the vmPFC seems to lead the hippocampus during memory and imagination processes, and there is evidence to suggest this region helps to facilitate a mismatch between prior and ongoing experience. Long et al. (2016) trained participants to associate words with images. Later, during an fMRI scan, images presented with the same words were either those expected from training, different but from the same category, or from another category entirely. They searched for evidence of predicted representations in a number of default mode network regions, including the vmPFC. The strength of predictions generated in the vmPFC was positively correlated with activation in the hippocampus when

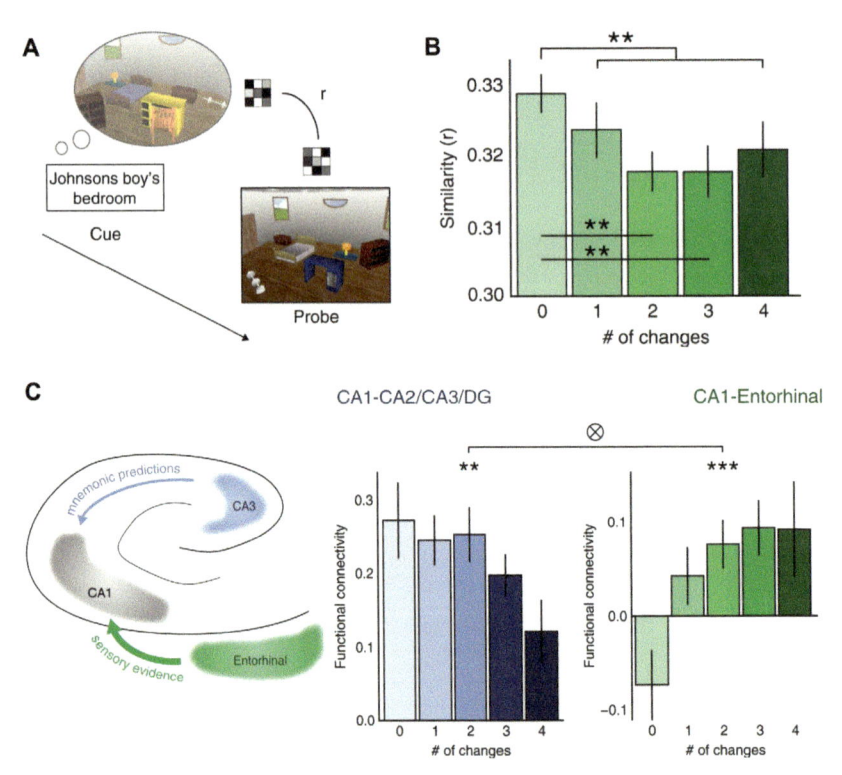

Figure 13.10 Mnemonic prediction errors in the hippocampus. (A) Participants retrieved memories of complex room images and were then presented with an identical or modified image. (B) Neural representations in CA1 were more dissimilar between the retrieved memory and the probe image when parts of the room were changed, consistent with a prediction error signal. (C) Functional connectivity between CA1 and CA3 decreased with the extent of prediction errors in memory, and connectivity between the entorhinal cortex and CA1 increased, reflecting the updating of new sensory information. (Reproduced with permission from Bein et al., 2020.)

unpredicted stimuli were encountered. This effect was observed for those trials during which the expected and perceived stimuli were similar, but not entirely different, suggesting the vmPFC may facilitate the recognition of minor deviations from predicted representations, and in doing so accurately disambiguate current from prior experience.

iEEG recordings have provided further insights into the neural processes underpinning the detection of unexpected information by the hippocampus. Axmacher et al. (2010) showed patients with implanted hippocampal electrodes a stream of images that were predominantly from one category (for example, faces), superimposed on a specific colored background (for example, red). These were interspersed with unexpected items (houses with a green background). The infrequent presentation of these unexpected items was associated with an initial increase in low-frequency theta power (3–8 Hz) between 200 and 400 ms, followed by a subsequent decrease. Higher-frequency gamma power (70–90 Hz) was also increased later in the trial. In addition, a late event-related potential in the hippocampus was observed in response to unexpected items at around 500 ms. This observed response later in the trial was associated with successful subsequent memory for these items. These results suggest that unexpected information is characterized by two stages of processing in the hippocampus. The first signal is related to the expected status of the presented stimuli, while the more delayed process likely facilitates the encoding of this novel information into memory.

While Axmacher et al. (2010) assessed contextual novelty, unexpected disruption to sequences of events is also associated with changes in hippocampal theta power. Chen et al. (2013) used a modified version of the task previously deployed by Kumaran and Maguire (2006b) with iEEG patients, where four items were presented in a sequence and subsequently re-experienced in either an entirely scrambled format, or where the last two stimuli were swapped around. This latter condition constituted a mismatch, where an expectation generated by the first two stimuli was violated. At the onset of this third unexpected stimulus, an increase in theta power in the hippocampus was observed, supporting a role for theta in sequence novelty as well as contextual novelty.

Garrido et al. (2015) also used the Kumaran and Maguire (2006b) task but this time in healthy participants during MEG in order to explicitly examine connectivity between the hippocampus and vmPFC. The expectation violation period constituted the time following the onset of the unexpected part of the sequence, and was associated with an increase in theta power in both the anterior hippocampus and vmPFC. An effective connectivity analysis showed that vmPFC drove the hippocampus during these unexpected events, suggesting that the hippocampal response to novelty is facilitated by input from the vmPFC. The prefrontal cortex may also help the hippocampus to shift from a predictive state into an encoding state during such novel events, as found by Gruber et al. (2018). They had patients with implanted hippocampal electrodes perform Axmacher et al.'s (2010) contextual novelty task, where faces and houses presented on colored backgrounds were presented with varying degrees of frequency to manipulate expected and unexpected events. They observed an increase in theta phase synchronization between hippocampal and prefrontal electrodes during the presentation of unexpected but not expected stimuli, consistent with the prior MEG results. In addition, phase synchronization for subsequently remembered unexpected items was higher

than those stimuli that were later forgotten. This is indicative of a hippocampal–prefrontal dialogue that switches from representing predictions to encoding novel stimuli when those predictions are not realized. In summary, the predictions generated from prior experience and used by the hippocampus not only serve to enhance processing of a known environment but also provide a backdrop against which novel salient information can stand out, and be highlighted as deserving attention and committal to memory.

13.6 Summarizing what we know

Our understanding of the functions of the human hippocampus has gathered pace over the last few decades. The most notable evolution in the literature is the acknowledgment that the hippocampus participates in a wide range of cognitive processes beyond episodic memory and retrieval. This region is actively involved in coordinating the visual exploration of our environment, whether we are static or moving through space. There is increasing evidence that maintaining complex, naturalistic information in working memory is heavily dependent on hippocampal integrity. The hippocampus also helps to support encoding sequences of events as they unfold, parceling ongoing experience into separate episodes, and committing these to memory. We know much more about the memory consolidation processes that occur shortly after an experience, when recent events are replayed in the hippocampus during rest and sleep. Such processes are essential in order to strengthen and reorganize information. Consolidation over time also facilitates the extraction of conceptual knowledge, and even benefits tasks that are not hippocampus-dependent. While the hippocampus is critical for the retrieval of rich, detailed memories, its contribution to mental life is not bound to the past. It is needed to construct a plausible future, imagine a fictitious scenario, and even contributes to day and sleep dreaming. The hippocampus is involved in aspects of navigating through an environment, including simulating possible routes. It is sensitive to positions in 2D and 3D environments, whether the space is physical or conceptual in nature. In summary, this brain structure plays a fundamental role in generating internal representations that help us anticipate our environment, direct our attention, and make decisions.

Advances in technology have helped to functionally dissect the human hippocampus, and there is a growing appreciation that the multiple subfields that constitute the hippocampal formation have unique roles to play in cognition. The DG separates out similar experiences during encoding and retrieval by orthogonalizing representations. A potentially important discovery relating to this region is its high neuronal turnover due to neurogenesis that may reflect dynamic functional changes across time in the hippocampal formation (see Chapter 9 for more on neurogenesis). Its close neighbor, CA3, appears to perform a complementary function, completing an entire representation from a partial input, and contributing to the precision of memory recall. Together, these regions appear to be biased toward particular attentional states to facilitate adaptive behavior. Area CA2 in the human hippocampus is not yet well studied, but may be involved in social memory as in animals. Area CA1 is involved in both the encoding and retrieval of memory, and helps to compute the overlap between expected and observed experience. The presubiculum and parasubiculum have received increasing attention due to their consistent involvement in tasks assessing autobiographical memory retrieval, future thinking, and the construction of scene imagery, highlighting these structures as potential hubs for scene-based cognition. Another consistent finding is the emergence of grid-like patterns of encoding in the entorhinal cortex, whether the task in question concerns physical or abstract space.

The segmentation of its subregions has also enabled us to start looking at intrinsic connectivity within the hippocampal formation, and connectivity between the entorhinal cortex and subfields such as the DG and CA1 appears to underlie memory encoding and retrieval. A coarser division of the hippocampus into its anterior and posterior segments has revealed some level of functional differentiation. The anterior hippocampus appears to be more engaged by the construction of scene imagery, decision-making, novelty detection, and computing distance in conceptual space. The posterior hippocampus appears to be more involved with working memory, navigation in physical space, and the retrieval of very remote memories.

A consistent theme across studies is that the hippocampus seems, on the face of it, to be specialized for processing stimuli that are spatial in nature. However, there is an interesting distinction that has emerged within this rubric, between scene processing and other types of spatial processing, and this gives rise to a tension in the literature that is particularly evident in relation to the human hippocampus. For instance, spatial information is undeniably strongly represented in the hippocampus during recall, and this is also apparent in anticipatory representations of the environment. The hippocampus is required in order to learn new spatial layouts of the environment, and there is evidence that goal locations and possible routes are simulated in the hippocampus. The hippocampus also tracks movement through space, and represents current spatial locations, whether these are in the horizontal or vertical plane. A central thesis here is that viewer-independent allocentric computations are necessary for these tasks, and that they predominate in the hippocampus. This spatial bias is particularly evident in the entorhinal cortex, where a grid-like structure of space is observed during viewing behavior, navigation through space, and imagined navigation, and is even manifested in the organization of conceptual space.

Despite these findings, however, it is now well established that some patients with selective bilateral hippocampal damage can in fact navigate effectively through environments learned long before the onset of amnesia, including describing possible detours. This is especially the case when the layout of environments is regular or major roads can be utilized. Particularly striking is the fact that such patients can also accurately complete other spatial tasks such as the estimation of distance and direction in these familiar settings, which rely on allocentric processing. Therefore, it appears that allocentric computations can be performed without a functioning hippocampus. By contrast, a more consistent deficit across hippocampal-damaged patients is an impaired ability, even during perception, to mentally construct and internally visualize specifically scene imagery. This deficit occurs regardless of whether past, present, future, or fictitious representations are involved. The perspective of scenes is egocentric in nature. This, coupled with fMRI findings that 3D space alone does not invariably engage the hippocampus, raises the possibility that egocentric hippocampal spatial representations may in fact underlie many of the aforementioned findings relating to navigation.

Much research has also focused on what happens to hippocampal representations between learning and retrieval, during offline states of rest and sleep. There is ample evidence showing that recent experience is replayed in the hippocampus, which generally helps to strengthen memory, reorganize it, and extract elements across multiple experiences. However, there is long-standing disagreement over the fate of hippocampal memory traces over the course of consolidation. While semantic memories can become independent of the hippocampus over time, it appears that autobiographical memories across the entire life span can be affected by hippocampal damage; however, the evidence is equivocal. The issue is complicated further by the discovery of high levels of neuronal turnover in the human hippocampus dentate gyrus, which calls into question the long-term viability of hippocampal memory traces. This has motivated an alternate perspective, that remote memories are reconstructed by the hippocampus—this accounts for the apparent need for the hippocampus in perpetuity, despite the lack of evidence for permanent memory traces residing there (see more on this and other perspectives in the next section). Furthermore, the distortion of remote memories and their vulnerability to misinformation aligns with this view. Evidence from fMRI studies supports a role for the hippocampus in the retrieval of detailed autobiographical memories across the life span, with some evidence that remote memories are represented even more strongly there, adding further credence to a reconstructive account, as remote memories may lean more heavily on reconstructive processes.

A recurrent observation about the human hippocampus is that its activity is closely coupled with that of the vmPFC across multiple domains. The vmPFC contains stronger representations of memories as they age, and appears to drive hippocampal activity during memory retrieval. A similar dynamic has also been observed during the imagination of novel scene imagery, with the vmPFC initiating scene construction. There is also evidence that the vmPFC structures information in a similar way to the hippocampal formation, as it contains grid-like representations of conceptual knowledge. Restructuring of this conceptual space is also facilitated by a dialogue between the vmPFC and hippocampus. The two regions appear to cooperate on a number of other tasks—connectivity is higher during decision-making, as the vmPFC facilitates the retrieval of memories to guide behavior. The vmPFC also enters an anticipatory attentional state relevant to task demands, similar to the hippocampus, and signals to the hippocampus when unexpected events are encountered.

Having attempted in this chapter to review decades of work that has examined the functions of the human hippocampus, and having distilled the points of particular note in this summary, we next consider how these findings are accommodated by extant theories of human hippocampal function.

13.7 Integrating the empirical and theoretical

Since the initial discovery that hippocampal damage results in profound anterograde and retrograde amnesia, a multitude of theories have been advanced to explain how the hippocampus is involved in the rapid formation and long-term retrieval of memories. An enduring perspective that forms the basis of many theories of hippocampal function is the indexing theory (Teyler and DiScenna, 1985). The basic tenet of this theory is that the hippocampus does not store a memory locally, but retains a record of the neocortical locations where the constituents of that memory reside. This view is motivated by the extensive afferent and efferent connections the hippocampus has with neocortical association areas. The proposal is that during the encoding of a new experience, a unique distributed pattern of activity forms across the neocortex. This is relayed to the hippocampus, where both the activated locations in the brain, and temporal dynamics of that event, are encoded in a unique neuronal ensemble. If part of this event is subsequently presented as a cue, this should lead to the hippocampal index being evoked, which in turn activates the relevant original locations in the neocortex to help recall the entire memory. In essence, the indexing theory maintains that efferent hippocampal connections are able to reaccess the cortical locations that originally communicated the event via its afferent connections.

While this idea has featured in many theories of hippocampal functioning (Eichenbaum et al., 1992; O'Keefe and Nadel, 1978; Schacter et al., 1998; Squire, 1992), there is still a lack of empirical data to support the existence of an index. Furthermore, memories become more reliant on different neuronal populations within the posterior hippocampus as time goes on (Bonnici, Chadwick, Lutti, et al., 2012; Bonnici et al., 2013), while the vmPFC assumes a greater role in supporting remote memories (Bonnici, Chadwick, Lutti, et al., 2012; Bonnici and Maguire, 2018), and drives hippocampal activity during retrieval (McCormick et al., 2020), features and processes for which the indexing theory cannot fully account.

Another controversial aspect of the indexing theory concerns how long such hypothetical traces persist within the hippocampus. This has relevance for a related prominent account of hippocampal function, the standard consolidation theory (Squire, 1992) that proposes the hippocampus rapidly encodes what is termed "declarative memory." This encompasses consciously accessible memories that can take many forms, such as an event, faces, spatial layouts, odors, or sounds, but also facts about the world. An important distinction is made between these representations and nondeclarative memories, which could still be learned in the absence of a functioning hippocampus, such as the acquisition of a motor skill (Milner, 1965; Brooks and Baddeley, 1976), eyeblink conditioning (Daum et al., 1989), and priming (Haist et al., 1991). Another important feature of the standard consolidation theory is that no distinction is made between recalling information freely from memory, and recognizing such information on its presentation, in terms of the level of hippocampal involvement.

However, the most controversial tenet of the standard consolidation theory is that the hippocampus only stores memory traces or memory indices for a period of time. This is supported by observations that patients with hippocampal damage cannot remember facts about the world (Manns et al., 2003), or personally experienced events (Kirwan et al., 2008) from a period of time just before the lesions occurred, but access to earlier memories is purported to be preserved. This loss of recent memories despite the apparent preservation of older memories is termed "temporally graded retrograde amnesia" (RA: Ribot, 1891). In the case of extensive hippocampal damage, the standard consolidation theory posits that the RA covers periods of at least one decade. It is also argued that over this lengthy period of time, a consolidation process occurs whereby connections between neocortical areas strengthen, and these new indices support the retrieval of older memories. The hippocampus is therefore deemed nonessential for accessing older memories, serving only as a temporary store.

However, a large number of patients with focal bilateral hippocampal damage have been identified whose behavioral deficits do not support a number of core predictions of the standard consolidation theory (e.g., Cipolotti et al., 2001; Rosenbaum et al., 2008; Maguire et al., 2006a; reviewed in Winocur and Moscovitch, 2011). Nadel and Moscovitch (1997) highlighted that retrograde amnesia for autobiographical memories often extends for many decades, or an entire lifetime. They not only deemed this length of time implausible for a consolidation process to occur but also noted that it also renders such a process redundant, as memories would retain their hippocampal dependence across most of a human life span. Therefore, the hippocampus is unlikely to operate as a temporary memory store.

A second observation of Nadel and Moscovitch (1997) is that memory for semantic information, such as public figures or events or facts about one's own life, tend to show a different temporal gradient, in that remote memories for this kind of information are less affected by hippocampal damage (Rempel-Clower et al., 1996). This challenges the view that all types of declarative memory are equivalently dependent on the hippocampus. The idea that memory is multifaceted was given particular impetus by Tulving's (1972) distinction between episodic memories, which relate to temporally dated events and the relationships between these events, and an independent system of semantic memories, which comprise words, rules, and concepts. This dichotomization maps well onto the different temporal profiles of hippocampal-related amnesia, in that episodic memories in particular appear to remain hippocampal-dependent over time.

Based on this evidence, Nadel and Moscovitch (1997) put forward the alternative multiple trace theory to characterize hippocampal function. According to this view, experiences are rapidly encoded as a neuronal ensemble in the hippocampus, which serves as an index to neocortical locations that represent the elements of experience. The hippocampus provides the spatial context to such an experience. When that memory is recalled later, a similar ensemble of neocortical and hippocampal neurons is activated, and thus a novel, but overlapping, index is formed in the hippocampus. The creation of these multiple indices to support an event are proposed to account for the patterns of deficits that are not explained by standard consolidation theory. Older memories, through many reactivations, contain multiple traces and are therefore more likely to survive partial hippocampal lesions but not more extensive damage. A semantic memory, which is derived from these episodes, can be extracted from multiple related traces, and is stored outside of the hippocampus.

A key feature of the multiple trace theory is that the spatial context of an event and all its related details are stored permanently in a hippocampal-neocortical ensemble. One challenge to multiple trace theory is that key aspects of remote spatial memory appears to be relatively unaffected by hippocampal damage (Maguire et al., 2006; Rosenbaum et al., 2000; Teng and Squire, 1999), which suggests that forms of contextual memory become hippocampus-independent. A subsequent evolution of this theory, the trace transformation hypothesis, attempts to address this by proposing that over the course of consolidation, a schematic, impoverished version of these memories form independently in the neocortex (Winocur and Moscovitch, 2011). While these memories can be retrieved in the absence of a functioning hippocampus, and superficially give the impression that the remote memories are unaffected by hippocampal damage, they are in fact stripped of their detailed spatial context when carefully probed.

Another prediction of multiple trace theory is that remote memories would be spared by smaller hippocampal lesions due to the multitude of traces supporting them. However, even highly selective lesions to the hippocampus can cause profound remote autobiographical memory loss (Miller et al., 2020). Another criticism of multiple trace theory is it does not adequately account for the phenomenon of forgetting. Contextual binding theory (Yonelinas et al., 2019) agrees with multiple trace theory in regarding the hippocampus as a permanent memory store, particularly for associations that are complex in nature (Yonelinas, 2013). However, this theory goes further by proposing that forgetting occurs when interfering information is presented during postencoding activity of the hippocampus (Tambini and Davachi, 2013). In a similar way, proponents of contextual binding theory propose that sleep actually preserves memory due to protecting against interference. However, the memory-enhancing effects of sleep suggest additional processes might be at work (see Schapiro et al., 2017). An additional challenge to both multiple trace and contextual binding theory, which both support a role for permanent hippocampal memory traces, is the mounting evidence that hippocampal representations are highly unstable over time, both functionally and structurally (Barry and Maguire, 2019a, 2019b; but see Moscovitch and Nadel, 2019).

While the debate concerning the stability of hippocampal memory traces continues, other theorists have focused on the flexibility of the memory representations themselves, and how this property supports adaptive behavior. Eichenbaum et al. (1992; see also Cohen and Eichenbaum, 1993) elaborated on prior theories which asserted that the hippocampus was responsible for declarative memory, or the encoding of both facts and events. They emphasized a core feature of hippocampal memory, namely that it concerns the relationships between multiple items and events. In addition, the hippocampus also stores the sequence in which these events occur (Eichenbaum, 2003). What emerges from these properties is a multidimensional "memory space," a conceptualization of hippocampal function shared by other theorists (e.g., Ekstrom and Ranganath, 2018). The nature of this highly interconnected space implies there are multiple ways in which the same memory can be accessed, such as by different kinds of external sensory or internal cues. The relational property of memory storage also allows for their flexible manipulation, in that what has been learned can be recombined, and transferred to a novel context to support adaptive responses. New experiences are rapidly woven into this existing knowledge store and, with the strengthening effects of repetition and re-exposure, they can endure for a lifetime. Another property of the complex web of memories stored in the hippocampus is that the activation of one memory can trigger the activation of another through their overlapping elements. Therefore, the idea is that we can transition easily from one episodic memory to another through these linking features.

Elaborating further on the different formats of relational memory, Eichenbaum (2017) proposed three structures on which memories in the hippocampus are organized. The first refers to the ability to infer associations across separate memories by realizing the common elements that link them together, a process purported to be hippocampus-dependent (Zeithamova et al., 2012). The second organizing principle is time, in that the hippocampus is necessary for the encoding of sequences of events (Dede et al., 2016). The third is schematic organization, where events that initially appear disconnected can become represented more similarly in the hippocampus as they are integrated via an overall narrative (Milivojevic et al., 2015).

A limitation of relational memory theory, and similar perspectives, is the core assumption that the hippocampus binds together arbitrary items and contexts, irrespective of their nature. This limitation is evident in the preferential hippocampal engagement observed during the learning of pairs of concrete as opposed to abstract words during fMRI suggests the hippocampus is geared toward highly imageable stimuli and not associative processing per se (Clark et al., 2018). Moreover, the mental construction of scenes composed of three objects and a 3D space compared with arrays that were composed of three objects and a 2D space gave rise to increased engagement of the anterior medial hippocampus (Dalton et al., 2018; see also Monk et al., 2021). The scene and array stimuli were highly matched in terms of content and the associative and constructive processes they evoked. This also suggests that more complex processes are at work than simply binding arbitrary items together.

Flexibility as a core feature of a useful memory system is a sentiment also shared by the constructive episodic simulation hypothesis of memory (Schacter et al., 1998). This approach takes into consideration the observation that memory is not a perfect reproduction of the original experience, but can be distorted and error prone. This view incorporates fundamental principles of other theories, namely that encoded experience consists of a range of features constituting an event that are widely distributed throughout the brain. Each novel representation is represented by a unique hippocampal index that binds these features together, while keeping them separate from other experiences. The retrieval of a specific memory relies on the proposed hippocampus-dependent process of pattern separation. However, memory retrieval is often flawed. Participants, simply through imagining an event, can find it difficult to distinguish it from an actual memory if it contains self-relevant details (Desjardins and Scoboria, 2007). Participants can also falsely endorse that they have heard an item that is semantically similar to those from a previous list (Roediger and McDermott, 1995).

According to the constructive episodic simulation hypothesis, these phenomena represent a failure of pattern separation, where previous memories lose their individuality and become gist-like, thus similar experiences will be falsely recognized as real. Accordingly, amnesic patients make fewer of these errors (Schacter et al., 1996). However, these distortions are thought to reveal a key property of episodic memory, that it is constructive in nature, in that the recall of the past involves the bringing together of various learned features. Furthermore, rather than being detrimental to daily functioning, the tendency of memory to become gist-like can be highly beneficial in situations where veridical retrieval of the past does not lead to optimal solutions. For example, we are often required to imagine alternative scenarios, or simulate a plausible future. Such a process, it is argued, requires the flexible recombination of previous memories into a new event. This self-projection across time is thought to be dependent on a core network of brain regions including the hippocampus. Hippocampal damage results in an inability to imagine one's future (Tulving et al., 1988; Hassabis et al., 2007a). Moreover, the hippocampus has been observed to be activated during recall of the past and imagination of the future (Addis et al., 2007), with some finding that it is more strongly recruited for future projection (Weiler et al., 2010).

However, the constructive episodic simulation hypothesis does not account for the deficits hippocampal-damaged patients display in constructing entirely fictitious scenes, rather than ones from their past or personal future that could not be a recombination of previous memory traces (Hassabis et al., 2007a). In addition, this theory does not adequately explain the frequent observation that the hippocampus is more sensitive to spatial as opposed to other kinds of stimuli, particularly in perceptual tasks where memory processes are not required (McCormick et al., 2017).

This apparent sensitivity to spatial information is a theme apparent throughout the literature on human hippocampal function. Separate lines of thought have converged on this as a fundamental organizing principle around which hippocampal representations are formed. The cognitive map theory is one such account (O'Keefe and Nadel, 1978). Echoing other theoretical positions, this theory proposes a dichotomy between memory for items that are stored independently of the spatial and temporal context in which they were encountered, and memory for events and items that are bound to a specific context. The latter kind of memory is proposed to be stored in the hippocampus, and multiple routes of access to a single memory, along with its time and place, are available. The key feature of this theory is that hippocampal memories are arranged in the form of a map. This is most obviously pertinent to memory for space, in that the physical environment is stored as an internal representation in which the spatial relationships between elements are encoded. More specifically, these representations are proposed to be stored in a way that is allocentric and so independent of the observer's perspective.

According to the cognitive map theory, we have the capacity to move items around the map, or recombine them, which underlies our capacity for imagination (Byrne et al., 2007; O'Keefe and Nadel, 1978). Our ability to reconstruct a scene from memory is proposed to involve accessing the spatial relationships between all the relevant items. However, nonspatial, or semantic maps are also proposed (O'Keefe and Nadel, 1978). These represent conceptual spaces, where an entity such as a person could be located, or move around. Thus, damage to the hippocampus is predicted to disrupt both kinds of cognitive maps, that is, the ability to learn and remember spatial environments and routes, and to reconstruct a verbal narrative of experience.

In line with some of the predictions of the cognitive map theory, patients with hippocampal damage fail to learn how to navigate new environments, even after years of exposure (Teng and Squire, 1999; Rosenbaum et al., 2000). Recent supporting evidence for semantic maps in the hippocampus has shown that the region helps navigation around, and distance estimation within, conceptual (Theves et al., 2019), semantic (Solomon et al., 2019), and social spaces (Tavares et al., 2015). However, the ability of some patients with focal bilateral hippocampal damage to use mental maps acquired long before the onset of their amnesia, and their preserved ability to perform challenging allocentric tasks, questions the idea that the hippocampus is a neural locus for allocentric maps of naturalistic spatial environments.

An alternate perspective has emerged on the role of the hippocampus that has been inspired by a more reliable deficit displayed by hippocampal-damaged patients that, while involving a spatial element, does not have space alone at its core. The capacity to mentally construct scene imagery is impaired following hippocampal damage (Hassabis et al., 2007a). As noted previously, a scene is defined as a naturalistic 3D spatially coherent representation of the world typically populated by objects and viewed from an egocentric perspective (Dalton et al., 2018; Maguire and Mullally, 2013). This deficit applies to the generation of completely novel scenes (so not a memory task per se), and is comparable whether the scene is generic in nature or a plausible one from the future. This indicates the impairment is unrelated to self-referential processing or the use of temporal information. It also stresses the egocentric nature of hippocampal representations, in contrast to the allocentric emphasis of the cognitive map theory. As patients have no difficulty imagining novel objects, their deficit is not related to the capacity to imagine per se, but rather to the specific ability to construct and internally visualize scene imagery.

Hassabis and Maguire (2007; see also Maguire and Mullally, 2013; Zeidman and Maguire, 2016) proposed that the hippocampus is responsible for the process of constructing scene imagery. Accordingly, the hippocampus is recruited in healthy controls during the recollection, imagination, or perception of scenes (Hassabis et al., 2007b; Zeidman and Maguire, 2016; Zeidman, Mullaly, et al., 2015; Zeidman, Lutti, et al., 2015). As noted above, Dalton et al. (2018; see also Monk et al., 2021) confirmed the scene-specificity of the hippocampal response by comparing scene and highly matched array construction. They found that it is specifically scene representations that consistently engage the hippocampus.

Scene construction as a process may address a number of the issues raised by ongoing theoretical debates into the function of the hippocampus. An inability to construct spatially coherent scenes may account for the flat gradient of retrograde amnesia commonly observed following hippocampal damage. As similar processes are proposed to underlie thinking about future, or fictitious events, these deficits are also predicted by the framework. Similarly, the association between spatial stimuli and the hippocampus could, in fact, reflect our lived experience of the world that comprises a series of scenes that are perceived between the interruptions imposed by eye blinks and saccades. In addition, the apparent preservation of allocentric information following hippocampal damage (Maguire et al., 2006; Rosenbaum et al., 2000; Teng and Squire, 1999) suggests hippocampal constructions may be egocentric in nature. Furthermore, recent evidence that hippocampal memory traces are temporary despite its continuing involvement in supporting remote memories (Barry and Maguire, 2019a, 2019b), necessitates an account of hippocampal functioning that is fundamentally constructive. Additional evidence in support of this theory arises from self-report measures of memory, prospection and navigation tasks, where individuals describe the use of scene imagery as their primary cognitive strategy (Clark et al., 2020a).

In summary, for many years, the hippocampus was conceptualized solely as a temporary store for declarative memory, however, as new evidence has emerged, our understanding of its functions has expanded beyond the mnemonic alone. The hippocampus appears to be involved in the reconstruction of memories regardless of their age, while also supporting various aspects of perception, imagination, navigation, and future thinking. Theoretical frameworks have also evolved and been newly developed to accommodate these discoveries, seeking to provide a perspective that can accommodate the totality of this new evidence. But of course, these vigorous theoretical debates expose the fact that many gaps in our knowledge still remain. In the next, and final, section we suggest several avenues that might be pursued in order to push our understanding of the functions of the human hippocampus even further.

13.8 Looking forward

In recent years there has been much focus on the functions of individual subfields of the human hippocampus, however, this has largely been limited to domains with which the hippocampus is conventionally associated, namely that of memory encoding and retrieval. More work is needed to establish their exact roles in other functions such as perception, attention, future thinking, decision-making, and navigation in various spaces. A particular barrier to progress in understanding human hippocampal subfield function is that they have been challenging to separately delineate in structural MRI brain scans. For example, the DG and CA3 are often analyzed together, despite the fact that quite different functional roles have been theoretically assigned to them. Likewise, the subiculum and presubiculum/parasubiculum are often difficult to differentiate and are therefore frequently analyzed as a unitary region. Addressing these issues involves developing improved subfield segmentation protocols, some of which are already available (e.g., Dalton et al., 2017; see also Yushkevich et al., 2015). Moreover, it is now also possible to automatically segement the hippocampal subfields (e.g., Hickling et al., 2024). However, further work, assisted by ultra-high-resolution (e.g., 7 T and above) MRI scanning, could help achieve a clearer understanding of the precise contributions of specific subfields to cognition (Figure 13.11).

Likewise, although some progress has been made in characterizing the intrinsic connectivity of hippocampal subfields during the performance of memory tasks and during rest, capturing the changes in this connectivity profile within the hippocampus across a range of tasks is necessary to understand how these regions cooperate in the service of cognition. In addition, the anterior and posterior hippocampus may display different intrinsic and extrinsic connectivity, which will further illuminate their differential functions.

Of particular interest is the connectivity between the hippocampus and medial prefrontal cortex, especially the vmPFC. Although the two regions cooperate to support many different functions, the functional connectivity between the vmPFC and hippocampus has yet to be systematically mapped out and understood, which may provide an insight into the underlying processes and whether they differ across cognitive domains. In particular, vmPFC, although often treated as such, is not unitary and comprises distinct subregions about which we know very little, let alone how they interact with specific hippocampal subfields. Ultra-high-resolution MRI will be invaluable here also, as it is now possible to examine BOLD activity within specific layers of the medial prefrontal cortex. Gaining insights into how the range of cognitive functions with which it has been linked play out within its microcircuitry could revolutionize our understanding of its contributions and, by extension, that of the hippocampus.

Ultra-high-resolution MRI may also help to advance long-standing debates. Contemporary theories of hippocampal function agree that the hippocampus is necessary for remote memories, however, there is also strong evidence that memory traces in the hippocampus are unstable over time. High-resolution functional imaging

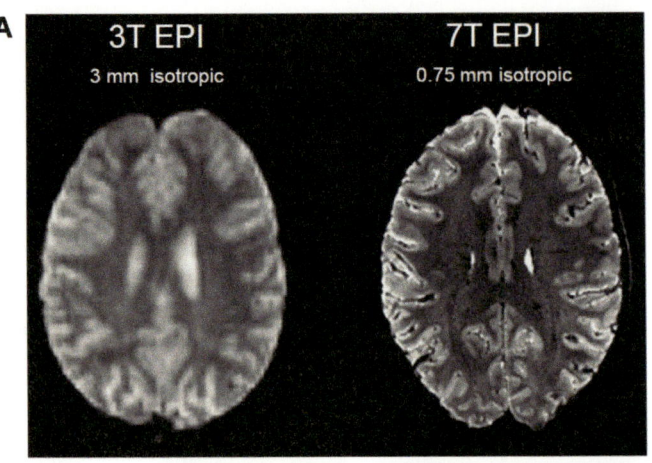

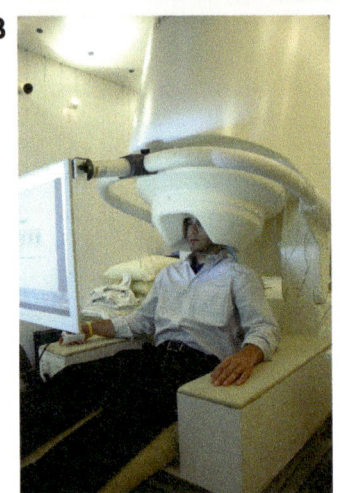
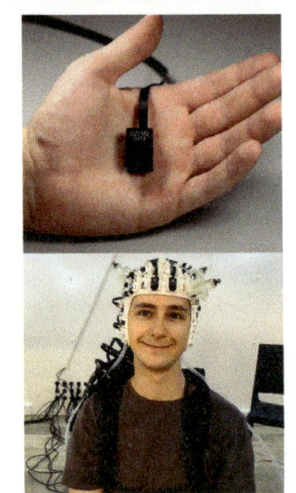

Figure 13.11 Advances in the methods used for studying human hippocampal function. (A) Standard 3T (left panel) and ultrahigh resolution 7T (right panel) axial echoplanar (EPI) functional MR images, with the greatly increased spatial resolution of the 7T image clearly evident. (Courtesy of Christina Triantafyllou, Siemens Healthcare GmbH.) (B) Standard SQUID magnetoencephalography (MEG) (left panel). (Courtesy of the National Institute of Mental Health, National Institutes of Health, Department of Health and Human Services.) Optically pumped MEG (right panel) with an example small, lightweight sensor (upper panel) and a full-head sensor array with the participant free to move (lower panel).

will yield detailed activity patterns related to individual memories that can be localized to hippocampal subfields, and vmPFC cortical layers, with high precision. This will allow us to track the signatures of remote memories over time in unprecedented detail, and reveal the extent to which older memories are reconstructed, particularly in regions such as the DG. This kind of high-resolution scanning brings us closer to the spatial specificity of animal research and helps to bridge the gap across species.

This gap can be closed further by technologies that mirror the precise interventions and measurements observed in rodent studies. Recordings from the hippocampus, vmPFC, and other cortical regions in patients with intracranial electrodes can help to characterize the responses of individual cells to stimuli, and measure the activity of groups of neurons with millisecond temporal accuracy. This approach can, for example, target hippocampal subfields with high spatial accuracy, and also harness a high temporal resolution to study processes such as memory reconstruction and the timing of medial prefrontal–hippocampal interactions. Using the same electrodes, disruptive stimulation can be administered to either the hippocampal formation or medial prefrontal cortex during task performance to provide a causal link with behavior. Other types of stimulation can also be used to help patients with progressive pathologies to improve memory and other functions of the hippocampus.

An exciting emerging technology that is now possible to execute using the same iEEG electrodes is electrochemistry (Kishida et al., 2011). This permits the in vivo measurement of neurotransmitter release in the human brain on a subsecond level (e.g., Bang et al., 2020). This will provide an even deeper insight into the neural processes underlying cognition in areas like the hippocampus and vmPFC, moving us to a level of analysis traditionally afforded only by animal studies. The precision of these types of approaches, coupled with the clear advantage of studying the hippocampus in humans with the ability to probe learned or generated representations with high precision through detailed interviews and feedback, offers a powerful means to progress the field.

One of the greatest challenges for studying the functions of the human hippocampus is that it is maximally engaged by tasks that are active, multisensory experiences, such as forming autobiographical memories and engaging in spatial navigation. These have been simulated with some success within the confines of conventional brain scanners, but exciting new technologies are developing that can take scientific discovery one step further. For example, wireless measurements from intracranial electrodes implanted in the hippocampus have already been achieved during navigation in virtual reality, which was previously only possible in animal research. In healthy people, noninvasive OP-MEG represents the next evolution of scanning capabilities that allows unrestricted and realistic movement in space (Figure 13.11). This permits participants to fully engage in tasks that tax the hippocampus in a naturalistic way, and will provide new insights about old debates. For example, we can examine whether the hippocampus is geared toward egocentric or allocentric spatial processing, probe how the hippocampus responds during active, embodied navigation, and we will be able to observe for the first time the encoding of real-world, immersive experiences in the hippocampal formation.

The rich literature on hippocampal function was initially inspired by a single patient study, H.M. The contribution of neuropsychological cases to our understanding of the roles of the hippocampus remains as critical as ever. With the advancement of technology, we have more sophisticated tools to understand the mapping between hippocampal damage and observed behavioral deficits. For example, high resolution imaging can help better characterize the precise nature of hippocampal lesions and attribute specific impairments to individual subregions. Likewise, expertise in fields such as navigation or memory can be studied in more detail in terms of the structural and functional changes that arise from knowledge acquisition and superior task performance. At the other end of the spectrum, the field is increasingly benefiting from large-scale data collection in healthy controls. These databases consist of hundreds of participants performing a wide range of tasks, or observing naturalistic stimuli such as movies. These are often accompanied by functional and structural brain scans. This approach will allow scientists to test a range of hypotheses and compare analytical approaches, with large sample sizes that lead to robust reproducible research.

The evidence outlined in this chapter places the hippocampus at the heart of our mental life, from our very perception of the world to our most creative flights of the imagination. Its vulnerability to many common pathologies adds urgency to the goal of understanding the mechanisms underlying its functions, if we are to ever have a chance of intervening in a principled way to manage or relieve memory impairments. By looking beyond memory and indeed beyond the hippocampus itself, and by deploying new technologies and analytic approaches, we believe our knowledge will continue to evolve at pace, and from this a theoretical consensus on human hippocampal function will emerge.

REFERENCES

Addis, D. R., Wong, A. T., Schacter, D. L. (2007). Remembering the past and imagining the future: common and distinct neural substrates during event construction and elaboration. *Neuropsychologia*, 45(7), 1363–1377. https://doi.org/10.1016/j.neuropsychologia.2006.10.016

Addis, D. R., Cheng, T., P. Roberts, R., Schacter, D. L. (2011). Hippocampal contributions to the episodic simulation of specific and general future events. *Hippocampus*, 21(10), 1045–1052. https://doi.org/10.1002/hipo.20870

Aggleton, J. P., Brown, M. W. (1999). Episodic memory, amnesia, and the hippocampal-anterior thalamic axis. *Behav Brain Sci*, 22(3), 425–444; discussion 444–489.

Aggleton, J. P., Vann, S. D., Denby, C., Dix, S., Mayes, A. R., Roberts, N., Yonelinas, A. P. (2005). Sparing of the familiarity component of recognition memory in a patient with hippocampal pathology. *Neuropsychologia*, 43(12), 1810–1823. https://doi.org/10.1016/j.neuropsychologia.2005.01.019

Aghajan, Z. M., Schuette, P., Fields, T. A., Tran, M. E., Siddiqui, S. M., Hasulak, N. R., ... Suthana, N. (2017). Theta oscillations in the human medial temporal lobe during real-world ambulatory movement. *Curr Biol.* https://doi.org/10.1016/j.cub.2017.10.062

Aghajan, Z. M., Villaroman, D., Hiller, S., Wishard, T. J., Topalovic, U., Christov-Moore, L., ... Suthana, N. (2019). Modulation of human intracranial theta oscillations during freely moving spatial navigation and memory. *bioRxiv*, 738807. https://doi.org/10.1101/738807

Aly, M., Ranganath, C., Yonelinas, Andrew P. (2013). Detecting changes in scenes: the hippocampus is critical for strength-based perception. *Neuron*, 78(6), 1127–1137. https://doi.org/10.1016/j.neuron.2013.04.018

Aly, M., Turk-Browne, N. B. (2016a). Attention promotes episodic encoding by stabilizing hippocampal representations. *Proc Natl Acad Sci U S A*, 113(4), E420–429. https://doi.org/10.1073/pnas.1518931113

Aly, M., Turk-Browne, N. B. (2016b). Attention stabilizes representations in the human hippocampus. *Cereb Cortex*, 26(2), 783–796. https://doi.org/10.1093/cercor/bhv041

Axmacher, N., Cohen, M. X., Fell, J., Haupt, S., Dümpelmann, M., Elger, C. E., ... Ranganath, C. (2010). Intracranial EEG correlates of expectancy and memory formation in the human hippocampus and nucleus accumbens. *Neuron*, 65(4), 541–549. https://doi.org/10.1016/j.neuron.2010.02.006

Axmacher, N., Henseler, M. M., Jensen, O., Weinreich, I., Elger, C. E., Fell, J. (2010). Cross-frequency coupling supports multi-item working memory in the human hippocampus. *Proc Natl Acad Sci U S A*, 107(7), 3228–3233. https://doi.org/10.1073/pnas.0911531107

Baddeley, A. (2003). Working memory: looking back and looking forwards. *Nat Rev Neurosci*, 4, 829–839.

Baddeley, A. (2010). Working memory. *Curr Biol*, **20**(4), R136–R140. https://doi.org/10.1016/j.cub.2009.12.014

Bakkour, A., Palombo, D. J., Zylberberg, A., Kang, Y. H. R., Reid, A., Verfaellie, M., … Shohamy, D. (2019). The hippocampus supports deliberation during value-based decisions. *Elife*, **8**, e46080. https://doi.org/10.7554/eLife.46080

Baldassano, C., Chen, J., Zadbood, A., Pillow, J. W., Hasson, U., Norman, K. A. (2017). Discovering event structure in continuous narrative perception and memory. *Neuron*, **95**(3), 709–721.e705. https://doi.org/10.1016/j.neuron.2017.06.041

Bang, D., Kishida, K. T., Lohrenz, T., White, J. P., Laxton, A. W., Tatter, S. B., et al. (2020). Sub-second dopamine and serotonin signalling in human striatum during perceptual decision-making. *Neuron*, **108**(5), 999–1010.

Bao, X., Gjorgieva, E., Shanahan, L. K., Howard, J. D., Kahnt, T., Gottfried, J. A. (2019). Grid-like neural representations support olfactory navigation of a two-dimensional odor space. *Neuron*, **102**(5), 1066–1075.e1065. https://doi.org/10.1016/j.neuron.2019.03.034

Barense, M. D., Henson, R. N. A., Lee, A. C. H., Graham, K. S. (2010). Medial temporal lobe activity during complex discrimination of faces, objects, and scenes: effects of viewpoint. *Hippocampus*, *20*(3), 389–401. https://doi.org/10.1002/hipo.20641

Barron, H. C., Garvert, M. M., Behrens, T. E. (2016). Repetition suppression: a means to index neural representations using BOLD? *Philos Trans R Soc Lond B Biol Sci*, **371**(1705). https://doi.org/10.1098/rstb.2015.0355

Barry, D. N., Barnes, G. R., Clark, I. A., Maguire, E. A. (2019). The neural dynamics of novel scene imagery. *J Neurosci*. https://doi.org/10.1523/jneurosci.2497-18.2019

Barry, D. N., Chadwick, M. J., Maguire, E. A. (2018). Nonmonotonic recruitment of ventromedial prefrontal cortex during remote memory recall. *PLoS Biol*, **16**(7), e2005479. https://doi.org/10.1371/journal.pbio.2005479

Barry, D. N., Clark, I. A., Maguire, E. A. (2021). The relationship between hippocampal subfield volumes and autobiographical memory persistence. *Hippocampus*, **31**(4), 362–374.

Barry, D. N., Maguire, E. A. (2019a). Remote memory and the hippocampus: a constructive critique. *Trends Cogn Sci*, **23**(2), 128–142. https://doi.org/10.1016/j.tics.2018.11.005

Barry, D. N., Maguire E. A. (2019b). Consolidating the case for transient hippocampal memory traces. *Trends Cogn Sci*, **23**, 635–636.

Bartsch, T., Alfke, K., Stingele, R., Rohr, A., Freitag-Wolf, S., Jansen, O., Deuschl, G. (2006). Selective affection of hippocampal CA-1 neurons in patients with transient global amnesia without long-term sequelae. *Brain*, **129**(11), 2874–2884. https://doi.org/10.1093/brain/awl248

Bartsch, T., Dohring, J., Rohr, A., Jansen, O., Deuschl, G. (2011). CA1 neurons in the human hippocampus are critical for autobiographical memory, mental time travel, and autonoetic consciousness. *Proc Natl Acad Sci U S A*, **108**(42), 17562–17567. https://doi.org/10.1073/pnas.1110266108

Bein, O., Duncan, K., Davachi, L. (2020). Mnemonic prediction errors bias hippocampal states. *Nat Commun*, **11**(1), 3451. https://doi.org/10.1038/s41467-020-17287-1

Ben-Yakov, A., Dudai, Y. (2011). Constructing realistic engrams: poststimulus activity of hippocampus and dorsal striatum predicts subsequent episodic memory. *J Neurosci*, **31**(24), 9032–9042. https://doi.org/10.1523/JNEUROSCI.0702-11.2011

Ben-Yakov, A., Henson, R. N. (2018). The hippocampal film editor: sensitivity and specificity to event boundaries in continuous experience. *J Neurosci*, **38**(47), 10057–10068. https://doi.org/10.1523/jneurosci.0524-18.2018

Bergmann, H. C., Daselaar, S. M., Beul, S. F., Rijpkema, M., Fernández, G., Kessels, R. P. C. (2015). Brain activation during associative short-term memory maintenance is not predictive for subsequent retrieval. *Front Hum Neurosci*, **9**(479). https://doi.org/10.3389/fnhum.2015.00479

Berron, D., Schütze, H., Maass, A., Cardenas-Blanco, A., Kuijf, H. J., Kumaran, D., Düzel, E. (2016). Strong evidence for pattern separation in human dentate gyrus. *J Neurosci*, **36**(29), 7569–7579. https://doi.org/10.1523/jneurosci.0518-16.2016

Bird, C. M., Vargha-Khadem, F., Burgess, N. (2008). Impaired memory for scenes but not faces in developmental hippocampal amnesia: a case study. *Neuropsychologia*, **46**(4), 1050–1059. https://doi.org/10.1016/j.neuropsychologia.2007.11.007

Blakemore, C. B., Falconer, M. A. (1967). Long-term effects of anterior temporal lobectomy on certain cognitive functions. *J Neurol Neurosurg Psychiatry*, **30**, 364–367.

Bonnici, H. M., Chadwick, M. J., Lutti, A., Hassabis, D., Weiskopf, N., Maguire, E. A. (2012). Detecting representations of recent and remote autobiographical memories in vmPFC and hippocampus. *J Neurosci*, **32**(47), 16982–16991. https://doi.org/10.1523/JNEUROSCI.2475-12.2012

Bonnici, H. M., Kumaran, D., Chadwick, M. J., Weiskopf, N., Hassabis, D., Maguire, E. A. (2012). Decoding representations of scenes in the medial temporal lobes. *Hippocampus*, **22**(5), 1143–1153. https://doi.org/10.1002/hipo.20960

Bonnici, H. M., Chadwick, M. J., Maguire, E. A. (2013). Representations of recent and remote autobiographical memories in hippocampal subfields. *Hippocampus*, **23**, 849–854. https://doi.org/10.1002/hipo.22155

Bonnici, H. M., Maguire, E. A. (2018). Two years later – autobiographical memory representations revisited in vmPFC and hippocampus. *Neuropsychologia*, **110**, 159–169. https://doi.org/10.1016/j.neuropsychologia.2017.05.014

Borders, A. A., Aly, M., Parks, C. M., Yonelinas, A. P. (2017). The hippocampus is particularly important for building associations across stimulus domains. *Neuropsychologia*, **99**, 335–342. https://doi.org/10.1016/j.neuropsychologia.2017.03.032

Boto, E., Holmes, N., Leggett, J., Roberts, G., Shah, V., Meyer, S. S., Muñoz, L. D., Mullinger, K. J., Tierney, T. M., Bestmann, S., Barnes, G. R., Bowtell, R., Brookes, M. J. (2018). Moving magnetoencephalography towards real-world applications with a wearable system. *Nature*, **555**(7698), 657–661. https://doi.org/10.1038/nature26147

Bottomley, P. A., Edelstein, W. A., Foster, T. H., Adams, W. A. (1985). In vivo solvent-suppressed localized hydrogen nuclear magnetic resonance spectroscopy: a window to metabolism? *Proc Natl Acad Sci U S A*, **82**(7), 2148–2152. https://doi.org/10.1073/pnas.82.7.2148

Brier, M. R., Gordon, B., Friedrichsen, K., McCarthy, J., Stern, A., Christensen, J., … Ances, B. M. (2016). Tau and Aβ imaging, CSF measures, and cognition in Alzheimer's disease. *Sci Transl Med*, **8**(338), 338ra366. https://doi.org/10.1126/scitranslmed.aaf2362

Brooks, D. N., Baddeley, A. D. (1976). What can amnesic patients learn? *Neuropsychologia*, **14**(1), 111–122. https://doi.org/10.1016/0028-3932(76)90012-9

Brown, T. I., Carr, V. A., LaRocque, K. F., Favila, S. E., Gordon, A. M., Bowles, B., … Wagner, A. D. (2016). Prospective representation of navigational goals in the human hippocampus. *Science*, **352**(6291), 1323–1326. https://doi.org/10.1126/science.aaf0784

Buckner, R. L., Vincent, J. L. (2007). Unrest at rest: default activity and spontaneous network correlations. *Neuroimage*, **37**(4), 1091–1096; discussion 1097–1099. https://doi.org/10.1016/j.neuroimage.2007.01.010

Burgess, N., Maguire, E. A., O'Keefe, J. (2002). The human hippocampus and spatial and episodic memory. *Neuron*, **35**, 625–641.

Bush, D., Bisby, J. A., Bird, C. M., Gollwitzer, S., Rodionov, R., Diehl, B., … Burgess, N. (2017). Human hippocampal theta power indicates movement onset and distance travelled. *Proc Natl Acad Sci U S A*. https://doi.org/10.1073/pnas.1708716114

Byrne, P., Becker, S., Burgess, N. (2007). Remembering the past and imagining the future: a neural model of spatial memory and imagery. *Psychol Rev*, **114**(2), 340–375. https://doi.org/10.1037/0033-295x.114.2.340

Cave, C. B., Squire, L. R. (1992). Intact verbal and nonverbal short-term memory following damage to the human hippocampus. *Hippocampus*, **2**(2), 151–163. https://doi.org/10.1002/hipo.450020207

Chadwick, M. J., Bonnici, H. M., Maguire, E. A. (2012). Decoding information in the human hippocampus: a user's guide. *Neuropsychologia*, **50**(13), 3107–3121. https://doi.org/10.1016/j.neuropsychologia.2012.07.007

Chadwick, M. J., Bonnici, H. M., Maguire, E. A. (2014). CA3 size predicts the precision of memory recall. *Proc Natl Acad Sci U S A*, **111**(29), 10720–10725. https://doi.org/10.1073/pnas.1319641111

Chadwick, M. J., Mullally, S. L., Maguire, E. A. (2013). The hippocampus extrapolates beyond the view in scenes: an fMRI study of boundary extension. *Cortex*, **49**(8), 2067–2079. https://doi.org/10.1016/j.cortex.2012.11.010

Chaieb, L., Leszczynski, M., Axmacher, N., Höhne, M., Elger, C. E., Fell, J. (2015). Theta-gamma phase-phase coupling during working memory maintenance in the human hippocampus. *Cogn Neurosci*, **6**(4), 149–157. https://doi.org/10.1080/17588928.2015.1058254

Chen, D., Kunz, L., Wang, W., Zhang, H., Wang, W. X., Schulze-Bonhage, A., … Wang, L. (2018). Hexadirectional modulation of theta power in human entorhinal cortex during spatial navigation. *Curr Biol*, **28**(20), 3310–3315.e3314. https://doi.org/10.1016/j.cub.2018.08.029

Chen, J., Dastjerdi, M., Foster, B. L., LaRocque, K. F., Rauschecker, A. M., Parvizi, J., Wagner, A. D. (2013). Human hippocampal increases in low-frequency power during associative prediction violations. *Neuropsychologia*, **51**(12), 2344–2351. https://doi.org/10.1016/j.neuropsychologia.2013.03.019

Chen, J., Olsen, R. K., Preston, A. R., Glover, G. H., Wagner, A. D. (2011). Associative retrieval processes in the human medial temporal lobe: hippocampal retrieval success and CA1 mismatch detection. *Learn Mem*, **18**(8), 523–528. https://doi.org/10.1101/lm.2135211

Cipolotti, L., Bird, C., Good, T., Macmanus, D., Rudge, P., Shallice, T. (2006). Recollection and familiarity in dense hippocampal amnesia: A case study. *Neuropsychologia*, **44**(3), 489–506. https://doi.org/10.1016/j.neuropsychologia.2005.05.014

Cipolotti, L., Shallice, T., Chan, D., Fox, N., Scahill, R., Harrison, G., … Rudge, P. (2001). Long-term retrograde amnesia...the crucial role of the hippocampus. *Neuropsychologia*, **39**(2), 151–172.

Clark, I. A., Hotchin, V., Monk, A., Pizzamiglio, G., Liefgreen, A., Maguire, E. A. (2019). Identifying the cognitive processes underpinning hippocampal-dependent tasks. *J Exp Psychol Gen*, **148**(11), 1861–1881. https://doi.org/10.1037/xge0000582

Clark, I. A., Kim, M., Maguire, E. A. (2018). Verbal paired associates and the hippocampus: the role of scenes. *J Cogn Neurosci*, 1–25. https://doi.org/10.1162/jocn_a_01315

Clark, I. A., Monk, A. M., Hotchin, V., Pizzamiglio, G., Liefgreen, A., Callaghan, M. F., Maguire, E. A. (2020b). Does hippocampal volume explain performance differences on hippocampal-dependant tasks? *Neuroimage*, **221**, 117211. https://doi.org/10.1016/j.neuroimage.2020.117211

Clark, I. A., Monk, A. M., Maguire, E. A. (2020a). Characterizing strategy use during the performance of hippocampal-dependent tasks. *Front Psychol*, **11**, 2119. https://doi.org/10.3389/fpsyg.2020.02119

Cohen, D. (1972). Magnetoencephalography: detection of the brain's electrical activity with a superconducting magnetometer. *Science*, **175**(4022), 664–666. https://doi.org/10.1126/science.175.4022.664

Cohen, N. J., Eichenbaum, H. (1993). Memory, Amnesia, and the Hippocampal System. Cambridge, MA: MIT Press.

Constantinescu, A. O., O'Reilly, J. X., Behrens, T. E. (2016). Organizing conceptual knowledge in humans with a gridlike code. *Science*, **352**(6292), 1464–1468. https://doi.org/10.1126/science.aaf0941

Corkin, S. (2002). What's new with the amnesic patient H.M.? *Nat Rev Neurosci*, **3**, 153–160.

Corkin, S. (2013). Permanent Present Tense: The Unforgettable Life of the Amnesic Patient, H. M. New York: Basic Books.

Cornwell, B. R., Johnson, L. L., Holroyd, T., Carver, F. W., Grillon, C. (2008). Human hippocampal and parahippocampal theta during goal-directed spatial navigation predicts performance on a virtual Morris water maze. *J Neurosci*, **28**(23), 5983–5990. https://doi.org/10.1523/JNEUROSCI.5001-07.2008

Cowan, E., Liu, A., Henin, S., Kothare, S., Devinsky, O., Davachi, L. (2020). Sleep spindles promote the restructuring of memory representations in ventromedial prefrontal cortex through enhanced hippocampal–cortical functional connectivity. *J Neurosci*, **40**(9), 1909–1919. https://doi.org/10.1523/jneurosci.1946-19.2020

Dalton, M. A., Zeidman, P., Barry, D. N., Williams, E., Maguire, E. A. (2017). Segmenting subregions of the human hippocampus on structural magnetic resonance image scans: an illustrated tutorial. *Brain Neurosci Adv*, **1**, 2398212817701448.

Dalton, M. A., Zeidman, P., McCormick, C., Maguire, E. A. (2018). Differentiable processing of objects, associations and scenes within the hippocampus. *J Neurosci*, **38**(38), 8146–8159. https://doi.org/10.1523/jneurosci.0263-18.2018

Dalton, M. A., Maguire, E. A. (2017). The pre/parasubiculum: a hippocampal hub for scene-based cognition? *Curr Opin Behav Sci*, **17**, 34–40. http://doi.org/10.1016/j.cobeha.2017.06.001

Daum, I., Channon, S., Canavan, A. G. (1989). Classical conditioning in patients with severe memory problems. *J Neurol Neurosurg Psychiatry*, **52**(1), 47–51. https://doi.org/10.1136/jnnp.52.1.47

Dede, A. J. O., Frascino, J. C., Wixted, J. T., Squire, L. R. (2016). Learning and remembering real-world events after medial temporal lobe damage. *Proc Natl Acad Sci U S A*, **113**(47), 13480–13485. https://doi.org/10.1073/pnas.1617025113

Denis, D., Schapiro, A., Poskanzer, C., Bursal, V., Charron, L., Morgan, A., Stickgold, R. (2020). The roles of item exposure and visualization success in the consolidation of memories across wake and sleep. *Learn Mem*, **27**(11), 451–456.

Desjardins, T., Scoboria, A. (2007). "You and your best friend Suzy put slime in Ms. Smollett's desk": producing false memories with self-relevant details. *Psychon Bull Rev*, **14**(6), 1090–1095

Doeller, C. F., Barry, C., Burgess, N. (2010). Evidence for grid cells in a human memory network. *Nature*, **463**, 657–661. https://doi.org/10.1038/nature0870

Douglas, D., Thavabalasingam, S., Chorghay, Z., O'Neil, E. B., Barense, M. D., Lee, A. C. (2017). Perception of impossible scenes reveals differential hippocampal and parahippocampal place area contributions to spatial coherency. *Hippocampus*, **27**(1), 61–76. https://doi.org/10.1002/hipo.22673

DuBrow, S., Davachi, L. (2016). Temporal binding within and across events. *Neurobiol Learn Mem*, **134** Pt A, 107–114. https://doi.org/10.1016/j.nlm.2016.07.011

Eichenbaum, H. (2003). The hippocampus, episodic memory, declarative memory, spatial memory ... where does it all come together? *Int Congr Series*, **1250**, 235–244. https://doi.org/10.1016/s0531-5131(03)00183-3

Eichenbaum, H. (2017). Memory: organization and control. *Annu Rev Psychol*, **68**, 19–45. https://doi.org/10.1146/annurev-psych-010416-044131

Eichenbaum, H., Otto, T., Cohen, N. J. (1992). The hippocampus: what does it do? *Behav Neural Biol*, **57**(1), 2–36

Eichenbaum, H., Yonelinas, A. P., Ranganath, C. (2007). The medial temporal lobe and recognition memory. *Annu Rev Neurosci*, **30**, 123–152. https://doi.org/10.1146/annurev.neuro.30.051606.094328

Ekstrom, A. D., Kahana, M. J., Caplan, J. B., Fields, T. A., Isham, E. A., Newman, E. L., Fried, I. (2003). Cellular networks underlying human spatial navigation. *Nature*, **425**(6954), 184–188. https://doi.org/10.1038/nature01964

Ekstrom, A. D., Ranganath, C. (2018). Space, time, and episodic memory: the hippocampus is all over the cognitive map. *Hippocampus*, **28**, 680–687. https://doi.org/10.1002/hipo.22750

Ellamil, M., Fox, K. C. R., Dixon, M. L., Pritchard, S., Todd, R. M., Thompson, E., Christoff, K. (2016). Dynamics of neural recruitment surrounding the spontaneous arising of thoughts in experienced mindfulness practitioners. *Neuroimage*, **136**, 186–196. https://doi.org/10.1016/j.neuroimage.2016.04.034

Fernandez, G., Morris, R. G. M. (2018). Memory, novelty and prior knowledge. *Trends Neurosci*, **41**, 654–659. https://doi.org/10.1016/j.tins.2018.08.006

Fuentemilla, L., Palombo, D. J., Levine, B. (2017). Gamma phase-synchrony in autobiographical memory: Evidence from magnetoencephalography and severely deficient autobiographical memory. *Neuropsychologia*, **110**, 7–13. https://doi.org/10.1016/j.neuropsychologia.2017.08.020

Gaffan, D. (1994). Scene-specific memory for objects: a model of episodic memory impairment in monkeys with fornix transection. *J Cogn Neurosci*, **6**, 305–320.

Garrido, M. I., Barnes, G. R., Kumaran, D., Maguire, E. A., Dolan, R. J. (2015). Ventromedial prefrontal cortex drives hippocampal theta oscillations induced by mismatch computations. *Neuroimage*, **120**, 362–370. https://doi.org/10.1016/j.neuroimage.2015.07.016

Garvert, M. M., Dolan, R. J., Behrens, T. E. (2017). A map of abstract relational knowledge in the human hippocampal-entorhinal cortex. *Elife*, **6, e17086**. https://doi.org/10.7554/eLife.17086

Geib, B. R., Stanley, M. L., Wing, E. A., Laurienti, P. J., Cabeza, R. (2017). Hippocampal contributions to the large-scale episodic memory network predict vivid visual memories. *Cereb Cortex*, **27**(1), 680–693. https://doi.org/10.1093/cercor/bhv272

Gluth, S., Sommer, T., Rieskamp, J., Buchel, C. (2015). Effective connectivity between hippocampus and ventromedial prefrontal cortex controls preferential choices from memory. *Neuron*, **86**(4), 1078–1090. https://doi.org/10.1016/j.neuron.2015.04.023

Goldfarb, E. V., Chun, M. M., Phelps, E. A. (2016). Memory-guided attention: independent contributions of the hippocampus and striatum. *Neuron*, **89**(2), 317–324. https://doi.org/10.1016/j.neuron.2015.12.014

Goyal, A., Miller, J., Watrous, A. J., Lee, S. A., Coffey, T., Sperling, M. R., ... Jacobs, J. (2018). Electrical stimulation in hippocampus and entorhinal cortex impairs spatial and temporal memory. *J Neurosci*, **38**(19), 4471–4481. https://doi.org/10.1523/jneurosci.3049-17.2018

Graham, K. S., Barense, M. D., Lee, A. C. H. (2010). Going beyond LTM in the MTL: a synthesis of neuropsychological and neuroimaging findings on the role of the medial temporal lobe in memory and perception. *Neuropsychologia*, **48**(4), 831–853. https://doi.org/10.1016/j.neuropsychologia.2010.01.001

Grande, X., Berron, D., Horner, A. J., Bisby, J. A., Duzel, E., Burgess, N. (2019). Holistic recollection via pattern completion involves hippocampal subfield CA3. *J Neurosci*, **39**(41), 8100–8111. https://doi.org/10.1523/jneurosci.0722-19.2019

Gruber, M. J., Hsieh, L.-T., Staresina, B. P., Elger, C. E., Fell, J., Axmacher, N., Ranganath, C. (2018). Theta phase synchronization between the human hippocampus and prefrontal cortex increases during encoding of unexpected information: a case study. *J Cogn Neurosci*, **30**(11), 1646–1656. https://doi.org/10.1162/jocn_a_01302 %M 29952700

Guitart-Masip, M., Barnes, G. R., Horner, A., Bauer, M., Dolan, R. J., Duzel, E. (2013). Synchronization of medial temporal lobe and prefrontal rhythms in human decision making. *J Neurosci*, **33**(2), 442–451. https://doi.org/10.1523/JNEUROSCI.2573-12.2013

Günseli, E., Aly, M. (2020). Preparation for upcoming attentional states in the hippocampus and medial prefrontal cortex. *Elife*, **9**, e53191. https://doi.org/10.7554/eLife.53191

Haist, F., Musen, G., Squire, L. R. (1991). Intact priming of words and nonwords in amnesia. *Psychobiology*, **19**(4), 275–285. https://doi.org/10.3758/BF03332081

Hannula, D. E., Ryan, J. D., Tranel, D., Cohen, N. J. (2007). Rapid onset relational memory effects are evident in eye movement behavior, but not in hippocampal amnesia. *J Cogn Neurosci*, **19**(10), 1690–1705. https://doi.org/10.1162/jocn.2007.19.10.1690

Hartley, T., Bird, C. M., Chan, D., Cipolotti, L., Husain, M., Vargha-Khadem, F., Burgess, N. (2007). The hippocampus is required for short-term topographical memory in humans. *Hippocampus*, **17**(1), 34–48. https://doi.org/10.1002/hipo.20240

Hassabis, D., Kumaran, D., Vann, S. D., Maguire, E. A. (2007a). Patients with hippocampal amnesia cannot imagine new experiences. *Proc Natl Acad Sci U S A*, **104**(5), 1726–1731. https://doi.org/10.1073/pnas.0610561104

Hassabis, D., Kumaran, D., Maguire, E. A. (2007b). Using imagination to understand the neural basis of episodic memory. *J Neurosci*, **27**(52), 14365–14374. https://doi.org/10.1523/JNEUROSCI.4549-07.2007

Hassabis, D., Maguire, E. A. (2007). Deconstructing episodic memory with construction. *Trends Cogn Sci*, **11**, 299–306. https://doi.org/10.1016/j.tics.2007.05.001

Hassabis, D., Maguire, E. A. (2009). The construction system of the brain. *Philos Trans R Soc Lond B Biol Sci*, **364**(1521), 1263–1271. https://doi.org/10.1098/rstb.2008.0296

Hayne, R., Meyers, R. Knott, J. R. (1949). Characteristics of electrical activity of human corpus striatum and neighboring structures. *J Neurophysiol*, **12**, 185–195.

Helfrich, R. F., Lendner, J. D., Mander, B. A., Guillen, H., Paff, M., Mnatsakanyan, L., ... Knight, R. T. (2019). Bidirectional prefrontal-hippocampal dynamics organize information transfer during sleep in humans. *Nat Commun*, **10**(1), 3572. https://doi.org/10.1038/s41467-019-11444-x

Hermans, E. J., Kanen, J. W., Tambini, A., Fernández, G., Davachi, L., Phelps, E. A. (2017). Persistence of amygdala–hippocampal connectivity and multi-voxel correlation structures during awake rest after fear learning predicts long-term expression of fear. *Cereb Cortex*, **27**(5), 3028–3041. https://doi.org/10.1093/cercor/bhw145

Hermiller, M. S., Chen, Y. F., Parrish, T. B., Voss, J. L. (2020). Evidence for immediate enhancement of hippocampal memory encoding by network-targeted theta-burst stimulation during concurrent fMRI. *J Neurosci*, **40**(37), 7155–7168. https://doi.org/10.1523/jneurosci.0486-20.2020

Heusser, A. C., Poeppel, D., Ezzyat, Y., Davachi, L. (2016). Episodic sequence memory is supported by a theta-gamma phase code. *Nat Neurosci*, 19(10), 1374–1380. https://doi.org/10.1038/nn.4374

Hickling, A. L., Clark, I. A., Wu, Y. I., Maguire, E. A. (2024). Automated protocols for delineating human hippocampal subfields from 3 Tesla and 7 Tesla magnetic resonance imaging data. *Hippocampus*, 34, 302–308. https://doi.org/10.1002/hipo.23606

Hindy, N. C., Avery, E. W., Turk-Browne, N. B. (2019). Hippocampal-neocortical interactions sharpen over time for predictive actions. *Nat Commun*, 10(1), 3989. https://doi.org/10.1038/s41467-019-12016-9

Hindy, N. C., Ng, F. Y., Turk-Browne, N. B. (2016). Linking pattern completion in the hippocampus to predictive coding in visual cortex. *Nat Neurosci*, 19(5), 665–667. https://doi.org/10.1038/nn.4284

Hodges, J. R., Warlow, C. P. (1990). Syndromes of transient amnesia: towards a classification. A study of 153 cases. *J Neurol Neurosurg Psychiatry*, 53(10), 834–843. https://doi.org/10.1136/jnnp.53.10.834

Hodgetts, C. J., Shine, J. P., Lawrence, A. D., Downing, P. E., Graham, K. S. (2016). Evidencing a place for the hippocampus within the core scene processing network. *Hum Brain Mapp*, 37(11), 3779–3794. https://doi.org/10.1002/hbm.23275

Hoffman, K. L., Dragan, M. C., Leonard, T. K., Micheli, C., Montefusco-Siegmund, R., Valiante, T. A. (2013). Saccades during visual exploration align hippocampal 3–8 Hz rhythms in human and non-human primates. *Front Syst Neurosci*, 7, 43.

Horner, A. J., Bisby, J. A., Bush, D., Lin, W. J., Burgess, N. (2015). Evidence for holistic episodic recollection via hippocampal pattern completion. *Nat Commun*, 6, 7462. https://doi.org/10.1038/ncomms8462

Horner, A. J., Bisby, J. A., Zotow, E., Bush, D., Burgess, N. (2016). Grid-like processing of imagined navigation. *Curr Biol*, 26(6), 842–847. https://doi.org/10.1016/j.cub.2016.01.042

Hou, G., Yang, X., Yuan, T.-F. (2013). Hippocampal asymmetry: differences in structures and functions. *Neurochem Res*, 38, 453–460.

Hrybouski, S., MacGillivray, M., Huang, Y., Madan, C. R., Carter, R., Seres, P., Malykhin, N. V. (2019). Involvement of hippocampal subfields and anterior-posterior subregions in encoding and retrieval of item, spatial, and associative memories: Longitudinal versus transverse axis. *Neuroimage*, 191, 568–586. https://doi.org/10.1016/j.neuroimage.2019.01.061

Intraub, H. (2020). Searching for boundary extension. *Curr Biol*, 30, R1463–R1464.

Intraub, H., Richardson, M. (1989). Wide-angle memories of close-up scenes. *J Exp Psychol Learn Mem Cogn*, 15(2), 179–187. https://doi.org/10.1037/0278-7393.15.2.179

Irish, M., Mothakunnel, A., Dermody, N., Wilson, N. A., Hodges, J. R., Piguet, O. (2017). Damage to right medial temporal structures disrupts the capacity for scene construction-a case study. *Hippocampus*, 27(6), 635–641. https://doi.org/10.1002/hipo.22722

Jacobs, J., Miller, J., Lee, S. A., Coffey, T., Watrous, A. J., Sperling, M. R., ... Rizzuto, D. S. (2016). Direct electrical stimulation of the human entorhinal region and hippocampus impairs memory. *Neuron*, 92(5), 983–990. https://doi.org/10.1016/j.neuron.2016.10.062

Javadi, A. H., Emo, B., Howard, L. R., Zisch, F. E., Yu, Y., Knight, R., ... Spiers, H. J. (2017). Hippocampal and prefrontal processing of network topology to simulate the future. *Nat Commun*, 8, 14652. https://doi.org/10.1038/ncomms14652

Jordan, J. T. (2020). The rodent hippocampus as a bilateral structure: A review of hemispheric lateralization. *Hippocampus*, 30, 278–292.

Kaplan, R., Friston, K. J. (2019). Entorhinal transformations in abstract frames of reference. *PLoS Biol*, 17(5), e3000230. https://doi.org/10.1371/journal.pbio.3000230

Kaplan, R., Bush, D., Bonnefond, M., Bandettini, P. A., Barnes, G. R., Doeller, C. F., Burgess, N. (2014). Medial prefrontal theta phase coupling during spatial memory retrieval. *Hippocampus*, 24(6), 656–665. https://doi.org/10.1002/hipo.22255

Karapanagiotidis, T., Bernhardt, B. C., Jefferies, E., Smallwood, J. (2017). Tracking thoughts: Exploring the neural architecture of mental time travel during mind-wandering. *Neuroimage*, 147, 272–281. https://doi.org/10.1016/j.neuroimage.2016.12.031

Kennepohl, S., Sziklas, V., Garver, K. E., Wagner, D. D., Jones-Gotman, M. (2007). Memory and the medial temporal lobe: hemispheric specialization reconsidered. *Neuroimage*, 36, 969–978.

Kim, M., Jeffery, K. J., Maguire, E. A. (2017). Multivoxel pattern analysis reveals 3D place information in the human hippocampus. *J Neurosci*, 37(16), 4270–4279. https://doi.org/10.1523/jneurosci.2703-16.2017

Kim, M., Maguire, E. A. (2019). Can we study 3D grid codes non-invasively in the human brain? Methodological considerations and fMRI findings. *Neuroimage*, 186, 667–678. https://doi.org/10.1016/j.neuroimage.2018.11.041

Kirwan, C. B., Bayley, P. J., Galvan, V. V., Squire, L. R. (2008). Detailed recollection of remote autobiographical memory after damage to the medial temporal lobe. *Proc Natl Acad Sci U S A*, 105(7), 2676–2680. https://doi.org/10.1073/pnas.0712155105

Kishida, K. T., Sandberg, S. G., Lohrenz, T., Comair, Y. G., Sáez, I., Phillips, P. E. M., Montague, P. R. (2011). Sub-second dopamine detection in human striatum. *PLoS One*, 6(8), e23291. https://doi.org/10.1371/journal.pone.0023291

Klooster, N. B., Duff, M. C. (2015). Remote semantic memory is impoverished in hippocampal amnesia. *Neuropsychologia*, 79, 42–52. https://doi.org/10.1016/j.neuropsychologia.2015.10.017

Knight, R. T. (1996). Contribution of human hippocampal region to novelty detection. *Nature*, 383(6597), 256–259. https://doi.org/10.1038/383256a0

Kok, P., Turk-Browne, N. B. (2018). Associative prediction of visual shape in the hippocampus. *J Neurosci*, 38(31), 6888–6899. https://doi.org/10.1523/jneurosci.0163-18.2018

Koster, R., Chadwick, M. J., Chen, Y., Berron, D., Banino, A., Duzel, E., ... Kumaran, D. (2018). Big-loop recurrence within the hippocampal system supports integration of information across episodes. *Neuron*, 99(6), 1342–1354.e1346. https://doi.org/10.1016/j.neuron.2018.08.009

Kumar, S., Joseph, S., Gander, P. E., Barascud, N., Halpern, A. R., Griffiths, T. D. (2016). A brain system for auditory working memory. *J Neurosci*, 36(16), 4492–4505. https://doi.org/10.1523/jneurosci.4341-14.2016

Kumaran, D., Maguire, E. A. (2005). The human hippocampus: cognitive maps or relational memory? *J Neurosci*, 25, 7254–7259. https://doi.org/10.1523/JNEUROSCI.1103-05.2005

Kumaran, D., Maguire, E. A. (2006a). The dynamics of hippocampal activation during encoding of overlapping sequences. *Neuron*, 49(4), 617–629. https://doi.org/10.1016/j.neuron.2005.12.024

Kumaran, D., Maguire, E. A. (2006b). An unexpected sequence of events: mismatch detection in the human hippocampus. *PLoS Biol*, 4(12), e424. https://doi.org/10.1371/journal.pbio.0040424

Kumaran, D., Summerfield, J. J., Hassabis, D., Maguire, E. A. (2009). Tracking the emergence of conceptual knowledge during human decision making. *Neuron*, 63(6), 889–901. https://doi.org/10.1016/j.neuron.2009.07.030

Kunz, L., Schroder, T. N., Lee, H., Montag, C., Lachmann, B., Sariyska, R., ... Axmacher, N. (2015). Reduced grid-cell-like representations in adults at genetic risk for Alzheimer's disease. *Science*, **350**(6259), 430–433. https://doi.org/10.1126/science.aac8128

Kunz, L., Wang, L., Lachner-Piza, D., Zhang, H., Brandt, A., Dümpelmann, M., … Axmacher, N. (2019). Hippocampal theta phases organize the reactivation of large-scale electrophysiological representations during goal-directed navigation. *Sci Adv*, **5**(7), eaav8192–eaav8192. https://doi.org/10.1126/sciadv.aav8192

Kwan, D., Craver, C. F., Green, L., Myerson, J., Rosenbaum, R. S. (2013). Dissociations in future thinking following hippocampal damage: evidence from discounting and time perspective in episodic amnesia. *J Exp Psychol Gen*, **142**(4), 1355–1369. https://doi.org/10.1037/a0034001

Le Bihan, D., Breton, E., Lallemand, D., Grenier, P., Cabanis, E., Laval-Jeantet, M. (1986). MR imaging of intravoxel incoherent motions: application to diffusion and perfusion in neurologic disorders. *Radiology*, **161**(2), 401–407. https://doi.org/10.1148/radiology.161.2.3763909

Lee, A. C., Bussey, T. J., Murray, E. A., Saksida, L. M., Epstein, R. A., Kapur, N., … Graham, K. S. (2005). Perceptual deficits in amnesia: challenging the medial temporal lobe "mnemonic" view. *Neuropsychologia*, **43**(1), 1–11. https://doi.org/10.1016/j.neuropsychologia.2004.07.017

Lega, B., Burke, J., Jacobs, J., Kahana, M. J. (2014). Slow-theta-to-gamma phase–amplitude coupling in human hippocampus supports the formation of new episodic memories. *Cereb Cortex*, **26**(1), 268–278. https://doi.org/10.1093/cercor/bhu23

Levine, B., Svoboda, E., Hay, J. F., Winocur, G., Moscovitch, M. (2002). Aging and autobiographical memory: dissociating episodic from semantic retrieval. *Psychology and Aging*, **17**(4), 677–689. https://doi.org/10.1037//0882-7974.17.4.677

Liang, J. C., Preston, A. R. (2017). Medial temporal lobe reinstatement of content-specific details predicts source memory. *Cortex*, **91**, 67–78. https://doi.org/10.1016/j.cortex.2016.09.011

Liu, W., Shi, Y., Cousins, J. N., Kohn, N., Fernández, G. (2022). Hippocampal-medial prefrontal event segmentation and integration contribute to episodic memory formation. Cereb Cortex, 32(5), 949–969. https://doi.org/10.1093/cercor/bhab258

Liu, Y., Dolan, R. J., Kurth-Nelson, Z., Behrens, T. E. J. (2019). Human replay spontaneously reorganizes experience. *Cell*, **178**(3), 640–652.e614. https://doi.org/10.1016/j.cell.2019.06.012

Liu, Z. X., Shen, K., Olsen, R. K., Ryan, J. D. (2017). Visual sampling predicts hippocampal activity. *J Neurosci*, **37**(3), 599–609. https://doi.org/10.1523/JNEUROSCI.2610-16.2016

Lohnas, L. J., Duncan, K., Doyle, W. K., Thesen, T., Devinsky, O., Davachi, L. (2018). Time-resolved neural reinstatement and pattern separation during memory decisions in human hippocampus. *Proc Natl Acad Sci U S A*, **115**(31), E7418–e7427. https://doi.org/10.1073/pnas.1717088115

Long, N. M., Lee, H., Kuhl, B. A. (2016). Hippocampal mismatch signals are modulated by the strength of neural predictions and their similarity to outcomes. *J Neurosci*, **36**(50), 12677–12687. https://doi.org/10.1523/JNEUROSCI.1850-16.2016

Lucas, H. D., Duff, M. C., Cohen, N. J. (2019). The hippocampus promotes effective saccadic information gathering in humans. *J Cogn Neurosci*, **31**(2), 186–201. https://doi.org/10.1162/jocn_a_01336 %M 30188777

Luettgau, L., Tempelmann, C., Kaiser, L. F., Jocham, G. (2020). Decisions bias future choices by modifying hippocampal associative memories. *Nat Commun*, **11**(1), 3318. https://doi.org/10.1038/s41467-020-17192-7

Mack, M. L., Love, B. C., Preston, A. R. (2016). Dynamic updating of hippocampal object representations reflects new conceptual knowledge. *Proc Natl Acad Sci U S A*, **113**(46), 13203–13208. https://doi.org/10.1073/pnas.1614048113

Mack, M. L., Preston, A. R. (2016). Decisions about the past are guided by reinstatement of specific memories in the hippocampus and perirhinal cortex. *Neuroimage*, **127**, 144–157. https://doi.org/10.1016/j.neuroimage.2015.12.015

Maguire, E. A. (2001). Neuroimaging studies of autobiographical event memory. *Philos Trans R Soc Lond B Biol Sci*, **356**, 1441–1451.

Maguire, E. A. (2014). Memory consolidation in humans: new evidence and opportunities. *Exp Physiol*, **99**(3), 471–486. https://doi.org/10.1113/expphysiol.2013.072157

Maguire, E. A., Burke, T., Phillips, J., Staunton, H. (1996). Topographical disorientation following unilateral temporal lobe surgery in humans. *Neuropsychologia*, **34**, 993–1001.

Maguire, E. A., Gadian, D. G., Johnsrude, I. S., Good, C. D., Ashburner, J., Frackowiak, R. S., Frith, C. D. (2000). Navigation-related structural change in the hippocampi of taxi drivers. *Proc Natl Acad Sci U S A*, **97**(8), 4398–4403. https://doi.org/10.1073/pnas.070039597

Maguire, E. A., Mullally, S. L. (2013). The hippocampus: a manifesto for change. *J Exp Psychol Gen*, **142**(4), 1180–1189. https://doi.org/10.1037/a0033650

Maguire, E. A., Nannery, R., Spiers, H. J. (2006). Navigation around London by a taxi driver with bilateral hippocampal lesions. *Brain*, **129**(Pt 11), 2894–2907. https://doi.org/10.1093/brain/awl286

Maguire, E. A., Spiers, H. J., Good, C. D., Hartley, T., Frackowiak, R. S., Burgess, N. (2003). Navigation expertise and the human hippocampus: a structural brain imaging analysis. *Hippocampus*, **13**(2), 250–259. https://doi.org/10.1002/hipo.10087

Manns, J. R., Hopkins, R. O., Squire, L. R. (2003). Semantic memory and the human hippocampus. *Neuron*, **38**(1), 127–133.

Mayes, A. R., Isaac, C. L., Holdstock, J. S., Hunkin, N. M., Montaldi, D., Downes, J. J., … Roberts, J. N. (2001). Memory for single items, word pairs, and temporal order of different kinds in a patient with selective hippocampal lesions. *Cogn Neuropsychol*, **18**(2), 97–123. https://doi.org/10.1080/02643290125897

Mayes, A. R., Holdstock, J. S., Isaac, C. L., Montaldi, D., Grigor, J., Gummer, A., … Norman, K. A. (2004). Associative recognition in a patient with selective hippocampal lesions and relatively normal recognition memory. *Hippocampus*, **14**, 763–784.

McCormick, C., Barry, D. N., Jafarian, A., Barnes, G. R., Maguire, E. A. (2020). vmPFC drives hippocampal processing during autobiographical memory recall regardless of remoteness. *Cereb Cortex*, **30**(11), 5972–5987. https://doi.org/10.1093/cercor/bhaa172

McCormick, C., Rosenthal, C. R., Miller, T. D., Maguire, E. A. (2016). Hippocampal damage increases deontological responses during moral decision making. *J Neurosci*, **36**(48), 12157–12167. https://doi.org/10.1523/JNEUROSCI.0707-16.2016

McCormick, C., Rosenthal, C. R., Miller, T. D., Maguire, E. A. (2018). Mind-wandering in people with hippocampal damage. *J Neurosci*, **38**, 2745–2754. https://doi.org/10.1523/JNEUROSCI.1812-17.2018

McCormick, C., Rosenthal, C. R., Miller, T. D., Maguire, E. A. (2017). Deciding what is possible and impossible following hippocampal damage in humans. *Hippocampus*, **27**(3), 303–314. https://doi.org/10.1002/hipo.22694

Milivojevic, B., Vicente-Grabovetsky, A., Doeller, C. F. (2015). Insight reconfigures hippocampal-prefrontal memories. *Curr Biol*, **25**(7), 821–830. https://doi.org/10.1016/j.cub.2015.01.033

Miller, G. A., Galanter, E., Pribram, K. H. (1960). Plans and the Structure of Behavior. New York: Holt, Rinehart and Winston, Inc.

Miller, T. D., Chong, T. T. J., Aimola Davies, A. M., Johnson, M. R., Irani, S. R., Husain, M., … Rosenthal, C. R. (2020). Human hippocampal

CA3 damage disrupts both recent and remote episodic memories. *Elife*, 9, e41836. https://doi.org/10.7554/eLife.41836

Miller, T. D., Chong, T. T.-J., Aimola Davies, A. M., Ng, T. W. C., Johnson, M. R., Irani, S. R., ... Rosenthal, C. R. (2017). Focal CA3 hippocampal subfield atrophy following LGI1 VGKC-complex antibody limbic encephalitis. *Brain*, 140(5), 1212–1219. https://doi.org/10.1093/brain/awx070

Milner, B. (1965). Physiologie de l'Hippocampe: Colloque International, No. 107, Editions du Centre National de la Recherche Scientifique, Paris, 1962. In: Pergamon.

Milner, B. (1968). Disorders of memory after brain lesions in man: preface: material-specific and generalized memory loss. *Neuropsychologia*, 6, 175–179.Monk, A. M., Dalton, M. A., Barnes, G. R., Maguire, E. A. (2021). The role of hippocampal-ventromedial prefrontal cortex neural dynamics in building mental representations. *J Cogn Neurosci*, 33, 89–103. https://doi.org/10.1162/jocn_a_01634

Montchal, M. E., Reagh, Z. M., Yassa, M. A. (2019). Precise temporal memories are supported by the lateral entorhinal cortex in humans. *Nat Neurosci*, 22(2), 284–288. https://doi.org/10.1038/s41593-018-0303-1

Mooneyham, B. W., Schooler, J. W. (2013). The costs and benefits of mind-wandering: a review. *Can J Exp Psychol*, 67(1), 11–18. https://doi.org/10.1037/a0031569

Moscovitch, M., Cabeza, R., Winocur, G., Nadel, L. (2016). Episodic memory and beyond: the hippocampus and neocortex in transformation. *Annu Rev Psychol*, 67, 105–134. https://doi.org/10.1146/annurev-psych-113011-143733

Moscovitch, M., Nadel, L. (2019). Sculpting remote memory: Enduring hippocampal traces and vmPFC reconstructive processes. *Trends Cogn Sci*, 23, 634–635.

Mullally, S. L., Intraub, H., Maguire, E. A. (2012). Attenuated boundary extension produces a paradoxical memory advantage in amnesic patients. *Curr Biol*, 22, 261–268. https://doi.org/10.1016/j.cub.2012.01.001

Mullally, S. L., Maguire, E. A. (2014). Counterfactual thinking in patients with amnesia. *Hippocampus*, 24(11), 1261–1266. https://doi.org/10.1002/hipo.22323

Munoz, M., Chadwick, M., Perez-Hernandez, E., Vargha-Khadem, F., Mishkin, M. (2010). Novelty preference in patients with developmental amnesia. *Hippocampus*, 21, 1268–1276.

Nadel, L., Moscovitch, M. (1997). Memory consolidation, retrograde amnesia and the hippocampal complex. *Curr Opin Neurobiol*, 7(2), 217–227.

Nadel, L., Winocur, G., Ryan, L., Moscovitch, M. (2007). Systems consolidation and hippocampus: two views. *Debates in Neuroscience*, 1(2–4), 55–66. https://doi.org/10.1007/s11559-007-9003-9

Nau, M., Navarro Schröder, T., Bellmund, J. L. S., Doeller, C. F. (2018). Hexadirectional coding of visual space in human entorhinal cortex. *Nat Neurosci*, 21(2), 188–190. https://doi.org/10.1038/s41593-017-0050-8

Nee, D. E., Jonides, J. (2011). Dissociable contributions of prefrontal cortex and the hippocampus to short-term memory: evidence for a 3-state model of memory. *Neuroimage*, 54(2), 1540–1548. https://doi.org/10.1016/j.neuroimage.2010.09.002

Nieuwenhuis, I. L., Takashima, A. (2011). The role of the ventromedial prefrontal cortex in memory consolidation. *Behav Brain Res*, 218(2), 325–334. https://doi.org/10.1016/j.bbr.2010.12.009

Norman, Y., Yeagle, E. M., Khuvis S., Harel, M., Mehta, A. D., Malach, R. (2019). Hippocampal sharp-wave ripples linked to visual episodic recollection in humans. *Science*, 365(6454), eaax1030. https://doi.org/10.1126/science.aax1030

O'Keefe, J., Nadel, L. (1978). The Hippocampus as a Cognitive Map. Oxford: Clarendon Press.

Ogawa, S., Tank, D. W., Menon, R., Ellermann, J. M., Kim, S. G., Merkle, H., Ugurbil, K. (1992). Intrinsic signal changes accompanying sensory stimulation: functional brain mapping with magnetic resonance imaging. *Proc Natl Acad Sci U S A*, 89(13), 5951–5955. https://doi.org/10.1073/pnas.89.13.5951

Okuda, J., Fujii, T., Ohtake, H., Tsukiura, T., Tanji, K., Suzuki, K., ... Yamadori, A. (2003). Thinking of the future and past: the roles of the frontal pole and the medial temporal lobes. *Neuroimage*, 19(4), 1369–1380. https://doi.org/10.1016/s1053-8119(03)00179-4

Olsen, R. K., Sebanayagam, V., Lee, Y., Moscovitch, M., Grady, C. L., Rosenbaum, R. S., Ryan, J. D. (2016). The relationship between eye movements and subsequent recognition: evidence from individual differences and amnesia. *Cortex*, 85, 182–193. https://doi.org/10.1016/j.cortex.2016.10.007

Pacheco Estefan, D., Sanchez-Fibla, M., Duff, A., Principe, A., Rocamora, R., Zhang, H., ... Verschure, P. (2019). Coordinated representational reinstatement in the human hippocampus and lateral temporal cortex during episodic memory retrieval. *Nat Commun*, 10(1), 2255. https://doi.org/10.1038/s41467-019-09569-0

Palombo, D. J., Keane, M. M., & Verfaellie, M. (2016). Does the hippocampus keep track of time? *Hippocampus*, 26(3), 372–379. https://doi.org/10.1002/hipo.22528

Park, S. A., Miller, D. S., Boorman, E. D. (2021). Inferences on a multidimensional social hierarchy use a grid-like code. *Nat Neurosci* 24(9):1292–1301. https://doi.org/10.1038/s41593-021-00916-3

Piefke, M., Weiss, P. H., Zilles, K., Markowitsch, H. J., Fink, G. R. (2003). Differential remoteness and emotional tone modulate the neural correlates of autobiographical memory. *Brain*, 126(Pt 3), 650–668.

Race, E., Keane, M. M., Verfaellie, M. (2011). Medial temporal lobe damage causes deficits in episodic memory and episodic future thinking not attributable to deficits in narrative construction. *J Neurosci*, 31(28), 10262–10269. https://doi.org/10.1523/JNEUROSCI.1145-11.2011

Rekkas, P. V., Constable, R. T. (2005). Evidence that autobiographic memory retrieval does not become independent of the hippocampus: an fMRI study contrasting very recent with remote events. *J Cogn Neurosci*, 17(12), 1950–1961.

Rempel-Clower, N. L., Zola, S. M., Squire, L. R., Amaral, D. G. (1996). Three cases of enduring memory impairment after bilateral damage limited to the hippocampal formation. *J Neurosci*, 16(16), 5233–5255.

Raichle, M. E., Snyder A. Z. (2001). A default mode of brain function: a brief history of an evolving idea. *NeuroImage*, 37, 1083–1090.

Rauchs, G., Feyers, D., Landeau, B., Bastin, C., Luxen, A., Maquet, P., Collette, F. (2011). Sleep contributes to the strengthening of some memories over others, depending on hippocampal activity at learning. *J Neurosci*, 31(7), 2563–2568. https://doi.org/10.1523/JNEUROSCI.3972-10.2011

Reif, P. S., Strzelczyk, A., Rosenow, F. (2016). The history of invasive EEG evaluation in epilepsy patients. *Seizure*, 41, 191–195.

Ribot, T. (1891). Les maladies de la mémoire. Baillière. Paris.

Roberts, B. M., Libby, L. A., Inhoff, M. C., Ranganath, C. (2018). Brain activity related to working memory for temporal order and object information. *Behav Brain Res*, 354:55–63. https://doi.org/10.1016/j.bbr.2017.05.068

Roediger, H. L., McDermott, K. B. (1995). Creating false memories: remembering words not presented in lists. *J Exp Psychol: Learn Mem Cogn*, 21(4), 803–814. https://doi.org/10.1037/0278-7393.21.4.803

Rolls, E. T., Kesner, R. P. (2006). A computational theory of hippocampal function, and empirical tests of the theory. *Prog Neurobiol*, 79(1), 1–48. https://doi.org/10.1016/j.pneurobio.2006.04.005

Rosenbaum, R. S., Köhler, S., Schacter, D. L., Moscovitch, M., Westmacott, R., Black, S. E., . . . Tulving, E. (2005). The case of KC: contributions of a memory-impaired person to memory theory. *Neuropsychologica*, 43, 989–1021.

Rosenbaum, R. S., Moscovitch, M., Foster, J. K., Schnyer, D. M., Gao, F., Kovacevic, N., ... Levine, B. (2008). Patterns of autobiographical memory loss in medial-temporal lobe amnesic patients. *J Cogn Neurosci*, 20(8), 1490–1506. https://doi.org/10.1162/jocn.2008.20105

Rosenbaum, R. S., Priselac, S., Köhler, S., Black, S. E., Gao, F., Nadel, L., Moscovitch, M. (2000). Remote spatial memory in an amnesic person with extensive bilateral hippocampal lesions. *Nat Neurosci*, 3, 1044. https://doi.org/10.1038/79867

Sargent, J. Q., Zacks, J. M., Hambrick, D. Z., Zacks, R. T., Kurby, C. A., Bailey, H. R., ... Beck, T. M. (2013). Event segmentation ability uniquely predicts event memory. *Cognition*, 129(2), 241–255. https://doi.org/10.1016/j.cognition.2013.07.002

Schacter, D. L., Addis, D. R. (2007). The cognitive neuroscience of constructive memory: remembering the past and imagining the future. *Philos Trans R Soc Lond B Biol Sci*, 362(1481), 773–786. https://doi.org/10.1098/rstb.2007.2087

Schacter, D. L., Norman, K. A., Koutstaal, W. (1998). The cognitive neuroscience of constructive memory. *Annu Rev Psychol*, 49, 289–318. https://doi.org/10.1146/annurev.psych.49.1.289

Schacter, D. L., Verfaellie, M., Pradere, D. (1996). The neuropsychology of memory illusions: false recall and recognition in amnesic patients. *J Mem Lang*, 35(2), 319–334. https://doi.org/10.1006/jmla.1996.0018

Schapiro, A. C., McDevitt, E. A., Chen, L., Norman, K. A., Mednick, S. C., Rogers, T. T. (2017). Sleep benefits memory for semantic category structure while preserving exemplar-specific information. *Sci Rep*, 7(1), 14869. https://doi.org/10.1038/s41598-017-12884-5

Schapiro, A. C., McDevitt, E. A., Rogers, T. T., Mednick, S. C., Norman, K. A. (2018). Human hippocampal replay during rest prioritizes weakly learned information and predicts memory performance. *Nat Commun*, 9(1), 3920. https://doi.org/10.1038/s41467-018-06213-1

Schapiro, A. C., Reid, A. G., Morgan, A., Manoach, D. S., Verfaellie, M., Stickgold, R. (2019). The hippocampus is necessary for the consolidation of a task that does not require the hippocampus for initial learning. *Hippocampus*, 29(11), 1091–1100. https://doi.org/10.1002/hipo.23101

Schapiro, A. C., Turk-Browne, N. B., Norman, K. A., Botvinick, M. M. (2016). Statistical learning of temporal community structure in the hippocampus. *Hippocampus*, 26(1), 3–8. https://doi.org/10.1002/hipo.22523

Schönauer, M., Alizadeh, S., Jamalabadi, H., Abraham, A., Pawlizki, A., Gais, S. (2017). Decoding material-specific memory reprocessing during sleep in humans. *Nat Commun*, 8, 15404. https://doi.org/10.1038/ncomms15404

Schuck, N. W., Niv, Y. (2019). Sequential replay of nonspatial task states in the human hippocampus. *Science*, 364(6447), eaaw5181. https://doi.org/10.1126/science.aaw5181

Scoville, W. B., Milner, B. (1957). Loss of recent memory after bilateral hippocampal lesions. *J Neurol Neurosurg Psychiatry*, 20(1), 11–21.

Sejnowski, T. J., Churchland, P. S., Movshon, J. A. (2014). Putting big data to good use in neuroscience. *Nat Neurosci*, 17(11), 1440–1441. https://doi.org/10.1038/nn.3839

Smallwood, J., Andrews-Hanna, J. (2013). Not all minds that wander are lost: the importance of a balanced perspective on the mind-wandering state. *Front Psychol*, 4, 441–441. https://doi.org/10.3389/fpsyg.2013.00441

Smith, C. N., Jeneson, A., Frascino, J. C., Kirwan, C. B., Hopkins, R. O., Squire, L. R. (2014). When recognition memory is independent of hippocampal function. *Proc Natl Acad Sci U S A*, 111(27), 9935–9940. https://doi.org/10.1073/pnas.1409878111

Solomon, E. A., Lega, B. C., Sperling, M. R., Kahana, M. J. (2019). Hippocampal theta codes for distances in semantic and temporal spaces. *Proc Natl Acad Sci U S A*, 116(48), 24343–24352. https://doi.org/10.1073/pnas.1906729116

Spalding, Kirsty L., Bergmann, O., Alkass, K., Bernard, S., Salehpour, M., Huttner, Hagen B., ... Frisén, J. (2013). Dynamics of hippocampal neurogenesis in adult humans. *Cell*, 153(6), 1219–1227. http://dx.doi.org/10.1016/j.cell.2013.05.002

Spanò, G., Weber, F. D., Pizzamiglio, G., McCormick, C., Miller, T. D., Rosenthal, C. R., Edgin, J. O., Maguire, E. A. (2020a). Sleeping with hippocampal damage. *Curr Biol* 30, 523–529.

Spanò, G., Pizzamiglio, G., McCormick, C., Clark, I. A., De Felice, S., Miller, T. D., ... Maguire, E. A. (2020b). Dreaming with hippocampal damage. *Elife*, 9, e56211. https://doi.org/10.7554/eLife.56211

Spiers, H. J., Burgess, N., Maguire, E. A., Baxendale, S. A., Hartley, T., Thompson, P., O'Keefe, J. (2001). Unilateral temporal lobectomy patients show lateralised topographical and episodic memory deficits in a virtual town. *Brain*, 124, 2476–2489.

Spiers, H. J., Maguire, E. A. (2006). Thoughts, behaviour, and brain dynamics during navigation in the real world. *Neuroimage*, 31(4), 1826–1840. https://doi.org/10.1016/j.neuroimage.2006.01.037

Spiers, H. J., Maguire, E. A., Burgess, N. (2001). Hippocampal amnesia. *Neurocase*, 7, 575–582.

Spreng, R. N., Gerlach, K. D., Turner, G. R., Schacter, D. L. (2015). Autobiographical planning and the brain: activation and its modulation by qualitative features. *J Cogn Neurosci*, 27(11), 2147–2157. https://doi.org/10.1162/jocn_a_00846

Squire, L. R. (1992). Memory and the hippocampus: a synthesis from findings with rats, monkeys, and humans. *Psychol Rev*, 99(2), 195–231. Squire, L. R., Alvarez, P. (1995). Retrograde amnesia and memory consolidation: a neurobiological perspective. *Curr Opin Neurobiol*, 5(2), 169–177.

Squire, L. R., Genzel, L., Wixted, J. T., Morris, R. G. (2015). Memory consolidation. *Cold Spring Harb Perspect Biol*, 7(8), a021766. https://doi.org/10.1101/cshperspect.a021766

Squire, L. R., Ojemann, J., Miezin, F., Petersen, S., Videen, T., Raichle, M. (1992). Activation of the hippocampus in normal humans: a functional anatomical study of memory. *Proc Natl Acad Sci U S A*, 89, 1837–1841. https://doi.org/10.1073/pnas.89.5.1837

Steemers, B., Vicente-Grabovetsky, A., Barry, C., Smulders, P., Schroder, T. N., Burgess, N., Doeller, C. F. (2016). Hippocampal attractor dynamics predict memory-based decision making. *Curr Biol*, 26(13), 1750–1757. https://doi.org/10.1016/j.cub.2016.04.063

Steinvorth, S., Corkin, S., Halgren, E. (2006). Ecphory of autobiographical memories: an fMRI study of recent and remote memory retrieval. *Neuroimage*, 30(1), 285–298. https://doi.org/10.1016/j.neuroimage.2005.09.025

Steinvorth, S., Levine, B., Corkin, S. (2005). Medial temporal lobe structures are needed to re-experience remote autobiographical memories: evidence from H.M. and W.R. *Neuropsychologia*, 43, 479–496.

Steinvorth, S., Wang, C., Ulbert, I., Schomer, D., Halgren, E. (2010). Human entorhinal gamma and theta oscillations selective for remote autobiographical memory. *Hippocampus*, 20(1), 166–173. https://doi.org/10.1002/hipo.20597

Strange, B. A., Dolan, R. J. (2001). Adaptive anterior hippocampal responses to oddball stimuli. *Hippocampus, 11*(6), 690–698. https://doi.org/10.1002/hipo.1084

Summerfield, J. J., Lepsien, J., Gitelman, D. R., Mesulam, M. M., Nobre, A. C. (2006). Orienting attention based on long-term memory experience. *Neuron, 49*(6), 905–916.

Suthana, N. A., Donix, M., Wozny, D. R., Bazih, A., Jones, M., Heidemann, R. M., ... Bookheimer, S. Y. (2015). High-resolution 7T fMRI of human hippocampal subfields during associative learning. *J Cogn Neurosci, 27*(6), 1194–1206. https://doi.org/10.1162/jocn_a_00772

Swallow, K. M., Barch, D. M., Head, D., Maley, C. J., Holder, D., Zacks, J. M. (2011). Changes in events alter how people remember recent information. *J Cogn Neurosci, 23*(5), 1052–1064. https://doi.org/10.1162/jocn.2010.21524 %M 20521850

Sweegers, C. C., Takashima, A., Fernandez, G., Talamini, L. M. (2014). Neural mechanisms supporting the extraction of general knowledge across episodic memories. *Neuroimage, 87*, 138–146. https://doi.org/10.1016/j.neuroimage.2013.10.063

Sweegers, C. C. G., Talamini, L. M. (2014). Generalization from episodic memories across time: A route for semantic knowledge acquisition. *Cortex, 59*, 49–61. https://doi.org/10.1016/j.cortex.2014.07.006

Symm, M., Jager, H. R., Schmierer, K., Yousry, T. A. (2004). A review of structural magnetic resonance imaging. *J Neurol Neurosurg Psychiatry, 75*, 1235–1244.

Tambini, A., Davachi, L. (2013). Persistence of hippocampal multivoxel patterns into postencoding rest is related to memory. *Proc Natl Acad Sci U S A, 110*(48), 19591–19596. https://doi.org/10.1073/pnas.1308499110

Tavares, R. M., Mendelsohn, A., Grossman, Y., Williams, C. H., Shapiro, M., Trope, Y., Schiller, D. (2015). A map for social navigation in the human brain. *Neuron, 87*(1), 231–243. https://doi.org/10.1016/j.neuron.2015.06.011

Taylor, K. J., Henson, R. N. A., Graham, K. S. (2007). Recognition memory for faces and scenes in amnesia: Dissociable roles of medial temporal lobe structures. *Neuropsychologia, 45*(11), 2428–2438. https://doi.org/10.1016/j.neuropsychologia.2007.04.004

Teng, E., Squire, L. R. (1999). Memory for places learned long ago is intact after hippocampal damage. *Nature, 400*(6745), 675–677. https://doi.org/10.1038/23276

Teyler, T. J., DiScenna, P. (1985). The role of hippocampus in memory: a hypothesis. *Neurosci Biobehav Rev, 9*(3), 377–389.

Theves, S., Fernandez, G., Doeller, C. F. (2019). The hippocampus encodes distances in multidimensional feature space. *Current Biology, 29*(7), 1226–1231.e1223. https://doi.org/10.1016/j.cub.2019.02.035

Titiz, A. S., Hill, M. R. H., Mankin, E. A., M Aghajan, Z., Eliashiv, D., Tchemodanov, N., ... Fried, I. (2017). Theta-burst microstimulation in the human entorhinal area improves memory specificity. *Elife, 6*, e29515. https://doi.org/10.7554/eLife.29515

Tranel, D., Jones, R. D. (2006). Knowing "what" and knowing "when." *J Clin Exp Neuropsychol, 28*(1), 43–66. https://doi.org/10.1080/13803390490919344

Tubridy, S., Davachi, L. (2011). Medial temporal lobe contributions to episodic sequence encoding. *Cereb Cortex, 21*(2), 272–280. https://doi.org/10.1093/cercor/bhq092

Tulving, E. (1972). Episodic and semantic memory. In: Organization of Memory (E. Tulving & W. Donaldson, eds.), pp 381–403. New York: Academic.

Tulving, E., Schacter, D. L., McLachlan, D. R., Moscovitch, M. (1988). Priming of semantic autobiographical knowledge: a case study of retrograde amnesia. *Brain Cogn, 8*(1), 3–20. Retrieved from http://www.ncbi.nlm.nih.gov/pubmed/3166816

van Kesteren, M. T., Fernandez, G., Norris, D. G., Hermans, E .J. (2010). Persistent scheme-dependent hippocampal-neocortical connectivity during memory encoding and postencoding rest in humans. *Proc Natl Acad Sci U S A, 107*, 7550–7555.

van Kesteren, M .T., Ruiter, D. J., Fernandez, G., Henson, R. N. (2012). How schema and novelty augment memory formation. *Trends Neurosci, 35*, 211–219.

Van Veen, B. D., van Drongelen, W., Yuchtman, M., Suzuki, A. (1997). Localization of brain electrical activity via linearly constrained minimum variance spatial filtering. *IEEE Trans Biomed Eng, 44*(9), 867–880. https://doi.org/10.1109/10.623056

Vargha-Khadem, F., Gadian, D. G., Watkins, K. E., Connelly, A., Van Paesschen, W., Mishkin, M. (1997). Differential effects of early hippocampal pathology on episodic and semantic memory. *Science, 277*(5324), 376–380

Viard, A., Piolino, P., Desgranges, B., Chetelat, G., Lebreton, K., Landeau, B., ... Eustache, F. (2007). Hippocampal activation for autobiographical memories over the entire lifetime in healthy aged subjects: an fMRI study. *Cereb Cortex, 17*(10), 2453–2467. https://doi.org/10.1093/cercor/bhl153

von Allmen, D. Y., Wurmitzer, K., Martin, E., Klaver, P. (2013). Neural activity in the hippocampus predicts individual visual short-term memory capacity. *Hippocampus, 23*(7), 606–615. https://doi.org/10.1002/hipo.22121

Wamsley, E. J., Stickgold, R. (2019). Dreaming of a learning task is associated with enhanced memory consolidation: Replication in an overnight sleep study. *J Sleep Res, 28*(1), e12749–e12749. https://doi.org/10.1111/jsr.12749

Warren, D. E., Duff, M. C., Jensen, U., Tranel, D., Cohen, N. J. (2012). Hiding in plain view: lesions of the medial temporal lobe impair online representation. *Hippocampus, 22*(7), 1577–1588. https://doi.org/10.1002/hipo.21000

Warren, D. E., Duff, M. C., Tranel, D., Cohen, N. J. (2011). Observing degradation of visual representations over short intervals when medial temporal lobe is damaged. *J Cogn Neurosci, 23*(12), 3862–3873. https://doi.org/10.1162/jocn_a_00089

Watrous, A. J., Miller, J., Qasim, S. E., Fried, I., Jacobs, J. (2018). Phase-tuned neuronal firing encodes human contextual representations for navigational goals. *Elife, 7*, e32554. https://doi.org/10.7554/eLife.32554

Watrous, A. J., Lee, D. J., Izadi, A., Gurkoff, G. G., Shahlaie, K., Ekstrom, A. D. (2013). A comparative study of human and rat hippocampal low-frequency oscillations during spatial navigation. *Hippocampus, 23*(8), 656–661. https://doi.org/10.1002/hipo.22124

Weiler, J. A., Suchan, B., Daum, I. (2010). When the future becomes the past: differences in brain activation patterns for episodic memory and episodic future thinking. *Behav Brain Res, 212*(2), 196–203. https://doi.org/10.1016/j.bbr.2010.04.013

Weisberg, S. M., Newcombe, N. S., & Chatterjee, A. (2019). Everyday taxi drivers: Do better navigators have larger hippocampi? *Cortex, 115*, 280–293. https://doi.org/10.1016/j.cortex.2018.12.024

West, K. L., Zuppichini, M. D., Turner, M. P., Sivakolundu, D. K., Zhao, Y., Abdelkarim, D., ... Rypma, B. (2019). BOLD hemodynamic response function changes significantly with healthy aging. *Neuroimage, 188*, 198–207. https://doi.org/10.1016/j.neuroimage.2018.12.012

Wilson, N.-A., Ramanan, S., Roquet, D., Goldberg, Z.-L., Hodges, J. R., Piguet, O., Irish, M. (2020). Scene construction impairments in frontotemporal dementia: evidence for a primary hippocampal contribution. *Neuropsychologia, 137*, 107327. https://doi.org/10.1016/j.neuropsychologia.2019.107327

Wimmer, G. E., Shohamy, D. (2012). Preference by association: how memory mechanisms in the hippocampus bias decisions. *Science, 338*(6104), 270. https://doi.org/10.1126/science.1223252

Winocur, G., Moscovitch, M. (2011). Memory transformation and systems consolidation. *J Int Neuropsychol Soc, 17*(5), 766–780. https://doi.org/10.1017/S1355617711000683

Woollett, K., Maguire, E. A. (2011). Acquiring "the Knowledge" of London's layout drives structural brain changes. *Curr Biol*, 21(24), 2109–2114. https://doi.org/10.1016/j.cub.2011.11.018

Woollett, K., Glensman, J., Maguire, E. A. (2008). Non-spatial expertise and hippocampal grey matter volume in humans. *Hippocampus*, 18, 981–984. https://doi.org/10.1002/hipo.20465

Yonelinas, A. P. (2002). The nature of recollection and familiarity: a review of 30 years of research. *J Mem Lang*, 46(3), 441–517. https://doi.org/10.1006/jmla.2002.2864

Yonelinas, A. P. (2013). The hippocampus supports high-resolution binding in the service of perception, working memory and long-term memory. *Behav Brain Res*, 254, 34–44. https://doi.org/10.1016/j.bbr.2013.05.030

Yonelinas, A. P., Ranganath, C., Ekstrom, A. D., Wiltgen, B. J. (2019). A contextual binding theory of episodic memory: systems consolidation reconsidered. *Nat Rev Neurosci*, 20(6), 364–375. https://doi.org/10.1038/s41583-019-0150-4

Yushkevich, P. A., Amaral, R. S., Augustinack, J. C., Bender, A. R., Bernstein, J. D., Boccardi, M., ... Zeineh, M. M. (2015). Quantitative comparison of 21 protocols for labeling hippocampal subfields and parahippocampal subregions in in vivo MRI: towards a harmonized segmentation protocol. *Neuroimage*, 111, 526–541.

Zacks, J. M., Speer, N. K., Swallow, K. M., Braver, T. S., Reynolds, J. R. (2007). Event perception: A mind-brain perspective. *Psychol Bull*, 133(2), 273–293. https://doi.org/10.1037/0033-2909.133.2.273

Zeidman, P., Mullally, S. L., Schwarzkopf, D. S., Maguire, E. A. (2012). Exploring the parahippocampal cortex response to high and low spatial frequency spaces. *Neuroreport*, 23, 503–507. https://dopi.org/10.1097/WNR.0b013e328353766a

Zeidman, P., Lutti, A., Maguire, E. A. (2015). Investigating the functions of subregions within anterior hippocampus. *Cortex*, 73, 240–256. https://doi.org/10.1016/j.cortex.2015.09.002

Zeidman, P., Maguire, E. A. (2016). Anterior hippocampus: the anatomy of perception, imagination and episodic memory. *Nat Rev Neurosci*, 17(3), 173–182. https://doi.org/10.1038/nrn.2015.24

Zeidman, P., Mullally, S. L., Maguire, E. A. (2015). Constructing, perceiving, and maintaining scenes: hippocampal activity and connectivity. *Cereb Cortex*, 25(10), 3836–3855. https://doi.org/10.1093/cercor/bhu266

Zeithamova, D., Dominick, A. L., Preston, A. R. (2012). Hippocampal and ventral medial prefrontal activation during retrieval-mediated learning supports novel inference. *Neuron*, 75(1), 168–179. https://doi.org/10.1016/j.neuron.2012.05.010

Zhang, H., Fell, J., Axmacher, N. (2018). Electrophysiological mechanisms of human memory consolidation. *Nat Commun*, 9(1), 4103. https://doi.org/10.1038/s41467-018-06553-y

Zola-Morgan, S., Squire, L. R., Amaral, D. G. (1986). Human amnesia and the medial temporal region: enduring memory impairment following a bilateral lesion limited to field CA1 of the hippocampus. *J Neurosci*, 6, 2950–2967.

14

Theories of Hippocampal Function

Sam McKenzie, Francesco Gobbo, and Richard G. M. Morris

14.1 The hippocampal formation as a memory machine

In his book *Vision* the mathematician David Marr argued that analysis of what a machine does and how it works should proceed at three levels (Marr, 1982). One level, which he referred to as the "computational" level, is about understanding its *function*. What does the machine do? The second *algorithmic* level of analysis focuses on a logical analysis of how its function is carried out. Applied to the brain, this level specifies how information associated with a specific computation is represented, and the logical procedures for performing the relevant manipulations. The *implementational* level zeroes in on how the algorithms are carried out in neurobiological terms. Marr warned that any bottom-up analysis was risky, arguing instead that these three steps should be carried out in sequence: function, *then* algorithm, *then* implementation.

Contemporary neuroscience is not, however, normally done in this way—instead proceeding at numerous levels of analysis simultaneously as graphically displayed in the famous Sejnowski and Churchland diagram (Chapter 1, Figure 1.3). Marr's analysis, building on his earlier MIT discussion paper with Tommy Poggio, was very influential but also controversial. A later reassessment argued that there needs to be more attention to how different levels of analysis interact (Poggio, 2012). Poggio also suggested that a cardinal problem for which the interaction between the three levels is vital is that of learning and the evolution of different types of learning and memory (Sherry and Schacter, 1987; Murray et al., 2016). In this chapter, we shall outline how theoretical ideas about hippocampal function and interventional studies in animals reflect and benefit from Marr's tripartite approach.

14.1.1 Function

The theoretical ideas outlined in this chapter all focus on the idea that the hippocampus is a special kind of "memory machine." The link between the hippocampus and memory has its roots in clinical and experimental observations on patients who sustained brain damage that included the hippocampus and who had memory problems (Chapter 2). Although damage often extended into other areas of the medial temporal lobe or midbrain, careful study of both the small number of patients with selective damage of the hippocampus and the data from contemporary neuroimaging (Chapter 13), provided further grounds for believing that the integrity of the hippocampal formation is involved in implementing some but not all types of memory. The contributions of animal studies outlined in this chapter have been pivotal in building evidence of a causal nature for theories that link function, algorithm, and neural implementation.

This chapter outlines foundational theories of hippocampal function and discusses how a new framework is emerging, based on the hypothesis that the hippocampal formation plays a vital role in the encoding of new "episodic-like" memory traces and in organizing the consolidation of such information. This perspective embraces ideas ranging from Tulving's (1972) concepts of episodic memory and mental time travel, through to ideas about the creation of and assimilation of newly acquired information into knowledge structures in the brain as considered in complementary learning systems theory (Tulving, 1972; McClelland et al., 1995).

Two foundational theories have dominated research on hippocampus-dependent memory (Figure 14.1). The *cognitive map theory*, emerging from observations first made during the recording of single-cell activity in freely moving rodents and the discovery of place and head-direction cells (Chapters 11 and 12), holds that the hippocampal formation is involved in spatial memory and navigation through space by both rodents (O'Keefe and Conway, 1978) and humans (Burgess et al., 2002; Epstein et al., 2017). The *declarative memory theory* asserts that the hippocampus is part of a medial temporal lobe memory system involved in the formation of memories for everyday facts and events that can be consciously recalled (Squire et al., 1992; Squire et al., 2004; Squire and Deed, 2015). We shall outline these theories in section 14.2, identify the reasons for their exceptional influence, and comment on why they are giving way to new ideas.

14.1.2 Algorithm

An algorithm is a set of rules that precisely defines a sequence of operations. Hebb's (1949) ideas about "cell-assemblies" are algorithmic in character, albeit prescient of neural implementation (Hebb, 1949). Examples of an "algorithm" relevant to the hippocampal formation include the process of "pattern separation" (to distinguish partially overlapping stimuli); "pattern-completion" (resurrecting a complete pattern from partial input), the detection of novel events, and the forming of "associations" between arbitrary stimuli. A key aspect of association is the notion of the "automatic binding" in memory of our experience of events to the spatiotemporal contexts in which they occur. This process lies at the heart of episodic-like memory.

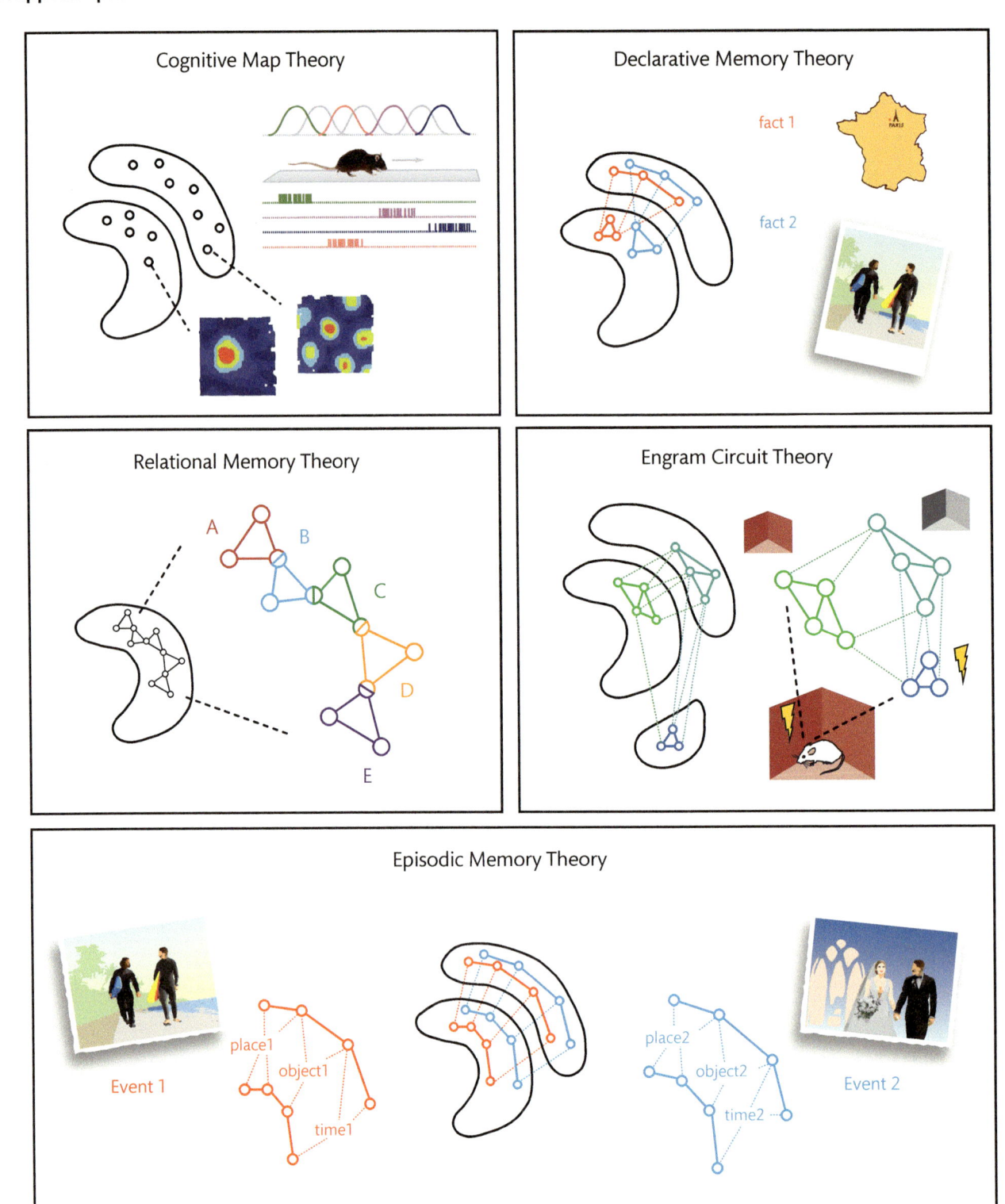

Figure 14.1 Two foundation theories of hippocampal function and later theories. The cognitive-mapping and declarative memory theories (top two panels) highlight different aspects of hippocampal function. One focuses on the representation of space in the form of cognitive maps and its role in spatial navigation, the other on information about facts (episodic or semantic)—distinguishing these from nondeclarative forms of memory; Other theories emerged (middle and bottom panels) including relational memory, engram cells and circuits, and episodic-like memory—to address issues that have arisen in the course of research over the past 30 years that are discussed in later sections of this chapter.

The original declarative memory framework contains no explicit statement about "algorithms," as its research focus was largely confined to building a trans-species model of amnesia and understanding the mystery of temporal gradients of retrograde amnesia. However, its fundamental distinction between declarative and procedural (nondeclarative) information processing is algorithmic in character. It echoes Ryle's philosophical distinction between *knowing that* vs. *knowing how* (Ryle, 1949). In contrast, the cognitive map theory is explicitly "algorithmic," as it asserts that the brain constructs a representation of the outside world that depends on, but is logically independent of, information derived from specific sensory/perceptual systems. In their book, O'Keefe and Nadel (1978) drew attention to debates among philosophers about the nature of mind, coming down firmly in favor of a nativist Kantian rather than an experiential and associationistic "Lockean" framework. Buzsáki adopts the same perspective (Buzsáki, 2019).

Another facet of the algorithmic approach is distinguishing four phases of memory processing: the *encoding* of information; the *storage* of memory traces; a *consolidation* process that is responsible for stability over time and the assimilation of new information within existing knowledge structures; and last, the subsequent *retrieval* and *reactivation* of memory during acts of *recognition* and *recall*.

Marr's original mathematical theory of hippocampal function (Marr, 1971), later developed and discussed by others (McNaughton and Morris, 1987; Willshaw and Buckingham, 1990; Rolls and Treves, 1998), proposed that the potential contribution of the hippocampus to memory could be to form random, orthogonal representations from correlated cortical inputs from sensory/perceptual systems. Once stored in memory, even partial cortical inputs should be able to cue the retrieval of the full-learned pattern of activity that then triggers successful recall. During an experience, which may be new or old, the hippocampus may either create a new and random pattern of active neurons (via pattern separation) and learn this novel constellation; or it may reactivate an existing pattern (pattern completion) and thereby recall past experience. This algorithmic model has been mapped, in terms of implementation, onto different anatomical subregions of hippocampal circuitry, but with a growing realization that the hippocampus sometimes achieves recall in conjunction with information already stored in neocortex.

14.1.3 Mechanism

Turning to *implementation* within the brain, we arrive at not only the diverse physiological, biochemical, and molecular mechanisms identified in earlier chapters of this book, but also the range of contemporary techniques now used to monitor or control the nervous system at different levels of analysis. A striking feature of the last 10 years has been that classical technical approaches (lesions, pharmacology, single-cell recording) are now complemented by new monitoring and interventional techniques, such as multiple single-cell recording, Ca^{2+} imaging, and cell-specific viral manipulations (Figure 14.2). Neuronal monitoring techniques began with extracellular field-potential recording or single-wire recording of single cells, and then moved on to recording hundreds of cells simultaneously, initially with stereotrodes and later tetrodes (McNaughton, O'Keefe, et al., 1983). These methods are now supplemented by multiple-electrode silicon probes (Berenyi et al., 2014). Such multichannel technology, with submillisecond resolution, also permits the recording of specific patterns such as sharp waves and other oscillatory rhythms, from which numerous discoveries about the dynamic operation of hippocampal processing have emerged (Figure 14.2). These recording techniques, with ever more sophisticated computational analyses, are also being complemented by slower but more inclusive Ca^{2+}-imaging techniques using miniature, head-mounted endoscopes in freely moving animals and 2-photon imaging of head-fixed animals moving in virtual reality (Ziv et al., 2013). As Scanziani and Häusser have aptly put it, electrophysiology has moved into "the age of light" (Scanziani and Häusser, 2009).

These techniques have been accompanied by the development of new behavioral techniques beyond those of an earlier generation of researchers who relied on a small corpus of tasks such as delayed nonmatching to sample, context fear conditioning or the watermaze. The past 10+ years have witnessed a technological transformation of behavioral neuroscience, such as the use of virtual reality in studies of behavior that permit awake, head-fixed animals to be monitored using multiphoton microscopy (Harvey et al., 2009). One wonders what Tolman would think if he were able to watch flashing calcium transients in the brain of a mouse on a trackball traversing a complex virtual maze. Like Miranda in Shakespeare's *The Tempest*, he might be tempted to say, "O brave new world!"

Two important qualifications arise. First, while the hippocampal formation and its component subareas have discrete functions, algorithms, or mechanisms, it does not operate in isolation from the rest of the brain. It operates, of course in conjunction with numerous other brain regions and networks, such that even a hippocampus specific function may require that interconnectivity. These include neocortical input structures, such as the parahippocampal, perirhinal, and entorhinal cortices (Chapter 12), and output structures such as the lateral septum, mammillary bodies, and the prefrontal, cingulate, and retrosplenial cortices (Chapter 3). Various subcortical structures containing neuromodulatory afferent systems (e.g., cholinergic and catecholaminergic inputs) also make major contributions to the effectiveness of its function, ranging from attentional salience to mediating the process of cellular consolidation.

The second qualification is work exploring whether the hippocampus has qualitatively distinct functions along its posterior-to-anterior axis (in humans) or corresponding dorsal-ventral axis (in rodents). Specifically, the anterior/ventral parts of the hippocampus may have functions beyond memory—such as a possible specialization of the ventral hippocampus in anxiety and fear (Gray, 1982; Bannerman et al., 2004), or in motivational context (Davidson and Jarrard, 2004). Moreover, the hippocampus is also thought to exert an influence on stress processing via the hypothalamic-pituitary-adrenal (HPA) axis—an issue pursued in Chapter 17. Greater attention to a wider variety of species in their natural habitats, and to the evolution of memory systems, lead us to consider alternatives about hippocampal function that are too often overlooked in the narrow confines of laboratory science (Sherry and Schacter, 1987; Clayton and Dickinson, 1998; Emery and Clayton, 2004; Jeffery, 2024).

14.1.4 Framework of the chapter

We now turn to outlining two foundational theories of hippocampal function. This is followed by sections on recognition memory, spatial memory, and relational-processing that collectively identified issues and problems associated with these earlier theories. The current contemporary framework of episodic and episodic-like memory is then outlined, followed by a section on engram cells and circuits, and then the puzzle of systems memory consolidation mediated by hippocampal-neocortical interactions.

14.2 The foundation stones of two rival theories

14.2.1 The cognitive-map theory–the hippocampus and space

The cognitive mapping theory is predicated on the central role of physical space in organizing memory. "Space," wrote John O'Keefe and Lynn Nadel in 1978 (p 5), "plays a role in all our behavior. We live in it, move through it, explore it, defend it [. . .] yet we find it

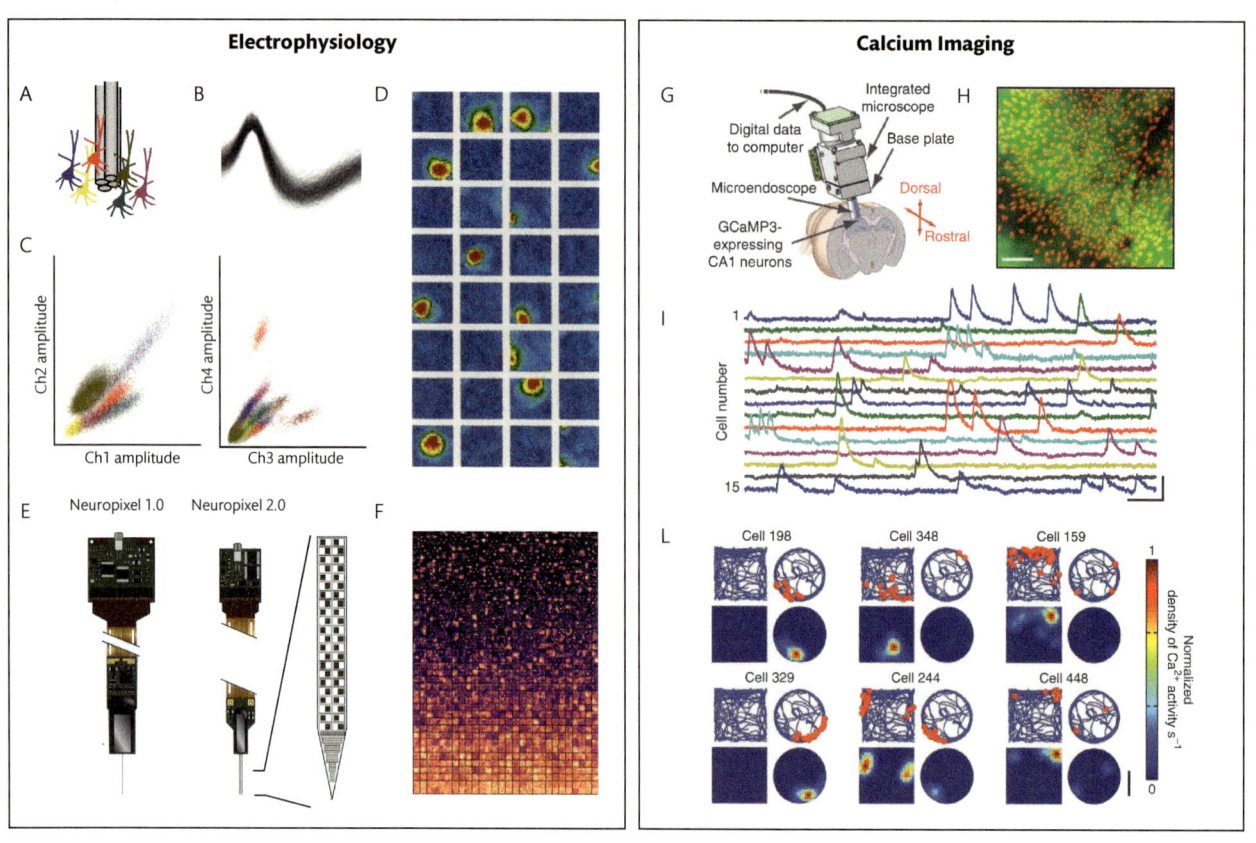

Figure 14.2 Novel technologies for activity recording in freely navigating animals. Traditionally, tetrode recordings (A) have been used to identify single units (B) that can be discriminated by their unique position in the 4-dimension space produced by the 4-channels amplitudes (C). Tetrodes have been used to identify multiple unique place cells. Panel (D) shows the results from Wilson and McNaughton (1993), who introduced the classical representation of action potential distribution in space. (E) Technological advancement has brought the introduction of Neuropixel 1.0, and later of Neuropixel 2.0, allowing the recording of thousands of individual neurons. (F) This panel shows an ensemble of thousands of cells recorded from the medial entorhinal cortex. (Image courtesy of Kavli Institute for Systems Neuroscience.) Conversely, (G) the introduction of miniature microscopes (commonly known in the field as "miniscopes") allows the imaging of neurons in the brain of freely moving animals. When coupled with fluorescent sensors of neuronal activity, such as the calcium indicators from the GCaMP series (Chen et al., 2013), it is possible to record the activity of hundreds of neurons with known identity over multiple days (H). The output is a series of activated calcium traces much like single-cell electrophysiological recordings (I). Note the repetition of units with rapid rise time and extended decay ("Calcium events"), due to the kinetics of the calcium sensor. The amplitude of the event is roughly proportional to the number of action potentials. L) By examining the correlation of calcium events and the animal's position, it is possible to record place-cell dynamics over multiple days. (Panels G–L derived from Ziv et al., 2013.)

extraordinarily difficult to come to grips with space." This engaging rhetoric, together with discussion of the philosophical concept of space, introduced a book called *The Hippocampus as a Cognitive Map* (O'Keefe and Nadel, 1978). Building on ideas long ago outlined by Tolman (1948), they introduced a neurobiological theory that has developed substantially over the past 45 years.

The discovery of "place cells" in the hippocampus of freely moving rats (O'Keefe and Dostrovsky, 1971) (Chapter 11) motivated the development of the cognitive mapping theory. Observations on place cells were quickly followed by the discovery that lesions of a major fiber tract into the hippocampal formation, the fimbria/fornix, resulted in an apparently selective deficit of spatial-learning, but not cue-learning by rats in a circular maze (Nadel et al., 1975). Taken together, these findings led to a theoretically motivated review of the literature, offering an imaginative reassessment of findings hitherto explained in other ways (O'Keefe and Nadel, 1978).

The architects of the cognitive map approach have since outlined various modifications to the theory, beginning with Nadel's work on "spatial context" (Nadel and Willner, 1980), through to ideas about "multiple memory traces" stored within hippocampus (Nadel and

Moscovitch, 1997). Neuroimaging findings on humans performing virtual navigation tasks (Burgess et al., 2002) extended the conclusions derived from rodent studies to the realm of human cognition. However, the cognitive map theory is not the only one that discusses spatial memory. Other spatially oriented theories include a "scene memory" approach to recognition memory (Gaffan, 1991), a "fragment assembly" hypothesis (Worden, 1992), and the idea that the hippocampal formation might be involved in a process we shall outline later called "path integration" (Taube et al., 1990; McNaughton et al., 1996; Whishaw, 1998). Others have, however, placed the path-integration system outside the hippocampus (Redish, 1999). Cell-types beyond place cells have been incorporated into the theory, including head-direction cells (Taube and Schwartzkroin, 1987; Taube, 1998) and grid cells (Fyhn et al., 2004; Hafting et al., 2005). There have also been ideas about the different "metrics" in which spatial information may be processed (Poucet, 1993), with the concept of metrics widely discussed following the discovery of the repetitive pattern of grid-cell firing. Several other cell types such as boundary-vector/border cells lurk at the side (Hartley et al., 2000). The discovery of place cells and grid cells was to earn the Nobel

1. *Learning and representation:* The vertebrate brain has a "locale" system that organizes the encoding and representation of perceived stimuli with respect to an allocentric "cognitive map," in which the position of objects and the observer is defined relative to the environment. Learning occurs automatically in the absence of reward, with the spatial locations of landmarks stored in a neural map of space during exploration.

2. *Retrieval and navigation:* Information is retrieved and used for spatial navigation. The various anatomical subregions of the hippocampal formation mediate different aspects of spatial information processing, with distinct classes of neurons responsive to an animal's place, head direction, and view and its movement through the metric of space. Different neural populations encode memories that take occur in different places. Path integration may contribute to location updating.

3. *Evolution and the laws of learning:* Spatial mapping evolved as one of the multiple memory systems of the vertebrate brain with its own distinctive learning rules. Other types of learning and memory include simpler associative mechanisms and certain geometric tasks that can be acquired using "taxon" strategies. These other systems obey different laws of learning from the locale system, specifically in requiring reward.

4. *Sites of storage:* Spatial maps are stored in the hippocampus. They were thought not to be consolidated elsewhere in the brain, although information stored in the hippocampus does interact with information stored elsewhere for the purpose of guiding navigation.

5. *Extension of the theory to humans:* Whereas the cognitive map is spatial in animals, it was proposed that it also subserves the storage and recall of linguistic information in humans. Lateralization enables the right hippocampus to maintain a primarily spatial function, while the left hippocampus incorporates the temporal sense and linguistic entities that together provide the basis for mediating episodic memory.

Box 14.2 The declarative memory theory

1. *Memory:* The primary function of the hippocampal formation is in memory.

2. *Selectivity:* The role of the hippocampal formation in memory is selective. It mediates the memory of facts and events—called "declarative memory." This is the type of memory that, in humans, can be consciously recalled.

3. *Memory systems:* The hippocampal formation is one of several structures that comprise a "medial temporal lobe memory system." While the components of this system may have distinct subfunctions, it operates collectively to mediate the formation and initial storage of declarative memories.

4. *Time-limited:* The role of the hippocampus in memory is time-limited. Memory is gradually reorganized as time passes after learning. The hippocampus contributes to a time-dependent systems-level consolidation process such that, once completed, long-term memory traces are stored in cortex and neural activity in the hippocampus is no longer required for or involved in recall.

Prize for John O'Keefe, and Edvard and May-Britt Moser, in 2014. The five main suppositions of the original theory (1978) are as follows (Box 14.1).

In contrast to the neuropsychological focus of the declarative memory theory, neurophysiological findings are the backbone of the cognitive map idea. The spatial-mapping theory of was largely developed using rodents, with bats recently flying into the picture (Ulanovsky and Moss, 2007, 2011; Ulanovsky, 2011). The theory's impact on human studies was initially modest compared with the declarative memory theory, but there has recently been an upsurge of interest in contexts, scenes and maps in humans as a substrate for diverse facets of memory (Chapter 13).

14.2.2 The declarative memory theory

The philosopher Gilbert Ryle, writing in 1949, suggested that knowledge should be categorically divided between "knowing that" and "knowing how" (Ryle, 1949). Inspired by this idea, Neal Cohen and Larry Squire suggested that the distinction between "declarative" and "procedural" information processing was both fundamental for understanding amnesia and likely to be reflected in the anatomical organization of the brain (Cohen and Squire, 1980). Squire went on to articulate a declarative memory theory that implicated the hippocampal formation and other structures of the medial temporal lobe in the formation of declarative memory (Squire and Cohen, 1984; Squire and Zola-Morgan, 1991; Squire, 1992; Squire et al., 2004), a theory he has continued to articulate (Squire and Deed, 2015).

The primary support for this theory came from detailed single-case neuropsychological assessments of amnesic subjects followed, when possible, by meticulous histological assessment of their brain damage. A number of amnesic subjects were identified with extremely restricted hippocampal damage (patients R.B. and E.P.) (Zola-Morgan et al., 1986; Teng and Squire, 1999). A comprehensive program of research was also undertaken using nonhuman primates motivated by the ambition of creating an animal model of amnesia. This was led by the National Institutes of Health group of Mortimer Mishkin and the San Diego group led by Larry Squire. The key achievement in that work was the demonstration of accelerated, time-dependent forgetting of a declarative memory task in lesioned monkeys in which normal perceptual function was demonstrated at zero or minimal delays; severe deficits in recognition memory were observed at time periods longer than the duration of short-term memory. There are four key propositions of the theory (Box 14.2).

14.2.3 Comparative evaluation of the "declarative memory" and "cognitive-mapping" theories

These two theories offer very different perspectives on the role of the hippocampus in memory. Both assert a selectivity of declarative/spatial memory formation respectively, and neither has an explicit role for reward or punishment (valence) in this process. The implication is that the learning rules of hippocampal memory encoding differ from those of other brain systems that, guided by reward expectancy, have been studied so intensively in the behavioral domain by animal learning theorists (such as action and habit learning).

The major difference between the two theories is their very distinct premise about the *nature of knowledge*. The declarative memory theory presupposes that information flows from sensory, through perceptual and attentional mechanisms, to a structure where a memory trace (or engram) about something that has just happened is then formed. The process is experientially driven. What is created in hippocampus are memory traces of experience, accessible to conscious awareness and available for linguistic declaration. The theory also asserts that such memory traces are stored as isolated entities; there need be no explicit framework at the outset (at least in hippocampus). This isolated entity subtext also re-emerges later in connection with the process of consolidation. In contrast, the cognitive-map theory asserts that structure exists within the brain that creates a framework, and specifically one defined by the physical dimensions of a three-dimensional (3D) world, into which information is then placed. Beyond place cells, the notion of a cognitive map became even clearer with the discovery of grid cells because the regular hexagonal pattern of repetitive firing in the medial entorhinal cortex is a tangible indication of just such an internal framework. This distinct perspective, extending from spatial to episodic-like memory, is captured well in Edvard Moser's reflection about: "a preconfigured or semi-preconfigured brain system for representation and storage of self-location relative to the external environment. In agreement with the general ideas of Kant, place cells and grid cells in the hippocampal and entorhinal cortices may determine how we perceive and remember our position in the environment as well as the events we experience in that environment" (Moser et al., 2008, p. 70).

Memory encoding within a structured framework is thought to happen, for example, as laboratory rats explore a novel environment; it occurs quickly, sometimes in one trial, with rats often pausing and rearing up to inspect distal cues. The analysis of exploratory behavior and reactions to novelty was central to O'Keefe and Nadel's 1978 book. According to the theory, curiosity-driven exploration involves more than mere perceptual learning about the identity of individual cues (such as objects, landmarks, and boundaries); specifically, the proposed hippocampal mapping system also encodes where landmarks are located in relation to each other in an explicitly geometric although not necessarily Euclidean framework. This "what and where" element of novelty detection became very relevant in later studies of novel object recognition.

The idea of an organized structure to memory is hardly unique to the cognitive map theory, as many other theories of human memory have embodied the same idea, including both artificial intelligence–derived theories of semantic memory (Collins and Quillian, 1969), connectionist theories of memory consolidation (McClelland et al., 1995; O'Reilly and Norman, 2002), and new models that embed specific learning rules into discrete subcomponents of hippocampal

circuitry (Zheng et al., 2022). In some respects, the complementary learning systems hypothesis of McClelland et al. (1995) spans the declarative and cognitive-mapping frameworks while also adding the mathematical precision argued for by Barry and Burgess in Chapter 16. Some form of memory organization would also be helpful for the encoding of one-time events in relation to static landmarks and, partly for this reason, the hippocampus in humans could be helpful for encoding information into episodic memory. The later recall of a specific event, such as what one did during a recent holiday, generally involves first remembering *where* one was, before proceeding to remembering what happened during it. Gaffan was the first to make this point explicitly (Gaffan, 1991), later building it into a "scene-specific" theory of episodic memory. Maguire (Chapter 13) discusses the notion of "scenes" extensively.

Separate from structure is the key question of how the brain uses a cognitive map and place cells to enable successful navigation (Figure 14.3A). O'Keefe and Nadel offered several early speculations about how vector operations could be implemented within the hippocampal formation (O'Keefe and Nadel, 1978), and a new behavioral task from O'Keefe's lab is designed to get at some of these issues (Wood et al., 2018). More recent neural modeling studies have modified and extended these ideas substantially (see Chapter 16). Notwithstanding these developments, the algorithmic description of the cognitive map theory has not yet been worked out in detail. For example, as a place cell is defined as a cell that fires if and only if an animal occupies a specific position in space, how can the mapping system access information pertaining to places that are located elsewhere (Morris, 1991)? That is, if a rat is at place A and wants to navigate to place B but not to place C, how does it at place A access information relevant to going to B rather than going to C? Place-cell firing on its own does not seem to help because the place cells corresponding to B and C cannot—by definition—fire until the animal gets to B or C respectively (Figure 14.3B). This puzzle has inspired a range of different modeling approaches.

What about the types of learning in which the hippocampal formation is *not* involved? For the cognitive map theory, these went

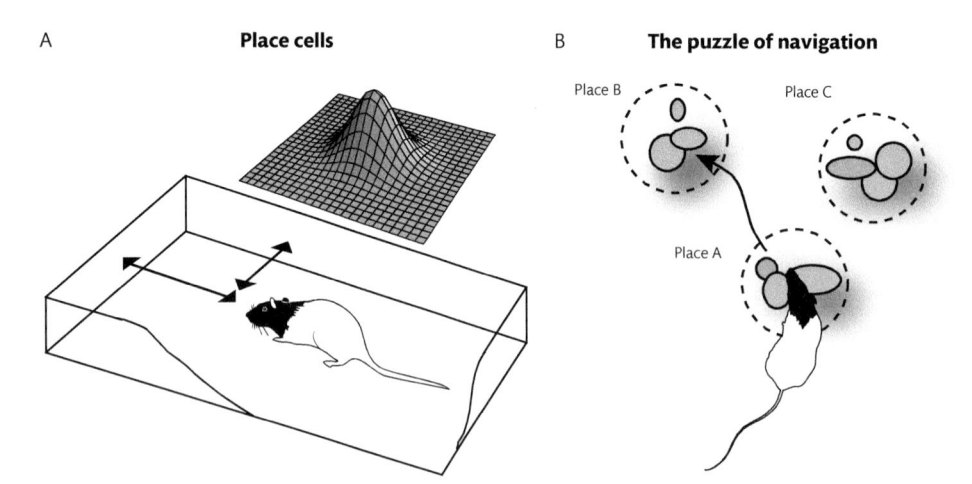

Figure 14.3 Place cells, cognitive mapping, and the puzzle of navigation. (A) The central concept of cognitive mapping theory is the existence of place cells that fire selectively at specific locations unmarked by any local cue. Place cells have different properties but some cells appear to encode vectors to specific boundaries in an environment. (B) A major puzzle concerns the role of place cells in navigation. Place A is defined by the firing of a constellation of cells, and distinct places B and C by the firing of different ensembles of cells. Given the definition of place cells, it is unclear how an animal at place A can access information about places B and C without their cells firing. This puzzle is discussed in detail in Chapter 16.

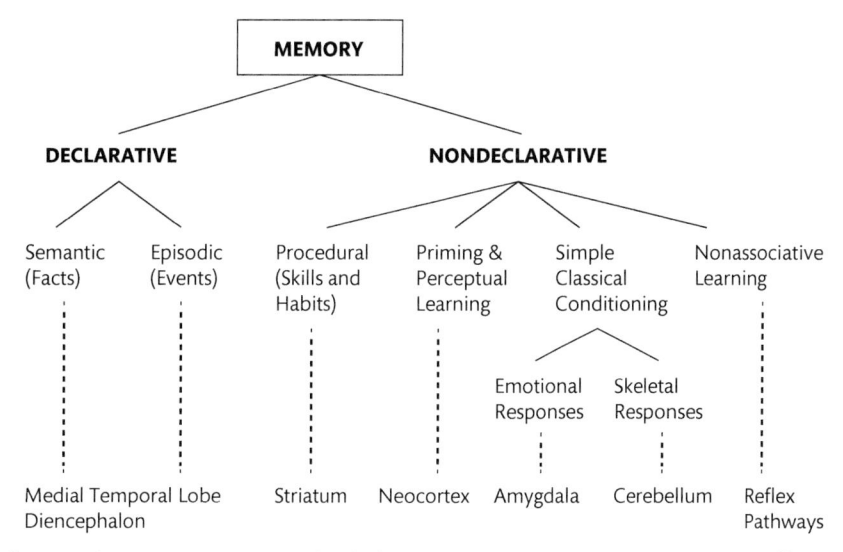

Figure 14.4 A taxonomy of mammalian memory systems. The declarative memory theory recognizes many different types of "memory system" and their mediation by distinct neural brain areas (listed below). The scheme was first introduced by Squire (1987) and has been updated many times since.

under the heading of "taxon strategies" that require actions to be performed relative to cues or beacons. However, for declarative memory, there has been a richer description of "nondeclarative" forms of learning and memory embraced within a wider framework of "multiple memory systems" (Figure 14.4). These nondeclarative forms are thought to reflect acquired information, habits, and learned dispositions that are expressed in behavior but cannot be "declared." One does not "declare" a tennis stroke, one simply makes one. Nor can a tennis stroke be "true" or "false," just good or bad. Initially called "procedural" (Squire and Cohen, 1984), a term first used in the field of artificial intelligence by Winograd (1975), nondeclarative learning is important in constituting "the dispositions, habits, attitudes, and preferences that are inaccessible to conscious recollection, yet are shaped by past events, influence our behavior and our mental life, and are a fundamental part of who we are" (Kandel and Squire, 2000). The declarative vs. nondeclarative distinction is fundamental to the theory. Procedures require sequential processing, whereas isolated memories do not. This idea has developed further in recent years with recognition that the sequential components of habits may develop from the learning of isolated actions that, through their explicit association with an intended goal or reward, include a declarative component that appears to be mediated by the prefrontal cortex (Balleine, 2019).

Moving on to Marr's level of *implementation*, the declarative memory theory asserts an anatomical organization of memory systems. The supposition that there are distinct brain systems for memory captured a lot of interest and became for many years a focus of much research. Different forms of memory have long been held to depend on anatomically distinct, albeit overlapping, brain regions. Moreover, different brain systems for memory probably evolved to mediate functionally incompatible purposes (Sherry and Schacter, 1987), though the lack of a "fossil record" for memory makes it extremely difficult to draw firm conclusions about how brain anatomy has been shaped by the evolutionary history of computational demands.

What about memory retention? This is a particularly important aspect of the declarative theory, but is barely discussed within cognitive mapping theory. The basic idea is that the hippocampal formation has a "time-limited" role in memory for an individual fact or event. Some interaction is held to take place between it and presumed long-term storage sites in the neocortex. Memory consolidation is described in section 14.8. A key issue in thinking about consolidation is understanding exactly what is temporarily stored in the hippocampal formation itself and what is stored elsewhere. If consolidation can be thought of (in Marr's terms) as a function, we may ask how this function could be realized algorithmically. There are several possibilities. One view was that detailed sensory/perceptual information is stored "in" the hippocampus for an intermediate period and then literally "shuttled" to the neocortex. Although reported in many textbooks, the "shuttling" idea is mostly apocryphal, as few theoretically minded neuroscientists had any confidence in it, and it should be put on record that it was not considered seriously by Squire at any time (as early as his 1987 book). Another idea is that hippocampal storage consists only of "pointers" or "indices" (Teyler and DiScenna, 1986). These representations do not contain detailed information—they are more like cartoons—but are thought to activate dispersed neocortical neurons at which traces representing detailed sensory/perceptual information are located (presumably through alterations in synaptic strength between interconnecting neurons).

The metaphor of neurons pointing at each other is imaginative, but it is unclear how such an addressing mechanism would be implemented. Contemporary theorists interested in indices, such as McNaughton, think that detailed sensory/perceptual information about facts or events may *never* need to be represented in the hippocampus. This implies that the hippocampus never acts alone. Declarative memory processing must involve simultaneous trace encoding in neocortex, albeit with cortical traces that would decay rapidly to baseline in the absence of consolidation signals from hippocampus. This implication was impossible to test experimentally with old-fashioned lesions, for it was essential to leave cortical areas intact for sensory/perceptual processing to occur and so provide afferent input to the hippocampus. Modern molecular-genetic techniques applied to systems neuroscience are coming to the rescue, but are not quite there yet.

Given that areas in the neocortex are the likely sites of perceptual processing and the eventual sites of storage, we might reasonably wonder why the hippocampus is ever needed. Why does the nervous system bother with such apparent duplication? One answer, due to McNaughton et al. (2003), is that the numerous neocortical interconnections which enable an associational framework of acquired knowledge are weak, slowly formed, and/or liable to rapid decay. It is essential to protect against "everything-becoming-connected-to-everything" during the long process of learning throughout development and adult life; such a situation would create catastrophic interference (McClelland et al., 1995). Memory consolidation was therefore asserted to be a gradual process precisely because it was thought that it had to be—ensuring that only the relevant connections are made across ensembles within and between cortical networks so that information about facts and events is represented accurately (O'Reilly and Norman, 2002). There is therefore no need for extensive long-term memory retention in hippocampus. Like forgotten movie stars, hippocampal pointers just fade away.

14.3 Recognition memory

As we go about our daily life, we experience new sensations, people, objects, and events. We recognize their novelty and distinguish novel stimuli immediately from the familiar aspects of everyday life. Whereas novelty commands attention, familiarity generally does not, although it sometimes does when an apparently new event feels eerily similar to something we have experienced before ("déjà vu"). Recognition and the distinct but related phenomenon of recall are both instances of the memory of prior occurrence—a form of declarative memory. We shall see, however, that the devil of "whether" the hippocampus is involved is embedded in the detail of the "how."

From a *functional* perspective, our primary focus in this section is the recognition of prior occurrence in its diverse forms (Mandler, 1980), often studied in standardized yes/no recognition memory paradigms in human neuropsychology (McCarthy and Warrington, 1990). Recognition and recall come in different flavors. In the simplest "vanilla" case, recognition is no more than familiarity. In other cases, recognition triggers a more detailed associative recollection. A problem in the field is that there has been a tendency to gloss over whether experiments designed to investigate memory involve one or both processes. It does not require recall to recognize that seeing a box of chocolates in the medicine cabinet is inappropriate; it simply evokes a feeling that something is wrong. In contrast, a full act of recall about something can involve saying something about an object (or event) that is presently *absent* from view, mediated by a rich associative structure. Recalling you put a chocolates box in the bathroom cabinet last month to hide it from your toddler would be such a case. In this instance, one has an episodic memory of what (the box), where (your bathroom) and of when (last month); such a memory definitively involves recollection. We shall turn to episodic memory in a later section but here assert only that simple forms of recognition and fully fledged associative recall are different beasts—and likely involving different circuitries.

From an *algorithmic perspective*, effective recognition memory implies the capacity to distinguish the novel from the familiar. Broadly speaking, two distinct algorithmic approaches have been

considered. In its simplest form, familiarity may just be a form of habituation in which the stimulus effectiveness wanes with repeated presentations, similarly to the gill and siphon reflex in *Aplysia* (Pinsker et al., 1970). However, recognition is often more complex than that with a comparator comparing the incoming stimulus with the remembered one, thereby permitting a *same* or *different* judgment by way of output (Horn, 1967, 2004; Vinogradova, 2001). Finally, algorithms for recall are yet different, because an event from the past must be brought to mind. Spatial recall of hidden locations is also like this—notably in the case of the watermaze (Morris, 1981).

It is important to see that the cognitive appraisal of same/different is logically separate from any response or action that is then evoked. Humans can be asked, and animals trained, to take different actions in response to such judgments. The training of animals, like the naming of cats, is a difficult matter. It generally takes time, which led some experimenters to prefer the monitoring of spontaneous responses to novelty such as eye movements or curiosity-driven exploration. Doing so obviates the need for extensive training, but it does so at the cost of the experimenter not really having a categorical yes/no answer of correct/incorrect. Well-habituated rodents generally prefer new objects, although the effect can be modest, quite apart from fearful or stressed animals typically withdrawing from novelty (Kim and Diamond, 2002), for example, by fleeing from a robot that enters an arena (Kim et al., 2016).

With respect to neural *implementation*, early animal work, primarily in monkeys and rodents, afforded the opportunity of making selective experimental damage to distinct structures within the medial temporal lobe. Brenda Milner's seminal work on patient Henry Molaison (H.M.) ignited decades of research as to how the hippocampus contributes to the conscious recollection of prior experience (Chapter 2). Milner noted that H.M. could "no longer recognize the hospital staff nor find his way to the bathroom, and he seemed to recall nothing of the day-to-day events of his hospital life" (Scoville and Milner, 1957). Over 50 years of research studying H.M. revealed that his anterograde declarative memory for stimuli of all modalities was severely impaired (Milner et al., 1968; Corkin, 2002) along with his ability to recall information up to 11 years prior to his surgery, including day-to-day occurrences, tunes, or news events (Corkin, 1984; Sagar et al., 1985). Subsequent research on other subjects with hippocampal-specific damage has confirmed both retrograde and anterograde memory declarative memory deficits supporting a role for the hippocampus in storing old memories and making new ones (Manns, Hopkins, Reed, et al., 2003; Bayley et al., 2006).

14.3.1 Nonhuman primate studies

To model recognition memory, Gaffan (1974) presented objects on trays to monkeys inside a so-called Wisconsin General Testing Apparatus (WGTA; see Figure 14.5) to test whether monkeys could discriminate between new and previously seen objects. During the sample phase, monkeys were rewarded for merely displacing one of these novel objects. After a delay (choice phase) a pair of objects was presented, one familiar and one new, and monkeys were rewarded again if they chose an identical of the object presented during the sample phase. The task was therefore called "delayed matching to sample with trial-unique cues" (DMS). Lesions of the fornix caused a striking delay-dependent impairment of memory (Figure 14.5B). Gaffan did not examine hippocampal lesions directly, but it was

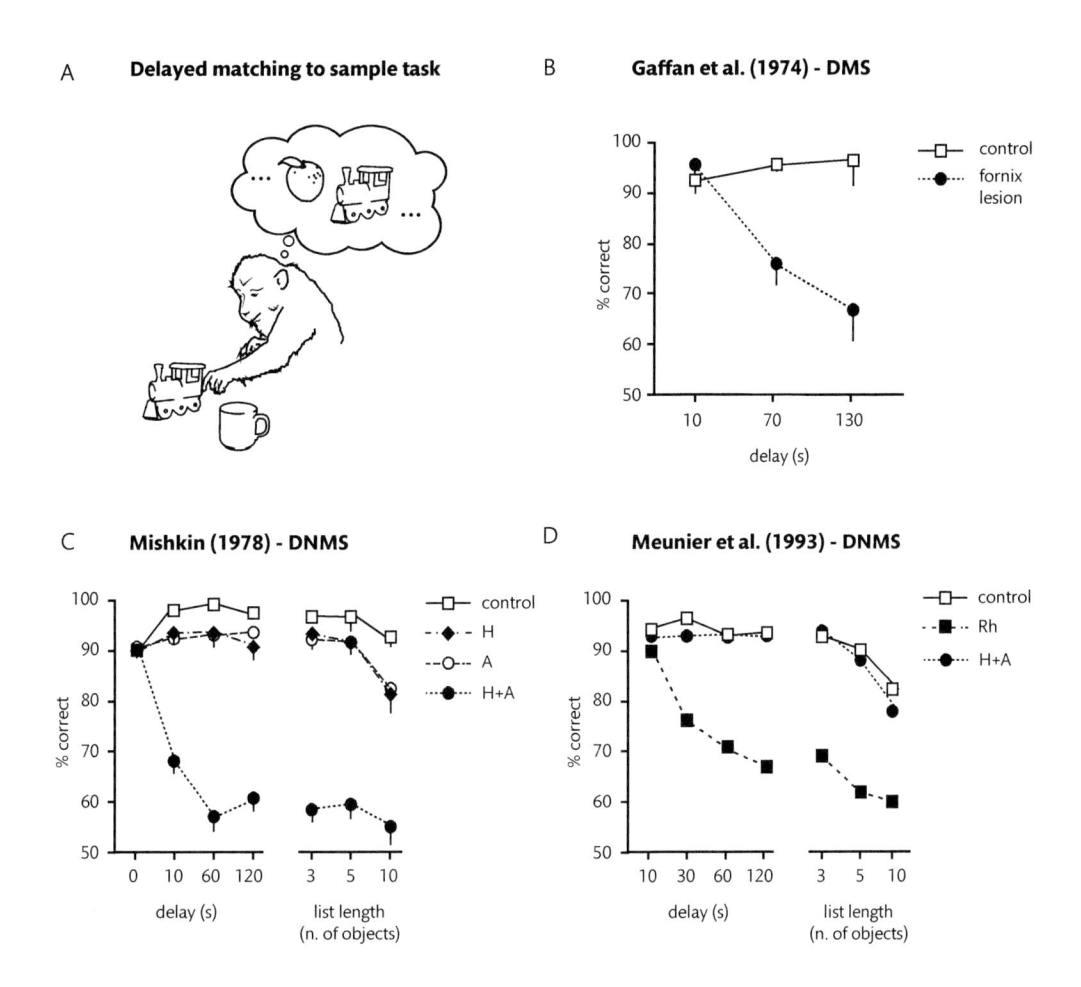

Figure 14.5 Standard procedures for testing recognition memory in nonhuman primates. (A) Cartoon of a monkey displacing objects in the Wisconsin General Testing Apparatus (WGTA). After being presented with a novel object in the sample phase, monkeys are rewarded in the choice phase (shown) if they recognize the distinction between a previously seen object and the novel one. (B) In delayed matching to sample (DMS), a trial consisted of a novel object in the initial sample phase, with monkeys rewarded in the choice phase of a trial if they reached for the now familiar object and not a different novel object (from Gaffan 1974). (C) In delayed nonmatching to sample (DNMS), the recognition memory judgment required of the monkeys was the same, but their task was always to reach for the novel object—in both the sample and choice phases of each trial. Performance across memory delays and list-lengths of control monkeys, or monkeys with hippocampal (H), amygdala (A), or both hippocampus and amygdala (H + A) lesions (from Mishkin, 1978). (D) By performing carefully controlled lesions, Meunier et al. (1993) demonstrated that the results obtained by Mishkin (1978) were due to the extent of lesion in the H + A group, which affected also the nearby areas. In fact, lesions limited to the hippocampal and amygdala lesion only did not affect the monkeys' performance in the DNMS task. However, monkeys with lesions to the rhinal cortex (Rh) were impaired.

reasonable to suppose that damaging this major afferent and efferent pathway would disrupt hippocampal function.

DMS was later superseded by the "delayed *non*-matching-to-sample" rule (DNMS). The rule for sample and choice was now matched, so that reward in both types of trial was given for reaching for the novel objects (Mishkin and Delacour, 1975). In a classic study, Mishkin (1978) showed that monkeys with a combined lesion to the hippocampus and amygdala, which was directly analogous to H.M.'s brain damage, were severely impaired. Groups with lesions confined to the hippocampus or to the amygdala performed indistinguishably from non-operated controls. Mishkin (1978) also found that the combined lesion group showed pronounced impairments in recognition memory when the delay between presentation and test, or the number of items in the list, increased (Figure 14.5C,D). This was a great step forward, and the paper is justly celebrated as a classic paper of 20th-century neuroscience (Aggleton, 1999).

DNMS rapidly emerged as the benchmark test of recognition memory. It was used in numerous studies by the NIH group (Mishkin, Bachevalier, Murray, Saunders, and others), and the San Diego group (Squire, Zola-Morgan, Amaral, Suzuki, and others). Summarizing many years of work, a delay-dependent deficit in recognition memory was observed after a combined lesion including the hippocampus, the underlying cortical structures of the posterior entorhinal cortex, the perirhinal cortex, and parahippocampal gyrus, providing apparently strong support for the declarative memory theory. DNMS was complemented by other tasks in a "test battery" held to be "declarative" in the sense that, with only a little suspension of disbelief, they could be seen as analogous to tasks given to people. The concurrent object discrimination task, in which monkeys learn which of a pair of objects predicts rewards, was thought to be analogous to learning a list of words; the delayed retention of object discriminations analogous to remembering a passage of prose, and so on.

However, the test battery was not widely adopted outside these two main laboratories and fell out of favor by the turn of the century because components of it were found to depend on other brain structures. For example, the deficit in the concurrent object discrimination task after large medial temporal lobe lesions was probably due to damage to area TE in the anterior inferotemporal cortex rather than hippocampus (Buffalo et al., 1998). This same task in humans also turned out to involve habit learning rather than declarative memory (Bayley et al., 2005). A related concern was the justification to consider a task "declarative" sometimes bordering on the circular, with tasks being named as "declarative" only if the outcome was affected by medial temporal lobe lesions (Squire, 1992). It came also to be appreciated that a single behavioral task can sometimes be learned using different strategies.

One way to avoid circularity is to come up with independent evidence that a particular strategy is being used, or that performance on one task correlates with that on another. For instance, in "reward devaluation," originally developed to distinguish actions and habits, pairing the reward with an unpalatable substance such as lithium chloride should make the animal less inclined to reach for the object if the reward-object association is learned as a "fact" (Adams and Dickinson, 1981). The animal would, in some sense, know that the reward was not worth having. However, if the animal had merely learned the habit of reaching for the object as a disposition, reward devaluation would not have an immediate effect on performance, because habits die hard.

Confidence in the benchmark test of DNMS therefore began to waver. One problem had to do with understanding what the test was measuring, the other with identifying the brain structures required for performance. These two problems are, of course, connected, but it was not seen that way at the time. A fundamental ambiguity in DNMS is what aspect of recognition memory was being tested—familiarity or recall? Most people now suspect that DNMS is primarily a test of familiarity. Moreover, different components of the medial temporal lobe were damaged by aspiration to identify the key areas whose integrity is essential for normal DMTS performance. These studies entailed lesions to the hippocampus or the amygdala (Figure 14.5C), but often the authors acknowledged that surgery required damage to other areas. With the wisdom of hindsight, there is a clear problem in the interpretation of the results. Later studies using more selective lesions demonstrated that deficits observed in the larger lesion group were largely due to damage to the entorhinal and perirhinal cortices (Figure 14.5D). In parallel, there were technical developments such as automated touchscreens in lieu of the WGTA (Gaffan, 1994, 2005) (Figure 14.6A), and the development of the visual paired-comparison (VPC) test, which looks at spontaneous rather than rewarded behavior (Pascalis and Bachevalier, 1999; Zola et al., 2000; Bachevalier et al., 2002) and which is also used with human subjects (Munoz et al., 2011) (Figure 14.6B,C). These were exciting times, with well attended symposia at the annual Society for Neuroscience meeting devoted to advances with respect to different bits of the puzzle. However, gradually, the sense of excitement

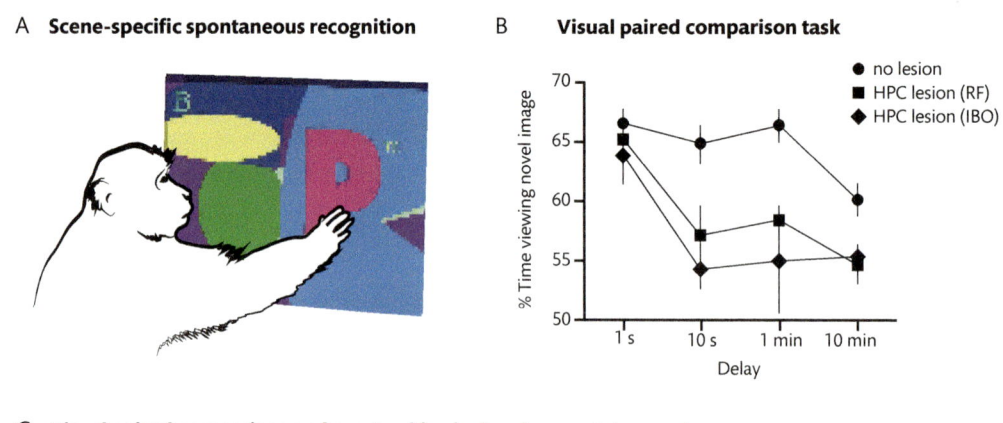

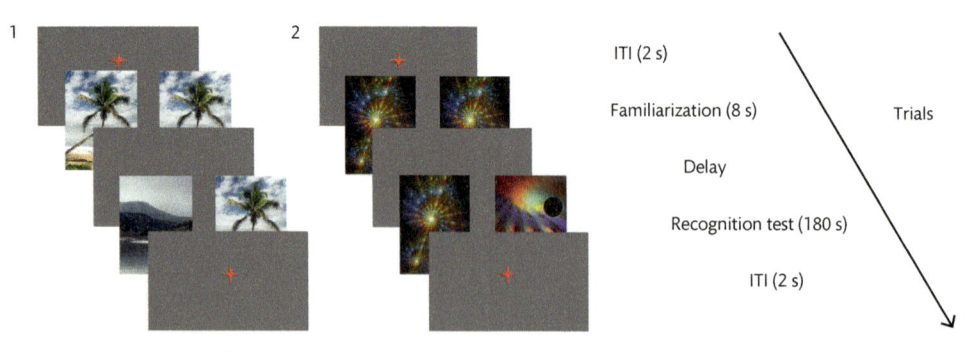

Figure 14.6 Developments in the testing of memory in nonhuman primates and humans. (A) Automated touchscreens, introduced by Gaffan, enabled analysis of associative learning and associative novelty recognition, using typographic characters placed against differing contextual backgrounds. (B) Spontaneous looking behavior in the visual paired-comparison task shows a memory deficit with delays in association with a discrete hippocampal lesion (after Zola et al, 2000). (C) As used in humans, images are presented successively across a large number of trials and eye-tracking is used to monitor what features of the two images on a choice-trial attract interest. A memory deficit is observed in developmental amnesia (after Munoz et al., 2011).

waned and the younger students listening to these symposia sought other pastures. The era of primate lesion experiments on recognition memory using DNMS drew to a close.

14.3.2 Recognition memory in rodents

14.3.2.1 Novel object recognition memory

In parallel with the primate work, work with rodents also explored variants of trained DMS and DNMS learning tasks using 3D objects as stimuli to be recognized (Aggleton, 1985; Mumby et al., 1990; Mumby et al., 1992; Otto and Eichenbaum, 1992; Kesner et al., 1993; Ramus and Eichenbaum, 2000). Performance was sustained by motivating the animals to secure reward. Selective lesions of the rodent hippocampus, which carefully avoided damage to these adjacent neocortical structures, had surprisingly little effect on performance, whereas deficits were seen after damage to perirhinal and frontal cortices.

An influential innovation in rodent work was the introduction by Ennaceur and Delacour (1988) of a task involving *spontaneous novel object recognition* (NOR). After habituation with the apparatus, rats (or mice) are given the opportunity to investigate two identical novel objects in the "sample" memory encoding phase for a short period, typically 2–5 min (Figure 14.7A). After a memory

retention interval (lasting a few seconds or even as long as 24 h), the subject is then put back into the testing chamber for the object recognition memory test—with the two objects now being a novel object and an identical copy of one of the sample-phase objects. Rodents preferentially investigate the novel rather than the now familiar object (Figure 14.7B) (Ennaceur and Delacour, 1988; Ennaceur, 2010).

It was soon found that the hippocampus itself is barely involved in novel object recognition. Numerous studies have repeatedly revealed relatively little or no effect of hippocampal lesions on NOR (Ennaceur and Aggleton, 1994; Warburton and Aggleton, 1999; Mumby et al., 2002; Winters et al., 2004; Forwood et al., 2005; Good et al., 2007; Langston and Wood, 2010; Barker and Warburton, 2011). In contrast, there is a clear effect of damage to the perirhinal cortex that is afferent to entorhinal cortex and thence to hippocampus (Ennaceur et al., 1996; Ennaceur and Aggleton, 1997; Bussey et al., 1999; Norman and Eacott, 2004; Winters et al., 2004; Barker et al., 2007) (Figure 14.7C). These data align with the conclusions from a body of work arising from studies in non-human primates on object novelty (Murray and Bussey, 1999), and fit better with the dual-process models of recognition in which the perirhinal cortex is involved in simple recognition (familiarity) whereas the hippocampus may only become involved in aspects

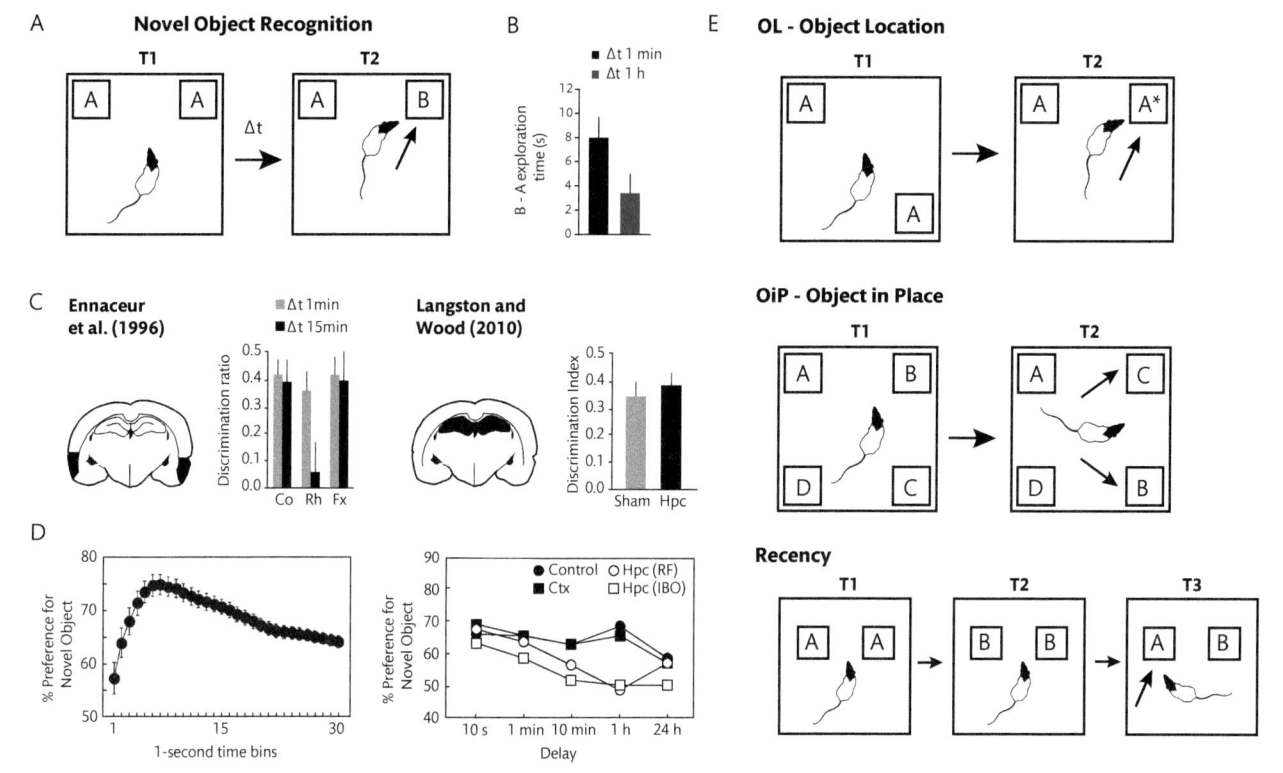

Figure 14.7 Various different protocols for spontaneous novelty tasks—object, location, and object-in-place. (A) Schematic of the NOR task. In the sample phase, animals are presented with two identical objects ("A"). After a delay period (Δt), the animal is put back in the arena and one of the two identical objects "A" has been substituted with a novel object ("B"). (B) The usual finding is that animals spend more time exploring the novel object rather than the now familiar one. This preference can be detected minutes or hours after the sample phase. Data from Ennaceur and Delacour (1988). (C) Experiments from Ennaceur et al. (1996) report that animals with lesions in the perirhinal cortex (Rh), but not in the fornix (Fx) are impaired in the NOR task, who perform comparably to that of control animals (Co). Langston and Wood (2010) report that animals with lesions of the hippocampus (Hpx) show no deficit in the NOR task. (D) Data from Clark et al. (2000) show the exploration preference of animals with 30-s bins. Animals with hippocampal lesions (H-RF and H-IBO) show an impairment in NOR starting 1 h after the sample phase relative to control animals (CON) and animals with lesions in the cortex above the hippocampus (CTX). (E) Evolution of novel object recognition protocols: object location, object-in-place, and recency. Object-in-place-in-context tasks have also been developed. These tests of associative recognition show deficits after hippocampal lesions.

of associative recognition—a dissociation that became one starting point of new theoretical approaches (Aggleton and Brown, 1999; Eichenbaum et al., 2007).

There are, however, numerous qualifications of the ostensibly tidy picture of differential perirhinal vs. hippocampal involvement in object recognition. The scientific literature is extensive, with a multitude of procedural differences across laboratories and—sadly—some discrepancies in the results. The apparently clear-cut nature of the differential sensitivity of the task to hippocampal and perirhinal lesions has been challenged, most recently with respect to variables including (a) time spent investigating the stimulus objects, (b) the completeness of lesions (an issue that could yet come to plague opto- or chemogenetic viral-infusion studies in neuroscience in the future), (c) short vs. long memory delays, (d) the difference between permanent lesions vs. temporary inactivation or blockade of the glutamatergic connectivity of hippocampus, and (e) a differential effect of anterograde vs. retrograde lesions on memory. In a comprehensive summary of numerous studies of NOR, Cohen and Stackman (2015) argue that only studies in which at least 30 s of initial object investigation has definitively occurred should be considered. They acknowledge that most studies using permanent lesions of HPC do *not* show a deficit in object recognition memory, but many report results after only a short memory delay. However, a deficit after HPC lesions is seen in some studies in which longer delays between sample and choice have been used (>10 min), thereby showing a time-dependent decay (Clark et al., 2000). However, other studies have come to the opposite conclusion. Barker and Warburton (2011) reported that a bilateral hippocampal lesion had no effect on NOR 24 hours after object exploration. Lurking in the details, however, is that lesion size averaged 89% in Clark et al. (2000) but only 58% in Barker and Warburton (2011). Could the residual hippocampal tissue in the later study have contributed to their seeing only a partial deficit? This comparison of just two critical experimental parameters of numerous studies on NOR illustrates that data variability remains seriously problematic in this field (Broadbent et al., 2010; Antunes and Biala, 2012; Denninger et al., 2018).

An intriguing question is whether brain damage in medial temporal lobe structures causes previously seen objects to appear *novel* or previously unseen objects to appear *familiar*. In both cases, recognition memory will fail. A heart-rending feature of a film made for BBC Television of the amnesic patient Clive Wearing, who lost the ability to form new memories after a severe form of encephalitis, were several encounters between him and his wife (https://en.wikipedia.org/wiki/Clive_Wearing). On every occasion shown, he expresses enormous surprise and delight at seeing her, hugging her and exclaiming that he hasn't seen her for ages. The loss of memory appeared to have turned his familiar wife into a person who was always novel.

14.3.2.2 Object-location, object-place, object-context, and other protocols for novelty detection and discrimination

Besides novel and familiar objects, there are other facets of novelty that we confront every day. We walk into a room to find that our favorite armchair has been moved from one side of the room to another. The room is familiar, the chair likewise, but its having moved is the surprise. Consider also the experience we may have had of walking on a beach, say on holiday, and seeing someone who feels familiar: "I know that person" you say to yourself. In this instance, the novelty of seeing the acquaintance in a novel setting is likely registered before identifying the person (this is an example of the "butcher-on-the-bus phenomenon"). The novelty associated with moving a piece of furniture is immediate and resolved in your mind straightaway; context novelty is different because the initial and immediate sense of surprise triggers a deliberate recall process that may take some time to resolve as the necessary associations are dredged up from long-term memory. Thus, some forms of novelty/familiarity detection may be only in the domain of "recognition" whereas others may trigger "recall."

A group led by Bruno Poucet in France began some of the early work on these aspects of spatial novelty (Poucet, 1989), but the main trigger to a wave of new studies was a report by Dix and Aggleton (1999), which laid out various protocols for object-location and object-in-place novelty. Figure 14.7 shows four different protocols, including one introducing a sequential order or time parameter—recency. The object location task is the experimental version of the chair example above. A rodent is given an opportunity to investigate two identical objects in an arena and then, soon after, put back into the arena with one of the two objects moved. Note that there is no need for explicit recognition of the object in this task. In the "object-in-place" task, the geometric arrangement of a set of four objects remains the same, but two objects swap places. The two moved objects typically trigger active curiosity. In this case, the identity of the objects does matter. In the recency task, animals may show greater interest in the earlier of two objects to be presented. These and other related tasks led by the groups in Cardiff and Bristol (UK) have done much to expand our understanding of recognition memory (Aggleton and Nelson, 2020). The object-location task, which introduces a a spatial element, is generally sensitive to lesions or inactivation of the hippocampus, or its extrinsic connections such as the fornix, as well as to other regions of the hippocampal formation such as the entorhinal cortex. Interestingly, the task is also sensitive to transient pharmacological disruption in the anterior cingulate and retrosplenial cortex (Ennaceur and Aggleton, 1997; de Landeta et al., 2020).

14.3.3 Social recognition memory

For a social species such as ourselves, and mammals in general, the historical failure to consider the social dimension of memory is a somewhat curious state-of-affairs. Social memory, social comparisons, and reciprocity have been a major driving forces in brain evolution, and the study of both social and parental behavior deserves much more attention (Wang et al., 2014; Kohl and Dulac, 2018). This experimental lacuna is now being put right in new animal studies of the hippocampus (and other brain regions) that seek to identify the neural mechanisms mediating the recognition of a familiar conspecific compared with a novel one.

A catalytic study for the field was conducted using mice, revealing a dissociation between normal *sociability* and impaired *social recognition memory* after inactivating area CA2 of the hippocampus (Hitti and Siegelbaum, 2014). They used an aptly named mouse line called *Amigo2-Cre* (mice speak Spanish!) which expresses Cre-recombinase in CA2 pyramidal neurons. To effectively silence the information transmission from CA2 neurons, they infused AAVs to transfer a transgene coding for a Cre-dependent tetanus light chain neurotoxin (or the fluorescent protein YFP as control) into the hippocampus, thereby restricting transgene expression to CA2. The behavioral effects were highly selective: locomotor activity,

A

Sociability

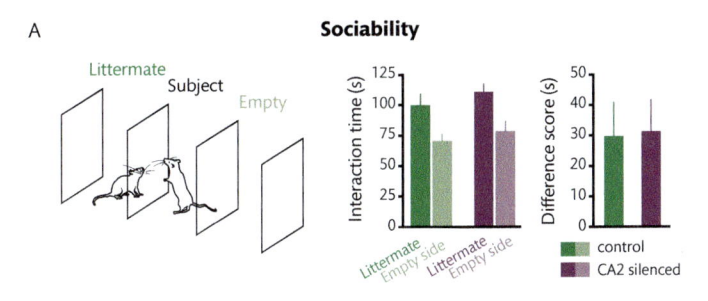

B

Social recognition

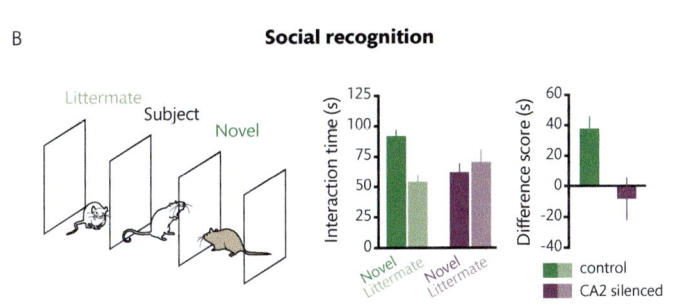

Figure 14.8 Silencing of area CA2 impairs social recognition memory without affecting sociability. (A) In a three-chamber test of sociability, the animal in the central chamber typically spends more time near the enclosure containing another rat. (B) In the test of social recognition memory, the animal in the center may spend more time near the novel animal instead of the animal it has already investigated. (After Hitti and Siegelbaum 2014.)

anxiety-like behavior, spatial learning, and context and cued fear conditioning were all unaffected. However, the mice showed a profound and apparently selective deficit in social recognition memory with no change in sociability (Figure 14.8). *Sociability* is measured in a two-choice paradigm as an enhanced predisposition to approach another animal rather than spend time investigating an empty cage (Panel A); *Social recognition memory* was indexed as the disposition to approach an unfamiliar animal rather than one who had been investigated thoroughly on a previous occasion (Panel B). A similar deficit in social recognition was also reported in a study using conventional lesions (Stevenson and Caldwell, 2014). The interpretation is that a potential role for CA2 neurons in social memory likely derives from its anatomical connectivity whereby it integrates input from the lateral entorhinal cortex (Hargreaves et al., 2005), serotoninergic afferents from the median raphe, and vasopressin from hypothalamic nucleus (Hensler, 2006; Young et al., 2006). All too often, detailed anatomy is a clue to function.

CA2 is a somewhat mysterious area of the hippocampus that has been rightfully drawing more attention recently in terms of function, connectivity, and plasticity (Dudek et al., 2016). Chronic CA2 silencing results in increased excitability of the recurrent CA3 network, while acute silencing has only a subtle effect on hippocampal physiology (Boehringer et al., 2017). This raises the possibility that the effect on social memory observed by Hitti and Siegelbaum (2014) is a secondary consequence of hyperexcitability emanating from CA2 disruption, which then affects other hippocampal subregions such as CA1. Meira et al. (2018) reported that acute DREADD-mediated inhibition of CA2 indeed impairs social recognition memory, but DREADD-induced inhibition is quite long-lasting. Debate about the possible differential effects of acute vs. chronic silencing of CA2 is exacerbated by separate reports indicating the

involvement of ventral CA1 in social memory (Okuyama, 2018). Acute optogenetically silencing of the ventral, but not the dorsal hippocampus, during social discrimination in the resident-intruder test (in which a familiar or a novel mouse is introduced in the cage of the test animal) impaired memory. Likewise, transient optogenetic perturbations in CA2 during the sleep after encountering a new conspecific reveal an essential role for the region in consolidating social memory (Oliva et al., 2020).

Anatomical projection studies show connectivity from the ventral hippocampus to other brain regions—the basolateral amygdala, olfactory bulb, and nucleus accumbens—but it turns out that, of these, the efferents to nucleus accumbens are the most critical for social memory. Selectively inhibiting the projections of the ventral CA1 (vCA1) to the shell region of the nucleus accumbens (NAc) when animals were near the familiar, but not the novel, animal in a social discrimination task removed the bias for the novel animal. Optogenetically activating the same projections while animals were near the novel animal also removed the bias. Together, these manipulations suggest that the sense of familiarity (or alternatively some identification of social identity) can be mediated by the vCA1-NAc pathway (Okuyama et al., 2016). The authors also found that cells representing the identity of an individual mouse are mediated in the vCA1 area, and when associated with positive or negative stimuli, form a sort of "social engram" akin to memory engrams (a topic that will be the focus of section 14.7).

On a final speculative note, the involvement of dorsal CA2 and ventral hippocampus in social recognition memory feels at first sight to be a very different function to that of spatial memory to which we turn next. However, identifying territorial boundaries would likely require both recognition of location and boundaries ("where") and of who occupies which space ("whose"). From the perspective of evolution, perhaps social and spatial memory are natural bedfellows.

14.3.4 Summary

Studies of recognition memory were, for many years, considered a "benchmark test" of declarative memory but, with the wisdom of hindsight, are now considered more difficult to interpret definitively due to a variety of factors. Do they really test "recognition" in a rich declarative manner or are they only tests of object novelty/familiarity? Why are there continuing disagreements about the critical brain structures and networks involved in processing different aspects of recognition memory—and specifically the necessity for hippocampal involvement? And is the use of spontaneous investigation of animals in tests of recognition memory in rodents sufficiently robust and reliable to draw firm conclusions? Opinions remain divided on these issues. A key point, however, is that sensitivity to hippocampal disruption appears to be greater for tasks that incorporate the element of spatial or context novelty.

14.4 Spatial memory

Spatial memory refers to memory for the locations of places, objects and landmarks. The study of spatial memory has always encompassed not only how location is represented but also how people and animals successfully navigate from one place to another. As such, the concept is central to the "cognitive map" theory of hippocampal function as one account of how navigation may be achieved (section 14.2). Spatial memory is also an intrinsically comparative topic with work on many species. Human studies of spatial memory, and the closely related concept of scene memory, are described in Chapter 13.

14.4.1 What is spatial memory and is the hippocampus involved?

Thinking about spatial memory includes fundamental questions about the nature of space and how it differs logically from, but cannot be completely independent of, sensory/perceptual processing. Adherents of the declarative memory perspective may look on spatial memory as another exemplar of declarative memory just like visual memory, auditory memory, olfactory memory, and so on. However, space is not a sensory modality; it is a construction of the mind that reflects what we believe to be "out there." A discrete set of regions of the brain has evolved to process information about space (O'Keefe and Nadel, 1978; White and McDonald, 2002) and, during brain development, the necessary neural circuitry is constructed (Moser et al., 2008; Farooq and Dragoi, 2019). It is unclear whether spatial memory can be adequately subsumed into the category of "declarative" and the perspective of this section is that it cannot.

Two strong but distinct intellectual traditions have permeated ideas about the hippocampus and space. One has to do with *navigation* and the other with *contextual binding*. The navigational tradition is concerned with getting from A to B to find food, seek shelter, or escape from a predator, all tasks for which there has been selection pressure in evolution. This tradition was captured in the metaphor used by the Nobel Foundation to describe the Nobel Prize in Physiology and Medicine of 2014—"discovery of the GPS system of the brain" (NobelPrize.org, 2014) (Figure 14.9). The

separate contextual binding tradition is to think of context, space, or scenes as essential backdrops for remembering events (Gaffan, 1994; Eichenbaum et al., 1999; Morris, 2006; Diana et al., 2012). The idea here is that events are not remembered in isolation—the "what" of an event is automatically bound to the "where" or to the "scene" where it happens. The automaticity of the binding of what and where is a point that we will expand on later when discussing episodic-like memory.

From the perspective of Marr's tripartite structure, the *computational* level is about where things are, about how navigation proceeds, and about space as a backdrop for remembering events. The *algorithmic* level entails reference to distinct mapping, navigational, and spatial representational systems. Last, *implementation* involves understanding the underlying physiology operating within the subset of anatomically connected brain areas, including those that express distinct place-, grid-, and head-direction-cell properties.

The discovery of place cells, followed by that of many other spatially tuned cells, points to world-centered (allocentric) spatial representations in the hippocampal formation and adjacent structures. We saw in section 14.2 that the idea that place cells constitute a map of space is not without difficulty; a map, on paper or on your phone, needs someone to be looking at it for it to be useful. How is the information about other places accessed when the animal is at a particular place? This conundrum, outlined many years ago (Morris, 1989), might find a solution in the context of navigation through "goal cells"—cells that signal the relative or absolute position of a target (Poucet et al., 2004). Ideas about the function of place-cell "replay" may also allow use of a map, as will be discussed below. Nyberg et al. (2022) outline model-free, topological, and

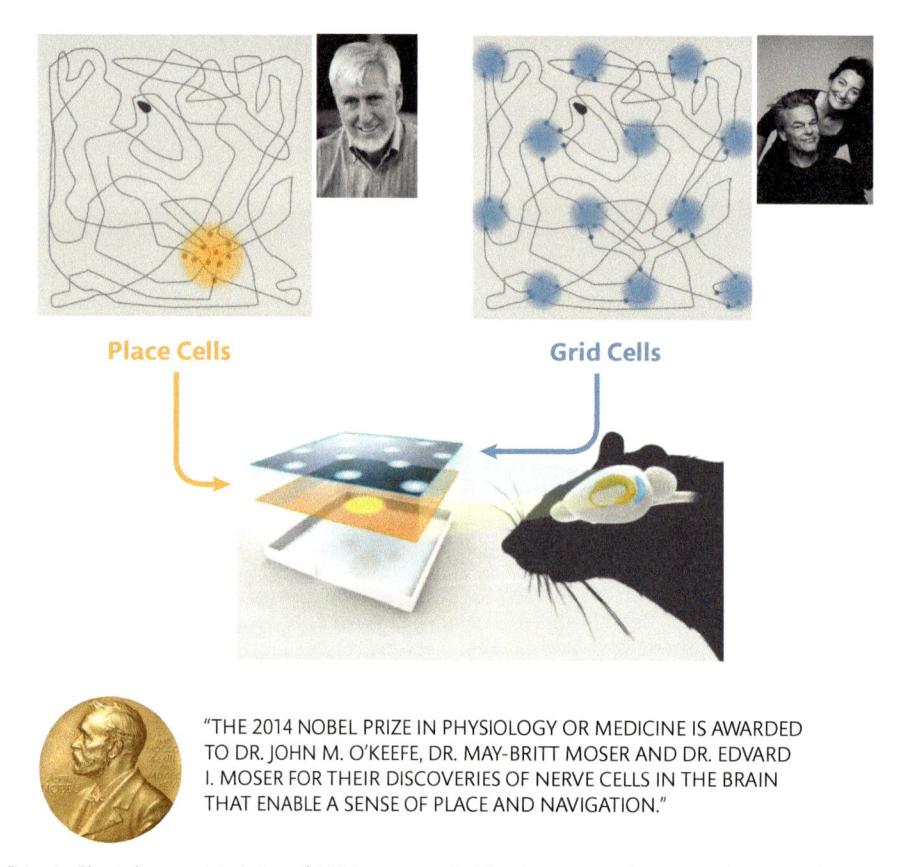

Place Cells　　　　　**Grid Cells**

"THE 2014 NOBEL PRIZE IN PHYSIOLOGY OR MEDICINE IS AWARDED TO DR. JOHN M. O'KEEFE, DR. MAY-BRITT MOSER AND DR. EDVARD I. MOSER FOR THEIR DISCOVERIES OF NERVE CELLS IN THE BRAIN THAT ENABLE A SENSE OF PLACE AND NAVIGATION."

Figure 14.9 The Nobel Prize in Physiology or Medicine of 2014 was awarded for discoveries about neural systems for spatial memory and navigation.

vector-based solutions to the general problem of goal planning and execution (see also Chapter 16).

O'Keefe and Nadel's (1978) original theory distinguished only between spatial memory and nonspatial associative learning. It asserted that a given environment should have a stable ensemble of hippocampal place cells representing specific locations. With respect to initial encoding and storage, interventions targeting normal hippocampal activity (lesions, drugs, or molecular-genetic interventions) should disrupt memory formation, storage, and/or retrieval. While qualified by such issues as the varying fidelity of both place and grid cells at different points along the longitudinal axis from dorsal to ventral (Jung et al., 1994; Brun, Solstad, et al., 2008; Stensola et al., 2012; Lyttle et al., 2013; Stensola and Moser, 2016), a large body of evidence using diverse techniques supports the idea of a major involvement of the hippocampal formation in spatial memory and navigation. The separate issue of whether the long-term consolidation of spatial information is in hippocampus or neocortex is discussed later in section 14.8.

Neocortical structures also process and store spatial information. Such regions include the retrosplenial cortex (Vann et al., 2009), the posterior parietal cortex (DiMattia and Kesner, 1988; Kesner, 1998), and the midline retrosplenial/cingulate cortex (Sutherland et al., 1988). Some work has pointed to differences between incidental processing of spatial cues, that is impaired by retrosplenial lesions, and more "active learning" over a series of training trials, for which no deficit is observed (Nelson et al., 2015). Kesner (2000) argued for parallel processing of spatial information in the hippocampus and parietal cortex, with the hippocampus being more important for "spatial events" and the parietal cortex part of a neocortical "knowledge" system. Hence, two possibilities include that (a) there are distinct forms of spatial representation in different brain areas, or (b) parallel memory encoding of spatial information occurs in both cortex and hippocampus, possibly with differing levels of fidelity and specificity.

Although the original cognitive map theory of hippocampal function was based largely on observations in rats, its extension to primate and human hippocampal function was recognized from the outset (Buffalo, 2015; Rolls, 2016). A key difference that then emerges is that primates can look at distal locations, they don't necessarily have to visit them, creating the possibility of "view cells." The later chapters of O'Keefe and Nadel's monograph also addressed the relevance of their ideas to human semantic memory and, specifically, the way in which spatial relationships are fundamental to certain linguistic prepositions that reflect knowledge representations (relationships such as "beside," "near," "above," and so on). While not originally influential in the human neuropsychology community, these ideas are now commanding greater interest in such domains as reasoning and abstract thought.

14.4.2 Representing spatial information: egocentric, allocentric, and idiothetic coding

There is something intrinsically stable about space. Even when landmarks can be seen, their appearance can change across the seasons (e.g., trees, riverbeds), but what does not change when a tree loses its leaves or a rock becomes covered in snow is their location. However, in what metric is this stability represented? The concept of "locale processing" of the original theory did not quite capture that the representation and storage of space may be "egocentric" or "allocentric" (Figure 14.10). The metric of egocentric space refers

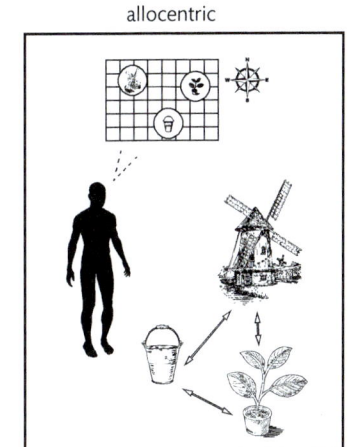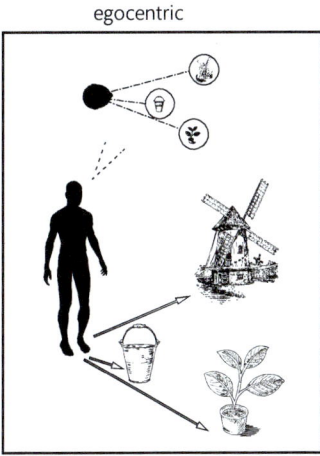

allocentric   egocentric

Figure 14.10 Egocentric and allocentric representations. In an allocentric representation, space is represented in a Euclidean-like way independent of the observer position and is anchored to landmarks and their relative position and distance from each other. In an egocentric representation instead, landmarks and objects are only encoded in relation to the observer.

to the locations of objects relative to a viewer—in front, to the left, or to the right—directions that will necessarily alter as the viewer moves around. This form of radial representation is essential if you want to hit a tennis ball, but beyond the immediacy of action, its virtues as a long-term storage representation are more limited, as it lacks stability beyond the immediate moment. Allocentric space, on the other hand, is a representation of spatial relationships within an absolute, quasi-Euclidean framework, and one that is shown clearly in the location of hippocampal place fields in simple open arenas, as first presented visually by Muller et al. (1987) (Figure 14.11A). Interestingly, Muller and Kubie (1987) observed that if a prominent cue card occupied an invariant location, place fields became anchored by it. If the cue card was then rotated, they would also rotate with it. Likewise, the stability of directionality without regard to location in a test arena is a key aspect of head-direction cells (Taube et al., 1990). Constellations of head-direction cells with differing preferred directionality work together like a corps de ballet; if one cell rotates its firing field when the extramaze cues of a recording arena are rotated, they all do.

There is, in short, a geometric "stability" about allocentric space. This can even be seen in the simplest of behavioral studies. Biegler and Morris (1993) trained rats in a large open arena to find food in hidden feeders whose cryptic location was defined by a directional vector from either of two highly discriminable landmarks (40 cm away). The contextual geometry of two landmarks was fixed for one group of animals, or these landmarks moved around relative to each other and the arena. Animals only learned to search correctly at the end of the 40 cm directional vector if the landmarks were in a fixed location, but not with landmarks whose arena location moved around (Figure 14.11B). The recent discovery of object-vector coding could be the basis of this observation (Høydal et al., 2019; Andersson et al., 2021). One possibility is that the entorhinal cortex processes object-centered distance and direction vectors whereas the hippocampus creates a stable frame of reference for such information with respect to multiple static objects. The need to build a map-like representation using stable landmarks that do not move is a fundamental concept that makes intuitive sense. Imagine,

A
Anchoring of place fields to landmarks

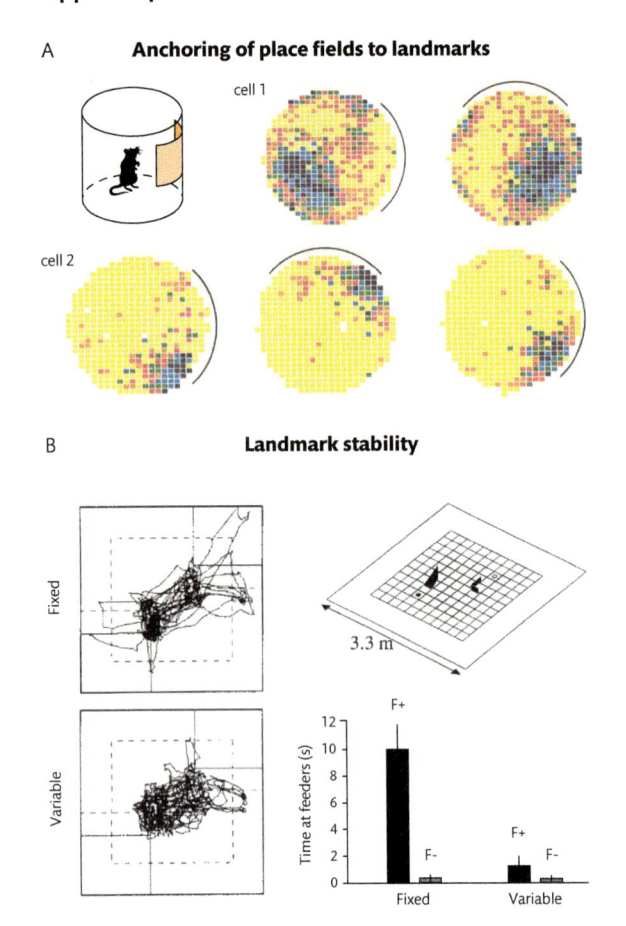

B
Landmark stability

Figure 14.11 Place-field and landmark stability. Whereas objects that we can recognize (such as a bicycle) may move around from place to place without it affecting our ability to recognize it, the same is not true of space. (A) Apparent place-field instability is observed when prominent cues move from location to location (after Muller and Kubie, 1987). The two cells shift their place fields when the cue is moved along the wall (black line near the firing maps). (B) Landmark stability in spatial learning. When rats were required to learn the location of a hidden reward, they could do this if the proximal landmark was, in a directionally polarized environment, in an invariant location relative to another prominent landmark but they failed to learn its location when the objects moved around. The relative valence of the two landmarks was acquired in both conditions, but location learning required stability (after Biegler and Morris, 1993, copyright 1993 Society for Neuroscience).

conversely, the absurdity of advising a lost tourist as follows: "Walk along the street until you see a red bicycle parked at a corner, then turn left until you come across a black dog."

The distinction between egocentric and allocentric space has not always been appreciated by critics of the cognitive map theory, with some failing to acknowledge that the 1978 theory does *not* predict that the hippocampal formation is functionally involved in any and all spatial learning tasks. Nadel and Hardt (2004) make this point emphatically. For example, a simple spatial task such as a T-maze is ambiguous because it can be solved using either an allocentric or an egocentric strategy. Inspired by Tolman's original studies (Tolman et al., 1946), a beautiful study by Packard and McGaugh (1996) illustrates this point (Figure 14.12). They trained rats to approach a goal to the left or right of a choice point in a T-maze, with the animals trained for a short period (8 days) or over a more extended period (16 days). In a critical test, the T-maze was turned into an X-maze with a new approach arm added opposite to the original

A
Place vs. Response test protocol

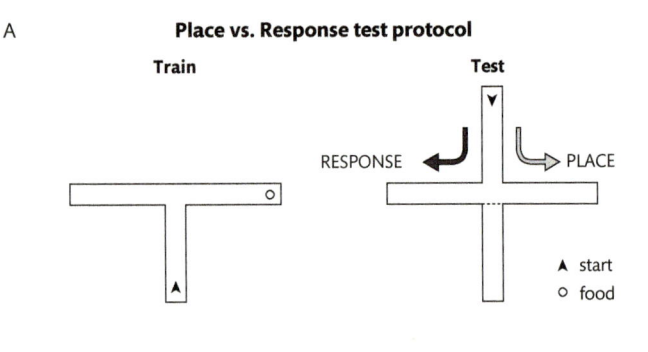

B
Impact of brain regions inactivation

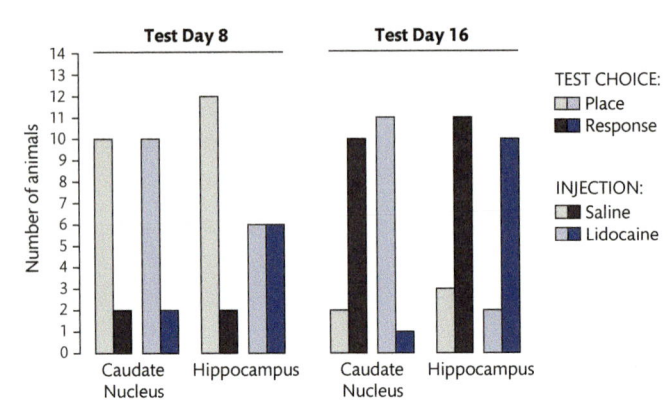

Figure 14.12 Place strategies and response strategies. (A) A famous study by Packard and McGaugh revealed that, in a simple T-maze, rats would first learn the location of reward with reference to its allocentric location in space (Day 8), but with overtraining, they would transition into an egocentric habit of turning in the correct direction, behavior that they would then execute incorrectly in a cross-maze (Day 16). (B) Pharmacological inactivation of the hippocampus or the caudate nucleus of the striatum indicates that the hippocampus is necessary for the allocentric representation at Day 8, while the caudate nucleus predominates at Day 16 (after Packard and McGaugh, 1996).

start arm. The experimental question was whether the animals had learned where the goal was in allocentric terms, which the authors called a place strategy, or which way to turn egocentrically (response strategy). After short periods of training, animals starting from the new position correctly turned toward the same place where reward had been available, i.e., continued to go toward the east arm; whereas after extended training, the animals adopted an egocentric turn, i.e., they continued to turn right. This finding has been replicated and extended by others (Yin and Knowlton, 2004; De Leonibus et al., 2011), who confirmed that the response strategy was mediated in the brain by the striatum (Yin and Knowlton, 2006), and the place strategy by the hippocampus (Ferbinteanu and Shapiro, 2003; Kosaki et al., 2018) (Figure 14.12B). Differential region-specific patterns of immediate early gene activation are also observed in this task when trials are started from novel locations by animals performing a place vs. response strategy (Rinaldi et al., 2020). Several experiments have demonstrated the partial independence of egocentric vs. allocentric information processing: for instance, inactivating the striatum impairs the consolidation of spatial information in an egocentric, but not an allocentric framework (De Leonibus et al., 2011). Conversely, lesioning the anterior thalamic nuclei affects the performance of rats in an allocentric task like the watermaze, but not in the egocentric radial-arm watermaze (Wolff et al., 2008).

The allocentric/egocentric distinction has traditionally been regarded in terms of a clear-cut dissociation between hippocampal (Morris et al., 1982; Eichenbaum et al., 1990) and striatal (Kesner et al., 1989; Packard and McGaugh, 1996) involvement respectively. But other brain areas play a role. A systematic attempt to elucidate the circuits involved in the conversion between the egocentric and the allocentric frameworks has been the object of intense research. Wilber et al. (2014) demonstrated that the posterior parietal cortex (PPC) contains both (allocentric) head-direction (HD) cells and egocentric cue direction (ECD) cells (Figure 14.13). These data suggest that the PPC is part of a network involved in coordinate transformations underlying landmark-vector cells in rodent entorhinal cortex (Høydal et al., 2019). Wang et al. (2018) suggested that one place where such a transformation may take place is at the level of the lateral and medial entorhinal cortex (LEC, MEC), part of the hippocampal formation, and afferent to DG, CA3, and CA1. They showed that single-cell firing in LEC is coded in egocentric coordinates whereas the MEC uses allocentric coordinates. Interestingly, cells in hippocampus appear to have object-vector memory correlates when objects occupy stable locations (Deshmukh and Knierim, 2013). The role of head-direction cells in the egocentric-to-allocentric conversion is supported by the finding that pure egocentric boundary cells (EBC) are found in the postrhinal cortex, in contrast with the conjunctive EBC x HD cells, which are found in the downstream areas of the MEC and the parasubiculum (Peyrache et al., 2017; Gofman et al., 2019). Conversely, allocentric-to-egocentric conversion of borders was found to involve an MEC to RSC communication (van Wijngaarden et al., 2020). The retrosplenial cortex contains border cells, which are sensitive to an animal's heading direction (Alexander et al., 2020); curiously, similar cells can be found in the striatum (Hinman et al., 2019). The current working model of information processing is the brain network presented by Wang et al. (2020) (Figure 14.13): the MEC processes allocentric information thanks to the presence of head-direction cells and grid cells, as well as the integration of self-motion cues, whereas the LEC creates an egocentric representation of locations. This information is integrated in the hippocampus to form a coherent map. Due to the presence of mixed cells integrating egocentric and allocentric modalities in their receptive field, the cortical areas of POR, RSC, and PPC are candidate regions to operate transformations between egocentric and allocentric coordinates. In this model, the hippocampus is considered to be largely involved in the processing and binding of allocentric information.

There is a further form of spatial representation called "idiothetic" in which positional information derives from an animal's own movements. Idiothetic processing includes keeping track of how far you are moving, of turns to the left and right, and other facets related to one's own movement. Such a system can work at night and during the day, and thus may be very helpful for nocturnal animals (such as rodents). Specifically, it seems that evolution worked out a distinction between "getting there" and "knowing where" (Whishaw, 1998). McNaughton et al. (1991) and Bures et al. (1998) joined others in noting the importance of path integration to aspects of navigation (Mittelstaedt and Mittelstaedt, 1982; Wehner et al., 1996; Etienne et al., 1998). Path integration operates using idiothetic cues, i.e., translational and rotational cues generated in the course of movement and has been studied extensively in ants. There have been numerous studies of path integration in many species, some of which make their point in rather amusing ways. For example,

altering the length of the legs in the *Cataglyphis fortis* desert ant by adding small stilts or clipping their extremeties during the return path to the nest results in an incorrect evaluation of the traveled distance (Wittlinger et al., 2007).

A controversial and, it turned out, incorrect proposal was that, in mammals at least, the hippocampus might also be involved in path navigation. (Wiener, 1993; McNaughton, 1996; McNaughton et al., 1996; Bures et al., 1998; Whishaw, 1998). In a series of studies, Whishaw and colleagues trained rats in an arena in which they spontaneously carried large food pellets back to nest boxes that were either visible or hidden at the edge of the arena (Whishaw and Tomie, 1997; Whishaw et al., 2001). Search paths from the home base were circuitous and marked by several pauses as the rats tried to find the cryptic food pellets, but the return path was much more direct. Return paths were disrupted in fimbria-fornix lesioned animals with respect to both direction and velocity—a finding interpreted as a deficit in path integration. However, Alyan and McNaughton (1999) cast doubt on this finding because rats with complete hippocampal lesions were able to home accurately in the dark.

That we may navigate from point A to point B by relying on a variety of strategies complicates simple assessments of structure-function relationships and necessitates carefully controlled behavioral experimentation. The richness of the navigational strategies used by human populations, from pathfinding across ocean waves by Pacific Islanders to GPS-aided navigation in the roads of bustling city centers, has been beautifully summarized in a recent review by Fernandez-Velasco and Spiers (2024).

14.4.3 Navigation in 3D environments and large spaces

Movement in three rather than two dimensions presents additional challenges, as identified in laboratory tasks with rats (Jeffery et al., 2013) and in bats (Finkelstein et al., 2015). One of the first 3D experiments relating to place cells was performed in absence of gravity in outer space during the 1998 Space Shuttle mission, during which three rats were recorded while moving along a three-sided 3D track (Figure 14.14A) (Knierim et al., 2000). The authors (and the astronauts) found no major disruption in the place-field system, with most cells having a single place field along the 3D track. Firmly grounded on terra firma, the Jeffery group used multiple 3D mazes. For example, Hayman et al. (2011) recorded from rats climbing up a vertical board with pegs, and observed that place fields resembled elongated ellipsoids, with the major axis in the vertical plane. Similarly, on helical stairs, place cells fired in multiple planes in corresponding vertical positions as seen from above. In both cases, grid cells behaved similarly, displaying elongated fields in the vertical plane (Figure 14.14B). Using a 3D lattice maze, Grieves et al. (2021) found that, in the rat, grid-cell firing fields did not make a geometrically regular pattern but instead formed irregular configurations of vertically elongated fields of variable size and spacing. Using the same apparatus, Grieves et al. (2020) found that 3D place cells are elongated in one direction (usually, the vertical one) and tend to be parallel to the maze axes (Figure 14.14C). Collectively, these findings point to little explicit representation of the vertical axis in rats.

In contrast, Yartsev and Ulanovsky (2013) found place cells in the hippocampus of Egyptian fruit bats (*Rousettus aegyptiacus*) that were roughly isometric in the three dimensions, and that such fields arising from an ensemble of cells can cover a complete 3D environment (Figure 14.14D). Furthermore, in the presubiculum and presubiculum of bats, head-direction cells tuned to the three spatial

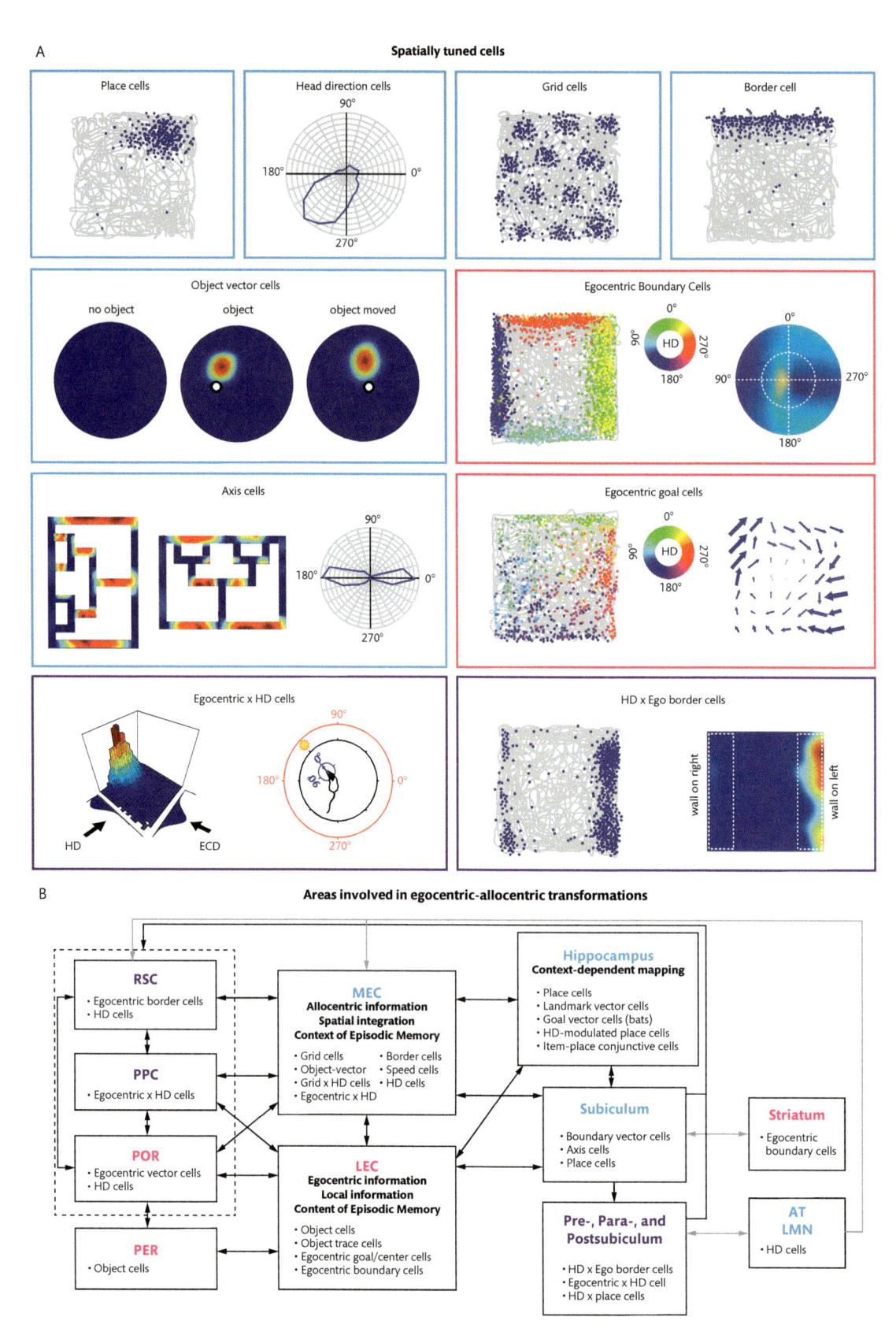

Figure 14.13 Types of cells identified in the brain with spatial fields. (A) Over the decades, several types of cells with responsiveness to space have been identified. Top row, "classical" spatial cells: place cells, head-direction cells, grid cells, and border cells. Conventionally, small dots represent neuronal activity, gray traces the space explored by animals. Recently, distinctive allocentric (blue boxes) or egocentric (red boxes) cells have been identified. Object vector cells in layer II of entorhinal cortex are cells that represent a specific distance and direction from objects, with these vectors being apparent even if the objects move (after Høydal et al., 2019). Smoothed density maps like this are a common way to represent neural activity in space. Egocentric boundary cells present in the RSC and striatum fire when the animal moves in a relative orientation and distance from a wall. Egocentric center and goal cells in the LEC fire when the animal is moving toward the center of the arena, or a goal, in egocentric coordinates, regardless of the direction with respect to fixed landmarks. Egocentric x HD cells in the parietal cortex are tuned to both egocentric and allocentric reference frames. HD x Ego cells in the presubiculum are HD cell influenced by the relative orientation of the animal with respect to the walls. (B) A provisional model of the brain areas involved in the representation of space and the conversion between egocentric and allocentric coordinates.

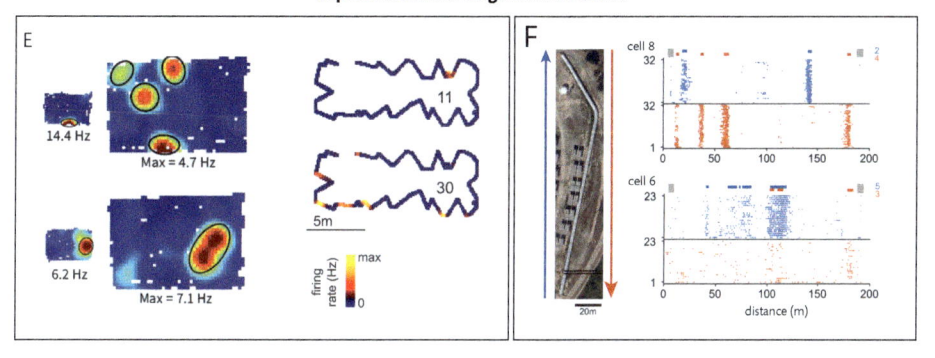

Figure 14.14 Spatial representations in 3D and large environments. (A) Record of place fields in absence of gravity in outer space. (B) Place cells and grid cells in multilayered environments show repeated place fields in the vertical dimensions in a quasicolumnar fashion. Blue are place cells, red are grid cells. (C) Place cells and grid cells in an isometric 3D reticular environment. See text for details. (D) Place fields recorded in flying bats show relatively homogeneous dimensions in the three axes. (E) Variable number of place fields in very large arenas and very long linear tracks. (F) Multiple place fields in bats flying along a 200 m linear environment. Cells show variable number and dimension of place fields.

angles (pitch, azimuth, and roll) can be detected, as well as head-direction cells with mixed orientation (Finkelstein et al., 2015). Curiously, when bats were turned upside-down, a 180° shift was observed in the pitch orientation preference for head-direction cells, though other shifts have been observed in the rat (Page et al., 2018; Shinder and Taube, 2019). These experiments suggest greater precision in processing the third dimension by bats compared to rats. This may be due to intrinsic adaptive differences in their systems or different exposure to a third dimension during their lifetime; in either case, future experiments should elucidate this topic. In this case, birds may provide a useful model system to extend this type of analysis, as they move in 3D environments and have been shown to have similar circuit mechanisms, including place cells (Payne et al., 2021). Further research should also focus on potential differences between multilayered navigation (i.e., when animals can move between multiple layers on one axis, but in each plane movements are essentially two-dimensional, akin to what happens on tree branches or in burrow systems) and volumetric navigation (i.e., when animals can move freely in three dimensions, e.g., bats flying in 3D).

The spaces we live in may be as small as a single room of an undergraduate dormitory or on the scale of the daily commute to work, typically measured in kilometers (Kung et al., 2014). How can a single spatial system handle environments that differ in size by

orders of magnitude? Most laboratory work on the neural representation of space has been done in the rodent equivalent of the cramped dorm room. Modestly expanding the length of a familiar space, while preserving its width, causes congruent expansion of place fields in the distorted axis; the reverse with compressions (O'Keefe and Burgess, 1996). In ethologically more relevant scales, such as when rats are permitted to run on long (48 m) linear tracks, some neurons showed the classic unimodal place field, while a minority encoded multiple fields (Rich et al., 2014) (Figure 14.14E). In general, both the number of place fields per cell and their size increased with the size of the to-be-encoded environment, as though more neural resources must be allocated to represent larger regions of space (Kjelstrup et al., 2008; Harland et al., 2021). The variability of subfield size was also greater in larger spaces, suggesting a multiscale representation of space. This is consistent with recordings from bats flying along a 200 m tunnel (Eliav et al., 2021) (Figure 14.14F). In the MEC, grid spacing changes as a function of the longitudinal axis in the entorhinal cortex with closer spacing in more dorsal locations, and then in incremental steps as recordings are taken toward ventral regions; this finding implies there may be discrete modules that can act semi-independently (Hafting et al., 2005; Brun, Solstad, et al., 2008; Stensola et al., 2012). The interaction and integration of these multiscale maps is a subject of current investigation.

Vector or Maps?

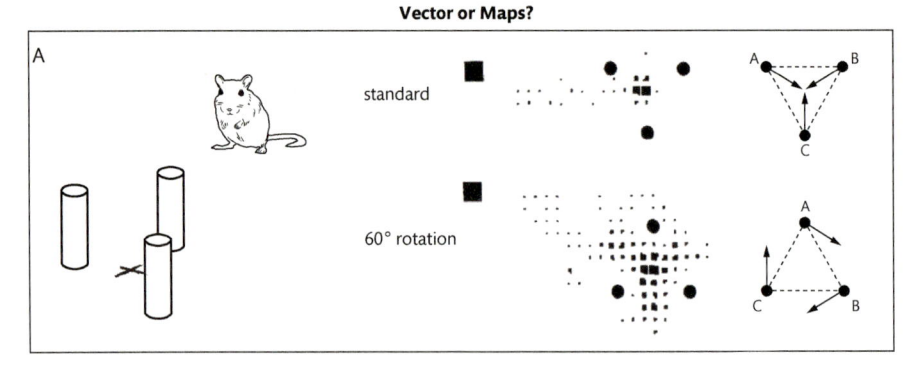

Local or Global Maps?

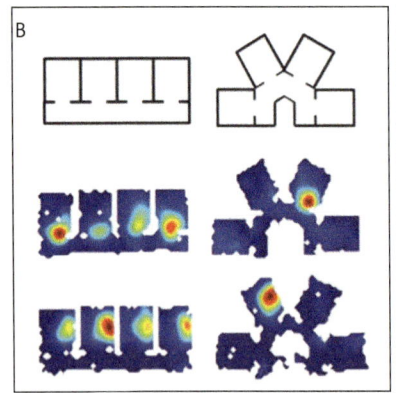
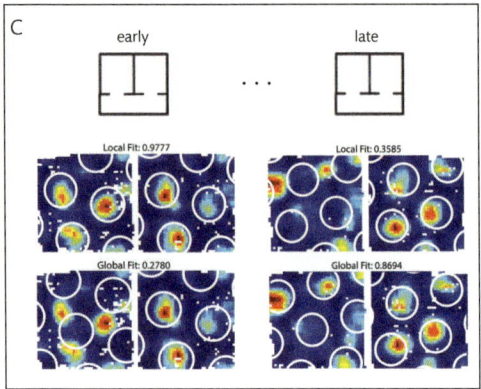

Figure 14.15 Local maps. (A) Collett et al. (1986) experimented with gerbils. After learning to retrieve a food reward in the center of an equilateral triangle of cues, rotating them by 60° led to animals digging both at the center (global reference map) and at the appropriate directional position outside the triangle (local reference map). (B) Repeated place fields in parallel compartments joined by a linear, but not an arched corridor. (C) Formation of a global grid-cell map over repeated sampling of a parallel two-chamber environment.

Local and global maps may occasionally come in conflict, as the lost wanderer in Venice's *calles* soon realizes. Collett et al. (1986) trained gerbils to search for sunflower seeds at the center of three cues disposed as a triangle. After rotating the object triads by 60°, the animals started searching in three separate positions outside the triangle, accurately referenced to each of the three cues in turn, rather than in the center of the triad, as before (Figure 14.15A). Grieves et al. (2016) discovered that repeated maps emerged when animals explored four boxes disposed in parallel and connected by a linear corridor (Figure 14.15B), but a global map preferentially emerged when the compartments were arranged in a different orientation. In a similarly connected environment with compartments in parallel, grid-cell patterns repeated local maps; with experience over time, the compartments started to merge into one, and a global grid map emerged (Carpenter et al., 2015) (Figure 14.15C).

14.4.4 Tasks developed to test whether the hippocampal formation or other brain regions are required for spatial memory

A variety of spatial memory tasks have been developed to investigate spatial representation, navigation, and event-context binding using interventional techniques rather than recording.

The widely used *radial maze* consists of radiating arms in which food is available that emerge from a central choice region (Olton and Samuelson, 1976) (Figure 14.16). In one variant, doors surround the central area, and, by arranging for only some arms to be rewarded, Olton et al. (1979) could distinguish between "reference memory"

(remembering which arms are ever rewarded) and "working-memory" (remembering if the arm has been visited already and the food reward taken)—the latter being closer to the concept of "episodic-like" memory. The *Barnes maze* consists of a large circular horizontal table on which rats (or mice) can move around searching for their home cage located below one of numerous circular holes at the periphery (Barnes, 1979) (Figure 14.16). It has proved very useful in studies of aging. The *watermaze* is a pool of water in which experimental animals swim to find a hidden escape platform under the water that they cannot see, hear, smell, or feel—until they have arrived at it (Morris, 1981) (Figure 14.16). The core concept behind this apparatus is the idea that place cells denote places rather than things—there is no local cue to be recognized. Rather than being a single task, the watermaze is a piece of apparatus in which different tasks can be scheduled: the platform can be made visible or hidden, maintained in the same position across days or its location changed from session to session.

The data secured from these procedures collectively pointed to the need for the integrity of the hippocampus and its extrinsic connections for normal allocentric spatial learning (see first edition). Learning to navigate accurately to the escape platform in the watermaze was found to depend on normal hippocampal function (Morris et al., 1982), but very little volume of hippocampus is necessary for successful learning: small "minislabs" of intact dorsal hippocampus are sufficient (E Moser et al., 1993; M Moser et al., 1995) (Figure 14.17). Rats with complete lesions of the hippocampal formation do show a severe deficit in learning, but it may not be

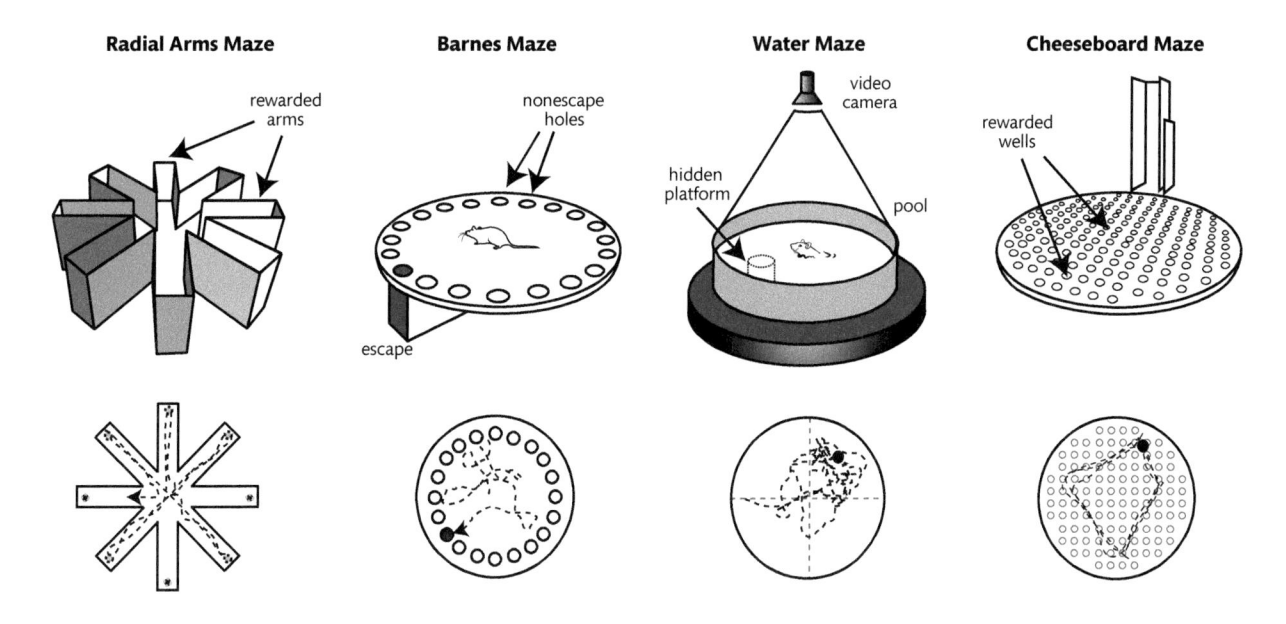

Figure 14.16 Widely used navigational tasks for rodents. The radial-maze (Olton and Samuelson, 1976). The animal's path is shown as a dotted line. Note that in the 18-arm version (and some 8-arm versions), some arms are consistently rewarded whereas others are not. The Barnes Maze (Barnes, 1979). The rat or mouse is typically released from a central holding location, and it must search for the hole at the edge of the table where it can enter its "burrow." With repeated training trials, the animals learn direct paths. Path-integration is not available, as the animal does not return to the central location unless carried there by the experimenter. The water maze is a circular pool of water (at approximately 26°C) in which the animals must search from any of multiple start locations to find an escape platform hidden underneath the cloudy water (Morris, 1981; Morris et al., 1982).

absolute, as overtraining on a reference memory protocol can be successful (Morris et al., 1990).

A novel series of tasks have been developed in the watermaze to model recent event-context binding, so-called everyday memories (such as where we put our glasses down). The focus of the memory-retrieval process has then to be on the most recently encoded information. Steele and Morris (1999) showed using the watermaze that everyday memory training resulted in widespread searching for the escape platform location on the first trial of the day, followed by relatively direct approaches to that day's correct location

on the subsequent and later trials of the day. It is, therefore, an "episodic-like" protocol with recall of the global context from long-term memory, but one-trial recency memory for the newly context-bound event information. Intrahippocampal infusion of D-AP5 at a volume and concentration sufficient to block induction of LTP1 before trial 1 impaired acquisition of memory for the escape location, with retrieval failing if trial 2 occurs 20 min or more after the end of trial 1. In later work in the watermaze, using a similar 4 trials/day training protocol, the introduction of the Atlantis Platform allowed a non-escape probe trial to be scheduled on trial 1 of every

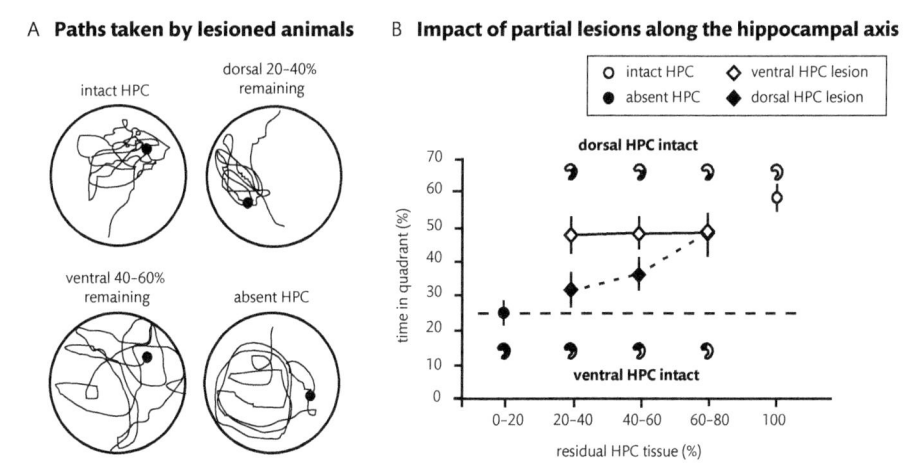

Figure 14.17 Partial lesions reveal a dissociation of function along the longitudinal axis of the hippocampus. (A) After training by animals with spared tissue volumes of different sizes that began at different ends of the longitudinal axis of the hippocampus, posttraining probe tests (hidden platform absent) revealed a graded change in animals in which only ventrally located tissue was intact, but good performance in animals with dorsal tissue. (B) Quantitative assessment of the probe tests show near normal performance of rats with as little as 20%–40% of dorsal hippocampus intact. Inset parasagittal diagrams of the hippocampus show the locations of intact (white) and lesioned (black) tissue along the longitudinal axis. (After Moser et al., 1995.)

day (Rossato et al., 2018). Thus, in the first 60 s of trial 1, with the platform deeply submerged and thus inaccessible, spatial memory for the previous day's location could be measured, showing modest but significant search in this area. Using successive blocks of three consecutive sessions, repeated many times over several weeks, they compared the impact of intrahippocampal infusion of D-AP5, CNQX, and low-dose muscimol on session 2 of each block. As expected, both CNQX and D-AP5 blocked memory updating, this being revealed on session 3. However, a very low dose of muscimol on session 2 blocked memory retrieval on that day, but still allowed memory updating on session 2, a phenomenon Rossato et al. (2018) called "silent learning." The muscimol dose was titrated such that it did not impair LTP1 despite blocking cell firing—hence the name.

14.4.4.1 Newer tasks to assess spatial memory

Many other dry-land place-finding tasks have been developed—of which an important one is *place avoidance*. Arguably, this is the mirror-image of place navigation, animals being trained stay *away* from various places in arena to avoid the punishment of mild footshock (Bures et al., 1998). The cheese board task developed by Kesner et al. (1989) and Dupret et al. (2010) is a dry, appetitive spatial memory assay, in which subjects may start from the perimeter of an open circular platform and learn which of several wells contain a hidden reward (Figure 14.16).

The *event arena* is likewise an appetitive spatial learning apparatus in which rats run from any of four start boxes at the side of a large arena to find and dig up food located at a fixed or varied position within sandwells placed in a 7 x 7 grid of locations within the large arena (Day et al., 2003; Bast et al., 2005). Digging up and carrying a large food reward is a critical aspect of the procedure as this constitutes the "event" with which the task is named. Broadbent et al. (2020) refined the task by introducing a "home base" to which the animal had to carry the food that they have successfully dug up, to render the task exclusively allocentric. In variants of these tasks, a modest number of daily training trials is given in the event arena each day, using a new starting location each session (Tse et al., 2022).

Last, various *virtual reality* tasks have been developed in which, typically, mice are permitted to run on an air-suspended "trackball" despite their head being held in a rigid frame (to allow intracellular physiological recording or confocal imaging). In front of and around the trackball are screens on which visual images may be projected, the image moving as a function of how the mouse runs on the ball. One motive for developing such tasks is to conduct more exacting physiological recording or imaging than is feasible with extracellular tetrode recording. Another motivation for VR is to develop better stimulus control (Ravassard et al., 2013). In the awake behaving subject, it can be difficult or impossible to know what stimuli are being attended to at any given moment. Not so in VR, as stimulus control allows for rapid transitions between environments ("teleporting"), control over optic flow (Acharya et al., 2016), and presentation of orienting landmarks (Zhao et al., 2020). There is, however, a price to be paid for this technical progress—namely that the animal cannot move around freely, thus fundamentally altering the normal and profound influence of vestibular inputs to the spatial mapping system.

14.4.5 Evidence that hippocampal place cells contribute to spatial memory

Since the first discovery of place-cell activity in the 1970s, place fields have been identified across the brain, including regions such as the claustrum (Jankowski and O'Mara, 2015) and S1 (Yin et al.,

2018; Long and Zhang, 2021); even neurons in V1 have tuning properties that are strongly modulated by the location of the subject to the degree that location information can be decoded from V1 neural activity (Saleem et al., 2018). Therefore, the existence of spatially tuned neurons does not immediately imply that a region computes or stores a mental map of physical space. With this caveat, what is the evidence that place-cell activity mediates spatial memory, a sense of space, or navigation?

Some of the first correlational evidence came from experiments that tracked a rat's spatial decision-making on plus mazes after orienting cues were removed (O'Keefe and Speakman, 1987). Rats learned to retrieve food rewards on a particular arm of the maze, then as they waited, orienting cues were eliminated; they were nonetheless able to navigate successfully from the start to the goal. Two important discoveries were made. First, place fields that were present with cues persisted in firing when these were removed. Second, when rats chose the wrong arm, place fields reflected the behavior of the subject, such that if a neuron fired on a goal arm with full cues, it would also fire on the chosen arm of the maze, even if that was physically in a different location. Such an observation is expected if rats made the wrong choice because they had rotated their mental map and place field activity defined that mental map.

If a place cell represents a place, and the set of active place cells represents a spatial context, then changes in spatial context should cause a large reorganization of the location of place fields. This is what is observed. The classic observation is that when either pairs or ensembles of neurons are recorded and the subject (usually a rat) is moved between one arena and another, different sets of neurons express place fields in the two environments. When neurons do express place fields in multiple spaces, the vector describing the spatial relationship between pairs of place field location is not preserved. This phenomenon is known as "global remapping," and it is generally believed that the activity patterns of hippocampal cells observed in one environment is not correlated with those observed in another (Muller and Kubie, 1987; Leutgeb et al., 2004; Leutgeb et al., 2005). This result was spectacularly shown by the Moser group who found 11 independent hippocampal maps for 11 different rooms (Alme et al., 2014).

When does a room become distinct enough to merit its own map? Studies have been conducted with rats exposed to a square-shaped arena and circular arena, or intermediaries whose shape is a blend or morph of the square and circle (Wills et al., 2005; Leutgeb and Leutgeb, 2007). The critical question was whether the hippocampus has either a map of the circular arena and the square arena or a place-field map that could ease gradually from one representation to the other? The answer depends on how the animal is trained. If the subject is given the opportunity to learn that it is impossible to simultaneously occupy the two spaces by being trained such that it can walk between the two environments, then the transition in the place-field remapping is sudden—the morphs are associated with either a circle or a square—consistent with a place representation that "pattern completes" to a learned attractor (discussed in section 14.6 and Chapter 15). On the other hand, if subjects are simply placed in the two environments before being exposed to the morphed intermediaries, then a smooth and gradual partial remapping is observed in square-like and circle-like spaces (Colgin et al., 2010). Even spaces with an identical layout can be represented by distinct hippocampal maps if maps if subjects can walk between them (one cannot occupy the same location after walking 10 m in a straight line), demonstrating that the place field is a conjunction of the visual scene and information about path integration (Skaggs and McNaughton, 1998; Harland et al., 2017).

Other studies cast some doubt on the isomorphism between a stable representation of place and a stable memory of space. If rats are placed in a square environment with white walls and trained to retrieve a food reward from a particular corner of the environment, place fields are readily apparent and stable across re-exposures to that arena. When that same enclosure is painted black and moved to a new room within the laboratory, place fields remap. However, the rat's behavior may be unaffected such that they readily retrieve reward from the correct location (Jeffery et al., 2003). If place fields stored the map of the hidden reward, and the place fields were completely altered, how was memory intact? Similar global remapping has been reported upon placing the rat in a familiar environment and then moving it to a neighboring room with another arena to explore, before bringing it back 1 hour later to the same space (McNaughton et al., 1996)! Longitudinal recordings of place field activity via endoscopic fluorescent recording of calcium reporters have also revealed "representational drift," where the same location becomes associated with different place-cell activity over days (Ziv et al., 2013). This mismatch between apparent mnemonic stability in the face of representational drift seems inconsistent with a simple conceptual mapping between place fields and place memory.

A neurobiological extension of the cognitive map theory is that the identity of place cells defines the spatial reference frame, the location of the firing fields dictates position within that reference frame, and the firing rate of the cells can correspond to nonspatial attributes of a specific position (Leutgeb et al., 2005; Lu et al., 2013; O'Keefe and Krupic, 2021). However, experimental manipulations that do not intuitively redefine the current spatial map (e.g., removing the animal and returning it to the same environment to do the same task; McNaughton et al., 1996) can also change the location in which a cell fires (e.g., Bostock et al., 1991; Markus et al., 1995; Eschenko and Mizumori, 2007; Bahar et al., 2011).

Notwithstanding, more recent evidence has shown a compelling causal role for place cells in forming the cognitive map that guides behavior. In one study, place fields were mapped in rats exploring a circular arena. Then, in subsequent sleep, the medial forebrain bundle was electrically stimulated every time a chosen place cell was active (such stimulation elicits appetitive behaviors in awake animals). The aim was to artificially form an association between the place field of the chosen cell, and a poorly specified but positive sensation. The rats indeed showed enhanced preference for being in the place field (Figure 14.18A) (de Lavilléon et al., 2015). If the firing of hippocampal neurons at a goal location signals to the rest of the brain that the animal has arrived at the right spot, then it should be possible to artificially activate those neurons and drive reward-related behaviors. Using all-optical technology, such an experiment was recently carried out by the Häusser lab (Robinson et al., 2020). Head-fixed mice were trained to stop and lick for water at a particular location on a virtual track. Hippocampal neurons expressing GCaMP6f and the red-shifted opsin C1V1 were imaged with a two-photon microscope, so that neuron imaging and excitation could be performed with two independent wavelengths, enabling the experimenters to see which neurons fired at the reward site in real time. Then, with holographic stimulation, Robinson et al. selectively stimulated these goal cells outside the virtual reward area; this caused an increase in the likelihood of the mouse stopping

and licking (Figure 14.18B). On stimulation trials, mice would also tend to skip the "real" reward site in favor of the rewarded "virtual" one. These behavioral results point to a causal role in the firing of specific hippocampal neurons in the expression of place-related behaviors—at least in virtual reality.

Another physiological phenomenon also points to a causal role of place-cell firing in memory—sharp wave ripples. It is unknown how the hippocampus accesses or expresses information for recall, but several pieces of evidence suggest that the hippocampal activity during rhythmic bursts of activity known as sharp wave ripples (SPW-Rs) constitute a physiological basis for recollection (Buzsáki et al., 1983; Chrobak et al., 2000; Foster and Wilson, 2006; Carr et al., 2011; Pfeiffer and Foster, 2013). Analysis of cell activity as rats run around linear tracks or open fields and then, subsequently, stop or sleep have shown that sequences of cells that were active during an experience are reactivated during ripples at compressed timescales during what are termed "replays" (Wilson and McNaughton, 1994; reviewed in Carr et al., 2011). Notably, this repetition has been reported both as inverted sequences (reverse replay) and in the same temporal orientation as the original sequence (forward replay) (Foster and Wilson, 2006; Diba and Buzsáki, 2007; Davidson et al., 2009; Gupta et al., 2010) (Figure 14.19A).

In principle, awake replay of events related to memory recall and planning can have either a *prospective* role, i.e., they are involved in planning the future path, or a *retrospective* role, i.e., they represent the animal accessing the past traversal of a part of the track akin to a memory recall (Krause and Drugowitsch, 2022). Replay events during SPW-Rs are commonly detected at starting or branch points of track mazes (Figure 14.19B) (Foster and Wilson, 2006; Gupta et al., 2010; Wu and Foster, 2014), and place cells corresponding to reward positions are strongly reactivated in SPW-Rs during sleep (Dupret et al., 2010). To show a causal role of SPW-Rs in behavior, Jadhav et al. (2012) detected and suppressed SPW-Rs as animals retrieved rewards alternating between the right and left arm from the central arm of a W-maze. Animals for which SPW-Rs were disrupted performed significantly worse in their choice of arm, suggesting that access to the memory of the traveled arm during SPW-Rs is necessary for correctly guiding the animals' behavior. Remarkably, optogenetically extending the duration of SPW-Rs enhances memory performance on a similar task (Fernandez-Ruiz et al., 2019). Correlative evidence suggests that the firing pattern of activity during ripples is also predictive of animal behavior. The Foster group showed that during a task involving an alternation between directed foraging from memory and random foraging in a two-dimensional arena, replays sometimes overrepresented paths ending at the location of the remembered destination (home base), and these trajectories reflected future behavioral paths taken by the animals. This suggests that replay events may be involved in planning possible future actions (Pfeiffer and Foster, 2013; Gillespie et al., 2021; Gobbo et al., 2022; Widloski and Foster, 2022).

14.4.5.1 Decision-making

As we have seen in this section, hippocampal replay of traversed space may be used to guide, or plan, future behavior. Are there other possibilities for animals to plan future actions? The discovery of splitter cells suggests that place-cell firing can be modulated by the past and future paths taken by the animal (see section 14.6). One intriguing possibility is that differential firing may be involved in guiding future behavior. Ainge et al. (2007) showed that

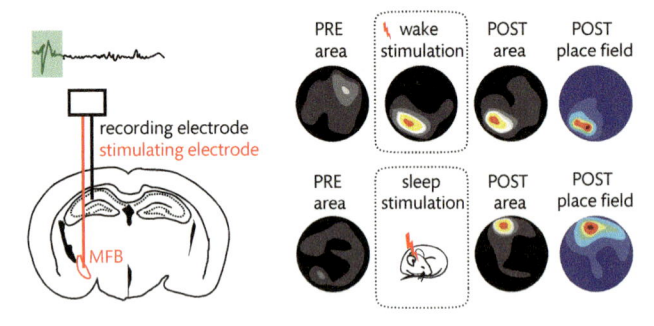

A   **Closed loop stimulation of MFB during PC activity**

recording electrode
stimulating electrode

MFB

PRE area | wake stimulation | POST area | POST place field

PRE area | sleep stimulation | POST area | POST place field

B   **Artificial reactivation of Reward zone place cells**

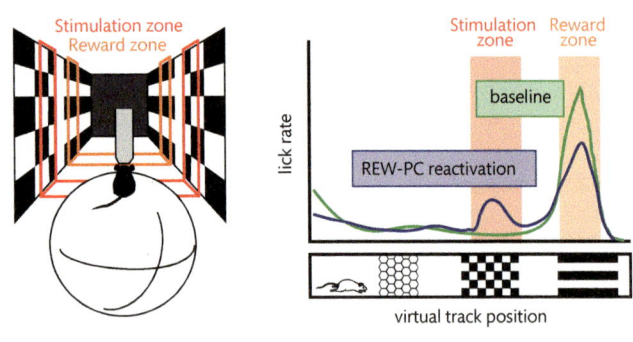

Stimulation zone
Reward zone

Stimulation zone   Reward zone

baseline

REW-PC reactivation

lick rate

virtual track position

Figure 14.18 Causality of place cells involvement in memory representation. (A) De Lavilléon et al. (2015) created an artificial link between selected place cells and positive stimulation by means of closed loop stimulation. This affected the animal's behavior, prompting them to spend more time in the place cells' field area. (B) Robinson et al. (2020) reactivated place cells out-of-field, showing that the animals display behavior consistent with the belief of being in the area corresponding to the place cells' field.

in a four-choice double-Y maze place-cell activity of well-trained animals differed in common parts of the track during journeys to different end-goal boxes. This modulation was more marked in the start box and after the first choice point. Overall, around half of the cells displayed modulated activity: in some cases, while some of the place cells behaved as splitter cells, others corresponding to the chosen end of the maze were preferentially reactivated in these choice points (Figure 14.19C).

In experiments in which two paths lead to the same goal, it has been shown that neural firing discriminates which route the subject takes to reach the common destination (Grieves et al., 2016) (Figure 14.19D). These results suggest that "splitter cells" code upcoming routes not goals, and that the output of this differential firing may be used to guide behavior.

14.4.6 What is the anatomical locus of spatial memory storage?

A spatial map is calculated from an integration of visual scenes, landmarks, a sense of direction, and an animal's own movements. Given the diversity of information that could be utilized, it is not surprising that tests of spatial memory falter after lesions to various structures beyond the hippocampus, e.g., retrosplenial cortex (Vann and Aggleton, 2002), medial entorhinal cortex (Nagahara et al., 1995), parietal cortex (Save and Poucet, 2009,) and postrhinal cortex (Schenk and Morris, 1985; Liu and Bilkey, 2002). Recordings from these structures also reveal neural firing patterns that correlate

with the spatial location of the subject. Given these observations, are there multiple maps or contributions to spatial maps stored across brain regions each serving a different role? If so, do they require hippocampal integrity for their construction or use? When spatial memory deficits emerge after an extrahippocampal lesion, is this due to elimination of the spatial map, or elimination of the computations required to use that map (e.g., destruction of the brain's compass)? The scientific field is currently grappling with such questions with analysis of the grid-cell map being a case in question.

The discovery of grid cells in the medial entorhinal cortex (Hafting et al., 2005) pointed to a kind of metric of spatial representation originally hypothesized to exist in the hippocampus. Neurons that fired in neat grids in every spatial context would allow a concept of distance and spatial relation independent of content (4 meters in Edinburgh = 4 meters in Padua ≈ 13.1 feet in Albuquerque). It was possible that hippocampal place fields would naturally emerge from integration of afferent grid cells, perhaps as some Fourier transform—but this was not the case. Lesion and inactivation studies have reliably shown that place fields exist in the absence of grid cells (Brun, Leutgeb, et al., 2008; Van Cauter et al., 2008; Hales et al., 2014; Rueckemann et al., 2016). In fact, grid cells require place cells for their spatial tuning (Bonnevie et al., 2013; Almog et al., 2019). The grid map and place map are also linked as remapping in one correlates with remapping in the other (Fyhn et al., 2007), the head-direction system likewise (Knierim et al., 1995). In addition, it is now becoming clear that the grid code is not actually uniform across environments. Changes in geometry can distort the grid spacing (T Stensola et al., 2015), as can overall experience in an environment (Barry et al., 2007), and grid-field activity is also modulated by what is occupying a given location (Navawongse and Eichenbaum, 2013; Boccara et al., 2019). Changes in spatial context can also affect firing rates within a grid field (Diehl et al., 2017). Therefore, both the medial entorhinal cortex and hippocampus encode information about place and the events happening within a place despite differences in the nature of the spatial code (McKenzie et al., 2016).

14.5 Relational memory theory

In the 1990s, it became clear that new theories of hippocampal function were needed and they were introduced. One was a fundamentally different vision for hippocampal function called "relational memory theory," developed by Cohen and Eichenbaum (1993). It took on two major issues of dissension that emerged in our two preceding sections: the distinction between recognition based on familiarity alone and associative recollection, and the question of whether spatial associations are special or could be subsumed within a broader category of cognitive associations.

Unlike other models that sought to account for the storage of dissociated snapshots, the relational memory theory stated that the hippocampus encodes memories as relationships between various distinct memory elements. The types of relation thought to be handled within the hippocampus certainly included spatial relationships but went beyond these to span multiple levels of abstraction. The relationships considered were also distinct from the conventional conditioned and unconditioned stimuli (CS-US) associations of learning theory in which a neural stimulus acquires value as a function of its probabilistic association with reward (Rescorla and Wagner, 1972; Pearce and Hall, 1980). For example, relational

Replay of past and future trajectories

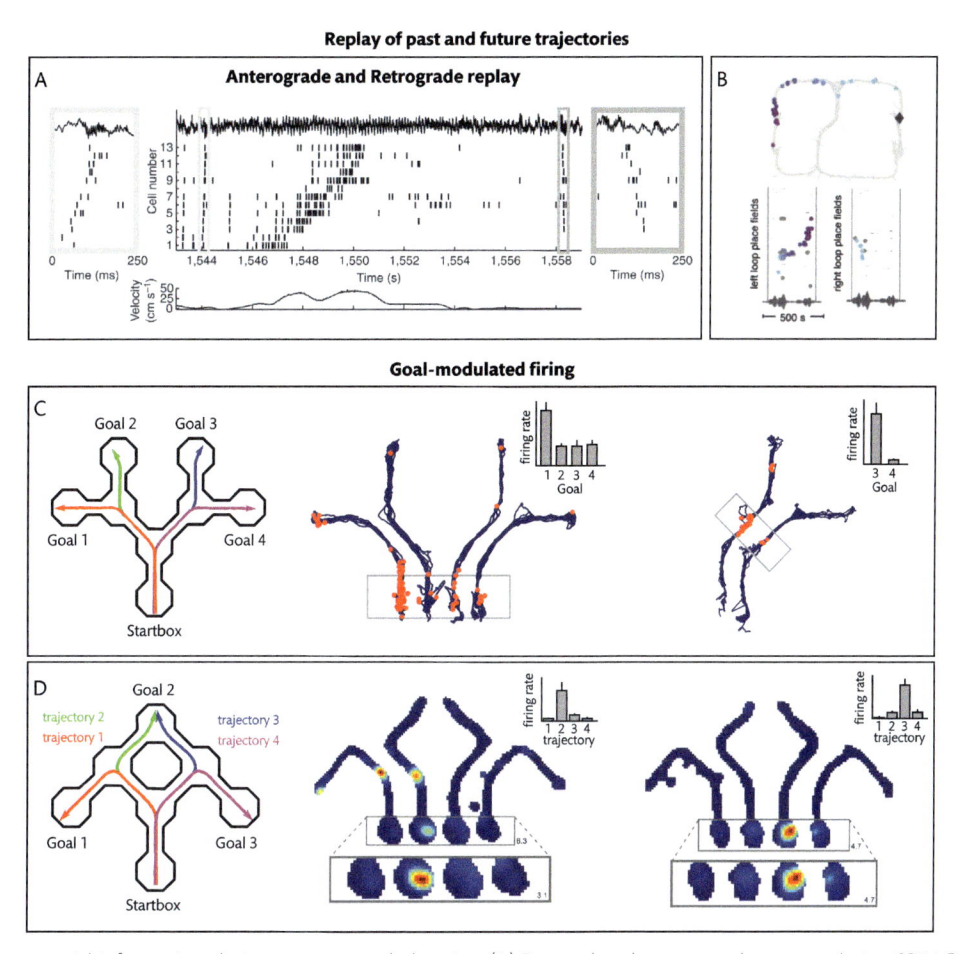

Figure 14.19 Access to spatial information during memory and planning. (A) Forward and reverse replay events during SPW-Rs. (From Diba and Buzsáki, 2007.) (B) Replay events for sequences of place cells away from the animal's position (diamonds). (From Gupta et al., 2010). (C, D) Goal-dependent and trajectory-dependent behavior of cells in double-Y mazes (From Ainge et al., 2007; Grieves, Wood, and Dudchenko, 2016).

memory sought to address patterns of co-occurrence, similarities in sensory features, hierarchical relationships, and both the spatial relationships that are central to the cognitive mapping theory and temporal relationships that would later become a central part of thinking about episodic memory. In terms of the elements that could be related, this process was thought to be independent of specific sensory modalities and could derive from any mental object as conceived in a Gestaltian sense such as abstract concepts. For instance, relationships might be represented by social hierarchies in family trees, obeying principles of transitive inference (e.g., a plane is faster than a car, a car is faster than a bike; therefore, a plane is faster than a bike), or by reciprocal spatial relationships (the Colisseum is east of the Tiber River and south of the Trevi Fountain). Key statements of the theory included that the hippocampus defines "multidimensional spaces that capture various possible relations" such that "representations can be accessible to and activated by all manner of processes and processing modules; and they can be manipulated and flexibly expressed in any number of novel situations" (Cohen and Eichenbaum, 1993). Accordingly, relational networks were proposed as being built up by "weaving new items into the existing organization of memory." Such a theory was computational and algorithmic in character (although not quantitative as in the Rescorla-Wagner equation), but it lacked detail about implementation beyond specifying the anatomical structures that performed various operations.

As originally proposed, the relational memory theory did not place any division of labor on episodic vs. semantic memory systems. Central to relational memory theory is the idea that, "the hippocampus contributes to semantic memory by the construction of relational networks that coordinate memories stored in the cerebral cortex" in support of the "flexibility of their expression through comparisons and generalizations across memories" (Eichenbaum, 2004). Historically, episodic memory only started to emerge later with consideration of temporal relations between memory elements, with the past and future differing primarily by the temporal order in which they occur rather than in terms of some absolute metric of time. That is, time was conceived of as more a matter of sequence than interval. You may remember that you went to school before you went to university, but your memory in a relational memory system does not necessarily induce any explicit sense of the passage of time.

14.5.1 Building relational memory networks in the laboratory

In most laboratory memory assessments, an experimentally naive subject is shaped to learn a simple association whose retention is then assessed after some delay or intervention. This is, however, not how memories work in normal everyday life. Almost no experience is totally novel, and we use what we have learned in the past to guide what we now learn and the meaning of those new associations, and

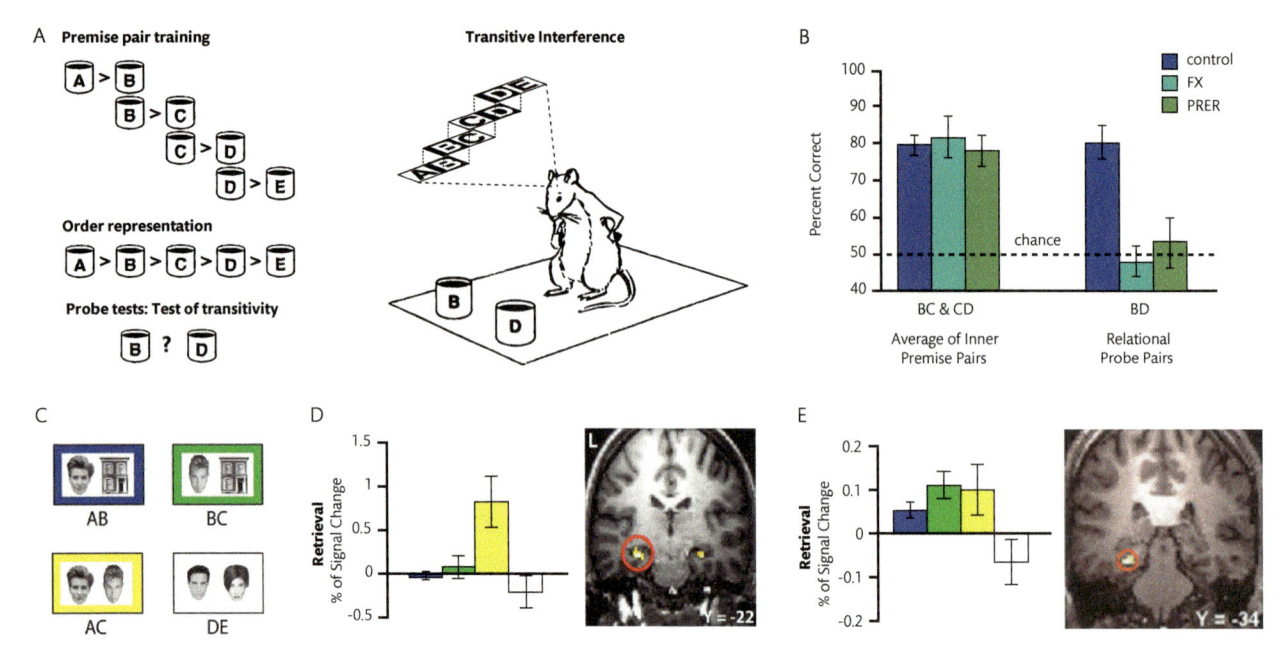

Figure 14.20 Relational memory tests in rats and people show a role for the hippocampus in flexible memory use. (A) Schematic of task design showing that subjects first learn a set of "premise pairs" in which a pair of scented sand wells is presented in which one contains a hidden food reward and one does not (e.g., A>B). Overlapping pairs are presented to build a theoretical hierarchical chain that should be used when rats are presented with a probe test of transitivity. (B) Pretraining lesions to either the fornix (FX) or the perirhinal/entorhinal cortices (PRER) did not prohibit rats from learning the premise pair associations. However, when challenged on the flexible memory probe (B>D), both lesion types produced a similar profound deficit. (C) Conceptually similar task design used to probe human memory where subjects learned pairs of images that could either be faces or houses. (D) Anterior hippocampal activity was observed during the inferential transitive probe (AC, yellow) but not during retrieval tests on the original premise pairs (AB, BC, DE). (E) Parahippocampal activity was observed during premise pairs that involved houses (AB/BC) but not those compose of just faces (DE). An inferential probe with just faces (AC, yellow) evoked parahippocampal activity presumably due to covert reactivation of the associated scene image.

these in turn influence future learning. Therefore, to study relational processing in the lab, new tasks were needed. The first set of relational tasks was closely modeled after Piaget's tests of inferential ability in human children, with similar faculties being reported in monkeys (McGonigle and Chalmers, 1977). Such experiments typically rely on two phases of learning, one in which specific associations are made, and another in which success depends on inferring relationships that could only be realized by combining information acquired over multiple experiences (Figure 14.20). These are examples of Jerome Bruner's classic phrase of "going beyond the information given" (Bruner, 2010).

For example, in one such experiment, rats had to dig through sandwells with different odors to secure reward. Rats first learned that odor A (e.g., coffee) predicted that reward would be only available when digging at odor B (e.g., turmeric), but not at odor Y. Odor B, in turn predicted reward only with odor C, but not with odor Z. Thus, a causal chain was potentially being created and stored in memory where A→B→C (Bunsey and Eichenbaum, 1996). In parallel, rats also learned that digging first at odor X predicted that reward would be available with odor Y (and not odor B), and that odor Y predicted reward with odor Z (and not odor C), forming a different associational chain X→Y→Z. Odors A, B, C, X, Y, and Z were equally familiar, and the spatial location of the sandwells was not a reliable cue; thus, neither task could be solved with respect to novelty or spatial cues. However, having set up these two distinct inferential chains of associations, a test for transitive inference was then given to determine whether rats could use them in novel ways. Rats were presented with odor A again and then challenged on

whether they could correctly predict reward association with odor C but not odor Z (A→C). Conversely, on presentation of odor X, could they correctly predict reward association with odor Z (X→Z)? The key findings were that, whereas hippocampal lesions did not affect rats' ability to learn the simple "premise pairs" of A→B and B→C, performance on the inference probe (A→C) was severely impaired (Bunsey and Eichenbaum, 1996). The hippocampus was required for flexible inference within relational networks, as the theory predicted. In another test of transitive inference, rat subjects were first given overlapping "premise pairs" of items in which they had to choose odor A and not odor B to secure reward, B and not C, C and not D, and then D and not E. This training might have led to isolated silos of object–reward associations (as in the classical concurrent discrimination task), or alternatively, have created a mental hierarchical space: A>B>C>D>E. This test had been successfully explored in monkeys (McGonigle and Chalmers, 1977; McGonigle and Margaret, 1992) but not yet in rodents. To test these alternatives, and as in the monkey experiments, rats were then probed with the novel combination of B and D to determine whether the relationships learned in separate, paired experiences could be integrated to make novel inferences. Disconnecting the hippocampus from its cortical or subcortical partners (via fornix lesions or lesions to the entorhinal/perirhinal cortices) prior to the start of training caused memory deficits specifically for the inferential probes (i.e., knowing that B is better than D) but left performance intact on the explicitly trained "premise pairs" e.g., B > C; (Dusek and Eichenbaum, 1997). Studies in mice have shown that hippocampal lesions made *after* completion of the initial training on the premise pairs also cause inference deficits on the inferential probe trial, revealing an important role for the hippocampus in flexible retrieval during inferential performance (Devito et al., 2010). A similar deficit has been found with optogenetic silencing of the hippocampus applied during the retrieval-based inference test (Barron et al., 2020).

Very different evidence for the relational memory hypothesis has been observed in human imaging studies that use BOLD signals to infer neural activation (Logothetis et al., 2001). Clever task designs have enabled testing whether memories for individual episodes become integrated during the encoding phase, or only during the inferential memory retrieval probes, a time at which hippocampal activation does not always correlate with performance (Shohamy and Wagner, 2008). Since images of faces and houses can activate different brain regions, tasks can be designed to infer whether subjects are thinking about one set of stimuli (e.g., houses) even when only another class (e.g., faces) is physically present. For example, human subjects could be asked to make an association between an image of a face (Item A) and a house (Item B) in the first phase of a study. In the second phase, the originally paired house image (Item B) could then be presented as subjects make a new association with a novel face image (Item C) (Figure 14.20C–E). With this task design, it is possible to ask whether, when presented with just a pair of faces (Item A and C), subjects show covert reactivation of the associated house image (Item B), which would manifest as BOLD activity in scene-related regions. Several studies using this type of design showed reactivation of the associated, though absent stimulus category, during this second stage of encoding (Preston et al., 2004; Shohamy and Wagner, 2008; Zeithamova, Dominick, et al., 2012). During learning, changes in hippocampal activity also correlate with the degree of associative reactivation which in turn correlated with inferential probe performance (association of Item A and Item C; Zeithamova, Dominick, et al., 2012). Successful retrieval of Item A, when learning to pair Items B and C is therefore critical for behavioral flexibility, showing a compelling role for the hippocampus and relational recall during learning. These results led to the integrative encoding hypothesis, which states that the representation encoded in a stored trace is dependent on both stimuli present at the time of training and other stimuli evoked in memory by the current situation (Gluck and Myers, 1993; Zeithamova and Preston, 2010; Zeithamova, Schlichting, et al., 2012).

Few studies have recorded single neurons to explicitly test predictions from the relational memory theory. Research from Dupret's group provides a critical link between rodent and human studies. In their experiments (Barron et al., 2020), mice and people learned a sensory preconditioning task in which subjects first learned that a complex natural sound X predicted a colored light Y, and then, in a separate phase, learned that the Y light predicted reward (Z). The inference required that subjects would infer that sound X, that had never been directly conditioned with Z, would also predict reward. In both species, the sensory preconditioning was established successfully—subjects displayed reward-seeking behavior when presented with the sounds. Silencing dorsal CA1 in the mouse eliminated the expected inference behavior during the sound presentation. To understand how activity during the inference trial could guide behavior, recordings of mouse neurons revealed that, on trials when mice appropriately sought reward, the pattern of activity during the sound presentation (X) correlated with the pattern of activity observed when the light stimulus (Y) was directly paired with reward, suggestive of a reactivation or association of the neural

codes for these related events that occurred at different moments (sound paired with light and light paired with reward). Moreover, during population bursts known as awake SPW-Rs, neurons that fired in response to the sound and to reward began firing together across learning. The firing patterns had a reverse-replay temporal order, with activity in the reward-responsive neurons (Z) preceding activity of the sound-responsive neurons (X) (Barron et al., 2020). These findings were strongly predicted by the relational memory theory. As these are not spatial associations, it is unclear how the cognitive map theory could predict such a result.

A potential difficulty is that transitive inference is a classic example of "devil-is-in-the-detail." This is true both conceptually and procedurally (McGonigle and Chalmers, 2003) because, like other ambiguous tasks, it may be solved in several ways. Van Elzakker et al. (2003) noted at least four different theoretical accounts of successful task performance and argued that a simple "excitatory stimulus value" account, not requiring inference, cannot be completely ruled out. This may seem surprising as, on the face of it, the novel B > D probe compares two stimuli that should be of equal "excitatory stimulus value" as they are equally often paired with reward and nonreward during training. However, there are some cryptic asymmetries to the training protocol that may render this assumption false. In learning D > E in the five-odor problem, the pairing is with a stimulus E that is *never* reinforced. D may therefore not need as high of an "excitatory stimulus value" before the difference between D and E crosses a theoretical threshold that drives choosing D over E. Similarly, A is always reinforced, and thus the A > B difference might also be realized quickly despite B gaining a high associative strength through its training with object C. Given this, the relative excitatory value of B may be higher than that of D, despite the ostensibly equal pairing with reward and non-reward that the training schedule was intended to set up. If that is true, one might then expect a B vs. D probe to be easier in a four-pair series (A > B, B > C, C > D, and D > E) than in a five-pair series in which an E > F problem is added. Exactly these results were found by Van Elzakker et al. (2003), who therefore queried whether relational processing and inferential memory retrieval was really being used to perform the task. Others have found that inferential performance is intact when premise pairs are presented physically one pair after another in a straight line. However, inference fails when premise pairs are presented (A>B>C>D>E) in a circle where A and E are presented in neighboring positions, although never on the same trial (Roberts and Phelps, 1994). These results show that a cognitive map of physical space in which the objects were located, and a hierarchical map learned during training, may interact in complex ways to guide behavior during probe trials.

14.5.2 Reframing aspects of spatial navigation in terms of relational memory

Spatial relationships are held to be the role of the hippocampus in the cognitive map theory but a specific instance of a more general kind of relation handled by the hippocampus is considered in the new approach. It was therefore of interest to reframe experiments on spatial navigation within relational memory theory and conduct relevant tests. For example, the ability of rats to find a hidden platform in the watermaze was known to depend on the hippocampus when rats must begin from a position that differs from that encountered during training (Morris et al., 1982). In contrast, "navigation" toward a single destination from a single start location might be accomplished without hippocampal processing, a prediction upheld in one study (Eichenbaum et al., 1990). Proponents of cognitive map theory were critical of this interpretation of these results, arguing that this "special case" was compatible with the original concept of "taxon" learning; approach from a single stable start location could be mediated by direct approach to a specific extramaze cue and need not involve a cognitive map. The supposition of the cognitive map theory is that hippocampus is only required for using stable knowledge about spatial relationships between room landmarks and the hidden goal when the navigating animal has to make novel inferences about the path, such as being confronted with a novel start location. Some of data concerning amnesic taxi-drivers is compatible with this apparent inflexibility of route planning (Maguire et al., 2006). Successful navigation in the absence of flexibility has since been confirmed in other studies testing relational memory in mice with hippocampal lesions on a radial-arm maze (Etchamendy et al., 2003). Nonetheless, these experiments may still be consistent with the hippocampus as a cognitive map, because one of its properties is to provide flexibility for inferring novel shortcuts from previously learned spatial relations (O'Keefe and Nadel, 1978).

A different challenge was that the relational memory theory must also give a satisfactory explanation for the origin and contribution of spatially tuned neurons such as place cells. Might such cells also encode more general relationships? In the canonical preparation to examine place-cell activity, animals forage in an open arena for bits of cereal reward scattered strategically around the floor to maximize the chance that the subject occupies each location. As we have seen, the classic observation is that hippocampal principal cells are tuned to particular locations in space and tend to fire irrespective of the running trajectory through that location. However, not all neurons display such invariance and changes in task demands can bias the likelihood of observing trajectory-dependent firing. For example,

training rats to run back and forth on a linear track generates strong directional dependencies (Navratilova et al., 2012).

A key new observation was that of "splitter cells" (E Wood et al., 2000) (Figure 14.21). These experiments were performed in rats trained to run around a figure-of Eight 8 maze and to turn alternately to the left on even runs and to the right on odd ones after running along the central arm. The key discovery was of neurons with "diversity of specificity," namely neurons that differentiated the journeys (the "splitter cells") that are distinct from cells showing location firing irrespective of trajectory ("place cells") (E Wood et al., 2000). It has been suggested that the cells that did not differentiate journeys "captured a set of regularities in stimulus relations that were common across both conditions—the nodal features" (Eichenbaum et al., 1999, p. 218). The splitter cells, on the other hand, were suggested to mark the unique aspects of a class of an episode (in this case, right vs. left turns). This is an important finding, and was the first of a range of papers from the Eichenbaum laboratory in which cells may at first appear to show only place correlates but, as training proceeded, came to display task-related correlates (e.g., Komorowski et al., 2009). Theoretically, there may exist neurons that fire in more and more restrictive conditions until there are those whose activity mark a unique episode. The relational memory theory predicts that invariant nodal cells that fire across a diversity of experience activate splitter cells (and those with more restrictive firing) to build a relational network linking episodic memories that occurred at different times in the same place (Eichenbaum et al., 1999). In such a network, "trajectory-independent" cells serve as the neurophysiological basis for the concept of a specific position divorced from the specific events that occur in that location. Conversely, "trajectory-dependent" cells represent a conjunction of position and task-demands. Linking distinct events that occurred in the same location would be possible through invariant nodal cell activity.

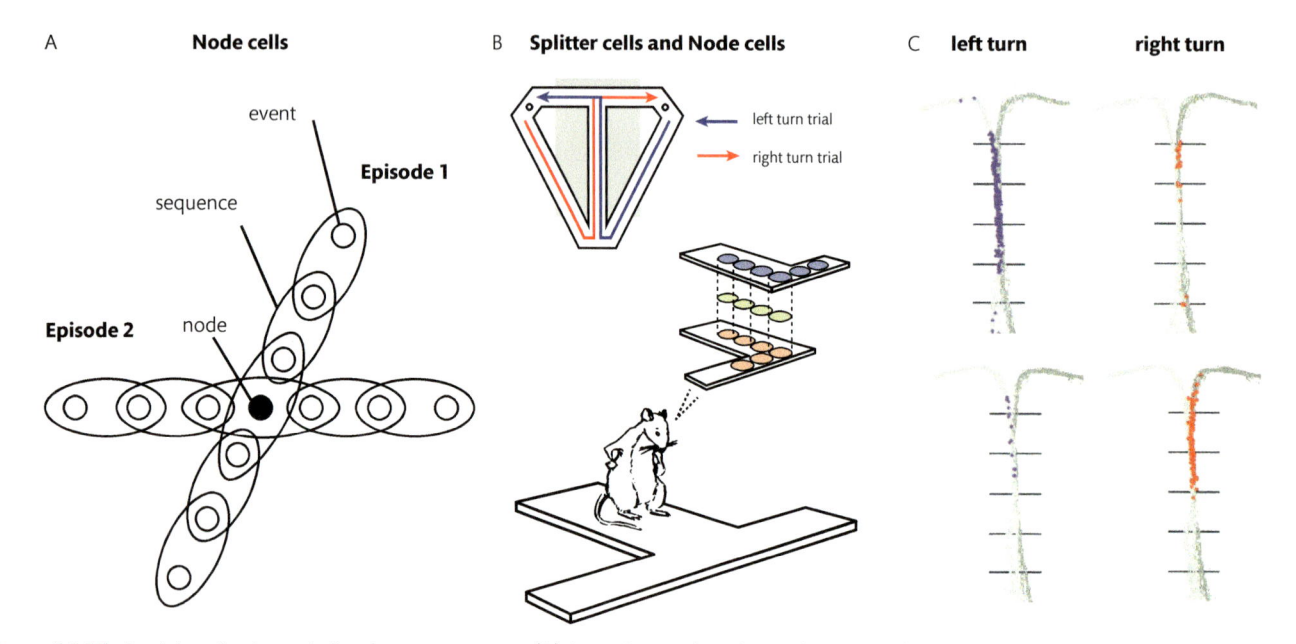

Figure 14.21 Spatial coding in a relational memory system. (A) According to the relational memory theory, the theoretical origin of direction invariance place cells comes from linking common elements of sequential paths that cross at common locations. A neuron that fires for Episode 1 and Episode 2 at the common location would be a node linking those experiences and that would display directional invariance. (B) Task design of an alternating T-maze, or Figure-of-eight maze, to assess the dependence on past and future actions on place coding. (C) Top, single CA1 neuron that fires on the central stem preferentially when the rat makes left-hand turns. Bottom, another CA1 neuron that fires when subjects turn right. (After Wood et al., 2000.)

The cognitive map theory nicely accounts for the existence of place fields, and even place fields modulated by other environmental factors (O'Keefe and Krupic, 2021). Chapter 12 of this book argues that there are few if any cases of complex correlates of hippocampal cell firing that are completely incompatible with the primary correlate being spatial. Others argue that the jury remains "out" on that issue. Perhaps a more compelling case for neurons that code for meaningful categories beyond spatial location comes from studies of functional equivalence in which the perceptual features of stimuli are distinct although their meaning is similar (Figure 14.22). The relational memory theory predicts that objects with functional equivalence come to be related by virtue of common neural activity across those conditions—the emergence of nodal cells that capture an associative regularity. Striking examples of "nodal cells" that show functional equivalence come from studies in human epileptic patients in whom cells increase their firing rate in response to pictures from the same category of stimuli such as houses or faces (Kreiman et al., 2000), or most remarkably cells that respond only to symbols that represent a specific person who rose to fame, such as the "Jennifer Aniston cell." Such cells respond to different color photographs, line drawings, and even the written name of famous individuals, such as the actors Jennifer Aniston or Halle Barry (Quiroga et al., 2005). They appear to be "concept cells." Just as nodal cells and splitter cells exist on a continuum of specificity, concept codes may also vary in the scope of stimuli they encode. For example, neurons that respond to the concept of the film character Luke Skywalker under multiple modalities (images, voice, text), are also found to respond to the related character of the Star Wars saga, Yoda (Quiroga et al., 2009). Similar category cells have been reported in the monkey during a delayed matching task (Hampson et al., 2004) in which neurons were observed responding generally to diverse images of people, or to color, but not black-and-white images. The existence of cells that reflect perceptually distinct though functionally equivalent stimuli show evidence that the correlational structure of memories has the potential to be represented within the hippocampus, but it is unclear whether they are stored in cortex and then retrieved to hippocampus, or stored in both structures (McClelland et al., 1995; Kumaran and McClelland, 2012).

14.5.3 Context can serve to set the occasion for retrieving specific associations

Though spatial context has a particular meaning in the cognitive map theory, the concept of context is much broader and can include aspects of the moment that are distinct from a visual scene or set of landmarks that differentiate one location from another. A context can, for example, be a specific mood. Importantly, contexts can also "set the occasion" for a particular cue having a particular significance or meaning. For example, the decision to eat depends on a realm of external cues (whether it is socially appropriate, whether there may be better options later), and internal cues (whether you are hungry). Although occasion-setting is not often discussed in texts on relational memory theory, there is a close link between the phenomenon of occasion-setting and the theory, as both require the

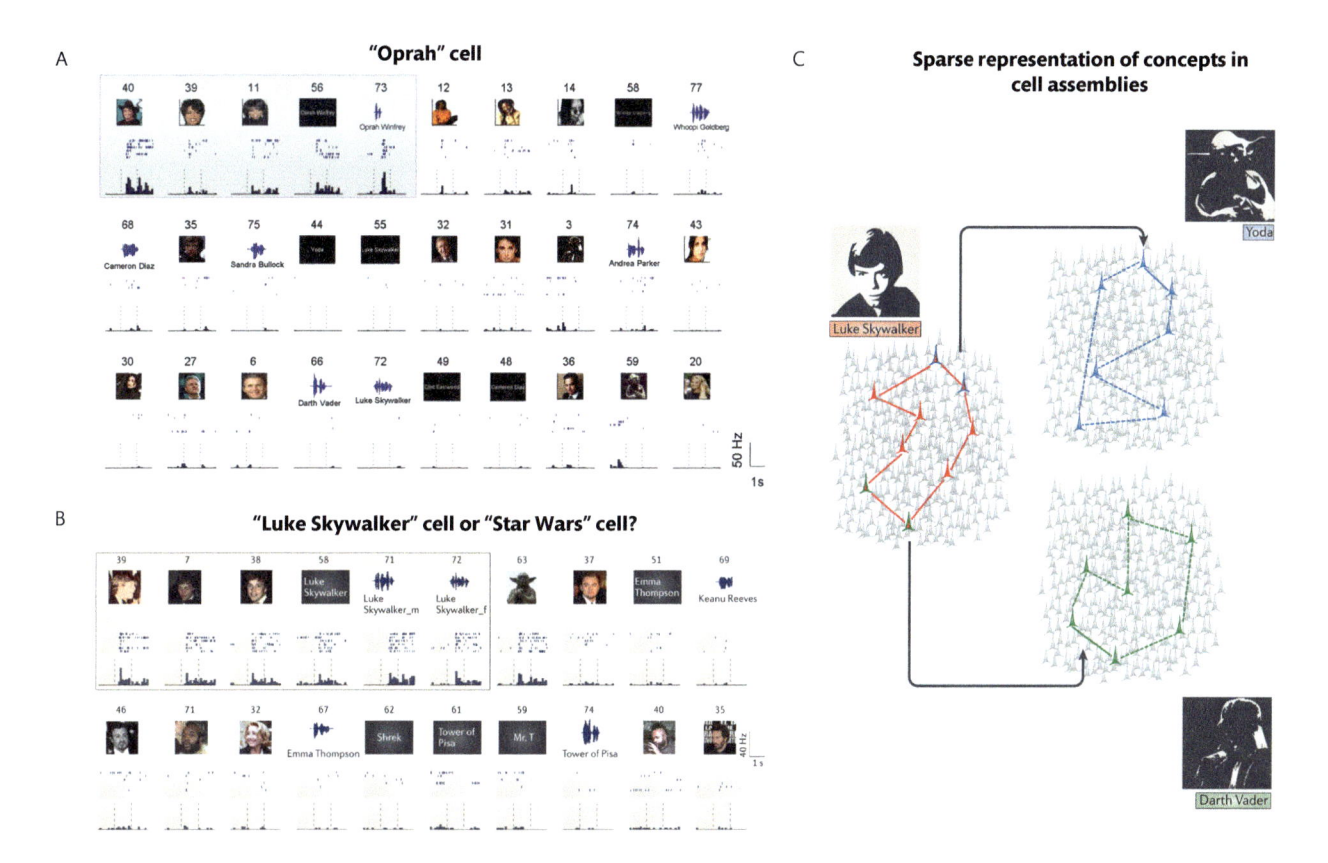

Figure 14.22 Concept cells in the human hippocampus. (A) Hippocampal neuron that fires in response to the American TV star Oprah Winfrey, whether it is her image, the sound of her voice, or her written name. (Reproduced from Quiroga et al., 2009.) (B) Neuron that fires in response to the *Star Wars* character "Luke Skywalker" also fires in response to another character from the same film series, "Yoda." (C) Rather than by individual cells, concepts are likely represented by concept "ensembles." Different, but related, concepts can therefore share some of these neurons while maintaining their individuality. (B,C adapted from Quiroga et al., 2012.)

construction of mental models about how elements of the world should interact and relate. Good and Honey (1991) developed the first satisfactory experimental design to investigate the role of the hippocampus in occasion-setting. Their protocol ensured that subjects became familiar with two separate contexts (operant conditioning chambers) and two distinct cues (tones and clickers) and were equally reinforced in relation to both sets of cues. Rats were trained in an appetitive paradigm (collecting food pellets) in which one discrete stimulus (A) was reinforced in one context X, whereas a second stimulus (B) was reinforced in context Y. The critical test of the ability of either context to retrieve the appropriate significance of these cues was to present—for the first time—A in the inappropriate context Y and B in context X. The phenomenon of "context specificity" was displayed as a reduction in the appetitive responses elicited by A and B in their now "inappropriate" contexts. Rats given electrolytic (Good and Honey, 1991) or neurotoxic (Honey and Good, 1993) hippocampal lesions failed to show this reduction of conditioned responding. This failure was not because the lesioned subjects could not discriminate the two contexts, because a separate experiment established that they had no difficulty in doing so when only one of the two contexts predicted the availability of reinforcement.

Internal cues can also be used to define a learning context. Early studies used spatial tasks in which a rat was required to perform one spatial response when hungry and a different one when thirsty. Rats could learn to do this, but any lesion-associated deficit could arise because of a failure to discriminate the different motivational states, to use this information to retrieve the appropriate response, or of spatial memory itself. Davidson and Jarrard (1993) examined a nonspatial task in which placement in an operant chamber was associated with footshock when the rats were hungry but not when satiated (or vice versa). Normal animals could learn this discrimination, whereas rats with neurotoxic lesions of the hippocampus could not.

Similarly, the extinction of a learned response can also come under the control of a learning context. In the extinction of classical fear conditioning, a tone (CS) that has previously predicted the imminent arrival of shock (US) is now followed by nothing, and the overt expression of the prior conditioning becomes weaker over successive extinction trials. An early supposition was that extinction is an "unlearning" process—a breaking of the associative bonds between cue and consequence. However, various phenomena discovered about the determinants of extinction have cast doubt on this unlearning idea, with extinction often being a new learning process in which contextual factors play a particularly important modulatory role—the extinction context altering what US memory is retrieved when the previously trained CS is presented (Bouton, 2004). In training, the CS comes to evoke a memory representation of the predicted US; in extinction, the CS may acquire a memory representation of "no-US" but, importantly, there may be no overwriting of the previous CS-US association. Which memory is retrieved will depend on the context of testing, with the nature of the environment and how it differs from other environments, the passage of time, or other factors influencing the operative "context" as perceived by the animal. As Bouton and Moody put it, "the fact that extinction is more context-dependent than conditioning is consistent with the idea that the animal codes extinction as a kind of conditional exception to the rule—one that depends on the current context" (Bouton and Moody, 2004, p 665).

New tasks are being developed to formalize how task regularities guide behavior and to investigate whether the hippocampal formation participates in these processes. Inspired by the reinforcement learning field, "agents" can make decisions about how to achieve reward based on information derived from multiple memory systems. For example, the brain can create and use mental models of the causal structure of the world to guide decision-making in model-based strategies. Alternatively, organisms may simply learn chains of stimulus response associations, or learn that certain stimuli possess value, without knowing how different stimuli predict and relate to one another. To test whether model-based learning relies on the integrity of the hippocampus, the Brody group at Princeton trained rats in a "two-step" task in which, in the first step of the task, the rat must make a choice between two nose ports, each of which leads to one of two reward ports becoming available with a probability of 80% (*common transition*), or to the other reward port with probability 20% (*uncommon transition*) (Miller et al., 2017). In the second step, the rat does not have a choice, but instead enters a single available port and either receives a reward or does not. The probability of reward delivery at each port changes at unpredictable intervals. To secure as much reward as possible, the hungry rats must learn which nose port currently is associated with the higher reward potential, and then select the choice port that is mostly likely to give subsequent access to that port. Remarkably, rats can learn this task and learn to switch choice ports when reward probabilities change. Without a model of the probability of transition from the first to second step of the task, rats should not be able to place extra value in learning when reward is delivered (or omitted) in the common transition conditions, as compared with placing less emphasis on learning reward outcomes after uncommon transition. Through analysis of response errors after changes in the reward probability, it is possible to infer how rats use the recent past to change behavioral strategies and to statistically assess whether knowledge of the "step-step" transition structure factors into how decisions change from one trial to the next. As expected, in the intact animals, repetition of a behavior is more likely if it was rewarded after a common transition. Rewards after uncommon transitions were less potent drivers in motivating repeated behaviors. Bilateral muscimol inactivation of the hippocampus decreased that bias, suggesting elimination of the storage, or use, of the relationships defining the transitions between the first and second stage of the task (Miller et al., 2017).

14.5.4 Assessment of the relational processing theory

The relational memory framework has been criticized for its lack of a formal definition of some key concepts such as "relational network," "memory element," and "memory flexibility" (Mackintosh, 2002). Unlike the computational theories that inspired the Hebb-Marr framework, the relational memory theory was developed as a functional theory without much linking to neurobiological implementation beyond an identification with the hippocampus as being critical and the use of nodal cells for making inferential leaps. The idea that the brain can do associative inference at the point of memory retrieval is interesting, but what is missing in implementational terms is what is actually happening in the dentate gyrus or areas CA3 and/or CA1 to achieve this. Is the re-entrant circuitry of CA3 amenable to serving as an inference engine?

The lack of computational implementation, and therefore precision of the relational memory theory, is also beginning to be addressed (Whittington et al., 2020). In their proposed "Tolman-Eichenbaum" machine model, the challenge posed by the relational memory theory is addressed by involving the complementary memory systems framework inspired by the functional anatomy of MEC, LEC, and its interactions with the hippocampus. A goal of the model is to infer which latent state the agent occupies at any given moment (see also Chapter 16). These states could map onto anything in the real world that has some kind of structural regularity, including positions in physical space, but also locations in other kinds of abstract graphs (like a family tree). On this view, the MEC stores the relational structure in the abstract (e.g., that family trees exist), the LEC provides inputs about particular perceptual details (e.g., the identity of a member of a family), and the hippocampus binds the particular item with the correct slot in the MEC schema (e.g., that a particular person belongs in a particular place in the family tree). As a case study, Whittington et al. (2020) made their model learn about family trees and they then found that some simulated MEC neurons learn to code for the concept of a father, and others the concept of a father's brother, and so on. LEC neurons then provide information about the particular family member and the hippocampus links that information with the correct MEC category. In this way learning is rapidly facilitated by leveraging the fact that families trees are in general very similar, or as Whittington et al. put it, "each world has the same underlying relational structure but with a different configuration of sensory observations, thus understanding a new world is simply a problem of relational memory" (Whittington et al., 2020, p. 1251). Critically, this view of the hippocampus is fundamentally distinct from that of an orthogonal memory space that minimizes memory interference, as preferred by the Hebb-Marr theories of episodic memory, the topic of the following section.

14.6 Episodic memory

The most widely accepted contemporary theory of hippocampal function, and one that this chapter espouses, is that it mediates episodic memory. The concept, as first introduced by Tulving (1972) and elaborated since (Tulving, 1983, 2004; Schacter and Tulving, 1994), refers to the memory of unique events and/or the temporal sequence of events making up an episode that collectively constitute our memory of lived experience. The early computational modeling of Marr (1971) was, in effect, the same claim. The content of episodic memory is a mental representation of "what" happened during an event, "where" it happened, and "when." Writing in 1983, Tulving asserted that episodic memory "receives and stores information about temporally-dated episodes or events, and temporal-spatial relations among these events" (Tulving, 1983, p 385). The idea that our everyday memories require the integrity of the hippocampal function emerged from the study of H.M. (Corkin, 2002) and other amnesic patients. The seminal neuropsychological studies of developmental amnesia (Vargha-Khadem et al., 1997) (see Chapter 13) added important evidence that hippocampal function is directly and specifically associated with episodic memory.

From an algorithmic perspective, contemporary computational models of hippocampal function take as their premise that episodic memory is the core function whose computational underpinnings are to be understood and they seek to explain how it may learn and store a large body of unique memories and then later enable their

recollection. The intrinsic circuitry of the hippocampus has inspired theoretical work mapping different computational subgoals intrinsic to episodic memory to different regions of the hippocampus. Key aspects, as we will see, are pattern separation of EC inputs by the dentate gyrus (DG) (McNaughton and Morris, 1987), and pattern completion by the CA3 autoassociative network receiving EC and DG inputs (O'Reilly and McClelland, 1994; Treves and Rolls, 1994), supported by activity-dependent plasticity.

The full hippocampal circuit is necessary for learning about *new* places and contexts, but events typically happen in spatial contexts with which we are completely familiar. If familiar context information, which rarely needs new processing, were to be stored outside the hippocampus, it could be projected in via the EC layer III input to CA1 where it could, using synaptic plasticity, realize the binding between events processed within other hippocampal regions, thus linking unique aspects of our experience with the context in which they have occurred. Morris (2006) developed this idea in distinguishing the potential role of the classical tri-synaptic circuit (for events) from that of the temporo-ammonic pathway (for context binding) respectively. The existence of both activity-dependent synaptic plasticity at each stage of this circuitry (DG, CA3, and CA1), and catecholaminergic neuromodulation (DA and NE), collectively builds the picture of the hippocampus being an ideal "episodic memory machine" that can store new information in a manner influenced by the relative novelty of new events.

A generic version of the episodic-memory theory of hippocampal function is as follows (Box 14.3).

Box 14.3 The hippocampus and episodic and episodic-like memory

1. *Conceptual issues:* Episodic memory encoding enables the later conscious recall, by humans, of discrete events that happened at a particular place and at a particular time or in a particular context. Such memory recall generally entails mental time travel.

2. *Specific behavioral protocols:* Episodic-like memory in animals is the memory of "what, where, and when" (www) (or "what, where, which") with respect to automatically encoded events, without any necessary reference to autonoetic consciousness.

3. *Hippocampal involvement:* The hippocampus is one of a network of brain structures that mediate the automatic encoding and subsequent retrieval of attended events and the contexts in which they occur. Distinct brain structures, including the prefrontal lobe, likely mediate other more volitional facets of this form of memory.

4. *Modeling and the differential role of hippocampal subcomponents:* Components of the hippocampal formation (DG, CA3, CA2, and CA1) are differentially involved in dissociable components of episodic-like memory such as pattern separation, pattern completion, possibly social recognition and event-context associations, building on ideas developed experimentally and in computational modeling.

5. *Neurobiological implementation:* The implementation of episodic-like memory includes associative links between www elements, mediated by synaptic plasticity with selective cellular consolidation mediated by synaptic tagging and capture (STC) as a necessary adjunct to automatic encoding.

6. *Awareness:* Episodic memory and episodic-like memory are distinguishable, as only the former requires "autonoetic" consciousness. Awareness of the strength of a memory could be an attribute of episodic-like memory in animals, such as metamemory, but establishing autonoetic awareness is presently beyond the feasibility of experimentation in animals.

14.6.1 Episodic memory as a distinct form of human memory

The memory of *what* you did on your last holiday, *where* you went and with whom, and having the feeling that these events happened to you in the past (*when*), would be an instance of episodic memory. This "www" definition of episodic memory captures an important feature that distinguishes it from other forms of declarative memory. Such remembering entails "mental time travel" to re-enact a past scene, distinguishing it from knowledge of facts (semantic memory). Tulving (1972) argued these two memory systems differ with respect to: (a) the sensory/perceptual systems that provide input, (b) the type and nature of information stored in the system, (c) the consequences of memory retrieval, and (d) the susceptibility of the memories to interference including retrieval-induced "transformations" of stored content. The status of spatial memory within Tulving's framework is unclear.

Although the theoretical divide between episodic and semantic memory was initially motivated by analyses at the cognitive level, later writings made clear that the hippocampus was the major neural substrate for the episodic memory system. The study of patient K.C. (Kent Cochrane), whose semantic memory was intact, but who suffered from lack of episodic memories of his entire past, as well as anterograde amnesia, was particularly influential for Tulving's thinking (although K.C.'s brain damage was not selectively hippocampal; Rosenbaum et al., 2005; Figure 14.23A,B). Given the close, bidirectional relationship between these two forms of memory, it is fair to ask whether dissociations could ever be observed. What evidence could falsify the episodic theory? Tulving answers this question directly: "the simplest and strongest case against the model [the hippocampus is required for episodic memory], one that would be sufficient for its rejection, would be made by patients with focal bilateral hippocampal pathology who have normal episodic memory but who cannot acquire new factual knowledge"

(Tulving and Markowitsch, 1998, p 203). No such patients have been reported, and indeed 25 years after episodic memory was first given an anatomical home, a large body of evidence validates the original conjecture. Though human studies are covered in more detail in Chapter 13, several important lines of work are described here to orient the animal studies on episodic-like memory that follow.

One important discovery relevant to episodic memory was that of *developmental amnesia*. Vargha-Khadem et al. (1997) focused on a case study of three young adults who, following perinatal medical events (such as anoxia), suffered brain damage ostensibly limited to the hippocampus (Figure 14.23C,D). These people show profound amnesia for everyday events, and they have limited ability, or are unable, to navigate familiar environments, learn new ones, or orient in time. They also show a delay-dependent deficit in the spontaneous preference for inspection of novel stimuli (Munoz et al., 2011). In contrast, their semantic memory is apparently good, they have normal verbal competency and show average performance on a test of verbal IQ for common-knowledge semantic information (Elward and Vargha-Khadem, 2018). Other studies that have specifically tested for episodic memory in subjects with damage to the hippocampus have also shown impairments (e.g., Steinvorth et al., 2005), although there is debate as to whether semantic memory is also affected (Manns, Hopkins, and Squire, 2003). There are also various divergent findings as to whether episodic memories remain dependent on hippocampal function for all times or only within a consolidation time window after learning (Kirwan et al., 2008, see Chapter 13).

Dual process models of memory posit that the hippocampus and associated diencephalic regions enable episodic recollection while the perirhinal cortex and other rhinal cortices support familiarity judgments. The observations of poor free recall (the ability to conjure learned material at will) with intact recognition (the ability to identify stimuli as familiar) is often considered evidence for

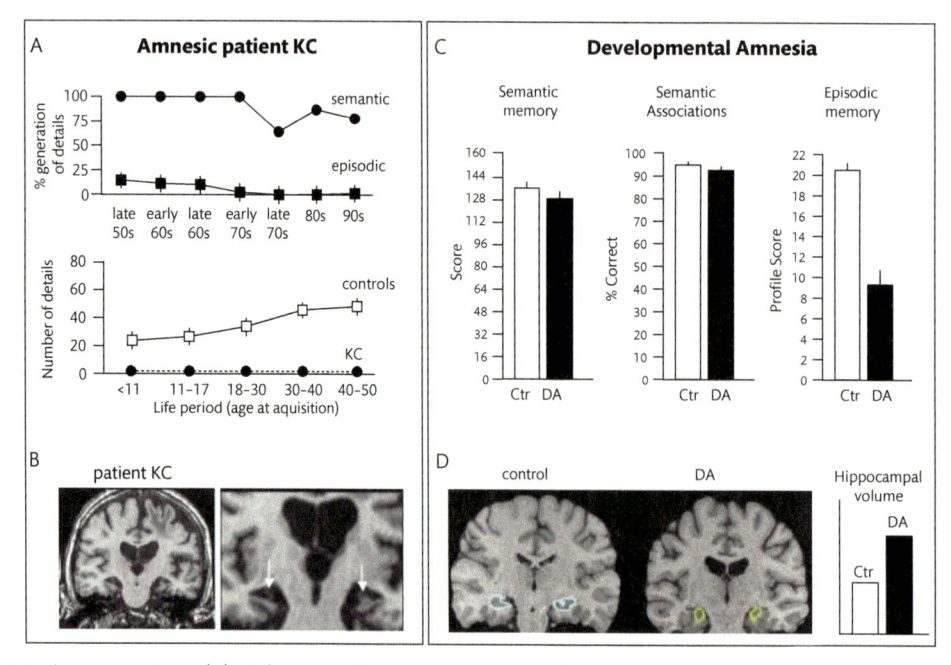

Figure 14.23 Amnesia in human patients. (A) Performance in semantic and episodic memory retrieval by amnesic patient KC as reviewed in Rosenbaum et al. (2005). Patient KC had severe lesions to the MTL as a consequence of a motorcycle accident, as seen in T1-weighted images of KC's brain. (B) Memory performance and brain lesion characterization in patients with developmental amnesia. (From Munoz et al., 2011.)

impaired recollection (Aggleton et al., 2005). For example, as discussed in Section 14.3, recognition can be supported by familiarity alone, whereas recall of paired associates cannot, and this latter faculty has been reported to be particularly sensitive to hippocampal damage (Vargha-Khadem et al., 1997; Mayes et al., 2004), as discussed in section 14.3 above. The dual process model is, nonetheless, controversial, with other papers reporting equivalent deficits in both recollection and familiarity in patients with damage limited to the hippocampus (Wais et al., 2006).

Can the role of the hippocampus be seen in both the process of encoding new memory traces and that of memory retrieval? It is impossible to tell from patients with permanent damage to the hippocampus, as intact encoding could be masked by deficits in retrieval. However, in support of the conclusion that hippocampal damage affects both encoding and retrieval of episodic details, disruption of the CA1 region of the hippocampus is associated with transient global amnesia (TGA) with retrograde episodic memory impairments lasting from hours to years for the events occurring during the transient episode (Bartsch et al., 2006). In contrast to patients with permanent retrograde amnesia, those with TGA regain their ability to form new memories with intact general retrieval of episodic information learned before and after the acute episode, while events that took place during the amnestic period remain forgotten (Sander and Sander, 2005). A similar pattern is seen in transient epileptic amnesia (TEA) (Butler et al., 2007). Furthermore, electrical stimulation of the medial temporal lobe of epileptic patients impairs encoding and subsequent retrieval of complex scenes (Halgren and Wilson, 1985). These studies show a clear role for the hippocampus in encoding and in retrieval of episodic information in humans.

14.6.2 Vertebrate animals have "episodic-like" memory

Tulving (2004) claimed that, as episodic memory relies on the capacity for mental time travel, episodic memory is unique to humans. Tulving posited that this requires a sense of self, or "autonoetic consciousness." Suddendorf and Corballis (1997) share this view, arguing that animals are forever mentally trapped in the present or, as Roberts (2000) put it, they are "stuck in time." This is a controversial claim, for biological scientists are rarely at ease with unsupported claims of human uniqueness. As it is unknown whether nonhuman subjects have a sense of self, the parallel concept of "episodic-like" memory was proposed to describe what lies beneath the behavioral manifestations of everyday memory in animals also. This respects the www feature of true episodic memory but finesses the need for autonoetic consciousness. Several lines of animal work suggest a preservation of function between humans and vertebrates within the domain of episodic-like memory, including lesion studies beginning with Gaffan (1994), avian studies of food caching by scrub jays (Clayton and Dickinson, 1998), and rodent and primate unit-recording studies (Wirth et al., 2003; Manns et al., 2007). The issue of whether animals have episodic memory has also attracted the interest of philosophers (e.g. Malinowski, 2016).

Clayton and her colleagues conducted numerous studies of food caching and recovery by hand-raised Californian scrub jays and, later, by crows. In a classic study, Clayton and Dickinson (1998) allowed scrub jays to cache food items in sand-filled ice-cube trays surrounded by distinctive visual objects. The two food items were (1) preferred but perishable wax moth larvae,

and (2) less-preferred but nonperishable peanuts. In two successive caching periods, separated by an interval of 5 days, the birds carried and then cached wax moths on one side of the caching tray, and peanuts on the other (Figure 14.24A,B). These caching periods constituted the opportunity for the animals to encode *what* food-item was being cached, *where*, and *when*. Recovery was permitted either 4 h or 124 h later, with both sides of the ice-cube tray available. Over several weeks, birds in a "degrade" group learned that wax moths retrieved after 4 h are tasty and well worth eating, whereas those retrieved after 124 h taste terrible. Birds assigned to a separate "replenish" control group always found fresh wax worms at recovery, whether this was scheduled at the short or the long recovery interval. The main finding of this ingenious study was that, in non-rewarded probe tests in which neither food was available, the scrub jays in the degrade group searched preferentially for wax moths when recovery occurred 4 h after caching but switched their search to peanuts when recovery occurred 124 h later (Figure 14.24B). This switch was not seen in the "replenish" group. This pattern of results implies that the birds can recollect what food item was stored where and when, at least in the sense of relative recency.

Long memory intervals excluded the use of short-term memory, and free recall at cache recovery obviates the use of familiarity. Clayton and Dickinson's fair claim that their 1998 study provided "the first conclusive behavioral evidence of 'episodic-like' memory in animals other than humans" (p 274) has been vindicated by later studies in which a number of detailed issues were taken further (Clayton et al., 2001; Clayton et al., 2003). Other studies have investigated prospective aspects of food caching in scrub jays called "forward planning" (Emery and Clayton, 2001), refined the criteria for identifying "mental time travel" in animals (Raby et al., 2007), and investigated both the impact of theft in studies of "pilfering" (Clayton et al., 2007) and the cues likely to be used to detect the threat of pilfering (Amodio et al., 2021).

Is the ability to track the recency of a food cache truly comparable to our mental time travel back to some moment past, a function thought to depend uniquely on hippocampal function? Jozet-Alves et al. (2013) challenge this notion by showing intact www memory recollection in organisms without a hippocampus. By teaching cuttlefish subjects that their favorite prey (shrimps) was replaced every 3 hours while their less preferred food (crabs) was replaced every hour, they showed that cuttlefish are able to keep track of the time by correctly searching in the shrimp-delivery area if 3 hours had passed from the first phase where they received shrimp, or in the crab-delivery area if only 1 hour had passed. Cuttlefish do not possess a hippocampal structure like vertebrates, but the vertical lobe presents similarities in connectivity and functionality with the hippocampus formation in vertebrates (Shomrat et al., 2015) and it would be interesting to see whether this structure serves some homologous function.

14.6.3 The role of the hippocampus in episodic-like memory

Other www tasks have been successfully developed for rodent studies building on the NOR tasks as described in section 14.3 above. However, all such tasks may depend on recognition rather than recall. One approach to investigate the neurobiology of recall in animals used the "event arena" (see section 14.4.4) to teach rats

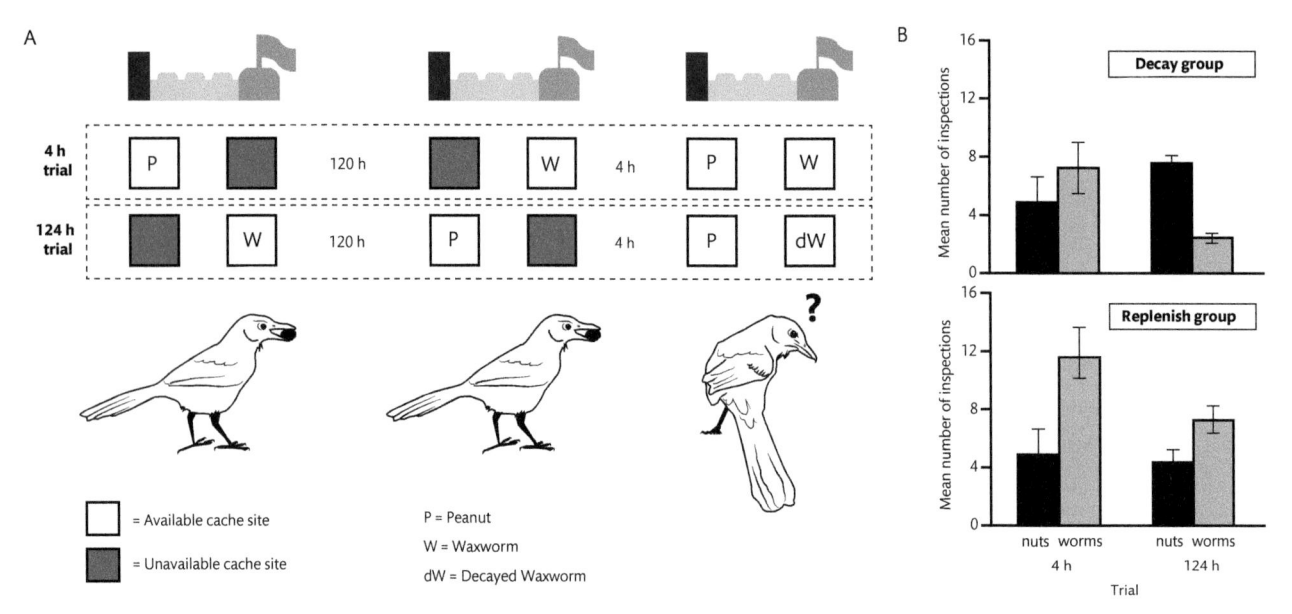

Figure 14.24 Memory for what, where, and when in California scrub-jays. (A) Experimental design for the training trials in which the birds in the "degrade" condition (shown) had the opportunity to learn that waxworms become unpalatable after a period of 4 days. (B) Results from the "degrade" group showing proportions of birds making their first pecks to the waxworm or peanut side of the caching tray. This effect was not seen in the "replenish" group, where decayed worms were changed with fresh worms by the experimenter. (After Clayton and Dickinson, 1998.)

the location of two different food rewards hidden within one of several identical-looking sandwells, with their position changing every day (Figure 14.25A) (Day et al., 2003). Bast et al. (2005) went on to observe that that blocking LTP with D-AP5 blocked memory encoding, but not memory recall, in such a recency recall task, whereas the AMPAR antagonist CNQX affected both.

If you ask someone about an event that happened when they were 20 years old, they most likely will *not* mentally time-travel themselves, but instead ask themselves where they were when aged 20, e.g. at university or in their first job. Easton et al. (2012) sought to model context rather than time as a www component using a series of distinct "what-where-which" tasks. The first was a modification of Ennaceur's novel object recognition (NOR) task for rats in which context, and object, and its place within the context were the triad of interest (Eacott and Norman, 2004). Rats had to learn that a specific object was in a specific location within a specific context, and then recognize any change in a subsequent test. Animals could recognize which of two identical objects was not in its proper context for periods of up to 15 min between the sample and test phase, and preferentially investigated it (Eacott and Norman, 2004). Performance was disrupted by lesions of the fornix, with no effect of either perirhinal or postrhinal cortex lesions. These lesions did not disrupt recognition performance in a simpler "object-location" task (what-where) in which context was not manipulated (Eacott and Gaffan, 2005). Similarly, a second set of tasks focused directly on recall, with rats running along an E-shaped maze to find a preferred object that had a specific place in each context (Eacott et al., 2005) (Figure 14.25B). Fornix lesions were reported to impair recollection but not familiarity (Easton et al., 2009). Eacott and Easton argue that identifying the context of an event ("which") may be more important than its point in time ("when").

Babb and Crystal (2006) developed a different www paradigm in the radial maze (Figure 14.25C). Animals were first presented with particularly palatable food pairs in two arms of the maze (e.g.,

chocolate-banana or berry-grape). These two arms were then empty, as the food had been eaten. After a short delay, a test was conducted with the remaining arms of the arm of maze having regular chow. Despite liking this food less, the animals preferentially visited these remaining arms, avoiding the empty ones. However, in a test conducted after a long delay, it was arranged that there would again be regular chow in the remaining arms, but the more desirable food options were again available in the original arms. Rats now visited the arms containing more palatable food options at longer delays. Their knowledge of the identity of the content of the arm was tested by using a taste devaluation procedure: rats chose not to visit a location where they had previously found a foodstuff that was now devalued with lithium chloride, preferring the other, nondevalued regular chow (Figure 14.25C).

14.6.4 A hippocampal neural code for episodic-like memory

Single-unit recording studies reveal that the "raw ingredients" for episodic-like memory formation are present in the hippocampus. The "where" component is almost universally assumed to be represented by place cells, and other spatially anchored cell types. Decades of work on the hippocampal cells and CA1 cells have shown preserved spatial correlates after an impressive number of neural manipulations (see section 14.4 and Chapter 11). As suggested by the lesion studies, there are multiple possible routes by which the "where" component may be computed and stored (assuming that the place field *is* the neurological basis for the spatial component). A large number of experimental factors influence changes in the position of a place field (global remapping) and the firing rate within a place field (rate remapping) such as the geometry or color of an open arena (Leutgeb et al., 2005), the identity of sampled item (Rolls et al., 1989; E Wood et al., 1999; Komorowski et al., 2009), conditioned stimuli (Moita et al., 2003), reward magnitude (Kobayashi et al., 1997), and running trajectory (McNaughton,

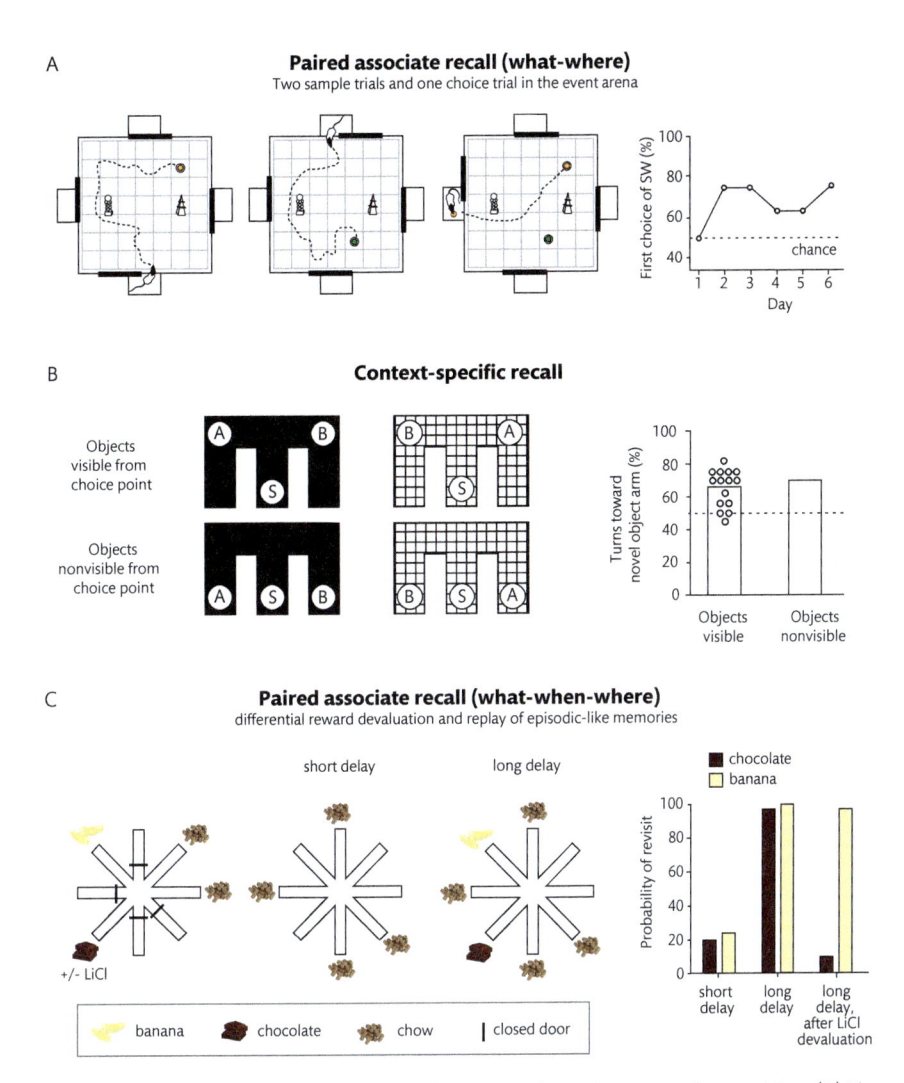

Figure 14.25 Testing the underlying mechanisms of recall requires different paradigms than tests of recognition. (A) The event-arena is a large 1.6 x 1.6 m arena divided according to a 7 x 7 grid into which sandwells can be placed where rats can dig up food. In this version of the tasks that can be trained in the event arena, rats had sample trials for each of two flavors (orange and green colors) and then a choice trial where, having been given one of the two flavors in the start box, was required to visit the same sandwell to secure more reward (win-stay). Choice performance was rapidly above chance, reflecting relatively automatic binding of what and when. (After Day et al., 2003.) (B) A rotated E-shaped maze was used to distinguish preferential visiting of objects (A, B) that had been displaced from their usual context-specific location. In a recognition version, the objects were visible at the choice-point but in a recall version were not. (After Eacott et al., 2005.) (C) Another approach involved placing different foodstuffs on distinct arms of an 8-arm radial maze that rats were allowed to explore. Standard chow was available at 6 of the arms (when access was permitted) but chocolate or banana at two other arms. After a long time-delay between trials, the animals preferentially visited the chocolate and banana arms. Devaluation of one of the flavors (chocolate) with lithium chloride caused approaches to chocolate to decline. After Babb and Crystal (2006).

Barnes, et al., 1983; E Wood et al., 2000) (see section 14.5). This work is consistent with place coding, but points to the possibility that hippocampal neurons can code much more than just *where* information.

What about the "what" and "when"? A prominent and, in our view, important example of object coding was reported by Komorowski et al. (2009) in the Eichenbaum lab (see also section 14.8.6). In the first of a series of studies, rats were trained to dig in terracotta pots filled with different digging media (e.g., beads or shredded paper) and scented with essential oils. Presented with two pots at a time, rats were to learn that one contained a buried food reward and the other did not. At first, hippocampal neurons looked like place cells: they fired when the rat occupied a particular position but the firing did not discriminate one object from another. As the rats learned, however, a large percentage of neurons that were

once place cells began to show firing that was well explained by the conjunction of a specific object present at a specific place.

Recent studies have also shown that the passage of time can drive changes in hippocampal activity, raising the prospect that the ever-evolving pattern of activity in the hippocampus sets a kind of "time-stamp" to allow for our understanding that certain events occur at a particular time point or in a particular order in our memories. The first animal study that showed this kind of dynamic was conducted in György Buzsáki's lab, where rats were trained to alternate on a Figure-of-8 maze, and then pause on a running wheel for a fixed amount of time before progressing to reward. In these experiments, when rats ran on the running wheel, neurons showed firing fields restricted to a specific time interval while running in a constant place (Pastalkova et al., 2008). Eichenbaum's group went on to characterize such "time cells" in greater detail in rats performing a delayed paired-associate task, where they first sampled an object, and then after a delay, sampled scented sand that had the potential to contain a concealed a hidden food reward, depending on the sampled object. MacDonald et al. (2011) set out to test what the hippocampus does during the delay to allow accurate performance. Like in the Buzsáki study, they identified "time cells" that fired at consistent but different intervals into the delay and were dependent on which of various objects was encountered recently, pointing to a kind of conjunctive object/duration representation that may be important for a memory system learning how to represent circumstances that precede and follow one another. Temporal coding in the hippocampus may extend even beyond the range of seconds. Electrophysiological recordings show that, especially in area CA2 and CA1, there is a constant "drift" in the pattern of neural activity in any given spot (Mankin et al., 2012). Over the course of hours, place fields that could be observed at a given location were observed to disappear, and cells that had been silent began to fire. Calcium imaging studies have further revealed that the drift occurs over multiple days and, unlike remapping, neurons fade in and out over days (Ziv et al., 2013). Though the physiological basis for this drift is not fully understood, it makes for an attractive neural basis for time coding in episodic memory (Howard et al., 2015). Temporal correlation in neural activity can also explain the association of memories observed with contextual fear conditioning (Cai et al., 2016). Overlapping ensembles represent memory closer in time (A and B), while distinct ensembles are recruited by memories learned several hours apart (A and C). If animals are fear conditioned in A, freezing is observed in context A, but also in context B, which was encountered in close temporal proximity to A, but not in context C at a more remote timepoint. Connections between the lateral entorhinal cortex (LEC) and the hippocampus seem to mediate the temporal component (Kitamura et al., 2015). For instance, reversible LEC inactivation after training impairs trace fear recall (Morrissey et al., 2012). Rather than elapsed time, LEC may code the beginning of noteworthy episodes or "epochs" providing support for the notion of temporal coding of an episode (Tsao et al., 2018).

Apart from time ("when"), events happen in places. Several studies correlate learning with changes in hippocampal cell firing. For example, accumulation of firing fields at goal areas has been observed as rats learn to swim to escape platforms (Hollup et al., 2001) or to find hidden food locations (Dupret et al., 2010). These results suggest that firing at goals reflects the long-term memory for the events that happened at those locations. However, overrepresentation with subsequent training generally decreases, but this does not reflect the elimination of the goal memory (Fyhn et al., 2002). Pharmacological blockade of NMDAR blocks the overrepresentation of goal sites in CA1 and causes a tendency for the animals to dwell at or revisit goal locations on non-rewarded probe trials (Dupret et al., 2010), suggesting a link between the memory and the overrepresentation. Place cells may fire outside of a primary place field at goal locations (Hok et al., 2007), and rewards can restructure the map of place cells in CA1 and of grid cells in the entorhinal cortex (Boccara et al., 2019; Butler et al., 2019). However, the relationship between remapping and memory is ambiguous (Jeffery et al., 2003).

Together, these correlative results suggest that the theoretical components of an episodic memory system are present in the hippocampal formation. However, there remains a large gulf between the aforementioned physiological observations and computational models of hippocampal function, the topic of the next sections.

14.6.5 Neural correlates of episodic memory recall

It is well known that, when people spontaneously recall a word from a studied list, the next word to be remembered is most likely to be that which appeared in the next serial position on the list, the next most likely is the word that preceded it, and so on (Howard and Kahana, 1999). Remarkably, this temporal contiguity effect holds over both short and long temporal intervals (Howard et al., 2008), suggesting a scale-free nature to the temporal organization of memory. Perhaps sequence matters more than time. This pattern of recall can be explained by models in which the present neural activity persists into the future and becomes the temporal context with which each word is learned; the neural activity is more correlated for word N and word N + 1 than word N and N + 2 (Sederberg et al., 2008). Recordings from human patients have found that recalling word N partially reinstates the pattern of hippocampal activity when word N was learned, as well as the neural activity for the surrounding words (Howard et al., 2012; Folkerts et al., 2018) as though recall of a specific word brings with it the temporal context in which the word was embedded, thus biasing the recall for neighboring words on the list. This is a possible implementation of Tulving's concept of mental time travel.

Recent studies on neuronal ripple activity in people have shown an increase in the frequency of ripples before free recall, and a change in cortical-hippocampal coupling prior to memory retrieval. These observations are consistent with the hippocampal ripple activity cueing the specific cortical representations (Norman et al., 2019; Vaz et al., 2019; Y Norman et al., 2021). Several studies have also examined episodic retrieval in epileptic patients with electrodes implanted into their hippocampi as well as other regions. In the first study to link activity of the human hippocampus with memory, researchers found cells that responded to conjunctions of facial expressions and facial identity. About 20% of cells fired differently for new and old images during a second presentation 10 hours later (Fried et al., 1997). Functional imaging studies have also showed impressive dissociations between episodic and semantic memory processing, and these are discussed in detail in Chapter 13.

Free recall studies have provided an important link between cells tuned to specific stimuli and memory. For example, neurons that were active while a patient viewed a movie fire again prior to voluntarily recall of the same movie clip (Gelbard-Sagiv et al., 2008). In another study, cells that fire when a patient occupies a virtual location in a first-person video game are preferentially reactivated when an item that was located in that "location" is remembered (Miller et al., 2013). As described, the pattern of activity observed during the repeated presentation of a stimulus reflects encoding of the perceptual details of the stimulus itself, as well as elements of the temporal context of the item during its first presentation: ensemble activity recorded during repeated presentations of a stimulus correlates significantly with activity recorded before, during, and after the item's original presentation (Howard et al., 2012). Together, these studies in humans link episodic encoding and retrieval with specific hippocampal firing patterns and suggest that reactivation of particular hippocampal cells active during learning elicits conscious memory recall of the associated episode. The psychological evaluation of animal recall is trickier; we will return to this aspect in section 14.7.

14.6.6 Modeling episodic-like memory formation and recall

With a core function of episodic or episodic-like memory, it stands to reason that the computational job to be solved is to store as many representations as possible with minimal interference, and to activate these representations appropriately during recall. Marr (1971) built on Donald Hebb's theory with information stored in a distributed manner via the pattern of synaptic connectivity strengths between neurons. He applied these principles to the anatomy and physiology of the hippocampus (Marr, 1971), a task elaborated extensively by others (McNaughton and Morris, 1987; O'Reilly and McClelland, 1994; Treves and Rolls, 1994; Hasselmo et al., 1996). Central to his model, and others that have built on that framework, is that the computational role of the hippocampus is to associate the www aspects of an experience into a memory trace. Importantly, though many experiences share common elements, the job of the hippocampus is to represent correlated inputs in independent networks which can be queried with partial input to reinstate the pattern of activity that was present during initial learning. This reinstatement constitutes the episodic memory.

McClelland et al. (1995) posited complementary roles for the hippocampus and the cortex, with the former being a fast memory system and the latter a slow one. Other theories model learning as changes in the connection strength between pre- and postsynaptic neurons that are coactive during learning. Studies on activity-dependent changes in synaptic strength such as LTP and LTD led to the hypothesis that associative learning contributes to adjusting connection strengths to create a weight matrix that defines the desired transform of the input patterns to the associated output patterns (McCulloch and Pitts, 1943; Kohonen, 1972; Anderson et al., 1977; Hopfield, 1982; Rumelhart and McClelland, 1986; Hinton, 1989; Oja, 1989; see Chapter 10).

One attractive feature of this Hebb-Marr framework is that it addresses what is known as the "plasticity-stability dilemma," which arises when learning occurs in networks that have already stored input/output associations. When multiple items are sequentially stored within the same set of synaptic weights, synaptic plasticity driven by the learning of new items can disrupt the ability of artificial neuron networks to recall previous associations. As interference is particularly detrimental for correlated patterns, one solution to the problem is to decorrelate the input patterns prior to storage (French, 1992). These conditions are remarkably similar to what appears to happen in the dentate gyrus: the large number of frequently silent cells in the dentate gyrus suggests that, at an early stage of hippocampal processing, "pattern separation" of correlated inputs occurs (McNaughton and Morris, 1987; O'Reilly and McClelland, 1994; Hasselmo and Wyble, 1997). Adult neurogenesis in the dentate may offer an additional mechanism by which to map inputs onto naive weight space, thereby ensuring minimal interference (Wiskott et al., 2006; see Chapter 9). The sparse dentate code is hypothesized to be the result of a "winner-take-all" computation in which a few cells fire *only* when specific conjunctions of stimuli (e.g., item in location) are present that, once active, inhibit their neighbors (Hasselmo and Wyble, 1997).

When a new pattern is established, it needs to be stored. According to the standard Hebb-Marr theory, the CA3 region is responsible.

Specifically, CA3 neurons send axons to many neighboring CA3 cells forming reciprocal autoassociative networks. CA3 receives inputs from dentate granule cells *and* the entorhinal cortices. This allows for an association of the cortical input with an orthogonalized signal arriving from the DG to foster a unique pattern of CA3 activity for that particular episode. Once a pattern of activity is stored within the weight matrix of synaptic connections, subsequent presentations of partial and even degraded inputs transmitted via the entorhinal cortex can associatively recall the original stored pattern, a process known as pattern completion (Kohonen, 1972; Anderson et al., 1977; Hopfield, 1982). Therefore, CA3 is hypothesized to be important for the recall of familiar memories from degraded inputs (O'Reilly and McClelland, 1994).

Within the hippocampal index theory (see "Cellular consolidation, systems consolidation, and memory assimilation" section 14.8 below), pattern completion also has profound ramifications. Activity patterns reflecting sensory detail in neocortical modules may generate a unique identifying pattern—a so-called index—(Teyler and DiScenna, 1987). This higher-level index is no longer "sensory" in a literal sense, but is stored associatively with other indices and the output fed back to neocortical modules via modifiable synapses. Activation of a cortical pattern (e.g., a specific flavor of food) could then result in activation of its index in the hippocampus. In turn, this enables retrieval of associated indices and thence the complementary pattern in the other cortical modules (e.g., where the food is found). Indirect associations enable memory retrieval between cortical modules that are too sparsely connected to do this directly.

In these models, there is a tension between recreating a pattern of activity stored during an earlier encoding experience and the formation of a new memory trace. As we will see, what route is taken may depend on several external and internal factors, and, in some instance, by stochastic fluctuations.

14.6.6.1 Neurobiological implementation of the computational models

We have seen that a key idea in Marr's original thinking (Marr, 1971) concerned the role of synaptic plasticity in storing information in hippocampus that might then be passed to neocortex. This idea has been incorporated into the thinking of several authors, including an implementational framework for the formation of "episodic-like" memory in hippocampus and experimental tests of its role by one of us (Morris and Frey, 1997; Morris et al., 2003; S Wang et al., 2010).

As discussed in Chapter 10, a possible facet of episodic memory learning is so-called *automatic encoding*. Information is stored temporarily in the pattern of synaptic weight changes mediated by LTP1, and its default destiny is to be lost relatively quickly. Under appropriate conditions, some of this information—be it as index or more detailed information—undergoes a protein-synthesis-dependent process that retains synaptic potentiation over much longer periods of time. The mechanism underlying local memory consolidation is thought to be synaptic tagging and capture (STC). Synaptic tags would also set automatically at the time of an event, irrespective of how trivial that event may be. During their transient existence, products of the somatic or dendritic synthesis of plasticity proteins (PRPs) could be captured whose role is to stabilize potentiation. The source of PRPs can be neural activation triggered by more important or surprising events before, during, or even after an event to be remembered. This capturing process renders the temporary indices in hippocampus more permanent and so allows sufficient time for systems-level consolidation to occur. Once stored, memory retrieval could be triggered by either exogenous reminder cues representing events, contexts, or places.

While most theories of consolidation consider longer memory retention intervals as desirable, the STC hypothesis argues instead that forgetting is vital for the selectivity of effective memory function and that forgetting is the default destiny of information unless a signal stating its novelty or relevance rescues it from oblivion. Without forgetting, an automatic encoding system would rapidly become saturated. Determining what matters would likely be a multidimensional process, with such factors as novelty, reward value, and relevance of new information to prior knowledge (among other factors) playing their role.

14.6.7 Awareness of memory

Experiments with animals that lay claim to revealing a "recollective" component of memory should somehow discriminate explicit and implicit processing. In seeking to understand the neural basis of recollective episodic-like memory, we should face up to the formidable problem of understanding the neurobiology of "awareness." One illustrative example of awareness, or lack thereof, is seminal work on "blindsight" in monkeys (Cowey and Stoerig, 1995). Blindsight is the ability to detect the location of a visual stimulus in space without being apparently aware that it is there, a dissociation that has been successfully achieved in nonhuman primates after unilateral lesions of area V1 of visual cortex and confirmed using signal-detection techniques (Stoerig and Cowey, 1995; Yoshida and Isa, 2015).

Linked to the problem of awareness is the concept of "metamemory"—knowing that we have remembered or knowing that we have forgotten. Monkeys have been shown to display awareness of whether they can remember (Hampton, 2001, 2009; Basile et al., 2015). Protocols for looking at "metamemory" vary, but a common feature is that the memory recall test itself is preceded by an initial step where the action required depends on the subject's confidence or uncertainty in answering correctly. Hence, the action undertaken reflects the animals' awareness of its own memory. For example, the main cognitive task may be a test of recognition memory, but in the secondary task, the animals are additionally given the opportunity to respond differentially as a function of their awareness, for example, by choosing to see the stimuli again or to proceed directly to the memory test. The goal for tests of nonhuman meta-cognition studies is to find an appropriate analogue to the "remember/know" distinction that is used in humans to assess recollection vs. familiarity. The challenge in developing these tasks—which is solved in Hampton's work—is to ensure that the monkeys do not just turn to the secondary task on the basis of simpler associative principles (i.e., because it is reinforced also).

The experimental protocols for realizing a cogent dissociation between an awareness vs. an associative explanation for reactions to uncertainty are among the most sophisticated behavioral studies of nonhuman animals that have ever been developed. In an illustrative behavioral study in rhesus monkeys (Templer et al., 2018), subjects were first presented with a study phase, in which a sequence of five images was presented. During a later phase, monkeys were required to report which of a pair of studied images appeared earlier in the sequence. Such a task models the "what" and "when" aspects of episodic memory. On a subset of trials, instead of an immediate memory assessment, monkeys were presented

with the pair of studied images and given the option to bow out and take a guaranteed smaller reward, or hang in there and take the test. The experimenters assumed that monkeys would choose the guaranteed smaller reward when memory confidence was low. Performance was systematically better when judgments were made for pairs of images presented at more distant positions within the study sequence; larger temporal intervals made the discrimination easier. However, before responding, the question arises of whether the monkeys were aware that they would likely be correct? The metacognition probe suggests—yes—because when monkeys were given the option to bow out and take the smaller reward, they did so more often when the number of intervening images was smaller, suggesting that they could anticipate the upcoming risk in taking a memory test for such challenging material (Templer et al., 2018).

These studies in the monkey show that an aspect of behavior that is consistent with awareness exists in nonhumans. We can never know if monkeys really have autonoetic awareness or can "travel back in time" to solve such a task or self-assess their memory confidence. Interpreting the consciousness of any other being requires the inference that should they behave as I do when I am aware, then they are likely aware too. No study can ever solve this "hard problem" in neuroscience, or as once put more prosaically, "we can never know what it is like to be a bat" (Nagel, 1974). With enough congruence between awareness-expected behaviors, we make the inference about our friends and family that they are conscious and aware just like ourselves. Such metacognition studies in animals are essential in showing us the reasonable bounds for extending this inference outside of the human sphere.

14.7 Engram cells or engram circuits?

We now turn to the discovery of "engram cells," achieved technically through the systematic introduction of synthetic molecular biology tools into the study of memory. It has been one of the most active fields in neuroscience of the last decade.

14.7.1 The engram in the molecular era

The acquisition of a new long-term memory occurs through the modification of one or more physical properties of neurons to create a representation of experience that can be reactivated during memory recall. The specific changes result in a new brain state collectively known as an "engram" or "memory trace." The physical substrate of a memory includes the ensemble of interconnected neurons, the changes in strength of their synaptic connections, other changes to the neurons themselves including their excitability, and perhaps changes in non-neuronal cells as well. Engrams are thus expressed in engram circuits.

Two distinct streams of thought permeate thinking on this issue. One stream incorporates ideas deriving from Cajal, Hebb, and others to the effect that changes in synaptic connectivity—potentiation and depression—are the primary physical basis of memory. This idea and how it has been tested is discussed at length in Chapter 10. A distinct stream argues that this focus on just synaptic changes is mistaken—one has also to think about the activity of the neurons themselves in what Hebb called "cell assemblies" but which are now commonly known as "engrams" or "engram circuits" (Josselyn and Tonegawa, 2020). One important reason for this distinct line of thought is that neuronal activity may participate in a recollective process even though these neurons' own synaptic connections may *not* have been changed during memory encoding. Moreover, as we shall see, neural activity itself plays a key role in how memory traces are allocated.

The idea that memories are "impressions" in the mind has a long history dating back to Plato's picture of the mind as a wax tablet, but the term "engram" was only coined in the 20th century by the philosopher Richard Semon (Schacter, 2001, pp 181–193). According to Semon, "all simultaneous excitations . . . within our organisms form a connected simultaneous complex of excitations which, as such, acts engraphically, that is to say leaves behind it a connected and, to that extent, unified engram-complex" (Semon, 1923, pp. 159–160). Although the engram was originally envisaged in psychophysiological terms, Schacter argues that Semon captured additional essential features. In his view, memories are not exact transcriptions of reality because distortions may be introduced at the time of storage. Furthermore, sensations reactivating elements of the engram can lead to reactivation of the whole engram-complex, bringing an experience back to mind.

The adoption of novel and ingenious techniques of molecular genetics and genetic engineering has heralded a breakthrough in the "search for the engram"—a phrase famously coined by Karl Lashley (1950). Interestingly, these molecular technologies are being used to answer *systems neuroscience* questions and not just molecular level questions. The school of thought pioneered by the groups of Josselyn, Mayford, and Tonegawa has proposed that engrams are allocated to specific groups of neurons in diverse regions of the brain. These are the so-called *engram cells*. However, a more comprehensive view emerging in recent papers refers to *engram circuits* as the likely basis of memory storage, making explicit the idea that memory traces are not in specific cells *per se* but embedded in the circuits composed of engram cells (broadly equivalent to Hebb's "cell assemblies"). Connections between engram cells may change as a function of a process such as activity-dependent synaptic plasticity, but importantly, they do not have to do so. We will initially focus on engram cells and then proceed to consider engram circuits.

14.7.2 Engram cell theory and initial experiments

The cellular engram hypothesis of the modern era was defined clearly by Tonegawa. Specifically, for a specific population of neurons to represent an engram complex, "multiple conditions must be met [. . .]. One must demonstrate that these cells are activated by learning, that they undergo enduring physical or chemical changes, and that their reactivation results in recall of the originally formed memory" (Tonegawa et al., 2015, p. 920). A theory of memory based on engram cells therefore assumes that (a) a defined set of cells is initially recruited into a particular memory trace at the time of memory formation, (b) this set of cells is necessary for the organism to recall the memory in question, and (c) their activity is sufficient for such memory to be recalled in the absence of the natural cues.

In their search for candidate engram cells, researchers initially focused on neurons expressing immediate early genes (IEGs) at the time of encoding. IEG are a class of genes comprising *cfos*, *arc*, *zif268/ergl*, and *npas-4*, whose expression is rapidly triggered by neuronal activation; their transcripts are detected within minutes of strong neural stimulation (Guzowski et al., 1999) (see also Chapter 15). IEG⁺ neurons at the time of memory satisfy a *correlation* principle, as their activation is temporally coincident with the animal learning or experiencing a new event. Furthermore, they display

a remarkable (although variable) consistency in their response to identical, repeated, stimulation, and could therefore provide a basis for the *stability* of representations (Guzowski et al., 1999).

With a clever use of IEGs and inducible promoters, experimenters could bend the IEG properties to their experiments. Hence, the advent of activity-tagging technology made it possible to test the role of specific neurons in memory by labeling neurons that are active during a time window controlled by the experimenter. An essential component of the technology is a combination of transgenes, expressed in knock-in lines or by viral vectors. For instance, in the TetTAG mouse line, the experimenter can selectively tag neurons that express cfos by controlling the bioavailability of doxycycline in the brain, usually delivered through the animal's diet (Reijmers et al., 2007). Here, the cfos promoter drives the expression of the transcription factor tTA that, in turn, can start the expression of a desired transgene (usually, a marker or a light- or compound-sensitive ion channels such as channelrhodopsin) but only in absence of tetracycline or its analogue doxycycline, which would otherwise block tTA function. This process is known as "tagging" (Figure 14.26). Once the transgenes are expressed in neurons, their excitation (or inhibition) can be controlled by researchers with light. The expression of the tag is long-lived or even indelible. The prediction is that, if this set of neurons is part of an engram, their artificial reactivation should result in artificial memory recall, while their inhibition during natural recall should impair memory accessibility. These two "gain-of-function" and "loss-of-function" tests respectively explore the *sufficiency* and *necessity* of candidate engrams respectively.

What of the behavioral side of the equation? If a memory is to be reactivated by light directed to neurons that now express channelrhodopsin, what tasks might be suitable to examine learning and subsequent recall? Most groups have so far used contextual fear conditioning and, to a lesser extent, place preference as experimental paradigms to begin the study of engram cells. These are behavioral experiences that entail Pavlovian context conditioning such as the association between an electrical shock and the context (or environment) the animal is currently in. The initial focus has been on the amygdala and the dentate gyrus of the hippocampal formation, with Mayford's group later pioneering the exploration of neocortical sites.

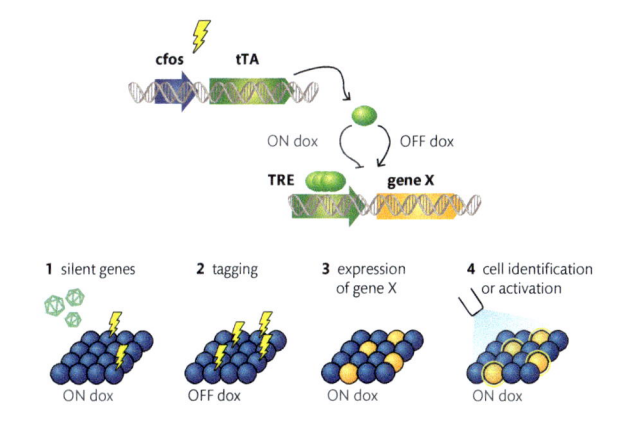

Figure 14.26 Schematic of the activity-tagging mechanism. tTA can drive transcription only in absence of doxycycline. Because tTA is only expressed in active cells from the IEG cfos promoter, only active cells during OFF dox period are tagged and express transgene X.

In two now classic papers, the TetTAG mouse line was used to test the existence and function of candidate engram cells (Garner et al., 2012; Liu et al., 2012). In the first of a series of experiments from the Tonegawa group, Liu et al. (2012) expressed TRE-ChR2 in the dentate gyrus (DG) of cfos-tTA mice. In absence of doxycycline ("off-dox"), animals were fear conditioned in a memorable context (called context A); this triggered cell-specific ChR2 expression in the subset of DG neurons active during fear conditioning. The following day, the animals were moved to a distinct context (context B). In this neutral non-fearful context, the onset of optical activation of the ChR2-labeled neurons elicited an immediate freezing response (Figure 14.27). In a control procedure, conducted after a similar cell-tagging process in a different context (context C) in which the animals did not experience shock, freezing was not observed, nor did it happen when the animals were returned to context B and the context C neurons were reactivated by light. Since only a small number (<5%) of DG neurons were tagged with ChR2 in the main experimental group, these findings suggest that activation of a sparse, distributed population of neurons, active during learning, can be sufficient to produce an apparent context-specific memory retrieval event. This study satisfies the *sufficiency* principle. In a complementary study, when a population of neurons was tagged during fear-conditioning and then *inactivated* by expressing a light-sensitive silencer, natural recall in the conditioned context (Context A) was impaired (Denny et al., 2014). This study satisfies the *necessity* principle.

These stunning results opened the entirely new field of artificial memory manipulations. One imaginative idea concerned whether an apparently "false memory" could be induced by carefully designing an optogenetic experiment that intersects natural and neural stimulation. Along with Garner et al. (2012) who first opened up this idea, Ramirez et al. (2013) explored the possibility of creating a false memory of the location in space where the mouse had experienced mild pain. On day 1, using TRE-ChR2/cfos-tTA mice, doxycycline was removed from the drinking water to open a tagging window. The next day, the animals were placed in a neutral Context A. A subset of DG neurons were active in this context and once tagged, were likely expressing ChR2. Doxycycline was then re-administered to close the tagging window. The following day, the animals were subject to fear conditioning in a distinct context—Context B. While this was happening, however, "Context A" neurons were activated optogenetically. While it is unclear what sort of perception animals may have had of their surrounding environment—a point we shall come back in section 14.7.5 ("Critique and open questions on engram cells")—two sets of DG neurons were active: those with spontaneous and endogenous responses to the current environment (Context B) and those of the previous day's Context A activated by light. This may have led to an association between the artificially activated Context A (CS) and footshock (US) even though the animals never experienced fear in Context A (Figure 14.28, top panel). Indeed, when the animals were later tested in Context A in the absence of light, they froze. Thus, a "false memory" was created, because the artificial reactivation caused the subset of neurons initially tagged during exploration of Context A to be associated with fear-responsive neurons in the basolateral amygdala (BLA) (Ramirez et al., 2013).

Garner et al. (2012) had performed the experiment in a similar manner, but unlike Ramirez et al. (2013), they tagged engram

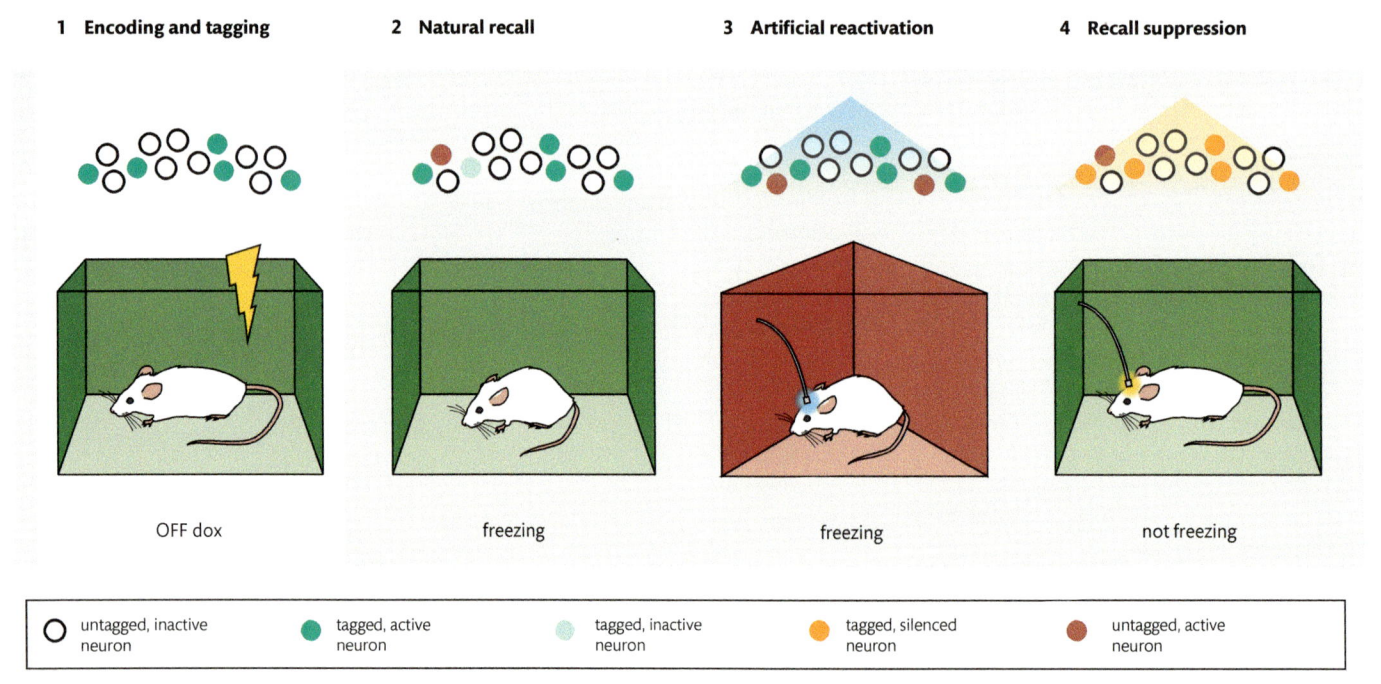

1 Encoding and tagging   **2 Natural recall**   **3 Artificial reactivation**   **4 Recall suppression**

OFF dox   freezing   freezing   not freezing

○ untagged, inactive neuron   ● tagged, active neuron   ● tagged, inactive neuron   ● tagged, silenced neuron   ● untagged, active neuron

Figure 14.27 Optogenetic tagging and reactivation. (1) While OFF dox, animals receive a footshock in context A (green), forming a contextual fear association. Labeled cells in the DG express an optogenetic activator (ChR2) or an optogenetic inhibitor (eNpHR3) (tagging). (2) Animals normally freeze when re-exposed to context A, showing that they have formed a CS-US association. (3) Artificially reactivating the fear engram with blue light (if the excitatory ChR2 is expressed during tagging) in a neutral context (context B, red) causes the animals to freeze (Liu et al., 2012). (4) Suppressing the activity of these neurons during natural recall with yellow light (if the express the inhibitory eNpHR3 is expressed during tagging) impairs recall in context A by natural cues (Denny et al., 2014). The transgene expressed during tagging depends of course on the choice of transgene X (see Figure 14.7.1)

Ramirez et al. (2013)

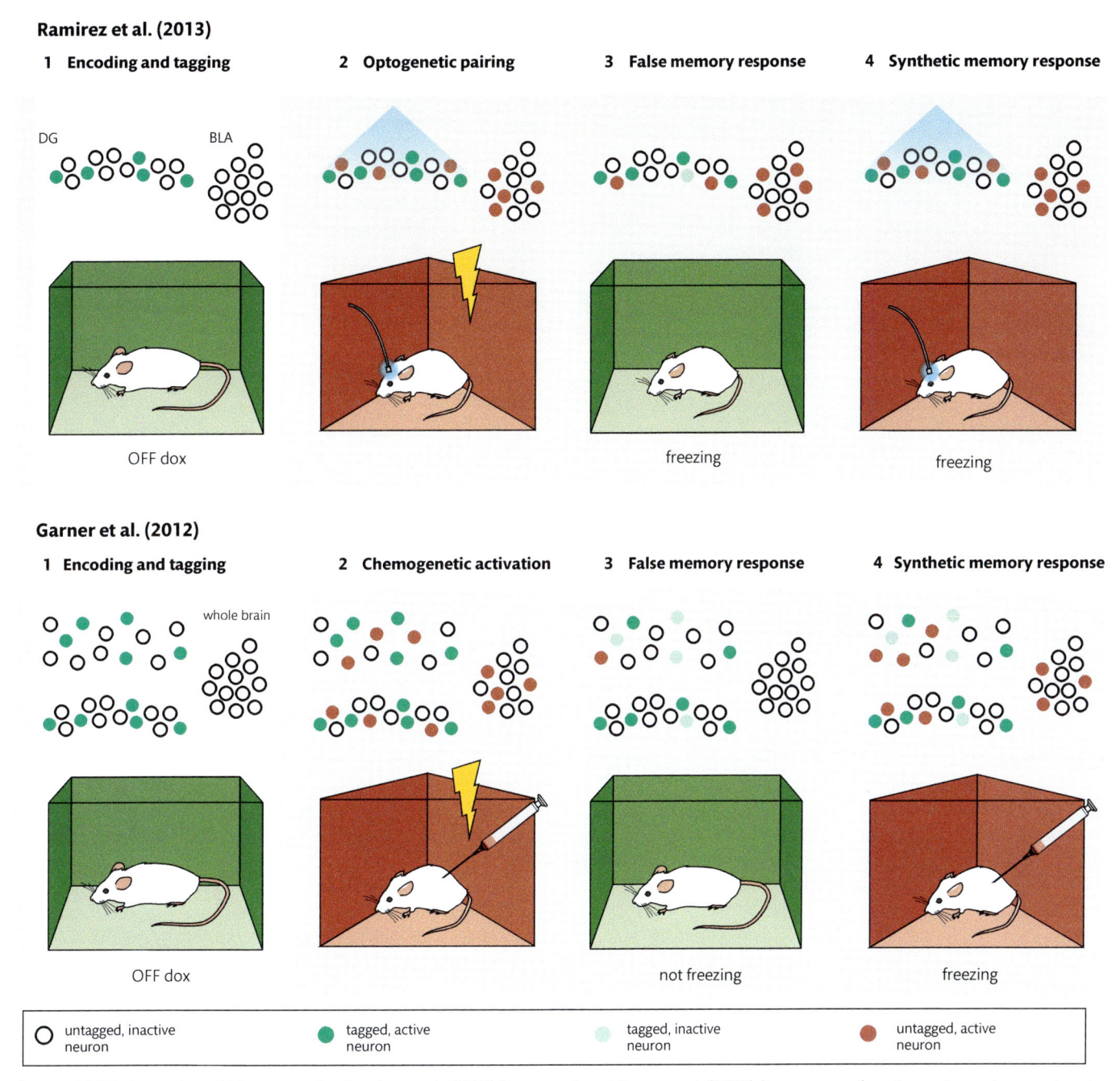

1 Encoding and tagging **2 Optogenetic pairing** **3 False memory response** **4 Synthetic memory response**

DG BLA

OFF dox

freezing

freezing

Garner et al. (2012)

1 Encoding and tagging **2 Chemogenetic activation** **3 False memory response** **4 Synthetic memory response**

whole brain

OFF dox

not freezing

freezing

○ untagged, inactive neuron   ● tagged, active neuron   ● tagged, inactive neuron   ● untagged, active neuron

Figure 14.28 Formation of false memories. Ramirez et al. (2013) (top panel) and Garner et al. (2012) (bottom panel) performed experiments aimed at creating artificial associations between a neutral context and an aversive stimulus using the TetTAG system. OFF dox tagging of the neutral context A (green) enabled Garner et al. to express the CNO-sensitive hM3Dq in active neurons in the whole brain, while Ramirez et al. expressed ChR2 in the DG region only. After exploration, mice were put back ON dox to close the tagging window. The following day, animals receive a footshock while in context B; at the same time, "context A" neurons are reactivated chemogenetically or optogenetically, respectively. When tested in context A the following day, mice froze in the Ramirez et al., but not in the Garnet et al., experiment. In both cases, mice froze significantly more when "context A" engram neurons were reactivated in the conditioned context B (synthetic memory response). See text for details.

cells in the whole brain (instead of the DG alone) and used chemogenetics as a tool to recall their activation during the artificial pairing. What they found is that animals responded by freezing to neither Context A nor Context B alone, but only in Context B if paired with the chemogenetic activation of "Context A." This suggests that the animals formed a hybrid "Context A/B" representation associated with the footshock (Figure 14.28, bottom panel). Taken together, it seems that the artificial activation of a sparse population of neurons can serve as a surrogate to represent

contextual information, and associations can be formed between these neurons and painful experience so that later presentations of the same context produce a behavioral response consistent with fear, i.e., the recall of a "false memory." Note that the false memory is not of the contexts per se, but of the association between the contexts and the experience of pain, an association that provokes fear and the fearful response of freezing.

While the DG has remained a popular area in the investigation of context memory, studies by numerous groups have also identified engram cells in other brain areas, including CA3, CA1, and the basal amygdala (Tonegawa et al., 2015). For instance, Cowansage et al. (2014) found engram cells in the retrosplenial cortex (RSC). The RSC receives outputs from the hippocampal formation and elsewhere, it projects to a wide variety of other cortical areas and is required for various forms of spatial and fear memories (Keene and Bucci, 2008). Mayford's group showed that, at the time of memory encoding, a neural ensemble representing the context is formed in the neocortex as well as the hippocampus. Optogenetic reactivation these RSC cells caused the animals to freeze even when the hippocampus was inactivated pharmacologically.

The Cowansage et al. (2014) result highlights a potential key problem with inferring that a tagged population of neurons is the site of the cellular engram if it is defined as "the population of cells whose activation produces a behavior consistent with recall." The circuit problem is that the same gain-of-function behavioral results could, in principle, be observed if the tagged neurons (the candidate engram cells) lie downstream of the neural population of engram cells that "contains" the encoded memory trace. Similarly, the tagged population could lie upstream of the locus of memory: for instance, Vetere et al. (2019) were able to express a completely artificial aversive memory by mimicking the activity elicited by an odorous compound with optogenetic activation of the olfactory sensory neurons expressing its receptors *and* brain pathways conveying negative or positive valence such as VTA. This ambiguity highlights the need to think in terms of engram circuits rather than just engram cells. The concept of engram cells conveys a sense of memory being "localized" in a manner that the circuit concept does not. Moreover, language counts; to say that "an engram has been created in the dentate gyrus during the process of fear conditioning" omits the fact that the engram created in the DG is likely only to do with the context in which the fear conditioning may later take place. It does not express the association between the context (CS) and the aversive experience (US)—an association that requires a wider circuit embracing the basolateral amygdala.

This crucial conceptual point is brought out by further key studies from the Tonegawa group that also collectively point to engram circuits being critical. It has long been known that the amygdala is central to the expression of fear memories (LeDoux, 2000). A key study showed that, in a place avoidance task, cfostTA mice could be taught to fear one of the chambers by creating an artificial memory (Redondo et al., 2014). This was achieved by optogenetically activating a footshock BLA engram every time mice entered one of the two chambers (Chamber A) of a place avoidance apparatus. This shifted the mice place preference away from chamber A toward chamber B. Tagging and reactivating the engram population in the DG had the same effect, and a symmetrical effect was observed when the male experimental animal was taught to seek a place associated with presentation of a desirable female mouse during the off-dox period. This also included the creation of an association in the BLA. In short, an engram circuit was set up between the hippocampal formation (the context engram) and the BLA (the context-US association engram) involving either positive or negative valence through use of access to a female (positive) or exposure to shock (negative).

Piece by piece, these and other studies have contributed to the dissection of the different "components" of engram circuits within the brain, providing a list of the areas where different kind of learning experiences lead to the tagging of cells, and starting to address the issue about how such cells in various brain areas are interconnected. Importantly, the various cell sets are not equivalent to each other and may show a hierarchical organization. In the aforementioned experiment of Redondo et al. (2014), the DG component of an engram circuit can be rewired to different emotional valences (for example, from the negative emotion of fear to the positive incentive of access to a female) by artificially reactivating it during the new relevant experience. However, the amygdala component, representing these two incentives, does not show this plasticity. Hence, subsets of BLA neurons are apparently hardwired to behavioral and autonomic expressions of fear on the one hand or joy on the other, and the connection between the DG and the BLA engram cells is directional (although not necessarily monosynaptic).

14.7.3 Relationship between engram circuits and engram cells

Tonegawa's defining criteria of *necessity* and *sufficiency* for memory recall have been demonstrated for specific cells across a circuit with distinct cells representing different components of the entire memory. An engram circuit contains cells within or across different parts of the brain, variably linked by local and interregional connections. Such a circuit is similar to Hebb's (1949) concept of cell assemblies with different parts of the assembly representing different facets of experience.

Experimentally, individual engrams can be linked in an associative form, and as we have seen sometimes create false memories (Ramirez et al., 2013; Ohkawa et al., 2015). Because the linking or "binding" of engrams is prevented by the application of either NMDA receptor antagonists or protein synthesis inhibitors, synaptic weight changes are likely to be involved. Connections at these nodes are therefore involved in creating memory representations. Moreover, once formed, selectively blocking synaptic transmission between engram cells after learning impairs the retrieval of the encoded memory (Matsuo, 2015). Synaptic plasticity and other modifications of the probability or strength of synaptic throughput provide one possible selection rule determining which and how engram cells are activated within the circuit (Nabavi et al., 2014; Lisman et al., 2018; Pignatelli et al., 2019). Several studies have detected LTP-like synaptic potentiation in the lateral amygdala with auditory fear conditioning (AFC) (Kim and Cho, 2017). Building on this, Nabavi et al. (2014) found that optogenetically inducing LTD in auditory cortex-amygdala connections reduced conditioned responding in mice performing an operant task after tone-frequency specific auditory fear conditioning. This could be reversed by optically inducing LTP on the same synaptic connections. Recent evidence suggests that interconnections between engram cells display enhanced synaptic potentiation: Ryan et al. (2015) observed an increase in excitatory postsynaptic current (EPSC) amplitude and in the ratio of AMPA/NMDA current relative to their negative neighbors in whole-cell recording (Ryan et al., 2015). Both observations are consistent with the potentiation of existing synapses linking components of an engram circuit.

However, in a key difference to the synaptic plasticity and memory (SPM) hypothesis, changes in the weights of existing connections may not be the only requirement for new memory representations. Specifically, engram cells have increased dendritic spine density, suggesting that structural plasticity may also contribute by enhancing or stabilizing synaptic potentiation. Choi et al. (2018) found that synapses between CA3 and CA1 engram cells had a significantly higher density than connections with nonengram neurons, and their spines were larger in volume and in diameter, both hallmarks of synaptic potentiation (Matsuzaki et al., 2004). Similarly, CA1 neurons expressing GFP-GluA1 under the cfos/tTA system showed accumulation of GFP-tagged AMPAR at mushroom spines at synapses following contextual fear conditioning or exploration of a new environment while off doxycycline (Matsuo et al., 2008; Takahashi et al., 2012). Engram theory, on the other hand, has no absolute requirement that every engram neuron within an engram circuit must itself have been subject to synaptic plasticity on its inputs, nor that every synapse involved undergoes potentiation.

A separate conceptual issue is that memory traces are often distributed but also overlapping. For example, two (or more) engram circuits can share a subpopulation of engram cells, but despite the overlap, the two representations can be maintained distinct by the differential connectivity of synaptic inputs onto these cells. Abdou et al. (2018) trained mice on auditory fear conditioning (AFC) using two different tones (7 kHz and 2 kHz) as the CSs to be associated with footshock (US) with a 5 h interval between the two training experiences (Figure 14.29). These experiences recruited two overlapping populations of neurons in the BLA from the different tonotopic afferents in the auditory cortex (AC). Despite the overlap, the two memories were successfully modified independently, with a

pharmacologically induced erasure of synaptic potentiation during recall of the 7 kHz memory which was achieved by interfering with reconsolidation. The erasure abolished subsequent fear responses to this frequency without affecting freezing in response to the 2 kHz tone. Moreover, optogenetically inducing LTD with 1 Hz blue-light stimulation (as in Nabavi et al., 2014) at the 7 kHz-engram cells terminals in the auditory cortex (AC) impaired freezing in response to the 7 kHz, but not to the 2 kHz tone (Figure 14.29, 3a). Conversely, the induction of optical LTP at the AC-BLA synapses after pharmacological erasure of preexisting plasticity in the 7 kHz-engram was able, at least partially, to restore fear responding (Figure 14.29, 3b and 4). This logically coherent set of experiments shows that synaptic efficiency can be one key regulator of the transmission of information between engram cells in the AFC paradigm and that two cellular AFC engrams that largely overlap at the cellular level in the BLA can be distinct at the afferent synapse level.

Other approaches to experimentally target active synaptic connections at the tagging stage are also starting to emerge (Gobbo and Cattaneo, 2020). Just as experiments have targeted the properties of engram cells, analogous questions can also be asked of engram synapses. Can the ensemble of synapses (synapsembles) involved in the formation of an engram be identified? Can the role of potentiated synapses be causally tested? Recent experiments have shown

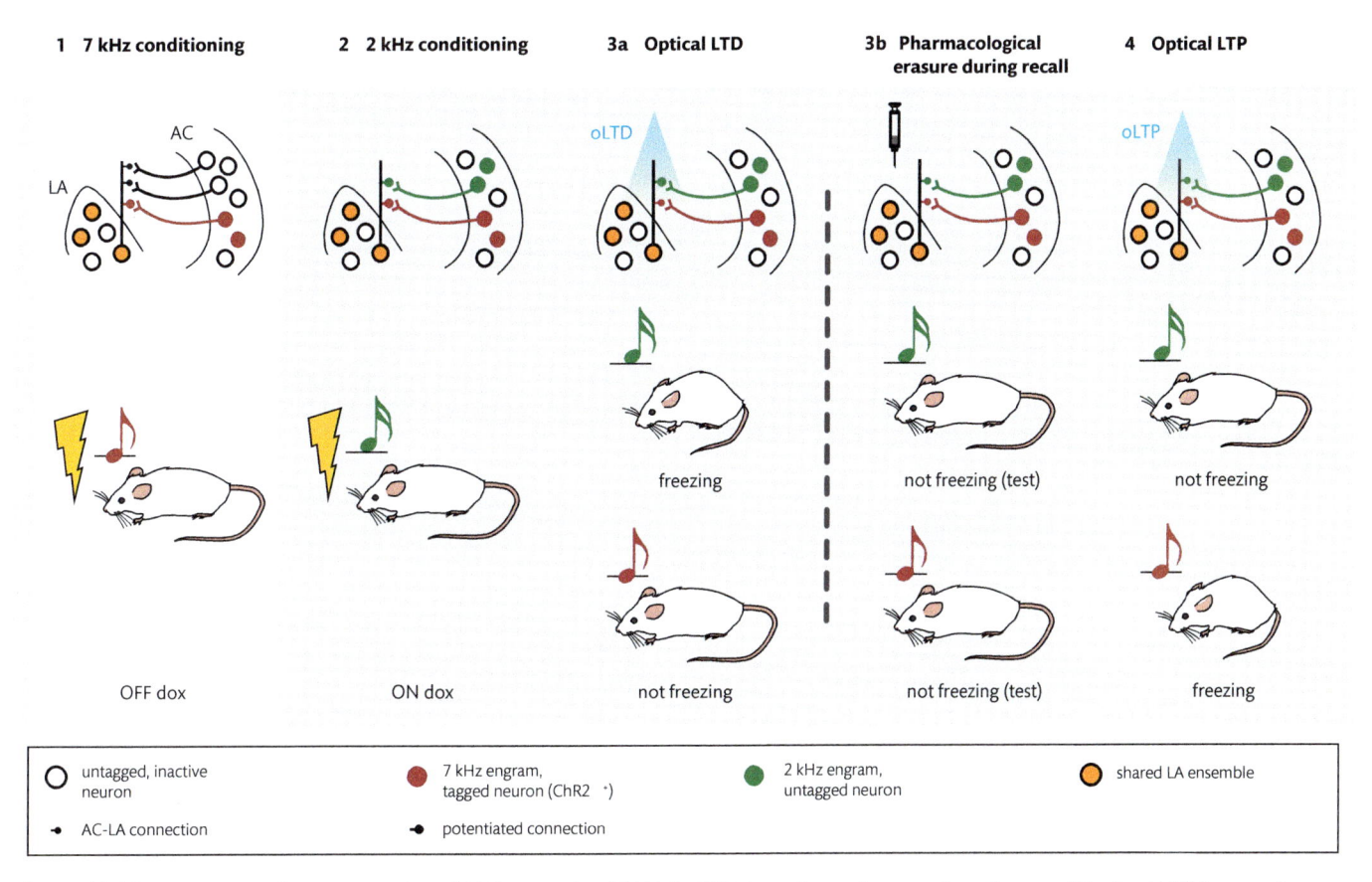

Figure 14.29 Synapse specific representation of AFC memories. (1) While OFF dox, mice undergo auditory fear conditioning (AFC) by coupling a 7 kHz tone with a footshock. 7 kHz engram cells in the auditory cortex (AC) are labeled to express ChR2. (2) Doxycycline is given to stop tagging, and after 5 h, the animals undergo AFC using a 2 kHz tone, which recruits a largely overlapping population in the lateral amygdala (LA). (3a) Inducing LTD between the 7 kHz AC engram cells and LA engram cells impairs the retrieval of the 7 kHz AFC, but spares the 2 kHz AFC association. (3b) Pharmacological treatment during recall of both memories erases synaptic potentiation. When tested afterward, animals do not freeze in response to either 2 kHz or 7 kHz tones. (4) Inducing LTP between the 7 kHz engram cells in the AC and engram cells in the LA by means of optogenetic high-frequency stimulation rescues the response to 7 kHz, but not 2 kHz.

that optically ablating synapses potentiated at the time of learning can effectively prevent or erase the encoding of motor or fear memories (Hayashi-Takagi et al., 2015; Takemoto et al., 2017; Goto et al., 2021). Together, this evidence suggests that synaptic plasticity is necessary for the formation and maintenance of engram circuits. Experimental modulation of specific synapses could provide a direct test of the hypothesis, such as the mimicry experiments envisaged in Chapter 10 (Gobbo and Cattaneo, 2020).

The synaptic plasticity and memory hypothesis states that "activity-dependent synaptic plasticity is induced at appropriate synapses during memory formation and is both necessary and sufficient for the information storage" (Martin et al., 2000). A potential challenge to this central tenet in neuroscience has arisen from two examples of successful artificial memory reactivation despite either the loss of synaptic potentiation or an impairment in its expression caused by a pharmacological treatment (Ryan et al., 2015) or by alterations induced in a molecular-genetic model of Alzheimer's disease (Roy et al., 2016). Both are key studies, but their interpretation is controversial. Ryan et al. (2015) conducted an important extension of the experiment by Liu et al. (2012) in administering anisomycin systemically during the tagging/contextual fear conditioning phase of training. This drug impairs protein synthesis and consequently inhibited the protein-synthesis-dependent stabilization of any synaptic change associated with learning (Frey and Morris, 1997), that had been confirmed to occur at the synapses between the entorhinal cortex and DG engram cells. The animals treated with anisomycin showed reduced freezing in the conditioned context when tested 24 h later, as the consolidation blocker disrupted late-phase LTP. However, in a striking result, the optical reactivation of DG engram cells expressing ChR2 still induced freezing. The optogenetic reactivation of the tagged cells apparently recruited a similar population of cells in CA3, CA1, and in the BLA as that activated by natural recall cues—leading the authors to propose that the tagged cells may still be the repository of "engrams" even when natural recall cues cannot elicit memory (Ryan et al., 2015).

This striking finding has led supporters of the engram cell theory to suggest that memories are stored as specific patterns of connectivity between engram cell ensembles distributed in multiple brain regions. Structural changes in the connectivity pattern are established during memory encoding and retained during consolidation in a protein synthesis-independent manner (Tonegawa et al., 2015). This assertion implies, however, that memory storage and memory retrieval can be dissociated. As outlined by Queenan and colleagues:

> When enhanced synaptic strength between engram cells is abolished, the memory is not. Gross synaptic strengthening can be excluded as a candidate mechanism for memory storage, though it seems essential for natural memory retrieval. [. . .] synaptic strength [is] a crucial determinant of memory accessibility or retrievability. When synapses are not operational, information—however stored—cannot be extracted from cells. [. . .] When the amnesic engram cells were directly stimulated with light, memory retrieval occurred, demonstrating the persistence of memory in a latent but reactivatable state. (Queenan et al., 2017, p. 115)

According to this view, memories are formed by establishing new or modified synaptic connections between neurons. Once formed, information would flow along this newly formed circuit.

If this argument is correct, the resulting engrams envisaged by this theory are in some way reminiscent of the reticular circuits imagined by Camillo Golgi, where each engram forms a separate reticulum. For the supporters of such a theory, synaptic weight plasticity would only ensure the smooth transmission of information along it. This would explain why, when transmission probability is weakened by the impaired synaptic plasticity, so is the ability to recall memories. The impairment may be due to pharmacological manipulations like anisomycin (Ryan et al., 2015) or to physiological decay (Ryan and Frankland, 2022). In support of this interpretation, it has been shown that optogenetically reactivating tagged DG engram cells can rescue infantile amnesia of CFC even months after the initial experience, and long after the animal has stopped responding in the conditioned context (Guskjolen et al., 2018). Engram cell theorists therefore regard forgetting as a process where these memories become progressively inaccessible with time (i.e., retrieval failure) rather than being permanently erased (i.e., storage failure).

An alternative possibility is that synaptic plasticity plays a bigger part in memory than this "reticular" perspective of engrams adequately conveys. For instance, the anisomycin administration used by Ryan et al. (2015) may have not blocked plasticity altogether. This would result in weaker connections so that the optogenetic re-exciting of DG engram cells would increase the probability of the reactivation of an engram circuit. This line of thought seems to be supported by later findings suggesting that anisomycin administration can cause the whole circuit connections to be weaker, requiring stronger light power to induce freezing (Roy et al., 2017). For such results to truly shake the foundation of the synaptic plasticity and memory hypothesis, future studies must conduct careful measurement of the extent to which protein synthesis was blocked, the time course of the block, and the effect on the persistence of connections in and between the different areas involved (see also Chapter 10).

To conclude this section, a meaningful definition of an "engram" must take into consideration both the structural connections between the engram cells *and* the synaptic rules that govern the probability of information transmission between neurons. The engram can be then described as a modified brain configuration of cellular and synaptic parameters. Structural changes in these connections may of course occur during memory formation and consolidation, and preexisting connectivity may in part dictate the end result of the connectivity between engram cells by limiting the space of possible connections (McKenzie et al., 2021). A broader "engram circuit theory" can arguably accommodate the aforementioned cases of impairment in memory retrieval from ostensibly silent engrams. As the animal displays only moderate freezing when it is re-exposed to the conditioned context under conditions of impaired plasticity, the encoded (weak) memory is expected to display some difference in its behavioral expression from that of the strong memory in the control group. A strictly cellular engram theory does not account for such difference, as there is no evident difference in the tagged set of neurons in the two groups. Hence, it is the engram circuit that is muted or silent, not the engram cells. The number of engram cells is remarkably consistent in a given brain region irrespective of memory strength (Morrison et al., 2016; Choi et al., 2018), which in turn is best described by the number and size of synapses between engram cells (Choi et al., 2018).

14.7.4 The changing engram

Engram circuits are not fixed features written inside the brain, but they can undergo significant evolution when they are recalled. Hence, engram circuits satisfy the *ecphory* principle of Semon's theory and, if extended beyond associative memories, Tulving's ideas about episodic memory: every time the silent trace of an engram is reactivated, it becomes liable to modification and it can change, expand, or merge with other engrams. When experiences are relived, they inevitably interact with other memories and with the rest of the brain in its new state. They can then be assimilated with experiences acquired between the last and current recall of the episode. This supposition is similar to the concept of reconsolidation.

Change can occur in the form of memory linking, often in the form of associations. These may be major changes to existing engrams, like false memories (Ramirez et al., 2013). Links between unrelated engrams can arise by coactivation, and these links are found to be sensitive to anisomycin and other treatments that disrupt synaptic plasticity (Ohkawa et al., 2015). Linking can also occur at the time of learning if multiple experiences occur in a relatively short time window due to partial coallocation (Cai et al., 2016; Rashid et al., 2016).

What engram experiments provide is a cellular snapshot of the IEG expression levels during the hours-long tagging interval. Different approaches have been taken to follow the evolution of such tagged neurons over time. For instance, two epochs can be compared by looking at the overlap between the labeled cells and an endogenous IEG protein product like cfos (e.g., Tayler et al., 2013), with two different systems to tag the epochs (like the cfos-tTA and TRAP system, e.g., DeNardo et al., 2019), or by looking at the expression of a fluorescent reporter from an IEG promoter (e.g., Attardo et al., 2018). These approaches have consistently shown that, although repeated presentations activate overlapping neuron populations, their overlap tends to fade over time. Combining calcium imaging with a photoswitchable reporter, Ghandour et al. (2019) showed that engram cell activity drifts between learning and retrieval of CFC, although at a lower rate than that of nonengram cells, a finding also suggested by the work of Tanaka et al. (2018). In particular, patterns or groups of engram cells that were also reactivated during sleep were more likely to be reactivated during recall, suggesting that consolidation plays a role in the selection of these neurons, a topic that will be discussed in section 14.8.

Representational drift has found experimental support from a variety of different sources (Ziv et al., 2013; DeNardo et al., 2019). In one experiment, after training animals in the auditory fear conditioning paradigm, the authors labeled engram cell populations in the prefrontal cortex during AFC (day 0) or during retrieval at different time points (day 1, 7, and 14 post training) (DeNardo et al., 2019) (Figure 14.30A). The temporal proximity of the tagging day to the retrieval session predicted the overlap of the tagged/cfos population. Consistently, a strong behavioral response was elicited when optogenetically stimulating engram cells that had been tagged in closer temporal proximity to the auditory conditioning (day 0 < day 1 < day 7 < day 14) (Figure 14.30A). Cho et al. (2021) observed an analogous drift in representation in the BLA engram after repeated AFC. The authors compared two groups of animals that received training on either day 1 or on day 1 and day 2. Day 2 retraining reduced the overlap between the tagged cells on day 1 and those activated by retrieval on day 3. While the reactivation of either the "day 1" or "day 2" engram was sufficient to induce freezing, only the "day 2" engram was necessary, as silencing the day 1 engram left retrieval intact. By day 4, the freezing response was impaired by optogenetically inhibiting neurons tagged on day 2, but not those on day 1.

Similar representational drift has been reported in RSC monitoring the expression of cfos-driven GFP (Figure 14.30B) (Milczarek et al., 2018). By longitudinally observing the pattern of cells expressing the Arc:GFP reporter in CA1, Attardo et al. (2018) also observed a continuous drift in the representation of space when mice were exposed repeatedly to the same environment. While the session-to-session variation would stabilize from earlier to later sessions, even later representations of the environment drifted away over time (Figure 14.30C). Similar considerations also apply to the stability of spatial fields of place cells (Figure 14.30D, see Chapter 11) (Mankin et al., 2012; Ziv et al., 2013; Hainmueller and Bartos, 2018; Gonzalez et al., 2019), with the caveat that the relationship between the cells in an engram circuit and the "place map" is unclear (Tanaka et al., 2018).

At the implementation level, the formation of an engram circuit produces a synaptic and cellular configuration that, following the perception of recall cues, results in the concerted activity of neurons that are responsible for the representation of a given memory—or, at least, for those aspects of a memory deemed relevant by the organism. Each individual synapse and individual neuron has a certain chance to participate in the recall of a particular memory governed by probability rules. Encoding experiences that involve large and distributed synaptic alterations facilitate robust future recall, while weak connections within the engram circuit may result in retrieval failures. This likely applies when memories are forgotten, as in the aforementioned cases of memory impairment (Ryan et al., 2015; Roy et al., 2017). Degradation of synaptic connections and of other stabilization mechanisms (or their partial impairment during encoding) makes the original memory no longer accessible because of the low probability of transitions across network states that normally depend on those weakened synapses; optogenetically stimulating a set of cells can facilitate network reactivation and potentially bypass parts of the larger engram circuit (Figure 14.31A).

A memory representation may stay close to its original state or may morph into a new representation that involves only a few of the neurons active during original learning. According to engram theory, the fidelity of retrieval depends on the ability of a recall cue to reinstate the original trace. Over time, engrams can undergo modifications that reshape the ensemble of active cells in a brain region but can also shift the relative involvement of brain areas to distinct memory recall events. This process is generally included within the domain of systems consolidation, the subject of the next section (14.8). This is a feature of engram circuits that can hardly be explained by an engram theory based on stable connectivity between engram cells. For example, with the potential exception of episodic memories, many remote memories rely on cortical activity more than recent memories, which are more dependent on hippocampus activity. Interestingly, the optogenetic reactivation of DG engram cells labeled at the time of learning can recall the memory long after its presumed dependence on the hippocampus has waned (Kitamura et al., 2017; Guskjolen et al., 2018), but is probably more telling of residual connections than of what happens physiologically in the brain (Figure 14.31B).

14.7.5 Critique and open questions on engram cells

There are a number of open questions about both theoretical and technical aspects. The former concern the definition and properties of engram cells, the nature of the recall experience and the relationship (if any) between the neuropsychologically defined theories

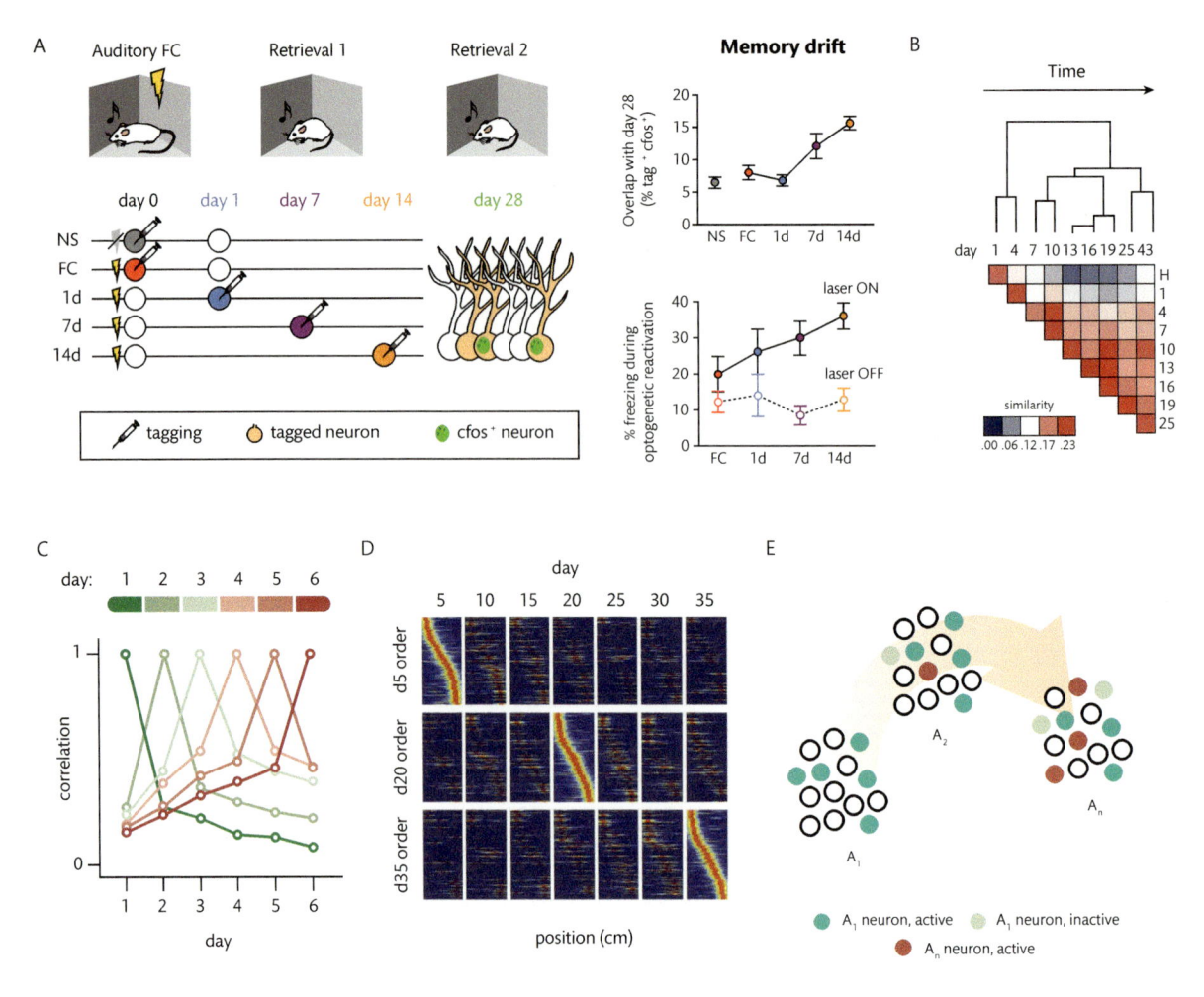

Figure 14.30 Drift of neural representations. (A) Cellular and functional drift of memory representation observed by DeNardo et al. (2019). Schematic of the experiment and results. (B) Over repeated learning sessions in a radial-arms maze, representation drifts over time, determined by comparing the expression of cfos on days 1 to 43. (Data from Milczarek et al., 2018.) (C) Attardo et al. (2018) compared the Arc-GFP engram representation over six consecutive days, showing that the correlation decreases the longer the time between two visits. (D) Similarly, the place map of a linear track changes in a continuous way with time. (Derived from Ziv et al., 2013.) (E) Representation of the same environment can drift over time. Similar sensory input will then result in the activation of a changing set of neurons. Some of the original neurons will not be active anymore, while others will be recruited to the engram.

and this new approach. The latter deal with the ability to refine the engram tag both spatially and temporally. We shall conclude by outlining two major issues.

One crucial aspect of the engram experiments relates to the congruence between neural underpinnings of natural recall and the experimental depolarization of tagged engram cells. Though the inner qualia cannot be known, we may wonder whether experimental engram reactivation drives bona fide recollection. Might the animal's experience be only a poorly anchored sense of fear that is independent of coherent contextual features? Is the subject experiencing a hallucination of the context rather than a memory of it? If we dare speak of beliefs in relation to mice, what does the animal *believe* it is experiencing? We take the somewhat radical view that it is very unlikely that the subject experiences anything like organic recall. The discrepancy between "perceptual equivalence" and merely "adequate reaction" arises because DG is not (as far as we know) a perceptual region. These considerations lead us to think more along the lines of "compulsion" than of "perception"—the animal may perceptually be experiencing nothing like a recollection of the

context where fear conditioning took place, but its brain is nonetheless compelled, by the laws of Pavlovian conditioning, to execute a defensive response.

Second, the protocols used to experimentally drive engram cells induce highly unnatural firing patterns—strong, rhythmic coactivation of every neuron that expressed an IEG over the course of a tagging period. To further complicate the matter, the standard tagging window with the current doxycycline-mediated tagging technique is generally 12–24 hours; as a consequence, a number of cells may be tagged during the resting activity of the brain outside the experimental context. This is thought to be low enough to observe an increase in tagged cells during any novel, memorable event happening during the time window—which in most cases is transfer from the boredom of the home cage to the opportunity to explore a new context and/or its association with a painful experience. However, this consideration currently prevents the engram cell approach from tackling issues like "event sequences" within an episodic-like memory. To do this, higher temporal resolution of tagging would be necessary that could rely on an optogenetic selection

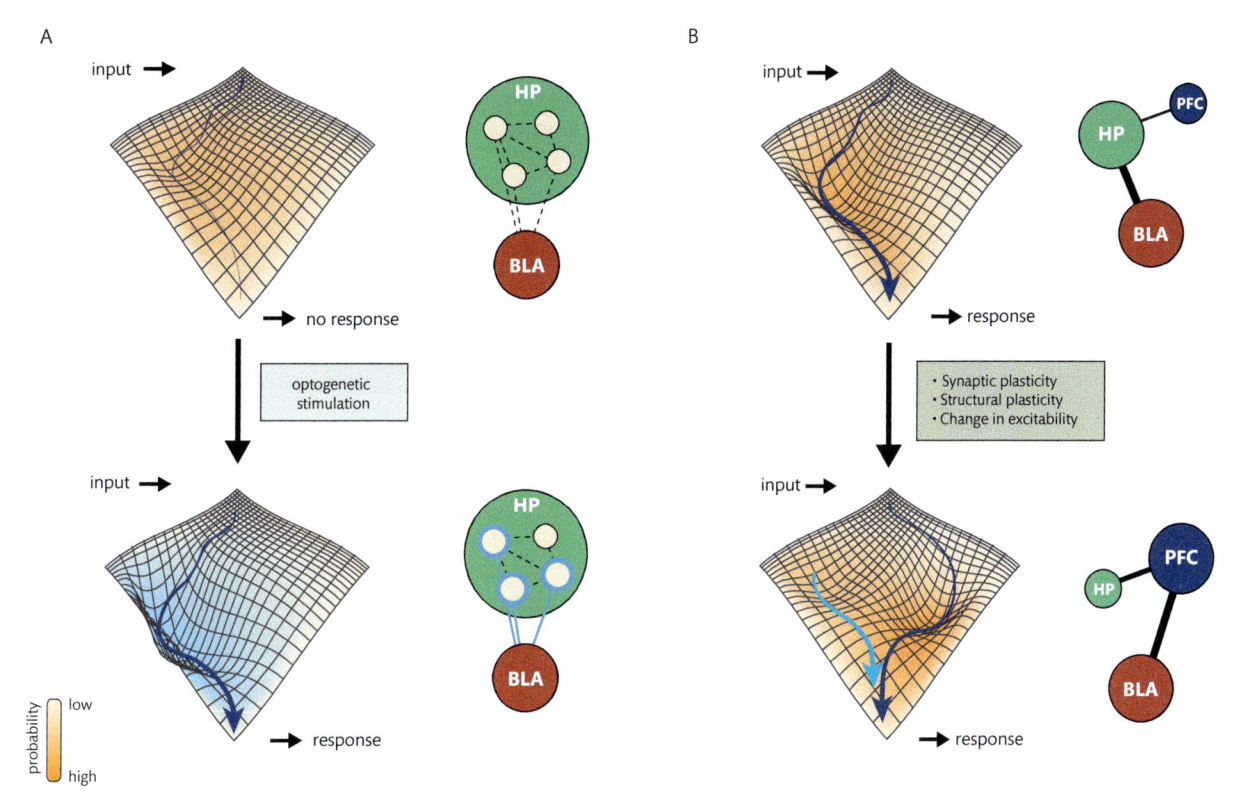

Figure 14.31 Impact of a probabilistic determination of brain states. (A) When plasticity is impaired (e.g., Ryan et al., 2015; Roy et al., 2017), an overall weaker circuit is formed during learning, so that natural inputs are not strong enough to drive the reactivation of the neurons involved in the memory expression. Optogenetic reactivation of engram cells in the hippocampus "boosts" the transition probability of the neural activity, resulting in the recall of the formed association. (B) At early time points following learning, the CFC engram circuit prevalently involves the activity of the hippocampus (HPC) and the amygdala (BLA). Over time, the unidirectional reorganization of the circuit alters the transition probabilities between brain statuses, so that natural recall preferentially activates neurons in the prefrontal cortex (PFC) and the amygdala (blue arrow). Artificial reactivation of the hippocampal engram (cyan arrow), however, can still result in freezing because of the remaining (although weakened) connections to the BLA. This, however, likely involves a different set of transitions than natural recall.

process at the time of tagging. An example of what is on the horizon are "read-and-reactivate" technologies with a much faster timescale (Marshel et al., 2019; Robinson et al., 2020).

Are engrams just *fata morganas* then? Probably not, but their artificial reactivation is unlikely to fully recapitulate what happens physiologically when episodic-like memory is recalled, nor how the learned information is normally accessed and utilized to guide decisions. We envisage that an exciting area of active research for the years to come will be aimed at understanding the role engram cells play physiologically, and how they can be employed by memory systems to guide behavior.

14.7.6 Concluding remarks

This section has summarized facets of the current status of the engram research in the hippocampal formation, amygdala, and associated areas. The recent history of engram research is a history of technological advancement—primarily the ability to tag and reactivate using sophisticated molecular engineering tools. It is witness to the service that these molecular-level tools are making to systems and cognitive-level questions. Along the way, engram research has revealed amazing and, in some cases, unforeseen properties of memory traces, including their remarkable propensity for modification (including "false memories"). Engram circuits are dynamic, ever-changing representations that can be updated every time they are reactivated. But the updating process can leave behind past

traces (such as cfos tags) that are no longer, or only partially used, by the animal. These remain as traces of bygone experience. In a sense, aspects of engram research reflect an "archaeology of memory."

A last comment concerns the relationship between engram cell/engram circuit theory and extant theories of hippocampal function such as declarative memory, cognitive mapping, or the episodic memory theory discussed in the preceding section. The engram theory does not easily incorporate or align selectively with these, but the findings are likely relevant. It has been shown that after contextual fear conditioning, engram cells are less likely to be place cells and provide less spatial information than nonengram cells (Tanaka et al., 2018), although they may provide a potentially more stable representation of the same environment across days (Ghandour et al., 2019). Hence, it would seem that engram cell representations and spatial representations can be disjoined—a finding that comes as no surprise. If that would be the case, engram cells could yet serve as an *index* pertaining to episodic information embedded in another population of neurons involved in scene representation such as place cells. This however raises the problem of how these two populations arise and how they differ in terms of information processing and transmission, or whether they differ a priori (or a posteriori) from a molecular point of view. This, however, could be due to the specific type of memory considered: it could be speculated that contextual fear conditioning is an association with the overall context and not a particular area of it. Possibly, engrams related to a more specific spatial component could show a higher correlation between engram cells and place cells.

If memory is in a constant flux then, is the destiny of every memory to be eventually forgotten or, at least, to lose its detail and become a general representation. In the words of Yadin Dudai, "the gist of the experience, or the processed and distilled mental narrative, is usually more important than the accuracy of the details. [. . .] In the process of forming mental narratives, engrams merge, losing much of their original individuality. They join the distributed, large and dynamic "society of engrams" that comes to constitute our memory. [. . .] In real life, engrams are palimpsests, reflecting physical traces of many layers of past events" (Dudai, 2010, p 38). This line of thought takes us naturally on the final theme of this chapter—memory consolidation.

14.8 Cellular consolidation, systems consolidation, and memory assimilation

The last issue to consider is the role of the hippocampus in the "keeping" of memory traces and, specifically, whether it is the site of long-term storage. Most neuroscientists believe that neocortical sites are more likely for lasting memory. However, the nature of the interactions between neural representations stored in hippocampus and neocortex and the process of consolidating such information have become major topics of investigation.

The topic can be divided into two separate but interacting processes—*cellular consolidation* and *systems consolidation* (Dudai and Morris, 2001; Klinzing et al., 2019). The former relates to mechanisms associated with the initial stabilization of memory storage at the very cells in which synaptic mechanisms have been engaged. Initial memory encoding and storage does not involve RNA translation, but cellular consolidation is dependent on translation. Systems consolidation, on the other hand, refers to network interactions between hippocampus and neocortex that create a lasting repository of information. Ordinarily, these two processes are bedfellows and work in conjunction with each other with cellular consolidation serving as a "low-pass" filter into overnight systems consolidation. We begin with the cellular side of the equation and then move on to the mystery of systems consolidation.

14.8.1 Cellular consolidation of memory

It is important to recognize that cellular consolidation is *not* required for initial learning. We saw in section 14.4 that the trigger for hippocampal memory trace encoding is the activation of hippocampal NMDA receptors with initial memory storage mediated by changes in AMPA receptor expression (postsynaptically) and changes in transmitter release (presynaptically). However, such traces decay rapidly over time unless cellular consolidation takes place.

Experiments in the event arena (Bast et al., 2005) offer specific behavioral support for the role of processes akin to LTP2 in cellular consolidation. If only LTP1 is engaged, synaptic potentiation decays over 3–24 h[1] and all information is lost. However, if the transition between LTP1 and LTP2 could be engaged it may be possible to

hold on to a subset of everyday memory for a longer time—at least a day (Figure 14.32A). This idea was tested by triggering cellular consolidation using unexpected, task-unrelated novelty. Environmental novelty is known to activate a range of immediate early genes in hippocampus (Guzowski, 2002), with these going on to activate downstream intracellular pathways triggering the synthesis of plasticity-related proteins in hippocampus. This should lead to an enhancement of memory retention by a synaptic-tagging-and-capture process (Morris and Frey, 1997).

Moncada and Viola (2007) were the first to show, in a brilliant paper, that novelty-enhancement of prior memory encoding of a hippocampus-dependent inhibitory avoidance learning task and the role of dopamine in this process. Wang et al. (2010) conducted a similar study in the event arena, finding that a spatial recency training protocol led to memory encoding and storage for a few hours but complete overnight forgetting (Figure 14.32B,C). However, the introduction of unrelated novelty exploration soon after memory encoding resulted in memory for 24 h (Figure 14.32D). The impact of novelty was blocked by anisomycin and, as in Moncada and Viola's (2007) study, by the D1/D5 receptor antagonist SH23390 (Figure 14.32E). Exposure to novelty also has been shown to change the induction threshold for late phases of LTP (Li et al., 2003) and LTD (Lemon and Manahan-Vaughan, 2006) through dopaminergic cAMP/PKA signaling. Takeuchi et al. (2016) used optogenetics in TH:*cre* mice to bypass environmental novelty and reveal, somewhat surprisingly, that the source of this dopaminergic signaling was the locus coeruleus (LC) rather than the VTA (Figure 14.32F). Corelease of dopamine and noradrenalin by the LC to the hippocampus was later confirmed by microdialysis and HPLC analysis (Kempadoo et al., 2016).

The behavioral significance of cellular consolidation in hippocampus is that a subset of recently encoded memories can have their lifetime extended in association with surprise or novelty. In this way, only some of what has been temporarily remembered during the day will be subject to systems consolidation. The rest will have been useful for a few hours and then lost.

14.8.2 The transition from cellular to systems consolidation: theories

An early idea about systems memory consolidation was that it is a kind of "fixing" process, analogous to applying the fixer solution during the classic photographic printing process in which a developer (creating the image on photographic paper) was followed by the fixer to ensure the newly formed image would last. The supposition was that, of these two facets, systems consolidation across brain networks was not only the fixing process (Alvarez and Squire, 1994), but one in which the time-course of consolidation was quite long—weeks, months, or even longer—based on evidence from humans and from animal models. However, this so-called standard model of systems consolidation ran into a range of difficulties, the first being conceptual. Is a putative brain process of consolidation lasting as long as 20+ years likely to be biologically plausible (Nadel and Moscovitch, 1997)? In a helpful development of the idea, called "complementary learning systems" (CLS), the supposition was that the developing process is in the fast-learning hippocampus and the fixing process involves a slower interaction between hippocampus and neocortex, but nothing like as slow as some of the human remote memory studies had suggested. There are several variations of the CLS framework, some implicating overnight

---

[1] In vitro brain slice physiology for STC experiments is typically conducted at 32°C, approximately 6°C lower than normal body temperature. The exact timing of LTP decay and information loss may be different in vivo.

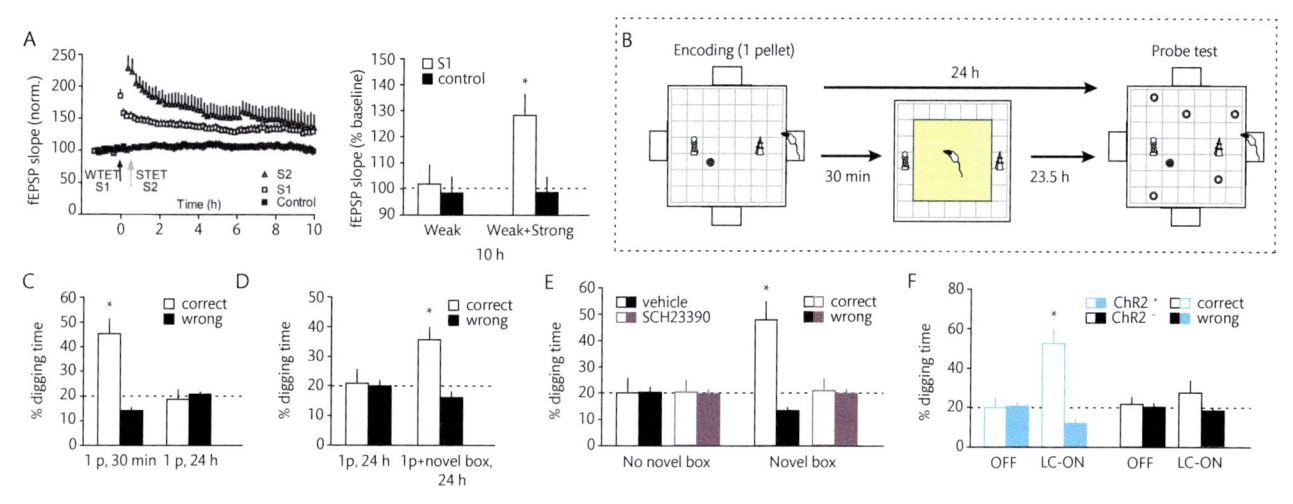

Figure 14.32 Cellular consolidation in the event arena. (A) Weak tetanus (WTET) on pathway S1 normally decays to baseline (Control level) within 3–4 h (right-hand panel). However, if followed within less than 90 min by strong tetanization on an independent pathway (S2, STET), the weakly tetanized pathway still displays LTP 10 h later (LTP2). (B) Schematic of the experimental protocol for behavioral tagging in the everyday arena; note that novel exploration may or may not memory encoding after 30 min. (C) After 1 pellet encoding, memory is retained at 30 min, but it decays over 24 h in the absence of novelty (D) Conversely, postencoding novelty stabilizes the weak memory so that it is retained 24 h later (E) Dependence of the novelty effect on D1/2 dopamine receptors. (Panels derived from Wang et al., 2010. (F) Takeuchi et al. (2016) identified the source of novelty stabilization in the activity of TH + neurons in LC. Optically stimulating LC fibers in the hippocampus prolongs memory lifetime in ChR2-expressing animals.

sleep, but all implying that cortex is the eventual site of lasting memory traces linked in networks that otherwise would have had only weak connections without the contribution of outputs from the fast-learning hippocampal system (Squire, 1992; McClelland et al., 1995; Frankland and Bontempi, 2005; Kumaran et al., 2016) (Figure 14.33).

In the computational model by McClelland et al, (1995), the slower rate of interaction with cortex serves to limit interference in neocortical storage. It might involve an explicit transfer of information from the fast site (hippocampus) to the slow one (neocortex), but an alternative perspective was of an interaction between brain structures that stabilizes otherwise unstable traces formed in distinct cortical regions during memory encoding, with the fast system serving more of an indexing role. The distinction between "transfer" of information from hippocampus to cortex and a "parallel encoding" perspective is often lost, with even textbooks referring to information transfer despite the earliest proposals about systems consolidation referring to parallel encoding (Squire, 1987; Frankland and Bontempi, 2005). In either case, however, a central aspect of the standard model and its derivatives is the notion that the dependence of memory storage on the hippocampus is limited in time.

Nadel and Moscovitch (1997) sought to make sense of the vast and at times contrasting literature the nature of human retrograde amnesia by proposing a "multiple trace" theory. Their suggestion was that, as episodic memories are recalled, or similar events reexperienced, multiple related traces are formed in the hippocampal and neocortex. Thus, older episodic memories would be associated with a greater number of hippocampal traces, which would make them more resilient to forgetting. In addition, systems consolidation differentiates distinct subtypes of declarative memory, with semantic information stored in cortex but at least facets of episodic and spatial information continuing to be stored in and always requiring the activity of the hippocampus for retrieval. This was later developed further to include the notion of

"trace transformation" (Winocur et al., 2010) (Figure 14.33) with the supposition that, as the content of memory traces became "semanticized" (by being stripped of their spatiotemporal tags and ephemeral details), they were transformed from less accurate and detail-rich episodes into more gist-like representations. Semantic consolidation is therefore not just a fixing process, but a kind of intelligent blurring process that extracts statistical regularities across multiple similar situations. Metaphorically, we may not remember the details of every birthday party we have attended, but we retain the gist-like memory that a birthday party has friends and relatives, a cake, maybe balloons if it is for a child, and so on (van Kesteren et al., 2012).

Storage is one thing but what about retrieval? It is all very well that memory traces are stored in a part of the brain that is permissive for lasting memory, but they may still be difficult to find. A library might achieve lasting protection of its books through appropriate air-conditioning and protection from the sun, but the library still needs an index so that users can find the book they are after. The index theory, first proposed nearly 40 years ago (Teyler and DiScenna, 1986) postulates that the role of the hippocampus is to form and retain an index of neocortical areas activated by experiential events. Although the index theory is not necessarily a theory of memory consolidation per se, the principle has been incorporated into many consolidation theories. The core principle is that, upon learning, the hippocampal index "points" to the appropriate cortical areas for memory representation. During later recall, partial stimulation activates the index, leading to the recruitment of the full cortical pattern (Teyler and Rudy, 2007; Figure 14.33). The electrophysiological techniques for testing this idea were not available at the time, but new molecular-genetic techniques offer one route into thinking about these via hippocampal engrams (Tayler et al., 2013; Goode et al., 2020). There is, consequently, a resurgence of interest in the indexing concept. Specifically, cell activity in one part of a larger engram circuit may have only part of the total information, but a pattern of activation from, for example, the DG identifies

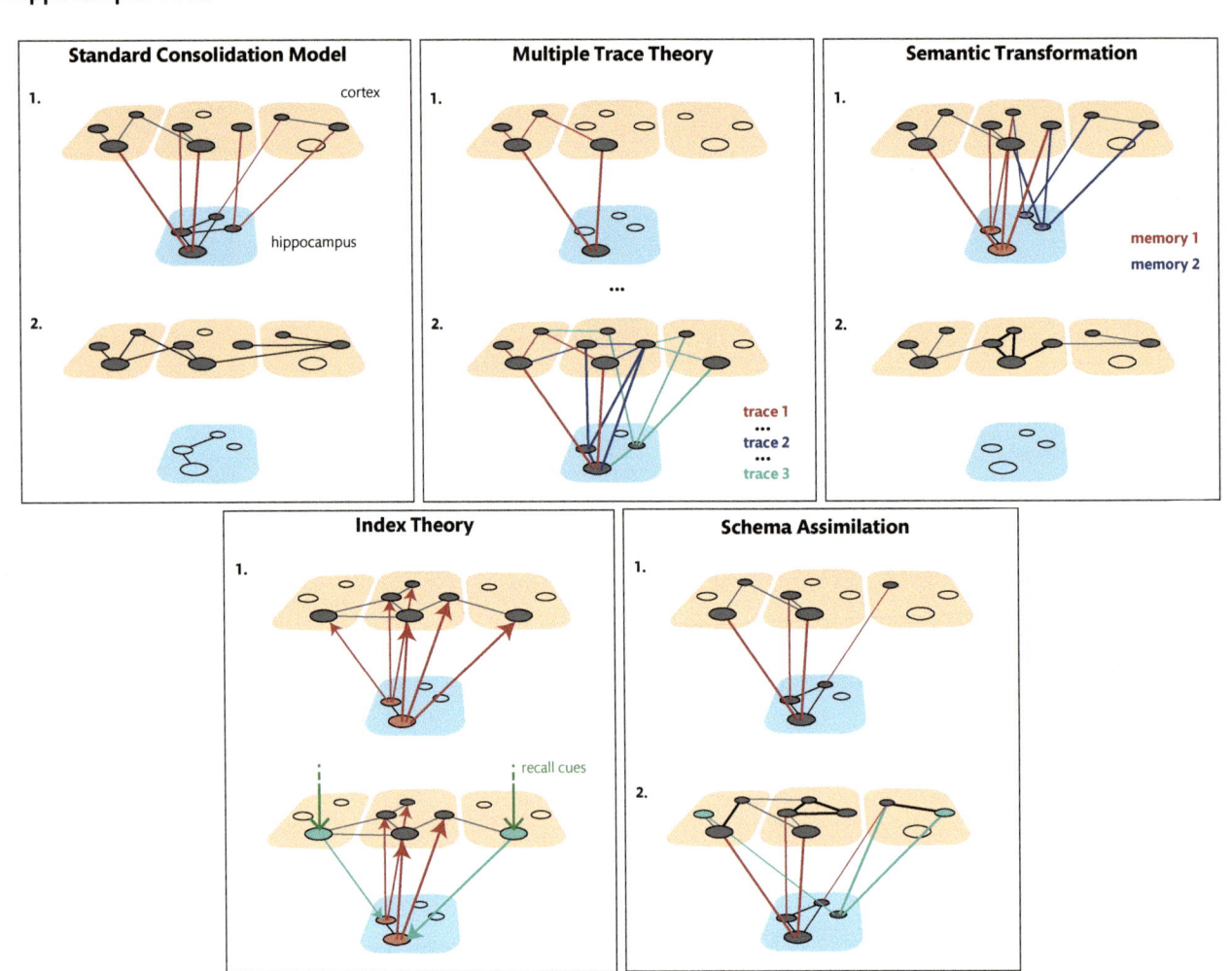

Figure 14.33 Theories of memory consolidation, showing how hippocampus and cortical areas interact during learning (1) and after consolidation (2). In the standard consolidation model the formation of stable cortical connections over time makes the hippocampal trace dispensable over time. In the multiple trace theory (MTT), repeated experiences or recall create additional traces. Over time, a single memory comes to be represented by numerous traces, making it more robust toward forgetting. In a variant of MTT, episodic memories can lose detail and become semanticized in the cortex, including generalized information common to multiple, related, experiences. In the index theory, the hippocampus stores "indices" or "pointers" to cortical areas. The presence of these indices enables the complete recall of the cortical population by means of their reactivation by sensory recall cues. The formation of schemas in cortex creates a cortical-guided framework that organized past information and guides the assimilation of new information. In the scene construction theory, cortical storage uses the hippocampus area to "project" its information and link various aspects of the memory into a coherent scenario.

the context in which an event happened but not itself specifying any details about the nature of the event or its valence (Redondo et al., 2014).

The range of thinking about memory consolidation over the years continues to be diverse, notably in relation to the implementational details of the process of semanticization of episodic memories. Its function is to strip them of their temporospatial attributes, as first raised by Nadel and Moscovitch (1997), but we do not yet have a really clear algorithmic understanding of such a process. Should a distinction be made between consolidation and semanticization? The former would allow the temporally persistent memory of discrete events and enable the recovered consciousness and mental time travel characteristic of episodic memory (Moscovitch, 1995). The latter would involve the process through which the statistical regularities that emerge from successive similar episodes are abstracted, and so add to a person's semantic knowledge. The later recall of such information would not require spatiotemporal tags (Winocur et al., 2005), the apocryphal

example being that few of us remember where or when we first learned that canaries are yellow.

However, effective long-lasting semantic memory is not just a matter of stripping away place and time tags, or forming gist-like memories, but also the creation of an appropriate and effective organization of information in long-term memory. Such a framework would provide a semantic structure of knowledge, sometimes called a "schema." The schema idea, originally proposed by Bartlett (1932) and extended to memory consolidation by McClelland et al. (1995), can be likened to the adage that "Rome wasn't built in day." Schemas develop gradually and become frameworks of knowledge, much more than just links between isolated memories.

An important recent revision of the CLS hypothesis encapsulates these principles to accommodate rapid assimilation when the consolidated framework in cortex is already appropriate for the new information (McClelland, 2013). In addition, the rediscovery in recent years of reconsolidation as a posttranslational memory process also raises the possibility of updating existing information via memory retrieval that brings long dormant information back to mind through reinstatement of neural activity. Originally described in the late 1960s (Lewis et al., 1968; Misanin et al., 1968), the reconsolidation idea suggests that, on their retrieval, items in long-term memory enter a transient and labile state, in which they are amenable to change (Dudai, 2004).

Systems consolidation appears straightforward but is a complex issue addressing the subtle distinction between memory and knowledge; as Steven Pinker wrote in connection with understanding the science of language: "it's a hard, easy problem."

14.8.3 Systems consolidation: experimental work

Hippocampal lesions produce profound anterograde amnesia in humans (i.e., inability to form new memories) (Figure 14.34A) but, importantly, also retrograde amnesia (i.e., inability to recall past memories) with either long or flat temporal gradients (Squire, 1992; Nadel and Moscovitch, 1997). A large body of work, using both monkeys and rodents, evaluated the existence of a retrograde gradient. A key prediction of the standard model was that systems consolidation was a drawn-out process taking place over weeks or longer (Alvarez and Squire, 1994). For example, Zola-Morgan and Squire (1990) trained monkeys on a series of 100 object discrimination problems. These were divided into 5 sets of 20 problems scheduled at intervals of 2, 4, 8, 12, and 16 weeks prior to giving the animals aspiration lesions of the hippocampus and surrounding parahippocampal cortex. Two weeks after surgery, they were retested on each of the 100 problems by presenting pairs of discriminanda just once (to examine retention uncontaminated by new learning). The lesioned monkeys were impaired relative to controls on the problems learned shortly before surgery, but the two groups performed at a comparable, above-chance level for problems learned 12 or 16 weeks earlier (Figure 14.34B). Control subjects did best on the most recent problems and but poorer on the older problems, reflecting gradual forgetting, but the lesioned monkeys did worse on the recent problems, pointing to a memory consolidation process that must have been taking place in normal animals which was interrupted by the creation of a hippocampal/parahippocampal lesion.

Studies of retrograde amnesia in nonprimate species have also been conducted using social transmission of food-preferences, cue- and context fear conditioning, trace-eyeblink conditioning, spatial learning, and object discrimination learning tasks (e.g., Winocur, 1990; Kim and Fanselow, 1992; Bolhuis et al., 1994; Anagnostaras et al., 1999; see Squire et al., 2001, for review). Temporal gradients of retrograde amnesia consistent with a gradual process of memory consolidation were observed in several early studies, including a now classic study of context fear conditioning (Figure 14.34C) (Kim and Fanselow, 1992). Complementing the lesion data, gradual time-dependent changes in 2-deoxyglucose utilization or immediate early-gene expression in the hippocampus and neocortex were observed after learning (Bontempi et al., 1999; Frankland et al., 2004; Maviel et al., 2004). These activity-dependent changes may constitute a physiological and molecular signature of the shifting focus from neural activity in hippocampus to activity in neocortex, providing a platform for new molecular engineering studies in mice.

However, difficulties in replicating these early findings were to emerge. For example, there are instances in which retrieval seems always to depend on an intact hippocampus. Specifically, flat temporal gradients (i.e., no gradient) are often observed for episodic memory (Nadel and Moscovitch, 1997) and, in the watermaze, for spatial memory (Bolhuis et al., 1994; Martin et al., 2005). Contextual fear conditioning is perhaps the most studied learning paradigm for assessment of systems consolidation, and even in this task flat gradients have now been seen after dorsal, ventral, partial, and complete hippocampal lesions (Figure 14.34D) (Lehmann et al., 2007; Sutherland et al., 2008; Ocampo et al., 2017). The potentially distinct effects of partial or complete lesions is interesting, especially in the retrograde domain. If learning takes place using the whole hippocampus, a distributed trace may be laid down along the full longitudinal axis. If a partial lesion is then made, it may be possible to retrieve something using pattern completion among the remaining neurons. The implication is that some information is still available in hippocampus. Moreover, a reminder of the learning experience delivered well after the consolidation window has passed (context re-exposure timed 45 days post conditioning) can render a memory trace to be vulnerable once more to hippocampal disruption, a phenomenon called reconsolidation (Debiec et al., 2002). That hippocampal involvement can be reignited through a reminder suggests a continuing hippocampal contribution to the memory beyond the time point when the standard systems consolidation window would have closed. This conclusion is bolstered by another study that used optogenetics and pharmacology (TTX/CNQX) to assess the hippocampal involvement in the storage and retrieval of old memories (Goshen et al., 2011). Silencing of the hippocampus pharmacologically revealed the standard model's predicted temporal amnesia gradient with memory deficits observed after hippocampal silencing 1 day post conditioning but intact contextual freezing when infusions and tests were given 45 days post conditioning. Optogenetic silencing of CA1 with eNpHR3.1, on the other hand, precisely timed during recall, had the quite different effect of blocking expression of both recent and remote memories—a flat amnesia gradient. However, with prolonged optogenetic silencing for 30 minutes before testing and during the test, the remote fear memory was once again preserved. These findings point to some temporal dynamics of the retrieval process of a systems nature. Other studies support a continued role for the hippocampus at remote time points, such as the finding that optogenetic silencing of the DG engram can impair freezing 2 weeks after CFC (Denny et al., 2014).

The dynamic nature of retrieval is complemented by work using engram tagging technology (see section 14.7) to study the role of cortical and hippocampal areas at different stages of consolidation (Kitamura et al., 2017). Results based on context fear conditioning suggest that "priming" of cortical areas may take place as early as the phase of initial learning (Figure 14.35). This early tag has been shown to involve NMDARs and to set in motion epigenetic changes which are required for long-term memory expression (Lesburgueres et al., 2011). A consistent finding is that, despite this early tag and later dependence, the activity of frontal circuits are sufficient but not necessary for retrieval of recent memories (Frankland et al., 2004; Kitamura et al., 2017). However, engram experiments have shown an interesting dichotomy between the necessity of neocortical circuits for recent memory expression and the sufficiency of those circuits to drive recall. For example, in line with inactivation and lesion studies, it was found that the engram cells tagged in the prefrontal cortex (PFC) during CFC were dispensable for the recall of recent memory but required for remote memory. However,

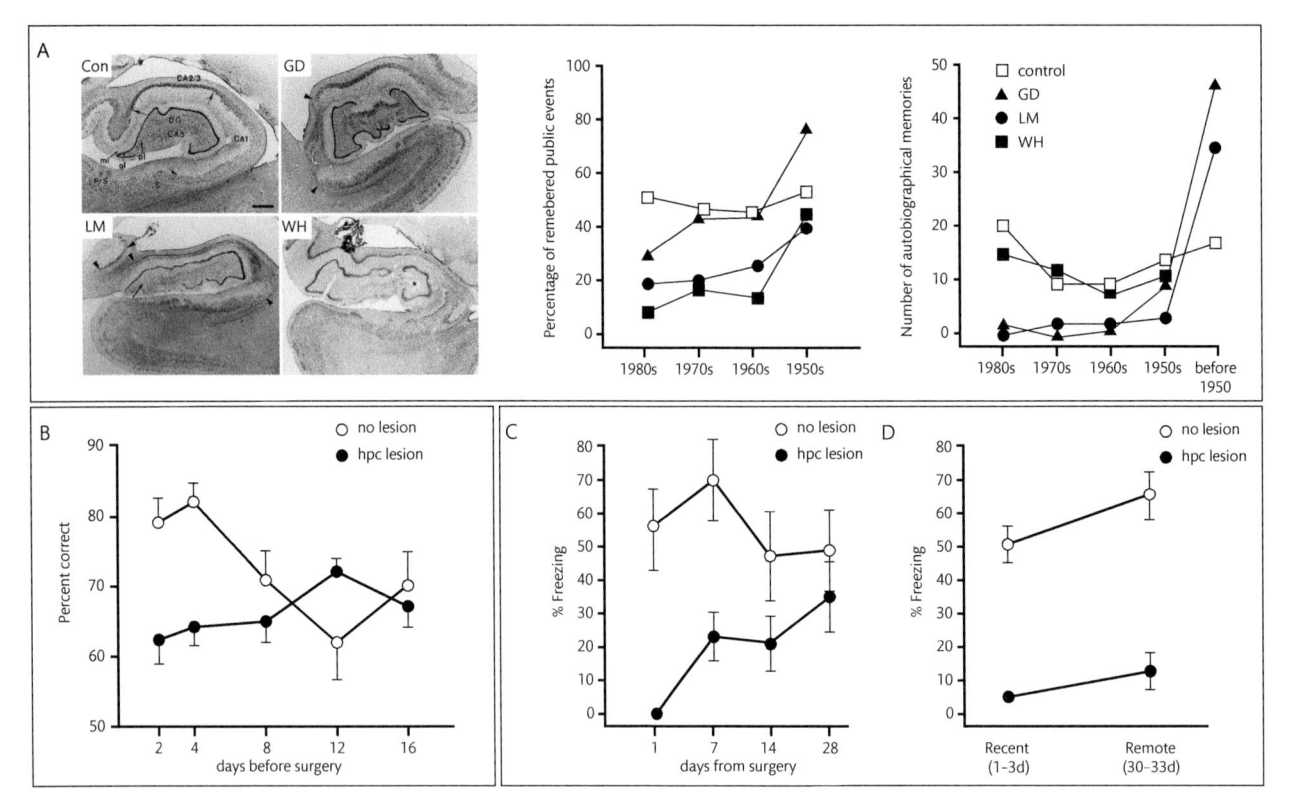

Figure 14.34 Retrograde amnesia and declarative memory theory. (A) Decade-long temporally graded retrograde amnesia for public facts and episodic memories is often reported in patients with MTL lesions. On the left, histological sections from a control subject (Con) and patients GD, LM and WH showing the extent of their hippocampal lesions. On the right, performance in memory retrieval as a function of memory age. Patient GD was born in 1940, so the Before 1950 time point was omitted because it represents episodes that occurred when he was younger than 10 years old. (Panels after Rempel-Clower et al., 1996, copyright 1996 Society for Neuroscience.) (B) Average performance during a single postsurgery probe trial for each of 100 object discrimination problems learned earlier. Problems learned 12 weeks before surgery are remembered better than those only 2 weeks beforehand. (From Zola-Morgan and Squire, 1990.) (C) Temporally graded retrograde amnesia in contextual fear conditioning in rats with hippocampal lesion, reported by Kim and Fanselow (1992). (D) Loss of retrograde amnesia gradient by hippocampal lesion on contextual fear conditioning of rats from Ocampo et al. (2017). The Remote group was lesioned 30–33 days after training, the Recent group 1–3 days after training.

optogenetic activation of these neurons induced freezing at both early and remote time points (Kitamura et al., 2017). Direct MEC to PFC connections were necessary for the allocation of engram cells in the PFC at the time of learning. The authors also showed that MEC-to-BLA connections were necessary for recent recall, whereas connections between PFC and BLA affected recall only at remote time points (Kitamura et al., 2017). Taken together, these results suggest that the hippocampus is initially essential for memory representations that support conditioned contextual fear; following consolidation, however, other brain areas that support a distinct and hippocampal-independent representation of that memory can be engaged during the pre-recall silencing of the hippocampus and elicit the freezing response. The Goshen et al. (2011) study pointed to the anterior cingulate as being one relevant extrahippocampal region, a structure that has also emerged in several consolidation studies in rodents and humans. Later work showed that new cells can be included in the CA1 engram as the memory consolidates, recruiting neurons receiving inputs from the entorhinal cortex and in turn increasing the projection of engram cells in the dorsal CA1 to the ACC (Refeli et al., 2023).

14.8.4 Sleep and memory consolidation

It is common experience that the world looks and feels different after a night of sleep. We spend one third of our lives asleep and

we are not alone in doing so; nearly all animals sleep (Tononi and Cirelli, 2014; Cirelli and Tononi, 2017). Sleep deprivation has devastating consequences on mood, cognition, memory, metabolism, thermoregulation, cardiovascular function, hormonal regulation, and the immune system. The longest confirmed period of time a person has stayed awake is just 11 days, in the famous experiment undertaken by Randy Gardner (Ross, 1965). However, notwithstanding that sleep is important for mental and bodily health, the reasons for this ubiquitous state are not fully understood. It likely serves multiple functions, of which one is connected to memory consolidation.

In Ebbinghaus's seminal experiments on the memorization of nonsense syllables, he found that retention was enhanced if subjects were permitted to sleep in between learning and retrieval (Ebbinghaus, 1885; Jenkins and Dallenbach, 1924) (Figure 14.36A). At the time, there was a belief that sleep was largely passive and the brain quiet; the observed enhancement after sleep was thought to be due to decreased retroactive memory interference due to the absence of other learning. According to this line of thinking, sleep does not play an active role in memory consolidation, but rather, the learning that occurs while awake can sometimes be a source of interference, with memory temporarily guarded during sleep by silencing the flow of new information. Contemporary thinking largely rejects this idea.

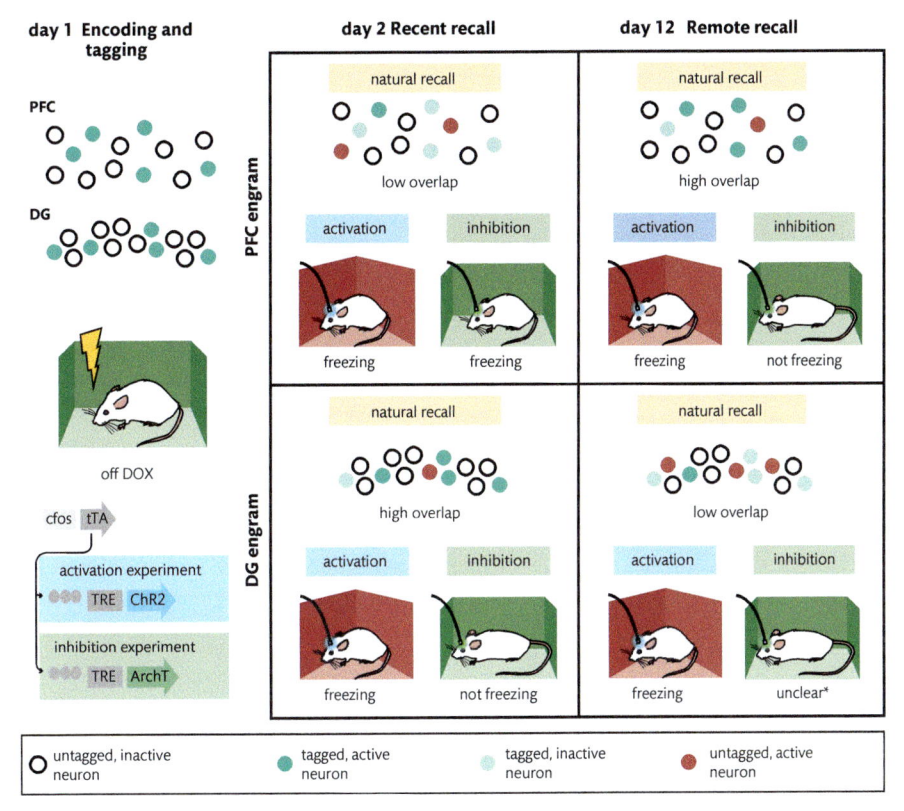

Figure 14.35 Engram cells and system consolidation. Summary of the results of the application of the activity-tagging technology to the study of system consolidation of contextual fear conditioning traces. (A) Using the cfos-tTA system, Kitamura et al. (2017) tagged engram population in the prefrontal cortex (PFC) or in the dentate gyrus (DG) during contextual fear conditioning to express either an inhibitory opsin (ArchT) or an excitatory opsin (ChR2). The results observed at recent or remote time points by activating or inhibiting the PFC or the DG engram are summarized in the figure, together with the observed overlap with the cells activated by the natural recall (cfos⁺). *The effect of inhibition of the DG engram at remote time points is unclear: Denny et al. (2014) showed that the inhibition of the DG engram 14 days after acquisition impairs memory retrieval. However, Goshen et al. (2011) reported that prolonged optogenetic or pharmacological silencing, but not acute optogenetic silencing, of the hippocampus has no effect on memory retrieval.

A fundamental challenge in sleep research is that if one conducts a causal experiment involving sleep deprivation, there will be wide-ranging consequences, not least stress. How is a researcher to make the definitive inference that it was sleep per se, or the lack of it, that contributed to memory performance? Moreover, sleep takes time and it normally occurs in humans at a fixed phase of the circadian cycles (it is somewhat different in experimental animals such as rodents). In designing exacting experiments, controls would therefore also be needed to control for the passage of time, and adequate assessment that any changes in memory retention were not due to encoding or retrieval occurring at different times of day. These considerations and the requisite controls are well recognized in the sleep field and it is not unusual to have studies with multiple experimental and control groups, and factorial designs to control for some of the issues. Consideration of these caveats led some to wonder if definitive experiments on the function of sleep were possible. One criticism was that studies often tested memory retention directly after sleep deprivation, i.e., at a time when subjects were acutely fatigued. Impaired performance might reflect impaired retrieval due to fatigue rather than the loss of sleep-dependent memory consolidation (Idzikowski, 1984).

Many things happen in the brain and body during sleep that could be the biological basis for these sleep-related changes in memory expression. First, sleep is not a single state and is composed, in humans, of multiple successive stages of slow-wave sleep (SWS, stages N1–N3) and then later periods of rapid-eye-movement (REM) sleep. Second, these two different patterns—SWS and REM—are associated with radically different electrophysiological and encephalographic patterns, including the inhibition of muscle tone during REM sleep. SWS is associated with specific electrical patterns such as sharp wave ripples in the hippocampus and cortical spindles in neocortex. We are now finally securing an understanding of how all these fit together (Klinzing et al., 2019).

A generation ago, following the discovery of REM sleep and the finding that waking people up during it revealed that they were often dreaming, led to human and animal studies of REM sleep deprivation. The work of Carlisle Smith emphasized the existence of a "paradoxical sleep window" in which REM sleep was thought to be necessary for normal sleep-dependent memory consolidation. In these experiments, REM sleep was diminished by placing rats on an inverted flower-pot in a tub of water, with standing on it requiring muscle tone for the animals to stay upright. Rats can engage in non-REM sleep and successfully balance on such a flower-pot; however the atonia during REM causes the rats to fall off into the water and thus awaken. By selectively giving the REM disruption at various time points after learning, a window of 5–8 h post encoding was found to be essential to recall the hidden escape position in a watermaze (Smith and Rose, 1996). That the timing of the window was defined post hoc and was influenced by species, strain, and even vendor of the animals did, however, call into question the reliability

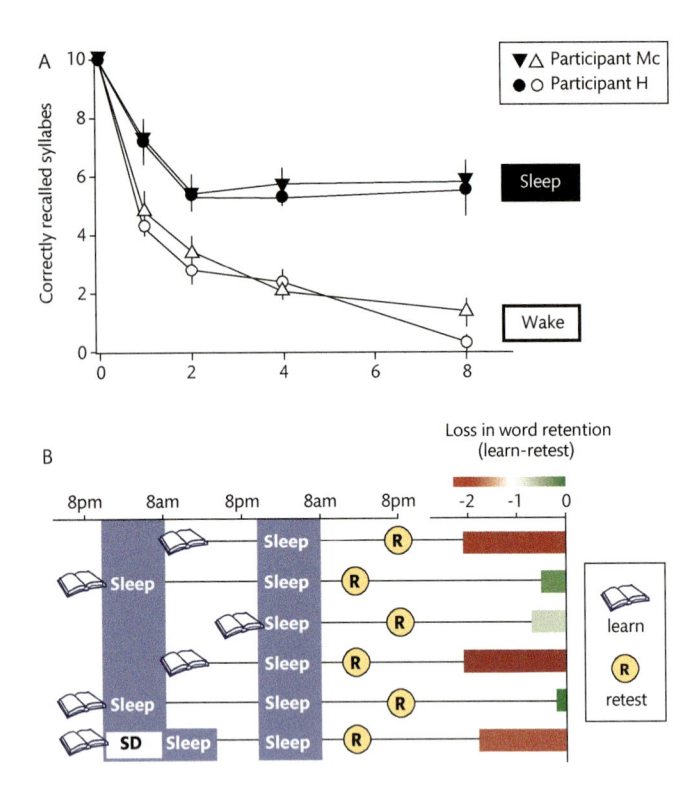

Figure 14.36 Effect of sleep on memory acquisition: (A) Ebbinghaus (1885) seminal experiment on the role of sleep on the memorization of nonsense syllables. (B) Gais et al. (2006) experiment on the memorization of German words by English-speakers studies the role of sleep on memory performance by controlling for multiple factors including the time of the day, and the elapsed time between learning and retest.

of the conclusions from this line of study (Siegel, 2001). But it is a striking result.

New experimental approaches were required, with one major step forward being a behavioral study of human subjects by Plihal and Born (1997), who showed that different stages of sleep benefited different types of memory, with early SWS boosting memory for paired-associates (declarative memory) but late REM sleep benefiting mirror tracing (a procedural skill). In another study (Gais et al., 2006), English-speaking high school students were asked to learn German vocabulary. The population was divided into six groups (Figure 14.36B) with some learning in the evening and some in the morning, some sleeping directly after learning and some remaining awake, and some deprived of sleep but others not. Critically, recall was always tested after a night of sleep (avoiding the fatigue concern). In this study, forgetting was unaffected by the interval between learning and test (24 vs. 36 h), or the time of day of recall (morning or night), but was strongly modulated by whether subjects were allowed to sleep directly after learning. Specifically, while forgetting was increased by depriving subjects of night-time sleep (and the associated ambiguities of doing this), but also by asking subjects to learn first thing in the morning and then spend several hours awake before being able to sleep. These results suggest that sleep directly aids the consolidation of declarative memory.

However, new technologies are raising questions about the relative importance of SWS and REM sleep. For example, contemporary optogenetic experiments have demonstrated a clear importance for

REM sleep that cannot be explained away by the caveats associated to the stress of losing a full night sleep. In the rodent hippocampus during REM, theta rhythms dominate; they can be eliminated by silencing the GABAergic neurons of the medial septum with the light-activated silencing opsin ArchT. Selectively inhibiting theta rhythms during REM sleep causes memory deficits in contextual fear conditioning and in a novel object-place recognition task (Boyce et al., 2016). These results show that hippocampal theta is essential for normal memory consolidation.

Of the three main memory functions of the hippocampus discussed in this chapter (declarative memory, spatial memory, and relational memory), all three have been found to benefit from a night of sleep (Ellenbogen et al., 2007; Wamsley et al., 2010). However, it seems that sleep does more than merely strengthen the persistence of declarative memories (the "fixing" process), but actually transforms the nature of the memory trace. Inspired by trace transformation theory (Winocur et al., 2010), one possibility is that the gist of a memory is extracted during SWS as the specific spatiotemporal details of an episodic memory are lost and the semantic details are integrated into cortical networks. Several research groups have tested this idea with the Deese-Roediger-McDermott paradigm, in which subjects are given a list of words related to a common gist word that is never presented. Subjects are later asked to recall, or recognize from a longer list, which words were on the list. The presence of gist vs. more exact episodic memory is revealed when subjects display a false memory for a nonpresented gist word. After a night of sleep, or daytime nap (which is exclusively a slow-wave state), memory for studied words was decreased, but false memory for gist words was found to increase relative to a control group that spent an equivalent time awake (J Payne et al., 2009; Darsaud et al., 2011). This supports the idea that gist can be extracted and assimilated into memory during consolidation.

Much recent focus has been centered on hippocampal-cortical dialogue during sharp wave ripples that occur during slow-wave sleep, and are almost completely absent during REM. Given the amount of work in this field and its integration into the CLS hypothesis, the next section is dedicated to this biological basis for how sleep contributes to memory consolidation. In passing, we must nonetheless note that other mechanisms are likely relevant, such as hormonal regulation (Plihal et al., 1999), synaptic up/down scaling (Tononi and Cirelli, 2014), and metabolic clearance through the glymphatic system (Xie et al., 2013).

14.8.5 Sharp wave ripples, hippocampal replay, and a putative teaching signal

Single-unit and field potential recordings in rodent (rats and mice) suggest that the hippocampus operates in two modes with distinct electrophysiological signatures: a theta mode observed during movement or exploration (see Chapter 11), and a separate mode dominated by large irregular activity (LIA) which is observed during both slow-wave sleep and quiet wakefulness. During LIA, "sharp wave ripples" (SPW-Rs) occur in bursts about every second. As the name suggests, the SPW-R event is composed of two components, the sharp wave—which is generated in stratum radiatum of CA1 due to strong inputs arriving from CA3 via the Schaffer collaterals—and the ripple, which is a high-frequency (140–200 Hz) burst of activity that reflects the rhythmic coupling between excitatory and inhibitory neurons, as feedback inhibition counteracts moments of strong depolarization. Buzsáki (1989) was the first to suggest that ripple activity could be a central component of a consolidation process involving the hippocampus, noting the temporal dissociation between ripples and active exploration, and the high-frequency nature of the ripple oscillation that felt a bit like the tetanus used in LTP experiments (Buzsáki, 1989). It was later suggested, in keeping with the CLS framework, that the neural activity observed during the ripple is the teaching signal that the fast learner (hippocampus) provides to the slow learner (cortex). This interpretation was based on the reliable observation that the neurons that are active during ripples, and the temporal ordering of those neurons, mirror the activity observed at other moments when subjects move about their environment. This match in the temporal structure of neural activity has led to the hypothesis that, during ripples, experiences are reactivated, or "replayed" and that this replay acts as an additional, virtual rehearsal from the perspective of the rest of the brain. Note that the time-course of events within a ripple is much faster than that of the events themselves.

The first hints of replay were made through the analysis of how place cells fired in the sleep before and after animals occupied a single neuron's place field (Pavlides and Winson, 1989). In a seminal paper using tetrode recording (Wilson and McNaughton, 1994), not only did individual neural excitability change with experience but also the synchronization of neural firing. Neurons that had overlapping place fields during a recent experience tended to continue to fire together during the subsequent sleep, an observation that was not observed for place cells within nonoverlapping fields (Wilson and McNaughton, 1994) (Figure 14.37A). Reactivation occurs not only at pairwise level but also at the sequence in which neural activity unfolds. The first observation of sequential replay was made by the Buzsáki group in rats that had run on a stationary "hamster wheel" and then slept. Reliable cell sequences could be observed during wheel running, and these were also seen during sleep-associated ripples, but the rate in which the sequences evolved during the ripples was faster (Nadasdy et al., 1999). This observation led to the hypothesis that replay during ripples is a temporally compressed version of our waking experience, with waking patterns compressed by a factor of about 10–15 times during sleep. Further studies revealed that temporally compressed replay events play out during both waking and sleep and, strikingly,

they can go in both the forward and reverse direction (Diba and Buzsáki, 2007).

Simultaneous monitoring of the hippocampus and the cortex has shown that, during sleep, ripples are embedded within and coupled to ongoing cortical dynamics, such as sleep spindles and up- and down-states (Siapas and Wilson, 1998; Sirota et al., 2003; Peyrache et al., 2009; Wang and Ikemoto, 2016), suggestive of a bidirectional flow of information between the cortex and the hippocampus. Cortical ensembles observed during waking are also reactivated around ripple onset (Peyrache et al., 2009; Jadhav et al., 2016), and this reactivation is synchronized with replay in the hippocampus (Ji and Wilson, 2007). Indeed, the reactivation of learned experience during sleep in the form of trajectories and goal locations is predictive of the subsequent performance in spatial memory tasks (Dupret et al., 2010). Studies in the nonhuman primate that combine electrophysiological recording of the hippocampus with BOLD imaging show widespread cortical and subcortical networks are modulated in their excitability around the time of the ripple (Logothetis et al., 2012), suggesting that these are special moments for interregional signaling. More recent studies in human patients with electrodes implanted for seizure diagnostics have found that hippocampal-cortical coupling around the time of ripples predicts the accuracy and even the content of episodic recall (Y Norman et al., 2019; Vaz et al., 2019; Y Norman et al., 2021). These important studies show (to the great relief of a generation of rodent researchers), the relevance of SPW-R activity to bona fide episodic memory retrieval.

Beyond this correlational evidence for the importance of ripples, intervention studies have shown that blocking ripples during rest periods after an experience impairs long-term (Girardeau et al., 2009) and short-term spatial memory (Jadhav et al., 2012; Roux et al., 2017). The key technical development was "ripple-killing" stimulation. In the first study of this kind (Girardeau et al., 2009), electrical stimulation of the ventral hippocampal commissure was delivered after rapid real-time detection of SPW-Rs during sleep periods after learning (Figure 14.37B). It effectively aborted the ripples and slowed the daily savings in reference-memory place learning in an eight-arm radial maze with three arms baited. Similar findings were observed when ripples and cortical spindles

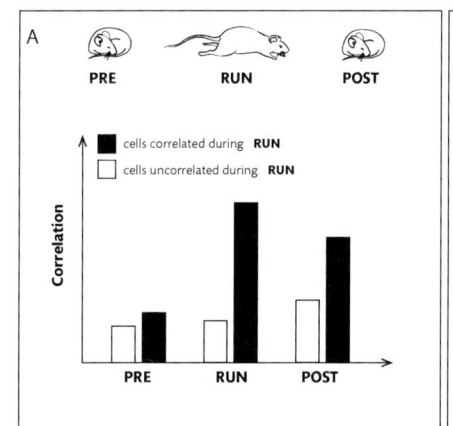
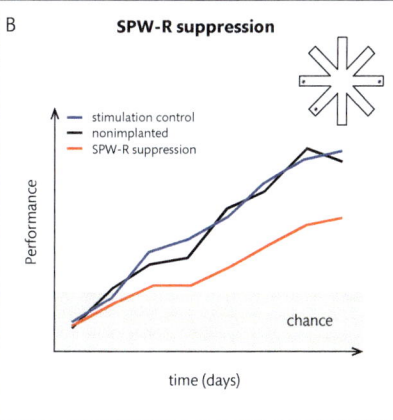
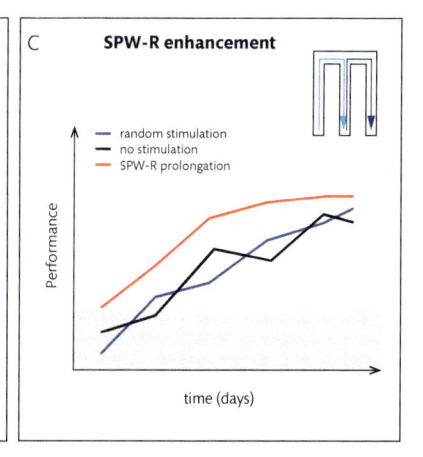

Figure 14.37 Replay during SPW-R and memory consolidation during sleep. (A) Wake experiences increase the correlation between specific neurons in the hippocampus, which is preserved in subsequent spontaneous reactivation events during sleep. (From Wilson and McNaughton, 1994.) (B) Optogenetic "ripple killing" of SPW-Rs during sleep significantly impairs the performance in retrieving food from specific arms of radial maze (Girardeau et al., 2009). Conversely, prolonging SPW-Rs duration during sleep increases memory performance (Fernandez-Ruiz et al., 2019).

were decoupled through ripple-triggered stimulation of the locus coeruleus (Novitskaya et al., 2016). Moreover, gain-of-function studies have shown that spatial memory can be improved by increasing the coupling rate of SPW-Rs to cortical delta waves and spindles (via electrical stimulation of the deep layers of the motor cortex) (Maingret et al., 2016) or by optogenetically prolonging ripples (Fernandez-Ruiz et al., 2019) (Figure 14.37C). Recent evidence has shown that disrupting MEC processing during learning, which in turn affects the fine-timescale of sequential activity of CA1 neurons normally embedded within theta rhythms, prevents the subsequent sequential replay of learning related patterns. Interestingly, the performance in learning reward positions in the cheeseboard maze (see section 14.4.4) was affected by this manipulation, but not learning a simpler place association task (Liu et al., 2023). Together these studies show a causal role for hippocampal-cortical coupling during SPW-Rs in the consolidation of spatial memory.

Which aspects of ripple-related activity are important? Several options exist—including the synchronous burst of hippocampal activity, the coordination of this burst with receptive brain regions downstream, the identity of which hippocampal neurons fire together during the ripple, and the sequence of those neurons relative to one another. From the perspective of the indexing model, the identity and order of the hippocampal neurons matter, as the set of neurons firing during the ripple likely defines a pointer to a particular cortical module, and the hippocampal sequence sets the order in which those cortical modules unfold. One recent study (Gridchyn et al., 2020) set out to causally test whether replay per se matters above and beyond the ripple event itself. In this study, the content of the ripple was decoded in real time to determine whether ripple activity was dominated by neurons with place fields active in each of two contexts (A and B) where mice had learned the location of hidden food rewards. Then, during "Context A" ripples, hippocampal neurons were optogenetically silenced by activating the inhibitory opsin ArchT. This content-specific silencing caused memory deficits for the recall of food location in Context A, but not for Context B, for which postlearning replay was allowed to proceed intact. This study using a discriminative paradigm showed, for the first time, a causal contribution of replay in postlearning memory consolidation. Importantly, place fields in Context A re-emerged after retraining, suggesting a role for strengthened synaptic connections as the basis for their maintenance.

This interpretation finds support in a recent study showing that the early phase of memory consolidation may rely on multiple synaptic plasticity events. Using optogenetic erasure of recently potentiated synapses, Goto et al., (2021) discovered that erasing synaptic plasticity shortly after learning, or during the later sleep phases, strongly impairs recall by mice in an inhibitory avoidance task. This provides evidence that a second round of plasticity occurs during sleep and is necessary for memory consolidation (Smith and Rose, 1996). Interestingly, Goto et al. (2021) also found that disrupting plasticity during online learning, or during subsequent sleep, had a different impact on place field stabilization. Online, but not offline, interference resulted in the decrease neuronal selectivity between the two compartments of the test apparatus; however, both online and offline disruption of plasticity reduced synchronous activity between neurons selective for the conditioned chamber, suggesting that offline plasticity is necessary to stabilize a circuit established during learning. Consolidation across brain areas follows hippocampal maturation because erasing new plasticity in the ACC

during sleep 1 day after learning, but neither on the day of learning nor 25 days later, impaired memory performance. It is commonly believed that ripples contribute to systems consolidation through virtual repeats of the earlier experiences. This thinking fits within the broad framework of the hippocampus as a fast-learning, episodic memory maker and the cortex as a slow-learning semantic memory integrator (McClelland et al., 1995).

Is replay the teaching signal? From a computational perspective, the signal is an appealing candidate. SPW-Rs occur during awake stillness and sleep, but rarely during active exploration—when learning should dominate. Ripples occur repetitively (Buzsáki et al., 1992), such that any change that they drive can afford to have a small effect that accumulates over time. Recent and remote experiences are both replayed in neighboring ripples (Gupta et al., 2010), providing a virtual and interleaved training protocol. SPW-Rs have a downstream effect in cortex (Nitzan et al., 2020), as they synchronize activity across the cortex as would be expected if a specific pattern of hippocampal activity acts as a pointer for a corresponding pattern of cortical activity. One analysis of how hippocampal and prefrontal cortex coordinate around ripples showed that hippocampal reactivations of different paths were often associated with similar PFC reactivations (Yu et al., 2018), suggesting a linking of a specific hippocampal representation to a more general trace in the cortex. The high frequency of neural activity during ripples is known to be a potent stimulus for inducing LTP (Laroche et al., 1990). Finally, the existence of replay shows that the firing patterns within the hippocampus can change rapidly after an experience, even after a single experience (Berners-Lee et al., 2022). Evidence consistent with an LTP induction perspective is that both knocking out the NR1 receptor in CA3 pyramidal cells (Dragoi and Tonegawa, 2013) or antagonizing NMDA receptors systemically during learning (Dupret et al., 2010; Silva et al., 2015) disrupt the replay of neural activity-patterns that occur with learning while simultaneously preserving the reactivation of neurons representing familiar spaces. In conclusion, if the brain needed a teaching signal, the pattern of activity observed during ripples would be ideal.

14.8.6 Schemas

One limitation with the ideas considered so far is that, with the exception of the CLS framework (McClelland et al., 1995), they offer few suggestions about the organization of information once consolidated in neocortex. They also assert that the driving force for systems consolidation is hippocampus, implying it is essentially a "bottom-up" process. A distinct neurobiological framework called "schemas," supported by both animal and human data, offers the suggestion of a "top-down" component driven by activated frameworks of prior knowledge (Fernandez and Morris, 2018). Schema theory asserts that the assimilation of new information into an existing structure may sometimes be achieved very rapidly (Figure 14.38).

Metaphors for the organizational process include "mental model," "cognitive map," and "schema." We are nervous about using the term "mental model" for an essentially neurobiological hypothesis, the term "cognitive map" is now generally reserved for a particular theory of hippocampus rather than cortex, and, if "schema" seems vague, it is at least a term that has been used for many years in experimental psychology (Bartlett, 1932; Bransford, 1979; Tse et al., 2007). The classic studies of Bransford and Johnson (1972) asserted the role of semantic links between concept units that collectively

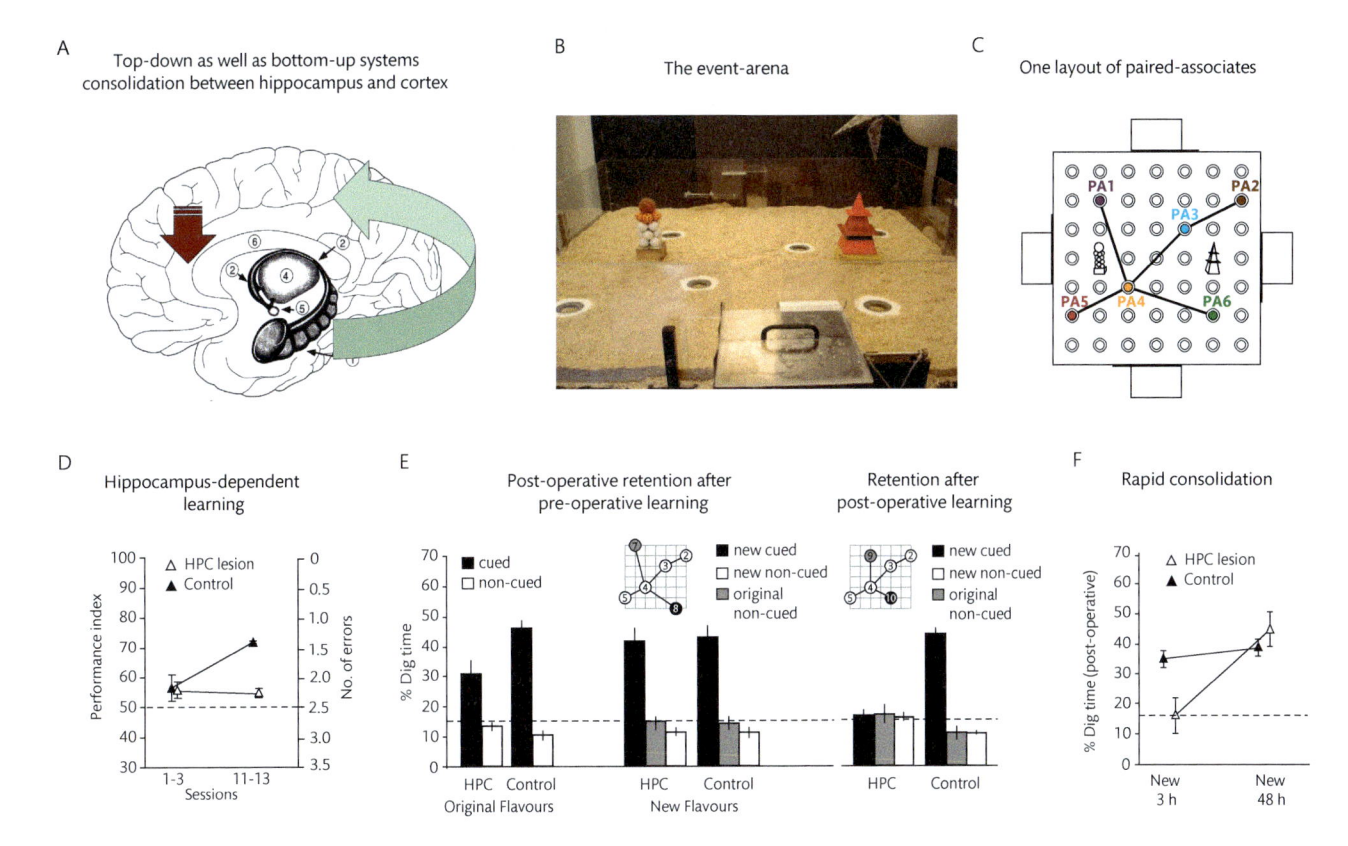

Figure 14.38 Top-down consolidation and schemas. (A) Systems consolidation is typically construed as a process by which information encoded in hippocampus is "transferred" to the neocortex. However, if relevant existing knowledge is present and activated, it may serve to guide the encoding of new information or its assimilation. (B) Photograph of the event arena showing two of the four start-boxes at "north" and "south," respectively, and six sandwells in the arena. (C) Cartoon of the 7 x 7 grid of possible sandwell locations and the placement of 6 paired-associates (PAs) that include different flavors of food. (D) Learning over about 3 weeks is hippocampus-dependent. (E) Different patterns of effect of hippocampal lesions are observed when learning occurs normally and the lesion made prior to recall, or an attempt is made to learn new PAs after the lesion. The original flavors can be remembered postoperatively, as can recently assimilated new flavors; however, the learning of new PAs requires the hippocampus to be intact. (F) Instead of taking as long as a month, consolidation of new PA information occurs within 48 h. (After Tse et al., 2007.)

realized a schematic story in memory retrieval. In a thoughtful essay, Ghosh and Gilboa (2014) sought to anchor the concept of schemas as an associative network structure that aids long-term memory during both encoding and retrieval. The more recent definition due to Fernandez and Morris (2018) is that a schema is "a framework of acquired knowledge, skills or attitudes implemented within a network of connected neurons in which the memory traces of associated information have been stored that, when activated, can alter the manner in which new information is processed, including memory encoding, consolidation and retrieval" (Fernandez and Morris, 2018, p. 657).

Tse et al. (2007) investigated paired-associate learning in animals from the perspective of the creation of a spatial structure for storing information. They used the event arena (which, as noted before, is an enclosure where events happen) to schedule paired-associates (PAs) consisting of foods of distinctive flavors occupying stable places at which the event of finding and digging up the different foods happened (Figure 14.38B,C). That is, Flavor 1 (F1) would, when available, only be available in Location 1 (L1), F2 only in L2, and so on. Over a period of 6–8 weeks, the animals learned each of six PAs at distinct places in the arena (hidden in sandwells with masking odors to rule out olfactory artifacts). The animals had to dig up the food, creating a "digging event" that likely aided location-event binding. Learning was slow, occurring over 15–20 sessions, but that

was not surprising with only 1 trial per PA per day. By asymptote, learning of the six PAs reached asymptote at well above chance levels in both choice and probe trials, and was hippocampus-dependent (Figure 14.38D). Once asymptotic performance had been achieved, two PAs were withdrawn on one session and replaced by two new PAs (new flavors in new but nearby locations). The new PAs were learned in a single trial—indicating that the prior knowledge of an already learned PA schema allowed rapid assimilation of relevant new information (Figure 14.38E). When an entirely new schema was introduced with six new flavors and locations (i.e., six new PAs), there was neither interference nor any synergistic effect on new learning, which took just as long this second time. It was as if flavor-place schemas act as self-contained frameworks for storing information. Hippocampal lesions within 3 h of training new PAs caused a total loss of memory for the new PAs, but an interval of as little as 48 h before such lesions was enough for successful neocortical assimilation and later hippocampal-independent retrieval of the new PAs given their flavor cue (Figure 14.38E,F). Thus, a rapid upward-gradient of systems consolidation over 48 h was observed. Moreover, whereas the creation of the initial six-PA schema took a minimum of 6 weeks (and 15–20 trials), the timescale for memory assimilation into this existing schema was much shorter. Thus, a cortical schema has a beneficial top-down influence on the learning of new information.

This animal study and the many human psychological and neuroimaging studies since point to something that makes intuitive sense (Fernandez and Morris, 2018). Prior knowledge has a profound influence on the acquisition and storage of new information. This is nothing to do with the anticipation of reward, it is not a "predictive-coding" issue in the usual sense of this concept, but a process underpinning the accumulation of knowledge. A biomedical science example might be expanding one's knowledge of the citric-acid cycle (sometimes called the Krebs cycle) which is notoriously detailed to the point of being daunting to learn. Adding extra information would be second nature to the experienced biochemist who would have learned about it carefully, whereas ordinary mortals would learn little.

Tse et al. (2007) was followed up by three causal studies from the same laboratory that pointed to the possible role of dopamine in memory retention within schema (Bethus et al., 2010), and the important of interactions between medial prefrontal cortex/anterior cingulate cortex and the hippocampus in the assimilation of PSs into an existing schema (Tse et al., 2011; Wang et al., 2012). Not only was plasticity-related immediate early gene (IEG) activation in mPFC quantitatively highest in association with assimilation success, rather than mere novelty, but also microinfusions of both an NMDA- and an AMPA-receptor antagonist into these cortical brain regions blocked assimilation. Thus, the interaction between hippocampus and at least these frontal regions of cortex required excitatory GluRA and GluRN receptor-mediated synaptic transmission. Takeuchi et al. (2022) have described cortical networks activated by schemas during new paired-associate encoding the event-arena task using immediate early-genes. These data and the electrophysiological findings (Karimi Abadchi et al., 2020) are consistent with the notion that, sometimes, cortex leads and hippocampus follows in terms of their interactions.

Physiological approaches have also been used to study sequential integration of related episodes. McKenzie et al. (2014) used tetrode recording to examine hippocampal cell firing in CA1 and CA3 during odor-reward association learning carried out in distinct contexts. In this paradigm, rats first learned that Object A was rewarded in Context 1 but not Object B, whereas the odor-reward relationships were reversed in Context 2. After 3 days of training, a novel set of objects was introduced into the same space, in which Object C was rewarded in Context 1 and Object D was rewarded in Context 2. This design established a functional equivalence between Objects A and C, and likewise between Objects B and D, in that they were always rewarded in the same contexts. Their findings indicated that there were hippocampal neural population firing patterns that constituted representations of multiple features of events, including the locations and contexts in which they occurred, as well as for object identity and reward potential. Strikingly, the neurons that had first fired for objects A and B rapidly generalized their firing to the functionally equivalent objects C and D. The new associations (Objects C/D) had presumably been stored within the networks dedicated to the related past (Objects A/B). These findings reveal neural mechanisms for the development and organization of relational representations, which are an important component of schemas (Figure 14.39A,B). The neural code that developed from learning this task contained information about object identity, reward potential, location, and context. Neurons in the hippocampus coded each of the task dimensions to various degrees, such that the context in which the animal was located (the variable that determined the reward

contingencies) dictated firing patterns most and the pattern of activity in one context was anticorrelated with activity in the other (Figure 14.39C). Consistent with the cognitive map hypothesis, location was the next most salient task dimension, followed by reward potential and finally object identity (see correlation dendrograms in Figure 14.39D). Such a code was not restricted to the hippocampus, but also found in the medial entorhinal cortex. The lateral entorhinal cortex and perirhinal cortex also showed hierarchical coding of task dimensions, though object identity rather than position was then the driving force (McKenzie et al., 2016). It is unknown whether these cortical schemas depend on the hippocampus or drive the hippocampal firing patterns. Longitudinal and inactivation studies are needed to understand how these correlational structures develop within and across regions.

14.9 Summary and future directions

The central argument of this chapter has been that an emerging consensus on function focusing on episodic memory (or "episodic-like" memory in animals) is well justified in terms of experimental work. Chapter 15 develops this idea from a computational perspective. We summarize our position in relation to Marr's three levels of understanding with which we began.

There is near universal agreement that the *functions* of the hippocampus include the encoding and later retrieval of episodic memories. It remains disputed to what extent the hippocampus is involved in the storage of memories in the long term. The existence of systems consolidation suggests a sharing of responsibilities between the hippocampus and other brain regions but the details remain elusive.

One puzzle concerns the constructive aspects of memory. Human memory is known to be a constructive process where retrieval is aided by our existing knowledge base about common co-occurrences and inference about cause and effect (Schacter and Addis, 2007). Getting at the neurobiology of this is difficult because, in general, animal models for reconstructive memory are lacking. Another puzzle is that, traditionally, memory and perception have been thought to be distinct processes, yet as outlined in Chapter 13, new research shows a role for the hippocampus in perceiving complex scene stimuli. This human perspective could be of clinical relevance.

Turning to *algorithm*, possible algorithmic computations performed by the hippocampus have focused on how the structure could support episodic memory processing and spatial memory. As discussed in sections 14.6 and 14.7, the Hebb-Marr framework for understanding episodic memory has been particularly influential and is now considered the standard model. According to this theory, the fundamental operations of the hippocampus are pattern separation, pattern completion, and signal comparison, which roughly map onto the DG, CA3, and CA1 areas, respectively. The pattern separation formalism, and the notion that ideally each memory is stored as independent memory traces has been influential, but there are important exceptions in the literature showing that multiple similarities between experiences are captured in the hippocampal codes for such experiences. In addition, CA1 receives a direct input from layer III of EC as well as event-related information processed in DG, CA3, and CA2—suggesting it as a likely site where the binding of events to context may occur.

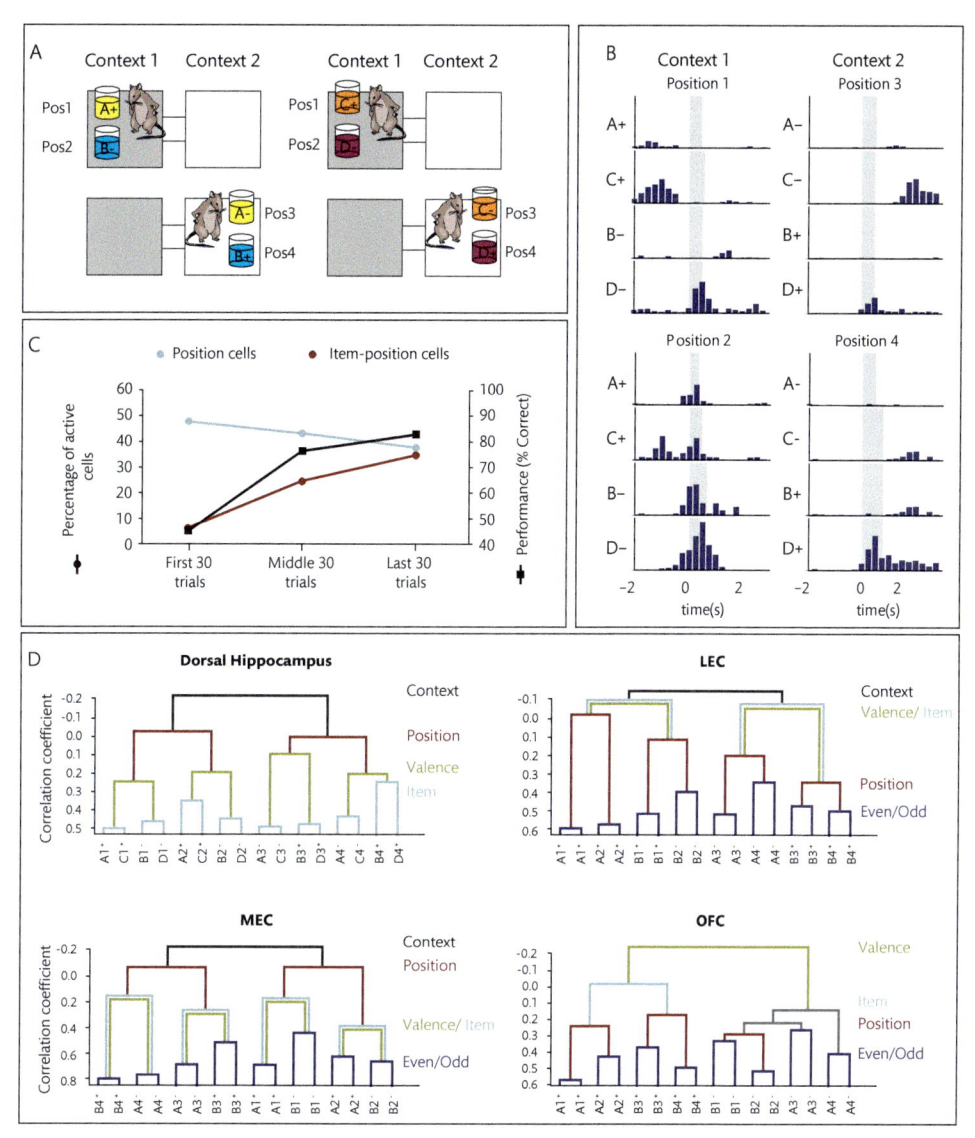

Figure 14.39 Schematic context representation in cell firing. (A) Schematic of the experiment by McKenzie et al. (2014). (B) Responses from a CA3 neuron that showed robust firing to Item D irrespective of position, and robust firing in Position 2 that was modulated by object and object valence. Gray shading indicates the minimum sampling period. (C) As performance increases on the conditional discrimination task, so does the number of recorded item-position cells. (From Komorowski et al., 2013.) (D) Dendrograms illustrating the representational similarity of related events. Neuronal activity recorded from each event type (object and place combination) was compared with correlation coefficients (r) of the population firing rate vector, which were hierarchically grouped according to the most similar event types. In the dorsal hippocampus, four objects were compared (A–D), while in other experiments only two objects (A, B) were tested, and for these experiments, the leaves of the dendrogram show an even/odd comparison. (After McKenzie et al., 2016.)

Frameworks of representation are also explicitly *algorithmic*. The information received from sensory modalities is intrinsically centered on the subject and therefore expressed in egocentric terms. However, this information is converted into an allocentric representation of space in a circuit involving the hippocampus and other brain areas involved in spatial representation (section 14.4). Much progress has been made in the recent years in linking the "unitary blocks" of space representations (place, grid, and head-direction cells) and the growing family of spatially tuned cells (see Chapters 11 and 12), and a system for the logical (inter) conversion between egocentric and allocentric frameworks is starting to emerge, but several aspects await elucidation and clarification. A further algorithmic question concerns how the brain can shift between representing current surroundings and separately accessing information

from the past. The future must also be prospectively imagined as a projection of what is expected to happen next. How can one system toggle between the past, present, and future?

Turning to the *implementational* aspects of memory, a decades-old question is the possible role of synaptic plasticity during learning. One puzzle is that connectionist models, with their focus on synaptic plasticity, may have limited our perspective in considering the plasticity-stability dilemma. Synaptic strength is often modeled as a scalar which changes at a fixed rate much more slowly than network spiking activity. However, the field of dendritic computation is pointing to synapses being dynamic across many timescales and modulated by the activity of dendritic domains, and backpropagation within the cells in which they are embedded. Point attractors are likely an exception in the brain. We do not yet have models for how information could be stored and retrieved in the face of such dynamics, nor do we have the neat proofs for the storage capacity of such dynamic networks.

The issue of synaptic plasticity has been addressed in detail in Chapter 10 and has resurfaced several times in this book, with new work pointing to unexpected facets such as calcium-permeable AMPA receptors and neuromodulation by nonglutamatergic neurons. In section 14.7.7, we saw that some experiments on engram cells have challenged some of the predictions of the SPM hypothesis. Such interpretations are not wholly convincing, and future work needs to elucidate how synaptic changes and nonsynaptic facets of activity (such as excitability) interact with each other in different forms of memory. Intriguingly, new evidence also points a role for nonneuronal cells, mainly astrocytes and microglia, in regulating, enabling, and supporting memory (Kol et al., 2020; Hösli et al., 2022). Glial biology is still conspicuously missing as a consideration in models of memory formation, and, to a lesser extent, this also applies to inhibitory neurons. Overall, future research must ground theories of hippocampal function into biological implementations from the systems through to the molecular level. Computational models, as we will see in the next chapter, will prove fundamental for testing these hypotheses, and the growing brain-wide systematic curation of data stored in public databases like those by the Allen Institute will help to provide the necessary information about the underlying biological networks (Abbott et al., 2020).

REFERENCES

Abbott LF, Bock DD, Callaway EM, Denk W, Dulac C, Fairhall AL, Fiete I, Harris KM, Helmstaedter M, Jain V, et al. (2020) The mind of a mouse. *Cell* 182:1372–1376.

Abdou K, Shehata M, Choko K, Nishizono H, Matsuo M, Muramatsu S-I, Inokuchi K (2018) Synapse-specific representation of the identity of overlapping memory engrams. *Science* 361:1227–1231.

Acharya L, Aghajan ZM, Vuong C, Moore JJ, Mehta MR (2016) Causal influence of visual cues on hippocampal directional selectivity. *Cell* 164:197–207.

Adams CD, Dickinson A (1981) Instrumental responding following reinforcer devaluation. *Quart J Exp Psychol* 33B:109–122.

Aggleton JP (1985) One-trial object recognition by rats. *Quart J Exp Psychol* 37B:279–294.

Aggleton JP (1999) Mapping recognition memory in the primate brain: why it's sometimes right to be wrong. *Brain Res Bull* 50:447–448.

Aggleton JP, Brown MW (1999) Episodic memory, amnesia, and the hippocampal-anterior thalamic axis. *Behav Brain Sci* 22:425–489.

Aggleton JP, Nelson AJD (2020) Distributed interactive brain circuits for object-in-place memory: a place for time? *Brain Neurosci Adv* 4:2398212820933471.

Aggleton JP, Vann SD, Denby C, Dix S, Mayes AR, Roberts N, Yonelinas AP (2005) Sparing of the familiarity component of recognition memory in a patient with hippocampal pathology. *Neuropsychologia* 43:1810–1823.

Ainge JA, Tamosiunaite M, Woergoetter F, Dudchenko PA (2007) Hippocampal CA1 place cells encode intended destination on a maze with multiple choice points. *J Neurosci* 27:9769–9779.

Alexander AS, Carstensen LC, Hinman JR, Raudies F, Chapman GW, Hasselmo ME (2020) Egocentric boundary vector tuning of the retrosplenial cortex. *Sci Adv* 6:eaaz2322.

Alme CB, Miao C, Jezek K, Treves A, Moser EI, Moser MB (2014) Place cells in the hippocampus: eleven maps for eleven rooms. *Proc Natl Acad Sci U S A* 111:18428–18435.

Almog N, Tocker G, Bonnevie T, Moser EI, Moser MB, Derdikman D (2019) During hippocampal inactivation, grid cells maintain synchrony, even when the grid pattern is lost. *Elife* 8:e47147.

Alvarez P, Squire LR (1994) Memory consolidation and the medial temporal lobe: a simple network model. *Proc Natl Acad Sci U S A* 91:7041–7045.

Alyan S, McNaughton BL (1999) Hippocampectomized rats are capable of homing by path integration. *Behav Neurosci* 113:19–31.

Amodio P, Farrar BG, Krupenye C, Ostojic L, Clayton NS (2021) Little evidence that Eurasian jays protect their caches by responding to cues about a conspecific's desire and visual perspective. *Elife* 10:e69647.

Anagnostaras SG, Maren S, Fanselow MS (1999) Temporally graded retrograde amnesia of contextual fear after hippocampal damage in rats: within-subjects examination. *J Neurosci* 19:1106–1114.

Anderson JA, Silverstein JW, Ritz SA, Jones RS (1977) Distinctive features, categorical perception, and probability learning: some applications of a neural model. *Psychol Rev* 84:413–451.

Andersson SO, Moser EI, Moser MB (2021) Visual stimulus features that elicit activity in object-vector cells. *Commun Biol* 4:1219.

Antunes M, Biala G (2012) The novel object recognition memory: neurobiology, test procedure, and its modifications. *Cogn Process* 13:93–110.

Attardo A, Lu J, Kawashima T, Okuno H, Fitzgerald JE, Bito H, Schnitzer MJ (2018) Long-term consolidation of ensemble neural plasticity patterns in hippocampal area CA1. *Cell Rep* 25:640–650, e642.

Babb SJ, Crystal JD (2006) Episodic-like memory in the rat. *Curr Biol* 16:1317–1321.

Bachevalier J, Nemanic S, Alvarado MC (2002) The medial temporal lobe structures and object recognition memory in nonhuman primates: In: Neuropsychology of Memory (Squire LR, Schacter DL, eds), pp 326–339. New York: The Guildford Press.

Bahar AS, Shirvalkar PR, Shapiro ML (2011) Memory-guided learning: CA1 and CA3 neuronal ensembles differentially encode the commonalities and differences between situations. *J Neurosci* 31:12270–12281.

Balleine BW (2019) The meaning of behavior: discriminating reflex and volition in the brain. *Neuron* 104:47–62.

Bannerman DM, Rawlins JN, McHugh SB, Deacon RM, Yee BK, Bast T, Zhang WN, Pothuizen HH, Feldon J (2004) Regional dissociations within the hippocampus—memory and anxiety. *Neurosci Biobehav Rev* 28:273–283.

Barker GR, Bird F, Alexander V, Warburton EC (2007) Recognition memory for objects, place, and temporal order: a disconnection analysis of the role of the medial prefrontal cortex and perirhinal cortex. *J Neurosci* 27:2948–2957.

Barker GR, Warburton EC (2011) When is the hippocampus involved in recognition memory? *J Neurosci* 31:10721–10731.

Barnes CA (1979) Memory deficits associated with senescence: a neurophysiological and behavioral study in the rat. *J Comp Physiol Psychol* 93:74–104.

Barron HC, Reeve HM, Koolschijn RS, Perestenko PV, Shpektor A, Nili H, Rothaermel R, Campo-Urriza N, O'Reilly JX, Bannerman DM, et al. (2020) Neuronal computation underlying inferential reasoning in humans and mice. *Cell* 183:228–243, e221.

Barry C, Hayman R, Burgess N, Jeffery KJ (2007) Experience-dependent rescaling of entorhinal grids. *Nat Neurosci* 10:682–684.

Bartlett FC (1932) Remembering. Cambridge: Cambridge University Press.

Bartsch T, Alfke K, Stingele R, Rohr A, Freitag-Wolf S, Jansen O, Deuschl G (2006) Selective affection of hippocampal CA-1 neurons in patients with transient global amnesia without long-term sequelae. *Brain* 129:2874–2884.

Basile BM, Schroeder GR, Brown EK, Templer VL, Hampton RR (2015) Evaluation of seven hypotheses for metamemory performance in rhesus monkeys. *J Exp Psychol Gen* 144:85–102.

Bast T, da Silva BM, Morris RGM (2005) Distinct contributions of hippocampal NMDA and AMPA receptors to encoding and retrieval of one-trial place memory. *J Neurosci* 25:5845–5856.

Bayley PJ, Frascino JC, Squire LR (2005) Robust habit learning in the absence of awareness and independent of the medial temporal lobe. *Nature* 436:550–553.

Bayley PJ, Hopkins RO, Squire LR (2006) The fate of old memories after medial temporal lobe damage. *J Neurosci* 26:13311–13317.

BBC (1998) Life without memory: the case of Clive Wearing. *Mind.* BBC series.

Berenyi A, Somogyvari Z, Nagy AJ, Roux L, Long JD, Fujisawa S, Stark E, Leonardo A, Harris TD, Buzsáki G (2014) Large-scale, high-density (up to 512 channels) recording of local circuits in behaving animals. *J Neurophysiol* 111:1132–1149.

Berners-Lee A, Feng T, Silva D, Wu X, Ambrose ER, Pfeiffer BE, Foster DJ (2022) Hippocampal replays appear after a single experience and incorporate greater detail with more experience. *Neuron* 110:1829–1842.

Bethus I, Tse D, Morris RG (2010) Dopamine and memory: modulation of the persistence of memory for novel hippocampal NMDA receptor-dependent paired associates. *J Neurosci* 30:1610–1618.

Biegler R, Morris RGM (1993) Landmark stability is a prerequisite for spatial but not discrimination learning. *Nature* 361:631–633.

Boccara CN, Nardin M, Stella F, O'Neill J, Csicsvari J (2019) The entorhinal cognitive map is attracted to goals. *Science* 363:1443–1447.

Boehringer R, Polygalov D, Huang AJY, Middleton SJ, Robert V, Wintzer ME, Piskorowski RA, Chevaleyre V, McHugh TJ (2017) Chronic loss of CA2 transmission leads to hippocampal hyperexcitability. *Neuron* 94:642–655, e649.

Bolhuis JJ, Stewart CA, Forrest EM (1994) Retrograde amnesia and memory reactivation in rats with ibotenate lesions to the hippocampus or subiculum. *Q J Exp Psychol B* 47:129–150.

Bonnevie T, Dunn B, Fyhn M, Hafting T, Derdikman D, Kubie JL, Roudi Y, Moser EI, Moser MB (2013) Grid cells require excitatory drive from the hippocampus. *Nat Neurosci* 16:309–317.

Bontempi B, Laurent_Demir C, Destrade C, Jaffard R (1999) Time-dependent reorganization of brain circuitry underlying long-term memory storage. *Nature* 400:671–675.

Bostock E, Muller RU, Kubie JL (1991) Experience-dependent modifications of hippocampal place cell firing. *Hippocampus* 1:193–205.

Bouton ME (2004) Context and behavioral processes in extinction. *Learn Mem* 11:485–494.

Bouton ME, Moody EW (2004) Memory processes in classical conditioning. *Neurosci Biobehav Rev* 28:663–674.

Boyce R, Glasgow SD, Williams S, Adamantidis A (2016) Causal evidence for the role of REM sleep theta rhythm in contextual memory consolidation. *Science* 352:812–816.

Bransford JD (1979) Human Cognition: Learning, Understanding and Remembering. Belmont, CA: Wadsworth.

Bransford JD, Johnson MK (1972) Contextual prerequisites for understanding: some investigations of comprehension and recall. *J Verb Learn Verb Behav* 11:717–726.

Broadbent N, Lumeij LB, Corcoles M, Ayres AI, Bin Ibrahim MZ, Masatsugu B, Moreno A, Carames JM, Begg E, Strickland L, et al. (2020) A stable home-base promotes allocentric memory representations of episodic-like everyday spatial memory. *Eur J Neurosci* 51:1539–1558.

Broadbent NJ, Gaskin S, Squire LR, Clark RE (2010) Object recognition memory and the rodent hippocampus. *Learn Mem* 17:5–11.

Brun VH, Leutgeb S, Wu HQ, Schwarcz R, Witter MP, Moser EI, Moser MB (2008) Impaired spatial representation in CA1 after lesion of direct input from entorhinal cortex. *Neuron* 57:290–302.

Brun VH, Solstad T, Kjelstrup KB, Fyhn M, Witter MP, Moser EI, Moser MB (2008) Progressive increase in grid scale from dorsal to ventral medial entorhinal cortex. *Hippocampus* 18:1200–1212.

Bruner J (2010) Beyond the Information Given. New York: Routledge.

Buffalo EA (2015) Bridging the gap between spatial and mnemonic views of the hippocampal formation. *Hippocampus* 25:713–718.

Buffalo EA, Stefanacci L, Squire LR, Zola SM (1998) A reexamination of the concurrent discrimination learning task: the importance of anterior inferotemporal cortex, area TE. *Behav Neurosci* 112:3–14.

Bunsey M, Eichenbaum H (1996) Conservation of hippocampal memory function in rats and humans. *Nature* 379:255–257.

Bures J, Fenton AA, Kaminsky Y, Wesierska M, Zahalka A (1998) Rodent navigation after dissociation of the allocentric and idiothetic representations of space. *Neuropharmacology* 37:689–699.

Burgess N, Maguire EA, O'Keefe J (2002) The human hippocampus and spatial and episodic memory. *Neuron* 35:625–641.

Bussey TJ, Muir JL, Aggleton JP (1999) Functionally dissociating aspects of event memory: the effects of combined perirhinal and postrhinal cortex lesions on object and place memory in the rat. *J Neurosci* 19:495–502.

Butler CR, Graham KS, Hodges JR, Kapur N, Wardlaw JM, Zeman AZ (2007) The syndrome of transient epileptic amnesia. *Ann Neurol* 61:587–598.

Butler WN, Hardcastle K, Giocomo LM (2019) Remembered reward locations restructure entorhinal spatial maps. *Science* 363:1447–1452.

Buzsáki G (1989) Two-stage model of memory-trace formation: a role for "noisy" brain states. *Neuroscience* 31:551–570.

Buzsáki G (2019) The Brain from Inside Out. New York: Oxford University Press.

Buzsáki G, Horvath Z, Urioste R, Hetke J, Wise K (1992) High-frequency network oscillation in the hippocampus. *Science* 256:1025–1027.

Buzsáki G, Leung LW, Vanderwolf CH (1983) Cellular bases of hippocampal EEG in the behaving rat. *Brain Res* 287:139–171.

Cai DJ, Aharoni D, Shuman T, Shobe J, Biane J, Song W, Wei B, Veshkini M, La-Vu M, Lou J, et al. (2016) A shared neural ensemble links distinct contextual memories encoded close in time. *Nature* 534:115–118.

Carpenter F, Manson D, Jeffery K, Burgess N, Barry C (2015) Grid cells form a global representation of connected environments. *Curr Biol* 25:1176–1182.

Carr MF, Jadhav SP, Frank LM (2011) Hippocampal replay in the awake state: a potential substrate for memory consolidation and retrieval. *Nat Neurosci* 14:147–153.

Chen TW, Wardill TJ, Sun Y, Pulver SR, Renninger SL, Baohan A, Schreiter ER, Kerr RA, Orger MB, Jayaraman V, et al. (2013) Ultrasensitive fluorescent proteins for imaging neuronal activity. *Nature.* 499:295–300.

Cho HY, Shin W, Lee HS, Lee Y, Kim M, Oh JP, Han JHJ, Jeong Y, Suh B, Kim E, et al. (2021) Turnover of fear engram cells by repeated experience. *Curr Biol* 31:5450–5461, e5454.

Choi JH, Sim SE, Kim JI, Choi DI, Oh J, Ye S, Lee J, Kim T, Ko HG, Lim CS, et al. (2018) Interregional synaptic maps among engram cells underlie memory formation. *Science* 360:430–435.

Chrobak JJ, Lorincz A, Buzsáki G (2000) Physiological patterns in the hippocampo-entorhinal cortex system. *Hippocampus* 10:457–465.

Cirelli C, Tononi G (2017) The sleeping brain. *Cerebrum* 2017:cer-07-17.

Clark RE, Zola SM, Squire LR (2000) Impaired recognition memory in rats after damage to the hippocampus. *J Neurosci* 20:8853–8860.

Clayton NS, Dally JM, Emery NJ (2007) Social cognition by food-caching corvids: the western scrub-jay as a natural psychologist. *Philos Trans R Soc Lond B Biol Sci* **362**:507–522.

Clayton NS, Dickinson A (1998) Episodic-like memory during cache recovery by scrub jays. *Nature* **395**:272–274.

Clayton NS, Griffiths DP, Emery N, Dickinson A (2001) Elements of episodic-like memory in animals. In: Episodic Memory: New Directions in Research.(Baddeley A, Conway M, Aggleton JP, eds), pp 232–248. Oxford: Oxford University Press.

Clayton NS, Yu KS, Dickinson A (2003) Interacting cache memories: evidence for flexible memory use by Western Scrub-Jays (*Aphelocoma californica*). *J Exp Psychol Anim Behav Processes* **29**:14–22.

Cohen NJ, Eichenbaum HE (1993) Memory, Amnesia and the Hippocampal System. Cambridge: MA, MIT Press.

Cohen NJ, Squire LR (1980) Preserved learning and retention of pattern-analyzing skill in amnesia: dissociation of knowing how and knowing that. *Science* **210**:207–210.

Cohen SJ, Stackman RW, Jr (2015) Assessing rodent hippocampal involvement in the novel object recognition task: a review. *Behav Brain Res* **285**:105–117.

Colgin LL, Leutgeb S, Jezek K, Leutgeb JK, Moser EI, McNaughton BL, Moser MB (2010) Attractor-map versus autoassociation based attractor dynamics in the hippocampal network. *J Neurophysiol* **104**:35–50.

Collett TS, Cartwright BA, Smith BA (1986) Landmark learning and visuo-spatial memories in gerbils. *J Comp Psychol A* **158**:835–851.

Collins AM, Quillian MR (1969) Retrieval time from semantic memory. *J Verbal Learning Verbal Behav* **8**:240–247.

Corkin S (1984) Lasting consequences of bilateral medial temporal lobectomy: clinical course and experimental findings in H.M. *Semin Neurol* **4**:249–259.

Corkin S (2002) What's new with the amnesic patient H.M.? *Nat Rev Neurosci* **3**:153–160.

Cowansage KK, Shuman T, Dillingham BC, Chang A, Golshani P, Mayford M (2014) Direct reactivation of a coherent neocortical memory of context. *Neuron* **84**:432–441.

Cowey A, Stoerig P (1995) Blindsight in monkeys. *Nature* **373**:247–249.

Darsaud A, Dehon H, Lahl O, Sterpenich V, Boly M, Dang-Vu T, Desseilles M, Gais S, Matarazzo L, Peters F, et al. (2011) Does sleep promote false memories? *J Cog Neurosci* **23**:26–40.

Davidson TJ, Kloosterman F, Wilson MA (2009) Hippocampal replay of extended experience. *Neuron* **63**:497–507.

Davidson TL, Jarrard LE (1993) A role for hippocampus in the utilization of hunger signals. *Behav Neural Biol* **59**:167–171.

Davidson TL, Jarrard LE (2004) The hippocampus and inhibitory learning: a "gray" area? *Neurosci Biobehav Rev* **28**:261–271.

Day M, Langston R, Morris RG (2003) Glutamate-receptor-mediated encoding and retrieval of paired-associate learning. *Nature* **424**:205–209.

Debiec J, LeDoux JE, Nader K (2002) Cellular and systems reconsolidation in the hippocampus. *Neuron* **36**:527–538.

de Landeta AB, Pereyra M, Medina JH, Katche C (2020) Anterior retrosplenial cortex is required for long-term object recognition memory. *Sci Rep* **10**:4002.

de Lavilléon G, Lacroix MM, Rondi-Reig L, Benchenane K (2015) Explicit memory creation during sleep demonstrates a causal role of place cells in navigation. *Nat Neurosci* **18**:493–495.

De Leonibus E, Costantini VJ, Massaro A, Mandolesi G, Vanni V, Luvisetto S, Pavone F, Oliverio A, Mele A (2011) Cognitive and neural determinants of response strategy in the dual-solution plus-maze task. *Learn Mem* **18**:241–244.

DeNardo LA, Liu CD, Allen WE, Adams EL, Friedmann D, Fu L, Guenthner CJ, Tessier-Lavigne M, Luo L (2019) Temporal evolution of cortical ensembles promoting remote memory retrieval. *Nat Neurosci* **22**:460–469.

Denninger JK, Smith BM, Kirby ED (2018) Novel object recognition and object location behavioral testing in mice on a budget. *J Vis Exp*. (141):10.3791/58593.

Denny CA, Kheirbek MA, Alba EL, Tanaka KF, Brachman RA, Laughman KB, Tomm NK, Turi GF, Losonczy A, Hen R (2014) Hippocampal memory traces are differentially modulated by experience, time, and adult neurogenesis. *Neuron* **83**:189–201.

Deshmukh SS, Knierim JJ (2013) Influence of local objects on hippocampal representations: landmark vectors and memory. *Hippocampus* **23**:253–267.

Devito LM, Kanter BR, Eichenbaum H (2010) The hippocampus contributes to memory expression during transitive inference in mice. *Hippocampus* **20**:208–217.

Diana RA, Yonelinas AP, Ranganath C (2012) Adaptation to cognitive context and item information in the medial temporal lobes. *Neuropsychologia* **50**:3062–3069.

Diba K, Buzsáki G (2007) Forward and reverse hippocampal place-cell sequences during ripples. *Nat Neurosci* **10**:1241–1242.

Diehl GW, Hon OJ, Leutgeb S, Leutgeb JK (2017) Grid and nongrid cells in medial entorhinal cortex represent spatial location and environmental features with complementary coding schemes. *Neuron* **94**:83–92, e86.

DiMattia BV, Kesner RP (1988) Role of the posterior parietal association cortex in the processing of spatial event information. *Behav Neurosci* **102**:397–403.

Dix SL, Aggleton JP (1999) Extending the spontaneous preference test of recognition: evidence of object-location and object-context recognition. *Behav Brain Res* **99**:191–200.

Dragoi G, Tonegawa S (2013) Development of schemas revealed by prior experience and NMDA receptor knock-out. *Elife* **2**:e01326.

Dudai Y (2004) The neurobiology of consolidations, or, how stable is the engram? *Annu Rev Psychol* **55**:51–86.

Dudai Y (2010) The engram revisited: on the elusive permanence of memory. In: The Memory Process: Neuroscientific and Humanistic Perspectives (Nalbantian S, Matthews PM, McClelland JL, eds), pp 29–40. Cambridge, MA: MIT Press.

Dudai Y, Morris RGM (2001) To consolidate or not to consolidate: what are the questions? In: Brain, Perception and Memory: Advances in Cognitive Sciences (Bolhuis J, ed), pp 147–162. Oxford, Oxford University Press.

Dudek SM, Alexander GM, Farris S (2016) Rediscovering area CA2: unique properties and functions. *Nat Rev Neurosci* **17**:89–102.

Dupret D, O'Neill J, Pleydell-Bouverie B, Csicsvari J (2010) The reorganization and reactivation of hippocampal maps predict spatial memory performance. *Nat Neurosci* **13**:995–1002.

Dusek JA, Eichenbaum H (1997) The hippocampus and memory for orderly stimulus relations. *Proc Natl Acad Sci U S A* **94**:7109–7114.

Eacott MJ, Easton A, Zinkivskay A (2005) Recollection in an episodic-like memory task in the rat. *Learn Mem* **12**:221–223.

Eacott MJ, Gaffan EA (2005) The roles of perirhinal cortex, postrhinal cortex, and the fornix in memory for objects, contexts, and events in the rat. *Q J Exp Psychol B* **58**:202–217.

Eacott MJ, Norman G (2004) Integrated memory for object, place, and context in rats: a possible model of episodic-like memory? *J Neurosci* **24**:1948–1953.

Easton A, Webster LA, Eacott MJ (2012) The episodic nature of episodic-like memories. *Learn Mem* **19**:146–150.

Easton A, Zinkivskay A, Eacott MJ (2009) Recollection is impaired, but familiarity remains intact in rats with lesions of the fornix. *Hippocampus* 19:837–843.

Ebbinghaus H (1885) Über das Gedächtnis. Leipzig: Dunker.

Eichenbaum H (2004) Hippocampus: cognitive processes and neural representations that underlie declarative memory. *Neuron* 44:109–120.

Eichenbaum H, Dudchenko P, Wood E, Shapiro M, Tanila H (1999) The hippocampus, memory, and place cells: is it spatial memory or a memory space? *Neuron* 23:209–226.

Eichenbaum H, Stewart C, Morris RGM (1990) Hippocampal representation in place learning. *J Neurosci* 10:3531–3542.

Eichenbaum H, Yonelinas AP, Ranganath C (2007) The medial temporal lobe and recognition memory. *Annu Rev Neurosci* 30:123–152.

Eliav T, Maimon SR, Aljadeff J, Tsodyks M, Ginosar G, Las L, Ulanovsky N (2021) Multiscale representation of very large environments in the hippocampus of flying bats. *Science* 372:eabg4020.

Ellenbogen JM, Hu PT, Payne JD, Titone D, Walker MP (2007) Human relational memory requires time and sleep. *Proc Natl Acad Sci U S A* 104:7723–7728.

Elward RL, Vargha-Khadem F (2018) Semantic memory in developmental amnesia. *Neurosci Lett* 680:23–30.

Emery NJ, Clayton NS (2001) Effects of experience and social context on prospective caching strategies by scrub jays. *Nature* 414:443–446.

Emery NJ, Clayton NS (2004) The mentality of crows: convergent evolution of intelligence in corvids and apes. *Science* 306:1903–1907.

Ennaceur A (2010) One-trial object recognition in rats and mice: methodological and theoretical issues. *Behav Brain Res* 215:244–254.

Ennaceur A, Aggleton JP (1994) Spontaneous recognition of object configurations in rats: effects of fornix lesions. *Exp Brain Res* 100:85–92.

Ennaceur A, Aggleton JP (1997) The effects of neurotoxic lesions of the perirhinal cortex combined to fornix transection on object recognition memory in the rat. *Behav Brain Res* 88:181–193.

Ennaceur A, Delacour J (1988) A new one-trial test for neurobiological studies of memory in rats. 1: Behavioral data. *Behav Brain Res* 31:47–59.

Ennaceur A, Neave N, Aggleton JP (1996) Neurotoxic lesions of the perirhinal cortex do not mimic the behavioural effects of fornix transection in the rat. *Behav Brain Res* 80:9–25.

Epstein RA, Patai EZ, Julian JB, Spiers HJ (2017) The cognitive map in humans: spatial navigation and beyond. *Nat Neurosci* 20:1504–1513.

Eschenko O, Mizumori SJ (2007) Memory influences on hippocampal and striatal neural codes: effects of a shift between task rules. *Neurobiol Learn Mem* 87:495–509.

Etchamendy N, Desmedt A, Cortes-Torrea C, Marighetto A, Jaffard R (2003) Hippocampal lesions and discrimination performance of mice in the radial maze: sparing or impairment depending on the representational demands of the task. *Hippocampus* 13:197–211.

Etienne AS, Maurer R, Berlie J, Reverdin B, Rowe T, Georgakopoulos J, Seguinot V (1998) Navigation through vector addition. *Nature* 396:161–164.

Farooq U, Dragoi G (2019) Emergence of preconfigured and plastic time-compressed sequences in early postnatal development. *Science* 363:168–173.

Ferbinteanu J, Shapiro ML (2003) Prospective and retrospective memory coding in the hippocampus. *Neuron* 40:1227–1239.

Fernandez G, Morris RGM (2018) Memory, novelty and prior knowledge. *Trends Neurosci* 41:654–659.

Fernandez-Ruiz A, Oliva A, Fermino de Oliveira E, Rocha-Almeida F, Tingley D, Buzsáki G (2019) Long-duration hippocampal sharp wave ripples improve memory. *Science* 364:1082–1086.

Fernandez-Velasco P, Spiers HJ (2024) Wayfinding across ocean and tundra: what traditional cultures teach us about navigation. *Trends Cogn Sci* 28:56–71.

Finkelstein A, Derdikman D, Rubin A, Foerster JN, Las L, Ulanovsky N (2015) Three-dimensional head-direction coding in the bat brain. *Nature, Nature Research* 517:159–164.

Folkerts S, Rutishauser U, Howard MW (2018) Human episodic memory retrieval is accompanied by a neural contiguity effect. *J Neurosci* 38:4200–4211.

Forwood SE, Winters BD, Bussey TJ (2005) Hippocampal lesions that abolish spatial maze performance spare object recognition memory at delays of up to 48 hours. *Hippocampus* 15:347–355.

Foster DJ, Wilson MA (2006) Reverse replay of behavioural sequences in hippocampal place cells during the awake state. *Nature* 440:680–683.

Frankland PW, Bontempi B (2005) The organization of recent and remote memories. *Nat Rev Neurosci* 6:119–130.

Frankland PW, Bontempi B, Talton LE, Kaczmarek L, Silva AJ (2004) The involvement of the anterior cingulate cortex in remote contextual fear memory. *Science* 304:881–883.

French RM (1992) Semi-distributed representations and catastrophic forgetting in connectionist networks. *Connect Sci* 4:365–377.

Frey U, Morris RGM (1997) Synaptic tagging and long-term potentiation. *Nature* 385:533–536.

Fried I, MacDonald KA, Wilson CL (1997) Single neuron activity in human hippocampus and amygdala during recognition of faces and objects. *Neuron* 18:753–765.

Fyhn M, Hafting T, Treves A, Moser MB, Moser EI (2007) Hippocampal remapping and grid realignment in entorhinal cortex. *Nature* 446:190–194.

Fyhn M, Molden S, Hollup S, Moser MB, Moser E (2002) Hippocampal neurons responding to first-time dislocation of a target object. *Neuron* 35:555–566.

Fyhn M, Molden S, Witter MP, Moser EI, Moser MB (2004) Spatial representation in the entorhinal cortex. *Science* 305:1258–1264.

Gaffan D (1974) Recognition impaired and association intact in the memory of monkeys after transection of the fornix. *J Comp Physiol Psychol* 86:1100–1109.

Gaffan D (1991) Spatial organization of episodic memory. *Hippocampus* 1:262–264.

Gaffan D (1994) Scene-specific memory for objects: a model of episodic memory impairment in monkeys with fornix transection. *J Cogn Neurosci* 6:305–320.

Gaffan D (2005) Neuroscience: widespread cortical networks underlie memory and attention. *Science* 309:2172–2173.

Gais S, Lucas B, Born J (2006) Sleep after learning aids memory recall. *Learn Mem* 13:259–262.

Garner AR, Rowland DC, Hwang SY, Baumgaertel K, Roth BL, Kentros C, Mayford M (2012) Generation of a synthetic memory trace. *Science* 335:1513–1516.

Gelbard-Sagiv H, Mukamel R, Harel M, Malach R, Fried I (2008) Internally generated reactivation of single neurons in human hippocampus during free recall. *Science* 322:96–101.

Ghandour K, Ohkawa N, Fung CCA, Asai H, Saitoh Y, Takekawa T, Okubo-Suzuki R, Soya S, Nishizono H, Matsuo M, et al. (2019) Orchestrated ensemble activities constitute a hippocampal memory engram. *Nature Commun* 10:1–14.

Ghosh VE, Gilboa A (2014) What is a memory schema? A historical perspective on current neuroscience literature. *Neuropsychologia* 53:104–114.

Gillespie AK, Astudillo Maya DA, Denovellis EL, Liu DF, Kastner DB, Coulter ME, Roumis DK, Eden UT, Frank LM (2021) Hippocampal replay reflects specific past experiences rather than a plan for subsequent choice. *Neuron* 109:3149–3163, e3146.

Girardeau G, Benchenane K, Wiener SI, Buzsáki G, Zugaro MB (2009) Selective suppression of hippocampal ripples impairs spatial memory. *Nat Neurosci* 12:1222–1223.

Gluck MA, Myers CE (1993) Hippocampal mediation of stimulus representation: a computational theory. *Hippocampus* 3:1–26.

Gobbo F, Cattaneo A (2020) Neuronal activity at synapse resolution: reporters and effectors for synaptic neuroscience. *Front Mol Neurosci* 13:572312.

Gobbo F, Mitchell-Heggs R, Tse D, Al Omrani M, Spooner PA, Schultz SR, Morris RGM (2022) Neuronal signature of spatial decision-making during navigation by freely moving rats by using calcium imaging. *Proc Natl Acad Sci U S A* 119:e2212152119.

Gofman X, Tocker G, Weiss S, Boccara CN, Lu L, Moser MB, Moser EI, Morris G, Derdikman D (2019) Dissociation between postrhinal cortex and downstream parahippocampal regions in the representation of egocentric boundaries. *Curr Biol* 29:2751–2757, e2754.

Gonzalez WG, Zhang H, Harutyunyan A, Lois C (2019) Persistence of neuronal representations through time and damage in the hippocampus. *Science* 365:821–825.

Good M, Honey RC (1991) Conditioning and contextual retrieval in hippocampal rats. *Behav Neurosci* 105:499–509.

Good MA, Barnes P, Staal V, McGregor A, Honey RC (2007) Context- but not familiarity-dependent forms of object recognition are impaired following excitotoxic hippocampal lesions in rats. *Behav Neurosci* 121:218–223.

Goode TD, Tanaka KZ, Sahay A, McHugh TJ (2020) An integrated index: engrams, place cells, and hippocampal memory. *Neuron* 107:805–820.

Goshen I, Brodsky M, Prakash R, Wallace J, Gradinaru V, Ramakrishnan C, Deisseroth K (2011) Dynamics of retrieval strategies for remote memories. *Cell* 147:678–689.

Goto A, Bota A, Miya K, Wang J, Tsukamoto S, Jiang X, Hirai D, Murayama M, Matsuda T, McHugh TJ, et al. (2021) Stepwise synaptic plasticity events drive the early phase of memory consolidation. *Science* 374:857–863.

Gray JA (1982) The Neuropsychology of Anxiety: An Enquiry into the Functions of the Septo-Hippocampal System. Oxford: Oxford University Press.

Gridchyn I, Schoenenberger P, O'Neill J, Csicsvari J (2020) Optogenetic inhibition-mediated activity-dependent modification of CA1 pyramidal-interneuron connections during behavior. *Elife* 9:e61106.

Grieves RM, Jedidi-Ayoub S, Mishchanchuk K, Liu A, Renaudineau S, Duvelle É, Jeffery KJ (2021) Irregular distribution of grid cell firing fields in rats exploring a 3D volumetric space. *Nat Neurosci* 24:1567–1573.

Grieves RM, Jedidi-Ayoub S, Mishchanchuk K, Liu A, Renaudineau S, Jeffery KJ (2020) The place-cell representation of volumetric space in rats. *Nature Commun* 11:789.

Grieves RM, Jenkins BW, Harland BC, Wood ER, Dudchenko PA (2016) Place field repetition and spatial learning in a multicompartment environment. *Hippocampus* 26:118–134.

Grieves RM, Wood ER, Dudchenko PA (2016) Place cells on a maze encode routes rather than destinations. *eLife* 5:e15986.

Gupta AS, van der Meer MA, Touretzky DS, Redish AD (2010) Hippocampal replay is not a simple function of experience. *Neuron* 65:695–705.

Guskjolen A, Kenney JW, de la Parra J, Yeung BrA, Josselyn SA, Frankland PW (2018) Recovery of "lost" infant memories in mice. *Curr Biol* 28:2283–2290, e2283.

Guzowski JF (2002) Insights into immediate-early gene function in hippocampal memory consolidation using antisense oligonucleotide and fluorescent imaging approaches. *Hippocampus* 12:86–104.

Guzowski JF, McNaughton BL, Barnes CA, Worley PF (1999) Environment-specific expression of the immediate-early gene Arc in hippocampal neuronal ensembles. *Nat Neurosci* 2:1120–1124.

Hafting T, Fyhn M, Molden S, Moser MB, Moser EI (2005) Microstructure of a spatial map in the entorhinal cortex. *Nature* 436:801–806.

Hainmueller T, Bartos M (2018) Parallel emergence of stable and dynamic memory engrams in the hippocampus. *Nature* 558:292–296.

Hales JB, Schlesiger MI, Leutgeb JK, Squire LR, Leutgeb S, Clark RE (2014) Medial entorhinal cortex lesions only partially disrupt hippocampal place cells and hippocampus-dependent place memory. *Cell Rep* 9:893–901.

Halgren E, Wilson CL (1985) Recall deficits produced by afterdischarges in the human hippocampal formation and amygdala. *Electroencephalogr Clin Neurophysiol* 61:375–380.

Hampson RE, Pons TP, Stanford TR, Deadwyler SA (2004) Categorization in the monkey hippocampus: a possible mechanism for encoding information into memory. *Proc Natl Acad Sci U S A* 101:3184–3189.

Hampton RR (2001) Rhesus monkeys know when they remember. *Proc Natl Acad Sci U S A* 98:5359–5362.

Hampton RR (2009) Multiple demonstrations of metacognition in nonhumans: converging evidence or multiple mechanisms? *Comp Cogn Behav Rev* 4:17–28.

Hargreaves EL, Rao G, Lee I, Knierim JJ (2005) Major dissociation between medial and lateral entorhinal input to dorsal hippocampus. *Science* 308:1792–1794.

Harland B, Contreras M, Souder M, Fellous JM (2021) Dorsal CA1 hippocampal place cells form a multi-scale representation of megaspace. *Curr Biol* 31:2178–2190, e2176.

Harland B, Grieves RM, Bett D, Stentiford R, Wood ER, Dudchenko PA (2017) Lesions of the head direction cell system increase hippocampal place field repetition. *Curr Biol* 27:2706–2712, e2702.

Hartley T, Burgess N, Lever C, Cacucci F, O'Keefe J (2000) Modeling place fields in terms of the cortical inputs to the hippocampus. *Hippocampus* 10:369–379.

Harvey CD, Collman F, Dombeck DA, Tank DW (2009) Intracellular dynamics of hippocampal place cells during virtual navigation. *Nature* 461:941–946.

Hasselmo ME, Wyble BP (1997) Free recall and recognition in a network model of the hippocampus: simulating effects of scopolamine on human memory function. *Behav Brain Res* 89:1–34.

Hasselmo ME, Wyble BP, Wallenstein GV (1996) Encoding and retrieval of episodic memories: role of cholinergic and GABAergic modulation in the hippocampus. *Hippocampus* 6:693–708.

Hayashi-Takagi A, Yagishita S, Nakamura M, Shirai F, Wu YI, Loshbaugh AL, Kuhlman B, Hahn KM, Kasai H (2015) Labelling and optical erasure of synaptic memory traces in the motor cortex. *Nature* 525:333–338.

Hayman R, Verriotis MA, Jovalekic A, Fenton AA, Jeffery KJ (2011) Anisotropic encoding of three-dimensional space by place cells and grid cells. *Nat Neurosci* 14:1182–1190.

Hebb DO (1949) The Organization of Behaviour. New York: Wiley.

Hensler JG (2006) Serotonergic modulation of the limbic system. *Neurosci Biobehav Rev* 30:203–214.

Hinman JR, Chapman GW, Hasselmo ME (2019) Neuronal representation of environmental boundaries in egocentric coordinates. *Nat Commun* 10:2772.

Hinton GE (1989) Connectionist learning procedures. *Artif Intell* 40:185–234.

Hitti FL, Siegelbaum SA (2014) The hippocampal CA2 region is essential for social memory. *Nature* 508:88–92.

Hok V, Lenck-Santini PP, Roux S, Save E, Muller RU, Poucet B (2007) Goal-related activity in hippocampal place cells. *J Neurosci* 27:472–482.

Hollup SA, Molden S, Donnett JG, Moser M-B, Moser EI (2001) Accumulation of hippocampal place fields at the goal location in an annular watermaze task. *J Neurosci* 21:1653–1644.

Honey RC, Good M (1993) Selective hippocampal lesions abolish the contextual specificity of latent inhibition and of conditioning. *Behav Neurosci* 107:22–33.

Hopfield JJ (1982) Neural networks and physical systems with emergent collective computational abilities. *Proc Natl Acad Sci U S A* 79:3088–3092.

Horn G (1967) Neuronal mechanisms of habituation. *Nature* 215:707–711.

Horn G (2004) Pathways of the past: the imprint of memory. *Nat Rev Neurosci* 5:108–120.

Hösli L, Binini N, Ferrari KD, Thieren L, Looser ZJ, Zuend M, Zanker HS, Berry S, Holub M, Möbius W, et al. (2022) Decoupling astrocytes in adult mice impairs synaptic plasticity and spatial learning. *Cell Rep* 38:110484.

Howard MW, Kahana MJ (1999) Contextual variability and serial position effects in free recall. *J Exp Psychol Learn Mem Cogn* 25:923–941.

Howard MW, Shankar KH, Aue WR, Criss AH (2015) A distributed representation of internal time. *Psychol Rev* 122:24–53.

Howard MW, Viskontas IV, Shankar KH, Fried I (2012) Ensembles of human MTL neurons "jump back in time" in response to a repeated stimulus. *Hippocampus* 22:1833–1847.

Howard MW, Youker TE, Venkatadass VS (2008) The persistence of memory: contiguity effects across hundreds of seconds. *Psychon Bull Rev* 15:58–63.

Høydal ØA, Skytoen ER, Andersson SO, Moser MB, Moser EI (2019) Object-vector coding in the medial entorhinal cortex. *Nature* 568:400–404.

Idzikowski C (1984) Sleep and memory. *Br J Psychol* 75(Pt 4):439–449.

Jadhav SP, Kemere C, German PW, Frank LM (2012) Awake hippocampal sharp-wave ripples support spatial memory. *Science* 336:1454–1458.

Jadhav SP, Rothschild G, Roumis DK, Frank LM (2016) Coordinated excitation and inhibition of prefrontal ensembles during awake hippocampal sharp-wave ripple events. *Neuron* 90:113–127.

Jankowski MM, O'Mara SM (2015) Dynamics of place, boundary and object encoding in rat anterior claustrum. *Front Behav Neurosci* 9:250.

Jeffery, KJ (2024). The mosaic structure of the mammalian cognitive map. *Learn Behav* 52:1–16.

Jeffery KJ, Gilbert A, Burton S, Strudwick A (2003) Preserved performance in a hippocampal-dependent spatial task despite complete place cell remapping. *Hippocampus* 13:175–189.

Jeffery KJ, Jovalekic A, Verriotis M, Hayman R (2013) Navigating in a three-dimensional world. *Behav Brain Sci* 36:523–543.

Jenkins JG, Dallenbach KM (1924) Obliviscence during sleep and waking. *Am J Psychol* 35:605–612.

Ji D, Wilson MA (2007) Coordinated memory replay in the visual cortex and hippocampus during sleep. *Nat Neurosci* 10:100–107.

Josselyn SA, Tonegawa S (2020) Memory engrams: recalling the past and imagining the future. *Science* 367:eaaw4325.

Jozet-Alves C, Bertin M, Clayton NS (2013) Evidence of episodic-like memory in cuttlefish. *Curr Biol* 23:R1033–1035.

Jung MW, Wiener SI, McNaughton BL (1994) Comparison of spatial firing characteristics of units in dorsal and ventral hippocampus of the rat. *J Neurosci* 14:7347–7356.

Kandel ER, Squire LR (2000) Neuroscience: breaking down scientific barriers to the study of brain and mind. *Science* 290:1113–1120.

Karimi Abadchi J, Nazari-Ahangarkolaee M, Gattas S, Bermudez-Contreras E, Luczak A, McNaughton BL, Mohajerani MH (2020) Spatiotemporal patterns of neocortical activity around hippocampal sharp-wave ripples. *Elife* 9:e51972.

Keene CS, Bucci DJ (2008) Involvement of the retrosplenial cortex in processing multiple conditioned stimuli. *Behav Neurosci* 122:651–658.

Kempadoo KA, Mosharov EV, Choi SJ, Sulzer D, Kandel ER (2016) Dopamine release from the locus coeruleus to the dorsal hippocampus promotes spatial learning and memory. *Proc Natl Acad Sci U S A* 113:14835–14840.

Kesner RP (1998) Neurobiological views of memory. In: Neurobiology of Learning and Memory (Martinez JL, Kesner RP, eds), pp 361–416. San Diego: Academic Press.

Kesner RP (2000) Behavioral analysis of the contribution of the hippocampus and parietal cortex to the processing of information: interactions and dissociations. *Hippocampus* 10:483–490.

Kesner RP, Bolland BL, Dakis M (1993) Memory for spatial locations, motor responses, and objects: triple dissociation among the hippocampus, caudate nucleus, and extrastriate visual cortex. *Exp Brain Res* 93:462–470.

Kesner RP, Farnsworth G, DiMattia BV (1989) Double dissociation of egocentric and allocentric space following medial prefrontal and parietal cortex lesions in the rat. *Behav Neurosci* 103:956–961.

Kim JJ, Choi J-S, Lee HJ (2016) Foraging in the face of fear: novel strategies for evaluating amygdala functions in rats. In: Living without an amygdala (Amaral DG, Adolphs RR, eds), pp 129–148. New York: Guilford Press.

Kim JJ, Diamond DM (2002) The stressed hippocampus, synaptic plasticity and lost memories. *Nat Rev Neurosci* 3:453–462.

Kim JJ, Fanselow MS (1992) Modality-specific retrograde amnesia of fear. *Science* 256:675–677.

Kim WB, Cho JH (2017) Encoding of discriminative fear memory by input-specific LTP in the amygdala. *Neuron* 95:1129–1146, e1125.

Kirwan CB, Bayley PJ, Galvan VV, Squire LR (2008) Detailed recollection of remote autobiographical memory after damage to the medial temporal lobe. *Proc Natl Acad Sci U S A* 105:2676–2680.

Kitamura T, Macdonald CJ, Tonegawa S (2015) Entorhinal-hippocampal neuronal circuits bridge temporally discontiguous events. *Learn Mem* 2:438–443.

Kitamura T, Ogawa SK, Roy DS, Okuyama T, Morrissey MD, Smith LM, Redondo RL, Tonegawa S (2017) Engrams and circuits crucial for systems consolidation of a memory. *Science* 356:73–78.

Kjelstrup KB, Solstad T, Brun VH, Hafting T, Leutgeb S, Witter MP, Moser EI, Moser MB (2008) Finite scale of spatial representation in the hippocampus. *Science* 321:140–143.

Klinzing JG, Niethard N, Born J (2019) Mechanisms of systems memory consolidation during sleep. *Nat Neurosci* 22:1598–1610.

Knierim JJ, Kudrimoti HS, McNaughton BL (1995) Place cells, head direction cells, and the learning of landmark stability. *J Neurosci* 15:1648–1659.

Knierim JJ, McNaughton BL, Poe GR (2000) Three-dimensional spatial selectivity of hippocampal neurons during space flight. *Nat Neurosci* 3:209–210.

Kobayashi T, Nishijo H, Fukuda M, Bures J, Ono T (1997) Task-dependent representations in rat hippocampal place neurons. *J Neurophysiol* 78:597–613.

Kohl J, Dulac C (2018) Neural control of parental behaviors. *Curr Opin Neurobiol* 49:116–122.

Kohonen T (1972) Correlation matrix memories. *IEEE Trans Comp* 100:353–359.

Kol A, Adamsky A, Groysman M, Kreisel T, London M, Goshen I (2020) Astrocytes contribute to remote memory formation by modulating hippocampal–cortical communication during learning. *Nat Neurosci* 23:1229–1239.

Komorowski RW, Garcia CG, Wilson A, Hattori S, Howard MW, Eichenbaum H (2013) Ventral hippocampal neurons are shaped by experience to represent behaviorally relevant contexts. *J Neurosci* 33(18):8079–8087.

Komorowski RW, Manns JR, Eichenbaum H (2009) Robust conjunctive item-place coding by hippocampal neurons parallels learning what happens where. *J Neurosci* 29:9918–9929.

Kosaki Y, Pearce JM, McGregor A (2018) The response strategy and the place strategy in a plus-maze have different sensitivities to devaluation of expected outcome. *Hippocampus* 28:484–496.

Krause EL, Drugowitsch J (2022) A large majority of awake hippocampal sharp-wave ripples feature spatial trajectories with momentum. *Neuron* 110:722–733, e728.

Kreiman G, Koch C, Fried I (2000) Category-specific visual responses of single neurons in the human medial temporal lobe. *Nat Neurosci* 3:946–953.

Kumaran, D, Hassabis, D, McClelland JL (2016) What learning systems do intelligent agents need? complementary learning systems theory updated. *Trends Cogn Sci* 20:512–534.

Kumaran D, McClelland JL (2012) Generalization through the recurrent interaction of episodic memories: a model of the hippocampal system. *Psychol Rev* 119:573–616.

Kung KS, Greco K, Sobolevsky S, Ratti C (2014) Exploring universal patterns in human home-work commuting from mobile phone data. *PloS One* 9:e96180.

Langston RF, Wood ER (2010) Associative recognition and the hippocampus: differential effects of hippocampal lesions on object-place, object-context and object-place-context memory. *Hippocampus* 20:1139–1153.

Laroche S, Redini-Del Negro C, Clements MP, Lynch MA (1990) Long-term activation of phosphoinositide turnover associated with increased release of amino acids in the dentate gyrus and hippocampus following classical conditioning in the rat. *Eur J Neurosci* 2:534–543.

Lashley KS (1950) In search of the engram. In: Society for Experimental Biology. Physiological mechanisms in animal behavior. (*Society's Symposium IV.*) (pp. 454–482). Academic Press.

LeDoux JE (2000) Emotion circuits in the brain. *Annu Rev Neurosci* 23:155–184.

Lehmann H, Lacanilao S, Sutherland RJ (2007) Complete or partial hippocampal damage produces equivalent retrograde amnesia for remote contextual fear memories. *Eur J Neurosci* 25:1278–1286.

Lemon N, Manahan-Vaughan D (2006) Dopamine D1/D5 receptors gate the acquisition of novel information through hippocampal long-term potentiation and long-term depression. *J Neurosci* 26:7723–7729.

Lesburgueres E, Gobbo OL, Alaux-Cantin S, Hambucken A, Trifilieff P, Bontempi B (2011) Early tagging of cortical networks is required for the formation of enduring associative memory. *Science* 331:924–928.

Leutgeb S, Leutgeb JK (2007) Pattern separation, pattern completion, and new neuronal codes within a continuous CA3 map. *Learn Mem* 14:745–757.

Leutgeb S, Leutgeb JK, Barnes CA, Moser EI, McNaughton BL, Moser MB (2005) Independent codes for spatial and episodic memory in hippocampal neuronal ensembles. *Science* 309:619–623.

Leutgeb S, Leutgeb JK, Treves A, Moser MB, Moser EI (2004) Distinct ensemble codes in hippocampal areas CA3 and CA1. *Science* 305:1295–1298.

Lewis DJ, Misanin JR, Miller RR (1968) Recovery of memory following amnesia. *Nature* 220:704–705.

Li S, Cullen WK, Anwyl R, Rowan MJ (2003) Dopamine-dependent facilitation of LTP induction in hippocampal CA1 by exposure to spatial novelty. *Nat Neurosci* 6:526–531.

Lisman J, Cooper K, Sehgal M, Silva AJ (2018) Memory formation depends on both synapse-specific modifications of synaptic strength and cell-specific increases in excitability. *Nat Neurosci* 21:309–314.

Liu C, Todorova R, Tang W, Oliva A, Fernández-Ruiz A (2023) Associative and predictive hippocampal codes support memory-guided behaviors. *Science* 382:eadi8237.

Liu P, Bilkey DK (2002) The effects of NMDA lesions centered on the postrhinal cortex on spatial memory tasks in the rat. *Behav Neurosci* 116:860–873.

Liu X, Ramirez S, Pang PT, Puryear CB, Govindarajan A, Deisseroth K, Tonegawa S (2012) Optogenetic stimulation of a hippocampal engram activates fear memory recall. *Nature* 484:381–385.

Logothetis NK, Eschenko O, Murayama Y, Augath M, Steudel T, Evrard HC, Besserve M, Oeltermann A (2012) Hippocampal-cortical interaction during periods of subcortical silence. *Nature* 491:547–553.

Logothetis NK, Pauls J, Augath M, Trinath T, Oeltermann A (2001) Neurophysiological investigation of the basis of the fMRI signal. *Nature* 412:150–157.

Long X, Zhang SJ (2021) A novel somatosensory spatial navigation system outside the hippocampal formation. *Cell Res* 31:649–663.

Lu L, Leutgeb JK, Tsao A, Henriksen EJ, Leutgeb S, Barnes CA, Witter MP, Moser MB, Moser EI (2013) Impaired hippocampal rate coding after lesions of the lateral entorhinal cortex. *Nat Neurosci* 16:1085–1093.

Lyttle D, Gereke B, Lin KK, Fellous JM (2013) Spatial scale and place field stability in a grid-to-place cell model of the dorsoventral axis of the hippocampus. *Hippocampus* 23:729–744.

MacDonald CJ, Lepage KQ, Eden UT, Eichenbaum H (2011) Hippocampal "time cells" bridge the gap in memory for discontiguous events. *Neuron* 71:737–749.

Mackintosh NJ (2002) Do not ask whether they have a cognitive map, but how they find their way about. *Psicologica* 23:165–185.

Maguire EA, Nannery R, Spiers HJ (2006) Navigation around London by a taxi driver with bilateral hippocampal lesions. *Brain* 129:2894–2907.

Maingret N, Girardeau G, Todorova R, Goutierre M, Zugaro M (2016) Hippocampo-cortical coupling mediates memory consolidation during sleep. *Nat Neurosci* 19:959–964.

Mandler G (1980) Recognizing: the judgement of previous occurrence. *Psychol Rev* 87:252–271.

Mankin EA, Sparks FT, Slayyeh B, Sutherland RJ, Leutgeb S, Leutgeb JK (2012) Neuronal code for extended time in the hippocampus. *Proc Natl Acad Sci U S A* 109:19462–19467.

Manns JR, Hopkins RO, Reed JM, Kitchener EG, Squire LR (2003) Recognition memory and the human hippocampus. *Neuron* 37:171–180.

Manns JR, Hopkins RO, Squire LR (2003) Semantic memory and the human hippocampus. *Neuron* 38:127–133.

Manns JR, Howard MW, Eichenbaum H (2007) Gradual changes in hippocampal activity support remembering the order of events. *Neuron* 56:530–540.

Markus EJ, Qin YL, Leonard B, Skaggs WE, McNaughton BL, Barnes CA (1995) Interactions between location and task affect the spatial and directional firing of hippocampal neurons. *J Neurosci* 15:7079–7094.

Marr D (1971) Simple memory: a theory for archicortex. *Philos Trans R Soc Lond B Biol Sci* 262:23–81.

Marr D (1982) Vision. Cambridge, MA: MIT Press.

Marshel JH, Kim YS, Machado TA, Quirin S, Benson B, Kadmon J, Raja C, Chibukhchyan A, Ramakrishnan C, Inoue M, et al. (2019) Cortical layer-specific critical dynamics triggering perception. *Science* 365:eaaw5202.

Martin SJ, de Hoz L, Morris RGM (2005) Retrograde amnesia: neither partial nor complete hippocampal lesions in rats result in preferential sparing of remote spatial memory, even after reminding. *Neuropsychologia* 43:609–624.

Martin SJ, Grimwood PD, Morris RG (2000) Synaptic plasticity and memory: an evaluation of the hypothesis. *Annu Rev Neurosci* 23:649–711.

Matsuo N (2015) Irreplaceability of neuronal ensembles after memory allocation. *Cell Rep* 11:351–357.

Matsuo N, Reijmers L, Mayford M, Myers RM (2008) Spine-type-specific recruitment of newly synthesized ampa receptors with learning. *Science* 319:1104–1107.

Matsuzaki M, Honkura N, Ellis-Davies GCR, Kasai H (2004) Structural basis of long-term potentiation in single dendritic spines. *Nature* 429:761–766.

Maviel T, Durkin TP, Menzaghi F, Bontempi B (2004) Sites of neocortical reorganization critical for remote spatial memory. *Science* 305:96–99.

Mayes AR, Holdstock JS, Isaac CL, Montaldi D, Grigor J, Gummer A, Cariga P, Downes JJ, Tsivilis D, Gaffan D, et al. (2004) Associative recognition in a patient with selective hippocampal lesions and relatively normal item recognition. *Hippocampus* 14:763–784.

McCarthy RA, Warrington EA (1990) Cognitive Neuropsychology. San Diego: Academic Press.

McClelland JL (2013) Incorporating rapid neocortical learning of new schema-consistent information into complementary learning systems theory. *J Exp Psychol Gen* 142:1190–1210.

McClelland JL, McNaughton BL, O'Reilly RC (1995) Why there are complementary learning systems in the hippocampus and neocortex: insights from the successes and failures of connectionist models of learning and memory. *Psychol Rev* 102:419–457.

McCulloch WS, Pitts W (1943) A logical calculus of the ideas immanent in nervous activity. *Bull Math Biophys* 5:115–133.

McGonigle B, Margaret C (1992) Monkeys are rational! *Q J Exp Psychol* 45:189–228.

McGonigle BO, Chalmers M (1977) Are monkeys logical? *Nature* 267:694–696.

McGonigle BO, Chalmers M (2003) The growth of cognitive structures in monkeys and men. In: Animal Cognition and Sequential Behavior: Behavioral, Biological and Computational Perspectives (Fountain SB, Bunsey MD, Danks JH, McBeath MK, eds), pp 269–314. Boston: Kluver Academic.

McKenzie S, Frank AJ, Kinsky NR, Porter B, Riviere PD, Eichenbaum H (2014) Hippocampal representation of related and opposing memories develop within distinct, hierarchically organized neural schemas. *Neuron* 83:202–215.

McKenzie S, Huszar R, English DF, Kim K, Christensen F, Yoon E, Buzsáki G (2021) Preexisting hippocampal network dynamics constrain optogenetically induced place fields. *Neuron* 109:1040–1054, e1047.

McKenzie S, Keene CS, Farovik A, Bladon J, Place R, Komorowski R, Eichenbaum H (2016) Representation of memories in the cortical-hippocampal system: results from the application of population similarity analyses. *Neurobiol Learn Mem* 134(Pt A):178–191.

McNaughton B (1996) Cognitive cartography. *Nature* 381:368–369.

McNaughton BL, Barnes CA, Battaglia FP, Bower MR, Cowen SL, Ekstrom AD, Gerrard JL, Hoffman KL, Houston FP, Karten Y, et al. (2003) Off-line reprocessing of recent memory and its role in memory consolidation: a progress report. In: Sleep and Synaptic Plasticity (Smith C, Maquet P, eds), pp 225–246. New York: Oxford University Press.

McNaughton BL, Barnes CA, Gerrard JL, Gothard K, Jung MW, Knierim JJ, Kudrimoti H, Qin Y, Skaggs WE, Suster M, et al. (1996) Deciphering the hippocampal polyglot: the hippocampus as a path integration system. *J Exp Biol* 199:173–185.

McNaughton BL, Barnes CA, O'Keefe J (1983) The contributions of position, direction, and velocity to single unit activity in the hippocampus of freely-moving rats. *Exp Brain Res* 52:41–49.

McNaughton BL, Chen LL, Markus EJ (1991) "Dead reckoning," landmark learning, and the sense of direction: a neurophysiological and computational hypothesis. *J Cogn Neurosci* 3:190–202.

McNaughton BL, Morris RGM (1987) Hippocampal synaptic enhancement and information storage within a distributed memory system. *TINS* 10:408–415.

McNaughton BL, O'Keefe J, Barnes CA (1983) The stereotrode: a new technique for simultaneous isolation of several single units in the central nervous system from multiple unit records. *J Neurosci Methods* 8:391–397.

Meira T, Leroy F, Buss EW, Oliva A, Park J, Siegelbaum SA (2018) A hippocampal circuit linking dorsal CA2 to ventral CA1 critical for social memory dynamics. *Nat Commun* 9:4163.

Meunier M, Bachevalier J, Mishkin M, Murray EA (1993) Effects on visual recognition of combined and separate ablations of the entorhinal and perirhinal cortex in Rhesus monkeys. *J Neurosci* 13:5418–5432.

Malanowski, S (2016) Is episodic memory uniquely human? Evaluating the episodic-like memory research program. *Synthese* 193:1433–1455.

Milczarek MM, Vann SD, Sengpiel F (2018) Spatial memory engram in the mouse retrosplenial cortex. *Curr Biol* 28:1975–1980, e1976.

Miller JF, Neufang M, Solway A, Brandt A, Trippel M, Mader I, Hefft S, Merkow M, Polyn SM, Jacobs J, et al. (2013) Neural activity in human hippocampal formation reveals the spatial context of retrieved memories. *Science* 342:1111–1114.

Miller KJ, Botvinick MM, Brody CD (2017) Dorsal hippocampus contributes to model-based planning. *Nat Neurosci* 20:1269–1276.

Milner B, Corkin S, Teuber HL (1968) Further analysis of the hippocampal amnesic syndrome: 14-year follow-up study of H.M. *Neuropsychologia* 6:215–234

Misanin JR, Miller RR, Lewis DJ (1968) Retrograde amnesia produced by electroconvulsive shock after reactivation of a consolidated memory trace. *Science* 160:554–555.

Mishkin M (1978) Memory in monkeys severely impaired by combined but not by separate removal of amygdala and hippocampus. *Nature* 273:297–298.

Mishkin M, Delacour J (1975) An analysis of short-term visual memory in the monkey. *J Exp Psychol Anim Behav Process* 1:326–334.

Mittelstaedt H, Mittelstaedt M (1982) Homing by path integration. In: Avian Navigation (Papi F, Wallraff HG, eds), pp 290–297. Berlin; Heidelberg: Springer-Verlag.

Moita MA, Rosis S, Zhou Y, LeDoux JE, Blair HT (2003) Hippocampal place cells acquire location-specific responses to the conditioned stimulus during auditory fear conditioning. *Neuron* 37:485–497.

Moncada D, Viola H (2007) Induction of long-term memory by exposure to novelty requires protein synthesis: evidence for a behavioral tagging. *J Neurosci* 27:7476–7481.

Morris RGM (1981) Spatial localisation does not depend on the presence of local cues. *Learning and Motivation* 12:239–260.

Morris RGM (1989) Does the hippocampus play a disproportionate role in spatial memory? In: FESN Study Group on Learning and Memory (Shimamura A, Squire LR, Mishkin M, eds), pp 39–45. Elsevier: Geneva.

Morris RGM (1991) Distinctive computations and relevant associative processes: hippocampal role in processing, retrieval, but not storage of allocentric spatial memory. *Hippocampus* 1:287–290.

Morris RGM (2006) Elements of a neurobiological theory of the hippocampus: the role of activity-dependent synaptic plasticity in episodic-like memory. *Eur J Neurosci* 23:2829–2846.

Morris RGM, Frey U (1997) Hippocampal synaptic plasticity: role in spatial learning or the automatic recording of attended experience? *Philos Trans R Soc Lond B Biol Sci* 352:1489–1503.

Morris RGM, Garrud P, Rawlins JN, O'Keefe J (1982) Place navigation impaired in rats with hippocampal lesions. *Nature* 297:681–683.

Morris RGM, Martin SJ, Moser EI, Riedel G, Sandin J, Day M, O'Carroll C (2003) Elements of a neurobiological theory of the hippocampus: the role of activity-dependent synaptic plasticity in memory. *Philos Trans R Soc Lond B Biol Sci* 358:773–786.

Morris RGM, Schenk F, Tweedie F, Jarrard LE (1990) Ibotenate lesions of hippocampus and/or subiculum: dissociating components of allocentric spatial learning. *Eur J Neurosci* 2:1016–1028.

Morrissey MD, Maal-Bared G, Brady S, Takehara-Nishiuchi K (2012) Functional dissociation within the entorhinal cortex for memory retrieval of an association between temporally discontiguous stimuli. *J Neurosci* 32:5356–5361.

Morrison DJ, Rashid AJ, Yiu AP, Yan C, Frankland PW, Josselyn SA (2016) Parvalbumin interneurons constrain the size of the lateral amygdala engram. *Neurobiol Learn Mem* 135:91–99.

Moscovitch M (1995) Recovered consciousness: a hypothesis concerning modularity and episodic memory. *J Clin Exp Neuropsychol* 17:276–290.

Moser EI, Moser MB, Anderson P (1993) Spatial learning impairment parallels the magnitude of dorsal hippocampal lesions, but is hardly present following ventral lesions. *J Neurosci* 13:3916–3925.

Moser EI, Kropff E, Moser MB (2008) Place cells, grid cells, and the brain's spatial representation system. *Annu Rev Neurosci* 31:69–89.

Moser MB, Moser EI, Forrest E, Andersen P, Morris RGM (1995) Spatial learning with a minislab in the dorsal hippocampus. *Proc Natl Acad Sci U S A* 92:9697–9701.

Muller RU, Kubie JL (1987) The effects of changes in the environment on the spatial firing of hippocampal complex-spike cells. *J Neurosci* 7:1951–1968.

Muller RU, Kubie JL, Ranck JB, Jr (1987) Spatial firing patterns of hippocampal complex-spike cells in a fixed environment. *J Neurosci* 7:1935–1950.

Mumby DG, Gaskin S, Glenn MJ, Schramek TE, Lehmann H (2002) Hippocampal damage and exploratory preferences in rats: memory for objects, places, and contexts. *Learn Mem* 9:49–57.

Mumby DG, Pinel JPJ, Wood ER (1990) Nonrecurring-items delayed nonmatching-to-sample in rats: a new paradigm for testing nonspatial working memory. *Psychobiology* 18:321–326.

Mumby DG, Wood ER, Pinel JP (1992) Object-recognition memory is only mildly impaired in rats with lesions of the hippocampus and amygdala. *Psychobiology* 20:18–27.

Munoz M, Chadwick M, Perez-Hernandez E, Vargha-Khadem F, Mishkin M (2011) Novelty preference in patients with developmental amnesia. *Hippocampus* 21:1268–1276.

Murray EA, Bussey TJ (1999) Perceptual-mnemonic functions of the perirhinal cortex. *Trends Cogn Sci* 3:142–151.

Murray EA, Wise SP, Graham KS (2016) The Evolution of Memory Systems. New York: Oxford University Press.

Nabavi S, Fox R, Proulx CD, Lin JY, Tsien RY, Malinow R (2014) Engineering a memory with LTD and LTP. *Nature* 511:348–352.

Nadasdy Z, Hirase H, Czurko A, Csicsvari J, Buzsáki G (1999) Replay and time compression of recurring spike sequences in the hippocampus. *J Neurosci* 19:9497–9507.

Nadel L, Hardt O (2004) The spatial brain. *Neuropsychology* 18:473–476.

Nadel L, Moscovitch M (1997) Memory consolidation, retrograde amnesia and the hippocampal complex. *Curr Opin Neurobiol* 7:217–227.

Nadel L, O'Keefe J, Black A (1975) Slam on the brakes: a critique of Altman, Brunner, and Bayer's response-inhibition model of hippocampal function. *Behav Biol* 14:151–162.

Nadel L, Willner J (1980) Context and conditioning: a place for space. *Physio Psychol* 8:218–228.

Nagahara AH, Otto T, Gallagher M (1995) Entorhinal-perirhinal lesions impair performance of rats on two versions of place learning in the Morris watermaze. *Behav Neurosci* 109:3–9.

Nagel T (1974) What is it like to be a bat? *Philos Rev* 83:435–450.

Navawongse R, Eichenbaum H (2013) Distinct pathways for rule-based retrieval and spatial mapping of memory representations in hippocampal neurons. *J Neurosci* 33:1002–1013.

Navratilova Z, Giocomo LM, Fellous JM, Hasselmo ME, McNaughton BL (2012) Phase precession and variable spatial scaling in a periodic attractor map model of medial entorhinal grid cells with realistic after-spike dynamics. *Hippocampus* 22:772–789.

Nelson AJ, Hindley EL, Pearce JM, Vann SD, Aggleton JP (2015) The effect of retrosplenial cortex lesions in rats on incidental and active spatial learning. *Front Behav Neurosci* 9:11.

Nitzan N, McKenzie S, Beed P, English DF, Oldani S, Tukker JJ, Buzsáki G, Schmitz D (2020) Propagation of hippocampal ripples to the neocortex by way of a subiculum-retrosplenial pathway. *Nat Commun* 11:1947.

NobelPrize.org. (2014). "The Nobel Prize in Physiology or Medicine 2014." Retrieved April 14, 2022, from https://www.nobelprize.org/prizes/medicine/2014/summary/.

Norman G, Eacott MJ (2004) Impaired object recognition with increasing levels of feature ambiguity in rats with perirhinal cortex lesions. *Behav Brain Res* 148:79–91.

Norman Y, Raccah O, Liu S, Parvizi J, Malach R (2021) Hippocampal ripples and their coordinated dialogue with the default mode network during recent and remote recollection. *Neuron* 109:2767–2780, e2765.

Norman Y, Yeagle EM, Khuvis S, Harel M, Mehta AD, Malach R (2019) Hippocampal sharp-wave ripples linked to visual episodic recollection in humans. *Science* 365:eaax1030.

Novitskaya Y, Sara SJ, Logothetis NK, Eschenko O (2016) Ripple-triggered stimulation of the locus coeruleus during post-learning sleep disrupts ripple/spindle coupling and impairs memory consolidation. *Learn Mem* 23:238–248.

Nyberg N, Duvelle E, Barry C, Spiers HJ (2022) Spatial goal coding in the hippocampal formation. *Neuron* 110:394–422.

Ocampo AC, Squire LR, Clark RE (2017) Hippocampal area CA1 and remote memory in rats. *Learn Mem* 24:563–568.

Ohkawa N, Saitoh Y, Suzuki A, Tsujimura S, Murayama E, Kosugi S, Nishizono H, Matsuo M, Takahashi Y, Nagase M, et al. (2015) Artificial association of pre-stored information to generate a qualitatively new memory. *Cell Rep* 11:261–269.

Oja E (1989) Neural networks, principal components, and subspaces. *Int J Neural Syst* 1:61–68.

O'Keefe J, Burgess N (1996) Geometric determinants of the place fields of hippocampal neurons. *Nature* 381:425–428.

O'Keefe J, Conway DH (1978) Hippocampal place units in the freely moving rat: why they fire where they fire. *Exp Brain Res* 31:573–590.

O'Keefe J, Dostrovsky J (1971) The hippocampus as a spatial map: preliminary evidence from unit activity in the freely-moving rat. *Brain Res* 34:171–175.

O'Keefe J, Krupic J (2021) Do hippocampal pyramidal cells respond to nonspatial stimuli? *Physiol Rev* 101:1427–1456.

O'Keefe J, Nadel L (1978) The Hippocampus as a Cognitive Map. Oxford: Clarendon Press.

O'Keefe J, Speakman A (1987) Single unit activity in the rat hippocampus during a spatial memory task. *Exp Brain Res* 68:1–27.

Oliva A, Fernández-Ruiz A, Leroy F, Siegelbaum SA (2020) Hippocampal CA2 sharp-wave ripples reactivate and promote social memory. *Nature* 587:264–269.

Okuyama T (2018) Social memory engram in the hippocampus. *Neurosci Res* 129:17–23.

Okuyama T, Kitamura T, Roy DS, Itohara S, Tonegawa S (2016) Ventral CA1 neurons store social memory. *Science* 353:1536–1541.

Olton DS, Becker JT, Handelmann GE (1979) Hippocampus, space, and memory. *Brain Behav Sci* 2:313–365.

Olton DS, Samuelson RJ (1976) Remembrance of places passed: spatial memory in rats. *J Exp Psychol Anim Behav Process* 2:97–116.

O'Reilly RC, McClelland JL (1994) Hippocampal conjunctive encoding, storage, and recall: avoiding a tradeoff. *Hippocampus* 6:661–682.

O'Reilly RC, Norman KA (2002) Hippocampal and neocortical contributions to memory: advances in the complementary learning systems framework. *Trends Cogn Sci* 6:505–510.

Otto T, Eichenbaum H (1992) Complementary roles of the orbital prefrontal cortex and the perirhinal-entorhinal cortices in an odor-guided delayed-nonmatching-to-sample task. *Behav Neurosci* 106:762–775.

Packard MG, McGaugh JL (1996) Inactivation of hippocampus or caudate nucleus with lidocaine differentially affects expression of place and response learning. *Neurobiol Learn Mem* 65:65–72.

Page HJI, Wilson JJ, Jeffery KJ (2018) A dual-axis rotation rule for updating the head direction cell reference frame during movement in three dimensions. *J Neurophysiol* 119:192–208.

Pascalis O, Bachevalier J (1999) Neonatal aspiration lesions of the hippocampal formation impair visual recognition memory when assessed by paired-comparison task but not by delayed nonmatching-to-sample task. *Hippocampus* 9:609–616.

Pastalkova E, Itskov V, Amarasingham A, Buzsáki G (2008) Internally generated cell assembly sequences in the rat hippocampus. *Science* 321:1322–1327.

Pavlides C, Winson J (1989) Influences of hippocampal place cell firing in the awake state on the activity of these cells during subsequent sleep episodes. *J Neurosci* 9:2907–2918.

Payne HL, Lynch GF, Aronov D (2021) Neural representations of space in the hippocampus of a food-caching bird. *Science* 373:343–348.

Payne JD, Schacter DL, Propper RE, Huang LW, Wamsley EJ, Tucker MA, Walker MP, Stickgold R (2009) The role of sleep in false memory formation. *Neurobiol Learn Mem* 92:327–334.

Pearce JM, Hall G (1980) A model for Pavlovian learning: variations in the effectiveness of conditioned but not of unconditioned stimuli. *Psychol Rev* 87:532–552.

Peyrache A, Khamassi M, Benchenane K, Wiener SI, Battaglia FP (2009) Replay of rule-learning related neural patterns in the prefrontal cortex during sleep. *Nat Neurosci* 12:919–926.

Peyrache A, Schieferstein N, Buzsáki G (2017) Transformation of the head-direction signal into a spatial code. *Nat Commun* 8:1752.

Pfeiffer BE, Foster DJ (2013) Hippocampal place-cell sequences depict future paths to remembered goals. *Nature* 497:74–79.

Pignatelli M, Ryan TJ, Roy DS, Lovett C, Smith LM, Muralidhar S, Tonegawa S (2019) Engram cell excitability state determines the efficacy of memory retrieval. *Neuron* 101:274–284, e275.

Pinsker H, Kupfermann I, Castellucci V, Kandel E (1970) Habituation and dishabituation of the gill-withdrawal reflex in Aplysia. *Science* 167:1740–1742.

Plihal W, Born J (1997) Effects of early and late nocturnal sleep on declarative and procedural memory. *J Cogn Neurosci* 9:534–547.

Plihal W, Pietrowsky R, Born J (1999) Dexamethasone blocks sleep induced improvement of declarative memory. *Psychoneuroendocrinology* 24:313–331.

Poggio T (2012) The levels of understanding framework, revised. *Perception* 41:1017–1023.

Poucet B (1989) Object exploration, habituation, and response to a spatial change in rats following septal or medial frontal cortical damage. *Behav Neurosci* 103:1009–1016.

Poucet B (1993) Spatial cognitive maps in animals: new hypotheses on their structure and neural mechanisms. *Psychol Rev* 100:163–182.

Poucet B, Lenck-Santini PP, Hok V, Save E, Banquet JP, Gaussier P, Muller RU (2004) Spatial navigation and hippocampal place cell firing: the problem of goal encoding. *Rev Neurosci* 15:89–107.

Preston AR, Shrager Y, Dudukovic NM, Gabrieli JD (2004) Hippocampal contribution to the novel use of relational information in declarative memory. *Hippocampus* 14:148–152.

Queenan BN, Ryan TJ, Gazzaniga MS, Gallistel CR (2017) On the research of time past: the hunt for the substrate of memory. *Ann N Y Acad Sci* 1396:108–125.

Quiroga RQ (2012) Concept cells: the building blocks of declarative memory functions. *Nat Rev Neurosci* 13:587–597.

Quiroga RQ, Kraskov A, Koch C, Fried I (2009) Explicit encoding of multimodal percepts by single neurons in the human brain. *Curr Biol* 19:1308–1313.

Quiroga RQ, Reddy L, Kreiman G, Koch C, Fried I (2005) Invariant visual representation by single neurons in the human brain. *Nature* 435:1102–1107.

Raby CR, Alexis DM, Dickinson A, Clayton NS (2007) Planning for the future by western scrub-jays. *Nature* 445:919–921.

Ramirez S, Liu X, Lin PA, Suh J, Pignatelli M, Redondo RL, Ryan TJ, Tonegawa S (2013) Creating a false memory in the hippocampus. *Science* 341:387–391.

Ramus SJ, Eichenbaum H (2000) Neural correlates of olfactory recognition memory in the rat orbitofrontal cortex. *J Neurosci* 20:8199–8208.

Rashid AJ, Yan C, Mercaldo V, Hsiang H-L, Park S, Cole CJ, De Cristofaro A, Yu J, Ramakrishnan C, Yeun Lee S, et al. (2016) Competition between engrams influences fear memory formation and recall. *Science* 353:383–387.

Ravassard P, Kees A, Willers B, Ho D, Aharoni DA, Cushman J, Aghajan ZM, Mehta MR (2013) Multisensory control of hippocampal spatiotemporal selectivity. *Science* 340:1342–1346.

Redish AD (1999) Beyond the Cognitive Map: From Place Cells to Episodic Memory. Cambridge, MA: MIT Press.

Redondo RL, Kim J, Arons AL, Ramirez S, Liu X, Tonegawa S (2014) Bidirectional switch of the valence associated with a hippocampal contextual memory engram. *Nature* 513:426–430.

Refeli R, Kreisel T, Groysman M, Adamsky A, Gosshen I (2023) Engram stability and maturation during systems consolidation. *Curr Biol* 33:3942–3950, e3.

Reijmers LG, Perkins BL, Matsuo N, Mayford M (2007) Localization of a stable neural correlate of associative memory. *Science* 317:1230–1233.

Rempel-Clower NL, Zola SM, Squire LR, Amaral DG (1996) Three cases of enduring memory impairment after bilateral damage limited to the hippocampal formation. *J Neurosci* **16**:5233–5255.

Rescorla RA, Wagner AR (1972) A theory of Pavlovian conditioning: the effectiveness of reinforcement and nonreinforcement. In: Classical Conditioning II: Current Research and Theory (Black AH, Prokasy WF, eds), pp 64–99. New York: Appleton-Century-Crofts.

Rich PD, Liaw HP, Lee AK (2014) Large environments reveal the statistical structure governing hippocampal representations. *Science* **345**:814–817.

Rinaldi A, De Leonibus E, Cifra A, Torromino G, Minicocci E, De Sanctis E, Lopez-Pedrajas RM, Oliverio A, Mele A (2020) Flexible use of allocentric and egocentric spatial memories activates differential neural networks in mice. *Sci Rep* **10**:11338.

Roberts WA (2000) Are animals stuck in time? *Psych Bulletin* **128**:473–489.

Roberts WA, Phelps MT (1994) Transitive inference in rats: a test of the spatial coding hypothesis. *Psychol Sci* **5**:368–374.

Robinson NTM, Descamps LAL, Russell LE, Buchholz MO, Bicknell BA, Antonov GK, Lau JYN, Nutbrown R, Schmidt-Hieber C, Häusser M (2020) Targeted activation of hippocampal place cells drives memory-guided spatial behavior. *Cell* **183**:1586–1599, e1510.

Rolls ET (2016) Cerebral Cortex: Principles of Operation. Oxford: Oxford University Press.

Rolls ET, Miyashita Y, Cahusac PM, Kesner RP, Niki H, Feigenbaum JD, Bach L (1989) Hippocampal neurons in the monkey with activity related to the place in which a stimulus is shown. *J Neurosci* **9**:1835–1845.

Rolls ET, Treves A (1998) Neural Networks and Brain Function. Oxford: Oxford University Press.

Rosenbaum RS, Kohler S, Schacter DL, Moscovitch M, Westmacott R, Black SE, Gao F, Tulving E (2005) The case of K.C.: contributions of a memory-impaired person to memory theory. *Neuropsychologia* **43**:989–1021.

Ross JJ (1965) Neurological findings after prolonged sleep deprivation. *Arch Neurol* **12**:399–403.

Rossato JI, Moreno A, Genzel L, Yamasaki M, Takeuchi T, Canals S, Morris RGM (2018) Silent learning. *Curr Biol* **28**:3508–3515, e3505.

Roux L, Hu B, Eichler R, Stark E, Buzsáki G (2017) Sharp wave ripples during learning stabilize the hippocampal spatial map. *Nat Neurosci* **20**:845–853.

Roy DS, Arons A, Mitchell TI, Pignatelli M, Ryan TJ, Tonegawa S (2016) Memory retrieval by activating engram cells in mouse models of early Alzheimer's disease. *Nature* **531**:508–512.

Roy DS, Muralidhar S, Smith LM, Tonegawa S (2017) Silent memory engrams as the basis for retrograde amnesia. *Proc Natl Acad Sci U S A* **114**:E9972–E9979.

Rueckemann JW, DiMauro AJ, Rangel LM, Han X, Boyden ES, Eichenbaum H (2016) Transient optogenetic inactivation of the medial entorhinal cortex biases the active population of hippocampal neurons. *Hippocampus* **26**:246–260.

Rumelhart DE, McClelland JL (1986) Parallel Distributed Processing: Explorations in the Microstructure of Cognition. Cambridge, MA: Bradford Books.

Ryan TJ, Frankland PW (2022) Forgetting as a form of adaptive engram cell plasticity. *Nat Rev Neurosci* **23**:173–186.

Ryan TJ, Roy DS, Pignatelli M, Arons A, Tonegawa S (2015) Engram cells retain memory under retrograde amnesia. *Science* **348**:1007–1013.

Ryle G (1949) The Concept of Mind. London: Hutchinson.

Sagar HJ, Cohen N, Corkin S, Growdon JH (1985) Dissociations among processes in remote memory. *Ann N Y Acad Sci* **444**:533–535

Saleem AB, Diamanti EM, Fournier J, Harris KD, Carandini M (2018) Coherent encoding of subjective spatial position in visual cortex and hippocampus. *Nature* **562**:124–127.

Sander K, Sander D (2005) New insights into transient global amnesia: recent imaging and clinical findings. *Lancet Neurol* **4**:437–444.

Save E, Poucet B (2009) Role of the parietal cortex in long-term representation of spatial information in the rat. *Neurobiol Learn Mem* **91**:172–178.

Scanziani M, Häusser M (2009) Electrophysiology in the age of light. *Nature* **461**:930–939.

Schacter DE, Tulving E (1994) Memory Systems. Cambridge, MA: MIT Press.

Schacter DL (2001) Forgotten Ideas, Neglected Pioneers. New York: Routledge.

Schacter DL, Addis DR (2007) The cognitive neuroscience of constructive memory: remembering the past and imagining the future. *Philos Trans R Soc Lond B Biol Sci* **362**:773–786.

Schenk F, Morris RG (1985) Dissociation between components of spatial memory in rats after recovery from the effects of retrohippocampal lesions. *Exp Brain Res* **58**:11–28.

Scoville WB, Milner B (1957) Loss of recent memory after bilateral hippocampal lesions. *J Neurol Neurosurg Psychiatry* **20**:11–21.

Sederberg PB, Howard MW, Kahana MJ (2008) A context-based theory of recency and contiguity in free recall. *Psychol Rev* **115**:893–912.

Semon R (1923) The Mneme. London: George Allen & Unwin.

Sherry DF, Schacter DL (1987) The evolution of multiple memory systems. *Psychol Rev* **94**:439–454.

Shinder ME, Taube JS (2019) Three-dimensional tuning of head direction cells in rats. *J Neurophysiol* **121**:4–37.

Shohamy D, Wagner AD (2008) Integrating memories in the human brain: hippocampal-midbrain encoding of overlapping events. *Neuron* **60**:378–389.

Shomrat T, Turchetti-Maia AL, Stern-Mentch N, Basil JA, Hochner B (2015) The vertical lobe of cephalopods: an attractive brain structure for understanding the evolution of advanced learning and memory systems. *J Comp Physiol A Neuroethol Sens Neural Behav Physiol* **201**:947–956.

Siapas AG, Wilson MA (1998) Coordinated interactions between hippocampal ripples and cortical spindles during slow-wave sleep. *Neuron* **21**:1123–1128.

Siegel JM (2001) The REM sleep-memory consolidation hypothesis. *Science* **294**:1058–1063.

Silva D, Feng T, Foster DJ (2015) Trajectory events across hippocampal place cells require previous experience. *Nat Neurosci* **18**:1772–1779.

Sirota A, Csicsvari J, Buhl D, Buzsáki G (2003) Communication between neocortex and hippocampus during sleep in rodents. *Proc Natl Acad Sci U S A* **100**:2065–2069.

Skaggs WE, McNaughton BL (1998) Spatial firing properties of hippocampal CA1 populations in an environment containing two visually identical regions. *J Neurosci* **18**:8455–8466.

Smith C, Rose GM (1996) Evidence for a paradoxical sleep window for place learning in the Morris watermaze. *Physiol Behav* **59**:93–97.

Squire LR (1987) Memory and Brain. Oxford: Oxford University Press.

Squire LR (1992) Memory and the hippocampus: a synthesis from findings with rats, monkeys, and humans. *Psychol Rev* **99**:195–231.

Squire LR, Clark RE, Knowlton BJ (2001) Retrograde amnesia. *Hippocampus* **11**:50–55.

Squire LR, Cohen NJ (1984) Human memory and amnesia. In: Neurobiology of Learning and Memory (Lynch G, McGaugh JL, Weinberger NM, eds), pp 3–64. New York: Gilford Press.

Squire LR, Deed AJO (2015) Conscious and unconscious memory systems: perspectives in learning and memory. *Cold Spring Harb Perspect Biol* **7**:a021667.

Squire LR, Ojemann JG, F.M. M, Petersen SE, Videen TO, Raichle ME (1992) Activation of the hippocampus in normal humans: a functional anatomical study of memory. *Proc Natl Acad Sci U S A* **89**:1837–1841.

Squire LR, Stark CE, Clark RE (2004) The medial temporal lobe. *Annu Rev Neurosci* **27**:279–306.

Squire LR, Zola-Morgan S (1991) The medial temporal lobe memory system. *Science* **253**:1380–1386.

Steele RJ, Morris RGM (1999) Delay-dependent impairment of a matching-to-place task with chronic and intrahippocampal infusion of the NMDA-antagonist D-AP5. *Hippocampus* **9**:118–136.

Steinvorth S, Levine B, Corkin S (2005) Medial temporal lobe structures are needed to re-experience remote autobiographical memories: evidence from H.M. and W.R. *Neuropsychologia* **43**:479–496.

Stensola H, Stensola T, Solstad T, Froland K, Moser MB, Moser EI (2012) The entorhinal grid map is discretized. *Nature* **492**:72–78.

Stensola T, Moser EI (2016) Grid cells and spatial maps in entorhinal cortex and hippocampus. In: Micro-, Meso- and Macro-Dynamics of the Brain (Buzsáki G, Christen Y, eds), pp 59–80. Springer: Cham (CH).

Stensola T, Stensola H, Moser MB, Moser EI (2015) Shearing-induced asymmetry in entorhinal grid cells. *Nature* **518**:207–212.

Stevenson EL, Caldwell HK (2014) Lesions to the CA2 region of the hippocampus impair social memory in mice. *Eur J Neurosci* **40**:3294–3301.

Stoerig P, Cowey A (1995) Visual perception and phenomenal consciousness. *Behav Brain Res* **71**:147–156.

Suddendorf T, Corballis MC (1997) Mental time travel and the evolution of the human mind. *Genet Soc Gen Psychol Monogr* **123**:133–167.

Sutherland RJ, O'Brien J, Lehmann H (2008) Absence of systems consolidation of fear memories after dorsal, ventral, or complete hippocampal damage. *Hippocampus* **18**:710–718.

Sutherland RJ, Whishaw IQ, Kolb B (1988) Contributions of cingulate cortex to two forms of spatial learning and memory. *J Neurosci* **8**:1863–1872.

Takahashi N, Kitamura K, Matsuo N, Mayford M, Kano M, Matsuki N, Ikegaya Y (2012) Locally synchronized synaptic inputs. *Science* **335**:353–356.

Takemoto K, Iwanari H, Tada H, Suyama K, Sano A, Nagai T, Hamakubo T, Takahashi T (2017) Optical inactivation of synaptic AMPA receptors erases fear memory. *Nat Biotech* **35**:38–47.

Takeuchi T, Duszkiewicz AJ, Sonneborn A, Spooner PA, Yamasaki M, Watanabe M, Smith CC, Fernandez G, Deisseroth K, Greene RW, et al. (2016) Locus coeruleus and dopaminergic consolidation of everyday memory. *Nature* **537**:357–262.

Takeuchi T, Tamura M, Tse D, Kajii Y, Fernandez G, Morris RGM (2022) Brain region networks for the assimilation of new associative memory into a schema. *Mol Brain* **15**:24.

Tanaka KZ, He H, Tomar A, Niisato K, Huang AJY, McHugh TJ (2018) The hippocampal engram maps experience but not place. *Science* **361**:392–397.

Taube JS (1998) Head direction cells and the neurophysiological basis for a sense of direction. *Prog Neurobiol* **55**:225–256.

Taube JS, Muller RU, Ranck JB, Jr (1990) Head-direction cells recorded from the postsubiculum in freely moving rats. II. Effects of environmental manipulations. *J Neurosci* **10**:438–447.

Taube JS, Schwartzkroin PA (1987) Intracellular-recording from hippocampal ca1 interneurons before and after development of long-term potentiation. *Brain Res* **419**:32–38.

Tayler KK, Tanaka KZ, Reijmers LG, Wiltgen BJ (2013) Reactivation of neural ensembles during the retrieval of recent and remote memory. *Curr Biol* **23**:99–106.

Templer VL, Brown EK, Hampton RR (2018) Rhesus monkeys metacognitively monitor memories of the order of events. *Sci Rep* **8**:11541.

Teng E, Squire LR (1999) Memory for places learned long ago is intact after hippocampal damage. *Nature* **400**:675–677.

Teyler TJ, DiScenna P (1986) The hippocampal memory indexing theory. *Behav Neurosci* **100**:147–154.

Teyler TJ, DiScenna P (1987) Long-term potentiation. *Ann Rev Neurosci* **10**:131–161.

Teyler TJ, Rudy JW (2007) The hippocampal indexing theory and episodic memory: updating the index. *Hippocampus* **17**:1158–1169.

Tolman EC (1948) Cognitive maps in rats and men. *Psychol Rev* **55**:189–208.

Tolman EC, Ritchie BF, Kalish D (1946) Studies in spatial learning; place learning versus response learning. *J Exp Psychol* **36**:221–229.

Tonegawa S, Liu X, Ramirez S, Redondo R (2015) Memory engram cells have come of age. *Neuron* **87**:918–931.

Tononi G, Cirelli C (2014) Sleep and the price of plasticity: from synaptic and cellular homeostasis to memory consolidation and integration. *Neuron* **81**:12–34.

Treves A, Rolls ET (1994) Computational analysis of the role of the hippocampus in memory. *Hippocampus* **4**:1–18.

Tsao A, Sugar J, Lu L, Wang C, Knierim JJ, Moser M-B, Moser EI (2018) Integrating time from experience in the lateral entorhinal cortex. *Nature* **561**:57–62.

Tse D, Langston RF, Kakeyama M, Bethus I, Spooner PA, Wood ER, Witter MP, Morris RG (2007) Schemas and memory consolidation. *Science* **316**:76–82.

Tse, D, Norton, AC, Spooner, PA, and Morris RG (2022) A behavioral task modeling "everyday memory" in an event arena to foster allocentric representations for rodents. *JoVE* 180:e63152.

Tse D, Takeuchi T, Kakeyama M, Kajii Y, Okuno H, Tohyama C, Bito H, Morris RG (2011) Schema-dependent gene activation and memory encoding in neocortex. *Science* **333**:891–895.

Tulving E (1972) Episodic and semantic memory. In: Organisation of Memory (Tulving E, Donaldson W, eds), pp 381–403. New York: Academic Press.

Tulving E (1983) Elements of Episodic Memory. New York: Oxford University Press.

Tulving E (2004) Episodic memory and autonoesis: uniquely human? In: The Missing Link in Cognition: Evolution of Self-Knowing Consciousness (Terrace H, Metcalfe J., eds), pp 3–56. New York: Oxford University Press.

Tulving E, Markowitsch HJ (1998) Episodic and declarative memory: role of hippocampus. *Hippocampus* **8**:198–204.

Ulanovsky N (2011) Neuroscience: how is three-dimensional space encoded in the brain? *Curr Biol* **21**:R886–888.

Ulanovsky N, Moss CF (2007) Hippocampal cellular and network activity in freely moving echolocating bats. *Nat Neurosci* **10**:224–233.

Ulanovsky N, Moss CF (2011) Dynamics of hippocampal spatial representation in echolocating bats. *Hippocampus* **21**:150–161.

van Cauter T, Poucet B, Save E (2008) Unstable CA1 place cell representation in rats with entorhinal cortex lesions. *Eur J Neurosci* **27**:1933–1946.

van Elzakker M, O'Reilly RC, Rudy JW (2003) Transitivity, flexibility, conjunctive representations, and the hippocampus. I. An empirical analysis. *Hippocampus* **13**:334–340.

van Kesteren MT, Ruiter DJ, Fernandez G, Henson RN (2012) How schema and novelty augment memory formation. *Trends Neurosci* **35**:211–219.

Vann SD, Aggleton JP (2002) Extensive cytotoxic lesions of the rat retrosplenial cortex reveal consistent deficits on tasks that tax allocentric spatial memory. *Behav Neurosci* **116**:85–94.

Vann SD, Aggleton JP, Maguire EA (2009) What does the retrosplenial cortex do? *Nat Rev Neurosci* **10**:792–802.

van Wijngaarden JB, Babl SS, Ito HT (2020) Entorhinal-retrosplenial circuits for allocentric-egocentric transformation of boundary coding. *Elife* 9:e59816.

Vargha-Khadem F, Gadian DG, Watkins KE, Connelly A, Van Paesschen W, Mishkin M (1997) Differential effects of early hippocampal pathology on episodic and semantic memory. *Science* **277**:376–380.

Vaz AP, Inati SK, Brunel N, Zaghloul KA (2019) Coupled ripple oscillations between the medial temporal lobe and neocortex retrieve human memory. *Science* **363**:975–978.

Vetere G, Tran LM, Moberg S, Steadman PE, Restivo L, Morrison FG, Ressler KJ, Josselyn SA, Frankland PW (2019) Memory formation in the absence of experience. *Nat Neurosci* **22**:933–940.

Vinogradova OS (2001) Hippocampus as comparator: role of the two input and two output systems of the hippocampus in selection and registration of information. *Hippocampus* **11**:578–598.

Wais PE, Wixted JT, Hopkins RO, Squire LR (2006) The hippocampus supports both the recollection and the familiarity components of recognition memory. *Neuron* **49**:459–466.

Wamsley EJ, Tucker MA, Payne JD, Stickgold R (2010) A brief nap is beneficial for human route-learning: the role of navigation experience and EEG spectral power. *Learn Mem* **17**:332–336.

Wang C, Chen X, Knierim JJ (2020) Egocentric and allocentric representations of space in the rodent brain. *Curr Opin Neurobiol* **60**:12–20.

Wang C, Chen X, Lee H, Deshmukh SS, Yoganarasimha D, Savelli F, Knierim JJ (2018) Egocentric coding of external items in the lateral entorhinal cortex. *Science* **362**:945–949.

Wang DV, Ikemoto S (2016) Coordinated interaction between hippocampal sharp-wave ripples and anterior cingulate unit activity. *J Neurosci* **36**:10663–10672.

Wang F, Kessels HW, Hu H (2014) The mouse that roared: neural mechanisms of social hierarchy. *Trends Neurosci* **37**:674–682.

Wang SH, Redondo RL, Morris RG (2010) Relevance of synaptic tagging and capture to the persistence of long-term potentiation and everyday spatial memory. *Proc Natl Acad Sci U S A* **107**:19537–19542.

Wang SH, Tse D, Morris RG (2012) Anterior cingulate cortex in schema assimilation and expression. *Learn Mem* **19**:315–318.

Warburton EC, Aggleton JP (1999) Differential deficits in the Morris watermaze following cytotoxic lesions of the anterior thalamus and fornix transection. *Beha Brain Res* **98**:27–38.

Wehner R, Lehrer M, Harvey WC (1996) Navigation: migration and homing. *J Exp Biol* **199**:1–260.

Whishaw IQ (1998) Place learning in hippocampal rats and the path integration hypothesis. *Neurosci Biobehav Rev* **22**:209–220.

Whishaw IQ, Hines DJ, Wallace DG (2001) Dead reckoning (path integration) requires the hippocampal formation: evidence from spontaneous exploration and spatial learning tasks in light (allothetic) and dark (idiothetic) tests. *Behav Brain Res* **127**:49–69.

Whishaw IQ, Tomie JA (1997) Perseveration on place reversals in spatial swimming pool tasks: further evidence for place learning in hippocampal rats. *Hippocampus* **7**:361–370.

White NM, McDonald RJ (2002) Multiple parallel memory systems in the brain of the rat. *Neurobiol Learn Mem* **77**:125–184.

Whittington JCR, Muller TH, Mark S, Chen G, Barry C, Burgess N, Behrens TEJ (2020) The Tolman-Eichenbaum machine: unifying space and relational memory through generalization in the hippocampal formation. *Cell* **183**:1249–1263, e1223.

Widloski J, Foster DJ (2022) Flexible rerouting of hippocampal replay sequences around changing barriers in the absence of global place field remapping. *Neuron* **110**:1547–1558.e8.

Wiener SI (1993) Spatial and behavioral correlates of striatal neurons in rats performing a self-initiated navigation task. *J Neurosci* **13**:3802–3817.

Wilber AA, Clark BJ, Forster TC, Tatsuno M, McNaughton BL (2014) Interaction of egocentric and world-centered reference frames in the rat posterior parietal cortex. *J Neurosci* **34**:5431–5446.

Wills TJ, Lever C, Cacucci F, Burgess N, O'Keefe J (2005) Attractor dynamics in the hippocampal representation of the local environment. *Science* **308**:873–876.

Willshaw DJ, Buckingham JT (1990) An assessment of Marr's theory of the hippocampus as a temporary memory store. *Philos Trans R Soc Lond B Biol Sci* **329**:205–215.

Wilson MA, McNaughton BL (1993) Dynamics of the hippocampal ensemble code for space. *Science* **261**:1055–1058.

Wilson MA, McNaughton BL (1994) Reactivation of hippocampal ensemble memories during sleep. *Science* **265**:676–679.

Winocur G (1990) Anterograde and retrograde amnesia in rats with dorsal hippocampal or dorsomedial thalamic lesions. *Behav Brain Res* **38**:145–154.

Winocur G, Moscovitch M, Bontempi B (2010) Memory formation and long-term retention in humans and animals: convergence towards a transformation account of hippocampal-neocortical interactions. *Neuropsychologia* **48**:2339–2356.

Winocur G, Moscovitch M, Fogel S, Rosenbaum RS, Sekeres M (2005) Preserved spatial memory after hippocampal lesions: effects of extensive experience in a complex environment. *Nat Neurosci* **8**:273–275.

Winograd T (1975) Frame representations and the procedural/declarative controversy. In: Representation and Understanding: Studies in Cognitive Science (Bobrow DG, Collins A, eds), pp 185–210. New York: Academic Press.

Winters BD, Forwood SE, Cowell RA, Saksida LM, Bussey TJ (2004) Double dissociation between the effects of peri-postrhinal cortex and hippocampal lesions on tests of object recognition and spatial memory: heterogeneity of function within the temporal lobe. *J Neurosci* **24**:5901–5908.

Wirth S, Yanike M, Frank LM, Smith AC, Brown EN, Suzuki WA (2003) Single neurons in the monkey hippocampus and learning of new associations. *Science* **300**:1578–1581.

Wiskott L, Rasch MJ, Kempermann G (2006) A functional hypothesis for adult hippocampal neurogenesis: avoidance of catastrophic interference in the dentate gyrus. *Hippocampus* **16**:329–343.

Wittlinger M, Wehner R, Wolf H (2007) The desert ant odometer: a stride integrator that accounts for stride length and walking speed. *J Exp Biol* **210**:198–207.

Wolff M, Gibb SJ, Cassel JC, Dalrymple-Alford JC (2008) Anterior but not intralaminar thalamic nuclei support allocentric spatial memory. *Neurobiol Learn Mem* **90**:71–80.

Wood ER, Dudchenko PA, Eichenbaum H (1999) The global record of memory in hippocampal neuronal activity. *Nature* **397**:613–616.

Wood ER, Dudchenko PA, Robitsek RJ, Eichenbaum H (2000) Hippocampal neurons encode information about different types of memory episodes occurring in the same location. *Neuron* **27**:623–633.

Wood RA, Bauza M, Krupic J, Burton S, Delekate A, Chan D, O'Keefe J (2018) The honeycomb maze provides a novel test to study hippocampal-dependent spatial navigation. *Nature* **554**:102–105.

Worden RP (1992) Navigation by fragment fitting: a theory of hippocampal function. *Hippocampus* **2**:165–187.

Wu X, Foster DJ (2014) Hippocampal replay captures the unique topological structure of a novel environment. *J Neurosci* **34**:6459–6469.

Xie L, Kang H, Xu Q, Chen MJ, Liao Y, Thiyagarajan M, O'Donnell J, Christensen DJ, Nicholson C, Iliff JJ, et al. (2013) Sleep drives metabolite clearance from the adult brain. *Science* **342**:373–377.

Yartsev MM, Ulanovsky N (2013) Representation of three-dimensional space in the hippocampus of flying bats. *Science* **340**:367–372.

Yin A, Tseng PH, Rajangam S, Lebedev MA, Nicolelis MAL (2018) Place cell-like activity in the primary sensorimotor and premotor cortex during monkey whole-body navigation. *Sci Rep* 8:9184.

Yin HH, Knowlton BJ (2004) Contributions of striatal subregions to place and response learning. *Learn Mem* 11:459–463.

Yin HH, Knowlton BJ (2006) The role of the basal ganglia in habit formation. *Nat Rev Neurosci* 7:464–476.

Yoshida M, Isa T (2015) Signal detection analysis of blindsight in monkeys. *Sci Rep* 5:10755.

Young WS, Li J, Wersinger SR, Palkovits M (2006) The vasopressin 1b receptor is prominent in the hippocampal area CA2 where it is unaffected by restraint stress or adrenalectomy. *Neuroscience* 143:1031–1039.

Yu JY, Liu DF, Loback A, Grossrubatscher I, Frank LM (2018) Specific hippocampal representations are linked to generalized cortical representations in memory. *Nat Commun* 9:2209.

Zeithamova D, Dominick AL, Preston AR (2012) Hippocampal and ventral medial prefrontal activation during retrieval-mediated learning supports novel inference. *Neuron* 75:168–179.

Zeithamova D, Schlichting ML, Preston AR (2012) The hippocampus and inferential reasoning: building memories to navigate future decisions. *Front Hum Neurosci* 6:70.

Zeithamova D, Preston AR (2010) Flexible memories: differential roles for medial temporal lobe and prefrontal cortex in cross-episode binding. *J Neurosci* 30:14676–14684.

Zhao X, Wang Y, Spruston N, Magee JC (2020) Membrane potential dynamics underlying context-dependent sensory responses in the hippocampus. *Nat Neurosci* 23:881–891.

Zheng Y, Liu XL, Nishiyama S, Ranganath C, O'Reilly RC (2022) Correcting the Hebbian mistake: toward a fully error-driven hippocampus. *Plos Comp Biol* 18:e1010589

Ziv Y, Burns LD, Cocker ED, Hamel EO, Ghosh KK, Kitch LJ, El Gamal A, Schnitzer MJ (2013) Long-term dynamics of CA1 hippocampal place codes. *Nat Neurosci* 16:264–266.

Zola SM, Squire LR, Teng E, Stefanacci L, Buffalo EA, Clark RE (2000) Impaired recognition memory in monkeys after damage limited to the hippocampal region. *J Neurosci* 20:451–463.

Zola-Morgan S, Squire LR (1990) The primate hippocampal formation: evidence for a time-limited role in memory storage. *Science* 250:288–290.

Zola-Morgan S, Squire LR, Amaral DG (1986) Human amnesia and the medial temporal region: enduring memory impairment following a bilateral lesion limited to field CA1 of the hippocampus. *J Neurosci* 6:2950–2967.

15

Aging and the Hippocampus

Sara N. Burke and Carol A. Barnes

15.1 Overview

Defining how aging impacts the neurobiology of structures critical for memory, like the hippocampus, has become a major area of study in the field of neuroscience over the past several decades. The importance of this area of research is highlighted by the fact that age is the single greatest risk factor for neurodegenerative diseases and loss of independent living. Studying the normative process of brain development across the lifespan is critical in its own right, as epidemiological investigations demonstrate. For example, Plassman et al. (2007) obtained data from a representative sample of individuals 70 years and older across the United States, including people living in rural and urban areas, of differing race/ethnicities and socioeconomic backgrounds. The results of this study of self-reported cognitive status (and disease diagnosis) suggests that 14% of individuals above 70 years of age in the United States have dementia—a terribly large number. By far the largest group of individuals with a neurodegenerative disease have a primary diagnosis of Alzheimer's disease, with the next most common form being vascular dementia. The prevalence of all dementias increases, of course, with increasing age—from 5% prevalence between 70 and 79 years, 24% prevalence between 80 and 89 years, and 37% prevalence at 90 years and above (Figure 15.1A). On the other hand, these data suggest that most individuals over 70 years of age are not demented. This chapter, therefore, reviews what is known about the aging hippocampus for the 86% of us that will age without dementia.[1]

Because the first edition of the *Hippocampus Book* did not include a chapter on aging, and considering the remarkable progress that has been made in the past 15 years in understanding the relationship between hippocampus-dependent behavioral and neurobiological alternations, we provide a comprehensive review that includes both older and contemporary experiments. We contend that it is critical to define normative changes in the aging brain to fully understand pathological conditions that tend to occur at older ages, such as Alzheimer's disease and related dementias (as reviewed in Chapter 20) that occur against the backdrop of an aging brain. This chapter will take a comparative approach to discuss what is currently known regarding the impact of normative aging on hippocampus structure and function across species, highlighting key areas that remain to be explored. While the hippocampus proper and dentate gyrus have been well studied, the entorhinal cortex, subiculum, presubiculum, and parasubiculum have not been extensively examined. We will include all regions of the hippocampus formation for which data from older age groups are available.

The chapter is divided into sections that summarize the impact of advanced age on different aspects of hippocampal structure, function, and dynamics that influence behavior. When possible, each section will integrate data obtained from rodents, monkeys, and humans. Even though the chronological age at which a given species is considered "old" can differ by an order of magnitude (Figure 15.1B), each animal exhibits brain and cognitive changes near the end of their lifespan. For many strains of rats and mice this is approximately 2 years, which corresponds to the age of 50% mortality. For nonhuman primates, this is approximately 22 years, which corresponds to a human equivalent age of 66 years (Tigges et al., 1988). For humans, 65 years is used to define the transition into old age in most studies of brain and cognitive aging.

Besides the definition of when each species is considered to be "old," the potential effects of housing conditions have also been considered. While social housing and environmental enrichment may boost cognition in all age groups, these conditions appear not to eliminate age differences. This has been explicitly examined in rodent models of aging. One study conducted using male Wistar rats reported that environment enrichment from weaning until the time of behavioral testing at 23 months did not reverse age differences in acquisition of an associative learning task (Soffié et al., 1999). Furthermore, when performance on a Hebb-Williams maze was examined in male Fischer344 (F344) rats that were either raised from weaning in a standard cage or an enriched environment until the time of testing at 2.5, 15, and 25 months, there remained substantial age-related learning deficits in both treatment groups (Kobayashi et al., 2002). Additionally, when female C57BL/6 mice were either single-housed in a standard cage or group-housed in an enriched environment from 10 to 20 months of age, no spatial memory differences between housing groups were detected at 20 months on the Morris watermaze (see section 15.2.1)

[1] The authors would like to dedicate this chapter to Dr. Brenda Milner, who has had a critical influence on both of us as an outstanding scientist role model. Fittingly, we finished the first complete draft of this chapter on aging on July 15, 2022, Dr. Milner's 104th birthday! She is the quintessential exemplar of successful aging, and she continues to inspire all of us to maintain our creative efforts in the field of neuroscience for as long as our brain and cognitive health can be sustained.

A Prevalence of dementia after 70 years of age in the United States

Age Group	No Dementia	All Dementias	Alzheimer's Disease Only	Vascular Dementia
71–79	95%	5%	2.3%	1%
80–89	76%	24%	18%	4%
90 and older	63%	37%	30%	6%

B Comparison of sexual maturity, life expectancy, and range of ages for young and old species reviewed in this chapter

	Humans	Nonhuman Primates (old world)	Rabbits	Rats	Mice
Average age of sexual maturity	12–14 years	3–4 years	6–7 months	2–3 months	2–3 months
Average life expectancy	76–81 years	26–30 years	5–8 years	24–36 months	24–32 months
Range for young in reviewed studies	17–52 years	4–14 years	2–6 months	1–13 months	1–12 months
Range for old in reviewed studies	60–104 years	22–33 years	2–4 years	18–36 months	18–33 months

Figure 15.1 Overview of normative aging. (A) The prevalence of normative aging versus aging with dementia after age 70 from Plassman et al. (2007). While the rates of Alzheimer's disease and other dementias increase after age 70, by far, most individuals will age without dementia. Even after age 90, almost two-thirds of individuals will not have dementia. (B) A comparison of the ages of sexual maturity (top row) and life expectancy (second row) for humans and common animal models of aging. The third row shows the range of ages used in the studies that are discussed in this chapter considered to be "young" for a particular species. The fourth row shows the range of ages used in the studies that are discussed in this chapter considered to be "aged" for a particular species.

(Kempermann et al., 2002). Another study that evaluated Morris watermaze performance in male C57BL/6 mice after a 6-week environmental enrichment intervention, reported that the enriched mice had faster swimming speeds, but were not more accurate in recalling the goal location (Bennett et al., 2006). More recently, it has been reported that young and old male Wistar rats raised with lifelong enrichment outperformed nonenriched animals, however, the old enriched animals were not as accurate as the young (Birch and Kelly, 2019).

Enriched housing conditions can both be more cognitively engaging and increase physical activity. With respect to exercise, there is a long experimental history of examining the impact of physical activity interventions on health and cognition. Although an active lifestyle for humans and other animals clearly has a positive effect on disease prevention and overall well-being (Damrongthai et al., 2021), obtaining objective evidence for a direct impact of long-term exercise programs on hippocampus-dependent cognition has remained elusive, despite evidence that it leads to volumetric increases in the hippocampus (Domingos et al., 2021). For example, the largest randomized clinical trial to date that manipulated physical activity found no differences between the group that was assigned a physical activity program and the control group that was assigned a health education program after 24 months of intervention (Sink et al., 2015). Even in a study in which a more physically demanding exercise program was implemented in a smaller sample size, no meaningful group differences were detected in spatial memory despite increases in hippocampus volume after 1 year of intervention (Erickson et al., 2011). Consistent with these human findings, another study that significantly increased VO_2 max following aerobic exercise in old rats, did not result in an improvement in spatial memory compared with animals that were housed without exercise (Barnes et al., 1991).

A number of studies that have explicitly examined the effect of cognitive training on older rodents and humans. An early study trained male Sprague Dawley daily between 6 and 26 months of age on an eight-arm radial maze task with a 5-hour delay imposed after the fourth arm was chosen (section 15.2.2). At 26 months, the rats' spatial memory was more accurate than when they were tested at 6 months, and also when they were compared with an independent group of rats that were 5 months old. When these old rats were trained in a separate room on the same problem, however, they acquired this spatial task more slowly than did the independent group of young animals. These data suggest that the old animals failed to transfer the trained skill to the new problem (Beatty et al., 1985). Analogous findings have been made in the human literature. For example, a recent meta-analysis reviewed 43 studies in which the efficacy of commercial training programs (BrainGymmer, BrainHQ, CogMed, CogniFit, Dakim, Lumosity, and MyBrainTrainer) was evaluated. While the older adults showed improvements in memory within a single game, there was no evidence for significant transfer of improved memory across testing situations. There was, however, an overall increase in processing speed, which parallels the faster swim speeds of aged rodents reared in enriched environments, as discussed above. Although "brain games" can be entertaining, there is insufficient evidence to date that general improvements in memory can be achieved by specific training programs (Nguyen et al., 2021).

It is important to keep in mind that all age-related hippocampus changes may not be detrimental—but can reflect compensatory processes or adaptive brain responses. Thus, this chapter will consider how we still need to distinguish between those changes that improve overall function versus those that are maladaptive (e.g., Gray and Barnes, 2015). Resolving this issue is critical for designing treatment strategies that optimize cognitive health outcomes. Finally, we will highlight gaps in our knowledge throughout this chapter with the goal of inspiring neuroscientists to understand and answer the extant questions regarding the aging hippocampus.

15.2 Cross-species hippocampus-dependent behaviors and aging

The involvement of the hippocampus in a broad range of higher cognitive functions has been extensively investigated in humans and other animals (Chapter 14). To summarize what is known regarding the impact of advanced age on hippocampus-dependent behaviors, this section will focus on research in which homologous behavioral tasks have been developed across species and tested in both young and old age groups within the same study. This criterion excludes studies that use language in the experimental design. With this criterion, the hippocampus-dependent behaviors that we will discuss can be broadly categorized into spatial behaviors, stimulus recognition and discrimination, and associative learning and conditioning. In most cases, the data collected across a large number of studies are in agreement that performance on hippocampus-dependent tasks changes across the lifespan.

15.2.1 Spatial behaviors

Hippocampus-dependent spatial navigational abilities have been examined across age and species (e.g., Schimanski and Barnes, 2015). Navigation can depend on an allocentric reference frame that does not change as one moves through space (Tolman, 1948), an egocentric reference frame that is from the perspective of the

navigator (Hartley et al., 2003), or a frame of reference based on stable features of the environment such as landmarks (Auger et al., 2012). Each of these strategies can be effective for solving navigation problems, but they rely on different brain structures. The hippocampus is more involved in allocentric navigation, while the parietal and superior temporal cortices as well as the basal ganglia participate more in egocentric solutions, and the anterior dorsal thalamus and retrosplenial cortex are associated with landmark-based strategies. While these generalizations are broadly true, each of these structures can participate across multiple strategies.

15.2.1.1 T-, Y-, and radial mazes

Age-related changes in spatial problem solving in both simple and complex T-mazes were described in male and female rats ranging in age from 1 to 30 months as early as 1929 across a variety of strains (Stone, 1929; Verzar-McDougall, 1957; Goodrick, 1968, 1972; Ingram et al., 1981; Skalicky et al., 1984; Goldman et al., 1987; Lohninger et al., 2001). Because none of these studies examined differences in strategy use, it is ambiguous whether the observed age deficits were due to hippocampal or extrahippocampal structures. One study explicitly examined strategy use in middle-aged (14 months) and aged (29 months) male Long Evans rats (Barnes et al., 1980). Figure 15.2 shows a schematic summary of how this experiment was conducted. A T-maze was used to train rats to move to a fixed reward location (Figure 15.2A). During training, young and aged rats acquired the task at a similar level of proficiency (Figure 15.2B). After 24 training trials, probe trials were used to determine what strategy was being implemented by individual rats for task solution (Figure 15.2C). This was accomplished by either

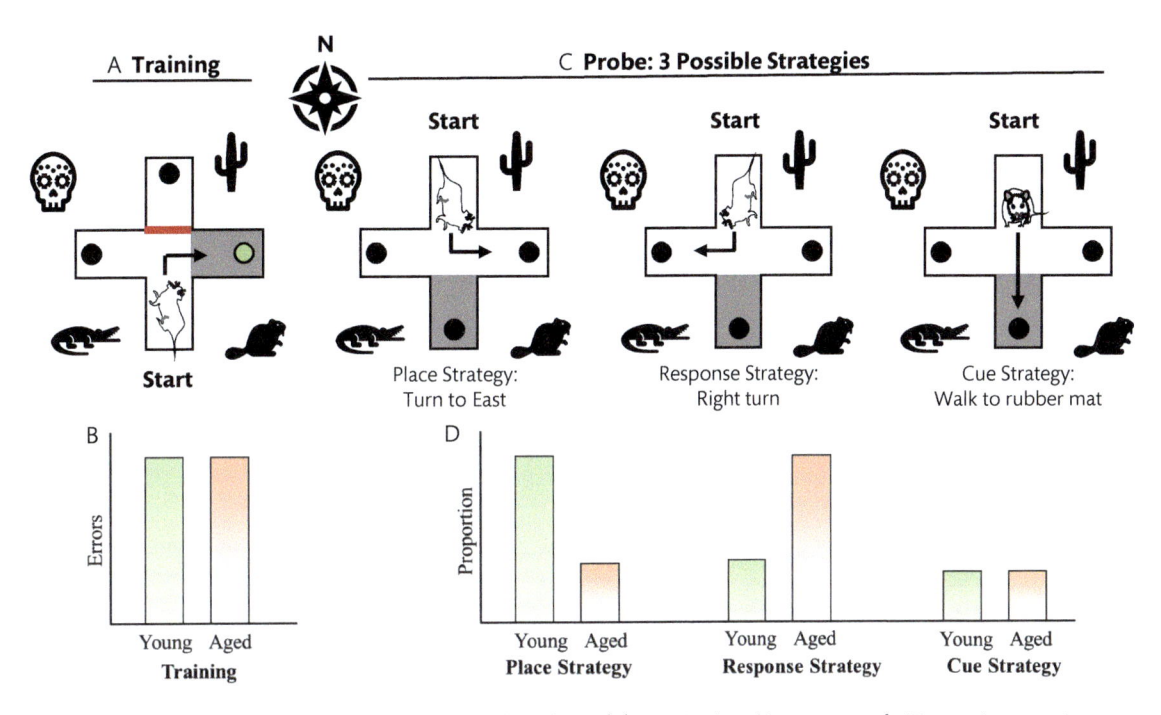

Figure 15.2 Strategy implementation in the T-maze in young and aged rats. (A) A rat is placed in one arm of a T-maze in an environment with distal visual cues (skull, cactus, alligator, beaver) to provide bearing. Over several trials, the rat is trained to the location of a reward (green circle). (B) Young and aged rats learn the reward location similarly, making comparable numbers of errors. (C) During a probe trial the start location is moved, and the rat's selection of an arm can be used to infer the animal's strategy. (*Left*) Turning to the same place in the room (that is, to the east) is consistent with an allocentric place strategy. (*Middle*) Turning in the same direction (that is, making a right turn) is consistent with an egocentric response strategy. (*Right*) Traversing to the rubber mat indicates the use of a cue strategy. (D) A higher proportion of young rats use an allocentric place strategy, while aged rats are more likely to use a response-based egocentric strategy.

moving the rubber mat to another arm or by flipping the start arm to the opposite coordinate. Performance strategy used by the rat was inferred as follows: (1) the rat could use a spatial allocentric solution by traveling to the same place in the environment defined by distal cues located around the maze; (2) the rat could use a response strategy by making a right turn, traversing to a different location in space; or (3) the rat could use a cue strategy, traversing to the arm with the rubber mat in a different location and requiring a different response (Barnes et al., 1980). For young rats, the majority of animals continued to go to the same place in the room, indicating the use of an allocentric place strategy. In contrast, for the aged rats, a majority continued to make a right turn even though this took them to a different location in the room (Figure 15.2D). This suggests the use of a response strategy by older animals to solve the problem. The authors interpreted this to mean that a compromised hippocampus in old rats provoked the use of strategies supported by other structures (Barnes et al., 1980). This hypothesis was later supported in a study in which the dorsal striatum was inactivated in young (4 months) and aged (25 months) male F344 rats. The dorsal striatum is a structure thought to mediate response-based behavior (Packard et al., 1989), and inactivation of this structure selectively provoked the use of a place-based strategy in old rats without altering behavior in young animals (Gardner, Gold, et al., 2020).

Age-related differences in strategy use have also been examined in humans in a virtual Y-maze task. As in the rodent studies, when the start location is changed in virtual space, older human participants (55–85 years) tend to use an egocentric response strategy whereas younger adults (18–35 years) were more likely to use a spatial allocentric strategy (Rodgers et al., 2012). Across studies, similar results are observed with more complex navigation tasks where older adults from different experiments ranged in age from 50 to 90 years compared with younger adults that ranged in age from 18 to 38 years. These studies reported that, compared with their younger counterparts, older adults are impaired at switching from the use of an egocentric to an allocentric strategy (Moffat et al., 2007; Iaria et al., 2009; Head and Isom, 2010; Etchamendy et al., 2012; Harris, Wiener, et al., 2012; Wiener et al., 2013; Harris and Wolbers, 2014; Schuck et al., 2015; Zhong and Moffat, 2016). Furthermore, it has been shown that older adults (53–85 years) that have a relatively smaller hippocampus are more likely to use response-based strategies than are older adults with larger hippocampal volumes (Moffat et al., 2007; Bohbot et al., 2012; Rodgers et al., 2012).

The eight-arm radial maze is another test of spatial behavior in which the use of multiple strategies between young and aged rats has been examined. Figure 15.3A schematically depicts this test of spatial behavior. In this maze a reward is placed at the end of each of eight arms, and an error is counted if the rat returns to a previously visited arm prior to retrieving all eight rewards (Potegal, 1969; Olton et al., 1977). Old male Long Evans rats (29 months) make significantly more errors than do 14-month-old animals (Barnes et al., 1980) (Figure 15.3B). Interestingly, neither age group used a serial response strategy in which adjacent arms were visited sequentially, suggesting that both young and old animals used an allocentric strategy to solve the task (Barnes et al., 1980). In a different experiment, local cues were placed on the eight arms (Figure 15.3C). Under these conditions, there was no difference in performance between 11- and 26-month-old male F344 rats (Figure 15.3D), showing that when old rats were allowed to use a cue-based strategy, presumably decreasing hippocampus involvement, they can perform as effectively as younger animals

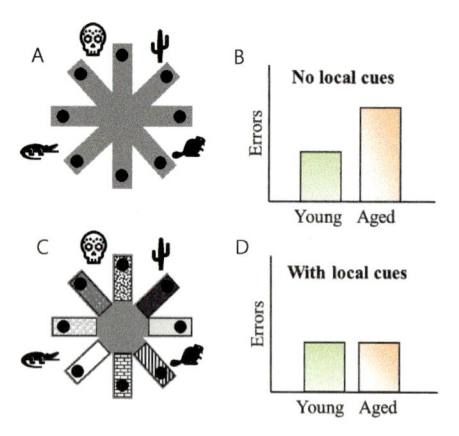

Figure 15.3 The eight-arm radial maze. (A) A rat is placed at the center of a radial maze and needs to visit each arm to retrieve a reward. In the spatial version of this task, all arms are identical, and the rat must use distal cues in the environment to facilitate performance. An error is counted if the animal returns to a previously visited arm before retrieving each reward from the different arms. (B) When a spatial strategy is required to complete the radial maze, aged rats make more errors than do their younger counterparts. (C) A different version of the eight-arm radial maze places distinct local cues in each arm. (D) When proximal cues are added to the maze to differentiate the arms, young and aged rats perform similarly.

(Barnes, Green, et al., 1987). A number of other studies have replicated the age-related impairment on the eight-arm radial maze when an allocentric strategy is required. This is true for male rats across F344, Sprague Dawley, and Long Evans strains between the ages of 1 and 33 months (Wallace et al., 1980; Beatty et al., 1985; Gallagher et al., 1985; Van Gool et al., 1985; Geinisman et al., 1986; deToledo-Morrell et al., 1988; Barnes et al., 1989; Mizumori et al., 1990; Caprioli et al., 1991; Mizumori et al., 1992; Mizumori et al., 1996; McLay et al., 1999; Templer et al., 2019).

Male and female mice across strains (C57Bl/6J, C57Bl/6, C57/bl6 Jico, CD-1, and Swiss Webster) between 2 and 28 months of age also show reduced performance accuracy on the radial eight-arm maze at older ages (Bernstein et al., 1985; Lebrun et al., 1990; Hoskins et al., 1991; Marighetto et al., 2000; Krazem et al., 2003; Touzani et al., 2003; Lohmann and Riepe, 2007). Likewise, in rhesus macaques, one study comparing young (6–8 years) to aged (23–33 years) animals (sex not specified), revealed age impairments with an eight-location spatial working memory task design (Rapp et al., 1997). The monkeys were tested on a circular platform that contained eight food wells around the edge. After each choice, the monkey was gently pulled by a collar back to the center of the platform for a delay, before being allowed to make an additional choice. Older rhesus macaques compared with younger animals, made more errors by returning to the food wells they had already visited (Rapp et al., 1997). Human participants have been tested in a virtual reality version of the eight-arm radial maze. In this study, performance accuracy in young (mean age 28 years) versus older adults (mean age 67 years) was equivalent (Bohbot et al., 2012). The reason for this discrepancy between humans and the nonhuman experiments remains to be determined.

15.2.1.2 Barnes maze and Morris watermaze

The Barnes maze (Barnes, 1979) and the Morris watermaze (Morris et al., 1982; Gage et al., 1984) require rats to use an allocentric

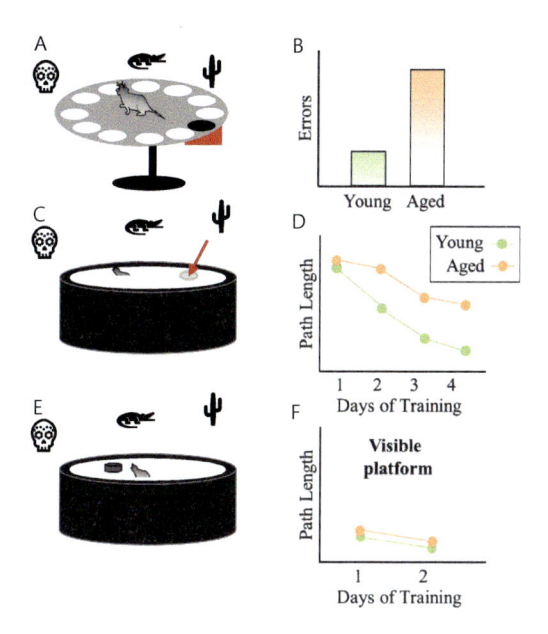

Figure 15.4 The Barnes maze and Morris watermaze. (A) In the Barnes maze, the rat or mouse is placed into a box in the center of a brightly lit circular platform that contains 18 holes around the perimeter. One of the holes leads to a dark escape tunnel (black hole above red box in this schematic), which is preferred over a brightly lit open space. The testing room contains distal cues to facilitate navigation. (B) Aged rats and mice make more errors before learning the location of the escape tunnel compared with younger animals. (C) In the Morris watermaze, a large pool of opaque cold water hides an escape platform just below the surface (indicated in this schematic with a red arrow). The animal is trained over days to find the hidden platform from different start locations. (D) On the first day of training, young and aged rodents perform similarly. Over days, while path lengths for both age groups shorten, aged rodents' path lengths remain longer than young. (E) To ensure that sensorimotor deficits are not confounding the results, rodents also perform a control task with a visible platform. (F) When animals are not blind or motor impaired and have no differences in motivation, young and aged rodents efficiently swim to the visible platform with similar path lengths.

strategy to solve these spatial tasks, and there are changes in performance accuracy across age. In the Barnes maze (Figure 15.4A), the animal is placed into a box in the center of a brightly lit circular platform that contains 18 holes around the perimeter. One of the holes leads to a dark escape tunnel, which is preferred over a brightly lit open space. When all distal cues are away from the maze edge, so they cannot be used as beacons, aged rats are less accurate than young at finding the escape tunnel (Figure 15.4B) (Barnes, 1979). It has been shown that both young (11 months) and aged (26 months) male F344 rats use an allocentric strategy to solve the Barnes maze. Specifically, when two of five cues in the surrounding environment were removed, the performance of young and aged rats was not affected. When all five cues were removed, however, performance deteriorated in both age groups (Barnes, 1987). This indicates that both young and aged animals use allocentric place strategies to solve the problem. Since it was first developed (Barnes, 1979), the Barnes maze has been used to show that male and female rats of the F344, Long Evans, Wistar, Sprague Dawley, Dark Agouti, and F344 x BN (BN) strains between the ages of 2 to 34 months show lower performance accuracy for finding the escape tunnel at the older ages (Barnes, 1979; Barnes et al., 1980; Barnes and McNaughton, 1985; Barnes et al., 1989; Markowska et al., 1989; Barnes et al.,

1990; McLay et al., 1999; Greferath et al., 2000; Barrett et al., 2009; Morel et al., 2015; Pardo et al., 2017; Hosseini et al., 2019; Jiménez-Rubio et al., 2020; Pan et al., 2020; dos Santos Cardoso et al., 2021; Scognamiglio et al., 2024). Similar age-associated impairments in spatial performance have been reported for male mice of the C57Bl/6J and SyG37 strains between the ages of 7 weeks and 30 months (Bach et al., 1999; for review, see Kennard and Woodruff-Pak, 2011; Pereda et al., 2019; Shoji and Miyakawa, 2019). In humans, a task similar to the Barnes maze was implemented in which study participants were asked to place a marker pole at one previously learned unmarked location in a room containing multiple distal cues. Much like the data discussed above from rats and mice, compared with younger adults (18–30 years), older adults (61–80 years) were less accurate at recalling the location (Newman and Kaszniak, 2000).

Tasks similar to the Barnes maze have been used to examine spatial behaviors in young and aged humans. In a real-world urban environment, spatial navigation was examined in young (26–45 years) and older (60–80 years) adults. Older participants had less accurate memory for the location of landmarks and relied more heavily on beacons for guiding navigation than did young adults (Evans et al., 1984). In another real-world task that tested spatial location recall for paintings in a museum, older adults (65–74 years) were less accurate at recalling the position of a painting on a map of the museum and less accurate at navigating to replace the painting at the correct location compared with younger participants (15–24 years; Uttl and Graf, 1993). The memory for locations of paintings has also been tested in a two-dimensional virtual reality task in which participants ambulated on a treadmill that was linked to the visual display. Again, the path lengths of older adults (60–70 years) for returning to a painting were longer and they required more trials to learn the locations of the paintings than did young adults (20–30 years; Lövdén et al., 2005).

A conceptually similar apparatus to the Barnes maze was developed independently by Richard Morris in the 1980s. In the Morris watermaze, a large pool of opaque cold water hides an escape platform just below the surface (Figure 15.4C). Rodents swim around the pool until they find the platform. Like the Barnes maze, the room contains distal spatial cues to facilitate allocentric-based navigation (Morris et al., 1982; Morris, 1984). A large body of literature consistently reports age-related spatial memory deficits in this task (Figure 15.4D) for male and female rats of the F344, Long Evans, F344 x BN, and Sprague Dawley rat strains between the ages of 1 and 32 months (Gage et al., 1984; Biegon et al., 1986; Rapp et al., 1987; Markowska et al., 1989; Lindner et al., 1992; Gallagher et al., 1993; Markus et al., 1994; Chouinard et al., 1995; Frick et al., 1995; Rapp and Gallagher, 1996; Barnes, Rao, et al., 1997; Barnes, Suster, et al., 1997; Lanahan et al., 1997; Lindner, 1997; Rosenzweig et al., 1997; Hebda-Bauer et al., 1999; Markowska, 1999; Markowska and Savonenko, 2002; Tombaugh et al., 2002; Bizon et al., 2004; Nicholson et al., 2004; Wilson et al., 2004; Tombaugh et al., 2005; Foster and Kumar, 2007; Adams et al., 2008; Gerrard et al., 2008; Krause et al., 2008; Bizon et al., 2009; Maei et al., 2009; Guidi et al., 2014; McQuail and Nicolle, 2015; Johnson et al., 2016; Rao et al., 2021; Koh et al., 2022; Gray et al., 2023; Chen et al., 2024). It has also been reported that aged male and female mice do not find the platform as efficiently as their younger counterparts in C57BL/6 and C57BL/6J strains between the ages of 3 and 24 months (Harburger et al., 2007; Pawlowski et al., 2009; Zhao et al., 2009; for review, see Kennard and Woodruff-Pak, 2011; Han et al., 2017; Shoji and

Miyakawa, 2019). Furthermore, aged (23 months) male and female C57Bl/6 x SJL F1 hybrid mice use cue-based over allocentric-based navigation strategies in the watermaze compared with younger (12 month) animals (Nicolle et al., 2003). This observation is consistent with age-related differences in strategy use observed on T-maze tasks described above. Once the platform location is learned in the watermaze, aged rats (Guidi et al., 2014), and mice (von Bohlen und Halbach et al., 2006) are also more likely to forget the location than are young animals.

It is worth mentioning a number of methodological considerations when testing spatial behaviors. It is critical to distinguish between age-related sensorimotor changes and age-related cognitive changes. Several methods have been used to accomplish this. The first method has been to include visual discrimination tests along with spatial memory acquisition trials. In the Barnes maze, this is accomplished, for example, by placing a beacon in the circular arena to indicate the location of the escape tunnel. For the Morris watermaze, the escape platform can be made visible to facilitate finding the goal location (Figure 15.4E). Aged animals without visual impairment typically learn cue-based tasks just as well as younger animals (Figure 15.4F). Additionally, the confounds of age-related motor slowing (e.g., Salthouse, 1976) can be eliminated by only looking at variables that are independent of motor performance, such as number of errors or total distance traveled (also referred to as path length). Studies in which latency values are presented as the primary measure of age differences should be viewed cautiously.

Another set of concerns involves the experimental procedures that are used to train animals and the age at which rodents are assessed for a given strain. The procedural factors include the number of trials administered per day, whether intermittent probe trials are used within the acquisition training across days, whether the cued training trials are included at the beginning or end of spatial training, how removed from the apparatus the distal cues are, and the number of distal cues available. Nonetheless, it should be pointed out that there is remarkable consistency across experiments that aged rodents perform more poorly on spatial tasks than do young animals. Another issue that arises is that an F344 rat is at its 50% mortality age at 24 months, whereas a Long Evans or F344 x BN is not at their 50% mortality age until past 30 months. In other words, 24 months is not an equivalent age across strains, which can impact the proportion of animals that appear to be impaired.

Virtual reality versions of the Morris watermaze have also been developed for humans. In the first study using this approach, young (<45 years), middle-aged (45–65), and older (>65 years) adults were tested for their ability to find a hidden goal location in virtual space (Moffat et al., 2001). The pathlength was greatest in the older adults, intermediate in the middle-aged group, and shortest for the young participants (Moffat et al., 2001). This pattern was also observed when pathlength and time spent in the target quadrant was measured in young (20–39), middle-aged (40–59), and older (>60) adults (Driscoll and Sutherland, 2005). When pathlength was examined across ages 25 to 93, there were small differences in path length between younger and older participants up to 65 years of age. The path lengths of individuals over 65, however, were longer than those observed in participants below 65 years (Moffat and Resnick, 2002). When a proximity measure to the platform was quantified, older adults (60–79) were less accurate than were young (18–30) (Zhong et al., 2017). Notably, in this study when the platform was visible,

there was no significant difference in pathlength across age. Older adults, however, were significantly slower in this cued condition, reinforcing the importance of controlling for age-related differences in movement speed.

In both young (mean age 27) and aged (mean age 68) participants, accuracy on the virtual Morris watermaze has been shown to correlate with the fMRI BOLD signal in the parahippocampal gyrus (Moffat et al., 2006). Moreover, another experiment compared young (mean 25 years) and older (mean 69 years) adults and replicated the age difference in virtual Morris watermaze performance (Moffat et al., 2007). A separate study also showed reduced navigation accuracy with age on a virtual Morris watermaze. In this study, the older individuals (64–79 years) showed no significant task-related hippocampus activation, while the young study participants (20–26 years) had significant activation bilaterally (Antonova et al., 2009). More recently, performance on the virtual Morris watermaze has been tested in a fully immersive three-dimensional virtual reality system with goggles, which requires ambulation to the goal location. Similar to the two-dimensional watermaze studies, older adults (66–82 years) remembered target locations less precisely than did the younger (18–28 years) adults (McAvan et al., 2021).

The precision of recalling a previously learned location on a background scene has also been shown to be reduced in older (59–80 years) compared with younger (18–33 years) adults (Nilakantan et al., 2018). Additionally, when asked to navigate to and locate specific items on a shopping list, older adults (61–77 years) took longer routes than younger adults (20–31 years) to locate the items. The authors conclude that this age difference was due to reduced knowledge of where items were located with respect to one another (Sjölinder et al., 2005).

Given the variety of tasks and procedures that have been used to examine hippocampus-dependent spatial behaviors in humans, nonhuman primates, and rodents, the consistency of the age-related changes in navigation accuracy is remarkable. Thus, it is not surprising that spatial behaviors have been a powerful tool for examining the cognitive consequences of age-related changes in hippocampus anatomy, connectivity, metabolic activity, neurophysiology, neurochemistry, and molecular signaling across species.

15.2.2 Recognition and discrimination

"Recognition" is used here to refer broadly to behaviors that involve the ability to recall a previously experienced stimulus or context. Central to this cognitive function is the ability to discriminate a novel stimulus from a familiar one. Because recognition cannot be achieved without effective discrimination, in this section, recognition-based behaviors will be discussed in relation to discrimination abilities. The term "pattern separation" (Marr, 1971; Rolls, 2013) is not used in the present section because pattern separation refers to a neuronal population-level mechanism for orthogonalizing overlapping inputs. This computation is theoretically used by the hippocampus and other networks (Kent et al., 2016) to reduce interference between similar episodes over time. While this process may support behavior, the term "discrimination" is more accurate than "behavioral pattern separation," because network computations cannot be assessed by behavior alone (Santoro, 2013).

15.2.2.1 Delayed non-matching-to-sample (DNMS) task

The DNMS task involves presenting a sample object after which a delay is imposed. The delay is followed by a test phase with two objects. One object is a copy of the sample object, while the other is new. The most common form of the task uses trial-unique objects, and the nonmatch rule requires the animal to remember the sample object and make the correct discrimination by selecting the novel object during test. Task difficulty can be manipulated by either increasing the length of the delay or increasing the number of sample stimuli presented prior to test. This task was first developed for testing the behavioral impact of hippocampus lesions in nonhuman primates (Mishkin and Delacour, 1975), and this structure has been implicated in supporting DNMS performance (Zola-Morgan and Squire, 1985; Leonard et al., 1995; Zola et al., 2000; Baxter and Murray, 2001b; Zola and Squire, 2001). Since its development, the DNMS task and similar tests of recognition have also been used to measure cognitive aging in primates and rodents. Moreover, age-related neurobiological changes in the hippocampus that will be discussed below have been correlated with DNMS performance. Prefrontal cortical (e.g., Bachevalier and Mishkin, 1986), perirhinal (e.g., Buffalo et al., 1999), and mixed rhinal cortical (e.g., Meunier et al., 1993) lesions, as well as functional disconnections between the prefrontal cortex and medial temporal lobe (Browning et al., 2013) have also been shown to impact DNMS performance accuracy. Thus, the hippocampus could serve as a critical hub of an integrated network that supports this behavior.

Early reports on the effects of age on DNMS task performance indicate a change in accuracy between young and older groups. Age-related differences were observed across increasing delays and increasing numbers of sample objects in 8 male and 11 female rhesus macaques ranging in age from 3 to 29 years (Presty et al., 1987). In a similar study, DNMS task performance was compared between young (4–5 years, $n = 6$) and aged (26–27 years, $n = 6$) male and female rhesus macaques using delays from 10 to 300 s, and for 1–10 different objects before test. Again, the aged monkeys made more errors under these conditions than did the younger animals (Moss et al., 1988). In another study, 5 aged (22–26 years) female rhesus macaques took more trials to reach criterion at a 10 s delay than did 4 young (9–11 years) animals (Rapp and Amaral, 1989). In a related study, aged monkeys (22–33 years) showed poorer performance than young monkeys out to 10-minute delays (Rapp and Amaral, 1991).

Differences in DNMS task performance across age have been replicated in subsequent studies, including one using 53 rhesus macaques (22 females and 31 males) between 4 and 31 years (Herndon et al., 1997). Additionally, later studies compared DNMS task performance between young (7–13 years) and aged (24–33 years) male and female rhesus macaques. Consistent with the studies discussed above, these aged monkeys took longer than their younger counterparts to learn the DNMS rule with a 10 s delay and made more errors when delays were increased from 30 to 600 seconds (Shamy et al., 2006; Bañuelos et al., 2023). In this study, the volume of the hippocampus was measured using structural MRI methods. Volume across the full rostrocaudal extent of the hippocampus differed between age groups by less than 6% and was not correlated with DNMS task performance. In these same monkeys, when cerebral blood volume (CBV) was examined in the entorhinal cortex, dentate gyrus, CA1, and subiculum, there was a region-selective reduction in metabolic activity in the dentate gyrus of the old animals compared with young. Additionally, within the old monkeys there was a significant positive correlation between the amount of CBV activity and DNMS task accuracy (Small et al., 2004). In a

more recent study, 15 young (7–14 years) and 20 old (24–30 years) rhesus macaques and 6 young (11–12 years) and 7 old (21–31 years) bonnet macaques were examined. The young bonnet and rhesus macaques acquired the task at similar rates. There was a species-by-age interaction, however, such that the aged bonnet macaques acquired the DNMS rule more rapidly than did the aged macaques. After criterion at a 10 s delay was achieved, however, aged bonnet and rhesus macaques showed similar reductions in task accuracy across longer delays up to 10 min (Comrie et al., 2018).

15.2.2.2 Digit recognition span test (DRST)

Another task that has been used to examine hippocampus dependent behavior in the nonhuman primate is the digit recognition span test (DRST). In this task, the animal is presented with an array of 18 food wells and the monkey must discriminate a new spatial location from a location in which food had previously been retrieved. Specifically, a location with a reward is marked by a small disc that the animal can displace to retrieve reward. After retrieval, the disc over the first location is replaced and a new identical disc at a different location on the array is then added. The monkey's task is to select the new location to retrieve a reward. Additional discs are added until the monkey makes an error. A new trial is begun at this point, and this is repeated for 10 trials to calculate an average recognition span score. For example, a recognition span of 2 means that the monkey made an error when there were three discs on the array. The DRST can also be implemented using different colors. In this version, a disk of a different color is added after each retrieval, but the location provides no information. In both versions of DRST, hippocampus lesions impair performance in young monkeys (Beason-Held et al., 1999). Age differences in performance of young and old rhesus macaques have been observed on both the spatial location and color versions of DRST. Young males (5–6 years) have significantly greater digit span recognition compared with aged male and female (25–27 years) rhesus macaques (Moss et al., 1997). This age-related impairment was replicated in a later study with 53 monkeys (22 females and 31 males) between the ages of 4 and 31 years (Herndon et al., 1997). As with the DNMS task, other structures such as the prefrontal cortex and parahippocampal region participate in task performance. The extent to which age-related changes in these regions contribute to observed deficits has yet to be examined.

15.2.2.3 Visual paired comparison (VPC) test

In addition to appetitive-based tests of discrimination, some tasks use an animal's natural tendency for viewing or exploring novel stimuli, such as the visual paired comparison (VPC) task, originally designed for visual discrimination in human infants (Fantz, 1964; Fagan, 1970). This task was later adapted for nonhuman primates, in which saccadic eye movements are monitored to measure the time spent viewing novel versus familiar images, which is shown in Figure 15.5A,B. While young primates spend more time viewing novel over familiar images, lesions of the hippocampus reduce this novelty preference (Zeamer et al., 2011). When male and female rhesus macaques were examined between 6 and 30 years of age, the older monkeys tended to have less of a preference for viewing the novel images (Insel et al., 2008) (Figure 15.5C). Using a similar protocol, the VPC task has also been used to measure the preference for viewing novel images in male and female human participants ranging in age from 18 to 99 years. Similar to observations made in

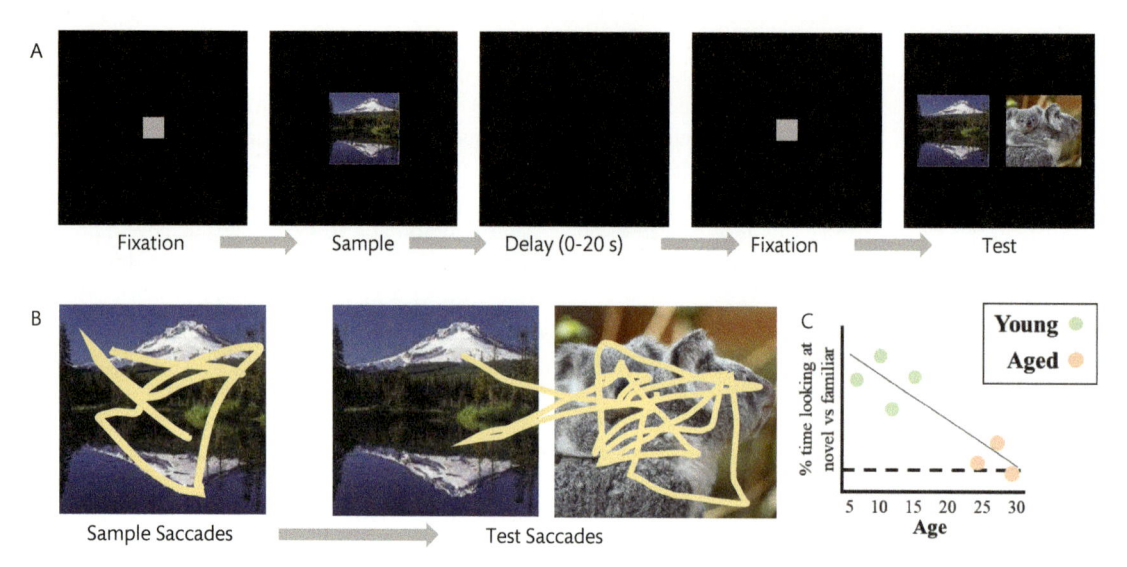

Figure 15.5 Human and nonhuman primate visual paired comparison (VPC) task. (A) Shows the phases of the VPC task. A study participant fixates on the center of a computer monitor, then a sample image appears, and saccades are monitored. After a delay, the fixation cue appears again, followed by the simultaneous presentation of the familiar sample image (mountain) and a novel image (koalas). (B) Example saccades (yellow lines) during the sample and test phases of the VPC task. (C) Younger study participants saccade more to the novel versus familiar image than do older monkeys and humans. Horizontal dashed line indicates no novelty preference.

nonhuman primates, older adults above 55 years showed less of a preference for viewing novel images (Whitehead et al., 2018).

A conceptually similar task was designed to examine discrimination performance in rodents in which exploration of a novel object (Ennaceur and Delacour, 1988), or spatial location (Ennaceur and Meliani, 1992) was compared with familiar objects and locations. Both the object and location variants of this task are shown in Figure 15.6A,B. While originally referred to as "spontaneous object recognition" or "spontaneous object location memory," these tasks are more commonly referred to as novel object recognition or novel location recognition. Similar to the VPC task used in primates, the acquisition of a learning rule is not required, and performance measurements are based on a rodent's natural preference for novelty. Also, like VPC, there is an initial familiarization phase, where the rodent explores a set of novel objects (that are usually identical). For the object recognition variant of the task, after a variable delay up to 24 hours, the test phase consists of presenting a third copy of the now familiar object and a novel object. For the location variant, the delay is followed by a test phase in which one of the familiar objects is moved to a novel location. Young rats

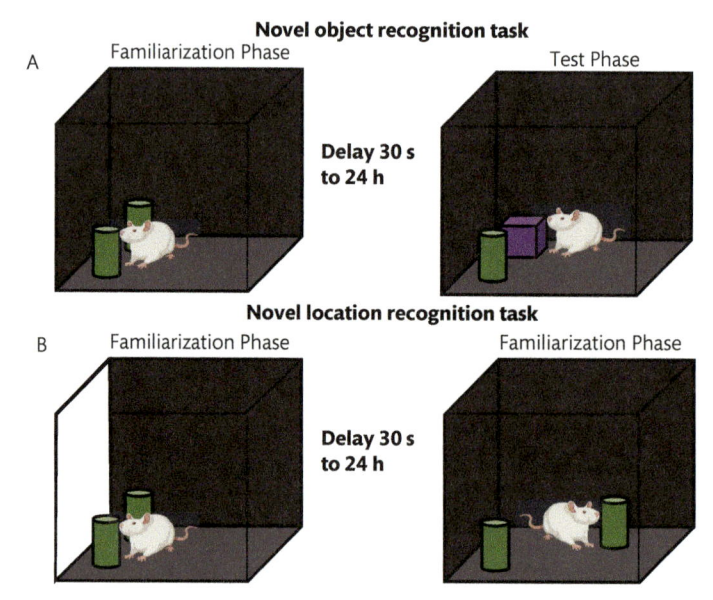

Figure 15.6 Novel object and novel location recognition tasks. (A) During the novel object recognition task, rodents first complete a familiarization phase in which they explore two identical novel objects in an arena. After a variable delay, the animal is returned to the arena for the test phase with a third copy of the original object from the familiarization phase, and a novel object. Young rodents spend more time exploring the novel over familiar object in the test phase. (B) The familiarization phase of the novel location task includes an orienting cue (for example, a white wall) in the arena while the rodent becomes familiar with the two identical objects. After the delay, the animal is returned to the arena in which one of the familiar objects has been moved to a novel location. Young rodents spend more time exploring the familiar object in the new location than do older animals.

spend more time exploring new objects or familiar objects in new locations (Ennaceur and Delacour, 1988; Ennaceur and Meliani, 1992). Under certain protocols, both variants of these recognition tasks require the hippocampus (e.g., Ennaceur and Aggleton, 1997; Ennaceur et al., 1997; Hammond et al., 2004; Cohen et al., 2013; Stackman et al., 2016). Although some studies have reported no effect of hippocampus lesions on novel object recognition (Mumby et al., 1992; Mumby, 2001; for review, see Aggleton and Nelson, 2020), other research has reported that the hippocampus is critical for object recognition (for review, see Cohen et al., 2013). This controversy aside, the perirhinal cortex is unequivocally critical for novel object recognition (Ennaceur and Aggleton, 1997; Mumby et al., 2002b).

The first study to evaluate performance on this task with respect to age examined male Wistar rats between 4 and 24 months. Up to a delay of 5 min, there was no age difference in the preference for a novel over a familiar object (Cavoy and Delacour, 1993). A similar lack of an age difference after a 3 min delay was recently reported for male Long Evans rats at 22–26 months compared with 4–6 months. Intact novel versus familiar object discrimination has also been reported with 5 min delay for male and female C57BL/6J mice between 3 and 20 months (Benice et al., 2006).

In later studies, using male rats of the Wistar, HsdCpb:WU, or CD-COBS strains between the ages of 3 and 25 months, a reduced preference for novelty was consistently found at older ages when a delay of 60 min between familiarization and test was used (Bartolini et al., 1996; Scali, Giovannini, Bartolini, et al., 1997; Scali, Giovannini, Prosperi, et al., 1997; Vannucchi et al., 1997; Pitsikas et al., 2005) (but see, de Lima et al., 2005). In one study that tested male C57Bl/6NIA mice 2–4 or 22–24 months, there was no difference in the exploration preference for a novel object between age groups with a delay of 24 hours (Wimmer et al., 2012). In a more recent study, however, aged male C57B7/6J mice (23 months) and middle-aged (13 months) mice were tested for novelty preference by measuring the number of nose touches to a new object. After only a 3 min delay, the middle-aged mice touched the novel object more than did the aged mice (Yanai et al., 2018). Several possibilities may explain these discrepancies, such as differences in the number of exploration trials and objects that are used. Other possibilities include measuring novelty preference by touching objects versus exploration times and whether raw data were analyzed, which allows for differentiation between exploring novel objects less versus familiar objects more (McTighe et al., 2010).

Another study also found differences in novelty preference between young (7–9 months) and old (24–25 months) male F344 rats for a delay interval as short as 15 min (Burke et al., 2010). This study examined raw exploration times of individual objects. Aged rats explored the novel object less than did their younger counterparts, while spending a similar amount of time exploring the familiar object. Thus, old animals behaved as if the novel object was familiar. At only a 2 min delay, exploration behavior was comparable between young and aged rats, ruling out overall age differences in motivation and sensorimotor impairments. This observation was replicated in a later study that used 4 objects, two of which were replaced during the test phase. Young (3 months) male Sprague Dawley rats were not different from the aged rats (18–24 months) at the 5 min delay, but the aged group explored novel objects less than did young animals at the 24-hour delay (Arias-Cavieres et al., 2017). In a more recent study, 18- to 22-month-old F344 rats were impaired and

novel versus familiar object discrimination compared with 2- to 4-month-old animals with a delay interval of 24 hours (Scognamiglio et al., 2024).

Discrimination of novel versus familiar locations of objects has also been examined across the lifespan, and this variation of a recognition task is unequivocally hippocampus-dependent (Ennaceur and Meliani, 1992; Ennaceur et al., 1997; Mumby et al., 2002a). Shukitt-Hale et al. (2001) made the observation that when familiar objects are moved to a new location, young (6 months), but not aged (22–24 months), male F344 rats increased their exploration of the displaced objects. In later studies, aged male Wistar rats (23–24 months) showed a reduced preference for a familiar object in a novel location for delays from 1.5 to 24 hours compared with young animals (3–4 months) (Bortolatto et al., 2012; Cechella et al., 2014). In another study, young (3 months) male Sprague Dawley rats were not different from the aged rats (18–24 months) at the 5 min delay, but the aged group explored objects in the novel locations less than did young animals did at the 24-hour delay (Arias-Cavieres et al., 2017).

In young (2–4 months) and old (22–24 months) male C57BL/6NIA mice, at a 3 min delay, there was no difference in the preference for the object in a novel location between age groups. At 24 hours, however, aged mice showed less of a preference for the novel location (Wimmer et al., 2012). A similar decrease in the exploration of an object that had been moved to a novel location has been reported in 18- to 20-month-old male C57BL/6JRj mice compared with 2.5-month-old mice (Gulmez Karaca et al., 2021), and for 22- to 24-month-old male C57Bl/6J mice compared with 3- to 6-month-old animals (Chen et al., 2023) with a 24-hour delay between sample and test. In male and female C57BL/6J mice at 3 and 20 months of age, older animals showed less preference for the object in a novel location after a 5 min delay than did the young animals (Benice et al., 2006). When nose touches were used to quantify differences in exploration, 13-month-old male C57BL/6J mice touched the object in a new location more than did the 23-month-old mice after a 3 min delay (Yanai et al., 2018).

The amount of object displacement can also affect novelty preference. In male C57BL/6J mice of 6 and 20 months of age, after a 3 min delay, objects were moved between 10 and 35 cm. At short distances of 10 or 15 cm, neither 6- nor 20-month-old mice showed a preference for the object in the new location. At 20 cm, the young mice had a significant novelty preference, but the aged animals did not. Both age groups showed a novelty preference when the object was displaced 35 cm (Cès et al., 2018). When mice at 3, 7, 11, 16, and 21 months were tested on the single 20 cm displacement condition, animals 11 months and older showed less of a novelty preference for the moved object (Cès et al., 2018).

A recent study examined the abilities of young (4–6 months) and aged (22–26 month) male Long Evans rats to recognize a familiar object in a different context (object-place-context task [OPC]) than it was originally experienced. All animals had been behaviorally assessed on the Morris watermaze. While there were no significant age differences on the OPC task, the aged rats with the lowest discrimination scores also showed worse performance on the spatial version of the watermaze (Chen et al., 2024).

Several factors can impact the interpretation of results from discrimination and recognition studies, including the delays that are imposed between sample and test, whether the animal is removed from the testing room during the delay, how many common features the test objects share, and how novel versus familiar object discrimination is quantified. Additionally, low levels of object exploration times can result in an inability to detect a novelty preference (e.g., Shukitt-Hale et al., 2001; Niewiadomska et al., 2006; Cechella et al., 2014; Kwapis et al., 2019; Gardner, Newman, et al., 2020).

Similar recognition and discrimination studies have been conducted with human participants. One example of this is an early study that used 20 objects placed in an array and participants were given 90 seconds to study the objects. During the test phase participants were first asked to freely recall the objects (which is cognitively more demanding than recognition), and then participants were asked to demonstrate recognition by discriminating each familiar object from 20 novel lures. Younger adults (17–30 years) recalled more objects than did older adults (60–80 years), but there was no difference in the probability of correctly discriminating the studied objects from the lures (Puglisi et al., 1985), suggesting that recognition was comparable between age groups. The lack of a difference in discrimination abilities between the young and old adults reported in Puglisi et al. (1985) is inconsistent with the rodent results discussed above, and other human experiments using images of objects, as reviewed below.

In many of the human experiments, differences in discrimination accuracy between novel and familiar stimuli between age groups have been reported, consistent with the rodent data. In a study that used images of objects, study participants were asked to discriminate between whether there was a new object or whether a familiar object was in a new location between sample and test presentations. Older adults (mean age 70 years, 11 male/1 female) were less accurate in both the change in object and change in object location conditions compared with the young group (mean age 25, 12 males) (Schiavetto et al., 2002). Consistent with this finding, two more recent studies, with identical behavioral testing procedures, presented participants with an array of objects and asked them to discriminate between a change in the array and no change in the array. There were two possible ways the array could be altered. One involved a condition in which a novel object replaced a familiar one, and the other involved a rearrangement of the objects in the array. In both of these studies, participants ranged in age from 20 to 79 years. Older participants (over 60 years) were less accurate than were younger adults (20–29 years) at detecting both the object and the location change (Muffato et al., 2019; Hilton et al., 2020). Among the older adults, individuals in their 70s performed more poorly than those in their 60s (Muffato et al., 2019). The apparent discrepancy between these studies, in which an age difference was detected, and Puligisi et al. (1985) could be accounted for by the fact that these more recent studies did not have a recall phase prior to discrimination testing. It is possible that recall before test served as a rehearsal that facilitated later discrimination.

In a longitudinal study of individuals initiated between the ages of 62 and 92, a procedurally similar task was administered to investigate the potential change in performance accuracy over a 4-year period. This experiment investigated discrimination of novel and familiar images of objects as well as objects in novel locations between a sample and test presentation. At the fourth and final test session in this longitudinal study, there was a significant decline in performance accuracy in both the object and location discrimination tests. It is not possible to say whether this effect was driven by participants who began testing in their 80s or 90s, as performance was not stratified by age at test onset (Haley et al., 2012). In a cross-sectional study, younger (mean age 21) and older (mean age 71) participants viewed an image of 12 objects in a room. During the test phase, participants were presented with 24 objects (12 familiar, and 12 lures) and asked to discriminate the 12 familiar objects from the 12 novel distractors. Older adults were less accurate than were young at selecting the target objects (Shih et al., 2012). In a more recent study, younger (mean age 24 years) and older (mean age 70 years) participants were asked to remember the identity of objects placed into a realistic virtual scene of Trinity College Dublin while navigating through familiar or less familiar routes on campus. During the test phase, 10 of these familiar objects were presented along with 10 novel lures. Older individuals did not discriminate between the familiar and lure objects as accurately as did the younger participants (Merriman et al., 2016).

15.2.2.4 Mnemonic similarity task

Similar to the VPC task, the "mnemonic similarity task" was also originally developed for humans. This task is designed to examine how feature similarity of familiar and novel stimuli impacts discrimination (Kirwan and Stark, 2007). Example stimuli used in this task are shown in Figure 15.7A. In humans, performance on this task is related to the intensity of medial temporal lobe BOLD signals (e.g., Kirwan and Stark, 2007; Yassa, Lacy, et al., 2010; Bakker et al., 2012; Bakker et al., 2015; Reagh et al., 2018). In rodents, disrupting hippocampal activity in young rats leads to an impairment in discriminating familiar objects from similar lures (Johnson et al., 2019). As in the DNMS task, in humans (Reagh et al., 2018; Nash et al., 2021), monkeys (Baxter and Murray, 2001a; Burke, Wallace, et al., 2011), and rats (Johnson et al., 2021), performance on the mnemonic similarity task also involves contributions from perirhinal and frontal cortical circuits.

Toner et al. (2009) was the first study to use the mnemonic similarity task to compare younger (mean age 19 years) and older (mean age 74 years) adults. Using a continuous recognition design with 108 images of everyday objects in each of 6 testing blocks, participants were asked to report whether the stimulus was "new," "old," or "similar" to a previously viewed object. The older adults were more likely to report that a novel lure stimulus was familiar than were the younger adults. This age difference was particularly evident when the lures shared similar features with a previously viewed stimulus (Toner et al., 2009). When encoding was increased, two later studies replicated this finding in young (mean age 21 years) and older adults (mean age 75 years) (Yassa, Lacy, et al., 2011; Holden et al., 2013). When participants were asked to determine whether an image was of an indoor or outdoor object, the older adults were more likely to report a similar novel lure as familiar (Yassa, Mattfeld, et al., 2011). In a later study, which also used indoor/outdoor judgments to facilitate encoding, a linear decrease in accuracy was found between the ages of 20 and 89 years in the ability to discriminate familiar stimuli from novel lures (Stark et al., 2013). Several studies have reported that even when the mnemonic similarity task is implemented in different ways (instructions to memorize the stimuli, self-paced or forced-choice responses, object or scene stimuli, and confidence ratings), a difference in discrimination accuracy between young (18–38 years) and older (59–89 years) adults is still consistently observed (Stark et al., 2015; Huffman and Stark, 2017; Stark and Stark, 2017; Trelle et al., 2017).

Variations of the mnemonic similarity task have been developed for testing young and old nonhuman primates and rats (Figure

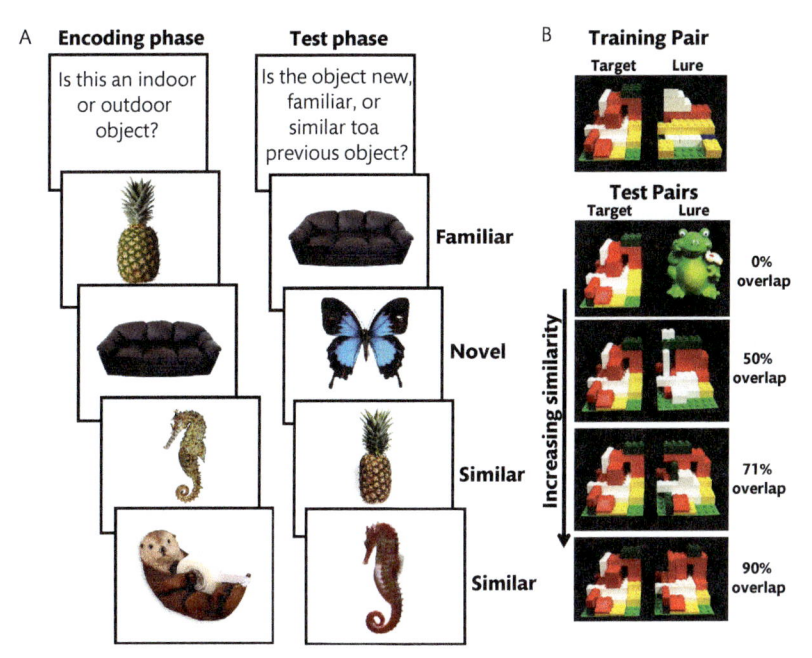

Figure 15.7 Mnemonic similarity task in humans and rodents. (A) The mnemonic similarity task has an encoding and test phase. During the encoding phase, human participants are presented with images of objects. In most variants of this task, incidental encoding occurs by asking the participant to determine whether the object would be found indoors or outdoors. During the test phase, participants are asked to report whether the object presented is "new," "old," or "similar" to a previously viewed object. Older participants are more likely than young are to incorrectly identify a similar novel lure as familiar. (B) In the rodent variant of the mnemonic similarity task, rats are first pretrained to discriminate the LEGO target object from a lure object that is also constructed from LEGO blocks, but is dissimilar from the target. After achieving criterion, rodents begin the testing phase in which the target (rewarded) object is presented with one of four possible lures that vary in similarity to the target. Young and aged rats are similarly accurate at discriminating between the target and lure when they share little to no features (feature overlap < 50%). When the target and lure LEGO objects have more than 50% feature overlap, the young rats are more accurate than the aged are at discrimination.

15.7B). In these versions, LEGO blocks have been used to manipulate the amount of feature overlap between a target and a lure object. In the nonhuman primate study, young (11–12 years) and aged (22–29 years) female bonnet macaques were trained to discriminate a target LEGO block object from a LEGO block lure. The feature overlap between target and lure ranged from 12.5% to 92%. All animals made more discrimination errors as feature overlap increased. The old animals, however, were less accurate compared with the young for the highest feature overlap conditions (>71%) (Burke, Wallace, et al., 2011). For the rat version of the mnemonic similarity task, animals were trained to discriminate a target LEGO block object from a dissimilar lure. Once accuracy was high under this condition, target and lure overlap was manipulated from 0% to 90%. Aged (24 months) male F344 x BN rats were less accurate than were young animals (4 months) at selecting the target object when there was greater feature overlap (Johnson et al., 2017). In rats, mnemonic discrimination abilities have also been tested using olfactory stimuli. Within a homologous chemical series (e.g., alcohols, aldehydes, or acids), feature overlap between two odorants can be manipulated by varying the number of carbon atoms between the two odorants. Young (6 months) and aged (24 months) male F344 rats had similar odor detection thresholds and discrimination accuracy for odorants of different chemical classes or when the carbon lengths of the two odorants varied by 5. When the carbon lengths only varied by 1 or 3, however, the aged rats were significantly less accurate than were the young (Yoder et al., 2017).

Discrimination abilities across the lifespan have also been tested by asking participants to identify whether an image is in a familiar or a new location. Stark et al. (2010) tested young (18–27 years) and cognitively normal aged adults (59–80 years) on a spatial version of the mnemonic similarity task. All participants completed the Rey auditory verbal learning task (RAVLT) and a continuous recognition task in which they studied 10 unique pairs of images and were told to remember their locations. During the test session, participants were told to indicate whether the pictures were in the same location as before or whether one of the pictures was in a different location by a small (10%–20% displacement), medium (25%–35% displacement), or large (40%–60% displacement) amount. Although all participants were less accurate at discriminating between locations when the amount of displacement was small, there was no effect of age on any of the displacement conditions used in this study. In the same study, the aged participants were stratified into impaired and unimpaired groups based on whether their performance on the RAVLT was within the range of young participants. The impaired older adults were more likely than the unimpaired old and young groups to report no change in location when the image had moved (Stark et al., 2010). In a conceptually similar task that employed a forced choice design during the test phase, young (mean age 20 years) and aged (mean age 75 years) participants were tested on accuracy for discriminating a target location from a lure. During the sample phase, a gray circle measuring 1.7 cm in diameter appeared on a computer screen in one of 18 possible locations. The participant was instructed to remember the location of the circle on the screen. During the test phase, two circles were displayed, one in the original location and a lure that was in a location to the left or right of the target. Participants were asked to select the circle in the original location. Distances between target and lure locations ranged from adjacent (but not touching) to 1.5 cm. Across all separations, the older adults were less accurate than were the young (Holden et al., 2012). Another study presented young (mean age 22 years) and aged (mean age 70 years) participants with an image in a location on a 5×7 grid on a computer monitor and asked them to make indoor/outdoor judgments. During test, the image was moved to the left or right by 1 to 4 grid spaces and the participants were asked to make "moved" or "not moved" judgments (Reagh et al., 2014). All participants performed near chance when the image was only moved by 1 grid space. Older adults, however, were less accurate than were the young at discriminating when the location change was 3 or 4 grid spaces (Reagh et al., 2014). Clearly, under some conditions, differences can be detected in the spatial discrimination ability of older compared with younger humans.

In the rat variant of this spatial discrimination task (Gilbert et al., 2001), aged (24 months) male F344 x BN rats were just as accurate as were the young animals (4 months) at discriminating between the target location when the lure was 88 cm or 48 cm from the target. At the 15 cm separation condition, both young and aged rats were at chance levels of performance (Johnson et al., 2016). This finding of no age difference in spatial discrimination performance is reminiscent of the Stark et al. (2010) study that detected no age difference in human participants on a similar task. These observations are consistent with the idea that age differences are particularly pronounced when discrimination is required of objects that share features compared with discrimination of changes in spatial location. Reagh et al. (2016) examined both the location and object versions of the mnemonic similarity task in young (mean age 21 years) and aged (mean age 74 years) humans. Both discrimination tests included an incidental encoding phase followed by same/different judgments. While older adults were less accurate than were the younger participants across both tasks, the effect size was larger for the object discrimination condition compared with location versions of the task. When the older participants were separated into impaired versus unimpaired on the RAVLT (as in Stark et al., 2010), the impaired older adults showed reduced performance on both object and location versions of the task. In contrast, the aged-unimpaired participants were only less accurate than the younger group for the object discrimination version (Reagh et al., 2016).

A wide variety of tasks and procedures have been used to test recognition and discrimination abilities across the lifespan in humans, monkeys, and rodents. A common thread across much of this work is that aged animals are less accurate than are young at discriminating novel from familiar stimuli. The difference in accuracy between age groups is particularly evident when the stimuli share features or when delays between familiarization and test are long. It is conceivable that long delays facilitate the accumulation of interference that then promotes false recognition during test. Thus, age-related changes in performance on DNMS, novel object recognition, and mnemonic similarity tasks may share some common mechanisms. While neurobiological alterations in the hippocampus are likely to make important contributions to these age-related deficits, it should be acknowledged that other structures (such as the entorhinal, perirhinal, and prefrontal cortices) are also likely to be involved in these cognitive changes over the lifespan.

15.2.3 Associative learning and conditioning

As far back as 1941, it was suggested that age-related changes in memory could be due to altered ability of older adults to form and retain associations between different elements of an event or episode (Gilbert, 1941). Following this early description, changes have been reported across a broad range of behaviors and species in the ability of older adults to form and retain associations. This section will focus on studies that have explicitly measured young and aged animals' abilities to create and retrieve links between items and contexts or locations. The extent to which a given memory task requires the creation or use of such associations has been hypothesized to predict the magnitude of older people's memory impairment (Naveh-Benjamin, 2000). While there is an enormous literature regarding associative learning and memory that use word-pairs, word-face pairs, or face-scene pairs in young and old human participants, we only review here those studies in which comparable human tasks have been implemented in rodent, rabbit, or nonhuman primate models. These studies include those that examine object-location binding, trace eyeblink conditioning, and fear conditioning.

15.2.3.1 Object-location binding

The ability to associate an object with a particular location is compromised in animals with lesions of the hippocampus (Lee and Solivan, 2008; Jo and Lee, 2010a) and is related to the intensity of the BOLD signal in the human hippocampus (e.g., Memel and Ryan, 2017). One of the first studies to directly measure the retention of object-location binding examined the ability of young (17–30 years) and older adults (60–80 years) to learn an association between real-world objects and their location on a grid with 40 possible locations. The participants were instructed to study the objects and their locations and then were presented with the empty grid and asked to return the object to the learned location. The young study participants were more likely to return objects to their correct location than were the older adults (Puglisi et al., 1985). A later series of studies tested young and older individuals' ability to recall object-location associations in a physical room, model reconstruction of a room, or on a map. Across three studies, younger adults (mean age 19 years) recalled more object locations than did older adults (mean age 71 years) (Sharps and Gollin, 1987, 1988; Park et al., 1990). The different conditions did not produce consistent age effects across studies, which Park et al. (1990) suggested could be due to demographic differences between study populations.

In contrast to the experiments discussed above, two studies have reported no age differences in object-location associations. When Gilbert et al. (2008) paired six objects with different locations, young (mean age 19 years) and aged (mean age 75 years) participants performed similarly. Another study also found no age difference in object-location associations of nine images located on a 3x3 grid in young (mean age 25 years) and older (mean age 65) participants (Meulenbroek et al., 2010). The discrepancy between these two studies and the earlier object-location results is likely due to only nine, or fewer, object-location associations being presented in the later studies compared with 20–50 associations in the earlier experiments. Odors have also been used to examine stimulus-location associations. Gilbert et al. (2008) paired six different odors with different spatial locations and found that older participants were less accurate than were young at recalling the odor location (Gilbert et al., 2008). In this case, even though a small stimulus set was used, an age difference was detected, suggesting that odor-location associations may be more vulnerable to aging effects than object-location associations.

Conceptually similar studies have used photos of rooms as test items. In one study, participants were shown photos of 5 rooms with

10 test objects in each room. After a learning phase, young participants (20–29 years) were more accurate in locating the objects in the rooms than were the aged (60–75 years) participants (Kessels et al., 2005). In a similar study, participants were shown an image of a room containing 12 objects. The younger (mean age 21 years) participants more accurately recalled the location of objects in the room than did the older (mean age 71 years) participants (Shih et al., 2012).

Associative memory in young and old participants has also been examined using images of objects located on a grid or embedded in a scene on a computer. In one study, young (mean age 19 years) and aged (mean age 71 years) participants were told to remember the location of images on a 7x7 grid. During test, the younger participants had more accurate memory for the object-location associations than did the older adults (Chalfonte and Johnson, 1996). A later study used eye tracking to measure exploration of objects embedded in a scene to infer the extent to which object-location associations had been formed. Ryan et al. (2007) found that young adults (mean age 24 years) saccade more to an area of the scene in which a novel object had appeared or had been moved. When performance of older adults (mean age 72 years) was assessed, they did not increase their saccades to the area of the scene that had a new or moved object to the same degree as did younger participants. This is consistent with other data indicating that the strength of associations between objects and locations in scenes is altered in aging.

In another study that used images of objects in scenes, young (mean age 24) and aged (mean age 71 years) participants were presented with a series of images of object-scene pairs and were told to remember each pair. To ensure that participants associated the object and the scene, they were asked to indicate whether the design of the object fit well with the décor of the scene. Older study participants were less accurate than were the younger adults at remembering the correct object-scene pairs (Memel and Ryan, 2017). A similar study measured the extent to which object-location memory could benefit from participants self-initiating the placement of the object versus being informed of the location. After the self-initiated and informed encoding conditions, older (mean age 69) and younger (mean age 25 years) participants were tested on object-location associations 30 minutes and 1 month after encoding. The older adults were less accurate in each condition than were the younger participants, but this difference was greater for the informed over the self-initiated condition. Accuracy was decreased at the 1-month time point in both age groups similarly (Berger-Mandelbaum and Magen, 2019).

Changes with age in recalling object-location associations have also been observed when study participants are required to place an object back into its original location in a scene presented on a computer monitor. Young (19–23 years old) and older adults (60–73 years old) viewed stimulus displays of three everyday objects in a scene and were told to memorize the identity and location of each of the objects. Older adults were less precise than were the young participants at placing the objects back into the correct location (Korkki et al., 2020).

Many tasks that have measured object-location associations in young and older adults have included an incidental or intentional encoding phase. In a recent study, participants were asked to complete a 2-back task of working memory in which a series of images of 50 objects were presented sequentially on a computer screen. Participants were instructed to indicate if the image was the same or different from the image presented two images ago. Following the 2-back task, young (mean age 24 years) and older (mean age 72 years) participants were surprised with a test that measured the accuracy of image-location memory from the previous working memory task. Older adults were less accurate than were the younger participants (Lugtmeijer et al., 2019). This finding is consistent with the idea that as long as a large stimulus set is used, regardless of intentional instructions or surprise memory retrieval conditions, older adults are less accurate at object-location associations compared with younger adults.

The object-place paired association task (Lee and Solivan, 2008; Jo and Lee, 2010a, 2010b) has been used to measure young and aged rats' ability to form these associations. In this task, a rat traverses between two different locations on a maze and is required to perform different object-location associations in these places. The same objects are used in both locations, but the correct choice is determined by location. Aged male F344 and F344 x BN rats (22–26 months old) take longer to acquire this object-location association than do young rats (4–6 months old) (Hernandez et al., 2015). When male and female F344 x BN rats were tested, aged (23–24 months) rats of both sexes made more errors than did the young rats (4–7 months) (Hernandez, Truckenbrod, et al., 2019).

Stimulus-location binding has also been examined using a version of the paired associates learning task (PAL), which is shown in Figure 15.8A. In the first experiment to use this test in the context of aging in humans, Robbins et al. (1994) examined a large sample of individuals (over 700) between 55 and 79 years of age. Participants were required to learn the location of 6 to 8 different colored stimuli on a computer monitor over 10 trials. When the error rate over 10 trials was examined in 55–64, 65–69, and 70–79 age categories, the oldest individuals showed the highest error rates, the 65–69 group showed an intermediate error rate, and the youngest group showed the fewest errors (Robbins et al., 1994). In a later study that used the same task to test stimulus-location binding in 184 participants ranging in age from 21 to 80 years, a significant negative correlation was found between association accuracy and age (Lee et al., 2013). One study has measured PAL in rats across age, using a task that was adapted from the original neuropsychological test used for human participants, which is depicted in Figure 15.8B. In a hippocampus-dependent rodent variant of this task (Kim et al., 2015), young (4 months) and aged (24 months) male F344 x BN rats were required to learn the location of three images on a computer monitor. Over 15 sessions of testing, the error rate was significantly higher in the older rats (Smith et al., 2021).

Regardless of the conditions under which object-location associations are tested (in a real room or maze, model room, map, or a location on a computer screen), it appears that older animals are disadvantaged in performing these tasks compared with younger animals. This is another example of a cross-species correspondence in the impact of age on hippocampus-dependent behavior.

15.2.3.2 Trace eyeblink conditioning

Eyeblink conditioning can be administered in several ways to measure an association between a tone (conditioned stimulus, CS) and a puff of air or mild shock that induces an eyeblink reflex (unconditioned stimulus, UCS). Young animals without brain damage will acquire an association between the CS and the UCS so that the CS alone will provoke an eyeblink. Hippocampus lesions do not produce deficits in a delay eyeblink conditioning paradigm (Solomon et al., 1983) (when there is no temporal gap between the

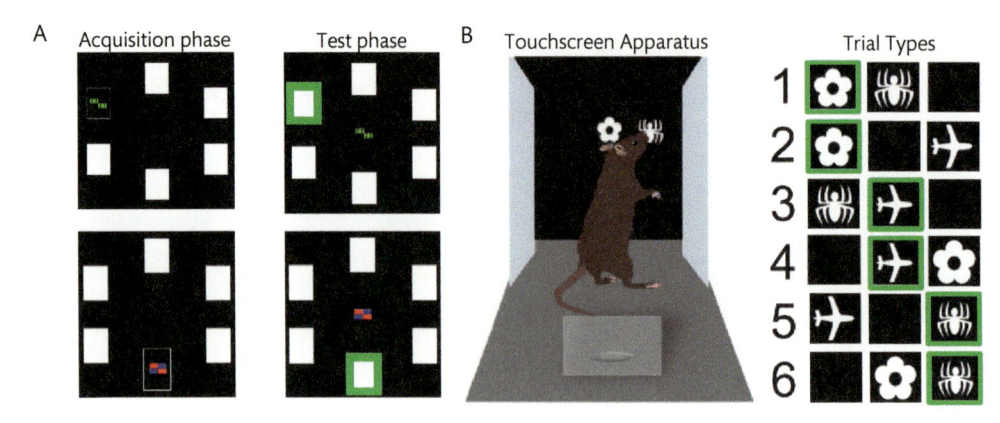

Figure 15.8 Human and rodent paired associates learning (PAL). (A) During the acquisition phase of the human PAL task, study participants are shown the location of an image in an array of six possible locations on a touchscreen tablet, marked by white rectangles. Six different images are shown in different trials. During the test phase, a learned image is presented in the center of the array. The participant is instructed to select the correct location from the acquisition phase (indicated here by green outline). (B) A schematic of the rodent touchscreen apparatus used for PAL testing. Images (flower, spider, or plane) are presented in one of three possible locations. The flower is the correct choice when in the left location, the plane is the correct choice when in the middle location, and the spider is the correct choice when in the right location (indicated by green outline). The rodent is rewarded if they select the image that is in the correct location. The six possible trial types for rodent PAL are shown on the right with green outline indicating the rewarded stimulus. (Rat drawing by Aleyna Ross, 2022.)

termination of the CS and the onset of the UCS), but hippocampus lesions do produce a deficit in the trace eyeblink conditioning version of this task (Solomon et al., 1986) (when a temporal gap is imposed between the termination of the CS and the onset of the UCS). Thus, we focus on the effects of advancing age on trace eyeblink conditioning here.

Many experiments that have examined trace eyeblink conditioning in the context of aging used New Zealand albino rabbits. These experiments consider rabbits between 2 and 6 months to be "young" and 26 and 42 months to be "aged." Because the age of sexual maturity is between 4 to 6 months and the mean lifespan is 5 to 8 years in this strain of rabbits (Figure 15.1B), in the experiments reported here the young rabbits are primarily at or below the age of sexual maturity and the aged rabbits could be considered late middle-age or early old-age. The first experiment that examined trace eyeblink conditioning across age measured differences in number of trials (or acquisition rate) that were necessary for a tone (the CS) to consistently elicit an eyeblink response (blinking to the tone in 4 of 5 trials) in young (6 months) and aged (36–60 months) New Zealand albino rabbits (sex not specified). For each trial, a 450 ms tone (CS) was presented, followed by a 500 ms trace interval during which no stimuli occurred prior to the delivery of a mild infraorbital shock (UCS). Although sensitivity to the tone stimulus and the shock was comparable across age groups, the aged rabbits took significantly longer than did the young animals to show acquisition of the CS (Graves and Solomon, 1985). This finding has been replicated in multiple experiments in young (2–6 months) and old (26–42 months) female New Zealand albino rabbits with a trace interval of 500 ms that precedes a shock or air puff to the eye (Thompson et al., 1996; Thompson and Disterhoft, 1997; Oh et al., 1999; Moyer et al., 2000; McEchron et al., 2001; Weible et al., 2004; Woodruff-Pak et al., 2007). In most of these experiments a pseudoconditioned group was also added to control for nonassociative age-dependent changes in performance. In this control, the tone and shock or air puff were unpaired and none of the animals in any age group acquired a conditioned response.

Differences in the acquisition of trace eyeblink conditioning with age have also been examined in rodents. Using male F344 x BN rats at 6, 18, 22–24, 28–29, and 34–35 months of age and a trace interval of 250 ms, there was no difference in acquisition performance between 6 and 24 months. At 28–29 months, there was a modest reduction in acquisition rate compared with the younger groups. The 34- to 35-month-old rats, however, showed slower acquisition compared with all other ages (Knuttinen, Gamelli, et al., 2001). Consistent with these findings, Matthews et al. (2009) found no difference in trace eyeblink conditioning with the same trace interval in male F344 x BNs in the age range of 3 to 31 months. Another study used a 500 ms trace interval to examine performance in male F344 x BN rats between 2 and 29 months of age. With this longer trace interval, the older animals acquired the conditioned response more slowly. In the aged rats only, slower acquisition was correlated with worse accuracy on the Morris watermaze (Curlik et al., 2014). The difference in performance accuracy between age groups using a 500 ms trace interval has been replicated using the same sex and strain of rat at 3–6 months and 26–32 months of age (Lin et al., 2020). A similar experiment was conducted in male C57bl/6J mice using a 500 ms trace interval in young (2 months), middle-aged (12 months), and aged (23 months) animals. For the young and middle-aged animals, trace conditioning acquisition performance was similar, and both age groups were different from the older mice who showed a substantially lower percent of conditioned responses (Kishimoto et al., 2001). The only other experiment to be conducted in mice used a trace interval of 250 ms in young (3 months), middle-aged (12 months), and aged (22 months) C57bl/6 mice (sex not specified). Two different trace conditioning procedures were used, one with an auditory CS and the other with a somatosensory CS (whisker movement). The young mice in the auditory trace conditioning paradigm acquired significantly more conditioned responses than either the middle-aged or old mice. For the whisker trace conditioning paradigm, the old mice showed significantly fewer conditioned responses than either the young or middle-aged mice (Galvez et al., 2011).

In male and female humans, trace eyeblink conditioning was first measured in adults between the ages of 17 and 81. Following 10 training blocks of 9 trials, with a trace interval of 1800 ms, the young (17–22 years), and middle-aged (39–52 years) participants displayed significantly more conditioned responses than did the older adults (64–81 years) (Finkbiner and Woodruff-Pak, 1991). An age difference in the acquisition of conditioned responses has also been reported for trace intervals of 500 ms and 1,000 ms in young (20–35 years) versus aged (60–75 years) adults, with the magnitude of the effect between age groups being larger for the longer trace interval (sex not specified) (Knuttinen, Power, et al., 2001). These observations were replicated using a 500 ms trace interval in a population of young (22 years) and old (64 years) male and female participants (Cheng et al., 2010).

In summary, an age difference in acquisition of trace eyeblink conditioning is consistently observed in rabbits, rats, mice, and humans. Furthermore, the magnitude of the difference in acquisition of conditioned responses between age groups appears to be greater when longer trace intervals are used.

15.2.3.3 Contextual and trace fear conditioning

There are several different fear conditioning paradigms that examine the degree to which a CS that can be an auditory cue or spatial context, becomes associated with an aversive shock (the USC) to produce a fear response. In rodents, fear responses are measured as a decrease in movement along with a crouched motionless posture (freezing) (Blanchard and Blanchard, 1969). When the conditioning is to a spatial context (Kim and Fanselow, 1992; Phillips and LeDoux, 1992), or there is a temporal interval inserted between the tone and the shock (McEchron et al., 1998), these fear conditioning tasks are dependent on the hippocampus.

The first study to examine fear conditioning in young (4 months), middle-aged (10 months), and aged (23 months) male F344 rats found no differences in shock sensitivity, or in conditioning to the tone CS when there was no interval between the tone and shock (Oler and Markus, 1998). Following three conditioning sessions (one tone-shock pairing in each session), conditioning to the context was examined by measuring freezing in the box without shock administration. There was no difference between age groups at 10 days following conditioning, but the oldest group showed less freezing in the conditioned context compared with the middle-aged and young rats at 52 days (Oler and Markus, 1998). The authors conclude that the aged rats were not able to maintain the context-shock association as well as the younger animals. Examining their data, however, another interpretation is possible. In the young and middle-aged rats, the level of freezing was increased between 10 and 52 days, while the level of freezing in the aged rats was only slightly lower. This suggests that the age effect could have, in part, been due to the younger groups showing an enhancement over time in the fear response that was not evident in the older animals. A subsequent study using the same sex and strain of rats at 3, 9, and 27 months of age, examined contextual fear conditioning to a tone at 1, 20, 40, and 60 days post conditioning with two sessions in which 4–8 tone-shock pairings were given. Consistent with the previous study, the magnitude of freezing behavior was similar between young and old rats 1 day after acquisition. In the 3- and 9-month-old rats, there was an increase in freezing behavior over the 60 days in the conditioning context (Houston et al., 1999). The observation of a strengthened suppression of movement is consistent with the concept of "incubation," first described by McAllister and McAllister (1967), which is a progressive increase in the strength of an aversive memory over time. This incubation effect was not evident in the old animals. When the young and middle-aged animals were placed into a different room in a different chamber, a similar suppression of movement accumulated over 60 days. This was also attenuated in the aged rats. Interestingly, when the conditioned tone was played in the novel context all age groups showed an enhanced suppression of movement (Houston et al., 1999), which is hippocampus-independent. When only one tone-shock pairings is used, age differences in fear conditioning can be observed at 2 days following conditioning in male F344 rats between 6 and 18 months (Mesches et al., 2004) and between 4 and 20 months of age (Gemma et al., 2004).

The hippocampus is also critical for fear conditioning to a tone when there is a sufficiently long trace between the tone and the shock. The first study to measure age differences in rats during trace fear conditioning used female young (4–6 months) and aged (23–25 months) F344 x BNs. All animals received one trace fear conditioning session that consisted of 10 tone-shock pairings with a 20 s interval separating the tone and shock. Conditioning was tested 24 hours later by placing the animals in a novel context and playing the tone. The aged rats showed significantly less freezing to the tone alone compared with the young animals. Additionally, the aged animals had less of an tone-induced increase in heart rate than did the younger rats (McEchron et al., 2004). This observation was replicated in young (2–4 months) and aged (22–24 months) male F344 rats with a 30 s trace interval. When rats of the same sex, age, and strain were tested on a delay version (no trace interval between tone and shock) of this task there was no difference in freezing behavior between age groups (Villarreal et al., 2004). This highlights that age differences in fear conditioning are more evident when the task is hippocampus dependent.

A subsequent study reported that age-related differences in trace fear conditioning are not observable until after late middle age. Male Sprague–Dawley rats at 3–6 months, 8–12 months, 16–20 months, and 24–33 months were tested for conditioning to tone following one session of 10 tone-shock pairings with a 15 s trace interval. The oldest age group was the only one that showed significantly less freezing compared with younger groups (Moyer and Brown, 2006). Normal trace fear conditioning in middle age but reduced freezing to tone in old age has also been reported for male F344 rats. Twenty-four hours after 10 tone-shock pairings with a 30 s trace interval, 3- and 15-month-old animals had similar levels of freezing to the tone in a novel context, while the 22-months-old rats showed less freezing (Dulka et al., 2020).

Studies of contextual fear conditioning in mice across the lifespan have not been designed to look at postshock interval that are long enough to capture the incubation effect, which is when age differences are observed in rats. In C57BL/6 or CBA mice between 2 and 24 months there are no age differences in freezing at 24 hours, 48 hours, 96 hours, and 1 week after training (Gould and Feiro, 2005; von Bohlen und Halbach et al., 2006; Woodruff-Pak et al., 2010; Shoji and Miyakawa, 2019). A more recent study, actually reported more freezing in the conditioned context in 18-month-old male C57BL/6 mice compared with 3-month-old animals (Evans et al., 2021). It remains to be examined whether are not incubation effects occur differentially in young and aged mice.

Only one study to date has measured trace fear conditioning in young and aged mice. Compared with young (4–6 months) male C57BL/6J mice, old (22–24 months) animals show lower levels of freezing to a tone in a novel context 24 hours after a single tone-shock pairing with a 15 s trace interval. Mice of the same sex and strain showed similar levels of conditioning when the there was no trace interval (Blank et al., 2003), which is consistent with reports in rats that trace, but not delay, fear conditioning is impaired in old age.

While there are ethical barriers to implementing fear conditioning studies in humans, one study has examined hippocampus-dependent contextual fear conditioning in younger and older adults. This study measured skin conductance (the unconditioned response) in study participants who viewed an image of a lamp or plant in a threatening context (Battaglia et al., 2018). In this condition, one image was paired with a shock for 60% of the trials (CS+) while the other image was neutral. The young (mean age ~25 years) and older adults (mean age ~66 years) showed similar increases in skin conductance during the acquisition of the CS+ image. Immediately after acquisition, the CS+ and neutral images were presented in a safe context in which neither were paired with a shock. In this safe context, both young and older adults had lower levels of skin conductance responses to the CS+ image. On the next day, the young adults had similar skin conductance responses to both images in the safe context, while the older adults showed an elevated response to the previously shocked CS+ image. When the images were presented in the threatening context, but without shock pairing, both age groups showed fear reinstatement (Battaglia et al., 2018). This is consistent with the majority of studies in rodents that report no difference between young and aged animals in the fear response elicited in the conditioned context when the time interval between training and test is less than several weeks.

15.2.4 Summary

In all mammals examined, age impacts most behaviors that are dependent on the integrity of hippocampus circuits. We broadly grouped hippocampus-dependent behaviors into three fundamental categories: spatial behaviors (section 15.2.1), recognition and discrimination behaviors (section 15.2.2), and associative learning and conditioning behaviors (section 15.2.3). Although distinct cellular- and systems-level mechanisms likely contribute to an animal's ability to accomplish solutions to the tasks discussed, it is stunning how consistent the data are across animals that live to different ages, are of different sexes and strains, and are often tested with different procedures. In all these conditions, clear differences in behavior can be observed at advanced ages. As will be discussed in subsequent sections, the underlying mechanisms that may contribute to these cognitive differences span many scales of analysis, including: anatomical (section 15.3), biophysical (section 15.4), synaptic (section 15.5), neuromodulatory (section 15.6), plastic modifiability (section 15.7), network dynamics (section 15.8), and gene expression (section 15.9). In the following sections, when possible, age-related alterations at these different scales will be linked to behavioral outcomes in the young and aged animals examined.

15.3 Hippocampus cell morphology, number, and phenotype

A common misconception about brain aging is that it results in profound reductions in brain weight (Brody, 1955) from substantial cell loss and deterioration of neuron morphology (e.g., Scheibel et al., 1976; Scheibel, 1979) (Figure 15.9A). While brain weight can decrease with age (Brody, 1955), it is now clear that widespread cell loss within the medial temporal lobe and other brain areas is not an obligatory facet of typical aging. Several improvements in experimental design and anatomical methodology that emerged in the late 1970s led to a more optimistic depiction of the morphology of the aged brain. These improvements include recognizing the importance of experimenters being blind to participant identity, differentiating between demented and nondemented aged individuals for study inclusion (Buell and Coleman, 1979; West et al., 1994), and incorporating mathematical approaches to cell counting that control for differences in histological preparation, an approach known as stereology (see Box 15.1 and corresponding Figure) (West, 1993a; West et al., 1994; Morrison and Hof, 1997; Long et al., 1999; Schmitz and Hof, 2005). This led to the consensus that, across species, the anatomical changes that do occur in the aged brain are subtle and subregion-selective (e.g., Morrison and Hof, 1997; Rosenzweig and Barnes, 2003; Burke and Barnes, 2006; Morrison and Baxter, 2012; Gray and Barnes, 2015).

15.3.1 Cell morphology and number in aged humans

The early reports that neurons showed substantial morphological deterioration in normative aging was questioned by a series of important papers published around 1980 that took into account the cognitive status of the aged individuals investigated. This seminal work found that there was extensive dendritic growth in layer II of the parahippocampal gyrus in nondemented individuals compared with young (Figure 15.9B). In the demented individuals on the other hand, a lack of growth was observed, and in some neurons frank atrophy (Buell and Coleman, 1979, 1981; de Ruiter and Uylings, 1987). Other investigations have reported increased dendritic extent in the dentate gyrus of old compared with middle-aged humans (Flood et al., 1985; Flood, Buell, et al., 1987). In other subregions of the human hippocampus, dendritic branching remains stable across age, including CA1 (Hanks and Flood, 1991), CA3 (Flood, Guarnaccia, et al., 1987) and the subiculum (Flood, 1991) (Figure 15.9B). Consistent with these observations, a study using high resolution structural MRI reported no difference between young (mean age 28 years) and old (mean age 70 years) participants in width of the apical dendritic tree of CA1 and the entire width of the entorhinal cortex (Kerchner et al., 2013).

Another aspect of cellular morphology that could be affected by aging is the density of dendritic spines, but this feature also seems to be stable in old age. Because the quantification of spine morphology is sensitive to postmortem delay (Uylings and de Brabander, 2002), there are few data regarding age-related changes in human spine density. One early study did report, however, that within the dentate gyrus there is no significant reduction in spine density in aged humans (Williams and Matthysse, 1986).

In the 1980s, when new stereological principles were developed (Box 15.1), it became possible to identify and eliminate many of the confounding factors of the previous studies that had indicated a profound decline in neuron number occurring in advanced age (West, 1993a). As a result of applying these new stereological methods, a body of data suggested that there is no significant decline in neuron number with age in many regions, including dentate gyrus, CA3 and CA1 (West et al., 1994). On the other hand, lower numbers of neurons were counted in the hilus and subiculum

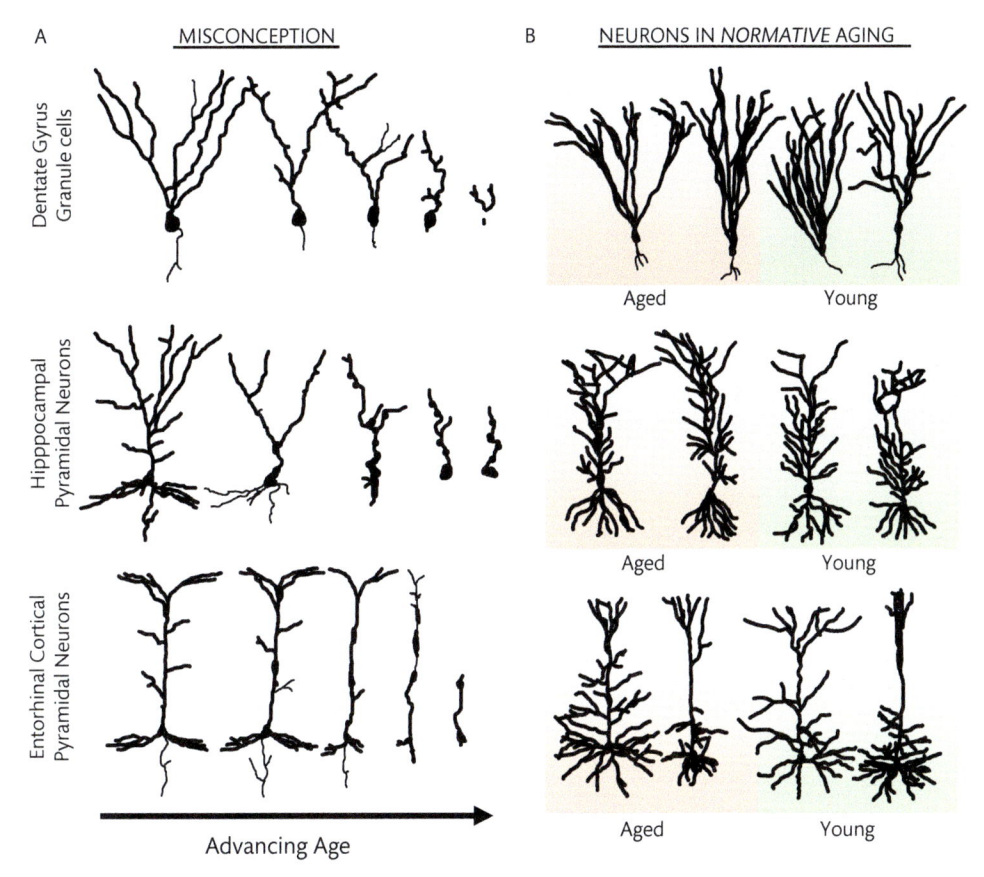

Figure 15.9 Misconceptions of aging hippocampus neurons. (A) Early ideas regarding the effects of advanced age on the morphology of neurons in the hippocampus centered around the notion that across the dentate gyrus, hippocampus proper, and entorhinal cortex there was deterioration. (B) We now understand this to be false. Across all subregions of the hippocampus, neurons continue to have elaborate dendritic arborizations, and there is no significant degeneration in normative aging.

in old compared with young individuals (West, 1993b; West et al., 1994). A careful examination of hilar cell number suggests that the primary age change is from adolescence to adulthood, with limited differences in cell number between the mid-30s through age 85. In contrast, for the subiculum, lower cell numbers are observed from 13 to 85 years of age (West, 1993b). While the stability of principal cell numbers in advancing age has been replicated in other species (i.e., DG, CA3, and CA1), the small change with age in hilar cell number and drastic decline in subicular neurons has not been replicated in other animals (Rasmussen et al., 1996; Spiegel et al., 2013) and warrants further consideration.

The relationship between age and entorhinal cortical cell numbers in humans is complex. One study, which did not use stereological methods, reported that there was no change in neuron number within layers II, III and V of entorhinal cortex between ages 35 and 75 years. None of these individuals had neurological or psychiatric diagnoses, but other aspects of cognitive status were not evaluated (Trillo and Gonzalo, 1992). In contrast, two studies using smaller sample sizes in cognitively uncharacterized individuals did find age-related difference in cell number with stereological methods (Heinsen et al., 1994; Simic et al., 2005). In another study that used stereological methods and considered cognitive status no cell number differences were detected between ages 60 and 89 years in normal adults. Individuals with mild clinically detectable dementia in the same age range, however, were found to have profound cell loss across all entorhinal cortical layers, but most notably in layer II

(Gómez-Isla et al., 1996). This suggests that the two studies that did report cell loss in the entorhinal cortex could have included individuals with mild cognitive impairment.

15.3.2 Cell morphology and number in aged nonhuman primates and rodents

Studies of dendritic extent in other animals have, in general, confirmed that there is no regression of dendrites with age. In the dentate gyrus of monkeys, while the vertical extent is slightly reduced with age in dentate gyrus granule cells, the total length, branching points, and transverse extent remain unchanged (Luebke and Rosene, 2003). Similarly, in rats there is no significant change in dendritic length of dentate gyrus granule cells between 3 and 30 months of age in F344 rats (sex not specified) (Flood, 1993). Unfortunately, the branching patterns of nonhuman primate and rodent CA3 neurons have not been investigated. While not yet measured in monkeys, the dendritic extent of CA1 neurons shows no change between young (2–3 months) and aged (24–26 months) female and male F344 rats (Turner and Deupree, 1991; Pyapali and Turner, 1996). There is some evidence that a small subset of CA1 neurons from 24-month-old male F344 rats have increased basilar dendritic length and branching compared with 2-month-old rats of the same sex and strain (Pyapali and Turner, 1996; but see, Markham et al., 2005). This observation is reminiscent of increased CA1 neuron branching with age observed in humans (Buell and Coleman, 1979). In the subiculum, there is one report in female

Box 15.1 How the advent of stereological methods changed how we think about the aging hippocampus

Early estimates of cell number in the young and aged hippocampus used biased density measures, resulting in the erroneous conclusion that massive cell loss in the hippocampus was a feature of normative aging. One of the problems with density-based measurements of cell number is the fact that tissue processing leads to shrinkage that can be inconsistent between different age groups (Long et al., 1999). Furthermore, corrections for density-based estimates rely on assumptions about the consistency of cell shape and size that are commonly violated (West, 1993a; Morrison and Hof, 1997; Schmitz and Hof, 2005). In the 1980s, stereological methods were developed that enabled accurate and unbiased estimates of cell counts. While there are many types of stereological methods, it is the *optical fractionator* method that enabled the fundamental breakthrough observation that there is no objective evidence for widespread cell loss in the aged hippocampus across species. The optical fractionator method employs four principles. The first is the use of systematic random sampling (A), which ensures that each cell in a structure has an equal probability of being counted. Panel A shows that if the full extent of the hippocampus is sectioned, an unbiased estimate can be obtained by counting cells on sampled sections of a fixed increment (in this example every 4th section, indicated in green). The second principle is the calculation of total number rather than densities (B). Panel B depicts how density measurements lead to biased estimates of cell number when the magnitude of tissue shrinkage during processing varies by age group. The third principle of the optical fractionator method is to count whole cells and not just their profiles on a single optical plane. This technique is called the optical dissector, and it involves creating a stack along the Z-axis (as seen in panel C) of a relatively thick section of tissue, typically 15–40 μm. In practice, this is accomplished by moving the focal plane of a high-power objective from the top to the bottom of the section and identifying and counting the leading edge of each cell. Cells that are not completely contained in the stack (that is, are cut at the top or bottom plane) are not counted, and each cell is only counted once regardless of the number of planes that it is visible on. The optical dissector ensures that all cells have an equal probability of being sampled, regardless of size, shape, or orientation (West, 1993a). Finally, the

optical fractionator method partitions the overall variance into that which is potentially due to biology (i.e., the group variance) and the variance of the individual estimate (i.e., the variance of the counts for sections sampled from the same subject) to determine the sampling precision (West et al., 1993a; Long et al., 1999). If the individual variance is high, then more samples from a single subject will be required to achieve adequate precision. If the group variance is high, then more subjects must be included in the study. This fourth principle revealed that in many early studies that reported differences in cell number between young and aged humans, the sample sizes were insufficient to account for the high group variance, and therefore misleading (West, 1993b).

Aged   Young

rhesus macaques between 7 and 28 years that demonstrated increases in dendritic branching and extent up to 20 years, followed by a reduction in these values in animals 27–28 years old (Uemura, 1985a). Dendritic properties of subicular neurons have not been examined in rodent models or in humans.

Similar to dendritic branching during aging, the data on spine density in animal models indicate that age-associated alterations are region-specific. In the outer molecular layer of the dentate gyrus, which receives synaptic input from the anterior lateral entorhinal cortex, there is no overall change in spine density between 10 and 30 years of age in female rhesus macaques (Hara, Punsoni, et al., 2012). While the CA3 and CA1 regions have not been examined in the nonhuman primate, there is some evidence from a nonstereological controlled study of reductions in spine density in the subiculum between the ages of 7 and 28 years in female rhesus macaques (Uemura, 1985b).

In rodents many more experiments have been conducted regarding spine density across the lifespan. Consistent with the human study, there are no differences in spine density in the dentate gyrus between 6 and 30 months of age in male Sprague Dawley rats (Curcio and Hinds, 1983), between 8 and 26 months in male Long Evans rats (Calhoun et al., 2008), or in male C57BL/6 mice between the ages of 6 and 22 months (von Bohlen und Halbach et al., 2006). A recent study, however, did report a lower density of spines in the dentate gyrus of 18–22-month-old male F344 rats compared with 2- to 4-month-old animals (Scognamiglio et al., 2024). While this study may appear to be an outlier, 2- to 4-month-old animals may still be developing and the higher spine density at this age could be related to a fixed developmental trajectory of decreasing spine numbers between 4 and 6 months of age.

Spine density in the CA3 subregion, as estimated by spinophilin immunohistochemistry, also did not change between 8 and 26 months in male Long Evans rats (Calhoun et al., 2008). In CA1, the effect of age on spine density depends on the dendritic field examined. Markham et al. (2005) reported no change in the numbers of spines within the CA1 stratum radiatum dendritic field between 3 and 24 months of age in both male and female Long Evans rats. Consistent with this finding von Bohlen und Halbach et al. (2006) found no change in the number of spines in the stratum radiatum between 6- and 22-month-old male C57BL/6 mice. They did, however, report a significant lowering in the numbers of basal dendritic spines with age (von Bohlen und Halbach et al., 2006). In contrast, the estimated spine density in the apical CA1 dendrites has been reported to be greater in aged compared with young male Long Evans rats (Calhoun et al., 2008). Clearly, a lifespan examination of spine density in the different subfields of CA1 pyramidal cells and the other principal cell types of the hippocampus will be necessary to clarify true aging effects on this morphological parameter.

In contrast to the experiments conducted with human post-mortem tissue, in monkeys, all studies to date concur that there is no cell loss in layer II of entorhinal cortex with aging (Gazzaley et al., 1997; Merrill et al., 2000). In a recent study, however, there was a reported decline in reelin-expressing stellate cells in layer II of the entorhinal cortex in old (27–38 years) memory-impaired rhesus macaques compared with young (8–10 years) animals (Long et al., 2020). Fewer reelin-positive stellate cells have also been reported in aged (24 months) spatial memory-impaired male Long Evans rats, compared with younger (6 months) animals (Stranahan et al., 2011). Additionally, in rats, there is no change in total cell number between 6 months and 27–28 months of age in the perirhinal cortex, postrhinal cortex (homologous to parahippocampal cortex in primates), lateral entorhinal, or medial entorhinal cortices of male Long Evans rats, even when the animals were impaired at spatial learning and memory (Rapp et al., 2002). Furthermore, monkeys and rodents show preserved neuron numbers in dentate gyrus, CA3, and CA1 (Rapp and Gallagher, 1996; Rasmussen et al., 1996; Calhoun et al., 1998; Merrill et al., 2001; Poe et al., 2001; Keuker et al., 2003). In contrast to the results of the West (1993b) study in humans, however, the numbers of cells in the hilus and the subiculum in monkeys and rats have not been observed to differ between age groups (Rasmussen et al., 1996; Spiegel et al., 2013). Further experiments will be necessary to clarify this discrepancy between species.

A complication that can arise in identifying which specific cell types are vulnerable with aging, is the fact that neurons can change their biochemical profiles across age. For example, while it has consistently been found in nonhuman primates and rodents that total cell number does not decline with age in any hippocampal subregion, the expression of GAD67, calcium-binding proteins, and neuropeptide cofactors do change within these cells in aging. In other words, these interneurons are changing their biochemical phenotype.

In nonhuman primates there is a specific decline in somatostatin-containing GABAergic neurons between middle- (13–18 years) and old-age (29–32 years) in CA3, with no age-related change in CA1 or perirhinal cortex (Thomé et al., 2016). By contrast, in the same animals, the number of parvalbumin-containing GABAergic neurons did not change with age in CA3 (Thomé et al., 2016). In rodents, altered GABAergic interneuron expression of the calcium-binding protein markers parvalbumin, calbindin, and calretinin was reported by A. Shetty and Turner (1998). They compared young (4–5 months) and aged (23–25 months) male F344 rats and found fewer GAD67-containing neurons in the dentate gyrus, CA3 and CA1 of older animals; however, they did not colabel all neurons using NeuN. When tissue was double labeled with NeuN and GAD67 in a later study, preserved total neuron numbers were apparent albeit with lower numbers of GAD67+ cells across all hippocampal subregions in both late-middle-aged and aged male F344 rats (Stanley and Shetty, 2004). In male F344 x BN rats, fewer numbers GAD67-expressing cells were observed between middle- and old-age in CA1 (Shi et al., 2004). It has also been observed that other markers of GABAergic interneurons, including neuropeptide Y in male Long Evans rats (Cadacio et al., 2003), calbindin in Sprague Dawley rats (sex not specified) (Potier et al., 2006), and somatostatin in male Wistar rats (Potier et al., 2006; Gavilán et al., 2007), decline between 3 and 28 months. Consistent with the nonhuman primate data,

Potier et al. (2006) reported no change with age in parvalbumin-positive GABAergic cell counts in male Sprague Dawley rats (Potier et al., 2006).

None of the above studies in rodents accounted for the behavioral status of the animals that were examined. In nonhuman primates, however, the number of somatostatin-positive GABAergic cells in CA3 positively correlated with behavior on a DNMS task (Thomé et al., 2016). In rodents, when performance on the Morris watermaze task was used to categorize animals, there were fewer numbers of GAD67-positive neurons in the hilus of spatial memory-impaired aged male Long Evans rats (24–29 months) compared with unimpaired and young (8-9 months) animals (Spiegel et al., 2013). This was a region-specific effect, as numbers of GAD67-positive cells were stable in CA1. There were lower numbers of GAD67-positive cells in the dentate gyrus and CA3 with age, however, these variables were not related to cognitive status (Spiegel et al., 2013). As in the nonhuman primate, it is the subset of GAD67 cells that are somatostatin-positive that are lower in aged-impaired animals (Spiegel et al., 2013). In a population of male diversity outbred mice, aged (18–24 months) memory-impaired mice also showed lower numbers of somatostatin-positive GABAergic neurons in the hilus compared with their young (4–8 months) counterparts and aged mice without impairment (Koh et al., 2014).

While there is good consensus in rodent and nonhuman primate models of aging that changes occur in calcium-binding proteins in interneuron populations, the examination of postmortem GABAergic neuron vulnerability in humans remains a major gap. That being said, the association between reduced CA3 somatostatin-containing interneurons and hyperexcitability in CA3 reported in nonhuman primates (Thomé et al., 2016), is consistent with the observation of an increased BOLD signal in the DG/CA3 region of the hippocampus in normal older adults with behavioral impairments (Yassa, Lacy, et al., 2010; Yassa, Mattfeld, et al., 2011; Carr et al., 2017). Furthermore, age-impaired rats that are treated with the antiepileptic medication levetiracetam show improved performance on the Morris watermaze and increased numbers of somatostatin-expressing interneurons in the hilus (Spiegel et al., 2013). Levetiracetam also attenuates the DG/CA3 fMRI BOLD signal and improves behavior in individuals with mild cognitive impairment (Bakker et al., 2012; Bakker et al., 2015). It remains to be established, however, whether the mechanism of levetiracetam's effect on cognition in humans involves alterations in somatostatin-containing interneurons. This highlights the need to define interneuron subpopulations that may be vulnerable in older humans.

15.3.3 Summary

Taken together, data from humans, nonhuman primates, and rodents all point to a relative preservation of neuron number and basic morphology in advanced age. This is encouraging because neurons are postmitotic and therefore cannot be replaced by any form of intervention. One goal of the neurobiology of cognitive aging field is to understand the aging brain well enough to identify targets that may allow optimization of cognitive health across the lifespan. Restoring the functional capacity to a network that has retained its basic cellular components is a tractable problem. For example, hippocampal networks that become hyperexcitable with aging, can be modified to perform similarly to younger circuits with the antiepileptic medication levetiracetam (Bakker et al., 2012; Spiegel et al., 2013; Bakker et al., 2015). Given the selective impact of age across neural circuits, and the individual differences that arise across populations, any optimization strategies for brain and cognitive health must be tailored precisely.

15.4 Basic biophysical properties

Even though there is no cell loss over the lifespan, it is possible that functional characteristics of individual cells may become compromised with age. The methods necessary to examine neuronal membrane dynamics and other cellular biophysical properties require invasive neurophysiological approaches. For this reason, animal models are crucial for answering these types of functional questions. Moreover, most experiments that examine basic biophysical properties of hippocampal neurons across the lifespan have, to date, relied on slice preparations by virtue of the electrophysiological techniques required to identify these properties. Nonhuman primate models are costly and often impractical. To date, only one experiment has reported on the biophysical properties of hippocampal neurons in aged monkeys compared with young animals, and it examined only dentate gyrus granule cells. These data will be discussed with comparable experiments in rodents. In many instances, the data obtained regarding the basic biophysiological characteristics of hippocampal neurons across the rodent lifespan are strikingly consistent across experimenters, as well as strains of rats and mice. In these cases, we will give examples citing sex, strain, and age, but will not provide exhaustive details for each study referenced.

15.4.1 Intrinsic membrane properties

Changes in biophysical characteristics critical for cell function could impact circuit dynamics to alter behavioral output. In all subregions of the hippocampus, however, most intrinsic membrane properties remain constant over the lifespan (e.g., Barnes, 1994). Remarkably, this consistency occurs across different rat strains, age ranges, and sexes, including male and female F344 rats between 1 and 30 months, male Long Evans rats between 12 and 30 months, male Sprague Dawley rats between 3 and 32 months, and male Wistar rats between 3 and 30 months. These properties include resting membrane potential for dentate gyrus granule cells (Barnes and McNaughton, 1980b; Barnes, Rao, et al., 1987; Baskys et al., 1987; Niesen et al., 1988; Foster et al., 1991; Barnes, Rao, and Houston, 2000; Krause et al., 2008), CA3 pyramidal cells (Barnes, Rao, et al., 1987; Simkin et al., 2015; Villanueva-Castillo et al., 2017), and CA1 pyramidal cells (Segal, 1982; Landfield and Pitler, 1984; Barnes, Rao, et al., 1987; Kerr et al., 1989; Turner and Deupree, 1991; Barnes et al., 1992; Potier et al., 1992; Potier et al., 1993; Rosenzweig et al., 1997; Kumar and Foster, 2002; Tombaugh et al., 2005; Kumar and Foster, 2007; Kumar et al., 2012b; Kumar et al., 2019). More recently, the resting membrane potential of CA1 pyramidal neurons was also reported to be similar between young (3–6 months) and aged (22–24 months) male C57Bl/6J mice (Chen et al., 2023). The consistency of these findings is striking.

Two studies in New Zealand albino rabbits, however, have reported that CA1 pyramidal cell membranes are slightly more hyperpolarized in aged (39 months) compared with young (4 months) animals (sex not specified; Moyer et al., 1992), and in female rabbits

examined at 2–3 and >36 months (Power et al., 2002). This could be a species difference.

One neuronal membrane change with age is an increase in gap junction connections between dentate gyrus granule cells, CA3, and CA1 pyramidal cells within both the soma and dendritic regions. This has been reported for male F344 rats examined at 9 and 24 months. On the one hand, this increase in ephaptic transmission could act as a shunt for current flow, in cases in which coupled cells are asynchronously activated. In contrast, when afferent input is synchronous, the spike from one cell could depolarize its neighboring cell from a resting state to a state closer to action potential discharge threshold, increasing excitability (Barnes, Rao, et al., 1987).

The somatic membrane time constant in dentate gyrus granule cells is not different between young (<11 years) and old (>24 years) male and female rhesus macaques (Luebke and Rosene, 2003), or between young (12 months) and old (28 months) male Long Evans rats (Barnes and McNaughton, 1980b), and male F344 rats between and 3 and 26 months (Krause et al., 2008). Consistent with this observation, when the passive electrical properties of granule cell dendrites were assessed in 3-, 12-, and 28-month-old Long Evans rats, the electrotonic relationship between synaptic input and location along the dendritic tree remained essentially constant across these ages (Barnes and McNaughton, 1979). Additionally, the membrane time constant is also unchanged with age in CA1 (Pitler and Landfield, 1990; Turner and Deupree, 1991), and CA3 pyramidal cells (Villanueva-Castillo et al., 2017). Basic action potential parameters in the dentate gyrus including current threshold (Barnes and McNaughton, 1980b; Niesen et al., 1988; Barnes, Rao, and Houston, 2000; Luebke and Rosene, 2003), peak amplitude (Barnes and McNaughton, 1980b; Niesen et al., 1988; Luebke and Rosene, 2003), and half width at threshold (Barnes and McNaughton, 1980b; Luebke and Rosene, 2003) are also unchanged in old male F344 rats and rhesus macaques. Although not extensively investigated, CA3 pyramidal cells also do not show significant changes in action potential threshold or amplitude in old compared with young rats (Simkin et al., 2015; Villanueva-Castillo et al., 2017). There is, however, a significantly lower half-width of CA3 action potentials in older compared with younger animals (Simkin et al., 2015).

CA1 pyramidal cell action potential characteristics are also consistent across age in male F344, Wistar, and Sprague Dawley rats, as well as rabbits. These characteristics include height (Segal, 1982; Barnes, Rao, et al., 1987; Kerr et al., 1989; Turner and Deupree, 1991; Moyer et al., 1992; Potier et al., 1992; Potier et al., 1993; Kumar and Foster, 2002; Tombaugh et al., 2005; Foster and Kumar, 2007; Kumar et al., 2012b), and half width at threshold (Segal, 1982; Turner and Deupree, 1991; Moyer et al., 1992; but see, Potier et al., 1993; Tombaugh et al., 2005). The data are equivocal, however, as to whether the threshold to elicit an action potential remains the same with age (Kerr et al., 1989; Tombaugh et al., 2005) or is higher (Landfield and Pitler, 1984; Turner and Deupree, 1991; Potier et al., 1992; Potier et al., 1993). This issue remains to be resolved. A recent paper did report, however, that CA1 pyramidal cells that were active during an epoch of object exploration recorded from male 3- to 6-month-old C57Bl/6J mice, fire more spikes in response to a depolarizing current than those cells that were inactive during behavior for the 5 hours following the experience. This behavior-induced increase in intrinsic excitability in CA1 pyramidal was not observed in 22- to 24-month-old animals (Chen et al., 2023). Because the data from young and aged mice were not directly compared in this manuscript, however, it is not clear that this finding is indicative of age differences in intrinsic membrane excitability.

Overall input resistance is also not different between young and aged granule cells in rats (Barnes and McNaughton, 1980b; Barnes, Rao, et al., 1987; Baskys et al., 1987; Niesen et al., 1988; Barnes, Rao, and Houston, 2000; Krause et al., 2008). In male and female nonhuman primates, while the intrinsic membrane properties are unaltered in old (>24 years) compared with young (<11 years) granule cells, there is a small significantly higher input resistance in older granule cells. Moreover, it is notable that for a range of hyperpolarizing and depolarizing current steps, the voltage measured between young and aged primate granule cells was similar (Luebke and Rosene, 2003). In CA3, the input resistance is also unchanged between young and aged rats (Barnes, Rao, et al., 1987; Simkin et al., 2015). Stable input resistance over the lifespan has also been reported for CA1 pyramidal neurons in rats (Segal, 1982; Landfield and Pitler, 1984; Barnes, Rao, et al., 1987; Kerr et al., 1989; Pitler and Landfield, 1990; Potier et al., 1992; Potier et al., 1993; Campbell et al., 1996; Rosenzweig et al., 1997; Kumar and Foster, 2002, 2007; Power et al., 2002; Kumar et al., 2012a). There is one report in rabbits that suggests a lower input resistance in aged (39 months) CA1 pyramidal cells compared with cells from 4-month-old rabbits (Moyer et al., 1992). Another report in rats suggests that aged spatial memory-impaired animals show a higher membrane resistance in CA1 pyramidal neurons compared with aged spatial memory-unimpaired and young animals (Tombaugh et al., 2005). Taken together, however, the majority of experiments do not indicate robust changes in intrinsic biophysical properties of aged hippocampal neurons.

15.4.2 Voltage-gated currents

While voltage-gated Na^+ currents are unchanged with age in granule cells, as discussed above, there is a reported lowering of voltage-gated L-type Ca^{2+} channel current amplitudes in old (26 months) compared with young (4 months) granule cells from male F344 rats. This difference can be reversed with intracellular injection of the Ca^{2+} chelator EGTA (Reynolds and Carlen, 1989), suggesting that channel number is unchanged with age. In fact, an autoradiographic study of the binding density of L-type Ca^{2+} channels in the dentate gyrus shows preserved channel numbers from 6 to 32 months of age in F344 x BN rats (Kelly et al., 2001). This is consistent with the observation that mRNA levels of the pore forming CaV1.2 and 1.3 subunits are unchanged in granule cells between young (4 months) and aged (25 months) male F344 rats (Herman et al., 1998). When male F344 x BN rats were examined at 3–4 months and 30–32 months, this stability with age was replicated (Núñez-Santana et al., 2014). Moreover, the protein levels in the granule cell membrane for the CaV1.2 subunit were unchanged with age (Núñez-Santana et al., 2014). There was also no age-related difference in CaV1.3 subunit expression in granule cells between 4 and 24 months in male F344 rats (Veng and Browning, 2002). Phosphorylation of surface-expressed CaV1.2, however, was higher in aged compared with young granule cells (Núñez-Santana et al., 2014). Increased phosphorylation is thought to augment Ca^{2+} influx (Gao et al., 1997), and could reflect one mechanism by which aged

granule cells achieve homeostasis in the face of the reduced amplitude of L-type Ca^{2+} channel currents.

One of the basic biophysical functions that L-type Ca^{2+} channels influence is the activation of potassium channels that are involved in repolarizing the neuron after action potentials are generated. In several cell types, this phenomenon can lead to a transient period of hyperpolarization referred to as the afterhyperpolarizing potential (AHP). In dentate gyrus granule cells this AHP amplitude is relatively modest (Barnes and McNaughton, 1980b; Baskys et al., 1987; Niesen et al., 1988) compared with CA1 and CA3 pyramidal neurons. Moreover, the AHP in granule cells does not change with age (Baskys et al., 1987; Niesen et al., 1988). Taken together, these data suggest that the reduced L-type Ca^{2+} channel current is due to altered function rather than loss of channels, but these alterations have minimal impact on the basic biophysical properties of granule cells.

In CA3, autoradiographic ligand binding of L-type Ca^{2+} channels showed no difference in binding density across age in rats (Kelly et al., 2001), nor does the CaV1.2 subunit show elevated phosphorylation, as was observed in the dentate gyrus (Núñez-Santana et al., 2014). In terms of the mRNA levels of these L-type Ca^{2+} channel subunits, there is no difference between young (~4 months) and old (>25 months) male F344 rats (Herman et al., 1998; Núñez-Santana et al., 2014); however, Herman et al. (1998) did observe lower CaV1.2 subunit mRNA expression in middle-aged rats (13 months) that was not evident in the other age groups. While the overall protein levels in CA3 cells of CaV1.2 and 1.3 subunits is lower in older animals (Núñez-Santana et al., 2014), when membrane fractions were examined in isolation, there was higher surface expression of CaV1.2 and 1.3 protein in aged CA3 pyramidal cells compared with young (Núñez-Santana et al., 2014). This change in surface expression is consistent with the observation of elevated binding of the L-type Ca^{2+} channel antagonist nimodipine in CA3 neurons from old male F344 rats (24 months) compared with neurons from younger animals (3 weeks to 18 months) (Araki, Kato, Shuto, and Itoyama, 1997).

In CA3 and CA1 pyramidal neurons, there are three components to the AHP, which are depicted in Figure 15.10A. A "fast" component, involving currents that are responsible for the repolarization phase of the action potential, which determines the rate of the initial hyperpolarization; a "medium" component that corresponds to the peak AHP amplitude; and a "slow" component reflecting the amplitude 1 s post a train of action potentials. While the medium and slow AHP are not altered with age in CA3 neurons, the fast component has a shorter latency to peak in aged compared with young animals following 50 Hz stimulation of the mossy fiber input from dentate gyrus granule cells (Simkin et al., 2015), illustrated in Figure 15.10B. Consistent with this finding, a more recent study showed that following a depolarizing voltage step, the initial interspike interval between the first two action potentials of CA3 pyramidal neurons was lower in 1.5- compared with 22-month-old Wistar rats (sex not specified) (Villanueva-Castillo et al., 2017). Evidence from electrophysiological recordings (Simkin et al., 2015) and gene expression studies (between 8 and 26 months in male Long Evans rats; Haberman et al., 2011) suggest that voltage-gated K^+ currents through the Kv4.2/4.3 A-type K^+ channels are elevated in aged compared with young CA3 neurons. These changes are presumably

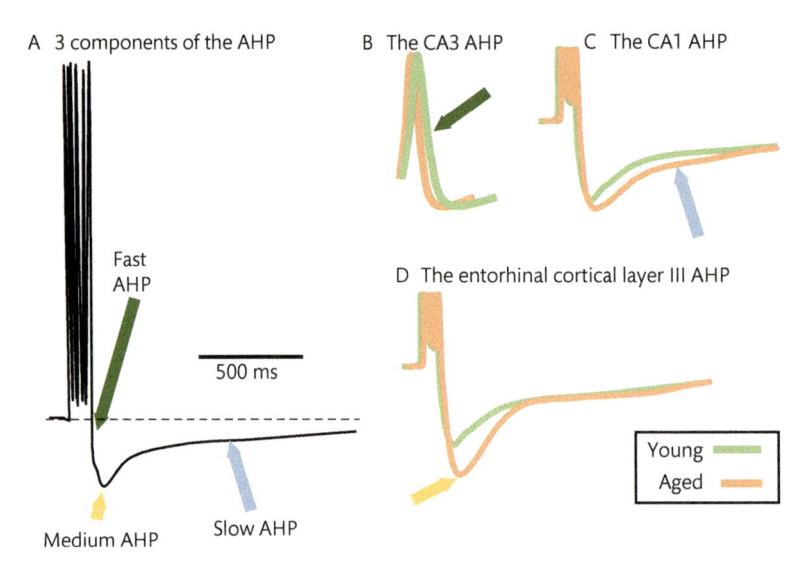

Figure 15.10 The afterhyperpolarization potential (AHP) in CA3, CA1, and entorhinal cortex layer III. (A) A depiction of the fast (green arrow), medium (yellow arrow), and slow (blue arrow) components of the AHP in CA3, CA1, and entorhinal cortical pyramidal neurons as described in the text. The dashed line indicates the resting membrane potential. (B) In CA3 pyramidal neurons, the fast component has a shorter latency to peak in aged compared with young animals, indicated by the green arrow. (C) In CA1 pyramidal neurons, the increase in L-type calcium channels triggers calcium-dependent K⁺ currents that are associated with a greater amplitude of the slow AHP, depicted by the blue arrow. (D) In layer III neurons of the entorhinal cortex, the medium AHP is increased in aged compared with young animals (yellow arrow).

responsible for the shorter latency fast AHP and reduced interspike interval in aged CA3 pyramidal cells.

Unlike dentate gyrus granule cells and CA3 pyramidal cells, CA1 neurons show higher numbers of L-type Ca^{2+} channels in aged (23–26 months) compared with young (12–14 months) CA1 neurons of male F344 rats, as inferred from single-channel recordings in CA1 pyramidal cells (Thibault and Landfield, 1996; but see, Kelly et al., 2001). Higher channel numbers are consistent with molecular data showing that mRNA levels for L-type Ca^{2+} channels are also higher in aged (24 to 32 months) compared with young (3–13 months) male F344 and F344 x BN rats (Herman et al., 1998; Veng and Browning, 2002; Núñez-Santana et al., 2014). Furthermore, the surface protein levels for the L-type Ca^{2+} channel pore-forming subunits are also higher in aged compared with young rats (Veng and Browning, 2002; Núñez-Santana et al., 2014). Functionally, these findings were predicted by the seminal work of Landfield and Pitler (1984). Using intracellular sharp electrode recording methods, they showed that the slow AHP was prolonged in CA1 pyramidal cells of aged (30 months) compared with young (5 months) male F344 rats, as depicted in Figure 15.10C. Later, it was reported in both rats and rabbits that all components of the AHP in CA1 neurons are increased with age (Moyer et al., 1992; Disterhoft et al., 1996; Oh et al., 1999; Weiss et al., 2000; Power et al., 2001; Power et al., 2002; Tombaugh et al., 2005; Kumar and Foster, 2007; Kumar et al., 2012a). While four distinct outward K⁺ currents involving different channels contribute to the AHP, whole-cell voltage-clamp recording experiments have shown that the slow outward calcium-activated potassium current is the primary current contributing to the enhanced AHP in aged CA1 pyramidal cells of rabbits (Power et al., 2001; Power et al., 2002). In line with this idea, blocking L-type Ca^{2+} channels with the antagonist nimodipine reduces the AHP in old rabbits, and improves performance on a trace

eyeblink conditioning task (Moyer et al., 1992; Disterhoft et al., 1996; Power et al., 2002). The layer III lateral entorhinal cortical neurons that project to CA1 also undergo an age-related reduction in excitability. In this case the medium, but not the slow, postburst AHP is increased in aged (26–32 months) male F344 x BN rats compared with young animals (3–6 months) (Lin et al., 2020), as shown in Figure 15.10D.

Interestingly, enriched environments (Kumar and Foster, 2007; Kumar et al., 2012a), exercise (Kumar et al., 2012a), new learning (Moyer et al., 2000), and better cognitive status (Thompson et al., 1996; Tombaugh et al., 2005) in aged animals are all associated with reductions in the AHP toward the range of young CA1 pyramidal cells. One way to view the function of the larger AHP in CA1 pyramidal cells of old animals is that it is adaptive (Gray and Barnes, 2015), and may protect CA1 neurons from the increased drive from CA3 input that has been reported in aged rats (Wilson et al., 2005; Robitsek et al., 2015), monkeys (Thomé et al., 2016), and humans (Yassa, Lacy, et al., 2010; Yassa, Mattfeld, et al., 2011). If the increased AHP indeed reflects a mechanism to compensate for hyperexcitability of CA3 neurons, then a direct prediction would be that nimodipine, new learning, enrichment, and better cognitive status in advanced age would normalize CA3 firing rates in aged animals. This hypothesis remains to be tested.

15.4.3 Calcium homeostasis

Regardless of whether the increase in the L-type voltage-gated calcium channels (L-type VGCC) reflects a primary insult or adaptive compensation (Gray and Barnes, 2015), it has the potential to significantly affect calcium homeostasis in the aged hippocampus. Khachaturian first proposed that altered regulation of cytosolic calcium could provide a common framework for understanding age-associated neuronal changes, as calcium signaling is critical for a number of cellular functions (Khachaturian, 1984). There are several mechanisms that converge to impact calcium homeostasis in hippocampal cells, including numbers of L-type VGCCs discussed above, levels of calcium-binding proteins, function of cellular organelles that sequester and release calcium (i.e., mitochondria and endoplasmic reticulum), and energy-dependent membrane extrusion pumps responsible for calcium transport (Khachaturian, 1991). Age-associated changes in several of these factors have been documented (e.g., Landfield, 1987; Khachaturian, 1989; Foster and Norris, 1997; Foster, 1999; Toescu and Verkhratsky, 2003; Nikoletopoulou and Tavernarakis, 2012; Chandran et al., 2017).

Calcium regulation within dentate gyrus or CA3 has not been widely studied. One report examining all three hippocampus subfields documented changes in two neuron-specific cytosolic calcium-binding proteins (hippocalcin and visinin-like calcium-binding protein 2; NVP2). Specifically, cells in all regions showed lower levels of NVP2 in 24-month-old male Sprague Dawley rats compared with 3-month-old animals. In contrast, hippocalcin levels were only lower in the older rats in dentate gyrus and CA3 cells (Furuta et al., 1999). It should be noted that while protein levels were lower within individual cells, the numbers of neurons that were positively labeled for these two markers were stable across age in the three hippocampus subfields (Furuta et al., 1999). Finally, while L-type calcium channel number was similar across age within dentate gyrus granule cells, one report indicates that the maximal transient intracellular calcium mobilization, elicited in response to elevated potassium, is greater in 2-month- compared with 18-month-old male F344 rats, and recovers more quickly (Kashiyae et al., 2009). This is consistent with lower L-type calcium channel currents observed in aged granule cells (Reynolds and Carlen, 1989), and implies blunted, but more sustained, calcium currents.

CA1 has a different pattern of calcium dyshomeostasis in aging than has been observed in dentate gyrus granule cells, with the numbers of L-type calcium channels being higher (Thibault and Landfield, 1996). The elevated numbers of these channels in aging could impact the timing and source of transient increases in cytosolic calcium, thus altering cellular function (Toescu and Verkhratsky, 2003; Toescu et al., 2004). In fact, within aged CA1 pyramidal neurons there is a shift in the source of intracellular calcium away from NMDA receptor currents (Kashiyae et al., 2009) to VGCCs. This shift presumably increases the activation of ryanodine receptors and the release of calcium from internal stores (Foster, 2007).

Three lines of evidence suggest that calcium currents through NMDA receptors are lower in aged CA1 neurons. First, GluN2B expression is decreased in older (26 years) male and female rhesus macaques compared with young (6 years) monkeys (Bai et al., 2004), but this is not observed in C57BL/6 mice (Magnusson, 2000). Relative to GluN2A, the GluN2B subunit has slower deactivation kinetics and higher calcium conductance (Monyer et al., 1992). Thus, lower numbers of GluN2B subunits may have the overall effect of lowering calcium currents through the NMDA receptor. Consistent with altered NMDA receptor subunit composition during aging, experiments using calcium imaging have shown that intracellular mobilization of calcium following application of NMDA is slower in old CA1 pyramidal neurons (Kashiyae et al., 2009). Finally, when NMDA receptor currents are isolated in single CA1 pyramidal neurons of male F344 rats aged 4–6 months and 24–26 months, the evoked NMDA receptor excitatory postsynaptic

potential (EPSP) amplitude is lower in the aged compared with young animals (Kumar and Foster, 2019; Kumar et al., 2019).

One factor that could contribute to age-related changes in calcium influx through NMDA receptors is higher oxidative stress known to occur within aged CA1 pyramidal neurons (Bodhinathan et al., 2010a; Kumar and Foster, 2013; Foster et al., 2017; A Kumar et al., 2018). Reactive oxygen species are known to both reduce NMDA receptor currents, as well as to increase the release of calcium from internal stores (Bodhinathan et al., 2010b; Bodhinathan et al., 2010a). Recently, using whole cell path clamp recordings in CA1 pyramidal neurons from male F344 rats 4–6 and 24–26 months of age, Kumar et al. (2019) reported that the lower NMDA receptor currents observed in aged rats could be reversed with the redox agent dithiothreitol. The mechanism for this enhancement was dependent on the GluNR2B receptor subunit as well as concentrations of calcium (Kumar et al., 2019).

While there is a lower calcium current amplitude through NMDA receptors, the increase in L-type VGCCs, discussed above, has the potential to increase overall calcium influx within aged CA1 neurons. In fact, peak calcium responses following 7 Hz stimulation is higher in 23-month-old male F344 rats compared with 12-month-old animals (Gant et al., 2006). Higher activity-induced calcium is hypothesized to trigger calcium-induced calcium release through both ryanodine and inositol 3-phosphate receptors on the endoplasmic reticulum. Because this has not been measured in the presence of an L-type VGCC blocker, it is not possible determine which receptor mechanism is affected in aging (Toescu and Verkhratsky, 2003). What is known, however, is that starting in middle age (12 months), high-dose ryanodine, which selectively locks ryanodine channels into a low conductance state, reverses the age-related change in the slow AHP amplitude. Moreover, ryanodine also eliminates age differences in spike frequency accommodation (Gant et al., 2006). Additional evidence that altered ryanodine receptor function in age contributes to calcium dyshomeostasis is the fact that *Fkbp1b* expression, which encodes a protein that inhibits ryanodine receptor-mediated calcium release, is downregulated with aging between 3 to 23 months in male F344 rats (Kadish et al., 2009). Consistent with the role of this protein in age-related calcium dyshomeostasis, is the observation that siRNA knockdown of *Fkbp1b* increases the slow AHP in hippocampal slices from young rats (Gant et al., 2011). Lastly, while it is also known that astrocyte-neuron signaling is important for overall calcium regulation, astrocyte-neuron interactions are reported to be preserved across age in male and female C57BL/6 mice when examined at 2 weeks, 5 months, 12 months, and 20 months (Gómez-Gonzalo et al., 2017).

The age-related differences in calcium homeostasis reviewed above can be interpreted in several ways. Among these, is the possibility that activity-driven increases in cytosolic calcium may represent a compensatory mechanism in response to reduced calcium currents through the NMDA receptor. In this view, increased VGCC and ryanodine receptor activity would balance reduced ionotropic receptor currents. Another possibility is that reduced calcium currents through the NMDA receptor could reflect a response to heightened levels of calcium in the cytosol that is protective of cellular function. A final possibility, of course, is that heightened VGCC and ryanodine receptor currents and decreased NMDA receptor currents with age occur through independent mechanisms. These potential alternatives remain to be evaluated.

15.4.4 Summary

In summary, not only are cell numbers preserved but most of the biophysical properties of old hippocampal granule cells, and CA3 and CA1 pyramidal cells are virtually unchanged in the aged hippocampus. The intriguing exception to these observations is the consistent enhancement of the AHP amplitude in aged CA1 pyramidal cells of old rats and rabbits, and the reduced onset latency of the fast AHP in aged CA3 pyramidal neurons. While altered AHP with age could be a symptom of changes in intrinsic excitability, the robust finding that the AHP in CA1 is modulated by experience also raises the possibility that this could be one means by which aged neurons adapt within the context of a dynamic hippocampal circuit.

15.5 Synapses

It is universally accepted that single neurons do not support behavior in isolation but rely on intricate connectivity patterns that permit intercellular communication. The concept that the brain consists of neurons that are unique elements rather than fused together may be traced back to a seminal study published by Santiago Ramón y Cajal in 1888, in which he proposed the "neuron doctrine" (Serrano-Castro and Garcia-Torrecillas, 2012). This influential work was the genesis for Cajal being invited to give a Croonian Lecture for the Royal Society in London 1894, where he met and had scientific exchanges with Sir Charles Sherrington. Shortly after this meeting, Sherrington coined the term "synapse" to describe the communication point of individual neurons (De Carlos and Molnár, 2019). The concept that neurons are individual entities communicating through synaptic connections was foundational for the field of modern neuroscience.

The importance of synaptic activity is highlighted by the fact that it uses a disproportionate amount of brain metabolic resources. For example, it is estimated that the reversal of ion fluxes through postsynaptic receptors alone accounts for 50% of the brain's ATP utilization (for review, see Harris, Jolivet, et al., 2012). Because points of synaptic contact are critical for hippocampal computations that support behavior, they may well become vulnerable in aging and contribute to cognitive decline. Importantly, distinct afferent inputs to the hippocampus terminate on different dendritic laminae (Chapter 3). Furthermore, synapses can have distinct morphological characteristics associated with the type of spine or dendritic shaft on which they terminate. It is therefore critical, when possible, to examine different synaptic input layers independently, as well as to consider the anatomical characteristics of affected synapses. While analysis of specific laminae has been difficult to achieve in primates, isolating distinct synaptic inputs in rodents has been more tractable and has resulted in the identification of distinct patterns of age-related vulnerability. Hippocampus synaptic morphology in young and aged rats is summarized schematically in Figure 15.11.

15.5.1 Synaptic integrity in aged humans

Much of what we know about synaptic alterations in advanced age is from animal models. While a number of studies have examined markers of synapse number in the postmortem hippocampus of humans, none of these studies have applied serial section electron microscopy (EM) or stereological methods that have been used in nonhuman species for synapse quantification. One study that examined synaptic density in the outer molecular layer of the dentate gyrus in young (25–52 years) and cognitively normal older participants (63–83 years) used antibodies against synapsin I, which is a synaptic terminal-specific phosphoprotein. With an average

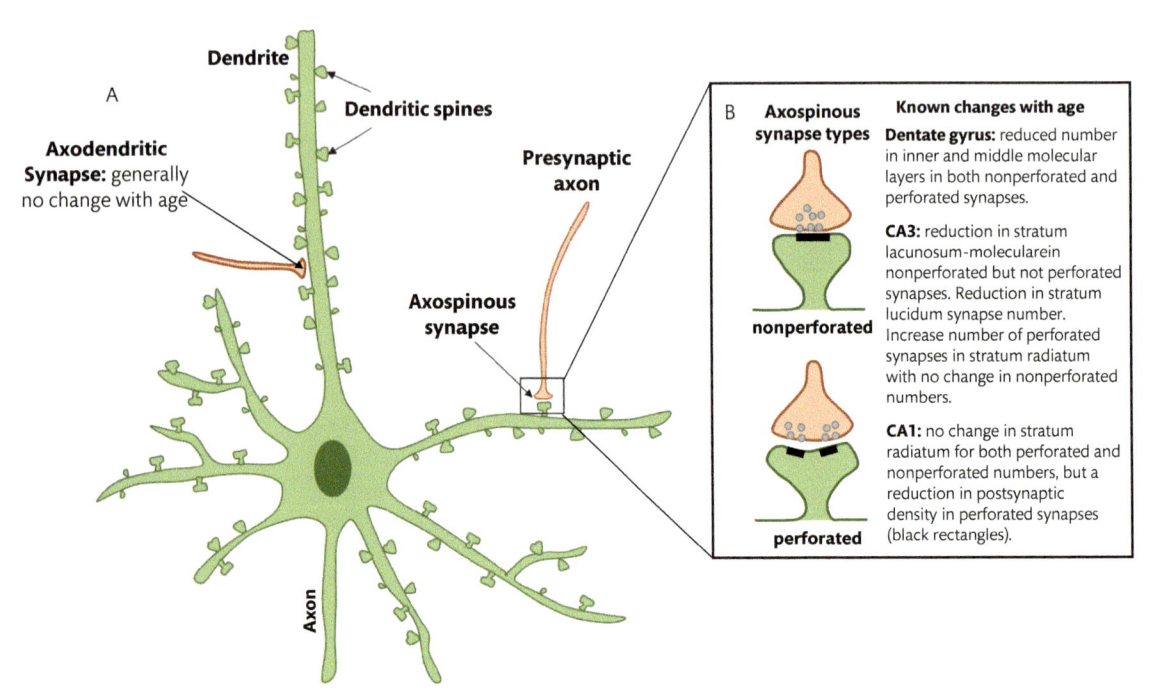

Figure 15.11 Synaptic morphology in the young and aged rat hippocampus. (A) Schematic of a pyramidal neuron showing axospinous versus axodendritic synapse types. (B) Summary of different types of synapses and known changes between young and aged animals in the dentate gyrus, CA3 and CA1.

postmortem interval of 6 hours, this study found no change in optical density in the dendritic layer that receives input from the anterolateral entorhinal cortex (Lippa et al., 1992). Another study focusing on normal human populations used the presynaptic terminal marker synaptophsyin to infer synapse numbers. In this thorough survey across the medial temporal lobe, including the dentate gyrus, CA3, CA1, and subiculum, they found no difference in the density of synaptophysin labeling (both protein and mRNA) between adults aged 34–43 compared with older individuals aged 68–86 across all regions examined (Eastwood et al., 2006).

Within studies that have focused on the impact of psychopathology on synapse markers, control groups spanning the age range of 19–79 years have also been examined for levels of synaptophysin across the dentate gyrus, CA3, CA1, and subiculum. In all but one of these experiments, stability of synapse markers with age has been reported. Specifically, no correlation between age and synaptophysin labeling in any of the regions examined in normal individuals was detected (Young et al., 1998; Eastwood and Harrison, 1999; Webster et al., 2001). In contrast to this, Eastwood et al. (1994) reported reductions in synapse markers across all hippocampal subregions as a function of increasing age between 22 and 84 years. Because shorter postmortem intervals are associated with higher levels of synaptophysin labeling (Eastwood et al., 1994; Eastwood and Harrison, 1999; Eastwood et al., 2006), the discrepant results on synapse numbers may be due to this variable.

The data that suggest no synapse change in the human hippocampus with age may be inconsistent with findings from human structural and diffusion tensor imaging (DTI) studies. For example, in memory-impaired older individuals, a number of studies indicate a reduction in white matter volume in the area of the perforant pathway, both by structural interrogation (Stoub et al., 2006; Rogalski et al., 2012a) and fractional anisotropy by DTI (Yassa, Muftuler, et al., 2010; Bennett and Stark, 2016). These authors concluded that the reduced white matter is consistent with fewer axon collaterals making synaptic contacts in the hippocampus. New experimental approaches for noninvasive in vivo measurements of inferred synapse number in humans are becoming available (Finnema et al., 2016; Prieto and Cotman, 2017), and these techniques may broaden our understanding of synaptic alterations over the human lifespan.

15.5.2 Synaptic integrity in aged nonhuman primates

Consistent with the observation of no synapse loss in the outer molecular layer of the dentate gyrus in humans (Lippa et al., 1992), Tigges et al. (1995) found no difference in total numbers of axospinous synapses between young (4–14 years) and aged (24–35 years) rhesus macaques (sex not specified) using serial EM methods to count synapses in this region. Furthermore, the depth of the granule cell molecular layer, the cross-sectional area of the synaptic terminals, and the length of the postsynaptic densities did not differ across age groups. Numbers and proportions of nonperforated and perforated synapses (Figure 15.11), reflecting contacts with single versus multiple discontiguous postsynaptic densities, respectively, were also similar across age in this dendritic region. In the same study when synaptic populations were separated into axospinous versus axodendritic synapses, they did find a statistically significant age-related loss in axodendritic contacts

in the outer molecular layer (which constitutes 13% of total synapses). Additionally, an age-related increase in dystrophic myelinated axons was observed in the dentate gyrus outer molecular layer (Tigges et al., 1995). These data may indicate compromised fibers arising from the anterolateral entorhinal cortex, which is consistent with human imaging data showing declines in white matter volume and integrity in this region of the perforant pathway (Stoub et al., 2006; Yassa, Muftuler, et al., 2010; Rogalski et al., 2012b; Bennett and Stark, 2016).

Hara et al. (2011) examined synaptic boutons in the outer molecular layer of the dentate gyrus of female young (9–11 years) and aged (22–35 years) rhesus macaques behaviorally characterized on the DNMS task. In contrast to human (Lippa et al., 1992) and monkey (Tigges et al., 1995) data from this region discussed above, these investigators did report differences between age groups. Namely, the older monkeys showed fewer presynaptic terminals associated with multiple postsynaptic densities on dendritic spines, and an increased number of synaptic terminals with no associated postsynaptic density (Hara et al., 2011). The number of axon terminals with single postsynaptic densities did not differ across age. The numbers of axon terminals correlated with poorer DNMS task performance across both age groups (Hara et al., 2011). A later report by these investigators, however, did not replicate the decline in axospinous synapses in the outer molecular layer of old female rhesus macaques (mean age 30 years) compared with young (mean age 10 years), although there was a trend toward fewer synapses with age (Hara, Punsoni, et al., 2012). More systematic investigation will be needed to clarify these discrepant findings.

Tigges et al. (1996) used stereological methods to estimate the numbers of synapses in the inner molecular layer of the dentate gyrus of young (5 male and 4 female) and aged (4 male and 2 female) rhesus macaques. There was no significant age-related difference in numbers of synapses, cross-sectional area of axon terminals, length of the postsynaptic density, or in the proportion of perforated versus nonperforated synapses on dendritic spines or shafts. The observation of preserved synaptic density in the inner molecular layer of the dentate gyrus was later replicated by another laboratory in young (2 male and 4 female; 9–14) and aged (2 male and 10 female; 22–35) macaques (Hara, Park, et al., 2012).

Hippocampus regions CA3 and CA1 have not been as extensively investigated in nonhuman primates. One study has looked across wide areas of the temporal lobe including the entorhinal cortex, dentate gyrus, CA3, and CA1 regions using immunofluorescence densitometry and Western blot analyses for synaptophysin in young (5–7 years), middle-aged (10–15 years), and old (23–31 years) male and female rhesus macaques. This study reported lower levels of immunofluorescence across all regions in the old animals compared with the adult and middle-aged monkeys. Lower expression of synaptophysin protein in the older animals was confirmed by Western blot analysis (Haley et al., 2010). This study, however, did not take into account potential dendritic layer-specific changes that have been reported using EM and stereological methodologies.

15.5.3 Synaptic integrity in aged rodents

In the rodent, careful structural and functional analyses of synaptic integrity have been quantified in different hippocampus subfields across the lifespan. While there do not appear to be large differences in spine density with age in the rodent hippocampus, alterations in axospinous synaptic density and function have been noted, which are summarized in Figure 15.11B. Because differential changes can occur in actual synapse numbers or in synaptic function across different hippocampus subregions and dendritic fields, it is optimal to analyze distinct termination zones separately. This is highlighted by the fact that there are no age differences in synaptic markers detected when whole hippocampus homogenates are used (Nicolle et al., 1999).

15.5.3.1 Dentate gyrus granule cell synaptic input, structure, and function

While the general laminar organization of the dentate gyrus is similar between rodents and primates, both monkey and human granule cells have basal as well as apical dendrites (Seress and Mrzljak, 1987). This anatomical feature has not been reported in rodents. The earliest EM investigations of the layer II medial entorhinal cortex projection to the middle molecular layer of dentate gyrus granule cells were not conducted stereologically, however, they did reveal that male F344 rats had ~27% fewer synapses on dendritic spines and 35% fewer synapses on dendritic shafts (Bondareff and Geinisman, 1976; Geinisman et al., 1977). A later study from this group, also not conducted stereologically, tested 6 young (4 months) and 12 aged (26 months) F344 male rats on a radial eight-arm maze to examine spatial working memory in relation to synapse density in the middle molecular layer of the dentate gyrus. There was a statistically significant lower number of perforated but not nonperforated synapses in the old memory-impaired rats compared with young or aged rats without memory deficits (Geinisman et al., 1986).

The first study to apply stereological EM methods to the question of age-related synapse loss was conducted in 1992. Geinisman et al. (1992a) used the optical dissector (Box 15.1) technique in 14 young (5 months) and 14 aged (28 months) male F344 rats to examine the numbers of synapses within the middle and inner molecular layers of the dentate gyrus. This study revealed no differences in number of axodendritic contacts as a function of age in either the inner or middle molecular layers. The number of axospinous synapses per neuron, however, was significantly lower in both layers by ~24% in aged compared with young rats (Geinisman et al., 1992a). While both perforated and nonperforated axospinous synapses were affected by age, it is the perforated synapses that have been linked to synaptic modification mechanisms that are implicated in learning and memory. In fact, stimulation that increases synaptic strength in the middle molecular layer leads to selective increases in the numbers of perforated synapses in both young (5 months) and old (28 months) male F344 rats (Geinisman et al., 1992b). While the aged rats showed a similar capacity for synaptic restructuring as did young, the absolute numbers of perforated synapses remained significantly lower in the older animals even after stimulation (Geinisman et al., 1992b; Geinisman et al., 1994). Another EM study also examined synaptic contacts in the middle molecular layer in F344 x BN rats and did not report a significant decline in number. When the individual synaptic numbers are taken into consideration, however, 4 of the 6 rats in the aged group did show a striking reduction compared with the young animals (Newton et al., 2008). As the rats were not behaviorally characterized in this study, it is possible that cognitive status may account for the discrepancy. Overall, the EM stereological investigations suggest that two major afferent projection systems show a significant loss in axospinous synapses with age: one involving the medial entorhinal cortex, the second the commissural and nonentorhinal cortical inputs. Although there is significant synaptic loss, the remaining synapses are anatomically modifiable. The outer molecular layer was not examined in these studies.

Synaptic protein analyses have also been implemented to estimate synaptic density across the lifespan in rodents. When the entire molecular layer of the dentate gyrus was examined in C57BL/6 mice 2 to 31 months of age, no difference was detected in the estimated numbers of synaptophysin-positive synaptic boutons (Calhoun et al., 1998). On the other hand, lower levels of synaptic proteins in the middle molecular layer of the dentate gyrus have been reported for aged (29 months) male F344 x BN rats compared with 10- and 18-month-old animals using quantitative Western blot analyses (Newton et al., 2008). Another study used the presynaptic marker synaptophysin to estimate synapse density in the inner, middle, and outer molecular layers of behaviorally characterized young (6 months) and aged (24–28 months) male Long Evans rats. The aged spatial memory-impaired rats (but not aged unimpaired) showed significantly lower synaptophysin immunoreactivity compared with young animals in the middle and outer molecular layers, but not in the inner layer (Smith et al., 2000). The lack of change in synaptic density in the inner molecular layer is not consistent with previous reports of EM counts in that region (Geinisman et al., 1992a), which could be due to a lack of quantification sensitivity.

Electrophysiological studies support the anatomical observation that there is a reduction in synapse number in the middle molecular layer of the dentate gyrus. Early studies used extracellular field potential recordings from the hilar region of the dentate gyrus in awake, chronically implanted rats with stimulation electrodes placed in medial perforant pathway fibers that synapse onto the middle molecular layer of dentate gyrus granule cells. Stimulation of this pathway elicits a field excitatory postsynaptic potential (fEPSP), which reflects the summed currents in granule cells from this synaptic activation. The fEPSP amplitudes recorded in the dentate gyrus of aged (30–32 months) and young (12 months) male Long Evans rats (Barnes, 1979) and aged (31 months) and young (10 months) male Wistar rats (Barnes and McNaughton, 1980b) was lower in the aged rats. This suggests weaker synaptic currents in the middle molecular layer elicited by equivalent intensity of medial perforant path stimulation. Lower fEPSP amplitudes in old compared with young animals has also been reported in male F344 rats (e.g., Foster et al., 1991; Barnes, Rao, and Houston, 2000; Krause et al., 2008; Sierra-Mercado et al., 2008; Yang et al., 2008). One study conducted in C57BL/6 mice (sex not specified) examined at 3 and 25 months of age has also reported a lower fEPSP amplitude in older mice in the outer molecular layer in response to equivalent stimulation intensity of the lateral perforant path (Froc et al., 2003).

Another component of the fEPSP that can be measured is the summed action potentials from entorhinal cortical axons of the perforant pathway, referred to as the presynaptic fiber potential. When the amplitude of this component was measured, older animals (31 months) also showed a lower amplitude of the presynaptic fiber

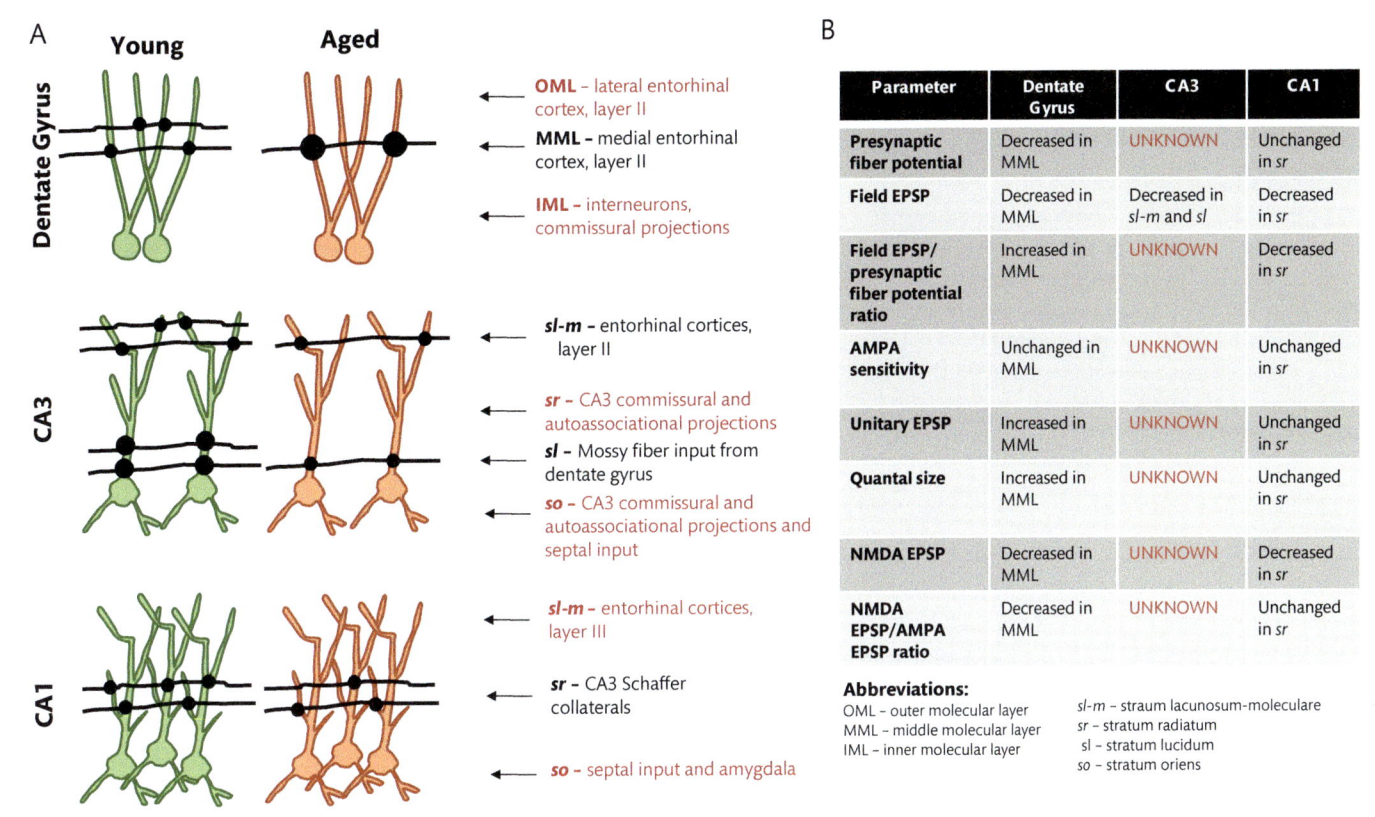

Figure 15.12 Synaptic function in the young and aged rat hippocampus. (A) Schematic summarizing the distinct synaptic inputs to the different laminae of the hippocampus. Red font indicates that synaptic function has not been examined in relation to age in rats. (B) Table summarizing known functional changes in hippocampal synapses between young and old rats by subregion.

potential response than did younger male Wistar rats (10 months) (Barnes and McNaughton, 1980b). A lower presynaptic fiber potential with age, has also been observed in old (24 months) compared with younger (5 and 8 months) male F344 rats (Foster et al., 1991). Because there is no loss of entorhinal cortical cells (Merrill et al., 2001; Rapp et al., 2002), the age-related change in fiber potential amplitude might be explained by fewer axon collaterals from layer II cells of the entorhinal cortex. In fact, the electrophysiological evidence for reduced axon collaterals from the entorhinal cortex is remarkably consistent with findings, discussed above, in nonhuman primate (Tigges et al., 1995) and human experiments (Stoub et al., 2006; Yassa, Muftuler, et al., 2010; Rogalski et al., 2012a; Bennett and Stark, 2016), suggesting a disruption across species of white matter pathways in this region. Functional changes in the perforant path-granule cell synapse are summarized in Figure 15.12.

Although the amplitude of the presynaptic fiber potential is smaller in old (30 months) compared with younger (12 months) male Long Evans rats, extracellularly recorded fEPSP amplitudes are larger for a given presynaptic fiber potential amplitude in the older animals (Barnes and McNaughton, 1980b). This suggests that the synapses that remain in aged rats are more powerful (Figure 15.12). This idea was directly confirmed in a later study using intracellular recording methods to measure the unitary EPSP amplitude in young (5–8 months) and old (24 months) male F344 rats. The unitary EPSP is the depolarization elicited by the stimulation of a single axon, and thus its amplitude reflects the strength of a single synapse. This experiment demonstrated that the depolarization

resulting from stimulation of a single fiber was larger in old rats (Foster et al., 1991). The increase in the amplitude of the unitary EPSP may be mediated by an increase in AMPA receptor currents. These enhanced currents may reflect a compensatory mechanism that increases postsynaptic sensitivity in response to the reduced medial perforant path input (Barnes and McNaughton, 1980b; Foster et al., 1991; Barnes, Rao, and Houston, 2000). In fact, when the NMDA receptor-mediated and AMPA receptor-mediated currents are isolated pharmacologically, aged rats show enhanced AMPA receptor-mediated currents at this synapse (Krause et al., 2008; Yang et al., 2008). On the other hand, the NMDA receptor-mediated fEPSP is smaller relative to young animals for a given fiber potential amplitude (Krause et al., 2008; Yang et al., 2008). This suggests that there is a shift in the ratio of AMPA to NMDA receptor currents in synapses of the dentate gyrus over the lifespan. This observation is consistent with the known age-related reduction in GluN2B NMDA receptor subunits (e.g., Magnusson et al., 2010). Remarkably, the AMPA receptor-to-NMDA receptor fEPSP response ratio is not altered by extensive environmental enrichment, which improves spatial memory in aged animals (although not to the accuracy of young animal performance). This unmodifiable trajectory of changing receptor ratios with age may therefore reflect a fixed developmental process (Yang et al., 2008).

While experiments have examined synapse numbers in the inner and outer molecular layers of the dentate gyrus, we are not aware of any functional assessments of the synaptic inputs to these dendritic layers. Furthermore, only one report in mice across age has examined the outer molecular layer. Going forward, it will be important to understand how each zone is modified by the aging process.

15.5.3.2 CA3 pyramidal cell synaptic input, structure, and function

CA3 pyramidal cells have both apical and basilar dendritic trees (Chapter 5). The apical dendrites receive interleaved medial and lateral entorhinal cortical input to the most distal outer regions, referred to as the stratum lacunosum-moleculare. The area of CA3 located in the limbs of the dentate gyrus (also known as CA3c) do not have a stratum lacunosum-moleculare, thus this area receives little to no direct input from entorhinal cortices (Amaral and Lavenex, 2007). Just below this layer is the stratum radiatum, which is the input zone for commissural projections from contralateral CA3, as well as autoassociational fibers from ipsilateral CA3 pyramidal cells (Witter, 2007; Chapter 3). Unlike in CA2 and CA1, the pyramidal cells of CA3 have a layer proximal to the cell body referred to as the stratum lucidum that contains the mossy fiber synaptic contacts from the granule cells of the dentate gyrus. For the basilar dendrites there is one layer referred to as the stratum oriens, which receives recurrent collaterals from ipsilateral CA3 axons, commissural projections from contralateral CA3, and input from the medial septum that largely targets GABAergic interneurons below the pyramidal cell layer (Witter, 2007; Chapters 3 and 7).

Pre- and postsynaptic protein markers of synapses have been examined using quantitative Western blots of whole CA3 homogenates in young (10–12 months), middle-aged (18–20 months), and aged (29–32 months) male F344 x BN rats. In both middle-aged and old rats, levels of synaptic proteins in CA3 were lower compared with the young group (Adams et al., 2008). Another study examined synaptophysin immunoreactivity specifically in the stratum lacunosum-moleculare in young (6 months) and old (24–28 months) male Long Evans rats. The aged animals with spatial learning impairments showed lower levels of immunoreactivity within this area (Smith et al., 2000b).

Another study examined synaptic contacts in the stratum lacunosum-moleculare of CA3b by three-dimensional serial EM reconstruction. This investigation observed lower numbers of synaptic contacts in CA3b of aged (29 months) compared with young (10 months) male F344 x BN rats (Adams et al., 2010), which is consistent with the immunohistochemical findings described above. In particular, Adams et al. (2010) reported that it was the axospinous nonperforated synapses, but not the perforated synapses, that changed in number with age (Figure 15.11B). The size of the synapse and postsynaptic density was not different between age groups in this region (Adams et al., 2010). It should be noted, however, that these rats were not behaviorally characterized.

The stratum lucidum of CA3 receives mossy fiber input from dentate gyrus granule cells. Two studies have reported that this dendritic region shows no synaptic change across age, one using synaptophysin immunoreactivity in male Long Evans rats examined at 6 and 28 months (Smith et al., 2000), and the other using stereological EM analysis in male F344 x BN rats examined at 4 and 29 months (Poe et al., 2001). With respect to the latter EM study, the rats were not behaviorally characterized and there were only 4 animals in each age group. This may not have provided sufficient power to detect differences in synapse numbers. In contrast to these studies, Ojo et al. (2013) found that total synaptic density with EM

stereological analysis in the stratum lucidum of male Wistar rats was lower in middle-aged (12 months) and aged (28 months) animals compared with the young (4 months) group (Ojo et al., 2013). Again, this latter study did not behaviorally characterize the animals and had a sample size of only 3 rats in each age group. It is, however, in agreement with a report by Villaneuva-Castillo et al. (2017), who conducted an electrophysiological examination of the mossy fiber to CA3 synapse in hippocampal slices with a robust sample size of over 20 animals in each age group. They found a lower amplitude of the extracellular fEPSP recorded from the stratum lucidum of CA3b in older (22-month) male Wistar rats compared with young (1.5-month) animals (Villanueva-Castillo et al., 2017). This "functional assay" supports the idea that there may be fewer mossy fiber synapses between the granule cells and CA3 pyramidal neurons (Figure 15.12). Finally, when the associational/commissural pathway in stratum radiatum was examined in male Long Evans rats of 6 and 24 months of age, no significant difference was found in the strength of this synapse between age groups (Yang et al., 2013).

In a recent study, serial EM stereology was used to examine synaptic contacts as well as AMPA and NMDA receptor expression in specific dendritic fields of CA3b/c, including proximal and distal stratum radiatum, and stratum lucidum in young (6–8 months) and aged (28–29 months) male F344 x BN rats. Animals were behaviorally characterized with two different hippocampus-dependent tasks (trace eyeblink conditioning and the Morris watermaze, section 15.2). Aged rats were characterized as being impaired if they performed out of range from the young group on both tasks. There were twice the number of perforated synaptic contacts in stratum radiatum in aged impaired animals compared with aged unimpaired and young adults, while unperforated synapses remained unchanged across groups (Buss et al., 2021). This is the first report of a region-selective increase in synaptic contacts in the aged brain. While the thorny excrescences of the mossy fiber projection from dentate gyrus granule cells could not be counted using the EM methods in this study, it was possible to examine AMPA and NMDA receptor expression using immunogold EM. While there was no change across age or cognitive status in NMDA receptor expression detected, AMPA receptor expression was highest in the perforated synapses of the stratum lucidum of aged unimpaired and young adults compared with age-impaired rats (Buss et al., 2021). The lower AMPA receptor expression in aged-impaired rats is consistent with functional studies showing weakened synaptic input from the mossy fibers to CA3 in aged animals (Villanueva-Castillo et al., 2017) and in a previous EM investigation (Ojo et al., 2013). While aged-impaired rats showed decreased AMPA receptor expression in stratum lucidum, they showed increased AMPA receptor expression in stratum radiatum compared with the aged-unimpaired and young rats. The authors suggest that the AMPA receptors may be redirected from the mossy fiber synapses to the commissural/associational projections in the stratum radiatum. This increase in AMPA receptor expression is also consistent with the observation of increased numbers of stratum radiatum perforated synapses in aged-impaired rats. These data (Buss et al., 2021), however, are not on the surface easy to reconcile with the findings of no functional change in the commissural/associational projections in CA3 with age (Yang et al., 2013).

Together, the data discussed above indicate reductions in synaptic contacts in the CA3 stratum lacunosum-moleculare of aged rats (Smith et al., 2000; Adams et al., 2008; Adams et al., 2010;

Buss et al., 2021). For the stratum radiatum on the other hand, aged-impaired rats show a twofold increase in perforated synaptic contacts compared with aged-unimpaired and young animals (Buss et al., 2021). While there have been some conflicting reports (Smith et al., 2000; Poe et al., 2001), for CA3 stratum lucidum there appears to be fewer synapses with age (Ojo et al., 2013), lower functional synaptic strength (Villanueva-Castillo et al., 2017), and lower AMPA receptor expression in perforated synapses of aged-impaired rats (Buss et al., 2021). One piece of the puzzle still missing is whether these layer-specific synaptic changes are consistent across the transverse axis of CA3, which receives different afferent inputs. Moreover, it has yet to be determined exactly how these age-related synaptic changes contribute to hyperactivity in CA3 neurons that is observed in vivo in rats (Wilson et al., 2005), monkeys (Thomé et al., 2016) and humans (Yassa, Mattfeld, et al., 2011).

15.5.3.3 CA1 pyramidal cell synaptic input, structure, and function

The CA1 subfield also has a laminar and transverse organizational structure that receives distinct synaptic inputs both in the apical and basilar portions of the dendritic tree (Chapter 3). The stratum lacunosum-moleculare is at the outer portion of the apical dendritic tree and receives input from layer III pyramidal cells of the entorhinal cortex as well as from the nucleus reuniens of the thalamus (Amaral and Lavenex, 2007; Chapter 3). In the CA1 region closest to CA2 (proximal), the projections originate from cells in the medial entorhinal cortex (Agster and Burwell, 2013). In the CA1 region near the subiculum (distal), the input is from cells in the lateral entorhinal (Amaral and Lavenex, 2007; Chapter 3) and perirhinal cortices (Naber et al., 1999; Agster and Burwell, 2013). There is also a direct projection from the postrhinal cortex to CA1, but it is unclear whether this terminates in more proximal versus distal areas of CA1 (Agster and Burwell, 2013). The Schaffer collateral axons from CA3 pyramidal neurons terminate in the stratum radiatum (proximal to the soma). The basilar dendrites in the stratum oriens of CA1 receive input from the medial septum and the amygdaloid complex.

Across apical and basilar dendrites of CA1, estimated synaptophysin-positive synaptic bouton number was reported to be comparable in 2- and 31-month-old C57BL/6 male mice (Calhoun et al., 1998). These data are consistent with the finding of no change in layer-specific synaptophysin density measured in the stratum lacunosum-moleculare and stratum radiatum of CA1 in 6- and 28-month-old male Long Evans rats (Smith et al., 2000). A more recent study using stereological EM synapse counts from behaviorally characterized young (6–8 months) and aged (28–29 months) male F344 x BN rats, also reported no change in synapse number across groups (Buss et al., 2021). Studies of CA3 Schaffer collateral synapses to the stratum radiatum of CA1 using stereological EM have suggested a preservation of total synapse numbers in 6- and 27-month-old male Long Evans rats (Geinisman et al., 2004; Nicholson et al., 2004), and 6- and 29-month-old male F344 x BN rats (Buss et al., 2021). Although synapse number in CA1 does not change with age, the postsynaptic density size of axospinous synapses in the stratum radiatum is lower in aged (27 months) behaviorally impaired male Long Evans rats compared with unimpaired and young (6 months) animals (Figure 15.11B). Importantly, the difference with age was observed in perforated, but not nonperforated synapses (Nicholson et al., 2004).

Electrophysiological data support the hypothesis that there is a loss of functional synapses in CA1. Although the unitary EPSP size (Barnes et al., 1992), and the amplitude of the Schaffer collateral presynaptic fiber potential is preserved with aging (Barnes, Rao, et al., 1997; Rosenzweig et al., 1997; Barnes, Rao, and Orr, 2000; Tombaugh et al., 2002), the fEPSP amplitude is lower in aged compared with young rats (Landfield et al., 1986; Barnes et al., 1992; Deupree et al., 1993; Tombaugh et al., 2002). Within male aged F344 (26 months) rats, but not younger age groups (<9 months), a lower fEPSP amplitude was significantly related to poorer Morris watermaze performance (Barnes, Rao, et al., 1996). Because total synapse number does not change in old animals (Calhoun et al., 1998; Smith et al., 2000; Geinisman et al., 2004), the reduced fEPSP amplitude in old age, with no change in unitary EPSP size (Barnes et al., 1992), suggests that some proportion of CA1 stratum radiatum synapses are silent in old animals (Figure 15.12).

15.5.4 Summary

Whether age-related changes in synapses are consistent across species cannot yet be determined, as rodent and nonhuman primate studies have focused on different dendritic laminae, and human experiments have not analyzed specific dendritic regions. In monkey studies, the focus has largely been on the dentate gyrus and specifically the outer molecular layer. Examination of the dentate gyrus in rodent studies, on the other hand, has focused on the inner and middle molecular layers. Figure 15.12 summarizes the known functional synaptic changes in the hippocampus of aged rats. Even in the rat, it is striking that a number of synaptic input layers across the different subregions have not been examined. With new imaging modalities under development and better human tissue preservation for EM stereological investigation, it may be possible to make direct cross-species comparisons. Until these methods are applied, however, a complete understanding of the hippocampus formation synaptic vulnerability or integrity across species is not possible.

15.6 Neuromodulation

The function and modification of synapses are powerfully regulated by neuromodulatory systems originating from nuclei in the midbrain and brainstem (Chapter 7). Specifically, neuromodulation can influence the window for plasticity, which can alter gene expression and support cognitive functions dependent on the hippocampus. Age-related alterations in hippocampus neuromodulation could therefore contribute to altered synaptic dynamics that ultimately manifest as behavioral impairments. There are several ways in which these systems could be altered, including loss of cell bodies in midbrain or brainstem nuclei, reduced axonal projections, changes in enzymatic activity in the terminal itself, or receptor modifications. Changes in any of these variables could result in altered physiological responses to neuromodulation within the hippocampus. When possible, the effects of advanced age on each of these variables will be considered.

15.6.1 Acetylcholine

Acetylcholine is synthesized by cell bodies located in basal forebrain nuclei. Of these nuclei it is primarily the medial septum and diagonal band complex that project diffusely throughout the hippocampus to activate both principal cells and interneurons. Bartus et al. (1982)

were the first to formalize the "cholinergic hypothesis" of cognitive decline in aging and dementia, and how the link between dysfunction of this system and behavioral impairment could be empirically tested. Before stereological methods were available, there were reports of cell loss in the basal forebrain in human postmortem tissue (e.g., Mann et al., 1984a; Mann et al., 1984b; Lowes-Hummel et al., 1989). Although other studies in humans did not detect a change in density or numbers of basal forebrain neurons during normative aging (e.g., Whitehouse et al., 1983; Chui et al., 1984; Bigl et al., 1987). As reviewed below, it is now clear that several aspects of cholinergic signaling are impaired in normative aging without frank cell loss (for review, see Decker, 1987).

15.6.1.1 The cholinergic system in young and aged humans

Early nonstereological studies examining cell number in the basal forebrain of younger and older humans reported lower numbers of cells when only neurons that exceeded 35 μm in diameter were included (Mann et al., 1984a; Mann et al., 1984b; Lowes-Hummel et al., 1989). When smaller neurons were included in counts, no age differences were detected (Whitehouse et al., 1983; Chui et al., 1984). Furthermore, cholinergic axon terminals appear to be intact in healthy older adults. In vivo single-photon emission computed tomography (PET) using [^{123}I]iodobenzovesamicol, which binds to the vesicular acetylcholine transporter to serve as a proxy for cholinergic axons, has shown no reduction in hippocampus binding density in individuals across the age range of 22 to 91 years (Kuhl et al., 1996). While the axons appear to be preserved in aging, there is lower synthesis of acetylcholine within hippocampus cholinergic terminals in late adulthood compared with middle age (Perry et al., 1977; Davies, 1978; Court et al., 1993). Consistent with these observations, when ChAT activity is inferred using radiolabeled acetyl-CoA, it was reported that acetylcholine synthesis and ChAT activity throughout the temporal lobe was systematically lower between 50 and 90 years (Allen et al., 1983). In another study, however, ChAT concentration within the hippocampus was not different between 58 to 83 years (Gottfries et al., 1983). The observation of stable ChAT levels with age was also replicated in individuals 18 to 95 years (Winblad et al., 1985). Although the synthesis of acetylcholine may be lower with age, the concentration of the enzyme responsible for its synthesis does not appear to change over the lifespan.

Postsynaptic acetylcholine receptors are broadly divided into muscarinic and nicotinic subtypes, both of which are expressed in the hippocampus. An early study using [^{3}H]-QNB ligands to label muscarinic acetylcholine receptors in the hippocampus, found lower binding at 85 years compared with 55, which was most prominent in the anterior hippocampus (Nordberg and Winblad, 1981). Note, that the anterior hippocampus in humans is homologous to the rodent ventral hippocampus. In agreement with this observation, [^{3}H]-QNB binding across the entire temporal lobe was shown to change linearly between 50 and 90 years (Allen et al., 1983). The observation of a lower hippocampal muscarinic receptor binding in old age was replicated in a larger study with 78 individuals ranging in age from 4 to 93 years (Rinne, 1987). The above findings from postmortem tissue have largely been consistent with in vivo studies using PET imaging of muscarinic receptor binding. One study using the [^{11}C]-N-methyl-4 piperidylbenzilate ligand showed a 40% lowering of hippocampal muscarinic acetylcholine receptor density in healthy individuals between the ages of 18 to 75 (Suhara et al., 1993). More recently, [^{123}I]-I-QNB binding measured by PET

in female participants ranging in age from 26 to 82 years confirmed a lower of muscarinic acetylcholine receptor density with age in the hippocampus in vivo (Norbury et al., 2005). In contrast to these studies, one autoradiographic study using tritiated scopolamine and other ligands that isolate different muscarinic receptor subtypes (M1, M2, M3, and M4) found no significant differences between young adulthood and older age within the hippocampus (Court et al., 1997). These discrepant findings might be due to a lack of consideration of cognitive status.

Autoradiographic binding assays using α-bungarotoxin to infer nicotinic acetylcholine receptor density from individuals ranging in age from 0 to 100 years showed changes across age in multiple hippocampus subregions. Although the most dramatic changes in nicotinic receptors occurred between birth and 10 years, there was a more modest lowering between 40 and 100 (Court et al., 1997). Consistent with this, a study using quantitative real time PCR to examine messenger RNA of α4 and β2 nicotinic acetylcholine receptor subtypes showed a lowering between 22 and 82 years of age in β2 but not α4 receptor subtype expression (Tohgi et al., 1998). In vivo imaging of nicotinic acetylcholine receptor density assessed by PET has been in general agreement with the biochemical assays conducted in human postmortem tissue. For example, the [^{18}F]-F-A-85830 ligand, which has a high affinity for nicotinic receptors, has been used to show a lowering of inferred density between 22 and 75 years (Lagarde et al., 2017). When the ^{18}F-(-)-JHU86428 PET ligand to α4β2 nicotinic acetylcholine receptors was measured across age, there was a negative correlation between inferred receptor density and age (from 30 to 82 years) (Coughlin, Slania, et al., 2018). Nicotinic receptor density of α7 within the hippocampus, measured using the [^{18}F]-ASEM PET ligand was positively correlated with age (between 21 and 86 years) (Coughlin, Du, et al., 2018). Thus, it does not appear that all cholinergic receptors subtypes are uniformly affected by advancing age.

15.6.1.2 The cholinergic system in young and aged nonhuman primates

Consistent with observations from human tissue, cell counts within the basal forebrain of rhesus macaques do not change in number between 9 to 33 years of age (Voytko et al., 1995). When the neurons in this region are labeled for ChAT immunoreactivity, however, there is a significant lowering of cells containing this enzyme (Stroessner-Johnson et al., 1992; Smith et al., 1999; Bañuelos et al., 2023). Importantly, the change in ChAT-expressing cells can be reversed by administration of nerve growth factor, indicating that the neurons are not lost but rather change their phenotypic expression profile with age (Smith et al., 1999).

Immunolabeling of the vesicular acetylcholine transporter in rhesus macaques can be used to identify cholinergic axons within the hippocampus. One study revealed that the length of axon fibers labeled was lower in old (28 years) compared with young (9 years) rhesus macaques. There was no significant relationship detected, however, between fiber length and memory on the DNMS task (Calhoun et al., 2004). No other studies have examined the integrity of basal forebrain cholinergic axons, acetylcholine synthesis, or enzymatic activity within the hippocampus of aged nonhuman primates.

Compared with experiments conducted in human tissue, relatively few studies have examined hippocampal acetylcholine receptor density in nonhuman primates. One PET study in which the [^{11}C]-(+)3-MPB ligand was used to measure muscarinic receptor density reported no change within the hippocampus in rhesus macaques between 6 and 19 years (comparable to humans 18 to 57 years in humans) (Tsukada, Kakiuchi, Nishiyama, Ohba, Sato, et al., 2001). Because the changes in receptor density in humans have been reported to be linear in cross-sectional samples over the lifespan, there is no apparent explanation for this discrepancy between species.

15.6.1.3 The cholinergic system in young and aged rodents

The literature on effects of aging on the rodent cholinergic system is quite extensive. While an early nonstereological study of neuron counts in the basal forebrain in male F344 rats at 3, 12, 16–18, 22–24, and 28–30 months reported lower cell numbers after 12 months (Fischer et al., 1992), the results were not replicated when differences in cell size were controlled for (e.g., Fischer et al., 1992; Smith et al., 1993; De Lacalle et al., 1996). Two other experiments in which stereological cell counts were conducted in male F344 rats produced conflicting results. Stereological cell counts from Nissl stained sections restricted to the horizontal limb of the nucleus basalis of Meynert showed lower cell numbers in 27 compared with 4-month-old male F344 rats (Smith and Booze, 1995). Another study reported no difference in NeuN-positive cells across the entire rostral basal forebrain in young (6 months) versus old (24 months) male F344 rats (Bañuelos et al., 2013). The discrepancy between these two studies may have arisen because of the differences in the regions examined and the staining procedures used. When cell counts are focused on ChAT-positive neurons, several studies have reported fewer ChAT-positive cells in older groups of male and female F344, Sprague Dawley, and Long Evans rats ranging in age from 2 to 33 months (Fischer et al., 1989; Armstrong et al., 1993; Smith et al., 1993; De Lacalle et al., 1996; Stemmelin et al., 2000; Baskerville et al., 2006; Bañuelos et al., 2013). Taken together, these data suggest that, as in the monkey, basal forebrain neurons of aged rats have altered phenotypic expression profiles.

When the axon projections to the hippocampus from basal forebrain neurons have been examined using vesicular acetylcholine transporter immunohistochemistry, the density is lower in 30- compared with 3-month-old male Wistar rats (Potier et al., 2006). These data are consistent with differences observed in whole hippocampus homogenates, as quantified by Western blot analysis in male Wistar rats ranging in age from 6 to 24 months (Canas et al., 2009). Since the transporter is found throughout the length of the axon, reduced levels in rodent studies could be consistent with shorter basal forebrain axon length within the hippocampus of nonhuman primates (Calhoun et al., 2004). In humans, however, the vesicular acetylcholine transporter has not been reported to change with age (Kuhl et al., 1996). This discrepancy could be due to reduced specificity or sensitivity of the PET ligand used in human studies relative to more quantitative analyses that are possible to evaluate in other animals.

Findings regarding the enzymatic activity in the cholinergic terminals of cells projecting to the hippocampus from the basal forebrain have been equivocal. A number of investigators have not detected a significant change in ChAT activity within the hippocampus across age in male and female Sprague Dawley, Wistar, F344, and Long Evans rats between 3 and 27 months (Strong et al., 1980; Ingram et al., 1981; Sherman et al., 1981; Fischer et al., 1989; Michalek et al., 1989; Baxter et al., 1999; Birthelmer et al., 2003) and male C57BL/6J mice at 6, 12, and 30 months (Strong et al., 1980). In contrast, another group of studies has reported less acetylcholine synthesis in male and female F344, Wistar, and Long Evans rats between 3 to 36 months (Dravid, 1983; Pintor et al., 1988; Araujo et al., 1990; Stemmelin et al., 2000). The latter group of experiments is consistent with what has been observed in the human hippocampus. Another important enzyme in the cholinergic synthesis and degradation pathway is acetylcholinesterase (AChE), which breaks acetylcholine into choline and acetate in the synaptic cleft. This enzyme has consistently been found to be lower in older male rats of F344 and Wistar strains between 3 and 26 months of age (Pintor et al., 1988; Fischer et al., 1989; Michalek et al., 1989). The reduction in AChE activity could either indicate a response to altered acetylcholine availability or it could reflect compensation to increase cholinergic signaling in the face of an impaired system.

Autoradiographic binding assays have also been used in rodents to examine hippocampus cholinergic receptor density. An early study measured binding of the muscarinic receptor ligand $[^3H]$-QNB in whole hippocampus homogenates in young (4 months) and older (22 months) male Long Evans rats. This study did not report a difference in receptor density or binding affinity at the ages examined (Morin and Wasterlain, 1980). Notably, Long Evans rats have a relatively long lifespan (>36 months), and 22 months may be more comparable to middle age. When older animals have been examined, however, the results have been conflicting. One study using $[^3H]$-QNB ligand binding and a muscarinic receptor agonist ($[^3H]$-CD) reported lower receptor binding for both ligands in old (26–28 months) compared with young (6–8 months) F344 rats (sex not specified) (Lippa et al., 1981). Another study using male Wistar rats reported that muscarinic receptor density was lower in the old groups (24 and 30 months) compared with the young (6 months) (London et al., 1985). Muscarinic receptor density was also observed to be lower in male F344 rats at 24–25 months compared with 3–4 months (Pintor et al., 1988). Finally, binding of the M_2 muscarinic receptor subtype, as assessed by the $[^3H]$-AF-DX 116 ligand, has been observed to be lower in 27-month-old male Long Evans rats compared with 3-month-old animals (Araujo et al., 1990). In contrast, another study that measured $[^3H]$-QNB binding in the hippocampus of male F344 rats found no difference in ages ranging from 3 to 30 months in muscarinic receptor density or binding affinity (Pedigo et al., 1984). The binding density of the M_1 muscarinic receptor subtype measured by $[^3H]$-pirenzepine ligand was reported to be stable in male Long Evans rats examined at 6 and 25 months (Aubert et al., 1995). Another study that used several different ligands to measure muscarinic receptor density also did not detect differences in binding in male Long Evans rats examined at 6 and 25 months of age (Smith et al., 1995). The reasons for these reported discrepancies remain to be discovered.

Autoradiographic binding assays for nicotinic acetylcholine receptors have also been conducted in the rodent hippocampus. An early study using the $[^3H]$-MCC ligand reported no change in binding affinity, but lower inferred receptor density in the hippocampus of 27-month-old male Long Evans rats compared with 3- and 9-month-old animals (Araujo et al., 1990). A later study that also examined overall nicotinic acetylcholine receptor binding using the $[^3H]$-Nic ligand in 6- to 25-month-old male Long Evans rats reported stability of receptor density across all hippocampus subregions (Smith et al., 1995). The observation of no change across age was replicated using α-bungarotoxin to interrogate general nicotinic receptor binding in male Wistar rats examined at 2 and 20 months of age (Tribollet et al., 2004). In the same study, α7 receptor binding was also shown to be stable in the hippocampus across age (Tribollet et al., 2004). Consistent with these observations, the threshold for inducing synaptic modification (section 15.7) in the CA1 subregion was lowered following acute or chronic nicotine treatment, as well as α7 receptor antagonism, in 19- to 21-month-old Sprague Dawley rats (Fujii and Sumikawa, 2001).

While there are inconsistencies regarding the effects of age on hippocampus acetylcholine receptor density, some aspects of cholinergic neurotransmission have been consistently reported. For example, when a nicotinic receptor agonist (MCC) is applied to hippocampal slices from 3-, 9-, and 27-month-old male Long Evans rats, there was less evoked release in the 27-month-old rats. Potassium evoked release of acetylcholine has also been observed to be lower in 27-month-old rats male Long Evans rats compared with younger groups. There was no age-related difference observed in acetylcholine release in response to application of the autoreceptor antagonist AF-DX 116, and no difference in spontaneous release of acetylcholine in older rats (Araujo et al., 1990). When acetylcholine is iontophoretically applied onto CA1 pyramidal neurons in hippocampal slices, firing rates increase in young animals (6 months), but this effect is blunted in old neurons from male F344 rats (28 months) (Lippa et al., 1981). This effect was replicated in male Wistar rats examined at 3 and 30 months (Segal, 1982). When the intracellularly recorded slow cholinergic excitatory postsynaptic potential (EPSP) was elicited in CA1 pyramidal cells by 20 to 30 Hz stimulation of cholinergic fibers from the medial septum, 32-month-old male Sprague Dawley rats had lower amplitudes relative to the 3-month-old group (Potier et al., 1992). Similarly, when 50 Hz stimulation of cholinergic fibers was applied to regions CA1, CA3, and the dentate gyrus, all subregions showed lower amplitude EPSP responses in 28-month-old male F344 rats compared with 1- and 9-month-old animals (Shen and Barnes, 1996). The lower cholinergic slow EPSP amplitude of old CA1 pyramidal neurons has also been confirmed using patch clamp methods (Potier et al., 2006). Furthermore, when acetylcholine release is measured in response to application of 3,4-diaminopyridine in whole hippocampal preparations, 27-month-old female Long Evans rats showed lower release compared with 3-month-old animals (Schweizer et al., 2003). This is consistent with the observed change in stimulated release of [^{3}H] choline in hippocampus slices from 3- to 27-month-old male Long Evans rats, regardless of behavioral status (Birthelmer et al., 2003).

In conclusion, across species a large body of work has examined the impact of age on cholinergic function. While the biochemical and receptor data have been equivocal, the functional data have consistently suggested that there is altered modulation of hippocampal cells by acetylcholine in old animals despite preservation of cell numbers in cholinergic nuclei across species. The observations that functional cholinergic transmission in the hippocampus is disrupted in old age might be considered to support Bartus' "original" cholinergic hypothesis of geriatric memory decline. A major difficulty for this hypothesis has arisen, however, because total lesions of hippocampal cholinergic input do not impact hippocampus-dependent memory (e.g., Baxter et al., 1995). This could suggest that other neuromodulatory systems are able to compensate for cholinergic defects.

15.6.2 Serotonin

Serotonin is synthesized by cells in the median and dorsal divisions of the raphe nuclei (Azmitia and Segal, 1978; Steinbusch, 1981; Vertes, 1991), which then project throughout the hippocampus.

This serotonergic input is most dense in the polymorphic layer of the dentate gyrus, less dense in CA3, and the least dense in CA1. These axons terminate preferentially, but not exclusively, onto GABAergic interneurons that contain the calcium-binding proteins calbindin and calretinin, but not parvalbumin (Freund et al., 1990; Acsády et al., 1993). Serotonin is hypothesized to act in parallel with the cholinergic projection to the hippocampus to modulate the balance between inhibition and excitation. As described below, the impact of age on hippocampus serotonergic neurotransmission is complex.

15.6.2.1 The serotonergic system in young and aged humans

Cell numbers in the raphe nuclei of humans remain stable between 5 and 82 years of age, when estimated with nonstereological methods (Klöppel et al., 2001). Additionally, when the concentration of serotonin (5-HT) and one of its metabolites (5-H1AA) was measured from postmortem hippocampus tissue, no detectable differences were reported between 18 and 95 years of age (Bucht et al., 1981). This observation was replicated in another population of individuals ranging in age from 17 to 100 years (Wester et al., 1984), and an additional population ranging in age from 58 to 83 years (Gottfries et al., 1983). The integrity of the axon projections from the median dorsal raphe nuclei to the hippocampus has been examined using [^{3}H]imipramine, which is a proxy for 5-HT fiber terminals. In individuals from 18 to 100 years, there was no reported change of 5-HT fiber terminals with age in the hippocampus (Marcusson et al., 1987). Additionally, when [^{3}H]5-HT uptake and binding was measured in the temporal lobe of individuals between 50 to 90 years, there was no relationship between age and either of these variables (Allen et al., 1983). Thus, in humans cell number in the median raphe nuclei and fiber terminals in the hippocampus may not change with age, but stereological counts are still needed. Consistent with these observations, the concentration of 5-HT in the hippocampus does not change between 18 and 95 years of age (Winblad et al., 1985). Finally, the enzyme that is responsible for 5-HT metabolism, monoamine oxidase A, also does not change from 2 to 95 years (Fowler et al., 1980).

When the overall density of postsynaptic 5-HT receptors has been examined with autoradiographic binding assays selective for the high affinity S-1 binding site in the hippocampus of human postmortem tissue in individuals 19 to 100 years, lower receptor densities have been reported at older ages (Marcusson, Oreland, et al., 1984). Density of the lower affinity S-2 binding site is also lower at older ages (Morgan, 1987). When this binding site is subdivided into the S-2A and S-2B subclasses, only the S-2A subclass was shown to have lower binding in individuals at older ages (Marcusson, Oreland, et al., 1984). There was no difference reported with age when the high affinity S-1 binding site was examined (Marcusson et al., 1987). There are, however, 14 subtypes of the 5-HT receptor (Hoyer and Martin, 1997), which are divided into 7 different classes (Hannon and Hoyer, 2008). The density of some of these receptor subtypes does appear to be affected in old age, but not every subtype has been examined in humans.

In the hippocampus the 5-HT$_{1A}$ receptor subtype is found on the dendrites and soma of both pyramidal neurons and granule cells (Riad et al., 2000). The activation of this receptor has been shown to hyperpolarize pyramidal neurons (Andrade and Nicoll, 1987). Autoradiographic analysis of the 5-HT$_{1A}$ receptor subtype in the hippocampus from postmortem tissue of individuals 15 to 81 years revealed lower binding with age in male, but not female study participants (Dillon et al., 1991). This age difference in males was replicated in vivo using PET to measure binding of the [^{11}C–carbonyl] WAY100635 ligand in study participants 21 to 80 years (Meltzer et al., 2001). Another PET imaging study that used the 5-HT$_{1A}$ ligand [^{3}H]8-OH-DPAT to quantify receptor density, however, detected a significant change in women, but not men between the ages of 32 and 83 (Palego et al., 1997). In contrast to these data, another report using the ligand [^{11}C]WAY-100635 found no change with age in either males or females between 19 to 70 years (Parsey et al., 2002). These discrepant results regarding 5-HT$_{1A}$ receptor binding could have arisen from the relatively small sample sizes (the largest included 28 individuals) across the lifespan, or differences in time of day of data acquisition known to affect receptor number and binding affinity.

In the hippocampus the 5-HT$_2$ receptor is found primarily on interneurons in all subregions, but less densely in the dentate gyrus (Morilak et al., 1994). An effect of age was not found between 17 to 100 years for 5-HT$_2$ receptor binding using an autoradiographic binding assay with the agonist [^{3}H]spiperone (Marcusson, Morgan, et al., 1984). When an autoradiagraphic binding assay using the ligand [^{3}H]ketaserin was used to detect overall 5-HT$_2$ binding, no change was found between 17 and 81 years (Gross-Isseroff et al., 1990). In contrast, 5-HT$_2$ receptor binding measured with the PET ligand [^{18}F]setoperone was shown to negatively correlate with age in study participants between 20 and 86 years (Blin et al., 1993). In another study, the total binding density of 5-HT$_2$ receptors in the hippocampus was similar between 19 and 100 years. When a competitive binding assay was performed using the selective 5-HT$_{2B}$ receptor antagonist methysergide to isolate the A and B subtypes, however, it was observed that there was a lower binding density selectively of the 5-HT$_{2A}$ receptor with age (Marcusson, Morgan, et al., 1984). The discrepancies among these investigations could have arisen from the sensitivity of the different PET ligands to 5-HT$_{2A}$ versus 5-HT$_{2B}$ receptors. There are no reports of the effects of advanced age on the density of 5-HT$_4$, 5-HT$_5$, or 5-HT$_6$ receptor binding in humans.

15.6.2.2 The serotonergic system in young and aged nonhuman primates

While no cell counts of raphe nuclei neurons are available, one study reported that pig-tail macaques 4 and 20 years old (sex not specified) had visible 5-HT histofluorescence throughout the processes of dorsal raphe nuclei cells in both age groups. Overall lower 5-HT histofluorescence intensity within the cells of the dorsal raphe nuclei, however, was observed in the older compared with the younger group (Sladek and Sladek, 1978). These data appear consistent with the observation in male tree shrews between 1 and 7 years (normal lifespan is 9–12 years) that the older animals have lower 5-HT immunoreactive fiber density in CA3 and CA1 stratum radiatum, and in the CA3 stratum oriens (Keuker et al., 2005). Moreover, the specific binding to the serotonin transporter has been reported to be significantly lower in the hippocampus of male rhesus macaques at 19 years compared with 6 years (Kakiuchi et al., 2001). No change has been reported in overall hippocampal 5-HT concentration in male and female rhesus macaques examined at 2 and 18 years (Goldman-Rakic and Brown, 1981). The oldest macaques in this study were middle-aged, equivalent to 54 human years. With respect to specific receptor subtypes, there were no changes observed in 5-HT$_{1A}$ receptor binding in the hippocampus

of male rhesus macaques examined at 6 and 19 years using the [^{11}C] WAY-100635 ligand with high-resolution PET methods (Tsukada, Kakiuchi, Nishiyama, and Ohba, 2001). There is, however, an aged-related change in [^{11}C]MDL100,907 binding to 5-HT$_{2A}$ receptors in the hippocampus of male rhesus macaques examined at 6 and 19 years (Kakiuchi et al., 2000). Lower serotonin transporter and 5-HT$_{2A}$ receptor binding in aged nonhuman primates is consistent with the data obtained from studies in humans. Moreover, the lack of an age-related change in 5-HT$_{1A}$ receptor binding is consistent with one human report (Parsey et al., 2002).

15.6.2.3 The serotonergic system in young and aged rodents

When nonstereological cell counts have been conducted in the dorsal raphe nuclei between 3 and 35 months in male Wistar rats, there is no loss of 5-HT-immunoreactive neurons (van Luijtelaar et al., 1992). This is consistent with nonstereological observations in humans. There are, however, changes in 5-HT fiber density within the hippocampus of aged Wistar rats and abnormal swollen varicosities (van Luijtelaar et al., 1988; van Luijtelaar et al., 1992; Venero et al., 1993). Fiber loss was also observed in male Wistar rats between 3 and 36 months throughout the dentate gyrus, which was particularly pronounced in the polymorphic layer (Nishimura et al., 1995). Overall levels of 5-HT in the hippocampus, however, have been reported to not change with age in male Wistar and Sprague Dawley rats from 1 to 35 months (Ponzio et al., 1982; van Luijtelaar et al., 1992; Lee et al., 1994; Míguez et al., 1999). When the biosynthesis of 5-HT has been quantified by examining overall 5-HT levels in addition to levels of its metabolite, 5-HIAA, overall biosynthesis is lower in 18-month-old male Fischer 344 rats compared with 4-month-old animals. When the ratio of 5-HIAA to 5-HT levels are examined, this ratio is also reported to change, suggesting lower monoamine oxidase activity in older rats (Miura et al., 2002). Because age-related lowering of biosynthesis is accompanied by weaker degradation of 5-HT, these two changes could effectively cancel each other out, resulting in no change of 5-HT availability.

Other studies have reported higher levels of 5-HT within the hippocampus in older rodents. In Wistar rats between 6 and 24 months, higher 5-HT concentrations within the hippocampus have been reported. This finding was interpreted as potentially indicating elevated 5-HT synthesis in older animals (Santiago et al., 1988). Consistent with this idea, the rate of accumulation of hippocampal 5-HT levels in response to the monoamine oxidase inhibitor pargyline is reported to be higher in male 26-month-old Wistar rats compared with 6-month-old animals (Venero et al., 1993). Similarly, 5-HIAA levels have been found to be greater in the hippocampus of 19-month-old male Sprague Dawley rats compared with 3-month-olds. These elevated levels of 5-HIAA, however, did not significantly vary with behavioral performance on the Morris watermaze (Lee et al., 1994).

In contrast to observations of no change or an increase in 5-HT levels, a modest lowering has been reported within the dorsal CA1 subregion of aged (25–26 months) female Fischer 344 rats compared with 4-month-old animals. However, all other hippocampus subregions were not altered (Luine et al., 1990). A lowering of overall hippocampus 5-HT levels with age has been reported for aged male BN rats examined at 5 and 32 months (Goudsmit et al., 1990), for male Wistar rats examined at 4 and 22 months (Gozlan et al., 1990; Saleem et al., 2014), and in Sprague-Dawley rats examined at 3 and 30 months (sex not specified) (Musumeci et al., 2015).

Several potential explanations could account for the discrepant findings including sex or time of day.

Overall, lower serotonergic receptor binding measured by autoradiography with [^{3}H]5-HT has been reported in 24-month-old male Wistar rats compared with 18-month-olds (Banerjee and Poddar, 2016). When specific receptor subtypes have been individually examined, however, the effects of age on receptor density are inconsistent. 5-HT$_{1A}$ receptor binding in the hippocampus, as measured by autoradiographic binding of the ligand [^{3}H]8-OH-DPAT, showed no change in male Wistar rats examined at 3 and 22 months (Gozlan et al., 1990). In a later study, using the same ligand in the same rat strain, lower binding was reported when examined at 3 and 30 months (Nyakas et al., 1997). The behavioral significance of changes in 5-HT$_{1A}$ receptor binding in old animals was directly examined in another study in which 32-month-old F344 x BN rats were tested on the spatial version of the Morris watermaze. While young animals were not included in this assay, overall 5-HT$_{1A}$ binding sites within the hippocampus were greater in the impaired compared with unimpaired old rats (Topic et al., 2007). In the same study, 5-HT$_2$ binding across all hippocampal subregions did not vary according to behavioral performance (Topic et al., 2007). In Syrian hamsters, ranging in age from 3 to 21 months (life expectancy 24–36 months), 5-HT$_7$ receptor binding in the hippocampus measured by autoradiography with the ligand [^{3}H]8-OH-DPAT did not change across age, but a significant relationship was found between receptor binding and time of day (Duncan et al., 2018).

When mRNA levels for 5-HT$_{1A}$, 5-HT$_{2A}$, 5-HT$_{2C}$, and 5-HT$_7$ have been quantified across hippocampal subregions no differences have been observed in male Lister Hooded rats when examined at 8 and 24 months (Yau et al., 1999). Another study also did not report a change with age in 5-HT$_7$ receptor mRNA in the dorsal CA3 region of the hippocampus in male BN rats, but they did observe lower 5-HT$_7$ mRNA at 12 and 24 months in ventral CA3 compared with 3 months (Kohen et al., 2000).

When serotonergic function has been examined in the young and aged hippocampus of rodents, several age-related changes have been documented. In hippocampal slices, the accumulation of [^{3}H]5-HT in response to 3 Hz stimulation is lower in 27-month-old female Long Evans rats compared with 3-month-olds (Birthelmer et al., 2003). Notably, this reduction in evoked 5-HT release did not differ between animals that were spatially impaired versus unimpaired on the Morris watermaze (Birthelmer et al., 2003). When the response of hippocampal cells to application of 5-HT was evaluated, alterations with age have also been noted. Intracellular recordings of dentate gyrus granule cells in F344 rats examined at 6 and 30 months have revealed that 5-HT evoked hyperpolarization was significantly attenuated in old compared with young cells (Baskys et al., 1987). Similarly, within the CA1 region, the hyperpolarization induced by application of 5-HT to single CA1 pyramidal cells in hippocampal slices was lower in 30-month-old male Wistar rats compared with 3-month-old animals (Segal, 1982). There was also an age-related lowering of the proportion of hippocampal pyramidal neurons that responded to the local application of 5-HT in 30-month-old male F344 rats compared with 3-month-old animals (Bickford-Wimer et al., 1988).

In conclusion, raphe nuclei cell numbers appear to be preserved in rodents and humans, but cell count studies have not been conducted in the monkey. While age-related changes in serotonergic function have been consistently observed within the rodent hippocampus, there appears to be no behavioral impact of the functional alterations as assessed by the Morris watermaze in the studies that did measure behavior. It is critical to also condsider the impact that activity levels across the day have on serotonergic function, as these variables are strongly related (Duncan et al., 2018). Moreover, circadian rhythms within the hippocampus can be disrupted by age (e.g., Fonken et al., 2016; Lacoste et al., 2017). Thus, measurements of serotoninergic function need to be tightly controlled to prevent potential confounds from arising.

15.6.3 Norepinephrine

Norepinephrine (NE) is synthesized by cells in the locus coeruleus (LC). In primates, most LC neurons contain the pigment neuromelanin making them easily identifiable without immunohistochemical or nuclear labeling (Mann, 1983). Neuromelanin is not present at birth in LC neurons and appears at around 15–18 years in humans (Scherer, 1939). Interestingly, rodent LC neurons are not pigmented (Goldman and Coleman, 1981). LC projections to the hippocampus primarily arise from the rostral portion of this structure and terminate in all subfields, although the densest terminal labeling has been observed in the hilus of the dentate gyrus, stratum lucidum of CA3, and in the molecular layer of the subiculum (Loy et al., 1980). Fluorescent varicosities often appear in perisomatic clusters rather than on the dendrites of granule and pyramidal cells (Loy et al., 1980). NE has multiple physiological effects within the hippocampus. In excitatory principal cells, activation of the β_1-receptor enhances excitability, whereas α_1 activation decreases evoked responses to afferent stimulation (for review, see Segal et al., 1991). Moreover, β-receptor activation can induce plasticity at the perforant path–granule cell synapse (Harley, 1991). Thus, LC input to the hippocampus could provide modulation that is critical for normal learning and memory (Mather and Harley, 2016).

15.6.3.1 The noradrenergic system in young and aged humans

Several studies have examined whether there is cell loss within the LC during aging. Early reports did not use unbiased stereological methods, and consistently reported reductions in the number of neuromelanin-containing LC neurons in individuals ranging in age from 11 to 103 years (Vijayashankar and Brody, 1979; Wree et al., 1980; Tomlinson et al., 1981; Tomonaga, 1983; Mann et al., 1984c; Lohr and Jeste, 1988; Marcyniuk et al., 1989). Notably, all pigmented LC neurons contain NE, but not all NE cells contain pigment. Thus, counts of LC cells immunolabeled with tyrosine hydroxylase (TH), which detects catecholamine-positive cells, tend to identify greater numbers of total NE neurons in this structure than looking at neuromelanin alone (Manaye et al., 1995). Across two studies examining individuals ranging in age from 1 to 104, TH-positive cell counts were reported to be lower in older individuals (Chan-Palay and Asan, 1989; Manaye et al., 1995). In contradiction to all the studies discussed above, when neuromelanin cells in the LC were counted semiautomatically in individuals 5 to 94 years old, there was no difference detected across age (Iwanaga et al., 1996).

There were a number of flaws in these early studies, and the idea that there is dramatic change in cell number with age in LC has not been supported when unbiased stereological or other correction methods have been applied. For example, Mouton et al. (1994) observed no difference in neuromelanin-containing cell numbers between 19 and 78 years of age in males. Consistent with this, using similar methods, Ohm et al. (1997) also found no correlation between cell number and age in males from 49 to 98 years. When the Abercrombie correction method was used to control for overestimates of counted cells, rather than stereological approaches, no age differences in the numbers of TH-positive LC neurons were reported in males and females ranging in age from 44 to 110 years (Kubis et al., 2000). In a case study of a 115-year-old woman, whose cognitive performance was comparable to healthy individuals of 60–80 years, LC cell number was counted with the Abercrombie correction method. Impressively, this individual did not show LC cell loss compared with 60–80-year-olds (den Dunnen et al., 2008). In a more recent study examining LC integrity (volume and stereological cell counts), no relationship was found with age in adults between 47 and 83 years that had little to no AD pathology (Theofilas et al., 2017). Interestingly, those individuals with significant levels of pathology, showed declines in LC TH-containing cell number and volume (Theofilas et al., 2017).

While stereological cell counts to date have not separated rostral versus caudal regions of LC when conducting age comparisons, recent MRI measurements have begun to make this distinction. Ex vivo postmortem imaging combined with histological sectioning of the same brains has shown a relationship between MRI signal intensity and neuromelanin- and TH cell counts in LC (Keren et al., 2015). In a large study of healthy adults from ages 18 to 88 years ($n = 605$), Liu et al. (2019) reported that the rostral region of the LC selectively showed reduced intensity at older ages, which was observed in both males and females (Liu et al., 2019). In a study using fewer participants ($n = 294$), LC intensity in the rostral portion was not different between young (mean age 32.5) and older (mean age 72.3) study participants. In the older adults, however, LC signal intensity correlated with memory performance on tasks that require the hippocampus (Dahl et al., 2019).

Noradrenergic fibers can be identified using immunolabeling for the enzyme dopamine β-hydroxylase (DBH), which is responsible for converting DA to NE. When this approach has been employed in human tissue from individuals 35 to 84 years, the distribution and orientation of DBH-immunoreactive fibers within the hippocampus appeared qualitatively similar (Powers et al., 1988). This is consistent with observations of little to no cell loss within the LC in normative aging (Mouton et al., 1994). Furthermore, one study reported that NE levels within the hippocampus did not change with age between 58 and 83 years (Gottfries et al., 1983).

Inferred receptor density of both the α_1 and α_2-adrenergic receptors has been examined across age within the hippocampus. Binding of the α_1-adrenergic receptor was quantified with the radioligand [^{125}I]2-(fl-4-hydroxyphenylethylamino-ethyltetralone) and showed no change in binding between 24 and 81 years (Kalaria, 1989). Binding of the α_2-adrenergic receptor in the hippocampus of aged individuals 50 to 81 years has revealed no difference in inferred receptor density across age using the ligand [^{3}H]para-aminoclonidine (Kalaria and Andorn, 1991). Using a different ligand that also binds to the α_2-adrenergic receptor, [^{3}H]UK-14304, another study reported a nonsignificant 37% lower binding in the CA1 subregion of individuals 19 to 84 years (Pascual et al., 1991).

15.6.3.2 The noradrenergic system in young and aged nonhuman primates

In an early nonstereological study conducted in two 4-year-old and four 20-year-old pig-tail macaques, lower numbers of TH-positive

LC neurons were reported in the older group using immunofluorescent methods (sex not specified) (Sladek and Sladek, 1978). In later studies, and consistent with the unbiased stereological studies in humans, when numbers of TH-positive cells within the LC were quantified using stereological methods, rhesus macaques ages 1–32 years exhibited no significant difference in cell number across this age range (Downs et al., 2007). While there was no change in cell number, TH mRNA levels within the LC were observed to be lower at the older ages (Downs et al., 2007). Although the possible effects of age on NE synthesis, release, uptake, and receptor density within the hippocampus has not been examined in the nonhuman primate, there is one report of no change in NE levels in 29 rhesus macaques between 2 and 18 years old (Goldman-Rakic and Brown, 1981). Clearly, the noradrenergic system in the aged nonhuman primate remains a potentially productive line of investigation.

15.6.3.3 The noradrenergic system in young and aged rodents

Two studies conducted without using stereological methods obtained contradictory results regarding LC cell numbers in old age. LC neuron number was reported to remain stable in male F344 rats between 12 and 32 months (Goldman and Coleman, 1981), whereas LC cell numbers counted in male ASH/TO mice ranging in age from 6 to 31 months were different between younger and older age groups (Sturrock and Rao, 1985). A more recent study using stereology observed stability in TH-positive neuron numbers within the LC between 6 and 22 months of age in male C57BL/6 mice (Mouton et al., 2012). This finding was recently replicated in male C57BL/6J mice examined at 4 and 19 months of age (Evans et al., 2021).

As discussed above, LC fiber integrity can be quantified by staining the processes with DBH and measuring immunoreactive varicosities in the hippocampus or by quantifying expression levels of the NE transporter. The density of DBH-labeled fiber varicosities in the dentate gyrus was lower in 27-month-old male F344 rats compared with 7-month-old animals (Ishida et al., 2000). In contrast, a later study reported that DBH-positive fibers within the hippocampus was higher in 13- compared with 6-month-old male F344 rats, with no further change at 25 months (Matsunaga et al., 2006). In these same animals, protein levels of the NE transporter showed the same pattern of an increase between 6 and 13 months with no further change at 25 months (Matsunaga et al., 2006). In a functional study, the antidromic response of LC neurons elicited by stimulation of the dentate gyrus, was reported to be stable between 7 and 27 months in male F344 rats, although the latencies of antidromic responses tended to be more variable in the older animals (Ishida et al., 2000). Thus, while there may be some changes in LC fibers over the lifespan, evidence to date suggests that LC projections to the hippocampus may be intact in old age.

While the literature is not completely consistent concerning the impact of age on LC cell number or fiber integrity, most studies quantifying concentrations of NE in the hippocampus have reported no change with age. Male Sprague-Dawley rats examined at 4 and 29 months had comparable concentrations of NE in the hippocampus as measured by high-pressure liquid chromatography (HPLC) with electrochemical detection (Ponzio et al., 1982). Similarly, using HPLC, no difference was observed in NE concentration in CA1 or the dentate gyrus in 3- and 25-month-old female F344 rats (Luine et al., 1990). Consistent with these studies, no differences in NE levels were found in the hippocampus of male Sprague-Dawley rats at 3 and 19 months (Lee et al., 1994), or at 3 and 24 months (Míguez et al., 1999). Also in line with no age effects on NE concentration, no differences were found in NE accumulation or turnover rate after MAO inhibition with pargyline in male Wistar rats at 6 and 26 months (Venero et al., 1993). Moreover, levels of NE and its metabolites in the hippocampus have also been reported to remain stable between 3 and 30 months in male Wistar rats (Santiago et al., 1988). Another study using female Long Evans rats at 3–5 and 25–27 months found no difference with age in NE accumulation, baseline outflow, or nicotine-evoked overflow in the hippocampus (Birthelmer et al., 2003). Importantly, when stimulated release of [³H]NE in hippocampal sections has been examined, concentration was comparable between 4- and 24-month-old male and female Wistar rats (Zsilla et al., 1994). This suggests no change in the releasable pool of NE with age.

In contrast to these reports of stability of hippocampus NE across age, there are several reports that do suggest changes. NE concentration measured using HPLC was reported to be lower in the dorsal and ventral hippocampus, but not the entorhinal cortex, of 26-month-old female Long Evans rats compared with 3-month-old animals (Stemmelin et al., 2000). Although Birthelmer et al. (2003) reported no functional change in evoked NE levels in the hippocampus with age, the same study reported lower concentrations of NE in old compared with young animals (Birthelmer et al., 2003). A more recent study also reported lower whole hippocampus NE concentrations in 16- and 30-month-old male Sprague Dawley rats compared with 2- and 8-month-old rats (Mei et al., 2015). In contrast to all studies cited above, Sirviö et al. (1994) reported higher hippocampus NE concentration in 22-month-old male Wistar rats compared with 4-month-old animals. The variability in the reported relationship between aging and the functional release of NE in the hippocampus highlights the complexities of this neuromodulatory system. In fact, NE release in the hippocampus can be evoked by other neurotransmitter systems. NMDA receptors exist on noradrenergic terminals in rat hippocampus where they can mediate the enhancement of NE release (Pittaluga and Raiteri, 1990). Studies using hippocampus slices (Gonzales et al., 1991; Scognamiglio et al., 2024) or synaptosome preparations (Pittaluga et al., 1993) with [³H]NE to measure release have reported that exposure to NMDA does not induce the same increase in NE concentration in 12- to 28-month-old male F344 rats compared with 3- to 5-month-old animals (Gonzales et al., 1991) and in male Wistar Kyoto rats at 12 and 24 months compared with 3-month-old animals (Pittaluga et al., 1993). The application of D-cycloserine, which mimics glycine and acts a positive modulator of the NMDA receptor, partially restored the NE response to NMDA (Pittaluga et al., 1993). A more recent study reported that the administration of the psychostimulant amphetamine was able to completely restore the glutamate-mediated release of NE in 18- and 22-month-old male F344 rats to the levels observed in 2- and 4-month-old animals (Scognamiglio et al., 2024).

Inferred receptor density within the hippocampus of both α- and β-adrenergic receptors has been examined across the lifespan using radioligand binding assays. No change was observed at 3, 18, and 28 months in male F344 rats in the competitive binding of [¹²⁵I] BE-2254 to the α_1 receptor. Moreover, the ability of NE to stimulate phosphoinositide hydrolysis was unaltered in these rats (Burnett et al., 1990). These data are consistent with a later study in which

[³H]prazosine binding to the α_1 receptor in male F344 rats examined at 5 and 24 months was found to remain stable in the dentate gyrus, hilus, and CA3 (Collier et al., 2004). Collier et al. (2004) also reported no change in α_2 receptor binding to [³H]Clonidine in the dentate gyrus at 24 compared with 4 months, whether or not the old rats were impaired or unimpaired on the Morris watermaze. In contrast, binding density in the hippocampus for the α_2 ligand [³H]rauwolscine has been reported to be lower in 24-month-old male Wistar rats compared with 4-month-old animals (Huguet and Tarrade, 1992). When the α_2 NE receptor was antagonized in young and middle-aged male and female Wistar rats (4 and 12 months), higher hippocampus NE levels were observed in response to electrical stimulation, while NE levels did not increase in the 24-month-old rats (Zsilla et al., 1994). Since α_2 is a presynaptic autoreceptor involved in negative feedback modulation of NE release, these data suggest that the availability of NE is lower in the aged hippocampus.

The binding density of [¹²⁵I]-Pindolol, a β-adrenergic receptor antagonist, has been reported to remain stable between 4 and 25 months in male F344 rats (Miller and Zahniser, 1988). In contrast, binding density of the β-adrenergic receptor to [³H]DHA has been shown to be lower in 22-month-old Wistar rats relative to 2- and 10-month-old animals (sex not specified) (Popova and Petkov, 1989). While these discrepant findings could be due to the different ligands used, a later study also reported no change in hippocampal binding density for β-adrenergic receptors in the dentate gyrus, hilus, and CA3. In this same study, stable receptor density was also observed when β_1- and β_2-adrenergic receptor subtypes were considered separately (Collier et al., 2004).

In male 3-month-old F344 rats, bath application of NE or the β-adrenergic receptor agonist isoproterenol leads to increased phosphorylation of synapsin I and II in the dentate gyrus, which can increase neurotransmitter release. In 26-month-old rats, the basal phosphorylation of synapsin I and II was elevated by twofold compared with younger animals, and application of NE and isoproterenol did not lead to additional phosphorylation. When phosphorylation levels were inhibited in aged rats, however, NE was able to enhance phosphorylation of synapsin I and II (Parfitt et al., 1991), suggesting decline with aging in the potential of NE to induce phosphorylation. Another study examined the electrophysiological impact of NE application within the CA1 region of the hippocampus of intact young and aged rats. In 6-month-old male F344 rats, spontaneous multiunit activity in CA1 was reported to decrease in a dose-dependent manner following application of NE from a micropipette at the recording site. In 28-month-old rats, however, there was an attenuation of the efficacy of NE to inhibit firing. This change in postsynaptic responsiveness to NE was detected starting at 18 months (Bickford-Wimer et al., 1988), suggesting that it could emerge as early as middle age.

Altered postsynaptic responsiveness of hippocampus neurons to NE could potentially impact LTP and behavior. In young rats, NE robustly enhances hippocampal LTP in both the dentate gyrus (Dahl and Sarvey, 1989; Harley, 1991) and CA1 (Thomas et al., 1996; Katsuki et al., 1997) through a mechanism that depends on β-adrenergic receptors and increased surface expression of GluR1-containing AMPA receptors (Hu et al., 2007). One study directly examined the modulation of CA1 LTP by NE in young and old rats (unspecified age, strain, and sex). Contextual fear conditioning was administered to young and old rats and the older animals exhibited normal acquisition of freezing behavior, but reduced retention at 2 and 24 hours. In response to fear conditioning, the aged rats showed an attenuated increase in hippocampal NE concentration and reduced surface expression of the GluR1 containing AMPA receptors compared with young rats. The maintenance of LTP 90 min after induction was also impaired in these older rats (Luo et al., 2015). Acute treatment with NE in the bath of hippocampal slices from aged rats, recovered CA1 LTP and increased surface expression of GluR1. Treatment with the NE reuptake blocker desipramine also rescued age-related deficits in the 24-hour retention of fear conditioning in a dose-dependent manner (Luo et al., 2015).

In conclusion, similar to the other neuromodulatory systems reviewed, cell numbers in the LC appear to be preserved across the lifespan in both primates and rodents. Moreover, in this system, most studies have reported no change with age in fiber projections, NE content, and receptor binding density across species. Several studies, however, have suggested differences in NE function within the aged hippocampus. These studies tend to suggest that with aging, NE may not modulate firing rates nor enhance phosphorylation of synaptic proteins to the same degree as occurs in young animals. Moreover, the enhancement of NE concentrations by behavior appears to be attenuated in older animals. Experimental elevation of NE, however, can rescue both plasticity mechanisms and behavior in aged rats. Interestingly in older adults, noninvasive measures show that NE integrity is related to cognitive function (Dahl et al., 2019), and it has been suggested that this neuromodulator may promote cognitive reserve (Mather and Harley, 2016). Thus, while most of the machinery for normal NE regulation of the hippocampus appears to be in place, the paradoxical observations of altered NE function during aging suggest that there is more to learn about the underlying mechanisms linking this neuromodulator to basic cell biology and plasticity.

15.6.4 Dopamine

There are three sources of dopamine (DA) to the hippocampus. One from the substantia nigra pars compacta (SN), a second from the ventral tegmental area (VTA), and a more recently described source from the LC (Kempadoo et al., 2016; Takeuchi et al., 2016). As discussed above, there is no significant loss of LC neurons with age in humans and rodents. Thus, this section will focus on the effects of aging on the SN and VTA. The DA output from these structures act at two groups of metabotropic G-protein-coupled receptors that can be broadly divided into subclasses of D1-like and D2-like. The D1-like family includes both the D1 and D5 receptors that mediate excitatory neurotransmission through adenylate cyclase to activate protein kinase A. The D2-like family includes D2, D3 and D4 G-protein-coupled receptors that are negatively coupled to this signaling cascade and mediate inhibitory neurotransmission. While the distribution of these different receptor subtypes varies across hippocampus subregions, inhibition of either D1/D5 or D2-like receptor activity in the hippocampus impairs memory (Bethus et al., 2010).

15.6.4.1 The dopaminergic system in young and aged humans

In early nonstereological studies of the numbers of TH- or neuromelanin-positive cells in the SN, fewer neurons were reported in the older compared with younger individuals between 10 and 91 years (McGeer et al., 1977; Mann and Yates, 1982; Fearnley and Lees, 1991). Stereological studies of neuron numbers in SN of individuals between 17 and 96 years consistently report lower numbers

at older ages (SY Ma, Röytt, et al., 1999; Cabello et al., 2002; Rudow et al., 2008). Differences in neuron volume at older ages, however, have been reported to either increase (Cabello et al., 2002; Rudow et al., 2008) or decrease (SY Ma, Röytt, et al., 1999). Dopaminergic neurons can also be identified by labeling the dopamine transporter (DAT). When stereological counts of DAT- and neuromelanin-positive cells have been obtained from individuals 6 to 85 years of age, there are fewer neuromelanin-positive cells darkly stained with DAT and more DAT-negative cells at the older ages (S Ma, Ciliax, et al., 1999). This observation suggests that DA neurons of the SN may undergo phenotypic changes with age. In humans, stereological counts of cell number in the VTA have not been conducted. Moreover, the axonal projections from the SN and VTA to the hippocampus have not been evaluated across the lifespan of humans.

In an early study, the concentration of DA in the hippocampus was reported to be lower in older individuals with an age range of 23 to 92 years (Adolfsson et al., 1979). Paradoxically, in these same individuals the concentration of homovanillic acid (HVA), a primary metabolite of DA, was not reported to change with age in the hippocampus (Adolfsson et al., 1979). A later report, however, did not detect a change in hippocampal DA or HVA concentration in individuals between 19 and 95 (Winblad et al., 1985).

While the concentrations of DA within the hippocampus appear to be relatively preserved across age, there are data suggesting that postsynaptic DA receptor density in the hippocampus is related to cognition and changes in advanced age. In fact, D2-like receptor binding has been found to positively correlate with episodic memory in adults aged 64–68 years (Nyberg et al., 2016). When the levels of RNA for D1, D2, D3, D4, and D5 receptors were examined in CA1 pyramidal neurons and layer II entorhinal cortical stellate cells, single cell gene expression for all 5 receptor subtypes was lower in CA1 neurons of older individuals ranging in age between 19 and 92 years. In contrast, no change in mRNA levels of these receptors were detected for stellate cells within layer II of the entorhinal cortex (Hemby et al., 2003). These findings are consistent with in vivo PET imaging studies. When male individuals 19 to 74 years of age were examined using the D2/D3 ligand [¹¹C]FLB457, Kaasinen et al. (2000) showed 10% less receptor binding within the hippocampus each decade. Inoue et al. (2001), using the same ligand in males aged 21–82 years found a significant negative relationship between binding and age corresponding to a 12.2% change per decade. The largest study conducted to date ($n = 132$ males and females) reported a stability in binding of the D2-like ligand [¹⁸F]Fallypride between ages 22 and 83 (Seaman et al., 2019). The discrepancy is not due to the inclusion of females in the study, because when the data were separated by sex, there were no age-related differences in either males or females. On the other hand, there was a modest loss of D2-like receptor binding in the parahippocampal gyri (i.e., the entorhinal, perirhinal, and parahippocampal cortices) (Seaman et al., 2019). While the hippocampal data are contradictory, it is notable that Seaman et al. (2019) corrected for potential volume changes with age while previous PET studies did not. Uncorrected age-related differences in volume can result in overestimates of the impact of aging on receptor binding (Smith et al., 2019).

15.6.4.2 The dopaminergic system in young and aged nonhuman primates

The first study to stereologically count SN neuron numbers reported no change overall between aged female rhesus macaques (23 years), compared with 7-year-old females. While the number of pigmented cells tended to go up, there was a lower number of nonpigmented cells in the old monkeys (Pakkenberg et al., 1995). In 3- to 27-year-old male and female rhesus macaques, Emborg et al. (1998) found that both TH- and DAT-positive SN neuron cell counts were lower in the older animals using stereological methods. Consistent with this observation, stereological analysis of total cell number in the SN was reported to negatively correlate with age in male and female rhesus macaques between 5 and 32 years (Siddiqi and Peters, 1999). When the numbers of TH-positive neurons in the ventral and dorsal tier of SN were quantified stereologically in rhesus macaques, fewer TH-positive neurons in the ventral, but not dorsal, tier of SN were found in male and female rhesus macaques 22–29 years compared with monkeys aged 9–17 years (Kanaan et al., 2007). When TH-positive cells have been counted stereologically throughout the entire extent of the SN no difference in number was detected in female rhesus macaques 8 to 31 years (Collier et al., 2007). In another study examining male and female squirrel monkeys, total numbers of cells in the SN (TH-positive and TH-negative) were observed to remain stable with age. When only the TH-positive cells were counted, however, there were lower numbers in the middle-aged (9–12 years) and aged (17–21 years) animals compared with 6-year-old monkeys. In the young monkeys, effectively all neuromelanin-positive cells were also TH-positive. In the older animals, however, the proportion of neuromelanin-positive cells that did not contain TH was increased. This observation suggests that a subset of neuromelanin-positive neurons in the SN lose their TH expression (McCormack et al., 2004), but there is no overall cell loss with age.

Few studies have examined VTA cell numbers across the lifespan of monkeys. One report suggests that the VTA paranigral region, but not the parabrachial pigmented region, shows fewer cell numbers in aged male and female rhesus macaques (26–35 years) compared with younger monkeys (3–11 years) using stereological methods (Siddiqi and Peters, 1999). When the number of TH-positive neurons across the entire VTA was quantified stereologically in rhesus macaques, no significant change was observed in males and females 22–29 years compared with 9- to 17-year-old animals (Kanaan et al., 2007). It is possible that there are subregion-specific changes in cell number across age that could not be detected when examining the entire VTA.

Only one study has examined the DA concentrations across age in the nonhuman primate, and the oldest animals were only middle aged (equivalent to 54 human years). This study reported no change in hippocampal DA levels in rhesus macaques between 2 and 18 years (Goldman-Rakic and Brown, 1981). Given the importance of DA for cognition, there are numerous opportunities to examine the impact of age on this system and how it modulates hippocampal function in nonhuman primates.

15.6.4.3 The dopaminergic system in young and aged rodents

Using stereological methods, the number of TH-positive cells in rostral SN has been reported to be lower in 24-month-old male Sprague Dawley rats compared with 5-month-old animals, with no change in intermediate and caudal portions (Gao et al., 2011). Consistent with the cell count data, this study also reported lower TH mRNA expression in the older animals (Gao et al., 2011). Numbers of TH-positive neurons counted stereologically in the SN and VTA of 22-month-old C57BL/6 mice also have been reported

to be lower compared with 6- and 14-month-old animals. Because the SN and VTA were analyzed together, it is not clear if one region is more dramatically affected than the other (Mouton et al., 2012). The observation of lower TH-positive cells in older rodents was also reported in a more recent study that evaluated the number of TH-positive neurons in the SN and VTA of male C57BL/6 mice at the ages of 1, 6, 9, 18, and 24 months. This study reported that numbers of TH+ cells in SN were lower after 9 months. In the VTA, a reduction of TH+ neurons began to occur at 6 months of age and reached the lowest number by 24 months (Shaerzadeh et al., 2020).

To date, there are no studies that examine the extent to which axonal projections from the SN, VTA, and LC to hippocampus potentially change with age. DA concentration within the hippocampus of rodents, however, has been examined. No significant age-associated change in DA levels in the CA1 subregion or entorhinal cortex (subregion not specified) were detected between 3- and 24-month-old female F344 rats (Luine et al., 1990). Similar stability for whole hippocampus was reported for male BN rats between 5 and 32 months (Goudsmit et al., 1990), male Wistar rats between 3 to 30 months (Santiago et al., 1988), and male Sprague Dawley rats between 3 and 19 months (Lee et al., 1994). Consistent with the possible stability of hippocampal DA concentration with age, no differences were found in DA accumulation or turnover rate after MAO inhibition with pargyline in male Wistar rats between 6 and 26 months (Venero et al., 1993).

Other studies, however, have detected age-related changes in DA concentrations in whole hippocampus of male Sprague Dawley rats from 1 to 24 months (Míguez et al., 1999), and male Wistar rats between 4 and 22 months (Saleem et al., 2014). In 3- and 26-month-old female Long Evans rats, DA concentrations measured with HPLC have been reported to be lower in the older animals in the dorsal hippocampus, but not ventral hippocampus or entorhinal cortex (Stemmelin et al., 2000). Hippocampus levels of the DA metabolite DOPAC showed an age-related change in male Sprague Dawley rats from 1 to 24 months (Míguez et al., 1999). DA turnover in the hippocampus has also been reported to be lower in 18-month-old male F344 rats compared with 3-month-old animals (Miura et al., 2002). Part of the problem with the interpretation of these data comes from a lack of understanding regarding the integrity of the three projection systems carrying DA to the hippocampus. While we know that cell numbers in the LC and axonal projections to the hippocampus are largely preserved, subregions of the SN do lose neurons with age. Critically, nothing is known about VTA cell numbers in old age or their projections to the hippocampus across the lifespan; nor have any of these biochemical measures been related to the cognitive status of the animal.

Although there is little information regarding the dopaminergic projections to the hippocampus, the density of postsynaptic receptors has been examined across the lifespan. In whole hippocampus homogenates, protein levels for the D1 receptor are lower in 20- to 24-month-old male C57BL/6n mice compared with 3- to 4-month-old animals (Guo et al., 2017). When 3- versus 25-month-old male Long Evans rats were examined using the D1-like receptor ligand [^{3}H]SCH 23390, there was no difference in binding detected across age (Hersi et al., 1995). Using the same ligand, Araki, Kato, Shuto, Fujiwara, et al. (1997) found no change in CA1, CA3, or the dentate gyrus in 6- compared with 24-month-old male F344 rats. On the other hand, Amenta et al. (2001), using the same ligand, showed lower D1-like receptor binding in the stratum oriens of CA1 in

24-month-old male Sprague Dawley rats compared with the 3- and 12-month-old groups. In the same study, the stratum oriens of CA3 showed a similar pattern at 24 months; however, they reported higher D1-like receptor binding in the cell body layer of CA3 (Amenta et al., 2001).

The D2-like receptor has been examined using two different ligands, [³H]Spiperone and [³H]Nemonapride, in 6- and 24-month-old male F344 rats. No change in binding with either ligand was detected (Araki, Kato, Shuto, Fujiwara, et al., 1997). Consistent with this observation, there was no reported change in hippocampus D2 receptor mRNA of 6- and 24-month-old Wistar Kyoto rats (Valerio et al., 1994). Another study, however, did report lower D2 mRNA levels in the hippocampus of 29-month-old Sprague Dawley rats compared with 2-month-old animals (Della Vedova et al., 1992). A study that also used the D2-like receptor ligand [³H]Spiperone to examine binding in male Sprague Dawley rats at 3, 12, and 24 months, found a pattern of results across age that was extremely variable (Amenta et al., 2001), precluding drawing a clear conclusion regarding the impact of age on this receptor subtype. This may point to the importance of targeting analyses of receptor binding to synaptic input fields that receive the densest dopaminergic fiber input. Among the receptor subtypes of the D2-like family, protein levels of the D4 receptor have been quantified in whole hippocampus homogenates with Western blot analysis. No changes were observed between 3–4 and 20–24 months in the male C57BL/6n mice (Guo et al., 2017). Finally, fewer CA1 uptake sites were found in 12- to 24-month-old male F344 rats compared with 6-month-old rats using the ligand [³H]Mazindol (Araki, Kato, Shuto, Fujiwara, et al., 1997). This suggests that DA change may occur in middle age.

In conclusion, the potential relationship between advanced age and the ability of dopamine signaling to modulate hippocampus function is an incomplete story. With respect to cell numbers of the three primary contributions of DA to the hippocampus, we know that the SN appears to lose neurons later in life, but the LC does not, and the VTA has not been examined to date. With respect to projection fibers, it appears that SN projections to the hippocampus are compromised, most available data indicate that LC input to the hippocampus is largely intact, and the VTA-hippocampus projections are sparse and unexplored in the context of aging. In humans and rodents, the data regarding DA receptor binding in the hippocampus are equivocal. There has been one study that examined the effect of application of the selective D4 receptor agonist, PD168077, in young and aged rats. While D4 receptor agonism did not affect CA1 LTP in young animals, it increased the magnitude of LTP in the aged mice (Guo et al., 2017). Given the critical role that dopamine plays in cognitive function, future work will be necessary to determine the relative contributions of the different dopamine projection systems to the hippocampus in relation to cognitive aging.

15.6.5 Neuropeptides

The balance between inhibition and excitation as well as functions of the cholinergic, noradrenergic, and dopaminergic systems are modulated by neuropeptides synthesized within neurons distributed throughout the brain, including in the hippocampus. These modulators influence a broad range of behaviors including those fundamentally controlled by networks in the hypothalamus involved in feeding, those in the amygdala related to affective states, and those in the hippocampus critical for behaviors discussed in section 15.2. While the neuropeptides and their respective receptor families are complex, one reason to attempt to understand their impact on aging is to disentangle the interactions that these systems have on hippocampus plasticity, circuit function, and behavioral outcomes across the lifespan. Surprisingly, relatively little is known in primates about how neuropeptides change with age. More work has been done in the rodent.

There are at least 11 primary neuropeptide families that could potentially impact hippocampus-dependent behaviors and have been examined in the context of aging. This is likely not a complete list, as new neuropeptides continue to be discovered. For example, adropin was first described in 2008 (Kumar et al., 2008) as a protein that regulates energy metabolism in liver and brain, and is potentially a twelfth neuropeptide group. Adropin has not been examined with respect to potential projections to the hippocampus, but levels in human plasma (Butler et al., 2012) and the cortex of rats (Yang et al., 2018) have been reported to decline with age. Below we describe each of the 11 neuropeptides that are known to impact hippocampus function to provide a framework for how these may be implicated in cognitive aging.

The first family, the tachykinins, comprises four peptides that include substance P, neurokinin A, neurokinin B, and hemokinin. These peptides act through three different receptors (NK1, NK2, and NK3). Some association between members of this family and DA and ACh transmission have been inferred (for review, see Borbély et al., 2013). Behavioral correlations have been established in a number of domains, for example, peripheral administration of substance P improves passive and active avoidance learning and appetitive learning of a T-maze (Schlesinger et al., 1983; Schlesinger et al., 1986). Moreover, acute administration of neurokinin B can promote performance in radial maze learning (Wenk et al., 1997).

The second neuropeptide family found in the hippocampus, somatostatin/cortistatin, acts through five G-protein-coupled receptors (sst₁₋₅). The two active forms of somatostatin are also called somatotropin release-inhibiting factor (SRIF), referred to as SST-14 and SST-28. In the hippocampus, the majority of somatostatin immunoreactive cells are colocalized with the enzyme necessary for GABA synthesis (GAD), suggesting that this peptide is located in interneurons (Kosaka et al., 1988). Interestingly, knockout mice for the sst₂ receptor show improved spatial memory and enhanced LTP (Dutar et al., 2002). Even though cortistatin works through similar receptors, increased levels of this neuropeptide worsen memory performance (Sánchez-Alavez et al., 2000) and impair LTP (Tallent et al., 2005).

The next family of neuropeptides includes vasoactive intestinal peptide (VIP) and pituitary andenylate cyclase-activating polypeptide (PACAP), which act on three different receptors: VPAC1, VPAC2, and PAC1. VIP and PACAP show similar affinities for VPAC1 and VPAC2, while PACAP has a higher affinity for PAC1 than for VIP. Both of these are known to have anti-inflammatory and neuroprotective effects and thus have been hypothesized to be promising therapeutic targets for neurodegenerative diseases (Chapter et al., 2010).

The fourth neuropeptide family is composed of calcitonin gene-regulated peptide (CGRP), which binds to the CGRP receptor-1 and has been shown to modulate hippocampus LTP (Liu et al., 2011). CGRP release can also lead to increased insulin-like growth factor (IGF-1), which has been shown to promote angiogenesis and neurogenesis (Harada et al., 2009).

The fifth family of hippocampal neuropeptides is neuropeptide Y (NPY). NPY is often colocalized with GAD in the hilus of the dentate gyrus (Freund and Buzsaki, 1996), and acts through five G-protein-coupled receptors (Y1, Y2, Y4, Y5, and Y6). The hippocampus is particularly rich in the Y2 receptor, but the Y5 receptor can also be detected in this region (Parker and Herzog, 1999). Interestingly, the Y2 receptor is present on mossy fibers that powerfully innervate CA3 pyramidal cells (Sperk et al., 2007), suggesting that NPY neurons in the hilus could play a modulatory role at this synapse. In addition, NPY is associated with the cholinergic system. The evidence for this is that there is a decrease in NPY immunoreactivity within the hilus of the dentate gyrus following cholinergic lesions with IgG-saporin (Milner et al., 1997).

The sixth family includes the opioid peptides enkephalins, dynorphins, endorphins, nociceptin, and hemorphins. These peptides act through a number of G-protein-coupled opioid receptors including delta, kappa, mu, nociceptin, sigma, zeta, and opioid growth factor (Borbély et al., 2013). Enkephalin acts primarily through the delta and mu opioid receptors (DOR), which are densely distributed throughout the hippocampus on GABAergic neuron axons that project to dendritic layers of glutamatergic pyramidal cells (Erbs et al., 2012). Activation of these receptors inhibits interneurons, which enhances pyramidal cell excitability (Masukawa and Prince, 1982; Svoboda et al., 1999), and facilitates LTP induction (Bramham et al., 1991; Bramham and Sarvey, 1996). In hippocampus, dynorphins are abundantly expressed on axons of the perforant path that run to the granule cell dendrites, and on the granule cell mossy fiber axons that project to CA3 dendrites (Schwarzer, 2009). The kappa opioid receptors are also found both pre- and postsynaptically. Presynaptically, these receptors are on lateral perforant path axons that project to the outer molecular layer of granule cells, and on the axons from the supramammillary input to the inner molecular layer of the granule cells. Postsynaptically, these receptors are found on hilar GABAergic interneurons, as well as CA3 and CA1 pyramidal cells (Schwarzer, 2009). Activating kappa opioid receptors with endogenously released dynorphins blocks the induction of hippocampal LTP (e.g., Wagner et al., 1993), and applying dynorphin can impair spatial learning (e.g., Sandin et al., 1998). Nociceptin is also found across the hippocampus and acts in this structure through the nociceptin/orphanin peptide receptor (NOP). The distribution of NOP receptor is dense in the human dentate gyrus, CA3, CA2, and CA1 regions (Berthele et al., 2003). In nonhuman primates these regions are also enriched with NOP receptor binding, as is the entorhinal cortex (Bridge et al., 2003). Interestingly, the nonhuman primate has higher levels of NOP receptor binding in the dentate gyrus and hilar regions, but less in CA2 compared with rodents. That being said, rodents also show extensive receptor binding throughout CA3, CA1, and the entorhinal cortex (Bridge et al., 2003). Nociceptin also appears to be involved in hippocampus-dependent behaviors and plasticity mechanisms. For example, deletion of the NOP receptor in transgenic mice enhances NMDA receptor-dependent LTP in CA1 (Manabe et al., 1998; Taverna et al., 2005), but the spatial receptive fields of CA1 pyramidal cells are disrupted (Taverna et al., 2005). Moreover, infusion of nociceptin into the hippocampus impairs spatial learning (e.g., Sandin et al., 1997). Interestingly, intracerebral infusion of nociceptin has been reported to reduce acetylcholine release in the rat hippocampus (Hiramatsu et al., 2008), and NOP receptor knockout mice show enhanced basal hippocampal acetylcholine release (Uezu et al., 2005).

The seventh family includes galanin, which exerts its effects through three G-protein-coupled receptors (GLA-R1, GLA-R2, and GLA-R3). GLA-R1 is densely distributed throughout the CA1 region of the ventral hippocampus (Burgevin et al., 1995), while GLA-R2 is distributed in both the dorsal and ventral hippocampus throughout the dentate gyrus granule cell layer. GLA-R3 is enriched throughout the longitudinal extent of the hippocampus in granule cells and pyramidal cell body layers of the dentate gyrus, CA3, CA1, and subiculum, as well as in the entorhinal cortex (Kolakowski et al., 1998). Infusion of galanin reduces the magnitude of LTP at the Schaffer collateral to CA1 synapse (Sakurai et al., 1996), and the perforant path to dentate gyrus granule cell synapse (Badie-Mahdavi et al., 2005; Kinney et al., 2009). Moreover, administration of galanin leads to impairments in the spatial version of the Morris watermaze (e.g., McDonald et al., 1998; Ögren et al., 2010). Of note, galanin interacts with several other neuromodulatory systems. Galanin coexists with acetylcholine in the medial septal projection to the hippocampus (Melander et al., 1985). It also coexists with noradrenergic cell bodies and fibers from the LC that project to the dentate gyrus and hilus (Xu et al., 1998).

The eighth family of neuropeptides is the Kallikrein-kinin system. This group is less well understood than the other peptide families, and includes bradykinin, kallidin, and vasodilators that act through two receptors (B_1 and B_2) (Raidoo and Bhoola, 1998). Although the kallikrein-kinin system has not been investigated in relation to hippocampus plasticity, direct infusion of a B_1, but not B_2, receptor antagonist into the hippocampus has been shown to improve performance on the spatial version of the Morris watermaze (Bitencourt et al., 2017).

The ninth family of neuropeptides is composed of orexin (also known as hypocretin), which originates from a cluster of cells in the lateral hypothalamus and perifornical area that project widely across the brain, including to the hippocampus (Chieffi et al., 2017). The orexins act through the OX_1 receptor, which is located in CA1, CA2, and CA3, and OX_2 receptor, which is in the dentate gyrus and CA3 (Trivedi et al., 1998). Orexin-A preferentially binds to OX_1, and Orexin-B shows greater affinity for the OX_2 receptor (Sakurai et al., 1998). Orexin knockout mice have reduced levels of phosphorylated CREB in the hippocampus and impaired long-term social memory (Yang et al., 2013).

The tenth family of neuropeptides is the gastrin family, which includes gastrin and cholecystokinin (CCK). Both of these peptides bind to G-protein-coupled receptors CCK_A and CCK_B. In the periphery, gastrins are released from the intestines and provide signals that regulate feeding behaviors (Williams and Elmquist, 2012). In the hippocampus, CCK is in basket cells that inhibit the soma of pyramidal neurons and in calbindin-positive interneurons that are found in the stratum radiatum (Cope et al., 2002). Activation of CCK-containing GABAergic neurons increases the inhibition of CA1 pyramidal cells and enhances performance on memory tasks, presumably by increasing the signal-to-noise ratio (Whissell et al., 2019).

The eleventh family of neuropeptides is composed of oxytocin and vasopressin. Oxytocin and vasopressin are two neuropeptides with many central actions related to social cognition. Neurons that synthesize and release vasopressin are found in the paraventricular nucleus, supraoptic nucleus, suprachiasmatic nucleus, bed nucleus of the stria terminalis, medial amygdaloid nucleus, dorsomedial hypothalamic nucleus, and locus coeruleus (Caffe and Van Leeuwen, 1983; van Leeuwen and Caffé, 1983). By contrast, oxytocin cells are found exclusively in the supraoptic and the paraventricular nuclei. These neuropeptides have recently garnered attention with regard to the hippocampus as more research is currently being conducted on the role of this structure in social cognition (Cilz et al., 2019). Importantly, oxytocin- and vasopressin-expressing fibers are abundant in the hippocampus, and receptors for both peptides are seen throughout the different subfields, suggesting that these neuropeptides may modulate hippocampus-dependent processes.

15.6.5.1 Neuropeptides in young and aged humans

Two of the 11 neuropeptide families have been examined in the human hippocampus with respect to the effects of age. One study examined the tackykinin receptor NK1, which has strong affinity for substance P, in young to middle-aged adults (19–55 years). Using the PET radioligand [^{18}F]SPA-RQ, which is an antagonist of the NK1 receptor, they found a negative association between age and NK1 receptor binding in both the hippocampus and parahippocampal gyrus within this age range (Nyman et al., 2007). Whether further declines continue throughout the lifespan remains to be determined.

The only other neuropeptide family to be examined in humans is the opioid peptides. In a small study examining four individual males ranging from 30 to 85 years, no differences in distribution or numbers of enkephalin immunoreactive neurons were detected with age (Kulmala, 1985). Consistent with these early findings, is an experiment using radio ligand binding for enkephalin receptors that examined 39 individuals ranging in age from 4 to 93 years. In this report, no relationship between age and receptor binding was observed (Rinne and Lo, 1993).

Given the importance of neuropeptides for modulating a number of other neurotransmitter systems and their involvement in a broad range of hippocampus-dependent behaviors, potential effects of advancing age on neuropeptide function is an area in which more investigation needs to be conducted.

15.6.5.2 Neuropeptides in young and aged nonhuman primates

Similar to humans, little is known regarding the impact of aging on neuropeptides in the nonhuman primate brain. Again, only two neuropeptide families have been examined with respect to changes across age in the hippocampus. In whole hippocampus homogenates, Hayashi et al. (1997) examined total somatostatin RNA in 10 Japanese macaques ranging in age from 2 to 33 years. They found that total RNA for somatostatin significantly declined by 60% over this age range (Hayashi et al., 1997). Consistent with this observation is the more recent finding that within CA3 of rhesus macaques, ranging in age from 13 to 32 years, there is a significant reduction in somatostatin-containing GABAergic neurons with no age-related change in CA1 or perirhinal cortex. This decline in somatostatin immunoreactive neurons with age in CA3 co-occurred with increases in CA3 excitability of the older monkeys, and with DNMS task performance (Thomé et al., 2016).

The VIP/PACAP family is the other class of neuropeptides that has been examined in the aged nonhuman primate hippocampus. In 24 male and female rhesus macaques ranging in age from 8 to 32 years, it was observed that overall immunostaining intensity for PACAP across the entire hippocampus was negatively correlated with the age of the animal, but was not related to DNMS task performance (Han et al., 2017).

15.6.5.3 Neuropeptides in young and aged rodents

In rats and mice, more data are available regarding the impact that advanced age has on neuropeptides. Within each neuropeptide family, however, there is not a complete understanding of the cell numbers, projections, enzymatic activity, or receptor function across the lifespan. Below we summarize the data that are available from the aged hippocampus for 10 of the 11 different neuropeptide families.

Of the tachykinin family, substance P as detected by radioimmunoassays of whole hippocampus homogenates did not change across 3-, 12-, and 22-month-old male Sprague Dawley rats (Wang et al., 1993).

In the somatostatin/cortistatin family, Wang et al., (1993) reported no change in somatostatin as detected by radioimmunohistochemical assays of whole hippocampus homogenates in male Sprague Dawley rats examined at 3, 12, and 22 months. Consistent with this observation, Sirvio et al. (1987) found no difference in binding of ^{125}I-monoiodinated Tyrl-somatostatin in the hippocampus across 1-, 8-, and 18-month-old male Wistar rats. This observation was replicated in male Wistar rats examined at 4, 18, and 26 months of age using a radioimmunohistochemical assay for somatostatin (Kowalski et al., 1992). In another study in which immunoreactivity to antisomatostatin was examined in the hilus, CA3, CA1, and entorhinal cortex, no difference was reported in any region for the number of somatostatin-positive cells in Wistar rats (sex not specified) examined at 3 and 26 months (Miettinen et al., 1993). There was, however, a trend for fewer somatostatin-positive cells in CA3 of the older animals. Cha et al. (1997) detected no differences in the number of somatostatin immunoreactive neurons in the dentate gyrus, CA3/CA1, and the subiculum between young (4–6 months) and older (20–29 months) Sprague Dawley rats (sex not specified). Because CA3 and CA1 were not examined separately, a different interpretation of these results can be drawn in the light of newer experiments that used stereological cell-counting methods. As discussed in section 15.3.2, these studies have shown that there are lower numbers of somatostatin-positive cells with age in CA3 of older rats and monkeys, and no change in CA1 (Spiegel et al., 2013; Koh et al., 2014; Thome et al., 2016). In a functional study that compared the efficacy of somatostatin application to stimulate 2-deoxyglucose uptake in whole hippocampus slices, Shibata et al. (1994) reported that uptake was enhanced to a similar extent in 2- and 22-month-old male Wistar rats. Without examining different subregions in isolation, it is not possible to clarify whether function in CA3 is disrupted.

With respect to the VIP/PACAP family of neuropeptides, one study reported stability of the number of VIP immunoreactive neurons in CA3/CA1 and subiculum but a lowering in numbers of immunoreactive cells in the dentate gyrus between 5- and 25-month-old Sprague Dawley rats (sex not specified) (Cha et al., 1997). In contrast, a qualitative reduction in VIP immunoreactivity in the pyramidal cell layers of the hippocampus was observed between 6 and 24 months in old Wistar Kyoto rats (sex not specified) (Andreose et al., 1994). Only one study has examined PACAP levels with respect to aging in the hippocampus of rodents. Enzyme-linked immunoassay was used to quantify PACAP in the hippocampus and surrounding cortical areas in C57BL/6 mice between 9 and 26 months, and no change was detected across age (Han et al., 2017). VIP and PACAP both bind to the $VPAC_1$ receptor. When $VPAC_1$ receptor immunoreactivity was examined in male Sprague Dawley rats 4 to 29 months of age, lower inferred receptor density was found across the whole hippocampus in the aged rats relative to the young group (Joo et al., 2004).

For the calcitonin gene-related peptide family (CGRP), qualitatively lower binding density of radiolabeled CGRP was observed using [^{125}I]Tyr-rat CGRP in 22- compared with 2-month-old male Sprague Dawley rats (Guidobono et al., 1989). Andreose et al. (1994) reported no change, however, in CGRP immunoreactive cells and fibers in the hippocampus of 6- to 12- compared with 18- to 24-month-old Wistar Kyoto rats (sex not specified).

For the NPY family, it has been reported that the number of NPY-positive neurons in the dentate gyrus, CA3/CA1, and subiculum does not significantly change between young (4–6 months) and old (20–29 months) Sprague Dawley rats (sex not specified) (Cha et al., 1997). Consistent with this observation, NPY-positive cells in these same regions were reported to not change in young (3–4 months) compared with aged (22–25 months) male Sprague Dawley rats (Croll et al., 1999). In contrast to these observations, a 50% lower number of NPY-positive cells was found in the dentate gyrus, CA3, and CA1 in 12- and 24-month-old male F344 rats compared with 4-month-old animals (Hattiangady et al., 2005). The densities of the Y_1, Y_2, and Y_5 NPY receptor subtypes have been examined in the hippocampus of 3- and 20-month-old male Sprague Dawley rats using radioligand labeling. Y_1 receptor binding was quantified using [^{125}I]GR231118 and observed to remain stable in the dentate gyrus and CA2 but was lower in the CA1 subregion of older rats. Y_2 receptor binding was quantified using [^{125}I]PYY(3-36) and no change was observed in the dentate gyrus, CA3, or CA2, but lower binding was observed in CA1 of old rats. Finally, inferred Y_5 receptor binding was observed to remain stable in dentate gyrus and CA1, but was lower in CA2 of aged rats (Veyrat-Durebex et al., 2013).

Within the opioid family, quite a few studies have examined how aging impacts different neuropeptides within the hippocampus. In an early study, whole hippocampus homogenates from male C57BL/6J mice were examined at 8–12 months compared with 28–32 months with respect to enkephalins. They used radioimmuno-assay with Leu^5-enkephalin and Met^5-enkephalin to create a total reactivity measure and no difference was observed across this age range (Rogers et al., 1985). Similarly, studies using quantitative radioimmunohistochemical assays to obtain methionine enkephalin concentrations in whole hippocampus homogenates, have not detected any significant changes when 4-, 18-, and 26-month-old male Wistar rats were compared (Kowalski et al., 1992). Consistent with this observation, using a similar approach Wang et al. (1993) found no change between 4-, 12- yo 13-, and 21- to 22-month-old male Sprague Dawley rats. In contrast, when quantitative densitometry for antibodies against leucine enkephalin was conducted in young (3–5 months), middle-aged (9–12 months), and old (~22 month) female Sprague Dawley rats, higher immunoreactivity was observed in both the dentate gyrus and CA3 in the older animals (Williams et al., 2011). In terms of cell function, the dose-dependent increase in CA3 firing rates in response to enkaphalin application in young (6–7 months) male F344 rats that was greatly attenuated in old animals (24–26 months). In CA1 neurons, there were no age-related differences in firing rate elevation elicited by the same application (Haigler et al., 1987).

Among the opioid family, dynorphins have also been examined with respect to the aged hippocampus. Both dynorphin A and B are in the hippocampus and largely act on kappa-opioid receptors, with dynophorphin A being more potent and selective for these receptors than B. In an early study, when dorsal and ventral hippocampal regions were separated and evaluated for tissue content of dynorphin, an elevation of radiolabeled dynorphin with the ligand dynorphin-A(1-8) was observed in aged male F344 rats (24 months) compared with 4-month-old animals in both the dorsal and ventral regions (Zhang et al., 1991). In another study using the same antibody, no change was observed between young (3–4 month) and old (22–25 months) male Sprague Dawley rats when immunoreactive cells were counted in the dentate gyrus and CA3 (Croll et al., 1999). Using an antibody to dynorphin B(1-13), the optical density of staining was lower in the dentate gyrus and CA3 of middle-aged (9–12 months) and aged (22 months) compared with young (3–5 months) female Sprague Dawley rats (Williams et al., 2011).

The final class of opioids that have been examined in the aged hippocampus is endorphin. In an early study, binding of β-endorphin in whole hippocampus homogenates from male Wistar rats at 4, 18, and 26 months was examined with radioimmunohistochemical assay to infer total content and no difference was observed across this age range (Kowalski et al., 1992). Using similar binding assays in whole hippocampus homogenates from male Sprague Dawley rats 3, 12, and 22 months of age, β-endorphin content was not different between age groups. Moreover, this stability occurred whether the animals were sacrificed during the light or dark phase of their diurnal cycle (Wang et al., 1993).

Many of the opioids discussed above bind to multiple receptor subtypes and not all of these have been examined across the lifespan in the hippocampus. When overall opioid receptor binding has been examined with autoradiography using the nonselective opioid antagonist [^{3}H]diprenorphine, in young (7–8 months) and aged (27–29 months) male Long Evans rats, a significant decline in overall binding was observed in the dorsal dentate gyrus with no age-related change in the ventral dentate gyrus or dorsal and ventral CA3 (Nagahara et al., 1996). In the same study, an agonist that is selective for the μ-opioid receptor ([^{3}H]$_D$-Ala^2, MePhe^4, Gly-01^5 enkephalin) also showed lower binding in the dorsal dentate gyrus of aged rats compared with young, but no changes in ventral dentate gyrus or dorsal and ventral CA3 (Nagahara et al., 1996). The only other opioid receptor to be measured in the aged hippocampus is the δ-opioid receptor. When the binding density of a selective ligand for the δ-opioid receptor ([D-PEN^2-D-PEN^5] enkephalin) was examined, there was no change observed in male Sprague Dawley rats when measured at 3 and 24 months (Dondi et al., 1992).

Although galanin is found in septohippocampal projection neurons and the ventral portion of the vertical limb of the diagonal band of Broca (e.g., Senut et al., 1989), and quite a bit is known regarding its interaction with acetylcholine and norepinephrine, there is little known about the potential role of galanin in cognitive aging. One study has examined the hippocampus in young (3–4 months) and aged (26–27 months) male Sprague Dawley rats for binding of [^{125}I]-Galanin to receptors throughout the hippocampus and surrounding cortex. In this study there were no changes in binding density found in the ventral dentate gyrus, CA3, or the dorsal subiculum. An age-related increase in binding was found in the perirhinal and entorhinal cortices, dorsal dentate gyrus, ventral CA1, and ventral subiculum (Krzywkowski et al., 1993).

For the orexin family of neuropeptides one study has examined the density of orexin-A immunopositive fibers in the CA1 subregion of the hippocampus in young (3–5 months) and old (26–30 months) male F344 x BN rats. Across all CA1 lamina (oriens, pyramidale, stratum radiatum, and lacunosum-moleculare) there was no significant age-related change (Stanley and Fadel, 2011). Orexin-B has not been examined. When mRNA levels were quantified in whole hippocampus for the two orexin receptor subtypes (OX_1 and OX_2) in male C57BL/6 mice at 3, 12, 18, and 24 months of age using quantitative PCR, the relationship with age group was complex. There was lower OX_1 receptor expression between 12 and 18 months with no further change at 24 months. The mRNA levels for the OX_2 receptor were lower between 3 and 24 months (Terao et al., 2002). In a functional assessment, orexin-A was directly infused into the CA1 subregion of the hippocampus through reverse microdialysis in young (3–5 months) and old (26–30 months) male F344 x BN rats. This study reported a dose-dependent increase in release of GABA and glutamate in response to orexin-A infusion. For GABA, there was more release to high doses of orexin-A in the aged animals compared with young, but no change across age was observed for glutamate release (Stanley and Fadel, 2011).

For the gastrin neuropeptide family, Wang et al. (1993) examined CCK levels within whole hippocampus homogenates with radioimmunohistochemical assays. In this study there was a time of day interaction with age such that in the dark phase of the diurnal cycle, CCK levels were reduced in 12- compared with 3-month-old, and in 22- compared with 12-month-old male Sprague Dawley rats (Wang et al., 1993). CCK-8 immunoreactivity was also examined in male Sprague Dawley rats at 3–4 months and 22–25 months. Immunoreactive fibers were counted in the hippocampus and observed to be lower in the older rats in the dentate gyrus, CA3, CA2, CA1, and subiculum. CCK in the dentate gyrus and subiculum was not related to spatial memory performance in these animals; however, there was a significant relationship between spatial behavior and CCK binding in CA3, CA2, and CA1 of the old animals (Croll et al., 1999). When CCK-8 receptor binding was examined across age in male Sprague Dawley rats at 2, 9, and 18 months, using the radioligand propionyl-(3H)CCK-8-sulphated, there was a significantly lower number of binding sites in 18-month-old compared with 2- or 9-month-old rats (Harro and Oreland, 1992).

An early study of hippocampus oxytocin levels reported a lower concentration with age, as measured by radioimmunohistochemical assay, in male Wistar Kyoto rats between 6 and 12 months. An additional decrease was observed between 12 and 18 months, with no further change at 24 months (Melis et al., 1992). In a later study, radiolabeled oxytocin was injected directly into the hippocampus to measure the rate of proteolysis. While the rate of oxytocin breakdown was similar in male Wistar Kyoto rats examined at 2, 6, 12, and 18 months, catabolism was 50% lower in 24-month-old rats compared with the younger groups (Stancampiano et al., 1994).

Similar to oxytocin, relatively little research has been conducted on hippocampus vasopressin levels over the lifespan. An early study using an antiserum assay in whole hippocampus homogenates reported that vasopressin immunoreactivity did not change when examined at 8–12 and 28–32 months in male C57BL/6J mice (Rogers et al., 1985). In contrast, the density of vasopressin immunolabeled fibers in the ventral hippocampus was lower in male BN rats at 33–35 months compared with 5 months (Fliers et al., 1985). The dorsal hippocampus was not examined in this study. These discrepant

observations could arise from the extent of the hippocampus that was examined or other methodological differences. Additional research is required to determine if hippocampal vasopressin levels are altered with age.

In conclusion, of the 11 neuropeptides families that are known to be present in the hippocampus, 10 have been examined across the lifespan. There are no data available in old animals of any species for the kallikrein-kinin family. Moreover, as the families that have been examined are not consistent across species, it is not possible at this time to make comparisons between humans, nonhuman primates, and rodents. The largest amount of data across the lifespan is available in rodents, and most of these experiments have focused on the opioid family. While there are a number of reports documenting changes (increases or decreases) in neuropeptide levels, receptors, and function with age in the hippocampus, there are just as many experiments that report stability across the lifespan. We will only get the full picture after more extensive work is done in this area.

15.6.6 Summary

How advanced age impacts neuromodulatory systems within the hippocampus is still an incomplete picture. Although cholinergic, serotonergic, noradrenergic, dopaminergic, and neuropeptide systems have all been examined across the lifespan, there is still no broad cross-species consensus regarding how these systems change later in life and how this is related to hippocampus-dependent behaviors. In fact, it is somewhat surprising, given the wealth of behavioral assays available (section 15.2), that so few studies involving hippocampus neuromodulators across the lifespan have examined the effects of age-related changes in relation to cognitive outcomes. Moreover, even within a species, there are still discrepancies between different studies as to exactly how receptor levels and neuromodulator metabolism are altered in aging. This may reflect the difficulty in using static measurements, such as binding assays, to interrogate dynamic systems that can rapidly fluctuate in response to circadian cycles, behavioral experience, and numerous other factors that may have not yet been identified.

15.7 Plasticity

Age-related impairments observed in hippocampus-dependent behaviors described in section 15.2 might find a mechanistic explanation in altered neural plasticity characteristics (for review, Rosenzweig and Barnes, 2003; Burke and Barnes, 2006). Numbers of hippocampus cells do not significantly decline with normative aging (section 15.3), and most biophysical properties of neurons are indistinguishable between old and young cells (section 15.4). Aging does, however, result in changes in numbers and functions of synapses (section 15.5), and neuromodulatory systems (section 15.6). These two latter factors alter the ability of the hippocampus network to respond and adapt to changes in sensory input. For example, a reduction in synapse number will interfere with the convergence requirements that are necessary to induce and maintain plasticity, while alterations in effective neuromodulation can change the synaptic modification window. Due to the difficulty of experimental examination of synaptic plasticity in humans and the limited data collected in nonhuman primates, this section will focus on data regarding synaptic plasticity that have been collected from rodents. Figure 15.13 summarizes the known age-related changes

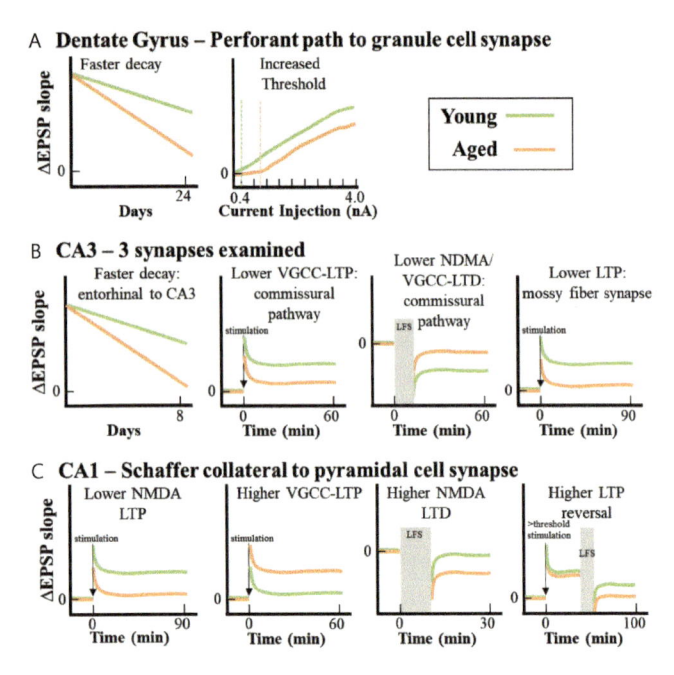

Figure 15.13 Summary of age-related changes in rat hippocampus plasticity. (A) Summary of age-related changes in LTP at the perforant path to dentate gyrus granule cell synapse. (Left) When young and aged rats have similar levels of LTP induced with suprathreshold stimulation parameters, LTP decay is faster in aged compared with young animals. (Right) When an intracellular depolarizing current is paired with perforant path fiber stimulation, aged granule cells have an increased threshold for LTP induction and show less of a potentiation for a given depolarizing current. Current thresholds are indicated for young (green) and aged (orange) rats with vertical dashed lines. (B) In CA3 age-related differences in plasticity have been documented at three synapses. (From left) At the perforant path to CA3 synapse, when suprathreshold stimulation parameters are used, LTP decays faster in aged compared with young rats. At the CA3 commissural pathway VGCC-dependent LTP is reduced in aged compared with young rats. At this same synapse, both NMDA- and metabotropic-dependent LTD is reduced in aged compared with young rats. Finally, at the mossy fiber to CA3 pyramidal cell synapse, aged rats have lower levels of LTP induction relative to young animals. (C) (From left) At the Schaffer collateral to CA1 synapse, when perithreshold stimulation parameters are used, aged rats show lower levels of NMDA receptor-dependent LTP induction, but higher levels of VGCC-dependent LTP. Aged rats also show higher levels of LTD, and greater LTP reversal than do younger animals.

in hippocampus plasticity across the dentate gyrus (Figure 15.13A), CA3 (Figure 15.13B), and CA1 (Figure 15.13C) that will be elaborated in this section.

15.7.1 Dentate gyrus

The notion that new learning results in a plastic modification of connections made between neurons enabling subsequent memory, has a long history. The term "plasticity" was first introduced by the Italian scientist Ernesto Lugaro in 1904 and was then translated into English in 1909 (Lugaro, 1909). Lugaro was heavily influenced by his teacher Eugenio Tanzi, who postulated that neuron interactions were facilitated by practice and experience, which promoted changes between functionally associated neurons. These ideas were clearly foundational to Donald Hebb's formalism of cell assembly formation (Hebb, 1949). It was not until 1966, however, that Terje Lømo, working in Per Andersen's laboratory in Oslo, observed a lasting enhancement of synaptic responses recorded

from the dentate gyrus granule cell region of rabbits that was durable enough to underlie the biological basis of memory. These data were presented at a Scandinavian Congress of Physiology meeting in 1966 (Lomo, 1966) (Chapters 2 and 10). When Lømo applied high-frequency stimulation to entorhinal cortical cell axons in the perforant pathway, he induced a short-term frequency potentiation in granule cells. Upon repeating this high-frequency stimulation, he noticed that synaptic responses become larger and lasted for hours. In his notes from that time, Lømo wrote, "if it is correct that the hippocampus is involved in memory function, this is a region where one should expect long lasting changes in synaptic efficiency to occur . . . and may have relevance to theories of learning" (p. 3) (Lømo, 2018). These findings were extended in collaboration with Tim Bliss and Tony Gardner-Medwin and published in 1973 (Bliss and Gardner-Medwin, 1973; Bliss and Lomo, 1973). In 1973, long-lasting potentiation was defined as synaptic modification lasting 30 min or more, as distinguished from shorter lasting frequency potentiation (Bliss and Gardner-Medwin, 1973; Bliss and Lomo, 1973). The terminology used today for this phenomenon of modified synaptic strength following patterned electrical or modulatory stimulation is "long-term potentiation" (LTP) (Douglas and Goddard, 1975).

Hebb (1949) suggested that durable changes in synaptic strength should function through a "cooperative mechanism," requiring the convergence of presynaptic input onto the postsynaptic cell. The first evidence that LTP was a cooperative process was provided by McNaughton, Douglas, and Graham Goddard (1978). Collingridge et al. (1983) later discovered the mechanism through which this co-operative phenomenon operated—namely the NDMA glutamate receptor. This receptor requires initial postsynaptic membrane depolarization through glutamatergic AMPA receptors. The depolarization releases the magnesium block from the NMDA receptor pore so that with glutamate ligand binding calcium entry is enabled.

The first study to investigate plasticity in the aged brain of rodents was conducted by Barnes in the mid-1970s. Young (13 months) and aged (32 months) male Long Evans rats were chronically implanted with recording electrodes in the hilus of the dentate gyrus and with stimulating electrodes in the medial perforant pathway. This enabled field excitatory postsynaptic potential (fEPSP) recordings in the awake state at precisely matched times of day through the animal's light/dark cycle in relation to behavioral status. The Barnes maze was developed (section 15.2.1) to examine the spatial memory capacity of each individual animal before conducting chronic electrophysiological recordings. Following high-frequency stimulation repeated on 3 consecutive days, the older animals showed faster decay of LTP over 14 days. This decay in synaptic response amplitude was significantly correlated with the accuracy of spatial memory in individual animals. The correlation held true in both young and old age groups. For example, the old animals with the best spatial memory had the most durable LTP in that age group, and the young animals with the least durable LTP had the worst memory in that age group (Barnes, 1979). In a follow-up study, LTP-inducing stimuli were delivered daily to young and old animals for 12 days, by the end of which young and aged rats showed comparable LTP magnitude. The young animals, however, reached asymptotic levels of synaptic modification in fewer days than did the older rats (~5 days for young versus ~10 days for aged) (Barnes and McNaughton, 1980a). The decay of the enhanced fEPSP amplitude was then followed for an additional 21 days. Even with matched LTP induction levels, the enhanced fEPSP amplitude of older animals decayed faster than that of the young rats (Barnes and McNaughton, 1985). This observation of preserved induction of LTP with faster decay in old animals, was replicated in another study with chronically implanted 4- and 27-month-old male F344 rats (deToledo-Morrell et al., 1988) using similar stimulation parameters as in Barnes (1979). Later reports, using the in vitro hippocampal slice preparation, confirmed the observation that when robust LTP-inducing stimulation parameters are used, the magnitude of granule cell synaptic strengthening could be comparable between age groups. These studies used young (6 months) and old (20 months) Sprague Dawley rats (sex not specified) (Diana, Domenici, et al., 1994; Diana, Scotti de Carolis, et al., 1994), which suggests consistency across rat strains.

When perithreshold LTP stimulation parameters are used to induce synaptic modification in young and aged rats under anesthesia, age-related differences in LTP induction have been observed in the dentate gyrus. For example, 3 trains of 250 Hz stimulation for a duration of 200 ms induced stronger LTP in 4- compared with 22-month-old female PVG hooded rats (Lynch and Voss, 1994), and in 4- compared with 20-month-old male Wistar rats (Mullany and Lynch, 1997). LTP induction equivalence was found in two other studies from this group, however, using the same preparation, strain, and stimulation parameters (Murray and Lynch, 1998; Dhanrajan et al., 2004), but old animals had faster decay over 40 min (Murray and Lynch, 1998). Chemical induction of LTP has also been examined with respect to aging, and BDNF-induced LTP resulted in increased granule cell synaptic responses in both young (2–4 months) and aged (20–24 months) male Wistar rats, but the magnitude was significantly lower in the older animals (Gooney et al., 2004).

The bulk of available evidence points to the conclusion that LTP induction in the dentate gyrus is impaired in advanced age. In addition to changes in neuromodulation discussed in section 15.6, another explanation for this is an increased depolarization threshold to achieve synaptic modification. This hypothesis was tested with an in vitro hippocampal slice preparation by Barnes et al. (2000a) in male F344 rats at 1, 9, and 26 months of age who were behaviorally characterized on the Morris watermaze. The spatial memory performance of the 26-month-old group was significantly worse than that of the two younger groups. The LTP threshold was tested by fixing the amplitude of the perforant path stimulation at 25 μA and ramping up an intracellular current injection pulse between 0 to 4 nA. This allowed determination of the point at which the paired depolarization and orthodromic stimulation produced elevated synaptic response amplitudes. The young and adult rats showed significantly lower LTP induction thresholds (0.6 and 0.8 nA, respectively), while the older animals did not exhibit LTP until the 1 nA pairing (Barnes, Rao, and Houston, 2000). These authors concluded that a change in LTP induction threshold in granule cells contributes to the greater difficulty to induce LTP in older animals using perithreshold stimulation parameters.

Several experiments have been conducted aimed at rescuing age-related LTP induction deficits. In adult animals, it is known that the hippocampal local field potential can modulate the probability of LTP induction. The hippocampal theta rhythm is a high-amplitude 4–12 Hz oscillation that is powerfully generated during movement in rats and other animals (Vanderwolf, 1969; Buzsaki et al., 1983). When LTP-inducing stimuli are introduced at the peak of the theta rhythm in young animals, there is greater synaptic modification compared with when stimuli are delivered at the trough of

this oscillation (Pavlides et al., 1988). One experiment examined whether delivering perithreshold stimulation parameters at the peak of theta in aged rats would overcome the deficits typically observed in LTP induction. Behaviorally characterized young (10 months) and aged (28 months) male F344 rats were given 2–4 bursts of 400 Hz stimulation at either the peak or the trough of the theta rhythm. The fEPSPs were then recorded across 72 h. Consistent with other studies, the magnitude of LTP was greater when induced at the peak of theta than at the trough, however, the older animals still showed reduced LTP induction levels compared with young rats (Orr et al., 2001). Another study using young (6 months) and old (23 months) male F344 rats examined whether perithreshold theta burst stimulation (parameters not specified) could produce more synaptic modification by exposing the older animals to a novel environment during LTP induction. When stimuli were delivered in the home cage, the theta burst parameters induced LTP in the young rats, but there was no synaptic modification apparent in the older animals (Sierra-Mercado et al., 2008). When older rats were given the same theta burst stimulation in a novel environment, LTP induction was comparable in amplitude to the LTP induced in young rats in the home cage condition, however, the synaptic modification decayed faster in the aged rats (Sierra-Mercado et al., 2008). Because no young rats were stimulated in the novel environment, it is not possible to conclude that the LTP induction deficit was completely overcome.

Another form of plasticity observed in the dentate gyrus that could impact cognitive aging is adult neurogenesis (e.g., Ming and Song, 2005; Li et al., 2009) (Chapter 9). One study has examined neurogenesis in humans using doublecortin as a marker of cell proliferation in postmortem brains ranging in age from 18 to 88. This study reported a significantly lower number of doublecortin positive cells in older compared with younger individuals (Mathews et al., 2017). Consistent with this, when neurogenesis in the subgranular zone of the dentate gyrus has been measured in young, middle-aged, and old rodents, a strikingly consistent pattern of results has been observed with a dramatic drop in proliferation between young and middle-aged animals and no further decline in old age. For example, this sharp decline from young to middle age is observed in female F344 rats (6, 12, and 27 months) (Kuhn et al., 1996), in male F344 x BNs (5, 18, and 28 months) (Lichtenwalner et al., 2001), in male Wistar rats (2 weeks, 6 weeks, 12 months, and 24 months) (Heine et al., 2004), male F344 rats (4, 12, and 24 months) (M Rao et al., 2005), and in male C57BL/6 mice (6 weeks, 9, 12, and 24 months) (Kronenberg et al., 2006). Remarkably, this pattern of altered proliferative capacity is also observed in hippocampal cell cultures generated from 2-, 9-, 15-, and 24-month-old rats, where a decline begins in middle-aged around 15 months with no further change in proliferation in older animals (Ray et al., 2018). Both in culture (Ray et al., 2018) and in vivo (Lichtenwalner et al., 2001; Heine et al., 2004; Rao et al., 2005), there is also a steep drop off in survival of the newborn granule cells in middle age that mirrors the proliferative change across the lifespan. Thus, it appears that age-related changes in neurogenesis proliferation and survival are a developmental effect of middle rather than old age. Because many cognitive deficits do not arise until older ages, it raises the question as to whether neurogenesis declines are responsible for memory impairments in old age. In fact, when neurogenesis has been directly related to cognitive status in aged rats, the old rats with the lowest neurogenesis rates in the dentate gyrus actually had better spatial memory as assessed by the Morris watermaze, compared with the old rats with the greatest number of new neurons (Bizon and Gallagher, 2003, 2005; Bizon et al., 2004). These data indicate that more neurogenesis does not result in better spatial cognition in old rats. One theoretical viewpoint consistent with this observation is that the functional significance of neurogenesis may not be for remembering, but for forgetting (Frankland et al., 2013; Ishikawa et al., 2016; Gao et al., 2018; Tran et al., 2019).

In summary, within the dentate gyrus, electrical or chemical induction of LTP declines in old age. Moreover, even when suprathreshold stimulation parameters are used to induce equivalent levels of LTP between age groups, the magnitude of synaptic change decays back to baseline levels more rapidly in the older animals. Furthermore, the decay rate is correlated with behavioral status, both at young and older ages. Thus, it appears that much of the machinery required to modify circuits in response to experience is reasonably preserved throughout the lifespan, but its optimal functionality may be compromised. Importantly, the alterations that occur in perithreshold LTP induction and LTP maintenance do appear to impact behavior, while adult neurogenesis does not.

15.7.2 CA3

Plasticity mechanisms over the lifespan have been examined at three different synapses in CA3 (entorhinal, commissural, and mossy fiber; Figure 15.13B). Plasticity changes with age have been noted in both the NMDA receptor-dependent form of LTP and in a voltage-gated calcium channel (VGCC)-dependent form of LTP (Grover and Teyler, 1990). Additionally, an NMDA receptor-dependent weakening of synaptic strength, called long-term depression (LTD) (Barrionuevo et al., 1980; Dudek and Bear, 1992) has also been observed to change in old age.

The medial entorhinal cortical projection to CA3 was examined in 7- and 23-month-old male F344 rats surgically implanted with recoding electrodes in CA3 and stimulating electrodes in the perforant pathway. Recordings were obtained while animals were awake and free to behave. Following suprathreshold LTP-inducing stimulation, the amplitude of LTP induction was comparable across a 2-hour period between age groups but declined faster over 8 days in the aged animals relative to young (Dieguez and Barea-Rodriguez, 2004). These data are reminiscent of the faster decay rates observed in the medial entorhinal cortical projection to dentate gyrus granule cells in aged rats (Barnes, 1979; Barnes and McNaughton, 1985).

For the commissural association projection to CA3, LTP induction has been measured in hippocampal slices from behaviorally characterized male Long Evans rats at 6 and 24 months. Following theta burst stimulation (10 trains of four pulses at 100 Hz; pulse interval of 200 ms delivered at 0.1 Hz) there was no difference in NMDA receptor-dependent LTP induction between young, aged behaviorally impaired, and aged behaviorally unimpaired rats (Yang et al., 2013). Under NMDA receptor blockade, VGCC-dependent LTP has been induced at CA3 commissural association synapses in slices from behaviorally characterized 6- and 24-month-old male Long Evans rats, using four 200 Hz stimulation epochs delivered at 0.2 Hz. Under these conditions, induction deficits were found in old rats with behavioral impairments on the Morris watermaze. Old behaviorally unimpaired rats, however, had levels of VGCC-dependent LTP induction that were comparable to the young animals (Yang et al., 2013).

At the CA3 commissural association pathway, NMDA receptor-dependent LTD has also been examined. It is hypothesized that in order to prevent network saturation, it is critical to have a mechanism that would reduce synapse strength to maintain a useful dynamic range for synaptic modification. The concept of homeostatic synaptic scaling was formalized in 1982 by Beinenstock, Cooper, and Munroe (Bienenstock et al., 1982; for review, see Cooper and Bear, 2012). Their model proposed that different patterns of input would dynamically regulate the total synaptic strength within a neuron and across circuits. The phenomena of LTP and LTD (Barrineuvo et al., 1980) could provide the mechanism for this homeostatic balance. Certain forms of LTD are NMDA glutamate receptor-dependent (Mulkey and Malenka, 1992), while others are metabotropic glutamate receptor-dependent (Palmer et al., 1997). For NMDA-receptor dependent LTD in the CA3 commissural association pathway, 24-month-old male Long Evans rats show lower LTD than did 6-month-old animals, but this occurred in both impaired and unimpaired aged rats (Yang et al., 2013). On the other hand, for metabotropic receptor-dependent LTD, there was a lower magnitude of LTD at older ages, but this only occurred in the aged behaviorally impaired group. The aged unimpaired animals had induction levels that were similar to young rats (Yang et al., 2013).

At the granule cell axon (mossy fibers) projection to CA3, LTP is opioid-receptor dependent rather than glutamatergic (e.g., Martin, 1983; Derrick et al., 1991). Plasticity at this synapse has been examined in 1.5- and 33-month-old Wistar rats (sex not specified). In hippocampal slices high-frequency electrical stimulation (100 pulses at 100 Hz, repeated 3 times at 10-second intervals) induced LTP at the CA3 mossy fiber synapse in both age groups. The magnitude of LTP, however, was lower at 30 min post induction in the old compared with the young rats (Villanueva-Castillo et al., 2017). When forskolin, an adenylyl cyclase cAMP-dependent activator of protein kinase A (PKA), was applied to slices to elicit LTP, no LTP was observed at 30 min in old rats, while this LTP was sustained for 2 hours in young rats (Villanueva-Castillo et al., 2017). This observation suggests that the adenylyl cyclase cAMP/PKA signaling cascade is disrupted in the mossy fiber to CA3 synapse of aged rats. Another potential mechanism for the age-related differences in plasticity at this synapse is the reduced binding to the mu-opioid receptor and increased binding to the kappa receptor in old compared with young rats (Nagahara et al., 1996). Because the mu receptor facilitates LTP (Bramham et al., 1991) and the kappa receptor reduces LTP (Wagner et al., 1993), this combination of receptor change could result in defective plasticity at the mossy fiber to CA3 synapse.

In summary, in CA3 multiple synaptic zones have been examined in young and old animals. While differences in LTP and LTD have been observed at some synaptic inputs in CA3, these studies should be replicated and extended before strong conclusions can be drawn.

15.7.3 CA1

Of all hippocampus areas, age-related changes in plasticity have been most extensively characterized in the CA1 subregion. Within CA1, NMDA receptor-dependent LTP, VGCC-dependent LTP, and LTD have been examined across the lifespan. These studies have exclusively interrogated the CA3 to CA1 Schaffer collateral synapse, which projects to both the stratum oriens and stratum radiatum. That being said, given the fibers of passage in this region, it is difficult to definitively isolate stimulation of only CA3 axon input to CA1. It is also worth noting that most research regarding age-related differences in CA1 plasticity have been conducted in the in vitro hippocampal slice preparation. In fact, to date no LTP data from CA1 have been obtained from chronically implanted, awake, behaving aged animals.

Early studies examining the effect of high-frequency stimulation in young and aged rats in CA1 failed to report measures of the fEPSP (synaptic strength), and only reported amplitudes of the population spike that reflect summed compound action potentials. While this measure can be related to changes in synaptic strength, it can also be influenced by changes in excitability independent of synaptic strength. This complicates the ability to precisely interpret these experimental observations. Landfield and Lynch (1977) recorded from hippocampal slices prepared from young (5 months) and aged (26 months) male F344 rats. Two different parameters of high-frequency stimulation were delivered: one at 15 Hz for 10 s, and another at 50 Hz for 5 s. There was a clear decrease in the proportion of slices that exhibited frequency potentiation, as well as a depression in the magnitude of the population spike following 15 Hz stimulation in old compared with young rats (Landfield and Lynch, 1977). While 50 Hz stimulation can result in long-lasting potentiation of both the fEPSP and the population spike, as originally shown by Bliss and Lømo (1973), Landfield and Lynch (1977) only examined the durability of this potentiation for 10 minutes. Within this time window, however, the magnitude was lower in old compared with young animals. Consistent with this report, a later study found that the magnitude of frequency potentiation of the population spike following 4 pulses of a 100 Hz stimulation was lower in aged (25 months) compared with young (3 months) male F344 rats at 10 minutes (Deupree et al., 1991). In another in vitro experiment in which 2- and 24-month-old male F344 rats were compared using 100–200 Hz stimulation for 1 s, old animals showed little change in the population spike amplitude, whereas the young animals had a significant increase that was maintained out to 25 min (Hori et al., 1992). In the only in vivo study conducted in aging animals in CA1, urethane-anesthetized male F344 rats (5 and 26 months) were given 100 Hz stimulation for 5 s. Under these experimental conditions, at the 30 min time point, both the young and aged rats had an increased population spike amplitude that did not differ between age groups (Landfield et al., 1978). When suprathreshold stimulation parameters were used (50 pulses at a 100 Hz), Deupree et al. (1991) reported that population spike amplitude increases in CA1 were initially comparable between age groups, but the amplitude decayed more rapidly at 60 min in old compared with young animals.

Later studies included measurements of the fEPSP amplitude in addition to the population spike amplitudes following a variety of stimulation parameters to induce LTP, ranging from weak (perithreshold) to very powerful (suprathreshold). Landfield et al. (1986) prepared hippocampal slices from young (5–8 months), and aged (27–29 months) male F344 rats and applied 7 Hz stimulation of Schaffer collateral inputs to CA1 for up to 45 sec. With this perithreshold stimulation procedure, slices prepared from young rats showed significant fEPSP LTP out to 30 min, whereas the amplitude of fEPSP for old rats was not significantly elevated at that time point. Interestingly, when Ca^{2+} was blocked by increasing levels of Mg^{2+}, the old rats did show significant LTP at 30 min (Landfield et al., 1986). This finding was consistent with the notion that Ca^{2+} dysregulation occurring during aging (section 15.4.3) may affect synaptic plasticity. In fact, a later study showed that the application of an L-type voltage-gated Ca^{2+} channel blocker affected LTP induction differently in old compared with young rats. Using parameters that do not reliably induce a durable LTP in slices from either young or aged male F344 rats (900 pulses at 5 Hz), this channel blocker resulted in an LTP-like increase in the fEPSP in aged (23 months) rats, but did not affect the young (5 months) rats (Norris et al., 1998). Furthermore, inhibition of Ca^{2+}-induced intracellular Ca^{2+} release through several pharmacological mechanisms has been observed to produce a similar effect in slices from old animals. For example, using three methods to reduce intracellular Ca^{2+}, Kumar and Foster (2004) showed that 5 Hz stimulation, which at baseline leads to little synaptic change, produced LTP in old (23 months) but not young (6 months) male F344 rats. The finding that manipulations of intracellular Ca^{2+} levels led to dissociable effects in slices from young and aged rats has been replicated using different LTP inducing stimuli. In hippocampal slices prepared from young (3 months) and old (25 months) rats, Tonkikh et al. (2006) delivered 100 Hz stimulation for 200 ms, repeated 5 times to CA1 afferent inputs. The younger rats showed greater fEPSP LTP than did the aged animals out to 60 min. Interestingly, when a Ca^{2+} chelator was applied to the slices, LTP was decreased in young rats, but augmented in the old animals (Tonkikh et al., 2006).

In addition to Ca^{2+}, another critical variable for unmasking potential age-related deficits in LTP induction is the stimulus parameters used to induce plasticity at the Schaffer collateral to CA1 synapse. A direct test of robust 1 s stimulation at 200 Hz versus weaker prime burst stimulation (1 pulse preceding 4 pulses at 200 Hz) was examined in slices prepared from aged (25 months) and young (4 months) male F344 rats. The fEPSP was increased at 20 min in both age groups following the robust stimulation parameters (Moore et al., 1993). In contrast, for the perithreshold stimulation parameter, a lower proportion of slices from old than young rats showed a significant increase in the fEPSP amplitude (Moore et al., 1993). Using the same prime burst stimulation parameter as in Moore et al. (1993), another study reported that slices from older F344 rats (24 months) showed less LTP induction than did those from young (9 months) animals (Rosenzweig et al., 1997). When a more robust stimulation parameter was used in this study (4 pulses at 100 Hz), the fEPSP amplitude did not differ between age groups at 40 min (Rosenzweig et al., 1997). Another study using perithreshold stimulus parameters (0.5 s of 30 Hz delivered 3 times) to induce LTP in slices, showed that aged (25 months) male F344 rats had impairments compared with young (5 months) animals when measured out to 180 minutes (Tombaugh et al., 2002). When more robust stimulation parameters were given (0.5 s at 70 Hz, repeated 3 times) old and young groups showed equivalent fEPSP LTP. In the same study, an intermediate stimulation parameter (30 s at 5 Hz) revealed a different pattern of results. Slices from the young and old behaviorally unimpaired rats had equivalent LTP of the fEPSP out to 40 minutes, while the old behaviorally impaired rats showed lower LTP (Tombaugh et al., 2002). Additionally, when LTP-inducing stimulation (5 trains of 4 pulses delivered at 100 Hz) was applied to CA1 Schaffer collateral fibers in slices from young (5 months) and old (26 months) male Wistar rats, the old rats showed no LTP. In contrast, the young animals exhibited LTP out to 60 min, the longest time point examined (Haxaire et al., 2012). Consistent with the observation that suprathreshold LTP induction parameters lead to similar levels of synaptic modification in young and old animals, the maximum capacity for synaptic change appears to be similar between age groups. When slices from young (6 months) and old (23 months) male BN rats were repeatedly stimulated with 4 pulses delivered at 100 Hz to achieve ceiling levels of LTP, no differences in fEPSP amplitudes were observed between age groups (Kumar et al., 2007).

In a study using behaviorally characterized male C57BL/6 mice at 3, 6, 12, and 18 months of age, when robust stimulation parameters were used, there was also no difference in the amplitude of the fEPSP following LTP between age groups. The 18-month-old mice, however, showed significantly faster decay of LTP across 1 to 3 hours. Furthermore, the magnitude of LTP at 3 hours in the 18-month-old animals was significantly correlated with spatial performance on the Barnes maze (Bach et al., 1999). Other experiments in mice have also shown intact LTP induction with age following robust stimulation. When theta-burst stimulation (1 pulse followed 200 ms later by 4 pulses at 100 Hz, repeated 5 times) was delivered to CA1, the amplitude of the fEPSP at 60 min was not different between 4- and 28-month-old mice (sex and strain not specified) (Larson et al., 1999). This lack of an age difference has also been observed in male C57BL/6 mice (3 and 24 months) following 1 s of 100 Hz stimulation, delivered twice (Watson et al., 2002). In another study, LTP was induced in slices from C57BL/6 mice (sex not specified) using robust parameters (150 pulses at 5 Hz) that induced LTP in both young (1.5 months) and old (26 months) animals that did not differ in magnitude (Watabe and O'Dell, 2003).

In contrast to the work described above, two studies have reported LTP deficits in aged rats using suprathreshold stimulation parameters. When slices were prepared from male Sprague Dawley rats at 4 and 25 months of age and trains of 4 pulses at 100 Hz repeated 5 times were delivered, the aged animals showed significantly lower fEPSP LTP compared with the young rats out to 60 min. This age difference was reversed by application of the D-cyloserine, an agonist of the glycine binding site on the NMDA receptor (Billard and Rouaud, 2007). In another study using slices from 1.5- versus 21-month-old male Wistar rats, 100 pulse trains were delivered 3 times at 100 Hz. With these parameters, LTP magnitude was lower in the aged compared with young animals (M Shetty et al., 2017). It is tempting to conclude, in spite of these two discrepant studies, that suprathreshold LTP induction is intact in older mice and rats.

One intracellular recording study has been conducted from CA1 pyramidal cells in three age groups of male F344 rats (1, 9, and 26 months). In this experiment, LTP was induced by pairing intracellular depolarization with 0.2 Hz orthodromic stimulation (repeated 10 times). Equivalent levels of synaptic enhancement were induced across age groups out to 45 min (Barnes, Rao, et al., 1996). This study also determined the intracellular threshold current necessary to elicit LTP induction across these three age groups. In contrast to what was observed for the dentate gyrus in which the depolarization threshold necessary to elicit LTP was elevated in aged animals (Barnes, Rao, and Houston, 2000), there was no threshold difference across age groups in CA1 (Barnes, Rao, et al., 1996). Because thresholds are the same, some other mechanisms must be responsible for age-related deficits in LTP induction observed with perithreshold stimulation parameters. At least one mechanism that could contribute to these deficits in older animals was identified by Rosenzweig et al. (1997). Specifically, patterned orthodromic stimulation resulted in greater summation of postsynaptic depolarization in CA1 pyramidal cells in young (9 months) compared with old (24 months) male F344 rats (Rosenzweig et al., 1997).

Suprathreshold stimulation parameters can overcome this age-related temporal summation deficit because of the greater overall depolarization produced under these conditions. The weaker stimulation parameters may not be able to reach the depolarization levels necessary to trigger LTP induction cascades in the old animals.

Another way to conceptualize the differences in LTP that arise during aging for perithreshold versus suprathreshold stimulation parameters is to consider the known contributions of NMDA receptor-dependent versus independent forms of LTP. With suprathreshold stimulation parameters, there are at least two ways that LTP can be induced. One is through the NMDA receptor and the other is through voltage-gated Ca^{2+} channels (VGCC), both of which result in increased intracellular Ca^{2+} levels that trigger cascades resulting in synaptic change. When VGCCs are blocked, it is possible to observe NMDA receptor-dependent LTP alone. Conversely, when NMDA receptors are blocked, VGCC-dependent LTP can be isolated. Importantly, perithreshold stimulation parameters do not engage the VGCC-mediated mechanism of LTP (Grover and Teyler, 1990).

The respective contributions to LTP during aging by NMDA versus VGCC mechanisms has been examined in a number of studies. In hippocampal slices prepared from 2- and 24-month-old male F344 rats, LTP was induced in control conditions using stimulation of 0.5 s trains of 200 Hz repeated 4 times. As in previous studies, these suprathreshold parameters produced the same levels of LTP in young and aged rats (Shankar et al., 1998). To examine the role of NMDA-dependent LTP, slices were bathed in nifedipine to block VGCC-mediated plasticity. In other slices, the NMDA receptor antagonist APV was added to the bath to eliminate NMDA-mediated plasticity. The young rats showed proportionally more contribution from the NMDA-dependent than the VGCC-dependent form of LTP, while the old animals showed the opposite relationship (Shankar et al., 1998). Consistent with this observation, when hippocampal slices were prepared from young (4 months) and aged (22 months) F344 rats (sex not specified) and stimulated with four 1 s trains of 100 Hz in the presence of nifedipine, the older rats showed lower fEPSP amplitude following LTP out to 60 min compared with the young animals (Coultrap et al., 2008). This study further demonstrates the greater contribution of the VGCC form of LTP, compared with NMDA form of LTP, for the older animals.

The enhanced VGCC LTP with aging could either reflect Ca^{2+} dysregulation or possible adaptation in the face of reduced function of NMDA-dependent LTP. One study has addressed these two possibilities directly in slices obtained from young (6 months) and old (24 months) male Long Evans rats that had been behaviorally characterized on the Morris watermaze. When LTP was induced with 10 trains of 4 pulses delivered at 100 Hz, fEPSP LTP was lower in both behaviorally impaired and unimpaired old animals compared with young (Boric et al., 2008). When NMDA-dependent LTP was blocked with APV to reveal VGCC-mediated LTP (using 0.5 s 200 Hz bursts of stimulation repeated four times), age-impaired old rats and young rats showed the same levels of this form of LTP. In contrast, age-unimpaired rats showed higher levels of VGCC-mediated LTP. The authors interpret these data to indicate that rats maintaining better spatial memory may achieve this through a process that increases VGCC-mediated LTP (Boric et al., 2008). Higher VGCC LTP in old animals has also been reported in mice. When LTP was induced in slices from C57BL/6 mice (sex not specified) using robust parameters (150 pulses at 5 Hz) in the presence of a

VGCC blocker to isolate NMDA receptor-dependent LTP, slices from young mice (1.5 months) showed little change. In contrast, for the old (26 months) animals, the VGCC blocker significantly reduced the fEPSP LTP, consistent with previous findings that there is a greater contribution from the VGCC-mediated mechanism in the older animals (Watabe and O'Dell, 2003).

As discussed above, to prevent network saturation there must be balancing mechanisms to reduce synaptic strength as well as to enhance it. Homosynaptic depression has been observed at the CA3 to CA1 Schaffer collateral synapse (Barrionuevo et al., 1980; Dudek and Bear, 1992). When stimulus parameters that reduce synaptic strength are applied to naive synapses, this is referred to as long-term depression (LTD). When these parameters are applied to previously potentiated synapses, this phenomenon is referred to as depotentiation (Barrionuevo et al., 1980). Both these types of synaptic modification have been examined across age.

The first study to demonstrate homosynaptic LTD and depotentiation in CA1 of aged rats was conducted in hippocampal slices prepared from young (7 month) and old (22 month) male F344 rats using 900 pulses delivered at 1 Hz. While the old rats showed strong LTD with these parameters out to 60 min, the young rats did not (Norris et al., 1996). For depotentiation (referred to as LTP reversal in this paper), both young and old rats were given robust high-frequency stimulation to induce comparable levels of LTP. When 900 pulses at 1 Hz were applied to the potentiated synapses, there was no difference in depotentiation between age groups. When 30 pulses were delivered at 1 Hz twice to these slices, both age groups showed depotentiation, but the slices from older animals showed a complete reversal of LTP, whereas the younger animals only showed a partial reversal (Norris et al., 1996). Thus, it appears that aging CA1 synapses are more susceptible to mechanisms that weaken synaptic strength than are younger animals. Interestingly, while LTD was not induced in the younger animals with the parameter mentioned above, when Ca^{2+} levels were increased in the bath, slices from young animals did show LTD. Conversely, LTD in slices from aged rats could be attenuated by blocking Ca^{2+} with elevated Mg^{2+} levels (Norris et al., 1996). These data are consistent with the idea that Ca^{2+} dysregulation in aging contributes to alterations in synaptic plasticity. Foster and Norris (1997) extended these data to show that low-frequency stimulation delivered at 3 Hz induced LTD in both young and aged rats. On the other hand, aged but not young rats showed LTD following 1 Hz stimulation. In line with the Ca^{2+} dysregulation hypothesis, LTD in aged rats following 15 min of 1 Hz stimulation was attenuated by blocking the release of Ca^{2+} from intracellular stores (Kumar and Foster, 2005). Although LTD is different between old and young animals under physiological conditions, the magnitude of LTD can be equivalent between age groups if the ratio of Ca^{2+} to Mg^{2+} is enhanced (Kumar et al., 2007). In contrast to the consistent finding of enhanced LTD in older animals, one study reported a lower LTD magnitude in old (25–27 months) male Sprague Dawley rats compared with young (3–5 months) animals following 900 pulses of 1 Hz stimulation (Billard and Rouaud, 2007). This study did use a slightly elevated Ca^{2+} to Mg^{2+} ratio compared with previous reports, which may explain the discrepancy.

15.7.4 Summary

A striking aspect of the available data regarding plasticity alterations in the aged hippocampus is the extent to which specific synapses have distinct vulnerabilities in advanced age (Figure 15.13).

For example, at the perforant path to dentate gyrus granule cell synapse there is an increased threshold of postsynaptic depolarization required to elicit LTP. This may account for the lower probability of inducing plasticity in old animals at this synapse. In contrast, at the Schaffer collateral to CA1 synapse, there are no threshold changes for LTP induction with age. Rather, old pyramidal cells have impaired temporal summation, reducing effective depolarization of the postsynaptic cell. In CA3, NMDA receptor-dependent LTP appears to be intact with age, while VGCC-dependent LTP is impaired in old rats with spatial memory deficits. A different pattern is observed in CA1, in which VGCC-dependent LTP is enhanced and NMDA receptor-dependent LTP is reduced with age. While the impact of advanced age on some synaptic inputs to the hippocampus have been examined, we have not yet begun to interrogate how plasticity mechanisms might be changed in synaptic outputs from the hippocampus to the subiculum, entorhinal cortex, as well as other cortical areas. It is likely that these outputs are critical for a number of cognitive functions that decline with age.

15.8 Behavior-induced neuron activity dynamics

Probing how old age impacts the ensemble properties of neuron populations in the hippocampus is critical for understanding age-related changes in hippocampus-dependent behaviors (section 15.2). Data examining ensemble properties during waking behaviors have mostly been obtained from rodent models of cognitive aging. While this section will primarily describe methodologies that enable single-cell or microcircuit resolution, human and non-human primate MRI studies will also be reviewed when they can be related to findings from rodents to facilitate cross-species comparisons. Thus, this section will include studies that have used in vivo electrophysiology, immediate early gene imaging, and MRI.

15.8.1 Dentate gyrus

To date, no age comparisons of the electrophysiological ensemble characteristics of dentate gyrus granule cells have been conducted. Rather, age differences in granule cell activity dynamics have been examined by evaluating behavior-induced expression patterns of immediate genes (IEGs). IEGs are a class of genes rapidly transcribed following neuron firing induced by seizure (Morgan et al., 1987), plasticity-inducing electrical stimulation (Cole et al., 1989; Worley et al., 1993), or waking behavior (Guzowski et al., 1999; Guzowski et al., 2001). The transcription kinetics of several IEGs have been particularly useful for identifying cell-specific network patterns between two distinct behavioral experiences across the entire hippocampus (Guzowski et al., 1999; Guzowski et al., 2001; Vazdarjanova et al., 2002). For example, *Arc* mRNA is visible in the nucleus 1–2 minutes after neuronal activity and moves to the cytoplasm within 25–30 minutes. Thus, the location of *Arc* mRNA within the cell can be used to infer whether a cell was active 5 minutes or 30 minutes before brain extraction (Figure 15.14). If two identical behavior treatments are given 30 and 5 minutes before brain extraction, one would expect to see one population of cells with no *Arc* expression (those that did not participate in the network reflecting this particular behavior), and another population of cells with *Arc* mRNA in both the nucleus and cytoplasm (the cells engaged during the behavior treatment) (Guzowski et al., 1999; Guzowski et al., 2001). The transcription factor *zif*268 shows transcription kinetics similar

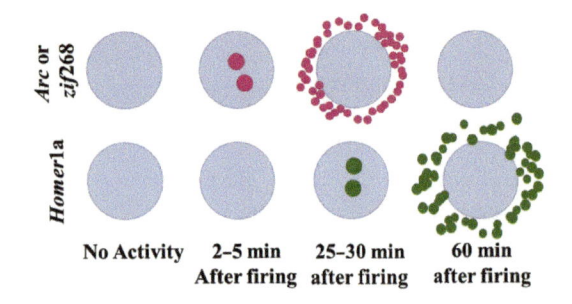

No Activity   **2–5 min After firing**   **25–30 min after firing**   **60 min after firing**

Figure 15.14 The temporal kinetics of *Arc*, *zif268*, and *Homer*1a mRNA expression. Blue circles indicate the nucleus of a neuron. (First column) When there is no activity during the 60 minutes prior to sacrifice, neither *Arc*, *zif268*, nor *Homer*1a show gene expression. (Second column) When fired action potentials associated with attentive behavior are fired 2–5 min prior to sacrifice, *Arc* and *zif268* are apparent at transcription foci in the nucleus of the neuron, but *Homer*1a is not. (Third column) When the neuron fired action potentials associated with attentive behavior 25–30 min prior to sacrifice, *Arc* and *zif268* are visible in the cytoplasm, whereas *Homer*1a appears in the nucleus. (Fourth column) Cell firing at 60 min prior to sacrifice is associated with no visible *Arc* or *zif268* in the cell body, while *Homer*1a is present at this time point in the cytoplasm.

to *Arc* (e.g., Marrone et al., 2011), while *Homer*1a does not appear in the nucleus until 30 minutes after cell activity, and in the cytoplasm at 1 hour (Vazdarjanova et al., 2002; Marrone et al., 2008). This molecular activity imaging approach was named cellular <u>c</u>ompartment <u>a</u>nalysis of <u>t</u>emporal activity by <u>f</u>luorescence <u>i</u>n <u>s</u>itu <u>h</u>ybridization (catFISH; Guzowski et al., 1999).

The first examination of behavior-driven granule cell activity using the catFISH method was conducted across three ages of male F344 rats (9, 15, and 24 months) following two 5-minute sessions of exploration of an environment separated by 20 minutes. This study reported an incremental decline in the proportion of active granule cells across age (Small et al., 2004). In the same study male and female rhesus macaques ranging in age from 7 to 31 years (21–93 human equivalent years) were imaged with high-resolution MRI methods to examine cerebral blood volume (CBV) within the dentate gyrus. CBV reflects resting metabolism and can be used as a proxy for activity. Consistent with the IEG results from the rat, the old monkeys showed lower CBV in the dentate gyrus, relative to young. Moreover, higher CBV within the dentate gyrus of the old age group was significantly correlated with better performance on a DNMS task (Small et al., 2004). Interestingly, in human participants (20 to 88 years), the older individuals showed lower CBV in this region of the hippocampus compared with younger participants (Small et al., 2002).

The general findings of lower dentate gyrus activity in older animals have been confirmed and extended in several additional studies. Using *Arc* catFISH, Penner et al. (2010b) found fewer granule cells active following behavior in old (32 months) compared with young (9 months) male F344 rats. Consistent with this, Marrone et al. (2011) found a lower proportion of dentate gyrus granule cells that transcribed *zif268* following exploration of two different environments, in old (23–27 months) compared with young (9–12 month) male F344 rats. A similar finding was reported, using the same ages and strain of male rats, following exploration of a single environment (Gheidi et al., 2013). When two sessions of environmental exploration are separated by 8 hours, dentate gyrus granule cells in young animals show sustained *Arc* transcription,

with most *Arc*-positive cells having both nuclear and cytoplasmic mRNA (Marrone et al., 2011). In this experiment the cytoplasmic *Arc* was associated with the remote experience 8 hours prior, and the nuclear *Arc* to the recent experience. In aged rats, both remote and recent *Arc* transcription is attenuated compared with the young animals (Marrone et al., 2011). Thus, activity in the aged dentate gyrus has consistently been observed to be reduced across different species and experimental procedures.

15.8.2 CA3

In this section we will discuss in vivo electrophysiological recordings, place-field properties, and imaging approaches that have been used to examine potential age effects on CA3 ensemble dynamics. As animals traverse an environment, hippocampus principal cells show receptive fields for spatial location. O'Keefe and Dostrovsky (1971) named this pattern of activity a "place field" (Chapter 11). When rodents visit the same environment twice, place fields are typically very stable and highly correlated between sessions, even when the sessions are separated by extended periods of time (Muller et al., 1987; Thompson and Best, 1990). When an animal is put into two different environments, on the other hand, place fields are uncorrelated (Muller and Kubie, 1987), which has been interpreted to reflect separate representations for different spaces (O'Keefe and Nadel, 1978).

One study has examined single-unit properties of CA3 pyramidal cells in male and female rhesus macaques. In this study in vivo recordings from CA3 and perirhinal cortex in 2 aged (30 and 32 years) and 3 middle-aged (14, 15, and 18 years) monkeys were obtained during quiet wakefulness. The firing rates of aged CA3 neurons, but not perirhinal cortical neurons, were elevated compared with middle-aged animals. This elevated firing rate was confirmed statistically when the analysis was done using all recorded neurons as the sample size as well as when animal number was used as the sample size (Thomé et al., 2016). The age-related firing rate difference was related to the expression of calcium-binding proteins in interneurons in CA3. When both parvalbumin- and somatostatin-containing GABAergic neurons were counted in the vicinity of the electrode, only somatostatin-containing interneurons were lower in the aged compared with younger animals. Moreover, lower numbers of somatostatin-containing interneurons were correlated with increased CA3 pyramidal cell firing rates in the older animals (Thomé et al., 2016). As discussed previously (section 15.3.2), it appears that the altered phenotypic expression of somatostatin in aged interneurons may have an important functional consequence for the CA3 network.

For rats, many of the initial recording experiments in young and old animals combined CA3 and CA1 data for their analyses (Tanila, Shapiro, Gallagher, et al., 1997; Tanila, Shapiro, and Eichenbaum, 1997; Tanila, Sapila, et al., 1997; Wilson et al., 2003; Wilson et al., 2004). We now understand that the firing rate properties, probability of being active, and modulation of place fields by context are distinct between CA3 and CA1 pyramidal neurons (Chapter 11; Guzowski et al., 2004; Lee, Yoganarasimha, et al., 2004; Leutgeb et al., 2004; Vazdarjanova and Guzowski, 2004). Moreover, as discussed in previous sections of this chapter, age impacts the structure and function of these subregions in dissociable ways. Because it is not possible to interpret the distinct contributions made by CA3 versus CA1 pyramidal cells in the studies cited above, they will not be considered here.

The first paper to focus on recordings from CA3 in behaving young (9–12 month) and spatial memory-impaired aged (24–27) male Long Evans rats reported that CA3 pyramidal neurons in old rats had elevated firing rates during behavior compared with young animals (Wilson et al., 2005). Furthermore, when the rats were moved between two different environments, place fields in young animals showed uncorrelated activity patterns. That is, they exhibited global remapping between the distinct environments. In contrast, the place fields of the old rats did not show remapping (Wilson et al., 2005). The information content of cell activity can be calculated (Skaggs et al., 1992) to quantify the extent that a neuron's place-field firing can predict the animal's spatial location. In CA3, the information content was significantly lower in old compared with young animals when they explored a novel, but not a familiar, environment (Wilson et al., 2005). In a more recent paper, similar findings were reported in the same strain, sex, and age of rat. That is, aged CA3 pyramidal cells had higher firing rates, lower information content, and reduced remapping of place fields between a familiar and a novel environment (Robitsek et al., 2015). This study also examined the extent to which these age effects could be reversed by the combined administration of antiepileptic medications levetiracetam and valproic acid. While this drug treatment reduced cell firing rates, and increased information content of cell spiking in aged rats, it did not restore normal place-field remapping dynamics. In fact, the overlap in place fields between two different environments was increased in both age groups, indicating that drug treatment did not reverse age impairments in remapping (Robitsek et al., 2015).

A recent mechanism that could impact excitation and network firing patterns in CA3 is the integrity of extracellular matrix proteins. Specifically, perineuronal nets that surround parvalbumin synapses onto CA3 pyramidal neurons are hypothesized to support synapse health in aging. In a recent study, aged male F344 rats (23–25 months) with greater numbers of CA3 perineuronal nets also showed better performance on the spatial version of the Morris watermaze compared with aged rats with lower numbers. In fact, the perineuronal net coverage of aged rats with intact watermaze performance was comparable to that of adult (7–13 months) and middle-aged (15–17 months) animals. One explanation for this effect is that perineuronal net integrity may aid in reducing hyperexcitability on CA3 pyramidal neurons (Gray et al., 2023).

A recent study to investigate CA3 single-unit activity in young (4–6 month), aged-unimpaired (22–26 month), and aged-impaired (22–26 month) male Long Evans rats, examined the firing rates across the CA3 transverse axis while rats performed a track running task for reward (Lee et al., 2021). The recordings were obtained from CA3c (which primarily receives input from the dentate gyrus), CA3b (an intermediate zone that receives input from the entorhinal cortex and dentate gyrus) and CA3a (that primarily receives input from the entorhinal cortex and CA3 recurrent collaterals). Relative to the young rats, the older animals, regardless of cognitive status, showed a firing rate increase in CA3c and a firing rate decrease in CA3a. When the firing rates were examined separately for those pyramidal cells that did not exhibit spatial selectivity, there was no age-related firing rate difference of this cell type in any CA3 region. While the firing rate increases in CA3c neurons were not associated with the cognitive status of the old rats, there were two differences noted between the aged-impaired and the aged-unimpaired and young rats in the CA3c region. The

first was lower information per spike, and the second was larger place-field sizes in the aged-impaired rats compared with aged unimpaired and young rats (Lee et al., 2021). A more recent follow-up study examined the remapping dynamics along the transverse axis of CA3 in young (4–6 month), aged-unimpaired (22–26 month), and aged-impaired (22–26 month) male Long Evans rats. In young and aged-unimpaired rats, when features of the environment were changed but the animal remained in the same room, there was more remapping in CA3c compared with CA3a. In contrast, aged-impaired rats showed reduced remapping in CA3c such that the remapping dynamics along the transverse axis was less distinct in the aged-impaired rats compared with the other groups. When rats were placed in different rooms, all rats showed remapping throughout the full extent of CA3 (Lee et al., 2022), which is inconsistent with earlier studies.

Because the rodent studies conducted have used cell numbers as sample size, these data should be interpreted with some causation. The reasons for this include that some animals can contribute disproportionately to the results, and it violates the assumption of independence of observations (Aarts et al., 2014). Only one of the studies conducted on CA3 ensemble dynamics in rats has attempted to address this. In Lee et al. (2021), the violation of the statistical assumption of independence was accounted for by using linear mixed effects models that control for correlations among cells from the same animal. The disproportionate contributions to the sample size from different animals, however, was not addressed.

There have only been two reports using the *Arc* catFISH method to evaluate CA3 cell activity in young and old animals. The first looked at *Arc* mRNA in the dorsal region of CA3c in male F344 rats at 9, 15, and 24 months following two 5-minute sessions of exploration of an environment separated by 20 minutes. No significant differences were observed in the proportion of *Arc*-positive CA3c cells in this region across age (Small et al., 2004). A later study examined *Arc* expression in a more ventral portion of CA3b and c, using the same catFISH approach in male F344 x BN rats (4 and 24 months). The aged rats with impairments on a rodent version of the mnemonic similarity task (section 15.2.2) had significantly more CA3 neurons that were *Arc*-positive in both the CA3b and c subregions. Old rats with behavioral performance comparable to young showed *Arc* expression patterns that were not different from the young animals (Maurer et al., 2017). It should be emphasized that *Arc* expression cannot be directly related to firing rate. The neuron has to show patterned bursting and reach a certain depolarization threshold for *Arc* induction to occur (Chawla et al., 2018). Thus, it is conceivable that aged CA3b/c pyramidal cells in more ventral regions of the hippocampus may be closer to that threshold than their younger counterparts. In Maurer et al. (2017), a retrograde tracer was injected into CA3 to identify the layer II projection neurons in lateral entorhinal cortex. Old behaviorally impaired rats showed more projection neurons with *Arc* expression than did the unimpaired and young rats.

It is difficult to isolate the BOLD signal generated from CA3 versus that from the dentate gyrus in human participants unless very high-resolution methods are employed. When the combined CA3/dentate gyrus BOLD signal has been examined in humans, however, multiple studies have reported that there is elevated activity in the CA3/dentate gyrus region, with no change detected in CA1 (Yassa, Lacy, et al., 2010; Yassa, Mattfeld, et al., 2011). If these data are interpreted in light of single-unit firing rate findings from rats (Wilson et al., 2005), and monkeys (Thomé et al., 2016), it is highly probable that the increased BOLD activity observed in older humans is generated from the CA3 region. Importantly, as discussed in section 15.2.2, this CA3 hyperactivity in human participants is related to both performance on the mnemonic similarity task (Yassa, Mattfeld, et al., 2011) and the degree of perforant pathway–fiber pruning (Yassa, Muftuler, et al., 2010). In a more recent study, activity in the CA3/dentate gyrus region was examined in young and old participants (mean age 21 and 74) in relation to anterolateral and posteriomedial entorhinal cortical activity (homologous to the rodent lateral and medial entorhinal cortex, respectively). The hyperactivity in CA3/dentate gyrus was replicated in the older individuals and reported to correlate with performance on the mnemonic similarity task (Reagh et al., 2018). Additionally, the increased activity in CA3/dentate gyrus was negatively correlated with BOLD activation in the anterolateral entorhinal cortex. In contrast, BOLD activity did not differ between age groups in CA1, or the posteriomedial entorhinal cortex (Reagh et al., 2018). Thus, there is evidence in rats and humans for an age-related vulnerability in the lateral entorhinal cortex-CA3 circuit that is related to behavioral outcomes.

To date, only one recent study has examined CA3 local field potential (LFP) activity in young and aged rats (DiCola et al., 2022). The LFP is the summation of inhibitory and excitatory synaptic activity across a population of neurons (Buzsaki et al., 2012), and different behavioral states are associated with distinct LFP frequencies. For example, it has been shown in the rat that the 4–12 Hz theta oscillation is prominent across all hippocampus subregions during locomotion and REM sleep (Vanderwolf, 1969; Vanderwolf et al., 1977). A higher-frequency (40–100 Hz) gamma rhythm is also observed during active behaviors (Bragin et al., 1995). In CA3 and CA1, spontaneous population discharges of pyramidal cells during rest and quiet wakefulness lead to even higher-frequency events (100–300 Hz) (Ylinen et al., 1995; Sullivan et al., 2011). This high-frequency event in CA3 produces an associated sharp-wave depolarization event (lasting ~40–100 ms; Vanderwolf, 1969) in the stratum radiatum and an associated high-frequency ripple in the CA1 pyramidal cell layer. Although sharp wave/ripples are most prominent during rest and quiet wakefulness (O'Keefe and Nadel, 1978; Ylinen et al., 1995), they can also be observed during pauses in behavior (O'Neill et al., 2006). Recently, high-frequency events during rest episodes before and after track running were quantified in young (4–8 months) and aged (24–26 months) male F344 x BN rats. The CA3 high-frequency events in aged rats had decreased amplitude and shorter duration compared with the young animals and were associated with a reduced current sink in the stratum radiatum, where the Schaffer collateral axons from CA3 terminate. The frequency and the rate of occurrence of these events, however, was comparable between age groups (DiCola et al., 2022). It is conceivable that disrupted inhibition within the CA3 circuit of old animals impairs the ability of pyramidal cells to synchronously discharge, leading to shorter higher-frequency events that are weaker.

15.8.3 CA1

In the only electrophysiological recording study from CA1 in young and aged nonhuman primates, LFP recordings were obtained from two female (13 and 31 years), and one male (14 years) rhesus macaque. Because the monkey recordings were obtained while the animal was in a primate restraint chair, movement-related theta was not obtained. Under these conditions, however, the older monkey had well-formed sharp wave/ripple events that reversed polarity in the pyramidal cell layer and coincided with the firing of both excitatory and inhibitory neurons (Skaggs et al., 2007). These data suggest that the ability of the LFP to organize spike timing may remain intact in older primates.

In rodents, a majority of studies have reported no changes in CA1 pyramidal cell in vivo firing rates between young and aged animals (Barnes et al., 1983; Barnes, Suster, et al., 1997; Oler and Markus, 2000a, 2000b; Wilson et al., 2005). In the studies that have detected significantly lower firing rates in aged compared with young rats (Shen et al., 1997; Sava and Markus, 2008), it is likely that this effect was due to behavioral rather than cellular changes. Because firing rate is known to increase with faster running velocity (McNaughton, Barnes, et al., 1983; Shen et al., 1997; Maurer et al., 2005), and aged rats tend to move more slowly than do young animals (Shen et al., 1997; Burke et al., 2014; Cowen et al., 2020), age-related firing rate differences could arise from differences in running speed. This idea is supported by the fact that CA1 neuron firing rates are not different during rest (Shen et al., 1997), nor when firing rates are obtained from similar running speed distributions across age groups (Barnes et al., 1983; Barnes, Suster, et al., 1997; Oler and Markus, 2000a, 2000b; Wilson et al., 2005; Schimanski et al., 2013). When firing rates have been examined when the animal is actively locomoting, and within- and out-of-field firing rates were assessed separately, the within-field rates were lower in older animals, while the out-of-field rates were not different (Crown et al., 2022). This suggests that in addition to controlling for differences in movement speed, it is also important to consider cellular activity both within and outside of the spatial receptive field when comparing firing rates between age groups. Additionally, while overall spatial information rate (Skaggs et al., 1992) was lower per cell in older rats, the information content per spike (Skaggs et al., 1992) was actually higher in the older rats (Crown et al., 2022). This indicates that age does not degrade information transmitted per spike. The reduced overall spatial information content in place cells of older rats may thus be due to the observed lower within-field firing rate. With respect to molecular markers of cell activity, the proportion of neurons expressing *Arc* as a result of a specific behavioral experience (Small et al., 2004; Penner, Roth, Chawla, et al., 2010; Hartzell et al., 2013; Hernandez et al., 2018), and BOLD activity levels (Yassa, Lacy, et al., 2010; Yassa, Mattfeld, et al., 2011; Reagh et al., 2018), do not change with age in CA1. There are, however, differences in behavior-driven ensemble dynamics of CA1 cells in old rodents as well as alterations in the LFP.

The first study to compare behavior-driven single-unit characteristics in CA1 examined young (10–14 months) and old (24–29 months) male F344 rats. Chronically implanted single-wire electrodes mounted on microdrives were used for precise placement in an intermediate zone of the CA1 pyramidal layer (Barnes et al., 1983). The transverse axis of CA1 receives different entorhinal cortical input. The region most proximal to CA2 gets direct afferent input from the medial entorhinal cortex, while the distal region closest to the subiculum receives input from the lateral entorhinal cortex (Amaral and Lavenex, 2007; Chapter 3). This anatomical organization follows a gradient such that the intermediate zone receives input from both entorhinal cortices. In the Barnes et al. (1983) study, rats traversed a radial eight-arm maze for food reward in conjunction with position tracking and recording of neuron spiking. The overall finding was that older rats showed less stability of their place fields than did younger animals, but did not show changes in firing rates (Barnes et al., 1983). It is important to note that animals were removed from the behavioral apparatus midway through the recording session so that the recording tether could be untangled (no commutator was available at the time). A later study reported that the information content of CA1 place fields recorded from aged male F344 rats (25 months) was comparable to those recorded from young animals (11 months) both when the room lights were on, and animals could orient to distal spatial cues, and when the lights were turned off. In both age groups, however, the information content between the lighted and dark conditions decreased, with place-field firing being less reliable in the dark (Markus et al., 1994). Another study comparing CA1 place-field activity in young (3–6 months) and aged (13–24 months) male C57xCD1 mice reported an increase in out of field firing in the aged group. In this study, the older animals spent a larger amount of time immobile, which was not accounted for in the analysis. Ripple activity, and associated cell firing, is likely to occur during these periods of inactivity (Jackson et al., 2006; O'Neill et al., 2006). This could account for the reduced specificity observed in CA1 place fields in these aged mice (Yan et al., 2003).

A later study used high channel count hyperdrives with tetrodes (four twisted wires that facilitate spike separation; McNaughton, O'Keefe, et al., 1983) to record larger ensembles of neurons in young (12 months) and aged (28 months) male F344 rats (Barnes, Suster, et al., 1997). With these methods, it was possible to record up to 100 cells simultaneously. The rats traversed a figure-8 maze twice in a day, with these sessions separated by an hour, and all analyses were conducted with rat number as the sample size. In this study the head stages for recording were connected to the hardware with a commutator so the tether could spin and not get tangled. Under these conditions, *within a session*, place-field stability was equivalent across age groups. When place-field stability was examined across the *two different recording sessions*, only the young animals had stable place-field representations. In contrast, one-third of the time the old rats tended to remap between sessions in the identical environment. Interestingly, the old rats that showed the most place-field remapping also showed the lowest spatial memory scores on the Morris watermaze. There were no differences in firing rate or spike amplitude between age groups (Barnes, Suster, et al., 1997). Given these results, the place-field instability within a session observed in Barnes et al. (1983) was likely due to a particular sensitivity of the old animals to being removed from the behavioral apparatus, which possibly resulted in remapping. Another study examined remapping in neurons recorded from proximal CA1 (and perhaps CA2) in middle-aged (14–18 months) and old (24–30 months) male Han Wistar rats and reported similar remapping between these groups (Hok et al., 2012). Because the middle-aged animals were relatively old, this could explain the lack of an age difference as was observed in Barnes, Suster, et al. (1997).

The higher probability of remapping between two daily sessions in the same environment in aged compared with young rats has been replicated when animals performed a spatial eyeblink conditioning task. Hyperdrives were implanted into the intermediate zone of the CA1 pyramidal cell layer in young (9–12 months) and aged (25–28 months) male F344 rats (Schimanski et al., 2013). During recordings, rats performed the spatial eyeblink conditioning task on two different sessions each day for 31 consecutive days. For this task, a brief electrical stimulus was delivered to the eyelid in association with two different unmarked locations along a circular track. The rats traversed this track in both clockwise and counterclockwise directions for food rewards on either side of a barrier. Stimuli at position 1 were delivered during the counterclockwise journey, and stimuli at position 2 were administered on the clockwise journey. There was no eyelid stimulus delivered during the first 10 laps of every session, and the probability of receiving a shock was 50% for the remaining laps. During the first recording day, animals were completely naïve to the requirements of the task and the environment. Young and aged rats rapidly learned the location of position 1 and 2 over the first 10 days of the experiment with no significant difference in performance between age groups. While 15,301 neurons were recorded in this experiment, all statistics were conducted with animal number as the sample size. As in other studies (Barnes et al., 1983; Barnes, Suster, et al., 1997; Oler and Markus, 2000a, 2000b; Wilson et al., 2005), there were no firing rate differences between CA1 cells in young and aged rats. There was also no remapping observed in any rat over the first 14 days of the study. Consistent with Barnes et al. (1997b), more old rats showed remapping between sessions after day 14 than did young rats, although a proportion of young rats also showed remapping. When the animals were divided by those who remapped versus those who remained stable (regardless of age), place-field stability positively correlated with Morris watermaze performance, and negatively correlated with place-conditioning performance (Schimanski et al., 2013). These data suggest that rats with place-field instability may use a behavioral strategy for place conditioning that does not require the hippocampus, such as a striatal-dependent response strategy, and this strategy is more likely to be used by old than by young rats (section 15.2.1).

The stability of CA1 activity patterns across sessions in the same environment has also been examined with the *Arc* catFISH method. Penner et al. (2011) found that when rats were exposed to a novel arena and then reintroduced a second time, separated by 20 min, the overlap in activation across sessions was comparable (~70%) between young (9–12 months) and aged (24–32 months) male F344 rats. This observation is consistent with Schimanski et al. (2013) in which place-field instability is not evident in any age group on the first day of exposure to a new environment. Hartzell et al. (2013) also examined overlap in behavior-induced *Arc* expression in young (7–9 months) and aged (24–26 months) male F344 rats. In this study, neurons were sampled from distal CA1 (closer to subiculum), which receives projections from lateral entorhinal cortex, and from proximal CA1 (closer to CA2), which receives projections from medial entorhinal cortex (Hafting et al., 2005; Hargreaves et al., 2005; Henriksen et al., 2010). In this study, rats were placed for 5 minutes in a novel arena containing 5 novel objects for exploration while their position was recorded. During a second session 20 minutes later, some rats were returned to the original arena with copies of the same objects (AA condition), while other rats were placed in a new arena that contained copies of the same objects (AB condition). For the AA condition, there was a slight decrease in the overlap of cell activity in aged compared with young rats in both proximal and distal CA1. This age difference in overlap was due to differences in exploration behavior between the age groups. Specifically, when the animals' paths through the arenas were compared across sessions, the young rats' exploration covered more of the arena, increasing the probability that the same sectors would be traversed in both epochs. The less extensive spatial exploration in the aged rats, resulted in less path overlap between epochs. For the AB condition, both the young and old animals showed *Arc* expression patterns that were consistent with global remapping in proximal CA1, although this remapping was weaker in the older animals. For distal CA1, the young animals showed considerable overlap in the ensemble activity patterns even though the environment changed, while old animals showed less overlap. Since objects are known to modulate activity in this region (Burke, Maurer, et al., 2011), presumably due object information from the lateral (Deshmukh and Knierim, 2011) and perirhinal cortices (Burke et al., 2012), the overlap of activity in distal CA1 between the A and B environments in young animals could be due to the influence of objects on place-field activity. In young rats there were differences in the extent of remapping between proximal and distal CA1 (greater remapping in proximal than distal), and this remapping difference was attenuated in the older animals (Hartzell et al., 2013). This implies that there are changes in the function of medial and lateral cortical inputs into CA1 of older animals.

Electrophysiological recordings from intermediate CA1 are also consistent with the idea that entorhinal cortical input is less effective at influencing place-field activity patterns. Young (10–13 months) and aged male (24–28 months) F344 rats were trained to pause at an unmarked location on a linear track for medial forebrain bundle stimulation reward (Rosenzweig et al., 2003). Although the track was uniform, the goal location could be found using distal landmarks in the environment. Across trials, the location of the start box was moved so that its distance from the goal location varied systematically from 107 to 46 cm, but the goal location remained stationary within the environment (as in Gothard et al., 1996). At the greatest distance from the goal location, the place fields were aligned to the start box. As the distance decreased to the goal, there was a point at which the place fields realigned to the room cues. For any individual rat, place-field realignments that occurred at shorter distances from the start box were predictive of greater accuracy to pause at the correct goal location. The aged rats showed delayed map realignment to the room, and were less accurate at stopping at the goal location (Rosenzweig et al., 2003).

When place fields are recorded from intermediate CA1 of young (6–8 months) and aged (25–27 months) male Long Evans rats in two distinctly different environments, place fields remap in young and old animals to the same extent between environments (Wilson et al., 2005). While place-field remapping in different environments is not altered by age, activity patterns in response to changes in task demands within an environment do differ between young and old animals. Mizumori et al. (1996) reported that old (24 months) male F344 rats had more directionally selective place fields than did young (9 months) on both a forced choice and spatial memory versions of an eight-arm radial maze. Another study examined CA1 place-field activity in young (12–16 months) and old (24–28 months) male F344 rats while animals traversed either a plus or a figure-8 maze in the same environment. The figure-8 maze was constructed by adding two bridges to the plus maze to connect the arms so that rats did not have to turn around, as they did in the plus maze configuration. When place-field activity in the common segments of the maze was compared, young rats showed more remapping than did the older animals (Oler and Markus, 2000a, 2000b). A later study, using a different maze configuration, replicated this age effect. Specifically, they showed that when one of two arms of

a maze was moved, the place fields in the unmoved arm changed more for young compared with aged rats (Sava and Markus, 2008), suggesting that CA1 place fields in young rats were more likely than aged to remap when task demands change. The differences in remapping with age found across these experiments could be explained by the fact that different variables were manipulated in each—cognitive load (Mizumori et al., 1996), versus movement requirements (Oler and Markus, 2000b; Sava and Markus, 2008). In the Sava and Markus (2008) study, they also included infusions of the cholinergic agonist carbachol into the medial septum. This disrupted place-field reliability in young rats, but improved reliability in older animals (Sava and Markus, 2008). These data may be consistent with an inverted U-shaped function, where augmenting normal homeostatic levels of cholinergic tone in young animals, past the optimal performance peak, worsens CA1 network function. In contrast, augmenting deficient cholinergic levels toward the performance peak is restorative in the old animals.

When a young rat repeatedly takes the same path, as when traversing a track for multiple laps, an experience-dependent form of place-field plasticity can be observed (Mehta et al., 1997). Specifically, place-field size asymmetrically increases, which shifts the center of mass location for maximal firing rate in the direction opposite to the movement of the rat (Mehta et al., 1997; Lee, Rao, et al., 2004). Consistent with an LTP-like mechanism, this behaviorally induced plasticity is dependent on the NMDA receptor (Ekstrom et al., 2001), and may provide a mechanism for sequence encoding in the hippocampus (Mehta et al., 1997; Shen et al., 1997). With respect to aging, the prediction was that experience-dependent plasticity would be impaired, as is experimentally induced LTP (e.g., Diana, Scotti de Carolis, et al., 1994; Rosenzweig et al., 1997). This prediction was confirmed by Shen et al. (1997) recording from the intermediate zone of CA1 in young (11–12 months) and aged (25–31 months) male F344 rats as they traversed a track. The young rats showed an increase in place-field size over the first 15 laps around the track, whereas the older animals showed minimal expansion of place-field size, which is schematically represented in Figure 15.15. Importantly, these investigators used a number of ways to quantify place-field size, all of which converged on the same conclusion. Due to the presumed LTP-like mechanism of place-field expansion plasticity, Burke et al. (2008) examined the effect of the noncompetitive NMDA receptor antagonist memantine in aged rats. Memantine binds to the receptor at a different site than does glutamate, reducing but not eliminating the CA^{2+} that enters the cell. This drug has also been shown to increase the durability of perforant path to granule cell LTP and improve spatial search patterns in the Morris watermaze (Barnes, Danysz, et al., 1996). In aged animals, memantine administration resulted in at least a partial restoration of experience-dependent place-field expansion (Burke et al., 2008).

Although there are a number of age-related changes in hippocampal activity during waking behaviors, the hippocampus is also active during rest or "offline" periods. For many decades it has been hypothesized that memory consolidation occurs during sleep or "offline" periods in which neuron activity patterns established during behavior are replayed. In theory, this replay would then lead to a strengthening of connections between cell ensembles involved in specific experiences (e.g., Sutherland and McNaughton, 2000). This reactivation occurs primarily during sharp wave/ripple events that arise in quiet rest and slow wave sleep (Wilson and McNaughton, 1994; Kudrimoti et al., 1999), and can be quantified

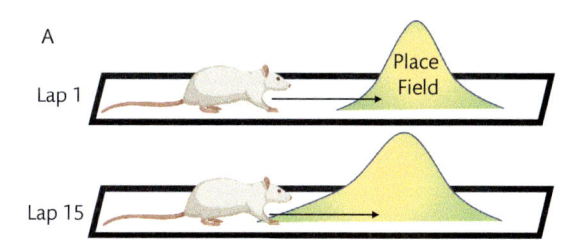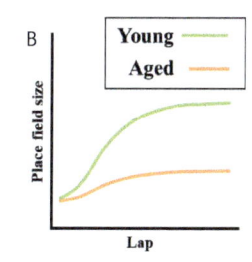

Figure 15.15 Place-field expansion plasticity in young and aged rats. (A) When a young rat repeatedly traverses the same path, an experience-dependent form of place-field plasticity can be observed. Plasticity can be measured as an asymmetrical increase in place-field size in the direction opposite to the movement of the rat. This is schematically illustrated by the size and shape of the place field on lap 1 (top) versus lap 15 (bottom) during the recording session. (B) Consistent with lower levels of LTP plasticity in aged compared with young rats, over repeated traversals of the track, the place fields of aged rats to do not expand to the same magnitude as observed in younger animals.

by measuring the correlations of activity patterns during behavior compared with activity patterns in the subsequent rest period (Wilson and McNaughton, 1994). The temporal order of activity patterns between behavior and sleep can also be examined (Skaggs and McNaughton, 1996). Gerrard et al. (2001) measured the reactivation of simple correlated activity patterns during rest following behavior in the intermediate zone of CA1 in young (11–12 months) and aged (25–31 months) male F344 rats. They found that reactivation of these activity patterns was comparable between young and aged animals (Gerrard et al., 2001). When the temporal order of the activity patterns was examined in a later study, however, aged (25–31 months) male F344 rats showed significantly weaker sequence reactivation compared with the young (11–12 months) animals. In both young and aged rats, the best performers on the Morris watermaze had the greatest amount of sequence reactivation during postbehavior rest (Gerrard et al., 2008). This observation supports the idea that successful sequence reactivation may be related to the accuracy of spatial memory.

Because reactivation occurs during sharp wave/ripple events, changes in the properties of this oscillation could impact hippocampal replay. The first study to assess ripple activity during rest periods in aging, compared young (11–12 months) and aged (25–31 months) male F344 rats (Smith et al., 2000). In this study the full extent of the LFP spectrum was analyzed, which included the spectral density for ripples (100–250 Hz). They found that aged rats had higher power in the ripple frequency band compared with the young rats, and a greater incidence of short latency interspike intervals, suggesting more burst firing in aged neurons. During behavior on the other hand, where ripples are less frequent, there was no difference in power across ripple frequencies or cell burstiness between age groups (A Smith et al., 2000). The observation that burst firing was more common in aged CA1 pyramidal neurons compared with what was observed in neurons from young rats was later confirmed with in vitro recordings in hippocampal slices from aged (~29 months) and young (~5 months) male Wistar rats (Kouvaros et al., 2015). The same study also observed reduced oscillatory frequency of spontaneous CA1 ripples in the aged compared with young rats (Kouvaros et al., 2015).

When using a different approach in which ripple and inter-ripple intervals were analyzed separately, Weigand et al. (2016) observed that CA1 cell bursting activity was less likely to occur during a ripple event in aged (25–28 months) compared with young (9–12 months) male F344 rats. This discrepancy with Smith et al. (2000) and Kouvaros et al., (2015) can be reconciled by the fact that both earlier

studies collapsed ripple and inter-ripple intervals in their analyses. Thus, the observed increase in power in the burst-frequency range of CA1 activity reported in these earlier papers, is likely due to more cell bursting during the inter-ripple interval in old compared with young animals. If this interpretation is correct, it could reflect deficits in neuron coordination and temporal summation in aged CA1 that is consistent with known age deficits in LTP (Rosenzweig et al., 1997). Wiegand et al. (2016) was also able to detect reduced oscillatory frequency of the ripple event in aged compared with young rats, consistent with observations from slice recordings (Kouvaros et al., 2015). Moreover, these sharp wave/ripple events occurred less often in aged compared with young rats following behavior, which could impact consolidation processes and memory stabilization in the aged brain. Weigand et al. (2016) also confirmed previous findings of Gerrard et al. (2001) that, when activity pattern reactivation was examined across the entire rest session, there was no difference between young and aged rats. When neuron spiking during wave/ripple events was examined, however, the young rats had more activity pattern reactivation than did the aged animals. Finally, aged CA1 neurons tended to fire at more consistent phases with respect to the ripple oscillation compared with young rats. These neurobiological differences could contribute to age-related impairments in hippocampus-dependent behaviors (section 15.2). Recently, the observation that the oscillatory frequency of CA1 ripple events during rest was reduced in aged (24–26 months) compared with young animals (4–8 months) was replicated in male F344 x BN rats. This study also reported that the sharp wave-associated current density in the stratum radiatum was lower in the aged compared with young rats (DiCola et al., 2022), which is consistent with reports of reduced evoked fEPSPs at the CA3 to CA1 Schaffer collateral synapse (Landfield et al., 1986; Barnes, Rao, and Orr, 2000). Despite the decreased current density in older animals, there was no difference in the probability of coincidence in high-frequency CA3 and CA1 sharp wave/ripple events between young and aged rats (DiCola et al., 2022).

Sharp wave/ripple events can also occur during periods of pauses of movement during behavior and reflect coordinated activity that is hypothesized to support learning and memory processes (Jackson et al., 2006; O'Neill et al., 2006). When these waking ripples have been examined in young (9–12 months) and aged (25–28 months) male F344 rats, aged rats have reduced ripple rates. The oscillatory frequency of the waking ripples, however, was indistinguishable between aged and young rats (Cowen et al., 2020). Interestingly, the older animals had more total ripple events over an entire behavioral session than did the young animals because they moved more slowly and paused more often (Cowen et al., 2020). The authors suggest that this could potentially give older animals more opportunity to replay task-relevant information. In fact, this may explain the comparable performance that aged and young rats displayed in acquiring eyeblink to place conditioning in this experiment.

As discussed in section 15.8.2, there are a number of other prominent oscillations in the hippocampal local field potential. The theta rhythm was first examined with respect to age in 1988 (Woodruff-Pak and Logan, 1988). Interestingly, in rabbits (unlike rats and mice) there is a pronounced theta oscillation even in the absence of locomotion. In head-fixed immobile rabbits between 3 months and 4 years, there were no differences in the frequency and power of the theta rhythm with age in spite of an impairment in trace eyeblink conditioning that was evident at 2.5 years (Woodruff-Pak and Logan, 1988). In adult animals, however, the amplitude and frequency of the theta rhythm is known to increase with faster running speeds (Vanderwolf, 1969). During freely moving behavior in rats, age differences in theta have been observed from intermediate CA1 recordings obtained from young (11–12 months) and old (25–31 months) male F344 rats (Shen et al., 1997). In this study, there were no differences observed in theta amplitude between age groups, but the sensitivity of theta frequency to movement speed was lower in old animals (Shen et al., 1997). When movement was eliminated as a variable, as during REM sleep, there were no differences in theta frequency between age groups (Shen et al., 1997). Consistent with these results, Jacobson et al. (2013) observed lower theta frequency in aged male F344 rats (23–28 months) compared with young rats (9–13 months). Other differences that have been noted between age groups are the impact of environmental novelty (Jacobson et al., 2013) and coherence between electrodes (Jacobson et al., 2015). The analyses in both of the Jacobsen et al. (2013, 2015) studies used recording sessions rather than animal number as the sample size. Moreover, they did not control for differences in movement speed between young and aged rats. Thus, it remains to be confirmed whether these variables change with age.

More recently, when differences in movement speed between young (9–12 months) and aged (25–28 months) male F344 rats were taken into consideration, the observation of reduced theta frequency for a given movement speed in aged compared with young rats was replicated. Unlike the results from Shen et al. (1997), in this study the increase in the theta frequency with movement speed was comparable between age groups (Crown et al., 2022).

O'Keefe and Recce (1993) reported that the phase of theta at which a hippocampal principal cell fires, advances gradually as the rat passes through a place field. They called this effect "phase precession." Skaggs et al. (1996) suggested that this process may provide a neural mechanism by which temporal sequences could be coded within individual theta cycles. CA1 pyramidal cells typically exhibit a phase advance of 360° within a place field. This results in different rates of phase precession for place fields of different sizes (Shen et al., 1997; Ekstrom et al., 2001; Maurer et al., 2006a; Maurer et al., 2006b). Shen et al. (1997) observed that the cell spiking in old rats precessed the full 360° of a theta cycle as the animals traversed place fields. Because of reduced place-field expansion plasticity in old rats, however, their place fields were smaller on average and thus the rate of precession was faster compared with the young animals.

This observation was comparable to the phase presession rate differences seen in young animals with NMDA receptor blockade that abolished place-field expansion (Ekstrom et al., 2001).

The gamma rhythm has also been examined in CA1 with respect to age. Power and peak frequency between 62 to 120 Hz was not different between young (9–12 months) and aged (25–28 months) male F344 rats (Insel et al., 2012). Consistent with these data, Jacobson et al. (2013) found that gamma power in the range of 65 to 140 Hz was not different between young (12 months) and aged (23 months) male F344 rats when animals traversed a familiar maze. More recently, Crown et al. (2022) also reported no difference in gamma frequency in the range of 30–120 Hz between young (9–12 months) and aged (25–28 months) male F344 rats during a spatial eyeblink conditioning task. Consistent with other studies (Ahmed and Mehta, 2012; Sheremet et al., 2018), gamma frequency was also found to be increased with running velocity in both young and old rats, although the rate of increase was slower in old compared with young animals (Crown et al., 2022). This occurred in conjunction with a decrease in the range of frequencies over which gamma was modulated by speed in the old animals. This study also reported that aged rats had increased phase-locking of pyramidal cell firing to the gamma rhythm compared with that observed in the young animals (Crown et al., 2022). This indicates that while the range of gamma frequencies observed in old animals is reduced, older neurons maintain a stronger phase relationship with the oscillation.

While gamma frequency in CA1 appears to be stable with age, there is one report that gamma power is lower in old animals under some circumstances. Specifically, when an arm of the maze was rotated to create a novel configuration, old rats showed lower gamma power relative to young (Jacobson et al., 2013). Because the relationship between gamma power and running speed (Ahmed and Mehta, 2012; Sheremet et al., 2018) was not taken into consideration, it is not possible to definitively conclude whether this effect was due to age differences in sensitivity to novelty or to running speed (Jacobson et al., 2013). The modulation of gamma by theta has also been investigated in young and aged animals. Jacobson et al., (2013) examined the depth of modulation of gamma power in relation to phase of theta and reported a reduced modulation index in aged compared with young animals across both novel and familiar maze configurations. Because theta-gamma coupling is also related to running speed (Ahmed and Mehta, 2012; Sheremet et al., 2018), these data are confounded.

15.8.4 Summary

Within the dentate gyrus the data are very consistent with respect to a decline in activity of aged granule cells across rats, nonhuman primates, and human studies. These observations have been conducted using imaging methodologies that include immediate early gene (IEG) activity markers in rats or MRI metabolic activity in primates. To date, there have been no electrophysiological recordings from the aged dentate gyrus that would enable evaluation of short timescale dynamics, oscillations in the LFP, or the relationship between cell spiking and hippocampus rhythms.

In CA3, there have been electrophysiological and imaging studies that have consistently reported an increase in activity with age in rats, nonhuman primates, and humans. In electrophysiological studies, individual CA3 pyramidal cells of old rats have been shown to have increased firing rates, decreased information content, and reduced place-field remapping between different environments compared with young rats. Recent data from rats suggests that age-related hyperactivity may be unique to CA3c pyramidal neurons, although this remains to be confirmed. Consistent with rodent data, CA3 pyramidal cells of nonhuman primates show increased firing rates with age and the BOLD signal in the CA3/dentate gyrus region of human participants is elevated in older adults. When IEG activity markers have been evaluated, there is no difference in the number of activated neurons in dorsal CA3, but more ventral regions show greater numbers of activated cells in old behaviorally impaired rats relative to young animals.

For CA1, both electrophysiological and imaging studies have been conducted. In nonhuman primates, sharp wave/ripple events are similar across age. All other electrophysiological studies have been conducted in rodents. Across several experiments, no age-related changes have been observed in awake firing rates, the numbers of cells positive for IEG activity markers in rats, and MRI metabolic activity in nonhuman primates or humans. When electrophysiology has been used to evaluate potential age differences in short timescale dynamics, aged rats have comparable firing rates, but less stable place fields across recording sessions, impairments in place-field expansion plasticity, a reduced ability to respond to changing task demands, and declines in the replay of activity patterns and sequences during rest that were established during the preceding behavior. With respect to the LFP, during waking behavior, theta frequency is reduced, and sharp wave/ripple occurrence is lower in aged compared with young rats. During rest, theta is intact in aged rats, but ripple frequency is lower and CA1 cells from aged rats are more likely to burst outside of the sharp wave/ripple event.

Many questions remain, particularly with regard to the impact of advanced age on the short timescale dynamics of the dentate gyrus and CA3. Another missing component that requires further investigation is how the activity patterns in the subiculum and other structures densely connected with the hippocampus change with age.

15.9 Gene expression

Alterations in gene expression in the hippocampus could potentially result from changes in epigenetic regulation of DNA, RNA transcription, or protein translation. Such age-related modifications in gene expression could play a pivotal role in directing functional outcomes. Experiments included in this review focus exclusively on research in which young and normal aged groups have been directly compared. Moreover, as discussed in sections 15.3–15.8, each hippocampus subregion undergoes a distinct pattern of age-related vulnerability. Thus, combining subregions for analysis obscures the true pattern of both circuit alterations and changes in gene expression. Thus, only studies that directly compare young and aged groups, as well as analyze subregions separately are included in this review. This greatly reduces the number of investigations included here from rodents, there are no nonhuman primate studies, and only one human experiment that met these criteria.

15.9.1 Gene expression in the dentate gyrus

The one study conducted in humans that compared young and old age groups used microarray to measure RNA levels and Western blot to quantify protein from 8 human brains free of significant pathology ranging in age from 33 to 88. They used standard Affymetrix microarrays to investigate gene expression in the dentate gyrus normalized to expression levels in the entorhinal cortex (Pavlopoulos et al., 2013). In the initial analysis, the expression levels in the dentate gyrus of 17 genes were significantly correlated with age. Of these genes, 9 were downregulated with age and 8 were upregulated. The gene that showed the strongest correlation with age was RbAp48, which plays multiple roles in histone acetylation and transcriptional regulation. It is also implicated in the cyclic adenosine monophosphate (cAMP)–protein kinase A (PKA)–cAMP response element–binding protein 1 (CREB1) pathway. As a validation study, 10 additional individuals were examined ranging in age from 41 to 89 years. The tissue was analyzed with quantitative Western blot to measure protein levels of RbAp48 in dentate gyrus, CA3, CA1, subiculum, and entorhinal cortex. The only region that showed significant reductions in RbAp48 with age was the dentate gyrus. The authors suggest that because RbAp48 is involved in histone acetylation, its downregulation with age may impact how synapses onto old granule cells can be modified by experience (Pavlopoulos et al., 2013).

As discussed in section 15.8, there is a class of genes whose transcription is dynamically regulated by behavior. These immediate early genes (IEGs) do not require de novo protein synthesis for their transcription and are therefore the first genomic event that occurs following patterned synaptic activity (Morgan et al., 1987). It is well documented that disruptions in IEG expression interfere with plasticity and memory (e.g., Guzowski et al., 2000). Thus, the regulation of IEG transcription could be a potential mechanism for age-related impairments in synaptic modification and cognition. Penner, Roth, Barnes, et al. (2010a) was the first to formalize a potential epigenetic hypothesis of IEG dysregulation in aging. They proposed that a disruption of chromatin regulation and DNA methylation might be a key driver of age-associated memory dysfunction. Initial support for this idea came from early reports of altered IEG expression with age from tissue samples that combined all hippocampus subregions (e.g., Blalock et al., 2003; Rowe et al., 2007). Several subsequent studies have tested this hypothesis by examining the dentate gyrus in isolation. The first among these studies examined the IEG Arc, which encodes an effector protein known to be important in synaptic plasticity and memory consolidation (Lyford et al., 1995; Lanahan et al., 1997; Guzowski et al., 2000; Chowdhury et al., 2006; Shepherd et al., 2006). The levels of behavior-induced Arc mRNA in the dentate gyrus were examined in young (9–12 months) and aged (24–32 months) male F344 rats using RT-PCR (Penner, Roth, Chawla, et al., 2010; Penner et al., 2011). Following behavior, Arc expression is elevated in granule cells of both young and aged rats. Expression levels in aged granule cells, however, was significantly reduced compared with levels in the young granule cells of the dentate gyrus. Additionally, direct bisulfite sequencing PCR was used to examine the methylation state of two loci of the Arc gene, one in the promoter region and another in a downstream CpG island. Within the promoter region, the methylation state following behavior was increased similarly in young and aged rats. In the downstream intragenic region, however, the young rats had reduced methylation following behavior. This suggests that Arc transcription was facilitated in the dentate gyrus of young animals. In contrast, the aged rats actually showed a significant increase in methylation at this site following behavior, which could account for lower Arc transcription levels (Penner et al., 2011). These findings are consistent with the hypothesis proposed by Penner, Roth, Barnes, et al. (2010) that alterations in epigenetic mechanisms may result in altered transcription that then contribute to cognitive impairment.

The transcription levels of *zif268*, an IEG that encodes a transcription factor important for learning and memory are elevated following behavior (Jones et al., 2001), and have also been examined with respect to age within the dentate gyrus. As with *Arc* expression, behavior-induced RNA levels of *zif268* were lower in aged (24–32 months) compared with young (9–12 months) granule cells from male F344 rats (Penner et al., 2016). To determine whether reduced expression levels of *zif268* were related to the methylation state of the gene, 20 different CpG sites were examined in young and old rats. In the young rats, there were no methylation differences at any site following behavior. In contrast, for the aged rats multiple *zif268* sites had reduced methylation following behavior. Unlike the IEG *Arc*, where decreased transcription was associated with increased methylation, for *zif268*, decreased transcription coincided with decreased methylation at multiple CpG sites. The factors that could account for this observed relationship have yet to be discovered (Penner et al., 2016). A more recent study also examined behavior-related induction of *zif268* in young (8 months) and aged (25 months) male Long Evans rats, in addition to a number of markers for inhibitory function (*GAD1*, *GAD2*, and GAD67 protein). These variables were assessed using quantitative in situ hybridization or immunohistochemistry (Branch et al., 2019). In this study, only aged rats that performed similar to young on the Morris watermaze were selected for inclusion. In both age groups, *zif268* was elevated following a change to the environment during behavior. In contrast, only the aged rats showed upregulation of inhibitory markers following environment change. The authors interpret this finding to mean that increased recruitment of inhibition may be a signature of successful aging (Branch et al., 2019).

Reduced mRNA levels in the dentate gyrus were also reported in aged rats for the IEGs *zif268*, *c-fos*, and *Homer1a* following behavior in young (6 months) and aged (24 months) male Long Evans rats (Myrum et al., 2020). Consistent with the finding for *c-fos*, Chawla et al. (2013) also detected lower levels of *c-fos* per cell using in situ hybridization and RT-PCR in aged (24 months) compared with young (9 months) male F344 rats. In the Myrum et al. (2020) study, no change was observed in the IEG *Narp/Nptx2* with age. In contrast to previous studies examining the IEG *Arc*, basal expression (that is, no behavior) within the dentate gyrus was elevated with age, and behaviorally induced expression was unchanged (Myrum et al., 2020). The discrepancy in the effect of age on basal *Arc* expression between studies remains to be determined, but could be related to differences between rat strains, behavioral methodologies, or epigenetic mechanisms that were differentially activated between studies.

The first microarray study in rats to investigate the dentate gyrus and other subregions separately examined young (8 months) versus aged (25 months) male Long Evans rats. While gene expression was upregulated in the dentate gyrus for 2 different prodynorphins, and other genes related to immune function, these changes did not discriminate between young, aged-impaired, and aged-unimpaired animals (Haberman et al., 2011). In another more recent study, the dentate gyrus of young (~5 months) and aged (~20 months) male F344 rats was examined using subregion-specific transcriptome profiling (Ianov et al., 2017). This RNA sequence analysis identified 161 genes that were differentially expressed between age groups. Of this total, 134 genes were upregulated and assessed using the DAVID functional annotation bioinformatics system. This analysis indicated that most of these genes were related to immune function. The expression levels of the upregulated genes did not stratify with behavioral performance on a variant of the Morris watermaze task (Ianov et al., 2017), consistent with the findings from Haberman et al. (2011). Another study used RT-PCR to focus on genes related to synaptic function. Of the 96 genes quantified in young (7 months) and aged (23 months) male F344 x BN rats, there were no significant effects of age in any of the transporter, receptor or signaling genes studied (Hernandez, Hernandez, et al., 2019). Another study using microarray analysis of the dentate gyrus in young (12 month) and old (26 month) male F344 x BN rats reported that 173 genes were differentially expressed between age groups. Of these, 81 were upregulated in older animals and 92 were downregulated (Masser et al., 2014), many of which were related to immune function. Of particular interest, this study explicitly examined the relationship between gene expression and Morris watermaze performance. Lower expression of the transporter transthyretin in the dentate gyrus was associated with worse performance on the Morris watermaze in the old animals (Masser et al., 2014).

15.9.2 Gene expression in CA3

Basal gene expression in the CA3 region has been examined in young (8 months) and aged (25 months) male Long Evans rats using Affymetrix microarray methods with molecular pathway analysis, as well as in situ hybridization. A specific decline with age in lipoprotein lipase, the gene encoding the α5 subunit of the $GABA_A$ receptor, chaperone/protein folding genes (e.g., Tcp1 complex), and the endoplasmic reticulum chaperone Hspa5/BiPi were found, but these changes were not related to Morris watermaze performance (Haberman et al., 2011). On the other hand, gene groups related to mitochondria and oxidative phosphorylation were decreased in CA3 of aged memory-impaired rats as evaluated with the Morris watermaze. Aged rats that performed better on the Morris watermaze had decreased expression of genes that could influence neuron excitability and plasticity, such as those encoding potassium channels and glutamate receptors (Haberman et al., 2011). Furthermore, RT-PCR of CA3 in aged (23 month) and young (7 month) male F344 x BN rats has shown lower expression of genes related to glutamatergic but not GABAergic signaling in the old animals (Hernandez, Hernandez, et al., 2019). In both the Haberman et al. (2011) and Hernandez, Hernandez, et al. (2019) studies expression patterns were only examined in animals that had been quietly maintained in their home cages without doing any behavior, that is, under basal conditions. While gene expression in CA3 is dramatically altered following behavior, no gene microarray study has directly compared the transcription landscape between basal and behavioral conditions in relation to age.

In another study, CA3 of young (~5 months) and aged (~20 months) male F344 rats was examined using subregion-specific transcriptome profiling (Ianov et al., 2017). This RNA sequence analysis identified 81 genes that were differentially expressed between age groups (61 upregulated), most were related to immune function, but none related to the behavioral status of the animal (Ianov et al., 2017). Another study using microarray analysis of CA3 in young (12 month) and old (26 month) male F344 x BN rats reported that 344 genes were differentially expressed between age groups (271 upregulated), many of which were related to immune function (Masser et al., 2014). When the relationship between gene expression and Morris watermaze performance was examined, similar to the dentate gyrus, lower expression of transthyretin in CA3 was associated with worse performance in the old animals (Masser et al., 2014).

The expression and translation of the IEG *Arc* has been examined in young (6 months) and aged (24 months) male Long Evans rats both with and without behavioral induction using radiolabeled in situ hybridization and immunoblot analyses (Fletcher et al., 2014). While there is an increase in expression of *Arc* mRNA following behavior in young and age unimpaired rats, aged rats with impaired Morris watermaze performance did not show this increase. Furthermore, regardless of age group and behavioral condition, there were no differences in levels of Arc protein in CA3, nor were there any correlations with watermaze performance (Fletcher et al., 2014). In a more recent study using RT-PCR of tissue from the same ages and strain of behaviorally characterized rats, a similar profile of increased expression of *Arc* following behavior was found for young and aged unimpaired rats. No change above basal levels of *Arc* expression following behavior was observed in aged-impaired rats (Myrum et al., 2020). In this study the IEGs *zif*268, *Homer*1a, and *Nptx2/Narp* were also examined using RT-PCR. *Zif*268 showed a similar expression profile with regard to age and behavioral induction as did *Arc*, while *Homer*1a and *Nptx*2 expression levels were not different across age or behavioral condition (Myrum et al., 2020). In this same study, the methylation state and histone marks for *Arc* were also examined for CA3. Behavior significantly increased methylation around the promoter region of the *Arc* gene in aged rats with watermaze impairments (Myrum et al., 2020). There were changes observed in two different histone marks under basal conditions in these rats. One was between young and aged-impaired groups (an increase in H3K9Me2 in the old rats), and an increase between aged-impaired compared with aged-unimpaired rats for H3K9AcS10p (Myrum et al., 2020).

Another study examined the transcription of *zif*268, *CamK2a*, and *Nlgn1* in young (8 months) and aged (25 months) male Long Evans rats. Only aged rats that were unimpaired on the Morris watermaze were compared with the young rats. In both the young and aged-unimpaired rats, expression of *zif*268, *CamK2a*, and *Nlgn1* were elevated following behavior in a novel maze configuration (Branch et al., 2019). *Gad1* mRNA and Gad67 protein were also elevated in this behavioral condition in the aged-unimpaired rats, but not in the young animals (Branch et al., 2019). Because aged-impaired rats were not examined in this study, it remains to be determined whether increased inhibitory markers are related to cognitive status.

15.9.3 Gene expression in CA1

The first study to examine gene expression in CA1 used Affymetrix microarrays in young (3 months) and aged (24 months) male F344 rats. Animals were behaviorally characterized on the Morris watermaze. To control for potential differences in physical activity, other groups of rats that only swam or underwent cued training were also included. The expression levels of 243 genes were significantly related to age but not of these changes were related to behavior (Burger et al., 2007). Another microarray study that directly compared young (12 months) and aged (23 months) male F344 rats found that 203 genes were differentially expressed between these ages, with 105 being upregulated and 98 being downregulated. The upregulated genes were involved in immune function and ribosome

biosynthesis/cell proliferation, while the downregulated genes were involved in cytoplasmic/vesicle cytoskeleton, GTP/ATP binding, and ion transport. Among each of these categories of genes, expression levels of several were related to Morris watermaze performance (Kadish et al., 2009), but the measurement used in this case was latency, which is confounded for the older age group.

Basal levels of gene expression in the CA1 region have been examined in young (8 months) and aged (25 months) male Long Evans rats using Affymetrix microarray methods. Overall expression levels of most genes examined did not differ between young, aged-unimpaired, and aged-impaired rats. Of the genes in which a change was detected, mitochondria and oxidative phosphorylation genes were increased in impaired rats compared with young and unimpaired groups (Haberman et al., 2011). Moreover, 20 genes associated with MAPK signaling were differentially expressed between impaired and unimpaired aged rats (Haberman et al., 2011). In another study using RT-PCR quantification for genes associated with synaptic transmission and neuronal signaling, there were no significant age differences in expression levels in CA1 of male F344 x BN rats (7 vs. 23 months; Hernandez, Hernandez, et al., 2019).

In another study, CA1 of young (~5 months) and aged (~20 months) male F344 rats was examined using subregion-specific transcriptome profiling. The expression of 286 genes was altered with age (182 genes upregulated in old rats), however, the expression patterns in CA1 were not evaluated with regard to cognitive function (Ianov et al., 2016). A study that did take into consideration Morris watermaze performance in young (12 month) and old (26 month) male F344 x BN rats reported that 350 genes were differentially expressed between age groups (161 upregulated in older animals). These genes were related to immune function, but none correlated with Morris watermaze performance (Masser et al., 2014). A more recent RNA sequence analysis identified 104 genes that were differentially expressed between age groups, 90 of the upregulated genes were related to immune function, the KEGG lysosome pathway, or MAPK signaling. In the aged rats only, gene expression patterns were compared between spatial memory unimpaired and impaired groups. The tissue was examined with both the Illumina and Ion Proton sequencing platforms. Of the genes that were differentially expressed between impaired and unimpaired aged rats, both analysis platforms identified 12 genes related to Ca^{2+} binding and 20 genes related to synaptic function (Ianov et al., 2017). In a recent metanalysis combining five different gene expression datasets (Burger et al., 2007; Haberman et al., 2011; Masser et al., 2014; Ianov et al., 2016; Ianov et al., 2017), Morris watermaze performance was compared with gene expression patterns in CA1. The authors hypothesized that there may be a pattern of gene expression that could predict cognitive reserve in old animals. While there were consistent age-associated changes in the expression of genes related to immune function, oxidative stress, and programmed cell death regulation, no straightforward relationship emerged in this meta-analysis between gene expression in CA1 and behavioral performance (Yegla and Foster, 2022).

The cell-specific expression of IEGs has also been examined in CA1 of young (9-12 months) and aged (24–32 months) male F344 rats. At rest, where few neurons are active, and following spatial behavior, where there is a dramatic increase in IEG expression, the same proportion of CA1 pyramidal cells express *Arc* in both age groups (Penner et al., 2011). When the amount of transcript was evaluated with RT-PCR, the old rats showed reduced transcription of *Arc* per cell (Penner et al., 2011). The methylation state of the promoter and an intragenic region of the *Arc* gene was also examined in these animals. In the promoter region, behavior led to a decrease in methylation in both young and aged rats, consistent with the enhanced expression of *Arc* following behavior. Paradoxically, while the old rats also showed decreased methylation following behavior in the intragenic region examined, the young rats exhibited an increase in methylation in that region (Penner et al., 2011). The explanation of this awaits further examination of other intragenic sites of the *Arc* gene. In another study that examined *Arc* transcription and translation at baseline and following behavior in young (6 months) and aged (24 months) male Long Evans rats, a different pattern of results was observed (Fletcher et al., 2014). When optical density measurements were used to infer *Arc* transcription levels across the entire CA1 region, aged-impaired rats showed elevated *Arc* signal compared with the young and age-unimpaired groups in the no behavior condition. Following behavior, the young and the aged-unimpaired rats showed a significant elevation in *Arc* signal. No further elevation of *Arc* was detected in aged-impaired rats following behavior. Quantitative Western blots confirmed these observations at the protein level. Translation-dependent decay mechanisms of *Arc* mRNA were not different between groups. The lack of increase in *Arc* expression following behavior in the age-impaired animals using the optical density method is not consistent with several other studies that reliably show increases following behavior in memory-impaired old animals when *Arc* expression per cell in taken into consideration (Small et al., 2004; Penner et al., 2011; Hartzell et al., 2013; Hernandez et al., 2018).

In a recent study, the transcription of several IEGs (*Arc*, *c-fos*, *Homer1a*, and *Nptx2/Narp*) were quantified using RT-PCR in young (6 month) and aged (24 month) male Long Evans rats. In this study, basal levels of *Arc* were elevated in aged-impaired rats compared with young and aged-unimpaired animals. Furthermore, only the young and aged-unimpaired rats showed elevated *Arc* expression following behavior (Myrum et al., 2020). These findings are in direct contradiction to the observations made from RT-PCR by Penner et al. (2011), and the in situ hybridization results from both Penner et al. (2011) and Fletcher et al. (2014). The reason for this discrepancy remains to be determined. For *Homer1a* and *Nptx2/Narp* there are no differences in baseline or behavioral conditions between age groups, nor did behavior increase expression. For *c-fos*, baseline expression was comparable across age groups, but the aged-impaired rats did not show a significant increase following behavior, while the other groups did (Myrum et al., 2020). Another study that examined *c-fos* in young (9 months) and aged (24 months) male F344 rats reported that at baseline the same numbers of cells transcribed *c-fos* in young and aged rats, but the amount of transcript per cell was reduced (Chawla et al., 2013). Spatial behavior led to an increase in *c-fos* expression with a similar proportion of pyramidal cells expressing *c-fos* between age groups. Again, the amount of mRNA per cell measured by RT-PCR was reduced in the old animals. This pattern of results is similar to what Penner et al. (2011) reported for *Arc* expression in young and aged rats. In this same study (Chawla et al., 2013), the investigators also induced ceiling levels of *c-fos* expression using maximal electroconvulsive shock stimulation. Thirty minutes after stimulation, similar proportions of cells were positive for *c-fos* in young and aged rats, although there was less transcript per cell in the aged rats. By 60 minutes post stimulation, the aged rats had a lower number of cells that were *c-fos* positive in addition

to the lower mRNA levels, suggesting more rapid degradation kinetics in aged animals (Chawla et al., 2013).

RNA levels and the methylation state of the *zif268* gene in CA1 have been examined in young (9–12 months) and aged (24–32 months) memory impaired male F344 rats. When animals were sacrificed without a behavioral experience, older rats showed reduced *zif268* mRNA per cell, but no change in the methylation state in over 20 different CpG sites compared with young rats (Penner et al., 2016). Following behavior, there were no significant differences in *zif268* mRNA levels per cell, but the aged rats had increased methylation at 3 CpG sites on the *zif268* gene relative to the young rats (Penner et al., 2016). The epigenetic regulation of *zif268* has also been examined in aged (~19 months) and young (~3 months) male and female C57BL/6J mice. Mice performed an object-location memory task, and behavior-induced gene expression was measured with RNA sequence analysis. Four genes were described as showing reduced behavior-induction that included *zif268*, *Per1*, *Nr4a1*, and *Tsc22d3* (Kwapis et al., 2018; Kwapis et al., 2019). Because the expression of each of these genes is regulated by the histone deacetylase HDAC3, the authors hypothesized that knocking down HDAC3 expression in dorsal CA1 could improve long-term memory on the object-location task and restore gene expression patterns in the old animals. This manipulation did in fact improve behavior and restore gene expression in old mice (Kwapis et al., 2019). A final study that examined the expression of *zif268* in young (8 months) and aged (25 months) male Long Evans rats only compared young to aged-unimpaired groups (Branch et al., 2019). Using quantitative in situ hybridization, the authors reported that a novel environmental configuration increased *zif268* expression in both age groups. Expression levels of *Gad1* were also measured and age group differences were reported. For the aged-unimpaired animals, *Gad1* levels increased after exploration, while levels decreased for the young rats (Branch et al., 2019). No explanation for these observations were offered by these authors.

15.9.4 Summary

There has been exponential growth in the number of approaches available for examining how aging alters gene expression. This has led to the potential for increased precision in identifying subregion and cellular specificity of age-related changes. Along with enhanced specificity, newer methods can provide insights simultaneously into DNA, RNA, and protein changes, offering an expansive landscape of the molecular networks that control cell function. The next challenge is going to be to discover how age-related alterations in identified gene pathways are associated with impaired cognition. In many ways, the new limitation becomes the necessity for investigators to develop and implement sophisticated bioinformatic approaches to aid in the interpretation and understanding of massive and complex datasets in the context of behavior.

15.10 Conclusions

The authors of this chapter took a comparative approach to comprehensively review documented cognitive changes in hippocampus-dependent behavior, and neurobiological alterations in the hippocampus during normative aging. It is truly astonishing the extent to which a consistent picture emerged of age-related changes in the hippocampus across widely different species. While we were confident that some cross-species consensus would be found, we did not imagine, at the beginning of writing this chapter 4 years ago, the consistency with which humans, monkeys, rabbits, and rodents would show fundamentally similar patterns of hippocampus preservation or vulnerability. In fact, given the remarkably different life expectancies, exposures, and disease vulnerabilities, a stronger initial hypothesis might have been that there would be dramatic and explicit differences in hippocampus changes between species with different lifespans. While fundamental aging processes appear to be similar across mammals, humans appear to be unique in our vulnerability to diseases that impact the hippocampus. A prime example is the fact that animals other than humans do not spontaneously show total hippocampus-dependent memory loss in the course of aging, as occurs during Alzheimer's disease and related dementias.

For the species in which data are available and reviewed here, there is no massive cell loss, deterioration of neuronal morphology, or biophysical changes in normative aging. Across these animals, there are subtle changes in synaptic contacts, receptor distribution, ensemble dynamics, and gene expression that relate to cognitive status on hippocampus-dependent tasks. Less than 50 years ago, it was believed that old age was associated with neurodegeneration that inevitably led to dementia. An important take-home message from this chapter is that age-related alterations are subtle and hippocampus-subregion-specific. In fact, the aged hippocampus retains a remarkable ability to undergo plastic change to support adaptive behaviors out to very old ages.

Acknowledgments

The authors would like to acknowledge and thank the McKnight Brain Research Foundation and the National Institute on Aging RO1AG003376, RO1AG081767, R01AG049722 and RF1AG060977 for their support.

REFERENCES

Aarts E, Verhage M, Veenvliet JV, Dolan CV, van der Sluis S (2014) A solution to dependency: using multilevel analysis to accommodate nested data. Nat Neurosci 17:491–496.

Acsády L, Halasy K, Freund T (1993) Calretinin is present in non-pyramidal cells of the rat hippocampus: III. Their inputs from the median raphe and medial septal nuclei. Neuroscience 52:829–841.

Adams MM, Donohue HS, Linville MC, Iversen EA, Newton IG, Brunso-Bechtold JK (2010) Age-related synapse loss in hippocampal CA3 is not reversed by caloric restriction. Neuroscience 171:373–382.

Adams MM, Shi L, Linville MC, Forbes ME, Long AB, Bennett C, Newton IG, Carter CS, Sonntag WE, Riddle DR, et al. (2008) Caloric restriction and age affect synaptic proteins in hippocampal CA3 and spatial learning ability. Exp Neurol 211:141–149.

Adolfsson R, Gottfries CG, Roos BE, Winblad B (1979) Post-mortem distribution of dopamine and homovanillic acid in human brain, variations related to age, and a review of the literature. J Neural Transm 45:81–105.

Aggleton JP, Nelson AJ (2020) Distributed interactive brain circuits for object-in-place memory: A place for time? Brain Neurosci Adv 4:2398212820933471.

Agster KL, Burwell RD (2013) Hippocampal and subicular efferents and afferents of the perirhinal, postrhinal, and entorhinal cortices of the rat. Behav Brain Res 254:50–64.

Ahmed OJ, Mehta MR (2012) Running speed alters the frequency of hippocampal gamma oscillations. J Neurosci 32:7373–7383.

Allen SJ, Benton JS, Goodhardt MJ, Haan EA, Sims NR, Smith CC, Spillane JA, Bowen DM, Davison AN (1983) Biochemical evidence of selective nerve cell changes in the normal ageing human and rat brain. J Neurochem 41:256–265.

Amaral DG, Lavenex P (2007) Hippocampal neuroanatomy. In: The Hippocampus Book (Andersen P, Morris RG, Amaral DG, Bliss TV, O'Keefe J, eds), pp 37–131. Oxford: Oxford University Press.

Amenta F, Mignini F, Ricci A, Sabbatini M, Tomassoni D, Tayebati SK (2001) Age-related changes of dopamine receptors in the rat hippocampus: a light microscope autoradiography study. Mech Ageing Dev 122:2071–2083.

Andrade R, Nicoll RA (1987) Pharmacologically distinct actions of serotonin on single pyramidal neurones of the rat hippocampus recorded in vitro. J Physiol 394:99–124.

Andreose JS, Fumagalli G, Clementi F (1994) On the effect of ageing on the distribution of vasoactive intestinal polypeptide and calcitonin gene-related peptide in the rat brain. Neurosci Lett 171:167–171.

Antonova E, Parslow D, Brammer M, Dawson G, Jackson S, Morris R (2009) Age-related neural activity during allocentric spatial memory. Memory 17:125–143.

Araki T, Kato H, Shuto K, Fujiwara T, Itoyama Y (1997) Effect of aging on dopaminergic receptors and uptake sites in the rat brain studied by receptor autoradiography. J Neurol Sci 148:131–137.

Araki T, Kato H, Shuto K, Itoyama Y (1997) Age-related changes in [3H]nimodipine and [3H]rolipram binding in the rat brain. J Pharm Pharmacol 49:310–314.

Araujo D, Lapchak P, Meaney M, Collier B, Quirion R (1990) Effects of aging on nicotinic and muscarinic autoreceptor function in the rat brain: relationship to presynaptic cholinergic markers and binding sites. J Neurosci 10:3069–3078.

Arias-Cavieres A, Adasme T, Sánchez G, Muñoz P, Hidalgo C (2017) Aging impairs hippocampal- dependent recognition memory and LTP and prevents the associated RyR up-regulation. Front Aging Neurosci 9:111.

Armstrong DM, Sheffield R, Buzsaki G, Chen KS, Hersh LB, Nearing B, Gage FH (1993) Morphologic alterations of choline acetyltransferase-positive neurons in the basal forebrain of aged behaviorally characterized Fisher 344 rats. Neurobiol Aging 14:457–470.

Aubert I, Rowe W, Meaney MJ, Gauthier S, Quirion R (1995) Cholinergic markers in aged cognitively impaired Long-Evans rats. Neuroscience 67:277–292.

Auger SD, Mullally SL, Maguire EA (2012) Retrosplenial cortex codes for permanent landmarks. PloS One 7:e43620.

Azmitia EC, Segal M (1978) An autoradiographic analysis of the differential ascending projections of the dorsal and median raphe nuclei in the rat. J Comp Neurol 179:641–667.

Bach ME, Barad M, Son H, Zhuo M, Lu YF, Shih R, Mansuy I, Hawkins RD, Kandel ER (1999) Age-related defects in spatial memory are correlated with defects in the late phase of hippocampal long-term potentiation in vitro and are attenuated by drugs that enhance the cAMP signaling pathway. Proc Natl Acad Sci U S A 96:5280–5285.

Bachevalier J, Mishkin M (1986) Visual recognition impairment follows ventromedial but not dorsolateral prefrontal lesions in monkeys. Behav Brain Res 20:249–261.

Badie-Mahdavi H, Behrens M, Rebek J, Bartfai T (2005) Effect of galnon on induction of long-term potentiation in dentate gyrus of C57BL/6 mice. Neuropeptides 39:249–251.

Bai L, Hof PR, Standaert DG, Xing Y, Nelson SE, Young AB, Magnusson KR (2004) Changes in the expression of the NR2B subunit during aging in macaque monkeys. Neurobiol Aging 25:201–208.

Bakker A, Albert MS, Krauss G, Speck CL, Gallagher M (2015) Response of the medial temporal lobe network in amnestic mild cognitive impairment to therapeutic intervention assessed by fMRI and memory task performance. Neuroimage Clin 7:688–698.

Bakker A, Krauss GL, Albert MS, Speck CL, Jones LR, Stark CE, Yassa MA, Bassett SS, Shelton AL, Gallagher M (2012) Reduction of hippocampal hyperactivity improves cognition in amnestic mild cognitive impairment. *Neuron* 74:467–474.

Banerjee S, Poddar MK (2016) Aging-induced changes in brain regional serotonin receptor binding: effect of Carnosine. *Neuroscience* 319:79–91.

Bañuelos C, Kittleson JR, LaNasa KH, Galiano CS, Roth SM, Perez EJ, Long JM, Roberts MT, Fong S, Rapp PR (2023) Cognitive aging and the primate basal forebrain revisited: disproportionate GABAergic vulnerability revealed. *J Neurosci* 43:8425–8441.

Bañuelos C, LaSarge CL, McQuail JA, Hartman JJ, Gilbert RJ, Ormerod BK, Bizon JL (2013) Age-related changes in rostral basal forebrain cholinergic and GABAergic projection neurons: relationship with spatial impairment. *Neurobiol Aging* 34:845–862.

Barnes CA (1979) Memory deficits associated with senescence: a neurophysiological and behavioral study in the rat. *J Comp Physiol Psychol* 93:74–104.

Barnes CA (1987) Neurological and behavioral investigations of memory failure in aging animals. *Int J Neurol* 21–22:130–136.

Barnes CA (1994) Normal aging: regionally specific changes in hippocampal synaptic transmission. *Trends Neurosci* 17:13–18.

Barnes CA, Danysz W, Parsons CG (1996) Effects of the uncompetitive NMDA receptor antagonist memantine on hippocampal long-term potentiation, short-term exploratory modulation and spatial memory in awake, freely moving rats. *Eur J Neurosci* 8:565–571.

Barnes CA, Eppich C, Rao G (1989) Selective improvement of aged rat short-term spatial memory by 3, 4-diaminopyridine. *Neurobiol Aging* 10:337–341.

Barnes CA, Forster M, Fleshner M, Ahanotu E, Laudenslager M, Mazzeo R, Maier S, Lal H (1991) Exercise does not modify spatial memory, brain autoimmunity, or antibody response in aged F-344 rats. *Neurobiol Aging* 12:47–53.

Barnes CA, Green EJ, Baldwin J, Johnson WE (1987) Behavioural and neurophysiological examples of functional sparing in senescent rat. *Can J Psychol* 41:131–140.

Barnes CA, Markowska A, Ingram D, Kametani H, Spangler E, Lemken V, Olton D (1990) Acetyl-1-carnitine 2: Effects on learning and memory performance of aged rats in simple and complex mazes. *Neurobiol Aging* 11:499–506.

Barnes CA, McNaughton BL (1979) Neurophysiological comparison of dendritic cable properties in adolescent, middle-aged, and senescent rats. *Exp Aging Res* 5:195–206.

Barnes C, McNaughton B (1980a) Spatial memory and hippocampal synaptic plasticity in senescent and middle-aged rats. *Psychobiol Aging: Problems and Perspectives* 253–272.

Barnes CA, McNaughton BL (1980b) Physiological compensation for loss of afferent synapses in rat hippocampal granule cells during senescence. *J Physiol* 309:473–485.

Barnes CA, McNaughton BL (1985) An age comparison of the rates of acquisition and forgetting of spatial information in relation to long-term enhancement of hippocampal synapses. *Behav Neurosci* 99:1040–1048.

Barnes CA, McNaughton BL, O'Keefe J (1983) Loss of place specificity in hippocampal complex spike cells of senescent rat. *Neurobiol Aging* 4:113–119.

Barnes CA, Nadel L, Honig WK (1980) Spatial memory deficit in senescent rats. *Can J Psychol* 34:29–39.

Barnes CA, Rao G, Foster TC, McNaughton BL (1992) Region-specific age effects on AMPA sensitivity: electrophysiological evidence for loss of synaptic contacts in hippocampal field CA1. *Hippocampus* 2:457–468.

Barnes CA, Rao G, Houston FP (2000) LTP induction threshold change in old rats at the perforant path—granule cell synapse. *Neurobiol Aging* 21:613–620.

Barnes CA, Rao G, McNaughton BL (1987) Increased electrotonic coupling in aged rat hippocampus: a possible mechanism for cellular excitability changes. *J Comp Neurol* 259:549–558.

Barnes CA, Rao G, McNaughton BL (1996) Functional integrity of NMDA-dependent LTP induction mechanisms across the lifespan of F-344 rats. *Learn Mem* 3:124–137.

Barnes CA, Rao G, Orr G (2000) Age-related decrease in the Schaffer collateral-evoked EPSP in awake, freely behaving rats. *Neural Plast* 7:167–178.

Barnes CA, Rao G, Shen J (1997) Age-related decrease in the N-methyl-D-aspartateR-mediated excitatory postsynaptic potential in hippocampal region CA1. *Neurobiol Aging* 18:445–452.

Barnes CA, Suster MS, Shen J, McNaughton BL (1997) Multistability of cognitive maps in the hippocampus of old rats. *Nature* 388:272–275.

Barrett GL, Bennie A, Trieu J, Ping S, Tsafoulis C (2009) The chronology of age-related spatial learning impairment in two rat strains, as tested by the Barnes maze. *Behav Neurosci* 123:533.

Barrionuevo G, Schottler F, Lynch G (1980) The effects of repetitive low frequency stimulation on control and "potentiated" synaptic responses in the hippocampus. *Life Sci* 27:2385–2391.

Bartolini L, Casamenti F, Pepeu G (1996) Aniracetam restores object recognition impaired by age, scopolamine, and nucleus basalis lesions. *Pharmacol Biochem Behav* 53:277–283.

Bartus RT, Dean RL, Beer B, Lippa AS (1982) The cholinergic hypothesis of geriatric memory dysfunction. *Science* 217:408–414.

Baskerville KA, Kent C, Nicolle MM, Gallagher M, McKinney M (2006) Aging causes partial loss of basal forebrain but no loss of pontine reticular cholinergic neurons. *Neuroreport* 17:1819–1823.

Baskys A, Niesen CE, Carlen PL (1987) Altered modulatory actions of serotonin on dentate granule cells of aged rats. *Brain Res* 419:112–118.

Battaglia S, Garofalo S, di Pellegrino G (2018) Context-dependent extinction of threat memories: influences of healthy aging. *Sci Rep* 8:1–13.

Baxter MG, Bucci DJ, Gorman LK, Wiley RG, Gallagher M (1995) Selective immunotoxic lesions of basal forebrain cholinergic cells: effects on learning and memory in rats. *Behav Neurosci* 109:714–722.

Baxter MG, Frick KM, Price DL, Breckler SJ, Markowska AL, Gorman LK (1999) Presynaptic markers of cholinergic function in the rat brain: relationship with age and cognitive status. *Neuroscience* 89:771–779.

Baxter MG, Murray EA (2001a) Impairments in visual discrimination learning and recognition memory produced by neurotoxic lesions of rhinal cortex in rhesus monkeys. *Eur J Neurosci* 13:1228–1238.

Baxter MG, Murray EA (2001b) Opposite relationship of hippocampal and rhinal cortex damage to delayed nonmatching-to-sample deficits in monkeys. *Hippocampus* 11:61–71.

Beason-Held LL, Rosene DL, Killiany RJ, Moss MB (1999) Hippocampal formation lesions produce memory impairment in the rhesus monkey. *Hippocampus* 9:562–574.

Beatty WW, Bierley RA, Boyd JG (1985) Preservation of accurate spatial memory in aged rats. *Neurobiol Aging* 6:219–225.

Benice TS, Rizk A, Kohama S, Pfankuch T, Raber J (2006) Sex-differences in age-related cognitive decline in C57BL/6J mice associated with increased brain microtubule-associated protein 2 and synaptophysin immunoreactivity. *Neuroscience* 137:413–423.

Bennett IJ, Stark CE (2016) Mnemonic discrimination relates to perforant path integrity: An ultra-high resolution diffusion tensor imaging study. *Neurobiol Learn Mem* 129:107–112.

Bennett JC, McRae PA, Levy LJ, Frick KM (2006) Long-term continuous, but not daily, environmental enrichment reduces spatial memory decline in aged male mice. *Neurobiol Learn Mem* 85:139–152.

Berger-Mandelbaum A, Magen H (2019) Self-initiated object-location memory in young and older adults. *Aging, Neuropsychol, and Cogn* 26:58–85.

Bernstein D, Olton DS, Ingram DK, Waller SB, Reynolds MA, London ED (1985) Radial maze performance in young and aged mice: neurochemical correlates. *Pharmacol Biochem Behav* 22:301–307.

Berthele A, Platzer S, Dworzak D, Schadrack J, Mahal B, Büttner A, Assmus H, Wurster K, Zieglgänsberger W, Conrad B (2003) [3H]-nociceptin ligand-binding and nociceptin opioid receptor mRNA expression in the human brain. *Neuroscience* 121:629–640.

Bethus I, Tse D, Morris RG (2010) Dopamine and memory: modulation of the persistence of memory for novel hippocampal NMDA receptor-dependent paired associates. *J Neurosci* 30:1610–1618.

Bickford-Wimer PC, Miller JA, Freedman R, Rose GM (1988) Age-related reduction in responses of rat hippocampal neurons to locally applied monoamines. *Neurobiol Aging* 9:173–179.

Biegon A, Greenberger V, Segal M (1986) Quantitative histochemistry of brain acetylcholinesterase and learning rate in the aged rat. *Neurobiol Aging* 7:215–217.

Bienenstock EL, Cooper LN, Munro PW (1982) Theory for the development of neuron selectivity: orientation specificity and binocular interaction in visual cortex. *J Neurosci* 2:32–48.

Bigl V, Arendt T, Fischer S, Werner M, Arendt A (1987) The cholinergic system in aging. *Gerontology* 33:172–180.

Billard JM, Rouaud E (2007) Deficit of NMDA receptor activation in CA1 hippocampal area of aged rats is rescued by D-cycloserine. *Eur J Neurosci* 25:2260–2268.

Birch AM, Kelly ÁM (2019) Lifelong environmental enrichment in the absence of exercise protects the brain from age-related cognitive decline. *Neuropharmacology* 145:59–74.

Birthelmer A, Stemmelin J, Jackisch R, Cassel JC (2003) Presynaptic modulation of acetylcholine, noradrenaline, and serotonin release in the hippocampus of aged rats with various levels of memory impairments. *Brain Res Bull* 60:283–296.

Bitencourt RM, de Souza ACG, Bicca MA, Pamplona FA, de Mello N, Passos GF, Medeiros R, Takahashi RN, Calixto JB, Prediger RD (2017) Blockade of hippocampal bradykinin B1 receptors improves spatial learning and memory deficits in middle-aged rats. *Behav Brain Res* 316:74–81.

Bizon JL, Gallagher M (2003) Production of new cells in the rat dentate gyrus over the lifespan: relation to cognitive decline. *Eur J Neurosci* 18:215–219.

Bizon JL, Gallagher M (2005) More is less: neurogenesis and age-related cognitive decline in Long-Evans rats. *Sci Aging Knowledge Environ* 2005:re2.

Bizon JL, LaSarge CL, Montgomery KS, McDermott AN, Setlow B, Griffith WH (2009) Spatial reference and working memory across the lifespan of male Fischer 344 rats. *Neurobiol Aging* 30:646–655.

Bizon JL, Lee HJ, Gallagher M (2004) Neurogenesis in a rat model of age-related cognitive decline. *Aging Cell* 3:227–234.

Blalock EM, Chen KC, Sharrow K, Herman JP, Porter NM, Foster TC, Landfield PW (2003) Gene microarrays in hippocampal aging: statistical profiling identifies novel processes correlated with cognitive impairment. *J Neurosci* 23:3807–3819.

Blanchard RJ, Blanchard DC (1969) Crouching as an index of fear. *J Comp Physiol Psychology* 67:370.

Blank T, Nijholt I, Kye M-J, Radulovic J, Spiess J (2003) Small-conductance, Ca 2+-activated K+ channel SK3 generates age-related memory and LTP deficits. *Nat Neurosci* 6:911–912.

Blin J, Baron JC, Dubois B, Crouzel C, Fiorelli M, Attar-Lévy D, Pillon B, Fournier D, Vidailhet M, Agid Y (1993) Loss of brain 5-HT2 receptors in Alzheimer's disease: in vivo assessment with positron emission tomography and [18F]setoperone. *Brain* 116(Pt 3): 497–510.

Bliss TV, Gardner-Medwin AR (1973) Long-lasting potentiation of synaptic transmission in the dentate area of the unanaesthetized rabbit following stimulation of the perforant path. *J Physiol* 232:357–374.

Bliss TV, Lomo T (1973) Long-lasting potentiation of synaptic transmission in the dentate area of the anaesthetized rabbit following stimulation of the perforant path. *J Physiol* 232:331–356.

Bodhinathan K, Kumar A, Foster TC (2010a) Intracellular redox state alters NMDA receptor response during aging through Ca2+/calmodulin-dependent protein kinase II. *J Neurosci* 30:1914–1924.

Bodhinathan K, Kumar A, Foster TC (2010b) Redox sensitive calcium stores underlie enhanced after hyperpolarization of aged neurons: role for ryanodine receptor mediated calcium signaling. *J Neurophysiol* 104:2586–2593.

Bohbot VD, McKenzie S, Konishi K, Fouquet C, Kurdi V, Schachar R, Boivin M, Robaey P (2012) Virtual navigation strategies from childhood to senescence: evidence for changes across the life span. *Front Aging Neurosci* 4:28.

Bondareff W, Geinisman Y (1976) Loss of synapses in the dentate gyrus of the senescent rat. *Am J Anat* 145:129–136.

Borbély E, Scheich B, Helyes Z (2013) Neuropeptides in learning and memory. *Neuropeptides* 47:439–450.

Boric K, Munoz P, Gallagher M, Kirkwood A (2008) Potential adaptive function for altered long-term potentiation mechanisms in aging hippocampus. *J Neurosci* 28:8034–8039.

Bortolatto CF, Wilhelm EA, Chagas PM, Nogueira CW (2012) p-Chloro-diphenyl diselenide, an organoselenium compound, with antidepressant-like and memory enhancer actions in aging male rats. *Biogerontology* 13:237–249.

Bragin A, Jandó G, Nádasdy Z, Hetke J, Wise K, Buzsáki G (1995) Gamma (40–100 Hz) oscillation in the hippocampus of the behaving rat. *J Neurosci* 15:47–60.

Bramham CR, Milgram N, Srebro B (1991) δ Opioid receptor activation is required to induce LTP of synaptic transmission in the lateral perforant path in vivo. *Brain Res* 567:42–50.

Bramham CR, Sarvey JM (1996) Endogenous activation of μ and δ-1 opioid receptors is required for long-term potentiation induction in the lateral perforant path: dependence on GABAergic inhibition. *J Neurosci* 16:8123–8131.

Branch A, Monasterio A, Blair G, Knierim JJ, Gallagher M, Haberman RP (2019) Aged rats with preserved memory dynamically recruit hippocampal inhibition in a local/global cue mismatch environment. *Neurobiol Aging* 76:151–161.

Bridge K, Wainwright A, Reilly K, Oliver K (2003) Autoradiographic localization of 125I [Tyr14] nociceptin/orphanin FQ binding sites in macaque primate CNS. *Neuroscience* 118:513–523.

Brody H (1955) Organization of the cerebral cortex: III. A study of aging in the human cerebral cortex. *J Comp Neurol* 102:511–516.

Browning PG, Baxter MG, Gaffan D (2013) Prefrontal-temporal disconnection impairs recognition memory but not familiarity discrimination. *J Neurosci* 33:9667–9674.

Bucht G, Adolfsson R, Gottfries C, Roos B-E, Winblad B (1981) Distribution of 5-hydroxytryptamine and 5-hydroxyindoleacetic acid in human brain in relation to age, drug influence, agonal status and circadian variation. *J Neural Transm* 51:185–203.

Buell SJ, Coleman PD (1979) Dendritic growth in the aged human brain and failure of growth in senile dementia. *Science* 206:854–856.

Buell SJ, Coleman PD (1981) Quantitative evidence for selective dendritic growth in normal human aging but not in senile dementia. *Brain Res* 214:23–41.

Buffalo EA, Ramus SJ, Clark RE, Teng E, Squire LR, Zola SM (1999) Dissociation between the effects of damage to perirhinal cortex and area TE. *Learn Mem* 6:572–599.

Burger C, Lopez MC, Feller JA, Baker HV, Muzyczka N, Mandel RJ (2007) Changes in transcription within the CA1 field of the hippocampus are associated with age-related spatial learning impairments. *Neurobiol Learn Mem* 87:21–41.

Burgevin M-C, Loquet I, Quarteronet D, Habert-Ortoli E (1995) Cloning, pharmacological characterization, and anatomical distribution of a rat cDNA encoding for a galanin receptor. *J Mol Neurosci* 6:33–41.

Burke SN, Barnes CA (2006) Neural plasticity in the ageing brain. *Nat Rev Neurosci* 7:30–40.

Burke SN, Maurer AP, Hartzell AL, Nematollahi S, Uprety A, Wallace JL, Barnes CA (2012) Representation of three-dimensional objects by the rat perirhinal cortex. *Hippocampus* 22:2032–2044.

Burke SN, Maurer AP, Nematollahi S, Uprety AR, Wallace JL, Barnes CA (2011) The influence of objects on place field expression and size in distal hippocampal CA1. *Hippocampus* 21:783–801.

Burke SN, Maurer AP, Nematollahi S, Uprety A, Wallace JL, Barnes CA (2014) Advanced age dissociates dual functions of the perirhinal cortex. *J Neurosci* 34:467–480.

Burke SN, Maurer AP, Yang Z, Navratilova Z, Barnes CA (2008) Glutamate receptor-mediated restoration of experience-dependent place field expansion plasticity in aged rats. *Behav Neurosci* 122:535–548.

Burke SN, Wallace JL, Hartzell AL, Nematollahi S, Plange K, Barnes CA (2011) Age-associated deficits in pattern separation functions of the perirhinal cortex: a cross-species consensus. *Behav Neurosci* 125:836–847.

Burke SN, Wallace JL, Nematollahi S, Uprety AR, Barnes CA (2010) Pattern separation deficits may contribute to age-associated recognition impairments. *Behav Neurosci* 124:559–573.

Burnett DM, Bowyer JF, Masserano JM, Zahniser NR (1990) Effect of aging on alpha-1 adrenergic stimulation of phosphoinositide hydrolysis in various regions of rat brain. *J Pharmacol Exp Ther* 255:1265–1270.

Buss EW, Corbett NJ, Roberts JG, Ybarra N, Musial TF, Simkin D, Molina-Campos E, Oh K-J, Nielsen LL, Ayala GD (2021) Cognitive aging is associated with redistribution of synaptic weights in the hippocampus. *Proc Natl Acad Sci U S A* 118:1–10.

Butler AA, Tam CS, Stanhope KL, Wolfe BM, Ali MR, O'Keeffe M, St-Onge M-P, Ravussin E, Havel PJ (2012) Low circulating adropin concentrations with obesity and aging correlate with risk factors for metabolic disease and increase after gastric bypass surgery in humans. *J Clin Endocrinol Metab* 97:3783–3791.

Buzsaki G, Anastassiou CA, Koch C (2012) The origin of extracellular fields and currents—EEG, ECoG, LFP and spikes. *Nat Rev Neurosci* 13:407–420.

Buzsaki G, Leung LW, Vanderwolf CH (1983) Cellular bases of hippocampal EEG in the behaving rat. *Brain Res* 287:139–171.

Cabello CR, Thune JJ, Pakkenberg H, Pakkenberg B (2002) Ageing of substantia nigra in humans: cell loss may be compensated by hypertrophy. *Neuropathol Appl Neurobiol* 28:283–291.

Cadacio CL, Milner TA, Gallagher M, Pierce JP, Cadiacio CL (2003) Hilar neuropeptide Y interneuron loss in the aged rat hippocampal formation. *Exp Neurol* 183:147–158.

Caffe AR, Van Leeuwen F (1983) Vasopressin-immunoreactive cells in the dorsomedial hypothalamic region, medial amygdaloid nucleus and locus coeruleus of the rat. *Cell Tissue Res* 233:23–33.

Calhoun ME, Fletcher BR, Yi S, Zentko DC, Gallagher M, Rapp PR (2008) Age-related spatial learning impairment is unrelated to spinophilin immunoreactive spine number and protein levels in rat hippocampus. *Neurobiol Aging* 29:1256–1264.

Calhoun ME, Kurth D, Phinney AL, Long JM, Hengemihle J, Mouton PR, Ingram DK, Jucker M (1998) Hippocampal neuron and synaptophysin-positive bouton number in aging C57BL/6 mice. *Neurobiol Aging* 19:599–606.

Calhoun ME, Mao Y, Roberts JA, Rapp PR (2004) Reduction in hippocampal cholinergic innervation is unrelated to recognition memory impairment in aged rhesus monkeys. *J Comp Neurol* 475:238–246.

Campbell LW, Hao SY, Thibault O, Blalock EM, Landfield PW (1996) Aging changes in voltage-gated calcium currents in hippocampal CA1 neurons. *J Neurosci* 16:6286–6295.

Canas PM, Duarte JM, Rodrigues RJ, Köfalvi A, Cunha RA (2009) Modification upon aging of the density of presynaptic modulation systems in the hippocampus. *Neurobiol Aging* 30:1877–1884.

Caprioli A, Ghirardi O, Giuliani A, Ramacci MT, Angelucci L (1991) Spatial learning and memory in the radial maze: a longitudinal study in rats from 4 to 25 months of age. *Neurobiol Aging* 12:605–607.

Carr VA, Bernstein JD, Favila SE, Rutt BK, Kerchner GA, Wagner AD (2017) Individual differences in associative memory among older adults explained by hippocampal subfield structure and function. *Proc Natl Acad Sci U S A* 114:12075–12080.

Cavoy A, Delacour J (1993) Spatial but not object recognition is impaired by aging in rats. *Physiol Behav* 53:527–530.

Cechella JL, Leite MR, Rosario AR, Sampaio TB, Zeni G (2014) Diphenyl diselenide-supplemented diet and swimming exercise enhance novel object recognition memory in old rats. *Age (Dordr)* 36:9666.

Cès A, Burg T, Herbeaux K, Héraud C, Bott JB, Mensah-Nyagan AG, Mathis C (2018) Age-related vulnerability of pattern separation in C57BL/6J mice. *Neurobiol Aging* 62:120–129.

Cha CI, Lee YI, Lee EY, Park KH, Baik SH (1997) Age-related changes of VIP, NPY and somatostatin-immunoreactive neurons in the cerebral cortex of aged rats. *Brain Res* 753:235–244.

Chalfonte BL, Johnson MK (1996) Feature memory and binding in young and older adults. *Mem Cogn* 24:403–416.

Chandran R, Kumar M, Kesavan L, Jacob RS, Gunasekaran S, Lakshmi S, Sadasivan C, Omkumar RV (2017) Cellular calcium signaling in the aging brain. *J Chem Neuroanat* 95:95–114.

Chan-Palay V, Asan E (1989) Quantitation of catecholamine neurons in the locus coeruleus in human brains of normal young and older adults and in depression. *J Comp Neurol* 287:357–372.

Chapter MC, White CM, DeRidder A, Chadwick W, Martin B, Maudsley S (2010) Chemical modification of class II G protein-coupled receptor ligands: frontiers in the development of peptide analogs as neuroendocrine pharmacological therapies. *Pharmacol Ther* 125:39–54.

Chawla MK, Gray DT, Nguyen C, Dhaliwal H, Zempare M, Okuno H, Huentelman MJ, Barnes CA (2018) Seizure-induced Arc mRNA expression thresholds in rat hippocampus and perirhinal cortex. *Front Syst Neurosci* 12:53.

Chawla MK, Penner MR, Olson KM, Sutherland VL, Mittelman-Smith MA, Barnes CA (2013) Spatial behavior and seizure-induced changes in c-fos mRNA expression in young and old rats. *Neurobiol Aging* 34:1184–1198.

Chen L, Francisco TR, Baggetta AM, Zaki Y, Ramirez S, Clem RL, Shuman T, Cai DJ (2023) Ensemble-specific deficit in neuronal intrinsic excitability in aged mice. *Neurobiol Aging* 123:92–97.

Chen Y, Branch A, Shuai C, Gallagher M, Knierim JJ (2024) Object-place-context learning impairment correlates with spatial learning impairment in aged Long-Evans rats. *Hippocampus* 34:88–99.

Cheng DT, Faulkner ML, Disterhoft JF, Desmond JE (2010) The effects of aging in delay and trace human eyeblink conditioning. *Psychol Aging* 25:684.

Chieffi S, Carotenuto M, Monda V, Valenzano A, Villano I, Precenzano F, Tafuri D, Salerno M, Filippi N, Nuccio F (2017) Orexin system: the key for a healthy life. *Front Physiol* 8:357.

Chouinard ML, Gallagher M, Yasuda RP, Wolfe BB, McKinney M (1995) Hippocampal muscarinic receptor function in spatial learning-impaired aged rats. *Neurobiol Aging* 16:955–963.

Chowdhury S, Shepherd JD, Okuno H, Lyford G, Petralia RS, Plath N, Kuhl D, Huganir RL, Worley PF (2006) Arc/Arg3.1 interacts with the endocytic machinery to regulate AMPA receptor trafficking. *Neuron* 52:445–459.

Chui HC, Bondareff W, Zarow C, Slager U (1984) Stability of neuronal number in the human nucleus basalis of Meynert with age. *Neurobiol Aging* 5:83–88.

Cilz NI, Cymerblit-Sabba A, Young WS (2019) Oxytocin and vasopressin in the rodent hippocampus. *Genes Brain Behav* 18:e12535.

Cohen SJ, Munchow AH, Rios LM, Zhang G, Asgeirsdottir HN, Stackman RW, Jr. (2013) The rodent hippocampus is essential for nonspatial object memory. *Curr Biol* 23:1685–1690.

Cole AJ, Saffen DW, Baraban JM, Worley PF (1989) Rapid increase of an immediate early gene messenger RNA in hippocampal neurons by synaptic NMDA receptor activation. *Nature* 340:474–476.

Collier TJ, Greene JG, Felten DL, Stevens SY, Collier KS (2004) Reduced cortical noradrenergic neurotransmission is associated with increased neophobia and impaired spatial memory in aged rats. *Neurobiol Aging* 25:209–221.

Collier TJ, Lipton J, Daley BF, Palfi S, Chu Y, Sortwell C, Bakay RA, Sladek JR, Kordower JH (2007) Aging-related changes in the nigrostriatal dopamine system and the response to MPTP in non-human primates: diminished compensatory mechanisms as a prelude to parkinsonism. *Neurobiol Dis* 26:56–65.

Collingridge GL, Kehl SJ, McLennan H (1983) The antagonism of amino acid-induced excitations of rat hippocampal CA1 neurones in vitro. *J Physiol* 334:19–31.

Comrie AE, Gray DT, Smith AC, Barnes CA (2018) Different macaque models of cognitive aging exhibit task-dependent behavioral disparities. *Behav Brain Res* 344:110–119.

Cooper LN, Bear MF (2012) The BCM theory of synapse modification at 30: interaction of theory with experiment. *Nat Rev Neurosci* 13:798–810.

Cope D, Maccaferri G, Marton L, Roberts J, Cobden P, Somogyi P (2002) Cholecystokinin-immunopositive basket and Schaffer collateral-associated interneurones target different domains of pyramidal cells in the CA1 area of the rat hippocampus. *Neuroscience* 109:63–80.

Coughlin JM, Du Y, Rosenthal HB, Slania S, Min Koo S, Park A, Solomon G, Vranesic M, Antonsdottir I, Speck CL, et al. (2018) The distribution of the alpha7 nicotinic acetylcholine receptor in healthy aging: An in vivo positron emission tomography study with. *Neuroimage* 165:118–124.

Coughlin JM, Slania S, Du Y, Rosenthal HB, Lesniak WG, Minn I, Smith GS, Dannals RF, Kuwabara H, Wong DF, et al. (2018) F-XTRA PET for enhanced imaging of the extrathalamic α4β2 nicotinic acetylcholine receptor. *J Nucl Med* 59:1603–1608.

Coultrap SJ, Bickford PC, Browning MD (2008) Blueberry-enriched diet ameliorates age-related declines in NMDA receptor-dependent LTP. *Age* 30:263–272.

Court J, Lloyd S, Johnson M, Griffiths M, Birdsall N, Piggott M, Oakley A, Ince P, Perry E, Perry R (1997) Nicotinic and muscarinic cholinergic receptor binding in the human hippocampal formation during development and aging. *Dev Brain Res* 101:93–105.

Court JA, Perry EK, Johnson M, Piggott MA, Kerwin JA, Perry RH, Ince PG (1993) Regional patterns of cholinergic and glutamate activity in the developing and aging human brain. *Brain Res Dev Brain Res* 74:73–82.

Cowen SL, Gray DT, Wiegand JL, Schimanski LA, Barnes CA (2020) Age-associated changes in waking hippocampal sharp-wave ripples. *Hippocampus* 30:28–38.

Croll SD, Chesnutt CR, Greene NA, Lindsay RM, Wiegand SJ (1999) Peptide immunoreactivity in aged rat cortex and hippocampus as a function of memory and BDNF infusion. *Pharmacol Biochem Behav* 64:625–635.

Crown LM, Gray DT, Schimanski LA, Barnes CA, Cowen SL (2022) Aged rats exhibit altered behavior-induced oscillatory activity, place cell firing rates, and spatial information content in the CA1 region of the hippocampus. *J Neurosci* 42:4505–4516.

Curcio CA, Hinds JW (1983) Stability of synaptic density and spine volume in dentate gyrus of aged rats. *Neurobiol Aging* 4:77–87.

Curlik DM, 2nd, Weiss C, Nicholson DA, Disterhoft JF (2014) Age-related impairments on one hippocampal-dependent task predict impairments on a subsequent hippocampal-dependent task. *Behav Neurosci* 128:676.

Dahl D, Sarvey JM (1989) Norepinephrine induces pathway-specific long-lasting potentiation and depression in the hippocampal dentate gyrus. *Proc Natl Acad Sci U S A* 86:4776–4780.

Dahl MJ, Mather M, Düzel S, Bodammer NC, Lindenberger U, Kühn S, Werkle-Bergner M (2019) Rostral locus coeruleus integrity is associated with better memory performance in older adults. *Nat Hum Behav* 3:1203–1214.

Damrongthai C, Kuwamizu R, Suwabe K, Ochi G, Yamazaki Y, Fukuie T, Adachi K, Yassa MA, Churdchomjan W, Soya H (2021) Benefit of human moderate running boosting mood and executive function coinciding with bilateral prefrontal activation. *Sci Rep* 11:22657.

Davies P (1978) Loss of choline acetyltransferase activity in normal aging and in senile dementia. *Adv Exp Med Biol* 113:251–256.

De Carlos JA, Molnár Z (2019) Cajal's interactions with Sherrington and The Croonian Lecture. *Anat Rec* 303:1181–1188.

Decker MW (1987) The effects of aging on hippocampal and cortical projections of the forebrain cholinergic system. *Brain Res* 434:423–438.

De Lacalle S, Cooper JD, Svendsen CN, Dunnett SB, Sofroniew MV (1996) Reduced retrograde labelling with fluorescent tracer accompanies neuronal atrophy of basal forebrain cholinergic neurons in aged rats. *Neuroscience* 75:19–27.

de Lima MN, Laranja DC, Caldana F, Bromberg E, Roesler R, Schroder N (2005) Reversal of age-related deficits in object recognition memory in rats with l-deprenyl. *Exp Gerontol* 40:506–511.Della Vedova F, Fumagalli F, Sacchetti G, Racagni G, Brunello N (1992) Age-related variations in relative abundance of alternative spliced D2 receptor mRNAs in brain areas of two rat strains. *Brain Res Mol Brain Res* 12:357–359.

den Dunnen WF, Brouwer WH, Bijlard E, Kamphuis J, van Linschoten K, Eggens-Meijer E, Holstege G (2008) No disease in the brain of a 115-year-old woman. *Neurobiol Aging* 29:1127–1132.

Derrick BE, Weinberger SB, Martinez Jr JL (1991) Opioid receptors are involved in an NMDA receptor-independent mechanism of LTP induction at hippocampal mossy fiber-CA3 synapses. *Brain Res Bull* 27:219–223.

de Ruiter JP, Uylings HB (1987) Morphometric and dendritic analysis of fascia dentata granule cells in human aging and senile dementia. *Brain Res* 402:217–229.

Deshmukh SS, Knierim JJ (2011) Representation of non-spatial and spatial information in the lateral entorhinal cortex. *Front Behav Neurosci* 5:69.

deToledo-Morrell L, Geinisman Y, Morrell F (1988) Age-dependent alterations in hippocampal synaptic plasticity: relation to memory disorders. *Neurobiol Aging* 9:581–590.

Deupree DL, Bradley J, Turner DA (1993) Age-related alterations in potentiation in the CA1 region in F344 rats. *Neurobiol Aging* 14:249–258.

Deupree DL, Turner DA, Watters CL (1991) Spatial performance correlates with in vitro potentiation in young and aged Fischer 344 rats. *Brain Res* 554:1–9.

Dhanrajan TM, Lynch MA, Kelly A, Popov VI, Rusakov DA, Stewart MG (2004) Expression of long-term potentiation in aged rats involves perforated synapses but dendritic spine branching results from high-frequency stimulation alone. *Hippocampus* 14:255–264.

Diana G, Domenici MR, Loizzo A, Scotti de Carolis A, Sagratella S (1994) Age and strain differences in rat place learning and hippocampal dentate gyrus frequency-potentiation. *Neurosci Lett* 171:113–116.

Diana G, Scotti de Carolis A, Frank C, Domenici MR, Sagratella S (1994) Selective reduction of hippocampal dentate frequency potentiation in aged rats with impaired place learning. *Brain Res Bull* 35:107–111.

DiCola NM, Lacy AL, Bishr OJ, Kimsey KM, Whitney JL, Lovett SD, Burke SN, Maurer AP (2022) Advanced age has dissociable effects on hippocampal CA1 ripples and CA3 high frequency events in male rats. *Neurobiol Aging* 117:44–58.

Dieguez D, Jr, Barea-Rodriguez EJ (2004) Aging impairs the late phase of long-term potentiation at the medial perforant path-CA3 synapse in awake rats. *Synapse* 52:53–61.

Dillon KA, Gross-Isseroff R, Israeli M, Biegon A (1991) Autoradiographic analysis of serotonin 5-HT1A receptor binding in the human brain postmortem: effects of age and alcohol. *Brain Res* 554:56–64.

Disterhoft JF, Thompson LT, Moyer JR, Jr, Mogul DJ (1996) Calcium-dependent afterhyperpolarization and learning in young and aging hippocampus. *Life Sci* 59:413–420.

Domingos C, Pêgo J, Santos N (2021) Effects of physical activity on brain function and structure in older adults: a systematic review. *Behav Brain Res* 402:113061.

Dondi D, Maggi R, Limonta P, Martini L, Piva F (1992) Binding characteristics of delta opioid receptors in different regions of the brain of young and old male rats as studied with the highly selective ligand [D-PEN 2-D-PEN 5] enkephalin. *Aging Clin Exp Res* 4:69–75.

dos Santos Cardoso F, Tavares CdSO, Araujo BHS, Mansur F, Lopes-Martins RÁB, da Silva SG (2021) Improved spatial memory and neuroinflammatory profile changes in aged rats submitted to photobiomodulation therapy. *Cell Mol Neurobiol* 42:1875–1886.

Douglas RM, Goddard GV (1975) Long-term potentiation of the perforant path-granule cell synapse in the rat hippocampus. *Brain Res* 86:205–215.

Downs JL, Dunn MR, Borok E, Shanabrough M, Horvath TL, Kohama SG, Urbanski HF (2007) Orexin neuronal changes in the locus coeruleus of the aging rhesus macaque. *Neurobiol Aging* 28:1286–1295.

Dravid A (1983) Deficits in cholinergic enzymes and muscarinic receptors in the hippocampus and striatum of senescent rats: effect of chronic hydergine treatment. *Arch Int Pharmacodyn Ther* 264:195–202.

Driscoll I, Sutherland RJ (2005) The aging hippocampus: navigating between rat and human experiments. *Rev Neurosci* 16:87–121.

Dudek SM, Bear MF (1992) Homosynaptic long-term depression in area CA1 of hippocampus and effects of N-methyl-D-aspartate receptor blockade. *Proc Natl Acad Sci U S A* 89:4363–4367.

Dulka BN, Pullins SE, Cullen PK, Moyer JR, Jr, Helmstetter FJ (2020) Age-related memory deficits are associated with changes in protein degradation in brain regions critical for trace fear conditioning. *Neurobiol Aging* 91:160–166.

Duncan MJ, Smith JT, Franklin KM (2018) Time of day but not aging regulates 5-HT. *Neurosci Lett* 662:306–311.

Dutar P, Vaillend C, Viollet C, Billard J-M, Potier B, Carlo A-S, Ungerer A, Epelbaum J (2002) Spatial learning and synaptic hippocampal plasticity in type 2 somatostatin receptor knock-out mice. *Neuroscience* 112:455–466.

Eastwood SL, Burnet PW, McDonald B, Clinton J, Harrison PJ (1994) Synaptophysin gene expression in human brain: a quantitative in situ hybridization and immunocytochemical study. *Neuroscience* 59:881–892.

Eastwood SL, Harrison PJ (1999) Detection and quantification of hippocampal synaptophysin messenger RNA in schizophrenia using autoclaved, formalin-fixed, paraffin wax-embedded sections. *Neuroscience* 93:99–106.

Eastwood SL, Weickert CS, Webster MJ, Herman MM, Kleinman JE, Harrison PJ (2006) Synaptophysin protein and mRNA expression in the human hippocampal formation from birth to old age. *Hippocampus* 16:645–654.

Ekstrom AD, Meltzer J, McNaughton BL, Barnes CA (2001) NMDA receptor antagonism blocks experience-dependent expansion of hippocampal "place fields." *Neuron* 31:631–638.

Emborg ME, Ma SY, Mufson EJ, Levey AI, Taylor MD, Brown WD, Holden JE, Kordower JH (1998) Age-related declines in nigral neuronal function correlate with motor impairments in rhesus monkeys. *J Comp Neurol* 401:253–265.

Ennaceur A, Aggleton JP (1997) The effects of neurotoxic lesions of the perirhinal cortex combined to fornix transection on object recognition memory in the rat. *Behav Brain Res* 88:181–193.

Ennaceur A, Delacour J (1988) A new one-trial test for neurobiological studies of memory in rats: 1: Behavioral data. *Behav Brain Res* 31:47–59.

Ennaceur A, Meliani K (1992) A new one-trial test for neurobiological studies of memory in rats: III. Spatial vs. non-spatial working memory. *Behav Brain Res* 51:83–92.

Ennaceur A, Neave N, Aggleton JP (1997) Spontaneous object recognition and object location memory in rats: the effects of lesions in the cingulate cortices, the medial prefrontal cortex, the cingulum bundle and the fornix. *Exp Brain Res* 113:509–519.

Erbs E, Faget L, Scherrer G, Kessler P, Hentsch D, Vonesch J-L, Matifas A, Kieffer B, Massotte D (2012) Distribution of delta opioid receptor-expressing neurons in the mouse hippocampus. *Neuroscience* 221:203–213.

Erickson KI, Voss MW, Prakash RS, Basak C, Szabo A, Chaddock L, Kim JS, Heo S, Alves H, White SM (2011) Exercise training increases size of hippocampus and improves memory. *Proc Natl Acad Sci U S A* 108:3017–3022.

Etchamendy N, Konishi K, Pike GB, Marighetto A, Bohbot VD (2012) Evidence for a virtual human analog of a rodent relational memory task: a study of aging and fMRI in young adults. *Hippocampus* 22:869–880.

Evans AK, Park HH, Saw NL, Singhal K, Ogawa G, Leib RD, Shamloo M (2021) Age-related neuroinflammation and pathology in the locus coeruleus and hippocampus: beta-adrenergic antagonists exacerbate impairment of learning and memory in aged mice. *Neurobiol Aging* 106:241–256.

Evans GW, Brennan PL, Skorpanich MA, Held D (1984) Cognitive mapping and elderly adults: verbal and location memory for urban landmarks. *J Gerontol* 39:452–457.

Fearnley JM, Lees AJ (1991) Ageing and Parkinson's disease: substantia nigra regional selectivity. *Brain* 114:2283–2301.

Finkbiner RG, Woodruff-Pak DS (1991) Classical eyeblink conditioning in adulthood: effects of age and interstimulus interval on acquisition in the trace paradigm. *Psychol Aging* 6:109–117.

Finnema SJ, Nabulsi NB, Eid T, Detyniecki K, Lin SF, Chen MK, Dhaher R, Matuskey D, Baum E, Holden D, et al. (2016) Imaging synaptic density in the living human brain. *Sci Transl Med* 8:348ra396.

Fischer W, Chen KS, Gage FH, Björklund A (1992) Progressive decline in spatial learning and integrity of forebrain cholinergic neurons in rats during aging. *Neurobiol Aging* 13:9–23.

Fischer W, Gage FH, Björklund A (1989) Degenerative changes in forebrain cholinergic nuclei correlate with cognitive impairments in aged rats. *Eur J Neurosci* 1:34–45.

Fletcher BR, Hill GS, Long JM, Gallagher M, Shapiro ML, Rapp PR (2014) A fine balance: regulation of hippocampal Arc/Arg3.1 transcription, translation and degradation in a rat model of normal cognitive aging. *Neurobiol Learn Mem* 115:58–67.

Fliers E, De Vries G, Swaab D (1985) Changes with aging in the vasopressin and oxytocin innervation of the rat brain. *Brain Res* 348:1–8.

Flood DG (1991) Region-specific stability of dendritic extent in normal human aging and regression in Alzheimer's disease: II. Subiculum. *Brain Res* 540:83–95.

Flood DG (1993) Critical issues in the analysis of dendritic extent in aging humans, primates, and rodents. *Neurobiol Aging* 14:649–654.

Flood DG, Buell SJ, Defiore CH, Horwitz GJ, Coleman PD (1985) Age-related dendritic growth in dentate gyrus of human brain is followed by regression in the "oldest old." *Brain Res* 345:366–368.

Flood DG, Buell SJ, Horwitz GJ, Coleman PD (1987) Dendritic extent in human dentate gyrus granule cells in normal aging and senile dementia. *Brain Res* 402:205–216.

Flood DG, Guarnaccia M, Coleman PD (1987) Dendritic extent in human CA2-3 hippocampal pyramidal neurons in normal aging and senile dementia. *Brain Res* 409:88–96.

Fonken LK, Kitt MM, Gaudet AD, Barrientos RM, Watkins LR, Maier SF (2016) Diminished circadian rhythms in hippocampal microglia may contribute to age-related neuroinflammatory sensitization. *Neurobiol Aging* 47:102–112.

Foster TC (1999) Involvement of hippocampal synaptic plasticity in age-related memory decline. *Brain Res Brain Res Rev* 30:236–249.

Foster TC (2007) Calcium homeostasis and modulation of synaptic plasticity in the aged brain. *Aging Cell* 6:319–325.

Foster TC, Barnes CA, Rao G, McNaughton BL (1991) Increase in perforant path quantal size in aged F-344 rats. *Neurobiol Aging* 12:441–448.

Foster TC, Kumar A (2007) Susceptibility to induction of long-term depression is associated with impaired memory in aged Fischer 344 rats. *Neurobiol Learn Mem* 87:522–535.

Foster TC, Kyritsopoulos C, Kumar A (2017) Central role for NMDA receptors in redox mediated impairment of synaptic function during aging and Alzheimer's disease. *Behav Brain Res* 322:223–232.

Foster TC, Norris CM (1997) Age-associated changes in Ca(2+)-dependent processes: relation to hippocampal synaptic plasticity. *Hippocampus* 7:602–612.

Fowler C, Wiberg Å, Oreland L, Marcusson J, Winblad B (1980) The effect of age on the activity and molecular properties of human brain monoamine oxidase. *J Neural Transm* 49:1–20.

Frankland PW, Köhler S, Josselyn SA (2013) Hippocampal neurogenesis and forgetting. *Trends Neurosci* 36:497–503.

Freund T, Gulyas A, Acsady L, Görcs T, Toth K (1990) Serotonergic control of the hippocampus via local inhibitory interneurons. *Proc Natl Acad Sci U S A* 87:8501–8505.

Freund TF, Buzsaki G (1996) Interneurons of the hippocampus. *Hippocampus* 6:347–470.

Frick KM, Baxter MG, Markowska AL, Olton DS, Price DL (1995) Age-related spatial reference and working memory deficits assessed in the water maze. *Neurobiol Aging* 16:149–160.

Froc DJ, Eadie B, Li AM, Wodtke K, Tse M, Christie BR (2003) Reduced synaptic plasticity in the lateral perforant path input to the dentate gyrus of aged C57BL/6 mice. *J Neurophysiol* 90:32–38.

Fujii S, Sumikawa K (2001) Nicotine accelerates reversal of long-term potentiation and enhances long-term depression in the rat hippocampal CA1 region. *Brain Res* 894:340–346.

Furuta Y, Kobayashi M, Masaki T, Takamatsu K (1999) Age-related changes in expression of hippocalcin and NVP2 in rat brain. *Neurochem Res* 24:651–658.

Gage FH, Dunnett SB, Bjorklund A (1984) Spatial learning and motor deficits in aged rats. *Neurobiol Aging* 5:43–48.

Gallagher M, Bostock E, King R (1985) Effects of opiate antagonists on spatial memory in young and aged rats. *Behav Neural Biol* 44:374–385.

Gallagher M, Burwell R, Burchinal M (1993) Severity of spatial learning impairment in aging: development of a learning index for performance in the Morris water maze. *Behav Neurosci* 107:618–626.

Galvez R, Cua S, Disterhoft JF (2011) Age-related deficits in a forebrain-dependent task, trace-eyeblink conditioning. *Neurobiol Aging* 32:1915–1922.

Gant JC, Chen KC, Norris CM, Kadish I, Thibault O, Blalock EM, Porter NM, Landfield PW (2011) Disrupting function of FK506-binding protein 1b/12.6 induces the Ca²+-dysregulation aging phenotype in hippocampal neurons. *J Neurosci* 31:1693–1703.

Gant JC, Sama MM, Landfield PW, Thibault O (2006) Early and simultaneous emergence of multiple hippocampal biomarkers of aging is mediated by Ca2+-induced Ca2+ release. *J Neurosci* 26:3482–3490.

Gao A, Xia F, Guskjolen AJ, Ramsaran AI, Santoro A, Josselyn SA, Frankland PW (2018) Elevation of hippocampal neurogenesis induces a temporally graded pattern of forgetting of contextual fear memories. *J Neurosci* 38:3190–3198.

Gao J, Miao H, Xiao CH, Sun Y, Du X, Yuan HH, Yu HL, Gao DS (2011) Influence of aging on the dopaminergic neurons in the substantia nigra pars compacta of rats. *Curr Aging Sci* 4:19–24.

Gao T, Yatani A, Dell'Acqua ML, Sako H, Green SA, Dascal N, Scott JD, Hosey MM (1997) cAMP-dependent regulation of cardiac L-type Ca2+ channels requires membrane targeting of PKA and phosphorylation of channel subunits. *Neuron* 19:185–196.

Gardner RS, Gold PE, Korol DL (2020) Inactivation of the striatum in aged rats rescues their ability to learn a hippocampus-sensitive spatial navigation task. *Neurobiol Learn Mem* 172:107231.

Gardner RS, Newman LA, Mohler EG, Tunur T, Gold PE, Korol DL (2020) Aging is not equal across memory systems. *Neurobiol Learn Mem* 172:107232.

Gavilán MP, Revilla E, Pintado C, Castaño A, Vizuete ML, Moreno-González I, Baglietto-Vargas D, Sánchez-Varo R, Vitorica J, Gutiérrez A, et al. (2007) Molecular and cellular characterization of the age-related neuroinflammatory processes occurring in normal rat hippocampus: potential relation with the loss of somatostatin GABAergic neurons. *J Neurochem* 103:984–996.

Gazzaley AH, Thakker MM, Hof PR, Morrison JH (1997) Preserved number of entorhinal cortex layer II neurons in aged macaque monkeys. *Neurobiol Aging* 18:549–553.

Geinisman Y, Bondareff W, Dodge JT (1977) Partial deafferentation of neurons in the dentate gyrus of the senescent rat. *Brain Res* 134:541–545.

Geinisman Y, de Toledo-Morrell L, Morrell F (1986) Aged rats need a preserved complement of perforated axospinous synapses per hippocampal neuron to maintain good spatial memory. *Brain Res* 398:266–275.

Geinisman Y, de Toledo-Morrell L, Morrell F, Persina IS, Rossi M (1992a) Age-related loss of axospinous synapses formed by two afferent systems in the rat dentate gyrus as revealed by the unbiased stereological dissector technique. *Hippocampus* 2:437–444.

Geinisman Y, de Toledo-Morrell L, Morrell F, Persina IS, Rossi M (1992b) Structural synaptic plasticity associated with the induction of long-term potentiation is preserved in the dentate gyrus of aged rats. *Hippocampus* 2:445–456.

Geinisman Y, deToledo-Morrell L, Morrell F (1994) Comparison of structural synaptic modifications induced by long-term potentiation in the hippocampal dentate gyrus of young adult and aged rats. *Ann N Y Acad Sci* 747:452–466.

Geinisman Y, Ganeshina O, Yoshida R, Berry RW, Disterhoft JF, Gallagher M (2004) Aging, spatial learning, and total synapse number in the rat CA1 stratum radiatum. *Neurobiol Aging* 25:407–416.

Gemma C, Stellwagen H, Fister M, Coultrap SJ, Mesches MH, Browning MD, Bickford PC (2004) Rosiglitazone improves contextual fear conditioning in aged rats. *Neuroreport* 15:2255–2259.

Gerrard JL, Burke SN, McNaughton BL, Barnes CA (2008) Sequence reactivation in the hippocampus is impaired in aged rats. *J Neurosci* 28:7883–7890.

Gerrard JL, Kudrimoti H, McNaughton BL, Barnes CA (2001) Reactivation of hippocampal ensemble activity patterns in the aging rat. *Behav Neurosci* 115:1180–1192.

Gheidi A, Azzopardi E, Adams AA, Marrone DF (2013) Experience-dependent persistent expression of zif268 during rest is preserved in the aged dentate gyrus. *BMC Neurosci* 14:100.

Gilbert JG (1941) Memory loss in senescence. *J Abnorm Soc Psychol* 36:73.

Gilbert PE, Kesner RP, Lee I (2001) Dissociating hippocampal subregions: double dissociation between dentate gyrus and CA1. *Hippocampus* 11:626–636.

Gilbert PE, Pirogovsky E, Ferdon S, Brushfield AM, Murphy C (2008) Differential effects of normal aging on memory for odor-place and object-place associations. *Exp Aging Res* 34:437–452.

Goldman-Rakic PS, Brown R (1981) Regional changes of monoamines in cerebral cortex and subcortical structures of aging rhesus monkeys. *Neuroscience* 6:177–187.

Goldman G, Coleman P (1981) Neuron numbers in locus coeruleus do not change with age in Fisher 344 rat. *Neurobiol Aging* 2:33–36.

Goldman H, Berman RF, Gershon S, Murphy SL, Altman HJ (1987) Correlation of behavioral and cerebrovascular functions in the aging rat. *Neurobiol Aging* 8:409–416.

Gómez-Gonzalo M, Martin-Fernandez M, Martínez-Murillo R, Mederos S, Hernández-Vivanco A, Jamison S, Fernandez AP, Serrano J, Calero P, Futch HS, et al. (2017) Neuron-astrocyte signaling is preserved in the aging brain. *Glia* 65:569–580.

Gómez-Isla T, Price JL, McKeel DW, Morris JC, Growdon JH, Hyman BT (1996) Profound loss of layer II entorhinal cortex neurons occurs in very mild Alzheimer's disease. *J Neurosci* 16:4491–4500.

Gonzales RA, Brown LM, Jones TW, Trent RD, Westbrook SL, Leslie SW (1991) N-methyl-D-aspartate mediated responses decrease with age in Fischer 344 rat brain. *Neurobiol Aging* 12:219–225.

Goodrick CL (1968) Learning, retention, and extinction of a complex maze habit for mature-young and senescent Wistar albino rats. *J Gerontol* 23:298–304.

Goodrick CL (1972) Learning by mature-young and aged Wistar albino rats as a function of test complexity. *J Gerontol* 27:353–357.

Gooney M, Messaoudi E, Maher FO, Bramham CR, Lynch MA (2004) BDNF-induced LTP in dentate gyrus is impaired with age: analysis of changes in cell signaling events. *Neurobiol Aging* 25:1323–1331.

Gothard KM, Skaggs WE, McNaughton BL (1996) Dynamics of mismatch correction in the hippocampal ensemble code for space: interaction between path integration and environmental cues. *J Neurosci* 16:8027–8040.

Gottfries CG, Adolfsson R, Aquilonius SM, Carlsson A, Eckernäs SA, Nordberg A, Oreland L, Svennerholm L, Wiberg A, Winblad B (1983) Biochemical changes in dementia disorders of Alzheimer type (AD/SDAT). *Neurobiol Aging* 4:261–271.

Goudsmit E, Feenstra MG, Swaab DF (1990) Central monoamine metabolism in the male Brown-Norway rat in relation to aging and testosterone. *Brain Res Bull* 25:755–763.

Gould TJ, Feiro OR (2005) Age-related deficits in the retention of memories for cued fear conditioning are reversed by galantamine treatment. *Behav Brain Res* 165:160–171.

Gozlan H, Daval G, Verge D, Spampinato U, Fattaccini CM, Gallissot MC, el Mestikawy S, Hamon M (1990) Aging associated changes in serotoninergic and dopaminergic pre- and postsynaptic neurochemical markers in the rat brain. *Neurobiol Aging* 11:437–449.

Graves CA, Solomon PR (1985) Age-related disruption of trace but not delay classical conditioning of the rabbit's nictitating membrane response. *Behav Neurosci* 99:88.

Gray DT, Barnes CA (2015) Distinguishing adaptive plasticity from vulnerability in the aging hippocampus. *Neuroscience* 309:17–28.

Gray DT, Zempare M, Carey N, Khattab S, Sinakevitch I, De Biase LM, Barnes CA (2023) Extracellular matrix proteoglycans support aged hippocampus networks: a potential cellular-level mechanism of brain reserve. *Neurobiol Aging* 131:52–58.

Greferath U, Bennie A, Kourakis A, Barrett G (2000) Impaired spatial learning in aged rats is associated with loss of p75-positive neurons in the basal forebrain. *Neuroscience* 100:363–373.

Gross-Isseroff R, Salama D, Israeli M, Biegon A (1990) Autoradiographic analysis of age-dependent changes in serotonin 5-HT2 receptors of the human brain postmortem. *Brain Res* 519:223–227.

Grover LM, Teyler TJ (1990) Two components of long-term potentiation induced by different patterns of afferent activation. *Nature* 347:477–479.

Guidi M, Kumar A, Rani A, Foster TC (2014) Assessing the emergence and reliability of cognitive decline over the life span in Fisher 344 rats using the spatial water maze. *Front Aging Neurosci* 6:2.

Guidobono F, Netti C, Bettica P, Sibilia V, Pagani F, Cazzamalli E, Pecile A (1989) Effects of age on binding sites for calcitonin gene related peptide in the rat central nervous system. *Neurosci Lett* 102:20–26.

Gulmez Karaca K, Brito DVC, Kupke J, Zeuch B, Oliveira AMM (2021) Engram reactivation during memory retrieval predicts long-term memory performance in aged mice. *Neurobiol Aging* 101:256–261.

Guo F, Zhao J, Zhao D, Wang J, Wang X, Feng Z, Vreugdenhil M, Lu C (2017) Dopamine D4 receptor activation restores CA1 LTP in hippocampal slices from aged mice. *Aging Cell* 16:1323–1333.

Guzowski JF, Knierim JJ, Moser EI (2004) Ensemble dynamics of hippocampal regions CA3 and CA1. *Neuron* 44:581–584.

Guzowski JF, Lyford GL, Stevenson GD, Houston FP, McGaugh JL, Worley PF, Barnes CA (2000) Inhibition of activity-dependent arc protein expression in the rat hippocampus impairs the maintenance of long-term potentiation and the consolidation of long-term memory. *J Neurosci* 20:3993–4001.

Guzowski JF, McNaughton BL, Barnes CA, Worley PF (1999) Environment-specific expression of the immediate-early gene Arc in hippocampal neuronal ensembles. *Nat Neurosci* 2:1120–1124.

Guzowski JF, McNaughton BL, Barnes CA, Worley PF (2001) Imaging neural activity with temporal and cellular resolution using FISH. *Curr Opin Neurobiol* 11:579–584.

Haberman RP, Colantuoni C, Stocker AM, Schmidt AC, Pedersen JT, Gallagher M (2011) Prominent hippocampal CA3 gene expression profile in neurocognitive aging. *Neurobiol Aging* 32:1678–1692.

Hafting T, Fyhn M, Molden S, Moser MB, Moser EI (2005) Microstructure of a spatial map in the entorhinal cortex. *Nature* 436:801–806.

Haigler HJ, Cahill LF, Crager MR, Charles E (1987) Met-enkephalin, age and anatomy: a microiontophoretic study in the hippocampus. *Life Sci* 40:203–213.

Haley GE, Berteau-Pavy F, Berteau-Pavy D, Raber J (2012) Novel image-novel location object recognition task sensitive to age-related cognitive decline in nondemented elderly. *Age (Dordr)* 34:1–10.

Haley GE, Kohama SG, Urbanski HF, Raber J (2010) Age-related decreases in SYN levels associated with increases in MAP-2, APOE, and GFAP levels in the rhesus macaque prefrontal cortex and hippocampus. *Age (Dordr)* 32:283–296.

Hammond RS, Tull LE, Stackman RW (2004) On the delay-dependent involvement of the hippocampus in object recognition memory. *Neurobiol Learn Mem* 82:26–34.

Han P, Nielsen M, Song M, Yin J, Permenter MR, Vogt JA, Engle JR, Dugger BN, Beach TG, Barnes CA (2017) The impact of aging on brain pituitary adenylate cyclase activating polypeptide, pathology and cognition in mice and rhesus macaques. *Front Aging Neurosci* 9:180.

Hanks SD, Flood DG (1991) Region-specific stability of dendritic extent in normal human aging and regression in Alzheimer's disease: I. CA1 of hippocampus. *Brain Res* 540:63–82.

Hannon J, Hoyer D (2008) Molecular biology of 5-HT receptors. *Behav Brain Res* 195:198–213.

Hara Y, Park CS, Janssen WG, Punsoni M, Rapp PR, Morrison JH (2011) Synaptic characteristics of dentate gyrus axonal boutons and their relationships with aging, menopause, and memory in female rhesus monkeys. *J Neurosci* 31:7737–7744.

Hara Y, Park CS, Janssen WG, Roberts MT, Morrison JH, Rapp PR (2012) Synaptic correlates of memory and menopause in the hippocampal dentate gyrus in rhesus monkeys. *Neurobiol Aging* 33:421, e417–428.

Hara Y, Punsoni M, Yuk F, Park CS, Janssen WG, Rapp PR, Morrison JH (2012) Synaptic distributions of GluA2 and PKMζ in the monkey dentate gyrus and their relationships with aging and memory. *J Neurosci* 32:7336–7344.

Harada N, Narimatsu N, Kurihara H, Nakagata N, Okajima K (2009) Stimulation of sensory neurons improves cognitive function by promoting the hippocampal production of insulin-like growth factor-I in mice. *Transl Res* 154:90–102.

Harburger LL, Nzerem CK, Frick KM (2007) Single enrichment variables differentially reduce age-related memory decline in female mice. *Behav Neurosci* 121:679.

Hargreaves EL, Rao G, Lee I, Knierim JJ (2005) Major dissociation between medial and lateral entorhinal input to dorsal hippocampus. *Science* 308:1792–1794.

Harley C (1991) Noradrenergic and locus coeruleus modulation of the perforant path-evoked potential in rat dentate gyrus supports a role for the locus coeruleus in attentional and memorial processes. *Prog Brain Res* 88:307–321.

Harris JJ, Jolivet R, Attwell D (2012) Synaptic energy use and supply. *Neuron* 75:762–777.

Harris MA, Wiener JM, Wolbers T (2012) Aging specifically impairs switching to an allocentric navigational strategy. *Front Aging Neurosci* 4:29.

Harris MA, Wolbers T (2014) How age-related strategy switching deficits affect wayfinding in complex environments. *Neurobiol Aging* 35:1095–1102.

Harro J, Oreland L (1992) Age-related differences of cholecystokinin receptor binding in the rat brain. *Prog Neuro-Psychopharmacol Biol Psychiatry* 16:369–375.

Hartley T, Maguire EA, Spiers HJ, Burgess N (2003) The well-worn route and the path less traveled: distinct neural bases of route following and wayfinding in humans. *Neuron* 37:877–888.

Hartzell AL, Burke SN, Hoang LT, Lister JP, Rodriguez CN, Barnes CA (2013) Transcription of the immediate-early gene Arc in CA1 of the hippocampus reveals activity differences along the proximodistal axis that are attenuated by advanced age. *J Neurosci* 33:3424–3433.

Hattiangady B, Rao MS, Shetty GA, Shetty AK (2005) Brain-derived neurotrophic factor, phosphorylated cyclic AMP response element binding protein and neuropeptide Y decline as early as middle age in the dentate gyrus and CA1 and CA3 subfields of the hippocampus. *Exp Neurol* 195:353–371.

Haxaire C, Turpin FR, Potier B, Kervern M, Sinet PM, Barbanel G, Mothet JP, Dutar P, Billard JM (2012) Reversal of age-related oxidative stress prevents hippocampal synaptic plasticity deficits by protecting d-serine-dependent NMDA receptor activation. *Aging Cell* 11:336–344.

Hayashi M, Yamashita A, Shimizu K (1997) Somatostatin and brain-derived neurotrophic factor mRNA expression in the primate brain: decreased levels of mRNAs during aging. *Brain Res* 749:283–289.

Head D, Isom M (2010) Age effects on wayfinding and route learning skills. *Behav Brain Res* 209:49–58.

Hebb DO (1949) The Organization of Behavior: A Neuropsychological Theory. New York, J. Wiley; Chapman & Hall.

Hebda-Bauer EK, Morano MI, Therrien B (1999) Aging and corticosterone injections affect spatial learning in Fischer-344× Brown Norway rats. *Brain Res* 827:93–103.

Heine VM, Maslam S, Joëls M, Lucassen PJ (2004) Prominent decline of newborn cell proliferation, differentiation, and apoptosis in the aging dentate gyrus, in absence of an age-related hypothalamus–pituitary–adrenal axis activation. *Neurobiol Aging* 25:361–375.

Heinsen H, Henn R, Eisenmenger W, Götz M, Bohl J, Bethke B, Lockemann U, Püschel K (1994) Quantitative investigations on the human entorhinal area: left-right asymmetry and age-related changes. *Anat Embryol (Berl)* 190:181–194.

Hemby SE, Trojanowski JQ, Ginsberg SD (2003) Neuron-specific age-related decreases in dopamine receptor subtype mRNAs. *J Comp Neurol* 456:176–183.

Henriksen EJ, Colgin LL, Barnes CA, Witter MP, Moser MB, Moser EI (2010) Spatial representation along the proximodistal axis of CA1. *Neuron* 68:127–137.

Herman JP, Chen KC, Booze R, Landfield PW (1998) Up-regulation of alpha1D Ca2+ channel subunit mRNA expression in the hippocampus of aged F344 rats. *Neurobiol Aging* 19:581–587.

Hernandez AR, Hernandez CM, Truckenbrod LM, Campos KT, McQuail JA, Bizon JL, Burke SN (2019) Age and ketogenic diet have dissociable effects on synapse-related gene expression between hippocampal subregions. *Front Aging Neurosci* 11:239.

Hernandez AR, Maurer AP, Reasor JE, Turner SM, Barthle SE, Johnson SA, Burke SN (2015) Age-related impairments in object-place associations are not due to hippocampal dysfunction. *Behav Neurosci* 129:599–610.

Hernandez AR, Reasor JE, Truckenbrod LM, Campos KT, Federico QP, Fertal KE, Lubke KN, Johnson SA, Clark BJ, Maurer AP, et al. (2018) Dissociable effects of advanced age on prefrontal cortical and medial temporal lobe ensemble activity. *Neurobiol Aging* 70:217–232.

Hernandez AR, Truckenbrod LM, Campos KT, Williams SA, Burke SN (2019) Sex differences in age-related impairments vary across cognitive and physical assessments in rats. *Behav Neurosci* 134:69–81.

Herndon JG, Moss MB, Rosene DL, Killiany RJ (1997) Patterns of cognitive decline in aged rhesus monkeys. *Behav Brain Res* 87:25–34.

Hersi AI, Rowe W, Gaudreau P, Quirion R (1995) Dopamine D1 receptor ligands modulate cognitive performance and hippocampal acetylcholine release in memory-impaired aged rats. *Neuroscience* 69:1067–1074.

Hilton C, Muffato V, Slattery TJ, Miellet S, Wiener J (2020) Differences in encoding strategy as a potential explanation for age-related decline in place recognition ability. *Front Psychol* 11:2182.

Hiramatsu M, Miwa M, Hashimoto K, Kawai S, Nomura N (2008) Nociceptin/orphanin FQ reverses mecamylamine-induced learning and memory impairment as well as decrease in hippocampal acetylcholine release in the rat. *Brain Res* 1195:96–103.

Hok V, Chah E, Reilly RB, O'Mara SM (2012) Hippocampal dynamics predict interindividual cognitive differences in rats. *J Neurosci* 32:3540–3551.

Holden HM, Hoebel C, Loftis K, Gilbert PE (2012) Spatial pattern separation in cognitively normal young and older adults. *Hippocampus* 22:1826–1832.

Holden HM, Toner C, Pirogovsky E, Kirwan CB, Gilbert PE (2013) Visual object pattern separation varies in older adults. *Learn Mem* 20:358–362.

Hori N, Hirotsu I, Davis P, Carpenter D (1992) Long-term potentiation is lost in aged rats but preserved by calorie restriction. *Neuroreport* 3:1085–1088.

Hoskins B, Peeler DF, Lawson K, Barnes AM, Ho K (1991) Effects of haloperidol on motor and cognitive functioning in aged mice. *Brain Res Bull* 27:279–281.

Hosseini L, Farokhi-Sisakht F, Badalzadeh R, Khabbaz A, Mahmoudi J, Sadigh-Eteghad S (2019) Nicotinamide mononucleotide and melatonin alleviate aging-induced cognitive impairment via modulation of mitochondrial function and apoptosis in the prefrontal cortex and Hippocampus. *Neuroscience* 423:29–37.

Houston FP, Stevenson GD, McNaughton BL, Barnes CA (1999) Effects of age on the generalization and incubation of memory in the F344 rat. *Learn Mem* 6:111–119.

Hoyer D, Martin G (1997) 5-HT receptor classification and nomenclature: towards a harmonization with the human genome. *Neuropharmacology* 36:419–428.

Hu H, Real E, Takamiya K, Kang M-G, Ledoux J, Huganir RL, Malinow R (2007) Emotion enhances learning via norepinephrine regulation of AMPA-receptor trafficking. *Cell* 131:160–173.

Huffman DJ, Stark CE (2017) Age-related impairment on a forced-choice version of the Mnemonic Similarity Task. *Behav Neurosci* 131:55.

Huguet F, Tarrade T (1992) Alpha 2-adrenoceptor changes during cerebral ageing: the effect of Ginkgo biloba extract. *J Pharm Pharmacol* 44:24–27.

Ianov L, De Both M, Chawla MK, Rani A, Kennedy AJ, Piras I, Day JJ, Siniard A, Kumar A, Sweatt JD (2017) Hippocampal transcriptomic profiles: subfield vulnerability to age and cognitive impairment. *Front Aging Neurosci* 9:383.

Ianov L, Rani A, Beas BS, Kumar A, Foster TC (2016) Transcription profile of aging and cognition-related genes in the medial prefrontal cortex. *Front Aging Neurosci* 8:113.

Iaria G, Palermo L, Committeri G, Barton JJ (2009) Age differences in the formation and use of cognitive maps. *Behav Brain Res* 196:187–191.

Ingram DK, London ED, Goodrick CL (1981) Age and neurochemical correlates of radial maze performance in rats. *Neurobiol Aging* 2:41–47.

Inoue M, Suhara T, Sudo Y, Okubo Y, Yasuno F, Kishimoto T, Yoshikawa K, Tanada S (2001) Age-related reduction of extrastriatal dopamine D2 receptor measured by PET. *Life Sci* 69:1079–1084.

Insel N, Patron LA, Hoang LT, Nematollahi S, Schimanski LA, Lipa P, Barnes CA (2012) Reduced gamma frequency in the medial frontal cortex of aged rats during behavior and rest: implications for age-related behavioral slowing. *J Neurosci* 32:16331–16344.

Insel N, Ruiz-Luna ML, Permenter M, Vogt J, Erickson CA, Barnes CA (2008) Aging in rhesus macaques is associated with changes in novelty preference and altered saccade dynamics. *Behav Neurosci* 122:1328–1342.

Ishida Y, Shirokawa T, Miyaishi O, Komatsu Y, Isobe K (2000) Age-dependent changes in projections from locus coeruleus to hippocampus dentate gyrus and frontal cortex. *Eur J Neurosci* 12:1263–1270.

Ishikawa R, Fukushima H, Frankland PW, Kida S (2016) Hippocampal neurogenesis enhancers promote forgetting of remote fear memory after hippocampal reactivation by retrieval. *Elife* 5:e17464.

Iwanaga K, Yamada M, Wakabayashi K, Ikuta F, Takahashi H (1996) A newly discovered age-related synaptic change in the human locus ceruleus: morphometric and ultrastructural studies. *Acta Neuropathologica* 91:337–342.

Jackson JC, Johnson A, Redish AD (2006) Hippocampal sharp waves and reactivation during awake states depend on repeated sequential experience. *J Neurosci* 26:12415–12426.

Jacobson TK, Howe MD, Schmidt B, Hinman JR, Escabi MA, Markus EJ (2013) Hippocampal theta, gamma, and theta-gamma coupling: effects of aging, environmental change, and cholinergic activation. *J Neurophysiol* 109:1852–1865.

Jacobson TK, Schmidt B, Hinman JR, Escabi MA, Markus EJ (2015) Age-related decrease in theta and gamma coherence across dorsal ca1 pyramidale and radiatum layers. *Hippocampus* 25:1327–1335.

Jiménez-Rubio G, Herrera-Pérez JJ, Martínez-Becerril HA, Márquez-Baltazar MS, Martínez-Mota L (2020) Age-dependent effects of testosterone on spatial memory in male rats. *Horm Behav* 122:104748.

Jo YS, Lee I (2010a) Disconnection of the hippocampal-perirhinal cortical circuits severely disrupts object-place paired associative memory. *J Neurosci* 30:9850–9858.

Jo YS, Lee I (2010b) Perirhinal cortex is necessary for acquiring, but not for retrieving object-place paired association. *Learn Mem* 17:97–103.

Johnson SA, Sacks PK, Turner SM, Gaynor LS, Ormerod BK, Maurer AP, Bizon JL, Burke SN (2016) Discrimination performance in aging is vulnerable to interference and dissociable from spatial memory. *Learn Mem* 23:339–348.

Johnson SA, Turner SM, Lubke KN, Cooper TL, Fertal KE, Bizon JL, Maurer AP, Burke SN (2019) Experience-dependent effects of muscimol-induced hippocampal excitation on mnemonic discrimination. *Front Syst Neurosci* 12:72.

Johnson SA, Turner SM, Santacroce LA, Carty KN, Shafiq L, Bizon JL, Maurer AP, Burke SN (2017) Rodent age-related impairments in discriminating perceptually similar objects parallel those observed in humans. *Hippocampus* 27:759–776.

Johnson SA, Zequeira S, Turner SM, Maurer AP, Bizon JL, Burke SN (2021) Rodent mnemonic similarity task performance requires the prefrontal cortex. *Hippocampus* 31:701–716.

Jones MW, Errington ML, French PJ, Fine A, Bliss TV, Garel S, Charnay P, Bozon B, Laroche S, Davis S (2001) A requirement for the immediate early gene Zif268 in the expression of late LTP and long-term memories. *Nat Neurosci* 4:289–296.

Joo KM, Chung YH, Kim MK, Nam RH, Lee BL, Lee KH, Cha CI (2004) Distribution of vasoactive intestinal peptide and pituitary adenylate cyclase-activating polypeptide receptors (VPAC1, VPAC2, and PAC1 receptor) in the rat brain. *J Comp Neurol* 476:388–413.

Kaasinen V, Vilkman H, Hietala J, Någren K, Helenius H, Olsson H, Farde L, Rinne J (2000) Age-related dopamine D2/D3 receptor loss in extrastriatal regions of the human brain. *Neurobiol Aging* 21:683–688.

Kadish I, Thibault O, Blalock EM, Chen KC, Gant JC, Porter NM, Landfield PW (2009) Hippocampal and cognitive aging across the lifespan: a bioenergetic shift precedes and increased cholesterol trafficking parallels memory impairment. *J Neurosci* 29:1805–1816.

Fagan JF 3rd (1970) Memory in the infant. *J Exp Child Psychol* 9:217–226.

Kakiuchi T, Nishiyama S, Sato K, Ohba H, Nakanishi S, Tsukada H (2000) Age-related reduction of [11C]MDL100,907 binding to central 5-HT(2A) receptors: PET study in the conscious monkey brain. *Brain Res* 883:135–142.

Kakiuchi T, Tsukada H, Fukumoto D, Nishiyama S (2001) Effects of aging on serotonin transporter availability and its response to fluvoxamine in the living brain: PET study with [(11)C](+) McN5652 and [(11)C](-)McN5652 in conscious monkeys. *Synapse* 40:170–179.

Kalaria RN (1989) Characterization of [125I] HEAT binding to α1-receptors in human brain: assessment in aging and Alzheimer's disease. *Brain Res* 501:287–294.

Kalaria RN, Andorn AC (1991) Adrenergic receptors in aging and Alzheimer's disease: decreased alpha 2-receptors demonstrated by [3H]p-aminoclonidine binding in prefrontal cortex. *Neurobiol Aging* 12:131–136.

Kanaan NM, Kordower JH, Collier TJ (2007) Age-related accumulation of Marinesco bodies and lipofuscin in rhesus monkey midbrain dopamine neurons: relevance to selective neuronal vulnerability. *J Comp Neurol* 502:683–700.

Fantz RL (1964) Visual experience in infants: decreased attention to familiar patterns relative to novel ones. *Science* 146:668–670.

Kashiyae Y, Kontani M, Kawashima H, Kiso Y, Kudo Y, Sakakibara M (2009) Arachidonic acid enhances intracellular calcium levels in dentate gyrus, but not CA1, in aged rat. *Neurosci Res* 64:143–151.

Katsuki H, Izumi Y, Zorumski CF (1997) Noradrenergic regulation of synaptic plasticity in the hippocampal CA1 region. *J Neurophysiol* 77:3013–3020.

Kelly KM, Kume A, Albin RL, Macdonald RL (2001) Autoradiography of L-type and N-type calcium channels in aged rat hippocampus, entorhinal cortex, and neocortex. *Neurobiol Aging* 22:17–23.

Kempadoo KA, Mosharov EV, Choi SJ, Sulzer D, Kandel ER (2016) Dopamine release from the locus coeruleus to the dorsal hippocampus promotes spatial learning and memory. *Proc Natl Acad Sci U S A* 113:14835–14840.

Kempermann G, Gast D, Gage FH (2002) Neuroplasticity in old age: sustained fivefold induction of hippocampal neurogenesis by long-term environmental enrichment. *Ann Neurol* 52:135–143.

Kennard JA, Woodruff-Pak DS (2011) Age sensitivity of behavioral tests and brain substrates of normal aging in mice. *Front Aging Neurosci* 3:9.

Kent BA, Hvoslef-Eide M, Saksida LM, Bussey TJ (2016) The representational-hierarchical view of pattern separation: not just hippocampus, not just space, not just memory? *Neurobiol Learn Mem* 129:99–106.

Kerchner GA, Bernstein JD, Fenesy MC, Deutsch GK, Saranathan M, Zeineh MM, Rutt BK (2013) Shared vulnerability of two synaptically-connected medial temporal lobe areas to age and cognitive decline: a seven tesla magnetic resonance imaging study. *J Neurosci* 33:16666–16672.

Keren NI, Taheri S, Vazey EM, Morgan PS, Granholm AC, Aston-Jones GS, Eckert MA (2015) Histologic validation of locus coeruleus MRI contrast in post-mortem tissue. *NeuroImage* 113:235–245.

Kerr DS, Campbell LW, Hao SY, Landfield PW (1989) Corticosteroid modulation of hippocampal potentials: increased effect with aging. *Science* 245:1505–1509.

Kessels RP, Te Boekhorst S, Postma A (2005) The contribution of implicit and explicit memory to the effects of errorless learning: a comparison between young and older adults. *J Int Neuropsychol Soc* 11:144–151.

Keuker JI, Keijser JN, Nyakas C, Luiten PG, Fuchs E (2005) Aging is accompanied by a subfield-specific reduction of serotonergic fibers in the tree shrew hippocampal formation. *J Chem Neuroanat* 30:221–229.

Keuker JI, Luiten PG, Fuchs E (2003) Preservation of hippocampal neuron numbers in aged rhesus monkeys. *Neurobiol Aging* 24:157–165.

Khachaturian Z (1984) Toward theories of brain aging. In: Handbook of Studies of Psychiatry and Old Age (Kay D, Burrows DG, eds), pp 7–30. Amsterdam.

Khachaturian ZS (1989) The role of calcium regulation in brain aging: reexamination of a hypothesis. *Aging (Milano)* 1:17–34.

Khachaturian ZS (1991) Calcium and the aging brain: upsetting a delicate balance? *Geriatrics* 46:78–79, 83.

Kim JJ, Fanselow MS (1992) Modality-specific retrograde amnesia of fear. *Science* 256:675–677.

Kinney JW, Sanchez-Alavez M, Barr AM, Criado JR, Crawley JN, Behrens MM, Henriksen SJ, Bartfai T (2009) Impairment of memory consolidation by galanin correlates with in vivo inhibition of both LTP and CREB phosphorylation. *Neurobiol Learn Mem* 92:429–438.

Kirwan CB, Stark CE (2007) Overcoming interference: an fMRI investigation of pattern separation in the medial temporal lobe. *Learn Mem* 14:625–633.

Kishimoto Y, Suzuki M, Kawahara S, Kirino Y (2001) Age-dependent impairment of delay and trace eyeblink conditioning in mice. *Neuroreport* 12:3349–3352.

Klöppel S, Kovacs GG, Voigtländer T, Wanschitz J, Flicker H, Hainfellner JA, Guentchev M, Budka H (2001) Serotonergic nuclei of the raphe are not affected in human ageing. *Neuroreport* 12:669–671.

Knuttinen M-G, Power J, Preston A, Disterhoft J (2001a) Awareness in classical differential eyeblink conditioning in young and aging humans. *Behav Neurosci* 115:747.

Knuttinen MG, Gamelli AE, Weiss C, Power JM, Disterhoft JF (2001b) Age-related effects on eyeblink conditioning in the F344 x BN F1 hybrid rat. *Neurobiol Aging* 22:1–8.

Kobayashi S, Ohashi Y, Ando S (2002) Effects of enriched environments with different durations and starting times on learning capacity during aging in rats assessed by a refined procedure of the Hebb-Williams maze task. *J Neurosci Res* 70:340–346.

Koh MT, McMahan RW, Gallagher M (2022) Individual differences in neurocognitive aging in outbred male and female Long-Evans rats. *Behav Neurosci* 136:13–18.

Koh MT, Spiegel AM, Gallagher M (2014) Age-associated changes in hippocampal-dependent cognition in diversity outbred mice. *Hippocampus* 24:1300–1307.

Kohen R, Heidmann DE, Anthony J, White SS, Hamblin MW, Szot P (2000) Changes in 5-HT(7) serotonin receptor mRNA expression with aging in rat brain. *Brain Res Mol Brain Res* 79:163–168.

Kolakowski LF, Jr, O'Neill GP, Howard AD, Broussard SR, Sullivan KA, Feighner SD, Sawzdargo M, Nguyen T, Kargman S, Shiao LL (1998) Molecular characterization and expression of cloned human galanin receptors GALR2 and GALR3. *J Neurochem* 71:2239–2251.

Korkki SM, Richter FR, Jeyarathnarajah P, Simons JS (2020) Healthy ageing reduces the precision of episodic memory retrieval. *Psychol Aging* 35:124.

Kosaka T, Wu J-Y, Benoit R (1988) GABAergic neurons containing somatostatin-like immunoreactivity in the rat hippocampus and dentate gyrus. *Exp Brain Res* 71:388–398.

Kouvaros S, Kotzadimitriou D, Papatheodoropoulos C (2015) Hippocampal sharp waves and ripples: effects of aging and modulation by NMDA receptors and L-type Ca2+ channels. *Neuroscience* 298:26–41.

Kowalski C, Micheau J, Corder R, Gaillard R, Conte-Devolx B (1992) Age-related changes in cortico-releasing factor, somatostatin, neuropeptide Y, methionine enkephalin and β-endorphin in specific rat brain areas. *Brain Res* 582:38–46.

Krause M, Yang Z, Rao G, Houston FP, Barnes CA (2008) Altered dendritic integration in hippocampal granule cells of spatial learning-impaired aged rats. *J Neurophysiol* 99:2769–2778.

Krazem A, Marighetto A, Higueret P, Jaffard R (2003) Age-dependent effects of moderate chronic ethanol administration on different forms of memory expression in mice. *Behav Brain Res* 147:17–29.

Kronenberg G, Bick-Sander A, Bunk E, Wolf C, Ehninger D, Kempermann G (2006) Physical exercise prevents age-related decline in precursor cell activity in the mouse dentate gyrus. *Neurobiol Aging* 27:1505–1513.

Krzywkowski P, Lagny I, Jazat F, Lamour Y, Epelbaum J (1993) Age-related increase in galanin-binding sites in the rat brain: correlation with behavioral impairment a. *Ann N Y Acad Sci* 695:249–253.

Kubis N, Faucheux B, Ransmayr G, Damier P, Duyckaerts C, Henin D, Forette B, Le Charpentier Y, Hauw J-J, Agid Y (2000) Preservation of midbrain catecholaminergic neurons in very old human subjects. *Brain* 123:366–373.

Kudrimoti HS, Barnes CA, McNaughton BL (1999) Reactivation of hippocampal cell assemblies: effects of behavioral state, experience, and EEG dynamics. *J Neurosci* 19:4090–4101.

Kuhl DE, Minoshima S, Fessler JA, Ficaro E, Wieland D, Koeppe RA, Frey KA, Foster NL (1996) In vivo mapping of cholinergic terminals in normal aging, Alzheimer's disease, and Parkinson's disease. *Annals of Neurology: Official Journal of the American Neurological Association and the Child Neurology Society* 40:399–410.

Kuhn HG, Dickinson-Anson H, Gage FH (1996) Neurogenesis in the dentate gyrus of the adult rat: age-related decrease of neuronal progenitor proliferation. *J Neurosci* 16:2027–2033.

Kulmala H (1985) Immunocytochemical localization of enkephalin-like immunoreactivity in neurons of human hippocampal formation: effects of ageing and Alzheimer's disease. *Neuropathol Appl Neurobiol* 11:105–115.

Kumar A, Foster T (2007) Environmental enrichment decreases the afterhyperpolarization in senescent rats. *Brain Res* 1130:103–107.

Kumar A, Foster TC (2002) 17beta-estradiol benzoate decreases the AHP amplitude in CA1 pyramidal neurons. *J Neurophysiol* 88:621–626.

Kumar A, Foster TC (2004) Enhanced long-term potentiation during aging is masked by processes involving intracellular calcium stores. *J Neurophysiol* 91:2437–2444.

Kumar A, Foster TC (2005) Intracellular calcium stores contribute to increased susceptibility to LTD induction during aging. *Brain Res* 1031:125–128.

Kumar A, Foster TC (2013) Linking redox regulation of NMDAR synaptic function to cognitive decline during aging. *J Neurosci* 33:15710–15715.

Kumar A, Foster TC (2019) Alteration in NMDA receptor mediated glutamatergic neurotransmission in the hippocampus during senescence. *Neurochem Res* 44:38–48.

Kumar A, Rani A, Tchigranova O, Lee WH, Foster TC (2012a) Influence of late-life exposure to environmental enrichment or exercise on hippocampal function and CA1 senescent physiology. *Neurobiol Aging* 33:828, e821–817.

Kumar A, Rani A, Tchigranova O, Lee WH, Foster TC (2012b) Influence of late-life exposure to environmental enrichment or exercise on hippocampal function and CA1 senescent physiology. *Neurobiol Aging* 33:828, e821–817.

Kumar A, Thinschmidt JS, Foster TC (2019) Subunit contribution to NMDA receptor hypofunction and redox sensitivity of hippocampal synaptic transmission during aging. *Aging (Albany NY)* 11:5140–5157.

Kumar A, Thinschmidt JS, Foster TC, King MA (2007) Aging effects on the limits and stability of long-term synaptic potentiation and depression in rat hippocampal area CA1. *J Neurophysiol* 98:594–601.

Kumar A, Yegla B, Foster TC (2018) Redox signaling in neurotransmission and cognition during aging. *Antioxid Redox Signal* 28(18):1724–1745.

Kumar KG, Trevaskis JL, Lam DD, Sutton GM, Koza RA, Chouljenko VN, Kousoulas KG, Rogers PM, Kesterson RA, Thearle M (2008) Identification of adropin as a secreted factor linking dietary macronutrient intake with energy homeostasis and lipid metabolism. *Cell Metab* 8:468–481.

Kwapis JL, Alaghband Y, Kramár EA, López AJ, Ciernia AV, White AO, Shu G, Rhee D, Michael CM, Montellier E (2018) Epigenetic regulation of the circadian gene Per1 contributes to age-related changes in hippocampal memory. *Nat Commun* 9:1–14.

Kwapis JL, Alaghband Y, López AJ, Long JM, Li X, Shu G, Bodinayake KK, Matheos DP, Rapp PR, Wood MA (2019) HDAC3-mediated repression of the Nr4a family contributes to age-related impairments in long-term memory. *J Neurosci* 39:4999–5009.

Lacoste MG, Ponce IT, Golini RL, Delgado SM, Anzulovich AC (2017) Aging modifies daily variation of antioxidant enzymes and oxidative status in the hippocampus. *Exp Gerontol* 88:42–50.

Lagarde J, Sarazin M, Chauviré V, Stankoff B, Kas A, Lacomblez L, Peyronneau M-A, Bottlaender M (2017) Cholinergic changes in aging and Alzheimer disease: an [18F]-FA-85380 exploratory PET study. *Alzheimer Dis Assoc Disord* 31:8–12.

Lanahan A, Lyford G, Stevenson GS, Worley PF, Barnes CA (1997) Selective alteration of long-term potentiation-induced transcriptional response in hippocampus of aged, memory-impaired rats. *J Neurosci* 17:2876–2885.

Landfield PW (1987) "Increased calcium-current" hypothesis of brain aging. *Neurobiol Aging* 8:346–347.

Landfield PW, Lynch G (1977) Impaired monosynaptic potentiation in in vitro hippocampal slices from aged, memory-deficient rats. *J Gerontol* 32:523–533.

Landfield PW, McGaugh JL, Lynch G (1978) Impaired synaptic potentiation processes in the hippocampus of aged, memory-deficient rats. *Brain Res* 150:85–101.

Landfield PW, Pitler TA (1984) Prolonged Ca2+-dependent afterhyperpolarizations in hippocampal neurons of aged rats. *Science* 226:1089–1092.

Landfield PW, Pitler TA, Applegate MD (1986) The effects of high Mg2+-to-Ca2+ ratios on frequency potentiation in hippocampal slices of young and aged rats. *J Neurophysiol* **56**:797–811.

Larson J, Lynch G, Games D, Seubert P (1999) Alterations in synaptic transmission and long-term potentiation in hippocampal slices from young and aged PDAPP mice. *Brain Res* **840**:23–35.

Lebrun C, Durkin TP, Marighetto A, Jaffard R (1990) A comparison of the working memory performances of young and aged mice combined with parallel measures of testing and drug-induced activations of septo-hippocampal and NBM-cortical cholinergic neurones. *Neurobiol Aging* **11**:515–521.

Lee A, Archer J, Wong CKY, Chen S-HA, Qiu A (2013) Age-related decline in associative learning in healthy Chinese adults. *PloS One* **8**:e80648.

Lee H, Wang Z, Tillekeratne A, Lukish N, Puliyadi V, Zeger S, Gallagher M, Knierim JJ (2022) Loss of functional heterogeneity along the CA3 transverse axis in aging. *Curr Biol* **32**(12):2681–2693.

Lee H, Wang Z, Zeger SL, Gallagher M, Knierim JJ (2021) Heterogeneity of age-related neural hyperactivity along the CA3 transverse axis. *J Neurosci* **41**:663–673.

Lee I, Rao G, Knierim JJ (2004) A double dissociation between hippocampal subfields: differential time course of CA3 and CA1 place cells for processing changed environments. *Neuron* **42**:803–815.

Lee I, Solivan F (2008) The roles of the medial prefrontal cortex and hippocampus in a spatial paired-association task. *Learn Mem* **15**:357–367.

Lee I, Yoganarasimha D, Rao G, Knierim JJ (2004) Comparison of population coherence of place cells in hippocampal subfields CA1 and CA3. *Nature* **430**:456–459.

Lee JM, Ross ER, Gower A, Paris JM, Martensson R, Lorens SA (1994) Spatial learning deficits in the aged rat: neuroanatomical and neurochemical correlates. *Brain Res Bull* **33**:489–500.

Leonard BW, Amaral DG, Squire LR, Zola-Morgan S (1995) Transient memory impairment in monkeys with bilateral lesions of the entorhinal cortex. *J Neurosci* **15**:5637–5659.

Leutgeb S, Leutgeb JK, Treves A, Moser MB, Moser EI (2004) Distinct ensemble codes in hippocampal areas CA3 and CA1. *Science* **305**:1295–1298.

Li Y, Mu Y, Gage FH (2009) Development of neural circuits in the adult hippocampus. *Curr Top Dev Biol* **87**:149–174.

Lichtenwalner R, Forbes M, Bennett S, Lynch C, Sonntag W, Riddle D (2001) Intracerebroventricular infusion of insulin-like growth factor-I ameliorates the age-related decline in hippocampal neurogenesis. *Neuroscience* **107**:603–613.

Lin C, Sherathiya VN, Oh MM, Disterhoft JF (2020) Persistent firing in LEC III neurons is differentially modulated by learning and aging. *eLife* **9**:e56816.

Lindner MD (1997) Reliability, distribution, and validity of age-related cognitive deficits in the Morris water maze. *Neurobiol Learn Mem* **68**:203–220.

Lindner MD, Balch AH, Vandermaelen CP (1992) Short forms of the "reference-" and "working-memory" Morris water maze for assessing age-related deficits. *Behav Neural Biol* **58**:94–102.

Lippa A, Critchett D, Ehlert F, Yamamura H, Enna S, Bartus R (1981) Age-related alterations in neurotransmitter receptors: an electrophysiological and biochemical analysis. *Neurobiol Aging* **2**:3–8.

Lippa CF, Hamos JE, Pulaski-Salo D, DeGennaro LJ, Drachman DA (1992) Alzheimer's disease and aging: effects on perforant pathway perikarya and synapses. *Neurobiol Aging* **13**:405–411.

Liu KY, Acosta-Cabronero J, Cardenas-Blanco A, Loane C, Berry AJ, Betts MJ, Kievit RA, Henson RN, Düzel E, Howard R, et al. (2019) In vivo visualization of age-related differences in the locus coeruleus. *Neurobiol Aging* **74**:101–111.

Liu X-D, Zhang J-J, Wang Y, Yu L-C (2011) Inhibitory effects of calcitonin gene-related peptide on long-term potentiation induced in hippocampal slices of rats. *Neurosci Lett* **494**:10–13.

Lohmann P, Riepe MW (2007) Neurotoxic effects of repetitive inhibition of oxidative phosphorylation in young adults surfacing with deficits of spatial learning in old age. *J Gerontol Series A: Biol Sci Med Sci* **62**:1352–1356.

Lohninger S, Strasser A, Bubna-Littitz H (2001) The effect of L-carnitine on T-maze learning ability in aged rats. *Arch Gerontol Geriatr* **32**:245–253.

Lohr JB, Jeste DV (1988) Locus ceruleus morphometry in aging and schizophrenia. *Acta Psychiatr Scand* **77**:689–697.

Lomo T (1966) Frequency potentiation of excitatory synaptic activity in dentate area of hippocampal formation. *Acta Physiol Scand* (p. 128).

Lømo T (2018) Discovering long-term potentiation (LTP)–recollections and reflections on what came after. *Acta Physiologica* **222**:e12921.

London ED, Waller SB, Ellis AT, Ingram DK (1985) Effects of intermittent feeding on neurochemical markers in aging rat brain. *Neurobiol Aging* **6**:199–204.

Long JM, Mouton PR, Jucker M, Ingram DK (1999) What counts in brain aging? design-based stereological analysis of cell number. *J Gerontol Series A: Biol Sci Med Sci* **54**:B407–B417.

Long JM, Perez EJ, Roberts JA, Roberts MT, Rapp PR (2020) Reelin in the years: decline in the number of reelin immunoreactive neurons in layer II of the entorhinal cortex in aged monkeys with memory impairment. *Neurobiol Aging* **87**:132–137.

Lövdén M, Schellenbach M, Grossman-Hutter B, Krüger A, Lindenberger U (2005) Environmental topography and postural control demands shape aging-associated decrements in spatial navigation performance. *Psychology and Aging* **20**:683.

Lowes-Hummel P, Gertz HJ, Ferszt R, Cervos-Navarro J (1989) The basal nucleus of Meynert revised: the nerve cell number decreases with age. *Arch Gerontol Geriatr* **8**:21–27.

Loy R, Koziell DA, Lindsey JD, Moore RY (1980) Noradrenergic innervation of the adult rat hippocampal formation. *J Comp Neurol* **189**:699–710.

Luebke JI, Rosene DL (2003) Aging alters dendritic morphology, input resistance, and inhibitory signaling in dentate granule cells of the rhesus monkey. *J Comp Neurol* **460**:573–584.

Lugaro E (1909) Modern Problems in Psychiatry. University Press.

Lugtmeijer S, de Haan EH, Kessels RP (2019) A comparison of visual working memory and episodic memory performance in younger and older adults. *Aging, Neuropsychol, and Cogn* **26**:387–406.

Luine V, Bowling D, Hearns M (1990) Spatial memory deficits in aged rats: contributions of monoaminergic systems. *Brain Res* **537**:271–278.

Luo Y, Zhou J, Li MX, Wu PF, Hu ZL, Ni L, Jin Y, Chen JG, Wang F (2015) Reversal of aging-related emotional memory deficits by norepinephrine via regulating the stability of surface AMPA receptors. *Aging Cell* **14**:170–179.

Lyford GL, Yamagata K, Kaufmann WE, Barnes CA, Sanders LK, Copeland NG, Gilbert DJ, Jenkins NA, Lanahan AA, Worley PF (1995) Arc, a growth factor and activity-regulated gene, encodes a novel cytoskeleton-associated protein that is enriched in neuronal dendrites. *Neuron* **14**:433–445.

Lynch M, Voss K (1994) Membrane arachidonic acid concentration correlates with age and induction of long-term potentiation in the dentate gyrus in the rat. *Eur J Neurosci* **6**:1008–1014.

Ma S, Ciliax B, Stebbins G, Jaffar S, Joyce J, Cochran E, Kordower J, Mash DC, Levey A, Mufson E (1999) Dopamine transporter-immunoreactive neurons decrease with age in the human substantia nigra. *J Comp Neurol* 409:25–37.

Ma SY, Röytt M, Collan Y, Rinne JO (1999) Unbiased morphometrical measurements show loss of pigmented nigral neurones with ageing. *Neuropathol Appl Neurobiol* 25:394–399.

Maei HR, Zaslavsky K, Teixeira CM, Frankland PW (2009) What is the most sensitive measure of water maze probe test performance? *Front Integr Neurosci* 3:4.

Magnusson KR (2000) Declines in mRNA expression of different subunits may account for differential effects of aging on agonist and antagonist binding to the NMDA receptor. *J Neurosci* 20:1666–1674.

Magnusson KR, Brim BL, Das SR (2010) Selective vulnerabilities of N-methyl-D-aspartate (NMDA) receptors during brain aging. *Front Aging Neurosci* 2:11.

Manabe T, Noda Y, Mamiya T, Katagiri H, Houtani T, Nishi M, Noda T, Takahashi T, Sugimoto T, Nabeshima T (1998) Facilitation of long-term potentiation and memory in mice lacking nociceptin receptors. *Nature* 394:577.

Manaye KF, McIntire DD, Mann DM, German DC (1995) Locus coeruleus cell loss in the aging human brain: a non-random process. *J Comp Neurol* 358:79–87.

Mann DM (1983) The locus coeruleus and its possible role in ageing and degenerative disease of the human central nervous system. *Mech Ageing Dev* 23:73–94.

Mann DM, Yates PO (1982) Pathogenesis of Parkinson's disease. *Arch Neurol* 39:545–549.

Mann DM, Yates PO, Marcyniuk B (1984a) Alzheimer's presenile dementia, senile dementia of Alzheimer type and Down's syndrome in middle age form an age related continuum of pathological changes. *Neuropathol Appl Neurobiol* 10:185–207.

Mann DM, Yates PO, Marcyniuk B (1984b) Changes in nerve cells of the nucleus basalis of Meynert in Alzheimer's disease and their relationship to ageing and to the accumulation of lipofuscin pigment. *Mech Ageing Dev* 25:189–204.

Mann DM, Yates PO, Marcyniuk B (1984c) Monoaminergic neurotransmitter systems in presenile Alzheimer's disease and in senile dementia of Alzheimer type. *Clin Neuropathol* 3:199–205.

Marcusson J, Oreland L, Winblad B (1984) Effect of age on human brain serotonin (S-1) binding sites. *J Neurochem* 43:1699–1705.

Marcusson JO, Alafuzoff I, Ba IT, Ericsoon E, Gottfries CG, Winblad B (1987) 5-Hydroxytryptamine-sensitive [3H] imipramine binding of protein nature in the human brain: II. Effect of normal aging and dementia disorders. *Brain Res* 425:137–145.

Marcusson JO, Morgan DG, Winblad B, Finch CE (1984) Serotonin-2 binding sites in human frontal cortex and hippocampus: selective loss of S-2A sites with age. *Brain Res* 311:51–56.

Marcyniuk B, Mann DMA, Yates PO (1989) The topography of nerve cell loss from the locus caeruleus in elderly persons. *Neurobiol Aging* 10:5–9.

Marighetto A, Touzani K, Etchamendy N, Torrea CC, De Nanteuil G, Guez D, Jaffard R, Morain P (2000) Further evidence for a dissociation between different forms of mnemonic expressions in a mouse model of age-related cognitive decline: effects of tacrine and S 17092, a novel prolyl endopeptidase inhibitor. *Learn Mem* 7:159–169.

Markham JA, McKian KP, Stroup TS, Juraska JM (2005) Sexually dimorphic aging of dendritic morphology in CA1 of hippocampus. *Hippocampus* 15:97–103.

Markowska AL (1999) Sex dimorphisms in the rate of age-related decline in spatial memory: relevance to alterations in the estrous cycle. *J Neurosci* 19:8122–8133.

Markowska AL, Savonenko AV (2002) Protective effect of practice on cognition during aging: Implications for predictive characteristics of performance and efficacy of practice. *Neurobiol Learn Mem* 78:294–320.

Markowska AL, Stone WS, Ingram DK, Reynolds J, Gold PE, Conti LH, Pontecorvo MJ, Wenk GL, Olton DS (1989) Individual differences in aging: behavioral and neurobiological correlates. *Neurobiol Aging* 10:31–43.

Markus EJ, Barnes CA, McNaughton BL, Gladden VL, Skaggs WE (1994) Spatial information content and reliability of hippocampal CA1 neurons: effects of visual input. *Hippocampus* 4:410–421.

Marr D (1971) Simple memory: a theory for archicortex. *Philos Trans R Soc Lond B Biol Sci* 262:23–81.

Marrone DF, Adams AA, Satvat E (2011) Increased pattern separation in the aged fascia dentata. *Neurobiol Aging* 32:2317, e2323–2317, e2332.

Marrone DF, Schaner MJ, McNaughton BL, Worley PF, Barnes CA (2008) Immediate-early gene expression at rest recapitulates recent experience. *J Neurosci* 28:1030–1033.

Martin MR (1983) Naloxone and long term potentiation of hippocampal CA3 field potentials in vitro. *Neuropeptides* 4:45–50.

Masser DR, Bixler GV, Brucklacher RM, Yan H, Giles CB, Wren JD, Sonntag WE, Freeman WM (2014) Hippocampal subregions exhibit both distinct and shared transcriptomic responses to aging and nonneurodegenerative cognitive decline. *J Gerontol Series A: Biol Sci Med Sci* 69:1311–1324.

Masukawa LM, Prince DA (1982) Enkephalin inhibition of inhibitory input to CA1 and CA3 pyramidal neurons in the hippocampus. *Brain Res* 249:271–280.

Mather M, Harley CW (2016) The locus coeruleus: essential for maintaining cognitive function and the aging brain. *Trends Cogn Sci* 20:214–226.

Mathews KJ, Allen KM, Boerrigter D, Ball H, Shannon Weickert C, Double KL (2017) Evidence for reduced neurogenesis in the aging human hippocampus despite stable stem cell markers. *Aging Cell* 16:1195–1199.

Matthews EA, Linardakis JM, Disterhoft JF (2009) The fast and slow afterhyperpolarizations are differentially modulated in hippocampal neurons by aging and learning. *J Neurosci* 29:4750–4755.

Matsunaga W, Isobe K, Shirokawa T (2006) Involvement of neurotrophic factors in aging of noradrenergic innervations in hippocampus and frontal cortex. *Neurosci Res* 54:313–318.

Maurer AP, Burke SN, Diba K, Barnes CA (2017) Attenuated activity across multiple cell types and reduced monosynaptic connectivity in the aged perirhinal cortex. *J Neurosci* 37(37):8965–8974.

Maurer AP, Cowen SL, Burke SN, Barnes CA, McNaughton BL (2006a) Organization of hippocampal cell assemblies based on theta phase precession. *Hippocampus* 16:785–794.

Maurer AP, Cowen SL, Burke SN, Barnes CA, McNaughton BL (2006b) Phase precession in hippocampal interneurons showing strong functional coupling to individual pyramidal cells. *J Neurosci* 26:13485–13492.

Maurer AP, Vanrhoads SR, Sutherland GR, Lipa P, McNaughton BL (2005) Self-motion and the origin of differential spatial scaling along the septo-temporal axis of the hippocampus. *Hippocampus* 15:841–852.

McAllister DE, McAllister WR (1967) Incubation of fear: an examination of the concept. *J Exp Res Per*.

McAvan A, Du Y, Oyao A, Doner S, Grilli M, Ekstrom A (2021) Older adults show reduced spatial precision but preserved strategy-use during spatial navigation involving body-based cues. *Front Aging Neurosci* 13:129.

McCormack AL, Di Monte DA, Delfani K, Irwin I, DeLanney LE, Langston WJ, Janson AM (2004) Aging of the nigrostriatal system in the squirrel monkey. *J Comp Neurol* **471**:387–395.

McDonald MP, Gleason TC, Robinson JK, Crawley JN (1998) Galanin inhibits performance on rodent memory tasks. *Ann N Y Acad Sci* **863**:305–322.

McEchron MD, Bouwmeester H, Tseng W, Weiss C, Disterhoft JF (1998) Hippocampectomy disrupts auditory trace fear conditioning and contextual fear conditioning in the rat. *Hippocampus* **8**:638–646.

McEchron MD, Cheng AY, Gilmartin MR (2004) Trace fear conditioning is reduced in the aging rat. *Neurobiol Learn Mem* **82**:71–76.

McEchron MD, Weible AP, Disterhoft JF (2001) Aging and learning-specific changes in single-neuron activity in CA1 hippocampus during rabbit trace eyeblink conditioning. *J Neurophysiol* **86**:1839–1857.

McGeer PL, McGeer EG, Suzuki JS (1977) Aging and extrapyramidal function. *Arch Neurol* **34**:33–35.

McLay R, Freeman S, Harlan R, Kastin A, Zadina J (1999) Tests used to assess the cognitive abilities of aged rats: their relation to each other and to hippocampal morphology and neurotrophin expression. *Gerontology* **45**:143–155.

McNaughton BL, Barnes CA, O'Keefe J (1983) The contributions of position, direction, and velocity to single unit activity in the hippocampus of freely-moving rats. *Exp Brain Res* **52**:41–49.

McNaughton BL, Douglas RM, Goddard GV (1978) Synaptic enhancement in fascia dentata: cooperativity among coactive afferents. *Brain Res* **157**:277–293.

McNaughton BL, O'Keefe J, Barnes CA (1983) The stereotrode: a new technique for simultaneous isolation of several single units in the central nervous system from multiple unit records. *J Neurosci Methods* **8**:391–397.

McQuail JA, Nicolle MM (2015) Spatial reference memory in normal aging Fischer 344 x Brown Norway F1 hybrid rats. *Neurobiol Aging* **36**:323–333.

McTighe SM, Cowell RA, Winters BD, Bussey TJ, Saksida LM (2010) Paradoxical false memory for objects after brain damage. *Science* **330**:1408–1410.

Mehta MR, Barnes CA, McNaughton BL (1997) Experience-dependent, asymmetric expansion of hippocampal place fields. *Proc Natl Acad Sci U S A* **94**:8918–8921.

Mei Y, Jiang C, Wan Y, Lv J, Jia J, Wang X, Yang X, Tong Z (2015) Aging-associated formaldehyde-induced norepinephrine deficiency contributes to age-related memory decline. *Aging Cell* **14**:659–668.

Melander T, Staines WA, Hökfelt T, Rökaeus Å, Eckenstein F, Salvaterra P, Wainer B (1985) Galanin-like immunoreactivity in cholinergic neurons of the septum-basal forebrain complex projecting to the hippocampus of the rat. *Brain Res* **360**:130–138.

Melis MR, Stancampiano R, Fratta W, Argiolas A (1992) Oxytocin concentration changes in different rat brain areas but not in plasma during aging. *Neurobiol Aging* **13**:783–786.

Meltzer CC, Drevets WC, Price JC, Mathis CA, Lopresti B, Greer PJ, Villemagne VL, Holt D, Mason NS, Houck PR (2001) Gender-specific aging effects on the serotonin 1A receptor. *Brain Res* **895**:9–17.

Memel M, Ryan L (2017) Visual integration enhances associative memory equally for young and older adults without reducing hippocampal encoding activation. *Neuropsychologia* **100**:195–206.

Merrill DA, Chiba AA, Tuszynski MH (2001) Conservation of neuronal number and size in the entorhinal cortex of behaviorally characterized aged rats. *J Comp Neurol* **438**:445–456.

Merrill DA, Roberts JA, Tuszynski MH (2000) Conservation of neuron number and size in entorhinal cortex layers II, III, and V/VI of aged primates. *J Comp Neurol* **422**:396–401.

Merriman NA, Ondřej J, Roudaia E, O'Sullivan C, Newell FN (2016) Familiar environments enhance object and spatial memory in both younger and older adults. *Exp Brain Res* **234**:1555–1574.

Mesches MH, Gemma C, Veng LM, Allgeier C, Young DA, Browning MD, Bickford PC (2004) Sulindac improves memory and increases NMDA receptor subunits in aged Fischer 344 rats. *Neurobiol Aging* **25**:315–324.

Meulenbroek O, Kessels RP, De Rover M, Petersson KM, Rikkert MGO, Rijpkema M, Fernández G (2010) Age-effects on associative object–location memory. *Brain Res* **1315**:100–110.

Meunier M, Bachevalier J, Mishkin M, Murray EA (1993) Effects on visual recognition of combined and separate ablations of the entorhinal and perirhinal cortex in rhesus monkeys. *J Neurosci* **13**:5418–5432.

Michalek H, Fortuna S, Pintor A (1989) Age-related differences in brain choline acetyltransferase, cholinesterases and muscarinic receptor sites in two strains of rats. *Neurobiol Aging* **10**:143–148.

Miettinen R, Sirviö J, Riekkinen Sr P, Laakso M, Riekkinen M, Riekkinen Jr P (1993) Neocortical, hippocampal and septal parvalbumin-and somatostatin-containing neurons in young and aged rats: correlation with passive avoidance and water maze performance. *Neuroscience* **53**:367–378.

Míguez JM, Aldegunde M, Paz-Valiñas L, Recio J, Sánchez-Barceló E (1999) Selective changes in the contents of noradrenaline, dopamine and serotonin in rat brain areas during aging. *J Neural Transm (Vienna)* **106**:1089–1098.

Miller JA, Zahniser NR (1988) Quantitative autoradiographic analysis of 125I-pindolol binding in Fischer 344 rat brain: changes in beta-adrenergic receptor density with aging. *Neurobiol Aging* **9**:267–272.

Milner TA, Wiley RG, Kurucz OS, Prince SR, Pierce JP (1997) Selective changes in hippocampal neuropeptide Y neurons following removal of the cholinergic septal inputs. *J Comp Neurol* **386**:46–59.

Ming GL, Song H (2005) Adult neurogenesis in the mammalian central nervous system. *Annu Rev Neurosci* **28**:223–250.

Mishkin M, Delacour J (1975) An analysis of short-term visual memory in the monkey. *J Exp Psychol Anim Behav Process* **1**:326–334.

Miura H, Qiao H, Ohta T (2002) Influence of aging and social isolation on changes in brain monoamine turnover and biosynthesis of rats elicited by novelty stress. *Synapse* **46**:116–124.

Mizumori SJ, Barnes CA, McNaughton BL (1990) Behavioral correlates of theta-on and theta-off cells recorded from hippocampal formation of mature young and aged rats. *Exp Brain Res* **80**:365–373.

Mizumori SJ, Barnes CA, McNaughton BL (1992) Differential effects of age on subpopulations of hippocampal theta cells. *Neurobiol Aging* **13**:673–679.

Mizumori SJ, Lavoie AM, Kalyani A (1996) Redistribution of spatial representation in the hippocampus of aged rats performing a spatial memory task. *Behav Neurosci* **110**:1006–1016.

Moffat SD, Elkins W, Resnick SM (2006) Age differences in the neural systems supporting human allocentric spatial navigation. *Neurobiol Aging* **27**:965–972.

Moffat SD, Kennedy KM, Rodrigue KM, Raz N (2007) Extrahippocampal contributions to age differences in human spatial navigation. *Cerebral Cortex* **17**:1274–1282.

Moffat SD, Resnick SM (2002) Effects of age on virtual environment place navigation and allocentric cognitive mapping. *Behav Neurosci* **116**:851.

Moffat SD, Zonderman AB, Resnick SM (2001) Age differences in spatial memory in a virtual environment navigation task. *Neurobiol Aging* **22**:787–796.

Monyer H, Sprengel R, Schoepfer R, Herb A, Higuchi M, Lomeli H, Burnashev N, Sakmann B, Seeburg PH (1992) Heteromeric

NMDA receptors: molecular and functional distinction of subtypes. *Science* **256**:1217–1221.

Moore CI, Browning MD, Rose GM (1993) Hippocampal plasticity induced by primed burst, but not long-term potentiation, stimulation is impaired in area CA1 of aged Fischer 344 rats. *Hippocampus* **3**:57–66.

Morel GR, Andersen T, Pardo J, Zuccolilli GO, Cambiaggi VL, Hereñú CB, Goya RG (2015) Cognitive impairment and morphological changes in the dorsal hippocampus of very old female rats. *Neuroscience* **303**:189–199.

Morgan DG (1987) The dopamine and serotonin systems during aging in human and rodent brain: a brief review. *Prog Neuropsychopharmacol Biol Psychiatry* **11**:153–157.

Morgan JI, Cohen DR, Hempstead JL, Curran T (1987) Mapping patterns of c-fos expression in the central nervous system after seizure. *Science* **237**:192–197.

Morilak DA, Somogyi P, Lujan-Miras R, Ciaranello RD (1994) Neurons expressing 5-HT2 receptors in the rat brain: neurochemical identification of cell types by immunocytochemistry. *Neuropsychopharmacology* **11**:157.

Morin AM, Wasterlain CG (1980) Aging and rat brain muscarinic receptors as measured by quinuclidinyl benzilate binding. *Neurochem Res* **5**:301–308.

Morris R (1984) Developments of a water-maze procedure for studying spatial learning in the rat. *J Neurosci Methods* **11**:47–60.

Morris RG, Garrud P, Rawlins JN, O'Keefe J (1982) Place navigation impaired in rats with hippocampal lesions. *Nature* **297**:681–683.

Morrison JH, Baxter MG (2012) The ageing cortical synapse: hallmarks and implications for cognitive decline. *Nat Rev Neurosci* **13**:240–250.

Morrison JH, Hof PR (1997) Life and death of neurons in the aging brain. *Science* **278**:412–419.

Moss MB, Rosene DL, Peters A (1988) Effects of aging on visual recognition memory in the rhesus monkey. *Neurobiol Aging* **9**:495–502.

Moss MB, Killiany RJ, Lai ZC, Rosene DL, Herndon JG (1997) Recognition memory span in rhesus monkeys of advanced age. *Neurobiol Aging* **18**:13–19.

Mouton PR, Kelley-Bell B, Tweedie D, Spangler EL, Perez E, Carlson OD, Short RG, deCabo R, Chang J, Ingram DK, et al. (2012) The effects of age and lipopolysaccharide (LPS)-mediated peripheral inflammation on numbers of central catecholaminergic neurons. *Neurobiol Aging* **33**:423, e427–436.

Mouton PR, Pakkenberg B, Gundersen HJ, Price DL (1994) Absolute number and size of pigmented locus coeruleus neurons in young and aged individuals. *J Chem Neuroanat* **7**:185–190.

Moyer JR, Jr, Brown TH (2006) Impaired trace and contextual fear conditioning in aged rats. *Behav Neurosci* **120**:612.

Moyer JR, Jr, Thompson LT, Black JP, Disterhoft JF (1992) Nimodipine increases excitability of rabbit CA1 pyramidal neurons in an age- and concentration-dependent manner. *J Neurophysiol* **68**:2100–2109.

Moyer JR, Power JM, Thompson LT, Disterhoft JF (2000) Increased excitability of aged rabbit CA1 neurons after trace eyeblink conditioning. *J Neurosci* **20**:5476–5482.

Muffato V, Hilton C, Meneghetti C, De Beni R, Wiener JM (2019) Evidence for age-related deficits in object-location binding during place recognition. *Hippocampus* **29**:971–979.

Mulkey RM, Malenka RC (1992) Mechanisms underlying induction of homosynaptic long-term depression in area CA1 of the hippocampus. *Neuron* **9**:967–975.

Mullany P, Lynch M (1997) Changes in protein synthesis and synthesis of the synaptic vesicle protein, synaptophysin, in entorhinal cortex following induction of long-term potentiation in dentate gyrus: an age-related study in the rat. *Neuropharmacology* **36**:973–980.

Muller RU, Kubie JL (1987) The effects of changes in the environment on the spatial firing of hippocampal complex-spike cells. *J Neurosci* **7**:1951–1968.

Muller RU, Kubie JL, Ranck JB, Jr. (1987) Spatial firing patterns of hippocampal complex-spike cells in a fixed environment. *J Neurosci* **7**:1935–1950.

Mumby DG (2001) Perspectives on object-recognition memory following hippocampal damage: lessons from studies in rats. *Behav Brain Res* **127**:159–181.

Mumby DG, Gaskin S, Glenn MJ, Schramek TE, Lehmann H (2002a) Hippocampal damage and exploratory preferences in rats: memory for objects, places, and contexts. *Learn Mem* **9**:49–57.

Mumby DG, Glenn MJ, Nesbitt C, Kyriazis DA (2002b) Dissociation in retrograde memory for object discriminations and object recognition in rats with perirhinal cortex damage. *Behav Brain Res* **132**:215–226.

Mumby DG, Wood ER, Pinel JP (1992) Object recognition memory is only mildly impaired in rats with lesions of the hippocampus and amygdala. *Psychobiology* **20**:18–27.

Murray CA, Lynch MA (1998) Dietary supplementation with vitamin E reverses the age-related deficit in long term potentiation in dentate gyrus. *J Biol Chem* **273**:12161–12168.

Musumeci G, Castrogiovanni P, Castorina S, Imbesi R, Szychlinska MA, Scuderi S, Loreto C, Giunta S (2015) Changes in serotonin (5-HT) and brain-derived neurotrophic factor (BDFN) expression in frontal cortex and hippocampus of aged rat treated with high tryptophan diet. *Brain Res Bull* **119**:12–18.

Myrum C, Kittleson J, De S, Fletcher BR, Castellano J, Kundu G, Becker KG, Rapp PR (2020) Survey of the arc epigenetic landscape in normal cognitive aging. *Mol Neurobiol* **57**:2727–2740.

Naber PA, Witter MP, Lopez da Silva FH (1999) Perirhinal cortex input to the hippocampus in the rat: evidence for parallel pathways, both direct and indirect: a combined physiological and anatomical study. *Eur J Neurosci* **11**:4119–4133.

Nagahara AH, Gill TM, Nicolle M, Gallagher M (1996) Alterations in opiate receptor binding in the hippocampus of aged Long-Evans rats. *Brain Res* **707**:22–30.

Nash MI, Hodges CB, Muncy NM, Kirwan CB (2021) Pattern separation beyond the hippocampus: a high-resolution whole-brain investigation of mnemonic discrimination in healthy adults. *Hippocampus* **31**:408–421.

Naveh-Benjamin M (2000) Adult age differences in memory performance: tests of an associative deficit hypothesis. *J Exp Psychol: Learn, Mem, and Cogn* **26**:1170.

Newman M, Kaszniak A (2000) Spatial memory and aging: performance on a human analog of the Morris water maze. *Aging, Neuropsychol Cogn* **7**:86–93.

Newton IG, Forbes ME, Linville MC, Pang H, Tucker EW, Riddle DR, Brunso-Bechtold JK (2008) Effects of aging and caloric restriction on dentate gyrus synapses and glutamate receptor subunits. *Neurobiol Aging* **29**:1308–1318.

Nguyen L, Murphy K, Andrews G (2021) A game a day keeps cognitive decline away? a systematic review and meta-analysis of commercially-available brain training programs in healthy and cognitively impaired older adults. *Neuropsychol Rev* **32**(3):601–630.

Nicholson DA, Yoshida R, Berry RW, Gallagher M, Geinisman Y (2004) Reduction in size of perforated postsynaptic densities in hippocampal axospinous synapses and age-related spatial learning impairments. *J Neurosci* **24**:7648–7653.

Nicolle MM, Gallagher M, McKinney M (1999) No loss of synaptic proteins in the hippocampus of aged, behaviorally impaired rats. *Neurobiol Aging* 20:343–348.

Nicolle MM, Prescott S, Bizon JL (2003) Emergence of a cue strategy preference on the water maze task in aged C57B6× SJL F1 hybrid mice. *Learn Mem* 10:520–524.

Niesen CE, Baskys A, Carlen PL (1988) Reversed ethanol effects on potassium conductances in aged hippocampal dentate granule neurons. *Brain Res* 445:137–141.

Niewiadomska G, Baksalerska-Pazera M, Gasiorowska A, Mietelska A (2006) Nerve growth factor differentially affects spatial and recognition memory in aged rats. *Neurochem Res* 31:1481–1490.

Nikoletopoulou V, Tavernarakis N (2012) Calcium homeostasis in aging neurons. *Front Genet* 3:200.

Nilakantan AS, Bridge DJ, VanHaerents S, Voss JL (2018) Distinguishing the precision of spatial recollection from its success: evidence from healthy aging and unilateral mesial temporal lobe resection. *Neuropsychologia* 119:101–106.

Nishimura A, Ueda S, Takeuchi Y, Sawada T, Kawata M (1995) Age-related decrease of serotonergic fibres and S-100 beta immunoreactivity in the rat dentate gyrus. *Neuroreport* 6:1445–1448.

Norbury R, Travis M, Erlandsson K, Waddington W, Owens J, Pimlott S, Ell P, Murphy D (2005) In vivo imaging of muscarinic receptors in the aging female brain with (R, R)[123I]-I-QNB and single photon emission tomography. *Exp Gerontol* 40:137–145.

Nordberg A, Winblad B (1981) Cholinergic receptors in human hippocampus—regional distribution and variance with age. *Life Sci* 29:1937–1944.

Norris CM, Halpain S, Foster TC (1998) Reversal of age-related alterations in synaptic plasticity by blockade of L-type Ca2+ channels. *J Neurosci* 18:3171–3179.

Norris CM, Korol DL, Foster TC (1996) Increased susceptibility to induction of long-term depression and long-term potentiation reversal during aging. *J Neurosci* 16:5382–5392.

Núñez-Santana FL, Oh MM, Antion MD, Lee A, Hell JW, Disterhoft JF (2014) Surface L-type Ca2+ channel expression levels are increased in aged hippocampus. *Aging Cell* 13:111–120.

Nyakas C, Oosterink BJ, Keijser J, Felszeghy K, de Jong GI, Korf J, Luiten PG (1997) Selective decline of 5-HT1A receptor binding sites in rat cortex, hippocampus and cholinergic basal forebrain nuclei during aging. *J Chem Neuroanat* 13:53–61.

Nyberg L, Karalija N, Salami A, Andersson M, Wåhlin A, Kaboovand N, Köhncke Y, Axelsson J, Rieckmann A, Papenberg G, et al. (2016) Dopamine D2 receptor availability is linked to hippocampal-caudate functional connectivity and episodic memory. *Proc Natl Acad Sci U S A* 113:7918–7923.

Nyman MJ, Eskola O, Kajander J, Vahlberg T, Sanabria S, Burns D, Hargreaves R, Solin O, Hietala J (2007) Gender and age affect NK1 receptors in the human brain–a positron emission tomography study with [18F] SPA-RQ. *Int J Neuropsychopharmacol* 10:219–229.

Ögren SO, Kuteeva E, Elvander-Tottie E, Hökfelt T (2010) Neuropeptides in learning and memory processes with focus on galanin. *Eur J Pharmacol* 626:9–17.

Oh MM, Power JM, Thompson LT, Moriearty PL, Disterhoft JF (1999) Metrifonate increases neuronal excitability in CA1 pyramidal neurons from both young and aging rabbit hippocampus. *J Neurosci* 19:1814–1823.

Ohm TG, Busch C, Bohl J (1997) Unbiased estimation of neuronal numbers in the human nucleus coeruleus during aging. *Neurobiol Aging* 18:393–399.

Ojo B, Davies H, Rezaie P, Gabbott P, Colyer F, Kraev I, Stewart MG (2013) Age-induced loss of mossy fibre synapses on CA3 thorns in the CA3 stratum lucidum. *Neurosci J* 2013:839535.

O'Keefe J, Dostrovsky J (1971) The hippocampus as a spatial map: preliminary evidence from unit activity in the freely-moving rat. *Brain Res* 34:171–175.

O'Keefe J, Nadel L (1978) The Hippocampus as a Cognitive Map. Oxford: Clarendon Press.

O'Keefe J, Recce ML (1993) Phase relationship between hippocampal place units and the EEG theta rhythm. *Hippocampus* 3:317–330.

O'Neill J, Senior T, Csicsvari J (2006) Place-selective firing of CA1 pyramidal cells during sharp wave/ripple network patterns in exploratory behavior. *Neuron* 49:143–155.

Oler JA, Markus EJ (1998) Age-related deficits on the radial maze and in fear conditioning: hippocampal processing and consolidation. *Hippocampus* 8:402–415.

Oler JA, Markus EJ (2000a) Age-related deficits in episodic memory may result from decreased responsiveness of hippocampal place cells to changes in context. *Ann N Y Acad Sci* 911:465–470.

Oler JA, Markus EJ (2000b) Age-related deficits in the ability to encode contextual change: a place cell analysis. *Hippocampus* 10:338–350.

Olton DS, Collison C, Werz MA (1977) Spatial memory and radial arm maze performance of rats. *Learning and Motivation* 8:289–314.

Orr G, Rao G, Houston FP, McNaughton BL, Barnes CA (2001) Hippocampal synaptic plasticity is modulated by theta rhythm in the fascia dentata of adult and aged freely behaving rats. *Hippocampus* 11:647–654.

Packard MG, Hirsh R, White NM (1989) Differential effects of fornix and caudate nucleus lesions on two radial maze tasks: evidence for multiple memory systems. *J Neurosci* 9:1465–1472.

Pakkenberg H, Andersen BB, Burns RS, Pakkenberg B (1995) A stereological study of substantia nigra in young and old rhesus monkeys. *Brain Res* 693:201–206.

Palego L, Marazziti D, Rossi A, Giannaccini G, Naccarato AG, Lucacchini A, Cassano GB (1997) Apparent absence of aging and gender effects on serotonin 1A receptors in human neocortex and hippocampus. *Brain Res* 758:26–32.

Palmer M, Irving A, Seabrook G, Jane D, Collingridge G (1997) The group I mGlu receptor agonist DHPG induces a novel form of LTD in the CA1 region of the hippocampus. *Neuropharmacology* 36:1517–1532.

Pan Z, He X, Zhou X, Li X, Rong B, Wang F (2020) Combination of ellagic acid and trans-cinnamaldehyde alleviates aging-induced cognitive impairment via modulation of mitochondrial function and inflammatory and apoptotic mediators in the prefrontal cortex of aged rats. *Chin J Physiol* 63:218.

Pardo J, Abba MC, Lacunza E, Francelle L, Morel GR, Outeiro TF, Goya RG (2017) Identification of a conserved gene signature associated with an exacerbated inflammatory environment in the hippocampus of aging rats. *Hippocampus* 27:435–449.

Park DC, Cherry KE, Smith AD, Lafronza VN (1990) Effects of distinctive context on memory for objects and their locations in young and elderly adults. *Psychology and Aging* 5:250.

Parker R, Herzog H (1999) Regional distribution of Y-receptor subtype mRNAs in rat brain. *Eur J Neurosci* 11:1431–1448.

Parsey RV, Oquendo MA, Simpson NR, Ogden RT, Van Heertum R, Arango V, Mann JJ (2002) Effects of sex, age, and aggressive traits in man on brain serotonin 5-HT1A receptor binding potential measured by PET using [C-11] WAY-100635. *Brain Res* 954:173–182.

Pascual J, del Arco C, González AM, Díaz A, del Olmo E, Pazos A (1991) Regionally specific age-dependent decline in α2-adrenoceptors: an autoradiographic study in human brain. *Neurosci Lett* 133:279–283.

Pavlides C, Greenstein YJ, Grudman M, Winson J (1988) Long-term potentiation in the dentate gyrus is induced preferentially on the positive phase of θ-rhythm. *Brain Res* **439**:383–387.

Pavlopoulos E, Jones S, Kosmidis S, Close M, Kim C, Kovalerchik O, Small SA, Kandel ER (2013) Molecular mechanism for age-related memory loss: the histone-binding protein RbAp48. *Sci Transl Med* **5**:200ra115–200ra115.

Pawlowski TL, Bellush LL, Wright AW, Walker JP, Colvin RA, Huentelman MJ (2009) Hippocampal gene expression changes during age-related cognitive decline. *Brain Res* **1256**:101–110.

Pedigo NW, Jr, Minor LD, Krumrei TN (1984) Cholinergic drug effects and brain muscarinic receptor binding in aged rats. *Neurobiol Aging* **5**:227–233.

Penner MR, Parrish RR, Hoang LT, Roth TL, Lubin FD, Barnes CA (2016) Age-related changes in Egr1 transcription and DNA methylation within the hippocampus. *Hippocampus* **26**:1008–1020.

Penner MR, Roth TL, Barnes CA, Sweatt JD (2010) An epigenetic hypothesis of aging-related cognitive dysfunction. *Front Aging Neurosci* **2**:9.

Penner MR, Roth TL, Chawla MK, Hoang LT, Roth ED, Lubin FD, Sweatt JD, Worley PF, Barnes CA (2010) Age-related changes in Arc transcription and DNA methylation within the hippocampus. *Neurobiol Aging* **32**:2198–2210.

Pereda D, Al-Osta I, Okorocha AE, Easton A, Hartell NA (2019) Changes in presynaptic calcium signalling accompany age-related deficits in hippocampal LTP and cognitive impairment. *Aging Cell* **18**:e13008.

Perry EK, Perry RH, Gibson PH, Blessed G, Tomlinson BE (1977) A cholinergic connection between normal aging and senile dementia in the human hippocampus. *Neurosci Lett* **6**:85–89.

Phillips R, LeDoux J (1992) Differential contribution of amygdala and hippocampus to cued and contextual fear conditioning. *Behav Neurosci* **106**:274.

Pintor A, Fortuna S, Volpe M, Michalek H (1988) Muscarinic receptor plasticity in the brain of senescent rats: down-regulation after repeated administration of diisopropyl fluorophosphate. *Life Sci* **42**:2113–2121.

Pitler TA, Landfield PW (1990) Aging-related prolongation of calcium spike duration in rat hippocampal slice neurons. *Brain Res* **508**:1–6.

Pitsikas N, Rigamonti AE, Cella SG, Sakellaridis N, Muller EE (2005) The nitric oxide donor molsidomine antagonizes age-related memory deficits in the rat. *Neurobiol Aging* **26**:259–264.

Pittaluga A, Fedele E, Risiglione C, Raiteri M (1993) Age-related decrease of the NMDA receptor-mediated noradrenaline release in rat hippocampus and partial restoration by D-cycloserine. *Eur J Pharmacol* **231**:129–134.

Pittaluga A, Raiteri M (1990) Release-enhancing glycine-dependent presynaptic NMDA receptors exist on noradrenergic terminals of hippocampus. *Eur J Pharmacol* **191**:231–234.

Plassman BL, Langa KM, Fisher GG, Heeringa SG, Weir DR, Ofstedal MB, Burke JR, Hurd MD, Potter GG, Rodgers WL (2007) Prevalence of dementia in the United States: the aging, demographics, and memory study. *Neuroepidemiology* **29**:125–132.

Poe BH, Linville C, Riddle DR, Sonntag WE, Brunso-Bechtold JK (2001) Effects of age and insulin-like growth factor-1 on neuron and synapse numbers in area CA3 of hippocampus. *Neuroscience* **107**:231–238.

Ponzio F, Calderini G, Lomuscio G, Vantini G, Toffano G, Algeri S (1982) Changes in monoamines and their metabolite levels in some brain regions of aged rats. *Neurobiol Aging* **3**:23–29.

Popova JS, Petkov VD (1989) Age-related changes in rat brain muscarinic receptors and beta-adrenoreceptors. *Gen Pharmacol* **20**:581–584.

Potegal M (1969) Role of the caudate nucleus in spatial orientation of rats. *J Comp Physiol Psychol* **69**:756–764.

Potier B, Jouvenceau A, Epelbaum J, Dutar P (2006) Age-related alterations of GABAergic input to CA1 pyramidal neurons and its control by nicotinic acetylcholine receptors in rat hippocampus. *Neuroscience* **142**:187–201.

Potier B, Lamour Y, Dutar P (1993) Age-related alterations in the properties of hippocampal pyramidal neurons among rat strains. *Neurobiol Aging* **14**:17–25.

Potier B, Rascol O, Jazat F, Lamour Y, Dutar P (1992) Alterations in the properties of hippocampal pyramidal neurons in the aged rat. *Neuroscience* **48**:793–806.

Power JM, Oh MM, Disterhoft JF (2001) Metrifonate decreases sI(AHP) in CA1 pyramidal neurons in vitro. *J Neurophysiol* **85**:319–322.

Power JM, Wu WW, Sametsky E, Oh MM, Disterhoft JF (2002) Age-related enhancement of the slow outward calcium-activated potassium current in hippocampal CA1 pyramidal neurons in vitro. *J Neurosci* **22**:7234–7243.

Powers R, Struble R, Casanova M, O'Connor D, Kitt C, Price D (1988) Innervation of human hippocampus by noradrenergic systems: normal anatomy and structural abnormalities in aging and in Alzheimer's disease. *Neuroscience* **25**:401–417.

Presty SK, Bachevalier J, Walker LC, Struble RG, Price DL, Mishkin M, Cork LC (1987) Age differences in recognition memory of the rhesus monkey (Macaca mulatta). *Neurobiol Aging* **8**:435–440.

Prieto GA, Cotman CW (2017) On the road towards the global analysis of human synapses. *Neural Regen Res* **12**:1586–1589.

Puglisi JT, Park DC, Smith AD, Hill GW (1985) Memory for two types of spatial location: effects of instructions, age, and format. *Am J Psychol* **98**:101–118.

Pyapali GK, Turner DA (1996) Increased dendritic extent in hippocampal CA1 neurons from aged F344 rats. *Neurobiol Aging* **17**:601–611.

Raidoo DM, Bhoola KD (1998) Pathophysiology of the kallikrein-kinin system in mammalian nervous tissue. *Pharmacol Ther* **79**:105–127.

Rao G, Lee H, Gallagher M, Knierim JJ (2021) Decreased investigatory head scanning during exploration in learning-impaired, aged rats. *Neurobiol Aging* **98**:1–9.

Rao MS, Hattiangady B, Abdel-Rahman A, Stanley DP, Shetty AK (2005) Newly born cells in the ageing dentate gyrus display normal migration, survival and neuronal fate choice but endure retarded early maturation. *Eur J Neurosci* **21**:464–476.

Rapp PR, Amaral DG (1989) Evidence for task-dependent memory dysfunction in the aged monkey. *J Neurosci* **9**:3568–3576.

Rapp PR, Amaral DG (1991) Recognition memory deficits in a subpopulation of aged monkeys resemble the effects of medial temporal lobe damage. *Neurobiol Aging* **12**:481–486.

Rapp PR, Deroche PS, Mao Y, Burwell RD (2002) Neuron number in the parahippocampal region is preserved in aged rats with spatial learning deficits. *Cereb Cortex* **12**:1171–1179.

Rapp PR, Gallagher M (1996) Preserved neuron number in the hippocampus of aged rats with spatial learning deficits. *Proc Natl Acad Sci U S A* **93**:9926–9930.

Rapp PR, Kansky MT, Roberts JA (1997) Impaired spatial information processing in aged monkeys with preserved recognition memory. *Neuroreport* **8**:1923–1928.

Rapp PR, Rosenberg RA, Gallagher M (1987) An evaluation of spatial information processing in aged rats. *Behav Neurosci* **101**:3.

Rasmussen T, Schliemann T, Sorensen JC, Zimmer J, West MJ (1996) Memory impaired aged rats: no loss of principal hippocampal and subicular neurons. *Neurobiol Aging* **17**:143–147.

Ray S, Corenblum MJ, Anandhan A, Reed A, Ortiz FO, Zhang DD, Barnes CA, Madhavan L (2018) A role for Nrf2 expression in defining the aging of hippocampal neural stem cells. *Cell Transplant* 27:589–606.

Reagh ZM, Ho HD, Leal SL, Noche JA, Chun A, Murray EA, Yassa MA (2016) Greater loss of object than spatial mnemonic discrimination in aged adults. *Hippocampus* 26:417–422.

Reagh ZM, Noche JA, Tustison NJ, Delisle D, Murray EA, Yassa MA (2018) Functional imbalance of anterolateral entorhinal cortex and hippocampal dentate/CA3 underlies age-related object pattern separation deficits. *Neuron* 97:1187–1198, e1184.

Reagh ZM, Roberts JM, Ly M, DiProspero N, Murray E, Yassa MA (2014) Spatial discrimination deficits as a function of mnemonic interference in aged adults with and without memory impairment. *Hippocampus* 24:303–314.

Reynolds JN, Carlen PL (1989) Diminished calcium currents in aged hippocampal dentate gyrus granule neurones. *Brain Res* 479:384–390.

Riad M, Garcia S, Watkins KC, Jodoin N, Doucet É, Langlois X, El Mestikawy S, Hamon M, Descarries L (2000) Somatodendritic localization of 5-HT1A and preterminal axonal localization of 5-HT1B serotonin receptors in adult rat brain. *J Comp Neurol* 417:181–194.

Rinne J (1987) Muscarinic and dopaminergic receptors in the aging human brain. *Brain Res* 404:162–168.

Rinne JO, Lo P (1993) Human brain methionine-and leucine-enkephalins and their receptors during ageing. *Brain Res* 624:131–136.

Robitsek J, Ratner MH, Stewart T, Eichenbaum H, Farb DH (2015) Combined administration of levetiracetam and valproic acid attenuates age-related hyperactivity of CA3 place cells, reduces place field area, and increases spatial information content in aged rat hippocampus. *Hippocampus* 25:1541–1555.

Rodgers MK, Sindone III JA, Moffat SD (2012) Effects of age on navigation strategy. *Neurobiol Aging* 33:202, e215–202, e222.

Rogalski E, Stebbins G, Barnes C, Murphy C, Stoub T, George S, Ferrari C, Shah R (2012a) Age-related changes in parahippocampal white matter integrity: a diffusion tensor imaging study. *Neuropsychologia* 50:1759–1765.

Rogalski E, Stebbins GT, Barnes CA, Murphy CM, Stoub TR, George S, Ferrari C, Shah RC, deToledo-Morrell L (2012b) Age-related changes in parahippocampal white matter integrity: a diffusion tensor imaging study. *Neuropsychologia* 50:1759–1765.

Rogers J, Shoemaker WJ, Morgan DG, Finch CE (1985) Senescent change in tissue weight and immunoreactive β-endorphin, enkephalin, and vasopressin in eight regions of C57BL/6J mouse brain and pituitary. *Neurobiol Aging* 6:1–9.

Rolls ET (2013) The mechanisms for pattern completion and pattern separation in the hippocampus. *Front Syst Neurosci* 7:74.

Rosenzweig ES, Barnes CA (2003) Impact of aging on hippocampal function: plasticity, network dynamics, and cognition. *Prog Neurobiol* 69:143–179.

Rosenzweig ES, Rao G, McNaughton BL, Barnes CA (1997) Role of temporal summation in age-related long-term potentiation-induction deficits. *Hippocampus* 7:549–558.

Rosenzweig ES, Redish AD, McNaughton BL, Barnes CA (2003) Hippocampal map realignment and spatial learning. *Nat Neurosci* 6:609–615.

Rowe WB, Blalock EM, Chen K-C, Kadish I, Wang D, Barrett JE, Thibault O, Porter NM, Rose GM, Landfield PW (2007) Hippocampal expression analyses reveal selective association of immediate-early, neuroenergetic, and myelinogenic pathways with cognitive impairment in aged rats. *J Neurosci* 27:3098–3110.

Rudow G, O'Brien R, Savonenko AV, Resnick SM, Zonderman AB, Pletnikova O, Marsh L, Dawson TM, Crain BJ, West MJ, et al. (2008) Morphometry of the human substantia nigra in ageing and Parkinson's disease. *Acta Neuropathol* 115:461–470.

Ryan JD, Leung G, Turk-Browne NB, Hasher L (2007) Assessment of age-related changes in inhibition and binding using eye movement monitoring. *Psychology and Aging* 22:239.

Sakurai E, Maeda T, Kaneko S, Akaike A, Satoh M (1996) Galanin inhibits long-term potentiation at Schaffer collateral-CA1 synapses in guinea-pig hippocampal slices. *Neurosci Lett* 212:21–24.

Sakurai T, Amemiya A, Ishii M, Matsuzaki I, Chemelli RM, Tanaka H, Williams SC, Richardson JA, Kozlowski GP, Wilson S (1998) Orexins and orexin receptors: a family of hypothalamic neuropeptides and G protein-coupled receptors that regulate feeding behavior. *Cell* 92:573–585.

Saleem S, Tabassum S, Ahmed S, Perveen T, Haider S (2014) Senescence related alteration in hippocampal biogenic amines produces neuropsychological deficits in rats. *Pak J Pharm Sci* 27:837–845.

Salthouse TA (1976) Speed and age: multiple rates of age decline. *Exp Aging Res* 2:349–359.

Sánchez-Alavez M, Gomez-Chavarın M, Navarro L, Jiménez-Anguiano A, Murillo-Rodrıguez E, Prado-Alcala RA, Drucker-Colin R, Prospero-Garcıa O (2000) Cortistatin modulates memory processes in rats. *Brain Res* 858:78–83.

Sandin J, Georgieva J, Schött PA, Ögren SO, Terenius L (1997) Nociceptin/orphanin FQ microinjected into hippocampus impairs spatial learning in rats. *Eur J Neurosci* 9:194–197.

Sandin J, Nylander I, Georgieva J, Schött P, Ögren S, Terenius L (1998) Hippocampal dynorphin B injections impair spatial learning in rats: a κ-opioid receptor-mediated effect. *Neuroscience* 85:375–382.

Santiago M, Machado A, Reinoso-Suárez F, Cano J (1988) Changes in biogenic amines in rat hippocampus during development and aging. *Life Sci* 42:2503–2508.

Santoro A (2013) Reassessing pattern separation in the dentate gyrus. *Front Behav Neurosci* 7:96.

Sava S, Markus EJ (2008) Activation of the medial septum reverses age-related hippocampal encoding deficits: a place field analysis. *J Neurosci* 28:1841–1853.

Scali C, Giovannini MG, Bartolini L, Prosperi C, Hinz V, Schmidt B, Pepeu G (1997) Effect of metrifonate on extracellular brain acetylcholine and object recognition in aged rats. *Eur J Pharmacol* 325:173–180.

Scali C, Giovannini MG, Prosperi C, Bartolini L, Pepeu G (1997) Tacrine administration enhances extracellular acetylcholine in vivo and restores the cognitive impairment in aged rats. *Pharmacol Res* 36:463–469.

Scheibel AB (1979) The hippocampus: organizational patterns in health and senescence. *Mech Ageing Dev* 9:89–102.

Scheibel ME, Lindsay RD, Tomiyasu U, Scheibel AB (1976) Progressive dendritic changes in the aging human limbic system. *Exp Neurol* 53:420–430.

Scherer H (1939) Melanin pigmentation of the substantia nigra in primates. *J Comp Neurol* 71:91–98.

Schiavetto A, Köhler S, Grady CL, Winocur G, Moscovitch M (2002) Neural correlates of memory for object identity and object location: effects of aging. *Neuropsychologia* 40:1428–1442.

Schimanski LA, Barnes CA (2015) Insights into age-related cognitive decline: coupling neurophysiological and behavioral approaches. In: The Maze Book, Heather Bimonte-Nelson (ed). pp 121–142. Springer: New York.

Schimanski LA, Lipa P, Barnes CA (2013) Tracking the course of hippocampal representations during learning: when is the map required? *J Neurosci* 33:3094–3106.

Schlesinger K, Lipsitz DU, Peck PL, Pelleymounter MA, Stewart JM, Chase TN (1983) Substance P enhancement of passive and active avoidance conditioning in mice. *Pharmacol Biochem Behav* 19:655–661.

Schlesinger K, Pelleymounter MA, van de Kamp J, Bader DL, Stewart JM, Chase TN (1986) Substance P facilitation of memory: effects in an appetitively motivated learning task. *Behav Neural Biol* 45:230–239.

Schmitz C, Hof P (2005) Design-based stereology in neuroscience. *Neuroscience* 130:813–831.

Schuck NW, Doeller CF, Polk TA, Lindenberger U, Li S-C (2015) Human aging alters the neural computation and representation of space. *Neuroimage* 117:141–150.

Schwarzer C (2009) 30 years of dynorphins—new insights on their functions in neuropsychiatric diseases. *Pharmacol Ther* 123:353–370.

Schweizer T, Birthelmer A, Lazaris A, Cassel J-C, Jackisch R (2003) 3, 4-DAP-evoked transmitter release in hippocampal slices of aged rats with impaired memory. *Brain Res Bull* 62:129–136.

Scognamiglio S, Aljohani YM, Olson TT, Forcelli PA, Dezfuli G, Kellar KJ (2024) Restoration of norepinephrine release, cognitive performance, and dendritic spines by amphetamine in aged rat brain. *Aging Cell* 23(4):e14087.

Seaman KL, Smith CT, Juarez EJ, Dang LC, Castrellon JJ, Burgess LL, San Juan MD, Kundzicz PM, Cowan RL, Zald DH, et al. (2019) Differential regional decline in dopamine receptor availability across adulthood: linear and nonlinear effects of age. *Hum Brain Mapp* 40:3125–3138.

Segal M (1982) Changes in neurotransmitter actions in the aged rat hippocampus. *Neurobiol Aging* 3:121–124.

Segal M, Markram H, Richter-Levin G (1991) Actions of norepinephrine in the rat hippocampus. *Prog Brain Res* 88:323–330.

Senut M, De Bilbao F, Lamour Y (1989) Age-related loss of galanin-immunoreactive cells in the rat septal area. *Neurosci Lett* 105:257–262.

Seress L, Mrzljak L (1987) Basal dendrites of granule cells are normal features of the fetal and adult dentate gyrus of both monkey and human hippocampal formations. *Brain Res* 405:169–174.

Serrano-Castro P, Garcia-Torrecillas J (2012) Cajal's first steps in scientific research. *Neuroscience* 217:1–5.

Shaerzadeh F, Phan L, Miller D, Dacquel M, Hachmeister W, Hansen C, Bechtle A, Tu D, Martcheva M, Foster TC, et al. (2020) Microglia senescence occurs in both substantia nigra and ventral tegmental area. *Glia* 68:2228–2245.

Shamy JL, Buonocore MH, Makaron LM, Amaral DG, Barnes CA, Rapp PR (2006) Hippocampal volume is preserved and fails to predict recognition memory impairment in aged rhesus monkeys (*Macaca mulatta*). *Neurobiol Aging* 27:1405–1415.

Shankar S, Teyler TJ, Robbins N (1998) Aging differentially alters forms of long-term potentiation in rat hippocampal area CA1. *J Neurophysiol* 79:334–341.

Sharps MJ, Gollin ES (1987) Memory for object locations in young and elderly adults. *J Gerontol* 42:336–341.

Sharps MJ, Gollin ES (1988) Aging and free recall for objects located in space. *J Gerontol* 43:P8–11.

Shen J, Barnes CA (1996) Age-related decrease in cholinergic synaptic transmission in three hippocampal subfields. *Neurobiol Aging* 17:439–451.

Shen J, Barnes CA, McNaughton BL, Skaggs WE, Weaver KL (1997) The effect of aging on experience-dependent plasticity of hippocampal place cells. *J Neurosci* 17:6769–6782.

Shepherd JD, Rumbaugh G, Wu J, Chowdhury S, Plath N, Kuhl D, Huganir RL, Worley PF (2006) Arc/Arg3.1 mediates homeostatic synaptic scaling of AMPA receptors. *Neuron* 52:475–484.

Sheremet A, Kennedy JP, Qin Y, Zhou Y, Lovett SD, Burke SN, Maurer AP (2018) Theta-Gamma cascades and running speed. *J Neurophysiol* 121(2):444–458.

Sherman KA, Kuster JE, Dean RL, Bartus RT, Friedman E (1981) Presynaptic cholinergic mechanisms in brain of aged rats with memory impairments. *Neurobiol Aging* 2:99–104.

Shetty AK, Turner DA (1998) Hippocampal interneurons expressing glutamic acid decarboxylase and calcium-binding proteins decrease with aging in Fischer 344 rats. *J Comp Neurol* 394:252–269.

Shetty MS, Sharma M, Sajikumar S (2017) Chelation of hippocampal zinc enhances long-term potentiation and synaptic tagging/capture in CA 1 pyramidal neurons of aged rats: implications to aging and memory. *Aging Cell* 16:136–148.

Shi L, Argenta AE, Winseck AK, Brunso-Bechtold JK (2004) Stereological quantification of GAD-67-immunoreactive neurons and boutons in the hippocampus of middle-aged and old Fischer 344 x Brown Norway rats. *J Comp Neurol* 478:282–291.

Shibata S, Tanaka T, Watanabe S (1994) Facilitatory effects of somatostatin on reduced uptake of 2-deoxyglucose in cerebral cortical and hippocampal slices from aged rats. *Eur J Pharmacol: Mol Pharmacol* 269:269–272.

Shih SI, Meadmore KL, Liversedge SP (2012) Aging, eye movements, and object-location memory. *PloS One* 7:e33485.

Shoji H, Miyakawa T (2019) Age-related behavioral changes from young to old age in male mice of a C57 BL/6J strain maintained under a genetic stability program. *Neuropsychopharmacol Rep* 39:100–118.

Shukitt-Hale B, Casadesus G, Cantuti-Castelvetri I, Joseph JA (2001) Effect of age on object exploration, habituation, and response to spatial and nonspatial change. *Behav Neurosci* 115:1059–1064.

Siddiqi ZA, Peters A (1999) The effect of aging on pars compacta of the substantia nigra in rhesus monkey. *J Neuropathol Exp Neurol* 58:903–920.

Sierra-Mercado D, Dieguez D, Jr, Barea-Rodriguez EJ (2008) Brief novelty exposure facilitates dentate gyrus LTP in aged rats. *Hippocampus* 18:835–843.

Simic G, Bexheti S, Kelovic Z, Kos M, Grbic K, Hof PR, Kostovic I (2005) Hemispheric asymmetry, modular variability and age-related changes in the human entorhinal cortex. *Neuroscience* 130:911–925.

Simkin D, Hattori S, Ybarra N, Musial TF, Buss EW, Richter H, Oh MM, Nicholson DA, Disterhoft JF (2015) Aging-related hyperexcitability in CA3 pyramidal neurons is mediated by enhanced A-Type K+ channel function and expression. *J Neurosci* 35:13206–13218.

Sink KM, Espeland MA, Castro CM, Church T, Cohen R, Dodson JA, Guralnik J, Hendrie HC, Jennings J, Katula J (2015) Effect of a 24-month physical activity intervention vs health education on cognitive outcomes in sedentary older adults: the LIFE randomized trial. *Jama* 314:781–790.

Sirvio J, Jolkkonen J, Pitkanen A, Riekkinen PJ (1987) Age dependence of somatostatin levels and somatostatin binding in the rat brain. *Comp Biochem Physiol A Comp Physiol* 87:355–357.

Sirviö J, Lahtinen H, Riekkinen P, Riekkinen PJ (1994) Spatial learning and noradrenaline content in the brain and periphery of young and aged rats. *Exp Neurol* 125:312–315.

Sjölinder M, Höök K, Nilsson L-G, Andersson G (2005) Age differences and the acquisition of spatial knowledge in a three-dimensional environment: evaluating the use of an overview map as a navigation aid. *Int J Hum Comput Stud* 63:537–564.

Skaggs W, McNaughton B, Gothard K (1992) An information-theoretic approach to deciphering the hippocampal code. *Adv Neural Inf Process Syst* 5.

Skaggs WE, McNaughton BL (1996) Replay of neuronal firing sequences in rat hippocampus during sleep following spatial experience. *Science* 271:1870–1873.

Skaggs WE, McNaughton BL, Permenter M, Archibeque M, Vogt J, Amaral DG, Barnes CA (2007) EEG sharp waves and sparse ensemble unit activity in the macaque hippocampus. *J Neurophysiol* 98:898–910.

Skalicky M, Bubna-Littitz H, Hofecker G (1984) The influence of persistent crowding on the age changes of behavioral parameters and survival characteristics of rats. *Mech Ageing Dev* 28:325–336.

Sladek JR, Sladek CD (1978) Relative quantitation of monoamine histofluorescence in young and old non-human primates. *Adv Exp Med Biol* 113:231–239.

Small SA, Chawla MK, Buonocore M, Rapp PR, Barnes CA (2004) Imaging correlates of brain function in monkeys and rats isolates a hippocampal subregion differentially vulnerable to aging. *Proc Natl Acad Sci U S A* 101:7181–7186.

Small SA, Tsai WY, DeLaPaz R, Mayeux R, Stern Y (2002) Imaging hippocampal function across the human life span: is memory decline normal or not? *Ann Neurol* 51:290–295.

Smith AC, Gerrard JL, Barnes CA, McNaughton BL (2000) Effect of age on burst firing characteristics of rat hippocampal pyramidal cells. *Neuroreport* 11:3865–3871.

Smith CT, Crawford JL, Dang LC, Seaman KL, San Juan MD, Vijay A, Katz DT, Matuskey D, Cowan RL, Morris ED, et al. (2019) Partial-volume correction increases estimated dopamine D2-like receptor binding potential and reduces adult age differences. *J Cereb Blood Flow Metab* 39:822–833.

Smith D, Roberts J, Gage F, Tuszynski M (1999) Age-associated neuronal atrophy occurs in the primate brain and is reversible by growth factor gene therapy. *Proc Natl Acad Sci U S A* 96:10893–10898.

Smith M, Booze R (1995) Cholinergic and GABAergic neurons in the nucleus basalis region of young and aged rats. *Neuroscience* 67:679–688.

Smith ML, Deadwyler SA, Booze RM (1993) 3-D reconstruction of the cholinergic basal forebrain system in young and aged rats. *Neurobiol Aging* 14:389–392.

Smith SM, Zequeira S, Ravi M, Johnson SA, Hampton AM, Ross AM, Pyon W, Maurer AP, Bizon JL, Burke SN (2021) Age-related impairments on the touchscreen paired associates learning (PAL) task in male rats. *Neurobiol Aging* 109:176–191.

Smith TD, Adams MM, Gallagher M, Morrison JH, Rapp PR (2000) Circuit-specific alterations in hippocampal synaptophysin immunoreactivity predict spatial learning impairment in aged rats. *J Neurosci* 20:6587–6593.

Smith TD, Gallagher M, Leslie FM (1995) Cholinergic binding sites in rat brain: analysis by age and cognitive status. *Neurobiol Aging* 16:161–173.

Soffié M, Hahn K, Terao E, Eclancher F (1999) Behavioural and glial changes in old rats following environmental enrichment. *Behav Brain Res* 101:37–49.

Solomon PR, Solomon SD, Schaaf EV, Perry HE (1983) Altered activity in the hippocampus is more detrimental to classical conditioning than removing the structure. *Science* 220:329–331.

Solomon PR, Vander Schaaf ER, Thompson RF, Weisz DJ (1986) Hippocampus and trace conditioning of the rabbit's classically conditioned nictitating membrane response. *Behav Neurosci* 100:729.

Sperk G, Hamilton T, Colmers WF (2007) Neuropeptide Y in the dentate gyrus. *Progress in Brain Res* 163:285–297.

Spiegel AM, Koh MT, Vogt NM, Rapp PR, Gallagher M (2013) Hilar interneuron vulnerability distinguishes aged rats with memory impairment. *J Comp Neurol* 521:3508–3523.

Stackman RW, Cohen SJ, Lora JC, Rios LM (2016) Temporary inactivation reveals that the CA1 region of the mouse dorsal hippocampus plays an equivalent role in the retrieval of long-term object memory and spatial memory. *Neurobiol Learn Mem* 133:118–128.

Stancampiano R, Melis MR, Fratta W, Argiolas A (1994) Brain proteolysis of oxytocin in vitro and in vivo changes during aging in male rats. *Neurobiol Aging* 15:185–189.

Stanley DP, Shetty AK (2004) Aging in the rat hippocampus is associated with widespread reductions in the number of glutamate decarboxylase-67 positive interneurons but not interneuron degeneration. *J Neurochem* 89:204–216.

Stanley EM, Fadel JR (2011) Aging-related alterations in orexin/hypocretin modulation of septo-hippocampal amino acid neurotransmission. *Neuroscience* 195:70–79.

Stark SM, Stark CEL (2017) Age-related deficits in the mnemonic similarity task for objects and scenes. *Behav Brain Res* 333:109–117.

Stark SM, Stevenson R, Wu C, Rutledge S, Stark CE (2015) Stability of age-related deficits in the mnemonic similarity task across task variations. *Behav Neurosci* 129:257–268.

Stark SM, Yassa MA, Lacy JW, Stark CE (2013) A task to assess behavioral pattern separation (BPS) in humans: data from healthy aging and mild cognitive impairment. *Neuropsychologia* 51:2442–2449.

Stark SM, Yassa MA, Stark CE (2010) Individual differences in spatial pattern separation performance associated with healthy aging in humans. *Learn Mem* 17:284–288.

Steinbusch HWM (1981) Distribution of serotonin-immunoreactivity in the central nervous system of the rat—cell bodies and terminals. *Neuroscience* 6:557–618.

Stemmelin J, Lazarus C, Cassel S, Kelche C, Cassel J-C (2000) Immunohistochemical and neurochemical correlates of learning deficits in aged rats. *Neuroscience* 96:275–289.

Stone CP (1929) The age factor in animal learning: I. Rats in the problem box and the maze. *Genet Psychol Monogr* 5:1–130.

Stoub TR, deToledo-Morrell L, Stebbins GT, Leurgans S, Bennett DA, Shah RC (2006) Hippocampal disconnection contributes to memory dysfunction in individuals at risk for Alzheimer's disease. *Proc Natl Acad Sci U S A* 103:10041–10045.

Stranahan AM, Haberman RP, Gallagher M (2011) Cognitive decline is associated with reduced reelin expression in the entorhinal cortex of aged rats. *Cerebral Cortex* 21:392–400.

Stroessner-Johnson H, Rapp P, Amaral D (1992) Cholinergic cell loss and hypertrophy in the medial septal nucleus of the behaviorally characterized aged rhesus monkey. *J Neurosci* 12:1936–1944.

Strong R, Hicks P, Hsu L, Bartus R, Enna S (1980) Age-related alterations in the rodent brain cholinergic system and behavior. *Neurobiol Aging* 1:59–63.

Sturrock R, Rao K (1985) A quantitative histological study of neuronal loss from the locus coeruleus of ageing mice. *Neuropathol Appl Neurobiol* 11:55–60.

Suhara T, Inoue O, Kobayashi K, Suzuki K, Tateno Y (1993) Age-related changes in human muscarinic acetylcholine receptors measured by positron emission tomography. *Neurosci Lett* 149:225–228.

Sullivan D, Csicsvari J, Mizuseki K, Montgomery S, Diba K, Buzsaki G (2011) Relationships between hippocampal sharp waves, ripples, and fast gamma oscillation: influence of dentate and entorhinal cortical activity. *J Neurosci* 31:8605–8616.

Sutherland GR, McNaughton B (2000) Memory trace reactivation in hippocampal and neocortical neuronal ensembles. *Curr Opin Neurobiol* 10:180–186.

Svoboda KR, Adams CE, Lupica CR (1999) Opioid receptor subtype expression defines morphologically distinct classes of hippocampal interneurons. *J Neurosci* 19:85–95.

Takeuchi T, Duszkiewicz AJ, Sonneborn A, Spooner PA, Yamasaki M, Watanabe M, Smith CC, Fernández G, Deisseroth K, Greene RW, et al. (2016) Locus coeruleus and dopaminergic consolidation of everyday memory. *Nature* 537:357–362.

Tallent MK, Fabre V, Qiu C, Calbet M, Lamp T, Baratta MV, Suzuki C, Levy CL, Siggins GR, Henriksen SJ, et al. (2005) Cortistatin overexpression in transgenic mice produces deficits in synaptic plasticity and learning. *Mol Cell Neurosci* 30:465–475.

Tanila H, Shapiro ML, Eichenbaum H (1997) Discordance of spatial representation in ensembles of hippocampal place cells. *Hippocampus* 7:613–623.

Tanila H, Shapiro M, Gallagher M, Eichenbaum H (1997) Brain aging: changes in the nature of information coding by the hippocampus. *J Neurosci* 17:5155–5166.

Tanila H, Sipila P, Shapiro M, Eichenbaum H (1997) Brain aging: impaired coding of novel environmental cues. *J Neurosci* 17:5167–5174.

Taverna FA, Georgiou J, McDonald RJ, Hong NS, Kraev A, Salter MW, Takeshima H, Muller RU, Roder JC (2005) Defective place cell activity in nociceptin receptor knockout mice with elevated NMDA receptor-dependent long-term potentiation. *J Physiol* 565:579–591.

Templer VL, Wise TB, Heimer-McGinn VR (2019) Social housing protects against age-related working memory decline independently of physical enrichment in rats. *Neurobiol Aging* 75:117–125.

Theofilas P, Ehrenberg AJ, Dunlop S, Alho ATDL, Nguy A, Leite REP, Rodriguez RD, Mejia MB, Suemoto CK, Ferretti-Rebustini REDL (2017) Locus coeruleus volume and cell population changes during Alzheimer's disease progression: a stereological study in human postmortem brains with potential implication for early-stage biomarker discovery. *Alzheimer's and Dementia* 13:236–246.

Terao A, Apte-Deshpande A, Morairty S, Freund YR, Kilduff TS (2002) Age-related decline in hypocretin (orexin) receptor 2 messenger RNA levels in the mouse brain. *Neurosci Lett* 332:190–194.

Thibault O, Landfield PW (1996) Increase in single L-type calcium channels in hippocampal neurons during aging. *Science* 272:1017–1020.

Thomas MJ, Moody TD, Makhinson M, O'Dell TJ (1996) Activity-dependent β-adrenergic modulation of low frequency stimulation induced LTP in the hippocampal CA1 region. *Neuron* 17:475–482.

Thomé A, Gray DT, Erickson CA, Lipa P, Barnes CA (2016) Memory impairment in aged primates is associated with region-specific network dysfunction. *Mol Psychiatry* 21:1257–1262.

Thompson LT, Best PJ (1990) Long-term stability of the place-field activity of single units recorded from the dorsal hippocampus of freely behaving rats. *Brain Res* 509:299–308.

Thompson LT, Disterhoft JF (1997) Age-and dose-dependent facilitation of associative eyeblink conditioning by {d}-cycloserine in rabbits. *Behav Neurosci* 111:1303.

Thompson LT, Moyer JR, Jr. and Disterhoft JF (1996) Trace eyeblink conditioning in rabbits demonstrates heterogeneity of learning ability both between and within age groups. *Neurobiol Aging* 17:619–629.

Tigges J, Gordon TP, McClure HM, Hall EC, Peters A (1988) Survival rate and life span of rhesus monkeys at the Yerkes Regional Primate Research Center. *Am J Primatol* 15:263–273.

Tigges J, Herndon JG, Rosene DL (1995) Mild age-related changes in the dentate gyrus of adult rhesus monkeys. *Acta Anat (Basel)* 153:39–48.

Tigges J, Herndon JG, Rosene DL (1996) Preservation into old age of synaptic number and size in the supragranular layer of the dentate gyrus in rhesus monkeys. *Acta Anat (Basel)* 157:63–72.

Toescu EC, Verkhratsky A (2003) Neuronal ageing from an intraneuronal perspective: roles of endoplasmic reticulum and mitochondria. *Cell Calcium* 34:311–323.

Toescu EC, Verkhratsky A, Landfield PW (2004) Ca2+ regulation and gene expression in normal brain aging. *Trends Neurosci* 27:614–620.

Tohgi H, Utsugisawa K, Yoshimura M, Nagane Y, Mihara M (1998) Age-related changes in nicotinic acetylcholine receptor subunits α4 and β2 messenger RNA expression in postmortem human frontal cortex and hippocampus. *Neurosci Lett* 245:139–142.

Tolman EC (1948) Cognitive maps in rats and men. *Psychol Rev* 55:189.

Tombaugh GC, Rowe WB, Chow AR, Michael TH, Rose GM (2002) Theta-frequency synaptic potentiation in CA1 in vitro distinguishes cognitively impaired from unimpaired aged Fischer 344 rats. *J Neurosci* 22:9932–9940.

Tombaugh GC, Rowe WB, Rose GM (2005) The slow afterhyperpolarization in hippocampal CA1 neurons covaries with spatial learning ability in aged Fisher 344 rats. *J Neurosci* 25:2609–2616.

Tomlinson BE, Irving D, Blessed G (1981) Cell loss in the locus coeruleus in senile dementia of Alzheimer type. *J Neurol Sci* 49:419–428.

Tomonaga M (1983) Neuropathology of the locus ceruleus: a semi-quantitative study. *J Neurol* 230:231–240.

Toner CK, Pirogovsky E, Kirwan CB, Gilbert PE (2009) Visual object pattern separation deficits in nondemented older adults. *Learn Mem* 16:338–342.

Tonkikh A, Janus C, El-Beheiry H, Pennefather PS, Samoilova M, McDonald P, Ouanounou A, Carlen PL (2006) Calcium chelation improves spatial learning and synaptic plasticity in aged rats. *Exp Neurol* 197:291–300.

Topic B, Willuhn I, Palomero-Gallagher N, Zilles K, Huston JP, Hasenöhrl RU (2007) Impaired maze performance in aged rats is accompanied by increased density of NMDA, 5-HT1A, and alpha-adrenoceptor binding in hippocampus. *Hippocampus* 17:68–77.

Touzani K, Marighetto A, Jaffard R (2003) Fos imaging reveals ageing-related changes in hippocampal response to radial maze discrimination testing in mice. *Eur J Neurosci* 17:628–640.

Tran LM, Josselyn SA, Richards BA, Frankland PW (2019) Forgetting at biologically realistic levels of neurogenesis in a large-scale hippocampal model. *Behav Brain Res* 376:112180.

Trelle AN, Henson RN, Green DAE, Simons JS (2017) Declines in representational quality and strategic retrieval processes contribute to age-related increases in false recognition. *J Exp Psychol Learn Mem Cogn* 43:1883–1897.

Tribollet E, Bertrand D, Marguerat A, Raggenbass M (2004) Comparative distribution of nicotinic receptor subtypes during development, adulthood and aging: an autoradiographic study in the rat brain. *Neuroscience* 124:405–420.

Trillo L, Gonzalo LM (1992) Ageing of the human entorhinal cortex and subicular complex. *Histol Histopathol* 7:17–22.

Trivedi P, Yu H, MacNeil DJ, Van der Ploeg LH, Guan XM (1998) Distribution of orexin receptor mRNA in the rat brain. *FEBS Lett* 438:71–75.

Tsukada H, Kakiuchi T, Nishiyama S, Ohba H, Harada N (2001) Effects of aging on 5-HT(1A) receptors and their functional response to 5-HT(1a) agonist in the living brain: PET study with [carbonyl-(11)C]WAY-100635 in conscious monkeys. *Synapse* 42:242–251.

Tsukada H, Kakiuchi T, Nishiyama S, Ohba H, Sato K, Harada N, Takahashi K (2001) Age differences in muscarinic cholinergic receptors assayed with (+) N-[11C] methyl-3-piperidyl benzilate in the brains of conscious monkeys. *Synapse* 41:248–257.

Turner DA, Deupree DL (1991) Functional elongation of CA1 hippocampal neurons with aging in Fischer 344 rats. *Neurobiol Aging* 12:201–210.

Uemura E (1985a) Age-related changes in the subiculum of Macaca mulatta: dendritic branching pattern. *Exp Neurol* 87:412–427.

Uemura E (1985b) Age-related changes in the subiculum of Macaca mulatta: synaptic density. *Exp Neurol* 87:403–411.

Uezu K, Sano A, Sei H, Toida K, Houtani T, Sugimoto T, Suzuki-Yamamoto T, Takeshima H, Ishimura K, Morita Y (2005) Enhanced hippocampal acetylcholine release in nociceptin-receptor knockout mice. *Brain Res* 1050:118–123.

Uttl B, Graf P (1993) Episodic spatial memory in adulthood. *Psychol Aging* 8:257–273.

Uylings HB, de Brabander JM (2002) Neuronal changes in normal human aging and Alzheimer's disease. *Brain Cogn* 49:268–276.

Valerio A, Belloni M, Gorno ML, Tinti C, Memo M, Spano P (1994) Dopamine D2, D3, and D4 receptor mRNA levels in rat brain and pituitary during aging. *Neurobiol Aging* 15:713–719.

Vanderwolf CH (1969) Hippocampal electrical activity and voluntary movement in the rat. *Electroencephalogr Clin Neurophysiol* 26:407–418.

Vanderwolf CH, Kramis R, Robinson TE (1977) Hippocampal electrical activity during waking behaviour and sleep: analyses using centrally acting drugs. *Ciba Found Symp* 199–226.

Van Gool W, Mirmiran M, Van Haaren F (1985) Spatial memory and visual evoked potentials in young and old rats after housing in an enriched environment. *Behav Neural Biol* 44:454–469.

van Leeuwen F, Caffé R (1983) Vasopressin-immunoreactive cell bodies in the bed nucleus of the stria terminalis of the rat. *Cell Tissue Res* 228:525–534.

van Luijtelaar MG, Steinbusch HW, Tonnaer JA (1988) Aberrant morphology of serotonergic fibers in the forebrain of the aged rat. *Neurosci Lett* 95:93–96.

van Luijtelaar MG, Tonnaer JA, Steinbusch HW (1992) Aging of the serotonergic system in the rat forebrain: an immunocytochemical and neurochemical study. *Neurobiol Aging* 13:201–215.

Vannucchi MG, Scali C, Kopf SR, Pepeu G, Casamenti F (1997) Selective muscarinic antagonists differentially affect in vivo acetylcholine release and memory performances of young and aged rats. *Neuroscience* 79:837–846.

Vazdarjanova A, Guzowski JF (2004) Differences in hippocampal neuronal population responses to modifications of an environmental context: evidence for distinct, yet complementary, functions of CA3 and CA1 ensembles. *J Neurosci* 24:6489–6496.

Vazdarjanova A, McNaughton BL, Barnes CA, Worley PF, Guzowski JF (2002) Experience-dependent coincident expression of the effector immediate-early genes arc and Homer 1a in hippocampal and neocortical neuronal networks. *J Neurosci* 22:10067–10071.

Venero JL, de la Roza C, Machado A, Cano J (1993) Age-related changes on monoamine turnover in hippocampus of rats. *Brain Res* 631:89–96.

Veng LM, Browning MD (2002) Regionally selective alterations in expression of the alpha(1D) subunit (Ca(v)1.3) of L-type calcium channels in the hippocampus of aged rats. *Brain Res Mol Brain Res* 107:120–127.

Vertes RP (1991) A PHA-L analysis of ascending projections of the dorsal raphe nucleus in the rat. *J Comp Neurol* 313:643–668.

Verzar-McDougall E (1957) Studies in learning and memory in ageing rats. *Gerontology* 1:65–85.

Veyrat-Durebex C, Quirion R, Ferland G, Dumont Y, Gaudreau P (2013) Aging and long-term caloric restriction regulate neuropeptide Y receptor subtype densities in the rat brain. *Neuropeptides* 47:163–169.

Vijayashankar N, Brody H (1979) A quantitative study of the pigmented neurons in the nuclei locus coeruleus and subcoeruleus in man as related to aging. *J Neuropath Exp Neur* 38:490–497.

Villanueva-Castillo C, Tecuatl C, Herrera-López G, Galván EJ (2017) Aging-related impairments of hippocampal mossy fibers synapses on CA3 pyramidal cells. *Neurobiol Aging* 49:119–137.

Villarreal JS, Dykes JR, Barea-Rodriguez EJ (2004) Fischer 344 rats display age-related memory deficits in trace fear conditioning. *Behav Neurosci* 118:1166.

von Bohlen und Halbach O, Zacher C, Gass P, Unsicker K (2006) Age-related alterations in hippocampal spines and deficiencies in spatial memory in mice. *J Neurosci Res* 83:525–531.

Voytko ML, Sukhov RR, Walker LC, Breckler SJ, Price DL, Koliatsos VE (1995) Neuronal number and size are preserved in the nucleus basalis of aged rhesus monkeys. *Dement Geriatr Cogn Disord* 6:131–141.

Wagner JJ, Terman GW, Chavkin C (1993) Endogenous dynorphins inhibit excitatory neurotransmission and block LTP induction in the hippocampus. *Nature* 363:451.

Wallace JE, Krauter EE, Campbell BA (1980) Animal models of declining memory in the aged: short-term and spatial memory in the aged rat. *J Gerontol* 35:355–363.

Wang Z, Man S, Tang F (1993) Age-related changes in the contents of neuropeptides in the rat brain and pituitary. *Neurobiol Aging* 14:529–534.

Watabe AM, O'Dell TJ (2003) Age-related changes in theta frequency stimulation-induced long-term potentiation. *Neurobiol Aging* 24:267–272.

Watson J, Khorasani H, Persson A, Huang KP, Huang F, O'Dell T (2002) Age-related deficits in long-term potentiation are insensitive to hydrogen peroxide: coincidence with enhanced autophosphorylation of Ca2+/calmodulin-dependent protein kinase II. *J Neurosci Res* 70:298–308.

Webster MJ, Shannon Weickert C, Herman MM, Hyde TM, Kleinman JE (2001) Synaptophysin and GAP-43 mRNA levels in the hippocampus of subjects with schizophrenia. *Schizophr Res* 49:89–98.

Weible AP, Oh MM, Lee G, Disterhoft JF (2004) Galantamine facilitates acquisition of hippocampus-dependent trace eyeblink conditioning in aged rabbits. *Learn Mem* 11:108–115.

Weiss C, Preston AR, Oh MM, Schwarz RD, Welty D, Disterhoft JF (2000) The M1 muscarinic agonist CI-1017 facilitates trace eyeblink conditioning in aging rabbits and increases the excitability of CA1 pyramidal neurons. *J Neurosci* 20:783–790.

Wenk GL, Zajaczkowski W, Danysz W (1997) Neuroprotection of acetylcholinergic basal forebrain neurons by memantine and neurokinin B. *Behav Brain Res* 83:129–133.

West MJ (1993a) New stereological methods for counting neurons. *Neurobiol Aging* 14:275–285.

West MJ (1993b) Regionally specific loss of neurons in the aging human hippocampus. *Neurobiol Aging* 14:287–293.

West MJ, Coleman PD, Flood DG, Troncoso JC (1994) Differences in the pattern of hippocampal neuronal loss in normal ageing and Alzheimer's disease. *Lancet* 344:769–772.

Wester P, Hardy J, Marcusson J, Nyberg P, Winblad B (1984) Serotonin concentrations in normal aging human brains: relation to serotonin receptors. *Neurobiol Aging* 5:199–203.

Whissell PD, Bang JY, Khan I, Xie Y-F, Parfitt GM, Grenon M, Plummer NW, Jensen P, Bonin RP, Kim JC (2019) Selective activation of cholecystokinin-expressing GABA (CCK-GABA) neurons enhances memory and cognition. *eNeuro* 6(1).

Whitehead JC, Li L, McQuiggan DA, Gambino SA, Binns MA, Ryan JD (2018) Portable eyetracking-based assessment of memory decline. *J Clin Exp Neuropsychol* 40:904–916.

Whitehouse PJ, Parhad IM, Hedreen JC, Clark AW, White CL, Struble RG, Price DL (1983) Integrity of the nucleus basalis of Meynert in normal aging: 10: 45 Am. *Neurology* 33:159.

Wiegand JP, Gray DT, Schimanski LA, Lipa P, Barnes CA, Cowen SL (2016) Age is associated with reduced sharp-wave ripple frequency and altered patterns of neuronal variability. *J Neurosci* 36:5650–5660.

Wiener JM, de Condappa O, Harris MA, Wolbers T (2013) Maladaptive bias for extrahippocampal navigation strategies in aging humans. *J Neurosci* 33:6012–6017.

Williams KW, Elmquist JK (2012) From neuroanatomy to behavior: central integration of peripheral signals regulating feeding behavior. *Nat Neurosci* 15:1350.

Williams RS, Matthysse S (1986) Age-related changes in Down syndrome brain and the cellular pathology of Alzheimer disease. *Prog Brain Res* 70:49–67.

Williams TJ, Mitterling KL, Thompson LI, Torres-Reveron A, Waters EM, McEwen BS, Gore AC, Milner TA (2011) Age-and hormone-regulation of opioid peptides and synaptic proteins in the rat dorsal hippocampal formation. *Brain Res* 1379:71–85.

Wilson IA, Ikonen S, Gallagher M, Eichenbaum H, Tanila H (2005) Age-associated alterarions in place cells are subregion specific. *J Neurosci* 25:6877–6886.

Wilson IA, Ikonen S, Gureviciene I, McMahan RW, Gallagher M, Eichenbaum H, Tanila H (2004) Cognitive aging and the hippocampus: how old rats represent new environments. *J Neurosci* 24:3870–3878.

Wilson IA, Ikonen S, McMahan RW, Gallagher M, Eichenbaum H, Tanila H (2003) Place cell rigidity correlates with impaired spatial learning in aged rats. *Neurobiol Aging* 24:297–305.

Wilson MA, McNaughton BL (1994) Reactivation of hippocampal ensemble memories during sleep. *Science* 265:676–679.

Wimmer ME, Hernandez PJ, Blackwell J, Abel T (2012) Aging impairs hippocampus-dependent long-term memory for object location in mice. *Neurobiol Aging* 33:2220–2224.

Winblad B, Hardy J, Bäckman L, Nilsson LG (1985) Memory function and brain biochemistry in normal aging and in senile dementia. *Ann N Y Acad Sci* 444:255–268.

Witter MP (2007) Intrinsic and extrinsic wiring of CA3: indications for connectional heterogeneity. *Learn Mem* 14:705–713.

Woodruff-Pak DS, Foy MR, Akopian GG, Lee KH, Zach J, Nguyen KPT, Comalli DM, Kennard JA, Agelan A, Thompson RF (2010) Differential effects and rates of normal aging in cerebellum and hippocampus. *Proc Natl Acad Sci U S A* 107:1624–1629.

Woodruff-Pak D, Logan C (1988) No apparent age differences in hippocampal theta frequency in rabbits aged 3–50 months. *Comprehensive Gerontology Section A, Clin Lab Sci* 2:24–28.

Woodruff-Pak DS, Seta SE, Roker LA, Lehr MA (2007) Effects of paradigm and inter-stimulus interval on age differences in eyeblink classical conditioning in rabbits. *Learn Mem* 14:287–294.

Worley PF, Bhat RV, Baraban JM, Erickson CA, McNaughton BL, Barnes CA (1993) Thresholds for synaptic activation of transcription factors in hippocampus: correlation with long-term enhancement. *J Neurosci* 13:4776–4786.

Wree A, Braak H, Schleicher A, Zilles K (1980) Biomathematical analysis of the neuronal loss in the aging human brain of both sexes, demonstrated in pigment preparations of the pars cerebellaris loci coerulei. *Anatomy and Embryology* 160:105–119.

Xu ZQD, Shi TJS, Hökfelt T (1998) Galanin/GMAP-and NPY-like immunoreactivities in locus coeruleus and noradrenergic nerve terminals in the hippocampal formation and cortex with notes on the galanin-R1 and-R2 receptors. *J Comp Neurol* 392:227–251.

Yan J, Zhang Y, Roder J, McDonald RJ (2003) Aging effects on spatial tuning of hippocampal place cells in mice. *Exp Brain Res* 150:184–193.

Yanai S, Ito H, Endo S (2018) Long-term cilostazol administration prevents age-related decline of hippocampus-dependent memory in mice. *Neuropharmacology* 129:57–68.

Yang C, DeMars KM, Candelario-Jalil E (2018) Age-dependent decrease in adropin is associated with reduced levels of endothelial nitric oxide synthase and increased oxidative stress in the rat brain. *Aging and Disease* 9:322.

Yang L, Zou B, Xiong X, Pascual C, Xie J, Malik A, Xie J, Sakurai T, Xie XS (2013) Hypocretin/orexin neurons contribute to hippocampus-dependent social memory and synaptic plasticity in mice. *J Neurosci* 33:5275–5284.

Yang S, Megill A, Ardiles AO, Ransom S, Tran T, Koh MT, Lee HK, Gallagher M, Kirkwood A (2013) Integrity of mGluR-LTD in the associative/commissural inputs to CA3 correlates with successful aging in rats. *J Neurosci* 33:12670–12678.

Yang Z, Krause M, Rao G, McNaughton BL, Barnes CA (2008) Synaptic commitment: developmentally regulated reciprocal changes in hippocampal granule cell NMDA and AMPA receptors over the lifespan. *J Neurophysiol* 99:2760–2768.

Yassa MA, Lacy JW, Stark SM, Albert MS, Gallagher M, Stark CE (2010) Pattern separation deficits associated with increased hippocampal CA3 and dentate gyrus activity in nondemented older adults. *Hippocampus* 21(9):968–979.

Yassa MA, Mattfeld AT, Stark SM, Stark CE (2011) Age-related memory deficits linked to circuit-specific disruptions in the hippocampus. *Proc Natl Acad Sci U S A* 108:8873–8878.

Yassa MA, Muftuler LT, Stark CE (2010) Ultrahigh-resolution microstructural diffusion tensor imaging reveals perforant path degradation in aged humans in vivo. *Proc Natl Acad Sci U S A* 107:12687–12691.

Yau JL, Olsson T, Noble J, Seckl JR (1999) Serotonin receptor subtype gene expression in the hippocampus of aged rats following chronic amitriptyline treatment. *Brain Res Mol Brain Res* 70:282–287.

Yegla B, Foster TC (2022) Operationally defining cognitive reserve genes. *Neurobiol Aging* 110:96–105.

Ylinen A, Bragin A, Nadasdy Z, Jando G, Szabo I, Sik A, Buzsaki G (1995) Sharp wave-associated high-frequency oscillation (200 Hz) in the intact hippocampus: network and intracellular mechanisms. *J Neurosci* 15:30–46.

Yoder WM, Gaynor LS, Burke SN, Setlow B, Smith DW, Bizon JL (2017) Interaction between age and perceptual similarity in olfactory discrimination learning in F344 rats: relationships with spatial learning. *Neurobiol Aging* 53:122–137.

Young CE, Arima K, Xie J, Hu L, Beach TG, Falkai P, Honer WG (1998) SNAP-25 deficit and hippocampal connectivity in schizophrenia. *Cereb Cortex* 8:261–268.

Zeamer A, Meunier M, Bachevalier J (2011) Stimulus similarity and encoding time influence incidental recognition memory in adult monkeys with selective hippocampal lesions. *Learn Mem* 18:170–180.

Zhang WQ, Mundy WR, Thai L, Hudson PM, Gallagher M, Tilson HA, Hong J (1991) Decreased glutamate release correlates with elevated dynorphin content in the hippocampus of aged rats with spatial learning deficits. *Hippocampus* 1:391–397.

Zhao H, Li Q, Pei X, Zhang Z, Yang R, Wang J, Li Y (2009) Long-term ginsenoside administration prevents memory impairment in aged C57BL/6J mice by up-regulating the synaptic plasticity-related proteins in hippocampus. *Behav Brain Res* 201:311–317.

Zhong JY, Magnusson KR, Swarts ME, Clendinen CA, Reynolds NC, Moffat SD (2017) The application of a rodent-based Morris water maze (MWM) protocol to an investigation of age-related differences in human spatial learning. *Behav Neurosci* **131**:470.

Zhong JY, Moffat SD (2016) Age-related differences in associative learning of landmarks and heading directions in a virtual navigation task. *Front Aging Neurosci* **8**:122.

Zola-Morgan S, Squire LR (1985) Medial temporal lesions in monkeys impair memory on a variety of tasks sensitive to human amnesia. *Behav Neurosci* **99**:22.

Zola SM, Squire LR (2001) Relationship between magnitude of damage to the hippocampus and impaired recognition memory in monkeys. *Hippocampus* **11**:92–98.

Zola SM, Squire LR, Teng E, Stefanacci L, Buffalo EA, Clark RE (2000) Impaired recognition memory in monkeys after damage limited to the hippocampal region. *J Neurosci* **20**:451–463.

Zsilla G, Zelles T, Mike A, Kékes-Szabó A, Milusheva E, Vizi ES (1994) Differential changes in presynaptic modulation of transmitter release during aging. *Int J Dev Neurosci* **12**:107–115.

Computational Models of Hippocampal Cognitive Function

Daniel Bush and Neil Burgess

16.1 Introduction

There have been many attempts to understand and quantify the contribution of the hippocampus to cognition. In this chapter we focus on models of the link between the cognitive ability of an animal and the action of individual cells and synapses. As reviewed in Chapter 14, lesion studies in a variety of mammals (including humans) have implicated the hippocampus in spatial navigation, while human neuropsychology has most notably implicated this region in episodic or declarative memory function (see Chapter 13). In addition to these data, a vast body of knowledge has been collected regarding neural representations of the spatial location and orientation of freely moving rodents (see Chapters 11 and 12). Hypotheses regarding the function of the hippocampus have traditionally been expressed in words. However, it is often possible to interpret verbal descriptions in more than one way, or to retrospectively change their interpretation to suit the facts. In addition, it can be difficult to tell whether the proposed explanation would actually work as described, and if so, difficult to make unambiguous quantitative predictions that can be used to test it. These problems become more acute where hypotheses address the question of how a putative function arises from the cooperative behavior of large numbers of neurons and synapses. One way around this is to express such a hypothesis in terms of equations or computer simulations, referred to as a computational model. An advantage of this approach is that all of the parameter values and assumptions necessary to generate the behavior concerned are made explicit; another is that the operation of the model is unambiguously specified. These advantages mean that computational modeling has an important role to play in the progress of scientific understanding, most importantly in its interaction with experimental investigation: by predicting critical experiments, undergoing revision to reflect their results, and then predicting further experiments. They are not a panacea for all ills, and the interpretation of a model, the way it works, and the values of its parameters can still be changed or disputed. At the most basic level a computational model can serve as an existence proof of the behavior that could result from a proposed mechanism, but more generally it can serve to properly define a theoretical understanding and provide a powerful framework in which the nature of a theory relating brain to behavior can be understood.

Computational modeling of the hippocampus initially followed two largely independent streams, one seeking to explain a general role in associative memory and the other focusing on its role in spatial cognition. More recently, however, broader theoretical frameworks have been proposed that attempt to account for both types of data. Models will usually start from as detailed a biophysical level as is useful for the level of the hypothesis they seek to investigate. While many models reviewed here involve detailed simulation of cellular and synaptic electrophysiology, the aim of this chapter is to explain the neural bases of spatial and mnemonic behavior—something that is made easier by focusing on the simplest level of description capturing the likely functional consequences of cellular and synaptic events: e.g., whether or not an action potential was fired. Thus, the activity (firing rate) of a neuron is often simply viewed as a monotonic function of the amount by which the net input to it exceeds some threshold value. The net input to a neuron is the sum of the activity of each neuron connected to it weighted by the strength of the connection (occasionally inhibitory inputs are modeled as a divisive term in the net input rather than a subtractive term). "Learning" corresponds to modification of the connection strengths. Most commonly learning is of a "Hebbian" nature (Hebb, 1949) such that simultaneous pre- and postsynaptic activity leads to increased connection strength, and is often used in explicit analogy to synaptic processes like long-term potentiation (LTP, see Chapter 10; Box 16.1). Other concepts are explained as and where necessary. Readers interested in neural computation more generally should see, e.g., (Rumelhart and McClelland, 1986; McClelland and Rumelhart, 1986; Hertz et al., 1990; Anderson, 1995; Gurney, 1997; Dayan and Abbott, 2001; Trappenberg, 2002.)

Since the anatomy of the hippocampal formation is similar in rodents, bats, primates, and humans, it seems sensible to start with neural models of the vast and well-established body of data regarding place and grid cells and the neural representation of space, drawing mostly on experimental data collected in rats. We next consider models that make use of these spatial representations to guide behavior. Together, models of the representation of location and orientation from sensory input and their service in spatial navigation provide one of the best quantitative accounts of the link between perception, cognition, and action and between cells, systems, and behavior. The next part of the chapter concerns attempts to

Box 16.1 Learning via synaptic modification: "Hebbian" learning rules

In the simplest type of neural network model, the firing rate or "activity" of a neuron (a) is simply a function (the "transfer function" f) of the net current coming into the neuron, which in turn is simply a weighted sum of the firing rates (u_i) of the neurons connecting to it. That is: $a = f(\sum_i w_i u_i)$, often written as: $a = f(w \cdot u)$, where w is the vector of connection "weights" modeling the strengths (e.g., net synaptic efficacy) of connections from the input neurons, and "." is the vector dot product. With the simplest, linear, transfer function, the activation is given by:

$$a = w.u \qquad \text{Equation 1}$$

In such networks, "learning" corresponds to modification of the connection weights w. Below we discuss some of the "Hebbian" learning rules mentioned in the rest of the chapter, and their effects, following the discussion in Dayan and Abbott (2001), where further details can be found.

A learning rule directly implementing Hebb's (1949) postulate of coincident firing leading to increased coupling between neurons describes the change in connection weights in terms of the product of pre- and postsynaptic firing rates:

$$\tau\frac{dw_i}{dt} = au_i, \quad \text{or} \quad \tau\frac{dw}{dt} = a\underline{u}, \qquad \text{Equation 2}$$

where τ gives the rate of change of connection weights with time. When this rule is applied to a "training set" of n example input patterns of activity $\underline{u}^\mu$, each presented for an equal duration over a total time T, we can integrate Equation 2 to see the total change in w:

$$\underline{w} \to \underline{w} + \frac{T}{\tau}\sum_\mu a^\mu \underline{u}^\mu, \qquad \text{Equation 3}$$

where $a^\mu = \underline{w} \cdot \underline{u}^\mu$ from Equation 1. If the connection weights are only updated after presentation of all of the input patterns then we can say:

$$\underline{w} \to \underline{w} + \frac{T}{\tau}\sum_\mu (\underline{w} \cdot \underline{u}^\mu)\underline{u}^\mu = \underline{w} + \frac{nT}{\tau}\mathbf{Q}\underline{w}, \qquad \text{Equation 4}$$

where $\mathbf{Q}$ is the correlation matrix of the input patterns ($\mathbf{Q}$ = $<\underline{u}\,\underline{u}>$ where $<>$ denotes the average over input patterns, and $\underline{u}\,\underline{u}$ is the outer product of $\underline{u}$ with itself). Thus simple Hebbian learning rules are also known as correlation-based learning rules. Inspection of Equation 4 indicates that the weight vector $\underline{w}$, if plotted in the same space as the input vectors $\underline{u}^\mu$, will eventually follow the principal eigenvector of the correlation matrix, i.e., it will lie along the direction from the origin to the mean input pattern ($<\underline{u}>$) or, if $<\underline{u}>$ is at the origin, along the first principal component of the set of input patterns. However, this learning rule is not stable: large weights produce large output activations, which produce large increases in weights, and so on. More formally, it can be seen from the dot product of $\underline{w}$ with Equation 2 that the length of the weight vector increases whenever the output neuron is active:

$$\frac{d|w|^2}{dt} = 2\underline{w} \cdot \frac{dw}{dt} = \frac{dw}{dt} = \frac{2aw.u}{\tau} = \frac{2a^2}{\tau} \qquad \text{Equation 5}$$

One way to introduce balance into the learning rule is to allow for a connection weight to increase or to decrease according to the levels of pre- and postconnection activity, by analogy with long-term potentiation and depression (LTP and LTD, see Chapter 10). In this way Equation 2 could become:

$$\tau\frac{dw}{dt} = (a - \theta)\underline{u}, \quad \text{or} \quad \tau\frac{dw}{dt} = a(\underline{u} - \underline{\varphi}), \qquad \text{Equation 6}$$

where either a postsynaptic threshold or a set of presynaptic thresholds are applied to determine the sense and size of weight changes (respectively: θ—the level postsynaptic activity must surpass for the connection to increase rather than decrease; or φ—the vector of activity levels each input neuron must surpass). The most obvious choice of threshold for the pre- or postsynaptic neuron is its average activity over the training set. In this case, following a similar derivation to Equation 4, both versions produce the same learning rule:

$$\underline{w} \to \underline{w} + \frac{nT}{\tau}\mathbf{C}\underline{w}, \qquad \text{Equation 7}$$

where $\mathbf{C}$ is the covariance matrix of the input patterns: $\mathbf{C}$ = $<(\underline{u}-<\underline{u}>)^2>$. These learning rules are also known as covariance rules. Inspection of Equation 7 indicates that the weight vector will eventually follow the principal eigenvector of the covariance matrix, i.e., it will lie along the direction of the first principal component of the set of input patterns. It should be noted that these rules are also not stable, in this case $d|w|^2/dt$ is proportional to the variance ($<a^2> - <a>^2$) of the output activity over the training set.

The BCM learning rule, derived from experimental investigation of visual cortical plasticity (Bienenstock et al., 1982), proposes that:

$$\tau\frac{dw}{dt} = a\underline{u}(a - \theta(a)). \qquad \text{Equation 8}$$

This requires both pre- and postsynaptic activity for modification of a connection weight (unlike the rules in Equation 6), and also involves a sliding postsynaptic threshold ($\theta(a)$), which varies with postsynaptic activity. So long as the postsynaptic threshold increases as a power of a greater than 1 (typically following a time-averaged estimate of a^2), it can ensure stability of the learning rule: effectively increasing the threshold to an overactive output neuron so that connection weights to it tend to be reduced.

The other common way in which Hebbian learning rules are stabilized (e.g., in Rumelhart and Zipser's 1986 "competitive learning" algorithm) is to use divisive normalization: explicitly constraining the length of the weight vector to remain constant during learning by dividing all weights by $|w|$. Although this is a nonlocal operation, since synaptic strengths must be altered according to the state of other, distant, synapses, a similar effect can be achieved by the local learning rule of Oja (1982):

$$\tau\frac{dw}{dt} = a\underline{u} - \beta a^2 \underline{w}. \qquad \text{Equation 9}$$

A similar analysis to Equation 5 shows that $|w|^2$ will tend to a value $1/\beta$ under repeated application of this rule.

As well as being stable, the BCM and normalized Hebbian learning rules involve competition between connections: increasing some of the connection weights onto a neuron will lead to a decrease in the others. Under the BCM rule this occurs due to increased activity leading to a higher postsynaptic threshold and thus an increased incidence of LTD versus LTP. With normalization this occurs directly due to the increase in the length of the weight vector. These learning rules tend to allow a neuron to become tuned to respond to specific patterns of input activation, see text. There is at least some evidence for competitive interaction between synapses such that increasing the strengths of one set of synapses leads to a decrease in the strengths of others so as to normalize the total synaptic strength onto the neuron (Royer and Pare, 2003). We note, however, that evidence for the dependence of synaptic plasticity on the precise timing of pre- and postsynaptic activity (see Chapter 10) changes the likely nature of learning rules based on LTP and LTD, as in the effects of temporal asymmetry noted in section 16.2.2.

model the more general role of the human hippocampus in memory for personal experience. As we shall see, the role of the recurrent collaterals in area CA3 of the hippocampus maintains a common point of contact between these models: in both the spatial and episodic memory frameworks they are assumed to perform an associative memory function. The chapter concludes with a discussion of theoretical attempts to reconcile these two streams of research (spatial and mnemonic). In particular, this unifying framework proposes that the hippocampus encodes efficient, low-dimensional representations of variables that are useful for planning and prediction, alongside representations that capture common structure in transitions or relationships across multiple task domains to support generalization. This framework goes some way to explaining experimental data across species in both the spatial and mnemonic domains and can be seen as implementing a cognitive map (Tolman, 1948; O'Keefe and Nadel, 1978; Eichenbaum and Cohen, 2014; Behrens et al., 2018).

16.2 The hippocampus and spatial representation

This section addresses the representation of spatial location and orientation at the level of single neurons in the hippocampal formation. These models take two structural forms: those relying predominantly on feedforward connections to capture the data, and those relying predominantly on recurrent connections. Models of the representation of location embodied by the firing of hippocampal place cells are considered first. Next, we consider the complementary representation provided by the firing of grid cells in medial entorhinal cortex (MEC). Importantly, it is not only the firing rates of place and grid cells that encode location but also the time of firing relative to the ongoing theta rhythm in the local field potential (LFP). Finally, we turn to the equally striking representation of the animal's orientation provided by head-direction cells, the nature of which has also been investigated by computational modeling.

16.2.1 Representing spatial location and orientation: data

A rich set of experimental data have been gathered on the neural representations of spatial behavior found in and around the hippocampus. Here we briefly summarize those results with the greatest relevance to the models described below (see Chapters 11 and 12 for more details). The firing of place cells in the hippocampi of freely moving rats encodes the location of the animal, each cell firing when the animal is within a particular portion of its environment (the corresponding "place field"). In smaller environments, place cells typically exhibit a single place field, but in larger environments they may exhibit several place fields with no apparent relationship between the location of each (Fenton et al., 2008; Alme et al., 2014; Rich et al., 2014). Cells with similar responses have also been observed in mice and gerbils (McHugh et al., 1996; Mankin et al., 2019); birds (Payne et al., 2021); bats (Ulanovsky et al., 2007; Yartsev and Ulanovsky, 2013); human (Ekstrom et al., 2003) and nonhuman primates (Hori et al., 2003; Ludvig et al., 2004; Courellis et al., 2019; Mao et al., 2021). In open environments through which the rat can move freely, firing rates are not influenced by the animal's orientation, while in environments in which movement direction is constrained (e.g., linear tracks, eight-arm mazes) firing is strongly modulated by the rat's direction of motion.

The location of the place-cell representation is controlled by "distal" cues at or beyond the edge of the environment (O'Keefe and Conway, 1978; Muller and Kubie, 1987) more than by those within it (Cressant et al., 1997). A place cell's spatially localized firing appears to be robust to the removal of subsets of cues, and indeed removal of all of the controlling visual cues while the rat remains in the environment (Muller and Kubie, 1987; O'Keefe and Speakman, 1987), although remaining uncontrolled cues may be important in these cases (Save et al., 2000). In addition, the peak firing rate of the place cell may change significantly when features of the environment are changed, a process known as "rate remapping"; while the location of a place field may change dramatically, the cell may stop firing altogether, or previously silent cells may begin to exhibit a place field when the environmental features are changed more significantly, a process known as "global remapping" (Muller and Kubie, 1987; Bostock et al., 1991). Finally, sequences of place-cell firing observed during active behavior are "replayed" on a compressed timescale during subsequent slow-wave sleep and quiescent waking periods (Wilson and McNaughton, 1994; Skaggs and McNaughton, 1996; Foster and Wilson, 2006).

In contrast, grid cells recorded in freely moving rodents fire action potentials at multiple spatial locations. These firing fields are typically arranged at the vertices of a regular triangular array covering the whole environment (Hafting et al., 2005). Grid cells were initially discovered in the superficial layers of rodent MEC (Hafting et al., 2005; Fyhn et al., 2008), but have since been identified in the deeper layers (Sargolini et al., 2006) and in pre- and parasubiculum (Boccara et al., 2010). Moreover, grid-like responses have been recorded in the parahippocampal cortices of the bat (Yartsev et al., 2011), human (Doeller et al., 2010; Jacobs et al., 2013), and nonhuman primate (Killian et al., 2012). Grid-cell firing patterns can be characterized by their scale (i.e., the distance between adjacent firing fields), orientation (of one principal grid axis relative to an external cue), and the phase or spatial offset of their firing fields. Grid scale has been shown to increase in discrete steps along the dorsoventral axis of MEC (Barry et al., 2007; Stensola et al., 2012), and evidence suggest that grid cells with a common scale form a single functional module (Stensola et al., 2012; Yoon et al., 2013). The scale, relative orientation, and offset of grid firing patterns within each module are generally conserved across environments (Fyhn et al., 2007), aside from a transient expansion of grid scale in novel environments that returns to baseline with experience (Barry et al., 2012). The spatial phases of individual grid cells are uniformly distributed across the environment but, importantly, the relative spatial phase of any two simultaneously recorded grid cells from the same module is conserved across all environments visited by the animal (Fyhn et al., 2007; Yoon et al., 2013).

The complementary representation of orientation independent of location is found in head-direction cells in the mammillary bodies, anterior thalamic nuclei, dorsal presubiculum, and MEC (Taube et al., 1990; Sargolini et al., 2006). These cells code for head-direction within an environment, each firing whenever the animal's head points in a specific direction, independently of the animal's location. The orientation of the head-direction representation is controlled by distal visual cues in the same way as the place-cell representation. The overall orientation of place, grid, and head-direction representations

> **Box 16.2** Population vectors
>
> Let us assume a population of neurons in which each fires according to the distance between some variable and a preferred value of that variable. This could be the case for place cells if, for example, we assume that the firing rates r_i are simply a Gaussian function of the distance between the animal's current location and preferred locations x_i. We can subsequently estimate or "decode" the animal's current location from the firing rate weighted average of this vector, also known as the "population vector" (following Georgopolous et al., 1986):
>
> $$\frac{\sum r_i x_i}{\sum r_i} \qquad \text{Equation 10}$$
>
> This estimate is simple to compute, requiring only the firing rates and preferred values, but will be biased unless the preferred values evenly cover the range of possible values. Such even coverage might be true for head-direction cells, but a population vector of place-cell firing recorded within an open arena will be biased toward the center (Muller et al., 1987). More generally, population vector estimates will be less accurate than methods that take into account the function relating firing rates to the encoded variable (i.e., the shape of the firing rate profile; see Dayan and Abbott, 2001).

may be disrupted by disorientation (rotating the rat in a covered container) and, when recorded simultaneously, all representations have remained in register with each other (Knierim et al., 1995; Sargolini et al., 2006). Interestingly, the firing rate of "conjunctive" grid cells in the deeper layers of MEC is also modulated by heading direction (Sargolini et al., 2006). In addition, the firing rate of place, grid, and head-direction cells (McNaughton et al., 1983; Sargolini et al., 2006; Hardcastle et al., 2017), as well as some MEC neurons that do not appear to encode any spatial variables (Kropff et al., 2015), are modulated by running speed.

Interestingly, while the firing rates of both place cells (e.g., Wilson and McNaughton, 1993) and grid cells (e.g., Fiete et al., 2008; Mathis et al., 2012) provide a population vector (Georgopoulos et al., 1986; see Box 16.2) that encodes the animal's location within a given environment, the times at which they fire relative to the LFP theta rhythm encodes additional information (see Chapter 11; O'Keefe and Recce, 1993; Skaggs et al., 1996; Jensen and Lisman, 2000; Hafting et al., 2008; Climer et al., 2013; Jeewajee et al., 2014). Specifically, these cells exhibit theta "phase precession," firing at a progressively earlier phase of each theta cycle as the firing field is traversed. Importantly, the initial phase of firing on entry to a place or grid field is typically consistent across cells and, as a result, phase precession generates "theta sequences" of place- and grid-cell firing across the population, whereby cells with receptive fields behind the animal fire early, and those ahead of the animal fire late, in each oscillatory cycle (Burgess et al., 1994; Skaggs et al., 1996; Johnson and Redish, 2007). Intriguingly, this phase code for location is conserved across species (Eliav et al., 2018; Qasim et al., 2021) but does not appear to rely on sustained rhythmicity in the theta band: place and grid cells in bats exhibit a phase code for location relative to LFP fluctuations that vary dynamically over a wide range of frequencies (Eliav et al., 2018).

16.2.2 Representing spatial location: feedforward models

Feedforward neural networks, in which activity propagates unidirectionally between successive layers of simulated neurons, have had great success in solving pattern recognition and classification problems—producing specific patterns of output activity (e.g., place- or grid-cell firing fields) given specific patterns of input (e.g., particular constellations of sensory features). Due to their limited internal dynamics, however, feedforward networks are typically unable to integrate the recent history of their inputs—to perform path integration by combining previous estimates of location with self-motion inputs, for example.

16.2.2.1 Place cells

Computational modeling of place-cell firing began with Zipser (1985). In this model, sensory details of the environment feedforward to landmark detectors, and thence to place cells. Landmark detectors are neurons specific to a unique place cell and aspect of the sensory scene (a "location parameter"). The output of these detectors is proportional to the match between the stored state of a location parameter and its currently perceived state. A place cell's activity corresponds to a thresholded sum of the strengths of the matches it receives from several landmark detectors. Interestingly, the most obvious location parameter—distance from a landmark—was rejected by the author, in favor of measures that scale with environmental size such as the retinal angle between two landmarks. As such, the model captures some of the motility of place fields in the presence of manipulations of environmental cues and some of their robustness to removal of subsets of cues, but (incorrectly) produces place fields that scale proportionately with environmental expansion (Muller and Kubie, 1987; O'Keefe and Burgess, 1996).

Sharp (1991) followed in the same vein of feedforward modeling of the response of place cells to sensory input from the environment, but with the incorporation of an element of "competitive learning" (Rumelhart and Zipser, 1986). Briefly, this involves neurons arranged into groups dominated by lateral inhibition such that only the neuron with the greatest input can fire. Normalized Hebbian learning is then applied (i.e., increasing the strengths of connections between simultaneously active neurons while decreasing the others so that the overall strength of connections to a neuron does not change, see Box 16.1). This learning results in specific neurons coming to represent specific patterns of sensory input: each neuron responding to a particular pattern, or to patterns similar to it. Her model envisaged two types of sensory input regarding each distal cue, one representing its distance from the rat and the other representing both its distance from the rat and its direction relative to the rat's heading. This sensory input passed forward to a layer of entorhinal cells and thence to a layer of place cells. Competitive learning at each layer causes the entorhinal cells and place cells to respond selectively to the pattern of sensory input present in a particular portion of the environment and produces reasonable robustness to cue removal. The successive layers of competition produce sharper tuning to position and greater robustness to cue removal in place cells than entorhinal cells.

Interestingly, place-cell firing in this model is initially directionally modulated, due to the partially directional sensory inputs. During random exploration in an open environment, competitive learning allows a given place cell to learn to respond to the sensory inputs occurring for different orientations at the place field, producing nondirectional firing. By contrast, this does not occur during constrained motion (i.e., back and forth in a single direction). This provides a simple account of the directionality of place-cell firing, although a more detailed look at the experimental data indicates that, if anything, place fields in open environments are initially nondirectional and become directional as a result of experience (Markus et al., 1995; Navratilova, Hoang, et al., 2012).

In a related model, Franzius et al. (2007) demonstrated that specific assumptions about the form of sensory inputs to place cells could be avoided by simply identifying the most slowly changing features of that input, motivated by the observation that sensory information typically varies much more quickly than behaviorally relevant features of the environment (Wiskott and Sejnowksi, 2002). This "slow feature analysis" (SFA) can produce both place- and head-direction-cell firing patterns from raw visual input, depending on the relative speed of translational movement and head rotation, and could be achieved by biologically plausible learning rules (Sprekeler et al., 2007). As in Sharp's model, place-cell responses in the output layer of the feedforward network are most realistic when SFA is combined with competitive learning.

More recently, it has been demonstrated that spatially modulated, feedforward excitatory and inhibitory inputs governed by different learning rules can also produce a variety of spatial firing patterns in an output neuron (Weber and Sprekeler, 2018). Specifically, if excitatory inputs are subject to a Hebbian learning rule while the strength of inhibitory inputs changes according to the product of the presynaptic firing rate and the difference between postsynaptic firing rate and a single, global target value (see Box 16.1), then the output neuron can learn to produce either place- or grid-cell firing patterns, depending on the relative spatial smoothness of those inputs. If inhibition is uniform across the environment, the output neuron produces a single place field; if inhibitory inputs are smoother than excitatory inputs, the output neuron produces a grid firing pattern by learning a center-surround input profile; and if inhibitory inputs are less smooth than excitatory inputs, the output neuron produces weakly spatially modulated firing.

In an attempt to derive the specific form of the sensory input to place cells, O'Keefe and Burgess (1996) systematically varied the shape and size of the rat's environment while recording from the same cells. The patterns of firing across environments included place fields that stretched or became bimodal when the environment expanded. These patterns were not consistent with previous models of place fields depending on the relative locations of discrete landmarks from the rat (e.g., Zipser, 1985; Sharp, 1991), but rather indicated continuous dependence on environmental boundaries. Specifically, place fields were viewed as a thresholded linear sum of inputs tuned to respond to the presence of a boundary at a given distance along a given allocentric direction (i.e., independent of the orientation of the rat, and probably determined relative to the head-direction system, see below; Figure 16.1). These hypothetical inputs were termed "boundary vector cells."

By fitting a place cell's firing pattern across several different environmental shapes, the model can predict its firing pattern in an environment of novel shape (Hartley et al., 2000). Indeed, recent studies have shown that this model provides a good fit to experimental data across environments of many different configurations (Grieves et al., 2018; Lee et al., 2023). In addition, the predicted boundary vector cells with allocentric firing patterns were later identified in the medial entorhinal cortex and subiculum (Solstad et al., 2008; Lever et al., 2009; Muessig et al., 2024), along with the related object-vector cells (Høydal et al., 2019). Importantly, however, the recent observation that place-cell firing is modulated by heading direction relative to some fixed reference point indicates that some egocentric influence remains (Jercog et al., 2019). In addition, place-cell activity must be at least partially determined by nonboundary related inputs, or firing patterns would be conserved across all geometrically identical environments. More generally, the feedforward models described above cannot account for the persistence of place-cell firing in darkness, when visual inputs are

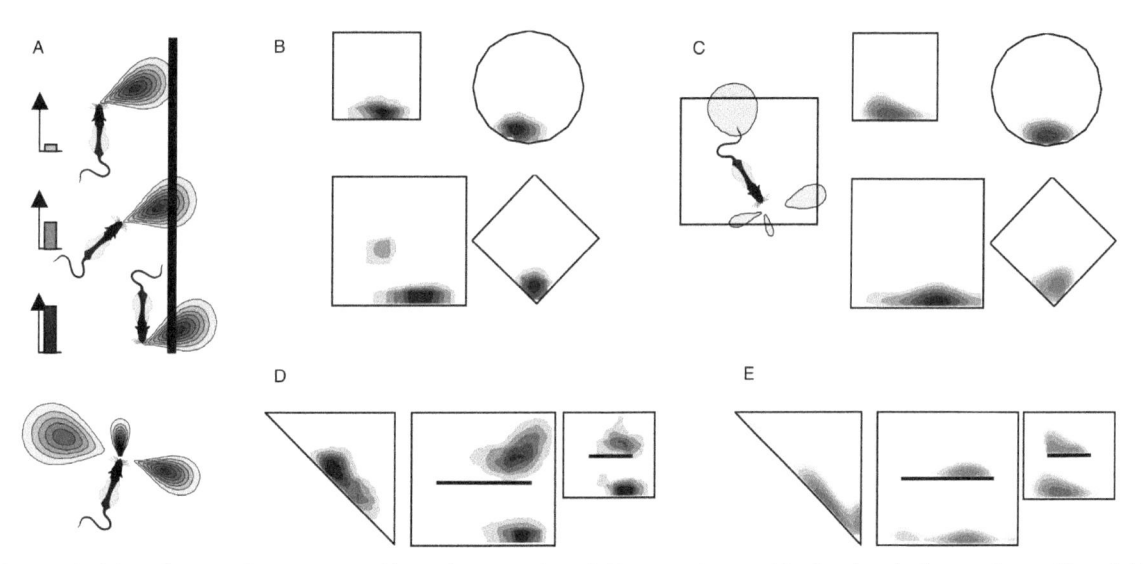

Figure 16.1 Model of the influence of environmental boundaries on place fields, assuming a stable directional reference frame. Place fields are composed from thresholded linear sums of the firing rates of "boundary vector cells" (BVCs). (A) Above: Each BVC has a Gaussian tuned response to the presence of a boundary at a given distance and bearing from the rat (independent of its orientation). Below: The sharpness of tuning of a BVC decreases as the distance to which it is tuned increases. The only free parameters of a BVC are the distance and direction of peak response. (B) Place fields recorded from the same cell in four environments of different shape or orientation relative to distal cues. (C) Simulation of the place fields in B by the best fitting set of 4 BVCs constrained to be in orthogonal directions (BVCs shown on the left, simulated fields on the right). The simulated cell can now be used to predict firing in novel geometrical configurations of boundaries. Real and predicted data from three novel configurations are shown in (D) and (E), respectively, showing good qualitative agreement. (Adapted from Burgess and Hartley, 2002.)

presumed to be absent and the updating of spatial representations is mediated by self-motion (i.e., "path integration") inputs.

Another phenomenon not addressed by the above models is the "remapping" of place-cell representations across different environments. This "remapping" can be both partial and incremental over time (e.g., Bostock et al., 1991; Skaggs and McNaughton, 1998; Lever et al., 2002), with the eventual creation of stable but distinct patterns of firing in the two environments. The factors influencing the speed and extent of remapping are currently not well understood (Sanders et al., 2020; see section 16.5.1), but one common change in an individual place cell is to continue to fire in the environment in which it fires most strongly, and to stop firing in the other. This aspect of remapping was addressed by Fuhs and Touretzky (2000) in a model of learning in the perforant path projection from entorhinal cortex to place cells in CA3. They found that the usual learning rules relating synaptic modification to the product of the pre- and postsynaptic activity (i.e., "Hebbian" learning), or to its covariance, were unable to reproduce this behavior. In the case of Hebbian learning, a place cell with strong firing in one environment and weak firing in the other will strengthen its firing in both environments. In the case of covariance learning, exposure to the second environment will tend to lead to loss of the place-cell representation in the first environment. By contrast, the BCM learning rule (Bienenstock et al., 1982; see Box 16.1), which explicitly makes the direction of synaptic modification dependent on the strength of postsynaptic activity, did produce the desired result: strong firing remaining stable and weak firing reducing with experience. This type of learning also captures the way place fields become more coherent with time, and the dynamics of their response to the introduction of a barrier into the environment (Barry and Burgess, 2007).

Evidence of experience-dependent change in place-cell firing also comes from experiments by Mehta et al. (1997; 2000). They found that, over the first few runs through a CA1 place field on a linear track, the spatial distribution of firing changes from roughly symmetrical to take on a slight asymmetry caused by additional firing at low rates earlier on the track. They suggest that this results from the known temporal asymmetry of LTP (which is greater when presynaptic activity precedes postsynaptic activity than vice versa, see, e.g., Bi and Poo, 1998) acting on the CA3 to CA1 pathway (see Chapter 10). Other models have implicated the recurrent connections within CA3 as responsible for this effect (see section 16.2.3). Interestingly, the theta phase precession of place-cell firing (see section 16.2.1 and Chapter 11 for data and section 16.2.4 for models) acts to increase the effect of temporal asymmetry in LTP: causing place cells with fields early on the path to fire before those with fields later along the path within each theta cycle.

Finally, following the discovery of grid cells, numerous theoretical models have demonstrated how input from grid modules of two or more spatial scales could be combined to generate place fields through an effective Fourier synthesis (e.g., Rolls et al., 2006; Solstad et al., 2006). Using either hardwired synaptic weights or some form of Hebbian learning rule, these models set the effective strength of grid-cell inputs to decline with their spatial offset from the output place field (Cheng and Frank, 2011). Grid- to place-cell models can produce either single or multiple place fields, although the secondary fields often exhibit sixfold symmetry—particularly when all grid inputs share a single orientation—in apparent contrast with empirical data. More restricted place-field firing can be generated by introducing some variation in firing rate between the receptive fields of each grid cell, in line with experimental data (Ismakov et al., 2017). Finally, making independent changes to the orientation and/or spatial phase of each grid module (Fyhn et al., 2007), and/or incorporating a "gating" input representing abstract contextual signals (Hayman and Jeffery, 2008), can account for the remapping of output place-field responses, while remapped field locations may reflect movements between the vertices of an underlying grid (Whittington et al., 2020). Several predictions of these models appear to be at odds with empirical data, however (Bush et al., 2014). Most notably, place-cell firing patterns appear to precede those of grid cells in the developmental timeline (Langston et al., 2010; Wills et al., 2010); and grid firing patterns are eliminated by inactivation of medial septum, with little effect on place-cell responses in either novel or familiar environments (Koenig et al., 2011; Brandon et al., 2014).

16.2.2.2 Grid cells

In addition to modeling place-cell responses, two main classes of grid-cell model suggest that their regular, periodic firing fields can be generated by feedforward input from other regions. Interestingly, the first class reverses the logic of grid- to place-cell models by suggesting that grid-cell firing patterns might be generated using feedforward input from the hippocampus through a process analogous to principal component analysis (PCA) of place-cell firing covariance (Castro and Aguiar, 2014; Dordek et al., 2016) or, relatedly, eigen decomposition of the transition matrix between place fields (Stachenfeld et al., 2017). These models build on the observations that a modified Hebbian learning rule acting on feedforward projections can approximate a process of PCA (Oja, 1982; see Box 16.1), that feedforward projections exist from CA1 to the deeper layers of MEC, and that grid-cell firing patterns appear to rely on stable place-cell activity (Bonnevie et al., 2013). Hence, employing this modified learning rule at feedforward projections from a population of simulated place cells—or approximating that process mathematically using nonnegative PCA—creates output units with grid-like firing patterns. This account bears some resemblance to earlier models, which suggested that feedforward input from place cells to a network of neurons with spike-frequency adaptation was also sufficient to generate grid-like firing patterns (Kropff and Treves, 2008; Si and Treves, 2013; D'Albis and Kempter, 2017).

In contrast, most theoretical models of grid-cell firing assume that their principal input is a self-motion signal, with periodic firing patterns resulting from the integration of that velocity signal over time, consistent with a proposed role in path integration (McNaughton et al., 2006; further discussion in the following section). In particular, following accounts of theta phase precession in place cells (O'Keefe and Recce, 1993; Lengyel et al., 2003; see section 16.2.4), the oscillatory interference (OI) model proposes that grid firing patterns can be accounted for at the single-cell level by constructive interference between two or more oscillatory inputs (Burgess and Hitch, 2005; Burgess et al., 2007; Blair et al., 2008; Burgess, 2008; Hasselmo, 2008). In its simplest one-dimensional (1D) form, one oscillation has a baseline frequency and the other "velocity controlled oscillator" (VCO) has a frequency that varies linearly from that baseline with the speed of movement (Burgess, 2008). In rodents, the baseline frequency is generally assumed to be the 5–12 Hz movement-related theta oscillation (Vanderwolf, 1969; O'Keefe and Nadel, 1978; Burgess et al., 2007).

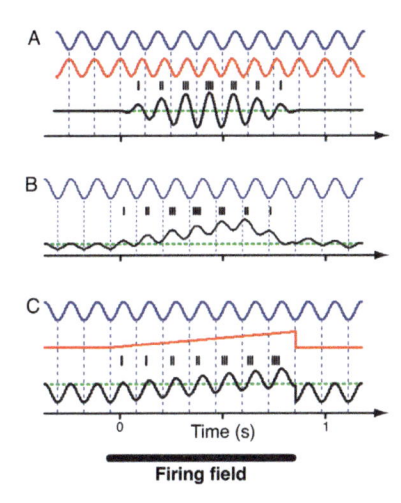

Firing field

Figure 16.2 Models of phase coding in place and grid cells. (A) The oscillatory interference (OI) model of phase precession and grid-cell firing in 1D environments. A baseline oscillation with frequency f_{base} (blue line) and a velocity-controlled oscillation (VCO) with frequency f_{VCO} (red line) that varies from f_{base} linearly with movement speed. Constructive interference between these two oscillations generates a spatially periodic activity pattern with a "carrier" frequency (black line) equal to their mean frequency $(f_{base} + f_{VCO})/2$ and an "envelope" equal to their difference in frequency $(f_{VCO} - f_{base})$. This activity pattern corresponds to spatially periodic firing fields within which spikes (black dashes) are fired at the peak of the membrane potential oscillation (MPO, black line) but progressively earlier phases of the baseline oscillation, as observed in grid cells. (B) Schematic representation of intracellular recording data from place (Harvey et al., 2010) and grid (Dominsoru et al., 2013; Schmidt-Hieber and Hausser, 2013) cells. The membrane potential (black line) shows a ramping depolarization but no increase in MPO amplitude within the firing field. Spikes (black dashes) are fired at the peak of MPOs but progressively earlier phases of the LFP theta oscillation (blue line). (C) The depolarizing ramp model of phase precession in place and grid cells. Ramp-like depolarization (red line) causes the membrane potential (black line) to exceed firing threshold (dashed green line) progressively earlier in each cycle of the LFP oscillation (blue line), such that spikes (black dashes) are fired at progressively earlier MPO phases (cf. panel B). (Adapted from Burgess and O'Keefe, 2011.)

These two signals generate grid-cell membrane potential oscillations (MPOs) modulated by an "envelope" frequency that is equal to the difference in baseline and VCO frequencies; and a "carrier" frequency between the baseline and active frequencies (see Figure 16.2A). The envelope corresponds to the grid-cell rate code—being spatially periodic and approximately Gaussian or cosine tuned; while the carrier corresponds to the temporal code—being higher in frequency than the baseline oscillation, and thus causing the grid cell to fire at progressively earlier phases of that baseline oscillation as the firing field is traversed (i.e., generating phase precession; see section 16.2.4). The scale of the resultant grid firing pattern is controlled by the slope of the VCO movement speed/burst firing frequency relationship, which determines how quickly the VCO and baseline oscillation move in and out of phase during movement.

The OI model accounts for two-dimensional (2D) grid firing patterns by incorporating input from multiple VCOs whose burst-firing frequencies vary linearly with movement speed along different preferred directions. Because distance is the time integral of velocity, and phase is the time integral of frequency, the phase of each VCO—if sampled at fixed intervals (i.e., at the peak or trough of the baseline oscillation)—encodes (periodic) displacement in its preferred direction. A grid cell that receives input from two or

more VCOs whose preferred directions differ by multiples of 60° will exhibit a triangular array of firing fields at locations where those VCO inputs are in phase. The specific location or offset of those firing fields can be manipulated by adding a constant phase-shift to one or more VCO inputs. Hence, the OI model proposes that each VCO performs path integration along different 1-D axes, while grid cells simply "read-out" the activity of multiple VCO inputs by firing whenever they are in phase.

The OI model accounts for both periodic firing patterns and theta phase precession in grid cells and is supported by the observation that a reduction in theta band activity caused either by passive transport of the animal (Winter et al., 2015) or inactivation of medial septum (Brandon et al., 2011; Koenig et al., 2011) leads to the loss of grid firing patterns. In addition, cells with VCO-like properties have been identified in the hippocampal formation (Welday et al., 2011). The OI model has been challenged by the observation that oscillatory activity with a relatively constant frequency is absent from the hippocampal formation of bats (Yartsev et al., 2011) and humans (Watrous et al., 2013). Importantly, however, it is the phase difference between VCO and baseline oscillations that encodes location, and the baseline frequency can therefore vary so long as this phase relationship is preserved (Burgess, 2008; Blair et al., 2014; Orchard, 2015; Bush and Burgess, 2020), e.g., if it is itself derived from the active frequencies (Burgess and Burgess, 2014). Indeed, models forming grid cells from path-integrating "stripe" or "band" cells (Mhatre et al., 2012; Horiuchi and Moss, 2015) are equivalent to oscillatory interference with a baseline frequency of 0 Hz. Nonetheless, the OI model alone cannot account for the strong interactions between grid cells from the same functional module that are clearly indicated by experimental data (Yoon et al., 2013), nor for the subthreshold membrane dynamics observed during movement through the grid field, which exhibit no change in the amplitude of theta band MPOs inside grid firing fields (see Figure 16.2B; Domnisoru et al., 2013; Schmidt-Hieber and Hausser, 2013).

16.2.3 Representing spatial location and orientation: feedback models

The long-range recurrent connections between pyramidal cells in area CA3 of the hippocampus have long been interpreted as enabling this region to work as an autoassociative neural network, see, e.g., (Marr, 1971; Hopfield, 1982; Amit, 1989). This type of network is most often used to provide a content-addressable memory, a subject explored in section 16.4. Elsewhere, it has been demonstrated that disynaptic recurrent inhibitory connections couple grid cells in MEC (Couey et al., 2013). In this section we consider the role played by recurrent collaterals in the spatial representations of place, grid and head-direction cells. Recurrent networks can take advantage of self-generated internal dynamics to imbue spatial representations with a dependence on the recent history of inputs. As such, these networks can readily account for path integration—that is, using self-motion signals to update previous estimates of self-location; as well as leveraging attractor dynamics (see Box 16.3) to ensure that spatial representations are robust to the withdrawal of a subset of sensory cues. Interestingly, direct experimental evidence for an associative function for CA3 has emerged, with indications that the NMDA receptors in this region are involved in making both the place fields and the rat's spatial memory robust to cue removal (Nakazawa et al., 2002). In parallel, attractor dynamics have been found in the place-cell representation of two environments of different shape after fast remapping caused by exposure to the two environmental shapes made of different materials (Wills et al., 2005), and analogous results have been obtained from the human hippocampus using fMRI (Steemers et al., 2016). In these representations, in contrast to those that have not fast-remapped (Leutgeb et al., 2005), the two shapes act as point attractors: all place cells in intermediate shaped environments coherently returning to one or other representation. Substantial evidence has also emerged for continuous attractor network dynamics in grid-cell firing patterns (Yoon et al., 2013; Gardner et al., 2022).

16.2.3.1 Continuous attractor models of head-direction cells

The simplest examples of the use of continuous attractors (see Box 16.3) to model spatial representations come from models of the representation of head direction rather than location. In many respects the literature on head-direction cells (HDCs) is much more straightforward than that on place or grid cells. The overall orientation of the head-direction representation can be controlled by sensory cues in a similar way to the place- and grid-cell representations. Unlike place cells, however, there have been no reports to date of HDCs changing their preferred orientations relative to each

---

Box 16.3 Attractors in memory, neural coding, and path integration

Point attractors and memory

A network of recurrently connected neurons can be arranged so that a finite number of discrete patterns of activation across the neurons are stable states or "attractors." This means that any pattern of activation similar enough to one of these attractors will evolve into that attractor pattern under the dynamics of the network. These patterns of activation are "stored" in the network in the sense that they will be "retrieved" from any initial pattern that is similar enough. Such networks are also referred to as "autoassociative" and are an example of a "content-addressable" memory, in that a pattern of activity is retrieved by a pattern of similar content rather than, say, an unrelated index term or the address of a storage location.

In one of the simplest models (Hopfield, 1982), activity of neuron i is modeled as $a_i = \pm 1$. Connections between neurons i and j are symmetric, with synaptic "weight" $w_{ij} = w_{ji}$. The dynamics of the network are given by: $a_i(t + 1) = \text{sign}(\sum_j w_{ij} a_j(t))$, such that the "energy" or Lyapunov function of the network:

$$E \propto -\sum_{ij} w_{ij} a_i a_j, \qquad \text{Equation 11}$$

can only reduce. If connection weights undergo a form of Hebbian learning when the to-be-stored patterns of activation ($\underline{a}^\mu$, say) are present, such that $w_{ij} \propto \sum_\mu a_i^\mu a_j^\mu$, then these representations will become attractors, so long as the number of stored patterns is not too large (less than around $0.14N$, where N is the number of neurons, in this case). That is, a similar enough pattern of activation will converge onto the stored pattern under the dynamics of the network (see also Cohen and Grossberg, 1983). This situation is often visualized by imagining how the "energy" of the network varies as a function of the network "state" $\underline{a} = (a_1, a_2, \ldots a_N)$—the attractor states being local minima of the energy surface to which nearby states will evolve under the network's dynamics (see Figure 16.3A). Similar behavior is also shown by more biologically realistic models (Amit, 1992; Treves and Rolls, 1992; McClelland et al., 1995; see also Figure 16.9). We note that "modern" Hopfield networks or "dense associative memories" (e.g., Krotov and Hopfield, 2016; Demircigil et al., 2017) exhibit much greater storage capacity, in addition to reduced interference between stored patterns, but biologically realistic implementations of those networks have yet to be proposed (but, see Krotov and Hopfield, 2020).

Line attractors and neural coding

The value of a continuous variable (or "stimulus" s) often seems to be represented in the firing rates of a population of neurons, each of which is tuned to respond preferentially to a single "preferred" value. For example, head-direction cells can be thought of in this way, with s representing the rat's heading. The pattern of activation of the population is often visualized by imagining the neurons arranged so that their location reflects their preferred values: showing a smooth bump of activity across the neurons peaked at the actual value of the stimulus. However, if the firing rates are noisy it will be difficult to estimate the precise value of the stimulus. The presence of recurrent connections between neurons, arranged so that the weight of the connection between each pair is simply a decreasing function of the difference in their preferred values (or physical separation

when arranged as above), can help by ensuring that the firing pattern takes the shape of a smooth bump (see Figure 16.3B; these patterns have low "energy" as activation is concentrated in nearby neurons, which have the strongest interconnections). With the appropriate choice of recurrent connections, such a network can perform optimal decoding (Latham et al., 2003), including the situation where the representation is formed from different unreliable sources of information (Deneve et al., 2001).

The patterns of activation composing a smooth bump can be thought of as a line in the N dimensional state space $\underline{a} = (a_1, a_2, \ldots a_N)$ of the network. Each point on the line corresponds to a different estimate of s (referred to as $\hat{s}$). Conversely, all of the possible noisy patterns of activation that end up producing the same $\hat{s}$ lie on an $N-1$ dimensional subspace within which the action of the recurrent connections corresponds to convergence onto the line (see Figure 16.3C). An important aspect of these networks is that, while the recurrent connections ensure that patterns of activation move onto the line attractor, movement along it, corresponding to changing $\hat{s}$, is not affected by the recurrent connections (since the connections between a pair of neurons depends only on the *difference* in their preferred values, not what those preferred values are).

Line attractors and path integration

Since the (symmetric) recurrent connections provide no resistance to motion of the bump of activity along the line attractor, its position is easily moved by asymmetric connections from each neuron to neighbors further along the line (Zhang, 1996; Skaggs et al., 1995). The strength of the asymmetric connections (which should correspond to the spatial derivative of the symmetric connections for the bump to move without changing shape; Zhang, 1996) compared with the symmetric ones dictates the movement of the bump (see Figures 16.3–16.5). Thus, if the strength of the asymmetric connections is proportional to angular velocity, the location of the bump of activity in a ring of head-direction cells will track the head direction of the animal—performing angular "path integration" (see Redish et al., 1996, for an alternative model using only neurons with conjunctive tuning to head direction and angular velocity).

As noted by Zhang (1996) and McNaughton et al. (1996), the angular path integration models of head-direction-cell firing can be extended to path integration models of place-cell firing. In this case, the place cells are imagined as a 2D array, so that the location of each neuron corresponds to the location of its place field in the environment (see Figure 16.4). Again, symmetrical connections decreasing in strength with the physical separation of the pre- and postsynaptic neurons can ensure that neural activity forms a single-peaked bump over the array, while asymmetric connections from each neuron to its neighbors along a given direction will cause the bump to shift in that direction (see Figures 16.3 and 16.4). In this case, to perform path integration of position, the strength of the asymmetric connections between a pair of neurons displaced in a given direction needs to be proportional to the velocity of the rat in that direction (see Samsonovich and McNaughton, 1997, for a more detailed model; Droulez and Berthoz, 1991; and Dominey and Arbib, 1992, for related earlier models; and Conklin and Eliasmith, 2005; Burak and Fiete, 2009, for accurate path integration using only neurons with conjunctive tuning to location and velocity).

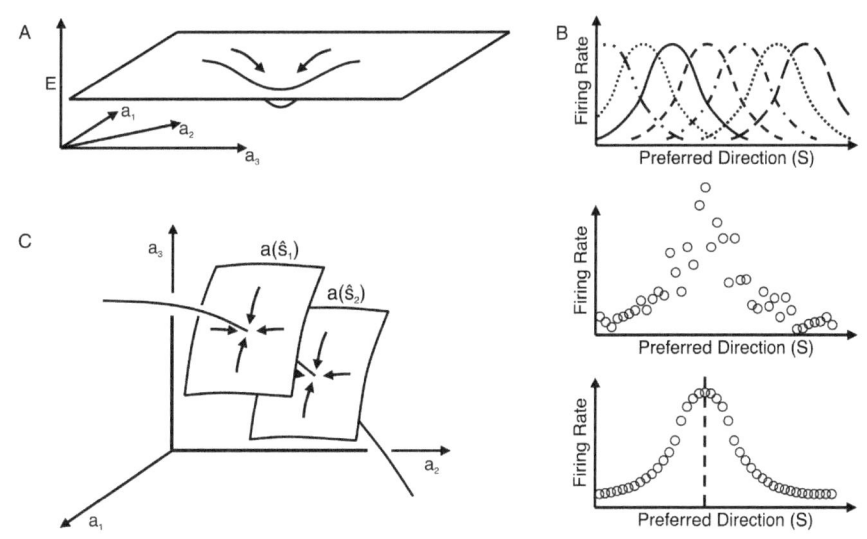

Figure 16.3 Point attractors and line attractors in neural systems (see Box 16.3). (A) A point attractor is a pattern of activation $a = (a_1, a_2, a_3 \ldots)$ into which other nearby patterns will evolve under the dynamics of the network (determined by the pattern of connection strengths, update rule, etc.). In some cases a function can be defined that can only decrease under the dynamics (a "Lyapunov" function, or the energy E of a physical system), so that attractor states lie at local minima of this function. (B) Population encoding and decoding (see Box 16.2). Neural populations can encode the current value of a variable in the pattern of activation across neurons, each of which is tuned to respond to a preferred value. These are often imagined to be laid-out so that the position of each neuron on the horizontal axis corresponds to its preferred value. For example, a set of head-direction cells might each be tuned to a different "preferred" direction (top). If firing rates are noisy, it may be difficult to estimate the actual value of the variable (middle). Recurrent connections can be organized so that all other patterns of activation evolve into a smooth bump-shaped patterns of activation (below). This process can provide an optimal way of decoding the value of the variable from the population (the peak of the bump—dashed line). (C) The set of smooth bump-shaped patterns of activation form a "line attractor": a continuous set of patterns of activity onto which other nearby patterns will evolve, but along which movement is unimpeded. Locations along the line attractor can be thought of as estimates of the variable ($\hat{S}$), and all of the patterns of activity that end up at a given estimate ($\hat{S}_1$, say) form a subspace $a(\hat{S})$ within which the intersection with the line is a point attractor. (Adapted from Latham et al., 2003.)

other (i.e., remapping). Even when the rat is disoriented, asleep, or in a symmetrical environment without polarizing cues, or if angular head velocity inputs are inhibited, the preferred directions of simultaneously recorded HDCs remain consistent—if they rotate, all rotate together (Peyrache et al., 2015; Butler et al., 2017; Bassett et al., 2018; Chaudhuri et al., 2019; but see Kornienko et al., 2018). This is analogous to grid-cell firing patterns, which preserve the spatial offset of their firing fields (or relative phase) across all environments visited by the animal (Fyhn et al., 2007; Yoon et al., 2013) and during sleep (Trettel et al., 2019; Gardner et al., 2019). For this reason all models of the head-direction system follow a similar basic mechanism of a 1D continuous attractor or "line attractor" (Skaggs et al., 1995; Redish et al., 1996; Zhang, 1996) from which the 2D continuous attractor models of place and grid cells developed (see Figures 16.3. 16.4 and 16.5, and Box 16.3).

If HDCs are imagined laid out in a ring with each cell's location corresponding to its preferred direction, and each is connected to its neighbors (see Box 16.3), then activity will be smoothly peaked at the current heading direction. Skaggs et al.'s model contains two further rings of cells, with each cell receiving connections from the corresponding HDC. One ring is composed of "left rotation" cells, which project back to the HDCs to the left (anticlockwise) of their location, while the other is composed of "right rotation" cells, which project back to HDCs to the right (clockwise) of their location. The left rotation cells corresponding to the current heading direction are activated when the rat is turning left, due to inputs from the vestibular system as well as the HDCs, causing the HDC activation to move leftward. Alternatively, a similar system can be formed of just two turn-modulated rings with offset connections (Redish

et al., 1996). In addition to these cells, the HDCs receive input from "sensory cells" ("visual cells" in Figure 16.5A) to become associated with those sensory inputs appearing at a stable bearing during exploration of a new environment. These sensory inputs subsequently prevent the cumulative errors that would otherwise occur in the integration of angular velocity.

This basic model has been implemented and extended in different ways, developing in hand with our knowledge of the operation of the head-direction system. This is now thought to involve a circuit from the mammillary bodies (MB) to anterior thalamic nuclei (ATN) to dorsal presubiculum (PS), with visual inputs arriving in PS via retrosplenial cortex (RSC). In this circuit, cells in the MB code for head direction further in the future (60 to 70 ms) than those in the ATN (20 to 30 ms), while those in the PS code for current or past head direction (0 to 10 ms; see Blair and Sharp, 1995; Taube and Muller, 1998; Taube, 1998; Blair et al., 1998). Various of the additional detailed properties of these systems, such as time advances and asymmetric responses during turning, have been incorporated, e.g., (Touretzky and Redish, 1996; Blair et al., 1997; Goodridge and Touretzky, 2000). In addition, some models have addressed the problem of parallax, whereby proximal sensory cues that present different orientations depending on location within the environment introduce errors into the head-direction circuit (Bicanski and Burgess, 2016) and head-direction coding in three dimensions (Page et al., 2018; Laurens and Angelaki, 2018). Finally, it is worth noting the incredible correspondence between the ring attractor model of head-direction coding and activity in the ellipsoid body of the fly brain (Seelig and Jayaraman, 2015; see Figure 16.5B). Here we focus on the hippocampus, however, and return to models of location.

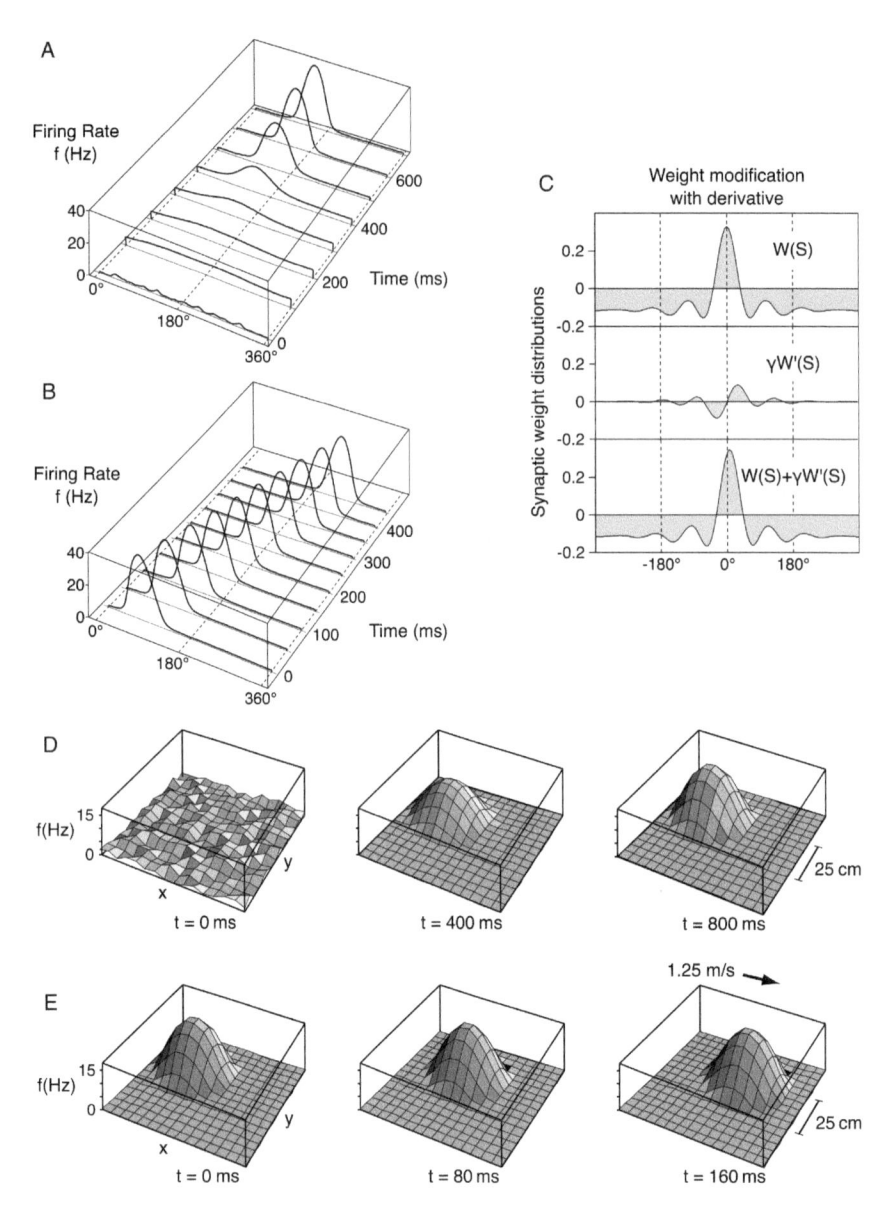

Figure 16.4 Continuous attractor networks of place and head-direction cells. (A) Emergence of a stable firing profile from an arbitrary initial state in a network of head-direction cells arranged as a 1-D continuous attractor. The cells are indexed by their preferred firing direction and connected by weights with a symmetrical distribution, i.e., an even function of the difference between cell's tuning directions (see C, top row). (B) Movement of the peak caused by an asymmetrical component in the weight distribution (see C, middle row). (C) Distribution of connection weights in a 1-D attractor network (bottom row), showing symmetrical component (top row) and additional asymmetric component (middle row). Note the slight asymmetry in the combined connection weights. The asymmetric component is the spatial derivative of the symmetric component along the direction of drift, and its size (γ) determines the speed of drift of the represented head-direction. (D) A 2-D place-cell network similar to the 1-D head-direction cell network, showing emergence of a stereotyped stable firing profile from an arbitrary initial state, using a symmetric weight distribution (a Gaussian with constant inhibitory background). (E) As with the 1-D network, the addition of an asymmetric component to the connection weights causes the represented location to drift (again, the asymmetric component is the spatial derivative along the direction of drift and its size determines the speed of drift). (Adapted from Zhang, 1996, copyright 1996 by Society for Neuroscience.)

16.2.3.2 Continuous attractor models of place cells

Samsonovich and McNaughton (1997) produced a detailed model of the place-cell representation as a continuous attractor, following (Zhang, 1996). In this model, the recurrent connections in CA3 are preconfigured to provide several different continuous attractor representations of location (termed "charts"). Each chart involves a different set of place cells, the relative positions of whose place fields are predetermined. The strength of the recurrent connection between two cells in a chart is set as a Gaussian function of the proximity of their place fields. The place cells connect with a "path integration"

(PI) system, originally hypothesized to reside in the subiculum, in which neurons respond to combinations of the rat's location and orientation (Sharp, 1996; Cacucci et al., 2004). Specifically, the place cells connect to PI neurons representing similar locations while the return projections connect back to place cells representing slightly different locations shifted along the rat's direction of orientation. The gain of this return projection is modulated by information relating to the rat's speed of self-motion (presumably carried by motor efference signals). This system, while demanding a highly specific set of hardwired connections, provides a self-consistent continuous

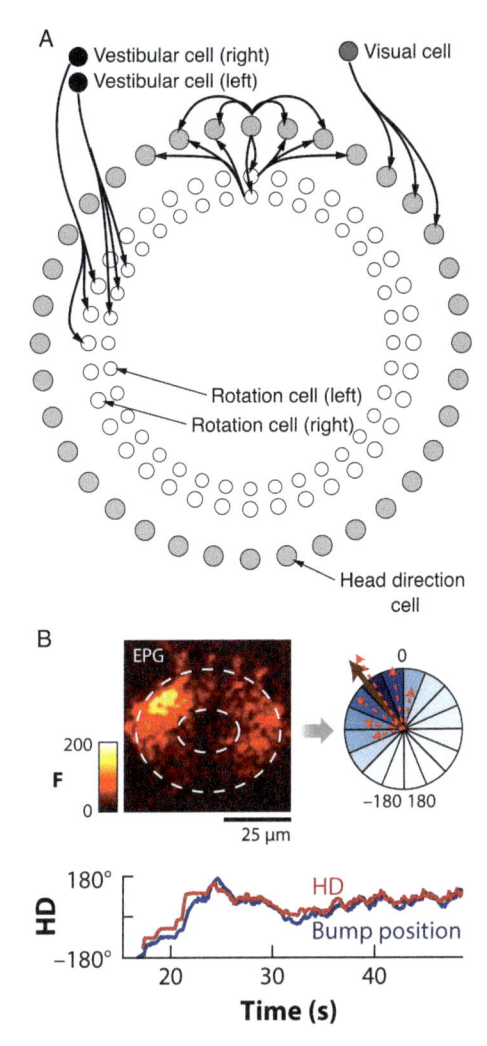

Figure 16.5 Ring attractor network model of head-direction cells and empirical data. (A) Skaggs et al.'s (1995) model of head-direction cells, showing the lateral connections among head-direction cells providing a continuous attractor, and connections from left or right rotation cells, visual inputs and vestibular inputs. The input from rotation cells serves the same purpose as the asymmetric component of lateral connections in Figure 16.4C. (Adapted from Skaggs et al., 1995.) (B) Empirical data from *Drosophila*. Snapshot of calcium activity (F) in EPG neurons of the ellipsoid body, showing a single activity bump (top left panel). This can be used to compute a resultant vector that tracks the angular position of the activity bump (top right panel). This angular position (blue line) maintains close correspondence with the fly's heading direction (HD, red line) while walking on a spherical treadmill. (Adapted from Turner-Evans et al., 2017.)

attractor representation of location that moves automatically with self-motion. Finally, the hippocampus also receives sensory input so that, when the rat is placed in an environment for the first time, associations between the sensory scene and the internal representation of location can be formed, which can then be used to periodically reset the system.

Overall, the model can be seen as a possible implementation of O'Keefe and Nadel's (1978, pp 220–230) view of the role of path integration in supporting short-term continuity in a cognitive map. Subsequent developments eliminated the need for a separate path integration system by incorporating direction and velocity modulation of place cells within the continuous attractor network (Conklin and Eliasmith, 2005). Samsonovich and McNaughton (1997) also

suggest that remapping reflects the system switching between uncorrelated charts. This is a reasonable model of the situation after global remapping, which is consistent with each chart acting as an attractor (Wills et al., 2005). However, the model is not consistent with situations in which individual place fields can move relative to each other in response to environmental change (e.g., O'Keefe and Burgess, 1996; Fenton et al., 2000), nor with slow (Lever et al., 2002) or partial remapping (e.g., Skaggs and McNaughton, 1998). To fit these data requires feedforward inputs to dominate, replacing the model's main feature.

Conversely, the Samsonovich and McNaughton (1997) model is consistent with data showing that the stability of the place-cell representation is dependent on NMDA receptors (Kentros et al., 1998); that place-field locations remain consistent with each other but slowly drift in the absence of anchoring sensory cues or if the rat is consistently disoriented before each trial (Knierim et al., 1995); and that the membrane potential of place cells exhibits a ramp-like depolarization as the firing field is traversed, presumably reflecting a release from recurrent inhibition (see Figure 16.2B; Harvey et al., 2010). In addition, the notion that synaptic connections between place cells are preconfigured is consistent with the "preplay" of place-cell sequences before the first visit to a new environment (Dragoi and Tonegawa, 2011). The involvement of some form of path integration is also suggested by the increased influence of the boundary the rat is running from compared with the one it is running toward (O'Keefe and Burgess, 1996; Gothard et al., 1996; Redish et al., 2000). We note that the important role played by path integration in updating the representation of spatial location does not necessarily imply that the hippocampus is required for behavior in all tests of path integration, as other brain regions may be sufficient to support this function. For example, in Alyan and McNaughton's (1999) experiment, hippocampal lesions did not prevent rats returning to the start of an outbound path in complete darkness.

Elsewhere, recurrent networks have also been used to examine place-field directionality, as modeled in a feedforward manner by Sharp (1991). In these models (Brunel and Trullier, 1998; Kali and Dayan, 2000) place-cell firing is initially derived from orientation-specific sensory input at each location (referred to as the "local view" from that location), while the dynamics of the network are strongly dependent on the recurrent connections in CA3. As with Sharp (1991), in these models, directionally constrained exploration results in orientation-dependent place fields. If exploration is unconstrained and random, however, then Hebbian learning in the recurrent collaterals of these models will result in a continuous attractor of the sort hardwired by Samsonovich and McNaughton (1997), and an orientation-independent place-cell representation of space. One caveat to this is that the Hebbian learning must be modulated by novelty to prevent inhomogeneity in exploration causing nonuniform weight profiles and unrealistic firing patterns (Kali and Dayan, 2000). Such novelty information has been suggested as a function for the cholinergic septal inputs to the hippocampus (Hasselmo et al., 1996; see section 16.4.4; but see Hasselmo and Fehlau, 2001). In addition, Kali and Dayan (2000) demonstrated how novelty-modulated learning could be used to control the formation of independent place-cell maps in environments that are sufficiently distinct—although this may not be sufficient to capture the complexities of all data concerning remapping. Like Sharp's (1991) model, these recurrent models are also inconsistent with data showing that place-cell firing in open fields is initially nondirectional but can become directional as a result of experience (Markus et al., 1995; Navratilova, Hoang, et al., 2012).

16.2.3.3 Continuous attractor models of grid cells

Although continuous attractor network models of place-cell firing are consistent with several aspects of the experimental data, they are generally unable to account for the heterogeneous changes in place-cell firing that follow various environmental manipulations (i.e., slow and partial remapping), and the conjunctive location by movement direction modulated "shifter" cells required to update place-cell firing patterns have remained elusive. Conversely, continuous attractor network models appear much better suited to account for grid-cell firing patterns (McNaughton et al., 2006). As direct recurrent excitatory connections between grid-cell candidate neurons in MEC are sparse, however, recurrent connectivity in most implementations is mediated by disynaptic inhibition from interneurons, which have been shown to densely innervate MEC principal neurons (Dhillon and Jones, 2000; Couey et al., 2013; Pastoll et al., 2013; Fuchs et al., 2016). Uniform excitatory input to such a network will generate one or more stable activity packets or "bumps," and self-motion information can then be used to translate the position of this activity packet across the neural sheet in accordance with the animal's movement in the real world (Fuhs and Touretzky, 2006; Guanella et al., 2007; Burak and Fiete, 2009). As with the continuous attractor models of place cells described above, most of these models suggest that the activity bump is shifted by asymmetric interactions between grid cells in the neural sheet. This can be achieved by rate-coded input from conjunctive grid x movement direction cells, which bear some relation to the conjunctive grid x head direction cells identified in the deeper layers of MEC (Sargolini et al., 2006). If the recurrent inhibitory input from these conjunctive cells to other cells in the network is shifted along the axis of their preferred firing direction, then their firing will shift the activity bump in the movement direction.

In the case of a single activity bump, a continuous attractor network model of grid-cell firing must exhibit a twisted torus topology, such that movement of a set distance in a direction corresponding to any multiple of 60° across the neural sheet will return it to its original position, thus accounting for the hexagonal symmetry of the grid firing pattern in the real world (Guanella et al., 2007; Pastoll et al., 2013). In the case of multiple bumps, the circular weight profile dictates that the location of activity bumps on the neural sheet exhibit sixfold symmetry through circular close packing. To ensure that activity bumps smoothly appear and disappear at the edges of the neural sheet, either periodic boundary conditions are imposed (which places constraints on the dimensions of the neural sheet) or, alternatively, the synaptic weights (Fuhs and Touretzky, 2006) or feedforward synaptic inputs (Burak and Fiete, 2009) are smoothly modulated to zero toward the edges of the neural sheet. Importantly, population activity is constrained by the synaptic connections between neurons such that grid-cell firing patterns can only ever encode a single location at any time. Hence, grid cells in the continuous attractor network effectively perform path integration, tracking the animal's location by integrating self-motion signals. Like any path integration system, this representation will accumulate noise over time, but this can be ameliorated by learned associations with sensory inputs that can "reset" the location estimate (as with models of place and head-direction firing patterns,

described above, and analogous to "pose cells" in robotics models of simultaneous localization and mapping, e.g., Milford and Wyeth, 2008). Incorporating associations with cells encoding the location of different landmarks, formed by slow Hebbian learning, also produces shifts and deformations of the grid firing pattern consistent with those observed during navigation in familiar environments (Ocko et al., 2018).

Continuous attractor network models of grid-cell firing readily account for the modular organization of grid cells (Barry et al., 2007; Stensola et al., 2012), for the consistent offset of firing patterns from corecorded grid cells across environments (Fyhn et al., 2007; Yoon et al., 2013), and for the apparently coherent drifts in grid firing patterns relative to the environment during active movement (Hardcastle et al., 2015; Chen et al., 2016; Perez-Escobar et al., 2016; Almog et al., 2019). In addition, subthreshold membrane potential recordings during the traversal of grid firing fields revealed a ramp depolarization (i.e., release from inhibition) predicted by continuous attractor network models (see Figure 16.2B; Domnisoru et al., 2013; Schmidt-Hieber and Hausser, 2013). However, these models generally predict that local interneurons should exhibit grid firing patterns, for which experimental evidence is lacking (Buetfering et al., 2014; but see Solanka et al., 2015; Shipston-Sharma et al., 2016). These models also struggle to account for distortions of the grid firing pattern (e.g., Krupic et al., 2015); for the rate modulation of different firing fields (e.g., Ismakov et al., 2017); and for the theta modulation and phase code for location exhibited by grid cells (Hafting et al., 2008) without relying on unrealistic subthreshold currents (Navratilova, Giocomo, et al., 2012; Pastoll et al., 2013), as discussed in the next section.

16.2.4 Modeling phase coding in place and grid cells

Most of the place- and grid-cell models described above focus on the rate code for location exhibited by these cells, while ignoring the concurrently expressed theta phase code for location within the firing field. Nonetheless, the origin of the phase coding of place- and grid-cell firing with respect to the concurrent theta rhythm of the EEG (O'Keefe and Recce, 1993; Hafting et al., 2008) has been the subject of several computational models. Before considering these models, we very briefly review the relevant experimental findings (see section 16.2.1 and Chapter 11 for more details).

The theta rhythm is a large amplitude LFP oscillation of around 6 to 10 Hz that is present whenever the rat is actively moving its head through the environment. As the rat traverses a place or grid field, the corresponding cell tends to fire spikes with a systematic phase relationship to the theta rhythm. On entering the field spikes are fired at a "late" phase, and as the rat passes through the field, spikes are fired at successively earlier phases so that, on exiting the field, the phase of firing may have "precessed" by up to 360 degrees (corresponding to an "early" phase). Interestingly, the phase of firing correlates better with the location of the rat within the place or grid firing field than with other variables such as the time spent within the field, or the instantaneous firing rate of the cell (Huxter et al., 2003; Climer et al., 2013; Jeewajee et al., 2014).

An appealingly simple feedforward model of the place-cell phase code assumes that excitatory synaptic input might increase as the rat runs through the place field, while the theta rhythm might reflect a sawtooth-shaped inhibitory input (i.e., inhibition decreasing through each cycle; see Figure 16.2C; Harris et al., 2002; Mehta et al., 2000). In this model, firing phase would advance simply because the increasing excitatory input manages to overcome the inhibitory input successively earlier in each cycle. The cause of the increasing excitatory input might reflect an exaggerated form of the asymmetry reported by (Mehta et al., 1997), or an increasing then decreasing input but with lack of firing on the decreasing portion due to effects such as habituation (Harris et al., 2002). Interestingly, this subthreshold "ramp" depolarization appears to be consistent with whole cell recordings from place cells during navigation in virtual reality environments (Harvey et al., 2010; see Figure 16.2B). These models also capture the observation that the phase shift becomes more reliable over the first few runs of a trial, as does the asymmetry of place fields (Mehta et al., 2002; Feng et al., 2015), and allow phase to be analyzed in terms of firing rate during nontranslational behaviors such as dreaming or wheel-running (Harris et al., 2002). However, they predict a relationship between firing rate and phase—both driven by the amplitude of subthreshold depolarization—which does not appear to exist in empirical data (Huxter et al., 2003), and go against the finding that, while the development of asymmetry in place fields over the first few runs of a trial is prevented by blockade of NMDA receptors, the phase shift phenomenon is unaffected by this manipulation (Ekstrom et al., 2001). In addition, the correlation between phase and location is stronger than that between phase and rate, and, on the linear track at least, the weaker correlation is a side effect of the stronger one (O'Keefe and Burgess, 2005).

As with models of place- and grid-cell firing, an alternative formulation stresses the role of recurrent connectivity as opposed to feedforward connections. Specifically, simulations of the Samsonovich and McNaughton (1997) model, in which net activation is made to oscillate at theta frequency, show something qualitatively similar to the phase shift, due to path integration occurring within each cycle. That is, the initially active set of place cells settles to those with fields centered on the rat and then expands to include those with fields centered ahead of the rat. The first quantitative model of this phase shift was proposed by Tsodyks et al. (1996). In this model, the recurrent connections between place cells in CA3 are asymmetrically arranged so that each place cell projects to place cells further along a learned path (see also Blum and Abbott, 1996). External input to a CA3 place cell arrives at a fixed (early) phase of theta, causing place-cell activity at this phase which in turn propagates through the recurrent connections to place cells with fields further along the path and causes them to fire. Overall activity is inhibited at the end of each theta cycle, preventing the further propagation of activity into the next cycle. Thus, when the rat enters a place field the corresponding cell starts to fire at a late phase due to propagated activity from cells with fields earlier on the path, and fires earlier within each cycle as the rat advances due to activity having to propagate through fewer cells, until finally firing at the early phase due solely to external inputs (see Kang and De Weese, 2019 for a related model in grid cells).

Several similar mechanisms, depending on the association of place cells firing earlier along a learned path to those firing later along it, have been proposed (Touretzky and Redish, 1996; Wallenstein and Hasselmo, 1997; Jensen and Lisman, 1996). The Jensen and Lisman (1996) model also makes interesting suggestions for the gamma rhythm, in separating the firing of cells corresponding to the current and successively further advanced locations, and for the dynamics of NMDA channels, in separating each route retrieval into successive cycles of the theta rhythm. Wallenstein and

Hasselmo (1997) emphasize the role of GABA$_B$ receptors in varying the relative influence of the inputs to CA1 from CA3 compared with those directly from EC over the theta cycle: allowing sensory (EC) input to dominate early and predictive input from CA3 to dominate late in the cycle (see also Chance, 2012). More recent models emphasize the role of spike-frequency adaptation in generating an activity bump that oscillates around the current location in a continuous attractor network (Chu et al., 2023; see Hopfield, 2010, for a related model of "mental exploration"). This can naturally account for theta phase precession, as well as several other features of place-cell firing, but faces the same issues as other continuous attractor network models of place-cell firing described above. It is also important to note that the apparent lack of direct excitatory connections between principal cells in superficial MEC suggest that these models could not explain phase precession in grid-cell firing. Instead, Navratilova, Giocomo, et al. (2012) suggest that after-spike dynamics could account for phase precession in an attractor network model of grid-cell firing, although it is difficult to see how these ionic currents might be coordinated by movement speed on the requisite timescale (i.e., to give a faster change in firing phase during faster runs through the place or grid field).

These models do, however, produce a phase shift that is limited to 360 degrees, more strongly correlated with position than time, and greater for well-learned paths than random exploration. Other aspects of these models are less consistent with empirical data. First, since the initial firing of a place cell depends on both the externally driven activity of other cells and its propagation through the network, it seems likely that, on a cell-by-cell and on a run-by-run basis, the initial phase of firing should be more variable than the (externally driven) final phase of firing, but this is not the case in the data (Skaggs et al., 1996; Huxter et al., 2003). Second, the observation that the theta phase preference of place-cell firing is maintained after transient perturbation of the hippocampus suggests that phase precession might be generated by external, rather than internal, mechanisms (Zugaro et al., 2005).

A third type of model stresses the inherent oscillatory nature of some cellular processes, as did Jensen and Lisman (1996), but for different reasons. Specifically, O'Keefe and Recce (1993) pointed out that the phase and amplitude characteristics of place-cell firing could be modeled as the interference pattern between an 11 Hz external input to the cell (perhaps the sensory input) and a 9 Hz external or internal oscillation corresponding to LFP theta (perhaps driven by the septal input). This produces an oscillation of 10 Hz corresponding to firing that shifts in phase relative to LFP theta and a 1 Hz envelope, one half-cycle of which corresponds to the place field. This model was subsequently extended (Lengyel et al., 2003), identifying the first input as a voltage-controlled oscillation of the membrane potential (see e.g., Hoppensteadt, 1987) in the dendrites, and the second as an inhibitory input to the soma of fixed frequency. The frequency of the dendritic oscillation was assumed to increase above that of the somatic oscillation proportionally to the strength of the dendritic input, which is assumed to be zero outside the place field and proportional to the rat's running speed within it (McNaughton et al., 1983; Ekstrom et al., 2001; Czurko et al., 1999; Huxter et al., 2003). Thus the two oscillations destructively interfere outside of the place field, while phase of firing relative to the somatic input within the field can shift more rapidly as the rat runs faster, preserving the relationship between phase and location. In addition, the dendritic oscillation must be weakly driven in antiphase to the somatic input so that, in the absence of any dendritic input, it ensures complete destructive interference.

Corroborative evidence for interference models comes from the observation that the increase in place-field size along the dorso-ventral axis of the hippocampus parallels a corresponding decrease in the intrinsic firing frequency of place cells—reducing toward LFP theta frequency in more ventral regions (Maurer et al., 2005). Similarly, the dorsoventral increase in grid-field size is matched by a corresponding gradient in h-current that reduces the res-onant frequency of stellate cells in MEC (Giocomo et al., 2011). Issues with the original model include why only one half cycle of the interference pattern is observed, and the demonstration that somatic and dendritic oscillatory processes cannot remain inde-pendent, but quickly phase lock in real neurons (Remme et al., 2010). As discussed above (section 16.2.2.2), however, it is pos-sible that the full interference pattern is expressed by the periodic firing fields of entorhinal grid cells; and that the interference pat-tern is generated entirely from feedforward inputs, rather than in-dependent processes in a single cell (Burgess et al., 2007; Burgess, 2008; Hasselmo, 2008). This raises the possibility that theta phase precession in hippocampal place cells might be inherited from grid-cell inputs (consistent with some empirical observations, e.g., Bonnevie et al., 2013; Schlesiger et al., 2015), and several models of such inheritance exist (e.g., Jaramillo et al., 2014). However, re-cent experiments have demonstrated that place fields artificially induced by optogenetic activation of CA1 pyramidal cells exhibit theta phase precession, suggesting that it is generated by local os-cillatory processes (Sloin et al., 2024). Another important point is that, to ensure that the moving representation of location gener-ated by the entire hippocampus within each theta cycle is coherent, phase precession must be coordinated across multiple grid- and place-field scales expressed along the dorsoventral axis, wherein theta oscillations act as a traveling wave (e.g., Lubenov and Siapas, 2009; Leibold and Monsalve-Mercado, 2017). Finally, it is im-portant to reiterate that interference models do not rely on any spe-cific assumptions about either the frequency or stationarity of the baseline (or "somatic") oscillation (which is generally equivalent to the dominant LFP frequency, see, e.g., Geisler et al., 2010): phase coding of location within the firing field arises from the difference between this and the active (i.e., velocity-controlled) oscillation. Hence, the baseline frequency does not need to occupy any par-ticular value, nor remain constant over time (Burgess, 2008; Blair et al., 2014; Orchard, 2015; Bush and Burgess, 2020).

16.2.5 Hybrid models of place- and grid-cell firing

In recent years, several groups have proposed hybrid models of place- and grid-cell firing that incorporate contributions from both feedforward and recurrent inputs to account for a greater body of experimental data; as well as models that emphasize the interactions between complementary spatial representations provided by place and grid cells, respectively. This is consistent with empirical data which indicates that place-cell firing patterns tend to be more strongly dictated by sensory inputs, and grid-cell firing patterns by self-motion (Chen et al., 2019). As such, it is possible that the path integration input to place cells, which accounts for stable activity patterns when sensory cues are diminished, arises from grid-cell in-puts; while the sensory input to grid cells, revealed by the "resetting" of accumulated error in grid-cell firing patterns during periods of running away from environmental boundaries or other prominent

sensory features, arises reciprocally from place-cell inputs. These models, building on earlier models of place- (e.g., Wan et al., 1994; Touretzky and Redish, 1996; Arleo and Gerstner, 2000) and grid- (e.g., Ocko et al., 2018) cell firing, emphasize the importance of interactions between place and grid cells to establish robust repre-sentations of location (e.g., Renno-Costa and Tort, 2017; Agmon and Burak, 2020), and also account for coherent remapping in the grid- and place-cell populations (Fyhn et al., 2007) and the hetero-geneity of grid-cell in-field firing rates (Ismakov et al., 2017).

Similarly, to account for a more complete body of empirical data relating to grid cells, several hybrid models of grid firing patterns that incorporate contributions of both feedforward and recurrent inputs have been proposed (Hasselmo and Brandon, 2012; Schmidt-Hieber and Hausser, 2013; Bush and Burgess, 2014). Specifically, these models make use of continuous attractor dynamics to ensure relative stability among the firing patterns of grid cells from within the same module; and oscillatory interference to shift the activity bump. As such, path integration is performed by VCO inputs to grid cells, rather than by conjunctive cells within the grid-cell net-work (Welday et al., 2011). This solves the problematic issue for continuous attractor network models that conjunctive cells in MEC are modulated by head, rather than movement, direction, which is not sufficient to support accurate path integration (Raudies et al., 2015). These hybrid models can therefore account for a greater body of experimental data, including both the rate and temporal firing pattern of grid cells, the relative stability of grid-cell firing patterns from the same module, and the subthreshold ramp depolarization of grid cells inside the firing field. Nonetheless, like all continuous attractor network models of grid-cell firing, they predict the exist-ence of interneurons with grid firing patterns in MEC, for which strong evidence has not yet been found (Buetfering et al., 2014; but see Solanka et al., 2015; Shipston-Sharma et al., 2016).

16.3 The hippocampus and spatial navigation

In this section we consider the contribution of hippocampal spa-tial representations to guiding behavior. We focus on large-scale navigation, the spatial behavior most commonly associated with the hippocampus and medial temporal lobes (see Chapter 14). This compares with planning movements in smaller-scale spaces and over shorter durations, such as visually guided reaching, which is most commonly associated with the posterior parietal lobe (see, e.g., Burgess et al., 1999). As with models of spatial representation, these models can be approximately divided into those stressing the role of feedforward connections, and those stressing the role of re-current connections.

16.3.1 Spatial navigation: data

Behavioral data indicate that rats learn about the spatial layout of their environment during exploration in the absence of explicit goals or rewards (e.g., Tolman, 1948) and can profit from being placed at the goal location without having explored the rest of the environ-ment (Keith and McVety, 1988). These processes are referred to as "latent learning." Rats also appear to be able to perform short cuts and detours. These abilities contributed to the idea that rats form a cognitive map of their environment as opposed to simply learning to associate individual stimuli with responses (see Tolman, 1948; O'Keefe and Nadel, 1978; but see Grieves and Dudchenko, 2013).

In the framework of reinforcement learning (RL), this corresponds to a "model-based" approach, whereby a model of the world is used to predict the outcomes of different actions. This world model may require extensive learning, but that can proceed in the absence of reward and subsequently support flexible planning. In contrast, "model-free" RL, whereby a value function that maps actions in each state to long-term cumulative reward is learned by trial and error, may be less computationally expensive but is more rigid: when the goal or the optimal route to the goal changes, learning must begin again from scratch. Stimulus-response associations undoubtedly play an important role in spatial navigation, such as when the goal is directly visible or a well-learned turn or sequence of turns is to be performed. However, there seems to be good evidence that these types of behavior are less dependent on the hippocampus than those associated with cognitive mapping (Morris et al., 1982; Packard and McGaugh, 1996; O'Keefe and Nadel, 1978; Doeller and Burgess, 2008; Vikbladh et al., 2019). These issues are discussed in more detail in Chapter 14. Of note, many models of navigation combine contributions from parallel model-based and model-free strategies alongside dynamic arbitration between the (sometimes conflicting) output of each strategy, to account for more behavioral data (Guazzelli et al., 1998; Arleo and Gerstner, 2000; Chavarriga et al., 2005; Dolle et al., 2010; Geerts et al., 2020). However, we focus specifically on models of hippocampal function here.

The initial spur to the association of the hippocampus with a cognitive map of the rat's environment was the discovery of place cells, whose activity is not easily described in terms of a simple response to a single stimulus (like that of concept cells in the human hippocampal formation; Quiroga et al., 2005). Indeed, some recent empirical studies have begun to demonstrate a causal role for rodent place cells in spatial behavior (de Lavilleon et al., 2015; Robinson et al., 2020). Nonetheless, an explanatory gap remains between the properties of place cells and the properties required of a system for spatial navigation. Three features of place-cell firing are particularly problematic. First, information about a place in an environment (i.e., the firing of the corresponding place cells) can only be accessed locally (by actually visiting that place). Although hippocampal replay events may allow nonlocal place-cell activity during quiescent waking or rest, it is not yet clear if these events are utilized during active navigation or can represent novel trajectories through known environments, rather than simply recapitulating previous experience (Gillespie et al., 2021; but see Gupta et al., 2010; Ólafsdóttir et al., 2015; Liu et al., 2023). An alternative solution to navigating with place cells may be provided by "spatial view cells" in the macaque hippocampus (Rolls et al., 1997) which fire as a function of where the monkey is looking rather than where it is physically located.

Second, there is limited evidence that place-field activity is modulated by the location of the current goal more than by the location of any other cue (e.g., Speakman and O'Keefe, 1990; Hok et al., 2007; Duvelle et al., 2019)—although there is some evidence that place (Hollup et al., 2001; Lee et al., 2006; Dupret et al., 2010; Mamad et al., 2017; Kaufman et al., 2020) and grid (Boccara et al., 2019; Butler et al., 2019) fields shift slightly toward persistently rewarded locations. That is, place cells appear to tell you where you currently are rather than where your goal is (particularly if that location is not where reward is delivered). Nonetheless, several recent empirical studies have described the modulation of place- and non-place-cell firing rates in the mammalian hippocampus by goal direction (e.g., Sarel et al., 2017; Kunz et al., 2021; Ormond and O'Keefe, 2022),

which could be used to support navigation (by selecting a movement direction that maximizes those firing rates), although the origin of this goal direction signal and manner in which it is learned are not yet clear. Similarly, place-cell theta sequences (see section 16.2.1) appear to dynamically explore different movement trajectories away from the current location (e.g., Johnson and Redish, 2007; Wikenheiser and Redish, 2015; Kay et al., 2020), akin to a process of deliberation or "vicarious trial and error" (VTE; Redish, 2016), but their potential role in navigation has not yet been explicitly modeled.

Third, the phenomenon of global remapping indicates that place cells do not provide any metric information about the relative location of their place fields, and therefore cannot be used to generalize information across environments (i.e., learning the relation between the place-field locations of two cells in one environment provides no information about their relative location in a second environment). The compact and efficient representation of large-scale space offered by grid cells appear better suited to support long-range navigation by computing direct vectors between start and goal locations (Fiete et al., 2008; Bush et al., 2015; Stemmler et al., 2015) or supporting generalization across relational structures, in a broader sense (Behrens et al., 2018). Nonetheless, these vectors may need further refinement in light of the sensory and affective properties of intermediate locations, which may be furnished by place cells or those encoding the presence of boundaries (e.g., Edvardsen et al., 2019).

16.3.2 Spatial navigation: feedforward models

Zipser's (1986) "view field" model built on the observation that, in some circumstances, place-cell firing is modulated by the orientation of the rat. In this model, a set of orientation dependent place cells or "view-field units" become associated to a set of "goal units," which encode the direction to the goal relative to the current heading direction. So long as the appropriate cells become associated, the population vector of directions represented by the goal units guide the rat to the goal, as goal units driven by place cells representing the current location will fire the most strongly. However, this model requires the direction toward the goal to be continuously maintained during initial exploration of the environment, perhaps as a path integration vector, in order for that direction to be associated with active place cells in each location. In a second ("beta coefficient") model, Zipser suggested that this could be avoided by calculating and storing the location of the goal relative to subsets of landmarks (as the coefficients of the linear sum of landmark locations that is equal to the goal location). In this model, learning at the goal location is sufficient to support navigation back to that location, although the neural mechanisms required to implement the desired calculations are not explained. A similar model was proposed by Wilkie and Palfrey (1987) but, again, this model was primarily heuristic and no biologically plausible implementation of the landmark distance matching procedure was provided. More importantly, it is not clear whether these models require an explicit representation of place, as they act directly on sensory input (analogous to models of insect navigation, e.g., Cartwright and Collett, 1983). Nonetheless, each of these models can account for the latent learning of goal locations, as well as behavioral search patterns following the movement or removal of prominent visual cues.

Several models have followed Zipser's view field model in associating places or local views to movements (see Trullier et al., 1997, for a wider review of biologically based artificial navigation systems). McNaughton and Nadel (1990) suggested that routes might be learned as a chain of associations from a local view to an action and thence to the next local view, and so on. This model was not actually simulated, and simply storing routes is insufficient to enable spatial navigation. Even if a given route can be correctly selected in terms of the locations to which it leads, navigational abilities such as generating novel shortcuts and detours will be beyond a simple route-based system. The task of accumulating route-independent spatial information faces several issues, including the "credit assignment" problem: deciding which actions along a route are critical in determining whether it eventually leads to the goal.

Brown and Sharp (1995) provided a more sophisticated model for associating locations with actions (see also Sharp et al., 1996). In their model, the possible actions in a place are represented by left turn and right turn cells (in nucleus accumbens) driven by each place cell. These "turn cells" receive modifiable connections from head-direction cells (HDCs), which support the rat's spatial learning. When the rat reaches the goal, connections between head-direction and turn cells are modified according to a recency-weighted index of their simultaneous activity. Thus, if turning left in a particular place when facing north leads immediately to the goal, then the HDC representing north becomes more strongly associated to the left turn cell driven by the corresponding place cell. The recency weighting of connection modification is designed to provide an approximate solution to the credit assignment problem (when applied over many trials) by effectively dividing credit according to the number of steps within which an action leads to finding the goal. This model successfully simulates learning in the Morris watermaze but does not show latent learning: performance would not be affected by whether the rat can look around from the goal location, and navigation to the goal would be strongly affected if stereotyped routes were used during learning.

A related way to think about spatial navigation is to imagine defining a surface over the environment on which gradient ascent leads to the goal, like the value function in RL (Dayan, 1991; Foster et al., 2000, see below). The simplest model of this sort has place cells connected to a goal cell via reward-modulated Hebb-modifiable connections such that encountering a goal causes the strengthening of its input connections from concurrently active place cells (see N Burgess and O'Keefe, 1996; Figure 16.6A). The activity of the goal cell will subsequently increase with proximity to the goal since the net activity of those place cells with strengthened connections will increase with the proximity to the goal. The task for the rat is then to move in the direction that increases the firing rate of the cell representing the desired goal (Figure 16.6B). This type of model qualitatively captures the rapid nature of learning a goal location once place-cell firing has become established and the ability to learn simply by being at the goal location as opposed to having to find it many times. However, finding the goal would involve the rat hunting around to determine the best direction in which to move. This VTE behavior is often observed at choice points but is less common in the open field (Redish, 2016). A second problem raised by this model is the range over which spatial information is accessible. If there are no place cells that fire at both the goal location and the current location of the rat, then there will be no gradient in the firing rate of the goal cell (being locally zero). Hence, this type of model requires the place-cell population to include some firing fields that have nonzero firing rates at any two points in the environment, however far apart.

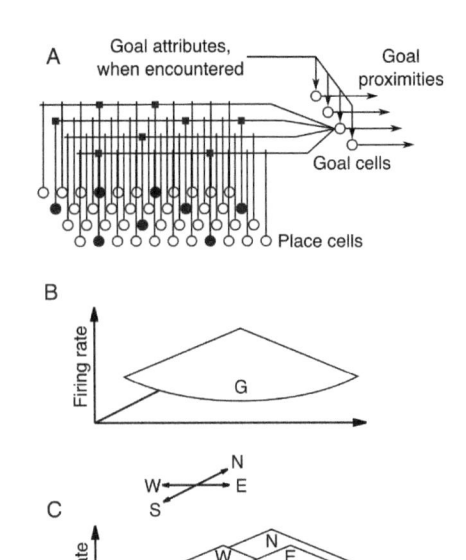

Figure 16.6 Simple model of navigation with place cells. (A) A "goal" cell stores a goal's location by taking a snapshot of place-cell activity via Hebbian synaptic modification when the goal cell is excited by the attributes of a particular goal location. Solid circles are active place cells; open circles are inactive place cells and solid squares mark potentiated synapses between place-cell axons and goal cell dendrites. (B) The firing rate map of the goal cell (roughly an inverted cone) during subsequent movements of the rat codes for the proximity of the goal (G). (C) The firing rate maps of four goal cells whose population vector codes for the goal location (G). Each is associated with the allocentric direction u_i in which the location of its peak firing rate is displaced from G; thus the vector sum of the directions $\underline{u}_i$ weighted by the instantaneous firing rates f_i of the goal cells (i.e., $\Sigma_i f_i \underline{u}_i / \Sigma_i f_i$) codes for the direction of the rat from the goal, and the net firing rate of the goal cells (i.e., $\Sigma_i f_i$) codes for the goal's proximity. (Adapted from Burgess and O'Keefe, 1996.)

Although larger place fields have been observed in ventral hippocampus (e.g., Jung et al., 1994; Kjelstrup et al., 2008), this places strong constraints on the spatial range over which goal-directed navigation might be feasible.

Burgess et al. (1994) proposed a biologically inspired navigation model that aimed to address both issues. First, to calculate the direction to the goal from any location after a single visit to that goal, this model made use of the empirical observation that place cells which fire at a late phase of the theta rhythm have fields peaked ahead of the rat (see section 16.2.1). Specifically, the model posits a set of goal cells that are each associated with a different head-direction and assumes that synaptic connections between place cells and each directional goal cell are only modified at late phases of the theta cycle (consistent with observations of theta phase dependent synaptic plasticity, e.g., Pavlides et al., 1988; Huerta and Lisman, 1995; Holscher et al., 1997). Hence, when the rat is at the goal and facing north, connections are formed between place cells slightly north of the goal (i.e., ahead of the rat) and the "north" goal cell; and turning to face each direction while located at the goal allows connections between place cells offset in each different direction from the goal and the corresponding goal cell to be learned (Figure 16.6C). This produces a set of directional goal cells with firing fields that are offset in the corresponding direction from the goal, such that the population vector of goal cell firing rates at any location within their firing fields indicates the direction of the goal. In addition, different sets of directional goal cells can be used to encode the location of (and thus support navigation to) different salient locations. Second, the range over which spatial information is available from place-cell firing was increased by interposing a set of subicular cells between the place and goal cells. Weaker inhibitory competition between subicular cells coupled with competitive learning in the inputs from place cells during exploration causes the subicular cells to build up larger firing fields, each one effectively composed of several place fields. This learning is goal-independent and corresponds to latent learning in preparing the ground for effective one-shot learning of the location of any goals, should they be encountered.

As described by Foster et al. (2000), another way to ameliorate the issue of navigational range being limited to the diameter of the largest place field is to make use of a temporal difference (TD) learning rule (R Sutton and Barto, 1988). Under this model-free RL formulation, place cells provide a representation of the task "state" (i.e., the rat's current location; Dayan, 1991) and its value reflects the expected number of steps needed to reach the goal (one unit of reward being received on reaching the goal). TD learning can be implemented by connecting place cells to "actor" and "critic" units with connections that are adjusted according to a modified Hebbian rule (see Arleo and Gerstner, 2000, for an alternative implementation that makes use of the Q-learning algorithm). The activation of the critic unit is equal to the expected future reward from the current state, discounted by distance into the future (see, e.g., Dayan and Abbott, 2001), a more principled analogue of the simple goal cell formulation above. The set of actor units, only one of which can be active at a given time, represent movement in different directions. At each step the connection weight from a place cell to the critic unit or to the active actor unit is adjusted by an amount proportional to the product of the place cell's firing rate and the amount by which the reward exceeds that expected from the change in the activity of the critic unit. This type of learning with reward prediction errors is consistent with a role

for dopaminergic modulation of LTP (e.g., Montague et al., 1996; Schultz et al., 1997). Over many routes to the goal, ideally involving performing all actions at all locations many times, this rule causes both the critic to provide an accurate estimation of value and the appropriate actions to be associated with each state (see Figure 16.7). For a given environmental configuration and goal location, this can provide the optimal strategy, which is not the case with the approximate recency weighting implemented by Brown and Sharp (1995) above (and Blum and Abbott, 1996, below) or, if obstacles are present, with goal cells simply indicating the physical proximity of the goal (Burgess et al., 1994). As mentioned earlier, however, learning is both experience-dependent and goal-dependent: knowing to head north from a given place results from this route having previously led to the goal, and there is no transfer of learning when the goal is moved. Like the Brown and Sharp (1995) model, therefore, navigation can be strongly influenced by taking stereotyped routes during learning and is inflexible to changes in reward location.

To simulate goal-independent learning over many trials in which the location of the goal changes, Foster et al. (2000) proposed that a second system learns to form a coordinate representation of the rat's position by using the rat's locally accurate ability to estimate self-motion (potentially foreshadowing the computational benefit and generative mechanisms of grid-cell firing patterns, see sections 16.3.4 and 16.2, respectively). The place cells are connected to two units that learn to estimate the x and y coordinate of the rat, again using TD learning to adjust connection weights. In this system, the change in a connection weight to the x unit is proportional to the place-cell activation times the amount by which the change in x, as estimated by self-motion, exceeds that estimated by the change in the activity of the x unit. The explicit representation of x and y coordinates enables accurate navigation after one exposure to the goal and so corresponds well with latent learning. No neural implementation of this vector navigation procedure was described, however.

As described by Dayan (1993), an alternative approach to making TD learning more flexible and support more efficient RL is to

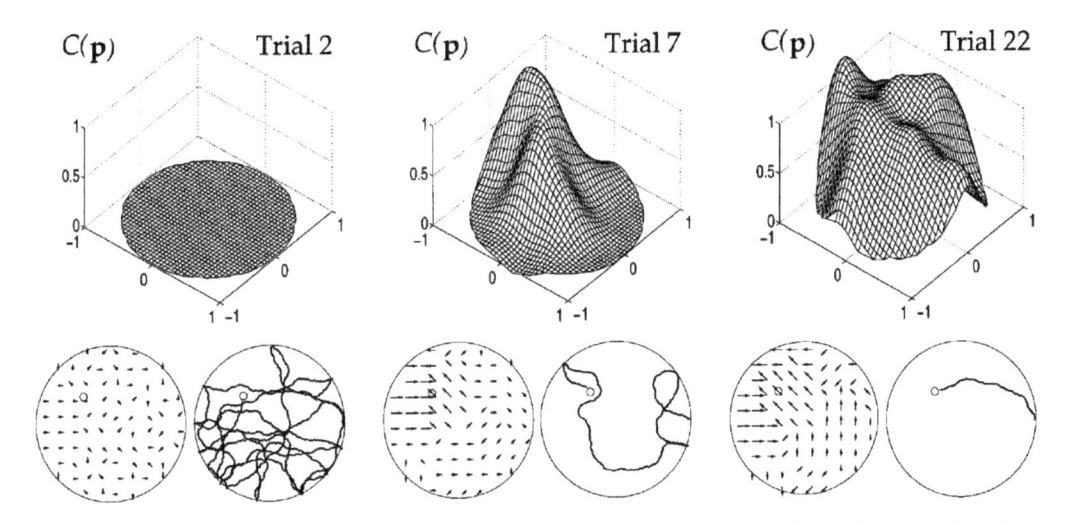

Figure 16.7 Learning in the actor-critic system in a water maze. The plots for each trial show the critic's value function C(p) (above), the preferred actions at various locations (below left, the length of each arrow is related to the probability that the particular action shown is taken by a logarithmic scale) and a sample path (below right). Trial 2: After a timed-out first trial, the critic's value function remains zero everywhere, the actions point randomly in different directions, and a long and tortuous path is taken to the platform. Trial 7: The critic's value function having peaked in the northeast quadrant of the pool, the preferred actions are correct for locations close to the platform, but not for locations further away. Trial 22: The critic's value function has spread across the whole pool, and the preferred actions are close to correct in most locations, so the actor takes a direct route to the platform. (Adapted from Foster et al., 2000.)

decompose the learned value function (i.e., the discounted sum of expected rewards at future states, given a specific action or policy) into a separate reward function and discounted expectancy of occupying each future state, or "successor representation" (see section 16.5.2). It has been hypothesized that the SR is the true variable encoded by place-cell activity (Stachenfeld et al., 2017; see also Gustafson and Daw, 2011). Under this formulation, place cells do not encode current location per se, but a predictive representation of future locations given the current location, which is learned as a function of the navigational history of the animal. The SR combines some advantages of both model-free and model-based approaches to navigation: it can be used to efficiently identify the optimal trajectory from current to goal locations, like model-free RL; but is flexible to changes in the goal location, like model-based RL, provided that the transition structure of the environment and policy remain unchanged. In addition, the notion that place cells may encode the SR accounts for various empirical observations, such as the increase in place-field asymmetry during repeated trajectories in the same direction of motion (Mehta et al., 2000); the local remapping of place fields close to a novel barrier in a linear maze (Alvernhe et al., 2011); and the skewing of place fields toward a repeatedly visited reward location (Markus et al., 1995; Hollup et al., 2001; see Stachenfeld et al., 2017, for further details). The SR is also consistent with some aspects of latent learning, as it can be learned during exploration of an environment prior to the introduction of any reward; and recent analyses suggest that some aspects of human and rodent navigation behavior can be best predicted by an SR formulation (de Cothi et al., 2022). Nonetheless, like many of the place-cell navigation models described above, navigation using the SR is limited to the diameter of the largest place field (beyond which the product of the reward function and SR will be zero); and will be biased by stereotyped movement patterns during exploration (which dictate the structure of the SR).

16.3.3 Spatial navigation: feedback models

As well as being linked with spatial representation and associative memory (see Box 16.3), the CA3 recurrent collaterals have been proposed to play a role in spatial navigation. The first model to formalize such a role was suggested by Muller et al. (1991, 1996) and focused on the Hebb-associative effects of LTP on the recurrent collaterals. If pre- and postsynaptic firing within a short time interval leads to a small increase in synaptic strength, then the firing of place cells as the rat moves around an environment will lead to the strength of a connection between two place cells depending on the proximity of their place fields. This occurs simply because the greater the overlap between place fields the more often they will fire near-coincidentally during random exploration. Muller et al. (1996) show that, after extensive exploration, the synaptic strengths represent a "cognitive graph": each approximately representing the minimum path-length between the centers of the place fields of the cells it connects. Their model proposes that the rat navigates by moving through the place fields of the cells most strongly connected to the cells with fields at the current and destination positions. This mechanism, reminiscent of a resistive grid (Connelly et al., 1990), works well but relies on a graph search. It is not easy to imagine how such a process could be implemented in a biologically plausible fashion given the apparent lack of influence of the goal location on the firing of place cells. One early suggestion was that activation corresponding to the goal location occurs in entorhinal cortex while activation corresponding to the current location occurs in CA3, and activation in each region spreads along the available paths (although more slowly in CA3 than entorhinal cortex) until a commonly activated location is detected in CA1 (Gorchetchnikov and Hasselmo, 2002). This location represents the next immediate destination for the rat, although how this information is interpreted in terms of whether to turn left or right is not described. More recent formulations have suggested that activation may spread backward from the goal location through cortical columns in prefrontal cortex that represent each action taken and state visited, thus providing the shortest sequence of actions needed to reach the goal (Hasselmo, 2005; see also Martinet et al., 2011).

In a related model, Blum and Abbott (1996) make use of the temporal asymmetry of LTP to strengthen recurrent connections from CA3 place cells that fire early on the rat's path to those that fire later along it (see also Gerstner and Abbott, 1997). This causes the activation of place cells to spread backward along the path, see also (Mehta et al., 1997; Mehta et al., 2000) and models of spatial representation above. If the firing of place cells is interpreted by systems downstream of CA3 as representing the location of the rat, this shift in firing (backward along the path) would be interpreted as a shift in the location of the rat forward along the path. Blum and Abbott suggested that navigation along a previously performed route could be performed by moving from the current location (e.g., read from CA1) to the shifted location represented in CA3, although how this could be implemented was not described. To enable navigation to a goal location the rules for synaptic change were modified to be proportional to the amount of pre- and postsynaptic activation weighted by how recently it occurred prior encountering the goal, i.e., a similar modification to that suggested by Brown and Sharp (1995), above.

It is interesting to note that the symmetric pattern of connection strengths learned in Muller et al.'s model resembles that used in continuous attractor models of place-cell firing, and so also serves to produce a consistent pattern of activity to represent each location. By contrast, the additional asymmetry in connection strengths learned in Blum and Abbott's model serve to shift the represented location along the learned route. Indeed this latter property has been shown to allow the represented location to move smoothly along the route over time, suggested as a model for mental replay during sleep (Redish and Touretzky, 1998; Bush et al., 2010). The goal-independent encoding of spatial proximity (as in the symmetric connections of Muller et al.'s cognitive graph) or of previously traveled routes (as in the asymmetric connections of the later models) correspond to latent learning. However, many visits are required to learn the synaptic weights that will incorporate any new goal location, which probably falls short of a rat's abilities. A further drawback associated with these models is that none makes clear the details of how the rat's brain might deduce the direction it should move in, or if it would be able to generate a shortcut or detour. They also assume place fields of fixed relative location but might still make some interesting predictions regarding the locus of search in environments that had changed in shape or size. To build up a true distance metric in complex environments would take a long time, in common with the RL approaches (see Foster et al., 2000; section 16.3.2).

These models can be viewed in the context of a more general set of higher-level algorithms for navigation based on directed graphs. Lieblich and Arbib (1982) describe a "world graph," in which locations are represented as nodes connected by (asymmetric) edges that represent the movement necessary to get from one node to the next. In terms of the navigation of autonomous agents, Scholkopf and Mallot (1995) describe a "view graph," in which the local view or sensory perception at given locations form the nodes, and the actions required to get from one view to the next form the edges (see also McNaughton and Nadel, 1990, for a description of how a view graph might be implemented in the hippocampus). Mallot and Gillner (2000) argue that such view graphs are a good model for human navigation despite their simplicity. One key requirement for building a world graph is to be able to decide whether to assign a new node to a location. This can be dictated on the basis of its familiarity (see Touretzky and Redish, 1996; Kali and Dayan, 2000) for models relating to this, or possibly on the basis of the sequence of actions that lead back to a location. Lieblich and Arbib (1982) further suggest that the nodes of a world graph might also represent a location's motivational valence and thus become a general model for goal-directed behavior, even though its creation might correspond to latent learning. Finally, George et al. (2021) describe how "clone structured cognitive graphs," in which nodes that correspond to a specific constellation of sensory inputs are cloned to disambiguate the recent history of inputs that led to that state, can account for a wide variety of data regarding hippocampal spatial representations and navigation behavior. Specifically, by separating behavioral states that are associated with equivalent sensory inputs but differ in their temporal context, the directed graphs that are learned by this framework during exploration can account for the existence of "splitter cells" (Frank et al., 2000; Wood et al., 2000; Grieves et al., 2016) and various remapping phenomena.

16.3.4 Models of navigation with grid cells

In contrast to place cells, grid cells exhibit several properties that naturally afford large-scale vector navigation and address many of the issues relating to place-cell navigation models described above. The regular periodic firing patterns of grid cells potentially provide a compact code that resembles a residue number system, encoding locations over a very large range that approaches the lowest common multiple of the spatial scales of all grid modules (Gorchetchnikov and Grossberg, 2007; Fiete et al., 2008; Sreenivasan and Fiete, 2011; Mathis et al., 2012). Importantly, grid cells generally fire in all environments visited by an animal and do not exhibit global remapping but tend to maintain a constant phase relationship across all environments (Fyhn et al., 2007; Yoon et al., 2013). Hence, the periodic firing patterns of grid cells appear to provide a framework with which to infer the vector between two locations, even when those locations are much farther apart than the largest grid scale and the intervening space has not been explored (Erdem and Hasselmo, 2012; Kubie and Fenton, 2012; Bush et al., 2015). The grid-cell population effectively provides an efficient coordinate system for large-scale space, which should theoretically allow the direction and distance between any two previously visited points (at which the grid-cell population activity is known) to be computed (Stemmler et al., 2015; Behrens et al., 2018). Consistent with this view, units with grid-like firing patterns emerge in some recurrent networks trained to perform vector navigation (Banino et al., 2018; Cuevas and Wei, 2018).

Several possible methods of computing navigational vectors from grid-cell population activity using realistic neural networks have been proposed. One possible solution is to perform "linear look ahead" by propagating sweeps of activity sequentially through the grid-cell population in different directions, beginning at the start location. The time taken for grid cells encoding the goal location to become active, or the activity of a neuron that integrates the total output of the grid-cell population during that time, subsequently provides an indication of the distance to the goal in that direction, which can be combined across any two noncollinear axes to produce a direct movement vector (Erdem and Hasselmo, 2012; Kubie and Fenton, 2012; Bush et al., 2015). Such activity sweeps are consistent with observations of grid-cell "replay" in MEC (Ólafsdóttir et al., 2016; O'Neill et al., 2017), and this model has the advantage of requiring no additional circuitry or mechanisms to solve the navigation problem, beyond those already in place to update the grid representation and its association with environmental sensory-driven place-cell representations during exploration. In addition, this model predicts that more time and greater metabolic activity within the hippocampal formation should be associated with the construction of longer vectors, consistent with some experimental data (Kosslyn et al., 1978; Sherrill et al., 2013; Howard et al., 2014).

Alternatively, the distance between different locations encoded in grid-cell population activity can be directly linearly decoded using a "distance cell" model, analogous to neural network models of the mental number line (Dehaene, 1997). Briefly, separate arrays of distance cells code for each direction of travel along two noncollinear axes and receive input from grid cells in each module with synaptic weights proportional to their mean firing rate at that location on that axis. Winner-take-all dynamics ensure that only a single distance cell in each array is active, and all distance cells provide input to a readout neuron with synaptic weights that increase in strength linearly with distance along the axis. Hence, the firing rate of that readout neuron signals the distance from the origin to that location along that directional axis, and the combined output of readout neurons stimulated, via the distance cells, by grid-cell population activity encoding the start and goal location is then directly proportional to the distance between those locations along that directional axis (Bush et al., 2015). Because distance and direction are decoded linearly, the distance cell model is rapid, and predicts no scaling of computational time or effort when decoding increasingly large vectors. However, it does require a significant amount of additional neural circuitry, and it is not clear how the fine-tuned weights of those connections may be learned during development or exploration.

In sum, although the properties of grid-cell firing fields appear to be perfectly suited to support vector navigation in large-scale space, and despite behavioral evidence that navigation in real (Chen et al., 2015) and virtual (Bellmund et al., 2020) environments is consistent with grid firing patterns, the exact mechanism by which this might be achieved has yet to be elucidated. Of note, this mechanism might not be restricted to support the navigation of an agent through the world—it has also been proposed to support the planning of saccades during visual exploration (Bicanski and Burgess, 2019), consistent with reports of grid-like responses in MEC during visual search (e.g., Killian et al., 2012; Nau et al., 2018; Julian et al., 2018). Indeed, it has been suggested that grid cells might be used throughout neocortex to encode the location of sensory features in different modalities using a consistent coordinate system (Hawkins et al., 2019). In spatial navigation, however, it seems likely that vector navigation would have to be combined with some other method for evaluating the sensory and affective properties of intervening locations during the planning of feasible routes through cluttered environments that prevent movement in a straight line between current and goal locations. One such method could involve generating potential trajectories by the firing of place cells influenced by grid vectors and the presence of boundaries (Edvardsen et al., 2019). This mechanism would be consistent with the recent observation that the replay of goal-directed place-cell sequences circumnavigates the current configuration of barriers (Widlowski and Foster, 2022). Overall, several plausible computational mechanisms have been proposed that utilize place cells to label specific locations and grid cells to encode the spatial relationship between those locations, but no one specific mechanism has so far have been conclusively endorsed by experimental data.

16.4 The hippocampus and associative memory

In contrast to the vast amount of animal work linking hippocampal damage to deficits in spatial cognition, the major impairment noted in humans following bilateral damage to the hippocampus is amnesia: a much more general impairment in memory. The extent of this impairment into various subdivisions of memory and into information acquired prior to the damage is a contentious issue. Here we briefly review the data on human hippocampal function in memory, introduce the canonical "complementary learning systems" model (McClelland et al., 1995) derived from Marr's seminal paper in 1971 and discuss various developments made to this framework over the years.

16.4.1 Hippocampus and memory: data

Substantial bilateral damage to the hippocampus and medial temporal lobes almost invariably leads to amnesia, characterized as a drop in the memory component of the intelligence quotient (MIQ) of at least 20 points relative to full-scale IQ. Since only a relatively small number of cases of damage restricted to the hippocampus have been studied (e.g., Kartsounis et al., 1995), it is difficult to draw general conclusions regarding its role in memory as opposed to the roles of surrounding cortical areas. However, some general points can be made (see Spiers et al., 2001; Squire et al., 2004; Squire and Wixted, 2011; and Chapter 13 for details). These include a ubiquitous deficit in long-term memory for personally experienced events that occur after the lesion (i.e., an "anterograde" deficit in "episodic" memory) alongside spared procedural and working memory. The extent of retrograde amnesia (loss of memory for information acquired prior to the lesion) appears to vary across patients and possibly across types of information (Nadel and Moscovitch, 1997; Winocur et al., 2010). Memory loss can extend over the entire lifetime or be restricted to shorter periods prior to the damage, but does seem to be relatively limited in the case of lesions to the fornix (Aggleton and Brown, 1999).

More controversial findings include the relative sparing of semantic memory (memory for facts) and of familiarity-based recognition in some cases of focal hippocampal damage (Vargha-Kardem et al., 1997; Manns et al., 2003). A relative sparing of recognition memory is consistent with findings in monkeys showing that this type of memory is more strongly dependent on nearby cortical areas (e.g., Zola-Morgan et al., 1994; Baxter and Murray, 2001; Gaffan, 1994; Aggleton and Brown, 1999). There is also some evidence for specific impairments in short-term memory for the relations among

co-occurring items or features (e.g., Hannula et al., 2006; Olson et al., 2006; Pertzov et al., 2013) and the topography of visual scenes (Lee et al., 2006; Hartley et al., 2007); while in animals, hippocampal lesions are associated with deficits in sequence learning (Fortin et al., 2002) and trace conditioning, in which a response must be made at a fixed delay after the disappearance of a cue (Solomon et al., 1986). Finally, it should be noted that the human hippocampus, particularly in the right hemisphere, is also involved in spatial navigation (Burgess et al., 2002) and model-based decision-making (Vikbladh et al., 2019); and that intact hippocampal function appears to be required for imagining new experiences (i.e., "scene construction" or "episodic future thinking"; Atance and O'Neill, 2001; Hassabis et al., 2007; Schacter et al., 2012; see Chapter 13).

16.4.2 Marr's (1971) model of long-term memory

Much of the modeling work on the role of the hippocampus in episodic or associative memory can be considered part of a long tradition reaching back to Marr (1971). In this section we sketch the main components that provide a common framework for subsequent models, and indicate how these components correspond to various aspects of the data on human memory (see also Willshaw and Buckingham, 1990; Burgess et al., 2001a; Norman et al., 2008). We refer to this as the canonical hippocamponeocortical model (see Figure 16.8) and note its extension as "complementary learning systems theory," following McClelland et al. (1995). We also note

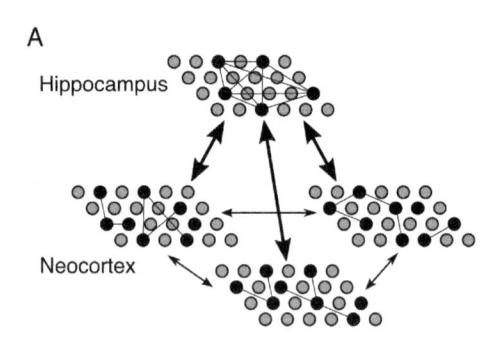

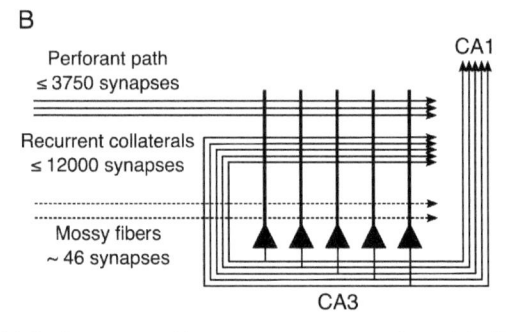

Figure 16.8 The canonical hippocamponeocortical model of long-term memory. (A) Illustration of the model (strong connections and active cells shown in black). Relatively dense recurrent connections and sparse representations in the hippocampus enable efficient pattern completion. Connections between neocortex and hippocampus allow the hippocampal representation of an event to be associated with its sensory details, including reactivation of the representations in different neocortical areas dealing with different sensory modalities. Abstracted semantic representations may also be learned over time in neocortex. The recurrent connections within each neocortical area allow unimodal recognition. (B) Anatomy of the inputs to CA3 pyramidal cells, showing the approximate number of synapses in the rat. (Adapted from Treves and Rolls, 1992.)

the related recent focus on the potential contribution of episodic memory to efficient RL, which is discussed in section 16.5.4.

In Marr's (1971) model, events in the outside world are represented by patterns of activity in neocortical areas. The role of the hippocampus is to store these representations over the short term so that relevant events can be categorized and stored for the long term in neocortex (see Marr's 1970 model of cerebral neocortex). This is achieved by mapping the neocortical representation of an event into a "simple representation" in hippocampus, with modifiable connections to and from the hippocampus storing the mappings between those (full and simple) representations. The CA3 recurrent collaterals are also modified to store the simple representation as an associative memory so that, if it is incompletely activated, the "collateral effect" will result in the full representation being recovered via a process of "pattern completion." Thus, partial activation of the neocortical representation of an event can lead to complete reactivation of its simple representation in the hippocampus, which can in turn reactivate the entire neocortical representation (e.g., Horner et al., 2015).

In Marr's view, the capacity of the hippocampal system should be enough to store a day's events so that the process of categorization and long-term storage in neocortex can take place during the following night's sleep. We note that this now seems at odds with the much larger extent of retrograde amnesia following hippocampal lesions, and the possibility that some types of information (e.g., episodic as opposed to semantic) remain forever dependent on the hippocampus (Nadel and Moscovitch, 1997; Winocur et al., 2010; see section 16.4.5). Marr further suggests that the simple representations need only reflect those parts of the event through which it will be addressed, and that they should be sparsely encoded to reduce possible interference between representations—i.e., undergo a process of "pattern separation." The sparsity of a representation refers to the fraction of neurons that are active: if this is very low, the chance of the same neuron being active in the representation of different events is small and interference between representations is minimized.

16.4.3 Associative memory and the hippocampus

Much of the development and analysis of this canonical model has followed from research on the associative properties of feedforward (e.g., Willshaw et al., 1969) and recurrent networks (Kohonen, 1972; Gardner-Medwin, 1976; Hopfield, 1982) based on Hebbian learning (see Figure 16.9). Initial developments concentrated on matching the major anatomical properties of the hippocampus (see Chapter 3 and Figure 16.8B) with constraints on the representations and learning mechanisms indicated by a functional analysis of associative memory (see Figure 16.10). The first major attempt of this sort (McNaughton and Morris, 1987) highlighted the potential contribution of the dentate gyrus (DG).

Specifically, the much larger number of projection cells in the DG (around one million granule cells in the rat) than in either entorhinal cortex (EC, around 200,000 layer II cells project into the hippocampus) or region CA3 (around 300,000 pyramidal cells) indicate that it could be used for "pattern separation" (Amaral et al., 1990). This means that distinct (i.e., nonoverlapping or orthogonal) patterns of activation will be created in DG despite similarity in patterns of EC activation representing similar events. Thus, pattern completion in CA3 will not lead to a novel event causing retrieval of the representation of similar, familiar events, which would lead to

interference between old and new memories. Of course, one cannot have perfect pattern completion *and* perfect pattern separation of incoming patterns of activity—there is a balance between recognizing new input as a noisy version of a stored pattern versus a new pattern to be stored in its own right. In this respect, the nature of the overlapping and distinct content may be as important as its absolute similarity (see section 16.4.4).

Second, the specific nature of the various synaptic inputs to CA3 pyramidal cells suggest different functions. The input from DG comes from a small number (around 46) of very large synapses proximal to the soma. A much larger number of connections are received further up the dendrites from within CA3 (up to 12,000) and on the distal apical dendrites from EC (up to 3,750). It was suggested that the powerful input from DG (via "detonator synapses") serve to impose a new pattern of activity to be learned in CA3 in the face of interference due to feedback via the recurrent connections, which will tend to cause the system to return to a previously stored pattern of activity (McNaughton and Morris, 1987). Once the representation of a new event has been imposed, Hebbian modification of both the recurrent connections and the connections from EC can occur. The large number of recurrent synapses per cell allow for a large autoassociative memory capacity, while the large number of synapses in the input from EC allow for a large heteroassociative memory capacity in associating the EC representation to the CA3 representation (Treves and Rolls, 1992; see Figure 16.8B).

Third, the requirements of Hebbian learning in the CA3 recurrent collaterals and the inputs from EC to CA3, but not those from DG, are consistent with the physiology of these various connections. The synapses in the former two pathways are thought to be capable of NMDA receptor dependent LTP, while the mossy fiber connections from DG show only non-Hebbian modification (see Chapter 10). Equally, the divisive normalization required by associative networks (Willshaw et al., 1969; see Box 16.3) is consistent with the action of interneurons providing inhibition by opening ion channels near to the soma to shunt input current in the dendrites (see Figure 16.9). Further analysis of autoassociative memory indicates that "progressive recall" improves performance (Gardner-Medwin, 1976). Under this model, inhibition is slowly reduced during retrieval so that the first few cells that become active are the most likely to be correct and feedback from their activation decreases the chances of subsequent erroneous activation. Such periodic fluctuation of inhibition (or equivalently, the firing threshold) may provide a functional interpretation for the theta rhythm (see also section 16.4.4). Finally, the canonical model has been elaborated to include separate input and output representations in the entorhinal cortex (in the superficial and deep layers, respectively). Many of these ideas have been reviewed or developed further in (McClelland et al., 1995; Amit, 1989; Rolls and Treves, 1997; Hasselmo and McClelland, 1999; Redish, 1999; Rolls and Kesner, 2006).

16.4.4 The hippocampal representation and novelty

The considerations of sparsity and pattern separation regarding the hippocampal representation of an event raise the issue of how these representations relate to the various elements of its content and context. First note that the conflicting processes of pattern separation and pattern completion serve to define the similarity space of retrieval, i.e., which dimensions a retrieval cue can vary along but still reinstate the event representation and which dimensions serve to discriminate different events. In the limit of complete

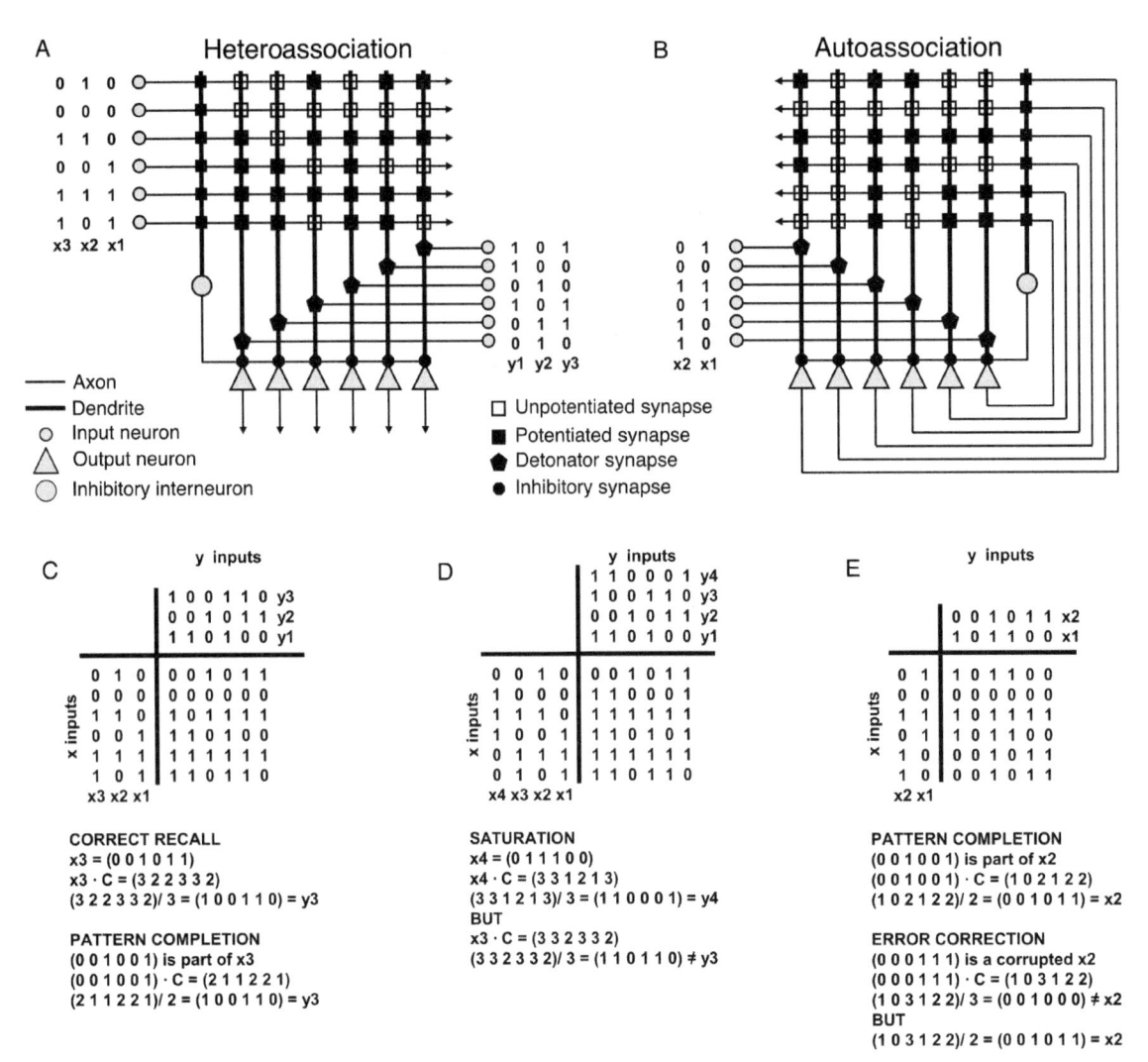

Figure 16.9 The biological implementation of associative memory in the hippocampus. (A) A heteroassociative network associates pattern of output activity Y1 with input X1, and Y2 with X2, etc., to form an associative memory (the matrix of connection weights shown in (A) is the result of successive presentations of input pattern X1 and output pattern Y1, X2 and Y2, X3 and Y3, to an initially blank matrix). This enables input X1 to reproduce activation Y1. Even an incomplete or corrupted version of X1 can reproduce Y1, see (C). Storing too much information leads to "saturation" of the system and retrieval failures, see (D). (B) An autoassociative network associates pattern X1 with itself, and X2 with itself, etc., to form an autoassociative memory. This enables an incomplete or corrupted pattern to be denoised, see (E). The essential functional components of these networks are: a set of powerful "detonator" synapses that can impose the pattern of activity to be stored; a set of extensively connected inputs with modifiable synapses; and a set of inhibitory interneurons whose role is to set a divisive threshold for the activity of the cells. (C–E) Details of associative memory using correlation matrix formalism (Willshaw et al., 1969; Kohonen, 1972). Pairs of binary vectors (e.g., X1, Y1) are presented to the system for storage. A Hebbian learning rule is used: a synaptic connection is strengthened (set to 1 from 0) given pre- and postsynaptic activity (i.e., both set to 1). Since the net input to a cell is the sum of inputs multiplied by the strength of the connections mediating them, the net input to a cell corresponds to the number of active inputs arriving via strengthened connections. To fire, the net input to a cell must equal the number of currently active inputs. Thus retrieval of a vector given its corresponding paired associate is achieved by matrix-vector multiplication (e.g., pattern Y3 in (A) is extracted by multiplying the matrix rows by corresponding elements of vector X3 and summing the columns) followed by integer division by the number of active bits in the input vector. Provided that not too many patterns have been stored, any unique subset of an X vector will recall the correct Y vector. The autoassociative case (B and E) work as the heteroassociative cases (A, C, D) with output Y1 = input X1, Y2 = X2, etc. (Adapted from McNaughton and Morris, 1987.)

orthogonalization in the dentate gyrus, the hippocampal representations are independent of the details of the events and can be thought of as simply an index for them (Teyler and DiScenna, 1986). However, as the hippocampal representation must initially be activated by inputs from neocortex, the overall memory system is still "content addressable" and its behavior (e.g., pattern separation or pattern completion) will depend on how different aspects of an event and its context contribute to the activation of its hippocampal representation. This relates to Marr's observation that

the hippocampal representation should include only those aspects of an event used for its retrieval.

In a simple associative memory, all elements of the representation of an event are equally associated with all other elements. As implied by Marr, however, it seems plausible that some aspects of an event are better able to cue associative retrieval than others, while other aspects of an event can be associatively retrieved more easily than others. Thus the "simple representations" envisaged for the hippocampus would reflect some aspects more than others. A related

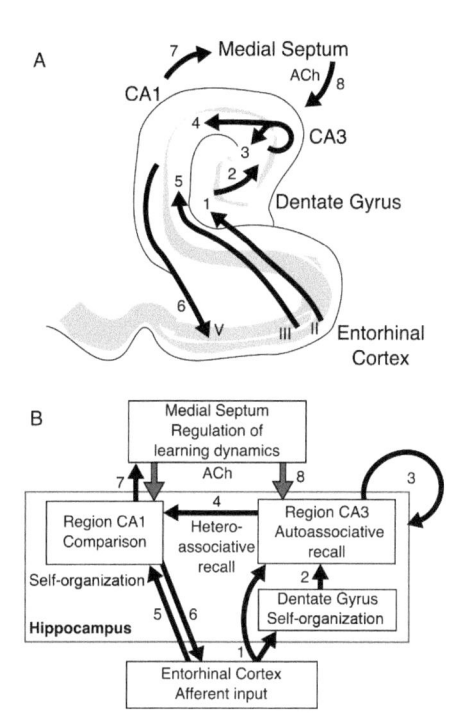

Figure 16.10 Schematic representation of (A) hippocampal anatomy and (B) computational models of hippocampal episodic memory function. Numbers label synaptic connections mediating various functions in the model. (1) Synapses of the perforant path fibers projecting from entorhinal cortex layer II to the dentate gyrus undergo sequential self-organization to form sparse, less overlapping representations of entorhinal activity patterns. Direct connections to CA3 may be used to cue recall. (2) Mossy fibers transfer sparse dentate gyrus activity to CA3. (3) Excitatory recurrent connections in region CA3 mediate autoassociative encoding and retrieval of the features of episodic memories. (4) Schaffer collaterals encode and retrieve associations between CA3 activity and activity patterns induced by entorhinal input to CA1. (5) Perforant path input to region CA1 undergoes self-organization, forming new representations of entorhinal cortex input for comparison with recall from CA3. (6) Projections from region CA1 to deep layers of the entorhinal cortex allow representations in CA1 to activate the associated patterns in entorhinal cortex. (7) Output from region CA1 to the medial septum regulates cholinergic modulation. (8) Cholinergic modulation from the medial septum sets appropriate dynamics for encoding in hippocampus. (Adapted from Hasselmo and McClelland, 1999.)

suggestion is that the hippocampal representation reflects efficient compression of the neocortical representations—extracting the distinguishing features of each event (Gluck and Myers, 1996). For example, the name of somebody you only met once is often a good cue to recalling the meeting but can be hard to retrieve, while the location of the meeting is often both a good cue and relatively easy to retrieve. Similarly, the sequential position of an item in a list is easier to use as a cue than it is to retrieve (Jones, 1976). Thus, even the simplest associative model of memory should include asymmetric associations between the elements of an event.

The nature of the hippocampal representation has also been elucidated by recordings of place cells in rodents and concept cells in humans (Quiroga et al., 2005; Quiroga, 2012). These data suggest that specific patterns of neural activity might consistently encode different elements of an event—a specific population of concept cells when perceiving Jennifer Aniston (a well-known US movie star), and a specific population of place cells when one occupies

a specific location, for example. These "invariant" responses to elements that may appear in multiple events challenge the idea that hippocampal representations of similar events are completely orthogonalized. However, it is also clear that place cells exhibit remapping (i.e., hippocampal representations change) when individual locations become associated with different task contingencies (e.g., Markus et al., 1995; Frank et al., 2000; Wood et al., 2000; Grieves et al., 2016). Whether the same is true for concept cells in the human hippocampus has yet to be established. As such, pattern separation may be driven by necessity—when new events must be dissociated from previous experiences that share overlapping features to support different behavioral outputs, consistent with the notion that the hippocampus encodes task relevant latent variables (see section 16.5.1).

Consideration of the different requirements of encoding and retrieval also raises some interesting questions. Notwithstanding the suggestion that "detonator synapses" from the DG can impose a new pattern of activation on CA3 in spite of the retrieval-related feedback from recurrent connections (McNaughton and Morris, 1987), there must be some mechanism to determine whether the system should be optimized for encoding or retrieval. One proposal is that the supply of acetylcholine (ACh) from the medial septum switches the hippocampus between encoding and retrieval modes (Hasselmo et al., 1995; Wallenstein and Hasselmo, 1997; Murre, 1996). In this model, elevated ACh increases the rate of synaptic modification of the recurrent connections in CA3 and suppresses the synaptic transmission of intrinsic activity (within CA3 and from CA3 to CA1), enabling new patterns of activity to be stored without interference from retrieved memories. Conversely, decreased ACh reduces the rate of synaptic modification and enhances synaptic transmission both within CA3 and from CA3 to CA1, providing favorable conditions for memory retrieval and output to neocortex (Hasselmo, 1999). The delivery of ACh is determined by the novelty of the neocortical input, as represented by direct activation of CA1 from EC, compared with the most similar previously stored event, as represented by the input to CA1 from CA3 after settling to a stored state. Specifically, if both CA3 and EC inputs to CA1 are matching (as with a familiar stimulus), strong activation of CA1 drives interneurons in the medial septum, which decrease the activity of cholinergic cells projecting to the hippocampus (see Figure 16.10). More generally, a medial temporal lobe circuit that can generate a novelty signal by comparing incoming sensory information with previous memories encoded in the recurrent connections of CA3 may be useful to enhance the encoding of salient or unexpected events.

Two types of evidence support this hypothesis. First, by emphasizing the connections between the hippocampus and medial septum, the model begins to address data showing the importance of the fornix, the large fiber bundle connecting the hippocampus with medial septum and other subcortical structures. In the model, sectioning the fornix will prevent the learning of new memories due to lack of ACh, which corresponds well to the effects of damage to the fornix in neuropsychological patients (see, e.g., Gaffan and Gaffan, 1991; Aggleton and Brown, 1999; Spiers et al., 2001). Second, blocking ACh receptors (by injecting scopolamine) impairs encoding—which impairs recollection more strongly than familiarity-based recognition, as the former relies on forming novel associations within the hippocampus (Hasselmo and Wyble, 1997). This will also be the case in the model, assuming that CA3 serves to associate events and their contexts, since recall is more reliant on these associations than recognition. However, disruption of the hippocampus might also impair recall more than recognition in many other models, e.g., due to disrupting associations with context (see section 16.4.6).

In addition, ACh enhances theta band activity, which has been proposed to dynamically schedule periods of encoding and retrieval within each oscillatory cycle by alternately inhibiting intrahippocampal connections and entorhinal inputs to the hippocampus, respectively (Hasselmo et al., 2002). Around the trough of the theta cycle (as measured at the hippocampal fissure), strong input from entorhinal cortex is paired with inhibition of synaptic transmission (but not plasticity) at recurrent collaterals within CA3 to produce favorable conditions for the encoding of new associations. Conversely, around the peak of the theta cycle, entorhinal input is inhibited while synaptic currents within hippocampus are enhanced to produce favorable conditions for the retrieval of existing associations. This model is supported by observations of a shift in the preferred firing phase of place cells toward the trough of the theta cycle during exposure to novel environments, consistent with the encoding of new information, which is disrupted by cholinergic antagonists (Douchamps et al., 2013). The dynamic scheduling of encoding and retrieval by the theta rhythm is also supported by the observation that LTP is preferentially induced at specific phases of the oscillatory cycle (Pavlides et al., 1988; Huerta and Lisman, 1995; Holscher et al., 1997).

16.4.5 Consolidation and cross-modal binding of events in memory

Ever since the initial reports of dense anterograde amnesia but weaker or temporally graded retrograde amnesia after bilateral medial temporal lobectomy (Scoville and Milner, 1957; see Chapter 13), researchers have considered how the hippocampus contributes to the long-term consolidation of memories. One hypothesis is that information is consolidated elsewhere in the brain, after which it can be recalled without the hippocampus. Marr's (1971) model follows this view, suggesting that the day's events are stored in the hippocampus before information deemed relevant to the animal's future is categorized and incorporated into the long-term store of knowledge in neocortex. However, experimental data regarding the gradient of retrograde amnesia (i.e., the sparing of memories acquired sufficiently long enough before the damage) is inconsistent and remains controversial in both animals (see Chapter 14 and Squire et al., 2015) and humans (see Chapter 13 and Spiers et al., 2001). One problem in the human data is that the amnesia often extends back to childhood, implying that the hippocampus stores several decades worth of information. Nonetheless, several arguments have been put forward for the transfer of information from the hippocampus into a consolidated form in neocortex. In particular, this hypothesis has been developed by complementary learning systems theory, which describes the benefits of combining a fast learning (hippocampal) system that can rapidly acquire the details of specific experiences with a slow learning (neocortical) system that can gradually extract structural or semantic knowledge from those experiences to support generalization (Marr, 1971; McClelland et al., 1995; McClelland, 2013; Kumaran et al., 2016).

Complementary learning systems theory is consistent with memory for the unique content and context of a specific event (i.e., episodic memory) depending on the hippocampus, but semantic memory depending on other neocortical areas (see, e.g., Graham and Hodges, 1997). It is also consistent with the suggestion of Nadel and Moscovich (1997) that semantic memories show a temporal gradient of retrograde amnesia while detailed episodic memories do not. The model is less obviously consistent with the suggestion that semantic information can be acquired despite early bilateral hippocampal pathology (Vargha-Khadem et al., 1997). However, the possibility of partial sparing of the hippocampus (Squire and Zola, 1998), or the use of external rehearsal of information (Baddeley et al., 2001), might provide explanations for these developmental cases within the framework of the model. The process of memory consolidation also has many parallels with the training of deep neural networks—e.g., those that use a fixed feedforward structure and error-driven learning rules to optimally extract the statistics of their inputs following the repeated and interleaved presentation of large numbers of training examples (Rumelhart et al., 1986; LeCun et al., 2015; Kumaran et al., 2016). We note that some consolidation processes might also occur within the hippocampus without transfer of information from one region to another—using protein synthesis to stabilize changes in the strength of individual synapses, for example (M Sutton and Schuman, 2006; Redondo and Morris, 2011).

Evidence for the replay of hippocampal activity patterns in the rodent hippocampus during quiescent waking periods and sleep led to the hypothesis that these events might mediate long-term memory consolidation (Wilson and McNaughton, 1994; Skaggs and McNaughton, 1996; Carr et al., 2011; Olafsdottir et al., 2018). Consistent with this view, hippocampal replay events are coordinated with increased neocortical activity (Siapas and Wilson, 1998; Sirota et al., 2003; Battaglia et al., 2004; Ji and Wilson, 2007); and disrupting replay events during rest or sleep impairs the acquisition of spatial memory tasks (Girardeau et al., 2009; Nakashiba et al., 2009; Ego-Stengel and Wilson, 2010). In addition, hippocampal replay appears to favor rewarded experiences (Ambrose et al., 2016), which aligns well with Marr's hypothesis that salient or statistically unusual events should be preferentially consolidated in order to direct future behavior. Indeed, one theoretical account suggests that the replay of different experiences is prioritized in order to optimize future reward (Mattar and Daw, 2018). Importantly, a number of studies have demonstrated that neural activity patterns observed during learning are also reactivated during rest in the human brain, and that reactivation is correlated with subsequent memory performance (e.g., Staresina et al., 2013; Deuker et al., 2013; Schapiro et al., 2018; Schreiner and Staudigl, 2020).

Early models of memory consolidation focused on the anatomical convergence of information from different sensory modalities onto the hippocampus. In the absence of dense long-range connections between different sensory cortical areas, associations between the elements of an event such as its sight, sound, and smell cannot be formed in the lower-level cortices. Thus, Damasio (1989) suggested that "convergence zones" must exist where these "cross-modal bindings" could be formed. Several models have extended this idea to include rapid learning of a hippocampal, or medial temporal lobe, representation reciprocally connected to all the unimodal cortical representations of the event that allows them to be associated to each other (Alvarez and Squire, 1994; Murre, 1996; Moll and Miikkulainen, 1997). These models also suggest that, after multiple rehearsals of a memory driven by the hippocampus, long-range associations can be learned directly between the unimodal representations, finally making the stored information independent of the hippocampus.

An interpretation of the experimental data regarding the gradient of retrograde amnesia associated with medial temporal lobe damage led Nadel and Moscovitch (1997) to a different conclusion regarding consolidation (see also Winocur et al., 2010). Noticing that, in many instances, retrograde amnesia extends back over a much longer time than that envisaged by Marr, they proposed that the hippocampus remains necessary for the retrieval of detailed episodic or spatial information. To account for both the common occurrence of a temporal gradient in memory for other types of information and the possibility of partial damage to the hippocampus, they proposed a new model. According to this "multiple trace theory," whenever a memory is rehearsed or reactivated, a new hippocampal representation is formed, again connected to all of the neocortical representations. The result of this is that, while a complete lesion of the medial temporal lobe impairs retrieval of all memories, the older the memory, the more robust it will be to partial damage by virtue of being represented in multiple locations within hippocampus (but see Teng and Squire, 1999; Rosenbaum et al., 2000, for evidence that early spatial memories become hippocampus independent).

Both the arguments regarding data abstraction and anatomical convergence were represented in a model by Kali and Dayan (2004). In this model, the hippocampus serves to aid the learning of a hierarchical semantic system, by being able to reinstate (i.e., replay) the top-level (i.e., entorhinal/perirhinal/parahippocampal) representation of events during sleep. The semantic system contains reciprocal connections between these top-level cortical areas and those below them in the hierarchy, but no direct connections between areas at the same level. Aided by the hippocampus, the neocortical system forms an associative representation of activity patterns in lower cortical areas. This is achieved by the top-level representations learning a "generative model" of representations lower in the hierarchy (e.g., Hinton and Sejnowski, 1999; see section 16.4.8). Thus these top-level representations (see also "latent state representations" in section 16.5.1) can be cued by input from a subset of lower cortical areas and then cause pattern completion in all lower areas via the reciprocal connections. In further simulations, Kali and Dayan (2004) note that regular reactivation of episodic hippocampal representations is required to maintain them in register with the slowly changing semantic representations. As such, the occasional replay or rehearsal of episodic information from the past may be required to maintain functional connections between the hippocampus and neocortex following the initial stages of memory consolidation.

Another argument for consolidation refers to the effects of interference. In deep neural networks, new information can interfere with previously stored information, sometimes "catastrophically," such that all information is lost (McCloskey and Cohen, 1989). This problem can also occur in associative memories (see Figure 16.9). McClelland et al. (1995) proposed a solution to this in which long-term consolidation involves random interleaved presentation of all previous knowledge along with newly acquired knowledge, to produce a single integrated neocortical representation of semantic knowledge. Note, however, that this mechanism requires the temporary store to have capacity for the entire dataset, although more recent studies have demonstrated that "generative replay" (in which replay sequences are constructed from a generative model, rather than replaying specific events; see section 16.4.8) can avoid this issue (Shin et al., 2017; van de Ven et al., 2020; Stoianov et al.,

2022). However, "modern" Hopfield networks (also known as dense associative memories, e.g., Krotov and Hopfield, 2016; Demircigil et al., 2017), which are not subject to the same capacity constraints as the canonical model, exhibit reduced interference between stored patterns and more rapid convergence. Biologically realistic implementations of these networks include a new memory unit for each pattern (Krotov and Hopfield, 2020), which might correspond to the observation of episode-specific neurons in the human hippocampus (Kolibius et al., 2023). This idea might also relate to neurogenesis in the rodent dentate gyrus and its potential role in learning (Deng et al., 2010), although the extent of neurogenesis in the adult human hippocampus remains controversial (e.g., Franjic et al., 2022).

Relatedly, experimental data indicate that new memories are consolidated more quickly if they are consistent with previously existing knowledge or "schema" (Tse et al., 2007; Squire et al., 2015). It is relatively straightforward to incorporate this feature into the canonical model, given that slow learning is only required when new information is inconsistent with existing knowledge and may therefore lead to catastrophic interference (McClelland, 2013). However, evidence also indicates that the hippocampus can support rapid generalization or "statistical learning" in some cases (e.g., Zeithamova et al., 2012; Schapiro et al., 2014), a role ascribed to neocortex in the canonical model. This is implicitly at odds with a process of pattern separation, by which overlapping sensory inputs are orthogonalized, reducing the representational overlap between related events and impairing generalization. This issue can be addressed by "big loop recurrence" at the point of memory retrieval (i.e., recursive interactions between the hippocampus and neocortex; Kumaran and McClelland, 2012), rather than within the hippocampus itself. Specifically, if hippocampal output is iteratively fed back as input to prompt further retrieval, and several retrieved memory patterns can be coactive within the hippocampus at any one time, then it is possible to perform rapid generalization and inference across the content of those related experiences. Alternatively, the CA1 region of the hippocampus can be cast in the role of neocortex, producing overlapping activity patterns for related events from the pattern separated output of CA3, and therefore supporting generalization and inference despite individual memory traces being stored in an orthogonal manner (Schapiro et al., 2017). This issue can also be addressed at the point of memory encoding, if one assumes that the constituent elements of related experiences are represented invariantly in the hippocampus (e.g., Quiroga et al., 2005; see section 16.4.4). This preserves the overlap between the representation of related events, supporting generalization and inference between those events, but places specific constraints on the process of pattern separation.

The need for interaction between the two "complementary learning systems" can be seen when trying to generalize from previous experience in novel circumstances. Here, memories of "unpredictable" events (i.e., those inconsistent with the statistical regularities extracted from wider experience) should be retained in the hippocampus, while memories of "predictable" events can be consolidated in neocortex (W Sun et al., 2023). This addresses an issue known as "overfitting" in machine learning, whereby extensive training to capture the statistics of even the most unpredictable exemplars impairs generalization. The (re)constructive nature of episodic memory and the possibility that the neocortical system is a deep generative network emphasizes how the two systems must interact. According to such a model (Spens and Burgess, 2024), in which events are represented as simple scenes, the generative network (a variational autoencoder; Kingma and Welling, 2014; see also sections 16.4.8 and 16.5.1) develops latent state representations of the contents of each scene. Briefly, this is achieved by training the network to reproduce input activity patterns in its output layer, after passing activity through a much smaller intermediate layer. Latent state representations in the intermediate layer (potentially, analogous to concept cells; Quiroga et al., 2005) can subsequently be used to generate new scenes in the output layer that are consistent with the statistics of all previously learned scenes. However, the hippocampus must also store any unique features of new scenes for addition to the generic scenes generated by the latent state representations. This framework extends the traditional model of systems consolidation to include imagery, novelty responses and gist-based distortions in human memory.

16.4.6 Hippocampal contributions to familiarity-based recognition

A distinction has been made between episodic memory, semantic memory, and familiarity-based recognition (see Chapter 13). Episodic memory is characterized by the ability to recall detailed information about an event and its context. Semantic memory is characterized by factual knowledge without recall of the individual events and contexts in which it was acquired. Familiarity-based recognition depends on an unattributable feeling of familiarity associated with a stimulus in the absence of detailed information about the event and context in which it was encountered. Of these three processes, the hippocampus has been most strongly associated with episodic memory (e.g., Aggleton and Brown, 1999). As described above, however, it has also been argued that the hippocampus is required to provide associations between representations in disparate cortical areas, while associations within each area can be formed locally. Thus, the familiarity of single stimuli might be supported by the association of elements within each neocortical area, independent of the hippocampus, while recognition of cross-modal associates among equally familiar distractors would require the hippocampus.

Consistent with this view, empirical evidence indicates that simple recognition memory does not depend on the hippocampus, but on nearby neocortical areas (Zhu et al., 1996; Murray and Mishkin, 1998; Wan et al., 1999; Aggleton and Brown, 1999; Baxendale et al., 1997; Baddeley et al., 2001; but see also Manns and Squire, 1999; Zola et al., 2000). In contrast, there is some evidence that recognition of cross-modal associations is impaired by bilateral damage restricted to the hippocampus (Holdstock et al., 2000; Vargha-Khadem et al., 1997), although more extensive unilateral damage may also impair the binding of elements within the same modality (Kroll et al., 1996). The logical extension of this idea is that episodic memory requires the full recollection of an event and its context in all its multimodal detail and so will require an intact hippocampus.

Much of the analysis of the differential role of the hippocampus in episodic retrieval (or "recollection") and familiarity-based recognition has focused on the idea that these two processes both contribute independently to the performance of recognition memory tests (see e.g., Yonelinas, 2002). In both forced choice and yes-no recognition paradigms, the recollective component is assumed to be "all or nothing" and "high-threshold." That is, the stimulus is recalled in great detail or not at all, and a novel foil is never falsely recalled. By contrast, the familiarity-based process is more like a signal-detection problem: the subject guesses whether the item is familiar or not informed by a noisy measure of familiarity. The hippocampus has been associated with the recollective component (Aggleton and Brown, 1999; Yonelinas et al., 2002) and so should provide a high-threshold, all-or-nothing mechanism in recognition memory tests (see Rugg and Yonelinas, 2003, for a review).

The hippocampal contribution to recognition memory (via "recollection") can be modeled by using the stimulus-driven medial temporal neocortical representation to retrieve a stored pattern of activation in CA3, and comparing the retrieved activation to the stimulus-driven activation in the EC (Norman and O'Reilly, 2003). By explicitly retrieving an entire stored pattern, the process is all-or-nothing, and even foils that resemble previously presented patterns are not falsely recognized. The use of sparse hippocampal representations, orthogonalized via the DG, serves to prevent interference between different stored events. By contrast, familiarity-based recognition is modeled as a "sharpening" of the neocortical representation. Under this model, while a new item is represented by weak activation of a large number of neocortical neurons, repeated presentation of the item results in strong activation of a smaller number of neocortical neurons via a competitive learning mechanism. The activation of neocortical neurons that fire in response to a given stimulus can then be used as a measure of familiarity-based recognition. A similar model holds that the hippocampus (or adjacent cortical regions) can also signal stimulus or event familiarity by probing the energy function of previously stored memories (Bogacz et al., 2001; Greve et al., 2010). If incoming sensory input is consistent with previously stored activity patterns, then network output will be boosted by strong recurrent connections between active neurons; while novel sensory input will produce lower network activity due to the absence of those connections. As such, simply monitoring overall network output during the initial presentation of a stimulus provides a measure of familiarity.

One advantage of this scheme is that repeated presentations of some items in a list will not impair recognition of the other items in the list, as seen experimentally (Ratcliff, 1990). A characteristic of this model is that hippocampal damage will specifically impair recognition memory when related lures (novel items that resemble previously seen items) are included in the test. The familiarity-based recognition mechanism would produce false alarms to these stimuli, while the hippocampal recollection mechanism would not, consistent with some empirical evidence (Holdstock et al., 2002).

16.4.7 Free recall and temporal context

One of the distinguishing features of episodic memory is the ability to retrieve the ongoing context within which an event occurs (Gardiner and Java, 1993; Tulving, 1993; Knowlton and Squire, 1995), and one suggestion for the role of the human hippocampus is that it provides the spatiotemporal context for episodic memory (O'Keefe and Nadel, 1978). Theoretical analyses of associative memory have also made the distinction between the content of an event and its context (e.g., Raaijmakers and Shiffrin, 1981) or between the record of an event and the "header" or index term used to reference it (e.g., Morton et al., 1985). One possibility is that the hippocampus serves to associate the content of an event with its context. A related possibility is that the hippocampus provides a representation of temporal context itself, e.g., dynamically varying patterns of activity generated by its own recurrent connectivity that serve to bind coactive neocortical representations (Buzsaki and Tingley, 2018). This type of model coincides with a considerable psychological literature describing models of memory in which the retrieval of stored items is held to depend, at least in part, on their association to a representation of context that changes slowly with time or experience. In some of these models the context representation changes independently of the stored items (Estes, 1955; Mensink and Raaijmakers, 1988; Davelaar et al., 2005), while in others the context representation is derived from the items themselves (Howard and Kahana, 2001; Howard et al., 2015). A given item will subsequently be retrieved according to the similarity between the context signal at retrieval and that associated with the item. In particular, these models are often used to address free recall paradigms, in which the cue for retrieval is not external (as is typically the case for the canonical model) but internally generated.

One of the first mechanistic models of this type was described by Levy (1996), who demonstrated that a recurrent network model of CA3 with Hebbian plasticity that is repeatedly exposed to sequential activity patterns (i.e., temporally correlated inputs) develops "context neurons." These do not form part of the sequential activity pattern but fire persistently during specific subsections of that pattern, providing a slowly varying context signal that supports sequence retrieval and allows sequences with overlapping sections to be disambiguated (see Figure 16.11). Wallenstein et al. (1998) described a similar model that uses context neurons to form associations between temporally discontiguous events (further apart in time than the timescale required for pre- and postsynaptic activity to induce LTP, i.e., more than around one hundred milliseconds, see Chapter 10) and can therefore account for the role of the hippocampus in trace conditioning. Indeed, this type of mechanism also provides a good model for short-term serial recall (Burgess and Hitch, 2005).

The temporal context model (Howard and Kahana, 2001) extended this framework to account for several additional features of experimental data from free recall paradigms. In this model, the context representation is derived from the presented or retrieved items themselves, becoming a recency-weighted sum of the context arising from each item. After a sequence of items has been presented, the context vector will be most similar to that associated with recent items, producing the well-known recency effect; and the context vector for consecutive items in the sequence will be more similar, producing the well-known temporal contiguity effect, both observed during free recall. Finally, because each item that is presented affects the context vector to which subsequent items are associated, the retrieval of immediately subsequent items in the list is more likely. This leads to an asymmetry such that forward associations within the list are stronger than backward associations, creating the characteristic forward-bias of free recall (e.g., Kahana, 1996).

Each of these models is supported by the observation of slow changes in hippocampal activity over time (e.g., Manns et al., 2007; Mankin et al., 2012; Ziv et al., 2013; Cai et al., 2016), and by evidence that representations of spatiotemporal context within the hippocampus are reinstated during retrieval (Manning et al., 2011; Howard et al., 2012; Miller et al., 2013). Intriguingly, it has been demonstrated that a generalized form of the temporal context model is equivalent to a temporal difference algorithm for learning the successor representation, hinting that spatial and episodic

context may share a common mechanism (Gershman et al., 2012; see section 16.3.2). Similarly, we note that the temporal context model has been extended to account for spatially tuned responses in the hippocampus (Howard et al., 2005; Howard et al., 2014).

In a related model of free recall, Romani et al. (2013) focused on accounting for a different feature of the experimental data—the relationship between the number of items studied and retrieved (e.g., Murray et al., 1976). They demonstrated that, following the encoding of an arbitrary number of discrete, sparse activity patterns in the asymmetric synaptic connections of a recurrent neural network, a combination of periodic inhibition and firing rate adaptation could be used to produce the sequential reinstatement of those activity patterns. Importantly, transitions tended to occur between activity patterns with the greatest representational overlap and be limited to a subset of activity patterns that followed a power law relationship with the total number of encoded items, as observed in experimental data. Transitions between activity patterns also tended to be cyclical, moving sequentially between the same subset of patterns, and recall was terminated when the system completed one loop. This is consistent with the observation that subjects tend not to recall any further words after they have erroneously recalled a studied item for the second time (Miller et al., 2012). However, this model cannot account for primacy, recency, or temporal contiguity effects.

16.4.8 The hippocampus as a generative model

It has long been known that episodic memory retrieval is reconstructive rather than veridical (e.g., Bartlett, 1932; Shacter and Addis, 2007) and that the hippocampus is implicated in the imagination of new experiences (e.g., "episodic future thinking" or "scene construction"; Atance and O'Neill, 2001; Hassabis et al., 2007; see Chapter 13). As noted earlier, hippocampal spatial representations can also be predictive (e.g., Skaggs et al., 1996; Mehta, et al., 1997; Stachenfeld et al., 2017) and—in some circumstances—represent behavioral trajectories that have never been experienced (e.g., Gupta et al., 2010; Dragoi and Tonegawa, 2011; Ólafsdóttir et al., 2015). These observations have led to the hypothesis that the hippocampus may function as a generative model (Kali and Dayan, 2004; Finnegan et al., 2017; Whittington et al., 2020; Spens and Burgess, 2024), making use of existing memories to simulate the sensory and reward contingencies of new experiences. As mentioned above, a generative memory system may offer several advantages for efficiently extracting the descriptive statistics of experience by optimizing the "training" of neocortex during long-term consolidation (Shin et al., 2017; van de Ven et al., 2020; Stoianov et al., 2022).

A detailed, neural level model of how the hippocampus might use episodic memories to generate complex visuospatial imagery was described by Becker and Burgess (2001) and subsequently developed by Byrne et al. (2007) and Bicanski and Burgess (2018; see Figure 16.12). This model explicitly makes use of the constraints associated with spatial information and our detailed knowledge of how it is represented in the brain. Specifically, the representations of spatial layout in long-term memory are assumed to be allocentric (e.g., independent of the orientation of the person) in contrast to the egocentric (i.e., body-centered) short-term representations involved in perception, action, and working memory (Goodale and Milner, 1992; Milner et al., 1999; Burgess et al., 1999). Transformation between these two reference frames is achieved by a

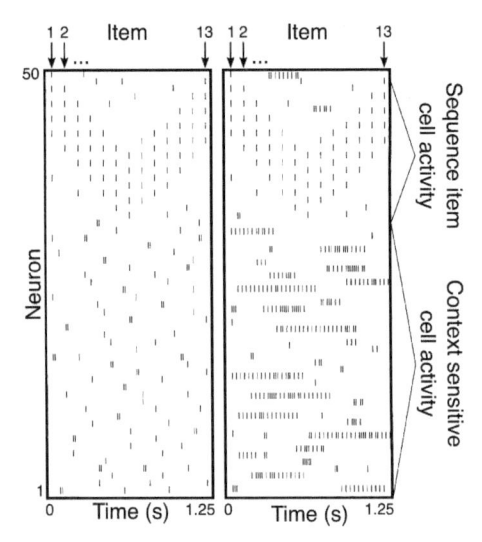

Figure 16.11 Context field development. Each rectangle shows a subset of 50 simulated pyramidal cells firing across time, each action potential represented by a vertical line. A unique group of five cells firing at the same time encodes a single item in a 13-item sequence, see the top portion of each rectangle ('sequence item cell activity'). This can be thought of as afferent activation of CA3 pyramidal cells due to a specific pattern of sensory events. (A) Notice the background firing during the first learning trial that does not encode sequence items directly. This stems from activity at recurrent excitatory synapses. Repeated exposure to the same sequence can lead to enhanced synaptic potentiation between cells firing in the background and cells that encode sequence items, due to a simple Hebbian learning rule. (B) After the fourth learning trial, this repeated potentiation leads to a condition where background cells begin to respond to the appearance of contiguous segments of the entire sequence. The portion of the full sequence to which the cell responds is called the "context field" of the cell. Because the context fields overlap, the entire sequence can be reconstructed by interdigitating them in the proper order. (Adapted from Wallenstein et al., 1998.)

head-direction-modulated gain-field circuit, hypothesized to reside in retrosplenial cortex, and analogous to the role proposed for gain-field neurons found in posterior parietal cortex (e.g., Pouget and Sejnowski, 1997). Again, it is worth noting the incredible correspondence between this model and synaptic connectivity in the fly brain (Lu et al., 2022; see Figure 16.12B).

During memory encoding, egocentric representations of the distance and direction to spatial boundaries and discrete objects from the current viewpoint are transformed, via the gain-field circuit, into allocentric boundary- and object-vector cell (BVC and OVC) representations in the medial temporal lobe. By extension from spatial models of the hippocampus (Hartley et al., 2000), BVCs are bidirectionally connected to place cells, which form a continuous attractor. When attending to a specific object, OVCs also become bidirectionally connected to the place cells encoding that location, head-direction cells encoding the current orientation, and perirhinal neurons encoding object identity. During subsequent memory retrieval—cued by activity in perirhinal neurons encoding object identity, for example, attractor dynamics reinstate activity in OVCs, place cells, and head-direction cells as well as BVCs. This allocentric representation of spatial context is transformed into egocentric spatial imagery via the gain-field circuit, with a viewing location and orientation dictated by reinstated place- and head-direction-cell activity to be consistent with that during encoding.

Importantly, in later versions of the model, mock motor efference from grid-cell inputs is also used to support dynamic imagery, planning, and the mental exploration of previously unexplored routes (Bicanski and Burgess, 2018). As such, this model provides a neural level framework for interpreting the role of hippocampus in reconstructive episodic memory retrieval, episodic future thinking, and scene construction.

This model is consistent with the observation of hemispatial neglect in imagery following parietal damage (e.g., Bisiach and Luzzatti, 1978) and functional imaging of the retrieval of spatial context (Burgess et al., 2001). It also provides an explanation for the involvement of Papez's circuit (see Chapter 3) in supporting both episodic memory (see Chapter 13) and the representation of head direction (see Chapter 11). In addition, several of the allocentric and egocentric spatial responses predicted by this model have subsequently been identified in the rodent brain (Deshmukh and Knierim, 2013; Wang et al, 2018; Hinman et al., 2019; Høydal et al, 2019; Alexander et al., 2020; see Bicanski and Burgess, 2020, for a review).

Finally, we note that the place cells in this model correspond to a latent variable representation of location to which different sensory inputs are mapped (during bottom-up encoding) and can be generated from (during top-down imagery). In addition, grid-cell inputs allow imagery to be dynamic and generated from new viewpoints, consistent with their proposed role in planning routes through real or conceptual spaces (Bush et al., 2015; Stemmler et al., 2015; Behrens et al., 2018). Intriguingly, a similar transformation circuit and set of allocentric spatial responses are learned by an agent tasked solely with predicting upcoming egocentric visual inputs (Uria et al., 2020). More often, however, generative models go beyond these networks (which predict a single set of inputs) by attempting to learn or approximate the probability distribution from which their inputs (or predicted outputs) are drawn (e.g., variational autoencoders; Kingma and Welling, 2014). Indeed, theta oscillations (George et al., 2024), systems consolidation (Spens and Burgess, 2024), or dreaming (Hoel, 2021) might correspond to the training of generative models that capture these distributions rather than specific examples.

16.5 Hippocampal function beyond space and memory

In recent years, theoretical models of the hippocampus have been reinvigorated by empirical findings that demonstrate coding for task-relevant nonspatial dimensions (e.g., Constantinescu et al., 2016; Aronov et al., 2017; Bao et al., 2019; Knudsen and Wallis, 2021; Nieh et al., 2021). This has led to a broader conceptualization of hippocampal function that encompasses and incorporates both spatial cognition and associative memory. As described below, these models propose that the hippocampus encodes low-dimensional cognitive maps (Tolman, 1948), which capture relational structure (Eichenbaum and Cohen, 2014) between task-relevant states and can be used to plan behavior, e.g., via model-based RL (Stachenfeld et al., 2017). This process is facilitated by the formation of efficient representations—both in terms of identifying and encoding the relevant dimensions and by capturing the underlying structure of experienced transitions or relationships between states to

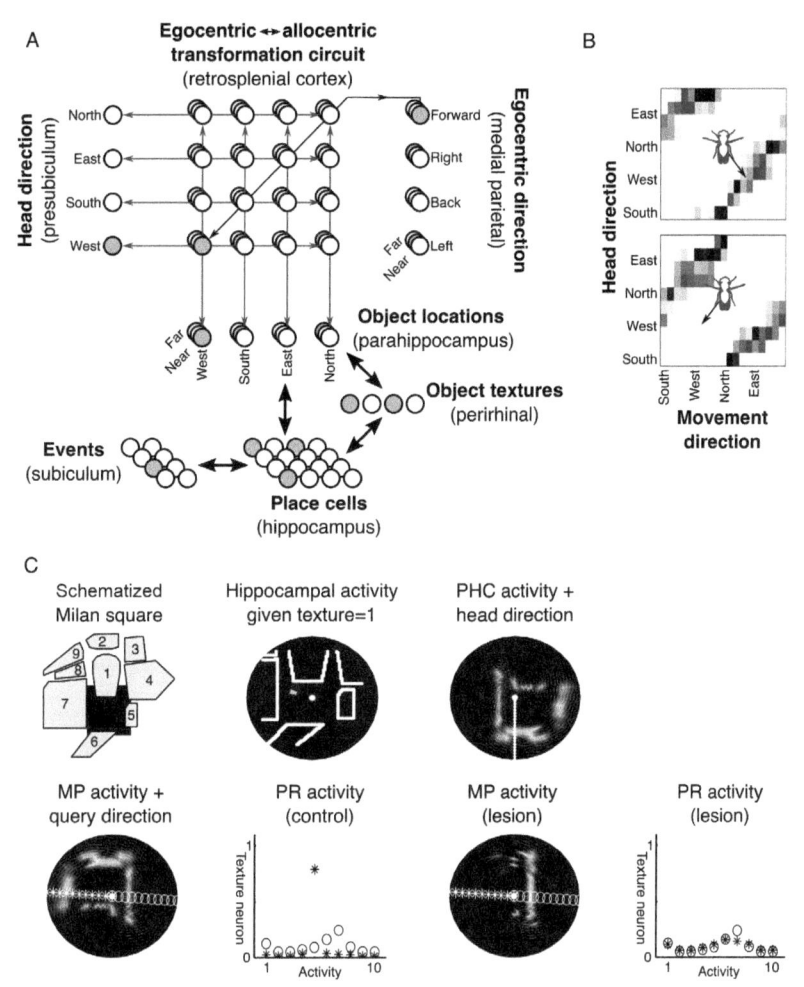

Figure 16.12 A model of episodic memory and visuospatial imagery. (A) Functional architecture of encoding and retrieving the spatial context of an event. Neurons shown in gray illustrate a possible pattern of activity, corresponding to an imagined location with extended landmarks nearby to the west, far away to the north and at an intermediate distance to the south. The imagined westerly heading direction means that these landmarks are imagined as far to the right, nearby straight ahead, and at an intermediate distance to the left. The transformation between egocentric (left, right, ahead) and allocentric (north, south, east, west) directions to landmarks occurs via a circuit linking these representations and head direction. (B) Empirical data from *Drosophila*, illustrating the strength of synaptic connections between neurons encoding head direction and allocentric movement direction, and projecting to regions that drive movement in specific egocentric directions (backward and right, top panel; backward and left, bottom panel). Note the correspondence with the diagonal synaptic weight matrix in the transformation circuit predicted by the model (shown in panel A). (Adapted from Lu et al., 2022.) (C) Simulation of the retrieval of spatial information in the Milan square experiment of Bisiach and Luzzatti (1978). (i) Training consists of simulated exploration of the square (shaded area, north is up). The system is cued to imagine being near to the Cathedral (i.e., the perirhinal cell for the texture of building 1 and parahippocampal cell for a building at a short distance north are activated) and the recurrently connected hippocampal-parahippocampal-perirhinal system settles. (ii) The hippocampus settles to a location in the northwest corner of the square (hippocampal cell activity shown as the brightness of the pixel corresponding to the location of each cell's place field). (iii) The parahippocampus correctly retrieves the locations of the other buildings (parahippocampal cell activity shown as the brightness of the pixel for the location encoded by each cell, relative to the subject at the center). A line indicates that the imagined heading direction is south. (iv) Medial parietal cell activity: the parahippocampal map has been correctly rotated given head-direction south (straight ahead is up), stars indicate a direction of inspection to the left, circles to the right. (v) Perirhinal cell activations correctly showing building 5 to the left and building 7 to the right. (vi) Effect of a right parietal lesion on the medial parietal representation (note lack of activation on the left) and perirhinal activations. (vii) Note decrease in activation of building 5 when inspection is to the left. (Adapted from Becker and Burgess, 2001.)

facilitate prediction, generalization and planning (Behrens et al., 2018; Whittington et al., 2022).

16.5.1 Low-dimensional latent state representations

Numerous recent experimental studies have demonstrated that the hippocampal formation can also code for location and movement direction along abstract, continuous dimensions beyond those that represent physical space. For example, Aronov et al. (2017) demonstrated that hippocampal pyramidal cells form receptive fields in auditory space (i.e., firing in response to specific tones) when

rodents were trained to manipulate sound frequencies using a joystick in order to obtain reward. Similarly, Nieh et al. (2021) showed that the same neurons jointly encoded location and the accumulation of visual evidence when reward was contingent on turning in the direction of the greatest number of visual cues distributed along the walls of a virtual T-maze. This has led to the theory that the hippocampus attempts to form efficient representations of the structure or "state space" (i.e., a cognitive map) of any given task to support ongoing behavior. Importantly, this requires identifying the "latent variables" (those that are not directly mapped to sensory inputs, such as location and head direction in the case of spatial navigation) that most efficiently and accurately describe the relevant task dimensions (Gershman and Niv, 2010; Niv, 2019; Radulescu et al., 2021). This formulation provides a unifying explanation for several features of both place-cell firing and single unit responses to nonspatial variables. We note, however, that in the rodent hippocampus at least, spatial variables appear to occupy a privileged position, in that they are reliably encoded even in the absence of reward (while responses to nonspatial variables tend to rely on the delivery of reward, potentially indicating task relevance). Indeed, it has been suggested that nonspatial variables are consistently encoded in conjunction with location (O'Keefe and Krupic, 2021; see Chapter 11). Whether this is because rodents consistently expect spatial structure to be task-relevant or reflects the evolutionary trajectory of the hippocampus (from coding for space to any task relevant variable) is not yet clear.

In either case, the idea that hippocampal cells code for task-relevant latent variables rather than purely location helps to explain several features of spatial firing patterns. For example, "splitter cells" fire in a specific location on the neck of a T-maze depending on whether the animal is about to turn right or left on a spatial alternation task (Frank et al., 2000; Wood et al., 2000; Grieves et al., 2016), thereby disambiguating identical sensory inputs depending on behavioral context. Similar responses have been observed when mice are rewarded on every fourth lap of a circular track, with hippocampal place cells conjunctively coding both location on the track and lap number (C Sun et al., 2020). Crucially, this conjunctive code was replaced by a purely spatial code when reward was provided on every lap of the track. Another example is provided by hippocampal remapping (Bostock et al., 1991; see Chapter 11), which can be triggered by changes in the task being executed within a specific environment (e.g., Markus et al., 1995), thereby forming a new representation to support a different behavior (Sanders et al., 2020; Geerts et al., 2024); or using the statistics of prior experience to produce an optimal estimate of the current context (Plitt and Giocomo, 2021). Each of these examples is consistent with the hippocampus identifying higher-level task structure that disambiguates perceptually identical visits to the same location according to prospective (or retrospective) behavior. Conversely, orientation-independent firing of place cells in an open field could be understood as resulting from a complementary process by which the hippocampus associates perceptually distinct inputs (i.e., the view in each head direction) with a task state that affords the same contingencies (i.e., a single spatial location). In the nonspatial domain, we note that the receptive fields of time cells—which fire at specific time points during delay periods in which spatial location is approximately constant (Eichenbaum, 2014; Umbach et al., 2020)—can also be understood as encoding latent states. Time is an implicitly latent variable, given that it cannot be directly observed, and these representations encode progress through a delay period prior to the receipt of reward (or in trace conditioning tasks, see section 16.4.7).

To efficiently encode task structure, hippocampal representations of latent variables should be low dimensional, with activity patterns varying according to changes in task-relevant variables but remaining insensitive to those which are not predictive of reward. Continuous attractor models of head-direction, place, and grid cells (which encode latent spatial variables) highlight how the firing patterns of very large numbers of neurons can be constrained to exist on a low dimensional manifold (i.e., surface) via specific patterns of recurrent connectivity (see section 16.2.3, Box 16.3). In those examples, the manifold corresponds directly to the physical variables of heading direction (a 1D ring) or the (2D) location of the moving animal on the surface of the ground. More generally, when the state-space of a behavioral task or function can be described in terms of a small number of latent variables, it would be efficient for the firing patterns of neurons supporting that function to form population codes for the values of those latent variables. Such codes, in which populations of neurons with localized tuning curves densely cover the range of values taken by a given latent variable, can encode probability distributions over values of that variable (Zemel et al., 1998) and facilitate appropriate generalization by being constrained to firing patterns with a correspondence to performance of the task.

How might task-relevant latent variables be identified? As described above, the hippocampal role in episodic memory can be framed as finding and storing compressed representations of sensory experience that can later be used to construct the full sensory representation (see section 16.4.4). In machine learning, the same problem is addressed by "autoencoders"—feedforward neural networks that are trained to reconstruct input patterns in the output layer via a much smaller intermediate layer of neurons (Hinton, 1989). Gluck and Myers (1993) extended this framework by describing the hippocampus as a "predictive autoencoder": a network that can reproduce the input pattern as well as classifying the "outcome" with which it is associated. This constrains the network to find internal representations that differentiate input patterns which predict different outcomes, serving to dissociate identical perceptual states that are associated with different actions and thus identify task relevant latent variables (see also Benna and Fusi, 2021).

More recent models have demonstrated similar functionality by incorporating representations of behavioral context. Specifically, latent variables can be identified by accounting for the prospective or retrospective behavior or neural activity associated with a specific perceptual input. For example, Recatanesi et al. (2021) demonstrated that training a recurrent neural network to predict upcoming sensory inputs produces representations of the low dimensional latent variables defining a range of different tasks, including place-cell-like responses during spatial tasks. Similarly, George et al. (2021) demonstrated that disambiguating sensory representations according to the recent history of activity successfully disambiguated latent states associated with the same perceptual inputs, accounting for the splitter cell and lap cell responses described above. It is also possible that extracting the most slowly varying features of sensory input may identify underlying statistical regularities which encode useful latent variables. As described earlier, this "slow feature analysis" has been used to account for the emergence of place, grid, and head-direction coding (i.e., account for the identification of latent spatial variables) from visual input (Franzius et al., 2007; see section 16.2.2.1).

16.5.2 Predicting future state occupancy

In the same way that spatial representations in the rodent hippocampus (see section 16.2) are believed to support navigation (see section 16.3), the purpose of the latent variable representations described above is to support efficient planning across a range of task domains by predicting the outcome of different actions. Ideally, the mechanisms that support planning should also generalize easily between domains to make the learning of novel tasks more efficient by leveraging previous experience. As discussed earlier, planning behavior in arbitrary state spaces has been formalized by RL (e.g., R Sutton and Barto, 1988), in which the "value" of states is estimated in terms of the expected future reward to be gained discounted by how far into the future it will be reached. In particular, it has been proposed that hippocampal pyramidal cells might encode a successor representation (SR; i.e., the expected discounted future occupancy of other states from each starting state) to facilitate straightforward planning in arbitrary spatial and nonspatial state spaces (Stachenfeld et al., 2017; see section 16.3.2). Importantly, the SR is more flexible than model-free RL because it can still be used to compute value if the distribution of rewards changes. However, the SR is biased by the transitions experienced during learning and therefore policy-dependent and sensitive to the distribution of previous rewards. If the agent's policy or the transition structure of the task changes, the SR will no longer reflect future state occupancy. One solution is to learn the SR under a default policy (e.g., random exploration) and use that "default representation" (DR) for planning under new goal-directed policies, taking account of deviations from the default policy, if those are not too great (Todorov, 2007; Piray and Daw, 2021). We also note the potential role for "predecessor" (Namboodiri and Stuber, 2021) and "first occupancy" (Moskovitz et al., 2021) representations in planning as alternatives to the SR.

However, if the hippocampus encodes the probability distribution of *future* state occupancy under a given policy, how does this relate to the idea that the hippocampus encodes the probability distribution of *current* state occupancy in these arbitrary spaces? Representations of current and predicted future state occupancy are related by the transition matrix of a given task and policy. Specifically, the predicted occupancy of states at the next time step can be estimated by taking the current state-occupancy distribution and multiplying it by the transition matrix (see Figure 16.13). Similarly, the SR (or DR) can be estimated by repeatedly multiplying the current state-occupancy distribution by the transition matrix and a temporal discount factor. We note that the transition matrix itself could reflect movements between locations in spatial navigation, or the relations between latent states in any cognitive map (Tolman, 1948; Eichenbaum and Cohen, 2014; Behrens et al., 2018). The models in this section assume that the transition matrix is implicitly encoded within the hippocampal representation of current state occupancy. Specifically, as noted in section 16.3.3, the covariance of state occupancy representations (e.g., place-cell firing patterns) effectively encodes the transition matrix between those states—cells encoding adjacent states are more likely to be coactive, and those with distal states less likely to be coactive. As discussed earlier (see section 16.2.2.2), there is also an apparent similarity between grid-cell firing patterns and the eigenvectors of the covariance matrix between place-cell firing patterns (Castro and Aguiar, 2014; Dordek et al., 2016).

Under this formulation, then, the hippocampus provides a probabilistic representation of state occupancy that closely resembles (and may be equivalent to) the SR (or DR), the covariance of this representation encodes the transition matrix between states during exploration, and grid cells represent the eigenvectors of that transition matrix. Appealingly, these eigenvectors have several features that could facilitate planning. Specifically, a weighted sum of their firing rates can represent the current state occupancy distribution (analogous to grid- to place-cell models; see section 16.2.2.1). In addition, multiplying the representation of state occupancy by the

transition matrix to compute future state occupancy simply corresponds to changing the weights from each grid cell by the eigenvalue corresponding to the eigenvector represented by its firing pattern (see Figure 16.13). Thus, a simple weighted sum of the firing of grid cells could estimate future state occupancy and compute the SR (or DR) for use in planning (Corneil and Gerstner, 2015; Stachenfeld et al., 2017; Baram et al., 2018). Importantly, this reweighting process does not necessarily involve changes in synaptic weights but could be implemented by simply modulating grid-cell firing rates. Indeed, several empirical studies have provided evidence of a role for grid firing patterns in planning movements through abstract state spaces. For example, Constantinescu et al. (2016) studied this kind of "conceptual navigation" using a task in which participants predicted the types of bird that would be reached by a trajectory through a 2D space of varying neck and leg length. They found patterns of metabolic activity with sixfold (or "hexadirectional") modulation in the entorhinal and medial prefrontal cortices that may be consistent with the presence of grid firing patterns, which are also observed during navigation through virtual spatial environments (Doeller et al., 2010).

A single transition structure—such as that resulting from random exploration—can be used for planning, as described above, but cannot predict the effects of multiple different actions, as in models of path integration in which grid-cell firing predicts the effects of successive directed actions on state occupancy. Indeed model-based RL, or dynamic programming, generally depends on exploring the effects of sequences of specific actions. One solution is to create multiple "first occupancy" representations corresponding to different policies, and search through the effects of sequentially combining them (Moskovitz et al., 2021). An alternative solution, using a single set of eigenvectors, is available for translation-invariant transition structures, in which a transition or action has the same effect irrespective of the current state, allowing perfectly factorized state and transition representations (see section 16.5.3). Fourier basis functions (i.e., plane waves of differing frequency and orientation) are eigenvectors for any translation-invariant transition matrices. Thus, a single Fourier set could act as eigenvectors for multiple translation invariant transition matrices corresponding to different actions, with different eigenvalues for each action; and sums of eigenvectors weighted by the appropriate eigenvalues could represent future state occupancy under different combinations of actions. This provides a potentially unifying framework for grid-cell models: both in facilitating prediction and planning, and as the effects of the complex eigenvalues on the phases of the Fourier components corresponds to oscillatory interference models of grid-cell firing, while the dynamics of the evolution of state occupancy is equivalent to continuous attractor models of path integration (Yu et al., 2020).

16.5.3 Factorizing states and transition structure for prediction

The rapid generalization of existing knowledge to new situations is a crucial skill. One way to approach this problem is to factorize tasks into the structure of transitions between states and the contents of each state. In this way, common structure can be learned across several tasks in parallel to the contents of each state which can vary from task to task (Behrens et al., 2018). According to the formulation described in the previous section, grid cells in MEC might represent abstract transition structure while environmental sensory inputs are conveyed via lateral entorhinal cortex (LEC),

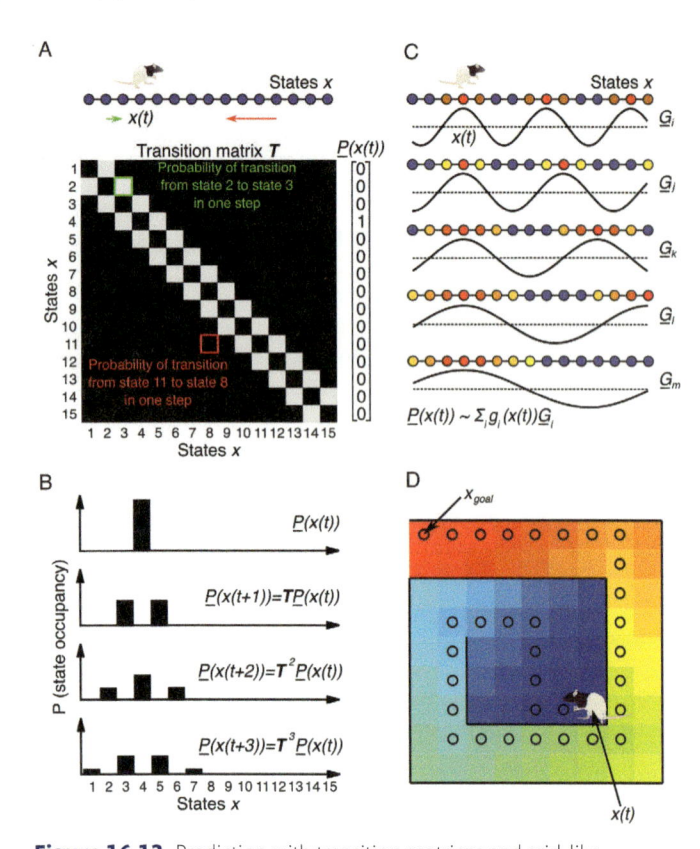

Figure 16.13 Prediction with transition matrices and grid-like eigenvectors. (A) Many (Markovian) tasks can be conceived as a set of discrete states (for example locations x) where the probability of transitions between states is captured by a transition matrix T. This is illustrated by the transition matrix T for a mouse with a policy of moving one step left or right along a linear track in each time step with equal probability. (B) Premultiplying the current state occupancy distribution $P(x(t))$ by T predicts state occupancy at the next time step $P(x(t+1))$, or at any subsequent time step. (C) Grid firing patterns could be eigenvectors of a diffusive transition matrix reflecting random movements (i.e., $TG_i = \lambda_i G_i$). In this case, using a grid-cell population vector (i.e., summing grid-cell firing profiles weighted by their firing rates $G_i(x(t))$ to represent current state occupancy (i.e., $P(x(t)) \sim \sum_i G_i(x(t))G_i$), means that premultiplying the current state occupancy $P(x(t))$ by the transition matrix simply reweights each grid cell's firing rate within the population vector by its eigenvalue (λ_i), so that: $P(x(t+1)) \sim \sum_i G_i(x(t))\lambda_i G_i$. This type of weighted sum could be performed by a single layer readout network. (D) The temporally discounted future state occupancy over multiple steps (i.e., the "successor representation") $P_\gamma(x(\tau \geq t))$ sums the effects of premultiplying by the transition matrix multiple times, each time weighted by the discount factor (γ), producing a power series whose value is again a simple reweighting of each grid cell's firing within the population vector. This example shows how the discounted future probability of a goal location x_{goal} is simply a weighted sum of the products of grid-cell firing rates at the current and goal locations: $P_\gamma(x(\tau \geq t) = x_{goal}) \sim \sum_i G_i(x(t))G_i(x_{goal})/(1-\gamma\lambda_i)$. It increases as the current location moves toward the goal and could therefore be used to guide navigation if T captures the transition structure of the environment under random exploration. (Adapted from Baram et al., 2018.)

and place cells represent the conjunction between transition-related and environment-related information (Manns and Eichenbaum, 2006; Knierim et al., 2006). This is consistent with results obtained in virtual environments wherein these two sources of (movement and sensory) input can be dissociated, showing that place-cell firing is more influenced by environmental visual inputs while grid-cell firing is more influenced by physical self-motion (Chen

et al., 2019), and generalizes those results to nonspatial tasks. The proposed factorization of transition structure and content applies most completely to situations in which the transition structure is translation-invariant and can therefore be learned and applied across both states and tasks.

The preeminent example of such a transition structure is Euclidean space, whose rules apply across all spatial environments (e.g., moving one step north, then east, then south, then west always brings you back to the same location). The place-, head-direction-, and grid-cell system may therefore have evolved to perform a factorization of structure and content under pressure to perform spatial navigation in familiar and new environments. This machinery provides a preconfigured representation of structure that can be used to organize external experience (McNaughton et al., 1996; Buzsaki and Tingley, 2018). For example, using the high-capacity code for spatial location provided by grid cells to "scaffold" factorized memory content could avoid issues of catastrophic forgetting and support efficient sequence learning alongside spatial navigation (Chandra et al., 2023). This mechanism could also confer rapid generalization across any tasks with a common relational structure, by attaching contents (or concepts) to locations whose transitions (or relationship) to all other locations are predefined, i.e., by constructing a cognitive map (see Tolman, 1948; O'Keefe and Nadel, 1978; Eichenbaum and Cohen, 2014). The formation of an efficient representation of these relationships over different sets of content allows rapid generalization of the prediction of future states to new situations with similar relational structure (as discussed in section 16.5.2), and the ability to form efficient structural representations corresponds to the representations of the states themselves lying on a low dimensional manifold (as discussed in section 16.5.1). These insights apply to continuous inputs and state spaces, but they should also apply more generally to any set of discrete states with graph-like transition structures. However, we note that learning to map a transition-driven structural representation onto a sensory-driven representation of state-content, when both representations may contain noise or uncertainty, can be difficult. This is a well-known problem in robotics (a.k.a. simultaneous localization and mapping) and may require nonlocal propagation of mismatch errors, which has been proposed as a potential role for hippocampal replay (Evans and Burgess, 2019).

The "Tolman-Eichenbaum Machine" ("TEM," Whittington et al., 2020) aimed to test the idea that optimizing neural network parameters for prediction of future state information could explain neural responses in the hippocampal formation (see also Uria et al., 2020) and demonstrate the value of factorizing transition structure and state content. This model comprised three components: an MEC network with action-dependent recurrent connectivity that encodes and updates an estimate of abstract location (in a manner similar to continuous attractor network models, see section 16.2.3); an LEC network that encodes sensory inputs; and a recurrently connected hippocampal network that encodes task specific representations of location as conjunctions of the inputs arriving from the MEC and LEC via Hebbian learning (as in models of associative memory, see section 16.4). The model was trained, in discrete graph-like state spaces, to predict sensory inputs at the next state given previous sensory inputs and actions (i.e., state transitions) via an error-correcting learning rule. Importantly, training was performed across multiple tasks with the same transition structure but different contents and applied to both spatial and nonspatial domains (see Figure 16.14). After random exploration of these state spaces, the TEM learns representations in the hippocampal network that resemble place-cell responses and representations in the MEC network that include grid-like firing patterns. Interestingly, if the agent systematically approaches objects, the firing patterns of some units in the MEC network also resemble object-vector cells (Høydal et al., 2019), while some units in the hippocampal network resemble landmark-vector cells (Deshmukh and Knierim, 2013; see Figure 16.14).

More generally, the ability to predict future state occupancy is important for efficient RL and has motivated models that go beyond the discounted average over all future time steps captured by the SR (or DR). Deep networks that learn from large numbers of training examples to map sensory inputs to actions that maximize return (e.g., Mnih et al., 2015) benefit from an ability to read and write to an external memory system when relevant information is only partially observable (Graves et al., 2016). In RL settings, however, such memory systems do not work well without a predictive internal model which ensures that the format of stored representations allows the prediction of future observations. For example, Wayne et al. (2018) combined an autoencoder with a recurrent network that can learn over long timescales (Hochreiter and Schmidhuber, 1997) in order to predict future sensory inputs from current observations. This necessitated the generation of latent variable representations that could be stored in memory and accessed by a separate policy network that learns to produce optimal actions. Importantly, the autoencoder network was trained to predict both the sensory inputs (requiring it to develop a model of sensory dynamics) and the estimated value of each state (i.e., discounted future reward). This strategy, similar to Gluck and Myers (1993), encourages the emergence of representations that emphasize features that are salient for future reward. This network could subsequently perform latent learning and flexible navigation within virtual environments. More generally, this work highlights the utility of developing mnemonic representations to predict future observations and rewards through unsupervised learning, complementing representations driven by direct reinforcement. Indeed, many of the models described in sections 16.5.1–3 stress the hippocampal contribution to this role. Importantly, it has recently been demonstrated that the same functionality can be achieved without the biologically implausible aspects of training deep networks (error backpropagation requiring a detailed record of nonlocal neural activity to guide synaptic change), by employing local learning rules across basal and apical dendrites that are modulated by the theta rhythm (George et al., 2024) following the predictive coding framework (Dayan et al., 1995; Rao and Ballard, 1999).

16.5.4 What is the role of episodic memory?

Although the models described above can account for hippocampal representations of both spatial and nonspatial state spaces to support planning, prediction, and generalization across tasks with similar structure, it is less clear how they relate to memory for individual events. Marr (1971) and related models of memory conceive the role of hippocampus in terms of storing and retrieving single episodes (using orthogonal representations to avoid interference), so that statistical structure across episodes could be extracted into semantic memory in neocortex (using invariant representations to support generalization). This dichotomy (between representing individual events and common structure) raises similar questions

as the debate concerning pattern separation, reflecting the theoretical advantages of orthogonal representations for disambiguating similar events versus the apparently invariant representations of event elements observed in place and concept cell recordings (see section 16.4.4). Hence, it is still unclear how to reconcile the two proposed roles of the hippocampal formation: in generating cognitive maps for planning and in storing the contents of individual episodes. It is possible that the region mediates both roles, as suggested by TEM, by extracting low-dimensional latent variable representations (such as those for space and time) across multiple events in entorhinal cortex, while making use of associative memory in the hippocampus proper (i.e., CA3) to store specific experiences as conjunctions of those variables with the sensory contents of each event. The hippocampus could subsequently aid the learning of latent variable representations by replaying specific events until their statistics are fully captured (see section 16.4.5). This would result in a separation of "predictable" episodes, which are consistent with prior experience and can be rapidly consolidated (e.g., Tse et al., 2007; Tse et al., 2011); and "unpredictable" episodes, which would degrade the generalization of entorhinal cognitive maps and should therefore be retained in the hippocampus proper (e.g., W Sun et al., 2023; Spens and Burgess, 2024).

Importantly, a similar process (i.e., the slow extraction of even longer-range statistical regularities) could operate from entorhinal cortex to more distant cortical structures (such as ventromedial prefrontal cortex) to explain "systems consolidation," by which knowledge becomes fully independent of the hippocampal formation. However, it is possible that use of the latent variables associated with space and time to fully reconstruct images of past events, or to imagine new experiences, remains dependent on the hippocampus, unlike more abstract semantic knowledge (Nadel and Moscovitch, 1997; see section 16.4.5). We note the similarity with theoretical models that examine the role of episodic memory in supporting planning within an RL framework. In particular, Lengyel and Dayan (2007) described how "episodic control" supports more efficient behavior than either model-free or model-based RL when the transition and reward structure of a task have been poorly sampled. Specifically, if an agent has discovered any sequence of actions that lead to reward and is under pressure to limit exploration of an environment, then repeating that sequence of actions is more advantageous than trying to construct and exploit a complex model or an incomplete value function (see also Zilli and Hasselmo, 2008; Gershman and Daw, 2017; Pritzel et al., 2017; Botvinick et al., 2019).

16.6 Conclusions

As in other areas of neuroscience, the ability to specify a proposed mechanism of hippocampal function as a computational model has been invaluable in many ways. First, it allows potential mechanisms to be described precisely, reducing the ambiguity and potential "hypothesis drift" that might afflict verbal descriptions. Second, it enables simulation of the resulting behavior that, at the very least, can serve as a demonstration of the viability of a given proposal. Beyond this it enables quantitative, falsifiable predictions regarding the effects of experimental manipulations to be made at the levels of cells, systems, and behavior. Some of the models reviewed here have been used to make such predictions and have also contributed to the design of experiments to test them. Nonetheless, the value of

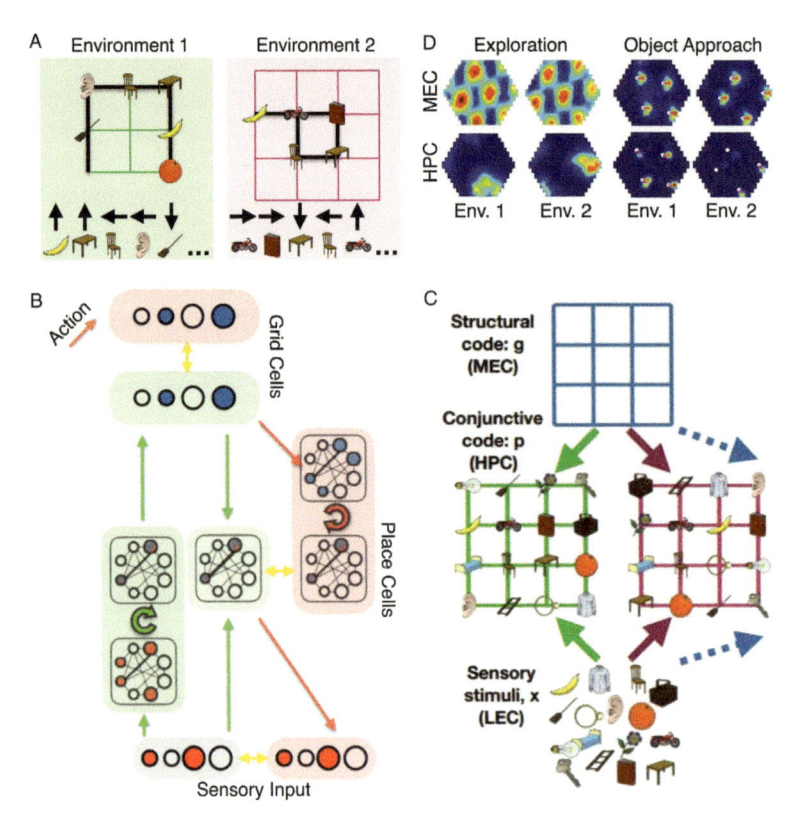

Figure 16.14 The Tolman-Eichenbaum machine. (A) The agent learns to predict the next item (e.g., banana, table, chair, etc.) as a function of the previous item and the transition/action taken (e.g., north, south, east, west) across several environments. The possible actions and underlying structure (i.e., the graph) remain constant, but the allocation of items to states (i.e., graph vertices) varies across environments. An object-location task is shown, but nonspatial structures, e.g., family trees, can also be learned. (B) The network architecture can be seen as a variational autoencoder in which "encoding" connections (shown in green) propagate a representation of recent sensory input up through a recurrent place-cell layer ("HPC") to a recurrent grid-cell layer ("MEC"), and "decoding" connections (shown in red) predict the next grid, place, and sensory representation. Recurrent connections between grid cells are action-dependent (allowing prediction, given the action taken in the previous time step, top left corner), and recurrent connections between place cells form a Hopfield-like memory for the item-state associations in the current environment. Yellow arrows show differences between "predicted" and "encoded" representations whose minimization drives learning. (C) The network develops representations that capture the transition structure in the MEC layer, and representations of states in the HPC layer determined by the conjunction of transitions and sensory information. (D) During random exploration, MEC neurons develop grid-like responses and HPC neurons develop place-like responses, but if systematically approaching objects, these become more like object vector cell and landmark vector cell responses, respectively. (Adapted from Whittington et al., 2020.)

a computational model lies in the insights it provides, just like other forms of scientific endeavor.

Numerous questions for future research are prompted by these models, not least how to resolve the apparent differences between the proposed hippocampal roles in cognitive mapping and episodic memory. Computational models have been invaluable in attempting to unify these two largely disparate streams of research. Specifically, by suggesting that the hippocampus encodes an index of features that identify the current event among perceptually similar events in episodic memory, consistent with representing the current "location" in a low-dimensional task-relevant latent state space during cognitive mapping. In addition, cognitive mapping models propose a role for entorhinal cortex in embedding these latent state representations within the structure of transitions or relationships between them. Beyond the efficient storage and retrieval of experience via latent states (i.e., a memory system), this supports planning: the ability to infer the effects of applying transition or relational operators to the latent state representations (equivalent to path integration in the spatial domain). In situations in which the transition or relational structure is conserved across states or tasks (spatial navigation being the preeminent example), the factorization of states and transitions allows rapid generalization. This framework is consistent with the original idea of the hippocampus providing a cognitive map or efficient representation of states or concepts and the relationships between them for planning and inference. Nonetheless, many questions remain—such as how this framework relates to the consolidation of mnemonic information. Future modeling will undoubtedly refine our understanding of the specific mechanisms at work, by informing empirical studies and being modified by their results.

Acknowledgments

The authors thank Andrej Bicanski, Jesse Geerts, Zilong Ji, Eleanor Spens, and Oliver Vikbladh for useful discussions and feedback during the preparation of this chapter.

REFERENCES

Aggleton JP, Brown MW (1999) Episodic memory, amnesia, and the hippocampal-anterior thalamic axis. *Behav Brain Sci* 22:425–490.

Agmon H, Burak Y (2020) A theory of joint attractor dynamics in the hippocampus and the entorhinal cortex accounts for artificial remapping and grid cell field-to-field variability. *eLife* 9:e56894.

Alexander AS, Carstensen LC, Hinman JR, Raudies F, Chapman GW, Hasselmo ME (2020) Egocentric boundary vector tuning of the retrosplenial cortex. *Sci Adv* 6(8):eaaz2322.

Alme CB, Miao C, Jezek K, Treves A, Moser EI, Moser M-B (2014) Place cells in the hippocampus: eleven maps for eleven rooms. *PNAS* 111(52):18428–18435.

Almog N, Tocker G, Bonnevie T, Moser EI, Moser MB, Derdikman D (2019) During hippocampal inactivation, grid cells maintain synchrony, even when the grid pattern is lost. *eLife* 8:e47147.

Alvarez P, Squire LR (1994) Memory consolidation and the medial temporal lobe: a simple network model. *PNAS* 91:7041–7045.

Alvernhe A, Save E, Poucet B (2011) Local remapping of place cell firing in the Tolman detour task. *Eur J Neurosci* 33(9):1696–705.

Alyan S, McNaughton BL (1999) Hippocampectomized rats are capable of homing by path integration. *Behav Neurosci* 113:19–31.

Amaral DG, Ishizuka N, Claiborne B (1990) Neurons, numbers and the hippocampal network. *Prog Brain Res* 83:1–11.

Ambrose RE, Pfeiffer BE, Foster DJ (2016) Reverse replay of hippocampal place cells is uniquely modulated by changing reward. *Neuron* 91(5):1124–1136.

Amit DH (1989) Modelling Brain Function. Cambridge, UK: Cambridge University Press.

Amit DJ (1992) Modeling Brain Function: The World of Attractor Neural Networks. Cambridge, UK: Cambridge University Press.

Anderson JA (1995) An Introduction to Neural Networks. Cambridge, MA, USA: MIT Press.

Arleo A, Gerstner W (2000) Spatial cognition and neuro-mimetic navigation: a model of hippocampal place cell activity. *Biol Cybern* 83(3):287–299.

Aronov D, Nevers R, Tank DW (2017) Mapping of a non-spatial dimension by the hippocampal-entorhinal circuit. *Nature* 543(7647):719–722.

Atance CM, O'Neill DK (2001) Episodic future thinking. *Trends Cogn Sci* 5(12):533–539.

Baddeley AD, Vargha-Khadem F, Mishkin M (2001) Preserved recognition in a case of developmental amnesia: implications for the acquisition of semantic memory? *J Cogn Neurosci* 13:357–369.

Banino A, Barry C, Uria B, Blundell C, Lillicrap T, Mirowski P, et al. (2018) Vector-based navigation using grid-like representations in artificial agents. *Nature* 557(7705):429–433.

Bao X, Gjorgieva E, Shanahan LK, Howard JD, Kahnt T, Gottfried JA (2019) Grid-like neural representations support olfactory navigation of a two dimensional odor space. *Neuron* 102:1066–1075.

Baram AB, Muller TH, Whittington JCR, Behrens TEJ (2018) Intuitive planning: global navigation through cognitive maps based on grid-like codes. *bioRxiv* 2018:421461.

Barry C, Burgess N (2007) Learning in a geometric model of place cell firing. *Hippocampus* 17:786–800.

Barry C, Ginsberg LL, O'Keefe J, Burgess N (2012) Grid cell firing patterns signal environmental novelty by expansion. *PNAS* 109:17687–17692.

Barry C, Hayman R, Burgess N, Jeffery KJ (2007) Experience-dependent rescaling of entorhinal grids. *Nat Neurosci* 10:682–684.

Bartlett FC (1932) Remembering: A Study in Experimental and Social Psychology. Cambridge, UK: Cambridge University Press.

Bassett JP, Wills TJ, Cacucci F (2018) Self-organized attractor dynamics in the developing head direction circuit. *Curr Biol* 28:609–615.

Battaglia FP, Sutherland GR, McNaughton BL (2004) Hippocampal sharp wave bursts coincide with neocortical "up-state" transitions. *Learn Mem* 11:697–704.

Baxendale SA, Van Paesschen W, Thompson PJ, Duncan JS, Shorvon SD, Connelly A (1997) The relation between quantitative MRI measures of hippocampal structure and the intracarotid amobarbital test. *Epilepsia* 38:998–1007.

Baxter MG, Murray EA (2001) Opposite relationship of hippocampal and rhinal cortex damage to delayed nonmatching-to-sample deficits in monkeys. *Hippocampus* 11:61–71.

Becker S, Burgess N (2001) A model of spatial recall, mental imagery and neglect. *Adv Neural Inf Process Syst* 13:96–102.

Behrens TEJ, Muller TH, Whittington JCR, Mark S, Baram AB, Stachenfeld KL, Kurth-Nelson Z (2018) What is a cognitive map? organizing knowledge for flexible behavior. *Neuron* 100(2):490–509.

Bellmund JLS, de Cothi W, Ruiter TA, Nau M, Barry C, Doeller CF (2020) Deforming the metric of cognitive maps distorts memory. *Nat Hum Behav* 4:177–188.

Benna MK, Fusi S (2021) Place cells may simply be memory cells: memory compression leads to spatial tuning and history dependence. *PNAS* 118(51):e2018422118.

Bi G-Q, Poo M-M (1998) Synaptic modifications in cultured hippocampal neurons: dependence on spike timing, synaptic strength, and postsynaptic cell type. *J Neurosci* 18(24):10464–10472.

Bicanski A, Burgess N (2016) Environmental anchoring of head direction in a computational model of retrosplenial cortex. *J Neurosci* 36(46):11601–11618.

Bicanski A, Burgess N (2018) A neural-level model of spatial memory and imagery. *eLife* 7:e33752.

Bicanski A, Burgess N (2019) A computational model of recognition memory via grid cells. *Curr Biol* 29:1–12.

Bicanski A, Burgess N (2020) Neuronal vector coding in spatial cognition. *Nat Rev Neurosci* 21:453–470.

Bienenstock EL, Cooper LN, Munro PW (1982) Theory for the development of neuron selectivity: orientation specificity and binocular interaction in visual cortex. *J Neurosci* 2:32–48.

Bisiach E, Luzzatti C (1978) Unilateral neglect of representational space. *Cortex* 14:129–133.

Blair HT, Cho J, Sharp PE (1998) Role of the lateral mammillary nucleus in the rat head direction circuit: a combined single unit recording and lesion study. *Neuron* 21:1387–1397.

Blair HT, Gupta K, Zhang K (2008) Conversion of a phase- to a rate-coded position signal by a three stage model of theta cells, place cells, and grid cells. *Hippocampus* 18:1239–1255.

Blair HT, Lipscomb BW, Sharp PE (1997) Anticipatory time intervals of head-direction cells in the anterior thalamus of the rat: implications for path integration in the head-direction circuit. *J Neurophysiol* 78:145–159.

Blair HT, Sharp PE (1995) Anticipatory head direction signals in anterior thalamus: evidence for a thalamocortical circuit that integrates angular head motion to compute head direction. *J Neurosci* 15:6260–6270.

Blair HT, Wu A, Cong J (2014) Oscillatory neurocomputing with ring attractors: a network architecture for mapping locations in space onto patterns of neural synchrony. *Philos Trans R Soc B* 369(1635):20120526.

Blum KI, Abbott LF (1996) A model of spatial map formation in the hippocampus of the rat. *Neural Comput* 8:85–93.

Boccara CN, Nardin M, Stella F, O'Neill J, Csicsvari J (2019) The entorhinal cognitive map is attracted to goals. *Science* 363(6434):1443–1447.

Boccara CN, Sargolini F, Thoresen VH, Solstad T, Witter MP, Moser EI, Moser MB (2010) Grid cells in pre- and parasubiculum. *Nat Neurosci* 13:987–994.

Bogacz R, Brown MW, Giraud-Carrier C (2001). Model of familiarity discrimination in the perirhinal cortex. *J Comput Neurosci* **10**:5–23.

Bonnevie T, Dunn B, Fyhn M, Hafting T, Derdikmann D, Kubie JL, Roudi Y, Moser EI, Moser M-B (2013) Grid cells require excitatory drive from the hippocampus. *Nat Neurosci* **16**:309–317.

Bostock E, Muller RU, Kubie JL (1991) Experience-dependent modifications of hippocampal place cell firing. *Hippocampus* **1**:193–205.

Botvinick M, Ritter S, Wang JX, Kurth-Nelson Z, Blundell C, Hassabis D (2019) Reinforcement learning, fast and slow. *Trends Cogn Sci* **23**(5):408–422.

Brandon MP, Bogaard AR, Libby CP, Connerney MA, Gupta K, Hasselmo ME (2011) Reduction of theta rhythm dissociates grid cell spatial periodicity from directional tuning. *Science* **332**:595–599.

Brandon MP, Koenig J, Leutgeb JK, Leutgeb S (2014) New and distinct hippocampal place codes are generated in a new environment during septal inactivation. *Neuron* **82**(4):789–96.

Brown MA, Sharp PE (1995) Simulation of spatial learning in the Morris water maze by a neural network model of the hippocampal formation and nucleus accumbens. *Hippocampus* **5**:171–188.

Brunel N, Trullier O (1998) Plasticity of directional place fields in a model of rodent CA3. *Hippocampus* **8**:651–665.

Buetfering C, Allen K, Monyer H (2014) Parvalbumin interneurons provide grid cell-driven recurrent inhibition in the medial entorhinal cortex. *Nat Neurosci* **17**(5):710–8.

Burak Y, Fiete IR (2009) Accurate path integration in continuous attractor network models of grid cells. *PLoS Comput Biol* **5**:e1000291.

Burgess CP, Burgess N (2014) Controlling phase noise in oscillatory interference models of grid cell firing. *J Neurosci* **34**:6224–6232.

Burgess N (2008) Grid cells and theta as oscillatory interference: theory and predictions. *Hippocampus* **18**:1157–1174.

Burgess N, Barry C, O'Keefe J (2007) An oscillatory interference model of grid cell firing. *Hippocampus* **17**:801–812.

Burgess N, Hartley T (2002) Orientational and geometric determinants of place and head-direction. *Adv Neural Inf Process Syst* **14**:165–172.

Burgess N, Hitch GJ (2005) Computational models of working memory: putting long term memory into context. *Trends Cogn Sci* **9**:535–541.

Burgess N, Jeffery KJ, O'Keefe J (1999) Integrating hippocampal and parietal functions: a spatial point of view. In: The Hippocampal and Parietal Foundations of Spatial Cognition (Burgess N, Jeffery KJ, O'Keefe J, eds), pp 3–29. Oxford, UK: Oxford University Press.

Burgess N, Maguire E, O'Keefe J (2002) The human hippocampus and spatial and episodic memory. *Neuron* **35**:625–641.

Burgess N, Maguire EA, Spiers HJ, O'Keefe J (2001) A temporoparietal and prefrontal network for retrieving the spatial context of lifelike events. *Neuroimage* **14**:439–453.

Burgess N, O'Keefe J (1996) Neuronal computations underlying the firing of place cells and their role in navigation. *Hippocampus* **6**:749–762.

Burgess N, O'Keefe J (2011) Models of place and grid cell firing and theta rhythmicity. *Curr Opin Neurobiol* **21**:734–744.

Burgess N, Recce M, O'Keefe J (1994) A model of hippocampal function. *Neural Netw* **7**:1065–1081.

Bush D, Barry C, Burgess N (2014) What do grid cells contribute to place cell firing? *Trends Neurosci* **37**:136–145.

Bush D, Barry C, Manson D, Burgess N (2015) Using grid cells for navigation. *Neuron* **87**:507–520.

Bush D, Burgess N (2014) A hybrid oscillatory interference/continuous attractor network model of grid cell firing. *J Neurosci* **34**(14):5065–5079.

Bush D, Burgess N (2020) Advantages and detection of phase coding in the absence of rhythmicity. *Hippocampus* **30**:745–762.

Bush D, Philippides A, Husbands P, O'Shea M (2010) Dual coding with STDP in an auto-associative network model of the hippocampus. *PLoS Comput Biol* **6**(7):e1000839.

Butler WN, Hardcastle K, Giocomo LM (2019) Remembered reward locations restructure entorhinal spatial maps. *Science* **363**:1447–1452.

Butler WN, Smith KS, van der Meer MA, Taube JS (2017) The head-direction signal plays a functional role as a neural compass during navigation. *Curr Biol* **27**:1259–1267.

Buzsáki G, Tingley D (2018) Space and time: the hippocampus as a sequence generator. *Trends Cogn Sci* **22**(10):853–869.

Byrne P, Becker S, Burgess N (2007) Remembering the past and imagining the future: a neural model of spatial memory and imagery. *Psychol Rev* **114**:340–375.

Cacucci F, Lever C, Wills TJ, Burgess N, O'Keefe J (2004) Theta-modulated place-by-direction cells in the hippocampal formation in the rat. *J Neurosci* **24**:8265–8277.

Cai DJ, Aharoni D, Shuman T, Shobe J, Biane J, Song W, et al. (2016) A shared neural ensemble links distinct contextual memories encoded close in time. *Nature* **534**(7605):115–118.

Carr MF, Jadhav SP, Frank LM (2011) Hippocampal replay in the awake state: a potential substrate for memory consolidation and retrieval. *Nat Neurosci* **14**:147–153.

Cartwright BA, Collett TS (1983) Landmark learning in bees. *J Comp Physiol* **151**:521–543.

Castro L, Aguiar P (2014) A feedforward model for the formation of a grid field where spatial information is provided solely from place cells. *Biol Cybern* **108**:133–143.

Chance FS (2012) Hippocampal phase precession from dual input components. *J Neurosci* **32**(47):16693–16703.

Chandra S, Sharma S, Chaudhuri R, Fiete I (2023) High-capacity flexible hippocampal associative and episodic memory enabled by prestructured "spatial" representations. *bioRxiv* 2023-11.

Chaudhuri R, Gercek B, Pandey B, Peyrache A, Fiete I (2019) The intrinsic attractor manifold and population dynamics of a canonical cognitive circuit across waking and sleep. *Nat Neurosci* **22**:1512–1520.

Chavarriaga R, Strösslin T, Sheynikhovich D, Gerstner W (2005) A computational model of parallel navigation systems in rodents. *Neuroinformatics* **3**:223–241.

Chen G, Lu Y, King JA, Cacucci F, Burgess N (2019) Differential influences of environment and self-motion on place and grid cell firing. *Nat Commun* **10**(1):1–11.

Chen G, Manson D, Cacucci F, Wills TJ (2016) Absence of visual input results in the disruption of grid cell firing in the mouse. *Curr Biol* **26**(17):2335–2342.

Chen X, He Q, Kelly JW, Fiete IR, McNamara TP (2015) Bias in human path integration is predicted by properties of grid cells. *Curr Biol* **25**(13):1771–1776.

Cheng S, Frank LM (2011) The structure of networks that produce the transformation from grid cells to place cells. *Neuroscience* **197**:293–306.

Chu T, Ji Z, Zuo J, Mi Y, Zhang W-H, Huang T, Bush D, Burgess N, Wu S (2023) Firing rate adaptation affords place cell theta sweeps, phase precession and procession. *eLife* **12**:RP87055.

Climer JR, Newman EL, Hasselmo ME (2013) Phase coding by grid cells in unconstrained environments: two-dimensional phase precession. *Eur J Neurosci* **38**(4):2526–2541.

Cohen MA, Grossberg S (1983) Absolute stability of global pattern formation and parallel memory storage by competitive neural networks. *IEEE Trans Sys Man and Cybernetics* **13**:815–821.

Conklin J, Eliasmith C (2005) A controlled attractor network model of path integration in the rat. *J Comput Neurosci* **18**:183–203.

Connelly CI, Burns JB, Weiss R (1990) Path planning using Laplace's equation. *IEEE Int Conf Robot Autom* **3**:2102–2106.

Constantinescu AO, O'Reilly JX, Behrens TEJ (2016) Organizing conceptual knowledge in humans with a gridlike code. *Science* **352**(6292):1464–1468.

Corneil DS, Gerstner W (2015) Attractor network dynamics enable preplay and rapid path planning in maze–like environments. *Adv Neural Inf Process Syst* **28**:1684–1692.

Couey JJ, Witoelar A, Zhang S-J, Zheng K, Ye J, Dunn B, Czajkowski R, Moser M-B, Moser EI, Roudi Y, et al. (2013) Recurrent inhibitory circuitry as a mechanism for grid formation. *Nat Neurosci* **16**:318–324.

Courellis HS, Nummela SU, Metke M, Diehl GW, Bussell R, Cauwenberghs G, et al. (2019) Spatial encoding in primate hippocampus during free navigation. *PLoS Biol* **17**(12):e300054.

Cressant A, Muller RU, Poucet B (1997) Failure of centrally placed objects to control the firing fields of hippocampal place cells. *J Neurosci* **17**:2531–2542.

Cueva CJ, Wei XX (2018) Emergence of grid-like representations by training recurrent neural networks to perform spatial localization. *ICLR*.

Czurko A, Hirase H, Csicsvari J, Buzsaki G (1999) Sustained activation of hippocampal pyramidal cells by "space clamping" in a running wheel. *Eur J Neurosci* **11**:344–352.

D'Albis T, Kempter R (2017) A single-cell spiking model for the origin of grid-cell patterns. *PLoS Comput Biol* **13**(10):e1005782.

Damasio AR (1989) The brain binds entities and events by multiregional activation from convergence zones. *Neural Comput* **1**:123–132.

Davelaar EJ, Goshen-Gottstein Y, Ashkenazi A, Usher M (2005) A context activation model of list memory: dissociating short-term from long-term recency effects. *Psychol Rev* **112**:34–53.

Dayan P (1991) Navigating through temporal difference. *Adv Neural Inf Process Syst* **3**:464–470.

Dayan P (1993) Improving generalization for temporal difference learning: the successor representation. *Neural Comput* **5**(4):613–624.

Dayan P, Abbott LF (2001) Theoretical Neuroscience. Cambridge, MA, USA: MIT Press.

Dayan P, Hinton GE, Neal RM, Zemel RS (1995) The Helmholtz machine. *Neural Comput* **7**(5):889–904.

de Cothi W, Nyberg N, Griesbauer E-M, Ghanamé C, Zisch F, Lefort JM, Fletcher L, Newton C, Renaudineau S, Bendor D, et al. (2022) Predictive maps in rats and humans for spatial navigation: the successor representation explains flexible behaviour. *Curr Biol* **32**(17):3676–3689.

Dehaene S (1997) The Number Sense: How the Mind Creates Mathematics. Oxford, UK: Oxford University Press.

de Lavilléon G, Lacroix MM, Rondi-Reig L, Benchenane K (2015) Explicit memory creation during sleep demonstrates a causal role of place cells in navigation. *Nat Neurosci* **18**:493–495.

Demircigil M, Heusel J, Löwe M, Upgang S, Vermet F (2017) On a model of associative memory with huge storage capacity. *J Stat Phys* **168**:288–299.

Deneve S, Latham PE, Pouget A (2001) Efficient computation and cue integration with noisy population codes. *Nat Neurosci* **4**:826–831.

Deng W, Aimone J, Gage F (2010) New neurons and new memories: how does adult hippocampal neurogenesis affect learning and memory? *Nat Rev Neurosci* **11**:339–350.

Deshmukh SS, Knierim JJ (2013) Influence of local objects on hippocampal representations: landmark vectors and memory. *Hippocampus* **23**(4):253–67.

Deuker L, Olligs J, Fell J, Kranz TA, Mormann F, Montag C, et al. (2013) Memory consolidation by replay of stimulus-specific neural activity. *J Neurosci* **33**(49):19373–19383.

Dhillon A, Jones R (2000) Laminar differences in recurrent excitatory transmission in the rat entorhinal cortex in vitro. *Neuroscience* **99**:413–422.

Doeller CF, Barry C, Burgess N (2010) Evidence for grid cells in a human memory network. *Nature* **463**(7281):657–661.

Doeller CF, Burgess N (2008) Distinct error-correcting and incidental learning of location relative to landmarks and boundaries. *PNAS* **105**:5909–5914.

Dollé L, Sheynikhovich D, Girard B, Chavarriaga R, Guillot A (2010) Path planning versus cue responding: a bio-inspired model of switching between navigation strategies. *Biol Cybern* **103**(4):299–317.

Dominey PF, Arbib MA (1992) A cortico-subcortical model for generation of spatially accurate sequential saccades. *Cereb Cortex* **2**:153–175.

Domnisoru C, Kinkhabwala AA, Tank DW (2013) Membrane potential dynamics of grid cells. *Nature* **495**:199–204.

Dordek Y, Soudry D, Meir R, Derdikman D (2016) Extracting grid cell characteristics from place cell inputs using non-negative principal component analysis. *eLife* **5**:e1009.

Douchamps V, Jeewajee A, Blundell P, Burgess N, Lever C (2013) Evidence for encoding versus retrieval scheduling in the hippocampus by theta phase and acetylcholine. *J Neurosci* **33**:8689–8704.

Dragoi G, Tonegawa S (2011) Preplay of future place cell sequences by hippocampal cellular assemblies. *Nature* **469**:397–401.

Droulez J, Berthoz A (1991) A neural network model of sensoritopic maps with predictive short-term memory properties. *PNAS* **88**:9653–9657.

Dupret D, O'Neill J, Pleydell-Bouverie B, Csicsvari J (2010) The reorganization and reactivation of hippocampal maps predict spatial memory performance. *Nat Neurosci* **13**:995–1002.

Duvelle E, Grieves RM, Hok V, Poucet B, Arleo A, Jeffery KJ, Save E (2019) Insensitivity of place cells to the value of spatial goals in a two-choice flexible navigation task. *J Neurosci* **39**:2522–2541.

Edvardsen V, Bicanski A, Burgess N (2019) Navigating with grid and place cells in cluttered environments. *Hippocampus* **30**(3):220–232.

Ego-Stengel V, Wilson MA (2010) Disruption of ripple associated hippocampal activity during rest impairs spatial learning in the rat. *Hippocampus* **20**:1–10.

Eichenbaum H (2014) Time cells in the hippocampus: a new dimension for mapping memories. *Nat Rev Neurosci* **15**:732–744.

Eichenbaum H, Cohen NJ (2014) Can we reconcile the declarative memory and spatial navigation views on hippocampal function? *Neuron* **83**(4):764–770.

Ekstrom AD, Kahana MJ, Caplan JB, Fields TA, Isham EA, Newman EL, Fried I (2003) Cellular networks underlying human spatial navigation. *Nature* **425**:184–188.

Ekstrom AD, Meltzer J, McNaughton BL, Barnes CA (2001) NMDA receptor antagonism blocks experience-dependent expansion of hippocampal "place fields." *Neuron* **31**:631–638.

Eliav T, Geva-Sagiv M, Yartsev MM, Finkelstein A, Rubin A, Las L, Ulanovsky N (2018) Nonoscillatory phase coding and synchronization in the bat hippocampal formation. *Cell* **175**(4):1119–1130.

Erdem UM, Hasselmo M (2012) A goal-directed spatial navigation model using forward trajectory planning based on grid cells. *Eur J Neurosci* **35**:916–931.

Estes WK (1955) Statistical theory of spontaneous recovery and regression. *Psychol Rev* **62**:145–154.

Evans T, Burgess N (2019) Coordinated hippocampal-entorhinal replay as structural inference. *Adv Neural Inf Process Syst* 32.

Feng T, Silva D, Foster DJ (2015) Dissociation between the experience-dependent development of hippocampal theta sequences and single-trial phase precession. *J Neurosci* **35**(12):4890–4902.

Fenton AA, Csizmadia G, Muller RU (2000) Conjoint control of hippocampal place cell firing by two visual stimuli: I. The effects of moving the stimuli on firing field positions. *J Gen Physiol* **116**:191–209.

Fenton AA, Kao HY, Neymotin SA, Olypher A, Vayntrub Y, Lytton WW, Ludvig N (2008) Unmasking the CA1 ensemble place code by exposures to small and large environments: more place cells and multiple, irregularly arranged, and expanded place fields in the larger space. *J Neurosci* **28**:11250–11262.

Fiete IR, Burak Y, Brookings (2008) What grid cells encode about rat location. *J Neurosci* **28**:6856–6871.

Finnegan R, Shaw M, Becker S (2017) Restricted Boltzmann machine models of hippocampal coding and neurogenesis. In: The Rewiring Brain: a Computational Approach to Structural Plasticity in the Adult Brain (Van Ooyen A, Butz-Ostendorf M, eds), pp 443–461. Cambridge, MA, USA: Academic Press.

Fortin NJ, Agster KL, Eichenbaum HB (2002) Critical role of the hippocampus in memory for sequences of events. *Nat Neurosci* **5**(5):458–62.

Foster DJ, Morris RG, Dayan P (2000) A model of hippocampally dependent navigation, using the temporal difference learning rule. *Hippocampus* **10**:1–16.

Foster DJ, Wilson MA (2006) Reverse replay of behavioural sequences in hippocampal place cells during the awake state. *Nature* **440**:680–683.

Franjic D, Skarica M, Ma S, Arellano JI, Tebbenkamp AT, Choi J, et al. (2022) Transcriptomic taxonomy and neurogenic trajectories of adult human, macaque, and pig hippocampal and entorhinal cells. *Neuron* **110**:452–469.

Frank LM, Brown EN, Wilson M (2000) Trajectory encoding in the hippocampus and entorhinal cortex. *Neuron* **27**:169–178.

Franzius M, Sprekeler H, Wiskott L (2007) Slowness and sparseness lead to place, head-direction, and spatial-view cells. *PLoS Comput Biol* **3**(8):e166.

Fuchs EC, Neitz A, Pinna R, Melzer S, Caputi A, Monyer H (2016) Local and distant input controlling excitation in layer II of the medial entorhinal cortex. *Neuron* **89**(1):194–208.

Fuhs MC, Touretzky DS (2000) Synaptic learning models of map separation in the hippocampus. *Neurocomputing* **32**:379–384.

Fuhs MC, Touretzky DS (2006) A spin glass model of path integration in rat medial entorhinal cortex. *J Neurosci* **26**:4266–4276.

Fyhn M, Hafting T, Treves A, Moser MB, Moser EI (2007) Hippocampal remapping and grid realignment in entorhinal cortex. *Nature* **446**:190–194.

Fyhn M, Hafting T, Witter MP, Moser EI, Moser MB (2008) Grid cells in mice. *Hippocampus* **18**:1230–1238.

Gaffan D (1994) Dissociated effects of perirhinal cortex ablation, fornix transection and amygdalectomy: evidence for multiple memory systems in the primate temporal lobe. *Exp Brain Res* **99**:411–422.

Gaffan D, Gaffan EA (1991) Amnesia in man following transection of the fornix. *Brain* **114**:2611–2618.

Gardiner JM, Java RI (1993) Theories of Memory. In: Recognising and Remembering (Collins A, Gathercole S, Morris P, eds), pp 168–188. Hillsdale, NJ: Erlbaum.

Gardner RJ, Hermansen E, Pachitariu M, Burak Y, Baas NA, Dunn BA, Moser MB, Moser EI (2022) Toroidal topology of population activity in grid cells. *Nature* **602**:123–128.

Gardner RJ, Lu L, Wernle T, Moser M-B, Moser EI (2019) Correlation structure of grid cells is preserved during sleep. *Nat Neurosci* **22**:598–608.

Gardner-Medwin AR (1976) The recall of events through the learning of associations between their parts. *Proc R Soc Lond B Biol Sci* **194**:375–402.

Geerts JP, Chersi F, Stachenfeld KL, Burgess N (2020) A general model of hippocampal and dorsal striatal learning and decision making. *PNAS* **117**(49):31427–31437.

Geerts JP, Gershman SJ, Burgess N, Stachenfeld KL (2024) A probabilistic successor representation for context-dependent learning. *Psychol Rev* **131**(2):578–597.

Geisler C, Diba K, Pastalkova E, Mizuseki K, Royer S, Buzsáki G (2010) Temporal delays among place cells determine the frequency of population theta oscillations in the hippocampus. *PNAS* **107**(17):7957–7962.

George D, Rikhye RV, Gothoskar N, Guntupalli JS, Dedieu A, Lázaro-Gredilla M (2021) Clone-structured graph representations enable flexible learning and vicarious evaluation of cognitive maps. *Nat Commun* **12**(1):1–17.

George TM, Stachenfeld KL, Barry C, Clopath C, Fukai T (2024) A generative model of the hippocampal formation trained with theta driven local learning rules. *Adv Neural Inf Process Syst* 36.

Georgopoulos AP, Schwartz AB, Kettner RE (1986) Neuronal population coding of movement direction. *Science* **233**:1416–1419.

Gershman SJ, Daw ND (2017) Reinforcement learning and episodic memory in humans and animals: an integrative framework. *Annu Rev Psychol* **68**:101–128.

Gershman SJ, Moore CD, Todd MT, Norman KA, Sederberg PB (2012) The successor representation and temporal context. *Neural Comput* **24**:1553–1568.

Gershman SJ, Niv Y (2010) Learning latent structure: carving nature at its joints. *Curr Opin Neurobiol* **20**:1–6.

Gerstner W, Abbott LF (1997) Learning navigational maps through potentiation and modulation of hippocampal place cells. *J Comput Neurosci* **4**(1):79–94.

Gillespie AK, Astudillo Maya DA, Denovellis EL, Liu DF, Kastner DB, Coulter ME, Roumis DK, Eden UT, Frank LM (2021) Hippocampal replay reflects specific past experiences rather than a plan for subsequent choice. *Neuron* **109**(19):3149–3163.

Giocomo LM, Hussaini SA, Zheng F, Kandel ER, Moser MB, Moser EI (2011) Grid cells use HCN1 channels for spatial scaling. *Cell* **147**(5):1159–1170.

Girardeau G, Benchenane K, Wiener SI, Buzsáki G, Zugaro MB (2009) Selective suppression of hippocampal ripples impairs spatial memory. *Nat Neurosci* **12**:1222–1223.

Gluck MA, Myers CE (1993) Hippocampal mediation of stimulus representation: a computational theory. *Hippocampus* **3**(4):491–516.

Gluck MA, Myers CE (1996) Integrating behavioral and physiological models of hippocampal function. *Hippocampus* **6**:643–653.

Goodale MA, Milner AD (1992) Separate visual pathways for perception and action. *Trends Neurosci* **15**:20–25.

Goodridge JP, Touretzky DS (2000) Modeling attractor deformation in the rodent head-direction system. *J Neurophysiol* **83**:3402–3410.

Gorchetchnikov A, Grossberg S (2007) Space, time and learning in the hippocampus: how fine spatial and temporal scales are expanded into population codes for behavioural control. *Neural Netw* **20**:182–193.

Gorchetchnikov A, Hasselmo ME (2002) A model of hippocampal circuitry mediating goal-driven navigation in a familiar environment. *Neurocomputing* 44–46:423–427.

Gothard KM, Skaggs WE, McNaughton BL (1996) Dynamics of mismatch correction in the hippocampal ensemble code for space: interaction between path integration and environmental cues. *J Neurosci* 16:8027–8040.

Graham KS, Hodges JR (1997) Differentiating the roles of the hippocampus complex and the neocortex in long-term memory storage: evidence from the study of semantic dementia and Alzheimer's disease. *Neuropsychology* 11:77–89.

Graves A, Wayne G, Reynolds M, Harley T, Danihelka I, Grabska-Barwińska A, et al. (2016) Hybrid computing using a neural network with dynamic external memory. *Nature* 538:471–476.

Greve A, Donaldson DI, van Rossum MCW (2010) A single-trace dual-process model of episodic memory: a novel computational account of familiarity and recollection. *Hippocampus* 20:235–251.

Grieves RM, Dudchenko PA (2013) Cognitive maps and spatial inference in animals: rats fail to take a novel shortcut, but can take a previously experienced one. *Learning and Motivation* 44(2): 81–92.

Grieves RM, Duvelle E, Dudchenko PA (2018) A boundary vector cell model of place field repetition. *Spat Cogn Comput* 18:217–256.

Grieves RM, Wood ER, Dudchenko PA (2016) Place cells on a maze encode routes rather than destinations. *eLife* 5:e15986.

Guanella A, Kiper D, Verschure P (2007) A model of grid cells based on a twisted torus topology. *Int J Neural Syst* 17:231–240.

Guazzelli A, Bota M, Corbacho FJ, Arbib MA (1998) Affordances: motivations, and the world graph theory. *Adapt Behav* 6(3–4): 435–471.

Gupta AS, van der Meer MAA, Touretzky DS, Redish AD (2010) Hippocampal replay is not a simple function of experience. *Neuron* 65(5):695–705.

Gurney K (1997) An Introduction to Neural Networks. London, UK: Taylor and Francis.

Gustafson NJ, Daw ND (2011) Grid cells, place cells, and geodesic generalization for spatial reinforcement learning. *PLoS Comput Biol* 7(10):e1002235.

Hafting T, Fyhn M, Bonnevie T, Moser MB, Moser EI (2008) Hippocampus-independent phase precession in entorhinal grid cells. *Nature* 453:1248–1252.

Hafting T, Fyhn M, Molden S, Moser MB, Moser EI (2005) Microstructure of a spatial map in the entorhinal cortex. *Nature* 436:801–806.

Hannula DE, Tranel D, Cohen NJ (2006) The long and the short of it: relational memory impairments in amnesia, even at short lags. *J Neurosci* 26(32):8352–8359.

Hardcastle K, Ganguli S, Giocomo LM (2015) Environmental boundaries as an error correction mechanism for grid cells. *Neuron* 86(3):827–839.

Hardcastle K, Maheswaranathan N, Ganguli S, Giocomo LM (2017) A multiplexed, heterogeneous, and adaptive code for navigation in medial entorhinal cortex. *Neuron* 94(2):375–387.

Harris KD, Henze DA, Hirase H, Leinekugel X, Dragoi G, Czurko A, Buzsaki G (2002) Spike train dynamics predicts theta-related phase precession in hippocampal pyramidal cells. *Nature* 417: 738–741.

Hartley T, Bird CM, Chan D, Cipolotti L, Husain M, Vargha-Khadem F, Burgess N (2007) The hippocampus is required for short-term topographical memory in humans. *Hippocampus* 17(1):34–48.

Hartley T, Burgess N, Lever C, Cacucci F, O'Keefe J (2000) Modeling place fields in terms of the cortical inputs to the hippocampus. *Hippocampus* 10:369–379.

Harvey CD, Collman F, Dombeck DA, Tank DW (2010) Intracellular dynamics of hippocampal place cells during virtual navigation. *Nature* 461:941–946.

Hassabis D, Kumaran D, Vann SD, Maguire EA (2007) Patients with hippocampal amnesia cannot imagine new experiences. *PNAS* 104(5):1726–1731.

Hasselmo ME (1999) Neuromodulation: acetylcholine and memory consolidation. *Trends Cogn Sci* 3:351–359.

Hasselmo ME (2005) A model of prefrontal cortical mechanisms for goal directed behavior. *J Cogn Neurosci* 17(7):1115–1129.

Hasselmo ME (2008) Grid cell mechanisms and function: contributions of entorhinal persistent spiking and phase resetting. *Hippocampus* 18:1116–1126.

Hasselmo ME, Bodelon C, Wyble BP (2002) A proposed function for hippocampal theta rhythm: separate phases of encoding and retrieval enhance reversal of prior learning. *Neural Comput* 14:793:817.

Hasselmo ME, Brandon MP (2012) A model combining oscillations and attractor dynamics for generation of grid cell firing. *Front Neural Circuits* 6:30.

Hasselmo ME, Fehlau BP (2001) Differences in time course of ACh and GABA modulation of excitatory synaptic potentials in slices of rat hippocampus. *J Neurophysiol* 86:1792–1802.

Hasselmo ME, McClelland JL (1999) Neural models of memory. *Curr Opin Neurobiol* 9:184–188.

Hasselmo ME, Schnell E, Barkai E (1995) Dynamics of learning and recall at excitatory recurrent synapses and cholinergic modulation in rat hippocampal region CA3. *J Neurosci* 15:5249–5262.

Hasselmo ME, Wyble BP (1997) Free recall and recognition in a network model of the hippocampus: simulating effects of scopolamine on human memory function. *Behav Brain Res* 89:1–34.

Hasselmo ME, Wyble BP, Wallenstein GV (1996) Encoding and retrieval of episodic memories: role of cholinergic and GABAergic modulation in the hippocampus. *Hippocampus* 6:693–708.

Hawkins J, Lewis M, Klukas M, Purdy S, Ahmad S (2019) A framework for intelligence and cortical function based on grid cells in the neocortex. *Front Neural Circuits* 12:121.

Hayman R, Jeffery K (2008) How heterogeneous place cell responding arises from homogeneous grids—a contextual gating hypothesis. *Hippocampus* 18:1301–1313.

Hebb DO (1949) The Organisation of Behavior. New York: Wiley.

Hertz J, Krogh A, Palmer R (1990) Introduction to the Theory of Neural Computation. New York, NY, USA: Perseus Books.

Hinman JR, Chapman GW, Hasselmo ME (2019) Neuronal representation of environmental boundaries in egocentric coordinates. *Nat Commun* 10(1):2772.

Hinton GE (1989) Connectionist learning procedures. *Artificial Intelligence* 40(1–3):185–234.

Hinton GE, Sejnowski TJ (1999) Unsupervised learning. Cambridge, MA, USA: MIT Press.

Hochreiter S, Schmidhuber J (1997) Long short-term memory. *Neural Comput* 9(8):1735–1780.

Hoel E (2021) The overfitted brain: dreams evolved to assist generalization. *Patterns* 2:100244.

Hok V, Lenck-Santini PP, Roux S, Save E, Muller RU, Poucet B (2007) Goal-related activity in hippocampal place cells. *J Neurosci* 27:472–482.

Holdstock JS, Mayes AR, Cezayirli E, Isaac CL, Aggleton JP, Roberts N (2000) A comparison of egocentric and allocentric spatial memory in a patient with selective hippocampal damage. *Neuropsychologia* 38:410–425.

Holdstock JS, Mayes AR, Roberts N, Cezayirli E, Isaac CL, O'Reilly RC, Norman KA (2002) Under what conditions is recognition spared relative to recall after selective hippocampal damage in humans? *Hippocampus* 12:341–351.

Hollup SA, Molden S, Donnett JG, Moser MB, Moser EI (2001) Accumulation of hippocampal place fields at the goal location in an annular watermaze task. *J Neurosci* 21:1635–1644.

Hölscher C, Anwyl R, Rowan MJ (1997) Stimulation on the positive phase of hippocampal theta rhythm induces long-term potentiation that can be depotentiated by stimulation on the negative phase in area CA1 in vivo. *J Neurosci* 17(16):6470–6477.

Hopfield JJ (1982) Neural networks and physical systems with emergent collective computational abilities. *PNAS* 79:2554–2558.

Hopfield JJ (2010) Neurodynamics of mental exploration. *PNAS* 107:1648–1653.

Hoppensteadt FC (1987) Frequency modulation dynamics in neural networks. *Ann N Y Acad Sci* 504:52–61.

Hori E, Tabuchi E, Matsumura N, Tamura R, Eifuku S, Endo S, Nishijo H, Ono T (2003) Representation of place by monkey hippocampal neurons in real and virtual translocation. *Hippocampus* 13:190–196.

Horiuchi TK, Moss CF (2015) Grid cells in 3-D: reconciling data and models. *Hippocampus* 25(12):1489–500.

Horner AJ, Bisby JA, Bush D, Lin W-J, Burgess N (2015) Evidence for holistic episodic recollection via hippocampal pattern completion. *Nat Commun* 6:7462.

Howard LR, Javadi AH, Yu Y, Mill RD, Morrison LC, Knight R, Loftus MM, Staskute L, Spiers HJ (2014) The hippocampus and entorhinal cortex encode the path and Euclidean distances to goals during navigation. *Curr Biol* 24:1331–1340.

Howard MW, Fotedar MS, Datey AV, Hasselmo ME (2005) The temporal context model in spatial navigation and relational learning: toward a common explanation of medial temporal lobe function across domains. *Psychol Rev* 112:75–116.

Howard MW, Kahana MJ (2001) A distributed representation of temporal context. *J Math Psychol* 46:269–299.

Howard MW, MacDonald CJ, Tiganj Z, Shankar KH, Du Q, Hasselmo ME, Eichenbaum H (2014) A unified mathematical framework for coding time, space, and sequences in the hippocampal region. *J Neurosci* 34(13):4692–4707.

Howard MW, Shankar KH, Aue WR, Criss AH (2015) A distributed representation of internal time. *Psychol Rev* 122:24–53.

Howard MW, Viskontas IV, Shankar KH, Fried I (2012) Ensembles of human MTL neurons "jump back in time" in response to a repeated stimulus. *Hippocampus* 22:1833–1847.

Høydal ØA, Skytøen ER, Andersson SO, Moser M-B, Moser EI (2019) Object-vector coding in the medial entorhinal cortex. *Nature* 568:400–404.

Huerta PT, Lisman JE (1995) Bidirectional synaptic plasticity induced by a single burst during cholinergic theta oscillation in CA1 in vitro. *Neuron* 15(5):1053–1063.

Huxter J, Burgess N, O'Keefe J (2003) Independent rate and temporal coding in hippocampal pyramidal cells. *Nature* 425:828–832.

Ismakov R, Barak O, Jeffery J, Derdikman D (2017) Grid cells encode local positional information. *Curr Biol* 27(15):2337–2343.

Jacobs J, Weidemann CT, Miller JF, Solway A, Burke JF, Wei X, Suthana N, Sperling MR, Sharan AD, Fried I, et al. (2013) Direct recordings of grid-like neuronal activity in human spatial navigation. *Nat Neurosci* 16:1188–1190.

Jaramillo J, Schmidt R, Kempter R (2014) Modeling inheritance of phase precession in the hippocampal formation. *J Neurosci* 34(22):7715–7731.

Jeewajee A, Barry C, Douchamps V, Manson D, Lever C, Burgess N (2014) Theta phase precession of grid and place cell firing in open environments. *Philos Trans R Soc B* 369:20120532.

Jensen O, Lisman JE (1996) Hippocampal CA3 region predicts memory sequences: accounting for the phase precession of place cells. *Learn Mem* 3:279–287.

Jensen O, Lisman JE (2000) Position reconstruction from an ensemble of hippocampal place cells: contribution of theta phase coding. *J Neurophysiol* 83:2602–2609.

Jercog PE, Ahmadian Y, Woodruff C, Deb-Sen R, Abbott LF, Kandel ER (2019) Heading direction with respect to a reference point modulates place-cell activity. *Nat Commun* 10:2333.

Ji D, Wilson MA (2007) Coordinated memory replay in the visual cortex and hippocampus during sleep. *Nat Neurosci* 10:100–107.

Johnson A, Redish AD (2007) Neural ensembles in CA3 transiently encode paths forward of the animal at a decision point. *J Neurosci* 27(45):12176–89.

Jones VJ (1976) A fragmentation hypothesis of memory: cued recall of pictures and of sequential position. *J Exp Psychol: Gen* 105:277–293.

Julian JB, Keinath AT, Frazzetta G, Epstein RA (2018) Human entorhinal cortex represents visual space using a boundary-anchored grid. *Nat Neurosci* 21(2):191–194.

Jung MW, Wiener SI, McNaughton BL (1994) Comparison of spatial firing characteristics of units in dorsal and ventral hippocampus of the rat. *J Neurosci* 14:7347–7356.

Kahana MJ (1996) Associative retrieval processes in free recall. *Mem Cogn* 24:103–109.

Kali S, Dayan P (2000) The involvement of recurrent connections in area CA3 in establishing the properties of place fields: a model. *J Neurosci* 20:7463–7477.

Kali S, Dayan P (2004) Off-line replay maintains declarative memories in a model of hippocampal-neocortical interactions. *Nat Neurosci* 7:286–294.

Kang L, De Weese MR (2019) Replay as wavefronts and theta sequences as bump oscillations in a grid cell attractor network. *eLife* 8:e46351.

Kartsounis LD, Rudge P, Stevens JM (1995) Bilateral lesions of CA1 and CA2 fields of the hippocampus are sufficient to cause a severe amnesic syndrome in humans. *J Neurol Neurosurg Psychiatry* 59(1):95–98.

Kaufman AM, Geiller T, Losonczy A (2020) A role for the locus coeruleus in hippocampal CA1 place cell reorganization during spatial reward learning. *Neuron* 105(6):1018–1026.

Kay K, Chung JE, Sosa M, Schor JS, Karlsson MP, Larkin MC, Liu DF, Frank LM (2020) Constant sub-second cycling between representations of possible futures in the hippocampus. *Cell* 180(3):552–567.

Keith JR, McVety KM (1988) Latent place learning in a novel environment and the influence of prior training in rats. *Psychobiology* 16:146–151.

Kentros C, Hargreaves E, Hawkins RD, Kandel ER, Shapiro M, Muller RV (1998) Abolition of long-term stability of new hippocampal place cell maps by NMDA receptor blockade. *Science* 280:2121–2126.

Killian NJ, Jutras MJ, Buffalo EA (2012) A map of visual space in the primate entorhinal cortex. *Nature* 491(7426):761–764.

Kingma DP, Welling M (2014) Auto-encoding variational bayes. *arXiv* 1312.6114.

Kjelstrup KB, Solstad T, Brun VH, Hafting T, Leutgeb S, Witter MP, Moser EI, Moser M-B (2008) Finite scale of spatial representation in the hippocampus. *Science* 321(5885):140–143.

Knierim JJ, Kudrimoti HS, McNaughton BL (1995) Place cells, head direction cells, and the learning of landmark stability. *J Neurosci* 15:1648–1659.

Knierim JJ, Lee I, Hargreaves EL (2006) Hippocampal place cells: parallel input streams, subregional processing, and implications for episodic memory. *Hippocampus* 16:755–764.

Knowlton BJ, Squire LR (1995) Remembering and knowing: two different expressions of declarative memory. *J Exp Psychol Learn Mem Cogn* 21:699–710.

Knudsen EB, Wallis JD (2021) Hippocampal neurons construct a map of an abstract value space. *Cell* 184(18):4640–4650.

Koenig J, Linder AN, Leutgeb JK, Leutgeb S (2011) The spatial periodicity of grid cells is not sustained during reduced theta oscillations. *Science* 332:592–595.

Kohonen T (1972) Correlation matrix memories. *IEEE Trans Comp C* 21:353–359.

Kolibius LD, Roux F, Parish G, Ter Wal M, Van Der Plas M, Chelvarajah R, et al. (2023) Hippocampal neurons code individual episodic memories in humans. *Nat Hum Behav* 7:1968–1979.

Kornienko O, Latuske P, Bassler M, Kohler L, Allen K (2018) Non-rhythmic head-direction cells in the parahippocampal region are not constrained by attractor network dynamics. *eLife* 7:e35949.

Kosslyn SM, Ball TM, Reiser BJ (1978) Visual images preserve metric spatial information: evidence from studies of image scanning. *J Exp Psychol: Hum Percept Perform* 4:47–60.

Kroll NE, Knight RT, Metcalfe J, Wolf ES, Tulving E (1996) Cohesion failure as a source of memory illusions. *J Mem Lang* 35:176–196.

Kropff E, Carmichael JE, Moser M-B, Moser EI (2015) Speed cells in the medial entorhinal cortex. *Nature* 523:419–424.

Kropff E, Treves A (2008) The emergence of grid cells: intelligent design or just adaptation? *Hippocampus* 18:1256–1269.

Krotov D, Hopfield JJ (2016) Dense associative memory for pattern recognition. *Adv Neural Inf Process Syst* 29:1172–1180.

Krotov D, Hopfield JJ (2020) Large associative memory problem in neurobiology and machine learning. *arXiv* 2008.06996.

Krupic J, Bauza M, Burton S, Barry C, O'Keefe J (2015) Grid cell symmetry is shaped by environmental geometry. *Nature* 518:232–235.

Kubie JL, Fenton AA (2012) Linear look-ahead in conjunctive cells: an entorhinal mechanism for vector-based navigation. *Front Neural Circuits* 6:20.

Kumaran D, Hassabis D, McClelland DL (2016) What learning systems do intelligent agents need? complementary learning systems theory updated. *Trends Cogn Sci* 20(7):512–334.

Kumaran D, McClelland JL (2012) Generalization through the recurrent interaction of episodic memories: a model of the hippocampal system. *Psychol Rev* 119(3):573–616.

Kunz L, Brandt A, Reinacher PC, Staresina BP, Reifenstein ET, Weidemann CT, et al. (2021) A neural code for egocentric spatial maps in the human medial temporal lobe. *Neuron* 109(17):2781–2796.

Langston RF, Ainge JA, Couey JJ, Canto CB, Bjerknes TL, Witter MP, Moser EI, Moser MB (2010) Development of the spatial representation system in the rat. *Science* 328:1576–1580.

Latham PE, Deneve S, Pouget A (2003) Optimal computation with attractor networks. *J Physiol Paris* 97:683–694.

Laurens J, Angelaki DE (2018) The brain compass: a perspective on how self-motion updates the head direction cell attractor. *Neuron* 97(2):275–289.

LeCun Y, Bengio Y, Hinton G (2015) Deep learning. *Nature* 521:436–444.

Lee I, Griffin AL, Zilli EA, Eichenbaum H, Hasselmo ME (2006) Gradual translocation of spatial correlates of neuronal firing in the hippocampus toward prospective reward locations. *Neuron* 51(5):639–650.

Lee JQ, Keinath AT, Cianfarano E, Brandon MP (2023) Identifying representational structure in CA1 to benchmark theoretical models of cognitive mapping. *bioRxiv* 2023-2010.

Leibold C, Monsalve-Mercado MM (2017) Traveling theta waves and the hippocampal phase code. *Sci Rep* 7(1):7678.

Lengyel M, Dayan P (2007) Hippocampal contributions to control: the third way. *Adv Neural Inf Process Syst* 20:889–896.

Lengyel M, Szatmary Z, Erdi P (2003) Dynamically detuned oscillations account for the coupled rate and temporal code of place cell firing. *Hippocampus* 13:700–714.

Leutgeb JK, Leutgeb S, Treves A, Meyer R, Barnes CA, McNaughton BL, Moser MB, Moser EI (2005) Progressive transformation of hippocampal neuronal representations in "morphed" environments. *Neuron* 48:345–358.

Lever C, Burton S, Jeewajee A, O'Keefe J, Burgess N (2009) Boundary vector cells in the subiculum of the hippocampal formation. *J Neurosci* 29:9771–9777.

Lever C, Wills T, Cacucci F, Burgess N, O'Keefe J (2002) Long-term plasticity in the hippocampal place cell representation of environmental geometry. *Nature* 416:90–94.

Levy WB (1996) A sequence predicting CA3 is a flexible associator that learns and uses context to solve hippocampal-like tasks. *Hippocampus* 6:579–590.

Lieblich I, Arbib MA (1982) Multiple representations of space underlying behavior. *Behav Brain Sci* 5:627–659.

Liu C, Todorova R, Tang W, Oliva A, Fernandez-Ruiz A (2023) Associative and predictive hippocampal codes support memory-guided behaviors. *Science* 382(6668):eadi8237.

Lu J, Behbahani AH, Hamburg L, Westeinde EA, Dawson PM, Lyu C, et al. (2022) Transforming representations of movement from body- to world-centric space. *Nature* 601:98–104.

Lubenov EV, Siapas AG (2009) Hippocampal theta oscillations are travelling waves. *Nature* 459(7246):534–539.

Ludvig N, Tang HM, Gohil BC, Botero JM (2004) Detecting location-specific neuronal firing rate increases in the hippocampus of freely-moving monkeys. *Brain Res* 1014:97–109.

Mallot HA, Gillner S (2000) Route navigating without place recognition: what is recognised in recognition-triggered responses? *Perception* 29:43–55.

Mamad O, Stumpp L, McNamara HM, Ramakrishnan C, Deisseroth K, Reilly RB, et al. (2017) Place field assembly distribution encodes preferred locations. *PLoS Biol* 15(9):e2002365.

Mankin EA, Sparks FT, Slayyeh B, Sutherland RJ, Leutgeb S, Leutgeb JK (2012) Neuronal code for extended time in the hippocampus. *PNAS* 109:19462–19467.

Mankin EA, Thurley K, Chenani A, Haas OV, Debs L, Henke J, Galinato M, Leutgeb JK, Leutgeb S, Leibold C (2019) The hippocampal code for space in Mongolian gerbils. *Hippocampus* 29(9):787–801.

Manning JR, Polyn SM, Litt B, Baltuch G, Kahana MJ (2011) Oscillatory patterns in temporal lobe reveal context reinstatement during memory search. *PNAS* 108:12893–12897.

Manns JR, Eichenbaum H (2006) Evolution of declarative memory. *Hippocampus* 16(9):795–808.

Manns JR, Hopkins RO, Squire LR (2003) Semantic memory and the human hippocampus. *Neuron* 37:127–133.

Manns JR, Howard MW, Eichenbaum H (2007) Gradual changes in hippocampal activity support remembering the order of events. *Neuron* 56(3):530–540.

Manns JR, Squire LR (1999) Impaired recognition memory on the Doors and People Test after damage limited to the hippocampal region. *Hippocampus* 9:495–499.

Mao D, Avila E, Caziot B, Laurens J, Dickman JD, Angelaki DE (2021) Spatial modulation of hippocampal activity in freely moving macaques. *Neuron* 109(21):3521–3534.

Markus EJ, Qin YL, Leonard B, Skaggs WE, McNaughton BL, Barnes CA (1995) Interactions between location and task affect the spatial and directional firing of hippocampal neurons. *J Neurosci* 15(11):7079–7094.

Marr D (1970) A theory for cerebral cortex. *Proc R Soc Lond B Biol Sci* **176**:161–234.

Marr D (1971) Simple memory: a theory for archicortex. *Philos Trans R Soc B* **262**:23–81.

Martinet L-E, Sheynikhovich D, Benchenane K, Arleo A (2011) Spatial learning and action planning in a prefrontal cortical network model. *PLoS Comput Biol* **7**(5):e1002045.

Mathis A, Herz AV, Stemmler M (2012) Optimal population codes for space: grid cells outperform place cells. *Neural Comput* **24**:2280–2317.

Mattar MG, Daw ND (2018) Prioritized memory access explains planning and hippocampal replay. *Nat Neurosci* **21**:1609–1617.

Maurer AP, Van Rhoads SR, Sutherland GR, Lipa P, McNaughton BL (2005) Self-motion and the origin of differential spatial scaling along the septo-temporal axis of the hippocampus. *Hippocampus* **15**:841–852.

McClelland JL (2013) Incorporating rapid neocortical learning of new schema-consistent information into complementary learning systems theory. *J Exp Psychol Gen* **142**:1190–1210.

McClelland JL, McNaughton BL, O'Reilly RC (1995) Why there are complementary learning systems in the hippocampus and neocortex: insights from the successes and failures of connectionist models of learning and memory. *Psychol Rev* **102**:419–457.

McClelland JL, Rumelhart DE (1986) Parallel Distributed Processing: Explorations in the Microstructure of Cognition: Vol 2. Psychological and Biological Models. Cambridge, MA, USA: MIT Press.

McCloskey M, Cohen NJ (1989) Catastrophic interference in connectionist networks: the sequential learning problem. *Psychol Learn Motiv* **24**:109–165.

McHugh TJ, Blum KI, Tsien JZ, Tonegawa S, Wilson MA (1996) Impaired hippocampal representation of space in CA1-specific NMDAR1 knockout mice. *Cell* **87**(7):1339–49.

McNaughton BL, Barnes CA, Gerrard JL, Gothard K, Jung MW, Knierim JJ, Kudrimoti H, Qin Y, Skaggs WE, Suster M, et al. (1996) Deciphering the hippocampal polyglot: the hippocampus as a path integration system. *J Exp Biol* **199**:173–185.

McNaughton BL, Barnes CA, O'Keefe J (1983) The contributions of position, direction, and velocity to single unit activity in the hippocampus of freely-moving rats. *Exp Brain Res* **52**:41–49.

McNaughton BL, Battaglia FP, Jensen O, Moser EI, Moser MB (2006) Path integration and the neural basis of the cognitive map. *Nat Rev Neurosci* **7**:663–678.

McNaughton BL, Morris RG (1987) Hippocampal synaptic enhancement and information storage within a distributed memory system. *Trends Neurosci* **10**:408–415.

McNaughton BL, Nadel L (1990) Hebb-Marr networks and the neurobiological representation of action in space. In: Neuroscience and Connectionist Theory (Gluck MA, Rumelhart DE, eds), pp 1–63. Hillsdale, NJ: Lawrence Erlbaum.

Mehta MR, Barnes CA, McNaughton BL (1997) Experience-dependent, asymmetric expansion of hippocampal place fields. *PNAS* **94**:8918–8921.

Mehta MR, Lee AK, Wilson MA (2002) Role of experience and oscillations in transforming a rate code into a temporal code. *Nature* **417**:741–746.

Mehta MR, Quirk MC, Wilson MA (2000) Experience-dependent asymmetric shape of hippocampal receptive fields. *Neuron* **25**:707–715.

Mensink GJ, Raaijmakers JG (1988) A model for interference and forgetting. *Psychol Rev* **95**:434–455.

Mhatre H, Gorchetchnikov A, Grossberg S (2012) Grid cell hexagonal patterns formed by fast self-organized learning within entorhinal cortex. *Hippocampus* **22**:320–334.

Milford MJ, Wyeth GF (2008) Mapping a suburb with a single camera using a biologically inspired SLAM system. *IEEE Trans Robotics* **24**(5):1038–1053.

Miller JF, Neufang M, Solway A, Brandt A, Trippel M, Mader I, Hefft S, Merkow M, Polyn SM, Jacobs J, et al. (2013) Neural activity in human hippocampal formation reveals the spatial context of retrieved memories. *Science* **342**:1111–1114.

Miller JF, Weidemann CT, Kahana MJ (2012) Recall termination in free recall. *Mem Cogn* **40**:540–550.

Milner AD, Dijkerman HC, Carey DP (1999) Visuospatial processing in a case of visual form agnosia. In: The Hippocampal and Parietal Foundations of Spatial Cognition (Burgess N, Jeffery KJ, O'Keefe J, eds), pp 443–466. Oxford: Oxford University Press.

Mnih V, Kavukcuoglu K, Silver D, Rusu AA, Veness J, Bellemare MG, et al. (2015) Human-level control through deep reinforcement learning. *Nature* **518**:529–533.

Moll M, Miikkulainen R (1997) Convergence-zone episodic memory: analysis and simulations. *Neural Netw* **10**:1017–1036.

Montague PR, Dayan P, Sejnowski TJ (1996) A framework for mesencephalic dopamine systems based on predictive Hebbian learning. *J Neurosci* **16**:1936–1947.

Morris RGM, Garrud P, Rawlins JN, O'Keefe J (1982) Place navigation impaired in rats with hippocampal lesions. *Nature* **297**:681–683.

Morton J, Hammersley RH, Bekerian DA (1985) Headed records: a model for memory and its failure. *Cognition* **20**:1–23.

Moskovitz T, Wilson SR, Sahani M (2021) A first-occupancy representation for reinforcement learning. *arXiv* 2109.13863.

Muessig L, Ribeiro Rodrigues F, Bjerknes TL, Towse BW, Barry C, Burgess N, Moser EI, Moser M-B, Cacucci F, Wills TJ (2024) Environment geometry alters subiculum boundary vector cell receptive fields in adulthood and early development. *Nat Commun* **15**:982.

Muller RU, Kubie JL (1987) The effects of changes in the environment on the spatial firing of hippocampal complex-spike cells. *J Neurosci* **7**:1951–1968.

Muller RU, Kubie J, Ranck JB (1987) Spatial firing patterns of hippocampal complex-spike cells in a fixed environment. *J Neurosci* **7**(7):1935–1950.

Muller RU, Kubie JL, Saypoff R (1991) The hippocampus as a cognitive graph (abridged version). *Hippocampus* **1**:243–246.

Muller RU, Stead M, Pach J (1996) The hippocampus as a cognitive graph. *J Gen Physiol* **107**:663–694.

Murray DJ, Pye C, Hockley WE (1976) Standing's power function in long-term memory. *Psychol Res* **38**:319–331.

Murray EA, Mishkin M (1998) Object recognition and location memory in monkeys with excitotoxic lesions of the amygdala and hippocampus. *J Neurosci* **18**:6568–6582.

Murre JM (1996) TraceLink: a model of amnesia and consolidation of memory. *Hippocampus* **6**:675–684.

Nadel L, Moscovitch M (1997) Memory consolidation, retrograde amnesia and the hippocampal complex. *Curr Opin Neurobiol* **7**:217–227.

Nakashiba T, Buhl DL, McHugh TJ, Tonegawa S (2009) Hippocampal CA3 output is crucial for ripple-associated reactivation and consolidation of memory. *Neuron* **62**:781–787.

Nakazawa K, Quirk MC, Chitwood RA, Watanabe M, Yeckel MF, Sun LD, Kato A, Carr CA, Johnston D, Wilson MA, et al. (2002) Requirement for hippocampal CA3 NMDA receptors in associative memory recall. *Science* **297**(5579):211–218.

Namboodiri VMK, Stuber GD (2021) The learning of prospective and retrospective cognitive maps within neural circuits. *Neuron* **109**(22):3552–3575.

Nau M, Navarro Schröder T, Bellmund JLS, Doeller CF (2018) Hexadirectional coding of visual space in human entorhinal cortex. *Nat Neurosci* 21:188–190.

Navratilova Z, Hoang LT, Schwindel CD, Tatsuno M, McNaughton BL (2012) Experience-dependent firing rate remapping generates directional selectivity in hippocampal place cells. *Front Neural Circuits* 6:6.

Navratilova Z, Giocomo LM, Fellous JM, Hasselmo ME, McNaughton BL (2012) Phase precession and variable spatial scaling in a periodic attractor map model of medial entorhinal grid cells with realistic after-spike dynamics. *Hippocampus* 22:772–789.

Nieh EH, Schottdorf M, Freeman NW, Low RJ, Lewallen S, Koay SA, Pinto L, Gauthier JL, Brody CD, Tank DW (2021) Geometry of abstract learned knowledge in the hippocampus. *Nature* 595(7865):80–84.

Niv Y (2019) Learning task-state representations. *Nat Neurosci* 22(10):1544–1553.

Norman KA, Detre G, Polyn SM (2008) Computational models of episodic memory. In: The Cambridge Handbook of Computational Psychology (Sun R, ed), pp 189–225 Cambridge, UK: Cambridge University Press.

Norman KA, O'Reilly RC (2003) Modeling hippocampal and neocortical contributions to recognition memory: a complementary-learning-systems approach. *Psychol Rev* 110:611–646.

Ocko SA, Hardcastle K, Giocomo LM, Ganguli S (2018) Emergent elasticity in the neural code for space. *PNAS* 115(50):11798–11806.

Oja E (1982) A simplified neuron model as a principal component analyzer. *J Math Biol* 15:267–273.

O'Keefe J, Burgess N (1996) Geometric determinants of the place fields of hippocampal neurons. *Nature* 381:425–428.

O'Keefe J, Burgess N (2005) Dual phase and rate coding in hippocampal place cells: theoretical significance and relationship to entorhinal grid cells. *Hippocampus* 15:853–866.

O'Keefe J, Conway DH (1978) Hippocampal place units in the freely moving rat: why they fire where they fire. *Exp Brain Res* 31:573–590.

O'Keefe J, Krupic J (2021) Do hippocampal pyramidal cells respond to nonspatial stimuli? *J Physiol* 101(3):1427–1456.

O'Keefe J, Nadel L (1978) The Hippocampus as a Cognitive Map. Oxford: Oxford University Press.

O'Keefe J, Recce ML (1993) Phase relationship between hippocampal place units and the EEG theta rhythm. *Hippocampus* 3:317–330.

O'Keefe J, Speakman A (1987) Single unit activity in the rat hippocampus during a spatial memory task. *Exp Brain Res* 68:1–27.

Ólafsdóttir HF, Barry C, Saleem AB, Hassabis D, Spiers HJ (2015) Hippocampal place cells construct reward related sequences through unexplored space. *eLife* 4:e06063.

Olafsdottir HF, Bush D, Barry C (2018) The role of hippocampal replay in memory and planning. *Curr Biol* 28:37–50.

Ólafsdóttir HF, Carpenter F, Barry C (2016) Coordinated grid and place cell replay during rest. *Nat Neurosci* 19(6):792–794.

Olson IR, Page K, Moore KS, Chatterjee A, Verfaellie M (2006) Working memory for conjunctions relies on the medial temporal lobe. *J Neurosci* 17:4596–4601.

O'Neill J, Boccara CN, Stella F, Schoenenberger P, Csicsvari J (2017) Superficial layers of the medial entorhinal cortex replay independently of the hippocampus. *Science* 355(6321):184–188.

Orchard J (2015) Oscillator-interference models of path integration do not require theta oscillations. *Neural Comput* 27(3):548–560.

Ormond J, O'Keefe J (2022) Hippocampal place cells have goal-oriented vector fields during navigation. *Nature* 607:741–746.

Packard MG, McGaugh JL (1996) Inactivation of hippocampus or caudate nucleus with lidocaine differentially affects expression of place and response learning. *Neurobiol Learn Mem* 65:65–72.

Page H, Wilson J, Jeffery KJ (2018) A dual-axis rule for updating the head direction cell reference frame during movement in three dimensions. *J Neurophysiol* 119(1):192–208.

Pastoll H, Solanka L, van Rossum MCW, Nolan MF (2013) Feedback inhibition enables theta-nested gamma oscillations and grid firing fields. *Neuron* 77:141–154.

Pavlides C, Greenstein YJ, Grudman M, Winson J (1988) Long-term potentiation in the dentate gyrus is induced preferentially on the positive phase of theta-rhythm. *Brain Res* 439(1–2):383–387.

Payne HL, Lynch GF, Aronov D (2021) Neural representations of space in the hippocampus of a food-caching bird. *Science* 373(6552):343–348.

Pérez-Escobar JA, Kornienko O, Latuske P, Kohler L, Allen K (2016) Visual landmarks sharpen grid cell metric and confer context specificity to neurons of the medial entorhinal cortex. *eLife* 5:e16937.

Pertzov Y, Miller TD, Gorgoraptis N, Caine D, Schott JM, Butler C, Husain M (2013) Binding deficits in memory following medial temporal lobe damage in patients with voltage-gated potassium channel complex antibody-associated limbic encephalitis. *Brain* 136(8):2474–2485.

Peyrache A, Lacroix MM, Petersen PC, Buzsáki G (2015) Internally organized mechanisms of the head direction sense. *Nat Neurosci* 18:569.

Piray P, Daw ND (2021) Linear reinforcement learning in planning, grid fields, and cognitive control. *Nat Commun* 12(1):4942.

Plitt MH, Giocomo LM (2021) Experience-dependent contextual codes in the hippocampus. *Nat Neurosci* 24(5):705–714.

Pouget A, Sejnowski TJ (1997) A new view of hemineglect based on the response properties of parietal neurones. *Philos Trans R Soc B* 352:1449–1459.

Pritzel A, Uria B, Srinivasan S, Puigdomènech A, Vinyals O, Hassabis D, Wierstra D, Blundell C (2017) Neural episodic control. *Proceedings of the 34th International Conference on Machine Learning, PMLR* 70:2827–2836.

Qasim SE, Fried I, Jacobs J (2021) Phase precession in the human hippocampus and entorhinal cortex. *Cell* 184(12):3242–3255.

Quiroga RQ (2012) Concept cells: the building blocks of declarative memory functions. *Nat Rev Neurosci* 13(8):587–597.

Quiroga RQ, Reddy L, Kreiman G, Koch C, Fried I (2005) Invariant visual representation by single neurons in the human brain. *Nature* 435(7045):1102–1107.

Raaijmakers JG, Shiffrin RM (1981) Search of associative memory. *Psychol Rev* 88:93–134.

Radulescu A, Shin YS, Niv Y (2021) Human representation learning. *Annu Rev Neurosci* 44:253–273.

Ratcliff R (1990) Connectionist models of recognition memory: constraints imposed by learning and forgetting functions. *Psychol Rev* 97:285–308.

Raudies F, Brandon MP, Chapman GW, Hasselmo ME (2015) Head direction is coded more strongly than movement direction in a population of entorhinal neurons. *Brain Res* 1621:355–67.

Rao RP, Ballard DH (1999) Predictive coding in the visual cortex: a functional interpretation of some extra-classical receptive-field effects. *Nat Neurosci* 2(1):79–87.

Recanatesi S, Farrell M, Lajoie G, Deneve S, Rigotti M, Shea-Brown E (2021) Predictive learning as a network mechanism for extracting low-dimensional latent space representations. *Nat Commun* 12(1):1–13.

Redish AD (1999) Beyond the Cognitive Map: From Place Cells to Episodic Memory. Cambridge, MA: MIT Press.

Redish AD (2016) Vicarious trial and error. *Nat Rev Neurosci* 17(3):147–159.

Redish AD, Elga AN, Touretzky DS (1996) A coupled attractor model of the rodent head direction system. *Netw: Comput Neural Syst* 7:671–685.

Redish AD, Rosenzweig ES, Bohanick JD, McNaughton BL, Barnes CA (2000) Dynamics of hippocampal ensemble activity realignment: time versus space. *J Neurosci* 20:9298–9309.

Redish AD, Touretzky DS (1998) The role of the hippocampus in solving the Morris water maze. *Neural Comput* 10:73–111.

Redondo R, Morris RGM (2011) Making memories last: the synaptic tagging and capture hypothesis. *Nat Rev Neurosci* 12:17–30.

Remme MW, Lengyel M, Gutkin BS (2010) Democracy-independence trade-off in oscillating dendrites and its implications for grid cells. *Neuron* 66(3):429–437.

Rennó-Costa C, Tort ABL (2017) Place and grid cells in a loop: implications for memory function and spatial coding. *J Neurosci* 37(34):8062–8076.

Rich PD, Liaw HP, Lee AK (2014) Place cells: large environments reveal the statistical structure governing hippocampal representations. *Science* 345(6198):814–817.

Robinson NT, Descamps LA, Russell LE, Buchholz MO, Bicknell BA, Antonov GK, et al. (2020) Targeted activation of hippocampal place cells drives memory-guided spatial behavior. *Cell* 183(6):1586–1599.

Rolls ET, Kesner RP (2006) A computational theory of hippocampal function, and empirical tests of the theory. *Prog Neurobiol* 79(1):1–48.

Rolls ET, Robertson RG, Georges-Francois P (1997) Spatial view cells in the primate hippocampus. *Eur J Neurosci* 9:1789–1794.

Rolls ET, Stringer SM, Elliot T (2006) Entorhinal cortex grid cells can map to hippocampal place cells by competitive learning. *Network* 17:447–465.

Rolls ET, Treves A (1997) Neural Networks and Brain Function. Oxford, UK: Oxford University Press.

Romani S, Pinkoviezky I, Rubin A, Tsodyks M (2013) Scaling laws of associative memory retrieval. *Neural Comput* 25(10):2523–2544.

Rosenbaum RS, Priselac S, Kohler S, Black SE, Gao F, Nadel L, Moscovitch M (2000) Remote spatial memory in an amnesic person with extensive bilateral hippocampal lesions. *Nat Neurosci* 3:1044–1048.

Royer S, Pare D (2003) Conservation of total synaptic weight through balanced synaptic depression and potentiation. *Nature* 422:518–522.

Rugg MD, Yonelinas AP (2003) Human recognition memory: a cognitive neuroscience perspective. *Trends Cogn Sci* 7:313–319.

Rumelhart DE, Hinton GE, Williams RJ (1986) Learning internal representations by error propagation. In: Parallel distributed programming: Vol 1. Foundations (Rumelhart DE, McClelland JL, eds), pp 318–364. Cambridge, MA, USA: MIT Press.

Rumelhart DE, McClelland JL (1986) Parallel Distributed Processing: Explorations in the Microstructure of Cognition: Vol I: Foundations. Cambridge, MA, USA: MIT Press.

Rumelhart DE, Zipser D (1986) Feature discovery by competitive learning. In: Parallel distributed programming: Vol 1. Foundations (Rumelhart DE, McClelland JL, eds), pp 151–193. MIT Press.

Samsonovich A, McNaughton BL (1997) Path integration and cognitive mapping in a continuous attractor neural network model. *J Neurosci* 17:5900–5920.

Sanders H, Wilson MA, Gershman SJ (2020) Hippocampal remapping as hidden state inference. *eLife* 9:e51140.

Sarel A, Finkelstein A, Las L, Ulanovsky N (2017) Vectorial representation of spatial goals in the hippocampus of bats. *Science* 355:176–180.

Sargolini F, Fyhn M, Hafting T, McNaughton BL, Witter MP, Moser MB, Moser EI (2006) Conjunctive representation of position, direction, and velocity in entorhinal cortex. *Science* 312:758–762.

Save E, Nerad L, Poucet B (2000) Contribution of multiple sensory information to place field stability in hippocampal place cells. *Hippocampus* 10:64–76.

Schacter DL, Addis DR (2007) The cognitive neuroscience of constructive memory: remembering the past and imagining the future. *Philos Trans R Soc B* 362(1481):773–786.

Schacter DL, Addis DR, Hassabis D, Martin VC, Spreng RN, Szpunar KK (2012) The future of memory: remembering, imagining, and the brain. *Neuron* 76:677–694.

Schapiro AC, Gregory E, Landau B, McCloskey M, Turk-Browne NB (2014) The necessity of the medial temporal lobe for statistical learning. *J Cogn Neurosci* 26(8):1736–1747.

Schapiro AC, McDevitt EA, Rogers TT, Mednick SC, Norman KA (2018) Human hippocampal replay during rest prioritizes weakly learned information and predicts memory performance. *Nat Commun* 9(1):3920.

Schapiro AC, Turk-Browne NB, Botvinick MM, Norman KA (2017) Complementary learning systems within the hippocampus: a neural network modelling approach to reconciling episodic memory with statistical learning. *Philos Trans R Soc B* 372(1711):20160049.

Schlesiger MI, Cannova CC, Boublil BL, Hales JB, Mankin EA, Brandon MP, Leutgeb JK, Leibold C, Leutgeb S (2015) The medial entorhinal cortex is necessary for temporal organization of hippocampal neuronal activity. *Nat Neurosci* 18(8):1123–1132.

Schmidt-Hieber C, Häusser M (2013) Cellular mechanisms of spatial navigation in the medial entorhinal cortex. *Nat Neurosci* 16:325–331.

Scholkopf B, Mallot HA (1995) View-based cognitive mapping and path planning. *Adapt Behav* 3:311–348.

Schreiner T, Staudigl T (2020) Electrophysiological signatures of memory reactivation in humans. *Philos Trans R Soc B* 375(1799):20190293.

Schultz W, Dayan P, Montague PR (1997) A neural substrate of prediction and reward. *Science* 275:1593–1599.

Scoville WB, Milner B (1957) Loss of recent memory after bilateral hippocampal lesions. *J Neurol Neurosurg Psychiatry* 20:11–21.

Seelig JD, Jayaraman V (2015) Neural dynamics for landmark orientation and angular path integration. *Nature* 521:186–191.

Sharp PE (1991) Computer simulation of hippocampal place cells. *Psychobiology* 19:103–115.

Sharp PE (1996) Multiple spatial/behavioral correlates for cells in the rat postsubiculum: multiple regression analysis and comparison to other hippocampal areas. *Cereb Cortex* 6:238–259.

Sharp PE, Blair HT, Brown M (1996) Neural network modeling of the hippocampal formation spatial signals and their possible role in navigation: a modular approach. *Hippocampus* 6:720–734.

Sherrill KR, Erdem UM, Ross RS, Brown TI, Hasselmo ME, Stern CE (2013) Hippocampus and retrosplenial cortex combine path integration signals for successful navigation. *J Neurosci* 33:19304–19313.

Shin H, Lee JK, Kim J, Kim J (2017) Continual learning with deep generative replay. *Adv Neural Inf Process Syst* 31:2994–3003.

Shipston-Sharman O, Solanka L, Nolan MF (2016) Continuous attractor network models of grid cell firing based on excitatory-inhibitory interactions. *J Physiol* 594(22):6547–6557.

Si B, Treves A (2013) A model for the differentiation between grid and conjunctive units in medial entorhinal cortex. *Hippocampus* 23(12):1410–1424.

Siapas AG, Wilson MA (1998) Coordinated interactions between hippocampal ripples and cortical spindles during slow-wave sleep. *Neuron* **21**(5):1123–1128.

Sirota A, Csicsvari J, Buhl D, Buzsáki G (2003) Communication between neocortex and hippocampus during sleep in rodents. *PNAS* **100**:2065–2069.

Skaggs WE, Knierim JJ, Kudrimoti H, McNaughton BL (1995) A model of the neural basis of the rat's sense of direction. In: Neural Information Processing Systems 7 (Hanson SJ, Cowan JD, Giles CL, eds), pp 173–180. Cambridge, MA, USA: MIT Press.

Skaggs WE, McNaughton BL (1998) Spatial firing properties of hippocampal CA1 populations in an environment containing two visually identical regions. *J Neurosci* **18**:8455–8466.

Skaggs WE, McNaughton BL (1996) Replay of neuronal firing sequences in rat hippocampus during sleep following spatial experience. *Science* **271**:1870–1873.

Skaggs WE, McNaughton BL, Wilson MA, Barnes CA (1996) Theta phase precession in hippocampal neuronal populations and the compression of temporal sequences. *Hippocampus* **6**:149–172.

Sloin HE, Spivak L, Levi A, Gattegno R, Someck S, Start E (2024) Local activation of CA1 pyramidal cells induces theta-phase precession. *Science* **383**(6682):551–558.

Solanka L, van Rossum MC, Nolan MF (2015) Noise promotes independent control of gamma oscillations and grid firing within recurrent attractor networks. *eLife* **4**:e06444.

Solomon PR, Vander Schaaf ER, Thompson RF, Weisz DJ (1986) Hippocampus and trace conditioning of the rabbit's classically conditioned nictitating membrane response. *Behav Neurosci* **100**(5):729–744.

Solstad T, Boccara CN, Kropff E, Moser MB, Moser EI (2008) Representation of geometric borders in the entorhinal cortex. *Science* **322**:1865–1868.

Solstad T, Moser EI, Einevoll GT (2006) From grid cells to place cells: a mathematical model. *Hippocampus* **16**:1026–1031.

Speakman A, O'Keefe J (1990) Hippocampal complex spike cells do not change their place fields if the goal is moved within a cue controlled environment. *Eur J Neurosci* **7**:544–555.

Spens E, Burgess N (2024) A generative model of memory construction and consolidation. *Nat Hum Behav.* **8**:526–543.

Spiers HJ, Maguire EA, Burgess N (2001) Hippocampal amnesia. *Neurocase* **7**:357–382.

Sprekeler H, Michaelis C, Wiskott L (2007) Slowness: an objective for spike-timing-dependent plasticity? *PLoS Comput Biol* **3**(6):e112.

Squire LR, Genzel L, Wixted JT, Morris RG (2015) Memory consolidation. *Cold Spring Harb Perspect Biol* **7**(8):a021766.

Squire LR, Stark CEL, Clark RE (2004) The medial temporal lobe. *Annu Rev Neurosci* **27**:279–306.

Squire LR, Wixted JT (2011) The cognitive neuroscience of human memory since HM. *Annu Rev Neurosci* **34**:259–288.

Squire LR, Zola SM (1998) Episodic memory, semantic memory, and amnesia. *Hippocampus* **8**:205–211.

Sreenivasan S, Fiete I (2011) Grid cells generate an analog error-correcting code for singularly precise neural computation. *Nat Neurosci* **14**:1330–1337.

Stachenfeld KL, Botvinick MM, Gershman SJ (2017) The hippocampus as a predictive map. *Nat Neurosci* **20**(11):1643–1653.

Staresina BP, Alink A, Kriegeskorte N, Henson RN (2013) Awake reactivation predicts memory in humans. *PNAS* **110**(52):21159–21164.

Steemers B, Vicente-Grabovetsky A, Barry C, Smulders P, Schröder TN, Burgess N, Doeller CF (2016) Hippocampal attractor dynamics predict memory-based decision making. *Curr Biol* **26**(13):1750–1757.

Stemmler M, Mathis A, Herz AV (2015) Connecting multiple spatial scales to decode the population activity of grid cells. *Sci Adv* **1**(11):e1500816.

Stensola H, Stensola T, Solstad T, Frøland K, Moser MB, Moser EI (2012) The entorhinal grid map is discretized. *Nature* **492**:72–78.

Stoianov I, Maisto D, Pezzulo G (2022) The hippocampal formation as a hierarchical generative model supporting generative replay and continual learning. *Prog Neurobiol* **217**:102329.

Sun C, Yang W, Martin J, Tonegawa S (2020) Hippocampal neurons represent events as transferable units of experience. *Nat Neurosci* **23**(5):651–663.

Sun W, Advani M, Spruston N, Saxe A, Fitzgerald JE (2023) Organizing memories for generalization in complementary learning systems. *Nat Neurosci* **26**:1438–1448.

Sutton MA, Schuman EM (2006) Dendritic protein synthesis, synaptic plasticity, and memory. *Cell* **127**(1):49–58.

Sutton RS, Barto AG (1988) Reinforcement Learning: An Introduction. Cambridge, MA, USA: MIT Press.

Taube JS (1998) Head direction cells and the neuropsychological basis for a sense of direction. *Prog Neurobiol* **55**:225–256.

Taube JS, Muller RU (1998) Comparisons of head direction cell activity in the postsubiculum and anterior thalamus of freely moving rats. *Hippocampus* **8**:87–108.

Taube JS, Muller RU, Ranck JB, Jr (1990) Head-direction cells recorded from the postsubiculum in freely moving rats: II. Effects of environmental manipulations. *J Neurosci* **10**:436–447.

Teng E, Squire LR (1999) Memory for places learned long ago is intact after hippocampal damage. *Nature* **400**:675–677.

Teyler TJ, DiScenna P (1986) The hippocampal memory indexing theory. *Behav Neurosci* **100**:147–154.

Todorov E (2007) Linearly-solvable Markov decision problems. *Adv Neural Inf Process Syst* **19**:1369–1376.

Tolman EC (1948) Cognitive maps in rats and men. *Psychol Rev* **55**:189–208.

Touretzky DS, Redish AD (1996) Theory of rodent navigation based on interacting representations of space. *Hippocampus* **6**:247–270.

Trappenberg T (2002) Fundamentals of Computational Neuroscience. Oxford, UK: Oxford University Press.

Trettel SG, Trimper JB, Hwaun E, Fiete IR, Colgin LL (2019) Grid cell co-activity patterns during sleep reflect spatial overlap of grid fields during active behaviors. *Nat Neurosci* **22**:609–617.

Treves A, Rolls ET (1992) Computational constraints suggest the need for two distinct input systems to the hippocampal CA3 network. *Hippocampus* **2**:189–199.

Trullier O, Wiener SI, Berthoz A, Meyer JA (1997) Biologically based artificial navigation systems: review and prospects. *Prog Neurobiol* **51**:483–544.

Tse D, Langston RF, Kakeyama M, Bethus I, Spooner PA, Wood ER, et al. (2007) Schemas and memory consolidation. *Science* **316**:76–82.

Tse D, Takeuchi T, Kakeyma M, Kajii Y, Okuno H, Tohyama C, Bito H, Morris RGM (2011) Schema-dependent gene activation and memory encoding in neocortex. *Science* **333**:891–895.

Tsodyks MV, Skaggs WE, Sejnowski TJ, McNaughton BL (1996) Population dynamics and theta rhythm phase precession of hippocampal place cell firing: a spiking neuron model. *Hippocampus* **6**:271–280.

Tulving E (1993) What is episodic memory? *Curr Perspect Psychol Sci* **2**:67–70.

Turner-Evans D, Wegener S, Rouault H, Franconville R, Wolff T, Seelig JD, Druckmann S, Jayaraman V (2017) Angular velocity integration in a fly heading circuit. *eLife* **6**:e23496.

Ulanovsky N, Moss CF (2007) Hippocampal cellular and network activity in freely moving echolocating bats. *Nat Neurosci* 10(2):224–233.

Umbach G, Kantak P, Jacobs J, Kahana M, Pfeiffer BE, Sperling M, Lega B (2020) Time cells in the human hippocampus and entorhinal cortex support episodic memory. *PNAS* 117(45):28463–28474.

Uria B, Ibarz B, Banino A, Zambaldi V, Kumaran D, Hassabis D, Barry C, Blundell C (2020) The spatial memory pipeline: a model of egocentric to allocentric understanding in mammalian brains. *bioRxiv* 2020:11.

Vanderwolf CH (1969) Hippocampal electrical activity and voluntary movement in the rat. *EEG Clin Neurophysiol* 26:407–418.

van de Ven GM, Siegelmann HT, Tolias AS (2020) Brain-inspired replay for continual learning with artificial neural networks. *Nat Commun* 11:4069.

Vargha-Khadem F, Gadian DG, Watkins KE, Connelly A, Van Paesschen W, Mishkin M (1997) Differential effects of early hippocampal pathology on episodic and semantic memory. *Science* 277:376–380.

Vikbladh OM, Meager MR, King J, Blackmon K, Devinsky O, Shohamy D, Burgess N, Daw ND (2019) Hippocampal contributions to model-based planning and spatial memory. *Neuron* 102(3):683–693.

Wallenstein GV, Eichenbaum H, Hasselmo ME (1998) The hippocampus as an associator of discontiguous events. *Trends Neurosci* 21:317–323.

Wallenstein GV, Hasselmo ME (1997) GABAergic modulation of hippocampal population activity: sequence learning, place field development, and the phase precession effect. *J Neurophysiol* 78:393–408.

Wan H, Aggleton JP, Brown MW (1999) Different contributions of the hippocampus and perirhinal cortex to recognition memory. *J Neurosci* 19:1142–1148.

Wan HS, Touretzky DS, Redish AD (1994) Towards a computational theory of rat navigation. *Proceedings of the 1993 Connectionist Models Summer School* 11–19.

Wang C, Chen X, Lee H, Deshmukh SS, Yoganarasimha D, Savelli F, Knierim JJ (2018) Egocentric coding of external items in the lateral entorhinal cortex. *Science* 362:945–949.

Watrous AJ, Lee DJ, Izadi A, Gurkoff GG, Shahlaie K, Ekstrom AD (2013) A comparative study of human and rat hippocampal low-frequency oscillations during spatial navigation. *Hippocampus* 23(8):656–661.

Wayne G, Hung CC, Amos D, Mirza M, Ahuja A, Grabska-Barwinska A, et al. (2018) Unsupervised predictive memory in a goal-directed agent. *arXiv* 1803.10760.

Weber SN, Sprekeler H (2018) Learning place cells, grid cells and invariances with excitatory and inhibitory plasticity. *eLife* 7:e34560.

Welday AC, Shlifer IG, Bloom ML, Zhang K, Blair HT (2011) Cosine directional tuning of theta cell burst frequencies: evidence for spatial coding by oscillatory interference. *J Neurosci* 31:16157–16176.

Whittington JCR, Muller TH, Mark S, Chen G, Barry C, Burgess N, Behrens TEJ (2020) The Tolman-Eichenbaum machine: unifying space and relational memory through generalization in the hippocampal formation. *Cell* 183(5):1249–1263.

Whittington JCR, McCaffary D, Bakermans JJW, Behrens TEJ (2022) How to build a cognitive map. *Nat Neurosci* 25(10):1257–1272.

Widlowski J, Foster DJ (2022) Flexible rerouting of hippocampal replay sequences around changing barriers in the absence of global place field remapping. *Neuron* 110:1547–1558.

Wikenheiser AM, Redish AD (2015) Hippocampal theta sequences reflect current goals. *Nat Neurosci* 18:289–294.

Wilkie DM, Palfrey R (1987) A computer simulation model of rat's place navigation in the Morris water maze. *Behav Res Meth Instrum Comput* 19:400–403.

Wills T, Lever C, Cacucci F, Burgess N, O'Keefe J (2005) Attractor dynamics in the hippocampal representation of the local environment. *Science* 308:873–876.

Wills TJ, Cacucci F, Burgess N, O'Keefe J (2010) Development of the hippocampal cognitive map in pre-weanling rats. *Science* 328:1573–1576.

Willshaw DJ, Buckingham JT (1990) An assessment of Marr's theory of the hippocampus as a temporary memory store. *Philos Trans R Soc B* 329:205–215.

Willshaw DJ, Buneman OP, Longuet-Higgins HC (1969) Non-holographic associative memory. *Nature* 222:960–962.

Wilson MA, McNaughton BL (1993) Dynamics of the hippocampal ensemble code for space. *Science* 261:1055–1058.

Wilson MA, McNaughton BL (1994) Reactivation of hippocampal ensemble memories during sleep. *Science* 265:676–679.

Winocur G, Moscovitch M, Bontempi JB (2010) Memory formation and long-term retention in humans and animals: convergence towards a transformation account of hippocampal-neocortical interactions. *Neuropsychologia* 48:2339–2356.

Winter SS, Mehlman ML, Clark BJ, Taube JS (2015) Passive transport disrupts grid signals in the parahippocampal cortex. *Curr Biol* 25(19):2493–2502.

Wiskott L, Sejnowski TJ (2002) Slow feature analysis: unsupervised learning of invariances. *Neural Comput* 14(4):715–770.

Wood ER, Dudchenko PA, Robitsek RJ, Eichenbaum H (2000) Hippocampal neurons encode information about different types of memory episodes occurring in the same location. *Neuron* 27(3):623–633.

Yartsev MM, Ulanovsky N (2013) Representation of three-dimensional space in the hippocampus of flying bats. *Science* 340:367–372.

Yartsev MM, Witter MP, Ulanovsky N (2011) Grid cells without theta oscillations in the entorhinal cortex of bats. *Nature* 479:103–107.

Yonelinas AP (2002) The nature of recollection and familiarity: a review of 30 years of research. *J Mem Lang* 46:441–517.

Yonelinas AP, Kroll NE, Quamme JR, Lazzara MM, Sauve MJ, Widaman KF, Knight RT (2002) Effects of extensive temporal lobe damage or mild hypoxia on recollection and familiarity. *Nat Neurosci* 5:1236–1241.

Yoon K, Buice MA, Barry C, Hayman R, Burgess N, Fiete IR (2013) Specific evidence of low-dimensional continuous attractor dynamics in grid cells. *Nat Neurosci* 16:1077–1084.

Yu C, Behrens TEJ, Burgess N (2020) Prediction and generalisation over directed actions by grid cells. *arXiv* 2006.03355.

Zeithamova D, Dominick AL, Preston AR (2012) Hippocampal and ventral medial prefrontal activation during retrieval-mediated learning supports novel inference. *Neuron* 75(1):168–179.

Zemel RS, Dayan P, Pouget A (1998) Probabilistic interpretation of population codes. *Neural Comput* 10(2):403–430.

Zhang K (1996) Representation of spatial orientation by the intrinsic dynamics of the head-direction cell ensemble: a theory. *J Neurosci* 16:2112–2126.

Zhu XO, McCabe BJ, Aggleton JP, Brown MW (1996) Mapping visual recognition memory through expression of the immediate early gene c-fos. *Neuroreport* 7:1871–1875.

Zilli EA, Hasselmo ME (2008) Analyses of Markov decision process structure regarding the possible strategic use of interacting memory systems. *Front Comput Neurosci* 2:6.

Zipser D (1985) A computational model of hippocampal place fields. *Behav Neurosci* **99**:1006–1018.

Zipser D (1986) Place recognition. In: Parallel Distributed Programming: Vol 2. Psychological and Biological Models (McClelland JL, Rumelhart DE, eds), pp 432–470. Cambridge, MA, USA: MIT Press.

Ziv Y, Burns LD, Cocker ED, Hamel EO, Ghosh KK, Kitch LJ, El Gamal A, Schnitzer MJ (2013) Long-term dynamics of CA1 hippocampal place codes. *Nat Neurosci* **16**(3):264–266.

Zola SM, Squire LR, Teng E, Stefanacci L, Buffalo EA, Clark RE (2000) Impaired recognition memory in monkeys after damage limited to the hippocampal region. *J Neurosci* **20**:451–463.

Zola-Morgan S, Squire LR, Ramus SJ (1994) Severity of memory impairment in monkeys as a function of locus and extent of damage within the medial temporal lobe memory system. *Hippocampus* **4**:483–495.

Zugaro MB, Monconduit L, Buzsáki G (2005) Spike phase precession persists after transient intrahippocampal perturbation. *Nat Neurosci* **8**:67–71.

17

Stress and the Hippocampus

Bruce S. McEwen and Sumantra Chattarji

17.1 Overview

The other chapters in this book cover hippocampal function across biological scales. Together these chapters reflect a powerful intellectual and methodological framework for studying the circuit, synaptic, and molecular basis of normal and pathological hippocampal function across levels of neural organization. However, there are other aspects to be considered, in particular how the brain and body interact with each other. It was the discovery of stress hormone receptors in the hippocampus (McEwen et al., 1968) that provided a gateway into recognition of ongoing structural and functional plasticity of the developing, adult, and aging brain regulated in part, by systemic factors, including sex and metabolic hormones and immune system mediators.

Diseases that affect hippocampal function such as depression and Type 2 diabetes, in turn, have provided a way of testing this brain-body framework. Furthermore, the same framework has been utilized for studies of other brain areas that interact with the hippocampus in the context of stress effects on the brain, such as the amygdala and prefrontal cortex. This chapter describes major findings that have given rise to a body of work that highlights the role of epigenetics in shaping individual characteristics and determining the trajectory of an animal's life course. These investigations have broadened the definition of stress and the biological processes that are involved. This includes the reciprocal interactions between brain and body and the many humoral mediators in addition to cortisol. It also includes acknowledging the constraining influences of the physical and social environment, and how our resulting life experiences epigenetically determine who we are by shaping both brain and body. Out of this is emerging a concept of "brain health".

The story began with the discovery of glucocorticoid and mineralocorticoid receptors (Reul and De Kloet, 1985) in the hippocampal formation of rodents and, later, rhesus monkeys. Along this path of discovery, additional influences of sex and metabolic hormones were discovered in the hippocampus and other brain regions. This work also reveals cellular and molecular mechanisms involving multiple comediators in the brain, and cooperation between events at the cell surface, and signaling to and from the cell nucleus. Together, these mediate structural as well as functional remodeling not only of hippocampus but also of other interacting brain regions as a result of stressful and other experiences. In turn, the remodeling and changing interactions of circuits within the brain alters its output via neuroendocrine, autonomic, metabolic, and immune systems, as well as health-promoting and health-damaging behaviors. In summarizing these advances, we shall describe key findings and formulation of influential concepts, as much as possible, in a chronological order (Figure 17.1), although many of the branches of this story emerged at the same time. This information, largely garnered from studies of animal models, is being echoed in findings on the human brain, with respect not only to mental and neurological disorders but also to the impact on the brain of systemic diseases such as Type 2 diabetes and to the understanding of how health-promoting behaviors such as physical activity and sleep benefit the brain and its interactions with the body. (See list of Milestone Papers at the end of this chapter for further reading, cited in Figure 17.1.)

17.2 Introduction

The fundamental discovery of the communication between hypothalamus and pituitary by Geoffrey Harris established the basis for understanding brain–body communication via the neuroendocrine system (Harris, 1970). Since the discovery of releasing factors in the hypothalamus that lead to the release of pituitary hormones and subsequent release of steroid hormones from the adrenals (e.g., Guillemin, 1978; Schally et al., 1973; Vale et al., 1981), the field of neuroendocrinology has flourished. At the same time, steroid hormones were shown to bind to intracellular receptors that regulate gene expression in tissues such as liver, or the prostate and uterus in the case of sex hormones (Jensen and Jacobson, 1962).

The recognition of the role of steroids in brain function began in the late 1960s with the serendipitous discovery of adrenal steroid, and, later, estrogen receptors, in the hippocampal formation of the rat (Gerlach and McEwen, 1972; Loy et al., 1988; McEwen and Plapinger, 1970; McEwen et al., 1968; Milner et al., 2001) using injections of tritium-labeled steroids into adrenalectomized or gonadectomized animals, followed by cell fractionation, and steroid autoradiography on brain sections (Figure 17.2). These findings were extended to the infrahuman primate brain (Gerlach et al., 1976; Figure 17.1) and to other regions of the brain involved in cognitive and emotional regulation, as will be described below.

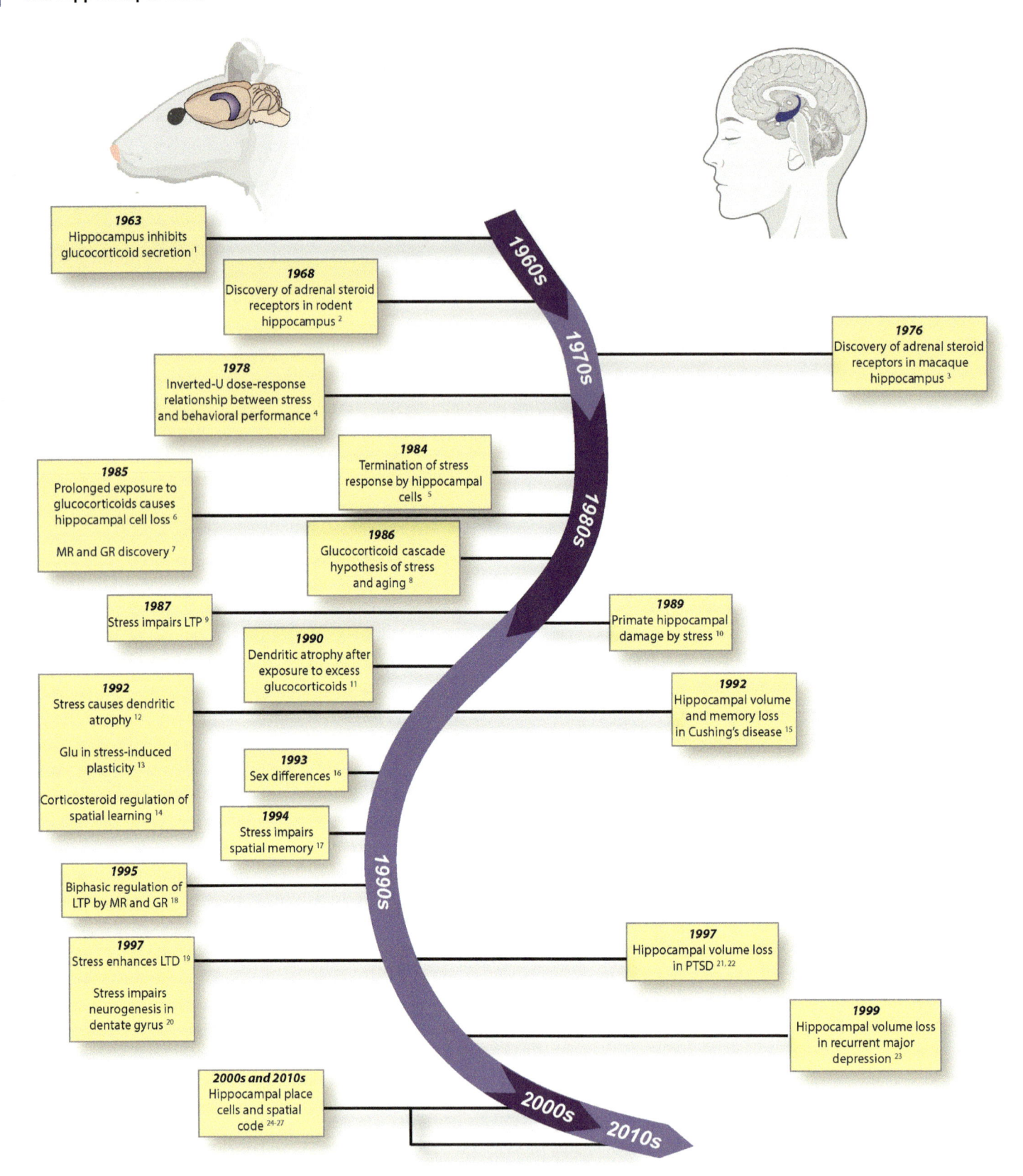

Figure 17.1 Timeline of key findings on the effects of stress on the hippocampus and hippocampal regulation of the stress response. Important findings in this field have emerged from animal models (*left*), as well as studies in humans and primates (*right*). Thus, both basic and clinical research coevolved over several decades giving rise to a powerful intellectual and methodological framework of analyses spanning multiple levels of neural organization from behavior to cells and molecules. Due to space constraints, only a few of the early papers in each area of investigation are listed here in chronological order. Notably, each of these reports subsequently paved the way for a series of important studies; these are discussed in the text and listed at the end of the chapter (Milestone papers), just before the References.

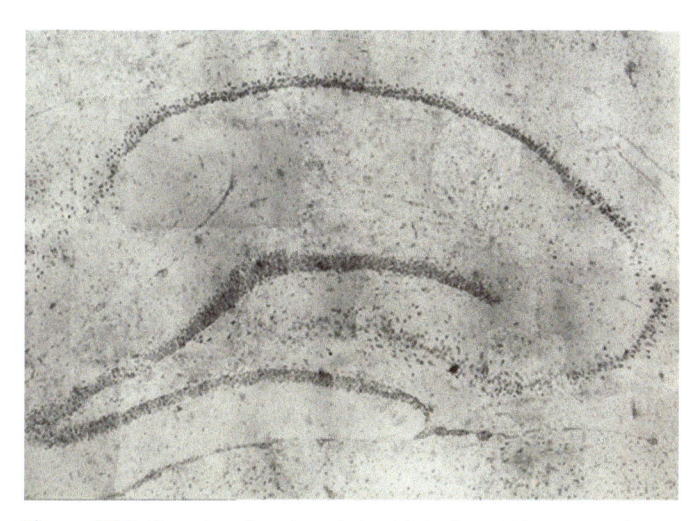

Figure 17.2 Receptors for adrenal steroids in the rat hippocampal formation. Autoradiogram shows uptake and retention of 3H-corticosterone by principal neurons of Ammon's horn and dentate gyrus of bilaterally adrenalectomized, adult rats (adapted from Gerlach and McEwen, 1972). Interestingly, the original image was constructed from individual photos by Louis Koster with methods used in aerial photography before the advent of satellites.

At that time, the focus of steroid hormone feedback to regulate neuroendocrine function was mainly on the pituitary and the hypothalamus, and this approach continued to uncover important aspects of neuroendocrine regulation (Meites, 1992). Yet, clinical observations on war veterans suffering from stress-related psychiatric disorders, such as PTSD, anxiety disorders, and depression (Mason, 1975; Sachar et al., 1973), revealed stress effects that impacted both behavior and systemic physiology. At that time, hormones were thought to affect a range of physiological functions, but little was known about potential effects on the brain until these observations on veterans brought the question into focus. The discovery of glucocorticoid receptors in the hippocampus bridged this gap, providing a gateway for studying the effects of stress and stress hormones on the hippocampus and paving the way for studies of the actions of sex and metabolic hormones on hippocampal function. This has catalyzed studies that look at actions of hormonal feedback on the brain, not only to regulate hypothalamic functions but also to influence neurological, cognitive, and emotional functions of the whole brain. Animal studies have led to insights into human brain function, in relation to aging, anxiety, mood disorders, PTSD, and the impact of the social environment, as will be discussed later in this chapter. We now describe some of the outcomes of these initial findings.

17.3. What is stress? Adaptation, allostasis and allostatic load, and damage

17.3.1 Glucocorticoids and damage

Regarding functional implications of the discovery of stress hormones in hippocampus, the initial focus was on damaging effects of glucocorticoids after stress and in aging. These detrimental effects include a loss of hippocampal CA3 neurons, neuronal corticosterone receptors and glial hyperplasia in rodents, and reduction of hippocampal volume in human subjects (Landfield et al., 1978;

Lupien et al., 1998; Sapolsky et al., 1983; Sapolsky et al., 1984; Sapolsky et al., 1985; Sapolsky et al., 1986a) as well as ischemic damage (Sapolsky and Pulsinelli, 1985) and seizures (Smith-Swintosky et al., 1996) via NMDA receptors (Armanini et al., 1990). The glucocorticoid cascade hypothesis (Figure 17.3) of stress and aging was an important conceptual contribution to understanding the negative impact of chronic stress on the aging process itself (Sapolsky et al., 1986a). According to this influential hypothesis, two key components—the cumulative impact of corticosterone in the hippocampus along with hippocampal regulation of corticosterone secretion—together create a feedforward cascade of degeneration with stress and age. These ideas were transferred to the effects of stress on the human brain (Lupien et al., 1998) as discussed further below (McEwen, 1998; McEwen and Stellar, 1993). The concepts of allostasis and allostatic load (Figure 17.4) that look across the life course at both the beneficial and deleterious actions of mediators of adaptation in which the brain is the central organ and communicates reciprocally with the body broadens the concept of "stress" to experiences in general (Figure 17.4).

17.3.2 What is stress?

Stress is an ambiguous word—good stress, tolerable stress, toxic stress—have different meanings, with the second two implying that stress is, to different degrees, out of control; in toxic stress lack of control leads more quickly to disease. Many experiences that affect stress levels are not conventionally called "stressful", including experiences like jet lag, shift work that perturbs circadian variation, loneliness, or living in an environment devoid of green space (Bowles et al., 2017; Cacioppo et al., 2011; Cho, 2001a; Cole et al., 2007; Evans et al., 2005; Kondo et al., 2018; Layden et al., 2017; Reynolds et al., 2017). A broader and more inclusive concept is that of "allostasis" and "allostatic load and overload" in which the mediators that promote adaptation (neuroendocrine, autonomic, metabolic, and immune) can also cause cumulative change (e.g., obesity) or pathophysiology (e.g., diabetes, cardiovascular disease) when they are overused and/or dysregulated both within and between each category (McEwen, 1998; McEwen and Stellar, 1993) (Figure 17.4). Damaging health behaviors resulting from daily experiences, like sleep deprivation, lack of exercise, comfort food, alcohol, smoking, contribute to allostatic load/overload and health-promoting behaviors can reduce the load.

Figure 17.5 depicts how patterns of response of stress mediators (e.g., cortisol or inflammatory cytokines) can lead to allostatic load.

The most efficient and effective response is to turn on the response when needed and turn it off when the stressor is over. Accumulating evidence from animal studies have characterized how the severity and duration of stressors leads to damaging or adaptive alterations in the hippocampus. Importantly, these stress effects are accompanied by a range of structural and functional changes across biological scales in the hippocampus, which are described in the following sections.

17.4 Neuronal correlates of stress: morphological and electrophysiological changes

Investigations into cellular mechanisms underlying stress-induced alterations have focused largely on two common metrics of hippocampal plasticity—one structural, and the other

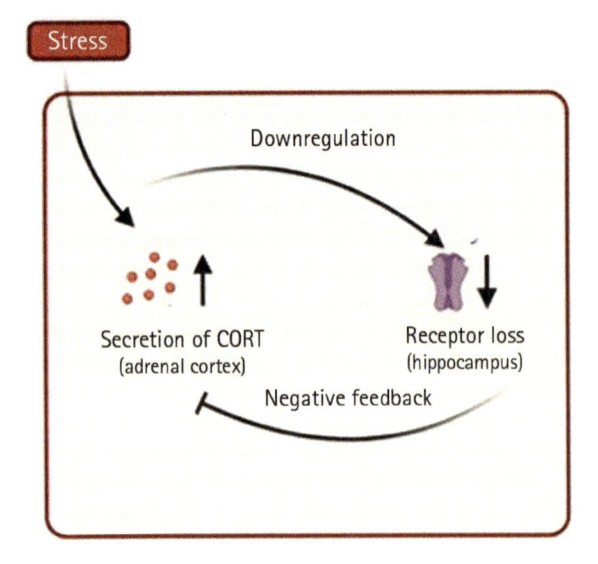

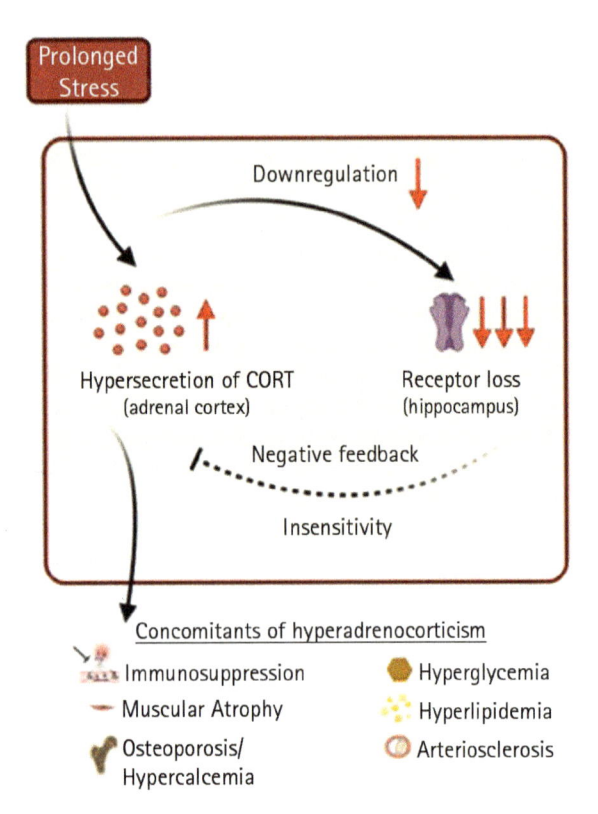

Concomitants of hyperadrenocorticism

- Immunosuppression
- Muscular Atrophy
- Osteoporosis/ Hypercalcemia
- Hyperglycemia
- Hyperlipidemia
- Arteriosclerosis

Figure 17.3 The glucocorticoid cascade hypothesis. The glucocorticoid cascade hypothesis, proposed in 1986 by Sapolsky and colleagues (Sapolsky et al., 1986a), provided a conceptual framework for understanding how glucocorticoids dynamically modulate hippocampal function with aging. This influential hypothesis proposed that two key components—the cumulative impact of corticosterone in the hippocampus along with hippocampal regulation of corticosterone secretion—together create a feedforward cascade of degeneration with age. (*Top*) Stress-induced hypersecretion of glucocorticoids leads to a downregulation of the number of glucocorticoid receptors in hippocampal neurons. Importantly, this process is self-correcting such that the loss of receptors is reversed when the stress and corticosterone hypersecretion ends. (*Bottom*) However, under conditions of prolonged and severe stress, this same adaptive feedback mechanism can become maladaptive when the downregulation of glucocorticoid receptors reaches sufficiently low levels. This impairs hippocampal feedback inhibition of the adrenocortical axis, resulting in further hypersecretion

electrophysiological. Here, we first describe the morphological changes triggered by various animal models of stress. This is followed by an overview of key findings emerging from electrophysiological analyses of stress-induced plasticity. A wide variety of rodent models of physical and psychosocial stressors have been used in these studies (see Box 17.1 for a summary).

17.4.1 Dendritic remodeling

At the time when the glucocorticoid cascade hypothesis was introduced as a progression toward damage (Sapolsky et al., 1986), alterations of neuronal structure were then thought of as "damage" (Uno et al., 1989). Indeed, chronic glucocorticoid administration to adult rats led to "neuronal atrophy" in the hippocampus (Sapolsky et al., 1990; Woolley et al., 1990) (Figure 17.6). Moreover, repeated restraint stress also caused apical dendrites of hippocampal CA3 neurons to become shorter and less branched, although basal dendrites did not change (Watanabe, Gould, and McEwen, 1992) (Figure 17.6). Another form of stress involving chronic immobilization, however, led to significant atrophy in both apical and basal dendrites of CA3 pyramidal cells (Vyas et al., 2002; Figure 17.6).

Further, the stress and glucocorticoid effects could be blocked by the anticonvulsant phenytoin (Watanabe, Gould, Cameron, et al., 1992; Figure 17.7) and by NMDA receptor antagonists (Magarinos and McEwen, 1995), indicating involvement of excitatory amino acids. However, a subsequent study (Conrad et al., 1999) reported recovery of dendrite shrinkage after termination of stress, indicating that this was not "brain damage" but a "reversible" shrinkage of the cytoskeleton. This led to call such changes being labeled as "remodeling" or "adaptive plasticity," which is likely to be protective, since later studies showed that long CA3 dendrites make the hippocampus more vulnerable to seizure damage (McCall et al., 2013).

Of relevance to this notion of "reversibility" is that watermaze training promotes recovery from stress-induced dendritic shrinkage after 2–3 days (Sandi et al., 2003). Moreover, studies on hibernating European hamsters revealed shorter apical dendritic trees of CA3 principal neurons with fewer branches and spines in hypothermic hamsters compared with active animals. Notably, these were rapid adaptive morphological changes wherein the apical dendritic lengths, branching patterns, and spine density returned to levels found in active, euthermic hamsters within 2 hours of arousal from torpor (Magarinos et al., 2006). The rapidity of these changes also pointed to cellular mechanisms involving cytoskeletal depolymerization and a role for a soluble phosphorylated form of tau (Arendt et al., 2003). Interestingly, in a study using the visible burrow system, both subordinate and dominant rats exhibited CA3 dendritic atrophy compared with unstressed controls (McKittrick et al., 2000). The similarity of the changes in dendritic arborization between both groups of animals, despite apparent differences

of corticosterone. This, in turn, precipitates further loss of receptors and even greater secretion of corticosterone, leading to permanent loss of hippocampal neurons. This downward spiral, according to the glucocorticoid cascade hypothesis, makes the hippocampus insensitive to further elevations in glucocorticoid levels. Consequently, this creates a runaway feedforward cycle of elevated glucocorticoids and irreversible hippocampal damage that is exacerbated by age. This degenerative cascade has been suggested to have a range of pathophysiological consequences in the brain and other organs, such as depression and Cushing's disease, steroid diabetes, muscle atrophy, arteriosclerosis, etc.

Box 17.1 Commonly used rodent models of stress

(A) Several stress procedures (acute stressors, blue; chronic stressors, red) have been used to study the effects of stress on neural plasticity in rodents. Widely used physical stressors include repeated exposure to immobilization and restraint stress. In contrast, a range of naturalistic or ethologically relevant stressors have also been used to trigger innate fear. These commonly used models of psychosocial stress include predator odor and exposure to bright elevated platform, as well as maternal separation and social defeat. (B) The examples depicted in (A) are part of a wider range of rodent models that have been widely used to examine the effects of stress on hippocampal structure and function. The unpredictable stress model (bottom) involves exposing rodents to multiple stressors across different episodes, often in random order. (Adapted from Chattarji et al., 2015; Tomar and McHugh, 2022)

in stressor severity, suggests that these alterations may be part of the normal adaptive response to chronic social stress. Some of the mediators of stress-induced neuronal remodeling, including some of the interactions from the cell surface to the cell nucleus, are described in Table 17.1.

The alterations in CA3 apical dendritic morphology after chronic stress are associated with changes in the mossy fiber projection from the dentate gyrus, which terminates on large dendritic spines, the so-called thorny excrescences, of stratum lucidum. Three-dimensional reconstructions of electron microscope images revealed retraction of thorny excrescences after chronic restraint stress, which was reversed after watermaze training (Stewart et al., 2005). Further, watermaze training alone enhances thorny excrescence volume as well as the number of thorns per thorny excrescence. In restrained rats that received watermaze training, a significant increase in postsynaptic density (PSD) volume and surface area was observed. Also, the proportion of perforated PSDs almost doubled after watermaze training and restraint stress. A related electron microscopic study of the glutamatergic mossy fiber terminals showed that, whereas terminals of control rats were packed with small, clear synaptic vesicles, terminals from stressed animals showed a marked rearrangement of vesicles, with more densely

packed clusters localized in the vicinity of active zones (Magarinos et al., 1997). Moreover, compared with controls, chronic restraint stress increased the area of the mossy fiber terminal occupied by mitochondrial profiles, reflecting what may be a larger, localized energy-generating capacity. A single stress session did not produce these changes either immediately after or the next day following the restraint session (Magarinos et al., 1997). The importance of excitatory amino acids in dendrite and synapse remodeling will be discussed further below.

17.4.2 Stress and neurogenesis in the dentate gyrus

Studies of the songbird brain showed that neurogenesis continues in adulthood (Nottebohm, 2002; Paton and Nottebohm, 1984) and raised the possibility that the same might be true in the mammalian brain. The work of Altman (Altman and Bayer, 1990a, 1990b), followed by that of Kaplan (Kaplan, 2001; Kaplan and Hinds, 1977), provided clues that this was indeed the case, at least in the hippocampus. A report that adrenalectomy caused extensive loss of neurons in the dentate gyrus (Sloviter et al., 1989) led to the discovery of naturally occurring cell death in the developing dentate gyrus (Gould, Wooley, and McEwen, 1991b) and then to the rediscovery of neurogenesis by Gould and Cameron (Gould,

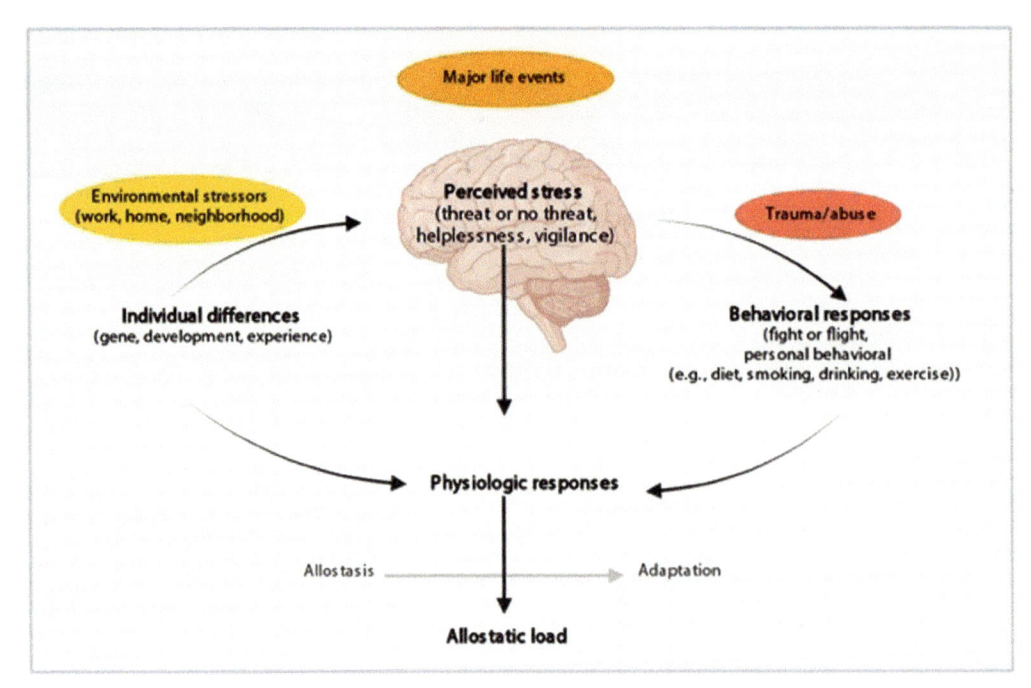

Figure 17.4 The stress response and development of allostatic load. The perception of stress is influenced by one's experiences, genetics, and behavior. When the brain perceives an experience as stressful, physiologic and behavioral responses are initiated, leading to adaptation and allostasis—the ability to achieve stability through change. The price of this accommodation to stress can lead to allostatic load, which is the wear and tear that results from chronic overactivity of allostatic systems. Over time, allostatic load can accumulate, and the overexposure to mediators of neural, endocrine, and immune stress can have adverse effects on various organ systems, leading to disease. Stressful experiences include major life events, trauma, and abuse and are sometimes related to the environment in the home, workplace, or neighborhood. Acute stress (in the sense of "fight or flight" or major life events) and chronic stress (the cumulative load of minor, day-to-day stresses) can both have long-term consequences. Two factors largely determine individual responses to potentially stressful situations: the way a person perceives a situation and a person's general state of physical health, which is determined not only by genetic factors but also by behavioral and lifestyle choices. Whether one perceives a situation as a threat, either psychological or physical, is crucial in determining the behavioral response—whether it is fleeing, fighting, or cowering in fear—and the physiologic response – calmness or heart palpitations and elevated cortisol levels. (Adapted from McEwen, 1998.)

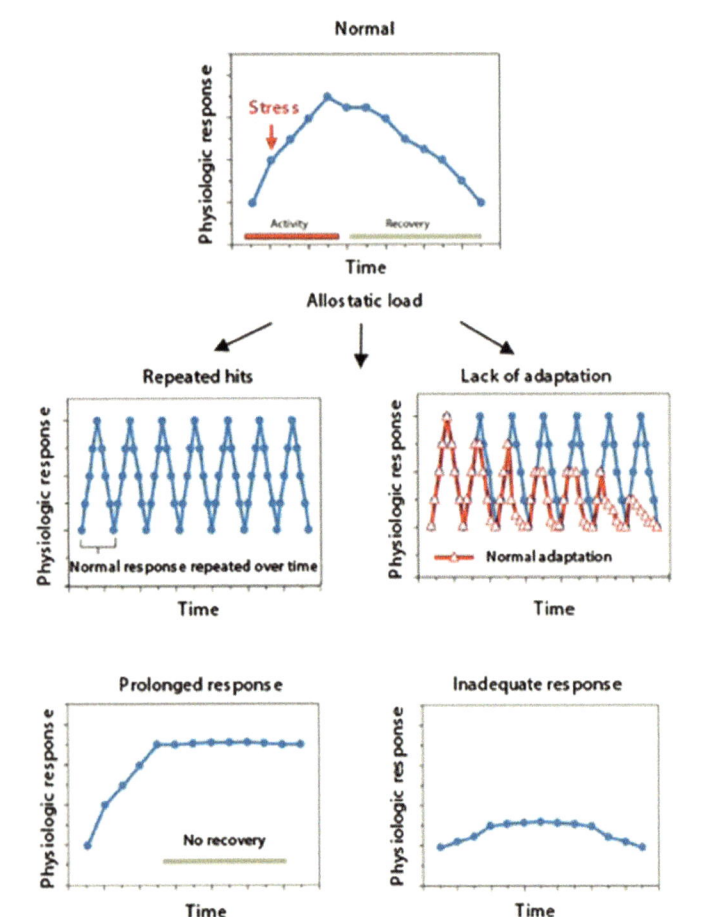

Wooley, and McEwen, 1991a; Gould, Wooley, Cameron, et al., 1991) (Figures 17.1 and 17.8).

Subsequently, a series of influential studies characterized the impact of stress on neurogenesis in the dentate gyrus. For example, exposure to acute psychosocial stress caused a rapid reduction in dentate neurogenesis in adult tree shrews. Overall, a growing body of work has shown stress to suppress neurogenesis (Figure 17A) (Schoenfeld and Gould, 2012; Briones and Gould, 2019). Stressful experiences also have differential effects on neurogenesis depending on the stage of adult neurogenesis, i.e., cell proliferation, neuronal differentiation, and cell death (Briones and Gould, 2019). Social disruption in rats also reduced the number of progenitors in the ventral dentate gyrus (Figure 17.8B,C), which in turn modulated social behavior in an adaptive manner that may also involve reduction in adult neurogenesis in the hippocampus (Opendak et al., 2016).

Pharmacological inhibition of NMDA receptors, on the other hand, led to an increase (Gould et al., 1997). In rats, adrenal steroids also regulated adult neurogenesis in the dentate gyrus (Cameron

Figure 17.5 Types of allostatic load. The top panel illustrates the normal allostatic response, in which a response is initiated by a stressor, sustained for an appropriate interval, and then turned off. The remaining panels illustrate four conditions that lead to allostatic load: repeated "hits" from multiple stressors; lack of adaptation; prolonged response due to delayed shutdown; and inadequate response that leads to compensatory hyperactivity of other mediators (e.g., inadequate secretion of glucocorticoids, resulting in increased concentrations of cytokines that are normally counterregulated by glucocorticoids). (Adapted from McEwen, 1998.)

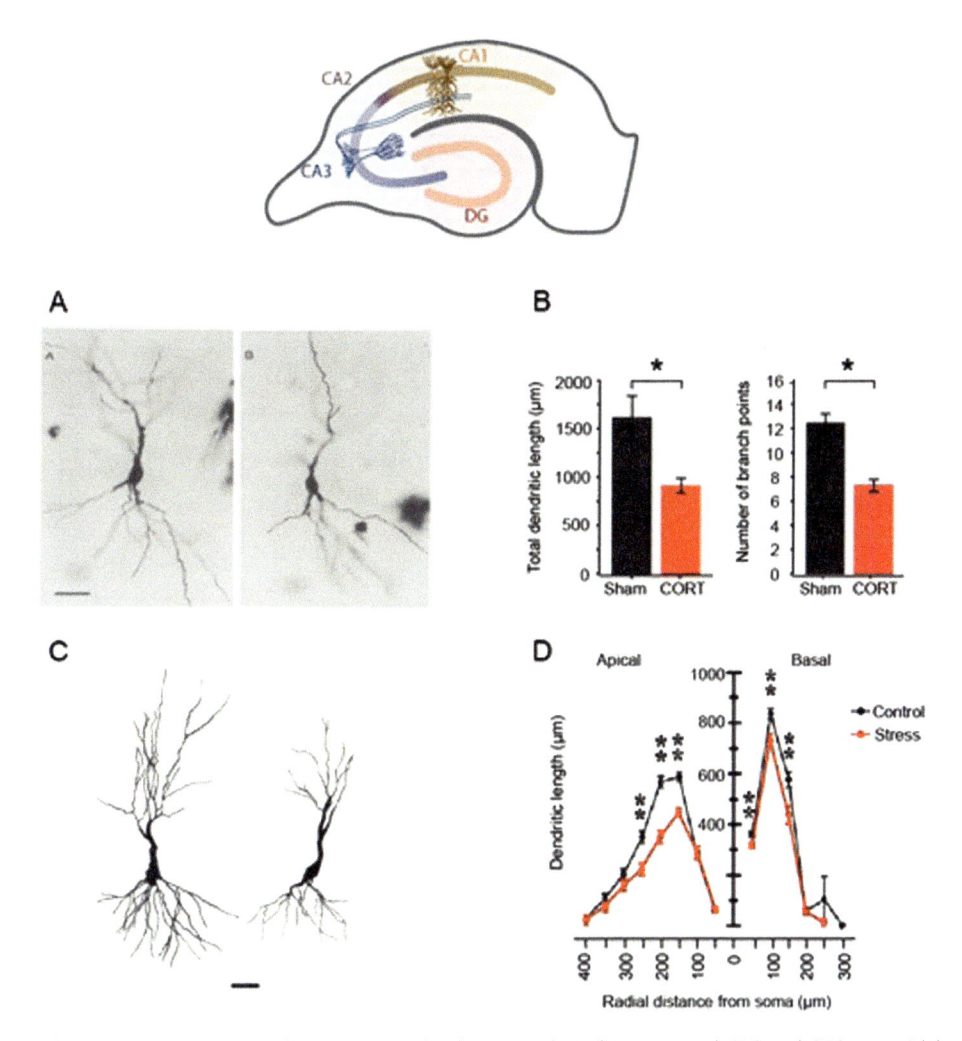

Figure 17.6 Exposure to chronic corticosterone and stress causes dendritic atrophy in hippocampal CA3 and CA1 pyramidal neurons. Daily injection of corticosterone (10 mg) for 21 days caused shrinkage of dendritic arbors in rat hippocampal CA3 pyramidal cells. (A) Golgi-impregnated CA3c pyramidal cells from brains of sham-injected (*left*) and CORT-injected (*right*) animals. Scale bar = 50 μm. (B) Quantification of decreased total apical dendritic length (*left*) and reduction in the numbers of apical dendritic branch points in CA3 pyramidal cells from sham-injected (*black*) and CORT-injected (*red*) animals (Woolley et al., 1990). (C) Chronic stress (2 h/day for 10 days) also causes dendritic atrophy in CA3 pyramidal cells in rats. Camera lucida drawings of representative Golgi-impregnated hippocampal CA3 pyramidal neurons from control (*left*) and stressed animals (*right*). Scale bar = 50 μm. (D) Effects of chronic stress on mean dendritic length for each successive 50 μm segment as a function of the radial distance of the corresponding segment from the soma. Changes in apical (*left*) and basal (*right*) dendrites are shown separately. (Adapted from Vyas et al., 2002.)

et al., 1998). Dentate gyrus neurogenesis was also seen in the macaque (Gould, Reeves, Fallah, et al., 1999; Gould, Reeves, Graziano, et al., 1999) and human (Eriksson et al., 1998) hippocampus, with some question as to how long it continues in adult life (Sorrells et al., 2018), along with methodological issues (Moreno-Jimenez et al., 2019). A key regulator of hippocampal neurogenesis is physical activity (van Praag et al., 1999) and daily physical activity of sedentary older adults increases the volume of the hippocampus within 6 to 12 months, although whether dentate gyrus neurogenesis is the reason for this is not known (Erickson et al., 2011b). Nevertheless, the extent of physical activity must be factored into any consideration of the amount of neurogenesis. Mediators of increased neurogenesis include circulating IGF1 (Aberg et al., 2003) and cathepsin B (Moon et al., 2016) and locally produced dihydrotestosterone (Okamoto et al., 2012), as well as BDNF (Kobilo et al., 2011) and possibly osteocalcin (Oury et al., 2013). Individual differences in physical activity among genetically identical mice develops over time, indicating that "factors unfolding or emerging during development

contribute to individual differences in structural brain plasticity and behaviour" (Freund et al., 2013) operating on the same genetic material and reflecting how nonshared environmental experiences contribute to individual differences in behavior. In contrast to exercise, chronic stress causes the hippocampus to become smaller, with fewer granule neurons and lower neurogenesis (Pham et al., 2003).

As to what neurogenesis in the dentate gyrus means for behavior, there are connections both to learning and to emotional regulation, based in large part on studies in which new neurons are deleted (Cameron and Glover, 2015). Associative learning tasks involving the hippocampus lead to a doubling of newly born granule neurons (Gould, Beylin, et al., 1999). Further studies revealed a role for the new neurons in a trace cue conditioning task, in which there is a 50 ms interval between the end of the cue and the unconditioned stimulus, but not in a delayed conditioning task in which the shock occurred during the last 100 ms of the auditory cue (Shors, Miesegaes, et al., 2001). A similar impairment was also found in freezing in a cued fear conditioning task with a trace interval but not

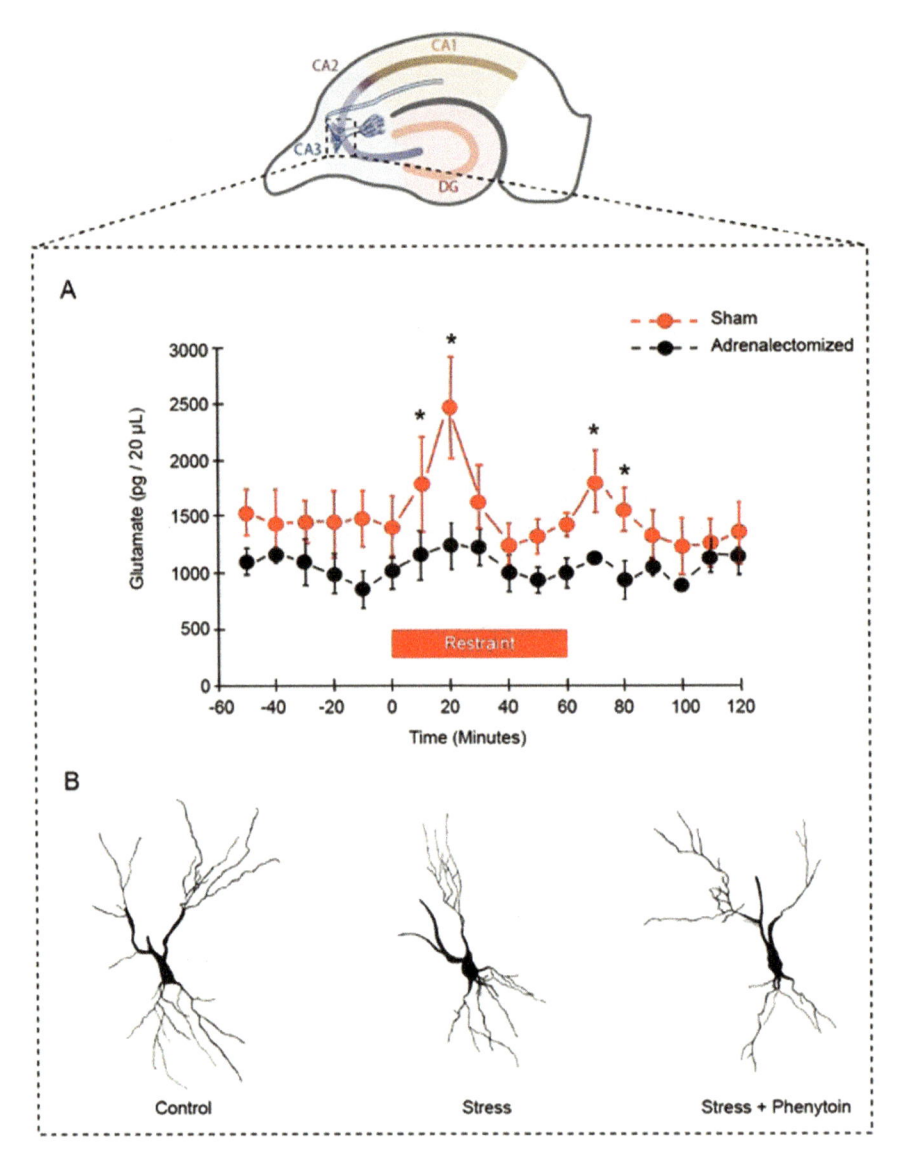

Figure 17.7 Stress, glutamate, and dendritic atrophy in CA3 pyramidal neurons. (A) Effect of 1-hour restraint stress on hippocampal extracellular concentrations of glutamate. Adrenalectomy attenuates this stress-induced elevation in extracellular glutamate concentrations in the rat hippocampus, suggesting a link between stress-induced release of excess glutamate and morphological changes; this has been tested using various pharmacological interventions, as shown in the next panel (Lowy et al., 1993). (B) Phenytoin, which is known to interfere with excitatory amino acid release and actions, prevents stress-induced atrophy of CA3 pyramidal neurons. Camera lucida drawings of representative Golgi-impregnated CA3 pyramidal neurons from control (*left*), stress (*center*), and stress + phenytoin (*right*) rats. Note the decrease in number of dendritic branch points after stress compared with both control and stress + phenytoin (Watanabe et al., 1992a).

in spatial maze learning, contextual fear conditioning, novel context exploration, or anxiety-like behavior in the elevated plus maze (Shors et al., 2002). Some but not all studies, reviewed by (Cameron and Glover, 2015), show evidence for a role of new neurons in recognition memory, spatial memory, and pattern separation, and in a number of nonmnemonic tasks.

As indicated by neuroanatomical studies of inputs to the hippocampus, particularly from the basolateral amygdala (Petrovich et al., 2001), dorsal and ventral hippocampus appear to have different functions involving cognition and mood (Kheirbek et al., 2013; Kheirbek and Hen, 2011). In relation to mood, basolateral amygdala stimulation increases anxiety, and antidepressants stimulate maturation of immature ventral dentate gyrus neurons (reviewed in (Cameron and Glover, 2015). Further, dentate gyrus neurogenesis is required for some (Santarelli et al., 2003) but not all antidepressant effects indicating that other cellular processes involving neuronal

remodeling may also play a role (Bessa et al., 2008). Moreover, consistent with an important role for dentate gyrus neurogenesis in mood regulation and depressive illness, ablation of new neurons revealed that glucocorticoid levels were slower to recover after moderate stress (Snyder et al., 2011), consistent with a role for the hippocampus in regulation of the hypothalamic-pituitary-adrenal (HPA) axis (Herman et al., 2003; Roozendaal et al., 2001).

Also consistent with an important role for dentate gyrus neurogenesis in mood regulation and depressive illness, following inhibition of adult neurogenesis using radiation and transgenic manipulations, glucocorticoid levels were slower to recover after moderate stress. Glucocorticoid levels were also less suppressed by dexamethasone in neurogenesis-deficient mice compared with intact mice. These observations are also consistent with a role for the hippocampus in regulation of the HPA axis (Figure 17.1). According to the authors (Snyder et al., 2011), "these findings identify a small

Table 17.1 Molecules that are necessary/permissive for stress-induced remodeling

A	Secreted signaling molecules		
	Molecule	**Function**	**Reference**
1	BDNF	Modulator of stress-induced plasticity	Bath et al., 2013 Chen et al., 2006 Govindarajan et al., 2006
2	CRF	Downregulates thin spines via RhoA signaling and regulated tPA release	Chen et al., 2013
3	tPA	Required for stress-induced spine loss in CA1 area and medial amygdala	Bennur et al., 2007 Matys et al., 2004 Pawlak et al., 2003, 2005
4	Lipocalin-2	Acute stress upregulates lipocalin-2 in hippocampus Genetic deletion of lipocalin-2 increases neuronal excitability and anxiety	Mucha et al., 2011 Skrzypiec et al., 2013
5	Endocannabinoids	Induced via glucocorticoids Regulates emotionality and HPA axis habituation Buffer against stress-induced remodeling	Gunduz-Cinar et al., 2013 Hill et al., 2013 Hill and McEwen, 2010 Hill et al., 2010
B	From the cell surface to nucleocytoplasmic interactions		
1	PSA-NCAM	Stress increases expression of PSA-NCAM Removal of PSA expands CA3 dendrites and eclipses stress-induced atrophy PSA removal also exacerbates stress-induced neurodegeneration and body weight loss	McCall et al., 2013 Rutishauser, 2008 Sandi, 2004
2	CAM	Chronic stress disrupts neuroligin-neurexin interaction Stress reduces nectin-3 Suppression of nectin-3 causes spine loss and spatial memory deficit	van der Kooij, Fantin, Kraev, et al., 2014 van der Kooij, Fantin, Rejmak, et al., 2014 Wang et al., 2013
3	NUP62	Chronic stress reduces expression in CA3 neurons Reduction of NUP-62 leads to dendrite shrinkage	Kinoshita et al., 2014

subset of neurons within the dentate gyrus that are critical for hippocampal negative control of the HPA axis and support a direct role for adult neurogenesis in depressive illness," as will be discussed below. We note that stress effects on dendritic branching and neurogenesis have been reported for many species in addition to the rat and mouse, such as the European Hamster, tree shrew, marmoset, rhesus monkey, and human.

17.4.3 Loss of hippocampal volume and spatial memory deficits

Several studies have shown significant hippocampal volume loss using different stress models (Kalisch et al., 2006; Lee et al., 2009; Rahman et al., 2016). One study that carried out longitudinal behavioral analyses during 10 days of chronic stress pointed to a delayed decline in spatial memory, the full impact of which was evident only after the end of stress (Figure 17.9). In contrast, concurrent volumetric measurements, using structural MRI, in the same animals revealed significant reduction in hippocampal volumes in stressed animals relative to their unstressed counterparts, as early as the third day of stress. Notably, animals that were behaviorally the worst affected at the end of chronic stress suffered the most pronounced early loss in hippocampal volume. Together, these findings support the view that smaller hippocampal volume is not only linked to stress-induced memory deficits but also may act as an early risk factor for the eventual development of impairments in spatial memory performance (Rahman et al., 2016).

17.4.4 Electrophysiological changes in synaptic transmission and plasticity

Effects of stressful experiences can also be measured electrophysiologically, guided by the hypothesis that stress causes deficits in hippocampal memory by disrupting synaptic transmission

and plasticity mechanisms. Accumulating evidence from electrophysiological recordings in different hippocampal subregions has established that exposure to stress and stress hormones affects synaptic plasticity in the hippocampus (McEwen, 1999; Kim and Diamond, 2002). The first evidence for stress-induced deficits in long-term potentiation (LTP) came from a study that subjected rats to unpredictable and restraint tailshock (Figure 17.1). *In vitro* electrophysiological recordings of population field potentials from hippocampal slices prepared from these animals exhibited a significant suppression of LTP at the Schaffer collateral inputs to area CA1 (Foy et al., 1987). This was followed by a series of reports on stress-induced suppression of LTP in the dentate gyrus (DG), as well as analyses of how long these effects last in area CA1 in both rats and mice (Shors et al., 1989; Shors et al., 1997; Garcia et al., 1997). Recordings from the intact CA1 area *in vivo*, as well as the DG in hippocampal slices, have shown that acute stress and acute elevation of glucocorticoid impairs LTP (Diamond and Rose, 1994; Diamond et al., 1992). Similarly, several physical stressors, such as repeated restraint stress, also suppress LTP in both the DG and area CA1.

Studies have also characterized the effects of stress on long-term depression (LTD) of synaptic strength. Interestingly, chronic stress has the complementary effect by enhancing LTD (Kim and Diamond, 2002). In a manner similar to chronic stress, a single episode of acute stress also impairs LTP, but enhances LTD (Figure 17.10; Kim et al., 2005; Kumar et al., 2014; Xu et al., 1997).

Studies on a close relative of LTP, primed-burst potentiation (PBP), have also revealed an interesting "dose-response" relationship. There is an inverted U-shaped dose-response curve (Figure 17.11), with low levels of corticosterone facilitating PBP and high levels inhibiting PBP in the CA1 region (Diamond et al., 1992). The effects of activation of the two types of adrenal steroid

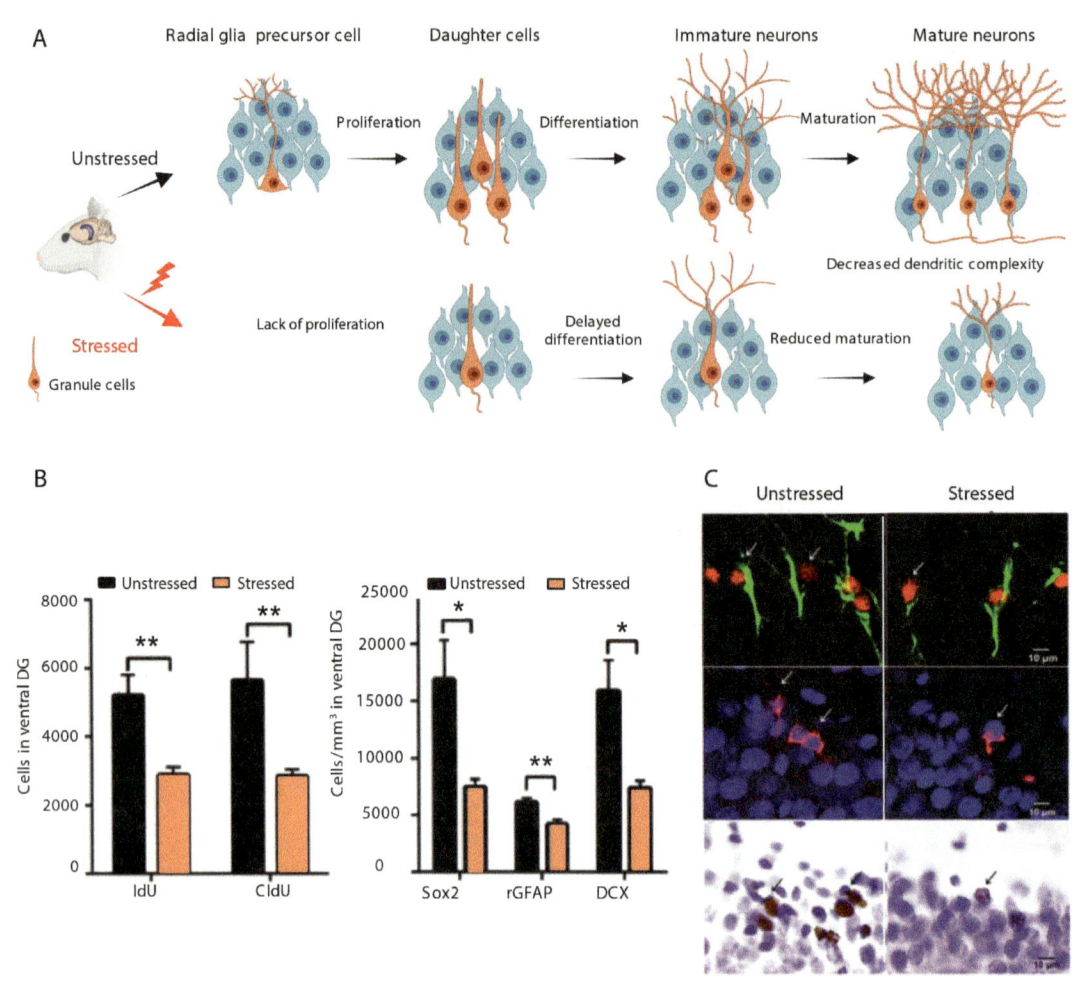

Figure 17.8 Stages of adult hippocampal neurogenesis and how stress can affect neurogenesis in the dentate gyrus continuously or at different stages. (A) This simplified schematic shows radial glia-like precursor cells proliferating and producing daughter cells, which then differentiate into immature granule neurons, in the dentate gyrus. A portion of these immature neurons will survive and become mature granule neurons, which have the potential to impact the hippocampal circuitry. Different stressors have been shown to affect adult neurogenesis by decreasing the number of proliferating cells, delaying neuronal differentiation, reducing the number of adult-born granule cells, and diminishing their dendritic complexity (adapted from Briones & Gould, 2019). (B) Graphs showing that social instability stress suppresses processes leading to adult neurogenesis at multiple levels, by reducing survival of adult-born granule cells (labeled with IdU or CldU), diminishing the proliferation of progenitor cells (labeled with Sox2 or rGFAP) as well as the numbers of immature adult-generated neurons (labeled with DCX) (adapted from Opendak et al., 2016). (C) Confocal images of progenitor cells (Sox2 (red)/rGFAP (green)—top panel), immature neurons (DCX (red)—middle panel) IdU labeled mature adult-born granule cells (brown)—bottom panel) in "unstressed" and "stressed" conditions (adapted from Opendak et al., 2016). IdU, iododeoxyuridine; CldU, chlorodeoxyuridine; Sox2, SRY-box 2; DCX, doublecortin; rGFAP, radial glial cells labeled with glial fibrillary acidic protein. (Courtesy: Prof. Elizabeth Gould, Princeton University.)

receptors—mineralocorticoid (MR) and glucocorticoid (GR) receptors—by adrenal steroids on synaptic plasticity in the CA1 area have also been examined in hippocampal slices. In slices prepared from adrenalectomized rats, application of aldosterone, a specific MR agonist, enhanced CA1 LTP (Pavlides et al., 1996). The specific GR agonist RU 28362, on the other hand, suppressed LTP. Unlike findings from *in vivo* recordings in animals receiving RU 28362 (see section 17.4.5 below), however, LTD was not seen in the CA1 area of hippocampal slices.

Although pyramidal neurons in area CA3 undergo robust dendritic atrophy with stress, less is known about how stress affects synaptic plasticity in this area. Studies using whole-cell recordings in CA3 pyramidal cells reported that brief social stress prevents induction of LTP by low-frequency tetanic stimulation (3 Hz for 3 minutes) of commissural–associational synapses even after a 21-day time delay (Kole, Costoli, et al., 2004). Following repeated stress, on the other hand, the same low-frequency tetanic stimuli tended to reverse the EPSP amplitude, resembling LTD (Kole, Czeh, et al., 2004). The involvement of excitatory amino acids and NMDA receptors, in hippocampal dendritic remodeling (Magarinos and McEwen, 1995b; McEwen, 1999), also offered insights into the underlying synaptic signaling mechanisms. Specifically, whole-cell recordings in CA3 pyramidal neurons showed that the same 21-day repeated restraint stress, which had been shown to cause CA3 dendritic atrophy, increased the amplitude and deactivation time-constant of the NMDA receptor-mediated currents, without affecting the AMPA/kainate-receptor-mediated currents at commissural–associational inputs (Kole et al., 2002). Such stress-induced increase in NMDA-receptor signaling, however, is a condition that is likely to facilitate, and not impair, LTP induction. Further, intracellular calcium, a key determinant of hippocampal LTP, is also enhanced by glucocorticoids (Kerr, Campbell, et al.,

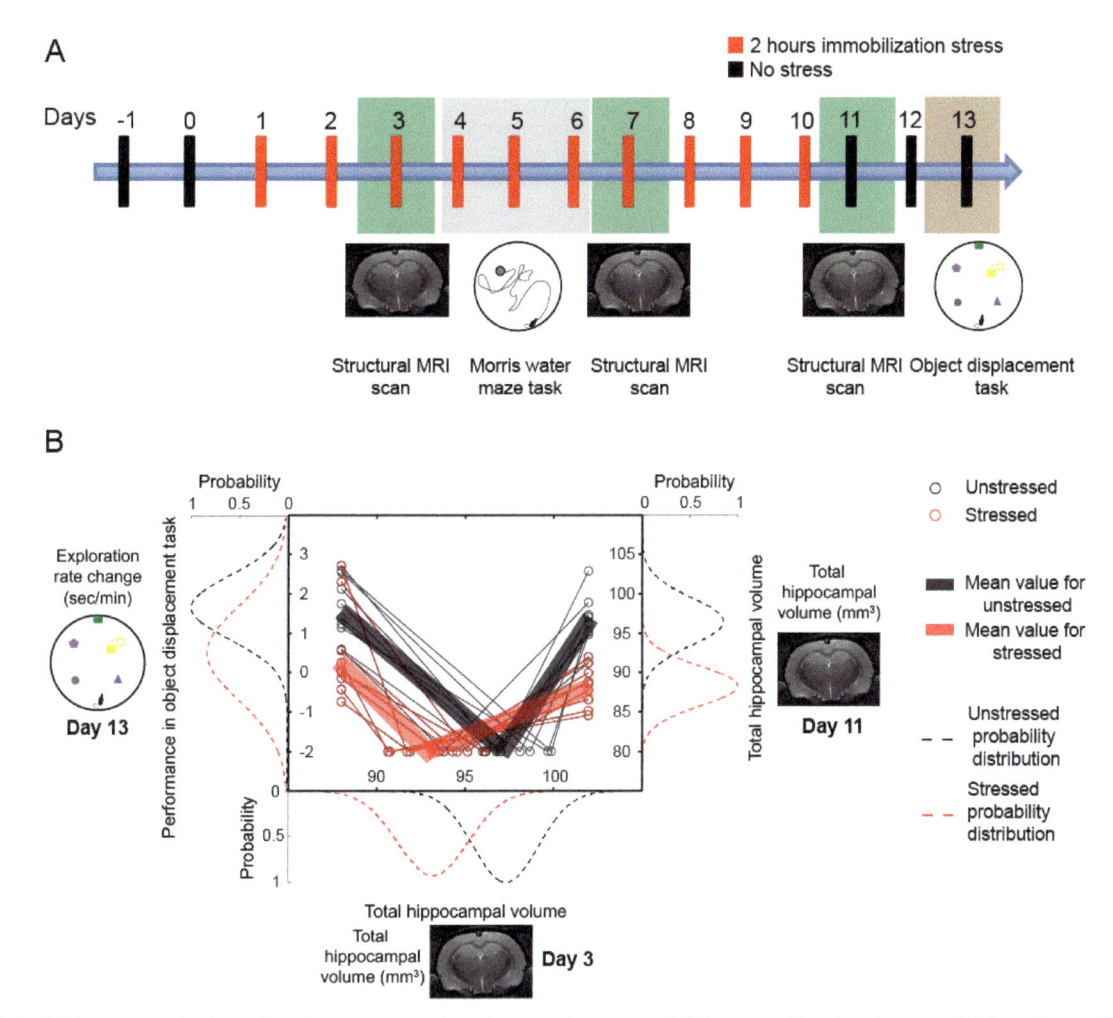

Figure 17.9 Early hippocampal volume loss in rats as a marker of eventual memory deficits caused by chronic stress. (A) Experimental design that combined volumetric measurements of the rat hippocampus using MRI with behavioral assays of hippocampus-based spatial memory tasks in the same animal longitudinally at multiple time points during and after a 10-day chronic immobilization stress paradigm. (B) Summary of the effect of stress on hippocampal volume and its correlation with spatial memory deficit. Each circle and line represents a single animal. The dotted lines denote the probability distribution of the stressed (red) and unstressed (black) group of rats. Stress caused a loss in hippocampal volume on Day 3 and Day 11 (indicated by the shift of the probability distribution of stressed animals in the bottom and right axes). Stress also led to impaired performance in a spatial memory task (indicated by the shift of the probability distribution of stressed animals in the left axis). Animals that had lower hippocampal volume on Day 3 also had lower hippocampal volume on Day 11, i.e., a day after the end of chronic stress. Notably, these animals also performed more poorly in the Object Displacement Task on Day 13. Light red and light black lines depict the average trend for the stressed and unstressed animals respectively. (Adapted from Rahman et al., 2016.)

1992; Joels and Vreugdenhil, 1998). These observations, therefore, are somewhat counterintuitive in light of the significant body of evidence for stress-induced impairment of LTP elsewhere in the hippocampus. In summary, accumulating evidence from a variety of models of stress (Box 17.1) have been shown to elicit a range of structural, neuroendocrine, synaptic plasticity, and behavioral alterations in rodents (Dos-Santos et al., 2023).

17.4.5 Electrophysiological changes in the intact hippocampus

In vivo recordings in the DG of anesthetized and freely behaving rats revealed that both acute and chronic administration of corticosterone leads to a suppression in LTP (Pavlides et al., 1993). Similar *in vivo* recordings in the DG were also used to demonstrate that activation of MR and GR receptors—elicit biphasic effects on synaptic plasticity. For example, in adrenalectomized rats, administration of aldosterone, a specific MR agonist, caused an enhancement in LTP.

By contrast, administration of RU 28362, a specific GR agonist, led to a significant reduction in the induction of LTP (Pavlides et al., 1995). In a separate study, high-frequency stimulation, which normally produces LTP, instead caused long-term depression (LTD) in rats that were administered the GR agonist RU 28362 (Pavlides et al., 1993). Notably, *in vivo* recordings in awake, behaving rodents have also revealed how exposure to mild naturalistic stressors can elicit changes in both the direction of and susceptibility to hippocampal synaptic plasticity (Xu et al., 1997, 1998). Specifically, brief behavioral stress, induced by exposing the animal to a brightly lit elevated platform, blocked LTP triggered by high-frequency stimuli in the CA1 area. On the other hand, LTD in area CA1, induced by low-frequency stimuli, was increased by the same stress. Furthermore, effects of this stress on *in vivo* LTP/LTD were reversed rapidly following acclimatization to, or removal from, the stressful conditions. Thus, stress appears to exert its detrimental effect on hippocampal synaptic plasticity by tilting the balance toward LTD—even as stress

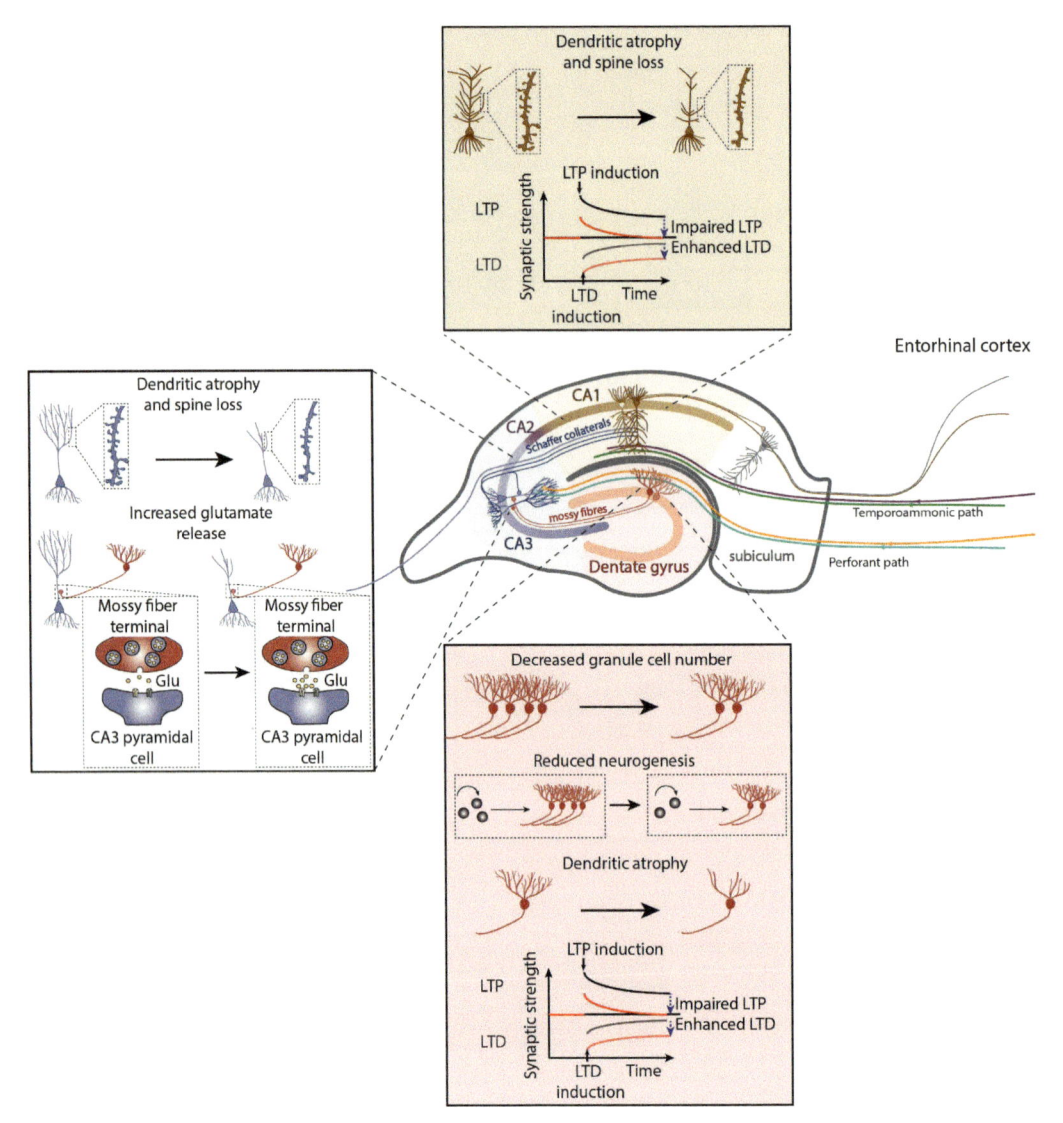

Figure 17.10 Cellular and synaptic alterations triggered by stress in subregions of the rodent hippocampus. Exposure to stress elicits a range of morphological and physiological changes, some of which share common features between subregions while others are distinct. In the DG, stress impairs LTP but facilitates LTD; similar stress-induced changes in LTP/LTD have also been reported in the CA1 area. Stress leads to reduced neurogenesis, as well as granule cell numbers, in the DG. Dendritic atrophy has been seen in all three areas—granule cells of the DG, and pyramidal neurons in areas CA1 and CA3. In addition, stress causes reduction in dendritic spine density in both CA1 and CA3 areas. Excess glutamate release from mossy fiber terminals onto thorny excrescences on apical dendrites of CA3 pyramidal cells is a key driver of excitotoxic damage in these cells.

impairs the capacity of these synapses to undergo activity-induced strengthening, it also creates conditions that favor further weakening of synaptic transmission.

17.5 Stress, glucocorticoids, and memory

The finding of stress-induced shrinkage of dendrites in CA3 pyramidal cells after 21 days of chronic restraint stress (CRS) (Watanabe, Gould, and McEwen, 1992) led to an investigation showing that this regimen impaired learning and performance in a radial maze, with recovery several weeks after the end of stress (Luine, Villegas, et al., 1994). Similarly, CRS led to impaired memory of the novel arm in a Y-maze; this effect was prevented by the antidepressant tianeptine, which also prevents stress-induced shrinkage of apical dendrites of CA3 pyramidal cells (Conrad et al., 1996b; Watanabe, Gould, Daniels, et al., 1992). However,

the simple relationship between dendrite shrinkage and memory impairment is challenged by the finding that attenuating corticosterone levels in chronically stressed rats at the time of memory assessment prevented chronic stress-induced impairments in spatial memory (Wright et al., 2006). The authors interpreted this as due to an altered HPA reactivity to the memory test and/or altered sensitivity of the receptors that respond to corticosterone, and not a direct effect that is solely due to dendritic atrophy, which has been shown to reverse 7 days after the end of repeated stress. It should be noted that both genomic and nongenomic mechanisms may also be involved.

As to the role of glucocorticoids in learning and recall, when tasks are minimally aversive, the glucocorticoid receptor (GR) mediates an inverted U-shaped relationship between glucocorticoid levels and hippocampal function, while the MR mediates attentional processes and/or reaction to novelty (Conrad, 2005). This inverted U-shaped relationship (Figure 17.11) during minimally

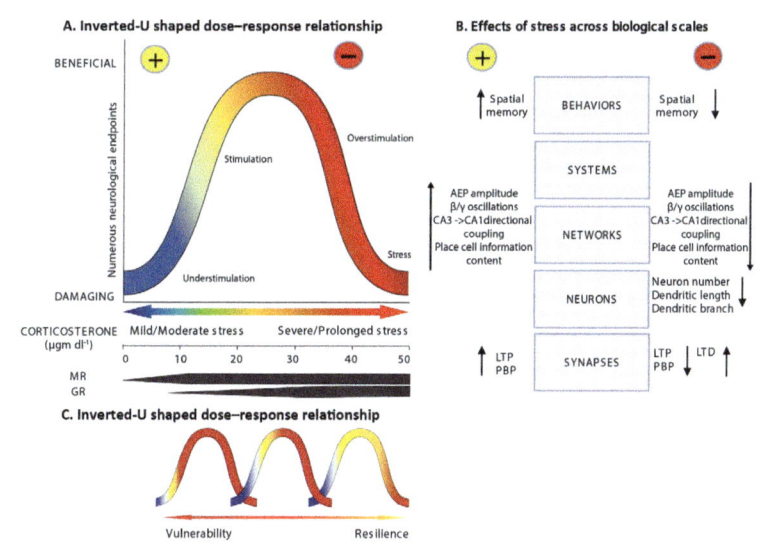

Figure 17.11 Inverted-U dose-response relationship between stress, stress hormones, and hippocampal function. (A) The inverted-U relationship offers a useful framework for assessing the beneficial and damaging effects of stress hormones and severity of stress on hippocampal function. Brief stressors associated with mild-to-moderate range of corticosterone, are considered to be stimulatory and lead to beneficial effect. On the other hand, both the complete absence of stress (understimulatory), and severe, prolonged and repeated stressors lead to damaging effects on various neurobiological endpoints. (B) This spectrum of alterations in hippocampal function is manifested in a range of neurobiological endpoints spanning multiple levels of neural organization, such as LTP at the synaptic level and spatial memory performance at the behavioral level. For example, low and high corticosterone levels cause deficits in LTP, while intermediate levels of corticosterone (approximately 10–20 μg/dl) are conducive for maximal LTP. Similar effects have been observed at the behavioral level in hippocampus-dependent memory tasks. In contrast, higher levels of corticosterone associated with severe/chronic stress lead to impaired LTP/PBP, enhanced LTD, reduction in neuronal number and dendritic atrophy, and spatial memory deficits. *In vivo* recordings from areas CA1 and CA3 in awake behaving animals showed that the amplitude of auditory evoked potentials (AEPs), the power of evoked beta/gamma oscillation and directional coupling from area CA3 to CA1 are all enhanced 1 hour after a single episode of acute immobilization stress. Yet, when the same stress is repeated for 10 days, there is a significant reduction in all of these parameters in the same animals (Figure 17.17). Further, a single episode of acute stress increased, but repeated stress decreased, place-cell information content, i.e. the ability of place-cell firing to predict information about the animal's location (see section 17.8). The dual receptor system for glucocorticoids offer a mechanistic basis for this inverted-U dose-response curve. While increasing occupancy of the high-affinity, low-capacity MRs (occurring at mild-to-moderate levels) contribute to the beneficial effects of corticosterone, the detrimental effects are mediated by the low-affinity, high-capacity GRs (occurring at severe-to-prolonged levels). (C) The inverted-U framework is also useful in understanding individual differences in responsiveness and vulnerability/resilience to stress. Thus, the same stressful experience can elicit different effects in different individuals. For instance, genetic/environmental factors and/or early life experiences can shift the Inverted-U curve to the left, thereby making an individual more vulnerable to subsequent stress, while a rightward shift can confer resilience. (Adapted from Sapolsky, 2015.)

aversive training paradigms describes glucocorticoid-mediated memory processing during both acquisition and consolidation. Findings on the modulation of hippocampal learning by stress and glucocorticoids suggest an inverted U-shaped dose-response relationship, similar to what has also been reported for changes in synaptic plasticity mechanisms like LTP. While very low and high levels may impair consolidation, moderate levels appear to enable efficient long-term encoding of information (Flood et al., 1978; Diamond et al., 1992,1999; Oitzl et al., 1994; Sandi and Rose, 1994a, 1994b; Vaher et al., 1994; Yau et al., 1995; Conrad et al., 1997; Pugh et al., 1997; Liu et al.,1999). For example, stress or high corticosterone levels, or stress administered before training or testing, caused deficits in spatial performance and memory (Diamond et al., 1996; de Quervain et al., 1998; Conrad et al., 1999). Consistent with this, adrenalectomy or blocking GRs that led to the removal of endogenous corticosterone, resulted in impaired performance in a spatial task and fear conditioning (Oitzl and de Kloet, 1992; Vaher et al., 1994; Pugh et al., 1997). Interestingly, the impact of stress *during* training is quite different. Rats trained for a massed spatial learning task in the watermaze in cold water showed elevated corticosterone levels and performed better than those trained in warmer water (Sandi et al., 1997). This led to subsequent analyses of whether manipulating the levels of corticosterone affects the

strength of spatial information acquisition and retention (Akirav et al., 2004). Rats were injected with different doses of the corticosterone synthesis inhibitor metyrapone, or with corticosterone, and then trained in a massed spatial task in either cold or warm water, the latter being less stressful. While vehicle-injected rats performed well in the spatial task in cold water, rats injected with an intermediate dose of metyrapone exhibited impaired performance in the same task. On the other hand, animals treated with vehicle performed poorly in warm water, but those injected with a lower corticosterone dose performed better. Together, these studies using corticosterone blockade and enhancement suggest that variations in the levels of corticosterone play an important role in the acquisition and retention of spatial learning task. In terms of clinical implications of these rodent studies, the work of Lupien is instructive. In a study elucidating a role for the corticosteroid system in declarative memory function (Maheu et al., 2005), human subjects were administered a placebo or metyrapone before a psychological stressor that consisted of a free speech and a mental arithmetic task performed in front of an audience (Kirschbaum et al., 1993). The subjects viewed a neutral story that was unrelated to the stressor immediately after the being subjected to the stressor. The placebo group showed significant stress-related increases in corticosteroid levels, which was prevented in subjects that received metyrapone.

> **Box 17.2** Epigenetic mechanisms
>
> Histone modifications are keys to epigenetic regulation of gene expression. Besides the acetylation of histones involved in the upregulation of mGlu2 gene expression described above, repressive epigenetic modifications of histones are also evident after acute and chronic stress. For example, acute stress dramatically increased the levels of H3K9 trimethylation (H3K9me3) in the dentate gyrus (DG) and CA1, while chronic restraint stress (CRS) for 21 days abolished this effect. Treatment with fluoxetine during CRS reversed the decrease in DG H3K9me3 (Hunter et al., 2009). Regarding the substantial, regionally specific, increase in hippocampal levels of the repressive histone H3 lysine 9 trimethylation (H3K9me3), chromosomal immunoprecipitation (ChIP) and sequencing of the DNA revealed that acute stress trapped certain transposon and retrotransposon elements of what used to be called junk DNA, which is derived from retroviruses that have become part of the mammalian genome. Since these elements may be rearranged within the genomic ("jumping genes"; McClintock, 1956) trapping them in the stress-induced H3K9 trimethyl immunoprecipitate suggests that acute stress promotes genomic stability (Hunter et al., 2012). In addition, the histone H3K9-specific methyltransferase Suv39h2 is upregulated by acute stress in the hippocampus, and this may explain the hippocampal specificity (Hunter et al., 2012). This response may represent a genomic stress response aimed at maintaining genomic and transcriptional stability in vulnerable brain regions such as the hippocampus, although the transposome might have adaptive functions at the level of both evolution and the individual organism (Hunter et al., 2013).

Compared with placebo, metyrapone impaired short-term (5 min after learning), but not long-term (1 week after learning), recall of declarative memory related to the story. Further, the sensitivity of neural systems to glucocorticoids on a target brain region of the hippocampus, the prefrontal cortex, also shifts with age (Lupien et al., 1997; Lupien et al., 2002).

It is also important to note that the role of glucocorticoid hormones in the regulation of memory consolidation and memory retrieval also depends on the level of emotional arousal induced by the training experience (Okuda et al., 2004). In rats that were not previously habituated to the experimental context, varying doses of corticosterone administered immediately after a 3-minute training trial enhanced 24-hour retention performance in an inverted-U shaped dose–response relationship. In contrast, corticosterone did not affect 24-hour retention of rats that received extensive prior habituation to the experimental context and, thus, had decreased novelty-induced emotional arousal during training. Additionally, immediate posttraining administration of corticosterone to nonhabituated rats, in doses that enhanced 24-hour retention, impaired object recognition performance at a 1-hour retention interval, whereas corticosterone administered after training to well-habituated rats did not impair 1-hour retention. Thus, these findings suggest that training-induced emotional arousal may be essential for glucocorticoid effects on object recognition memory (Okuda et al., 2004).

17.6 Epigenetics, brain plasticity, stress, and damage

As the first extrahypothalamic brain structure recognized to have receptors for adrenal steroids (McEwen et al., 1968), the hippocampus has been an important gateway for understanding the epigenetic effects of glucocorticoids and stress on gene expression in the brain (see Box 17.2).

At first recognized for their epigenetic effects as regulators of gene transcription, glucocorticoids are now known to have multiple nongenomic effects at the synapse, in mitochondria, and at the cell surface (Figure 17.12). Recent technological advances have allowed high-throughput analysis of changes in gene expression in response to stress (Musazzi et al., 2023; Rubin et al., 2014). For example, a microarray analysis of whole hippocampus after acute stress, chronic stress, and stress recovery in mice revealed that acute and chronic stress modulate a core set of genes, but that numerous changes are exclusive to each condition, highlighting how duration and intensity of stress alters reactivity (Gray et al., 2014). Furthermore, corticosterone injections do not yield the same expression profile as acute stress, suggesting that *in vivo* stressors activate a diverse set of pathways independent of glucocorticoid receptor (GR) activation (Gray et al., 2014). Finally, characterization of expression profiles after extended recovery from 21 days of chronic stress showed that, despite a normalization of anxiety-related behaviors, recovery did not represent a return to the stress-naive baseline, but rather represents a new state in which reactivity to a novel stressor produces a unique expression profile (Gray et al., 2014).

Studies in rats confirm that gene expression profiles can vary significantly from the immediate end of stress to 24 hours later (K Wang et al., 2010), and that chronic stress can alter the transcriptional response to an acute corticosterone injection in the dentate gyrus (Datson et al., 2013). Together, these studies demonstrate that a history of stress exposure can have a lasting impact on future stress reactivity and hippocampal function. In other words, the life course is a one-way street! Rather than focusing only on the reversibility of the effects of stress on the brain, we should think rather in terms of "recovery" and "resilience." It seems logical to assume that this generalizes to all experiences that we have, whether or not we call them "stress. Moreover, it is evident that experiences of many types can alter brain architecture in a healthy brain. This emerging view has been greatly stimulated by findings on the effects of stress in remodeling of dendrites and synapses, as well as by its effects on neurogenesis in the dentate gyrus.

17.7 Central role of glutamate and other mediators in stress-induced plasticity and damage

17.7.1 Glucocorticoid-glutamate interactions at the core of adaptive plasticity

Excitatory amino acids, particularly glutamate, play a key role in structural as well as functional changes in the brain, since glutamate is the major excitatory transmitter, while, at the same time, excess glutamate causes damage and inflammation (McEwen, 1999b). This is represented as an inverted-U dose relationship in both dose and time, as described in the previous section (Figure 17.11). The shrinkage of apical dendrites of CA3 pyramidal neurons produced by chronic corticosterone treatment or repeated restraint stress can both be blocked by the antiepileptic drug phenytoin, implicating excitatory amino acid release and excitatory synaptic transmission

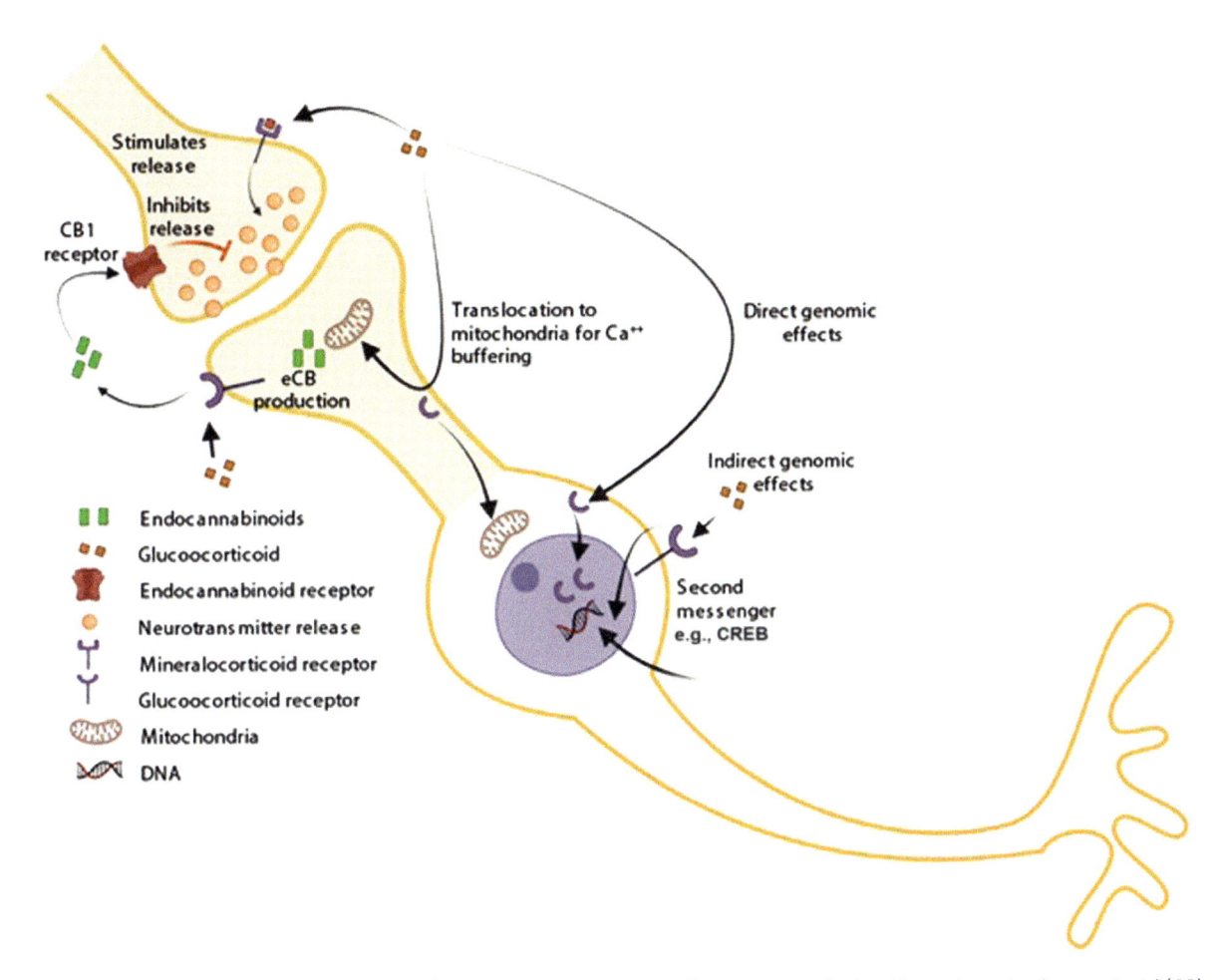

Figure 17.12 Glucocorticoids produce direct and indirect genomic actions as well as nongenomic signaling actions via glucocorticoid (GR) and mineralocorticoid (MR) receptors. Glucocorticoids (GCs) exert their effects in the CNS through a variety of mechanisms. The classical glucocorticoid receptors, mineralocorticoid (MR) and glucocorticoid receptor (GR), both belong to the family of nuclear receptors, which modulate transcription of responsive genes upon binding to GCs (Popoli et al., 2012; McEwen et al., 2015; Musazzi et al., 2023). These genomic effects of steroid activity have a slow time course. GCs also elicit non-genomic rapid effects (timescales of seconds to minutes), which have subsequently been shown to be mediated by membrane-bound receptors for GCs (Popoli et al., 2012; McEwen et al., 2015). These receptors are transcriptional variants of the nuclear receptors (Pietras et al., 2001). For instance, corticosterone increases the release probability of the glutamate-containing vesicles in CA1 pyramidal cells via rapid nongenomic mechanisms, mediated by membrane bound MRs (Karst et al., 2005). Membrane-associated receptors, however, also mediate genomic effects indirectly by recruiting second messengers (Popoli et al., 2012; McEwen et al., 2015).

In the hippocampus, GR activation by corticosterone (and acute restraint stress) increases endocannabinoid (eCB) levels, which in turn dampens GABAergic neurotransmitter release onto CA1 pyramidal cells (Wang et al., 2012). In the dentate gyrus (DG), release of eCBs from granule cells suppresses excitatory synaptic transmission and LTP induction at mossy cell inputs (Jensen et al., 2021). Although MRs and GRs are abundantly present in the DG (Joëls, 2007), involvement of GCs in this region has not been investigated yet. CB1 receptors have also been shown to be present in hippocampal mitochondria and activation of these receptors leads to reduced mitochondrial activity and synaptic depression (Hebert-Chatelain et al., 2016). Translocation of GRs into the mitochondria have been shown to have a dose-dependent effect on mitochondrial function and calcium buffering in cortical cultures (Du et al., 2009). Interaction between GCs and BDNF signaling plays a key role in maintaining neuronal response to stress. In hippocampal and cortical neuronal cultures, GCs can selectively activate tropomyosin receptor kinase B (TrkB), independently of BDNF (Jeanneteau et al., 2008). Concurrently, in the presence of GCs, BDNF phosphorylates GR, facilitating its translocation to the nucleus for regulation of gene transcription (Arango-Lievano et al., 2015). This creates a positive feedback loop between glucocorticoids and BDNF, each potentiating the other's activity (McEwen, 2015). (Adapted from McEwen, 2015).

(Watanabe, Gould, Cameron, et al., 1992; McEwen, 2016; Figure 17.7). Indeed, acute restraint stress elevates extracellular glutamate levels via a process that is blocked in adrenalectomized animals, implicating the adrenal cortex and possible direct effects of adrenal steroids on glutamate release (Lowy et al.,1993; Figure 17.7). Corticosterone was subsequently shown to act directly via membrane-associated MR and GR to cause glutamate release (Karst et al., 2005; Treccani et al., 2014) (Figure 17.12). Blocking NMDA receptors prevents stress-induced dendritic remodeling, as does blockade of adrenal steroid synthesis (Magarinos and McEwen, 1995; Watanabe, Gould, and McEwen, 1992). A stress-induced NMDAR-dependent dendritic remodeling has also been reported in medial prefrontal cortex and basolateral amygdala neurons (Martin and Wellman, 2011; Yasmin et al., 2016). Glutamate overactivity also suppresses dentate gyrus neurogenesis (Cameron et al., 1995).

An unregulated overflow of glutamate (Figure 17.13) appears to play a role in depressive-like behavior in various animal models of stress, in which in addition to shrinkage of dendrites in the

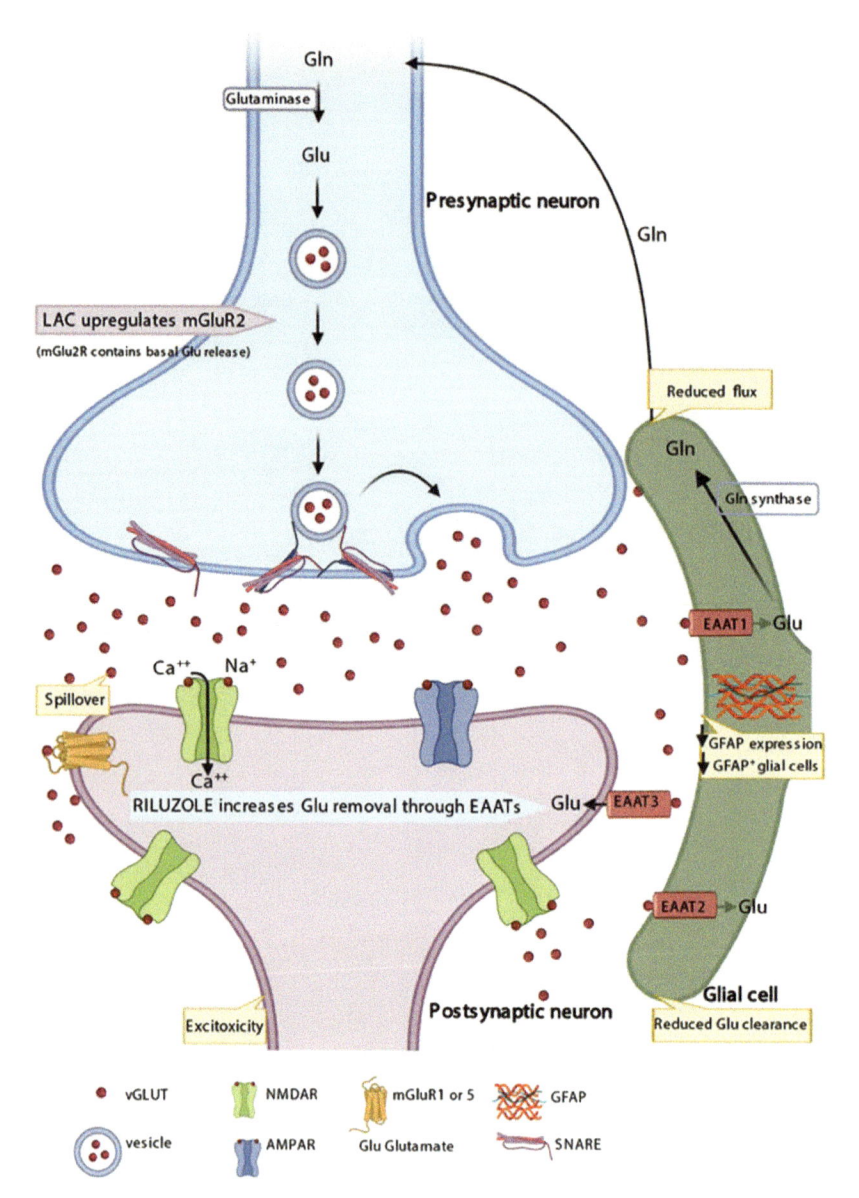

Figure 17.13 Stress, glutamate metabolism, and pharmacological targets for reducing excess glutamate. Chronic stress elevates glutamate levels at excitatory synapses of the hippocampus, a process that involves significant changes in glial cell function. Reduction in the expression of glial fibrillary acid protein (GFAP) and in the number of GFAP-expressing glial cells in the hippocampus after chronic stress (Banasr and Duman, 2008). Chronic stress may also cause deficits in the efficient clearance of synaptic glutamate (Glu) through glial excitatory amino acid transporters (EAATs). This, in turn, is likely to contribute to excess glutamate, thereby enhanced activation of extrasynaptic glutamate receptors, and eventually excitotoxic damage caused by repeated stress (Banasr et al., 2010). Finally, chronic stress may decrease the rates of flux through the glutamate–glutamine (Gln) cycle, resulting in reduced glutamate metabolism. These stress-induced effects on the glutamatergic synapse also suggest potential pharmacological interventions against stress-related psychiatric disorders. For example, riluzole, which indirectly facilitates glutamate transport into glia, has neuroprotective and antidepressant-like effects (Banasr et al., 2010). Further, dampening of the group II mGluR-mediated inhibition of presynaptic glutamate release could provide a mechanism of antidepressant drug action. Acetyl-L-carnitine (LAC), a natural molecule that acts on mGluR2, is deficient in animals that show depressive-like behavior in rodent models (Bigio et al., 2016; Nasca et al., 2013). Further, mGluR5 in hippocampal CA1 pyramidal neurons have also been show to mediate stress-induced anxiety-like behavior (Li et al., 2023).

AMPAR, AMPA receptor; mGluR, metabotropic glutamate receptor; NMDAR, NMDA receptor; vGluT, vesicular glutamate transporter; EAAT, excitatory amino acid transporter; Gln, glutamine. (Adapted from Popoli et al., 2012.)

hippocampus and suppression of neurogenesis, a range of changes occur in intracellular signal pathways (Li, Teng, et al., 2023). For instance, acetyl-L-carnitine (LAC), a natural molecule that is deficient in animals exhibiting depressive-like behavior, rapidly upregulates the metabotropic glutamate receptor, mGluR2, via an epigenetic mechanism involving acetylation of lysine 27 on histone H3. This is mimicked by histone deacetylase (HDAC) inhibitors and by selective serotonin-reuptake inhibitors (SSRIs) that act more slowly (Nasca et al., 2013, Nasca et al., 2015) (Figure 17.13). Thus, LAC is a putative rapidly acting antidepressant candidate as shown in several animal models that have a deficiency of LAC with normal levels of carnitine (Bigio et al., 2016, Nasca et al., 2013). Moreover, LAC deficiency is also associated with insulin resistance that can be corrected by LAC supplementation (Bigio et al., 2016).

This has led to investigations on human major depression (Nasca et al., 2018). Metabolic hormone effects are discussed further in section 17.11.

17.7.2 Glutamate overflow in the hippocampus, aging, and dementia

Unregulated glutamate overflow is also implicated in aging and dementia. During aging in the rat, treatment with riluzole, which is known to prevent glutamate release and promote glutamate reuptake by astrocytes, retards aging in the hippocampus as measured by preservation of spatial memory and thin spines that are found in young hippocampal neurons (Pereira et al., 2014). Moreover, assessing gene expression changes associated with aging in rodents using RNA-sequencing, riluzole prevented many of the changes in hippocampal age-related gene expression. Further, a comparison of the effects of riluzole in rats against human AD datasets revealed that many of the gene changes in AD are reversed by riluzole (Pereira et al., 2016) (Figure 17.13).

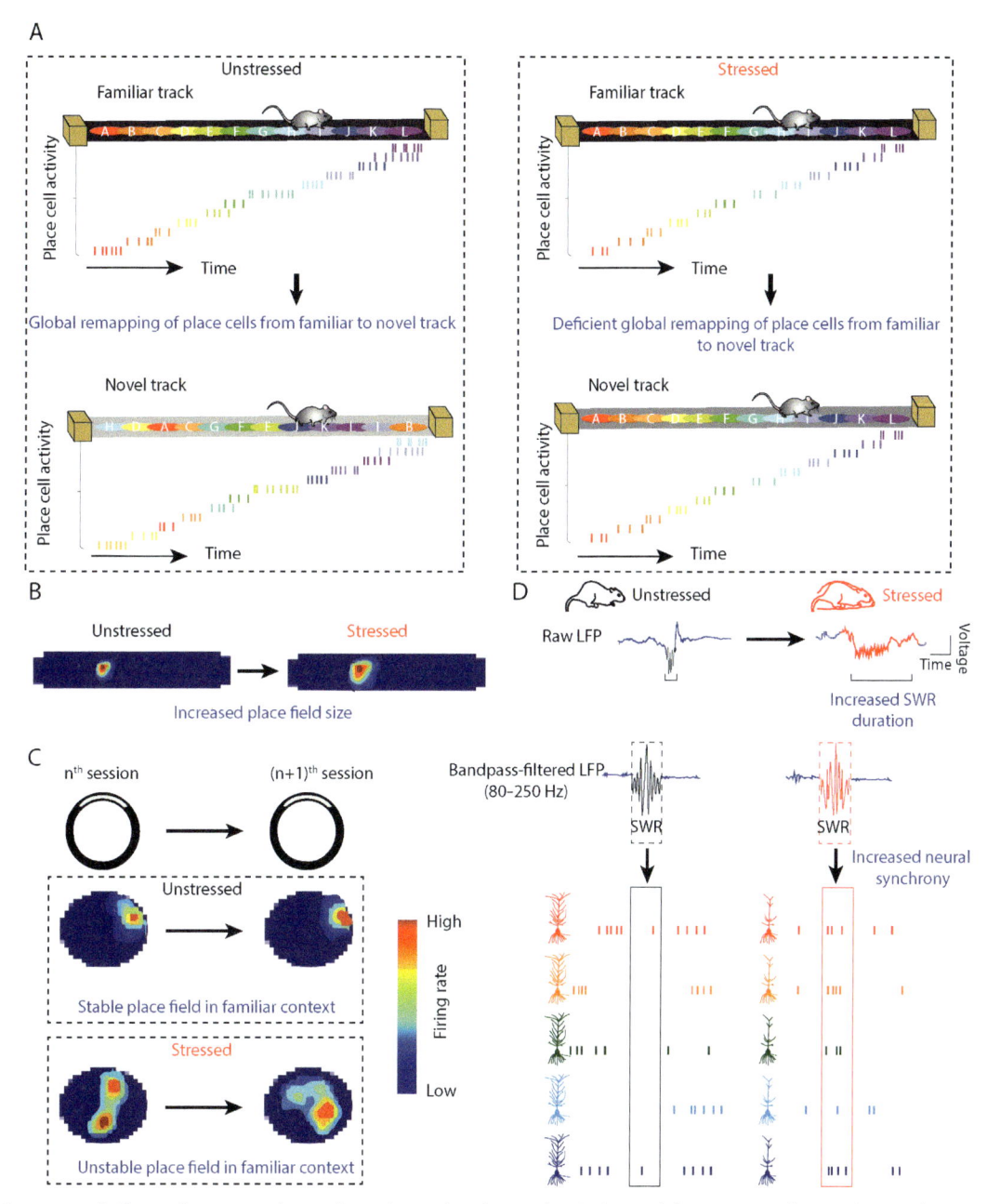

Figure 17.14 Summary of effects of stress on place cells and spatial coding in the CA1 area. (A) In unstressed control mice, the exposure to a novel track leads a familiar track's place-cell ensemble to undergo change in firing rate and location of place fields (global remapping) resulting in encoding of a novel place map (left). In stressed mice, introduction to a novel track leads to deficient global remapping (right), impairing formation of the novel map (Tomar et al., 2015). (Adapted from Joo & Frank, 2018.) (B) Schematic representation depicting enlarged CA1 place fields in mice before (left) and after (right) exposure to chronic stress, as described in Tomar et al. (2021). (C) In a familiar context, stable CA1 place-field representations are maintained across sessions in unstressed mice (top), but in stressed mice these representations are less stable across sessions (bottom). (Adapted from Park et al., 2015.) (D) Schematic depiction of raw LFP traces showing prolonged sharp wave ripple (SWR) events in the CA1 sub-region of stressed mice during immobilization stress (top). CA1 pyramidal neurons show increased SWR-specific coactivity both during immobilization stress as well as during awake-immobility/sleep after the termination of the chronic stress protocol. (Adapted from Tomar et al., 2021.)

Besides glutamate and glucocorticoids, there are other mediators that participate in experience-dependent structural and functional remodeling of brain circuits, as summarized in Table 17.1. These include BDNF, tissue plasminogen activator, lipocalin 2, and corticotrophin-releasing factor. Moreover, as shown in Table 17.1, a number of cellular processes are involved in dendritic remodeling following stress, including cytoskeletal depolymerization caused by a soluble phosphorylated tau (Arendt et al., 2003) and a reduction in expression of a cell nuclear pore complex protein (Kinoshita et al., 2014), suggesting that ongoing gene expression may be involved in maintaining the dendritic tree. Excess glutamatergic activity, without adequate reuptake in the aftermath of trauma from seizures, ischemia, or head trauma, leads to permanent neuronal loss in the hippocampus by a process that is exacerbated by glucocorticoids (Sapolsky et al., 1986).

17.8 From cells and molecules to networks: effects of stress on hippocampal place cells

The studies described above provide snapshots, through postmortem analyses at fixed time points, of stress-induced physiological and structural plasticity in the hippocampus. Thus, the functional effect of stress is inferred from analysis at the cellular and behavioral levels without any online readout of dynamic changes in neuronal activity in the intact animal. This section describes more recent studies using *in vivo* recordings of spatially receptive fields of hippocampal place cells, the firing of which occurs in a specific location in the environment of the rodent (O'Keefe, 1979; Eichenbaum et al., 1999; Moser et al., 2008) (see Chapter 11). These recordings, thereby, link stress-induced memory deficits to changes in neuronal physiology at the level of the intact hippocampal network in a behaving animal.

One of the first studies examined the effects of acute audiogenic stress on hippocampal "place cells" (Kim, Lee et al., 2007). Audiogenic stress impaired the stability of firing rates of CA1 place cells recorded in rats foraging freely around a novel open-field platform. These observations raised the possibility that stress-induced impairment in synaptic plasticity may block the storage of stable "rate maps" by hippocampal place cells, and this may in turn underlie spatial memory deficits triggered by stress (Kim, Lee, et al., 2007). A series of more recent studies carried out a detailed analysis of the cumulative and dynamic effect of chronic immobilization stress on the hippocampal spatial map *in vivo* (Tomar et al., 2015) (Figure 17.14). Stress-induced modulation of hippocampal CA1 place cells was characterized as mice explored familiar and novel spatial contexts after 5 and 10 days of immobilization stress. This study found that the impact of chronic stress, spanning 10 days, on the *in vivo* physiology of the hippocampus is not a stationary process, but rather a dynamic one that parallels other hormonal and structural modifications taking place over the course of repeated stress. For instance, after 5 days of immobilization stress (2 hours/day), CA1 pyramidal cells showed a decrease in excitability and increased rate variability across contexts, effects similar to what have been reported following episodes of acute stress. However, following 10 days of the same stress, these deficits recovered, suggesting the structural changes associated with chronic stress may be an adaptive response to changes in neuronal excitability. Surprisingly, only subtle changes were found in spatial encoding after both 5 and 10 days of chronic

stress. Place cells recorded on novel tracks on days 6 and 11 were largely similar in stressed and control mice, despite the fact that synaptic plasticity at CA3-to-CA1 Schaffer collateral synapses is compromised by repeated stress (Shors et al., 1989; Pavlides et al., 2002). This is reminiscent of earlier genetic and pharmacological studies showing that the formation of place fields can occur in the complete absence of CA1 plasticity (McHugh et al., 1996; Kentros et al., 1998) or even when CA3 transmission is impaired (Brun et al., 2002; Nakashiba et al., 2008).

In the same study (Tomar et al., 2015), detailed analyses of the ability of the hippocampus to distinguish novel from familiar contexts revealed that at the level of individual neurons, there was no difference in spatial remapping between control and stressed mice. However, despite the lack of change at the single neuron level, investigation of the ensemble representation pointed to enhanced correlation between the novel and familiar tracks on both day 6 and day 11 in the stressed mice. These findings suggest that stress may limit the capacity of the CA1 pyramidal population to properly distinguish the novel track from the familiar one (Figure 17.14). In other words, the mice exhibited deficient context discrimination, wherein both short-term and chronic stress impaired the ability of the CA1 pyramidal population to unambiguously distinguish novel and familiar environments. This, in turn, is consistent with a growing body of evidence that behavioral changes observed in chronically stressed animals can be attributed to the generalization of aversive events to unrelated contexts or cues (Conrad et al., 1999) and its adverse effects on decision-making (Dias-Ferreira et al., 2009). Indeed, overgeneralization is a key feature of the behavioral symptoms of PTSD.

How could such rigidity be brought about by chronic stress? One influential idea in the field, the "glucocorticoid cascade hypothesis" (Figure 17.3), suggests that the long-term impact of sustained elevation in stress hormones is akin to premature aging of the brain (Sapolsky et al., 1986; McEwen, 1999). Interestingly, a similar rigidity in spatial representation has been seen in the hippocampus of aged rats (Wilson, 2005), perhaps as a result of a suppression of plasticity in the hippocampus. Together, these results suggest that a loss of network flexibility may underlie some of the behavioral deficits, such as overgeneralization, accompanying chronic stress. Interestingly, a recent study also reported that hippocampal place-cell activity was modulated even by perturbations that were significantly less severe than physical stressors such as chronic immobilization. The presence of a predatory threat while foraging for food caused remapping of place fields, as the animals got closer to the threat. Furthermore, amygdala lesions prevented these *in vivo* physiological effects in the hippocampus, suggesting a pivotal role for threat-associated signals from the amygdala in modulating the stability of hippocampal place maps (Kim et al., 2015). This, in turn, highlights the importance of network interactions between the hippocampus and other brain areas, which is discussed in later sections.

A subsequent study analyzed the effects of the same chronic immobilization stress on sharp wave ripples (SPW-Rs) (Tomar, Polygalov, Chattarji, McHugh, 2021), high-frequency oscillation transients crucial for memory consolidation. *In vivo* tetrode recordings revealed that although there was a net decrease in pyramidal cell activity in stressed animals, a greater fraction of spikes in the CA1 area occurred specifically during SPW-Rs, leading to enhanced neuronal synchrony. Strikingly, following exposure to chronic stress, some of these changes were evident during rest even in the absence of stress. Together, these studies provide new

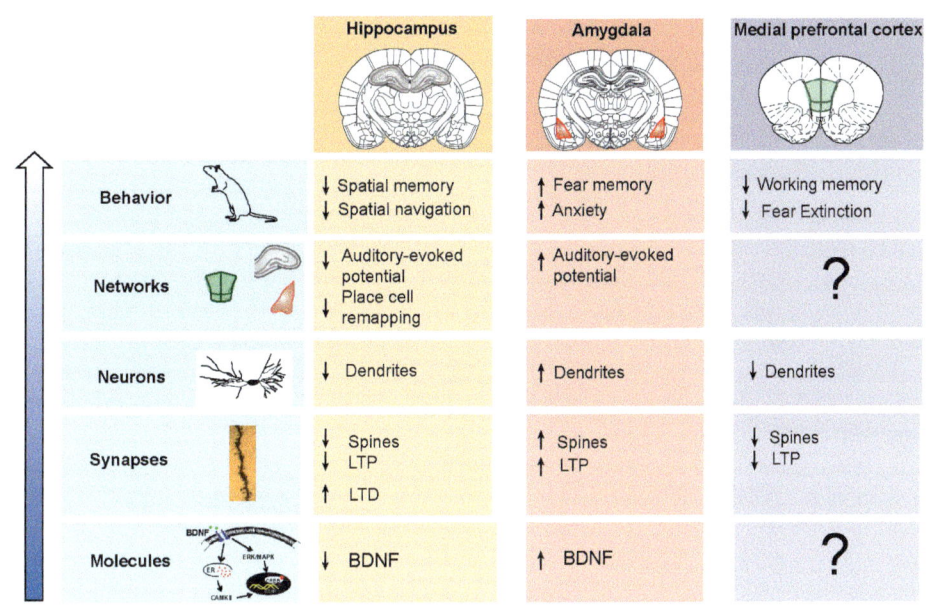

Figure 17.15 Contrasting patterns of stress-induced plasticity across brain areas. At the behavioral level, chronic stress enhances fear and anxiety while impairing spatial and working memory and fear extinction. At the network level, stress causes an increase in neural activity in the amygdala, whereas it has the opposite effect in the hippocampus. At the levels of neurons and synapses, repeated stress leads to growth of dendrites and spines in the amygdala, but loss of dendritic arbors and spines in the hippocampus and mPFC. These morphological changes are accompanied by enhanced LTP in the amygdala, as well as by impaired and/or reduced LTP in the hippocampus and mPFC. At the molecular level, BDNF protein is increased in the amygdala, but decreased in the hippocampus. In the mPFC, certain forms of stress increase BDNF mRNA expression, whereas others do not. The effect of chronic stress on BDNF protein levels in the mPFC is not known. (Adapted from Chattarji et al., 2015.)

insights into stress-induced alterations in ripple-spike interactions and potential mechanisms through which chronic stress may interfere with subsequent information processing (Tomar and McHugh, 2022) (Figure 17.14). Interestingly, SPW-Rs in the ventral hippocampus have also been shown to underlie stress susceptibility in mice (Kuga et al., 2023)

17.9 From local to distributed effects of stress: interactions between the hippocampus and other brain areas

The preceding sections describe how a combination of behavioral, morphological, electrophysiological, pharmacological, and molecular techniques have enabled detailed analyses of the effect of stress on plasticity at multiple levels of neural organization in the hippocampus. The effect of stress on plasticity mechanisms are manifested as behavioral effects at one end of the spectrum, and as cellular effects at the level of neurons, synapses, and molecules at the other. Although much of the early evidence on stress-induced plasticity emerged primarily from studies on the hippocampus, subsequent research has been extended to studies of other brain areas that interact with the hippocampus, such as the amygdala and medial prefrontal cortex (mPFC). Hence, the next section provides a brief description of the divergent patterns of stress-induced plasticity across the amygdala and mPFC, and how they compare with those seen in the hippocampus (Figure 17.15).

17.9.1 Stress-induced plasticity in the prefrontal cortex (PFC) shares some similarities with the hippocampus

Similar to the hippocampus, the mPFC is also involved in shutting off the HPA stress response. And the effects of stress on the mPFC, in

turn, appears to be similar to that seen in the hippocampus (Arnsten, 2015; Goldwater et al., 2009). Further, structural plasticity elicited by stress varies between layers and subregions in the mPFC (Cook and Wellman, 2004; Liston et al., 2006; Radley et al., 2006; Radley et al., 2004). For instance, repeated stress (3 hours or 6 hours per day for 21 days) and repeated treatment with corticosterone causes structural remodeling in the infralimbic (IL) region of the mPFC, as evidenced by a shortening of dendritic length and a simplification of dendritic branching in layer II/III pyramidal neurons (Cook and Wellman, 2004; Radley et al., 2004; Wellman, 2001) There is also a reduction in spine density on the apical dendrites of these layer II/III neurons after 21 days of repeated restraint stress. Together, the combined effect of these morphological changes is estimated to be a decrease of 40% in synaptic inputs to the mPFC. Compared with the hippocampus, less is known about the *in vitro* electrophysiological correlates of stress-induced changes in synaptic plasticity. The same 21 days of restraint stress that causes apical dendritic atrophy and spine loss in the IL-mPFC also impairs catecholaminergic facilitation of LTP in the IL (Arnsten, 2015; Goldwater et al., 2009). Poststress recovery for 21 days reversed this effect. In the mPFC, however, the efficacy of the same poststress recovery in countering stress-induced structural plasticity varies with dendritic location. In another study, application of local tetanic stimuli, in the presence of bath-applied serotonin, elicited LTD at excitatory inputs to layer V/VI pyramidal neurons in the mPFC (Zhong et al., 2008). This form of LTD, mediated by 5-HT2A/C receptors, was substantially impaired in brain slices taken from animals exposed to acute stress; this marks a difference with the hippocampus, where stress has been shown to enhance LTD (Holderbach et al., 2007; Xu et al., 1997). Although stress-induced structural and functional plasticity in the PFC and hippocampus appear to share similarities in that both are negatively modulated by stress (for example, loss of dendrites and spines, impaired LTP), more detailed analysis is needed to investigate the links between morphological and physiological changes elicited by stress in the PFC.

17.9.2 The impact of stress is strikingly different in the amygdala compared with the hippocampus

The impetus for the search for cellular correlates of stress in the amygdala came from findings that highlight the contrasting manner in which the hippocampus and amygdala affect the stress response and how their behavioral outputs in turn are modulated by stress. First, there are anatomical data showing that limbic inputs to the paraventricular nucleus (PVN) of the hypothalamus and to hypothalamic GABAergic neurons can be either excitatory from the hippocampus and thereby enhance GABAergic tone or inhibitory from the amygdala and thereby reduce GABAergic tone (Herman and Cullinan, 1997; Herman et al., 1989; Jacobson and Sapolsky, 1991; Pitkanen and Amaral, 1994; Sapolsky et al., 1991). A recent study has provided more direct functional evidence for ventral hippocampal efferents attenuating acute stress responses through disynaptic inhibition of corticotropin-releasing factor (CRF) cells in the paraventricular nucleus of the hypothalamus (PVN), thereby contributing to a net inhibition of the HPA axis (Cole et al., 2022). This implies that whereas enhanced hippocampal input would suppress the HPA axis, enhanced amygdalar input could have the opposite effect on HPA activity. Second, stress was shown to facilitate aversive learning but impair spatial learning in rodents (Luine, Villegas, et al., 1994; Shors et al., 1992). Although repeated stress that produces dendritic atrophy in the CA3 region impairs hippocampus-dependent learning (Conrad et al., 1996), the basolateral nucleus of the amygdala (BLA) has been shown to be essential for stress-induced facilitation of aversive learning (Liang et al., 1994; Shors and Mathew, 1998). Taken together, these observations highlighted the need to examine the cellular effects of stress in the amygdala, and how they compare to those observed in the hippocampus.

Applying the same tools of morphometric analysis of Golgi-stained neurons that were earlier used in the hippocampus, the first cellular evidence for contrasting patterns of stress-induced structural plasticity was found in the BLA (Chattarji et al., 2015; Vyas et al., 2002). For instance, chronic immobilization stress (2 hours per day for 10 days) induced dendritic atrophy and debranching in hippocampal CA3 pyramidal neurons (Vyas et al., 2002), which is consistent with earlier reports using other forms of repeated stress (McEwen, 1999a). In the basolateral amygdala (BLA), by contrast, chronic stress triggered the opposite effect by strengthening the structural basis of synaptic connectivity through dendritic growth and spinogenesis (Figure 17.15) (Chattarji et al., 2015; Mitra et al., 2005, Roozendaal et al., 2009; Vyas et al., 2002). Stress-induced dendritic remodeling in these two brain areas differs not only in polarity but also in terms of their temporal persistence. For instance, exposure to 10 days of chronic immobilization stress elicits dendritic hypertrophy in BLA principal neurons that lasts till at least 21 days after the termination of stress. Hippocampal CA3 atrophy, on the other hand, is reversible within the same period of poststress recovery (Vyas et al., 2004). Interestingly, the unique temporal features of stress-induced changes in the BLA are not limited to chronic stress alone. The temporal pattern of structural plasticity in the BLA can also be modulated by the duration of the stressor. A much shorter duration of the same stress, such as a single 2-hour

episode of immobilization, that fails to affect spine density or dendritic arborization 1 day later, leads to a significant increase in spine density 10 days later (Mitra et al., 2005). Together, these studies have helped identify novel features of stress-induced plasticity in the amygdala that are quite distinct from those observed in the hippocampus (Chattarji et al., 2015; Roozendaal et al., 2009).

These divergent patterns between the hippocampus and the amygdala also extend to the molecular level. For example, the same chronic stress that elicits hippocampal dendritic atrophy also reduces levels of the neurotrophin brain-derived neurotrophic factor (BDNF) in the rodent hippocampus (Nibuya et al., 1995; Smith et al., 1995). Conversely, chronic administration of antidepressants prevents stress-induced decrease in BDNF levels and dendritic atrophy in the hippocampus (Chen et al., 2001; Nibuya et al., 1995). Together these and other findings have contributed to the "neurotrophic hypothesis," which states that symptoms associated with stress-related disorders such as depression are a result of decreased neurotrophic support in the hippocampus, and conversely, that increasing neurotrophic support would lead to the correction of these symptoms (Duman and Monteggia, 2006; Nestler et al., 2002). This hypothesis has received support from several studies including a report that direct BDNF infusion into the rodent hippocampus produces antidepressant effects (Shirayama et al., 2002; Siuciak et al., 1997). Also, transgenic overexpression of the neurotrophin BDNF has antidepressant effects and prevents chronic stress-induced hippocampal atrophy in mice (Govindarajan et al., 2006). Interestingly, in the same transgenic mice, overexpression of BDNF also causes spinogenesis in the BLA. Moreover, BLA spinogenesis is also triggered by chronic stress in control mice but is occluded by BDNF overexpression. Thus, structural changes in the amygdala and hippocampus, caused by genetic manipulation of the same molecule BDNF, gave rise to contrasting effects on anxiety and depressive symptoms, both of which are major behavioral correlates of stress disorders (Govindarajan et al., 2006). Furthermore, acute and chronic stress trigger opposite effects on BDNF levels in the BLA and the CA3 area, and these divergent changes also follow distinct temporal profiles (Lakshminarasimhan and Chattarji, 2012).

Impaired NMDA receptor (NMDAR)-dependent LTP and dendritic atrophy are believed to be key factors contributing to chronic stress-induced deficits in hippocampal learning and memory (Diamond et al., 2007; Luine, Villegas, et al., 1994; McEwen, 1999a; Sandi and Pinelo-Nava, 2007) Notably, NMDAR-dependent LTP in the lateral amygdala (LA) is also pivotal for classical fear conditioning (Bauer et al., 2002; LeDoux, 2000). Why then does repeated stress facilitate amygdala-dependent fear learning, when previous studies report stress-induced suppression of NMDAR-dependent LTP in the hippocampus (Cordero et al., 2003; Rau et al., 2005; Rodrigues et al., 2009, Shors et al., 1992)? In rats subjected to 10 days of chronic immobilization stress, whole-cell patch-clamp recordings in amygdala slices showed NMDAR-mediated synaptic responses to be enhanced in principal neurons of the lateral amygdala (LA) (Suvrathan et al., 2014). This creates permissive conditions for LA neurons to undergo NMDAR-mediated synaptic plasticity, the consequences of which maybe manifested in several ways. First, this increase in NMDAR currents provides a synaptic substrate that is primed to undergo further strengthening through LTP, a prediction that was confirmed by several studies. Second, this also implies that any behavioral output that relies on NMDAR-dependent LTP in the

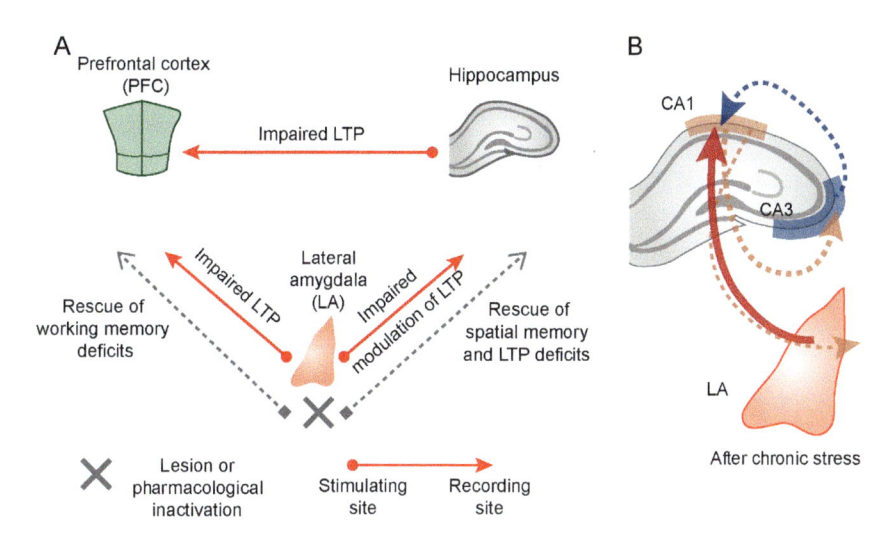

Figure 17.16 Interactions and interdependence of stress-induced plasticity between the hippocampus and other brain areas. (A) Stress impairs in vivo LTP in the BLA–mPFC and hippocampus–mPFC pathways. Stress also suppresses the modulation of hippocampal LTP by the BLA. Origin of the red arrow indicates the location of stimulation and arrowhead indicates site of recording of changes in plasticity. Lesion or inactivation (X) of the BLA rescues behavioral deficits in spatial (hippocampus) and working memory (mPFC) caused by stress. These BLA manipulations also reverse stress-induced LTP deficits in the hippocampus. (B) Granger causality graphs, based on analysis of hippocampal and amygdalar time series, depicting the modulation of directional influence. Chronic stress causes a persistent impairment of directional coupling from hippocampal area CA3 to CA1. In contrast, directional coupling from the LA to area CA1 is enhanced after chronic stress. The strength of Granger spectral causality values are coded by the thickness of lines between the three recording sites. The arrowheads indicate the direction of Granger causal influence. Solid and dotted lines indicate presence and absence of dominant directional influence, respectively. (Adapted from Chattarji et al., 2015.)

LA, such as conditioned fear, would also be amplified by chronic stress (Figure 17.15).

In summary, findings on structural and physiological plasticity induced by chronic stress highlight important differences between the hippocampus, amygdala, and PFC. Principal neurons in specific subregions of the hippocampus and PFC, both part of the stress-inhibitory circuitry, undergo structural and functional deficits. In contrast, the physiological and structural basis of synaptic connectivity grows stronger in the BLA following chronic stress.

Finally, what might be the functional consequences of the opposite directions of stress-induced plasticity in the hippocampus versus the amygdala? Intriguing possibilities emerged from an earlier study (Conrad et al., 1999a) that tested the prediction that stress would enhance auditory cued conditioning (which depends on the amygdala and where plasticity is enhanced by stress), but not context conditioning (which depends on both the amygdala and hippocampus, with plasticity in the latter being suppressed by stress). Surprisingly, this study reported that repeated restraint stress facilitates both tone and context fear conditioning independently of causing hippocampal CA3 dendritic atrophy. Antidepressant treatment failed to block enhanced fear conditioning and anxiety-like behavior after stress, despite preventing CA3 atrophy in the hippocampus (Conrad et al., 1999a). Thus, chronic stress may have a powerful enhancing effect on the amygdala that could override any influence of the hippocampus. Stress hormones released as a result of stress-induced amygdala activity can strengthen the excitatory drive in the BLA and thereby influence subsequent information processing by the amygdala and its downstream targets. This suggests that chronic stress could lead to an imbalance in HPA axis function through a gradual loss of hippocampal/PFC inhibitory control as well as a gain in excitatory control exerted by the amygdala. As described later, in vivo electrophysiological analyses offer further insights into these processes.

17.9.3 Interconnectivity and interdependence–beyond the hippocampus

As informative as these results have been in constructing a useful intellectual and experimental framework for animal models of stress, in the majority of these studies, stress-induced plasticity has been viewed as stand-alone effects intrinsic to each area. However, neuroanatomical data point to extensive interconnections between these brain areas (Petrovich et al., 2001; Pikkarainen et al., 1999; Pitkänen et al., 1997). This raises the intriguing possibility that some of the structural and physiological changes triggered by stress in the hippocampus may, at least in part, be influenced by changes in other brain areas (Figure 17.16). Several lines of investigation have addressed this question in the broader context of the influence of stress on the spatiotemporal dynamics of neural activity in awake, behaving animals. Early evidence suggesting that neuronal activity in one brain area can influence stress-induced plasticity in other areas came from seminal work by McGaugh and colleagues. Their work revealed that in vivo pharmacological manipulations of synaptic transmission and neuromodulators in the amygdala impair or facilitate the formation of hippocampal memory (McGaugh, 2000; Packard et al., 1994; Roozendaal et al., 2003). Lesions and drug infusions targeting the amygdala, as well as stimulation of the amygdala, have also been shown to modulate the magnitude of LTP in the DG (Abe, 2001). On the other hand, accumulating behavioral evidence shows that inactivation of the amygdala can rescue stress-induced deficits in hippocampal spatial memory (Kim et al., 2001; Roozendaal and McGaugh, 1996). Taken together, these findings imply that amygdalar activity may be involved in mediating the effects of stress on hippocampal function. Consistent with this prediction, electrolytic lesions of the amygdala before exposure to uncontrollable stress prevents hippocampal LTP and spatial memory deficits in rats (Roozendaal and McGaugh, 1996; Kim et al.,

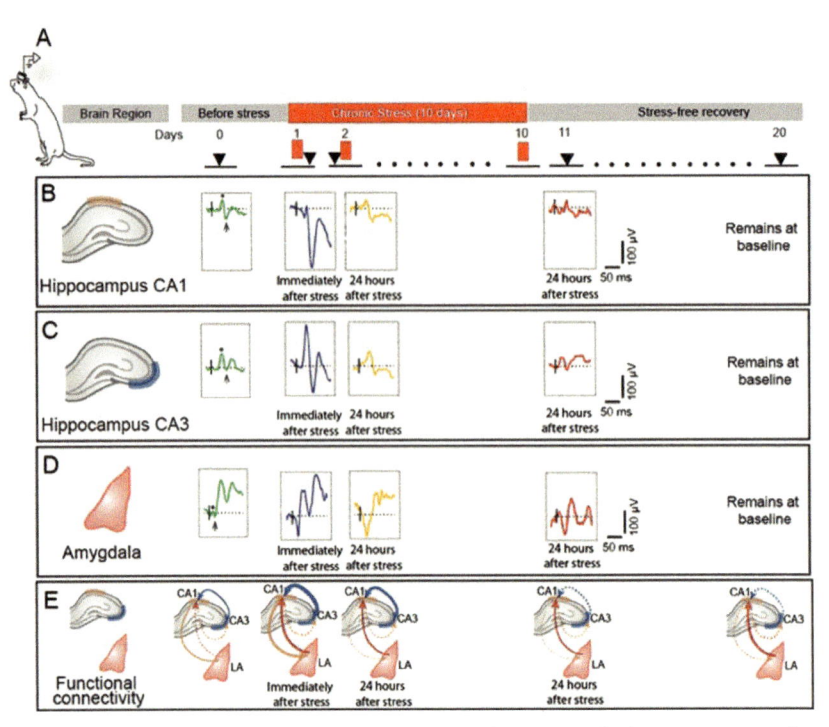

Figure 17.17 Temporal features of the impact of chronic stress on in vivo neuronal activity in the hippocampus and amygdala in awake, behaving rodents. During 10-day chronic immobilization stress, AEPs were simultaneously monitored in areas CA1 (B), CA3 (C), and LA (D). On day 1, 1 h (indicated by black inverted triangle) after a single exposure to acute stress, AEP amplitudes were enhanced in all three areas. This increase was evident even 1 day later in the lateral amygdala (LA), but not in the CA1 and CA3 areas. 1 day after the 10th day of chronic stress, AEP amplitudes were back to baseline in the CA1 and CA3 areas, whereas a significant increase was still visible in the LA. This enhancement returns to baseline after a 10-day stress free recovery. (E) Chronic stress causes a gradual impairment of directional coupling from hippocampal areas CA1 to CA3 and a gradual enhancement from the LA to CA1. 1 h after the first episode of acute stress (day 1), functional coupling was strengthened between CA3–CA1, CA1–LA, and LA–CA1. 24 h after the 10th day of stress, only LA–CA1 connectivity continued to be strong. This persisted even after a 10 day stress-free recovery. The strength of Granger spectral causality values are coded by the thickness of lines between the three recording sites. The arrowheads indicate the direction of Granger causal influence. Solid and dotted lines indicate presence and absence of dominant directional influence, respectively. Taken together, these findings suggest that while functional connectivity from the lateral amygdala to the hippocampus grows stronger after chronic stress, it becomes weaker from the CA3 to CA1 area in the same animals. (Adapted from Ghosh et al., 2013; Chattarji et al., 2015.)

2001). Furthermore, targeted inactivation of the amygdala with microinfusions of the GABA$_A$ receptor agonist muscimol prevents stress-induced suppression of LTP in ex vivo hippocampal slices (Kim et al., 2001). Muscimol infusions into the amygdala immediately after stress, however, do not rescue stress-induced deficits in LTP and spatial memory (Kim et al., 2001). These behavioral and physiological data identify an important role for amygdalar activity in the impairment of hippocampal synaptic plasticity and memory caused by stress.

Insights into how behavioral stress affects dynamic changes and interactions in neuronal activity across the hippocampal-amygdala-PFC network have emerged recently from simultaneous *in vivo* recordings of activity of neuronal populations located in these brain areas. For instance, a recent study simultaneously monitored *in vivo* auditory-evoked potentials (AEPs) from hippocampal areas CA1 and CA3, as well as the LA, in rats during and after the 10-day chronic immobilization stress protocol described earlier (Ghosh et al., 2013). The amplitude of AEPs in the hippocampus increased transiently after a single episode of 2-hour stress. But this enhancement reversed to control levels when the same stress was repeated for 10 consecutive days, which is suggestive of an adaptive response that builds up in response to repeated stress. In contrast, both acute and chronic stress caused a persistent increase in AEPs in the LA. Chronic stress also elicited a reduction in the evoked power

of gamma and beta frequencies in the hippocampus. Moreover, beta and gamma synchrony were reduced between areas CA1 and CA3, but enhanced between the LA and hippocampus after chronic stress. Stress-induced increase in the power spectra and phase synchrony in beta/gamma oscillations raised the possibility that these oscillations within the amygdala–hippocampal network may be coupled (Ghosh et al., 2013). Therefore, this study also examined how stress modulates the directionality of these oscillations across the LA–CA3–CA1 network using Granger causality analysis (Granger, 1969; Geweke, 1982). Granger causality has been used to measure whether a time series is causally related to another by assessing whether past values of the former are able to predict future values of the latter. This method has been applied to study directionality in neuronal interactions by analysing neurophysiological data in both the frequency and time domains (Bernasconi and Konig, 1999; Bernasconi et al., 2000; Hesse et al., 2003), including studies in primates and rodents to analyze the directionality of interactions between various brain areas under different behavioral conditions (Brovelli et al., 2004; Gregoriou et al., 2009; Popa et al., 2010). When this was applied to the 10-day chronic stress data obtained from simultaneous *in vivo* AEP recordings (Ghosh et al., 2013), a strong directional influence from the LA to area CA1 was revealed that persisted throughout, and even 10 days after, chronic stress. In contrast, the same chronic stress caused a persistent suppression of oscillatory coupling from area CA3 to CA1 within the hippocampus (Figure 17.17). These findings suggest that lateral amygdalar influence on the hippocampus becomes dominant during chronic stress (Ghosh et al., 2013). Specifically, repeated stress appears to shift control over area CA1 from the CA3 area to LA. Importantly, some of these changes persist even 10 days after the cessation of stress, raising the possibility of a prolonged rewiring of the amygdala–hippocampal network. However, it should be noted that the Granger causality framework is statistical in nature, and thus these results by themselves do not prove that a neuronal assembly in the LA directly activates another in the hippocampus. But, significant neuroanatomical data, showing robust interconnectivity across the LA–CA3–CA1 network, raises the intriguing possibility that these changes observed in Granger causality analysis echo stress-induced modifications in functional interactions between neuronal populations across this network. Thus, future studies will need to investigate the role of amygdalar projection neurons and their outputs in modulating stress-induced plasticity mechanisms in the hippocampus. Underscoring the importance of such interactions between brain regions, a recent study combined *in vivo* optogenetic- and biosensor-based methods to show that stress-induced endocannabinoid (eCB) release at ventral hippocampus (vHPC)-basolateral amygdala (BLA) synapses helps to cope with the adverse behavioral consequences of stress exposure (Kondev et al., 2023).

Stress-induced modulation of interactions across the hippocampal-amygdala-PFC network is also manifested as changes in synaptic plasticity between these areas. For example, in addition to affecting LTP and LTD *within* individual brain regions, stress also modulates synaptic plasticity at pathways *between* the three brain areas. Using extracellular field recordings, chronic unpredictable stress was found to reduce *in vivo* LTP in the prelimbic (PL) region of the mPFC induced by high-frequency stimulation of the CA1 area in the ventral hippocampus (Cerqueira et al., 2007). The same chronic stress also disrupted working memory and behavioral flexibility, in addition to causing volume loss in specific layers of the mPFC (Cerqueira et al., 2007). Analyses of the effects of stress on hippocampal LTP and how it is modulated by amygdalar activity has relied on a combination of *in vivo* manipulations of the BLA in conjunction with *in vivo* electrophysiological recordings in the dentate gyrus (DG). These studies by Richter-Levin and colleagues used high-frequency stimulation (HFS) of the perforant path inputs to induce LTP in the DG. Interestingly, priming, consisting of tetanic stimulation of the BLA 30 s before the HFS was applied to the perforant path, leads to enhanced LTP in the DG. This priming-induced enhancement was blocked by exposure to a combination of behavioral stressors, as well as systemic treatment with corticosterone (Akirav and Richter-Levin, 1999, 2002).

17.10 Sex differences in stress

So far in this chapter, we have not considered how men and women differ in their response to life stressors. Sex differences in the brain have emerged as more widespread than previously believed. There is accumulating evidence for significant differences between males and females in both health and disease (McCarthy et al., 2012). Brain and body sex differences are produced not only by hormones during phases of development but also by genetic sex interacting with experience throughout the human life course. These have important effects on the response to stressors. It is now well recognized that men and women typically handle stress in different ways, and often with equal success. This is evident in an imaging study on men and women during tests of emotional sensitivity, where men and women scored equally well but showed marked differences in the brain regions activated by the same tasks (Derntl et al., 2010). Also, women are more prone to depression after toxic stress while men show more antisocial behavior as their response (Eme, 2007; Kessler et al., 1994; Kessler et al., 1993). Besides the hypothalamus, sex hormones act on the hippocampus and virtually every extrahypothalamic brain region to affect a wide range of neurological and behavioral processes (McEwen et al., 2012; McEwen and Milner, 2007, 2017). Indeed, there are receptors for estradiol, androgens, and progestins in regions of both the male and female brain that regulate memory, pain, coordinated movement, and cognitive functions. Developmentally and genetically programmed sex differences in the brain affect the way it responds to stressors and other experiences.

In the hippocampus of male rats, 21 days of chronic restraint stress (CRS) cause apical dendrites of CA3 neurons to retract and a loss of ~30% of the parvalbumin-expressing neurons in the dentate gyrus. These changes, however, do not occur following CRS in female rats (Galea et al., 1997, Milner et al., 2013). Interestingly, chronic stress affects hippocampus-dependent memory in opposite directions in male and female rats, with males showing impairment and females showing enhancement or no effect (Bowman et al., 2003; Luine et al., 1996; Luine, Villegas, et al., 1994). Moreover, exposure of male and female rats to restraint, along with intermittent tail shock, has opposite effects on classical eyeblink conditioning, inhibiting it in females and enhancing it in males; in females, this effect is abolished by ovariectomy and is therefore estradiol-dependent (Shors, Chua, et al., 2001; Wood and Shors, 1998). A morphological correlate of this in the hippocampus is the finding that acute stress inhibits estradiol-dependent spine formation in hippocampal CA1 neurons in the female rat, whereas the same acute stressors enhance spine density in CA1 neurons in the male, possibly by increasing testosterone secretion (Shors, Chua, et al., 2001), on which spine formation in area CA1 of the male rat is dependent (Leranth et al., 2003). Neonatal masculinization of females made them respond positively, like genetic males, to the shock stressor (Shors, 2016). Moreover, in females, depending on reproductive status and previous experience, the negative effects of stress were altered, e.g., it was absent in mothers and virgin females that had had experience with infants (Shors, 2016).

Another interesting facet of sex difference has emerged as subregion-specific contrasts—between areas CA1 and CA3—within the hippocampus (McLaughlin et al., 2005). A study on the impact of stress on ovariectomized female rats revealed that dendritic spine shape on CA1 pyramidal neurons, following chronic restraint stress (6 h/day/21 days), may parallel spatial memory in female rats despite robust CA3 dendritic atrophy. Chronic restraint stress caused CA3 apical dendritic retraction in both short- and long-shafted neurons, while it reduced basal dendritic arbors only in long-shafted neurons. Yet the same stress did not affect CA1 dendritic arborization, although it increased the proportion of mature CA1 spines compared with controls (McLaughlin et al., 2005). Further, spatial memory on the Y-maze was found to be intact, or even enhanced, despite CA3 dendritic retraction. Strikingly, performance on the Y-maze exhibited a positive correlation with the proportion of mature CA1 spines. Thus, unlike male rats, CA3 morphology was not a reliable predictor of spatial memory performance in female rats. Taken together, these results suggest that the CA1 area may play a more important role in spatial memory, compared with the CA3 region, following chronic stress in females (McLaughlin et al., 2005).

The effects of stress on the amygdala are also different between males and females. The neurons in the BLA of female rats undergo dendritic hypotrophy and increased action potential firing following the same chronic stress that triggers hypertrophy, but reduced firing, in male BLA neurons (Blume et al., 2019). Further, 10 days of chronic immobilization stress (2 h/day) enhances anxiety-like behavior in male rats but not in female rats (Mitra et al., 2005, Vyas et al., 2002). This could be due to baseline morphological and physiological differences between male and female LA neurons, such as higher firing rates and spine density in female compared with male rats (Blume et al., 2017). These neurons also function in a different microenvironment, as indicated by lower extracellular levels of serotonin and dopamine in the female BLA (Mitsushima et al., 2006). Sex differences have also been seen in the delayed impact of acute stress on the amygdala (Gupta and Chattarji, 2021). Ten days after 2-hour acute immobilization stress, there was enhanced excitatory, but reduced inhibitory, synaptic transmission in lateral amygdala principal neurons in male rats. In female rats, by contrast, the same acute stress failed to elicit either of these synaptic changes 10 days later. This stress-induced tilt in the balance in favor of synaptic excitation over inhibition was also accompanied by a delayed but increased anxiety-like behavior in male but not female rats 10 days later. Further, stress induces sex-specific variations in neurotrophin expression in the brain (Bath et al., 2013). For example, BDNF expression in the hippocampus increases in female rats (Lin et al., 2009), but not in male rats after acute stress (Lakshminarasimhan and Chattarji, 2012; Lin et al., 2009).

Among possible mechanisms for these sex differences, the corticotrophin-releasing factor (CRF) receptor stands out in the hippocampus. There are sex differences in the association of the CRF1 receptor with G proteins and beta-arrestin 2, which make females more adaptable to acute stress, but less to chronic stress, due to compromised CRF1 internalization (Valentino et al., 2013). Thus, the failure of female rats and mice to show spine loss and dendritic shrinkage (Galea et al., 1997; Pawlak et al., 2005) may be related to this sex difference; in particular, the role of CRF-activated tissue plasminogen activator (tPA) secretion in causing stress-induced CA1 spine loss may be compromised in females as it is in tPA knockout mice (Pawlak et al., 2005).

While the majority of rodent studies have focused on the effects of chronic stress in adults, less is known about the impact of chronic stress during the juvenile and adolescent period. A study using a rat model of chronic juvenile stress (restraint 6 h daily from postnatal day 20–41), reported that chronic stress caused significant and immediate alterations in both males and females during this developmental window (Eiland et al., 2012). In both male and female adolescent rats, chronic stress altered HPA reactivity and elicited depressive-like behavior. In striking contrast to what has been seen in adult rats, there was not a significant effect of sex on stress-induced dendritic remodeling. During adolescence, both male and female rats subjected to chronic stress showed significant dendritic atrophy in area CA3 and prefrontal cortex, but dendritic hypertrophy in the

basolateral amygdala. However, restraint stress in adolescents suppresses neurogenesis in females but not in males (Barha et al., 2011).

Sex differences in responses to hormones are also evident in the hippocampus. In male rats, synapse formation in the hippocampus is stimulated by androgens but not by estradiol (Leranth et al., 2003). However, males respond to estradiol if sexual differentiation is blocked at birth by aromatase inhibitors (Lewis et al., 1995). Further, testosterone, but not estradiol, increases hippocampal neurogenesis through increased cell survival in the DG by an androgen-receptor-dependent mechanism (Hamson et al., 2013; Spritzer and Galea, 2007). Similar to the actions of estrogens in female rats, androgens too can affect dendritic spine density in the CA1 area of the male rat hippocampus (Leranth et al., 2003). Light microscopic analyses showed that androgen receptors (ARs) are present in the nuclei of CA1 pyramidal neurons (Kerr et al., 1995; Tabori et al., 2005). Electron microscopy revealed AR-immunoreactivity at several extranuclear sites in all subregions of the hippocampus. Specifically, AR-immunoreactivity was observed in dendritic spines on pyramidal and granule cell dendrites. Together, these findings suggest that ARs may serve as both a genomic and nongenomic transducer of androgen action in the hippocampus (Kerr et al., 1995, Tabori et al., 2005). Other sex differences in hormone action have been documented by Cahill (2017).

These sex differences occur throughout the brain and not just in brain regions like the hypothalamus that are involved in reproduction (McEwen and Milner, 2017). In fact, more recent research indicates that, at the molecular level, male and female responses to stress in the hippocampus, can be strikingly different (Marrocco and McEwen, 2016). For example, RNA sequencing of ribosome-bound RNA from a single neuron type, hippocampal CA3 pyramidal neurons, revealed remarkable qualitative sex differences (Marrocco et al., 2017). Exposure to acute forced-swim stress

Table 17.2 Translation to human hippocampus: negative and positive effects

A	Decreased volume	
1	Depression	Bremner et al., 2000 MacQueen et al., 2003 Sheline et al., 1996
2	Cushing's syndrome	Starkman et al., 1992 Starkman, 2003
3	PTSD	Bremner et al., 1997 Gilbertson et al., 2002 Gurvits et al., 1996, 1997
4	Jet lag	Cho, 2001
5	Aging associated with higher corticosterone	Lupien et al., 1998
6	Low self-esteem	Pruessner et al., 2005
7	Diabetes	Convit, 2005 Gold et al., 2007 Yau et al., 2012
8	Chronic inflammation	Marsland et al., 2008
9	Dementia	DeLeon and Miller, 2018
B	Increased volume	
1	Exercise	Erickson et al., 2011
2	Intense learning	Draganski et al., 2006
3	Postmenstrual phase vs. premenstrual phase	Protopopescu et al., 2008

activated two immediate early genes, *Fos* and *Arc*, in both males and females. But, there was significant sexual dimorphism in the expression of other genes. Importantly, the same genes that were found to be upregulated by stress in males were downregulated in females, or vice versa. Additional gene ontology analysis revealed that those genes were implicated in synaptic function, transcription regulation, glycosylation, and ion channel formation. Moreover, heterozygous BDNF Val66Met mice, a model that is genetically susceptible to stress, recapitulated the effects of acute stress on mRNA levels in wildtype mice without any applied stress (a "prestress" state) (Marrocco et al., 2017). However, like wildtype mice, heterozygous BDNF Val66met mice only displayed transcription of immediate early genes when actually stressed. This phenotype included the expression of genes related to glutamatergic and glucocorticoid pathways. Behaviorally, only heterozygous BDNF Val66Met females exhibited spatial memory impairment, regardless of acute stress, and this effect was not observed in ovariectomized heterozygous BDNF Val66Met females, suggesting that circulating ovarian hormones induce cognitive impairment in Val66Met carriers. Cognitive deficits were not observed in males of either genotype, which instead showed impaired memory only after stress. This work sheds additional light on ways that genes, environment, and sex interact to affect the transcriptome, furthering our understanding of sexually dimorphic molecular mechanisms that underlie the response to stress in the male and female organism, and the ongoing reciprocal interactions between the brain and the rest of the body.

17.11 Translation to the human hippocampus and connected regions

17.11.1 Mood disorders—Cushing's disease, depression, PTSD

Recognition in animal models that hormones play an important role in modulating brain structure and function has opened the way to studies of how circulating hormones contribute to human brain disorders when their normal functions to promote adaptation go awry. Here we describe how studies in the hippocampus have provided valuable examples of translation, as well as reverse translation. The range of techniques that can be used, and endpoints assessed, are obviously constrained in the study of humans; nonetheless, this literature demonstrates that, as in animal models, sustained stress and/or glucocorticoid exposure has adverse effects on the hippocampus and hippocampal-dependent function.

As might be expected, the most frequent endpoint used in human studies has been volumetric analyses of the hippocampus, using structural brain imaging. Table 17.2 shows examples of hippocampal shrinkage in major depression, Cushing's disease, PTSD (Gurvits et al., 1996, 1997), diabetes, and dementia. Loss of hippocampal volume has also been seen as a result of chronic inflammation, in aging individuals with higher glucocorticoid levels, in individuals with extended histories of perceived stress, individuals with self-reported low self-esteem, and in individuals with long histories of circadian phase changes with little time given for recovery, producing chronic jet lag.

The sheer heterogeneity of human disorders associated with hippocampal atrophy allows for important insights about the phenomenon. One issue to raise is whether the disorder/atrophy correlation is a case of reverse causality. For example, could a small hippocampus predispose individuals toward major depressive disorders, an increased vulnerability for PTSD, more perceived stress, and lower self-esteem? There are some data in support of this, particularly regarding PTSD in response to single traumas (Pitman et al., 2006). However, other examples of the hippocampal atrophy clearly show the same direction of causality as in lab animals. For example, there is no plausible route by which a small hippocampus predisposes toward tumor formation in the pituitary, lungs, or adrenals, producing Cushing's disease, or toward autoimmune disorders that require chronic treatment with high-dose synthetic steroids. In addition, it is even less plausible that there is a route linking a small hippocampus with increased likelihood of taking a job producing chronic jet lag (i.e., being a flight attendant on international, rather than domestic flights).

Another issue is whether hippocampal volume reduction in response to these disorders is progressive. This appears to be the case with both major depressive illness as well as in Cushing's disease. Moreover, it is the duration of the illness (and number of depressive episodes), and not the age of the subjects, that predicts a progressive reduction in volume of the hippocampus (Drevets et al., 1997; MacQueen et al., 2003; Sheline et al., 1998; Sheline et al., 1999; Starkman et al., 1992).

These longitudinal studies on the progressive loss of hippocampal volume over the course of a history of major depression are particularly interesting (Sheline et al., 2019). Loss of volume in CA2, CA3, and CA4 subfields is evident even in patients with first-episode depression (Roddy et al., 2019). With repeated depressive episodes, the dentate gyrus, CA1, and subiculum also exhibit volume loss, which thus encompasses the entire trisynaptic circuit. This pattern is quite similar to the emergence of dendritic atrophy and dendritic spine loss seen in animal models.

Another issue raised by the array of findings in Table 17.2 is whether it is indeed an excess of glucocorticoids that is responsible for the hippocampal atrophy. This is difficult to answer in the case of disorders in which there are extensive neurochemical and neuroendocrine abnormalities along with adrenocortical changes (such as in major depression or PTSD). However, the commonality among the different tumor locations that can give rise to Cushing's disease is the elevation of glucocorticoid concentrations; the same is obviously the case in instances in which autoimmune disorders are treated with synthetic glucocorticoids.

A final issue concerns what happens when the disorder abates—does the progressive atrophy halt at that point, or even reverse? This is obviously not possible to answer in a case where it is ambiguous whether the disorder ever does, in fact, abate. For example, a general clinical perception is that few, if any, PTSD sufferers are ever "cured" of the disease; instead, with luck, the individual gains the means to contain it. The clearest evidence that volume loss can be halted and even reversed comes with Cushing's disease, following surgical correction of the hypercortisolemia (Murphy, 1991; Starkman et al., 1981). Moreover, as evidence of a positive side (Table 17.2), increased hippocampal volume is reported as a result of regular physical activity, intense learning, and the follicular phase of the ovulatory cycle (Chaddock et al., 2010; Erickson et al., 2011a; Lisofsky et al., 2015).

Thus, a variety of human disorders, psychological states and life-history situations are associated with hippocampal volume loss in a

Box 17.3 Metabolic hormones in the brain

These are transported into the brain and have multiple functions in the healthy brain. Besides glucocorticoids and excitatory amino acids, a number of protein hormones have been shown to affect the hippocampus. The hippocampus has receptors for IGF-1 and insulin and it responds to circulating insulin to translocate glucose transporters to cell membranes (Dore et al., 1997; Piroli et al., 2007). Circulating IGF-1 is a key mediator of the ability of physical activity to increase neurogenesis in the dentate gyrus of the hippocampal formation (Åberg et al., 2000; Carro et al., 2001). IGF-1 is taken up into brain via a transport system different from that which transports insulin, although there is some overlap (Banks et al., 2012). IGF-1 is a member of the growth hormone family, and growth hormone is implicated in cognitive function and mood regulation (Donahue et al., 2006). Growth hormone is expressed in the hippocampus, where it is upregulated by acute stress. Furthermore, circulating ghrelin, a proappetitive hormone, has been shown to increase synapse formation in hippocampal pyramidal neurons and to improve hippocampus-dependent memory (Diano et al., 2006). Ghrelin is transported into brain via a saturable system (Banks et al., 2002) and receptors for ghrelin are expressed in hippocampus, as well as in other regions of the brain (Zigman et al., 2006). Another metabolic hormone, leptin, has been found to exert antidepressant effects when infused directly into the hippocampus (Lu et al., 2006). Leptin is transported into the brain and is also expressed in the hippocampus (Yook et al., 2019), and both glucose and insulin mediate the ability of fasting to increase leptin transport into the brain (Kastin and Akerstrom, 2001). Leptin receptors are found in hippocampus among other brain regions and leptin has actions in hippocampus, via excitatory amino acid receptors, that reduce the probability of seizures and enhance aspects of cognitive function (Harvey et al., 2005).

way that is commensurate with the damaging effects of stress and glucocorticoid excess in animal models. Furthermore, in at least some of these instances, the atrophy is caused by glucocorticoid excess, is progressive as the disorder persists, but is potentially reversible.

Given the central role of the hippocampus in aspects of declarative memory, and the literature concerning the adverse effects of stress and glucocorticoids on hippocampus-dependent cognition in animal studies, one would expect that these human disorders are associated with cognitive impairments. This is indeed the case. Major depression is well-documented to be associated with a variety of cognitive impairments, as is Cushing's disease; moreover, in both instances, duration of disease, extent of hippocampal volume loss, and extent of cognitive impairments all covary. Tightening this relationship further, surgical correction of the hypercortisolemia in Cushing's disease leads to recovery of the cognitive impairments, along with recovery of the hippocampal atrophy (Murphy, 1991; Starkman et al., 1981). In addition, prolonged high-dose treatment with synthetic glucocorticoids gives rise to cognitive deficits (Belanoff et al., 2001). Moreover, the chronic occupational jet lag that gives rise to hippocampal volume loss also gives rise to hippocampus-dependent cognitive problems as well (Cho, 2001b).

As might be expected, these disorders associated with hippocampal atrophy also increase the risk of major depressive disorders. Chronic treatment with high-dose synthetic glucocorticoids increase the risk of depression, particularly of the psychotic subtype (Kenna et al., 2011). Similarly, Cushing's disease is associated with depressive symptoms as well, and surgical correction of the disorder leads to abatement of the symptoms (Murphy, 1991; Starkman et al., 1981). On the flip side, stress-reducing regular physical exercise improves both cognition and mood (Erickson et al., 2011).

As reviewed earlier, there are by now considerable insights into the cellular mechanisms by which stress and glucocorticoid excess

damage the hippocampus in animal models. Obviously, it has been difficult to examine the same endpoints in humans, but what little is known is commensurate with the animal studies. Notably, a recent study offered a strategy for using transcriptomic data from animal models together with human data to examine the effects of environmental influences on mental health (Arcego et al., 2024). These results are consistent with the hypothesis that hippocampal glucocorticoid-related transcriptional activity underlies the effects of early-life adversity on neural mechanisms implicated in stress-related psychiatric disorders.

The brain is renowned, of course, for its unfortunate combination of disproportionately large energy demands and limited energy storage capacity, and this vulnerability certainly pertains to the hippocampus. As one example, when the hippocampus is activated by a cognitive task, its utilization of glucose is greatly increased (McNay et al., 2000), and as a measure of that limited storage capacity, the hippocampus must directly mobilize peripheral metabolic compensation (by way of cholinergically mediated activation of the liver) to meet those demands (Uemura et al., 1989).

Such metabolic vulnerability (see Box 17.3) exacts an allostatic cost for the hippocampus, especially during aging. The capacity of the hippocampus to mobilize energy utilization during a cognitive task declines with age (Gold, 1987; McNay and Gold, 2001), and the extent of this impairment predicts the extent of subsequent cognitive decline (De Leon et al., 2001). In addition, Type 1 and Type 2 diabetes, as well as explicit insulin resistance, all increase the risk of dementia (De Leon et al., 2001; Haan, 2006; Ott et al., 1996; Rasgon et al., 2001). Furthermore, poor glucose regulation in the form of insulin resistance is a predictor of more hippocampal volume loss and more severe memory deficits in aged individuals with "mild cognitive impairment" (MCI) (Gold et al., 2007; McIntyre et al., 2010; Rasgon et al., 2011). Energetically compromised cells are less capable of resistance to and repair of damage caused by reactive oxygen species, and an oxidative stress and inflammatory cascade has been suggested as a pathway from insulin resistance to the neuropathology of Alzheimer's disease (AD) (Gold et al., 2013; Manolopoulos et al., 2010). This constitutes a striking example of an allostatic overload (McEwen and Wingfield, 2003) (see Box 17.3).

Stress and glucocorticoids intersect with the energetics of hippocampal vulnerability. As noted, both decrease glucose uptake and glucose transporter concentrations in the rodent hippocampus; consequences include the hippocampus then being impaired in the costly tasks of containing excesses of glutamate neurotransmission, cytosolic calcium accumulation, and generation of reactive oxygen species (Sapolsky, 1992). Importantly, the same broad picture holds in humans as well, in that pharmacological doses of cortisol cause significant reductions in glucose utilization in the human hippocampus, and on the same scale as in rodent studies (~15%) (De Leon et al., 1997; De Leon et al., 1988). The preferential vulnerability of the hippocampus is shown by the fact that no such decline in seen in the lateral temporal, parietal, or frontal lobe, nor in the midbrain (De Leon et al., 1997). Interestingly, cortisol does not cause a similar decline in hippocampal glucose utilization in individuals with AD. At first glance, this might reflect some manner of compensatory defense in such hippocampi, certainly a plausible explanation. However, the failure of cortisol to have this effect in AD patients reflects a floor effect; the disease involves elevated basal concentrations of cortisol, and basal glucose utilization is already decreased 30% in AD patients, relative to age-matched controls (De Leon et al., 1997).

To summarize, excesses of glucocorticoids or stress in an array of human circumstances give rise to hippocampal volume loss and cognitive impairments, much as in animal models. Moreover, this appears to reflect some of the same underlying mechanisms as in animals; specifically, glucocorticoids impair the ability of the already energetically vulnerable hippocampus to meet energy demands during challenges.

17.12 Conclusions

Over the past several decades, accumulating evidence on how stressful experiences affect hippocampal structure and function has offered valuable insights across biological scales, from the debilitating symptoms of stress-related psychiatric disorders on the one hand to molecular and physiological changes on the other. Further, these findings have served as a useful framework for validating the relationships between the various aspects of hippocampal function described in other chapters in this book. For instance, stress-induced impairment in hippocampus-dependent learning and memory is accompanied by a reduction in LTP in various subfields of the rodent hippocampus. These observations, in turn, are consistent with reports of stress-induced disruption in a range of synaptic and molecular signaling mechanisms, such as those involving NMDA receptors and BDNF, that underlie both synaptic plasticity and memory. As revealing as these observations have been in understanding various facets of stress-induced changes in the hippocampus, they have also opened up new and unexpected lines of inquiry that go beyond the original focus on the hippocampus.

First, studies on the hippocampus described here also provide a useful template for elucidating how the effects of stress vary across other brain regions that interact with the hippocampus, such as the amygdala and prefrontal cortex. Second, the actions of factors external to the brain, such as the stress and metabolic hormones, also play a key role in regulating stress-induced plasticity in the adult brain. Furthermore, while the vast majority of earlier research was centered around neural mechanisms, there is growing appreciation that many of these effects are not just limited to the brain, but can have wider implications for the overall health of the organism, including immune and metabolic function. Thus, what began as a somewhat reductionist investigation into how stressful experiences exert their influence on various aspects of hippocampal function at multiple levels of neural organization, has eventually led to an extension of the boundaries of how we think of "brain health" as a whole.

Looking at the interactions between stress hormones and the hippocampus and finding adaptive structural plasticity mediated, in part, by circulating hormones has been a gateway to recognizing a number of important biological concepts that apply to the hippocampus and beyond. First, we now have an increased understanding of how the hippocampus and other brain regions communicate reciprocally with the rest of the body in both health and disease, involving sex and metabolic as well as stress hormones and immune system mediators, among other influences. This understanding includes how these systemic mediators enter the brain, bind to receptors, and participate in structural and functional changes that continue throughout the life course. For example, regular physical activity enlarges the aging, as well as young human and rodent, hippocampus and improves mood. Importantly, exercise-induced increases in neurogenesis in the dentate gyrus require the participation of IGF-1 from liver as well as factors from muscle and body (Aberg et al.,

2002, 2003). In contrast, insulin and leptin resistance occur in the hippocampus and are associated with impaired cognitive function and mood regulation and with increased risk of dementia; thus, Type 2 diabetes is as much a brain as a systemic disorder.

Second, this path of discovery has broadened the understanding of stress via introduction of the concepts of "allostasis" and "allostatic load/overload" to include adaptations and adjustments of the brain and body to a changing environment and to health-promoting and health-damaging behaviors, whether or not we refer to these events as "stressors." The basic idea behind "allostasis" and "allostatic load/overload" is that the same interacting mediators that facilitate adaptation can also accelerate disease when overused and dysregulated among themselves—thus, nonlinearity in the form of inverted-U-shaped dose–response curves are often the best way to describe what is going on. Events in the hippocampus were among the first to illustrate this nonlinearity, particularly in relation to adaptive plasticity, but also in the irreversible damage mediated by excitatory amino acids and glucocorticoids.

This framework facilitates our understanding of the many ways that our experiences and our health-related behaviors shape both the brain and body epigenetically over our life span, where there is no "turning back the clock" but, rather, the possibility of positive or negative redirection at any stage of the life course owing to the adaptive plasticity as well as vulnerability of the brain. The field of epigenetics, subsuming the study of gene x environment interactions, increases our appreciation of how individual differences develop among identical twins and how experiences shape brain function and physiology. Finally, and of great importance, is the recognition that there are widespread sex differences in the actions of sex and stress hormones not only in the hippocampus but also throughout the rest of the brain (McEwen and Milner, 2017). This paves the way for a more nuanced understanding of how biological sex differences, sex and other hormones, and experiences interact epigenetically to affect individual behavior and physiology, and how these impact on vulnerability for stress disorders that affect mood and cognitive well-being.

Acknowledgments

S.C. is grateful to Tim Bliss, Robert Sapolsky, Richard Morris, and Karen Bulloch for helpful comments and suggestions on earlier drafts of the chapter. S.C. also thanks Ashutosh Shukla, Rakhi Pal, M.M. Rahman, Kanika Gupta, Prabahan Chakraborty, Zubin Rashid, and Anupratap Tomar for extensive help with preparing figures and with the text. Elizabeth Gould kindly provided material for one of the figures. Finally, S.C. is deeply indebted to his coauthor, the late Bruce McEwen, for being a kind and caring mentor, and for his warm friendship.

Milestone papers

1. Mandell A, Chapman L, Rand R, Walter R (1963) Plasma corticosteroids: changes in concentration after stimulation of hippocampus and amygdala. *Science* 139:1212–1213.
2. McEwen BS, Weiss J, Schwartz L (1968) Selective retention of corticosterone by limbic structures in rat brain. *Nature* 220:911–912.
3. Gerlach J, McEwen BS, Pfaff DW, Moskovitz S, Ferin M (1976) Cells in regions of rhesus monkey brain and pituitary retain radioactive estradiol, corticosterone and cortisol differently. *Brain Res* 103:603–612.
4. Flood JF, Vidal D, Bennett EL, Orme AE, Vasquez S, Jarvik ME (1978) Memory facilitating and anti-amnesic effects of corticosteroids. *Pharmacol Biochem Behav* 8:81–87.

5. Sapolsky R, Krey L, McEwen BS (1984) Glucocorticoid-sensitive hippocampal neurons are involved in terminating the adrenocortical stress response. *Proc Natl Acad Sci USA* 81:6174–6177.

6. Sapolsky R, Krey L, McEwen BS (1985) Prolonged glucocorticoid exposure reduces hippocampal neuron number: implications for aging. *J Neurosci* 5:1222–1227.

7. Reul JMHM, De Kloet ER (1985) Two receptor systems for corticosterone in rat brain: microdistribution and differential occupation. *Endocrinology* 117:2505–2511.

8. Sapolsky R, Krey L, McEwen BS (1986) The neuroendocrinology of stress and aging: the glucocorticoid cascade hypothesis. *Endocr Rev* 7:284–301.

9. Foy MR, Stanton ME, Levine S. Thompson, RF (1987) Behavioral stress impairs long-term potentiation in rodent hippocampus. *Behav Neural Bio* 48:138–149.

10. Shors TJ, Seib TB, Levine S, Thompson RF (1989) Inescapable versus escapable shock modulates long-term potentiation in the rat hippocampus. *Science* 244:224–226.

11. Woolley C, Gould E, McEwen BS (1990) Exposure to excess glucocorticoids alters dendritic morphology of adult hippocampal pyramidal neurons, *Brain Res* 531:225–231.

12. Watanabe Y, Gould E, McEwen BS (1992) Stress induces atrophy of apical dendrites of hippocampal CA3 pyramidal neurons. *Brain Res* 588:341–344.

13. Watanabe Y, Gould E, Cameron HA, Daniels DC, McEwen BS (1992) Phenytoin prevents stress- and corticosterone-induced atrophy of CA3 pyramidal neurons. *Hippocampus* 2:431–436.

14. Oitzl MS and de Kloet RE (1992) Selective corticosteroid antagonists modulate specific aspects of spatial orientation learning. *Behav Neurosci* 106(1):62–71.

15. Starkman MN, Gebarski SS, Berent S, Schteingart DE (1992) Hippocampal formation volume, memory dysfunction, and cortisol levels in patients with Cushing's syndrome. *Biol Psychiatry* 32:756–765.

16. Farabollini F, Albonetti ME, Aloisi AM, Facchinetti F, Grasso G, Lodi L, Lupo C, Muscettola M (1993) Immune and neuroendocrine response to restraint in male and female rats. *Psychoneuroendocrinology* 18:175–182.

17. Luine V, Villegas M, Martinez C, McEwen BS (1994). Repeated stress causes reversible impairments of spatial memory performance. *Brain Res* 639:167–170.

18. Pavlides C, Watanabe Y, Margarinos AM, McEwen BS (1995) Opposing roles of type I and type II adrenal steroid receptors in hippocampal long-term potentiation. *Neuroscience* 68:387–394.

19. Xu L, Anwyl R, Rowan MJ (1997) Behavioural stress facilitates the induction of long-term depression in the hippocampus. *Nature* 387:497–500.

20. Gould E, McEwen BS, Tanapat P, Galea LA, Fuchs E (1997) Neurogenesis in the dentate gyrus of the adult tree shrew is regulated by psychosocial stress and NMDA receptor activation. *J Neurosci* 17:2492–2498.

21. Bremner JD, Randall P, Vermetten E, Staib L, Bronen RA, Mazure C, Capelli S, McCarthy G, Innis RB, Charney DB (1997) Magnetic resonance imaging-based measurement of hippocampal volume in posttraumatic stress disorder related to childhood physical and sexual abuse—a preliminary report. *Biol Psychiatry* 41(1):23–32.

22. Gurvits TV, Shenton ME, Hokama H, Ohta H, Lasko NB, Gilbertson MW, Orr SP, Kikinis R, Jolesz FA, McCarley RW, Pitman RK (1996) Magnetic resonance imaging study of hippocampal volume in chronic, combat-related posttraumatic stress disorder. *Biol Psychiatry* 40(11):1091–1099.

23. Sheline YI, Sanghavi M, Mintun MA, Gado MH (1999) Depression duration but not age predicts hippocampal volume loss in medically healthy women with recurrent major depression. *J Neurosci* 19:5034–5043.

24. Kim JJ, Lee HJ, Welday AC, Song EY, Cho J, Sharp PE, Jung MW, Blair HT (2007) Stress-induced alterations in hippocampal plasticity, place cells and spatial memory. *Proc Natl Acad Sci USA* 104:18297–18302.

25. Tomar A, Polygalov D, Chattarji S, McHugh TJ (2015) The dynamic impact of repeated stress on the hippocampal spatial map. *Hippocampus* 25: 38–50.

26. Tomar A, Polygalov D, Chattarji S, McHugh TJ (2021) Stress enhances hippocampal neuronal synchrony and alters ripple-spike interaction. *Neurobiol Stress* 14: 100327.

27. Tomar A, McHugh TJ (2022) The impact of stress on the hippocampal spatial code. *Trends Neurosci* 45: 120–132.

REFERENCES

Abe K (2001) Modulation of hippocampal long-term potentiation by the amygdala: a synaptic mechanism linking emotion and memory. *Japanese J Clin Pharmacol Ther* 86:18–22.

Aberg MAI, Åberg ND, Hedbäcker H, Oscarsson J, Eriksson PS (2002) Peripheral infusion of IGF-I selectively induces neurogenesis in the adult rat hippocampus. *J Neurosci* 20:2896–2903.

Aberg MAI, Aberg D, Palmer TD, Alborn A-M, Carlsson-Skwirut C (2003) IGF-1 has a direct proliferative effect in adult hippocampal progenitor cells. *Mol Cell Neurosci* 24:23–40.

Akirav I, Kozenicky M, Tal D, Sandi C, Venero C, Richter-Levin G (2004) A facilitative role for corticosterone in the acquisition of a spatial task under moderate stress. *Learn Mem* 11(2):188–195.

Akirav I, Richter-Levin G (1999) Biphasic modulation of hippocampal plasticity by behavioral stress and basolateral amygdala stimulation in the rat. *J Neurosci* 19:10530–10535.

Akirav I, Richter-Levin G (2002) Mechanisms of amygdala modulation of hippocampal plasticity. *J Neurosci* 22:9912–9921.

Altman J, Bayer SA (1990a) Migration and distribution of two populations of hippocampal granule cell precursors during the perinatal and postnatal periods. *J Comp Neurol* 301:365–381.

Altman J, Bayer SA (1990b) Mosaic organization of the hippocampal neuroepithelium and the multiple germinal sources of dentate granule cells. *J Comp Neurol* 301:325–342.

Arango-Lievano M, Lambert WM, Bath KG, Garabedian MJ, Chao MV, Jeanneteau F (2015) Neurotrophic-priming of glucocorticoid receptor signaling is essential for neuronal plasticity to stress and antidepressant treatment. *Proc Natl Acad Sci USA* 112(51):15737–15742.

Arcego DM, Buschdorf JP, O'Toole N, Wang Z, Barth B, Pokhvisneva I, Rayan NA, Patel S, de Mendonça Filho EJ, Lee P, et al. (2024) A glucocorticoid-sensitive hippocampal gene network moderates the impact of early-life adversity on mental health outcomes. *Biol Psychiatry* 95:48–61.

Arendt T, Stieler J, Strijkstra AM, Hut RA, Rudiger J (2003) Reversible paired helical filament-like phosphorylation of tau is an adaptive process associated with neuronal plasticity in hibernating animals. *J Neurosci* 23:6972–6981.

Armanini MP, Hutchins C, Stein BA, Sapolsky RM (1990) Glucocorticoid endangerment of hippocampal neurons is NMDA-receptor dependent. *Brain Res* 532:7–12

Arnsten AFT (2015) Stress weakens prefrontal networks: molecular insults to higher cognition. *Nat Neurosci* 18:1376–1385.

Banasr M, Chowdhury GMI, Twewilliger R, Newton SS, Duman RS, Behar KL, Sanacora G (2010) Glial pathology in an animal model of depression: reversal of stress-induced cellular, metabolic and behavioral deficits by the glutamate-modulating drug riluzole. *Mol Psychiatry* 15(5):501–511.

Banasr M, Duman RS (2008) Glial loss in the prefrontal cortex is sufficient to induce depressive-like behaviors. *Biol Psychiatry* 64(10):863–870.

Banks WA, Owen JB, Erickson MA (2012) Insulin in the brain: there and back again. *Pharmacol Ther* 136:82–93.

Banks WA, Tschöp M, Robinson SM, Heiman ML (2002) Extent and direction of Ghrelin transport across the blood-brain barrier is determined by its unique primary structure. *J Pharmacol Exp Ther* 302:822–827.

Barha CK, Brummelte S, Lieblich SE, Galea LA (2011) Chronic restraint stress in adolescence differentially influences hypothalamic-pituitary-adrenal axis function and adult hippocampal neurogenesis in male and female rats. *Hippocampus* 21:1216–1227.

Bath K, Schilit A, Lee F (2013) Stress effects on BDNF expression: effects of age, sex, and form of stress. *Neuroscience* **239**:149–156.

Bauer EP, Schafe GE, LeDoux JE (2002) NMDA receptors and L-type voltage-gated calcium channels contribute to long-term potentiation and different components of fear memory formation in the lateral amygdala. *J Neurosci* **22**:5239–5249.

Belanoff JK, Gross K, Yager A, Schatzberg AF (2001) Corticosteroids and cognition. *J Psychiatr Res* **35**:127–145.

Bennur S, Shankaranarayana Rao BS, Pawlak R, Strickland S, McEwen BS, Chattarji S (2007) Stress-induced spine loss in the medial amygdala is mediated by tissue-plasminogen activator. *Neuroscience* **144**:8–16.

Bernasconi C, König P (1999) On the directionality of cortical interactions studied by structural analysis of electrophysiological recordings. *Biol Cybern* **81**:199–210.

Bernasconi C, von Stein A, Chiang C, König P (2000) Bi-directional interactions between visual areas in the awake behaving cat. *Neuroreport* **11**:689–692.

Bessa JM, Ferreira D, Melo I, Marques F, Cerqueira JJ (2008) The mood-improving actions of antidepressants do not depend on neurogenesis but are associated with neuronal remodeling. *Mol Psychiatry* **14**(8):764–773.

Bigio B, Mathe AA, Sousa VC, Zelli D, Svenningsson P (2016) Epigenetics and energetics in ventral hippocampus mediate rapid antidepressant action: Implications for treatment resistance. *Proc Natl Acad Sci USA* **113**:7906–7911.

Blume SR, Freedberg M, Vantrease JE, Chan R, Padival M (2017) Sex- and estrus-dependent differences in rat basolateral amygdala. *J Neurosci* **37**:10567–10586.

Blume SR, Padival M, Urban JH, Rosenkranz JA (2019) Disruptive effects of repeated stress on basolateral amygdala neurons and fear behavior across the estrous cycle in rats. *Sci Rep* **9**:1–18.

Bowles NP, McEwen BS, Boutin-Foster C (2017) Trouble in transit: organizational barriers to workers' health. *Am J Ind Med* **60**:350–367.

Bowman RE, Beck KD, Luine VN (2003) Chronic stress effects on memory: sex differences in performance and monoaminergic activity. *Horm and Behav* **43**:48–59.3

Bremner JD, et al. (2000) Hippocampal volume reduction in major depression. *Am J Psychiatry* **157**(1):115–118.

Bremner JD, Randall P, Vermetten E, Staib L, Bronen RA, Mazure C, Capelli S, McCarthy G, Innis RB, Charney DS (1997) Magnetic resonance imaging-based measurement of hippocampal volume in posttraumatic stress disorder related to childhood physical and sexual abuse—a preliminary report. *Biol Psychiatry* **41**:23–32.

Briones BA, Gould E (2019) Adult neurogenesis and stress. In: Stress: Physiology, Biochemistry, and Pathology: Handbook of Stress Series, Vol 3 (Fink G, ed). Academic Press.

Brovelli A, Ding M, Ledberg A, Chen Y, Nakamura R, Bressler SL (2004) Beta oscillations in a large-scale sensorimotor cortical network: directional influences revealed by Granger causality. *Proc Natl Acad Sci USA* **101**:9849–9854.

Brun VH, Otnæss MK, Molden S, Steffenach H-A, Witter MP, Moser M-B, Moser EI (2002) Place cells and place recognition maintained by direct entorhinal-hippocampal circuitry. *Science* **296**:2243–2246.

Cacioppo JT, Hawkley LC, Norman GJ, Berntson GG (2011) Social isolation. *Ann N Y Acad Sci* **1231**:17–22.

Cahill L (2017) An issue whose time has come. *J Neurosci Res* **95**:12–13.

Cameron HA, Glover LR (2015) Adult neurogenesis: beyond learning and memory. *Annu Rev Psychol* **66**:53–81.

Cameron HA, McEwen BS, Gould E (1995) Regulation of adult neurogenesis by excitatory input and NMDA receptor activation in the dentate gyrus. *J Neurosci* **15**:4687–4692.

Cameron HA, Tanapat P, Gould E (1998) Adrenal steroids and N-methyl-D-aspartate receptor activation regulate neurogenesis in the dentate gyrus of adult rats through a common pathway. *Neuroscience* **82**:349–354.

Carro E, Trejo JL, Busiguina S, Torres-Aleman I (2001) Circulating insulin-like growth factor I mediates the protective effects of physical exercise against brain insults of different etiology and anatomy. *J Neurosci* **21**:5678–5684.

Cerqueira JJ, Mailliet F, Almeida OFX, Jay TM, Sousa N (2007) The prefrontal cortex as a key target of the maladaptive response to stress. *J Neurosci* **27**:2781–2787.

Chaddock L, Erickson KI, Prakash RS, Kim JS, Voss MW (2010) A neuroimaging investigation of the association between aerobic fitness, hippocampal volume, and memory performance in preadolescent children. *Brain Res* **1358**:172–183.

Chattarji S, Tomar A, Suvrathan A, Ghosh S, Rahman MM (2015) Neighborhood matters: divergent patterns of stress-induced plasticity across the brain. *Nat Neurosci* **18**:1364–1375.

Chen B, Dowlatshahi D, MacQueen GM, Wang J-F, Young LT (2001) Increased hippocampal BDNF immunoreactivity in subjects treated with antidepressant medication. *Biol Psychiatry* **50**:260–265.

Chen Y, Kramár EA, Chen LY, Babayan AH, Andres AL, Gall CM, Lynch G, Baram TZ (2013) Impairment of synaptic plasticity by the stress mediator CRH involves selective destruction of thin dendritic spines via RhoA signaling. *Mol Psychiatry* **18**:485–496.

Chen Z-Y, Jing D, Bath KG, Ieraci A, Khan T, Siao C-J, Herrera DG, Toth M, Yang C, McEwen BS, et al. (2006) Genetic variant BDNF (Val66Met) polymorphism alters anxiety-related behavior. *Science* **314**:140–143.

Cho K (2001) Chronic "jet lag" produces temporal lobe atrophy and spatial cognitive deficits. *Nat Neurosci* **4**:567–568.

Cole AB, Montgomery K, Bale TL, Thompson SM (2022) What the hippocampus tells the HPA axis: hippocampal output attenuates acute stress responses via disynaptic inhibition of CRF+ PVN neurons. *Neurobiol Stress* **20**:100473.

Cole SW, Hawkley LC, Arevalo JM, Sung CY, Rose RM, Cacioppo JT (2007) Social regulation of gene expression in human leukocytes. *Genome Biol* **8**:R189.

Conrad CD (2005) The relationship between acute glucocorticoid levels and hippocampal function depends upon task aversiveness and memory processing stage. *Nonlinearity Biol Toxicol Med* **3**:57–78.

Conrad CD, Galea LA, Kuroda Y, McEwen BS (1996) Chronic stress impairs rat spatial memory on the Y maze, and this effect is blocked by tianeptine pretreatment. *Behav Neurosci* **110**:1321–1334.

Conrad CD, LeDoux JE, Magariños AM, McEwen BS (1999) Repeated restraint stress facilitates fear conditioning independently of causing hippocampal CA3 dendritic atrophy. *Behav Neurosci* **113**:902–913.

Conrad CD, Lupien SJ, Thanasoulis LC, McEwen BS (1997) The effects of Type I and Type II corticosteroid receptor agonists on exploratory behavior and spatial memory in the Y-maze. *Brain Res* **759**:76–83.

Convit A (2005) Links between cognitive impairment in insulin resistance: an explanatory model. *Neurobiol Aging* **26**:31–35.

Cook SC, Wellman CL (2004) Chronic stress alters dendritic morphology in rat medial prefrontal cortex. *J Neurobiol* **60**:236–248.

Cordero MI, Venero C, Kruyt ND, Sandi C (2003) Prior exposure to a single stress session facilitates subsequent contextual fear conditioning in rats: evidence for a role of corticosterone. *Horm Behav* **44**:338–345.

Datson NA, van den Oever JM, Korobko OB, Magarinos AM, de Kloet ER, McEwen BS (2013) Previous history of chronic stress changes the transcriptional response to glucocorticoid challenge in the dentate gyrus region of the male rat hippocampus. *Endocrinology* 154:3261–3272.

De Leon M, Convit A, Wolf O, Tarshish C, DeSanti S (2001) Prediction of cognitive decline in normal elderly subjects with 2-[18F] fluoro-2-deoxy-D-glucose/positron-emission tomography (FDG/PET). *Proc Natl Acad Sci USA* 98:10966–10971.

De Leon M, McRae T, Rusinek H, Convit A, De Santi S (1997) Cortisol reduces hippocampal glucose metabolism in normal elderly, but not in Alzheimer's disease. *J Clin Endocrinol Metab* 82:3251–3259.

De Leon M, Mcrae T, Tsai J, George A, Marcus D (1988) Abnormal cortisol response in Alzheimer's disease linked to hippocampal atrophy. *Lancet* 332:391–392.

DeLeon J, Miller BL (2018) Frontotemporal dementia. *Handb Clin Neurol* 148:409–430.

de Quervain DJ-F, Roozendaal B, McGaugh JL (1998) Stress and glucocorticoids impair retrieval of long-term spatial memory. *Nature* 394:787–790.

Derntl B, Finkelmeyer A, Eickhoff S, Kellermann T, Falkenberg DI (2010) Multidimensional assessment of empathic abilities: neural correlates and gender differences. *Psychoneuroendocrinology* 35:67–82.

Diamond DM, Bennett MC, Fleshner M, Rose GM (1992) Inverted-U relationship between the level of peripheral corticosterone and the magnitude of hippocampal primed burst potentiation. *Hippocampus* 2:421–430.

Diamond DM, Campbell AM, Park CR, Halonen J, Zoladz PR (2007) The temporal dynamics model of emotional memory processing: a synthesis on the neurobiological basis of stress-induced amnesia, flashbulb and traumatic memories, and the Yerkes-Dodson law. *Neural Plast* 2007:60803.

Diamond DM, Fleshner M, Ingersoll N, Rose G (1996) Psychological stress impairs spatial working memory: relevance to electrophysiological studies of hippocampal function. *Behav Neurosci* 110:661–672.

Diamond DM, Park CR, Heman KL, Rose GM (1999) Exposing rats to a predator impairs spatial working memory in the radial arm water maze. *Hippocampus* 9:542–552.

Diamond DM, Rose GM (1994) Stress impairs LTP and hippocampal-dependent memory. *Ann N Y Acad Sci* 746:411–414.

Diano S, Farr SA, Benoit SC, McNay EC, da Silva I, Horvath B, Gaskin FS, Nonaka N, Jaeger LB, Banks WA, et al. (2006) Ghrelin controls hippocampal spine synapse density and memory performance. *Nat Neurosci* 9:381–388.

Dias-Ferreira E, Sousa JC, Melo I, Morgado P, Mesquita AR, Cerqueira JJ, Costa RM, Sousa N (2009) Chronic stress causes frontostriatal reorganization and affects decision-making. *Science* 325:621–625.

Donahue AN, Aschner M, Lash LH, Syversen T, Sonntag WE (2006) Growth hormone administration to aged animals reduces disulfide glutathione levels in hippocampus. *Mech Ageing Dev* 127:57–63.

Dore S, Kar S, Quirion R (1997) Insulin-like growth factor I protects and rescues hippocampal neurons against -amyloid- and human amylin-induced toxicity. *Proc Natl Acad Sci USA* 94:4772–4777.

Dos-Santos RC, Sweeten BL, Stelly CE, Tasker JG (2023) The neuroendocrine impact of acute stress on synaptic plasticity. *Endocrinology* 164:bqad149.

Draganski B, Gaser C, Kempermann G, Kuhn HG, Winkler J, Buchel C, May A (2006) Temporal and spatial dynamics of brain structure changes during extensive learning. *J Neurosci* 26:6314–6317.

Drevets WC, Price JL, Simpson JR, Todd RD, Reich T (1997) Subgenual prefrontal cortex abnormalities in mood disorders. *Nature* 386:824–827.

Du J, McEwen B, Manji HK (2009) Glucocorticoid receptors modulate mitochondrial function: a novel mechanism for neuroprotection. *Commun Integr Biol* 2:350–352.

Duman RS, Monteggia LM (2006) A neurotrophic model for stress-related mood disorders. *Biol Psychiatry* 59:1116–1127.

Eichenbaum H, Dudchenko P, Wood E, Shapiro M, Tanila H (1999) The hippocampus, memory, and place cells. *Neuron* 23(2):209–226.

Eiland L, Ramroop J, Hill MN, Manley J, McEwen BS (2012) Chronic juvenile stress produces corticolimbic dendritic architectural remodeling and modulates emotional behavior in male and female rats. *Psychoneuroendocrinology* 37(1):39–47.

Eme RF (2007) Sex differences in child-onset, life-course-persistent conduct disorder: a review of biological influences. *Clin Psychol Rev* 27:607–627.

Erickson KI, Voss MW, Prakash RS, Basak C, Szabo A (2011) Exercise training increases size of hippocampus and improves memory. *Proc Natl Acad Sci USA* 108:3017–3022.

Eriksson PS, Permlieva E, Bjork-Eriksson T, Alborn A-M, Nordborg C (1998) Neurogenesis in the adult human hippocampus. *Nat Med* 4:1313–1317.

Evans GW, Gonnella C, Marcynyszyn LA, Gentile L, Salpekar N (2005) The role of chaos in poverty and children's socioemotional adjustment. *Psychol Sci* 16:560–565.

Flood JF, Vidal D, Bennett, EL, Orme AE, Vasquez S, Jarvik ME (1978) Memory facilitating and anti-amnesic effects of corticosteroids. *Pharmacol Biochem Behav* 8:81–87.

Foy MR, Stanton ME Levine, Levine S, Thompson, RF (1987) Behavioral stress impairs long-term potentiation in rodent hippocampus *Behav Neural Biol* 48(1):138–149.

Freund J, Brandmaier AM, Lewejohann L, Kirste I, Kritzler M (2013) Emergence of individuality in genetically identical mice. *Science* 340:756–759.

Galea LAM, McEwen BS, Tanapat P, Deak T, Spencer RL, Dhabhar FS (1997) Sex differences in dendritic atrophy of CA3 pyramidal neurons in response to chronic restraint stress. *Neuroscience* 81:689–697.

Garcia, R, Musleh, W, Tocco, G, Thompson, RF, Baudry, M (1997) Time-dependent blockade of STP and LTP in hippocampal slices following acute stress in mice. *Neurosci Lett* 233(1):41–44.

Gerlach J, McEwen BS (1972) Rat brain binds adrenal steroid hormone: radioautography of hippocampus with corticosterone. *Science* 175:1133–1136.

Gerlach J, McEwen BS, Pfaff DW, Moskovitz S, Ferin M (1976) Cells in regions of rhesus monkey brain and pituitary retain radioactive estradiol, corticosterone and cortisol differently. *Brain Res* 103:603–612.

Geweke J (1982) Measurement of linear dependence and feedback between multiple time series. *J Am Stat Assoc* 77:304–313.

Ghosh S, Laxmi TR, Chattarji S (2013) Functional connectivity from the amygdala to the hippocampus grows stronger after stress. *J Neurosci* 33:7234–7244.

Gilbertson MW, Shenton ME, Ciszewski A, Kasai K, Lasko NB, Orr SP, Pitman RK (2002) Smaller hippocampal volume predicts pathologic vulnerability to psychological trauma. *Nat Neurosci* 5:1242–1247.

Gold PE (1987) Sweet memories. *Am Sci* 75:151–155.

Gold PW, Licinio J, Pavlatou M (2013) Pathological parainflammation and endoplasmic reticulum stress in depression: potential translational targets through the CNS insulin, klotho and PPAR-γ systems. *Mol Psychiatry* 18:154–165.

Gold S, Dziobek I, Sweat V, Tirsi A, Rogers K, Bruehl H, Tsui W, Richardson S, Javier E, Convit A. (2007) Hippocampal damage and memory impairments as possible early brain complications of type 2 diabetes. *Diabetologia* 50:711–719.

Goldwater DS, Pavlides C, Hunter RG, Bloss EB, Hof PR, McEwen BS, Morrison JH (2009) Structural and functional alterations to rat medial prefrontal cortex following chronic restraint stress and recovery. *Neuroscience* 164:798–808.

Gould E, Beylin A, Tanapat P, Reeves A, Shors TJ (1999) Learning enhances adult neurogenesis in the hippocampal formation. *Nat Neurosci* 2:260–265.

Gould E, McEwen BS, Tanapat P, Galea LAM, Fuchs E (1997) Neurogenesis in the dentate gyrus of the adult tree shrew is regulated by psychosocial stress and NMDA receptor activation. *J Neurosci* 17:2492–2498.

Gould E, Reeves AJ, Fallah M, Tanapat P, Gross CG, Fuchs E (1999) Hippocampal neurogenesis in adult Old World primates. *Proc Natl Acad Sci USA* 96:5263–5267.

Gould E, Reeves AJ, Graziano MS, Gross CG (1999) Neurogenesis in the neocortex of adult primates. *Science* 286:548–552.

Gould E, Woolley CS, Cameron HA, Daniels DC, McEwen BS (1991) Adrenal steroids regulate postnatal development of the rat dentate gyrus: II. Effects of glucocorticoids and mineralocorticoids on cell birth. *J Comp Neurol* 313:486–493.

Gould E, Woolley C, McEwen BS (1991a) Adrenal steroids regulate postnatal development of the rat dentate gyrus: I. Effects of glucocorticoids on cell death. *J Comp Neurol* 313:479–485.

Gould E, Woolley C, McEwen BS (1991b) Naturally occurring cell death in the developing dentate gyrus of the rat. *J Comp Neurol* 304:408–418.

Govindarajan A, Rao BSS, Nair D, Trinh M, Mawjee N, Tonegawa S, Chattarji S (2006) Transgenic brain-derived neurotrophic factor expression causes both anxiogenic and antidepressant effects. *Proc Natl Acad Sci USA* 103:13208–13213.

Granger CWJ (1969) Investigating causal relations by econometric models and cross-spectral methods. *Econometrica* 37:424–438.

Gray JD, Rubin TG, Hunter RG, McEwen BS (2014) Hippocampal gene expression changes underlying stress sensitization and recovery. *Mol Psychiatry* 19:1171–1178.

Gregoriou GG, Gotts SJ, Zhou H, Desimone R (2009) High-frequency, long-range coupling between prefrontal and visual cortex during attention. *Science* 324:1207–1210.

Guillemin R (1978) Peptides in the brain: the new endocrinology of the neuron. *Science* 202:390–402.

Gunduz-Cinar O, Hill MN, McEwen BS, Holmes A (2013) Amygdala FAAH and anandamide: mediating protection and recovery from stress. *Trends Pharmacol Sci* 34:637–644.

Gupta K, Chattarji S (2021) Sex differences in the delayed impact of acute stress on the amygdala. *Neurobiol Stress* 14:100292.

Gurvits TV, Shenton ME, Hokama H, Ohta H, Lasko NB, Gilbertson MW, Orr SP, Kikinis R, Jolesz FA, McCarley RW, et al. (1996) Magnetic resonance imaging study of hippocampal volume in chronic, combat-related posttraumatic stress disorder *Biol Psychiatry* (11):1091–1099.

Gurvits TV, Shenton ME, Hokama H, Ohta H, Lasko NB, Gilbertson MW, Orr SP, Kikinis R, Jolesz FA, McCarley RW, et al. (1997) Magnetic resonance imaging-based measurement of hippocampal volume in posttraumatic stress disorder related to childhood physical and sexual abuse—a preliminary report. *Biol Psychiatry* 41(1):23–32.

Haan MN (2006) Therapy Insight: type 2 diabetes mellitus and the risk of late-onset Alzheimer's disease. *Nat Clin Pract Neurol* 2:159–166.

Hamson DK, Wainwright SR, Taylor JR, Jones BA, Watson NV, Galea LA (2013) Androgens increase survival of adult-born neurons in the dentate gyrus by an androgen receptor-dependent mechanism in male rats. *Endocrinology* 154:3294–3304.

Harris GW (1970) Effects of the nervous system on the pituitary-adrenal activity. *Prog Brain Res* 32:86–88.

Harvey J, Shanley LJ, O'Malley D, Irving AJ (2005) Leptin: a potential cognitive enhances? *Biochem Soc Trans* 33(5):1029–1032.

Hebert-Chatelain E, Desprez T, Serrat R, Bellocchio L, Soria-Gomez E, Busquets-Garcia A, Pagano Zottola AC, Delamarre A, Cannich A, Vincent P, et al. (2016) A cannabinoid link between mitochondria and memory. *Nature* 539:555–559.

Herman JP, Cullinan WE (1997) Neurocircuitry of stress: central control of the hypothalamo–pituitary–adrenocortical axis. *Trends Neurosci* 20:78–84.

Herman JP, Figueiredo H, Mueller NK, Ulrich-Lai Y, Ostrander MM, Choi DC, Cullinan WE (2003) Central mechanisms of stress integration: hierarchical circuitry controlling hypothalamo-pituitary-adrenocortical responsiveness. *Front Neuroendocrin* 24:151–180.

Herman JP, Schafer M, Young EA, Thompson R, Douglass J, Akil H, Watson SJ (1989) Evidence for hippocampal regulation of neuroendocrine neurons of the hypothalamo-pituitary-adrenocortical axis. *J Neurosci* 9:3072–3082.

Hesse W, Möller E, Arnold M, Schack B (2003) The use of time-variant EEG Granger causality for inspecting directed interdependencies of neural assemblies. *J Neurosci Methods* 124:27–44.

Hill MN, Bierer LM, Makotkine I, Golier JA, Galea S, McEwen BS, Hillard CJ, Yehuda R (2013) Reductions in circulating endocannabinoid levels in individuals with post-traumatic stress disorder following exposure to the world trade center attacks. *Psychoneuroendocrinology* 38:2952–2961.

Hill MN, McEwen BS (2010) Involvement of the endocannabinoid system in the neurobehavioural effects of stress and glucocorticoids. *Prog Neuropsychopharmacol Biol Psychiatry* 34:791–797.

Hill MN, Patel S, Campolongo P, Tasker JG, Wotjak CT, Bains JS (2010) Functional interactions between stress and the endocannabinoid system: from synaptic signaling to behavioral output. *J Neurosci* 30:14980–14986.

Holderbach R, Clark K, Moreau J-L, Bischofberger J, Normann C (2007) Enhanced long-term synaptic depression in an animal model of depression. *Biol Psychiatry* 62:92–100.

Hunter RG, McCarthy KJ, Milne TA, Pfaff DW, McEwen BS (2009) Regulation of hippocampal H3 histone methylation by acute and chronic stress. *Proc Natl Acad Sci USA* 106(49):20912–20917.

Hunter RG, McEwen BS, Pfaff DW (2013) Environmental stress and transposon transcription in the mammalian brain. *Mob Genet Elements* 3(2):e24555.

Hunter RG, Murakami G, Dewell S, Seligsohn M, Baker ME, Datson NA, McEwen BS, Pfaff DW (2012) Acute stress and hippocampal histone H3 lysine 9 trimethylation, a retrotransposon silencing response. *Proc Natl Acad Sci USA* 109(43):17657–17662.

Jacobson L, Sapolsky R (1991) The role of the hippocampus in feedback regulation of the hypothalamic-pituitary-adrenocortical axis. *Endocr Rev* 12:118–134.

Jeanneteau F, Garabedian MJ, Chao MV (2008) Activation of Trk neurotrophin receptors by glucocorticoids provides a neuroprotective effect. *Proc Natl Acad Sci USA* 105:4862–4867.

Jensen E, Jacobson H (1962) Basic guides to the mechanism of estrogen action. *Rec Prog Horm Res* 18:387–408.

Joëls, M (2007) Role of corticosteroid hormones in the dentate gyrus. *Prog Brain Res* 163:355–370.

Joels M, Vreugdenhil E (1998) Corticosteroids in the brain: cellular and molecular actions. *Mol Neurobiol* 17:87–108.

Joo, HR, Frank, LM (2018) The hippocampal sharp wave–ripple in memory retrieval for immediate use and consolidation. *Nat Rev Neurosci* 19(12):744–757.

Kalisch R, Schubert M, Jacob W, Kessler MS, Hemauer R, Wigger A, Landgraf R, Auer DP (2006) Anxiety and hippocampus volume in the rat. *Neuropsychopharmacol* 31:925–932.

Kaplan MS (2001) Environment complexity stimulates visual cortex neurogenesis: death of a dogma and a research career. *Trends Neurosci* 24:617–620.

Kaplan MS, Hinds JW (1977) Neurogenesis in the adult rat: electron microscopic analysis of light radioautographs. *Science* 197:1092–1094.

Karst H, Berger S, Turiault M, Tronche F, Schutz G, Joels M (2005) Mineralocorticoid receptors are indispensable for nongenomic modulation of hippocampal glutamate transmission by corticosterone. *Proc Natl Acad Sci USA* 102:19204–19207.

Kastin AJ, Akerstrom V (2001) Pretreatment with glucose increases entry of urocortin into mouse brain. *Peptides* 22:829–834.

Kenna HA, Poon AW, de los Angeles CP, Koran LM (2011) Psychiatric complications of treatment with corticosteroids: review with case report. *Psychiatry Clin Neurosci* 65:549–560.

Kentros C, Hargreaves E, Hawkins RD, Kandel ER, Shapiro M, Muller RV (1998) Abolition of long-term stability of new hippocampal place cell maps by NMDA receptor blockade. *Science* 280:2121–2126.

Kerr DS, Campbell LW, Thibault O, Landfield PW (1992) Hippocampal glucocorticoid receptor activation enhances voltage-dependent Ca2+ conductances: relevance to brain aging. *Proc Natl Acad Sci (USA)* 89(18):8527–8531.

Kerr JE, Allore RJ, Beck SG, Handa RJ (1995) Distribution and hormonal regulation of androgen receptor (AR) and AR messenger ribonucleic acid in the rat hippocampus. *Endocrinology* 136:3213–3221.

Kessler RC, McGonagle KA, Nelson CB, Hughes M, Swartz M, Blazer DG (1994) Sex and depression in the National Comorbidity Survey: II. Cohort effects. *J Affect Disord* 30:15–26.

Kessler RC, McGonagle KA, Swartz M, Blazer DG, Nelson CB (1993) Sex and depression in the National Comorbidity Survey: I. Lifetime prevalence, chronicity and recurrence. *J Affect Disord* 29:85–96.

Kheirbek MA, Drew LJ, Burghardt NS, Costantini DO, Tannenholz L, Ahmari SE, Zeng H, Fenton AA, Hen R (2013) Differential control of learning and anxiety along the dorsoventral axis of the dentate gyrus. *Neuron* 77:955–968.

Kheirbek MA, Hen R (2011) Dorsal vs ventral hippocampal neurogenesis: implications for cognition and mood. *Neuropsychopharmacol* 36:373–374.

Kim JJ, Diamond DM (2002) The stressed hippocampus, synaptic plasticity and lost memories. *Nat Rev Neurosci* 3:453–462.

Kim JJ, Hongjoo LJ, Adam CW, EunYoung S, Jeiwon C, Patricia ES, Min WJ, Hugh TB (2007) Stress-induced alterations in hippocampal plasticity, place cells and spatial memory. *Proc Natl Acad Sci USA* 104:18297–18302.

Kim JJ, Lee HJ, Han J-S, Packard MG (2001) Amygdala is critical for stress-induced modulation of hippocampal long-term potentiation and learning. *J Neurosci* 21:5222–5228.

Kim JJ, Koo JW, Lee HJ, Han JS (2005) Amygdalar inactivation blocks stress-induced impairments in hippocampal long-term potentiation and spatial memory. *J Neurosci* 25(6):1532–1539.

Kim JJ, Lee HJ, Welday AC, Song EY, Cho J, Sharp PE, Jung MW, Blair HT (2007) Stress-induced alterations in hippocampal plasticity, place cells and spatial memory. *Proc Natl Acad Sci USA* 104: 18297–18302.

Kim EJ, Park M, Kong M-S, Park SG, Cho J, Kim JJ (2015) Alterations of hippocampal place cells in foraging rats facing a "predatory" threat. *Curr Biol* 25:1362–1367.

Kinoshita Y, Hunter RG, Gray JD, Mesias R, McEwen BS, Benson DL, Kohtz DS (2014) Role for NUP62 depletion and PYK2 redistribution in dendritic retraction resulting from chronic stress. *Proc Natl Acad Sci USA* 111:16130–16135.

Kirschbaum C, Pirke KM, Hellhammer DH (1993) The "Trier Social Stress Test"—a tool for investigating psychobiological stress responses in a laboratory setting. *Neuropsychobiology* 28:76–81.

Kobilo T, Liu QR, Gandhi K, Mughal M, Shaham Y, van Praag H (2011) Running is the neurogenic and neurotrophic stimulus in environmental enrichment. *Learn Mem* 18:605–609.

Kole MHP, Costoli T, Koolhaas JM, Fuchs E (2004) Bidirectional shift in the cornu ammonis 3 pyramidal dendritic organization following brief stress. *Neuroscience* 125:337–347.

Kole MHP, Czéh B, Fuchs E (2004) Homeostatic maintenance in excitability of tree shrew hippocampal CA3 pyramidal neurons after chronic stress: CA3 excitability properties after chronic stress. *Hippocampus* 14:742–751.

Kole MHP, Swan L, Fuchs E (2002) The antidepressant tianeptine persistently modulates glutamate receptor currents of the hippocampal CA3 commissural associational synapse in chronically stressed rats: tianeptine modulates glutamate transmission. *Eur J Neurosci* 16:807–816.

Kondev V, Najeed M, Yasmin F, Morgan A, Loomba N, Johnson K, Adank DN, Dong A, Delpire E, Li Y, et al. (2023). Endocannabinoid release at ventral hippocampal-amygdala synapses regulates stress-induced behavioral adaptation. *Cell Rep* 42:113027

Kondo MC, Fluehr JM, McKeon T, Branas CC (2018) Urban green space and its impact on human health. *Int J Environ Res Public Health* 15(3):445.

Kuga N, Nakayama R, Morikawa S, Yagishita H, Konno D, Shiozaki H, Honjoya N, Ikegaya Y, Sasaki T (2023) Hippocampal sharp wave ripples underlie stress susceptibility in male mice. *Nat Commun* 14:2105.

Kumar P, Berghorst LH, Nickerson LD, Dutra SJ, Goer FK, Greve DN, Pizzagalli DA (2014) Differential effects of acute stress on anticipatory and consummatory phases of reward processing. *Neuroscience* 266:1–12.

Lakshminarasimhan H, Chattarji S (2012) Stress leads to contrasting effects on the levels of brain derived neurotrophic factor in the hippocampus and amygdala. *PLoS One* 7(1):e30481.

Landfield PW, Waymire JC, Lynch G (1978) Hippocampal aging and adrenocorticoids: quantitative correlations. *Science* 202:1098–1102.

Layden EA, Cacioppo JT, Cacioppo S, Cappa SF, Dodich A, Falini A, Canessa N (2017) Perceived social isolation is associated with altered functional connectivity in neural networks associated with tonic alertness and executive control. *Neuroimage* 145:58–73.

LeDoux JE (2000) Emotion circuits in the brain. *Annu Rev Neurosci* 23:155–184.

Lee T, Jarome T, Li S-J, Kim JJ, Helmstetter FJ (2009) Chronic stress selectively reduces hippocampal volume in rats: a longitudinal MRI study. *Neuroreport* 20:1554–1558.

Leranth C, Petnehazy O, MacLusky NJ (2003) Gonadal hormones affect spine synaptic density in the CA1 hippocampal subfield of male rats. *J Neurosci* 23:1588–1592.

Lewis C, McEwen BS, Frankfurt M (1995) Estrogen-induction of dendritic spines in ventromedial hypothalamus and hippocampus: effects of neonatal aromatase blockade and adult castration. *Dev Brain Res* 87:91–95.

Li X, Du ZJ, Xu JN, Liang ZM, Lin S, Chen H, Li SJ, Li XW, Yang JM, Gao TM (2023) mGluR5 in hippocampal CA1 pyramidal neurons mediates stress-induced anxiety-like behavior. *Neuropsychopharmacology* 48:1164–1174.

Li X, Teng T, Yan W, Fan L, Liu X, Clarke G, Zhu D, Jiang Y, Xiang Y, Yu Y, et al. (2023) AKT and MAPK signaling pathways in hippocampus reveals the pathogenesis of depression in four stress-induced models. *Transl Psychiatry* 13:200.

Liang KC, Hon W, Davis M (1994) Pre-and posttraining infusion of N-methyl-D-aspartate receptor antagonists into the amygdala impair memory in an inhibitory avoidance task. *Behav Neurosci* 108:241.

Lin Y, Ter Horst GJ, Wichmann R, Bakker P, Liu A, Li X, Westenbroek C (2009) Sex differences in the effects of acute and chronic stress and recovery after long-term stress on stress-related brain regions of rats. *Cereb Cortex* 19:1978–1989.

Lisofsky N, Mårtensson J, Eckert A, Lindenberger U, Gallinat J, Kühn S (2015) Hippocampal volume and functional connectivity changes during the female menstrual cycle. *Neuroimage* 118:154–162.

Liston C, Miller MM, Goldwater DS, Radley JJ, Rocher AB, Hof PR, Morrison JH, McEwen BS (2006) Stress-induced alterations in prefrontal cortical dendritic morphology predict selective impairments in perceptual attentional set-shifting. *J Neurosci* 26:7870–7874.

Liu L, Tsuji M, Takeda H, Takada K, Matsumiya T (1999) Adrenocortical suppression blocks the enhancement of memory storage produced by exposure to psychological stress in rats. *Brain Res* 821:134–140.

Lowy MT, Gault L, Yamamoto BK (1993) Adrenalectomy attenuates stress-induced elevations in extracellular glutamate concentrations in the hippocampus. *J Neurochem* 61:1957–1960.

Loy R, Gerlach J, McEwen BS (1988) Autoradiographic localization of estradiol-binding neurons in rat hippocampal formation and entorhinal cortex. *Dev Brain Res* 39:245–251.

Lu X-Y, Kim CS, Frazer A, Zhang W (2006) Leptin: a potential novel antidepressant. *Proc Natl Acad Sci USA* 103(5):1593–1598.

Luine V, Martinez C, Villegas M, Magarinos AM, McEwen BS (1996) Restraint stress reversibly enhances spatial memory performance. *Physiol Behav* 59:27–32.

Luine V, Villegas M, Martinez C, McEwen BS (1994) Repeated stress causes reversible impairments of spatial memory performance. *Brain Res* 639:167–170.

Lupien SJ, de Leon M, de Santi S, Convit A, Tarshish C, Nair NP, Thakur M, McEwen BS, Hauger RL, Meaney MJ (1998) Cortisol levels during human aging predict hippocampal atrophy and memory deficits. *Nat Neurosci* 1:69–73.

Lupien SJ, Gaudreau S, Tchiteya BM, Maheu F, Sharma S, Nair NP, Hauger RL, McEwen BS, Meaney MJ (1997) Stress-induced declarative memory impairment in healthy elderly subjects—relationship to cortisol reactivity. *J Clin Endo Metab* 82:2070–2075.

Lupien SJ, Wilkinson CW, Briere S, Menard C, Kin NMKNY, Nair NPV (2002) The modulatory effects of corticosteroids on cognition: studies in young human populations. *Psychoneuroendocrinology* 27:401–416.

MacQueen GM, Ramakrishnan K, Ratnasingan R, Chen B, Young LT (2003) Desipramine treatment reduces the long-term behavioural and neurochemical sequelae of early-life maternal separation. *Intl J Neuropsychopharmacol* 6:391–396.

Magarinos AM, McEwen BS (1995) Stress-induced atrophy of apical dendrites of hippocampal CA3c neurons: involvement of glucocorticoid secretion and excitatory amino acid receptors. *Neuroscience* 69:89–98.

Magarinos AM, McEwen BS, Saboureau M, Pevet P (2006) Rapid and reversible changes in intrahippocampal connectivity during the course of hibernation in European hamsters. *Proc Natl Acad Sci USA* 103:18775–18780.

Magarinos AM, Verdugo Garcia JM, McEwen BS (1997) Chronic restraint stress alters synaptic terminal structure in hippocampus. *Proc Natl Acad Sci USA* 94:14002–14008.

Maheu FS, Joober R, Lupien, SJ (2005) Declarative memory after stress in humans: differential involvement of the β-adrenergic and corticosteroid systems. *J Clin Endocrinol Metab* 90(3):1697–1704.

Mandell A, Chapman L, Rand R, Walter R (1963) Plasma corticosteroids: changes in concentration after stimulation of hippocampus and amygdala. *Science* 139:1212–1213.

Manolopoulos K, Karpe F, Frayn K (2010) Gluteofemoral body fat as a determinant of metabolic health. *Int J Obes* 34:949–959.

Marrocco J, McEwen BS (2016) Sex in the brain: hormones and sex differences. *Dialogues Clin Neurosci* 18:373–383.

Marrocco J, Petty GH, Ríos MB, Gray JD, Kogan JF, Waters EM, Schmidt EF, Lee FS, McEwen BS (2017) A sexually dimorphic pre-stressed translational signature in CA3 pyramidal neurons of BDNF Val66Met mice. *Nat Comm* 8:1–15.

Martin KP, Wellman CL (2011) NMDA receptor blockade alters stress-induced dendritic remodeling in medial prefrontal cortex. *Cereb Cortex* 21:2366–2373.

Marsland AL, Gianaros PJ, Abramowitch SM, Manuck SB, Hariri AR (2008) Interleukin-6 covaries inversely with hippocampal grey matter volume in middle-aged adults. *Biol Psychiatry* 64:484–490.

Mason JW (1975) A historical view of the stress field. *J Human Stress* 1:6–12.

Matys T, Pawlak R, Matys E, Pavlides C, McEwen BS, Strickland S (2004) Tissue plasminogen activator promotes the effects of corticotropin-releasing factor on the amygdala and anxiety-like behavior. *Proc Natl Acad Sci USA* 101:16345–16350.

McCall T, Weil ZM, Nacher J, Bloss EB, El Maarouf A, Rutishauser U, McEwen BS (2013) Depletion of polysialic acid from neural cell adhesion molecule (PSA-NCAM) increases CA3 dendritic arborization and increases vulnerability to excitotoxicity. *Exp Neurol* 241:5–12.

McCarthy MM, Arnold AP, Ball GF, Blaustein JD, De Vries GJ (2012) Sex differences in the brain: the not so inconvenient truth. *J Neurosci* 32:2241–2247.

McClintock B (1956) Controlling elements and the gene. *Cold Spring Harbor Symp Quant Biol* 21:197–216.

McEwen, BS (2015) Preserving neuroplasticity: role of glucocorticoids and neurotrophins via phosphorylation. *Proc Natl Acad Sci USA* 112(51):15544–15545.

McEwen BS (2016) Stress-induced remodeling of hippocampal CA3 pyramidal neurons. *Brain Res* 1645:50–54.

McEwen BS (1998) Protective and damaging effects of stress mediators. *New England J Med* 338:171–179.

McEwen BS (1999) Stress and hippocampal plasticity. *Annu Rev Neurosci* 22:105–122.

McEwen BS, Akama KT, Spencer-Segal JL, Milner TA, Waters EM (2012) Estrogen effects on the brain: actions beyond the hypothalamus via novel mechanisms. *Behav Neurosci* 126:4–16.

McEwen, BS, Bowles, NP, Gray, JD, Hill, MN, Hunter, RG, Karatsoreos, IN, Nasca, C (2015) Mechanisms of stress in the brain. *Nat Neurosci* 18(10):1353–1363.

McEwen BS, Milner TA (2007) Hippocampal formation: shedding light on the influence of sex and stress on the brain. *Brain Res Rev* 55:343–355.

McEwen BS, Milner TA (2017) Understanding the broad influence of sex hormones and sex differences in the brain. *J Neurosci Res* 95:24–39.

McEwen BS, Plapinger L (1970) Association of corticosterone-1,2 3H with macromolecules extracted from brain cell nuclei. *Nature* 226:263–264.

McEwen BS, Stellar E (1993) Stress and the Individual: mechanisms leading to disease. *Arch Intern Med* 153:2093–2101.

McEwen BS, Weiss J, Schwartz L (1968) Selective retention of corticosterone by limbic structures in rat brain. *Nature* 220:911–912.

McEwen BS, Wingfield JC (2003) The concept of allostasis in biology and biomedicine. *Horm Behav* 43:2–15.

McGaugh JL. 2000. Memory—a century of consolidation. *Science* 287:248–251.

McHugh TJ, Blum KI, Tsien JZ, Tonegawa S, Wilson MA (1996) Impaired hippocampal representation of space in CA1-specific NMDAR1 knockout mice. *Cell* 87:1339–1349.

McIntyre RS, Kenna HA, Nguyen HT, Law CW, Sultan F, Woldeyohannes HO, Adams AK, Cheng JSH, Lourenco M, Kennedy SH, et al. (2010) Brain volume abnormalities and neurocognitive deficits in diabetes mellitus: points of pathophysiological commonality with mood disorders? *Adv Ther* 27:63–80.

McKittrick CR, Magarinos AM, Blanchard DC, Blanchard RJ, McEwen BS, Sakai RR (2000) Chronic social stress reduces dendritic arbors in CA3 of hippocampus and decreases binding to serotonin transporter sites. *Synapse* 36:85–94.

McLaughlin KJ, Baran SE, Wright RL, Conrad CD (2005) Chronic stress enhances spatial memory in ovariectomized female rats despite CA3 dendritic retraction: possible involvement of CA1 neurons. *Neuroscience* 135:1045–1054.

McNay EC, Fries TM, Gold PE (2000) Decreases in rat extracellular hippocampal glucose concentration associated with cognitive demand during a spatial task. *Proc Natl Acad Sci USA* 97:2881–2885.

McNay EC, Gold PE (2001) Age-related differences in hippocampal extracellular fluid glucose concentration during behavioral testing and following systemic glucose administration. *J Gerontol A Biol Sci Med Sci J* 56:B66–B71.

Meites J (1992) Short history of neuroendocrinology and the International Society of Neuroendocrinology. *Neuroendocrinology* 56:1–10.

Milner TA, Burstein SR, Marrone GF, Khalid S, Gonzalez AD, Williams TJ, Schierberl KC, Torres-Reveron A, Gonzales KL, McEwen BS, et al. (2013) Stress differentially alters mu opioid receptor density and trafficking in parvalbumin-containing interneurons in the female and male rat hippocampus. *Synapse* 67:757–772.

Milner TA, McEwen BS, Hayashi S, Li CJ, Reagen L, Alves SE (2001) Ultrastructural evidence that hippocampal alpha estrogen receptors are located at extranuclear sites. *J Comp Neurol* 429:355–371.

Mitra R, Jadhav S, McEwen BS, Vyas A, Chattarji S (2005) Stress duration modulates the spatiotemporal patterns of spine formation in the basolateral amygdala. *Proc Natl Acad Sci USA* 102:9371–9376.

Mitsushima D, Yamada K, Takase K, Funabashi T, Kimura F (2006) Sex differences in the basolateral amygdala: the extracellular levels of serotonin and dopamine, and their responses to restraint stress in rats. *Eur J Neurosci* 24:3245–3254.

Moon HY, Becke A, Berron D, Becker B, Sah N, Benoni G, Janke E, Lubejko S, Greig N, Mattiosn J, et al. (2016) Running-induced systemic cathepsin B secretion is associated with memory function. *Cell Metab* 24:332–340.

Moreno-Jimenez EP, Flor-Garcia M, Terreros-Roncal J, Rabano A, Cafini F, Pallas-Bazarra, Avila J, Llorens-Martin M (2019) Adult hippocampal neurogenesis is abundant in neurologically healthy subjects and drops sharply in patients with Alzheimer's disease. *Nat Med* 25:554–560.

Moser, EI, Kropff, E and Moser, MB (2008) Place cells, grid cells, and the brain's spatial representation system. *Annul Rev Neurosci* 31(1):69–89.

Mucha M, Skrzypiec AE, Schiavon E, Attwood BK, Kucerova E, Pawlak R (2011) Lipocalin-2 controls neuronal excitability and anxiety by regulating dendritic spine formation and maturation. *Proc Natl Acad Sci USA* 108:18436–18441.

Murphy BEP (1991) Steroids and depression. *J Steroid Biochem Mol Biol* 38:537–559.

Musazzi L, Mingardi J, Ieraci A, Barbon A, Popoli M (2023) Stress, microRNAs, and stress-related psychiatric disorders: an overview. *Mol Psych* 28:4977–4994.

Nakashiba T, Young JZ, McHugh TJ, Buhl DL, Tonegawa S (2008) Transgenic inhibition of synaptic transmission reveals role of CA3 output in hippocampal learning. *Science* 319:1260–1264.

Nasca C, Bigio B, Lee FS, Young SP, Kautz MM, Albright A, Beasley J, Millington DS, Mathe AA, Kociss JH, et al. (2018) Acetyl-l-carnitine deficiency in patients with major depressive disorder. *Proc Natl Acad Sci USA* 115:8627–8632.

Nasca C, Xenos D, Barone Y, Caruso A, Scaccianoce S, Matrisciano F, Battaglia G, Mathe AA, Pittaluga A, Lonetto L, et al. (2013) L-acetylcarnitine causes rapid antidepressant effects through the epigenetic induction of mGlu2 receptors. *Proc Natl Acad Sci USA* 110:4804–4809.

Nasca C, Zelli D, Bigio B, Piccinin S, Scaccianoce S, Nistico R, McEwen BS (2015) Stress dynamically regulates behavior and glutamatergic gene expression in hippocampus by opening a window of epigenetic plasticity. *Proc Natl Acad Sci USA* 112:14960–14965.

Nestler EJ, Barrot M, DiLeone RJ, Eisch AJ, Gold SJ, Monteggia LM (2002) Neurobiology of depression. *Neuron* 34:13–25.

Nibuya M, Morinobu S, Duman RS (1995) Regulation of BDNF and trkB mRNA in rat brain by chronic electroconvulsive seizure and antidepressant drug treatments. *J Neurosci* 15:7539–7547.

Nottebohm F (2002) Why are some neurons replaced in adult brain? *J Neurosci* 624–628.

Oitzl, MS, de Kloet RE (1992) Selective corticosteroid antagonists modulate specific aspects of spatial orientation learning. *Behav Neurosci* 106(1):62–71.

Oitzl MS, Fluttert M, Ron de Kloet E (1994) The Effect of corticosterone on reactivity to spatial novelty is mediated by central mineralocorticosteroid receptors. *Eur J Neurosci* 6:1072–1079.

Okamoto M, Hojo Y, Inoue K, Matsui T, Kawato S, McEwen BS, Soya H (2012) Mild exercise increases dihydrotestosterone in hippocampus providing evidence for androgenic mediation of neurogenesis. *Proc Natl Acad Sci USA* 109:13100–13105.

O'Keefe, J (1979) A review of the hippocampal place cells. *Prog Neurobiol* 13(4):419–439.

Okuda S, Roozendaal B, McGaugh JL (2004) Glucocorticoid effects on object recognition memory require training-associated emotional arousal. *Proc Natl Acad Sci USA* 101:853–858.

Opendak M, Offit L, Monari P, Schoenfeld TJ, Sonti AN, Cameron HA, Gould E (2016) Lasting adaptations in social behavior produced by social disruption and inhibition of adult neurogenesis. *J Neurosci* 36(26):7027–7038.

Ott A, Stolk R, Hofman A, van Harskamp F, Grobbee D, Breteler M (1996) Association of diabetes mellitus and dementia: the Rotterdam Study. *Diabetologia* 39:1392–1397.

Oury, F, Khrimian, L, Denny, CA, Gardin, A, Chamouni, A, Goeden, N, Huang, Y, Lee, H, Srinivas, P, Gao, XB, et al. (2013) Maternal and offspring pools of osteocalcin influence brain development and functions. *Cell* 155(1):228–241.

Packard MG, Cahill L, McGaugh JL (1994) Amygdala modulation of hippocampal-dependent and caudate nucleus-dependent memory processes. *Proc Natl Acad Sci USA* 91:8477–8481.

Park M, Kim CH, Jo S, Kim EJ, Rhim H, Lee CJ, Kim JJ, Cho J (2015) Chronic stress alters spatial representation and bursting patterns of place cells in behaving mice. *Sci Rep* 5(1):16235.

Paton JA, Nottebohm FN (1984) Neurons generated in the adult brain are recruited into functional circuits. *Science* 225:1046–1048.

Pavlides C, Nivón LG, McEwen BS (2002) Effects of chronic stress on hippocampal long-term potentiation: effects of stress on LTP. *Hippocampus* 12:245–257.

Pavlides C, Ogawa S, Kimura A, McEwen BS (1996) Role of adrenal steroid mineralocorticoid and glucocorticoid receptors in long-term potentiation in the CA1 field of hippocampal slices. *Brain Res* 738:229–235.

Pavlides C, Watanabe Y, Margarinos AM, McEwen BS (1995) Opposing roles of type I and type II adrenal steroid receptors in hippocampal long-term potentiation. *Neuroscience* 68:387–394.

Pavlides C, Watanabe Y, McEwen BS (1993) Effects of glucocorticoids on hippocampal long-term potentiation. *Hippocampus* 3:183–192.

Pawlak R, Magarinos AM, Melchor J, McEwen B, Strickland S (2003) Tissue plasminogen activator in the amygdala is critical for stress-induced anxiety-like behavior. *Nat Neurosci* 6:168–174.

Pawlak R, Rao BSS, Melchor JP, Chattarji S, McEwen B, Strickland S (2005) Tissue plasminogen activator and plasminogen mediate stress-induced decline of neuronal and cognitive functions in the mouse hippocampus. *Proc Natl Acad Sci USA* 102:18201–18206.

Pereira AC, Gray JD, Kogan JF, Davidson RL, Rubin TG, Okamoto M, Morrison JH, McEwen BS (2016) Age and Alzheimer's disease gene expression profiles reversed by the glutamate modulator riluzole. *Mol Psychiatry* 22(2):296–305.

Pereira AC, Lambert HK, Grossman YS, Dumitriu D, Waldman R, Jannetty SK, Calakos K, Janssen WG, McEwen BS, Morrison JH (2014) Glutamatergic regulation prevents hippocampal-dependent age-related cognitive decline through dendritic spine clustering. *Proc Natl Acad Sci USA* 111:18733–18738.

Petrovich GD, Canteras NS, Swanson LW (2001) Combinatorial amygdalar inputs to hippocampal domains and hypothalamic behavior systems. *Brain Res Rev* 38:247–289.

Pham K, Nacher J, Hof PR, McEwen BS (2003) Repeated, but not acute, restraint stress suppresses proliferation of neural precursor cells and increases PSA-NCAM expression in the adult rat dentate gyrus. *J Neurosci* 17:879–886.

Pietras RJ, Nemere I, Szego CM (2001) Steroid hormone receptors in target cell membranes. *Endocrine* 14(3):417–428.

Pikkarainen M, Rönkkö S, Savander V, Insausti R, Pitkänen A (1999) Projections from the lateral, basal, and accessory basal nuclei of the amygdala to the hippocampal formation in rat. *J Comp Neurol* 403:229–260.

Piroli GG, Grillo CA, Reznikov LR, Adams S, McEwen BS, Charron MJ, Reagan LP (2007) Corticosterone impairs insulin-stimulated translocation of GLUT4 in the rat hippocampus. *Neuroendocrinology* 85:71–80.

Pitkanen A, Amaral DG (1994) The distribution of GABAergic cells, fibers, and terminals in the monkey amygdaloid complex: an immunohistochemical and in situ hybridization study. *J Neurosci* 14:2200–2224.

Pitkänen A, Savander V, LeDoux JE (1997) Organization of intra-amygdaloid circuitries in the rat: an emerging framework for understanding functions of the amygdala. *Trends Neurosci* 20:517–523.

Pitman RK, Gilbertson MW, Gurvits TV, May FS, Lasko NB, Metzger LJ, Shenton ME, Yehuda R, Orr SP, Harvard/VA PTSD Twin Study Investigators (2006) Clarifying the origin of biological abnormalities in AKT through the study of identical twins discordant for combat exposure. *Ann N Y Acad Sci* 1071:242–254.

Popa D, Duvarci S, Popescu AT, Léna C, Paré D (2010) Coherent amygdalocortical theta promotes fear memory consolidation during paradoxical sleep. *Proc Natl Acad Sci USA* 107:6516–6519.

Popoli M, Yan Z, McEwen BS, Sanacora G (2012) The stressed synapse: the impact of stress and glucocorticoids on glutamate transmission. *Nat Rev Neurosci* 13(1):22–37.

Protopopescu X, Butler T, Pan H, Root J, Altemus M, Polanecsky M, McEwen B, Silbersweig D, Stern E (2008) Hippocampal structural changes across the menstrual cycle. *Hippocampus* 18:985–988.

Pruessner JC, Baldwin MW, Dedovic K, Renwick R, Mahani NK, Lord C, Meaney M, Lupien S (2005) Self-esteem, locus of control, hippocampal volume, and cortisol regulation in young and old adulthood. *NeuroImage* 28:815–826.

Pugh CR, Tremblay D, Fleshner M, Rudy JW (1997) A selective role for corticosterone in contextual-fear conditioning. *Behav Neurosci* 111:503–511.

Radley JJ, Rocher AB, Miller M, Janssen WGM, Liston C, Hof PR, McEwen BS, Morrison JH (2006) Repeated stress induces dendritic spine loss in the rat medial prefrontal cortex. *Cereb Cortex* 16:313–320.

Radley JJ, Sisti HM, Hao J, Rocher AB, McCall T, Hof PR, McEwen BS, Morrison JH (2004) Chronic behavioral stress induces apical dendritic reorganization in pyramidal neurons of the medial prefrontal cortex. *Neuroscience* 125:1–6.

Rahman MM, Callaghan CK, Kerskens CM, Chattarji S, O'Mara SM (2016) Early hippocampal volume loss as a marker of eventual memory deficits caused by repeated stress. *Sci Rep* 6:1–15.

Rasgon NL, Kenna HA, Wroolie TE, Kelley R, Silverman D, Brooks J, Williams KE, Powers BN, Hallmayer J, Reiss A (2011) Insulin resistance and hippocampal volume in women at risk for Alzheimer's disease. *Neurobiol Aging* 32:1942–1948.

Rasgon NL, Small GW, Siddarth P, Miller K, Ercoli LM, Bookheimer SY, Lavretsky H, Huang SC, Barrio JR, Phelps ME (2001) Estrogen use and brain metabolic change in older adults: a preliminary report. *Psychiatry Res* 107:11–18.

Rau V, DeCola JP, Fanselow MS (2005) Stress-induced enhancement of fear learning: an animal model of posttraumatic stress disorder. *Neurosci Biobehavi Rev* 29:1207–12023.

Reul JMHM, De Kloet ER (1985) Two receptor systems for corticosterone in rat brain: microdistribution and differential occupation. *Endocrinology* 117:2505–2511.

Reynolds AC, Paterson JL, Ferguson SA, Stanley D, Wright KP, Jr, Dawson D (2017) The shift work and health research agenda: considering changes in gut microbiota as a pathway linking shift work, sleep loss and circadian misalignment, and metabolic disease. *SleepMed Rev* 34:3–9.

Roddy DW, Farrell C, Doolin K, Roman E, Tozzi L, Frodl T, O'Keane V, O'Hanlon E (2019) The hippocampus in depression: more than the sum of its parts? Advanced hippocampal substructure segmentation in depression. *Biol Psychiatry* 85:487–97.

Rodrigues SM, LeDoux JE, Sapolsky RM (2009) The influence of stress hormones on fear circuitry. *Annu Rev Neurosci* 32:289–313.

Roozendaal B, Griffith QK, Buranday J, Dominique J-F, McGaugh JL (2003) The hippocampus mediates glucocorticoid-induced impairment of spatial memory retrieval: dependence on the basolateral amygdala. *Proc Natl Acad Sci USA* 100:1328–33.

Roozendaal B, McEwen BS, Chattarji S (2009) Stress, memory and the amygdala. *Nat Rev Neurosci* 10:423–33.

Roozendaal B, McGaugh JL (1996) Amygdaloid nuclei lesions differentially affect glucocorticoid-induced memory enhancement in an inhibitory avoidance task. *Neurobiol Learn Mem* 65:1–8.

Roozendaal B, Phillips RG, Power AE, Brooke SM, Sapolsky RM, McGaugh JL (2001) Memory retrieval impairment induced by

prevents chronic stress-induced impairments in spatial memory. *Eur J Neurosci* **24**:595–605.

Xu L, Anwyl R, Rowan MJ (1997) Behavioural stress facilitates the induction of long-term depression in the hippocampus. *Nature* **387**:497–500.

Xu L, Holscher C, Anwyl R, Rowan MJ (1998) Glucocorticoid receptor and protein/RNA synthesis-dependent mechanisms underlie the control of synaptic plasticity by stress. *Proc Natl Acad Sci USA* **95**:3204–3208.

Yasmin F, Saxena K, McEwen BS, Chattarji S (2016) The delayed strengthening of synaptic connectivity in the amygdala depends on NMDA receptor activation during acute stress. *Physiol Rep* **4**(20):e13002.

Yau JLW, Olsson T, Morris RGM, Meaney MJ, Seckl JR (1995) Glucocorticoids, hippocampal corticosteroid receptor gene expression and antidepressant treatment: relationship with spatial learning in young and aged rats. *Neuroscience* **66**:571–581.

Yau PL, Castro MG, Tagani A, Tsui WH, Convit A (2012) Obesity and metabolic syndrome and functional and structural brain impairments in adolescence. *Pediatrics* **130**:e856–e864.

Yook JS, Rakwal R, Shibato J, Takahashi K, Koizumi H, Shima T, Ikemoto MJ, Oharomari LK, McEwen BS, Soya H (2019) Leptin in hippocampus mediates benefits of mild exercise by an antioxidant on neurogenesis and memory. *Proc Natl Acad Sci USA* **116**:10988–10993.

Zhong P, Liu W, Gu Z, Yan Z (2008) Serotonin facilitates long-term depression induction in prefrontal cortex via p38 MAPK/Rab5-mediated enhancement of AMPA receptor internalization. *J Physiol* **586**:4465–4479.

Zigman JM, Jones JE, Lee CE, Saper CB, Elmquist JK (2006) Expression of ghrelin receptor mRNA in the rat and the mouse brain. *J Comp Neurol* **494**:528–548.

18

Mesial Temporal Lobe Epilepsy

Matthew C. Walker, Maria Thom, and Umesh Vivekananda

18.1 Introduction

Epilepsy is the propensity to have seizures and is one of the most common serious neurological conditions, affecting 0.6% of the world's population (Beghi, 2020). There are approximately 60/100,000 new cases per year (Beghi, 2020), and the lifetime chance of developing epilepsy is 3%–4% (Hesdorffer et al., 2011). Seizure types can be divided into focal seizures, "originating within networks limited to one hemisphere," and generalized seizures, "originating at some point within, and rapidly engaging, bilaterally distributed networks," and the epilepsies are similarly defined by their seizure types into focal or generalized (Berg et al., 2010; Scheffer et al., 2017). Focal epilepsies constitute approximately 70% of newly diagnosed epilepsy (Beghi, 2020). The clinical manifestation of a seizure depends not only on where the seizure starts but also on the speed and pattern of seizure spread. Epilepsy type is determined by seizure type, and EEG abnormalities, and epilepsy syndromes are determined by specific patterns of seizure types, clinical features, EEG features, and imaging abnormalities. In the most recent classification of the epilepsies, etiology (structural, genetic, infectious, metabolic, immune, and unknown) and comorbidities are also included within the framework. Importantly, an epilepsy can have more than one etiology. Differing epilepsy syndromes can have different pathophysiologies and mechanisms; in this chapter we are solely concerned with mesial temporal lobe epilepsy, and we will focus on mesial temporal lobe epilepsy with hippocampal sclerosis, which can be considered as a specific epilepsy syndrome.

Temporal lobe epilepsy represents over 60% of all focal epilepsies (Semah et al., 1998). The commonest neuropathological lesion identified in patients with temporal lobe epilepsy is hippocampal sclerosis, or Ammon's horn sclerosis (Blumcke et al., 2017). Other major pathologies include focal cortical dysplasia, vascular malformations, malformations of cortical development, and glioneuronal tumors. Hippocampal sclerosis is present in approximately 10% of adults with new-onset focal epilepsy (Van Paesschen et al., 1998). Moreover, hippocampal sclerosis often causes refractory epilepsy and is the sole pathology in about a third of all surgical resections for epilepsy and is found with an associated pathology (so-called dual pathology) in approximately 1.5% (Blumcke et al., 2017).

18.1.1 History

The first description of hippocampal sclerosis dates back 200 years. In 1825, Bouchet and Cazauvielh presented their findings on 18 autopsied patients in a thesis that attempted to establish the relationship between epilepsy, "l'épilepsie," and insanity, "l'aliénation mentale" (Bouchet and Cazavieilh, 1825). They noted that in five cases where there were changes in the cornu ammonis, four were characterized by induration and one had softening. Sommer further described in detail the neuropathological finding of hippocampal sclerosis in the brains of patients with chronic epilepsy (Sommer, 1880). He noted gliosis and pyramidal cell loss in predominantly the CA1 region of the hippocampus, and he proposed that these lesions were the cause of the epilepsy. In the same year, Pfleger described hemorrhagic lesions in the mesial temporal lobe of a patient dying in status epilepticus and concluded that neuronal necrosis was the result of impaired blood flow or metabolic disturbances that occurred during the seizure (Pfleger, 1880). Since that time, it has been well established that hippocampal sclerosis can be the cause or result of seizures.

That hippocampal sclerosis is a cause of epilepsy is indicated by three lines of evidence. First, hippocampal sclerosis is closely associated with a particular seizure semiology, the psychomotor seizure—a seizure type first recognized by John Hughlings Jackson in the 19th century. Second, EEG evidence points to a seizure onset in the sclerosed hippocampus. Third, surgical resection of the sclerosed hippocampus can result in seizure remission.

18.2 Clinical features of mesial temporal lobe epilepsy

There is a typical course and anamnesis for temporal lobe epilepsy with hippocampal sclerosis (Figure 18.1A). Often, there is an antecedent history of a brain insult, most commonly febrile seizures (see below), but also meningitis, encephalitis, traumatic brain injury, and birth trauma, followed by a gap (a latent period) before seizures begin many years later (French et al., 1993).

These seizures often prove resistant to treatment and are associated with an increased risk of mortality. There is also an increased risk of comorbidities including psychiatric problems (depression, psychosis), and neuropsychological deficits that relate to the side of

A

History
A 32 year old man presented with refractory partial epilepsy. He had a prolonged febrile seizure at the age of 18 months, and spontaneous seizures began at the age of 8 years.
These seizures have continued despite trying all available antiseizure medications.
The seizures take the form of focal seizures in which he perceives a sense of fear rising from his stomach, and then, on occasions, he loses touch with his surroundings. During the loss of awareness, he is described as making chewing movements, his right hand is postured and he fiddles with his clothes with his left hand. This type of seizure lasts a couple of minutes, and he is then confused and has trouble finding words afterwards for approximately 5 minutes.

B

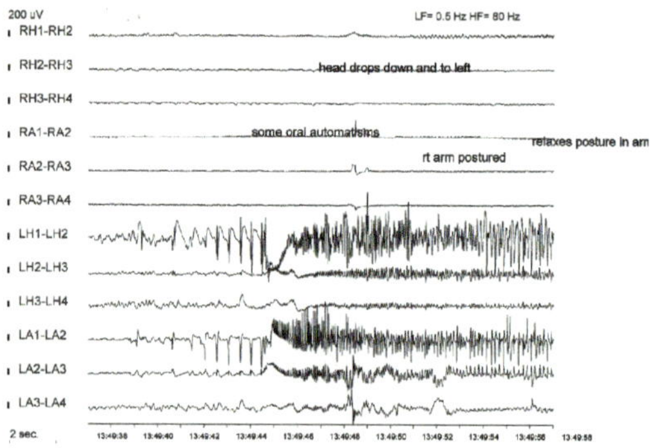

C

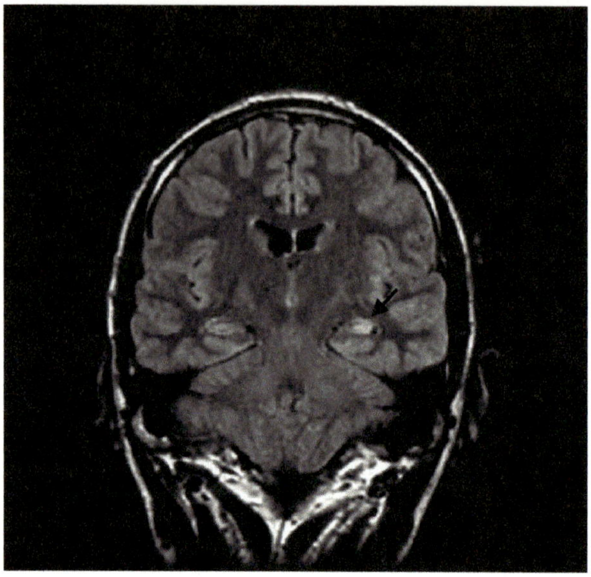

D

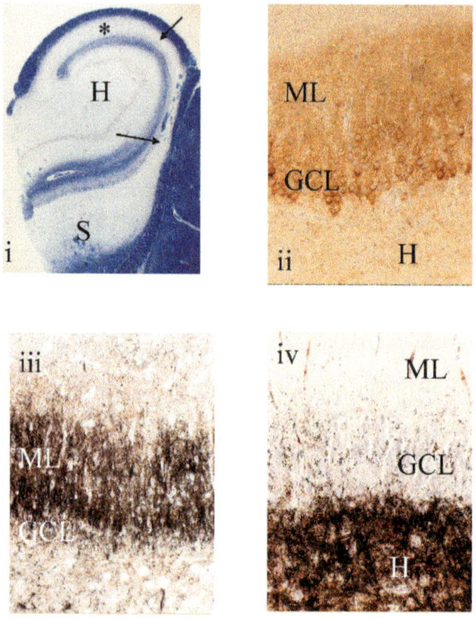

Figure 18.1 Typical case of hippocampal sclerosis. (A) Case history. (B) Intracranial EEG with electrodes into right hippocampus (RH), right amygdala (RA), left hippocampus (LH), and left amygdala (LA). Lower numbers are deeper, with 1&2 lying in hippocampi or amygdala. The seizure begins in left hippocampus and amygdala with high amplitude spikes, followed by a DC shift and a buildup of fast activity. (C) MRI, T2 coronal image demonstrating small left hippocampus (arrow) with high T2 signal, typical for hippocampal sclerosis. (D) (i) Typical pattern of neuronal loss in a surgical specimen of HS with neuronal loss in the hilar region (H) and CA1 (arrowed) with collapse of the pyramidal cell layer in contrast to the relative preservation of neurons in CA2 (asterisk) and the subiculum (S). (ii) Timm staining in a patient with minor hippocampal hilar neuronal loss shows positive granules in the Hilar region (H) and little staining in the molecular layer (ML) and granule cell layer (GCL). (iii) Dynorphin immunostaining shows mossy fiber sprouting in the GCL and ML in hippocampal sclerosis which is also seen in the same case with a similar distribution with Timm staining.

the hippocampal sclerosis (verbal memory deficits with dominant temporal lobe involvement, and nonverbal memory deficits with nondominant temporal lobe involvement).

18.2.1 Seizure semiology

Mesial temporal lobe seizures usually take the form of focal impaired awareness seizures (previously termed complex partial seizures), and less commonly focal aware seizures (previously termed simple partial seizures). These usually occur a few times per month. The seizure usually has a gradual evolution over 1–2 minutes (longer than extratemporal seizures) and lasts longer (2–10 minutes) than focal impaired awareness seizures originating in extratemporal sites (Chowdhury et al., 2021). The commonest aura is that of a rising sensation from the stomach. Other gastrointestinal auras can occur, especially nausea, stomach rumbling, and belching. Auras can also consist of olfactory-gustatory hallucinations (intense, often unpleasant, smells and tastes), affective symptoms, and dysmnestic symptoms. Affective symptoms typically take the form of fear (the commonest, and often very intense), depression, anger, and irritability. Euphoria and erotic thoughts have also been described. Dreamy states and feelings of depersonalization commonly occur. Déjà vu, déjà vécu, jamais vu, déjà entendu, and other dysmnestic symptoms such as recollections of childhood or even former lives are also specific for mesial temporal lobe epilepsy.

In the early stages, autonomic phenomena such as apnea (cessation of breathing), flushing pupillary dilatation, piloerection, and tachycardia (rapid heart rate) can occur. After the aura, motor arrest and absence are prominent. Typically, this is followed by marked automatisms. The automatisms of mesial temporal lobe epilepsy can be prolonged and are typically oroalimentary (e.g., lip-smacking, chewing) and/or gestural (e.g., fidgeting, undressing, walking). Typically, the automatisms are more marked ipsilaterally and can be associated with contralateral posturing. There may be some apparent responsiveness, and "conscious behavior" can occur, especially during nondominant temporal lobe seizures, although the person is amnesic for the episode. During the seizure, speech with recognizable words lateralizes the focus to the nondominant temporal lobe. Progression to bilateral tonic-clonic seizures (convulsions) is less common than in extratemporal lobe epilepsy. Postictal confusion is typical, and postictal dysphasia can occur following dominant temporal lobe seizures. Postictal headache and postictal psychosis have also been described.

18.2.2 EEG characteristics

Scalp EEG recordings usually demonstrate interictal epileptiform abnormalities (spikes, sharp waves) over the mid/anterior temporal region, but it is common for these epileptiform abnormalities to occur bilaterally or independently over both temporal regions (Williamson et al., 1993). Temporal intermittent rhythmic delta activity, sinusoidal trains of <4 Hz activity over the temporal regions, is also commonly seen and may be specific for mesial temporal lobe epilepsy (Di Gennaro et al., 2003). Recordings from electrodes placed into the hippocampus (depth electrode recordings) have revealed spikes originating from the hippocampi and surrounding structures. In addition, high-frequency oscillations (HFOs) from the abnormal temporal lobe can also be detected (Bragin et al., 1999). HFOs need to be differentiated from physiological oscillations such as sharp wave–ripples and from EEG noise. HFOs have been demonstrated to accurately localize the epileptogenic zone (Zijlmans et al., 2012), and the resection of HFO-generating areas is associated with seizure-free outcome (Jacobs et al., 2010). Perhaps an even more sensitive biomarker for epileptogenicity has been the co-occurrence of HFOs with interictal epileptiform discharges (Ren et al., 2015). The mechanisms generating these interictal abnormalities are discussed later.

During the seizure, scalp EEG recordings usually demonstrate a buildup of 5–10 Hz sharp activity localized to the mid/anterior temporal region. Because activity in the hippocampus is not, or is poorly, detected by scalp EEG, this activity is likely to represent propagation of seizure activity to lateral temporal regions. This activity can remain localized or commonly spreads to involve a wider field including the contralateral temporal lobe. Depth electrode studies have confirmed the electrographic origin of these seizures in the hippocampal formation (King and Spencer, 1995). Although interictal spikes may occur independently either from the hippocampus or from extrahippocampal sites, the ictal discharges are usually relatively well localized initially. Preictal abnormalities can occur with well localized 1–2 Hz spikes that recur over seconds or minutes (Figure 18.1B). With clinical seizure onset, there is a 10–15 Hz low-amplitude discharge that is initially confined to hippocampal electrodes (Figure 18.1B) but grows in amplitude and then spreads to other regions (King and Spencer, 1995). A second pattern has also been described in which the seizure begins as a low-amplitude, high-frequency discharge without the preictal spiking. These two types of onsets can occur in the same patient. The exact location for seizure onset can vary not only from patient to patient but also within the same patient. This suggests that seizure onset and generation are not from a single area within mesial temporal structures, but from a more distributed network.

18.2.3 Hippocampal resection

Surgery has provided the most compelling evidence of hippocampal sclerosis as the substrate for the epilepsy. Surgical outcome for intractable temporal lobe epilepsy is most successful when mesial temporal structures are included in the resection. In patients with drug-resistant epilepsy in whom there is concordance between neuroimaging, electroclinical characteristics of the seizure, and neuropsychological tests, there is >70% chance of seizure freedom with mesial temporal lobe resection in the first 2 years. However, the percentage seizure-free decreases with time, so that by 5 years this has decreased to fewer than 60% of people seizure-free following epilepsy surgery (Janszky et al., 2005). Predictors for effectiveness of surgery are length of time with epilepsy and removal of other brain regions such as piriform cortex and entorhinal cortex and disconnection of temporal, frontal, and limbic regions (Gleichgerrcht et al., 2022). Moreover, even when seizure-free, many people cannot come off medication and some of the "seizure-free" group in these studies remain having nondisabling auras. These observations, along with structural MRI studies showing subtle abnormalities in other brain regions including thalamus, suggest that temporal lobe epilepsy with hippocampal sclerosis is a network condition involving areas outside the hippocampus and that the extent of that network may expand with time and predict the success of hippocampal resection (see below).

18.3 What is and what causes hippocampal sclerosis?

"Hippocampal sclerosis" has been recognized to comprise more than one neuropathological entity (Blümcke et al., 2013). Older systems of grading the severity of cell loss in hippocampal sclerosis have been superseded by a system that recognizes that it is not just the severity of cell loss that is important but also the pattern of that cell loss. The new ILAE classification grades hippocampal sclerosis as:

1. type 1, with cell loss throughout the hippocampus, but primarily involving CA1 and CA4, and occurring in 60%–80% of resections previously termed 'classical hippocampal sclerosis' (Figure 18.1D);
2. type 2, CA1 predominant sclerosis, occurring in 5%–10%;
3. type 3, also termed "end-folium sclerosis" (mainly involving CA4 and dentate gyrus), occurring in 4%–7%;
4. gliosis without hippocampal sclerosis, which may be seen in up to 20% of temporal lobe resections.

The classification is clinically important because it may relate to surgical outcome (Thom et al., 2010). In a retrospective analysis, 70% of people with type 1 hippocampal sclerosis were seizure free 2 years after surgery, compared with ~40% with CA1 predominant sclerosis (type 2) or gliosis without hippocampal sclerosis. Advances in MRI technology will hopefully permit accurate presurgical classification, which would facilitate a prospective study to validate these findings (Sone et al., 2016). Another important issue is whether the pattern of damage relates to the nature of the precipitating event, age at the time of the precipitating event, duration of epilepsy, and seizure frequency. Interestingly, seizure frequency and duration of epilepsy had minimal impact on the type of hippocampal sclerosis. However, events before the age of 3 years tended to be associated with type 1 hippocampal sclerosis. Type 3 and gliosis without hippocampal sclerosis were less strongly associated with the occurrence of identifiable preceding events, which tended to happen later, during adolescence (Blümcke et al., 2013).

Epilepsy with hippocampal sclerosis, however, is a syndrome in which abnormalities are not restricted to the hippocampal formation. Neuronal loss and gliosis, albeit to a milder degree, often extends locally beyond the hippocampus and affects amygdala, parahippocampal gyrus, and entorhinal cortex (Yilmazer-Hanke et al., 2000; Bernasconi et al., 2003). Moreover, hippocampal sclerosis is also associated with brain abnormalities further afield with neuronal loss reported in subcortical structures such as the thalamus (Sinjab et al., 2013). Indeed, thalamic atrophy seems to be a common finding in medial temporal lobe epilepsy (Barron et al., 2012). Although these more widespread structural and functional abnormalities associated with hippocampal sclerosis could be due to the underlying etiology, there is also some evidence that they can result from secondary involvement of these regions, possibly due to the activity generated from mesial temporal structures. In support of this hypothesis, measurements of the epileptogenicity index (an EEG measure of abnormal brain activity) of the lateral neocortex are greater in people who have had mesial temporal lobe epilepsy for longer (Bartolomei et al., 2008). Also, animal experiments have demonstrated an increase in the extent of epileptogenic EEG abnormalities over time in a model of mesial temporal lobe epilepsy and that this expansion can be prevented by early but not late "silencing" of the hippocampus using the sodium channel inhibitor, tetrodotoxin (Sheybani et al., 2018). This expansion of the epileptogenic network with time should result in a delay of resective surgery negatively correlating with outcome, but this has not been consistently observed (Janszky et al., 2005; Lamberink et al., 2020).

Are these more widespread abnormalities epiphenomena or do they play a role in seizure generation? Structural abnormalities of the thalamus detected by MRI predict poorer surgical outcomes (Keller et al., 2015), and removal or disconnection of more widespread areas of cortex predict better surgical outcome (Gleichgerrcht et al., 2022), suggesting that abnormal areas beyond the hippocampus contribute to epileptogenesis.

It has long been appreciated that hippocampal sclerosis can result from different insults to the brain, such as prolonged seizures, infection, inflammation, and traumatic brain injury. The etiology of hippocampal sclerosis, however, is more likely a more complex interplay between genetic background and environmental insults. We discussed earlier that the potential vulnerability of the hippocampus to damage by seizures was first suggested over 100 years ago (Pfleger, 1880; Sommer, 1880) and this has gained support more recently from human and animal studies (Meldrum and Brierley, 1973; DeGiorgio et al., 1992). Yet, a later unselected postmortem series identified patients who had had a long history of seizures and even episodes of status epilepticus with no evidence of damage in the hippocampus; this indicates that prolonged seizures or multiple seizures are not sufficient to cause hippocampal damage and that other factors may be important (Thom et al., 2005). Nevertheless, a significant cerebral insult/injury occurring early in life is often reported in people with hippocampal sclerosis (between 30%–50% of cases but up to 80% in one retrospective surgical series of patients). Thus, although such injuries do not inevitably result in hippocampal damage, when such damage is present, they are the likely cause (French et al., 1993).

The commonest precipitating cause is febrile seizures. Febrile seizures occur in 3%–8% of the population, usually with fevers over 38°C, between the ages of 6 months and 6 years (Sadleir and Scheffer, 2007). Few people with simple febrile seizures go on to develop epilepsy—2.4% versus 1.4% for the general population by 25 years (Annegers et al., 1987). The risk of epilepsy is increased if the febrile seizure is complex (i.e., has one of the following features: longer than 15 minutes, multiple seizures within 24 hours, or focal features). One such feature increases the risk of later epilepsy to 6%–8% (Annegers et al., 1987). The etiology of febrile seizures is unclear with evidence for the involvement of environmental factors such as viral infection, genetic predisposition, and subtle developmental abnormalities of the hippocampus (Sawires et al., 2022). Serial neuroimaging has demonstrated that hippocampal sclerosis can develop following prolonged febrile convulsions, but that hippocampal sclerosis is not an inevitable consequence (Lewis et al., 2014). Approximately 10% of children with febrile seizures lasting longer than 30 minutes (febrile status epilepticus) have an associated high T2 signal in the hippocampus with later evolution to hippocampal sclerosis in most. In the other 90%, there was evidence of decreased hippocampal growth, suggesting subtle hippocampal injury. The importance of the seizure rather than the fever is emphasized by the observation that hippocampal damage is not restricted to those who have had febrile status epilepticus but can occur following any cause of convulsive status epilepticus (Yoong et al., 2013) in childhood. There appears to be an age-specific sensitivity for this injury, with more severe neuronal loss occurring when the febrile seizures occur at a younger age (Davies et al., 1996).

Head injury can also result in hippocampal sclerosis, even when the traumatic brain injury is remote to the hippocampus. Traumatic brain injury to the neocortex can be reproduced in rat models using fluid percussion injury to the dura, which results in interneuron loss in the hippocampus, which can progress over time (Lowenstein et al., 1992). The neuronal loss is accompanied by enhanced excitability of the hippocampus and, eventually, spontaneous seizures. The mechanisms underlying this progression are unclear. In humans, traumatic brain injury can be associated with covert limbic status epilepticus, which is later accompanied by hippocampal injury (Vespa et al., 2010).

Lastly, infections and inflammation can cause hippocampal sclerosis. One of the commonest causes of epilepsy worldwide, neurocysticercosis, can be associated with hippocampal sclerosis, although the extent to which the infection is causal is still unclear (Singh et al., 2013). Viral encephalitis often targets mesial temporal structures with the evolution to bilateral hippocampal sclerosis and profound memory difficulties. Acute limbic encephalitis due to autoantibodies directed against extracellular proteins/receptors, such as LGI1 and NMDA receptors, have been associated with the later development of hippocampal sclerosis (Finke et al., 2016; van Sonderen et al., 2016).

The above observations indicate that hippocampal injury can occur following a variety of "brain insults," but they also raise the question of why these insults result in hippocampal sclerosis in the minority of patients. Indeed, such observations indicate that other factors must be involved. Although temporal lobe epilepsy is generally regarded as an acquired disorder with only a small genetic contribution, there are common genetic variants that predispose to hippocampal sclerosis. Polymorphisms in a region of the genome encoding sodium channel subunits, in particular SCN1A, have been associated with the occurrence of febrile seizures and hippocampal sclerosis (Kasperaviciute et al., 2013). In addition, an underlying maldevelopment of the hippocampus could predispose to hippocampal sclerosis and also to febrile seizures (Fernández et al., 1998; Baulac et al., 1998; Blümcke et al., 2002); this may partly explain why hippocampal sclerosis is often a unilateral disease. Subtle preexisting hippocampal abnormalities have been reported in MRI studies of families with familial febrile convulsions. MRI studies have also reported alterations of hippocampus size and shape in unaffected relatives of patients with mesial temporal lobe epilepsy with hippocampal sclerosis (Long et al., 2020). This has been argued as an "endophenotype" or genetic predisposition for a preexisting abnormality that predisposes to hippocampal sclerosis, although pathological correlates are not available. Although there are anecdotal cases of association, there is no evidence that acquired hippocampal sclerosis in epilepsy is mechanistically linked with preexisting incomplete hippocampal inversion (also known as "malrotation") (Bernasconi et al., 2005).

A further argument supporting a developmental basis for hippocampal sclerosis comes from the observation that hippocampal sclerosis is often observed in association with subtle cytoarchitectural malformations in the neocortex, previously termed "microdysgenesis" (Hardiman et al., 1988) and now referred to as "mild malformations of cortical development" (Blümcke et al., 2011). It has been argued that these "abnormalities" represent acquired postdevelopmental reorganization linked with the etiology of the hippocampal sclerosis. However, hippocampal sclerosis is also well recognized to occur in association with more severe cortical malformations, vascular malformations, and low-grade glioneuronal tumors as a "dual" pathology (Cendes et al., 1995), leading to the hypothesis that the extrahippocampal lesion generates seizures or subclinical seizure activity that results in neuronal loss in the hippocampus. In a large European cohort, 1.5% of cases with hippocampal sclerosis had a dual pathology including ganglioglioma, glial scars, focal cortical dysplasia, dysembryoplastic neuroepithelial tumor, and cavernous hemangiomas (Blumcke et al., 2017). In such patients (i.e., those with dual pathology), removal of both the lesion and the abnormal hippocampus has the best outcome in terms of seizure control, emphasizing the role of the hippocampus in temporal lobe seizures even when a second pathology is present (Li et al., 1999). Hippocampal sclerosis has also been described to be progressive in some patients (Briellmann et al., 2002), suggesting a paradigm in which an epileptogenic hippocampus generates seizures, which then cause further damage to the hippocampus and more widespread structures including contralateral hippocampus.

Together, these findings point to the idea that a "brain insult" induces damage in a "predisposed" hippocampus. They also indicate that seizures or seizure activity outside the hippocampus can over time result in damage to the hippocampus. Furthermore, in some people, damage to the hippocampus continues over time and hippocampal sclerosis can be a progressive rather than static condition.

18.4 Models and mechanisms of hippocampal sclerosis and epileptogenesis

18.4.1 Animal models

The interpretation of many of the pathological findings, and electrophysiologic studies in human postsurgical specimens is confounded by (1) the influence of treatment; (2) the difficulty in differentiating cause from effect (i.e., it is possible that the changes are the result not the cause of the seizures), and (3) the lack of adequate control tissue for comparison. To overcome these handicaps, animal models of mesial temporal lobe epilepsy are used—the most commonly used are the kindling model and the post-status-epilepticus models, which we discuss further below. Intrahippocampal injection of tetanus toxin also results in spontaneous seizures even after clearance of the toxin, and this model has also contributed to our understanding of the pathophysiology of mesial temporal lobe epilepsy (Mellanby et al., 1977). This model does not result in hippocampal sclerosis, and the seizures usually abate, in contrast to the human condition (Walker et al., 2017). Also models of traumatic brain injury can result in hippocampal changes, in particular loss of hippocampal interneurons, which are remote to the site of primary injury with the eventual development of seizures that involve the hippocampus (Kharatishvili et al., 2006; Huusko et al., 2015).

Kindling is the repetition of stimuli that initially evoke afterdischarges but not seizures (Goddard, 1967; McNamara et al., 1993). However, repetition of the same stimuli results in a gradual lengthening of the afterdischarges, eventually leading to seizures (which then become more severe with each stimulation), analogous to the help kindling wood provides at a bonfire. Once an animal has been kindled, the heightened response to the stimulus seems to be permanent, and spontaneous seizures can occur (McNamara et al., 1993). The hippocampus and amygdala are easily kindled, resulting in a well-described progression of limbic seizures. Kindling shares several characteristics with NMDA-dependent long-term potentiation (LTP) of excitatory synaptic transmission. This has led to the suggestion that kindling and LTP have similar underlying mechanisms. In support of this, the rate at which kindling occurs is retarded in rodents treated with NMDA receptor antagonists. There are, however, several differences between kindling and LTP. For example, although NMDA receptor antagonists can completely block the induction of LTP, they are unable to block kindling completely (Cain et al., 1992). Perhaps a more fundamental difference is that the kindling process requires afterdischarges; the repeated induction of LTP without afterdischarges does not induce kindling. LTP of glutamatergic synaptic transmission may contribute to kindling by increasing the excitatory synaptic drive and the likelihood of evoking afterdischarges but is alone insufficient to explain the cellular mechanisms of kindling (Cain et al., 1992). Kindling can also be induced through optogenetically stimulating excitatory neurons in the hippocampus, and combined with fMRI in rats has been used to demonstrate expansion of the brain-wide network engaged during kindling, even when the response at the site of kindling is unchanged (Choy et al., 2022).

Kindling alone is unlikely to explain the occurrence of hippocampal sclerosis in association with other pathology in humans, because kindling itself usually results in no or minimal hippocampal damage and sclerosis (Tuunanen and Pitkänen, 2000). Kindling could, however, explain the progression of mesial temporal epilepsy. Eventually spontaneous seizures in the kindling model do result in progressive neuronal loss within the hippocampus (Cavazos et al., 1994). Indeed, even following single seizures there is evidence of both apoptotic cell death and also neurogenesis in the dentate granule cell layer (Bengzon et al., 1997). This would suggest that recurrent seizures may cause further structural and functional changes in the hippocampus. Human evidence for this has mainly been indirect. Epilepsy duration correlates with hippocampal volume loss and progressive neuronal loss and dysfunction (Theodore et al., 1999). Overall, notwithstanding methodological problems, imaging studies seem to indicate that there is progressive hippocampal atrophy with time in patients with hippocampal sclerosis (Caciagli et al., 2017).

Seizures are usually self-terminating and brief. Occasionally seizures can persist unabated, or repeated seizures can occur without recovery; this situation is termed "status epilepticus." While status epilepticus may occur in individuals with preexisting epilepsy, more than half of patients who present with status epilepticus have no history of seizures (DeLorenzo et al., 1996). In these patients, the status epilepticus is often acutely precipitated by infection, cerebral vascular accident, hypoxia, or alcohol. The probability of then developing epilepsy (unprecipitated seizures) is 41% within 2 years compared with 13% of those with acute symptomatic seizures but no status epilepticus (Hesdorffer et al., 1998). This suggests a relationship between the prolonged seizures of status epilepticus and subsequent epileptogenesis, although a relationship between the length of seizure and the nature and severity of the precipitant cannot be discounted. In humans, status epilepticus has been shown to result in hippocampal damage and subsequent hippocampal sclerosis. The hippocampus thus has a dichotomous role as the substrate for epilepsy, and as the structure susceptible to damage by prolonged seizures. Animal models of generalized convulsive as well as limbic status epilepticus have supported these findings. Limbic status epilepticus has been induced by the systemic or local administration of kainic acid, systemic administration of pilocarpine (a muscarinic receptor agonist) or protocols using electrical stimulation of limbic areas (Reddy and Kuruba, 2013; Lévesque et al., 2016). Status epilepticus in these models results in hippocampal damage in adult animals that is similar to that observed in humans. Following these acute episodes of limbic status epilepticus many of the animals go on to develop spontaneous limbic seizures after a quiescent period lasting days to weeks.

18.4.2 Mechanisms of hippocampal sclerosis

Seizures and epilepsy can originate in the hippocampus with minimal associated damage as is observed in kindling and tetanus toxin models of mesial temporal epilepsy, and in some people with mesial temporal lobe epilepsy (King et al., 1996). However, most people with mesial temporal lobe epilepsy have associated hippocampal sclerosis. Insights into the mechanisms underlying the development of hippocampal sclerosis have largely been derived from animal models of status epilepticus (Collins, Lothman, et al., 1983; Meldrum, 1991). These have shown that, although a certain amount of neuronal damage is secondary to physiological compromise that occurs during status epilepticus such as hypoxia, hypoglycemia, and hypotension, a large proportion of the damage is independent of these factors. This neuronal damage is due to excitotoxicity in which the presence of epileptic activity mediates neuronal death through the activation of glutamate receptors. Excessive influx of calcium through primarily NMDA receptors, but also through AMPA receptors lacking the GluA2 subunit, results in a cascade of reactions leading to cell death (Lipton and Rosenberg, 1994; Weiss and Sensi, 2000; Tanaka et al., 2000; Rajasekaran et al., 2012). Downstream from activation of NMDA receptors and calcium entry, there are interrelated putative pathogenic mechanisms that underlie neuronal death, synaptic reorganization, and alterations in channels and receptors that lead to the development of epilepsy and other comorbidities. Importantly, other brain insults that lead to hippocampal sclerosis and epilepsy, such as traumatic brain injury, encephalitis and infection, have shared mechanisms resulting in an "epileptic" hippocampus but the sequence and relative role of distinct processes may differ (Klein et al., 2018).

Key common related processes include inflammation, the generation of reactive oxygen species, release of adenosine and activation of purinergic receptors, and leakage of the blood-brain barrier (Figure 18.2).

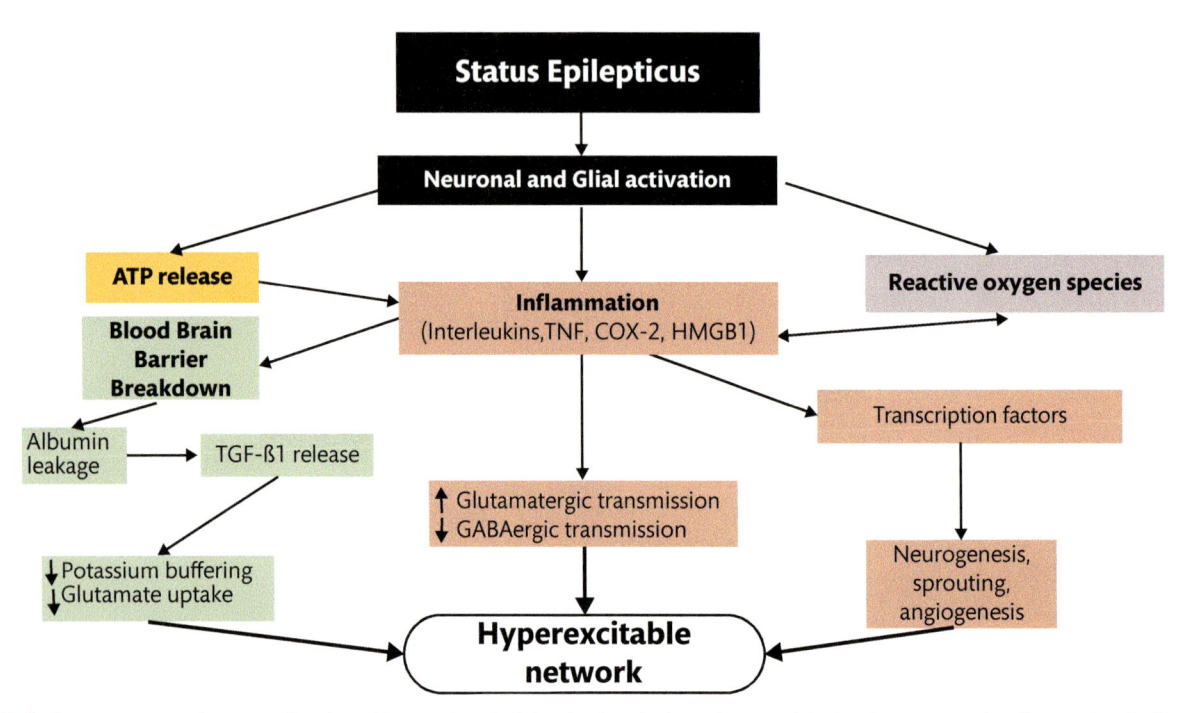

Figure 18.2 Consequences of status epilepticus. Neuronal and glial activation during seizure activity leads to a cascade of interrelated effects including inflammation, ATP release, generation of reactive oxygen species, and blood-brain barrier breakdown. These consequently lead to proexcitatory changes resulting in a hyperexcitable network.

Activation of microglia and neuroinflammatory processes (in particular those involving interleukin-1β, interleukin-6, cyclooxygenase-2, tumor necrosis factor-α, and high mobility group box protein-1) have been shown to occur during the epileptogenic process in the hippocampus and to increase excitation; consequently, anti-inflammatory therapies have disease-modifying effects following status epilepticus (Maroso et al., 2010; van Vliet et al., 2018). Excessive reactive oxygen species generation also occurs early in the epileptogenic process and enhancing endogenous antioxidants through activation of nuclear factor erythroid 2-related factor 2 (Nrf2) following status epilepticus reduces neuronal death, neuroinflammatory intermediaries, cognitive deficits, and seizure frequency (Shekh-Ahmad et al., 2018; Pauletti et al., 2019). Adenosine triphosphate release and later decreased expression of adenosine kinase results in the increased activation of purinergic receptors (in particular the P2X7 receptor), increasing inflammation and loss of adenosine regulation of excitatory transmission (Beamer et al., 2021). Decreased ATP can also have an epigenetic effect through altering DNA methylation, and this may also contribute to epileptogenesis (Williams-Karnesky et al., 2013). Lastly, disruption of the blood-brain barrier occurs in epilepsy (and epilepsy associated pathology), resulting in extravasation of serum albumin into the brain and activation of transforming growth factor beta (TGF-β), among other, proinflammatory pathways (Swissa et al., 2019). In support of this, inhibition of TGF-β with losartan has been shown to be an effective therapy against epileptogenesis (Bar-Klein et al., 2014).

Downstream of these processes are programmed necrosis through the activation of caspases (Niquet et al., 2005), changes in gene expression, and widespread modifications to protein expression, which may be secondary to changes in the expression of certain transcription factors such as NRSF (McClelland et al., 2011) and the proconvulsant gene regulator sestrin 3 (Johnson et al., 2015). Abnormalities of posttranscriptional mechanisms that regulate gene expression, including microRNA and messenger RNA polyadenylation, have also been implicated in epileptogenesis, and modifying these has been shown to have antiepileptogenic effects (Jimenez-Mateos et al., 2012; Parras et al., 2020).

However, it is important to recognize that transcriptional changes may also have an antiseizure effect (Hu et al., 2011). Indeed, a remarkable aspect of temporal lobe epilepsy is that seizures usually occur infrequently, suggesting that many of the changes observed in the "epileptic" hippocampus are compensatory rather than proepileptic.

18.5 The neurophysiology of interictal and ictal events in the hippocampus

It is important to distinguish seizures, interictal activity, and epilepsy. An epileptic seizure is a transient paroxysm of excessive discharges of neurons in the cerebral cortex causing a clinically discernible event. Brief synchronous activity of a group of neurons leads to the interictal spike, and as we will discuss, this shares some mechanisms with seizure generation; the interictal spike should, however, be recognized as a distinct phenomenon. Epilepsy, on the other hand, is the propensity to have seizures, and the concept of epileptogenesis comprises both the development of a neuronal network in which spontaneous seizures occur and also the extension of that network with time.

18.5.1 The interictal spike

Epileptiform interictal EEG abnormalities include spikes, which are fast electrographic transients lasting less than 70 ms, and sharp waves, which last 70–200 ms (Kane et al., 2017). That these are pathological is supported by their very rare occurrence (< 1%) in healthy adults (Gregory et al., 1993), and their strong association with epilepsy (Marsan and Zivin, 1970). Spikes and sharp waves are followed by a slow wave lasting hundreds of milliseconds. As discussed below, this slow wave probably represents a period of relative refractoriness. It was first established through concomitant field-potential and intracellular recordings from in vivo brain tissue, that the intracellular correlate of the interictal spike is the paroxysmal depolarizing shift (PDS) (Matsumoto and Marsan, 1964), a slow depolarizing potential, "up to 30 mV or occasionally more" with "durations from 40 up to 400 ms or more," with a high-frequency (> 200 Hz) burst of action potentials. PDS (and consequently interictal spikes) can occur in clusters (Zhou et al., 2007).

PDSs are proposed to be due to alterations in intrinsic neuronal properties along with aberrant synaptic activity. Experimentally, PDS-like events can be evoked by manipulating neurotransmission (increasing potassium, reducing magnesium) (Zuckermann and Glaser, 1968; Anderson et al., 1986), and inhibiting GABA$_A$ receptors (Straub et al., 1990). In addition, calcium homeostasis, in particular potentiated L-type calcium channel-mediated Ca^{2+} influx (Stiglbauer et al., 2017), and NMDA-receptor activation (Jones, 1988) appear to have a key role in the generation of PDS. Indeed, one hypothesized pathway for PDS generation starts with a network-driven giant excitatory postsynaptic potential (EPSP) triggered by AMPA receptor-mediated fast neurotransmission (early phase) and subsequently a depolarizing plateau, mediated by NMDA receptor channel currents and currents through L-type calcium channels (Hotka and Kubista, 2019).

Thus, the generation of interictal spikes is dependent on two phenomena: the intrinsic burst properties of neurons, and the synchronization of neuronal populations. Within the hippocampus, pyramidal cells in area CA3 and some in area CA1 demonstrate burst properties. The bursting in CA3 pyramidal cells appears to be dependent on regenerative dendritic potentials secondary to activation of calcium and sodium channels (Traub et al., 1994), and regulated by dendritic potassium (Kv2) and hyperpolarization-activated cyclic nucleotide-gated (HCN) channels (Raus Balind et al., 2019). The effect of a burst of action potentials is to increase synaptic reliability; within the excitatory network of the CA3 pyramidal cells, burst-firing in a single CA3 pyramidal cell can generate a synchronized burst throughout the whole network (Miles and Wong, 1983). Because of the propensity for the CA3 pyramidal cells to generate this synchronized burst, this region has often been considered as the "pacemaker" for seizure activity. Synchronized bursts can, however, also occur within the CA1 in epilepsy during epileptogenesis. This is likely due to an increase in the proportion of burst-firing CA1 pyramidal cells during epileptogenesis due to upregulation of a T-type calcium channel, Cav3.2 (Becker et al., 2008). Synchronization can also occur through a combination of nonsynaptic mechanisms including gap junctions, ephaptic transmission, and changes in the extracellular milieu. The importance of these nonsynaptic mechanisms in neuronal synchronization has been emphasized by the "zero" calcium model of ictal discharges, in which reducing extracellular calcium in a hippocampal slice preparation below that necessary for synaptic transmission results in synchronized epileptiform discharges due to increased axonal excitability and ephaptic transmission (Jefferys, 1995). Furthermore, decreasing the extracellular space (indirectly increasing ephaptic transmission) can promote bursting (Roper et al., 1992). Even when the conditions for an interictal spike are present, it is still unclear what initiates the spike. Observations indicate that the spike may be preceded by a burst of activity in local parvalbumin interneurons and then initiated by a collapse of this inhibition (Karlócai et al., 2014). During the spike itself, there is then the widespread recruitment of GABAergic interneurons, which reduce pyramidal cell firing and so potentially have an antiseizure effect (Muldoon et al., 2015). The interictal spike is terminated by GABAergic inhibition, and calcium-dependent potassium currents (Alger and Nicoll, 1980; Domann et al., 1994).

Spikes are, thus, intrinsically different from a seizure, and spikes that precede a seizure may differ from other interictal spikes as they are larger, driven more by focal glutamatergic transmission (Huberfeld et al., 2011). Depth EEG recordings in humans suggest that the interictal spike can originate from a much wider field than the ictal zone. Thus, it is not uncommon to find spikes originating in both hippocampi, often independently, even when seizure activity is confined to one hippocampus. These observations indicate that a seizure is not the evolution of spike discharges but is a distinct phenomenon. Critical experiments in entorhinal cortex-hippocampal slice preparations, in which there is partial preservation of the trisynaptic loop, have confirmed the antiepileptic potential of spikes. Spike discharges generated in CA3 inhibited epileptic activity in the entorhinal cortex, so that sectioning of the Schaffer collaterals led to potentiation of entorhinal cortex seizure activity (Barbarosie and Avoli, 1997).

18.5.2 High-frequency oscillations (HFOs)

Interest in HFOs has grown with studies demonstrating that they are a marker of epileptogenic tissue. It has been debated whether they are more specific than spikes or may give more information when used in combination with interictal spikes (Roehri et al., 2018). In humans, HFOs have been related to both physiological and pathological functions. Physiological HFOs, or "ripples," are thought to represent the summation of activity from interneuronal cell subpopulations regulating principal cell activity (Buzsáki et al., 1992). The role of ripples, particularly when coupled with sharp waves, within the hippocampus is thought to be primarily for transfer of information to associated neocortical structures, especially during memory consolidation (see Chapter 14). Pathological HFOs in epilepsy may represent abnormally synchronous firing from cohorts of pyramidal cells, resulting in population spiking (Engel et al., 2009). Recently, this has been confirmed in recordings from individual neurons in humans with the use of hybrid macro/microelectrodes, with HFOs coupled with interictal spikes, being associated with increased neuronal firing (Guth et al., 2021). These observations suggest why HFOs coupled with interictal spikes may be a better marker of epileptogenic tissue than either event alone, as the HFO-interictal spike discharge combination probably distinguishes the area where the interictal spike is generated from propagation of the interictal spike. This is because EEG largely represents the summation of excitatory postsynaptic potentials in an area rather than neuronal firing in that area, and so the HFO-interictal spike combination indicates both a large glutamatergic input/output and excessive neuronal firing.

18.5.3 Ictal events

Seizures have conventionally been considered to be secondary to the excessive and synchronous firing of neurons brought about by a shift in the excitatory-inhibitory balance toward excitation, and so manipulations, which either increase excitation (using glutamate agonists) or decrease inhibition (using GABA(A) receptor antagonists or potassium channel inhibitors), will induce seizures. Since these manipulations determine the brain area and time of initiation, they have been used in most of the studies of seizure generation (ictogenesis). However, although they have given useful insights, it is unclear how the mechanisms of these acutely precipitated seizures relate to the human condition in which seizures occur spontaneously. The study of spontaneous seizures is complicated by a number of factors including: (1) temporal lobe seizures occur spontaneously and randomly and often infrequently; (2) seizure initiation needs to be differentiated from seizure propagation, which can be difficult to differentiate using EEG, which generally represents the input to an area rather than neuronal firing (Schevon et al., 2012; Smith et al., 2016); (3) there can be different patterns of initiation in the same person, suggesting possibly different mechanisms; (4) seizures can initiate from different areas of the hippocampus in the same person; and (5) in most studies in humans and rodents only a limited area of cortex can be investigated at the cellular level.

Although studies have reported on the patterns of neuronal firing in the brain at the initiation of the seizures, many of these studies are probably reporting on propagated activity, and in vitro and in vivo studies in rodents and humans have indicated that the mechanisms underlying propagation and initiation differ (Schevon et al., 2012). Propagation seems to be determined by a substantial synaptic input into an area from the ictal wavefront (the area of excessive and synchronous neuronal firing). Interneuronal activity prevents seizure penetration into the area but, at some point, this inhibitory restraint breaks down, enabling recruitment of the area into the ictal wavefront. There have been a number of putative mechanisms suggested to underlie this failure of GABAergic inhibition including: (1) failure of synaptic transmission, for example, through the inhibition of postsynaptic GABA(A) receptors by excessive zinc release (Buhl et al., 1996); (2) potassium accumulation during excessive neuronal firing resulting in depolarizing block of interneurons while increasing pyramidal cell excitability (Călin et al., 2021); and (3) sustained GABAergic interneuron activity "chloride loading" neurons leading to a depolarizing reversal potential for GABA(A) receptors, i.e., when GABA(A) receptors open, chloride flows out of neurons, leading to depolarizing (excitable) GABAergic currents (Magloire et al., 2019).

Although experimental work is beginning to unravel the mechanisms underlying seizure propagation, the mechanisms of seizure initiation remain uncertain. Clinical evidence favors varying sites of seizure onset, but are the same groups of neurons within those sites involved in seizure initiation? The "hub" theory of seizure onset and propagation favors a paradigm in which there are a small number of hyperconnected "hub" neurons that can drive network activity; this hypothesis is supported by analysis of neuronal firing dynamics following chemoconvulsant-induced seizures (Hadjiabadi et al., 2021). The relevance of this for spontaneous seizures has been challenged in an in vitro model of spontaneous seizure activity, in which seizure initiation involved different

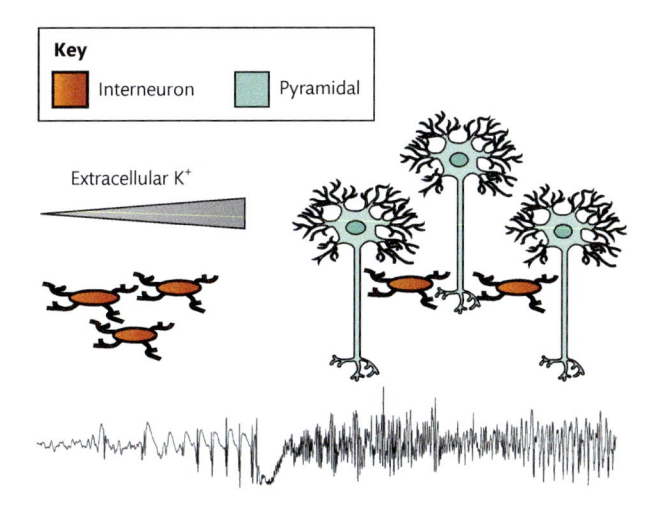

Figure 18.3 The initiation of a seizure. At the start of a seizure, it has been speculated that excessive interneuronal activity occurs during which there is an accumulation of extracellular potassium (through the potassium/chloride pump and potassium shifts from excessive neuronal firing). This leads to increased excitability of pyramidal cells, which are then recruited into the seizure.

populations of neurons from seizure to seizure (Lau et al., 2022). How these contradictory studies translate to human epilepsy is unresolved. Interestingly, it was observed in the second of these studies that interneuronal activity seemed to be driving seizure initiation, similar to studies of interictal activity. This observation is also supported by evidence from chemoconvulsant models, which indicate that ictogenesis begins with excessive activation of interneurons, accumulation of extracellular potassium, and then recruitment of pyramidal cells (Figure 18.3) (Sessolo et al., 2015; Librizzi et al., 2017).

Multiple mechanisms, including depolarizing block, vesicular depletion, energy failure, release of GABA, adenosine and neuropeptides, internal neuronal acidification, and inhibition from subcortical structures, have been proposed to terminate seizures (Lado and Moshé, 2008). It is likely that seizure termination may vary not only from person to person but also from seizure to seizure.

Although seizures can occur in any person under appropriate circumstances, there are changes to the neurons and networks that reduce the threshold for seizure activity in people with mesial temporal lobe epilepsy, resulting in spontaneous seizures. To understand how a network becomes "epileptic," it is paramount to consider the changes that occur within the hippocampus during epileptogenesis. One problem with much that has been described is that it is associational (i.e., changes are observed and are assumed to contribute to the epileptogenic process). However, many of the changes are likely compensatory (i.e., changes that protect against the epileptogenic process). In support of this, is the observation that even in someone in whom the seizures are frequent (e.g., daily), over 99.9% of the time the brain is not seizing, i.e., the network is stable for the majority of the time. Unfortunately, it has been difficult to distinguish between compensatory and proseizure changes, and we are far from a comprehensive model of epileptogenesis. Moreover, epileptogenesis results in other comorbidities such as depression and cognitive deficits, and it is unlikely that identical changes underlie each of these elements.

18.6 Pathological change in hippocampal sclerosis

As previously detailed, a host of different pathological insults along with a genetic predisposition probably contribute to the development of hippocampal sclerosis, and hippocampal sclerosis leads to epilepsy, which is often refractory to drug treatment. Notwithstanding the observation that cortical areas outside the hippocampus, including the amygdala, subiculum, insular, perirhinal cortex, entorhinal cortex, and piriform cortex, and subcortical areas, including the thalamus, probably participate in the network that underlies temporal lobe epilepsy with hippocampal sclerosis, we will focus here on the changes that occur in the hippocampus and how they may contribute to the epileptogenic process (Figure 18.4). The changes that occur can be divided into structural change, changes in neurotransmission, and changes in neuronal properties.

18.6.1 Structural change

18.6.1.1 Neuronal loss

Hippocampal sclerosis in human temporal lobe epilepsy is typically a unilateral process, affecting either hemisphere equally, and can vary in extent along the long axis of the hippocampus to involve the entire head to tail or cause more focal atrophy in the hippocampal body (Van Paesschen et al., 1997). However, it can sometimes also lead to bilateral sclerosis. The ILAE system for classification of hippocampal sclerosis subtypes is discussed above, based on qualitative evaluation of the patterns of subfield neuronal loss and gliosis.

Typical histological features of hippocampal sclerosis include the relative preservation of neurons in CA2 subfield, an abrupt transition of the sclerotic CA1 with the preserved adjacent subiculum, granule cell dispersion, and synaptic reorganization, particularly in the dentate gyrus (Figure 18.4D,E). In some cases, extensive neuronal loss is seen in all hippocampal subfields (old term "total hippocampal sclerosis") (Figure 18.4H).

A dense, chronic fibrillary gliosis accompanies the neuronal loss, particularly in CA1 region (Figure 18.4J). A more cellular gliosis in CA4 and radial gliosis in the dentate gyrus can be observed. Enlarged hilar neurons with enhanced neurofilament labeling and mTOR pathway activation can be prominent in some cases. It has been questioned whether such cytopathology in mesial temporal epilepsy represents true dysplasia in addition to sclerosis or secondary cytopathic phenomena. Furthermore, mesial infiltration by a low grade glioneuronal tumor needs to be excluded in the presence of aberrant hippocampal cytomorphology. Deposits of corpora amylacea may be pronounced in some cases of hippocampal sclerosis in the collapsed stratum pyramidale and proliferation of the microvasculature as well as atrophic vessels with increased pericytes have been reported (Thom, 2014).

Neuronal loss and gliosis may also be present in adjacent limbic structures, including the amygdala (Yilmazer-Hanke et al., 2000) and parahippocampal gyrus, which, along with hippocampal sclerosis, are collectively referred to as mesial temporal sclerosis (Figure 18.4S,T). Enlargement of the amygdala has also been increasingly recognized as a quantitative or qualitative MRI finding. A recent systematic review of 361 cases emphasized the heterogeneity of associated amygdala pathology, which included reports of astrogliosis, oligodendrogliosis, dysplasia (neuronal

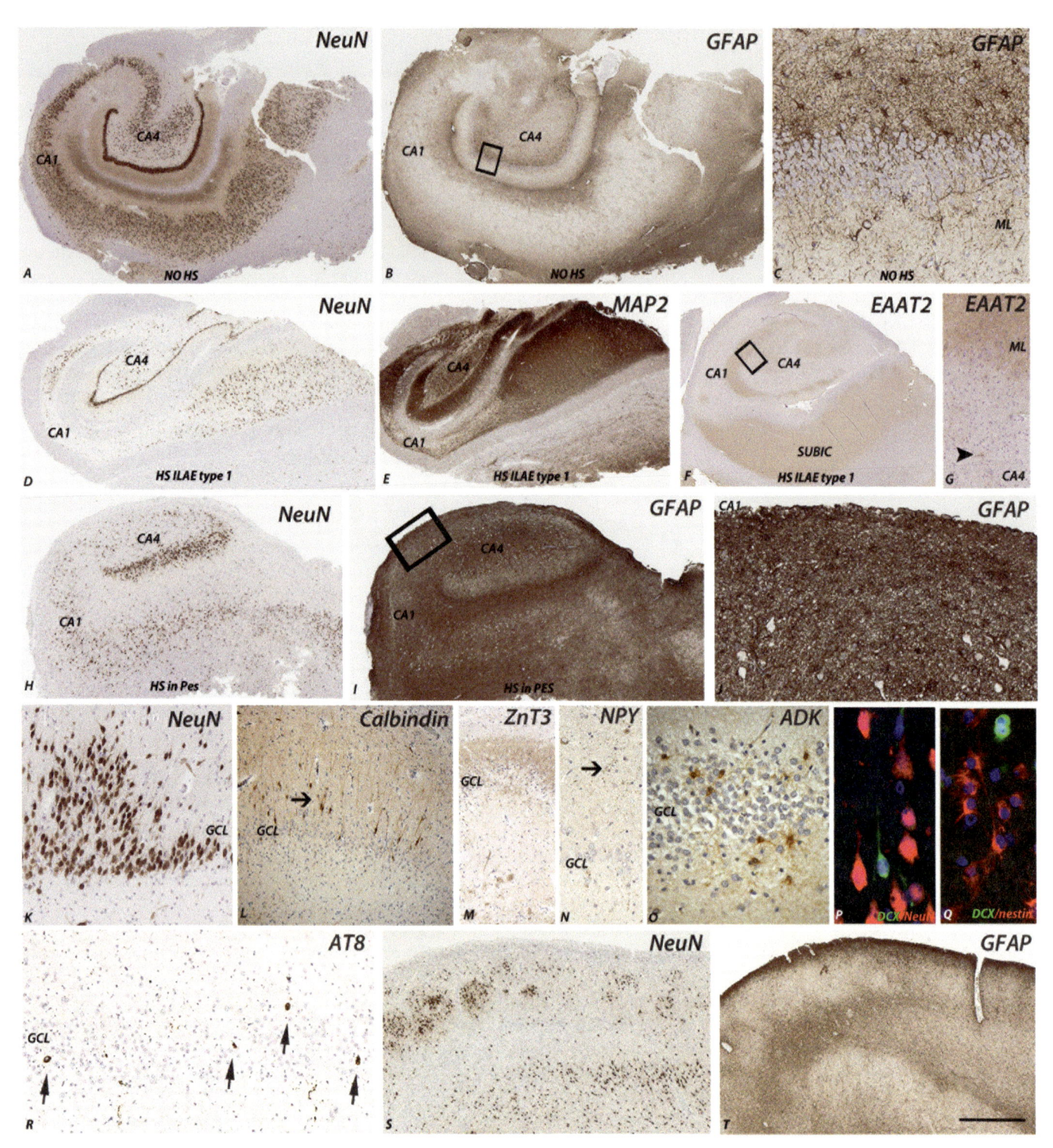

Figure 18.4 Histology of hippocampal sclerosis. (A) NeuN immunohistochemistry in a coronal hippocampal section from a patient with temporal lobe epilepsy where no evidence of hippocampal neuronal loss was observed; small heterotopia were noted in the white matter. (B) The same case stained with GFAP confirming a lack of significant gliosis through the stratum pyramidale; gliosis in the subgranular zone/polymorphic cell layer is a common finding in epilepsy patients but, without clear evidence of neuronal cell loss, does not amount to hippocampal sclerosis in the current ILAE 2013 classification system. This region shown in the box is highlighted in (C) at higher magnification where the compact granule cell layer is also apparent. (D) Temporal lobe epilepsy surgical resection in a patient with ILAE type 1 HS showing neuronal loss in CA1 and CA4 regions and relative preservation of neurones in CA2 and the subiculum. (E) The same case show with MAP2 labeling (neurones and dendrites) confirming greater neuronal loss in CA1 than CA4 but with preserved granule cell layer and subiculum. (F) A further HS type 1 cased labeled for astrocyte glutamate transporter EAAT2, which shows a pattern of loss of expression in astrocytes in the damaged and gliotic region of the hippocampus (CA1 and CA4); the region in the box is shown in higher magnification in (G) and scant positive astrocytes in CA4 arrowed. (H) The anterior part of the hippocampus, the pes hippocampus, can also show sclerosis and often a more diffuse pattern of neuronal loss from CA4 to CA1 is noted with more diffuse gliosis (I) and granule cell dispersion and mossy fiber sprouting is often significant. The region of CA1 outlined on the GFAP section is shown at higher magnification in (J) showing dense fibrillary gliosis. (K) Dispersion of the granule cell layer can be a frequent and dramatic finding in all types of HS

enlargement), low grade tumors, and autoimmune-related encephalitis (Chakravarty et al., 2021).

The parahippocampal gyrus, the more anterior entorhinal cortex, perirhinal, piriform, periamygdala cortex (allocortical regions), and parasubiculum have reciprocal connections with the hippocampus and may act as circuit "hubs" in mesial temporal lobe epilepsy, and inclusion of these regions in surgical resections can influence outcome (Galovic et al., 2019). However, there are limited correlative pathology studies of all these regions in surgical cases. Neocortical neuronal loss in the temporal lobe can be observed. "Temporal lobe sclerosis" has been used to describe a distinctive pattern of neuronal loss and gliosis in the superficial cortical layers of the lateral temporal lobe seen in 10% of cases (Meyer et al., 1954; Thom, Eriksson, et al., 2009); although likely an early acquired process, it is often accompanied by cytoarchitectural abnormalities and therefore has also been classified as part of the spectrum of abnormalities in focal cortical dysplasia type 3a. There is no clear evidence that the presence of temporal lobe (neocortical) sclerosis is predictive of a poorer postsurgical outcome following resection of mesial temporal lobe structures, raising the question of the role it plays in epileptogenesis.

18.6.1.2 Specific neuronal vulnerability in hippocampal sclerosis

Loss of the principal pyramidal cells in hippocampal sclerosis is established, but it is difficult conceptually to conceive how removal of principal excitatory neurons can contribute to a state of hyperexcitability. Undoubtedly neuronal loss may contribute to synaptic rearrangements and perhaps increased connectivity, but more important perhaps is the vulnerability of specific subsets of inhibitory interneurons within the hippocampal formation, which may influence the intrinsic circuitry of the hippocampus and seizure propagation. Most interneurons contain the neurotransmitter GABA, but can be further subdivided according to their location, connectivity, morphology, calcium-binding protein content, and neurotransmitter receptor status, which closely correlates with their functional status (Freund and Buzsáki, 1996). For example, parvalbumin and cholecystokinin (CCK) interneurons influence perisomatic or axon initial segment inhibition of principal neurons, whereas somatostatin, neuropeptide Y, and calretinin neurons influence dendritic inhibition. Although the diagnosis of hippocampal sclerosis is based on patterns of pyramidal cell loss, alterations to interneuronal cell types also occur and can show stereotypical patterns (Thom et al., 2012). Regional loss of interneuronal

groups can also be accompanied by hypertrophy and sprouting in residual neurons as a compensatory change, which can also manifest in abnormal synchronization of neuronal groups (Wittner et al., 2005; Maglóczky, 2010).

Neuropeptide Y (NPY)- and somatostatin-containing inhibitory interneurons are normally numerous in the hilus and form a dense plexus of fibers in the outer molecular layer of the dentate gyrus, which colocalizes with the GABA synthesizing enzyme glutamic acid decarboxylase (GAD) (Amaral and Campbell, 1986). Loss of these interneuronal subtypes in the hilus was noted in hippocampal sclerosis (de Lanerolle et al., 1989). Following status epilepticus, those animals that develop spontaneous seizures have greater hilar interneuronal loss, perhaps resulting in decreased inhibitory drive (van Vliet et al., 2004). NPY-containing axons also appeared to be reorganized in the dentate molecular layer in hippocampal sclerosis and ectopic expression of NPY in granule cells has been observed following seizures (Vezzani et al., 1999). This is likely to represent plasticity in NPY inhibitory mechanisms in the epileptogenic hippocampus.

The calcium-binding proteins—calbindin D-28-K, parvalbumin, and calretinin—label different and nonoverlapping subsets of inhibitory hippocampal interneurons, and the resistance or susceptibility of these cell populations in hippocampal sclerosis may directly affect hippocampal epileptogenesis. The normal distribution of calbindin is not restricted to interneurons but is also present in the dentate gyrus granule cells and mossy fibers, and CA2 pyramidal cells, whereas parvalbumin and calretinin are present only in interneurons. Common alterations of calbindin-expressing neurons in hippocampal sclerosis include hypertrophy and increased dendritic lengths and spine number of CA1 and CA4 neurons with reduced expression in dentate granule cells (Figure 18.4L) (Wittner et al., 2005; Maglóczky, 2010; Thom et al., 2012; You et al., 2017). Somatostatin-expressing interneurons in CA1 divide into groups that are calbindin positive or negative. The oriens-lacunosum-moleculare interneurons (calbindin-negative somatostatin interneurons) are lost during epileptogenesis with loss of distal dendritic inhibition; there is, however, preservation and increased connectivity of basket cells (Figure 18.6A) (Cossart et al., 2001). Basket cells make multiple perisomatic and somatic synapses and have extensive axonal arborizations leading to connection of one basket cell with many pyramidal cells. By synchronously modulating the excitability of a group of pyramidal neurons, one basket cell can synchronize pyramidal cell activity (Cobb et al., 1995). A shift of inhibition from dendrites to soma

---

Figure 18.4 Continued

and the breadth of the granule cell layer can in regions measure over 300 microns, as in this case. (L) Calbindin is normally expressed in granule cell neurones and the mossy fiber pathway in addition to interneurons; in many HS cases calbindin expression in granule cells is lost but in some cases residual expression is maintained in the dispersed granule cells but not the basal cells. (M) Mossy fiber axonal sprouting into the molecular layer can be demonstrated with Zinc transporter 3 protein (ZnT3) immunohistochemistry together with loss of the normal mossy fiber pathway in HS. (N) Neuropeptide Y in HS also demonstrates aberrant axonal sprouting into the molecular layer. (O) Adenosine kinase (ADK) expression in astrocytes in HS in the granule cell layer in an HS type 1 case. (P) Immature neurones expressing doublecortin and (Q) proliferative astrocytes expressing nestin have been reported in HS cases in various mesial temporal regions, as shown here from the temporal pole and amygdala respectively. (R) Increased phosphorylated tau can be seen in some patients with HS type 1, particularly over 50 years, and with patterns different from that in AD and normal aging, with early accumulation in granule cells neurones (arrows) and mossy fiber axons. (S) Neuronal loss in HS patients can extend to regions beyond the hippocampus, as shown here in the parahippocampal gyrus with neuronal loss in midlayers and corresponding gliosis on GFAP shown in (T). (Thanks to Joan Liu, Alicja Mrzyglod, and Smriti Patodia, who carried out the immunostaining.) Bar in (T) is equivalent to approximately 2 mm in A, B, D, E, F, H, and I; 250 microns in C, G, J, K, O, and R; 500 microns in L, M, and N; 100 microns in P and Q; 2.5 mm in S and T.

could thus have a synchronizing role (Cossart et al., 2001). The importance of GABAegic interneuronal loss/deficits in the hippocampus for the generation of seizures has further been emphasized by observations that inhibitory neuron transplantation into the hippocampus of adult epileptic mice has an antiseizure effect (Hunt et al., 2013).

Selective loss of hilar mossy cells, an excitatory interneuron with distinctive dendritic arborizations, has been described in hippocampal sclerosis cases compared with patients with generalized seizures (Blümcke, Suter, et al., 2000). Mossy cells are so called because of their characteristic proximal thorny spine excrescences akin to moss growing on a tree; they are glutamatergic neurons, projecting to the dentate gyrus, both granule cells and inhibitory neurons, orchestrating both network excitation and inhibition in the hilus. The loss of inhibition in the dentate gyrus on stimulation of the ipsilateral perforant path, despite the relative preservation of basket cells and their recruitment by the contralateral perforant path, led to the "dormant basket cell" hypothesis, in which the disinhibition was ascribed to failure of mossy cells to recruit inhibitory interneurons (Sloviter, 1991). Recent experiments support this concept and demonstrate direct roles of mossy cell dysfunction in convulsive seizures as well as spatial memory (Bui et al., 2018). They appear highly vulnerable in mesial temporal lobe epilepsy models (Sloviter et al., 2003; Hester and Danzer, 2013), and loss of these cells has also been proposed as a trigger for mossy fiber sprouting (Hester and Danzer, 2013).

Although neuronal damage/loss can play a crucial role in epileptogenesis and redressing neuronal loss is sufficient to treat epilepsy, the observation from animal models (kindling and tetanus toxin) and human tissue indicate that neuronal loss is not necessary for the development of epilepsy.

18.6.1.3 Granule cell dispersion and neurogenesis

In mesial temporal lobe epilepsy, there can be disorganization or dispersion of granule cells into the molecular layer of the dentate gyrus in hippocampal sclerosis marked by dispersed granule cells appearing separated from the normally compact cell layer, which gives an impression of an undulated irregular border with the molecular layer (Figure 18.4H,K) (Houser, 1990). In some cases, the deep (hilar border) of the granule cell layer is also ill-defined. The dispersed cells often appear elongated or fusiform in shape, reminiscent of migrating neurons. Less often a bilaminar arrangement of granule cells is observed. The incidence of granule cell dispersion in hippocampal sclerosis surgical series is of the order of 50%, and it can be observed with all subtypes of sclerosis (Houser, 1990). There is no clear evidence that dispersion in hippocampal sclerosis correlates with a better outcome postsurgery, but it has been linked with early onset of epilepsy and febrile seizures and correlates with a longer duration of epilepsy (Duarte et al., 2018).

It was initially considered that granule cell dispersion may represent a neuronal migration disorder or an underlying hippocampal malformation, as there are occasional reports of granule cell dispersion in association with cortical malformations in the absence of a history of seizures and with bilateral hippocampal involvement (Harding and Thom, 2001). However, there is now overwhelming evidence indicating that it is an acquired process. The ontogenesis of the human dentate gyrus has a prolonged postnatal developmental period and has also been recognized as a location for ongoing nonperiventricular adult neurogenesis in mammals, likely

of relevance to this observed reorganization. Dramatic dispersion occurs in some temporal lobe epilepsy models, for example, in the kainic acid model of status epilepticus but not the pilocarpine model (Moura et al., 2021); dispersion first appears at about 4 days following seizures, increasing over 8 weeks and persisting for at least 6 months (Suzuki et al., 2005). There has been extensive discussion regarding whether the dispersion is related to migration of newly generated neurons and astrocytes, enhanced by seizures (Figure 18.4P,Q). There is experimental evidence that acute seizures can increase neurogenesis in animal models and new neurons migrate to abnormal or ectopic positions, integrate into existing networks and acquire proepileptogenic physiology (Parent et al., 1997; Shapiro and Ribak, 2005; Pierce et al., 2005; Cameron et al., 2011; Hester and Danzer, 2013). Neurogenesis, itself, can enhance epileptogenesis, and chemogenetic silencing of newly born dentate granule cells can suppress seizures (Zhou et al., 2019). However, there is conflicting data regarding the significance and contribution of ongoing neurogenesis in the adult human dentate (Abbott and Nigussie, 2020). In real-time studies, migration was also shown to involve mature neurons by a process termed "somatic translocation." In surgical samples of hippocampal sclerosis, an age-dependent decline in cell cycle marker MCM2 and doublecortin (DCX) expression was observed in the granule cell layer, which was independent of the extent of dispersion, arguing against a significant contribution of neurogenesis to granule cell dispersion (Fahrner et al., 2007). Moreover, proteomic analysis of granule cells in human hippocampal sclerosis failed to identify progenitor cell markers such as SOX2, DCX, PAX6, TBR1, TBR2; however, Ras homologous (Rho) family of GTPases were upregulated in dispersed cells; these have known roles in regulating polarized cell migration, likely suggesting that it is not neurogenesis that leads to granule cell dispersion but rather abnormal cellular migration (Liu et al., 2020).

Attention has also been given to reelin protein as the cause of granule cell dispersion. This extracellular matrix protein, secreted by Cajal-Retzius cells and GABAergic neurons acts as a stop signal for migrating neurons, and decreased reelin protein and reelin-expressing cells have been shown in hippocampal sclerosis (Frotscher et al., 2003) as well as methylation of the reelin promoter gene (Kobow et al., 2009).

Excitatory neurotransmitter receptor activation has also been implicated in dispersion. In animal models, dispersion was prevented by application of glutamate receptor antagonists and $GABA_A$ receptor agonists (Hester and Danzer, 2013), and more recently a combination of NMDA and AMPA glutamate receptor antagonists significantly retarded epileptogenesis and also reduced dispersion (Schidlitzki et al., 2017). Together, these studies suggest that dentate granule cell reorganization and neurogenesis play a role in epileptogenesis but that they are likely separate processes.

18.6.1.4 Mossy fiber sprouting

In 1974, using Golgi techniques, Scheibel and colleagues identified aberrant axons from granule cell neurons ascending into the molecular layer of the dentate gyrus in hippocampal specimens from patients with epilepsy (Figures 18.1D and 18.4M,N) (Scheibel et al., 1974). Axonal sprouting is a common feature of the developing brain and also occurs in response to seizures, resulting in remodeling of neuronal networks (Maglóczky, 2010). This capacity for plasticity, revived in adult tissue, is presumably a reparative response but may ultimately prove proepileptogenic. It has been

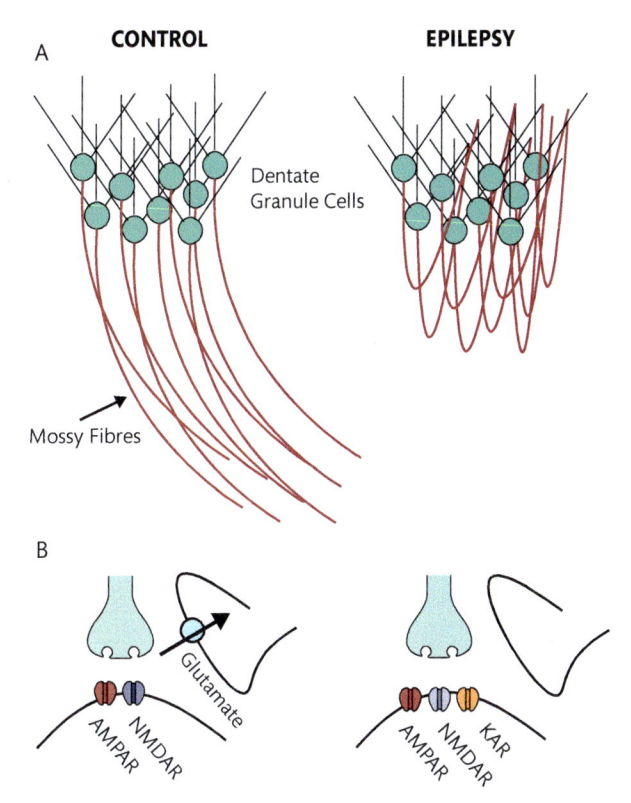

Figure 18.5 Changes in glutamatergic transmission in epilepsy. (A) Mossy fibers (the axons of dentate granule cells) normally project into the hilus, but in hippocampal sclerosis there is sprouting of mossy fibers into the molecular layer of the hippocampus, where they synapse with interneurons but also the dendrites of dentate granule cells, forming recurrent excitatory circuits. (B) There are synaptic changes including increased release probability and also changes in postsynaptic ionotropic receptors with changes in AMPA and NMDA receptors and the appearance of new kainate receptors. Glutamate uptake by perisynaptic glia is also decreased.

considered that reorganization of the excitatory glutamatergic mossy fiber pathway is a key event in the development of chronic seizures (Sutula et al., 1989). Mossy fiber sprouting in human hippocampal sclerosis specimens results in aberrant innervations of other granule cells (Figure 18.5A) (Babb et al., 1991), that also extends to CA2 (Freiman et al., 2021). In addition, aberrant mossy fibers in animal models also innervate interneurons, suggesting that new inhibitory circuits are established (Kotti et al., 1997).

Mossy fiber sprouting in the supragranular layer of the dentate gyrus can be demonstrated using the Timms histochemical method, which highlights the zinc-rich mossy fiber synaptic terminals (Babb et al., 1991), or with dynorphin or Zinc transporter 3 immunohistochemistry (Figure 18.1D, Figure 18.4M,N) (Houser et al., 1990).

Mossy fiber sprouting (MFS) has been such a striking histopathological feature of mesial temporal lobe epilepsy, but three critical questions arise: (1) why does it occur, (2) what functional roles does it play, and (3) is it necessary for epileptogenesis? It has been proposed that loss of specific neurons, in particular hilar mossy cells (the cellular targets for mossy fiber axons), stimulates this recurrent innervation. However, mossy fiber sprouting can occur after brief seizures and in the absence of neuronal loss (Koyama and Ikegaya, 2018). Seizure-induced neurogenesis was argued to underlie the sprouting (Cameron et al., 2011). However, ablating

neurogenesis did not affect the extent of sprouting (Hester et al., 2016) and both newly generated and adult granule cells can give rise to sprouting, albeit diminished in mature neurons (Hendricks et al., 2017). Mossy fiber axon branching and reverse projections are guided by a whole host of signaling molecules including BDNF, netrin-1, semaphorin3a, extracellular matrix proteins (such as tenascin-C, laminin, fibronectin, phosphacan, and neurocan), N-cadherin and GAP-43 expression (Proper et al., 2000; Holtmaat et al., 2003; Heck et al., 2004; Koyama et al., 2004; Lin et al., 2011). In addition, mTOR complex activation, perhaps as a "master controller," has also been implicated; this has regulatory roles in axonal growth, dendritic arborization, and synaptic plasticity. Moreover, mTOR pathway antagonists have been shown to rescue mossy fiber sprouting (Buckmaster et al., 2009). There has been long-standing controversy regarding the significance of mossy fiber sprouting in hippocampal epileptogenesis and the question of whether mossy fiber sprouting is "epileptogenic" or simply "restorative" still remains controversial (Cavarsan et al., 2018). The dentate granule cells of the hippocampus probably act as a brake against seizure propagation through limbic circuitry (Collins, Tearse, et al., 1983). This is mediated by the relative inexcitability of dentate granule cells through strong tonic GABAergic inhibition and relatively hyperpolarized membrane potentials (Nusser and Mody, 2002). Dentate granule cells do not show the burst properties characteristic of hippocampal pyramidal cells in response to a reduction of GABAergic inhibition, perhaps due to low calcium conductances (Fricke and Prince, 1984). Furthermore, dentate granule cell synchronization is difficult to achieve due to the low rate of connectivity between the granule cells. Thus, recurrent innervation by mossy fibers could contribute to hyperexcitability and disrupt this "brake." Even though sprouted mossy fiber synapses depress on repetitive activation (in contrast to dentate granule cell to CA3 synapses), selective optogenetic activation of sprouted fibers triggers reverberating network activity (in part due to decreased adenosine inhibition) (Hendricks et al., 2017). However, inhibition of mossy fiber sprouting does not necessarily prevent epileptogenesis (Buckmaster et al., 2009), the emergence of axonal sprouting is not always associated with seizure development (Nissinen et al., 2001), and spouted fibers also synapse with inhibitory interneurons and play a role in recruiting inhibitory networks (Frotscher et al., 2006). In operated patients with mesial temporal lobe epilepsy, mossy fiber sprouting is not always present and does not correlate with seizure-free outcomes, and, in postmortem epilepsy studies, mossy fiber sprouting has been demonstrated bilaterally in patients with long-term cessation of seizure activity, suggesting it may be an epiphenomenon (Thom, Martinian, et al., 2009). These results, similar to other changes observed with hippocampal sclerosis, indicate that mossy fiber sprouting can contribute to hippocampal hyperexcitability but is neither necessary for nor correlates well with epileptogenesis.

Importantly, there are other aberrant excitatory connections during epileptogenesis including sprouting of CA1 pyramidal cell axons, resulting in an increase in interconnectivity that results in increased excitability of the CA1 subfield (Esclapez et al., 1999). In addition, the temporoammonic pathway, a direct input from the cortex into the hippocampus, is highly enhanced, resulting in massive propagation of excitatory transmission into the hippocampus (Ang et al., 2006). Sprouting of excitatory axons, leading to increased interconnectivity, may be a powerful means of generating hyperexcitable circuits that can maintain and propagate epileptic activity.

18.6.1.5 Astroglia and extracellular matrix

Hippocampal sclerosis is associated with a reactive gliosis in which there are not only a proliferation of astrocytes but also changes in astrocytic morphology and gene expression (Figure 18.4I,J,Q) (Sofroniew and Vinters, 2010). This reactive gliosis reduces the extracellular space and promotes ephaptic transmission. With reactive gliosis, aquaporin expression shifts from astrocyte end feet (i.e., their perivascular location) to a more diffuse expression (Binder et al., 2012). This can result in abnormal water regulation, astrocyte swelling, and a decrease in the extracellular space, which promotes ephaptic transmission. Breakdown of the blood-brain barrier and accumulation of albumin within glia also leads to a reduction in glial inward-rectifying potassium channel expression, and so decreased buffering of potassium rises (David et al., 2009). A decrease in gap junction coupling between astrocytes further contributes to this dysregulation of extracellular potassium and has been suggested to play an important role in epileptogenesis (Bedner et al., 2015).

Astrocytes also play a key role in metabolism and neurotransmitter synthesis, both of which are altered during epileptogenesis. There is an increase in the expression of adenosine kinase and along with astrocytosis (Figure 18.4O), this leads to decreased adenosine levels with epileptogenesis (Boison, 2012). There are decreased levels of glutamine synthetase, and a consequent decrease in the glutamate-GABA shunt, resulting in decreased inhibitory transmission (Coulter and Eid, 2012). Indeed, a specific reactive gliosis mediated by transfection with a viral vector has been shown to have no effect on the intrinsic excitability of neighboring neurons, but selectively decreases inhibitory transmission, leading to an inhibitory deficit and increased propagation of excitatory transmission (Ortinski et al., 2010). Moreover, there is evidence in human epileptic tissue of a change in glial glutamate transporter expression and from rodent studies of epileptogenesis, decreased efficacy of glutamate uptake (Proper et al., 2002; David et al., 2009). Lastly, glial metabotropic receptors are upregulated in epilepsy (Aronica et al., 2000), which may promote increases in intracellular astrocyte calcium, and contribute to the generation of seizure activity in vitro and in vivo (Gómez-Gonzalo et al., 2010). There is, therefore, burgeoning evidence of a key role for astrocytes in the generation of seizures and the development of epilepsy.

The extracellular matrix (ECM) consists of molecules that are secreted both by neurons and glia, which aggregate in the extracellular space. About 20% of the volume of the adult brain consists of extracellular matrix, predominantly proteoglycans, glycosaminoglycans (and, in particular, hyaluronic acid), and glycoproteins of the tenascin family. There are also proteins that link the extracellular matrix to molecules on neurons and glia (Dityatev et al., 2010). There has been growing recognition that the extracellular matrix can play a key role in neuronal and network plasticity. Importantly, the extracellular matrix can undergo remodeling, which is dependent on a series of serine proteases, such as plasminogen activators (in particular urokinase-type plasminogen activator), thrombin, metalloproteinases, and reelin. All of these have been implicated in neuronal and network plasticity (Dityatev, 2010). Alterations and remodeling of perineuronal nets permit neuronal reorganization following brain damage and seizures, and

during development. There are persistent changes in multiple components of the extracellular matrix during the development of epilepsy. Perineuronal net components, including aggrecan, neurocan, hyaluronan, tenascin-R, and some of the linking proteins, decrease during epileptogenesis; a progressive decrease in perineuronal nets is associated with a progressive decrease in synaptic inhibition and the occurrence of hippocampal seizures following traumatic brain injury (Pavlov et al., 2011). In addition, degradation of the extracellular matrix may permit aberrant neuronal and synaptic reorganization. Extracellular matrix remodeling and the increased secretion of proteases may also contribute to this process. There is robust evidence that expression of metalloproteinases is increased during epileptogenesis, and inhibition of these have antiseizure and antiepileptogenic effects in kindling and post-status-epilepticus models (Broekaart et al., 2021). Other serine proteases are also upregulated in epilepsy including urokinase-type plasminogen activator (uPA) and its receptor (uPAR). Intriguingly, uPAR upregulation may be protective, as uPAR knockouts develop a more severe epilepsy phenotype following status epilepticus (Ndode-Ekane and Pitkänen, 2013). This indicates that some of the changes of extracellular matrix during epileptogenesis may be adaptive rather than pathogenic.

Lastly, an extracellularly secreted molecule, leucine-rich glioma-inactivated 1 (LGI1) is strongly associated with epilepsy and participates in the regulation of neuronal excitability in the hippocampus (Lugarà et al., 2020). Knockout of LGI1 results in spontaneous seizures that originate in the hippocampus (Chabrol et al., 2010). LGI1 interconnects presynaptic disintegrin and metalloproteinase domain-containing protein 23 (ADAM23) to postsynaptic ADAM22 at the synaptic cleft. LGI1 is important for trafficking and kinetics of a presynaptic potassium channel, Kv1.1 (Schulte et al., 2006), and also for trafficking of postsynaptic AMPA receptors (Fukata et al., 2006). In humans, autoantibodies directed against LGI1 have been shown to underlie limbic encephalitis and temporal lobe seizures in humans (Irani et al., 2010), while mutations in the *LGI1* gene are associated in humans with neocortical temporal lobe epilepsy (Nobile et al., 2009).

18.6.2 Neurotransmitter systems

As detailed above, there are considerable structural rearrangements of excitatory and inhibitory pathways that take place during epileptogenesis. An attractive hypothesis is that many of the changes that occur are homeostatic responses to damage with increased connectivity of excitatory neurons in response to neuronal loss/dysfunction and modification of inhibition to compensate for both neuronal loss and increased excitation (Swann and Rho, 2014). Indeed, the "success" of compensatory and homeostatic changes is, to some extent, supported by the observation that seizures are infrequent events and that the brain can still support learning and memory, although to a diminished extent. Unsurprisingly, in addition to structural changes, there are also marked functional changes with changes in receptor and ion channel expression.

18.6.2.1 Glutamatergic mechanisms

In addition to increased connectivity (Figure 18.5A), glutamatergic synaptic transmission is increased (Figure 18.5B). In studies, employing in situ hybridization techniques, it has been shown that there is an increase in pyramidal and granule cell AMPA receptor mRNA, in granule cell NMDAR1 and 2 subunit mRNA, which is also supported by autoradiographic studies (Brines et al., 1997; Mathern et al., 1997). NMDA receptor responses are prolonged in post-status-epilepticus and kindling models and in human tissue (Köhr et al., 1993; Lieberman and Mody, 1999; Scimemi, Schorge, et al., 2006). This has been ascribed to long-lasting posttranslational modifications in the function of dentate granule cell NMDA receptor channels, leading to increases in the mean open time, and to burst and cluster duration, and to decreases in the channel blocking effect by magnesium (Köhr et al., 1993). The modification of the NMDA receptor channels probably results from a decrease in the activity of intracellular phosphatases, leading to an increased phosphorylation of the receptors (Köhr et al., 1993; Lieberman and Mody, 1999).

There is more uncertainty concerning changes in AMPA receptor neurotransmission. Changes in AMPA receptor subunit composition are seen in animal models prior to neurodegeneration following status epilepticus. There is a decrease in the expression of the GluA2 subunit during and after status epilepticus, resulting in the increased expression of calcium-permeable AMPA receptors (Grooms et al., 2000; Rajasekaran et al., 2012). In chronic mesial temporal lobe epilepsy, there is also evidence of an increased proportion of AMPA receptor lacking the GluA2 subunit (Egbenya et al., 2018). There may also be an increase in postsynaptic kainate receptor currents at the recurrent mossy fiber synapses, which are longer than AMPA receptor currents and may contribute to the generation of seizures (Epsztein et al., 2005; Peret et al., 2014). Upregulation of excitatory metabotropic glutamate receptors (mGluR1 subunit) has also been observed in the dentate gyrus in both human and animal models of hippocampal sclerosis, and this could contribute to the development of chronic seizures through increased excitatory transmission (Blümcke, Becker, et al., 2000).

As detailed in the glia section, glial glutamate uptake is decreased during epileptogenesis (Figures 18.4F and 18.5B) (Proper et al., 2002; David et al., 2009), and this could have an important role in epileptogenesis. This could explain higher baseline glutamate concentrations in the epileptic hippocampus detected in humans using in vivo microdialysis (During and Spencer, 1993). In this study, a marked rise in extracellular glutamate was recorded prior to seizure onset, leading to the suggestion that this could be an initiating factor in spontaneous seizures (During and Spencer, 1993). These findings are consistent with rodent studies, in which knockout mice for the glial glutamate transporter GLT-1 (EAAT2) have lethal spontaneous seizures (Tanaka et al., 1997). The mechanisms of these effects may be through the excessive activation of NMDA receptors through glutamate "spillover" (Rusakov and Kullmann, 1998; Scimemi, Schorge, et al., 2006).

18.6.2.2 GABAergic mechanisms

The "GABA" hypothesis proposes that a deficit in inhibitory GABAergic transmission is implicated in seizures. Overall, what is found in epilepsy is not a decrease in GABAergic inhibition but a change of inhibition (Figure 18.6). As described earlier, changes in interneuronal survival underlies a shift of inhibition from dendrites to soma in CA1 (Figure 18.6A), perhaps maintaining inhibition at the expense of the potential for increased neuronal synchronization (Cossart et al., 2001). Indeed, many alterations in GABAergic transmission may represent an adaptive mechanism in the brain in response to repetitive seizures. Increased expression of $GABA_A$ receptors have frequently been documented in animal models

of epilepsy as a compensatory mechanism (Fritschy et al., 1999). During epileptogenesis in the dentate granule cells, there is an increase in the number of $GABA_A$ receptors per synapse, leading to increased quantal size (Nusser et al., 1998). Overall, however, the most notable changes are shifts in $GABA_A$ receptor subunit expression that occur during epileptogenesis (Schwarzer et al., 1997; Brooks-Kayal et al., 1998). This results in different pharmacological responses of the $GABA_A$ receptors in hippocampal sclerosis (Brooks-Kayal et al., 1998). Importantly this shift in $GABA_A$ receptor subunit expression has an impact on tonic $GABA_A$ receptor-mediated currents (Figure 18.6B). Tonic $GABA_A$ receptor currents are generated by extrasynaptic $GABA_A$ receptors that have a high affinity for GABA, so are able to detect the low ambient GABA that surrounds neurons (Belelli et al., 2009). Tonic $GABA_A$ receptor currents are maintained or increased during epileptogenesis (Scimemi et al., 2005; Zhang et al., 2007; Zhan and Nadler, 2009). This is not due to an increase in extracellular GABA concentrations, but rather is the result of a change in $GABA_A$ subunit expression and/or translocation of synaptic receptors to extrasynaptic sites. This

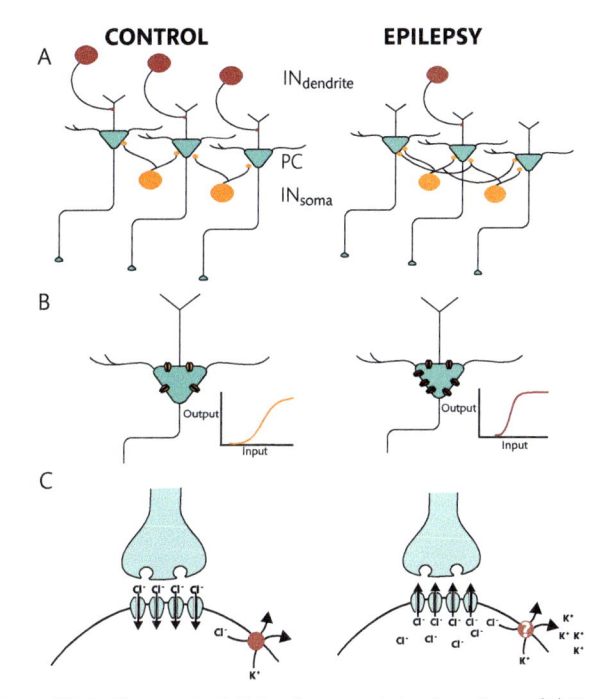

Figure 18.6 Changes in GABAergic transmission in epilepsy. (A) There is a selective loss of dendritic targeting interneurons ($IN_{dendrite}$) but an increase in perisomatic inhibition from somatic targeting interneurons (IN_{soma}). Although this maintains inhibitory tone, it can increase the synchronous activity of pyramidal cells (PC). (B) During the development of epilepsy, there is a change in the expression of $GABA_A$ receptor subunits which leads to increased tonic inhibition. With a loss of synaptic inhibition, the tonic inhibition maintains the offset of pyramidal cell input-output curves but increases the slope (gain), potentially leading to a less stable and more excitable network. (C) During $GABA_A$ receptor activation, there is chloride accumulation inside pyramidal cells. This is pumped out by the potassium/chloride transporter, KCC2. With excessive $GABA_A$ receptor activation, excessive chloride accumulation can result in depolarization of the chloride reversal potential, resulting in chloride efflux with $GABA_A$ receptor activation ("depolarizing GABA") and also extracellular potassium accumulation due to KCC2 activity. Thus, both up- (increasing potassium accumulation) and down- (increasing intracellular chloride accumulation) regulation of KCC2 could theoretically have proepileptic effects.

preservation of tonic currents is also evident in resected tissue from patients with mesial temporal lobe epilepsy (Scimemi, Andersson, et al., 2006). In CA1, there is a notable shift from synaptic $GABA_A$ receptor inhibition toward tonic inhibition (Scimemi et al., 2005; Pavlov et al., 2011). The network implications of this are unclear, but evidence indicates that an increase in tonic inhibition and a decrease in synaptic inhibition will have two major effects. First, there will be an increase in neuronal gain but a maintenance or increase in the offset of the input-output curve (Pavlov et al., 2009). Second, the decrease in synaptic currents will result in inadequate fast compensatory changes during increases in neuronal firing. These two sequelae will result in a network that responds adequately under baseline conditions but is inherently unstable during rapid increases in network activity. Such changes provide suitable conditions for the occurrence of seizures.

As previously described under the section on the generation of ictal activity, a further way in which $GABA_A$ receptor mediated inhibition can fail is through the accumulation of chloride within neurons, resulting in a change in the chloride reversal potential and depolarizing GABA(A) receptor mediated potentials. The hyperpolarizing chloride gradient in neurons is maintained by the $K+/Cl-$ cotransporter, KCC2, which pumps chloride out of neurons with potassium (Figure 18.6C). During excessive interneuronal activity, the chloride accumulation in neurons can result in a secondary increase in extracellular potassium, which may contribute to seizure initiation (Viitanen et al., 2010). There is some controversy surrounding the expression of KCC2 in epilepsy, with some proposing a downregulation of KCC2 in certain hippocampal/parahippocampal areas to explain apparent depolarizing $GABA_A$ receptor potentials recorded from human and rodent tissue (Cohen et al., 2002). However, in the human epileptic hippocampus, there is probably an upregulation of KCC2 (Karlócai et al., 2016), and it is likely that, in most neurons, this maintains a hyperpolarizing GABA(A) receptor-mediated potential but may contribute to the potassium accumulation that results in seizure generation.

$GABA_B$ receptor changes have also been demonstrated in human hippocampal sclerosis tissue. $GABA_B$ receptors inhibit neurotransmitter release from presynaptic terminals, and lead to a lasting postsynaptic hyperpolarizing potential through the activation of potassium currents (Marshall, 2008). Increased expression of $GABA_B$ receptors has been shown in the subiculum of hippocampal sclerosis cases and in surviving CA1 neurons and granule cells with augmented receptor binding in CA3 (Billinton et al., 2001a, 2001b), although functional interpretation of these findings is difficult. The upregulation could represent a greater number of inhibitory synapses, an increase in postsynaptic $GABA_B$ receptors, or an increase in presynaptic $GABA_B$ receptors leading to decreased neurotransmitter release mainly from inhibitory axonal terminals.

18.6.2.3 Other neurotransmitters

Alterations of many other transmitter systems have been described in association with acute limbic seizures, and also with hippocampal sclerosis. Many of these transmitters may play a role in seizure termination, and acute alterations have been implicated in the progression of seizures to status epilepticus. Adenosine, opioids, NPY, and galanin have all been proposed to play an important role in seizure termination (Vezzani and Sperk, 2004; Loacker et al., 2007; Lerner et al., 2008; Boison, 2012), while the accumulation of substance P has a proepileptogenic effect (Liu et al., 1999).

Adenosine is a potent inhibitor of neurotransmitter release and has been shown to be effective at terminating brief seizures. Indeed, accumulation of adenosine could play a prominent role in seizure termination, as seizures promote adenosine release in rodents and humans (During and Spencer, 1992; Berman et al., 2000). Adenosine antagonists shorten the stimulation protocol or lessen the chemoconvulsant dose necessary to induce status epilepticus (Young and Dragunow, 1994). There is also an acute downregulation in A1 receptor activity during prolonged seizures that promotes the progression of seizures into status epilepticus (Hamil et al., 2012).

Opioid release has also been suggested to be a major mechanism underlying the termination of seizures. The observed loss of dynorphin-like immunoreactivity in the hippocampus during sustained seizure activity is consistent with a loss of a potent endogenous antiepileptic (Mazarati et al., 1999). Knockout of prodynorphin lowers seizure threshold, which can be redressed using a kappa-opioid agonist, indicating a critical role for dynorphin and kappa opioid receptors in the regulation of hippocampal excitability (Loacker et al., 2007).

In addition to opioids, there are a variety of other modulatory neuropeptides. NPY is such a peptide; it has potent effects on neurotransmission. In human hippocampal sclerosis, there is increased NPY, upregulated presynaptic Y2 receptors that inhibit neurotransmitter release, and downregulated Y1 receptors that are expressed postsynaptically and are excitatory (Furtinger et al., 2001). Gene therapy overexpressing NPY in the hippocampus retards the development of seizures, and this is especially effective if both NPY and the Y2 receptors are overexpressed (Noè et al., 2008; Szczygieł et al., 2020).

Galanin is another bioactive peptide that is widely distributed throughout the CNS. Galanin in the hippocampus is predominantly inhibitory, decreasing the release of excitatory amino acids. In the hippocampus, galanin immunoreactivity is confined to axons; the bulk of these are the axons of medial septal neurons, and loss of galanin promotes the progression of seizure to status epilepticus (Lerner et al., 2008). Overexpressing galanin within the hippocampus using an adenoassociated viral vector increased the threshold for seizures and protected against neuronal death (Haberman et al., 2003).

18.6.3 Changes in neuronal properties

Although most recent research into epileptogenesis and seizure generation has concentrated on changes in the neuronal network, alterations in intrinsic neuronal properties also contribute to these processes. Importantly ion channel mutations in which there may only be subtle changes in the kinetics of ion channels can result in epilepsy, suggesting that the regulation of cortical excitability is nonlinear with small changes resulting in the generation of spontaneous seizures and conversely antiseizure therapies need only have a modest effect on their targets to be effective.

As discussed in the section on the interictal spike, CA3 pyramidal cells can generate burst-firing, while few pyramidal cells in CA1 demonstrate such firing properties. Alterations in intrinsic membrane properties can dramatically affect the firing properties of CA1 pyramidal cells and could promote burst-firing. Such burst-firing within a dense excitatory network has the potential to generate synchronized bursts, and may thus promote epileptic activity. In a post-status-epilepticus model of epileptogenesis, the proportion of bursting CA1 pyramidal cells increases dramatically, such that over half demonstrate bursting properties (Su et al., 2002). This may be due to an upregulation of a T-type calcium channel, Cav3.2, that can produce a significant calcium tail current following an action potential resulting in a significant afterdepolarization (Su et al., 2002). Persistent sodium currents may also contribute to this propensity to bursting behavior by maintaining neuronal depolarization (Chen et al., 2011). The importance of the increased excitability of pyramidal neurons in the hippocampus in the development of epilepsy is illustrated by the potent antiseizure effect of overexpressing an endogenous potassium channel, Kv1.1, using gene therapy and suppressing neuronal excitability using chemogenetics (Snowball et al., 2019; Desloovere et al., 2022).

There are also marked changes in dendritic excitability. Downregulation of dendritic A-type potassium channels has been found in a post-status-epilepticus epilepsy model (Bernard et al., 2004). This downregulation is partly due to increased channel phosphorylation by extracellular signal-regulated kinase but is also due to decreased transcription. These potassium channels limit the backpropagation of action potentials from the soma into the distal dendrites. The functional consequence of backpropagating action potentials is likely to be an amplification of EPSPs, and thus increased excitation. The effect of a downregulation of A-type potassium channels on dendritic calcium spikes and burst-firing is unknown.

Hyperpolarization-activated, cyclic-nucleotide gated (HCN) channels also play an important role in regulating dendritic excitability. HCN channels underlie the h-current, which is different from other voltage-gated ion currents in many features. The h-current is a mixed inward current carried by sodium and potassium ions that develops slowly upon hyperpolarization to potentials that are more negative than –60 mV. Upon sustained hyperpolarization, the h-current does not inactivate, whereas it slowly deactivates upon depolarization. The effect in the dendrite is to reduce EPSP summation, and its loss results in increased EPSP summation and consequently increased neuronal excitability (Shah et al., 2004). Downregulation and mislocalization to the soma of HCN1 is observed in CA1 pyramidal cell dendrites, leading to greater EPSP summation and hyperexcitability (Jung et al., 2007; Shin et al., 2008), and HCN1 expression may be downregulated because of seizure-induced changes in NRSF (McClelland et al., 2011). Animals with knockout of HCN1 are thus more susceptible to both seizures and the development of epilepsy (Huang et al., 2009). Such HCN channels are also critical for generating theta rhythms, and the loss of HCN may also have an impact on memory and learning (Marcelin et al., 2009). Epileptogenesis thus leads to an acquired channelopathy in neurons that may promote burst-firing and hyperexcitability.

18.7 The role of the hippocampus in the comorbidities of epilepsy

Mesial temporal lobe epilepsy is strongly associated with cognitive dysfunction, and this relates to the pattern of hippocampal atrophy (Postma et al., 2020). It is unsurprising that the considerable structural and functional changes detailed above are associated with memory dysfunction (Witt et al., 2014). The hippocampus with its well-studied mnemonic functions has been closely studied in relation to clinically defined memory deficits in presurgical psychometric testing. Memory impairment frequently accompanies hippocampal sclerosis with a dominant role for the left intact

hippocampus in verbal memory and the right in visual-spatial memory (Baxendale et al., 1998). Dysregulation of neurogenesis has also been proposed to play a role in memory dysfunction in mesial temporal lobe epilepsy. In an intriguing observation, the proliferative capacity of stem cells isolated from the human dentate gyrus correlated with memory performance (Coras et al., 2010). Moreover, in a rodent model of mesial temporal lobe epilepsy reversal of the neurogenic deficit with the antidepressant fluoxetine restored spatial learning (Barkas et al., 2012).

Although neuronal damage plays a critical role in cognitive deficits, memory problems can also be evident when there is minimal damage, suggesting that alterations in neuronal and network processes, short of overt damage, may contribute to cognitive deficits in temporal lobe epilepsy. One such mechanism is the epileptic activity itself. Interictal epileptiform activity in humans, such as interictal spikes and bursts of spike and wave discharges, have long been associated with impairments in cognition and memory (Rausch et al., 1978; Aarts et al., 1984). In humans, undergoing depth electrode EEG recordings, hippocampal interictal epileptiform discharges (IEDs) have been demonstrated to affect performance in working memory (Krauss et al., 1997) and delayed free recall (Kleen et al., 2013; Horak et al., 2017). At a neuronal level, micro/macroelectrode depth recording has revealed that hippocampal IEDs transiently modulate firing of hippocampal neurons and disrupt selectively the retrieval of declarative memories (Reed et al., 2020). The predominant recruitment of GABAergic interneurons, leading to suppression of principal cell firing, by interictal spikes is also likely to underlie the pathological impact on memory (Muldoon et al., 2015). Conversely, performance of hippocampal specific tasks can promote increased interictal spiking within the region (Vivekananda et al., 2019). A further mechanism of memory disruption by hippocampal IEDs is through the generation of aberrant cortical spindle oscillations (Gelinas et al., 2016).

There is also evidence that there can be progressive cognitive decline in people with hippocampal sclerosis, not dissimilar to that observed in Alzheimer's disease. Cognitive decline represents a significant comorbidity in epilepsy, particularly in the over-65-year age group (Helmstaedter and Witt, 2017). Longitudinal neuroimaging in epilepsy studies also support the concept of accelerated, progressive age-associated atrophy (Fuerst et al., 2003). The mechanisms of this are unclear (Tai et al., 2018). However, several studies of postsurgical tissue have reported phosphorylated tau (pTau) and Alzheimer's-like pathology in a proportion of patients; some studies also show a correlation between phosphorylated tau load and memory decline (Tai et al., 2016; Gourmaud et al., 2020). There is evidence that increased neuronal activity rapidly increases extracellular tau in the brain (Figure 18.4R) (Peng et al., 2020). Inhibition of tau phosphorylation following status epilepticus in rodents inhibits epileptogenesis and cognitive decline (Liu et al., 2016). In human hippocampal sclerosis tissue, there are also features that suggest tau phosphorylation is activity-driven, with prominent labeling in excitatory granule cells and sprouted mossy fiber axons (Tai et al., 2016). Since subclinical, covert seizures have been observed in people with Alzheimer's, it has been suggested that this epileptiform activity may accelerate the neurodegenerative process (Lam et al., 2017). There have been multiple mechanisms proposed for the generation of phosphorylated tau with epileptiform activity, including activation of the mTor pathway, production of reactive oxygen species, and neuroinflammation.

Depression and anxiety are also notable features of people with mesial temporal lobe epilepsy. There is also an increased incidence of psychosis which can occur between seizures (interictal psychosis) or shortly after a seizure (postictal psychosis) (Kanner and Rivas-Grajales, 2016). Each has been proposed to have a different mechanism, with the interictal psychosis being the result of the network and neuronal changes associated with epileptogenesis, while postictal psychosis seems to be related to the seizure activity itself, leading to transient cortical dysfunction. There is evidence that BDNF may play an important role in the depression associated with hippocampal sclerosis, with low BDNF levels prior to status epilepticus in a rodent model, predisposing to a reduced threshold for status epilepticus, accelerated epileptogenesis, and once epilepsy was established, depression and cognitive deficits (Becker et al., 2015).

18.8 Conclusion

Although the studies and findings described above focus on different facets of mesial temporal lobe epilepsy with hippocampal sclerosis, it is possible to create a unifying narrative. Seizures can occur in any of us if brain excitability is sufficiently increased (as occurs with alcohol withdrawal and electroconvulsive therapy), or if the brain is disinhibited (such as occurs with the ingestion of certain toxins). For each of us, there is a threshold of increased excitation/decreased inhibition at which we will have a seizure. Following a cortical insult, such as traumatic brain injury, status epilepticus, or hypoxia/ischemia, multiple mechanisms contribute to neuronal damage. In response to this and in order to maintain function, processes are in place that result in increased connectivity of principal excitatory cells and that strengthen excitatory synapses. To prevent continuous seizure activity, there are compensatory inhibitory changes, but, due to a reduction in specific interneuronal subtypes, there is a shift from dendritic to somatic inhibition and from synaptic inhibition to tonic inhibition. Although these compensatory inhibitory changes are sufficient most of the time to prevent seizure activity, they create a network that is less stable, resulting in sporadic seizures. These changes in the hippocampus also result in other comorbidities such as cognitive deficits and depression. Moreover, there is gathering evidence that, in some people, hippocampal sclerosis is a progressive condition.

REFERENCES

Aarts JH, Binnie CD, Smit AM, Wilkins AJ (1984) Selective cognitive impairment during focal and generalized epileptiform EEG activity. *Brain* **107**:293–308.

Abbott LC, Nigussie F (2020) Adult neurogenesis in the mammalian dentate gyrus. *Anat Histol Embryol* **49**:3–16.

Alger BE, Nicoll RA (1980) Epileptiform burst afterhyperolarization: calcium-dependent potassium potential in hippocampal CA1 pyramidal cells. *Science* **210**:1122–1124.

Amaral DG, Campbell MJ (1986) Transmitter systems in the primate dentate gyrus. *Hum Neurobiol* **5**:169–180.

Anderson WW, Anderson WW, Lewis DV, Scott Swartzwelder H, Wilson WA (1986) Magnesium-free medium activates seizure-like events in the rat hippocampal slice. *Brain Res* **398**:215–219.

Ang CW, Carlson GC, Coulter DA (2006) Massive and specific dysregulation of direct cortical input to the hippocampus in temporal lobe epilepsy. *J Neurosci* **26**:11850–11856.

Annegers JF, Hauser WA, Shirts SB, Kurland LT (1987) Factors prognostic of unprovoked seizures after febrile convulsions. *N Engl J Med* **316**:493–498.

Aronica E, van Vliet EA, Mayboroda OA, Troost D, da Silva FH, Gorter JA (2000) Upregulation of metabotropic glutamate receptor subtype mGluR3 and mGluR5 in reactive astrocytes in a rat model of mesial temporal lobe epilepsy. *Eur J Neurosci* **12**:2333–2344.

Babb TL, Kupfer WR, Pretorius JK, Crandall PH, Levesque MF (1991) Synaptic reorganization by mossy fibers in human epileptic fascia dentata. *Neuroscience* **42**:351–363.

Barbarosie M, Avoli M (1997) CA3-driven hippocampal-entorhinal loop controls rather than sustains in vitro limbic seizures. *J Neurosci* **17**:9308–9314.

Barkas L, Redhead E, Taylor M, Shtaya A, Hamilton DA, Gray WP (2012) Fluoxetine restores spatial learning but not accelerated forgetting in mesial temporal lobe epilepsy. *Brain* **135**:2358–2374.

Bar-Klein G, Cacheaux LP, Kamintsky L, Prager O, Weissberg I, Schoknecht K, Cheng P, Kim SY, Wood L, Heinemann U, et al. (2014) Losartan prevents acquired epilepsy via TGF-β signaling suppression. *Ann Neurol* **75**:864–875.

Barron DS, Fox PM, Laird AR, Robinson JL, Fox PT (2012) Thalamic medial dorsal nucleus atrophy in medial temporal lobe epilepsy: a VBM meta-analysis. *NeuroImage Clin* **2**:25–32.

Bartolomei F, Chauvel P, Wendling F (2008) Epileptogenicity of brain structures in human temporal lobe epilepsy: a quantified study from intracerebral EEG. *Brain* **131**:1818–1830.

Baulac M, De Grissac N, Hasboun D, Oppenheim C, Adam C, Arzimanoglou A, Semah F, Lehéricy S, Clémenceau S, Berger B (1998) Hippocampal developmental changes in patients with partial epilepsy: magnetic resonance imaging and clinical aspects. *Ann Neurol* **44**:223–233.

Baxendale SA, van Paesschen W, Thompson PJ, Connelly A, Duncan JS, Harkness WF, Shorvon SD (1998) The relationship between quantitative MRI and neuropsychological functioning in temporal lobe epilepsy. *Epilepsia* **39**:158–166.

Beamer E, Kuchukulla M, Boison D, Engel T (2021) ATP and adenosine—two players in the control of seizures and epilepsy development. *Prog Neurobiol* **204**:102105.

Becker AJ, Pitsch J, Sochivko D, Opitz T, Staniek M, Chen C-C, Campbell KP, Schoch S, Yaari Y, Beck H (2008) Transcriptional upregulation of Cav3.2 mediates epileptogenesis in the pilocarpine model of epilepsy. *J Neurosci* **28**:13341–13353.

Becker C, Bouvier E, Ghestem A, Siyoucef S, Claverie D, Camus F, Bartolomei F, Benoliel J-J, Bernard C (2015) Predicting and treating stress-induced vulnerability to epilepsy and depression. *Ann Neurol* **78**:128–136.

Bedner P, Dupper A, Hüttmann K, Müller J, Herde MK, Dublin P, Deshpande T, Schramm J, Häussler U, Haas CA, et al. (2015) Astrocyte uncoupling as a cause of human temporal lobe epilepsy. *Brain* **138**:1208–1222.

Beghi E (2020) The epidemiology of epilepsy. *Neuroepidemiology* **54**:185–191.

Belelli D, Harrison NL, Maguire J, Macdonald RL, Walker MC, Cope DW (2009) Extrasynaptic GABAA receptors: form, pharmacology, and function. *J Neurosci* **29**:12757–12763.

Bengzon J, Kokaia Z, Elmér E, Nanobashvili A, Kokaia M, Lindvall O (1997) Apoptosis and proliferation of dentate gyrus neurons after single and intermittent limbic seizures. *Proc Natl Acad Sci U S A* **94**:10432–10437.

Berg AT, Berkovic SF, Brodie MJ, Buchhalter J, Cross JH, van Emde Boas W, Engel J, French J, Glauser TA, Mathern GW, et al. (2010) Revised terminology and concepts for organization of seizures and epilepsies: report of the ILAE Commission on Classification and Terminology, 2005-2009. *Epilepsia* **51**:676–685.

Berman RF, Fredholm BB, Aden U, O'Connor WT (2000) Evidence for increased dorsal hippocampal adenosine release and metabolism during pharmacologically induced seizures in rats. *Brain Res* **872**:44–53.

Bernard C, Anderson A, Becker A, Poolos NP, Beck H, Johnston D (2004) Acquired dendritic channelopathy in temporal lobe epilepsy. *Science* **305**:532–535.

Bernasconi N, Bernasconi A, Caramanos Z, Antel SB, Andermann F, Arnold DL (2003) Mesial temporal damage in temporal lobe epilepsy: a volumetric MRI study of the hippocampus, amygdala and parahippocampal region. *Brain* **126**:462–469.

Bernasconi N, Kinay D, Andermann F, Antel S, Bernasconi A (2005) Analysis of shape and positioning of the hippocampal formation: an MRI study in patients with partial epilepsy and healthy controls. *Brain* **128**:2442–2452.

Billinton A, Baird VH, Thom M, Duncan JS, Upton N, Bowery NG (2001a) GABA(B) receptor autoradiography in hippocampal sclerosis associated with human temporal lobe epilepsy. *Br J Pharmacol* **132**:475–480.

Billinton A, Baird VH, Thom M, Duncan JS, Upton N, Bowery NG (2001b) GABA(B(1)) mRNA expression in hippocampal sclerosis associated with human temporal lobe epilepsy. *Brain Res Mol Brain Res* **86**:84–89.

Binder DK, Nagelhus EA, Ottersen OP (2012) Aquaporin-4 and epilepsy. *Glia* **60**:1203–1214.

Blümcke I, et al. (2011) The clinicopathologic spectrum of focal cortical dysplasias: a consensus classification proposed by an ad hoc task force of the ILAE Diagnostic Methods Commission. *Epilepsia* **52**:158–174.

Blümcke I, et al. (2013) International consensus classification of hippocampal sclerosis in temporal lobe epilepsy: a task force report from the ILAE Commission on Diagnostic Methods. *Epilepsia* **54**:1315–1329.

Blumcke I, et al. (2017) Histopathological findings in brain tissue obtained during epilepsy surgery. *N Engl J Med* **377**:1648–1656.

Blümcke I, Becker AJ, Klein C, Scheiwe C, Lie AA, Beck H, Waha A, Friedl MG, Kuhn R, Emson P, et al. (2000) Temporal lobe epilepsy associated up-regulation of metabotropic glutamate receptors: correlated changes in mGluR1 mRNA and protein expression in experimental animals and human patients. *J Neuropathol Exp Neurol* **59**:1–10.

Blümcke I, Suter B, Behle K, Kuhn R, Schramm J, Elger CE, Wiestler OD (2000) Loss of hilar mossy cells in Ammon's horn sclerosis. *Epilepsia* **41**(Suppl 6):S174–180.

Blümcke I, Thom M, Wiestler OD (2002) Ammon's horn sclerosis: a maldevelopmental disorder associated with temporal lobe epilepsy. *Brain Pathol Zurich Switz* **12**:199–211.

Boison D (2012) Adenosine dysfunction in epilepsy. *Glia* **60**:1234–1243.

Bouchet C, Cazavieilh J (1825) De L'epilepsie consideree dans ses rapports avec l'alienation mentale: recherche sur la nature et le siege de ces deux maladies. *Arch Gen Med* **9**:510–542.

Bragin A, Engel J, Wilson CL, Fried I, Mathern GW (1999) Hippocampal and entorhinal cortex high-frequency oscillations (100–500 Hz) in human epileptic brain and in kainic acid–treated rats with chronic seizures. *Epilepsia* **40**:127–137.

Briellmann RS, Berkovic SF, Syngeniotis A, King MA, Jackson GD (2002) Seizure-associated hippocampal volume loss: a longitudinal magnetic resonance study of temporal lobe epilepsy. *Ann Neurol* **51**:641–644.

Brines ML, Sundaresan S, Spencer DD, de Lanerolle NC (1997) Quantitative autoradiographic analysis of ionotropic glutamate receptor subtypes in human temporal lobe epilepsy: up-regulation in reorganized epileptogenic hippocampus. *Eur J Neurosci* **9**:2035–2044.

Broekaart DW, et al. (2021) The matrix metalloproteinase inhibitor IPR-179 has antiseizure and antiepileptogenic effects. *J Clin Invest* **131**:138332.

Brooks-Kayal AR, Shumate MD, Jin H, Rikhter TY, Coulter DA (1998) Selective changes in single cell GABA(A) receptor subunit expression and function in temporal lobe epilepsy. *Nat Med* **4**:1166–1172.

Buckmaster PS, Ingram EA, Wen X (2009) Inhibition of the mammalian target of rapamycin signaling pathway suppresses dentate granule cell axon sprouting in a rodent model of temporal lobe epilepsy. *J Neurosci* **29**:8259–8269.

Buhl EH, Otis TS, Mody I (1996) Zinc-induced collapse of augmented inhibition by GABA in a temporal lobe epilepsy model. *Science* **271**:369–373.

Bui AD, Nguyen TM, Limouse C, Kim HK, Szabo GG, Felong S, Maroso M, Soltesz I (2018) Dentate gyrus mossy cells control spontaneous convulsive seizures and spatial memory. *Science* **359**:787–790.

Buzsáki G, Horváth Z, Urioste R, Hetke J, Wise K (1992) High-frequency network oscillation in the hippocampus. *Science* **256**:1025–1027.

Caciagli L, Bernasconi A, Wiebe S, Koepp MJ, Bernasconi N, Bernhardt BC (2017) A meta-analysis on progressive atrophy in intractable temporal lobe epilepsy: time is brain? *Neurology* **89**:506–516.

Cain DP, Boon F, Hargreaves EL (1992) Evidence for different neurochemical contributions to long-term potentiation and to kindling and kindling-induced potentiation: role of NMDA and urethane-sensitive mechanisms. *Exp Neurol* **116**:330–338.

Călin A, Ilie AS, Akerman CJ (2021) Disrupting epileptiform activity by preventing parvalbumin interneuron depolarization block. *J Neurosci* **41**:9452–9465.

Cameron MC, Zhan R-Z, Nadler JV (2011) Morphologic integration of hilar ectopic granule cells into dentate gyrus circuitry in the pilocarpine model of temporal lobe epilepsy. *J Comp Neurol* **519**:2175–2192.

Cavarsan CF, Malheiros J, Hamani C, Najm I, Covolan L (2018) Is mossy fiber sprouting a potential therapeutic target for epilepsy? *Front Neurol* **9**:1023.

Cavazos JE, Das I, Sutula TP (1994) Neuronal loss induced in limbic pathways by kindling: evidence for induction of hippocampal sclerosis by repeated brief seizures. *J Neurosci* **14**:3106–3121.

Cendes F, Cook MJ, Watson C, Andermann F, Fish DR, Shorvon SD, Bergin P, Free S, Dubeau F, Arnold DL (1995) Frequency and characteristics of dual pathology in patients with lesional epilepsy. *Neurology* **45**:2058–2064.

Chabrol E, Navarro V, Provenzano G, Cohen I, Dinocourt C, Rivaud-Péchoux S, Fricker D, Baulac M, Miles R, Leguern E, et al. (2010) Electroclinical characterization of epileptic seizures in leucine-rich, glioma-inactivated 1-deficient mice. *Brain* **133**:2749–2762.

Chakravarty K, Ray S, Kharbanda PS, Lal V, Baishya J (2021) Temporal lobe epilepsy with amygdala enlargement: a systematic review. *Acta Neurol Scand* **144**:236–250.

Chen S, Su H, Yue C, Remy S, Royeck M, Sochivko D, Opitz T, Beck H, Yaari Y (2011) An increase in persistent sodium current contributes to intrinsic neuronal bursting after status epilepticus. *J Neurophysiol* **105**:117–129.

Chowdhury FA, Silva R, Whatley B, Walker MC (2021) Localisation in focal epilepsy: a practical guide. *Pract Neurol* 21:481–491.

Choy M, Dadgar-Kiani E, Cron GO, Duffy BA, Schmid F, Edelman BJ, Asaad M, Chan RW, Vahdat S, Lee JH (2022) Repeated hippocampal seizures lead to brain-wide reorganization of circuits and seizure propagation pathways. *Neuron* 110:221–236, e4.

Cobb SR, Buhl EH, Halasy K, Paulsen O, Somogyi P (1995) Synchronization of neuronal activity in hippocampus by individual GABAergic interneurons. *Nature* 378:75–78.

Cohen I, Navarro V, Clemenceau S, Baulac M, Miles R (2002) On the origin of interictal activity in human temporal lobe epilepsy in vitro. *Science* 298:1418–1421.

Collins RC, Lothman EW, Olney JW (1983) Status epilepticus in the limbic system: biochemical and pathological changes. *Adv Neurol* 34:277–288.

Collins RC, Tearse RG, Lothman EW (1983) Functional anatomy of limbic seizures: focal discharges from medial entorhinal cortex in rat. *Brain Res* 280:25–40.

Coras R, Siebzehnrubl FA, Pauli E, Huttner HB, Njunting M, Kobow K, Villmann C, Hahnen E, Neuhuber W, Weigel D, et al. (2010) Low proliferation and differentiation capacities of adult hippocampal stem cells correlate with memory dysfunction in humans. *Brain* 133:3359–3372.

Cossart R, Dinocourt C, Hirsch JC, Merchan-Perez A, De Felipe J, Ben-Ari Y, Esclapez M, Bernard C (2001) Dendritic but not somatic GABAergic inhibition is decreased in experimental epilepsy. *Nat Neurosci* 4:52–62.

Coulter DA, Eid T (2012) Astrocytic regulation of glutamate homeostasis in epilepsy. *Glia* 60:1215–1226.

David Y, Cacheaux LP, Ivens S, Lapilover E, Heinemann U, Kaufer D, Friedman A (2009) Astrocytic dysfunction in epileptogenesis: consequence of altered potassium and glutamate homeostasis? *J Neurosci* 29:10588–10599.

Davies KG, Hermann BP, Dohan FC, Foley KT, Bush AJ, Wyler AR (1996) Relationship of hippocampal sclerosis to duration and age of onset of epilepsy, and childhood febrile seizures in temporal lobectomy patients. *Epilepsy Res* 24:119–126.

DeGiorgio CM, Tomiyasu U, Gott PS, Treiman DM (1992) Hippocampal pyramidal cell loss in human status epilepticus. *Epilepsia* 33:23–27.

de Lanerolle NC, Kim JH, Robbins RJ, Spencer DD (1989) Hippocampal interneuron loss and plasticity in human temporal lobe epilepsy. *Brain Res* 495:387–395.

DeLorenzo RJ, Hauser WA, Towne AR, Boggs JG, Pellock JM, Penberthy L, Garnett L, Fortner CA, Ko D (1996) A prospective, population-based epidemiologic study of status epilepticus in Richmond, Virginia. *Neurology* 46:1029–1035.

Desloovere J, Boon P, Larsen LE, Goossens M-G, Delbeke J, Carrette E, Wadman W, Vonck K, Raedt R (2022) Chemogenetic seizure control with Clozapine and the novel ligand JHU37160 outperforms the effects of Levetiracetam in the intrahippocampal kainic acid mouse model. *Neurother J Am Soc Exp Neurother* 19:342–351.

Di Gennaro G, Quarato PP, Onorati P, Colazza GB, Mari F, Grammaldo LG, Ciccarelli O, Meldolesi NG, Sebastiano F, Manfredi M, et al. (2003) Localizing significance of temporal intermittent rhythmic delta activity (TIRDA) in drug-resistant focal epilepsy. *Clin Neurophysiol* 114:70–78.

Dityatev A (2010) Remodeling of extracellular matrix and epileptogenesis. *Epilepsia* 51(Suppl 3):61–65.

Dityatev A, Seidenbecher CI, Schachner M (2010) Compartmentalization from the outside: the extracellular matrix and functional microdomains in the brain. *Trends Neurosci* 33:503–512.

Domann R, Westerhoff CH, Witte OW (1994) Inhibitory mechanisms terminating paroxysmal depolarization shifts in hippocampal neurons of rats. *Neurosci Lett* 176:71–74.

Duarte JTC, Jardim AP, Comper SM, De Marchi LR, Gaça LB, Garcia MTFC, Sandim GB, Assunção-Leme IB, Carrete H, Centeno RS, et al. (2018) The impact of epilepsy duration in a series of patients with mesial temporal lobe epilepsy due to unilateral hippocampal sclerosis. *Epilepsy Res* 147:51–57.

During MJ, Spencer DD (1992) Adenosine: a potential mediator of seizure arrest and postictal refractoriness. *Ann Neurol* 32:618–624.

During MJ, Spencer DD (1993) Extracellular hippocampal glutamate and spontaneous seizure in the conscious human brain. *Lancet* 341:1607–1610.

Egbenya DL, Hussain S, Lai Y-C, Xia J, Anderson AE, Davanger S (2018) Changes in synaptic AMPA receptor concentration and composition in chronic temporal lobe epilepsy. *Mol Cell Neurosci* 92:93–103.

Engel J, Bragin A, Staba R, Mody I (2009) High-frequency oscillations: what is normal and what is not? *Epilepsia* 50:598–604.

Epsztein J, Represa A, Jorquera I, Ben-Ari Y, Crépel V (2005) Recurrent mossy fibers establish aberrant kainate receptor-operated synapses on granule cells from epileptic rats. *J Neurosci* 25:8229–8239.

Esclapez M, Hirsch JC, Ben-Ari Y, Bernard C (1999) Newly formed excitatory pathways provide a substrate for hyperexcitability in experimental temporal lobe epilepsy. *J Comp Neurol* 408:449–460.

Fahrner A, Kann G, Flubacher A, Heinrich C, Freiman TM, Zentner J, Frotscher M, Haas CA (2007) Granule cell dispersion is not accompanied by enhanced neurogenesis in temporal lobe epilepsy patients. *Exp Neurol* 203:320–332.

Fernández G, Effenberger O, Vinz B, Steinlein O, Elger CE, Döhring W, Heinze HJ (1998) Hippocampal malformation as a cause of familial febrile convulsions and subsequent hippocampal sclerosis. *Neurology* 50:909–917.

Finke C, Kopp UA, Pajkert A, Behrens JR, Leypoldt F, Wuerfel JT, Ploner CJ, Prüss H, Paul F (2016) Structural hippocampal damage following anti-N-methyl-D-aspartate receptor encephalitis. *Biol Psychiatry* 79:727–734.

Freiman TM, Häussler U, Zentner J, Doostkam S, Beck J, Scheiwe C, Brandt A, Haas CA, Puhahn-Schmeiser B (2021) Mossy fiber sprouting into the hippocampal region CA2 in patients with temporal lobe epilepsy. *Hippocampus* 31:580–592.

French JA, Williamson PD, Thadani VM, Darcey TM, Mattson RH, Spencer SS, Spencer DD (1993) Characteristics of medial temporal lobe epilepsy: I. Results of history and physical examination. *Ann Neurol* 34:774–780.

Freund TF, Buzsáki G (1996) Interneurons of the hippocampus. *Hippocampus* 6:347–470.

Fricke RA, Prince DA (1984) Electrophysiology of dentate gyrus granule cells. *J Neurophysiol* 51:195–209.

Fritschy JM, Kiener T, Bouilleret V, Loup F (1999) GABAergic neurons and GABA(A)-receptors in temporal lobe epilepsy. *Neurochem Int* 34:435–445.

Frotscher M, Haas CA, Förster E (2003) Reelin controls granule cell migration in the dentate gyrus by acting on the radial glial scaffold. *Cereb Cortex* 13:634–640.

Frotscher M, Jonas P, Sloviter RS (2006) Synapses formed by normal and abnormal hippocampal mossy fibers. *Cell Tissue Res* 326:361–367.

Fuerst D, Shah J, Shah A, Watson C (2003) Hippocampal sclerosis is a progressive disorder: a longitudinal volumetric MRI study. *Ann Neurol* 53:413–416.

Fukata Y, Adesnik H, Iwanaga T, Bredt DS, Nicoll RA, Fukata M (2006) Epilepsy-related ligand/receptor complex LGI1 and ADAM22 regulate synaptic transmission. *Science* 313:1792–1795.

Furtinger S, Pirker S, Czech T, Baumgartner C, Ransmayr G, Sperk G (2001) Plasticity of Y1 and Y2 receptors and neuropeptide Y fibers in patients with temporal lobe epilepsy. *J Neurosci* 21:5804–5812.

Galovic M, et al. (2019) Association of piriform cortex resection with surgical outcomes in patients with temporal lobe epilepsy. *JAMA Neurol* 76:690–700.

Gelinas JN, Khodagholy D, Thesen T, Devinsky O, Buzsáki G (2016) Interictal epileptiform discharges induce hippocampal-cortical coupling in temporal lobe epilepsy. *Nat Med* 22:641–648.

Gleichgerrcht E, Drane DL, Keller SS, Davis KA, Gross R, Willie JT, Pedersen N, Bezenac C de, Jensen J, Kuzniecky R, et al. (2022) Association between anatomical location of surgically induced lesions and postoperative seizure outcome in temporal lobe epilepsy. *Neurology* 98:E141–E151.

Goddard GV (1967) Development of epileptic seizures through brain stimulation at low intensity. *Nature* 214:1020–1021.

Gómez-Gonzalo M, Losi G, Chiavegato A, Zonta M, Cammarota M, Brondi M, Vetri F, Uva L, Pozzan T, de Curtis M, et al. (2010) An excitatory loop with astrocytes contributes to drive neurons to seizure threshold. *PLoS Biol* 8:e1000352.

Gourmaud S, Shou H, Irwin DJ, Sansalone K, Jacobs LM, Lucas TH, Marsh ED, Davis KA, Jensen FE, Talos DM (2020) Alzheimer-like amyloid and tau alterations associated with cognitive deficit in temporal lobe epilepsy. *Brain* 143:191–209.

Gregory RP, Oates T, Merry RT (1993) Electroencephalogram epileptiform abnormalities in candidates for aircrew training. *Electroencephalogr Clin Neurophysiol* 86:75–77.

Grooms SY, Opitz T, Bennett MV, Zukin RS (2000) Status epilepticus decreases glutamate receptor 2 mRNA and protein expression in hippocampal pyramidal cells before neuronal death. *Proc Natl Acad Sci U S A* 97:3631–3636.

Guth TA, Kunz L, Brandt A, Dümpelmann M, Klotz KA, Reinacher PC, Schulze-Bonhage A, Jacobs J, Schönberger J (2021) Interictal spikes with and without high-frequency oscillation have different single-neuron correlates. *Brain* 144:3078–3088.

Haberman RP, Samulski RJ, McCown TJ (2003) Attenuation of seizures and neuronal death by adeno-associated virus vector galanin expression and secretion. *Nat Med* 9:1076–1080.

Hadjiabadi D, Lovett-Barron M, Raikov IG, Sparks FT, Liao Z, Baraban SC, Leskovec J, Losonczy A, Deisseroth K, Soltesz I (2021) Maximally selective single-cell target for circuit control in epilepsy models. *Neuron* 109:2556–2572, e6.

Hamil NE, Cock HR, Walker MC (2012) Acute down-regulation of adenosine A(1) receptor activity in status epilepticus. *Epilepsia* 53:177–188.

Hardiman O, Burke T, Phillips J, Murphy S, O'Moore B, Staunton H, Farrell MA (1988) Microdysgenesis in resected temporal neocortex: incidence and clinical significance in focal epilepsy. *Neurology* 38:1041–1047.

Harding B, Thom M (2001) Bilateral hippocampal granule cell dispersion: autopsy study of 3 infants. *Neuropathol Appl Neurobiol* 27:245–251.

Heck N, Garwood J, Loeffler J-P, Larmet Y, Faissner A (2004) Differential upregulation of extracellular matrix molecules associated with the appearance of granule cell dispersion and mossy fiber sprouting during epileptogenesis in a murine model of temporal lobe epilepsy. *Neuroscience* 129:309–324.

Helmstaedter C, Witt J-A (2017) Epilepsy and cognition: a bidirectional relationship? *Seizure* 49:83–89.

Hendricks WD, Chen Y, Bensen AL, Westbrook GL, Schnell E (2017) Short-term depression of sprouted mossy fiber synapses from adult-born granule cells. *J Neurosci* 37:5722–5735.

Hesdorffer DC, Logroscino G, Benn EKT, Katri N, Cascino G, Hauser WA (2011) Estimating risk for developing epilepsy. *Neurology* 76:23–27.

Hesdorffer DC, Logroscino G, Cascino G, Annegers JF, Hauser WA (1998) Incidence of status epilepticus in Rochester, Minnesota, 1965–1984. *Neurology* 50:735–741.

Hester MS, Danzer SC (2013) Accumulation of abnormal adult-generated hippocampal granule cells predicts seizure frequency and severity. *J Neurosci* 33:8926–8936.

Hester MS, Hosford BE, Santos VR, Singh SP, Rolle IJ, LaSarge CL, Liska JP, Garcia-Cairasco N, Danzer SC (2016) Impact of rapamycin on status epilepticus induced hippocampal pathology and weight gain. *Exp Neurol* 280:1–12.

Holtmaat AJGD, Gorter JA, De Wit J, Tolner EA, Spijker S, Giger RJ, Lopes da Silva FH, Verhaagen J (2003) Transient downregulation of Sema3A mRNA in a rat model for temporal lobe epilepsy. a novel molecular event potentially contributing to mossy fiber sprouting. *Exp Neurol* 182:142–150.

Horak PC, Meisenhelter S, Song Y, Testorf ME, Kahana MJ, Viles WD, et al. (2017) Interictal epileptiform discharges impair word recall in multiple brain areas. *Epilepsia* 58:373–380.

Hotka M, Kubista H (2019) The paroxysmal depolarization shift in epilepsy research. *Int J Biochem Cell Biol* 107:77–81.

Houser CR (1990) Granule cell dispersion in the dentate gyrus of humans with temporal lobe epilepsy. *Brain Res* 535:195–204.

Houser CR, Miyashiro JE, Swartz BE, Walsh GO, Rich JR, Delgado-Escueta AV (1990) Altered patterns of dynorphin immunoreactivity suggest mossy fiber reorganization in human hippocampal epilepsy. *J Neurosci* 10:267–282.

Hu X-L, Cheng X, Cai L, Tan G-H, Xu L, Feng X-Y, Lu T-J, Xiong H, Fei J, Xiong Z-Q (2011) Conditional deletion of NRSF in forebrain neurons accelerates epileptogenesis in the kindling model. *Cereb Cortex* 21:2158–2165.

Huang Z, Walker MC, Shah MM (2009) Loss of dendritic HCN1 subunits enhances cortical excitability and epileptogenesis. *J Neurosci* 29:10979–10988.

Huberfeld G, Menendez de la Prida L, Pallud J, Cohen I, Le Van Quyen M, Adam C, Clemenceau S, Baulac M, Miles R (2011) Glutamatergic pre-ictal discharges emerge at the transition to seizure in human epilepsy. *Nat Neurosci* 14:627–634.

Hunt RF, Girskis KM, Rubenstein JL, Alvarez-Buylla A, Baraban SC (2013) GABA progenitors grafted into the adult epileptic brain control seizures and abnormal behavior. *Nat Neurosci* 16:692–697.

Huusko N, Römer C, Ndode-Ekane XE, Lukasiuk K, Pitkänen A (2015) Loss of hippocampal interneurons and epileptogenesis: a comparison of two animal models of acquired epilepsy. *Brain Struct Funct* 220:153–191.

Irani SR, Alexander S, Waters P, Kleopa KA, Pettingill P, Zuliani L, Peles E, Buckley C, Lang B, Vincent A (2010) Antibodies to Kv1 potassium channel-complex proteins leucine-rich, glioma inactivated 1 protein and contactin-associated protein-2 in limbic encephalitis, Morvan's syndrome and acquired neuromyotonia. *Brain* 133:2734–2748.

Jacobs J, Zijlmans M, Zelmann R, Chatillon C-E, Hall J, Olivier A, Dubeau F, Gotman J (2010) High-frequency electroencephalographic oscillations correlate with outcome of epilepsy surgery. *Ann Neurol* 67:209–220.

Janszky J, Janszky I, Schulz R, Hoppe M, Behne F, Pannek HW, Ebner A (2005) Temporal lobe epilepsy with hippocampal sclerosis: predictors for long-term surgical outcome. *Brain* 128:395–404.

Jefferys JG (1995) Nonsynaptic modulation of neuronal activity in the brain: electric currents and extracellular ions. *Physiol Rev* 75:689–723.

Jimenez-Mateos EM, Engel T, Merino-Serrais P, McKiernan RC, Tanaka K, Mouri G, Sano T, O'Tuathaigh C, Waddington JL, Prenter S, et al. (2012) Silencing microRNA-134 produces neuroprotective and prolonged seizure-suppressive effects. *Nat Med* 18:1087–1094.

Johnson MR, Behmoaras J, Bottolo L, Krishnan ML, Pernhorst K, Santoscoy PLM, et al. (2015) Systems genetics identifies Sestrin 3 as a regulator of a proconvulsant gene network in human epileptic hippocampus. *Nat Commun* 6:6031.

Jones RS (1988) Epileptiform events induced by GABA-antagonists in entorhinal cortical cells in vitro are partly mediated by N-methyl-D-aspartate receptors. *Brain Res* 457:113–121.

Jung S, Jones TD, Lugo JN, Sheerin AH, Miller JW, D'Ambrosio R, Anderson AE, Poolos NP (2007) Progressive dendritic HCN channelopathy during epileptogenesis in the rat pilocarpine model of epilepsy. *J Neurosci* 27:13012–13021.

Kane N, Acharya J, Benickzy S, Caboclo L, Finnigan S, Kaplan PW, Shibasaki H, Pressler R, van Putten MJAM (2017) A revised glossary of terms most commonly used by clinical electroencephalographers and updated proposal for the report format of the EEG findings: revision 2017. *Clin Neurophysiol Pract* 2:170–185.

Kanner AM, Rivas-Grajales AM (2016) Psychosis of epilepsy: a multi-faceted neuropsychiatric disorder. *CNS Spectr* 21:247–257.

Karlócai MR, Kohus Z, Káli S, Ulbert I, Szabó G, Máté Z, Freund TF, Gulyás AI (2014) Physiological sharp wave-ripples and interictal events in vitro: what's the difference? *Brain* 137:463–485.

Karlócai MR, Wittner L, Tóth K, Maglóczky Z, Katarova Z, Rásonyi G, Erőss L, Czirják S, Halász P, Szabó G, et al. (2016) Enhanced expression of potassium-chloride cotransporter KCC2 in human temporal lobe epilepsy. *Brain Struct Funct* 221:3601–3615.

Kasperaviciute D, Catarino CB, Matarin M, Leu C, Novy J, Tostevin A, et al. (2013) Epilepsy, hippocampal sclerosis and febrile seizures linked by common genetic variation around SCN1A. *Brain* 136:3140–3150.

Keller SS, Richardson MP, Schoene-Bake J-C, O'Muircheartaigh J, Elkommos S, Kreilkamp B, Goh YY, Marson A, Elger C, Weber B (2015) Thalamotemporal alteration and postoperative seizures in temporal lobe epilepsy. *Ann Neurol* 77:760–774

Kharatishvili I, Nissinen JP, McIntosh TK, Pitkänen A (2006) A model of posttraumatic epilepsy induced by lateral fluid-percussion brain injury in rats. *Neuroscience* 140:685–697.

King D, Spencer S (1995) Invasive electroencephalography in mesial temporal lobe epilepsy. *J Clin Neurophysiol* 12:32–45.

King D, Spencer SS, Bouthillier A, Kim J, de Lanerolle N, Bronen RA, McCarthy G, Luby M, Spencer DD (1996) Medial temporal lobe epilepsy without hippocampal atrophy. *J Epilepsy* 9:291–297.

Kleen JK, Scott RC, Holmes GL, Roberts DW, Rundle MM, Testorf M, Lenck-Santini P-P, Jobst BC (2013) Hippocampal interictal epileptiform activity disrupts cognition in humans. *Neurology* 81:18–24.

Klein P, Dingledine R, Aronica E, Bernard C, Blümcke I, Boison D, et al. (2018) Commonalities in epileptogenic processes from different acute brain insults: do they translate? *Epilepsia* 59:37–66.

Kobow K, Jeske I, Hildebrandt M, Hauke J, Hahnen E, Buslei R, Buchfelder M, Weigel D, Stefan H, Kasper B, et al. (2009) Increased reelin promoter methylation is associated with granule cell dispersion in human temporal lobe epilepsy. *J Neuropathol Exp Neurol* 68:356–364.

Köhr G, De Koninck Y, Mody I (1993) Properties of NMDA receptor channels in neurons acutely isolated from epileptic (kindled) rats. *J Neurosci* 13:3612–3627.

Kotti T, Riekkinen PJ, Miettinen R (1997) Characterization of target cells for aberrant mossy fiber collaterals in the dentate gyrus of epileptic rat. *Exp Neurol* 146:323–330.

Koyama R, Ikegaya Y (2018) The molecular and cellular mechanisms of axon guidance in mossy fiber sprouting. *Front Neurol* 9:382.

Koyama R, Yamada MK, Fujisawa S, Katoh-Semba R, Matsuki N, Ikegaya Y (2004) Brain-derived neurotrophic factor induces hyperexcitable reentrant circuits in the dentate gyrus. *J Neurosci* 24:7215–7224.

Krauss GL, Summerfield M, Brandt J, Breiter S, Ruchkin D (1997) Mesial temporal spikes interfere with working memory. *Neurology* 49:975–980.

Lado FA, Moshé SL (2008) How do seizures stop? *Epilepsia* 49:1651–1664.

Lam AD, Deck G, Goldman A, Eskandar EN, Noebels J, Cole AJ (2017) Silent hippocampal seizures and spikes identified by foramen ovale electrodes in Alzheimer's disease. *Nat Med* 23:678–680.

Lamberink HJ, Otte WM, Blümcke I, Braun KPJ, group EEBB writing, group study and EpiCARE ERN (2020) Seizure outcome and use of antiepileptic drugs after epilepsy surgery according to histopathological diagnosis: a retrospective multicentre cohort study. *Lancet Neurol* 19:748–757.

Lau LA, Staley KJ, Lillis KP (2022) In vitro ictogenesis is stochastic at the single neuron level. *Brain* 145:531–541.

Lerner JT, Sankar R, Mazarati AM (2008) Galanin and epilepsy. *Cell Mol Life Sci* 65:1864–1871.

Lévesque M, Avoli M, Bernard C (2016) Animal models of temporal lobe epilepsy following systemic chemoconvulsant administration. *J Neurosci Methods* 260:45–52.

Lewis DV, Shinnar S, Hesdorffer DC, Bagiella E, Bello JA, Chan S, et al. (2014) Hippocampal sclerosis after febrile status epilepticus: the FEBSTAT study. *Ann Neurol* 75:178–185.

Li LM, Cendes F, Andermann F, Watson C, Fish DR, Cook MJ, Dubeau F, Duncan JS, Shorvon SD, Berkovic SF, et al. (1999) Surgical outcome in patients with epilepsy and dual pathology. *Brain* 122:799–805.

Librizzi L, Losi G, Marcon I, Sessolo M, Scalmani P, Carmignoto G, de Curtis M (2017) Interneuronal network activity at the onset of seizure-like events in entorhinal cortex slices. *J Neurosci* 37:10398–10407.

Lieberman DN, Mody I (1999) Properties of single NMDA receptor channels in human dentate gyrus granule cells. *J Physiol* 518:55–70.

Lin H, Huang Y, Wang Y, Jia J (2011) Spatiotemporal profile of N-cadherin expression in the mossy fiber sprouting and synaptic plasticity following seizures. *Mol Cell Biochem* 358:201–205.

Lipton SA, Rosenberg PA (1994) Excitatory amino acids as a final common pathway for neurologic disorders. *N Engl J Med* 330:613–622.

Liu H, Mazarati AM, Katsumori H, Sankar R, Wasterlain CG (1999) Substance P is expressed in hippocampal principal neurons during status epilepticus and plays a critical role in the maintenance of status epilepticus. *Proc Natl Acad Sci U S A* 96:5286–5291.

Liu JYW, Dzurova N, Al-Kaaby B, Mills K, Sisodiya SM, Thom M (2020) Granule cell dispersion in human temporal lobe epilepsy: proteomics investigation of neurodevelopmental migratory pathways. *Front Cell Neurosci* 14:53.

Liu S-J, Zheng P, Wright DK, Dezsi G, Braine E, Nguyen T, Corcoran NM, Johnston LA, Hovens CM, Mayo JN, et al. (2016) Sodium selenate retards epileptogenesis in acquired epilepsy models reversing changes in protein phosphatase 2A and hyperphosphorylated tau. *Brain* 139:1919–1938.

Loacker S, Sayyah M, Wittmann W, Herzog H, Schwarzer C (2007) Endogenous dynorphin in epileptogenesis and epilepsy: anticonvulsant net effect via kappa opioid receptors. *Brain* 130:1017–1028.

Long L, Galovic M, Chen Y, Postma T, Vos SB, Xiao F, Wu W, Song Y, Huang S, Koepp M, et al. (2020) Shared hippocampal abnormalities in sporadic temporal lobe epilepsy patients and their siblings. *Epilepsia* 61:735–746.

Lowenstein DH, Thomas MJ, Smith DH, McIntosh TK (1992) Selective vulnerability of dentate hilar neurons following traumatic brain injury: a potential mechanistic link between head trauma and disorders of the hippocampus. *J Neurosci* 12:4846–4853.

Lugarà E, Kaushik R, Leite M, Chabrol E, Dityatev A, Lignani G, Walker MC (2020) LGI1 downregulation increases neuronal circuit excitability. *Epilepsia* 61:2836–2846.

Maglóczky Z (2010) Sprouting in human temporal lobe epilepsy: excitatory pathways and axons of interneurons. *Epilepsy Res* 89:52–59.

Magloire V, Cornford J, Lieb A, Kullmann DM, Pavlov I (2019) KCC2 overexpression prevents the paradoxical seizure-promoting action of somatic inhibition. *Nat Commun* 10:1225.

Marcelin B, Chauvière L, Becker A, Migliore M, Esclapez M, Bernard C (2009) h channel-dependent deficit of theta oscillation resonance and phase shift in temporal lobe epilepsy. *Neurobiol Dis* 33:436–447.

Maroso M, Balosso S, Ravizza T, Liu J, Aronica E, Iyer AM, Rossetti C, Molteni M, Casalgrandi M, Manfredi AA, et al. (2010) Toll-like receptor 4 and high-mobility group box-1 are involved in ictogenesis and can be targeted to reduce seizures. *Nat Med* 16:413–419.

Marsan CA, Zivin LS (1970) Factors related to the occurrence of typical paroxysmal abnormalities in the EEG records of epileptic patients. *Epilepsia* 11:361–381.

Marshall FH (2008) The role of GABA(B) receptors in the regulation of excitatory neurotransmission. *Results Probl Cell Differ* 44:87–98.

Mathern GW, Pretorius JK, Kornblum HI, Mendoza D, Lozada A, Leite JP, Chimelli LM, Fried I, Sakamoto AC, Assirati JA, et al. (1997) Human hippocampal AMPA and NMDA mRNA levels in temporal lobe epilepsy patients. *Brain* 120:1937–1959.

Matsumoto H, Marsan CA (1964) Cortical cellular phenomena in experimental epilepsy: interictal manifestations. *Exp Neurol* 9:286–304.

Mazarati A, Liu H, Wasterlain C (1999) Opioid peptide pharmacology and immunocytochemistry in an animal model of self-sustaining status epilepticus. *Neuroscience* 89:167–173.

McClelland S, Flynn C, Dubé C, Richichi C, Zha Q, Ghestem A, Esclapez M, Bernard C, Baram TZ (2011) Neuron-restrictive silencer factor-mediated hyperpolarization-activated cyclic nucleotide gated channelopathy in experimental temporal lobe epilepsy. *Ann Neurol* 70:454–464.

McNamara RK, Kirkby RD, dePape GE, Skelton RW, Corcoran ME (1993) Differential effects of kindling and kindled seizures on place learning in the Morris water maze. *Hippocampus* 3:149–152.

Meldrum B (1991) Excitotoxicity and epileptic brain damage. *Epilepsy Res* 10:55–61.

Meldrum BS, Brierley JB (1973) Prolonged epileptic seizures in primates: ischemic cell change and its relation to ictal physiological events. *Arch Neurol* 28:10–17.

Mellanby J, George G, Robinson A, Thompson P (1977) Epileptiform syndrome in rats produced by injecting tetanus toxin into the hippocampus. *J Neurol Neurosurg Psychiatry* 40:404–414.

Meyer A, Falconer MA, Beck E (1954) Pathological findings in temporal lobe epilepsy. *J Neurol Neurosurg Psychiatry* 17:276–285.

Miles R, Wong RK (1983) Single neurones can initiate synchronized population discharge in the hippocampus. *Nature* 306:371–373.

Moura DMS, de Sales IRP, Brandão JA, Costa MR, Queiroz CM (2021) Disentangling chemical and electrical effects of status epilepticus-induced dentate gyrus abnormalities. *Epilepsy Behav* 121:106575.

Muldoon SF, Villette V, Tressard T, Malvache A, Reichinnek S, Bartolomei F, Cossart R (2015) GABAergic inhibition shapes interictal dynamics in awake epileptic mice. *Brain* 138:2875–2890.

Ndode-Ekane XE, Pitkänen A (2013) Urokinase-type plasminogen activator receptor modulates epileptogenesis in mouse model of temporal lobe epilepsy. *Mol Neurobiol* 47:914–937.

Niquet J, Liu H, Wasterlain CG (2005) Programmed neuronal necrosis and status epilepticus. *Epilepsia* 46(Suppl 5):43–48.

Nissinen J, Lukasiuk K, Pitkänen A (2001) Is mossy fiber sprouting present at the time of the first spontaneous seizures in rat experimental temporal lobe epilepsy? *Hippocampus* 11:299–310.

Nobile C, Michelucci R, Andreazza S, Pasini E, Tosatto SCE, Striano P (2009) LGI1 mutations in autosomal dominant and sporadic lateral temporal epilepsy. *Hum Mutat* 30:530–536.

Noè F, Pool A-H, Nissinen J, Gobbi M, Bland R, Rizzi M, Balducci C, Ferraguti F, Sperk G, During MJ, et al. (2008) Neuropeptide Y gene therapy decreases chronic spontaneous seizures in a rat model of temporal lobe epilepsy. *Brain* 131:1506–1515.

Nusser Z, Hájos N, Somogyi P, Mody I (1998) Increased number of synaptic GABA(A) receptors underlies potentiation at hippocampal inhibitory synapses. *Nature* 395:172–177.

Nusser Z, Mody I (2002) Selective modulation of tonic and phasic inhibitions in dentate gyrus granule cells. *J Neurophysiol* 87:2624–2628.

Ortinski PI, Dong J, Mungenast A, Yue C, Takano H, Watson DJ, Haydon PG, Coulter DA (2010) Selective induction of astrocytic gliosis generates deficits in neuronal inhibition. *Nat Neurosci* 13:584–591.

Parent JM, Yu TW, Leibowitz RT, Geschwind DH, Sloviter RS, Lowenstein DH (1997) Dentate granule cell neurogenesis is increased by seizures and contributes to aberrant network reorganization in the adult rat hippocampus. *J Neurosci* 17:3727–3738.

Parras A, de Diego-Garcia L, Alves M, Beamer E, Conte G, Jimenez-Mateos EM, Morgan J, Ollà I, Hernandez-Santana Y, Delanty N, et al. (2020) Polyadenylation of mRNA as a novel regulatory mechanism of gene expression in temporal lobe epilepsy. *Brain* 143:2139–2153.

Pauletti A, Terrone G, Shekh-Ahmad T, Salamone A, Ravizza T, Rizzi M, Pastore A, Pascente R, Liang L-P, Villa BR, et al. (2019) Targeting oxidative stress improves disease outcomes in a rat model of acquired epilepsy. *Brain* 142:e39.

Pavlov I, Huusko N, Drexel M, Kirchmair E, Sperk G, Pitkänen A, Walker MC (2011) Progressive loss of phasic, but not tonic, GABAA receptor-mediated inhibition in dentate granule cells in a model of post-traumatic epilepsy in rats. *Neuroscience* 194:208–219.

Pavlov I, Savtchenko LP, Kullmann DM, Semyanov A, Walker MC (2009) Outwardly rectifying tonically active GABAA receptors in pyramidal cells modulate neuronal offset, not gain. *J Neurosci* 29:15341–15350.

Peng C, Trojanowski JQ, Lee VM-Y (2020) Protein transmission in neurodegenerative disease. *Nat Rev Neurol* 16:199–212.

Peret A, Christie LA, Ouedraogo DW, Gorlewicz A, Epsztein J, Mulle C, Crépel V (2014) Contribution of aberrant GluK2-containing kainate receptors to chronic seizures in temporal lobe epilepsy. *Cell Rep* 8:347–354.

Pfleger L (1880) Beobachtungen uber schrumpfung und Sclerose des Ammonshornes bei Epilepsie. *Allg Z Für Psychiatr* 36:359–365.

Pierce JP, Melton J, Punsoni M, McCloskey DP, Scharfman HE (2005) Mossy fibers are the primary source of afferent input to ectopic granule cells that are born after pilocarpine-induced seizures. *Exp Neurol* 196:316–331.

Postma TS, Cury C, Baxendale S, Thompson PJ, Cano-López I, de Tisi J, Burdett JL, Sidhu MK, Caciagli L, Winston GP, et al. (2020) Hippocampal shape is associated with memory deficits in temporal lobe epilepsy. *Ann Neurol* **88**:170–182.

Proper EA, Hoogland G, Kappen SM, Jansen GH, Rensen MGA, Schrama LH, van Veelen CWM, van Rijen PC, van Nieuwenhuizen O, Gispen WH, et al. (2002) Distribution of glutamate transporters in the hippocampus of patients with pharmaco-resistant temporal lobe epilepsy. *Brain* **125**:32–43.

Proper EA, Oestreicher AB, Jansen GH, Veelen CW, van Rijen PC, Gispen WH, de Graan PN (2000) Immunohistochemical characterization of mossy fibre sprouting in the hippocampus of patients with pharmaco-resistant temporal lobe epilepsy. *Brain* **123**:19–30.

Rajasekaran K, Todorovic M, Kapur J (2012) Calcium-permeable AMPA receptors are expressed in a rodent model of status epilepticus. *Ann Neurol* **72**:91–102.

Raus Balind S, Magó Á, Ahmadi M, Kis N, Varga-Németh Z, Lőrincz A, Makara JK (2019) Diverse synaptic and dendritic mechanisms of complex spike burst generation in hippocampal CA3 pyramidal cells. *Nat Commun* **10**:1859.

Rausch R, Lieb JP, Crandall PH (1978) Neuropsychologic correlates of depth spike activity in epileptic patients. *Arch Neurol* **35**:699–705.

Reddy DS, Kuruba R (2013) Experimental models of status epilepticus and neuronal injury for evaluation of therapeutic interventions. *Int J Mol Sci* **14**:18284–18318.

Reed CM, Mosher CP, Chandravadia N, Chung JM, Mamelak AN, Rutishauser U (2020) Extent of single-neuron activity modulation by hippocampal interictal discharges predicts declarative memory disruption in humans. *J Neurosci* **40**:682–693.

Ren L, Kucewicz MT, Cimbalnik J, Matsumoto JY, Brinkmann BH, Hu W, Marsh WR, Meyer FB, Stead SM, Worrell GA (2015) Gamma oscillations precede interictal epileptiform spikes in the seizure onset zone. *Neurology* **84**:602–608.

Roehri N, Pizzo F, Lagarde S, Lambert I, Nica A, McGonigal A, Giusiano B, Bartolomei F, Bénar C-G (2018) High-frequency oscillations are not better biomarkers of epileptogenic tissues than spikes. *Ann Neurol* **83**:84–97.

Roper SN, Obenaus A, Dudek FE (1992) Osmolality and nonsynaptic epileptiform bursts in rat CA1 and dentate gyrus. *Ann Neurol* **31**:81–85.

Rusakov DA, Kullmann DM (1998) Extrasynaptic glutamate diffusion in the hippocampus: ultrastructural constraints, uptake, and receptor activation. *J Neurosci* **18**:3158–3170.

Sadleir LG, Scheffer IE (2007) Febrile seizures. *BMJ* **334**:307–311.

Sawires R, Buttery J, Fahey M (2022) A review of febrile seizures: recent advances in understanding of febrile seizure pathophysiology and commonly implicated viral triggers. *Front Pediatr* **9**:801321

Scheffer IE, Berkovic S, Capovilla G, Connolly MB, French J, Guilhoto L, Hirsch E, Jain S, Mathern GW, Moshé SL, et al. (2017) ILAE classification of the epilepsies: position paper of the ILAE Commission for Classification and Terminology. *Epilepsia* **58**:512–521.

Scheibel ME, Crandall PH, Scheibel AB (1974) The hippocampal-dentate complex in temporal lobe epilepsy: a Golgi study. *Epilepsia* **15**:55–80.

Schevon CA, Weiss SA, McKhann G, Goodman RR, Yuste R, Emerson RG, Trevelyan AJ (2012) Evidence of an inhibitory restraint of seizure activity in humans. *Nat Commun* **3**:1060.

Schidlitzki A, Twele F, Klee R, Waltl I, Römermann K, Bröer S, Meller S, Gerhauser I, Rankovic V, Li D, et al. (2017) A combination of NMDA and AMPA receptor antagonists retards granule cell dispersion and epileptogenesis in a model of acquired epilepsy. *Sci Rep* **7**:12191.

Schulte U, Thumfart J-O, Klöcker N, Sailer CA, Bildl W, Biniossek M, Dehn D, Deller T, Eble S, Abbass K, et al. (2006) The epilepsy-linked Lgi1 protein assembles into presynaptic Kv1 channels and inhibits inactivation by Kvbeta1. *Neuron* **49**:697–706.

Schwarzer C, Tsunashima K, Wanzenböck C, Fuchs K, Sieghart W, Sperk G (1997) GABA(A) receptor subunits in the rat hippocampus II: altered distribution in kainic acid-induced temporal lobe epilepsy. *Neuroscience* **80**:1001–1017.

Scimemi A, Andersson A, Heeroma JH, Strandberg J, Rydenhag B, McEvoy AW, Thom M, Asztely F, Walker MC (2006) Tonic GABA(A) receptor-mediated currents in human brain. *Eur J Neurosci* **24**:1157–1160.

Scimemi A, Schorge S, Kullmann DM, Walker MC (2006) Epileptogenesis is associated with enhanced glutamatergic transmission in the perforant path. *J Neurophysiol* **95**:1213–1220.

Scimemi A, Semyanov A, Sperk G, Kullmann DM, Walker MC (2005) Multiple and plastic receptors mediate tonic GABAA receptor currents in the hippocampus. *J Neurosci* **25**:10016–10024.

Semah F, Picot MC, Adam C, Broglin D, Arzimanoglou A, Bazin B, Cavalcanti D, Baulac M (1998) Is the underlying cause of epilepsy a major prognostic factor for recurrence? *Neurology* **51**:1256–1262.

Sessolo M, Marcon I, Bovetti S, Losi G, Cammarota M, Ratto GM, Fellin T, Carmignoto G (2015) Parvalbumin-positive inhibitory interneurons oppose propagation but favor generation of focal epileptiform activity. *J Neurosci* **35**:9544–9557.

Shah MM, Anderson AE, Leung V, Lin X, Johnston D (2004) Seizure-induced plasticity of h channels in entorhinal cortical layer III pyramidal neurons. *Neuron* **44**:495–508.

Shapiro LA, Ribak CE (2005) Integration of newly born dentate granule cells into adult brains: hypotheses based on normal and epileptic rodents. *Brain Res Brain Res Rev* **48**:43–56.

Shekh-Ahmad T, Eckel R, Dayalan Naidu S, Higgins M, Yamamoto M, Dinkova-Kostova AT, Kovac S, Abramov AY, Walker MC (2018) KEAP1 inhibition is neuroprotective and suppresses the development of epilepsy. *Brain* **141**:1390–1403.

Sheybani L, Birot G, Contestabile A, Seeck M, Kiss JZ, Schaller K, Michel CM, Quairiaux C (2018) Electrophysiological evidence for the development of a self-sustained large-scale epileptic network in the kainate mouse model of temporal lobe epilepsy. *J Neurosci* **38**:3776–3791.

Shin M, Brager D, Jaramillo TC, Johnston D, Chetkovich DM (2008) Mislocalization of h channel subunits underlies h channelopathy in temporal lobe epilepsy. *Neurobiol Dis* **32**:26–36.

Singh G, Burneo JG, Sander JW (2013) From seizures to epilepsy and its substrates: neurocysticercosis. *Epilepsia* **54**:783–792.

Sinjab B, Martinian L, Sisodiya SM, Thom M (2013) Regional thalamic neuropathology in patients with hippocampal sclerosis and epilepsy: a postmortem study. *Epilepsia* **54**:2125–2133.

Sloviter RS (1991) Permanently altered hippocampal structure, excitability, and inhibition after experimental status epilepticus in the rat: the "dormant basket cell" hypothesis and its possible relevance to temporal lobe epilepsy. *Hippocampus* **1**:41–66.

Sloviter RS, Zappone CA, Harvey BD, Bumanglag AV, Bender RA, Frotscher M (2003) "Dormant basket cell" hypothesis revisited: relative vulnerabilities of dentate gyrus mossy cells and inhibitory interneurons after hippocampal status epilepticus in the rat. *J Comp Neurol* **459**:44–76.

Smith EH, Liou J, Davis TS, Merricks EM, Kellis SS, Weiss SA, Greger B, House PA, McKhann GM, Goodman RR, et al. (2016) The ictal wavefront is the spatiotemporal source of discharges during spontaneous human seizures. *Nat Commun* **7**:11098.

Snowball A, Chabrol E, Wykes RC, Shekh-Ahmad T, Cornford JH, Lieb A, Hughes MP, Massaro G, Rahim AA, Hashemi KS, et al. (2019) Epilepsy gene therapy using an engineered potassium channel. *J Neurosci* **39**:3159–3169.

Sofroniew MV, Vinters HV (2010) Astrocytes: biology and pathology. *Acta Neuropathol (Berl)* **119**:7–35.

Sommer W (1880) Erkrankung des Ammonshornes als aetiologisches Moment der Epilepsie. *Arch Psychiatr Nervenkr* **10**:631–675.

Sone D, Sato N, Maikusa N, Ota M, Sumida K, Yokoyama K, Kimura Y, Imabayashi E, Watanabe Y, Watanabe M, et al. (2016) Automated subfield volumetric analysis of hippocampus in temporal lobe epilepsy using high-resolution T2-weighed MR imaging. *NeuroImage Clin* **12**:57–64.

Stiglbauer V, Hotka M, Ruiß M, Hilber K, Boehm S, Kubista H (2017) Cav 1.3 channels play a crucial role in the formation of paroxysmal depolarization shifts in cultured hippocampal neurons. *Epilepsia* **58**:858–871.

Straub H, Speckmann EJ, Bingmann D, Walden J (1990) Paroxysmal depolarization shifts induced by bicuculline in CA3 neurons of hippocampal slices: suppression by the organic calcium antagonist verapamil. *Neurosci Lett* **111**:99–101.

Su H, Sochivko D, Becker A, Chen J, Jiang Y, Yaari Y, Beck H (2002) Upregulation of a T-type Ca2+ channel causes a long-lasting modification of neuronal firing mode after status epilepticus. *J Neurosci* **22**:3645–3655.

Sutula T, Cascino G, Cavazos J, Parada I, Ramirez L (1989) Mossy fiber synaptic reorganization in the epileptic human temporal lobe. *Ann Neurol* **26**:321–330.

Suzuki F, Heinrich C, Boehrer A, Mitsuya K, Kurokawa K, Matsuda M, Depaulis A (2005) Glutamate receptor antagonists and benzodiazepine inhibit the progression of granule cell dispersion in a mouse model of mesial temporal lobe epilepsy. *Epilepsia* **46**:193–202.

Swann JW, Rho JM (2014) How is homeostatic plasticity important in epilepsy? *Adv Exp Med Biol* **813**:123–131.

Swissa E, Serlin Y, Vazana U, Prager O, Friedman A (2019) Blood-brain barrier dysfunction in status epileptics: mechanisms and role in epileptogenesis. *Epilepsy Behav* **101**:106285.

Szczygieł JA, Danielsen KI, Melin E, Rosenkranz SH, Pankratova S, Ericsson A, Agerman K, Kokaia M, Woldbye DPD (2020) Gene therapy vector encoding neuropeptide Y and its receptor Y2 for future treatment of epilepsy: preclinical data in rats. *Front Mol Neurosci* **13**:232.

Tai XY, Bernhardt B, Thom M, Thompson P, Baxendale S, Koepp M, Bernasconi N (2018) Review: neurodegenerative processes in temporal lobe epilepsy with hippocampal sclerosis: clinical, pathological and neuroimaging evidence. *Neuropathol Appl Neurobiol* **44**:70–90.

Tai XY, Koepp M, Duncan JS, Fox N, Thompson P, Baxendale S, Liu JYW, Reeves C, Michalak Z, Thom M (2016) Hyperphosphorylated tau in patients with refractory epilepsy correlates with cognitive decline: a study of temporal lobe resections. *Brain* **139**:2441–2455.

Tanaka H, Grooms SY, Bennett MV, Zukin RS (2000) The AMPAR subunit GluR2:still front and center-stage. *Brain Res* **886**:190–207.

Tanaka K, Watase K, Manabe T, Yamada K, Watanabe M, Takahashi K, Iwama H, Nishikawa T, Ichihara N, Kikuchi T, et al. (1997) Epilepsy and exacerbation of brain injury in mice lacking the glutamate transporter GLT-1. *Science* **276**:1699–1702.

Theodore WH, Bhatia S, Hatta J, Fazilat S, DeCarli C, Bookheimer SY, Gaillard WD (1999) Hippocampal atrophy, epilepsy duration, and febrile seizures in patients with partial seizures. *Neurology* **52**:132–136.

Thom M (2014) Review: hippocampal sclerosis in epilepsy: a neuropathology review. *Neuropathol Appl Neurobiol* **40**:520–543.

Thom M, Eriksson S, Martinian L, Caboclo LO, McEvoy AW, Duncan JS, Sisodiya SM (2009) Temporal lobe sclerosis associated with hippocampal sclerosis in temporal lobe epilepsy: neuropathological features. *J Neuropathol Exp Neurol* **68**:928–938.

Thom M, Liagkouras I, Elliot KJ, Martinian L, Harkness W, McEvoy A, Caboclo LO, Sisodiya SM (2010) Reliability of patterns of hippocampal sclerosis as predictors of postsurgical outcome. *Epilepsia* **51**:1801–1808.

Thom M, Liagkouras I, Martinian L, Liu J, Catarino CB, Sisodiya SM (2012) Variability of sclerosis along the longitudinal hippocampal axis in epilepsy: a post mortem study. *Epilepsy Res* **102**:45–59.

Thom M, Martinian L, Catarino C, Yogarajah M, Koepp MJ, Caboclo L, Sisodiya SM (2009) Bilateral reorganization of the dentate gyrus in hippocampal sclerosis: a postmortem study. *Neurology* **73**:1033–1040.

Thom M, Zhou J, Martinian L, Sisodiya S (2005) Quantitative postmortem study of the hippocampus in chronic epilepsy: seizures do not inevitably cause neuronal loss. *Brain* **128**:1344–1357.

Traub RD, Jefferys JG, Miles R, Whittington MA, Tóth K (1994) A branching dendritic model of a rodent CA3 pyramidal neurone. *J Physiol* **481**:79–95.

Tuunanen J, Pitkänen A (2000) Do seizures cause neuronal damage in rat amygdala kindling? *Epilepsy Res* **39**:171–176.

Van Paesschen W, Duncan JS, Stevens JM, Connelly A (1998) Longitudinal quantitative hippocampal magnetic resonance imaging study of adults with newly diagnosed partial seizures: one-year follow-up results. *Epilepsia* **39**:633–639.

Van Paesschen W, Revesz T, Duncan JS, King MD, Connelly A (1997) Quantitative neuropathology and quantitative magnetic resonance imaging of the hippocampus in temporal lobe epilepsy. *Ann Neurol* **42**:756–766.

van Sonderen A, Thijs RD, Coenders EC, Jiskoot LC, Sanchez E, de Bruijn MAAM, van Coevorden-Hameete MH, Wirtz PW, Schreurs MWJ, Sillevis Smitt PAE, et al. (2016) Anti-LGI1 encephalitis: clinical syndrome and long-term follow-up. *Neurology* **87**:1449–1456.

van Vliet EA, Aronica E, Tolner EA, Lopes da Silva FH, Gorter JA (2004) Progression of temporal lobe epilepsy in the rat is associated with immunocytochemical changes in inhibitory interneurons in specific regions of the hippocampal formation. *Exp Neurol* **187**:367–379.

van Vliet EA, Aronica E, Vezzani A, Ravizza T (2018) Review: neuroinflammatory pathways as treatment targets and biomarker candidates in epilepsy: emerging evidence from preclinical and clinical studies. *Neuropathol Appl Neurobiol* **44**:91–111.

Vespa PM, McArthur DL, Xu Y, Eliseo M, Etchepare M, Dinov I, Alger J, Glenn TP, Hovda D (2010) Nonconvulsive seizures after traumatic brain injury are associated with hippocampal atrophy. *Neurology* **75**:792–798.

Vezzani A, Sperk G (2004) Overexpression of NPY and Y2 receptors in epileptic brain tissue: an endogenous neuroprotective mechanism in temporal lobe epilepsy? *Neuropeptides* **38**:245–252.

Vezzani A, Sperk G, Colmers WF (1999) Neuropeptide Y: emerging evidence for a functional role in seizure modulation. *Trends Neurosci* **22**:25–30.

Viitanen T, Ruusuvuori E, Kaila K, Voipio J (2010) The K+-Cl cotransporter KCC2 promotes GABAergic excitation in the mature rat hippocampus. *J Physiol* **588**:1527–1540.

Vivekananda U: Bush D, Bisby JA, Diehl B, Jha A, Nachev P, Rodionov R, Burgess N, Walker MC (2019) Spatial and episodic memory tasks promote temporal lobe interictal spikes. *Ann Neurol* **86**:304–309.

Walker MC, Jefferys JGR, Wykes RC (2017) Tetanus toxin. In: Models of Seizures and Epilepsy, Second Edition (Pitkänen A, Buckmaster PS, Galanopoulou AS, Moshé SL, eds) pp 589–598. Academic Press.

Weiss JH, Sensi SL (2000) Ca2+ -Zn2+ permeable AMPA or kainate receptors: possible key factors in selective neurodegeneration. *Trends Neurosci* **23**:365–371.

Williams-Karnesky RL, Sandau US, Lusardi TA, Lytle NK, Farrell JM, Pritchard EM, Kaplan DL, Boison D (2013) Epigenetic changes induced by adenosine augmentation therapy prevent epileptogenesis. *J Clin Invest* 123:3552–3563.

Williamson PD, French JA, Thadani VM, Kim JH, Novelly RA, Spencer SS, Spencer DD, Mattson RH (1993) Characteristics of medial temporal lobe epilepsy: II. Interictal and ictal scalp electroencephalography, neuropsychological testing, neuroimaging, surgical results, and pathology. *Ann Neurol* 34:781–787.

Witt J-A, Coras R, Schramm J, Becker AJ, Elger CE, Blümcke I, Helmstaedter C (2014) The overall pathological status of the left hippocampus determines preoperative verbal memory performance in left mesial temporal lobe epilepsy. *Hippocampus* 24:446–454.

Wittner L, Eross L, Czirják S, Halász P, Freund TF, Maglóczky Z (2005) Surviving CA1 pyramidal cells receive intact perisomatic inhibitory input in the human epileptic hippocampus. *Brain* 128:138–152.

Yilmazer-Hanke DM, Wolf HK, Schramm J, Elger CE, Wiestler OD, Blümcke I (2000) Subregional pathology of the amygdala complex and entorhinal region in surgical specimens from patients with pharmacoresistant temporal lobe epilepsy. *J Neuropathol Exp Neurol* 59:907–920.

Yoong M, Martinos MM, Chin RF, Clark CA, Scott RC (2013) Hippocampal volume loss following childhood convulsive status epilepticus is not limited to prolonged febrile seizures. *Epilepsia* 54:2108–2115.

You JC, Muralidharan K, Park JW, Petrof I, Pyfer MS, Corbett BF, LaFrancois JJ, Zheng Y, Zhang X, Mohila CA, et al. (2017) Epigenetic suppression of hippocampal calbindin-D28k by ΔFosB drives seizure-related cognitive deficits. *Nat Med* 23:1377–1383.

Young D, Dragunow M (1994) Status epilepticus may be caused by loss of adenosine anticonvulsant mechanisms. *Neuroscience* 58:245–261.

Zhan R-Z, Nadler JV (2009) Enhanced tonic GABA current in normotopic and hilar ectopic dentate granule cells after pilocarpine-induced status epilepticus. *J Neurophysiol* 102:670–681.

Zhang N, Wei W, Mody I, Houser CR (2007) Altered localization of GABA(A) receptor subunits on dentate granule cell dendrites influences tonic and phasic inhibition in a mouse model of epilepsy. *J Neurosci* 27:7520–7531.

Zhou J-L, Lenck-Santini P-P, Zhao Q, Holmes GL (2007) Effect of interictal spikes on single-cell firing patterns in the hippocampus. *Epilepsia* 48:720–731.

Zhou Q-G, Nemes AD, Lee D, Ro EJ, Zhang J, Nowacki AS, Dymecki SM, Najm IM, Suh H (2019) Chemogenetic silencing of hippocampal neurons suppresses epileptic neural circuits. *J Clin Invest* 129:310–323.

Zijlmans M, Jiruska P, Zelmann R, Leijten FSS, Jefferys JGR, Gotman J (2012) High-frequency oscillations as a new biomarker in epilepsy. *Ann Neurol* 71:169–178.

Zuckermann EC, Glaser GH (1968) Hippocampal epileptic activity induced by localized ventricular perfusion with high-potassium cerebrospinal fluid. *Exp Neurol* 20:87–110.

19

Schizophrenic Psychosis and the Hippocampus: Schizophrenia Mechanisms in the Hippocampus

The Role of Hippocampal Hyperactivity

Carol A. Tamminga, Daniel Scott, and Elena I. Ivleva

19.1 Introduction

19.1.1 Schizophrenia

Schizophrenia is a chronic psychotic disorder most prominently characterized by continuous or episodic manifestations including hallucinations (in any sensory modality), delusions, and/or thought disorder. Schizophrenia can also include some level of cognitive dysfunction, particularly in verbal memory and attention (Carpenter and Buchanan, 1994). [Box 19.1]. Once schizophrenia has its onset with a florid episode of psychosis, the person's mental status is often never the same, i.e., the psychotic mental manifestations rarely go away entirely, even with treatment.

The disorder characteristically begins in late adolescence or young adulthood. Childhood onset before 10 years of age represents less than 5% of the population and late onset (> 40 years) has approximately the same prevalence. Onset at any age leads to an illness with similar clinical characteristics and pharmacology. Once the psychosis begins, it customarily extends through the rest of the individual's lifetime. Cures are rare (Greenberg, 1964), even though symptoms can fade. Treatments are troublesome and incomplete (Correll, Martin, et al., 2022). Florid psychotic symptoms can be blunted, but not fully erased. Cognitive manifestations and negative symptoms are often worsened by antipsychotic treatment. The cognitive and negative symptoms can precede the first full psychotic episode by as much as 5–10 years (Velthorst, Fett, et al., 2017).

Box 19.1 Psychosis description

Psychosis is a brain disorder with persistent psychotic manifestations, variable cognitive dysfunction, and inevitable psychosocial impairment. The psychotic manifestations include delusions, hallucinations, and thought disorder. The most severe cognitive dysfunction is in relational memory.

A delusion is an incorrect belief that is firmly held against all reason. The false belief itself (i.e., a delusion) is a complex idea that is not true, often unreasonable, odd, and not based on previous experience. It resembles a memory and could use the brain's memory mechanisms in hippocampus to establish itself. A delusional individual with schizophrenia commonly has one or two recurring delusions, but not delusions that vary continuously. With each person, the same content is modified only slightly over time and held with various degrees of tenacity, and characteristically it involves the same storyline. There is wide variability across individuals in the content of delusions. Such a person might believe that their brain is being used by the US government as a surveillance tool on the Mexican-American border to gather data for generals in Washington; or, that their mother is trying to poison them with specific foods in their diet. A delusion appears as a fixed, odd, unlikely, and/or false memory. Even when psychosis is treated pharmacologically, delusions tend to resolve slowly, resulting in variable degrees of delusional symptoms and insight overtime. Even the most stable psychotic persons retain the memory of the delusion but may not think it is important anymore.

Hallucinations are sensory experiences that are not actually taking place. Hallucinatory experiences can use any of the sensory categories, including auditory, visual, olfactory, and/or somatosensory. When a psychotic person hears voices, it is a consistent storyline, not typically a different person or topics across time, but the voices remain the same, with great variability in content across individuals. People with psychosis hear a characteristic set of voices, with distinct identities and fixed levels of affect (e.g., complimentary, accusatory, threatening, pleasing, etc.); some hallucinations are ill-formed sounds; commonly hallucinations are a single voice talking, while some hallucinations include multiple voices talking with each other and to the affected person. Individuals with schizophrenia have somatosensory hallucinations, feeling a spider in their brain or touch on their arm. These kind of delusional and hallucinatory elements of psychotic thinking could be based on dysfunctional hippocampal activity playing on memory materials, albeit incorrectly associated, using usual mechanisms of memory, but without the relationship to reality testing that we rely on for normal memories. Thought disorder is reflected in speech that is illogical, contrived, and contradictory, such that thoughts do not fit together. This review will develop the evidence that the hippocampus contributes, in part, to the genesis and persistence of psychotic thinking in humans.

There are many different courses of illness (Ciompi, 1980), but the trajectory is downward in the main, in terms of brain function and psychosocial performance (Andreasen, Liu, et al., 2013; Kotov, Fochtmann, et al., 2017; Velthorst, Fett, et al., 2017). Rarely do longitudinal studies report recovery, but some individuals prevail and can live gainful, sometimes remarkable, lives (Saks, 2007). The actual variability in outcomes is high; heterogeneity in signs and symptoms is similarly broad. It has been only since schizophrenia genetics has shown broad heterogeneity in its associations that speculations have been raised that some variants could represent distinct pathophysiology (Lee, Ripke, et al., 2013). All of the outcome reports since 1950 have included affected individuals treated chronically with antipsychotic drugs (Correll, Solmi, et al., 2023). However, there are occasional populations to whom antipsychotic drugs have been unavailable. Here, the psychosocial outcome and brain measures of these never-treated individuals deteriorate more extensively than in treated persons, suggesting that antipsychotic treatment could protect brain through unknown mechanisms in some psychotic persons (Zhao, Zhang, et al., 2022).

19.1.2 Current treatments

Delnay and Deniker, two French psychiatrists responsible for a hospital of psychotic persons in 1950 Paris, heard of a new presurgical anesthetic that caused sedation and forgetfulness in normal people. They thought that this kind of sedation might help people with schizophrenia be more oblivious to psychotic symptoms. So, they administered chlorpromazine (Thorazine) to affected individuals and made the transformational observation not only that the drug was sedative but also that it selectively reduced psychotic symptoms (Lopez-Munoz, Alamo, et al., 2005). The treatment swept the world, emptied out mental hospitals, and brought hope to many people. Then, only 10 years later, Carlsson and Lindqvist (1963) discovered the antidopaminergic properties of Thorazine and parallel actions at other amine receptors. This allowed innovative pharmacologists like Paul Janssen (1967) to make additional antidopaminergic drugs to increase efficacy and reduce side effects, and soon there were not only first- but also second-generation antipsychotic drugs. The early antipsychotic drugs were within the same drug class as Thorazine (phenothiazines) and mimicked their putative mechanism of action as dopamine receptor antagonists. The follow-ons became highly potent at antagonizing dopamine receptors, all called first-generation antipsychotic drugs. After 20 years there again came an innovation; the antidopaminergic action of the most potent drug, haloperidol, was linked with a serotonin antagonist to broaden its action and relieve motor side effects, and risperidone was born (Leysen, Gommeren, et al., 1988), a second-generation drug. Soon, the pharmacology advanced further with the demonstration that agonists for the presynaptic dopamine receptors actually reduce the synthesis and release of dopamine and are antipsychotic (Tamminga and Carlsson, 2002); they act as indirect dopamine antagonists, often called partial dopamine agonists. And with the advent of more antidopaminergic treatment compounds (Creese, Manian, et al., 1978), Snyder and colleagues were able to demonstrate a tight correlation between the affinity of a drug for the dopamine receptor and its antipsychotic potency, connecting a dampening of the dopamine system in the human disorder with its antipsychotic effect. Throughout this whole time, there was one drug that performed the best of any antipsychotic (Woerner, Robinson, et al., 2003), yet with many serious side effects and a very complex pharmacology (Coward, 1992), called clozapine; it remains the broadest acting and most effective antipsychotic drug in 2024.

19.1.3 Mechanisms of schizophrenia: classical and long-standing formulations

At one time, there were many fantastical mechanisms proposed to account for psychosis. These ranged from demon possession to prophet status, from bad genes to immune dysfunction, from a frontal lobe disorder to altered synaptic function (Tamminga, 2020). The discovery of Thorazine (Lopez-Munoz, Alamo, et al., 2005) and its antidopaminergic mechanisms as postulated by Carlsson and Lindqvist (1963), motivated thinking to the dopamine hypothesis. Based on this biological clue, scientists studied available aspects of dopamine regulation, in an attempt to demonstrate this hypothesis of schizophrenia (Correll and Howes, 2021). While there have been subtle and undeniable dopaminergic hyperfunction characteristics discovered in this 50-year search (McCutcheon, Abi-Dargham, et al., 2019), these have been more modest than anticipated.

In addition, with time, it has become apparent that a dopamine antagonist, even if it is used at correct doses and with regular administration, does not reverse schizophrenia, even though it can modify psychotic symptoms. Neither is there any effect of the antidopaminergic drugs on cognition or negative symptoms, and often the best treatment outcomes coexist with residual psychosis. So, gradually, scientists have started proposing additional and new hypotheses of pathophysiology. Based on the demonstration of the psychotomimetic action of ketamine and its psychosis-stimulation properties in schizophrenia (Lahti, Koffel, et al., 1995), the glutamatergic hypothesis was born (Tamminga, 1998). Glutamatergic drugs are difficult to develop (Adams, Kinon, et al., 2013) and are associated with target changes and neuroplasticity, and therapeutics are still inadequate, despite many clever hypotheses and integrated theories (Lisman, Coyle, et al., 2008). The situation has encouraged psychosis investigators to identify other elements in brain to explain psychosis pathophysiology. This has included the proposal that the hippocampus might have a role in psychotic disorders (Tamminga, Stan, et al., 2010), with the tentative suggestion that hippocampal hyperactivity is involved. This is supported by added evidence of its anatomic, molecular, genetic and functional alterations in schizophrenia (Heckers, Rauch, et al., 1998; Tamminga, 1998; Medoff, Holcomb, et al., 2001; Schobel, Lewandowski, et al., 2009; Coyle, Balu, et al., 2010; Schobel, Chaudhury, et al., 2013; Heckers and Konradi, 2015; Kätzel, Wolff, et al., 2020).

19.1.4 How could schizophrenia mechanisms include the hippocampus?

Since the early days of biological studies in psychotic disorders, particularly in schizophrenia, there has been considerable interest in hippocampal pathology, both as underlying the episodic memory dysfunction in schizophrenia and as having a role in psychotic manifestations themselves (Stevens, 1973; Kovelman and Scheibel, 1984; Benes, 1989; Javitt and Zukin, 1990; Saykin, Gur, et al., 1991; McCarley, Shenton, et al., 1993; Tamminga, 1998; Weinberger, 1999; Tamminga, Stan, et al., 2010; Tamminga and Zukin, 2015). Early investigators theorized a parallel between behaviors of persons with psychosis and the gross behavior of persons with other kinds of hippocampal dysfunctions like epilepsy. Modern neuroscience techniques have provided high-resolution brain imaging, postmortem genetic and protein expression studies, and animal model experiments applied to the hippocampus, and the resulting advances have provided testable hypotheses of psychosis pathophysiology. With this have emerged several clear, even prescient, observations over recent decades, that focus on the presence of hippocampal hyperactivity as a critical pathological feature in psychosis, especially in early psychosis.

19.2 Hippocampal hyperactivity in schizophrenia

19.2.1 What is hippocampal hyperactivity?

Hyperactivity in the hippocampal formation, whether of a regular neuronal firing pattern or of a complex, integrated neural signal, has been reliably detected in individuals with schizophrenic psychosis across several laboratories (Figure 19.1). First demonstrated using positron emission tomography (PET) (Medoff, Holcomb, et al., 2001), then recorded with resting-state functional magnetic resonance imaging (fMRI) (Lahti, Weiler, et al., 2006; Malaspina, Corcoran, et al., 2009; Lui, Yao, et al., 2015) and the high-resolution MRI/Vascular-Active-Occupancy (VASO) technique (Heckers, Zalesak, et al., 2004), the hippocampus, bilaterally, represents the primary brain region in schizophrenia, where neuronal activity is *increased*. While the hippocampus appears to be *hyper*active in schizophrenic psychosis, other affected regions of brain in the same individuals (e.g., prefrontal cortex, thalamus) typically show *hypo*activity (Lui, Yao, et al., 2015). It is not known whether all regional activity alterations in schizophrenia are related or whether

distinct changes are independent and support independent cerebral dysfunctions (Samudra, Ivleva, et al., 2015). The increased hippocampal activity captured with PET/^{15}O-water or VASO appears to be partially sensitive to antipsychotic medication (Medoff, Holcomb, et al., 2001; Lahti, Weiler, et al., 2006)and correlates with the magnitude of cognitive dysfunction (Tregellas, Smucny, et al., 2014). These functional alterations have focused experimental molecular and cellular models of schizophrenia onto the hippocampus. While these formulations do not postulate that the hippocampus must be the *only* region involved, we have proposed that HH perverts a memory in the process of consolidation into a psychotic construct which is ten consolidated as a normal memory. The possibility that this kind of perverted memory could be experienced as a psychotic memory underlies the potential involvement of the hippocampus in psychotic disorders.

19.2.2 How is hyperactivity detected and located to distinct subfields?

The high-resolution cerebral blood volume (CBV) techniques have provided the most valuable tools to assess regional activity within hippocampal subfields. This technique measures CBV, as opposed to the cerebral blood flow measured by conventional blood-oxygen-level-dependent (BOLD) fMRI (Lu and van Zijl, 2012; Talati, Rane, et al., 2015). The ability to use this technique to collect high-resolution data from the hippocampal subfields underscores its importance to hippocampal studies. Several early CBV studies localized the hippocampal hyperactivity in psychosis to the CA1

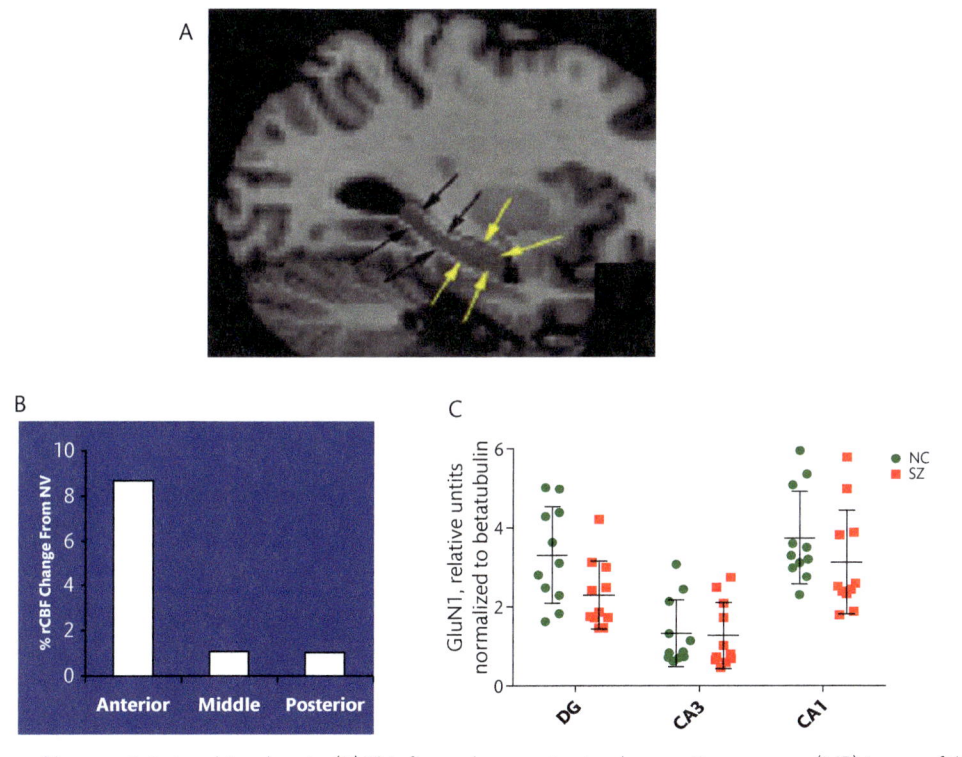

Figure 19.1 Hippocampal hyperactivity in schizophrenia. (A) This figure shows a structural magnetic resonance (MR) image of the human hippocampus. The anterior hippocampus is identified with yellow arrows, while the posterior hippocampus is shown with black arrows. (B) Regional hyperactivity in humans with schizophrenia predominantly involves the anterior portion, as shown in this graph, with the zero line being the activity values of the normal controls (NC) and the regional activities depicted in the anterior, middle, and posterior bars, as the change in schizophrenia from the NV baseline. (D) The final frame shows that the quantity of GluN1 protein (which is the necessary subunit of the NMDA receptor) in schizophrenia brain tissue (orange) is reduced significantly from normal (green) in DG but is not changed in CA3 and CA1; this could presumably account for downstream changes in hippocampus in schizophrenia.

subfield (Schobel, Lewandowski, et al., 2009; Schobel, Chaudhury, et al., 2013; Talati, Rane, et al., 2014). This hyperactivity in schizophrenia is almost entirely localized to the anterior hippocampus (McHugo, Talati, et al., 2019) and is most strongly detected in early psychosis. What draws special attention to the clinical importance of hippocampal hyperactivity is the correlation between hippocampal hyperactivity and psychotic phenomena in persons with schizophrenia (Lahti, Weiler, et al., 2006; Malaspina, Corcoran, et al., 2009; Schobel, Lewandowski, et al., 2009; Schobel, Chaudhury, et al., 2013), especially in individuals without antipsychotic medication (Medoff, Holcomb, et al., 2001), done early in disease course. These observations support the idea that hippocampal hyperactivity could be an essential element in the emergence of psychosis. In psychosis, the increase in hippocampal activity observed in some MRI studies could represent runaway excitatory neuronal activity in the hippocampus (Lawrence and McBain, 2003) critically impacting memory, resulting in mistaken memory products—memories with abnormal associations and even psychotic content. These functional abnormalities invite a molecular/cellular model for testing the disease mechanisms.

19.2.3 Changes in hippocampal structure and function in schizophrenia are potential correlates of hippocampal hyperactivity

19.2.3.1 Are anatomic and functional imaging changes in the hippocampus related to hippocampal hyperactivity?

Hippocampal size is reduced in schizophrenic psychosis, albeit modestly (Suddath, Casanova, et al., 1989; Bogerts, Ashtari, et al., 1990; Bilder, Bogerts, et al., 1995; Becker, Elmer, et al., 1996), and the reduction begins early in psychosis while individuals are still treatment naive (Briend, Nelson, et al., 2020) and implicates the hippocampus more often in schizophrenia and more consistently across laboratories than any other brain region (Honea, Crow, et al., 2005; Steen, Mull, et al., 2006). While the magnitude of the reduction is small (2%–4%), it is consistent across studies, some with substantial subject numbers (Arnold, Ivleva, et al., 2015). The reduction in size can be seen early, in the prodrome phase, and also during the first episode of illness (Szeszko, Goldberg, et al., 2003; Narr, Thompson, et al., 2004), and can progress modestly during early illness (Chakos, Schobel, et al., 2005; Velakoulis, Wood, et al., 2006). The volume reduction is said to be independent of antipsychotic medication (Panenka, Khorram, et al., 2007) and may be greater in individuals without genetic risk for psychosis (Tanskanen, Veijola, et al., 2005), in the schizophrenia prodrome (before the onset of florid symptoms) (Lawrie, Whalley, et al., 2001; van Erp, Saleh, et al., 2004), and in some but not all (Arnold, Ivleva, et al., 2015) studies in people with psychotic bipolar disorder (Strasser, Lilyestrom, et al., 2005). Individuals with psychosis show the greatest volume reduction in the CA3/2 regions compared with controls (Mathew, Gardin, et al., 2014). Regional changes in hippocampal shape occur in people with schizophrenia (Csernansky, Wang, et al., 2002) as they do in unaffected siblings of psychosis probands (Tepest, Wang, et al., 2003). The correlations between hippocampal volume reduction and memory dysfunction as well as psychotic symptoms (Mathew, Gardin, et al., 2014; Arnold, Ivleva, et al., 2015; McHugo, Talati, et al., 2019) suggest their clinical relevance.

In vivo brain imaging of hippocampus using memory paradigms and fMRI reveals a pathological reduction in activation in hippocampus and related memory circuits during memory tasks (Heckers, Rauch, et al., 1998; Eyler-Zorrilla, Jeste, et al., 2002; Jessen, Scheef, et al., 2003; Weiss, Schacter, et al., 2003; Heckers, Zalesak, et al., 2004; Weiss, Zalesak, et al., 2004; Achim, Bertrand, et al., 2007; Thermenos, Seidman, et al., 2007). In addition, individuals with psychosis often fail to activate essential brain regions outside of hippocampus for the performance of memory tasks (Collier, Wolf, et al., 2014) and show reduced habituation to memory stimuli and inadequate novelty recognition (Williams, Blackford, et al., 2013). Changes in memory-driven activation have been observed across the disease course in schizophrenia, with increased activation in temporal, parietal, and frontal regions found in early-course psychosis (Cao, McEwen et al., 2019) and, reduced activation in chronic psychosis (Lepage, Montoya, et al., 2006; Ragland, Blumenfeld, et al., 2012). Furthermore, both at rest and during task, connectivity between hippocampus and prefrontal cortex is reduced in schizophrenia (Fletcher, 1998; Meyer-Lindenberg, Olsen, et al., 2005; Molina, Sanz, et al., 2005), especially in genotypes vulnerable to psychosis, where connectivity between the two regions predicts working memory dysfunction (Liu, Zhang, et al., 2014).

19.2.3.2 Are cognitive and molecular alterations in schizophrenia related to hippocampal hyperactivity?

There are additional abnormal characteristics of schizophrenic psychosis that could be the consequence of hippocampal hyperactivity. For example, declarative memory performance—the hallmark function of the hippocampus—is selectively impaired in schizophrenia (Guo, Ragland, et al., 2019). If the hippocampus is firing at an abnormally elevated level, it would be plausible that memory function would be compromised. Indeed, McHugh (2019) has already demonstrated an association between hippocampal hyperactivity in schizophrenia, as measured with MRI/VASO, and a reduction in the verbal memory function of the same individuals (McHugo, Talati, et al., 2019). Changes in hippocampal size, shape, and memory-driven in vivo imaging functions have all been described in schizophrenia potentially related to hippocampal hyperactivity (Titone, Ditman, et al., 2004; Weiss, Zalesak, et al., 2004; Shohamy, Mihalakos, et al., 2010; Tamminga, Stan, et al., 2010) (Box 19.2). Data detailing alterations in hippocampal dysfunction in schizophrenia revealed sensory deception in early psychotic symptoms and behavioral similarities between psychosis and temporal lobe epilepsy (Maier, Mellers, et al., 2000; Gaitatzis, Trimble, et al., 2004). There have even been some reports of a proliferation of abnormal nonepileptic EEG activity over the temporal lobe during psychotic experiences (Stevens, 1973). A recent meta-analysis of the association between psychosis and epilepsy found the prevalence

---

Box 19.2 The hippocampus is significantly altered in schizophrenia

- There is a consistent but small (2-4%), reduction in hippocampal volume in SZ.
- Impairments in memory performance are characteristic of SZ, particularly in relational memory and pattern separation.
- There is an <u>increase</u> in the hippocampal perfusion at rest.
- There is an <u>activation deficit</u> during declaration declaration memory tasks, which is related to increased perfusion.
- These changes correlate with psychotic symptoms, and thus, appear functionally relevant.

of psychotic illness in temporal lobe epilepsy to be as high as 7% (Clancy, Clarke, et al., 2014).

Molecular abnormalities have been reported in whole hippocampus, albeit not yet replicated (Simpson, Slater, et al., 1989; Harrison, McLaughlin, et al., 1991; Cotter, Wilson, et al., 2000; East, Burnet, et al., 2002). Already, the dentate gyrus (DG) has been examined productively in schizophrenia for molecular alterations, and has shown evidence for decreased neurogenesis, reductions in GRIM3 and CACNA1AC, and reduced GluN1 message (Knable, Barci, et al., 2004; Altar, Jurata, et al., 2005). More recently, in a hypothesis-testing framework, distinct molecular changes have been found in postmortem tissue in human hippocampal subfields and subsequently cast into animal paradigms for reverse translational analyses, to inform schizophrenia mechanisms.

19.2.3.3 Human tissue measures of whole hippocampus

Human postmortem studies in schizophrenia have contributed to identifying pathology associated with the disorder. Often, in postmortem tissue, causative postmortem pathology is difficult to distinguish from an effect of chronic psychotic illness or an effect of chronic antipsychotic treatments, so findings need to be validated. In whole hippocampus (in contrast to subfield samples), studies have already reported evidence of dysfunctional GABAergic transmission, using as evidence downregulation of

GAD1, and genes in the GAD1 regulatory network. This work was recently advanced by showing altered methylation levels within the genes of the GAD1 regulatory network; specifically, methylation changes were found enriched in several GAD1 genes, like MSW1, in CCND2, and in DAXX within hippocampal tissue from cases with schizophrenia and bipolar disorder (Tao, Davis, et al., 2018).

As well, a transcriptomic study of a small number of cases, albeit across several conventional diagnoses and multiple brain regions, shows that across serious mental illness diagnoses, schizophrenia stands out as being strongly associated with inflammatory markers, and this observation is most striking in hippocampus (compared with the prefrontal cortex and striatum) (Lanz, Reinhart, et al., 2019). A study focusing on the hippocampus alone used schizophrenia and healthy control cases to observe a reduced density of neurons and oligodendrocytes in the DG and in CA4/hilus, implicating reduced DG neurogenesis in schizophrenia pathology. And, pertinent to potential novel treatments for psychosis, the M4, but not the M1 muscarinic cholinergic receptor is reduced in the hippocampus in schizophrenia cases (Crook, Tomaskovic-Crook, et al., 2000). While some constructs may be equally affected throughout the hippocampus, considering the well-known structural and functional diversity of the subfields, it remains possible that target molecular entities are subfield-specific.

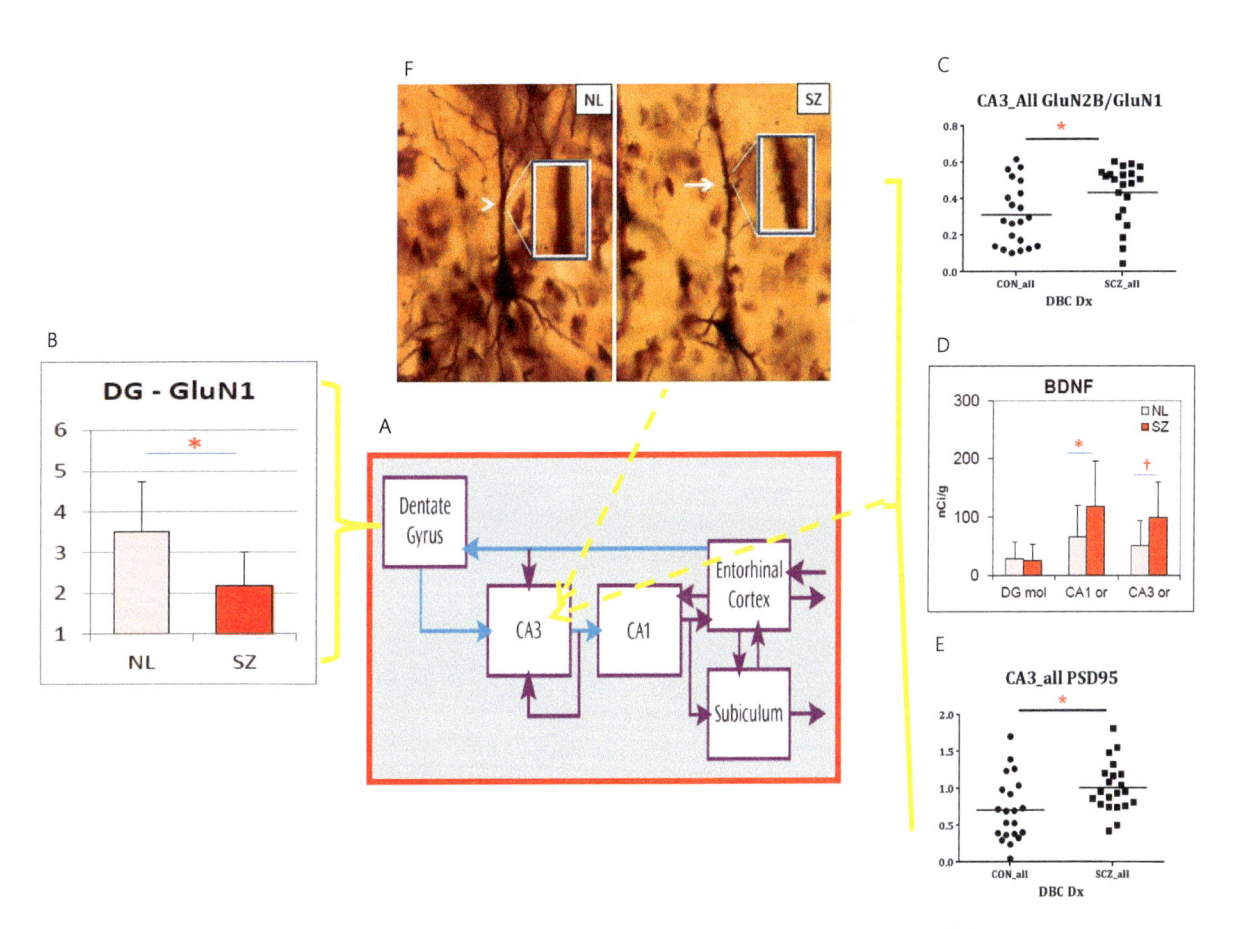

Figure 19.2 Contrasting schizophrenia protein in hippocampal subfield tissue from postmortem human cases. (A) Hippocampal structures, including the trisynaptic pathway (turquoise) and other microcircuits (purple) and the subfields, DG, CA3, and CA1, sequentially are related to each other. Tissue from these regions was analyzed for a selection of excitatory/inhibitory proteins. In schizophrenia, (B) DG shows significantly *reduced* GluN1, while (C) CA3 shows significantly *increased* numbers of the GluN2B receptor in schizophrenia (the hyperresponsive NMDA receptor), (D) shows increased BDNF in CA3 and CA1 stratum oriens, and (E) shows increased PSD95 in CA3. (F) The molecular picture of CA3/CA1 hyperactivity is corroborated by evidence of increased numbers of thorny excrescences (TE) in schizophrenia when examined with Golgi (Li, 2016).

19.3 Mechanisms of hippocampal hyperactivity in schizophrenia based on studies in hippocampal subfields

Studies designed to uncover the mechanism(s) that underlie a critical biomarker like hippocampal hyperactivity, should include a look at subfield function and cell populations within specific subfields. Previous investigations have speculated detailed microcircuit-level molecular alterations (Katzel, Wolff, et al., 2020).

19.3.1 Postmortem studies in schizophrenia by subfield

Based on the kinds of data presented so far, which implicate widespread hippocampal dysfunctions in psychosis along with hippocampal hyperactivity, a study assessing hippocampal proteins by subfield, especially general excitatory and inhibitory (E/I) synaptic biomarkers in psychosis, has been done. In this study, each subfield was individually addressed, generating hippocampal pathological outcomes in schizophrenia by the DG, CA3, and CA1 subfields. Hippocampal subfield tissue samples were taken from people with schizophrenia and healthy donors and microdissected into enriched samples of DG, CA3, CA1, and subiculum (Li, Ghose, et al., 2015). The outcomes were consistent with hippocampal hyperactivity (Figure 19.2). Specifically, in DG, GluN1 protein was reduced in schizophrenia cases, implicating a *reduction*, not an increase, in excitatory transmission in that subfield. Yet, in downstream subfields like CA3 and CA1, examination showed a significant *increase* in several excitation-associated proteins (specifically, GluN2B-containing NMDA receptors, BDNF, and PSD-95 proteins) in CA3, without a significant change in proteins involved in inhibition. In CA1, none of these abnormal E/I synaptic proteins were altered, but there was an increase in tissue BDNF, indicating hyperactivity. The strongest marker of synaptic remodeling in CA3 was alteration of synaptic anatomy showing an increase in dendritic spines on the apical dendrite of the CA3 pyramidal neuron in the schizophrenia cases at the insertion of the mossy fiber pathway onto CA3 pyramidal neurons in the human tissue, using Golgi staining (Figure 19.3) (Li, Ghose, et al., 2015). It is apparent that the three hippocampal subfields have molecular characteristics distinct from each other in schizophrenia, in that the molecular alterations associated with the disease were distinct by subfield. Consistent with these findings, a genetic analysis of RNA expression by subfield showed (1) a reduced neurogenesis signal in DG, (2) increased excitatory protein signals in CA3, and (3) both increased inhibitory and decreased excitatory protein synthesis in CA1, as if in compensation for its increased afferent signal (Perez, Berto, et al., 2020).

To explore the subfield data further and to specify the molecular determinants in the trisynaptic microcircuit in schizophrenia and understand the mechanisms of hippocampal hyperactivity, the preclinical literature became crucial. A unique synapse at the mossy fiber–CA3 pyramidal cell interface, purportedly critical in modifying CA3 function, is described by Lee et al. (Lee, Queenan, et al., 2013) and Laurence and McBain (2003). In light of their findings and the subfield-specific schizophrenia vs. healthy control outcomes, the model, focusing on reduced excitatory signaling from DG to CA3 in the mossy fiber pathway with a hyperactivity response in CA3/CA1, became plausible and is consistent with the

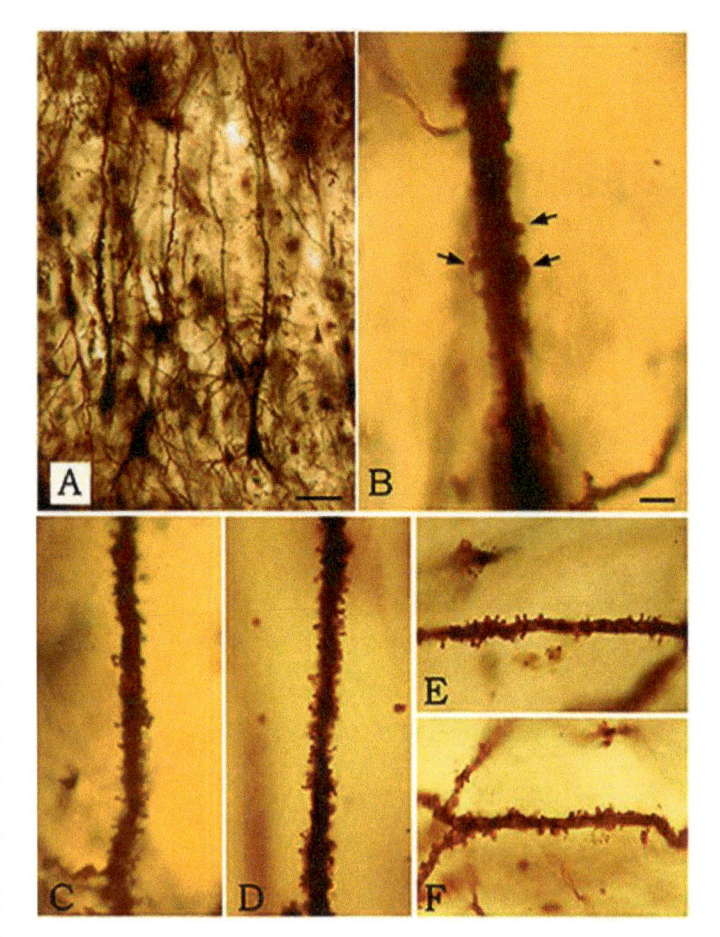

Figure 19.3 Golgi staining shows increased thorny excrecenses (TE) in CA3. (A) Apical dendrites of CA3 pyramidal neurons at the level of the first bifurcation, which occurs just at the insertion of the afferent DG fibers. (B) Increased resolution of the TEs in the schizophrenia tissue showing the increased size of these TEs and the presumed initiation of hyperactivity in response to reduction of afferent stimulation. (C) Normal and (D) schizophrenia cases, showing typical apical dendrites in these postmortem cases with the noticeable and significant differences between the normal (low) and the schizophrenia (high) TE size and density (Li et al., 2015). (E) NC and (F) schizophrenia recurrent collateral fibers in the same cells show no difference in the TEs in these cellular circuits, despite the hyperactivity driven by the exaggerated apical dendrite response to reduced afferent stimulation, suggesting a pyramidal cell hyperactivity in hippocampus in schizophrenia.

schizophrenia tissue data; here, the paradoxical increase in excitatory activity in CA3 is represented by (1) an increase in GluN2B-containing NMDAR, (2) an increase in PSD-95, and (3) an increase in BDNF RNA in CA3 (Li, Ghose, et al., 2015), all developed secondary to reduced afferent stimulation from DG. The strongest marker of synaptic remodeling in CA3 was alteration of synaptic anatomy showing an increase in dendritic spines on the apical dendrite of the CA3 pyramidal neuron in the schizophrenia cases at the insertion of the mossy fiber pathway onto CA3 pyramidal neurons in the human tissue (Figure 19.4) (Li, Ghose, et al., 2015). Although there were no such changes in CA1, genetic markers of hyperactivity were apparent in both CA3 and CA1 (Perez, Berto, et al., 2020). There were no alterations in GAD67 detected in any of the subfields; nonetheless, significantly more studies are needed

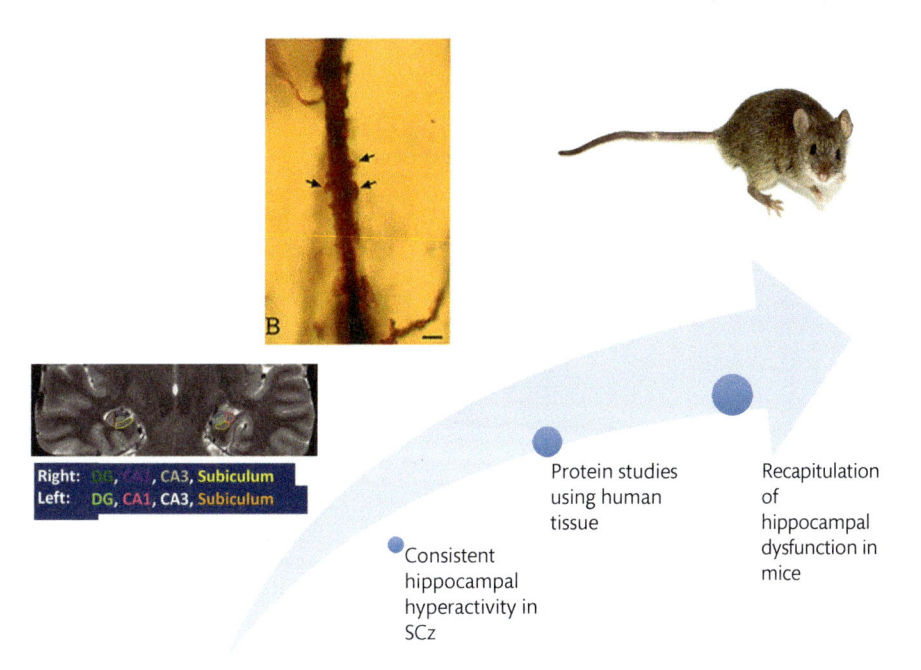

Figure 19.4 Taking the hyperactivity hypothesis to a reverse translation animal model. Starting with the discovery of hippocampal hyperactivity in human schizophrenia person (left) and generating the novel protein outcomes in subfields of hippocampal tissue by subfield analyses (middle), we turned to an animal model (right) to ask how a reduction of GluN1 in dentate gyrus can change regional neural activity in these and downstream subfields. The first comparative studies were done with the DG-selective GluN1 knockout mouse (McHugh et al., 2007). Mouse studies have also been repeated in a granule cell-specific inhibitory DREAD (Segev, 2018). In mouse the mere reduction of GluN1 in the DG, generates hyperactivity in CA3 and CA1; this hyperactivity is also associated with a downstream circuit of extrahippocampal regions, including amygdala, anterior cingulate cortex, and nucleus accumbens.

here to define molecular inhibition supporting hyperactivity at this synapse.

Jaffe (Jaffe, Hoeppner, et al., 2019) compared RNA expression outcome data from laser-captured granule cells from DG with RNA expression outcomes of whole hippocampal transcriptome sequencing, to show the advantage of laser-captured cell sequencing and, in relief, the molecular differences across cell types and brain regions. They found that GRIM3 and CACNA1AC emerged as differentially expressed genes in schizophrenia vs. the healthy control DG tissue. This study highlights the molecular diversity of tissues and regions within hippocampus.

19.3.2 Reverse translation of hippocampal pathology into mice to extend the molecular pathology

To explore these clues more fully, the human pathology model of psychosis described above was back-translated into two related mouse models (Segev, Yanagi, et al., 2020): (1) the DG-selective GluN1 knockout mouse from S. Tonegawa (McHugh, Jones, et al., 2007) and (2) a DG-placed granule cell-specific inhibitory DREADD (Scott and Tamminga, 2023) (Figure 19.4). Both models are based on different approaches to lesioning DG, reducing its efferent activity, and both resulted in hippocampal hyperactivity in CA3/CA1. The back-translated feature of each model, with reduction of DG granule cell activity, facilitated the study of hyperactivity mechanisms, *by subfield*, using E/I protein biomarkers. The models recapitulate potential human-specific schizophrenia pathology in a mouse in hippocampus (McHugh, Jones, et al., 2007). Specifically, in the GluN1 KO mouse, the analyses showed remarkably reduced glutamate release from the mossy fiber pathway onto CA3

pyramidal cells, which correlated with psychosis-like mouse behaviors. Moreover, AMPAR- and NMDAR-mediated postsynaptic excitatory currents were potently upregulated at the DG-CA3 synapse. These experiments document that *reduced* glutamate release onto CA3 pyramidal neurons in the DG-selective GluN1 knockout mouse can be associated with *increased* glutamatergic synaptic strength in CA3, on the surface, a paradoxical action. The downstream effects of GluN1 loss in DG with hyperactivity in CA3 also resulted in hyperactivity in CA1, as measured by increases in the number of cFos-positive excitatory neurons in CA1 and CA3. And, putatively related projection areas, including basolateral amygdala, medial prefrontal cortex, and nucleus accumbens, showed concurrent hyperactivity which implicates these regions in a circuit impacted by hippocampal hyperactivity (Suzuki and Amaral, 2003) and other areas already implicated in schizophrenia. The significant increase in cFos-positive cells in the knockout animal was prominent only in the ventral hippocampus (analogous to anterior hippocampus in human) in both CA3 and CA1, mimicking hippocampal hyperactivity in human schizophrenia (Medoff, Holcomb, et al., 2001; Schobel, Lewandowski, et al., 2009; Schobel, Chaudhury, et al., 2013). It is tempting to see these as links in a forward excitatory circuit from CA3 through the hippocampus then to basolateral amygdala and to medial prefrontal cortex, associated with nucleus accumbens, as a reflection of the extent of the influence of hippocampal hyperactivity within the cerebral cortex and on dopamine signaling pathways.

The GluN1 knockout mouse further displayed a psychosis-like behavioral phenotype. This manifested in specific alterations in hippocampal-mediated and memory-associated behaviors,

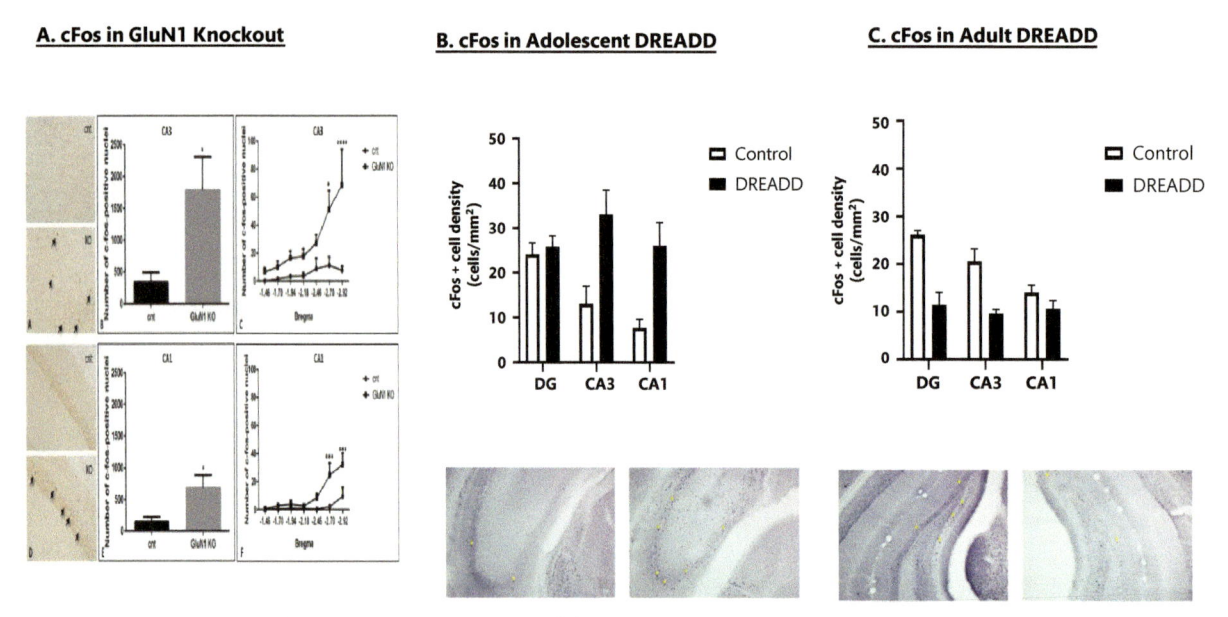

A. cFos in GluN1 Knockout   **B. cFos in Adolescent DREADD**   **C. cFos in Adult DREADD**

Figure 19.5 Extending the details of the model with animal data. (A) in the DG-selective GluN1 KO mouse, it is only the KO animals that show increased cFos activity (the hyperactivity marker) in hippocampal CA3 and CA1 with an animal whose only alteration is a GluN1 deficit in DG. It only shows hyperactivity in the anterior portions of the hippocampal regions, just as the hyperactivity in human schizophrenia. (B) In the animals with inhibitory DG granule cell DREADD, hyperactivity follows in CA3 and CA1 (i.e., elevated cFos-postive neurons), on the condition that the animals receive the DG inhibition during adolescent age (<10 weeks of age). (C) If the mouse is over 10 weeks and manipulated with inhibitory DG DREADD, the response in CA3 and CA1 is no longer paradoxical, but shows a reduction in activity CA3/CA1, without any overactivation. We will be testing this further with chronic local field potential (LFP) recordings using an indwelling probe in both the adolescent- and the adult-lesioned mice.

including impaired social cognition and spatial memory, reduced prepulse inhibition and exaggerated fear memory. Of interest, these behaviors share face validity with behaviors seen in humans with psychosis. Moreover, exogenously induced hippocampal hyperactivity, generated with an excitatory CA3 DREADD in the wild-type mouse, generated these behaviors in a mouse. (12).

19.3.3 Hippocampal hyperactivity and behavioral pharmacology

While confirming these findings in the DG-inhibitory DREADD mouse model, a developmental *risk window* for hippocampal hyperactivity in the mouse became apparent. The data show that the DREADD mouse inhibited during adolescence, but not those inhibited during adulthood, exhibited hippocampal hyperactivity. The DREADD inhibition of DG during adulthood *fails* to generate hyperactivity or induce a psychosis-like behavioral phenotype (Figure 19.5B,C). Whereas, the DREADD inhibition of DG during adolescence generates the same picture as the DG-selective GluN1 knockout mouse. Because this risk window is parallel to the characteristic clinical risk period for psychosis during adolescence, this may be of particular importance. This animal is a tool for future experiments to causally define the mechanisms underlying DG inhibition leading to hippocampal hyperactivity, limited by adolescent age. It will allow the testing of the precise timing of pharmacological agents known to modulate activity specifically in hippocampus, as novel treatments for schizophrenia.

19.4 Conclusions: hippocampal hyperactivity and psychosis

The role of the hippocampus in the psychosis of schizophrenia has a long and rich history. The precision of implicated molecular mediators has expanded with years of study. Mimicking the role of the hippocampus in memory, the role of the hippocampus in psychosis could be to develop the initial psychotic construct in memory and in reinforcing the psychotic construct when the memory is reactivated, but not in maintaining the psychotic memory complex within its bounds. As in normal memory, the hippocampus does not act in isolation, in that these pathological functions are supported by related hippocampal-cortical networks and circuits. The hippocampal subfield microcircuitry could be engaged pathologically to generate odd and mistaken memories without a basis in reality; then the maintenance of those psychotic thoughts would rely on neocortex and medial temporal lobe–neocortical interactions. There are many specific determinants of crystallized psychotic ideas that have yet to be discovered. The psychosis-related processes described here could be associated with hippocampal hyperactivity. If correct, this association could be used for novel drug targeting (Katzel, Wolff, et al., 2020), for prophylaxis of psychosis generation in very early years, and for the discovery of molecular targets overall. The development of anatomy and physiology of systems and circuits in the hippocampus is extremely important to the ideas of the involvement of this brain region in psychosis itself, indicating that the research to understand hippocampal function has been generative in psychosis research and schizophrenia.

REFERENCES

Achim AM, MC Bertrand, H Sutton, A Montoya, Y Czechowska, AK Malla, R Joober, JC Pruessner, M Lepage (2007) Selective abnormal modulation of hippocampal activity during memory formation in first-episode psychosis. *Arch Gen Psychiatry* **64**(9):999–1014.

Adams DH, BJ Kinon, S Baygani, BA Millen, I Velona, S Kollack-Walker, DP Walling (2013) A long-term, phase 2, multicenter, randomized, open-label, comparative safety study of pomaglumetad methionil (LY2140023 monohydrate) versus atypical antipsychotic standard of care in patients with schizophrenia. *BMC Psychiatry* **13**:143.

Altar CA, LW Jurata, V Charles, A Lemire, P Liu, Y Bukhman, TA Young, J Bullard, H Yokoe, MJ Webster, et al. (2005) Deficient hippocampal neuron expression of proteasome, ubiquitin, and mitochondrial genes in multiple schizophrenia cohorts. *Biol Psychiatry* **58**(2):85–96.

Andreasen NC, D Liu, S Ziebell, A Vora, BC Ho (2013) Relapse duration, treatment intensity, and brain tissue loss in schizophrenia: a prospective longitudinal MRI study. *Am J Psychiatry* **170**(6):609–615.

Arnold SJ, EI Ivleva, TA Gopal, AP Reddy, H Jeon-Slaughter, CB Sacco, AN Francis, N Tandon, AS Bidesi, B Witte, et al. (2015) Hippocampal volume is reduced in schizophrenia and schizoaffective disorder but not in psychotic bipolar I disorder demonstrated by both manual tracing and automated parcellation (freesurfer) *Schizophr Bull* **41**(1):233–249.

Becker T, K Elmer, F Schneider, M Schneider, W Grodd, M Bartels, S Heckers, H Beckmann (1996) Confirmation of reduced temporal limbic structure volume on magnetic resonance imaging in male patients with schizophrenia. *Psychiatry Res* **67**:135–143.

Benes FM (1989) Myelination of cortical-hippocampal relays during late adolescence. *Schizophr Bull* **15**(4):585–593.

Bilder RM, B Bogerts, M Ashtari, H Wu, JM Alvir, D Jody, G Reiter, L Bell, JA Lieberman (1995) Anterior hippocampal volume reductions predict frontal lobe dysfunction in first episode schizophrenia. *Schizophr Res* **17**:47–58.

Bogerts B, M Ashtari, G Degreef, JM Alvir, RM Bilder, JA Lieberman (1990) Reduced temporal limbic structure volumes on magnetic resonance images in first episode schizophrenia. *Psychiatry Res* **35**(1):1–13.

Briend F, EA Nelson, O Maximo, WP Armstrong, NV Kraguljac, AC Lahti (2020) Hippocampal glutamate and hippocampus subfield volumes in antipsychotic-naive first episode psychosis subjects and relationships to duration of untreated psychosis. *Transl Psychiatry* **10**(1):137.

Cao H, SC McEwen, Y Chung, OY Chen, CE Bearden, J Addington, B Goodyear, KS Cadenhead, H Mirzakhanian, BA Cornblatt, et al. (2019) Altered brain activation during memory retrieval precedes and predicts conversion to psychosis in individuals at clinical high risk. *Schizophr Bull* **45**(4):924–933.

Carlsson A, M Lindqvist (1963) Effect of chlorpromazine or haloperidol on formation of 3methoxytyramine and normetanephrine in mouse brain. *Acta Pharmacol Toxicol (Copenh)* **20**:140–144.

Carpenter WT, Jr, RW Buchanan (1994) Schizophrenia. *N Engl J Med* **330**(10):681–690.

Chakos MH, SA Schobel, H Gu, G Gerig, D Bradford, C Charles, JA Lieberman (2005) Duration of illness and treatment effects on hippocampal volume in male patients with schizophrenia. *Br J Psychiatry* **186**:26–31.

Ciompi L (1980) The natural history of schizophrenia in the long term. *Br J Psychiatry* **136**:413–420.

Clancy MJ, MC Clarke, DJ Connor, M Cannon, DR Cotter (2014) The prevalence of psychosis in epilepsy; a systematic review and meta-analysis. *BMC Psychiatry* **14**:75.

Collier AK, DH Wolf, JN Valdez, RE Gur, RC Gur (2014) Subsequent memory effects in schizophrenia. *Psychiatry Res* **224**(3):211–217.

Correll CU, OD Howes (2021) Treatment-resistant schizophrenia: definition, predictors, and therapy options. *J Clin Psychiatry* **82**(5): MY20096AH1C.

Correll CU, A Martin, C Patel, C Benson, R Goulding, J Kern-Sliwa, K Joshi, E Schiller, E Kim (2022) Systematic literature review of schizophrenia clinical practice guidelines on acute and maintenance management with antipsychotics. *Schizophrenia (Heidelb)* **8**(1):5.

Correll CU, M Solmi, S Cortese, M Fava, M Højlund, HC Kraemer, RS McIntyre, DS Pine, LS Schneider, JM Kane (2023) The future of psychopharmacology: a critical appraisal of ongoing phase 2/3 trials, and of some current trends aiming to de-risk trial programmes of novel agents. *World Psychiatry* **22**(1):48–74.

Cotter D, S Wilson, E Roberts, R Kerwin, IP Everall (2000) Increased dendritic MAP2 expression in the hippocampus in schizophrenia. *Schizophr Res* **41**(2):313–323.

Coward DM (1992) General pharmacology of clozapine. [Review] [56 refs]. *Br J Psychiatry - Supplement* **17**(17):5–11.

Coyle JT, D Balu, M Benneyworth, A Basu, A Roseman (2010) Beyond the dopamine receptor: novel therapeutic targets for treating schizophrenia. *Dialogues Clin Neurosci* **12**(3):359–382.

Creese I, AA Manian, TD Prosser, SH Snyder (1978) 3H-Haloperidol binding to dopamine receptors in rat corpus striatum: influence of chlorpromazine metabolites and derivatives. *Eur J Pharmacol* **47**(3):291–296.

Crook JM, E Tomaskovic-Crook, DL Copolov, B Dean (2000) Decreased muscarinic receptor binding in subjects with schizophrenia: a study of the human hippocampal formation. *Soc Biol Psychiatry* **48**:381–388.

Csernansky JG, L Wang, D Jones, D Rastogi-Cruz, JA Posener, G Heydebrand, JP Miller, MI Miller (2002) Hippocampal deformities in schizophrenia characterized by high dimensional brain mapping. *Am J Psychiatry* **159**(12):2000–2006.

East SZ, PW Burnet, RW Kerwin, PJ Harrison (2002) An RT-PCR study of 5-HT(6) and 5-HT(7) receptor mRNAs in the hippocampal formation and prefrontal cortex in schizophrenia. *Schizophr Res* **57**(1):15–26.

Eyler-Zorrilla, LT, DV Jeste, MP Paulus, GG Brown (2002) Functional abnormalities of medial temporal cortex during novel picture learning among patients with chronic schizophrenia. *Schizophr Res* **59**:187–198.

Fletcher P (1998) The missing link: a failure of fronto-hippocampal integration in schizophrenia. *News and Views* **1**(4):266–267.

Gaitatzis A, MR Trimble, JW Sander (2004) The psychiatric comorbidity of epilepsy. *Acta Neurol Scand* **110**(4):207–220.

Green H. (1964) I Never Promised You a Rose Garden. New York, Holt, Rinehart & Winston.

Guo JY, JD Ragland, CS Carter (2019) Memory and cognition in schizophrenia. *Mol Psychiatry* **24**(5):633–642.

Harrison PJ, D McLaughlin, RW Kerwin (1991) Decreased hippocampal expression of a glutamate receptor gene in schizophrenia. *Lancet* **337**(8739):450–452.

Heckers S, C Konradi (2015) GABAergic mechanisms of hippocampal hyperactivity in schizophrenia. *Schizophr Res* **167**(1–3):4–11.

Heckers S, SL Rauch, D Goff, CR Savage, DL Schacter, AJ Fischman, NM Alpert (1998) Impaired recruitment of the hippocampus during conscious recollection in schizophrenia. *Nat Neurosci* **1**(4):318–323.

Heckers S, M Zalesak, AP Weiss, T Ditman, D Titone (2004) Hippocampal activation during transitive inference in humans. *Hippocampus* 14(2):153–162.

Honea R, TJ Crow, D Passingham, CE Mackay (2005) Regional deficits in brain volume in schizophrenia: a meta-analysis of voxel-based morphometry studies. *Am J Psychiatry* 162(12):2233–2245.

Jaffe A, D Hoeppner, T Saito, L Blanpain, J Ukaigwe, E Burke, R Tao, K Tajinda, A Deep-Soboslay, J Shin, et al. (2019) Cell type-specific genetic regulation of expression in the granule cell layer of the human dentate gyrus. *bioRxiv*:612200.

Janssen PA (1967) The pharmacology of haloperidol. *Int J Neuropsychiatry* 3(Suppl 1):10–18.

Javitt DC, SR Zukin (1990) The role of excitatory amino acids in neuropsychiatric illness [Review]. *J Neuropsychiatry Clin Neurosci* 2(1):44–52.

Jessen F, L Scheef, L Germeshausen, Y Tawo, M Kockler, K-U Kuhn, W Maier, HH Schild, R Heun (2003) Reduced hippocampal activation during encoding and recognition of words in schizophrenia patients. *Am J Psychiatry* 160:1305–1312.

Kätzel D, AR Wolff, AM Bygrave, DM Bannerman (2020) Hippocampal hyperactivity as a druggable circuit-level origin of aberrant salience in schizophrenia. *Front Pharmacol* 11:486811.

Knable MB, BM Barci, MJ Webster, J Meador-Woodruff, EF Torrey (2004) Molecular abnormalities of the hippocampus in severe psychiatric illness: postmortem findings from the Stanley Neuropathology Consortium. *Mol Psychiatry* 9(6):609–620, 544.

Kotov R, L Fochtmann, K Li, M Tanenberg-Karant, EA Constantino, J Rubinstein, G Perlman, E Velthorst, AJ Fett, G Carlson, et al. (2017) Declining clinical course of psychotic disorders over the two decades following first hospitalization: evidence from the Suffolk County Mental Health Project. *Am J Psychiatry* 174(11):1064–1074.

Kovelman JA, AB Scheibel (1984) A neurohistological correlate of schizophrenia. *Biol Psychiatry* 19(12):1601–1621.

Lahti AC, B Koffel, D LaPorte, CA Tamminga (1995) Subanesthetic doses of ketamine stimulate psychosis in schizophrenia. *Neuropsychopharmacology* 13(1):9–19.

Lahti AC, MA Weiler, HH Holcomb, CA Tamminga, WT Carpenter, R McMahon (2006) Correlations between rCBF and symptoms in two independent cohorts of drug-free patients with schizophrenia. *Neuropsychopharmacology* 31(1):221–230.

Lanz TA, V Reinhart, MJ Sheehan, SJ S Rizzo, SE Bove, LC James, D Volfson, DA Lewis, RJ Kleiman (2019) Postmortem transcriptional profiling reveals widespread increase in inflammation in schizophrenia: a comparison of prefrontal cortex, striatum, and hippocampus among matched tetrads of controls with subjects diagnosed with schizophrenia, bipolar or major depressive disorder. *Transl Psychiatry* 9(1):151.

Lawrence JJ, CJ McBain (2003) Interneuron diversity series: containing the detonation—feedforward inhibition in the CA3 hippocampus. *Trends Neurosci* 26(11):631–640.

Lawrie SM, HC Whalley, SS Abukmeil, JN Kestelman, L Donnelly, P Miller, JJ Best, DG Owens, EC Johnstone (2001) Brain structure, genetic liability, and psychotic symptoms in subjects at high risk of developing schizophrenia. *Biol Psychiatry* 49(10):811–823.

Lee KJ, BN Queenan, AM Rozeboom, R Bellmore, ST Lim, S Vicini, DT Pak (2013) Mossy fiber-CA3 synapses mediate homeostatic plasticity in mature hippocampal neurons. *Neuron* 77(1):99–114.

Lee SH, S Ripke, BM Neale, SV Faraone, SM Purcell, RH Perlis, BJ Mowry, A Thapar, ME Goddard, JS Witte, et al. (2013) Genetic relationship between five psychiatric disorders estimated from genome-wide SNPs. *Nat Genet* 45(9):984–994.

Lepage M, A Montoya, M Pelletier, AM Achim, M Menear, S Lal (2006) Associative memory encoding and recognition in schizophrenia: an event-related fMRI study. *Biol Psychiatry* 60(11):1215–1223.

Leysen JE, W Gommeren, A Eens, D de Chaffoy de Courcelles, JC Stoof, PA Janssen (1988) Biochemical profile of risperidone, a new antipsychotic. *J Pharmacol Exp Ther* 247(2):661–670.

Li W, S Ghose, K Gleason, A Begovic, J Perez, J Bartko, S Russo, AD Wagner, L Selemon, CA Tamminga (2015) Synaptic proteins in the hippocampus indicative of increased neuronal activity in CA3 in schizophrenia. *Am J Psychiatry* 172(4):373–382.

Lisman JE, JT Coyle, RW Green, DC Javitt, FM Benes, S Heckers, AA Grace (2008) Circuit-based framework for understanding neurotransmitter and risk gene interactions in schizophrenia. *Trends Neurosci* 31(5):234–242.

Liu B, X Zhang, B Hou, J Li, C Qiu, W Qin, C Yu, T Jiang (2014) The impact of MIR137 on dorsolateral prefrontal-hippocampal functional connectivity in healthy subjects. *Neuropsychopharmacology* 39(9):2153–2160.

Lopez-Munoz, F, C Alamo, E Cuenca, WW Shen, P Clervoy, G Rubio (2005) History of the discovery and clinical introduction of chlorpromazine. *Ann Clin Psychiatry* 17(3):113–135.

Lu H, PC van Zijl (2012) A review of the development of Vascular-Space-Occupancy (VASO) fMRI. *NeuroImage* 62(2):736–742.

Lui S, L Yao, Y Xiao, SK Keedy, JL Reilly, RS Keefe, CA Tamminga, MS Keshavan, GD Pearlson, Q Gong, et al. (2015) Resting-state brain function in schizophrenia and psychotic bipolar probands and their first-degree relatives. *Psychol Med* 45(1):97–108.

Maier M, J Mellers, B Toone, M Trimble, MA Ron (2000) Schizophrenia, temporal lobe epilepsy and psychosis: an in vivo magnetic resonance spectroscopy and imaging study of the hippocampus/amygdala complex. *Psychol Med* 30(3):571–581.

Malaspina D, C Corcoran, SA Schobel, SA Small, D Kimby, N Lewandowski (2009) Hippocampal hyperactivity is associated with positive symptoms. *Schizophr Bull* 35(Suppl 1):160.

Mathew I, TM Gardin, N Tandon, S Eack, AN Francis, LJ Seidman, B Clementz, GD Pearlson, JA Sweeney, CA Tamminga, et al. (2014) Medial temporal lobe structures and hippocampal subfields in psychotic disorders: findings from the bipolar-schizophrenia network on intermediate phenotypes (B-SNIP) study. *JAMA Psychiatry* 71(7):769–777.

McCarley, RW, ME Shenton, BF O'Donnell, PG Nestor (1993) Uniting Kraepelin and Bleuler: the psychology of schizophrenia and the biology of temporal lobe abnormalities. *Harv Rev Psychiatry* 1(1):36–56.

McCutcheon, RA, A Abi-Dargham, OD Howes (2019) Schizophrenia, dopamine and the striatum: from biology to symptoms. *Trends Neurosci* 42(3):205–220.

McHugh, TJ, MW Jones, JJ Quinn, N Balthasar, R Coppari, JK Elmquist, BB Lowell, MS Fanselow, MA Wilson, S Tonegawa (2007) Dentate gyrus NMDA receptors mediate rapid pattern separation in the hippocampal network. *Science* 317(5834):94–99.

McHugo, M, P Talati, K Armstrong, SN Vandekar, JU Blackford, ND Woodward, S Heckers (2019) Hyperactivity and reduced activation of anterior hippocampus in early psychosis. *Am J Psychiatry* 176(12):1030–1038.

Medoff DR, HH Holcomb, AC Lahti, CA Tamminga (2001) Probing the human hippocampus using rCBF: contrasts in schizophrenia. *Hippocampus* 11(5):543–550.

Meyer-Lindenberg, AS, RK Olsen, PD Kohn, T Brown, MF Egan, DR Weinberger, KF Berman (2005) Regionally specific disturbance of dorsolateral prefrontal-hippocampal functional connectivity in schizophrenia. *Arch Gen Psychiatry* 62(4):379–386.

Molina V, J Sanz, F Sarramea, C Benito, T Palomo (2005) Prefrontal atrophy in first episodes of schizophrenia associated with limbic metabolic hyperactivity. *J Psychiatr Res* **39**(2):117–127.

Narr KL, PM Thompson, PR Szeszko, D Robinson, S Jang, RP Woods, S Kim, KM Hayashi, D Asunction, AW Toga, et al. (2004) Regional specificity of hippocampal volume reductions in first-episode schizophrenia. *NeuroImage* **21**:1563–1575.

Panenka WJ, B Khorram, AM Barr, GN Smith, DJ Lang, LC Kopala, RA Vandorpe, WG Honer (2007) A longitudinal study on the effects of typical versus atypical antipsychotic drugs on hippocampal volume in schizophrenia. *Schizophr Res* **94**(1–3):288–292.

Perez JM, S Berto, K Gleason, S Ghose, C Tan, TK Kim, G Konopka, CA Tamminga (2020) Hippocampal subfield transcriptome analysis in schizophrenia psychosis. *Mol Psychiatry*.

Ragland JD, RS Blumenfeld, IS Ramsay, A Yonelinas, J Yoon, M Solomon, CS Carter, C Ranganath (2012) Neural correlates of relational and item-specific encoding during working and long-term memory in schizophrenia. *Neuroimage* **59**(2):1719–1726.

Saks ER (2007) The Center Cannot Hold: My Journey through Madness. Hyperion.

Samudra N, EI Ivleva, NA Hubbard, B Rypma, JA Sweeney, BA Clementz, MS Keshavan, GD Pearlson, CA Tamminga (2015) Alterations in hippocampal connectivity across the psychosis dimension. *Psychiatry Res* **233**(2):148–157.

Saykin AJ, RC Gur, RE Gur, PD Mozley, LH Mozley, SM Resnick, DB Kester, P Stafiniak (1991) Neuropsychological function in schizophrenia: selective impairment in memory and learning. *Arch Gen Psychiatry* **48**(7):618–624.

Schobel SA, NH Chaudhury, UA Khan, B Paniagua, MA Styner, I Asllani, BP Inbar, CM Corcoran, JA Lieberman, H Moore, et al. (2013) Imaging patients with psychosis and a mouse model establishes a spreading pattern of hippocampal dysfunction and implicates glutamate as a driver. *Neuron* **78**(1):81–93.

Schobel SA, NM Lewandowski, CM Corcoran, H Moore, T Brown, D Malaspina, SA Small (2009) Differential targeting of the CA1 subfield of the hippocampal formation by schizophrenia and related psychotic disorders. *Arch Gen Psychiatry* **66**(9):938–946.

Scott D, C Tan, J Yamamoto, CA Tamminga (2023) Hippocampal hyperactivity associated with dentate gyrus (DG) insufficiency in adolescent mouse. [Under review].

Segev A, M Yanagi, D Scott, SA Southcott, JM Lister, C Tan, W Li, SG Birnbaum, S Kourrich, CA Tamminga (2020) Reduced GluN1 in mouse dentate gyrus is associated with CA3 hyperactivity and psychosis-like behaviors. *Mol Psychiatry* **25**(11):2832–2843.

Shohamy D, P Mihalakos, R Chin, B Thomas, AD Wagner, C Tamminga (2010) Learning and generalization in schizophrenia: effects of disease and antipsychotic drug treatment. *Biol Psychiatry* **67**(10):926–932.

Simpson MD C, P Slater, JF W Deakin, MC Royston, WJ Skan (1989) Reduced GABA uptake sites in the temporal lobe in schizophrenia. *Neurosci Lett* **107**:211–215.

Steen RG, C Mull, R McClure, RM Hamer, JA Lieberman (2006) Brain volume in first-episode schizophrenia: systematic review and meta-analysis of magnetic resonance imaging studies. *Br J Psychiatry* **188**:510–518.

Stevens JR (1973) An anatomy of schizophrenia? *Arch Gen Psychiatry* **29**(2):177–189.

Strasser HC, J Lilyestrom, ER Ashby, NA Honeycutt, DJ Schretlen, AE Pulver, RO Hopkins, JR Depaulo, JB Potash, B Schweizer, et al. (2005) Hippocampal and ventricular volumes in psychotic and nonpsychotic bipolar patients compared with schizophrenia patients and community control subjects: a pilot study. *Biol Psychiatry* **57**(6):633–639.

Suddath RL, MF Casanova, TE Goldberg, DG Daniel, JR Kelsoe, Jr, DR Weinberger (1989) Temporal lobe pathology in schizophrenia: a quantitative magnetic resonance imaging study. *Am J Psychiatry* **146**(4):464–472.

Suzuki W, DG Amaral (2003) Perirhinal and parahippocampal cortices of the macaque monkey: cytoarchitectonic and chemoarchitectonic organization. *J Comp Neurol* **463**:67–91.

Szeszko PR, E Goldberg, H Gunduz-Bruce, M Ashtari, D Robinson, AK Malhotra, T Lencz, J Bates, DT Crandall, JM Kane, et al. (2003) Smaller anterior hippocampal formation volume in antipsychotic-naive patients with first-episode schizophrenia. *Am J Psychiatry* **160**:2190–2197.

Talati P, S Rane, S Kose, JU Blackford, J Gore, MJ Donahue, S Heckers (2014) Increased hippocampal CA1 cerebral blood volume in schizophrenia. *Neuroimage Clin* **5**:359–364.

Talati P, S Rane, J Skinner, J Gore, S Heckers (2015) Increased hippocampal blood volume and normal blood flow in schizophrenia. *Psychiatry Res* **232**(3):219–225.

Tamminga CA (1998) Schizophrenia and glutamatergic transmission. *Crit Rev Neurobiol* **12**(1–2):21–36.

Tamminga CA, A Carlsson (2002) Partial dopamine agonists and dopaminergic stabilizers, in the treatment of psychosis. *Curr Drug Targets CNS Neurol Disord* **1**(2):141–147.

Tamminga CA, AD Stan, AD Wagner (2010) The hippocampal formation in schizophrenia. *Am J Psychiatry* **167**(10):1178–1193.

Tamminga CA, J van Os, U Reininghaus, E Ivleva (eds) (2020) Psychotic Disorders: Comprehensive Conceptualization and Treatments. Oxford University Press, New York.

Tamminga CA, RS Zukin (2015) Schizophrenia: evidence implicating hippocampal GluN2B protein and REST epigenetics in psychosis pathophysiology. *Neuroscience* **309**:233–242.

Tanskanen P, JM Veijola, UK Piippo, M Haapea, JA Miettunen, J Pyhtinen, ET Bullmore, PB Jones, MK Isohanni (2005) Hippocampus and amygdala volumes in schizophrenia and other psychoses in the Northern Finland 1966 birth cohort. *Schizophr Res* **75**(2–3):283–294.

Tao R, KN Davis, C Li, JH Shin, Y Gao, AE Jaffe, MC Gondré-Lewis, DR Weinberger, JE Kleinman, TM Hyde (2018) GAD1 alternative transcripts and DNA methylation in human prefrontal cortex and hippocampus in brain development, schizophrenia. *Mol Psychiatry* **23**(6):1496–1505.

Tepest R, L Wang, MI Miller, P Falkai, JG Csernansky (2003) Hippocampal deformities in the unaffected siblings of schizophrenia subjects. *Soc Biol Psychiatry* **54**:1234–1240.

Thermenos HW, LJ Seidman, RA Poldrack, NK Peace, JK Koch, SV Faraone, MT Tsuang (2007) Elaborative verbal encoding and altered anterior parahippocampal activation in adolescents and young adults at genetic risk for schizophrenia using FMRI. *Biol Psychiatry* **61**(4):564–574.

Titone D, T Ditman, PS Holzman, H Eichenbaum, DL Levy (2004) Transitive inference in schizophrenia: impairments in relational memory organization. *Schizophr Res* **68**(2–3):235–247.

Tregellas JR, J Smucny, JG Harris, A Olincy, K Maharajh, E Kronberg, LC Eichman, E Lyons, R Freedman (2014) Intrinsic hippocampal activity as a biomarker for cognition and symptoms in schizophrenia. *Am J Psychiatry* **171**:549–556.

van Erp TG, PA Saleh, M Huttunen, J Lonnqvist, J Kaprio, O Salonen, L Valanne, VP Poutanen, CG Standertskjold-Nordenstam, TD Cannon (2004) Hippocampal volumes in schizophrenic twins. *Arch Gen Psychiatry* **61**(4):346–353.

Velakoulis D, SJ Wood, MT Wong, PD McGorry, A Yung, L Phillips, D Smith, W Brewer, T Proffitt, P Desmond, et al. (2006) Hippocampal and amygdala volumes according to psychosis stage and diagnosis: a magnetic resonance imaging study of chronic schizophrenia, first-episode psychosis, and ultra-high-risk individuals. *Arch Gen Psychiatry* **63**(2):139–149.

Velthorst E, AJ Fett, A Reichenberg, G Perlman, J van Os, EJ Bromet, R Kotov (2017) The 20-year longitudinal trajectories of social functioning in individuals with psychotic disorders. *Am J Psychiatry* **174**(11):1075–1085.

Weinberger DR (1999) Cell biology of the hippocampal formation in schizophrenia. *Biol Psychiatry* **45**(4):395–402.

Weiss AP, DL Schacter, DC Goff, SL Rauch, NM Alpert, AJ Fischman, S Heckers (2003) Impaired hippocampal recruitment during normal modulation of memory performance in schizophrenia. *Biol Psychiatry* **53**(1):48–55.

Weiss AP, M Zalesak, I DeWitt, D Goff, L Kunkel, S Heckers (2004) Impaired hippocampal function during the detection of novel words in schizophrenia. *Biol Psychiatry* **55**(7):668–675.

Williams LE, JU Blackford, A Luksik, I Gauthier, S Heckers (2013) Reduced habituation in patients with schizophrenia. *Schizophr Res* **151**(1–3):124–132.

Woerner MG, DG Robinson, JM Alvir, BB Sheitman, JA Lieberman, JM Kane (2003) Clozapine as a first treatment for schizophrenia. *Am J Psychiatry* **160**(8):1514–1516.

Zhao Y, Q Zhang, C Shah, Q Li, JA Sweeney, F Li, Q Gong (2022) Cortical thickness abnormalities at different stages of the illness course in schizophrenia: a systematic review and meta-analysis. *JAMA Psychiatry* **79**(6):560–570.

20

Alzheimer's Disease

Dennis Chan, Tara Spires-Jones, Frank Provenzano, Elizabeth BC Glennon, and Karen Duff

20.1 Introduction

Alzheimer's disease (AD) is a progressive neurodegenerative disease that leads to cognitive decline, and it is the most common cause of dementia worldwide. The *World Alzheimer Report 2015* estimated that there are more than 46 million people with dementia, 70% of whom are considered to have AD. This number is projected to double approximately every 20 years, to 75 million by 2030 and 132 million by 2050, with the midcentury numbers being driven by markedly higher dementia prevalence in low- and middle-income countries (Prince et al., 2013). Dementia is associated with an economic cost in excess of US$800 billion. In recent years, it has become clear that the earliest stages of AD impact the hippocampal formation, later spreading to other brain areas. The prevalence of AD and the associated social and economic costs underline the importance of understanding hippocampal dysfunction, both for understanding the mechanistic underpinings, and for early diagnosis and possibly treatment.

20.2 Pathology of AD

AD is defined at postmortem by the accumulation of two hallmark pathologies: extracellular plaques composed of aggregated β-amyloid (Aβ) peptide and intracellular neurofibrillary tangles composed of hyperphosphorylated, aggregated tau protein (Figure 20.1).

20.2.1 Amyloid plaques and the accumulation of Aβ peptides

Amyloid plaques begin to accumulate many years before symptom onset, initially in the neocortex, followed by the hippocampus, then more subcortical regions as the disease progresses (Thal et al., 2002). Amyloid plaques are composed predominantly of the Aβ peptide along with a variety of other proteins, and they are located extracellularly. They are visualized either by immunohistochemistry using an antibody to Aβ or by use of silver stains. There are two types of amyloid plaque, neuritic plaques and diffuse plaques. The crucial difference between the two types of plaque is the form of amyloid. Neuritic plaques have a dense insoluble β-sheet amyloid core that stains with amyloid-binding dyes such as Congo red and thioflavin S. They are surrounded by oligomeric Aβ and activated glia and dystrophic neurites, suggesting degenerating processes. By contrast, diffuse plaques have few amyloid fibrils and they do not stain with amyloid-binding dyes; rather, they are composed of homogeneous deposits of fibrillar material (Koffie et al., 2012; Serrano-Pozo et al., 2011). Amyloid plaques are observed mainly in the neocortex, with only small numbers seen in hippocampal structures during the early stages of AD. Plaque density in the cortex increases with disease severity, and plaques progress from the neocortex through the hippocampus, basal ganglia, brainstem, and cerebellum (Thal et al., 2002).

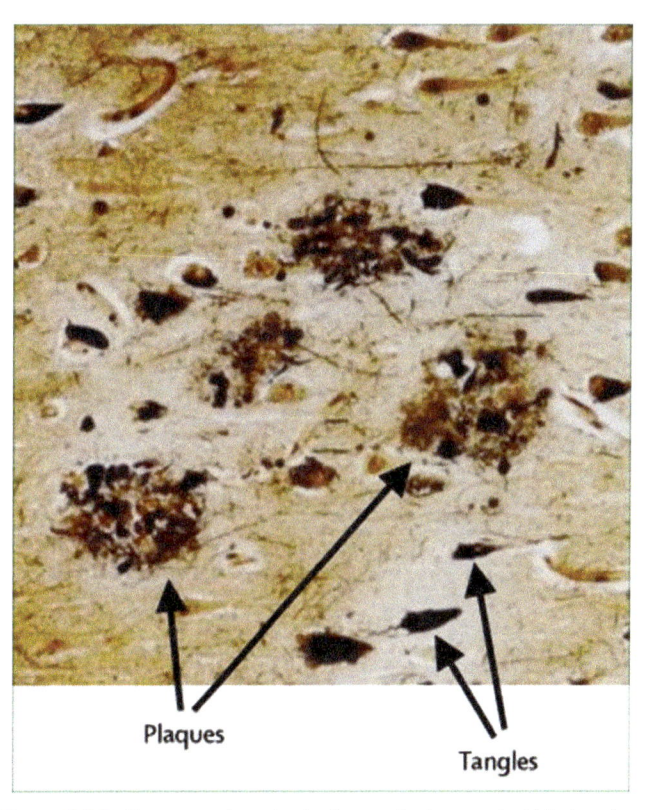

Plaques

Tangles

Figure 20.1 Plaques and tangles in the cerebral cortex in Alzheimer's disease. Plaques are extracellular deposits of Aβ surrounded by dystrophic neurites, reactive astrocytes, and microglia, whereas tangles are intracellular aggregates composed of a hyperphosphorylated form of the microtubule-associated protein tau. (From Blennow et al., 2006.)

20.2.2 Neurofibrillary tangles

Neurofibrillary tangles (NFTs) are primarily composed of the protein tau and they are found in the somatodendritic compartment of neurons. They are flame-shaped and can be visualized with the Bielschowsky silver stain, certain dyes, or by immunohistochemistry using antibodies to the tau protein itself. NFTs are usually intraneuronal but occasionally extracellular, where they represent the insoluble remains of a dead neuron (the "ghost tangle"). NFTs are primarily composed of tau arranged into paired helical filaments, which consist of several proteins including tau, Aβ, ubiquitin, and neurofilament.

20.2.3 Staging of AD

Overt tau pathology (tauopathy) manifests very early in the disease process, first in the entorhinal cortex, then the hippocampus, with increasing involvement of the neocortex as the disease progresses (Braak and Braak, 1991; Braak and Del Tredici, 2015). The distribution of NFTs in the cerebral cortex has been used as a staging system for AD progression called Braak staging (Braak and Braak, 1991) Most people accumulate small amounts of tau pathology in the brainstem during aging (Braak et al., 2011), but this appears to not be associated with a neurodegenerative disease process, which seems to start when tau pathology reaches the medial temporal lobe (Spires-Jones, Attems, and Thal, 2017). In early AD, the first neurons to exhibit substantial NFTs and neuropil threads (straight and paired helical filaments composed of abnormally phosphorylated tau protein) are found in hippocampal structures, the entorhinal cortex, the hippocampal CA1 region, and the transentorhinal cortex, which bridges the entorhinal cortex and the isocortex. These early stages are called the transentorhinal stages and they correspond to Braak stages I and II. The limbic stages, Braak stages III and IV, are characterized by increased numbers of NFTs in the hippocampal structures involved in stages I and II, as well as by low numbers of NFTs in adjacent regions, including CA4 of the hippocampus, the

subiculum, and the parasubiculum. In Braak stages V and VI (the "isocortical stages"), all hippocampal subfields and isocortical association areas are severely affected (Braak and Braak 1991, Braak and del Tredici 2015). The progression of these pathological changes is shown in Figure 20.2.

20.3 Vulnerability of the hippocampal formation in AD

20.3.1 Tau pathology is initiated in the entorhinal cortex

Within the entorhinal cortex, stellate cells of layer II are the first to exhibit NFTs and neuropil threads (NTs). This seems to be an invariant feature of the disease as in one study of patients with a pathological diagnosis of definite AD, severe infiltration of stellate cells by NFTs was observed in 100% of cases (Hyman, Van Hoesen, and Damasio, 1990). Degenerative changes are accompanied by neuronal loss, which is prominent even in the early stages of AD (Gomez-Isla et al., 1996). By late AD, severe loss of layer II cells occurs. Several associated changes are seen in the perforant path, including myelin cuffing and increased acetylcholinesterase staining.

Of the other layers of the entorhinal cortex, NFT formation is observed in most of the pyramidal cells of the Pri-α layer, deep to the cell-sparse lamina dissecans. By contrast, significantly fewer NFTs are seen in layers III, V, and VI. In layer III, the superficial layer of neurons is more severely affected, compounding disruption of the perforant path input to the hippocampus.

Assessment of neuritic plaque density reveals a different pattern of laminar involvement, with most plaques being present in layer III. Plaque density is similar in layers IV, V, and VI, but relatively few plaques are seen in layer II. Neither NFTs nor neuritic plaques are seen in layer I.

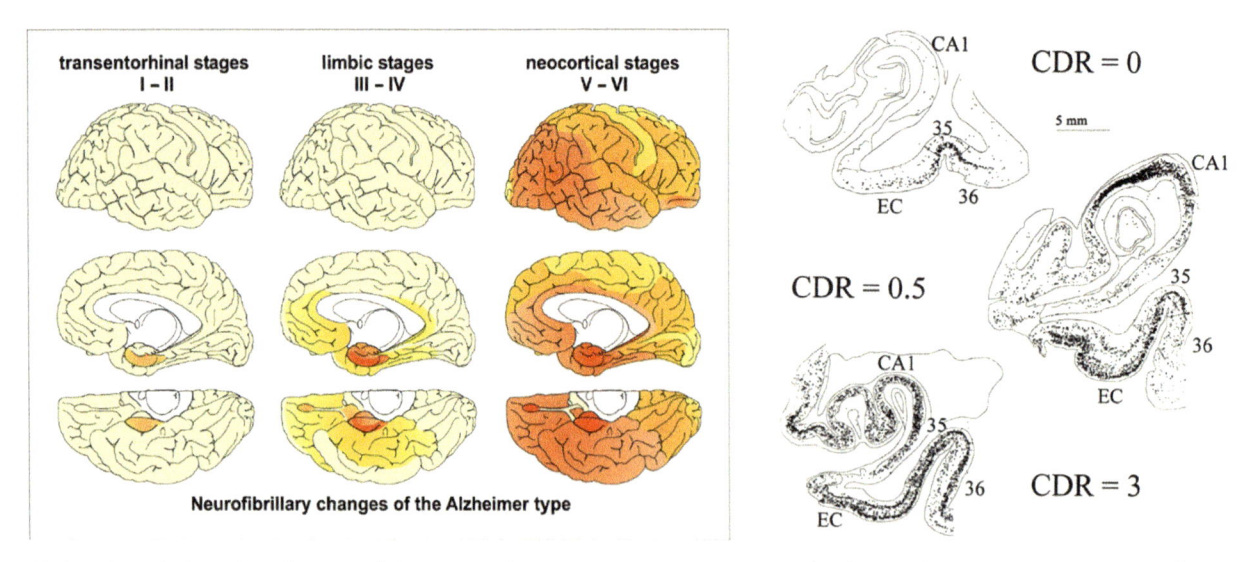

Figure 20.2 Early pathological involvement of the entorhinal cortex and hippocampus in AD. (Left) Neurofibrillary tangles consisting of pathological tau are initially seen in the entorhinal cortex, with subsequent infiltration of the hippocampus and neocortex. (From Braak and Braak 1991.) (Right) Loss of entorhinal cortex (EC) and transentorhinal cortex neurons in asymptomatic individuals (clinical dementia rating [CDR] score 0), with 60% loss of layer II entorhinal cortex neurons by the time of symptom onset (CDR 0.5). (From Gomez-Isla et al., 1996.) Black dots indicate tangle density. (Copyright 1996 Society for Neuroscience.)

Box 20.1 Other pathologies in AD

These pathologies are found in other neurodegenerative disorders and sometimes in normal ageing, so are not specific markers of AD. However, the common occurrence of copathologies may be important as mechanistic links have been observed between pathological proteins, including coseeding and coaggregation (Spires-Jones, Attems, and Thal 2017).

- **Inclusions of TAR DNA-binding protein 43 (TDP-43)** in the cytoplasm are observed in approximately 50% of AD cases (Spires-Jones, Attems, and Thal 2017). The relevance of this pathology to disease symptoms remains unclear. Alpha-synuclein pathology, which is classically associated with Lewy body diseases (LBD; Parkinson's and dementia with Lewy bodies), is also seen in more than 40% of AD cases. The coaccumulation of alpha-synuclein and AD pathologies is associated with aggravated disease progression compared with AD or LBD pathologies in isolation (Spires-Jones, Attems, and Thal 2017).
- **Granulovacuolar degeneration** is seen in up to 50% of AD cases. Vacuoles (3–5 μm diameter) are found in the cytoplasm of pyramidal neurons, either singly or in combination. In marked contrast to the widespread distribution of amyloid plaques and NFTs, granulovacuolar degeneration is restricted primarily to one neuronal population, pyramidal cells of the hippocampus.
- **Hirano bodies** are ovoid eosinophilic inclusions about 10–30 μm long. They are most commonly observed adjacent to hippocampal pyramidal cells, where they indent the neuronal cell body, although they can also be found in isolation in the stratum lacunosum of AD patients at postmortem.
- **Lipid droplets** are cytoplasmic accumulations of lipids in the cell body. Lipid droplets were first observed in retinal ganglion cells, glia, and vessel wall cells in the AD brain by Alois Alzheimer, but have received significantly less research attention than amyloid plaques and NFTs (Foley 2010). Increased numbers of larger lipid droplets are seen in microglia of the aged compared with the young brain (Marschallinger et al. 2020), and they are highly prevalent in the hippocampus of aged mice (Marschallinger et al. 2020). In aged mice, lipid droplets are mainly composed of glycerolipids and are formed in response to inflammatory stimulation of microglia. Microglia harboring lipid droplets show dysregulated expression of genes associated with phagocytosis and lysosomal pathways. Cells containing lipid droplets show impaired phagocytosis of particles (Marschallinger et al. 2020), which may contribute to the accumulation of pathological proteins.

20.3.2 Tau pathology spreads to the hippocampus

Of the hippocampal subfields, NFT and amyloid plaque density is highest in CA1 and the subiculum. The CA1/subiculum interface zone is particularly affected, with a large number of plaques and tangles observed in all cases. Only small numbers of plaques and tangles are seen in CA3 and CA4 (the part of CA3 inserting between the horns of the dentate gyrus). The outer two-thirds of the molecular layer of the dentate gyrus is heavily infiltrated by NFTs and neuritic plaques, and NFTs are also seen in dentate granule cells. Few pathological changes are seen in the mossy fiber zone. In contrast to the subiculum, the presubiculum is largely free of NFTs and plaques. In terms of the hierarchical staging of AD pathology, CA1 pyramidal cells are the first hippocampal neurons to exhibit changes and represent the second neuronal population to be affected in AD, after stellate cells of the entorhinal cortex. Large multipolar cells in CA4 and subicular neurons are the next to be affected; the granule cell layer of the dentate gyrus, CA3, and the presubiculum are involved only in the late stages of AD. Interestingly, NFTs are

seen in the inner third of the dentate molecular layer in the most severely affected AD cases, which suggests that in the late disease stages there is additional deafferentation of the input to the dentate gyrus from hilar cells. Although the hippocampus is affected throughout its extent, the number of neurons exhibiting NFTs and granulovacuolar degeneration is particularly high in the posterior hippocampus (Ball, 1987).

Pathological forms of tau spread from the entorhinal cortex and hippocampus through neural circuits of the brain in a stereotypical fashion. Data from mouse models and cell culture systems indicate that this spread of tau occurs via synaptic connections (de Calignon et al., 2012; Harris et al., 2012; Liu, Drouet, et al., 2012). For example, in the EC-tau mouse, which expresses disease-associated mutant human tau at high levels in the entorhinal cortex (medial and lateral, layer 2 and 3 neurons) reproducing the pathology seen in the early stages of human AD, tau first accumulates in axons projecting from the entorhinal cortex neurons expressing human tau; as the mice age, tauopathy spreads to CA pyramidal cells (especially CA1, reminiscent of human AD), into the deeper layers of the cortex, and throughout the neocortex (de Calignon et al., 2012; Liu, Drouet, et al., 2012). As tauopathy impacts the same regions of the brain affected in the earliest stages of AD (the entorhinal cortex), and then spreads to the hippocampus in a predictable fashion, this mouse line has been frequently used to correlate the spread of pathology with neurodegeneration including of specific cell types such as excitatory cells (Fu, Hardy, and Duff, 2018), functional decline as assessed by fMRI (Fung et al., 2020; Khan et al., 2014) and cognitive impairment (Fu et al., 2019).

The degree of overall hippocampal pyramidal cell loss in postmortem AD brains is estimated to be around 43%–47%, with increasing neuronal loss correlating with disease severity (Davies et al., 1992; Doebler et al., 1987). Some disagreement exists with regard to the distribution of neuronal loss affecting the hippocampus. Some observers have reported that the bulk of neuronal loss occurs in CA1, with additional neuronal loss in CA4, the subiculum, and the presubiculum and relative sparing of the dentate granule cells and neurons in CA3 and CA2 (Doebler et al., 1987; West et al., 1994). In a later study, no significant difference was noted in the amount of cell loss in CA1 in AD and normal aging; instead, the greatest differences in neuronal numbers were observed in the granule cell layer and the subiculum (Simic et al., 1997) An inverse correlation exists between hippocampal neuronal density and the number of neurons with NFT infiltration or granulovacuolar degeneration. In terms of the clinical significance of the severity of hippocampal involvement, the degree of neuronal loss in CA1, CA4, and the subiculum is found to correlate with greater severity of AD.

Interestingly, the hippocampal formation may be at the crux of the amyloid-dependent and -independent phases of the disease. Early studies using combined amyloid and tau-PET imaging suggest that, in the presence of amyloid, tau accumulation is exacerbated over time (Koychev et al., 2017). Cross-sectional PET imaging suggests that when amyloid pathology reaches the hippocampal formation, tau pathology then spreads through the brain (Hanseeuw et al., 2019), killing neurons in the process.

20.3.3 Cells of the hippocampal formation vary in their vulnerability

It is of great interest to understand the factors underlying why some cell types are more vulnerable than others in AD. These factors can be generally divided into two groups: cell-autonomous factors, which operate independently of each cell, and non-cell-autonomous factors, which are dependent on the status of other cells. Both types of factors seem to contribute to neuronal vulnerability in AD (Acosta et al., 2018; Wang et al., 2020). Many cell-autonomous factors fall under the umbrella of homeostatically regulated processes such as oxidative stress, metabolic and energy demands, intracellular calcium levels, excitotoxicity, proteolytic stress and protein folding, inflammatory reactions, unconventional translation, and aging (Fu, Hardy, and Duff, 2018; Gan et al., 2018; Muddapu et al., 2020). Non-cell-autonomous processes are primarily associated with the transsynaptic spread of pathological proteins from one cell to another (Vogels et al., 2020), but also include environmental factors such as vasculature, inflammation, immune response, blood-brain barrier disruptions, and glial biology (Henstridge, Tzioras, and Paolicelli, 2019; Saxena and Caroni, 2011).

To narrow down or unify these contributions, researchers often compare cell types and regions of differential vulnerability for common properties. Although no staging system exists that explicitly measures cell death in AD, Braak staging for NFTs is known to correlate well with selective damage, cognitive decline, and atrophy (Del Tredici and Braak, 2020). As mentioned previously, large pyramidal neurons of the CA1 and subiculum are commonly regarded as the earliest cells to accumulate NFTs after those in the entorhinal cortex, and those with long-range and sparsely myelinated or unmyelinated axons (Braak et al., 2006), and those that are neurofilament-rich (Morrison, Hof, and Morrison, 1998) are particularly vulnerable.

Several differences between CA1 neurons and others in the hippocampus may explain their initial vulnerability. Firstly. broad cell type composition differs across regions, with CA1 and the subiculum (as well as the less vulnerable CA3) being primarily composed of pyramidal neurons, although significant heterogeneity between and within these populations is being increasingly uncovered through new high-throughput cell-typing methods (Cembrowski and Spruston, 2019). In contrast, CA2 has been shown to contain larger numbers of calcium-buffering/binding protein (CBP) and reelin-positive interneurons in rodent studies (Botcher et al., 2014), which may confer a protective effect. The dentate gyrus and hilus contain a disparate population of cell types, being composed mainly of granule cells and mossy cells, respectively. Cell type differences are also seen along the rostral/caudal axis of the hippocampus; in induced pluripotential stem cells derived from patients with an AD-causing mutation, rostral neurons, which contain a mix of excitatory and inhibitory neurons, are more vulnerable than caudal neurons, which are more frequently inhibitory (Muratore et al., 2017). In general, inhibitory neurons are far less vulnerable to tauopathy than excitatory neurons, and their transcriptomes are characterized by higher levels of transcripts coding for aggregation-protecting factors, fewer transcripts coding for aggregation-promoting factors, and high levels of CBP transcripts (Fu et al., 2019). In addition, inhibitory neurons are rarely neurofilament-reactive (Morrison, Hof, and Morrison, 1998). However, specific inhibitory subpopulations still appear to be vulnerable, particularly parvalbumin-expressing interneurons such as chandelier cells (Braak and Del Tredici, 2015; Solodkin, Veldhuizen, and Van Hoesen, 1996).

Regions and cell types of the hippocampus have been shown in rodent models of AD to differ in their response to pathology, compared with later affected hippocampal areas. For example,

CA1 neurons exhibit higher reactive oxygen species and superoxide production (Wang et al., 2005; Wilde et al., 1997), a greater abundance of activated glial cells (Rodriguez, Noristani, et al., 2013), differential expression of N-methyl-D-aspartate (NMDA) receptors, including overexpression of the apoptosis-inducing NR2B subunit (Liu, Lv, et al., 2012), high Ca^{2+} influx through L-type voltage-gated calcium channels (Wang and Mattson, 2014), upregulation of certain kinases alongside downregulation of phosphatases (Gerschutz et al., 2014), and impaired autophagic lysosome function (Bordi et al., 2016). In humans, MRI studies in individuals with AD and MCI have shown preferential atrophy and blood-brain barrier breakdown in CA1 (Montagne et al., 2016). CA1 is also vascularized solely by the ventral arteries, while CA2–4 and the dentate gyrus are supplied by a mix of other arterial groups (Duvernoy, 2005). Human studies have also demonstrated that earlier-affected cells carry a greater proportion of tau inclusions composed of tau containing three repeat domains compared with four repeat domains (Hara et al., 2013; Iseki et al., 2006), but the significance of this is unknown. Some AD studies in humans have combined laser capture microdissection with RNA sequencing to study individual cells; for example, Ginsberg et al. found that genes associated with synapses, the cytoskeleton, dopamine receptors, glutamate receptors, phosphatases, and kinases were downregulated in NFT-bearing neurons from CA1 compared with the same neurons without tangles from age-matched non-AD controls (Ginsberg et al., 2006; Ginsberg et al., 2000). A recent study in non-NFT-bearing neurons identified upregulation of amyloid precursor protein in AD and altered expression of genes related to cell death, metabolic processes, mitochondria and synapses (Deng et al., 2019). Research in aging and stress-related conditions has also produced valuable insights into selective vulnerability in AD (Chapters 15 and 17). In rodents, compared with CA3 neurons, CA1 neurons show a greater reduction of calbindin during aging (Potier et al., 1994) and exhibit more severe mitochondrial damage postischemia (Radenovic et al., 2011) and from calcium-induced mitochondrial swelling (Mattiasson et al., 2003). Similarly, CA1 neurons experience greater calcium influx and calcium deposition into mitochondria after prolonged glutamate stimulation (Stanika et al., 2010).

These studies have identified several factors potentially underlying selective vulnerability, although more work is needed to incorporate them into a unified model. This will require the use of emerging tools for high-throughput molecular analysis within a spatial context to understand the contributions of regions within the hippocampus and other areas more accurately. Improvements in spatial and single cell transcriptomics and proteomics, coupled with computational, systems biology is now providing a wealth of information about the physiology of individual cell types, and their role in disease.

20.3.4 Hippocampal circuit vulnerability

Circuit dynamics and anatomical connectivity within the hippocampus are another important consideration, particularly when considering the ability of tau pathology to spread from region to region. Differentially vulnerable regions of entorhinal cortex and hippocampal subfields innervate one another in a highly organized fashion as described in Chapters 3, 6, and 12. There is evidence that CA3 becomes hyperactive in AD (Haberman, Branch, and Gallagher, 2017), which may be a mechanism for CA1 excitotoxicity.

Interestingly, in a normal physiological state, overall CA1 firing rate is higher than that of CA3 (Mizuseki et al., 2012) but this relationship reverses in aging (Kanak et al., 2013) (Oh, Simkin, and Disterhoft, 2016) (see also Chapters 3 and 6).

20.3.5 Defining AD based on pathophysiology

The definitive diagnosis of AD is dependent on the histopathological identification of amyloid plaques and neurofibrillary tangles, with diagnostic criteria for AD based on determination of neuritic plaque density, quantitative assessment of both plaques and tangles, and more recently on the number of tangles and neuropil threads in the cerebral cortex (Hyman et al., 2012; Hyman and Trojanowski, 1997).

Macroscopically, the correlate of AD neurodegeneration is brain atrophy, which is apparent on visual examination of the postmortem brain and manifests primarily as enlargement of ventricles, in particular the late ventricles, and a widening of sulci. In later stages of disease, there is generalized atrophy of the cerebral cortex, within which damage to the medial temporal lobe structures is manifest most notably as reduction of amygdala and hippocampal volumes, expansion of the temporal horns of the lateral ventricles and widening of the collateral sulcus due to atrophy of the entorhinal cortex and adjacent perirhinal cortex. It is however important to note that whole brain and even medial temporal lobe neurodegeneration and atrophy are not specific to AD but can occur—though typically to a lesser extent—in other neurodegenerative diseases such as Lewy body dementia (LBD) as well as nonneurodegenerative conditions including depression.

The events that lead to amyloid plaque and neurofibrillary tangle pathology are associated with synaptic dysfunction, gliosis, neurodegeneration, and network imbalance, but the contribution of each to dementia, and the cause-and-effect relationships, remain unclear. However, though our understanding of causality at present remains imprecise, the robustness of knowledge regarding the associations between molecular pathology and the clinical condition has prompted efforts to shift the emphasis from AD as a disease diagnosed purely on clinical grounds to one that is defined biologically. To encompass not just the presence of the two defining molecular pathologies of AD but also the occurrence of

neurodegeneration as the resultant disease process, a new research framework developed by the National Institute on Aging/Alzheimer's Association (NIA-AA) defined AD based on a tripartite "AT(N)" classification, requiring evidence of Aβ (A), tau (T), and neurodegeneration (N). It is hoped that taking these three features into account will improve diagnostic accuracy and serve as a template for understanding the interaction between these disparate pathological entities and their contribution to AD onset and progression (Jack et al., 2018) (Figure 20.3).

20.3.6 Pathological changes of the hippocampus can also occur in normal aging

Amyloid plaques and NFTs are also observed in the brains of aged individuals without dementia. Diffuse plaques and small numbers of neuritic plaques are found throughout the cerebral cortex, amygdala, entorhinal cortex, and CA1, and neuritic plaques appear enriched in the medial temporal lobe. Like neuritic plaques, NFTs are enriched in medial temporal lobe structures, including the hippocampus (where NFTs in CA1 correlate with age) and parahippocampal regions such as the entorhinal cortex. This has led to the suggestion that some "normal" elderly subjects may in fact have preclinical AD. However, the observation that hippocampal subregions are differentially vulnerable to normal aging and AD suggests that the two are separate pathways (Small et al., 2011; Small et al., 2004). The demonstration of AD-type pathology in "normal" elderly individuals and the concomitant difficulty in distinguishing these changes from those seen in the earliest stages of AD mirrors the clinical challenge of differentiating between individuals exhibiting age-related minor cognitive decline and patients manifesting the earliest symptoms of AD.

20.4 Clinical features of AD

20.4.1 Stages of AD

The diagnosis of AD was initially based on clinical features and the presence of dementia, as outlined in the National Institute of Neurological and Communicative Diseases and Stroke/Alzheimer's Disease and Related Disorders Association (NINCDS-ADRDA)

Syndromal Cognitive Stage				
Biomarker Profile		Cognitively unimpaired	MCI	dementia
	A⁻ T⁻ (N)⁻	normal AD biomarkers, cognitively unimpaired	normal AD biomarkers with MCI	normal AD biomarkers with dementia
	A⁺ T⁻ (N)⁻	Preclinical Alzheimer's pathologic change	Alzheimer's pathologic change with MCI	Alzheimer's pathologic change with dementia
	A⁺ T⁻ (N)⁺	Alzheimer's and concomitant suspected non-Alzheimer's pathologic change, cognitively unimpaired	Alzheimer's and concomitant suspected non-Alzheimer's pathologic change with MCI	Alzheimer's and concomitant suspected non-Alzheimer's pathologic change with dementia
	A⁺ T⁺ (N)⁻	Preclinical Alzheimer's disease	Alzheimer's disease with MCI (Prodromal AD)	Alzheimer's disease with dementia
	A⁺ T⁺ (N)⁺			

Figure 20.3 Tripartite AT(N) classification of AD. (From Jack et al., 2018.)

criteria (McKhann et al., 1984). However, AD diagnosis has been re-evaluated, following advances in understanding the AD phenotype and the advent of biomarkers able to detect evidence of Aβ and tau pathology or neurodegeneration using biofluid assays (cerebrospinal fluid [CSF], serum) and/or neuroimaging (section 20.6 below). Current guidelines for the diagnosis of AD have therefore been extended in two ways. First, they consider AD as a disease continuum ranging from an initial asymptomatic stage through to the clinical end-stage characterized by the presence of dementia. Second, they acknowledge the value of using biomarkers to provide evidence of AD as the underlying pathological disorder. This is reflected in the introduction of updated NIA-AA diagnostic guidelines in 2011, which divided AD into three stages. Preclinical AD refers to the presymptomatic stage when there is biomarker evidence of AD pathology but without associated cognitive decline (Sperling et al., 2011). Clinical AD, following the onset of symptoms, was split into two stages. "Mild cognitive impairment due to AD" describes the state when individuals are symptomatic, but the severity of cognitive decline is insufficient to compromise activities of daily living or functional independence (Albert et al., 2011). "AD dementia" refers to the clinical stage when there is widespread cognitive impairment affecting multiple cognitive domains, typically accompanied by significant changes in personality and behavior, with affected individuals needing significant care input (McKhann et al., 2011). A similar diagnostic framework was published by the International Working Group (IWG) for New Research Criteria for the Diagnosis of AD. It also acknowledged the preclinical stages of AD and the role of biomarkers but used the term "prodromal AD" to describe the early symptomatic stage, analogous to "mild cognitive impairment due to AD" (Dubois et al., 2010; Dubois et al., 2014). Importantly, both sets of revised guidelines emphasize the distinction between a diagnosis of AD that can be made by clinicians on clinical grounds alone, which is crucial given the varying access to specialized investigations in different clinical settings worldwide, and the more stringent criteria required for AD diagnosis in the context of research and clinical trials.

20.4.2 Memory impairments are characteristic symptoms of AD

Impairment of episodic memory (see Chapters 13 and 14) represents the archetypal presenting symptom of AD, typically with an insidious onset and subsequent gradual progressive decline over months and often several years. This takes various forms, such as difficulty recalling recent events and information from day to day, problems remembering conversations, and a tendency of affected individuals to repeat themselves. These impairments may be accompanied by a reduced ability to remember the storylines of television programs or recently read books. These symptoms are frequently intermixed with other reports of "poor memory," which may reflect impairment of other cognitive functions, such as attention (exemplified by a tendency to misplace items or to enter a room and forget why) or retrieval processes (manifest as a difficulty finding words or remembering names, with recollection occurring only belatedly or on prompting). "Getting lost" is another symptom frequently listed as a problem with "memory," which likely reflects the involvement of the hippocampal formation in spatial memory (Chapters 11 and 13). At the outset, people may have difficulty finding their way around unfamiliar places when on holiday or when driving. As the disease progresses, navigational difficulties can extend to familiar

environments such as home neighborhoods. In end-stage AD, patients may have problems finding their way around their own homes, although by this stage, navigation is also significantly complicated by profoundly impaired higher visual processing.

Further questioning in a clinic will often reveal impairment affecting other cognitive and behavioral domains at an early stage. Executive dysfunction may be represented by impaired decision-making and problem-solving, accompanied by loss of organizational ability. Such problems can impact professional work and disrupt domestic activities such as managing finances and other household duties. Changes in behavior or personality can occur alongside, or even predate, cognitive symptoms and may take various forms including apathy, anxiety, mood disturbance, irritability, agitation, and altered social conduct (although these are not specific to AD dementia). The observation that the early occurrence of these features can predict the onset of dementia has given rise to the notion of a "mild behavioral impairment" syndrome, in parallel with mild cognitive impairment, as a manifestation of prodromal AD (Ismail et al., 2016). Other studies have suggested that mild behavioral impairment may predate the onset of cognitive symptoms in early AD (Pink et al., 2015) and that it is associated with Aβ but not tau pathology (Lussier et al., 2020).

The progression from mild behavioral and cognitive impairment to frank dementia is associated with the loss of functional independence and impaired activities of daily living. This clinical decline mirrors the progressive pathological infiltration of the cerebral cortex, with all brain regions affected in late-stage disease, albeit with relatively lower disease burden in primary motor and sensory cortices (Braak and Braak, 1991). Consistent with this, multiple cognitive domains are severely impaired in later stages, with additional subcortical dysfunction characterized by reduced speed of information processing and motoric features such as imbalance and gait disorder. Significant care input is needed, aggravated by the loss of insight in affected individuals. In final stages, regular nursing is required, often in institutional settings, and medical complications such as sepsis or malnutrition may hasten death.

20.4.3 Presymptomatic stages of AD

Neuropathological changes in AD (and therefore biochemical changes within the brain) predate the onset of symptoms by many years. The advent of biomarkers, serving as surrogates of this pathology, has facilitated attempts to determine the preclinical stages of sporadic AD. As biomarker positivity is considered indicative but not confirmatory of AD, and thus merely predictive of future clinical progression, the International Working Group tasked with updating AD diagnostic criteria distinguished two categories of preclinical AD (Dubois et al., 2014). "Asymptomatic at risk for AD" describes those individuals without the symptomatology associated with AD but with positive AD biomarkers. "Presymptomatic AD" refers to those individuals with evidence of an AD autosomal dominant genetic mutation but without any accompanying clinical phenotype at the time of evaluation. Together, these two categories attempt to encompass both sporadic and familial forms of preclinical AD, as well as highlighting their differences in terms of diagnostic certainty. In both forms of AD, additional investigations have identified cognitive deficits, primarily in the domains of episodic memory and allocentric spatial memory (Insel et al., 2020; K Ritchie et al., 2018), consistent with the early pathological involvement of the hippocampal formation. Neuroimaging studies have shown evidence of additional neurodegeneration, manifest as either hypometabolism or atrophy, occurring up to 15 years before the anticipated age of symptom onset in a familial AD cohort (Bateman et al., 2012) and 20 years before dementia onset in a cohort at risk of sporadic AD (O'Brien et al., 2020) (section 20.6).

20.4.4 Mild cognitive impairment

The term "mild cognitive impairment" (MCI, Box 20.2) was introduced to address the need to define a state of cognitive decline that is insufficiently severe to warrant the diagnosis of dementia. The hope was that MCI would, in turn, aid efforts to identify AD in its earlier stages. The stipulation of memory as the primary cognitive domain of interest reflected the opinion that AD was the predominant disease underlying MCI. Subsequent definitions of MCI have expanded the construct to encompass the possibility that MCI may also represent the prodromal phase of non-AD dementias, in which nonmemory cognitive domains are more affected. This has led to the subdivision of MCI into amnestic and nonamnestic MCI, with a further categorization into single-domain and multidomain MCI, depending on the extent of cognitive impairment, in order to help predict the type of dementia into which MCI could evolve (Petersen, 2004).

While "MCI" is at present the most widely adopted term in both clinical and research settings, alternative terminologies have been used to describe a similar cognitive state. The 2013 *Diagnostic and Statistical Manual for Mental Disorders* (DSM-5) uses the term "mild neurocognitive disorder" to describe cognitive decline that is different from normal aging but not as severe as in dementia, with diagnostic criteria that are very similar to those previously outlined for MCI.

People with MCI may remain clinically stable, progress to dementia (AD or non-AD) or improve (Matthews et al., 2008). With respect to the second of these, rates of progression from MCI to dementia vary greatly across studies. A meta-analysis of 41 studies (Mitchell and Shiri-Feshki, 2009) identified annual rates of progression of 10% in specialist settings and 5% in community-based settings, with the former reflecting a study cohort enriched for the presence of underlying pathology by comparison with prospective community studies. With respect to possible improvement, reversion to normal cognition is a frequently described outcome of MCI, with anything from 6% to 55% of those diagnosed with MCI returning to a state of objectively normal cognition at annual follow up (Ganguli et al., 2011; Koepsell and Monsell, 2012; Sachdev et al., 2013).

Box 20.2 Mild cognitive impairment

The term "mild cognitive impairment" (MCI) is used to describe a loss of cognitive capacity beyond that expected in normal aging but not so severe to warrant a diagnosis of dementia. In its first iteration, the criteria for MCI were:

- Self- or informant-reported memory decline
- Objective evidence of cognitive impairment
- Relatively preserved functional independence
- Preserved activities of daily living
- Absence of dementia

(From Petersen et al. 1999.)

20.4.5 Pathological changes in MCI largely affect hippocampal structures

Postmortem analyses have revealed that the pathological changes associated with MCI primarily affect the entorhinal cortex and hippocampus. Patients with very mild dementia at the time of death exhibit severe neuronal loss primarily affecting EC layer II, with neuronal numbers being reduced by almost 60% (Gomez-Isla et al., 1996). In EC layer IV, neuronal numbers are reduced by 40%, whereas layers I, III, and V are less affected. The degree of neuronal loss is greater in cases of severe dementia, with the drop in neuronal counts in layers II and IV rising to about 90% and 70%, respectively. These reductions in neuronal numbers are accompanied by increased deposition of NFTs and neuritic plaques. A comparison of the severity of entorhinal cortex pathology in MCI and AD reveals that AD is associated with greater volume loss affecting layer II.

The distribution of pathological damage in the entorhinal cortex in people with MCI is similar to the initial stages of tau pathology described in AD (Braak stages I and II). For Aβ, the burden in MCI varies in density and cortical distribution but largely appears to lie at an intermediate level between that seen in healthy aging and AD dementia (Markesbery et al., 2006; Jicha et al., 2006).

20.4.6 Typical AD involves the hippocampal formation, whereas atypical presentations of AD affect other regions

In addition to the typical amnestic presentation, in which there is early pathological involvement of the entorhinal cortex and hippocampus, several atypical presentations of AD are now recognized in which the dominant initial symptom is not that of memory decline but instead impairment of higher visual processing, speech production, or executive function. These atypically presenting cases share the same underlying Aβ and tau pathology as typical AD, but the molecular pathology initially affects non-medial temporal lobe (MTL) cortical regions though with pathological spread ultimately leading to widespread cortical damage—including MTL regions—and global dementia with multiple cognitive domains affected. Imaging studies indicate that these variants are associated with differing patterns of cerebral hypometabolism and Aβ deposition, and potentially the spread of pathology within different functional brain networks (Lehmann et al., 2014).

20.4.7 Subjective cognitive decline often precedes AD and other dementias

The diagnostic criteria for MCI provide objective evidence of cognitive impairment, complementing reports of subjective cognitive decline. By extension, this raises the possibility of an earlier stage of AD characterized by the subjective report of cognitive difficulties (for example, an elderly person complaining of "just not feeling right") occurring prior to the identification of significant deficits on objective testing. This has given rise to the formulation of "subjective cognitive decline" (SCD) as an entity distinct from both normal cognitive function and MCI. While there is significant evidence that SCD is a clinical manifestation of a pre-MCI stage of AD that is associated with an increased risk of developing dementia (Glodzik-Sobanska et al., 2007; Reisberg et al., 2010; Visser et al., 2009), SCD is also seen in numerous non-AD states. This includes normal aging (the prevalence of SCD is 50%–80% in people aged over 70 years (van Harten et al., 2018)), psychiatric conditions such as anxiety and depression, and a wide range of other medical conditions. To aid characterization of SCD as a pre-MCI stage of AD, a working group developed a conceptual framework defining the core clinical aspects of SCD and described features associated with an increased probability of underlying AD. These included age of onset >60 years, reported decline in memory rather than another cognitive domain, and the presence of the apolipoprotein E4 (APOE4) genotype or biomarker evidence of AD (Jessen et al., 2020; Jessen et al., 2014). A comparison of SCD features and AD biomarkers has shown that a reported decline in memory and language are associated with lower CSF Aβ levels, which is thought to reflect greater retention of Aβ in the brain as amyloid plaques form (Miebach et al., 2019).

Individuals with SCD due to AD have a 40%–62% risk of progressing to MCI or dementia within 3 years (van Harten et al., 2013; Wolfsgruber et al., 2017). Imaging work has revealed evidence of early neurodegeneration within the medial temporal lobe, including hippocampal atrophy (Saykin et al., 2006) or hypometabolism (Vannini et al., 2017). SCD is associated with tau pathology in the entorhinal cortex and increased global amyloid burden (Buckley et al., 2017), reinforcing the opinion that SCD may in some instances represent the initial, pre-MCI, symptomatic stage of AD.

20.4.8 Cognitive testing in early AD

Numerous cognitive tests are used to diagnose AD, with the choice of test(s) determined by various factors, including operator experience and training, stage of AD under evaluation, and test setting (primary care general practice, specialist memory clinic, clinical trial, or research program). Tests range from brief pen-and-paper tests of general cognitive function, such as the Mini Mental State Examination (Folstein, Folstein, and McHugh, 1975) through to test batteries encompassing a range of cognitive domains and applied by trained neuropsychologists. While brief cognitive tests are widely used in clinical practice to detect dementia, due to their low cost and ease of use, they lack diagnostic specificity for different types of dementia and diagnostic sensitivity is low for predementia stages of disease. Their lack of diagnostic specificity is associated with a poor ability to predict cognitive decline, as evidenced by a Cochrane Database systematic review showing a summary sensitivity of 40% for predicting conversion from MCI to dementia at a median specificity of 88% (Arevalo-Rodriguez et al., 2015).

20.4.8.1 Cognitive testing focuses on detecting hippocampal dysfunction

Consistent with the early involvement of the medial temporal lobe in the AD disease process and with memory decline as the hallmark presenting symptom, tests of episodic memory are the most widely used in diagnostic practice (Maruta et al., 2011) and are applied at all stages of AD. While nonmemory tests such as the Trail Making Test and the Digit Symbol Test, both considered to measure attention, executive function, and speed of information processing, are sensitive to early AD and incorporated within cognitive test batteries for use in clinical trials (Donohue et al., 2014), most tests used clinically and in research focus on assessment of verbal and nonverbal memory.

20.4.8.2 Testing of episodic memory

Assessment of word-list recall is the most commonly applied test of episodic memory in AD (Box 20.3). These tests can generate a

---

Box 20.3 Verbal recall tasks

Verbal recall tasks are used to assess episodic memory. Examples of standalone verbal recall tasks include:

- Free and Cued Selective Reminding Test (Buschke 1984)
- Hopkins Verbal Learning Test (Brandt and Benedict 2001)
- California Verbal Learning Test (Delis et al. 1987)
- Rey Auditory Verbal Learning Test (Rey 1941)

Verbal recall tests may also form part of cognitive test batteries such as:

- Alzheimer's Disease Assessment Scale—cognition (ADAS-cog) (Mohs, Rosen, and Davis 1983)
- Repeatable Battery for the Assessment of Neuropsychological Status (RBANS) (Randolph et al. 1998)
- Wechsler Memory battery (http://www.pearsonclinical.com/)

Abbreviated recall subtests are embedded within short global cognitive assessment tools designed primarily for use in memory clinics. These include:

- Mini-Mental State Examination (MMSE)
- Test Your Memory (TYM) task (Brown et al. 2009)
- Montreal Cognitive Assessment (Nasreddine et al. 2005)
- Addenbrooke's Cognitive Examination—Revised (Mioshi et al. 2006)

---

number of outcomes, including immediate recall (% of items correctly recalled immediately after a learning phase), delayed free and cued recall (% of items correctly recalled after an interval, with and without cueing), and retention (difference between items correctly recalled immediately and after a delay).

Verbal recall can also be tested in the form of short story recall, such as the logical memory test within the Wechsler Memory Scale, which can again generate data on both immediate and delayed recall. Tasks used to assess nonverbal recall include the Rey figure recall (Osterrieth, 1944), involving delayed recall of a complex visual figure, and tests of the ability to recall an item and its location.

These memory tests have an extensive historical pedigree, some dating back to the first half of the 20th century and thus predating the original work linking the hippocampus to memory functions (Scoville and Milner, 1957). More recently introduced memory tests have therefore been designed around current understanding of the involvement of the hippocampal formation, and hippocampal subfields, in specific processes within memory formation. Examples of these tests include tests of visual short-term memory binding, pattern separation, and pattern completion (Figures 20.4 and 20.5).

20.4.8.3 Neuroimaging studies show links between hippocampal damage and performance in episodic memory tests.

Numerous imaging studies have shown correlations between memory impairment in AD and alterations in the medial temporal lobe. There is evidence of lateralization, with left and right hippocampal damage associated with impaired performance on tests of verbal and nonverbal memory, respectively (Kohler et al., 1998; Sarazin et al., 2010). Various magnetic resonance imaging (MRI) and positron emission tomography (PET) studies have found correlations between performance on memory tasks and hippocampal volume (Visser et al., 1999), metabolism (Chetelat et al., 2003), structural connectivity (Mielke et al., 2012), and functional connectivity (Berron et al., 2020), with imaging changes predictive of future clinical progression from the earliest, presymptomatic stages of AD (Fox et al., 1996). More recent hippocampal structure–function studies

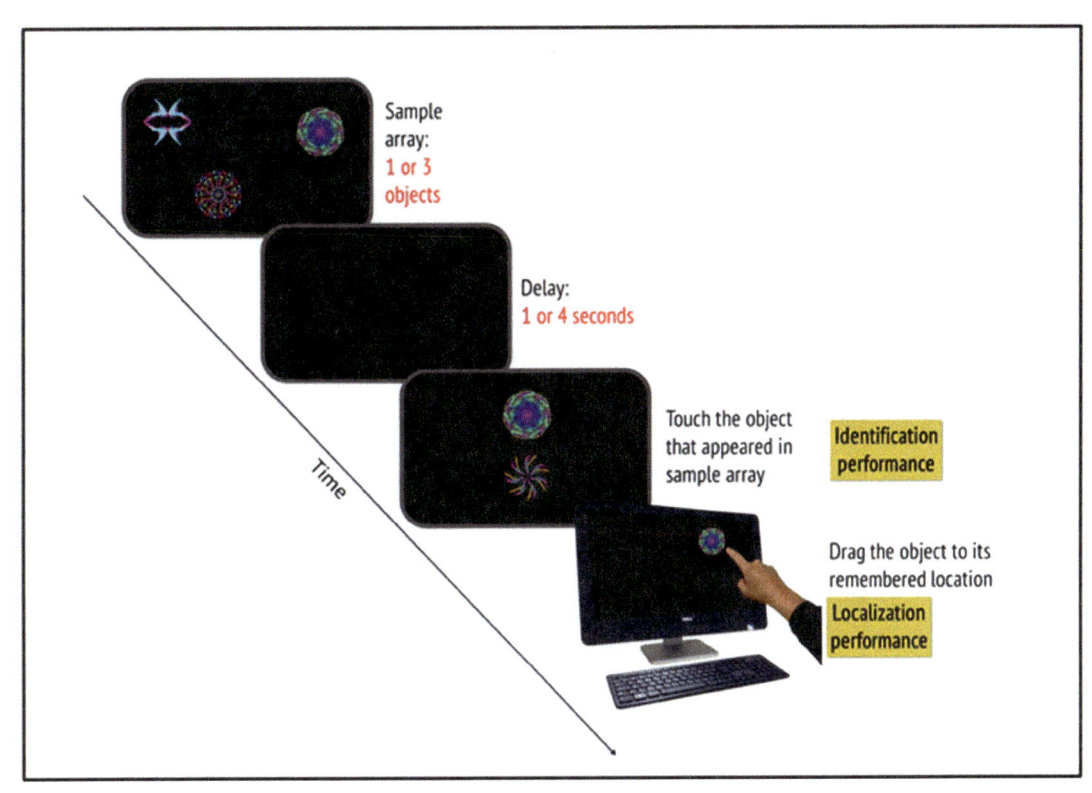

Figure 20.4 "What was where?" test of visual short-term memory binding. Participants are asked to remember the nature and on-screen location of one or three fractal images are presented at random locations on a touchscreen. After a 1 s or 4 s interval, two fractal objects are presented, one previously shown and one foil object. Participants are asked to touch the fractal they remember as initially shown and to drag it to its remembered on-screen location. (From Liang et al., 2016.)

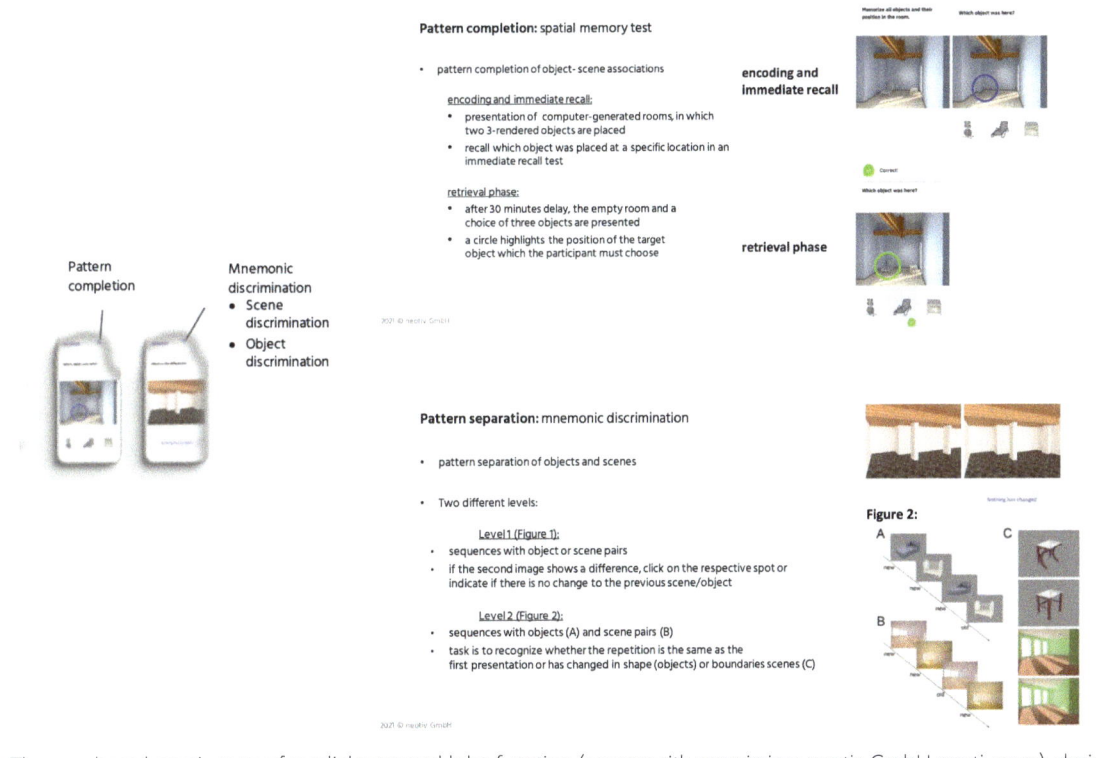

Figure 20.5 The app-based neotiv tests of medial temporal lobe function (source with permission: neotiv GmbH neotiv.com), designed for remote testing.

in AD have utilized advances in MRI hardware, notably ultra-high-field 7T scanning, and image-acquisition protocols to determine changes at the level of hippocampal subfields. In patients with prodromal AD, prospective and retrospective memory were associated with volumes of CA1 and CA3, respectively (Nurdal et al., 2020), while analysis of a birth cohort identified reduced presubiculum volume in cognitively intact individuals with preclinical AD (Parker et al., 2019). Notably, this subregion shows early convergence of Aβ and tau pathology (Jacobs et al., 2020).

20.4.8.4 Memory tests for the diagnosis of AD

The plethora of available tests of episodic memory and their differing methodologies raises challenges for clinical practice and research in terms of establishing those test(s) with greater diagnostic sensitivity and specificity for early AD and superior ability to predict cognitive decline and progression to dementia. While test choice to some extent will reflect individual experience and operational issues (time available to test, availability and cost of test materials), there is accumulating evidence on the diagnostic utility of tests, and protocols have been developed to maximize the diagnostic value of cognitive testing.

Systematic reviews and meta-analyses confirm that tests of episodic memory have high accuracy for diagnosing AD, with higher sensitivity and specificity for discriminating AD dementia from controls than MCI from controls. For MCI diagnosis, delayed recall tests are typically superior to immediate recall, and word-list recall is superior to story recall, memory retention, and recognition (Weissberger et al., 2017). However, the plethora of available tests and their deployment in cross-sectional and longitudinal studies with differing methodologies confounds attempts to identify individual tests with greatest diagnostic sensitivity and specificity for early AD and/or greatest ability to predict progression to dementia.

The validation of cognitive tests for diagnosis of prodromal AD in clinical practice requires a multistage process of test evaluation and subsequent incorporation within clinical settings as part of best practice guidelines. To this end, an international task force has created a roadmap for implementation of biomarker-based tests within routine clinical practice (Frisoni et al., 2017). The specific roadmap pertaining to cognitive tests (Cerami et al., 2017) focused on delayed recall as the modality of choice, in recognition of the International Working Group diagnostic criteria for AD. These describe memory impairment in prodromal AD as "objective evidence of significantly impaired episodic memory on testing, generally consisting of a recall deficit that does not improve significantly with cueing or recognition testing after effective encoding of information has been controlled" (Dubois et al., 2014). With this in mind, the test evaluation component of the roadmap used available evidence to select tests of word list recall. Short story recall and paired associative learning tests were excluded from the evaluation due to their different neuropsychological constructs, while more recently introduced tests of short-term memory binding (Parra et al., 2009; Parra et al., 2010), visual recognition (Barbeau et al., 2004), and allocentric spatial memory (Hartley et al., 2007; Moodley et al., 2015) were regarded as having potential diagnostic value for prodromal AD but lacking a sufficient evidence base for incorporation. However, with sufficient supporting evidence, these tests could be incorporated into future roadmap iterations, alongside newer tests probing specific aspects of entorhinal–hippocampal function, such as spatial tests (see below) and tests of pattern separation and pattern completion (Ally et al., 2013; Sinha et al., 2018), used in conjunction with novel delivery methodologies (e.g., tablets, smartphone apps, and virtual reality devices).

20.4.8.5 Testing of spatial navigation and memory can provide more information on entorhinal-hippocampal dysfunction in AD

The application of spatial behavioral tests for the diagnosis of early AD confers several theoretical and practical advantages over currently used cognitive tests. First, evidence that tau pathology spreads transneuronally within the entorhinal–hippocampal circuit in mouse models of disease (Ahmed et al., 2014; de Calignon et al., 2012; Liu, Drouet, et al., 2012), with subsequent neocortical infiltration, highlights the potential value of using tests of entorhinal cortex and hippocampal function to track disease progression from initial disease stages. Second, the extensive evidence indicating that grid- and place-cell activity is functionally coupled to spatial navigation and memory provides a physiological mechanism for understanding the behavioral changes occurring in humans with early AD, with attendant implications for translational research. This is underscored by work showing impaired grid-cell and place-cell activity in transgenic mouse models of AD-related pathology, with disruption of place-cell function correlated with performance on an alternation T-maze spatial behavioral task and with hippocampal amyloid burden (Cacucci et al., 2008; Fu et al., 2017). Third, testing of spatial navigation and memory represents an evaluation of a real-life behavior, conferring with the tests an ecological validity that is absent from the currently used pen-and-paper tests of cognition. The use of analogous spatial test paradigms facilitates cross-species comparison of AD-related behavioral change across animal models of disease and human cohorts, providing translatable outcome measures for comparing the effect of treatment across preclinical and clinical components of anti-AD treatment trials. Finally, spatial tests are less affected by the educational and linguistic confounds that compromise usage and interpretation of legacy cognitive tests, facilitating their application in different cultural settings.

20.4.8.6 Hippocampal-dependent spatial memory dysfunction is specific to AD

One difficulty with using episodic memory as a key test is that impairment of episodic memory is not specific to AD but is also seen in physiological age-associated memory impairment (Buckner, 2004), anxiety and depression (Zhou, Wang, et al., 2017), and non-AD dementias, including frontotemporal dementia and vascular dementia (Sachdev et al., 2014; Yew et al., 2013). By comparison, wayfinding difficulty and "getting lost" are symptoms that have greater specificity for AD, with spatial disorientation being less common in normal aging (Lithfous, Dufour, and Despres, 2013) or FTD (Tu et al., 2015). However, it is prevalent in Parkinson's disease dementia and Lewy body dementia, consistent with occipitoparietal damage in these disorders (Metzler-Baddeley, 2007).

People with early AD are impaired on tests of both allocentric and egocentric spatial memory, consistent with pathology in the medial temporal and medial parietal lobes respectively. Consistent with early Aβ deposition in the retrosplenial cortex (Mattsson, Palmqvist, et al., 2019) and the proposed role of this region

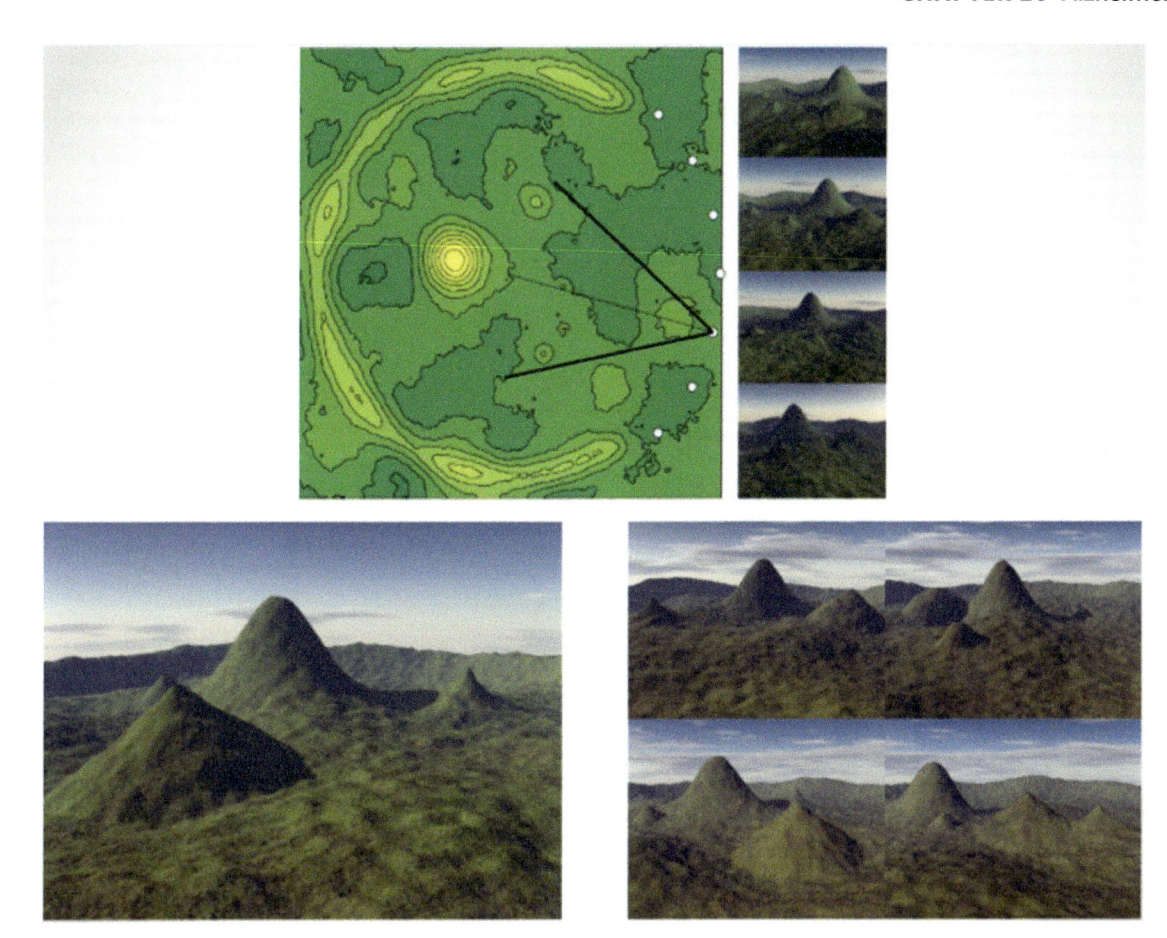

Figure 20.6 The Four Mountains Test of allocentric spatial memory. (Top) A schematic of the test. Viewers are shown an artificial landscape containing four mountains and for the recall test they are asked to identify the landscape but viewed from a different angle. (Bottom). A landscape is shown for 2 s (left). After a 10 s delay, the same landscape is presented but viewed from a different angle, alongside three foil images (right). The correct image in this case is the bottom left of the four images. (From Hartley et al., 2007.)

in egocentric–allocentric viewpoint transformation (Dhindsa et al., 2014), patients with early AD show impairments in shifting from allocentric to egocentric spatial representations (Morganti, Stefanini, and Riva, 2013).

Tests of allocentric spatial memory and navigation, designed to reflect hippocampal function, have been performed at different clinical stages of AD. They have been based on a variety of tasks using different platforms, ranging from apps running on tablets through to navigation within real-world environments. In patients with mild AD dementia, performance on the Four Mountains Test (Hartley et al., 2007; see Figure 20.6), a brief hippocampus-sensitive task assessing memory for computer-generated landscapes, differentiates patients with AD from those with FTD (Bird et al., 2010). Similarly, a variety of topographical memory tests were found to distinguish AD patients from those with semantic dementia, a clinical variant of FTD in which there is predominant temporal lobe pathology, with a desktop-based test of virtual navigation found to have the greatest diagnostic sensitivity and specificity (Pengas et al., 2010). Interestingly, the hippocampus is not spared in FTD. However, pathology is largely restricted to the anterior hippocampus, raising the possibility that the selective deficit of AD patients on these spatial tasks relates to damage within the posterior hippocampus, which corresponds to the dorsal hippocampus in rodents, where place-cell recording is typically conducted.

Subsequent studies concentrated on the application of spatial tests earlier in the disease course. Performance on the Four Mountains Test identified people with MCI with and without underlying AD pathology, as determined by CSF biomarker studies (Moodley et al., 2015), with performance correlating with hippocampal volume and being predictive of future progression from MCI to dementia (Wood et al., 2016). Studies involving path integration and spatial memory within real-world environments, the latter using a test paradigm designed to be analogous to the Morris watermaze, have shown impaired performance in people with MCI (Laczo et al., 2014; Mokrisova et al., 2016). The advent of immersive virtual reality (VR) technology, using commercially available headsets, has provided the opportunity to test navigation within virtual environments with provision of locomotor and proprioceptive feedback but without the logistical limitations of real-world tasks. A VR test of path integration, designed to reflect medial entorhinal cortex function, differentiates AD biomarker-positive MCI patients from biomarker-negative patients with high sensitivity and specificity (see Figure 20.7) and with a classification accuracy superior to that of gold-standard tests of verbal and nonverbal episodic memory (Howett et al., 2019). MCI biomarker-positive and biomarker-negative patients were also differentiated using a VR task involving use of both allocentric and egocentric route-planning strategies (Schoberl et al., 2020).

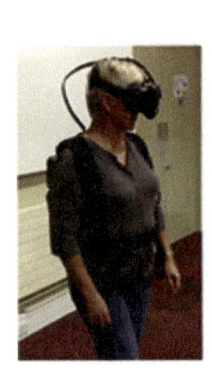
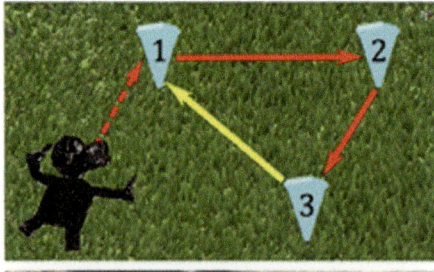
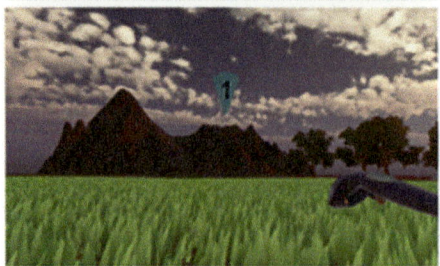

Figure 20.7 An entorhinal cortex-based VR path-integration task. (*Left*) Participant wearing VR headset, with (above) schematic of the task and (below) a screenshot of the VR environment as seen by participants. (*Right*) VR test performance—measured in terms of the Euclidean distance error between real and estimated location of Cone 1 (y-axis, in meters)—differentiates MCI patients with (MCI+) and without (MCI-) underlying AD with near-total group separation. (From Howett et al. 2019.)

20.4.8.7 Testing of hippocampus-dependent spatial memory could help diagnose preclinical AD

The effectiveness of spatial tests in MCI patients has raised the possibility of using these tests to detect entorhinal–hippocampal dysfunction in the preclinical stages of AD, prior to the onset of symptoms. Several studies, using different test paradigms, have provided the first evidence to support such usage. People with preclinical AD, defined by the presence of abnormal CSF biomarkers, showed impairments on a VR navigation task, and diagnostic classification accuracy was greater than that seen with the Selective Reminding Test of episodic memory (Allison et al., 2016). A follow-on longitudinal study found that performance on the cognitive mapping subtest of this VR task, involving acquisition of an allocentric spatial representation, was significantly predictive of clinical progression in individuals with preclinical AD, in contrast to performance on the egocentric route-learning subtest and tests of episodic memory (Levine et al., 2020).

Other work provides further evidence that spatial tests may detect the first behavioral changes in asymptomatic, at-risk populations. Performance on the Four Mountains Test correlated with dementia risk score (a composite measure encompassing risk factors for AD including age, gender, educational attainment, APOE status, systolic blood pressure, and body mass index) in a cohort aged 40–59 years who were on average 24 years younger than estimated age of dementia diagnosis. By comparison, no correlation was found between dementia risk score (DRS) and performance on a global battery of cognitive tests (K Ritchie et al., 2018). More recently, application of a VR path integration test to the same middle-aged cohort has found that people with risk factors for AD (positive family history of AD, high DRS, or presence of the ApoE4 allele) had subtle behavioral impairments relating primarily to defective angular distance estimation (Newton et al., 2024), consistent with

the purported role of the EC and hippocampus in vector computation (Bush et al., 2015; Ormond and O'Keefe, 2022). These behavioral studies are complemented by neuroimaging studies showing that young ApoE4-positive individuals had altered grid cell-like activation within the entorhinal cortex when performing a functional MRI navigation task, with fMRI changes associated with behavioral alterations in the form of impaired object-location memory (Kunz et al., 2015).

In summary, as well as their advantages over traditional cognitive tests in terms of ecological validity and value for translational research, tests of spatial behavior show promise for use in detection of preclinical AD. However, at present such tests have yet to be incorporated into routine clinical practice. Future work will need to focus on standardization of test methodologies, validation against AD biomarkers, and operational issues such as scalability and ease of use.

20.4.9 Digital diagnostics: future perspectives

As attention turns increasingly toward detection of early AD, prior to the onset of symptoms, when future application of disease-modifying drugs and other interventions may be most effective in delaying or preventing the onset of dementia, the clinical diagnostic approach is undergoing re-evaluation. Current cognitive tests used in routine clinical practice, such as the Mini Mental State Examination (MMSE; Folstein, Folstein, and McHugh, 1975) or Addenbrookes Cognitive Examination—Revised (Mioshi et al., 2006), are designed for detection of dementia and lack specificity and sensitivity for early AD, as exemplified by systematic reviews showing an approximate 50% ability of the MMSE to predict progression from MCI to dementia (Arevalo-Rodriguez et al., 2015). While tests probing entorhinal-hippocampal function have superior diagnostic capability for early AD, as outlined above, there is considerable interest in the use of digital wearable devices to detect early disease. Such digital tests have various potential advantages over legacy cognitive tests. First, the ability to capture data on a range of real-life activities known to be affected in early disease—such as sleep, navigation, and mobility—not only increases diagnostic sensitivity and specificity but also overcomes the limitations of pen-and-paper cognitive testing in terms of low ecological validity and restriction of testing to selected cognitive domains. The expansion of testing to encompass noncognitive functions will additionally improve understanding of disease phenotype and awareness of disease impact on everyday life, which in turn will enhance future clinical management. Second, the ability to track behaviors on an individual basis offsets the traditional drawbacks of interpreting data from traditional cognitive testing in light of demographic confounds (notably educational, linguistic, and cultural differences) and identification of impairment by comparison against historically collected normative data. Third, the ability of wearables to acquire data on multiple behaviors at a much higher frequency than is possible within the relatively infrequent assessments typically available in clinical practice will not only generate many more data points but also yield high throughput multidimensional datasets of sufficient size to enable application of machine-learning algorithms to extract additional diagnostic signals that that would be invisible to current data analysis methods.

These new approaches come with considerable opportunities and challenges, all of which will need to be mapped out and addressed before new tools can be adopted in clinical practice and research. Benefits include scalability at low cost to population-level usage without the need for trained testers, high ecological validity, the absence of educational and cultural confounds that hinder the application of current cognitive tests, and the ability to track cognitive trajectories within an individual in manner akin to personalized diagnostics (Kourtis et al., 2019). Challenges include front-end software engineering issues, such as application programming interfaces, heterogeneity of commercial devices, and risks of obsolescence associated with continual hardware and software upgrades. Back-end challenges include data issues such as acquisition and curation as well as the complexity associated with integrating data outputs generated from disparate software platforms running on diverse devices.

Finally, issues relating to data privacy and the ethics of testing for preclinical disease will need to be addressed. Passive sensing of behaviors such as navigation and sleep would raise concerns in users about the risk of leakage of personally sensitive information, and these will need to be mitigated using a variety of approaches including implementation of security systems such as two-factor identification, anonymization systems, and on-device analytics involving initial data analysis using the CPUs of the users' own devices, such that only de-identified data are sent on to remote servers for further diagnostic analysis.

Any proposed deployment at scale of digital devices for early detection of AD will need to be accompanied by an ongoing consideration of the ethical context of such deployment in the absence of effective treatments. Such conversations will need to encompass several issues, including the psychosocial advantages and disadvantages of a prediction of future dementia, stigmatization, and broader social issues such as equity of care.

20.5 Synaptic deficits and cognitive decline

As has been discussed in previous chapters (e.g., Chapter 10), synaptic plasticity is essential for memory. Thus, it is not surprising that synapse loss is the strongest neuropathological correlate of the memory symptoms observed in AD (de Wilde et al., 2016; Spires-Jones and Hyman, 2014). The association between synapse loss and cognitive decline was first described in the early 1990s using two independent methods, measurement of synaptic protein concentrations (Terry et al., 1991) and estimations of synapse numbers using electron microscopy of human brain tissue from biopsy and post-mortem samples (DeKosky and Scheff, 1990; DeKosky, Scheff, and Styren, 1996; Scheff, DeKosky, and Price, 1990). The importance of synapse loss in AD brain has been consistently replicated over the years, and data from animal models have begun to elucidate molecular mechanisms of synapse dysfunction and degeneration.

20.5.1 Aβ oligomers alter synaptic function in the hippocampus

Soluble oligomeric forms of Aβ (OAβ) are particularly synaptotoxic and lead to disruption of synaptic plasticity and loss of synapses in cultured neurons, rodent brain slices, and mice and rats in vivo (Cleary et al., 2005; Lambert et al., 1998; Shankar et al., 2008; Walsh et al., 2002). Of relevance to the hippocampus, OAβ inhibits hippocampal long-term potentiation (LTP) and facilitates

hippocampal long-term depression (LTD), when exogenously applied or expressed in transgenic mice (Larson et al., 1999; Li et al., 2009; Shankar et al., 2008; Spires-Jones and Hyman, 2014; Walsh et al., 2002). Synapses around plaques in transgenic mice accumulate OAβ and collapse, processes that can be reversed by removing oligomers with an antibody (Koffie et al., 2009; Spires et al., 2005; Spires-Jones et al., 2009). OAβ likely impairs synaptic plasticity by causing internalization of synaptic receptors essential for plasticity, including NMDA and α-amino-3-hydroxy-5-methyl-4-isoxazolepropionic acid (AMPA) receptors (Hsieh et al., 2006; Lacor et al., 2007; Snyder et al., 2005), and by interfering with calcium signaling at the synapse (Busche et al., 2008; Kuchibhotla et al., 2008). In model systems, the effects of OAβ on synaptic dysfunction and collapse appear to be mediated by binding of OAβ to synaptic receptors. Many candidate receptors have been identified in neuronal culture systems and in mouse models, including cellular prion protein (PrPC), leukocyte immunoglobulin-like receptor subfamily B2 (LilrB2), Nogo-66 receptor 1 (NgR1), ephrin type-B receptor 2 (EphB2), receptor for advanced glycation end products (RAGE) sigma-2 receptor, neuronal acetylcholine receptor subunit a7, and insulin receptor (Benilova and De Strooper, 2013; Smith and Strittmatter, 2017).

There is also evidence for OAβ-induced synapse loss in human AD. There is an association of OAβ accumulation in human brain with dementia symptoms (Mc Donald et al., 2010). Interestingly, people with high levels of plaque and tangle pathology who do not have dementia symptoms have lower burdens of OAβ-containing plaques than people with similar amounts of plaque and tangle pathology who do have expected dementia symptoms (Perez-Nievas et al., 2013). This further implicates OAβ in contributing to cognitive decline. In addition, high-resolution array tomography has identified OAβ accumulation within synaptic terminals around plaques in human AD brain tissue, which is exacerbated by the genetic risk gene variant, apolipoprotein 4 (Koffie et al., 2012). Which synaptic receptor/OAβ interactions at the synapse are relevant to human disease remains unclear. However, the drug CT1812, which removes OAβ from the sigma-2 receptor, is currently being tested in clinical trials (Grundman et al., 2019; Izzo et al., 2021).

20.5.2 Pathological tau alters synaptic function

Pathological forms of tau also contribute to synapse dysfunction and degeneration. In mouse models that overexpress human tau containing FTD-causing mutations, neurofibrillary pathology accumulates, and neurons are lost (Jankowsky and Zheng, 2017; Polydoro et al., 2009; Santacruz et al., 2005; Spires et al., 2006). Synapse dysfunction and loss are also common features of tauopathy mouse models and usually precede tangle formation and neurodegeneration (Busche et al., 2019; Kopeikina et al., 2013; Menkes-Caspi et al., 2015; Yoshiyama et al., 2007). Many groups have shown that synaptic dysfunction is not driven by the neurofibrillary tangles themselves; rather, soluble oligomeric forms of tau contribute to toxicity (Ghag et al., 2018; Kuchibhotla et al., 2014; Lasagna-Reeves et al., 2011; Rocher et al., 2010).

The mechanisms leading from tau pathology to synapse dysfunction and loss are not fully understood but likely include both loss of normal tau function and toxic gain of function. During the course of AD, aggregation of tau into tangles leads to loss of tau binding to microtubules. This likely impairs intracellular transport to synapses, which will impair synaptic function, including mitochondrial function (Kopeikina et al., 2011; Pickett et al., 2018). In addition to the well-known microtubule-stabilizing role of tau, there are data indicating tau has a physiological role in both pre- and postsynaptic terminals (A Ittner and Ittner, 2018; McInnes et al., 2018; L Zhou, McInnes, et al., 2017), and these normal functions are likely impaired in AD.

In human AD brain, phosphorylated tau has been observed in pre- and postsynaptic terminals (McInnes et al., 2018; L Zhou, McInnes, et al., 2017; Tai et al., 2012). Accumulation of phosphorylated tau in synapses is significantly higher in the brains of people with AD than in those from people with high levels of plaque and tangle pathology but no dementia symptoms (Perez-Nievas et al., 2013), implicating synaptic tau in cognitive decline.

20.5.3 Aβ, tau, and glia are involved in synapse loss in the hippocampus

Interactions between Aβ and tau in synaptic degeneration have been implicated in AD pathogenesis, indicating that the cascade of events that can result may be at least in part occurring in synapses. Removing endogenous mouse tau ameliorates synaptic plasticity phenotypes in plaque-bearing mouse models and in brain slices exposed to OAβ (Roberson et al., 2007; Shipton et al., 2011). OAβ activation of NMDARs has also been reported to cause excitotoxicity in a tau-dependent manner in mice, with recruitment of Fyn kinase to the postsynaptic density (L Ittner et al., 2010; Roberson et al., 2011). Data from a mouse model expressing familial AD genes and human wild-type tau indicate that amyloid pathology drives an inflammatory gene-expression phenotype that is associated with behavioral dysfunction only in mice that also express tau in synapses. Importantly, lowering tau levels in these mice ameliorates behavioral and gene-expression phenotypes (Pickett et al., 2019). The transsynaptic spread of tau is also accelerated by Aβ pathology in mice (Pooler et al., 2015), and human longitudinal PET imaging data similarly indicate that the presence of Aβ pathology is associated with accelerated spread of tau through the brain (Pontecorvo et al., 2019; Tosun et al., 2017).

In addition to the direct effects of Aβ and tau on synapses, recent data indicate that glia may be involved in synapse loss in AD (Henstridge, Tzioras, and Paolicelli, 2019; see Figure 20.8). APOE4, the most potent genetic risk factor for sporadic AD, is predominantly expressed in astrocytes in healthy brain and is upregulated in microglia in mouse models of AD (Keren-Shaul et al., 2017; Tzioras et al., 2019). APOE4 is associated with accelerated synapse loss around plaques and increased accumulation of OAβ in synapses both in mouse models and human AD brain (Hudry et al., 2013; Hudry et al., 2019; Koffie et al., 2012; Tzioras et al., 2019), and APOE4 exacerbates tau-mediated neurodegeneration in a mouse model of tauopathy (Shi, Yamada, et al., 2017). Other risk genes for AD, including triggering receptor expressed on myeloid cells 2 (*TREM2*), *CD33* and complement receptor 1 (*CR1*), are predominantly expressed in microglia, where they may influence synapse degeneration by increasing synaptic phagocytosis. Microglia prune synapses in a complement-dependent fashion during development as a normal part of circuit refinement (Stevens et al., 2007). In AD animal models, the complement system is involved in synapse loss, with tagging of synapses with C1q seen in both Aβ and tau models, resulting in CR3-mediated microglial phagocytosis of synapses (Dejanovic et al., 2018; Hong et al., 2016; Litvinchuk et al., 2018; Shi, Chowdhury, et al., 2017).

Synaptic changes are an attractive therapeutic target because, in animal models, the effects of AD pathology on synaptic function are reversible. In mice, lowering OAβ or tau levels through either genetic manipulations or immunotherapy leads to recovery of synaptic plasticity and cognition (Bittar, Sengupta, and Kayed, 2018; Janus et al., 2000; Santacruz et al., 2005; Schenk et al., 1999; Spires-Jones et al., 2009; Sydow et al., 2011) (see Figure 20.9).

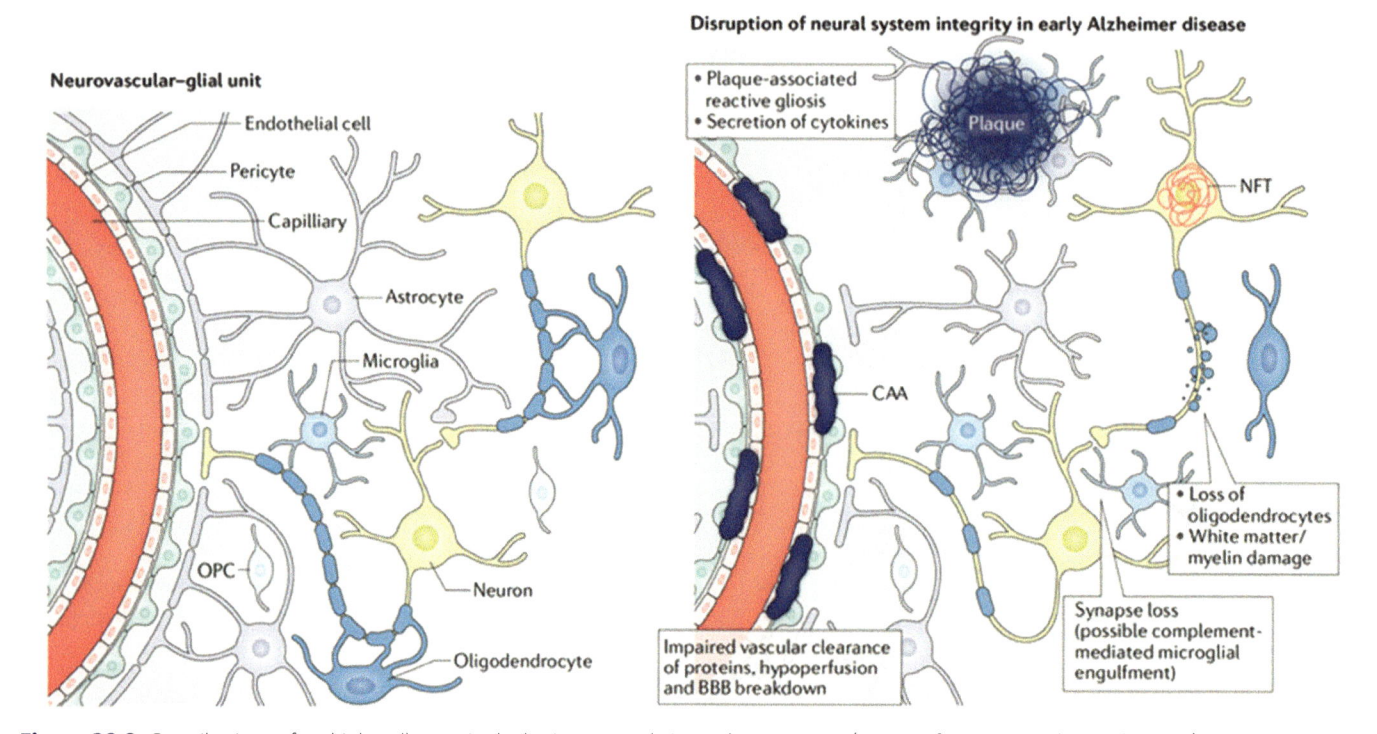

Figure 20.8 Contributions of multiple cell types in the brain to neural circuit degeneration. (Figure 2 from Henstridge et al., 2019.)

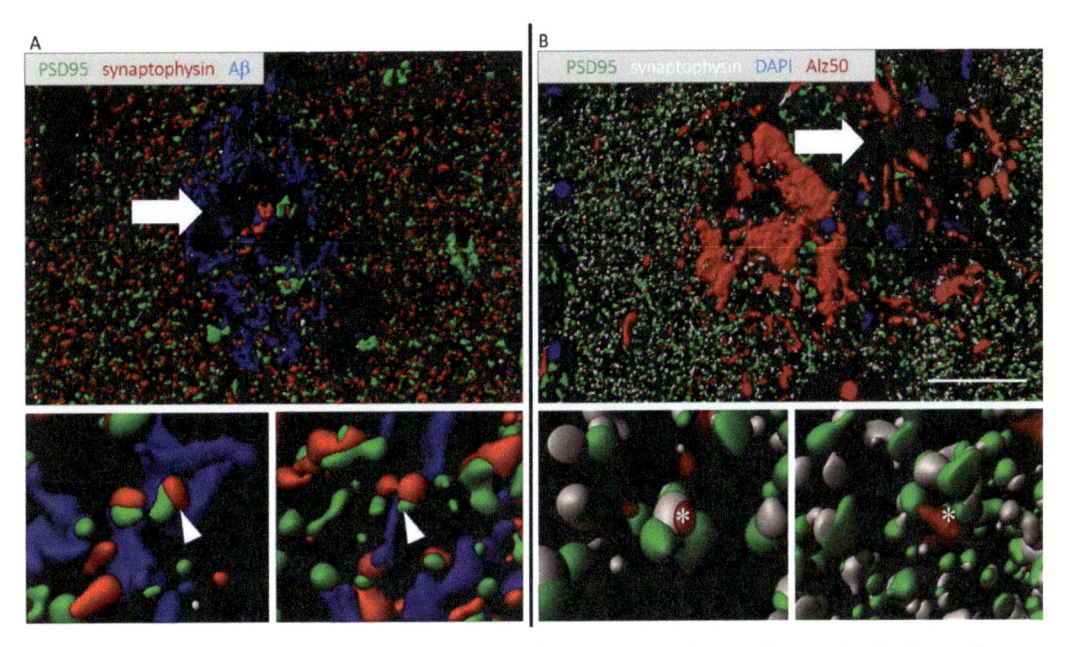

Figure 20.9 Using high-resolution array tomography imaging to examine human temporal cortex. Synapse loss is observed near amyloid plaques labeled with Aβ (blue, A) and identified by surrounding neuropil threads labeled with misfolded tau ALZ50 antibody (red, B). Arrows indicate loss of pre- and postsynaptic markers in plaques. Zooming in on these 3D reconstructions of neuropil surrounding plaques (bottom panels) shows both Aβ (arrowheads, A) and misfolded tau (asterisks, B) within pre- and postsynaptic terminals. Scale bar represents 20 μm.

Images courtesy Dr Declan King, Dr Carmen Montero and Dr Caitlin Davies. Use of human tissue for postmortem studies has been reviewed and approved by the Edinburgh Brain Bank ethics committee and the ACCORD medical research ethics committee, AMREC (approval number 15-HV-016; ACCORD is the Academic and Clinical Central Office for Research and Development, a joint office of the University of Edinburgh and NHS Lothian). The Edinburgh Brain Bank is a Medical Research Council funded facility with research ethics committee (REC) approval (11/ES/0022).

20.6 Biomarkers

20.6.1 Imaging biomarkers

A range of brain-imaging techniques are used to detect and track changes in AD pathology (Box 20.4).

Ligand PET provides evidence of AD molecular pathology, while markers of neurodegeneration (hippocampal atrophy on MRI, temporoparietal hypometabolism on fluorodeoxyglucose (FDG)-positron emission tomography (PET), or CSF total tau levels) may represent downstream evidence of an AD pathological process, although they are not specific to AD and may occur in other disorders causing brain injury.

Although AD is characterized by marked cerebral atrophy throughout the course of the disease, changes in the structure of the medial temporal lobe have been a particular area of focus for diagnosing and tracking disease progression. Regardless of the methods used to determine structural changes, neuronal loss as observed through either MRI, PET, or CSF biomarker levels is a core feature of the diagnostic criteria for the disease (McKhann et al., 2011).

20.6.1.1 Structural MRI has revealed characteristic trajectories of brain atrophy in AD

The imaging modality most used in AD is structural MRI, which yields submillimeter-resolution scans in minutes. The Alzheimer's Disease Neuroimaging Initiative (ADNI) has established criteria for longitudinal MRI and PET studies, and other clinical criteria, to promote harmonization of protocols across sites (Jack et al., 2008).

Accelerated hippocampal atrophy and whole-brain atrophy independently predict conversion to AD in people with or without MCI (Henneman et al., 2009). Furthermore, multimodal segmentation and ultra-high-field (7T or higher) MRI of the medial temporal lobe has provided volumetric estimates of both the entire hippocampus and of hippocampal subfields throughout the course of AD. Compared with controls and people with MCI, AD patients show broad volumetric reduction within the subiculum, CA1, CA3, DG/CA4 volumes, and entorhinal cortex; in addition, increasing age is associated with smaller CA1 and DG/CA4 volumes (Wisse et al., 2014). Longitudinal studies have shown that the volume of the entorhinal cortex is also significantly reduced in preclinical AD, with reductions starting in the lateral aspect and continuing

---

Box 20.4 Commonly used imaging modalities

The most commonly used brain-imaging techniques are structural and functional magnetic resonance imaging (MRI) and positron emission tomography (PET).

- **Structural MRI:** Structural MRI provides volumetric information about brain regions, generating insights into patterns of brain atrophy.
- **Functional MRI (fMRI):** fMRI measures regional variation in blood oxygen levels, which act as a proxy of neuronal activity. fMRI can therefore be used to assess and track changes in regional brain activity.
- **Positron emission tomography (PET):** PET is used to visualize metabolic processes or the distribution of particular biomolecules, through the use of radioactively labeled tracer compounds (radiotracers). Of particular relevance to AD are tracers that can be used to visualize the presence of Aβ and tau in the brain.
- **Diffusion tensor imaging (DTI):** DTI is a type of structural MRI that can provide insight into the structural integrity of tissues by extracting information related to the movement of water molecules. The most common measure derived from this technique is known as fractional anisotropy, which characterizes the degree to which water molecules are free to diffuse through space. DTI is commonly used to map white matter tracts in the brain.

medially (Miller et al., 2015). This is in line with neuropathology implicating the transentorhinal cortex, which is sometimes defined as the border zone between the lateral aspect of the entorhinal cortex and the perirhinal sulcus. However, while hippocampal atrophy can be used to distinguish people with MCI from healthy controls for initial diagnostic classification, it is less able to differentiate early AD from non-AD dementia cases due to hippocampal involvement in vascular dementia and non-AD neurodegenerative diseases (Chan et al., 2001; Harper et al., 2016). With regard to the specific issue of identifying MCI due to AD using structural MRI, a Cochrane Collaboration systematic review determined that the hippocampus, rather than whole brain or medial temporal lobe, was the most widely reported region of interest but that measurement of hippocampal volume had low diagnostic sensitivity and specificity and was not recommended for use as a standalone test for diagnosis of early AD (Lombardi et al., 2020). Instead, hippocampal atrophy may have greater utility to stratify cohorts in AD research studies and clinical trials (Jack et al., 2015).

20.6.1.2 Functional MRI has revealed altered connectivity of the hippocampal formation in AD

Blood oxygenation level-dependent (BOLD) functional MRI (fMRI) has provided many insights into both task-related and resting-state changes in neural activity in subjects with a variety of neurological and psychiatric conditions. Relatively high temporal resolution MRI imaging is used alongside established fMRI paradigms (usually but not limited to memory tasks) while the patient is located within the scanner. Although there is significant variance when accounting for preprocessing and acquisition of fMRI, one of the most convergent findings in AD is hypoactivation within the medial temporal lobe, and in particular the hippocampus (Machulda et al., 2003). The default mode network is frequently used as a baseline for comparing disease state (Raichle et al., 2001). Abnormal default mode network activity has been seen in AD patients, implicating dysfunction in both the posterior cingulate cortex and the hippocampus (Greicius et al., 2004).

20.6.1.3 FDG-PET imaging

18F-fluorodeoxyglucose (FDG) PET imaging is a powerful imaging technique across neurology, neuro-oncology, and psychiatry. Useful in determining overall absolute and relative glucose uptake (as a proxy measure of neuronal activity), it generates whole-brain values controlled for the injected dose of the radioligand. AD is typically characterized by reduced glucose uptake in the posterior cingulate cortex and throughout parietal, frontal, and temporal lobes, with generalized sparing of the occipital and sensory motor cortices, reflective of overall suspected neuronal loss (Matsuda, 2001). As with MRI, FDG-PET shows good sensitivity and specificity for differentiating people with MCI from controls (Frisoni et al., 2013), but appears overall superior to MRI in terms of differentiating between AD and non-AD dementia cases (Foster et al., 2007; Minoshima et al., 2001). However, a systematic review of FDG-PET usage in MCI has identified marked variability in its ability to predict progression from MCI to dementia, with sensitivity values of 25%–100% and specificity values of 24%–100%. Crucially, measurement technique has a significant impact, with studies using voxel-based methods to quantify hypometabolism associated with sensitivity and specificity both above 75% (Smailagic et al., 2018). Patterns of FDG-PET are useful in distinguishing AD-related dementias from other dementias due to specific imaging signatures, although

nonmetabolic radioligands (e.g., amyloid and tau) are increasingly used to track disease progression. FDG-PET imaging has been useful in distinguishing FTD from AD. FTD is characterized by reduced uptake in the anterior frontotemporal areas of the brain, whereas in AD reduced meta-analyses of longitudinal MCI studies have shown that abnormal amyloid-PET scans, validated as an in vivo surrogate marker of brain Aβ deposits, have a pooled sensitivity of 96% and specificity of 72% for predicting progression from MCI to dementia (Ma et al., 2014). This predictive ability is superior to that of tests of episodic memory and measurement of hippocampal atrophy on MRI (Ma et al., 2014).

MRI- and FDG-PET-based assessments complement the use of amyloid/tau biomarkers, with MRI typically used in clinical practice as the first-line diagnostic investigation for reasons of cost, availability, and patient acceptability. While not being specific to the Aβ and tau pathology of AD, both imaging modalities show good predictability (Yuan, Gu, and Wei, 2009). Uptake of tracer is also seen within posterior regions, including posterior cingulate cortex and posterior parietal lobes. Although other PET techniques are available for different biomarkers, FDG-PET is still a valuable imaging modality due to its utility in providing spatial information across a variety of diseases.

20.6.1.4 Amyloid-PET and tau-PET imaging can reveal sites of Aβ and tau aggregation

One advantage that PET has over other neuroimaging modalities is the availability of novel radiotracer compounds that selectively bind to specific molecules of interest. Chief among these are amyloid-targeting and tau-targeting ligands. Pittsburgh compound B (PiB), a thioflavin T histological dye analogue, was the first to be studied (Klunk et al., 2004). However, practical limitations (e.g., a short 20-minute half-life for 11C) have led to the development of a variety of radioligands based on the longer half-life 18F radionuclide, such as florbetapir and flutemetamol (Johnson et al., 2013). Regardless of compound, in AD, patterns of tracer uptake can be diffuse throughout the frontal, parietal, and occipital cortices; precuneus; striatum; and lateral temporal cortex. The patterns observed in amyloid PET reflect suspected Aβ plaque deposition known to occur throughout the brain in AD (Schilling et al., 2016) and can also be useful in distinguishing other suspected dementias, such as FTD.

20.6.1.5 Tau-PET has revealed pathology in the hippocampal formation in AD

While use of PET ligands for imaging tau within neurofibrillary tangles has revealed patterns of tau deposition that are consistent with Braak pathological staging (Lohith et al., 2019), their limited use to date means that too few data are available for systematic reviews or meta-analyses of their diagnostic accuracy in prodromal AD or predictive ability. However, an initial tau-PET study in the Harvard Brain Aging Cohort showed that increased neocortical deposition of tau was more closely associated with cognitive decline in a predementia cohort than baseline amyloid-PET or baseline tau-PET (Hanseeuw et al., 2019).

The characterization and spread of tau pathology is also a target for radioligand research and PET imaging. Tracers must both cross the blood-brain barrier and selectively bind to tau, which is challenging due to its intracellular location. AV-1451, THK-5351, THK-5317, PBB3, THK-5105, THK-5117, and MK-6240 have all shown varying utility in either autoradiography, in vivo studies, or both in targeting neurofibrillary tangles. The nature of tau binding in vivo, especially with tauopathy associated with FTD, is currently being explored. One noted limitation is that some tracers show uptake within the choroid plexus and striatum, with the former possibly impacting hippocampal uptake values.

One valuable aspect of tau imaging is the potential to map, in vivo, *where* tangles occur. During the progression of AD, elevated tau tracer uptake is seen within the neocortex, inferior temporal, fusiform gyrus, posterior cingulate, parahippocampal gyrus, and entorhinal cortex (Johnson et al., 2016). However, one limitation is that voxel sizes are generally higher than those achievable through MRI, so mapping uptake within a region as small as the entorhinal cortex (where tau deposition is known to vary nonuniformly between individuals) is challenging. Regardless, tau-PET is a promising approach, and longitudinal tau-PET imaging has confirmed increases in tau associated with cognitive decline (Hanseeuw et al., 2019; Pontecorvo et al., 2019). As well as fMRI and PET, many other imaging modalities have been applied to AD (Box 20.5). These are used in research to provide further insights into the progression and pathology of AD, but are rarely used to aid diagnosis.

Box 20.5 Additional imaging approaches to detecting AD-related atrophy or dysfunction

- **Imaging iron deposition:** Quantitative susceptibility mapping exploits changes in magnetic properties due to iron accumulation, either from iron overload or a reduction in myelin in white matter (Kim et al. 2017). Increased iron deposition is thought to be related to AD, and quantitative susceptibility mapping has identified changes in the hippocampus, amygdala, precuneus, and thalamus, with the precuneus also being an indicator of early change from amnestic MCI to controls.

- **Mapping cellular integrity and neural tract**s: Diffusion tensor imaging (DTI) can provide insight into the structural integrity of tissues, particularly white matter tracts. Two common approaches to DTI analysis exist: (1) region of interest (ROI)–based analyses, which restrict statistical analyses to previously identified regions or "skeletons" that conform to existing white matter tracts, or (2) voxel-based analyses. Through the tract-based spatial statistics approach, reductions in fractional anisotropy have been found in parahippocampal white matter, bilateral uncinate fasciculus, fornix, inferior and superior longitudinal fasciculus, cingulum, genu, and splenium of corpus callosum (Liu et al. 2011). Such techniques can provide insight into aberrations of cellular integrity within the medial temporal lobe as it relates to corresponding network dysfunction.

- **Vascular imaging:** Vascular changes, including microcerebrovascular impairment, are being considered a core biomarker of AD. The identification and location of these changes are also identified by MRI techniques. Specifically, white matter hyperintensities as determined by hyperintense signal on fluid-attenuated inversion recovery T2-weighted or similar MRI have been shown to independently confer a risk of developing AD, when compared with PiB PET imaging (Provenzano et al. 2013).

- **Imaging metabolic changes:** Magnetic resonance spectroscopy (MRS) is used to measure metabolite concentrations in vivo using an MRI machine. Through MRS, concentrations can be determined within a voxel larger than that used in conventional imaging. Metabolites analyzed include n-acetylaspertate and glutamate–glutamine (often measured against concentrations of reference compounds such as creatine or water). MRS can provide information about aberrations in a neurotransmitter pathway in brain regions. Alterations in the gray and white matter of the posterior cingulate cortex and precuneus have shown thresholds of such values can accurately classify asymptomatic FAD carriers using both choline and glutamate–glutamine measurements (Londono et al. 2014).

20.6.1.6 Imaging synaptic biomarkers

Synapse loss correlates very strongly with cognitive decline in AD, and a new PET ligand that binds synaptic glycoprotein 2A in presynaptic vesicles is a promising way to track synapse loss over time in vivo (Finnema et al., 2016). This may prove to be an excellent readout for clinical trials, as even a small study found that five AD patients had reduced hippocampal synapse PET signal compared with control subjects (Chen et al., 2018).

20.6.2 Fluid biomarkers

20.6.2.1 Fluid biomarkers correlate with pathology and hippocampal decline in AD

Work relating to CSF AD biomarkers relates primarily to Aβ, total tau, and phosphorylated tau (Blennow et al., 2010), the levels of which are highly correlated with amyloid plaque and neurofibrillary tangle pathology. CSF biomarker interpretation is complicated by differences in assay methodologies, diurnal variation, and age-related differences in normative values. Overall, however, there is evidence supporting the ability of CSF biomarkers to predict progression from MCI to dementia (Olsson et al., 2016). With regard to CSF biomarker combinations, the Aβ/phosphorylated tau ratio has higher diagnostic specificity than either biomarker alone with respect to the risk of misclassifying non-AD as AD. A systematic review has shown that the CSF Aβ/phosphorylated tau ratio is associated with sensitivities of 80%–96% and specificities of 33%–95%, indicating that the value of current CSF biomarkers in clinical practice is primarily in identifying MCI patients at low risk of progression to dementia (C Ritchie et al., 2017).

The invasiveness of lumbar puncture and need for specialist clinical settings and trained clinical staff have prompted research into AD biomarkers within more accessible biofluids, particularly blood-based biomarkers. Initial studies centered on plasma Aβ species, facilitated by high-precision ultrasensitive assays that can detect cerebral amyloid pathology with 70%–90% accuracy (Palmqvist et al., 2019), near that of CSF assays. Plasma phosphorylated tau levels predict the presence of brain tau and pathology with up to 90% accuracy and correlate with both hippocampal atrophy and cognitive decline (Karikari et al., 2020). The added diagnostic value of other proteins associated with neurodegeneration, such as neurofilament light (NF-L) chain (Forgrave et al., 2019), and of proteomic panels (Westwood et al., 2020), above that of amyloid/tau measurements, has yet to be established. Blood NF-L levels have been shown to correlate with FDG-PET imaging biomarkers in sporadic AD (Benedet et al., 2019), and a longitudinal study showed that levels correlate with CSF phosphorylated tau, hippocampal atrophy, and ATN score, and increase with disease progression (Mattsson, Cullen, et al., 2019). Blood NF-L is the result of axonal degeneration and is not unique to AD, so as a biomarker it would need to be used in combination with AD-specific measures (Massa et al., 2019). These early studies, showing abnormalities in blood-based biomarkers from preclinical stages of disease and with increasing biomarker changes correlating with disease progression, may herald their future implementation as diagnostic tests for early AD at a scale and level of acceptability that is beyond current CSF and ligand-PET capabilities.

Aβ and phosphorylated tau are also detectable in saliva (Ashton et al., 2019) and levels are abnormal in patients with AD. However, sensitivity and specificity are low due to large variation in levels

(Pekeles et al., 2019). While salivary testing has some operational advantages, at present there is insufficient data regarding the validation of salivary biomarkers against other in vivo biomarkers or gold-standard neuropathology. Potential confounds such as the effects of age, concomitant illnesses, medication usage, and possible differences between tests would also need to be considered.

20.6.2.2 Fluid synaptic biomarkers

As well as their therapeutic potential, readouts of synapse damage are emerging as potential biomarkers for tracking disease progression in clinical trials. Since synapse loss in the brain is the closest correlate of dementia symptoms, and cognitive readouts are variable and can be affected by the state of the person on the day of testing, much work is being done to accurately measure synapse loss as a more sensitive readout of disease progression. The appearance of fragments of the synaptic protein neurogranin in CSF is specific to AD (Portelius et al., 2018) and correlates with cognitive decline and brain atrophy (Kvartsberg et al., 2015). Other synaptic proteins also accumulate in CSF of AD patients, likely reflecting loss of synapses in the brain (Bereczki et al., 2018; Brinkmalm et al., 2014; Lleo et al., 2019). Although levels of these CSF biomarkers of synapse loss are variable in cross-sectional studies, they may be valuable when measured longitudinally in clinical trials, particularly in combination with markers of Aβ, tau, and neuron loss (Colom-Cadena et al., 2020).

20.6.3 Biomarkers: perspective

Given that biomarkers represent surrogate measures of different aspects of AD pathology, studies have examined the diagnostic and predictive value of combination biomarker testing. These have tended to show that combination testing delivers added predictive power compared with single biomarker tests, although to varying degrees. One study found that the combination of CSF $A\beta_{1-42}$, FDG-PET, and MRI was highly predictive of progression: all MCI patients with positive biomarkers across all modalities progressed to dementia, whereas no MCI patients with all-negative biomarkers developed dementia within the study period (Prestia et al., 2013). Subsequent work has shown that the predictive ability of biomarkers is dependent in part on age of onset, with FDG-PET in particular having higher prognostic value for younger-onset AD (Altomare et al., 2019). For imaging biomarkers alone, the combination of amyloid-PET plus structural MRI is associated with the best predictive accuracy (Trzepacz et al., 2014).

20.7 Risk factors: age, modifiable risk factors, and genes

20.7.1 The risk of AD increases with age

Age is the most substantial risk factor for AD. Dementia incidence increases with age, doubling every 6.3 years from 3.9 per 1,000 person-years at age 60–64 to 105 per 1,000 person-years for ages 90+, resulting in approximately 10 million new cases of dementia annually worldwide. Meta-analyses indicate that the incidence of dementia in low- and middle-income countries is approximately 10% lower than in high-income countries. Recent studies suggest that the incidence of dementia is declining in high-income countries (Chibnik et al., 2017; Roehr et al., 2018), with this decline

being attributed to reductions in vascular risk factors, as well as improved population health and levels of educational attainment across society (Matthews et al., 2016). One hippocampus-specific age-related change that is likely relevant to AD pathophysiology is the breakdown of the hippocampal blood-brain barrier (Montagne et al., 2015) (see also Chapter 15).

20.7.2 Risk factors associated with comorbidities

Both risk and protective factors for AD have been identified. Type 2 diabetes, hypertension, obesity, and smoking are all associated with increased risk of AD (Reitz, Brayne, and Mayeux, 2011) but also represent risk factors for cerebrovascular disease and vascular dementia. A history of prior traumatic brain injury (TBI) is also associated with a higher risk of dementia (Fleminger et al., 2003). The mechanistic relationship between these risk factors and AD is unclear, although there is evidence that cardiovascular risk factors may result in increased Aβ deposition, possibly as a result of increased oxidative stress and cytokine release. TBI is associated with tau deposition (Hawkins et al., 2013), which may then constitute a "second hit" when age-related Aβ pathology is present (Spires-Jones, Attems, and Thal, 2017).

Several protective factors for AD are associated with increased cognitive reserve, such as education and occupation (Richards and Deary, 2005). Crucially for public-health-led initiatives aimed at primary prevention of dementia, increased levels of physical, social, and intellectual activity also contribute to cognitive reserve and reduced dementia risk. The neural basis for this effect remains unclear, although there is emerging evidence to suggest that it may be mediated via alterations in brain functional connectivity (Stern, 2017). Relevant to the hippocampus, one of the putative protective mechanisms of exercise is the increase in brain-derived neurotrophic factor (BDNF) and hippocampal neurogenesis (Choi et al., 2018; Spires-Jones and Ritchie, 2018).

It is unclear whether diets high in antioxidants and polyunsaturated fatty acids are protective, with inconsistent study findings, although a recent meta-analysis suggested a possible association between high intake of a Mediterranean-style diet and reduced dementia risk (Wu and Sun, 2017). While the data around diet and risk remain controversial, a study in 2017 concluded that lifestyle interventions to increase exercise, education, and social engagement and to reduce smoking, diabetes, and obesity have the potential to delay or prevent one-third of dementia cases (Livingston et al., 2017).

20.7.3 Genetic risk factors

In addition to age and lifestyle factors, genetics contributes substantially to AD risk (Figure 20.10). Most AD cases are sporadic (SAD), i.e., not caused by a single-gene mutation, with familial AD (FAD) accounting for less than 5% of all cases. Apart from the earlier age at onset (typically before the age of 65 years) for FAD, no consistent differences in the clinical features of sporadic and familial AD have been identified. This similarity in clinical presentation has underpinned the belief that greater understanding of the consequences of the mutations associated with familial AD will, in turn, yield key insights into the mechanisms of disease in sporadic AD.

Familial AD mutations inevitably lead to AD but are rare, while some sporadic AD risk variants confer a moderate increase in risk and are more frequent (e.g., APOE4, TREM2). However, most AD risk variants are common and confer a low risk of AD.

20.7.3.1 Large effect AD-associated risk genes were the first to be identified

20.7.3.1.1 Early-onset AD genes

The first familial AD-associated mutations reported were those in the amyloid precursor protein (*APP*) gene on chromosome 21 (Chartier-Harlin et al., 1991). The exact function of the APP remains undetermined, although roles in growth promotion, signaling mechanisms, and cell adhesion have been suggested (Breen, Bruce, and Anderton, 1991; De Strooper and Annaert, 2000; Milward et al., 1992). *APP* mutations account for only a small proportion of early-onset FAD. Most of these cases are caused by mutations of the *PS1* gene on chromosome 14, coding for the protein presenilin 1 (PS1) (Campion et al., 1995). Shortly after the discovery of the *PS1* gene, a second presenilin gene, *PS2*, on chromosome 1 was identified (Levy-Lahad et al., 1995; Rogaev et al., 1995). PS1 and PS2 both form part of the γ-secretase complex, which cleaves APP to form Aβ (De Strooper et al., 1999; Wolfe et al., 1999; Zhang et al., 2000; Zoltowska and Berezovska, 2018). More than 100 different presenilin mutations have been linked to AD.

20.7.3.1.2 Late-onset AD genes

The first and most studied gene to be linked to late-onset AD was *APOE*. In families with late-onset FAD, a susceptibility gene was mapped to chromosome 19 (Pericak-Vance et al., 1991). This gene was found to code for apolipoprotein E (APOE), a 299-amino-acid lipid transport protein that mediates the intracellular uptake of lipids through binding to the low-density lipoprotein (LDL) receptor. Three alleles of the *APOE* gene exist: *APOE2, APOE3* (the most common form), and *APOE4*. The likelihood of developing AD correlates with the number of *APOE4* genes (Corder et al., 1993); *APOE4* heterozygotes have a greater risk and earlier disease onset than non-*APOE4* individuals, and *APOE4* homozygotes have the greatest risk of all. Homozygous *APOE4* patients have more amyloid plaques than patients homozygous for the *APOE3* allele. When compared with age-matched normal controls (in whom the *APOE4* allele is found in 16% of people), the *APOE4* allele is more

frequent in both late-onset AD with a positive family history (52% of cases) and sporadic AD (40% of cases). Further studies have suggested that APOE plays a role in a variety of processes, influencing the accumulation of both amyloid and tau. It also affects a wide range of other processes, including inflammatory responses, synaptic function, blood-brain barrier integrity, and metabolism (Yamazaki et al., 2019).

20.7.3.2 Multiple sporadic AD-associated risk factors of small effect have been identified

A host of genetic polymorphisms have been linked to disease risk, although how they contribute to disease is not clear cut. Some are described in section 20.9.

20.8 Pathogenic mechanisms

20.8.1 Familial AD-associated mutations have provided key insights into disease mechanisms

APP is cleaved at its N- and C-termini by β- and γ-secretases (Figure 20.11), respectively, to produce the peptide Aβ, comprising 40 to 42 amino acids, which is the main constituent of the amyloid plaques in AD (De Strooper et al., 1998; Vassar et al., 1999). Despite the uncertainty over the function of APP, its role in the pathogenesis of AD appears unequivocal; all currently identified disease-associated mutations of the APP gene result in increased levels of Aβ or Aβ fragments containing 41 or 42 amino acids, which are more amyloidogenic and therefore more likely to form amyloid plaques. Further, in 2012 the A673T *APP* mutation, which results in reduced Aβ generation, was found to be associated with lower risk of AD in the Icelandic population (Jonsson et al., 2012).

Nearly all (90%) of AD-linked presenilin mutations lead to a reduction in total Aβ generation, suggesting that presenilin mutations are pathogenic loss-of-function mutations. However, many of the mutations also increase the Aβ42:Aβ40 ratio, resulting in a relative increase in the levels of longer and therefore more aggregation-prone

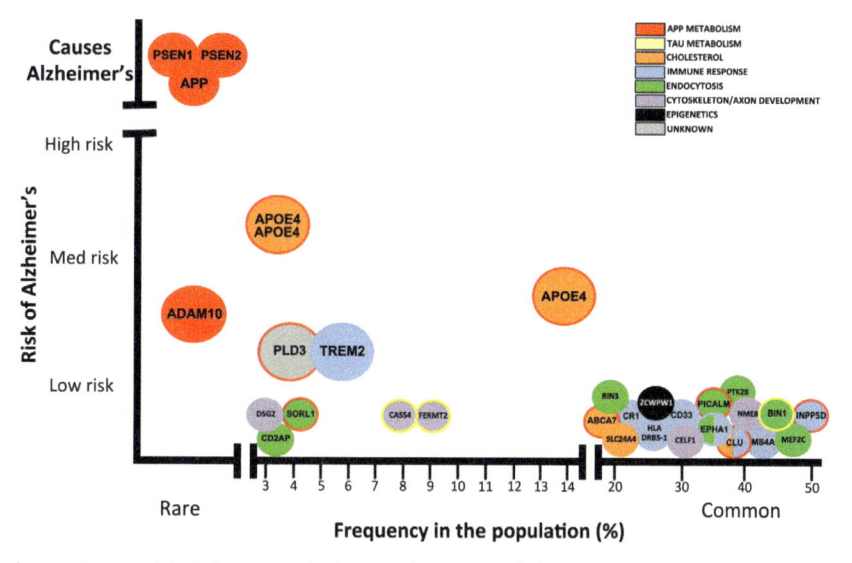

Figure 20.10 AD-associated mutations and their frequency in the population. Familial AD-causing mutations in APP and PS proteins are rare. Mutations or polymorphisms in genes linked to sporadic AD are more frequent in the population but confer a low risk of developing AD. There are a few polymorphisms (e.g., TREM2) that, although not as rare as causative familial AD mutations, are less common than most SAD polymorphisms and have a larger effect on AD risk. For the APOE4 gene, the risk depends on copy number with the less common genotype of two copies of the gene resulting in an increased risk of AD. (From Karch and Goate, 2015).

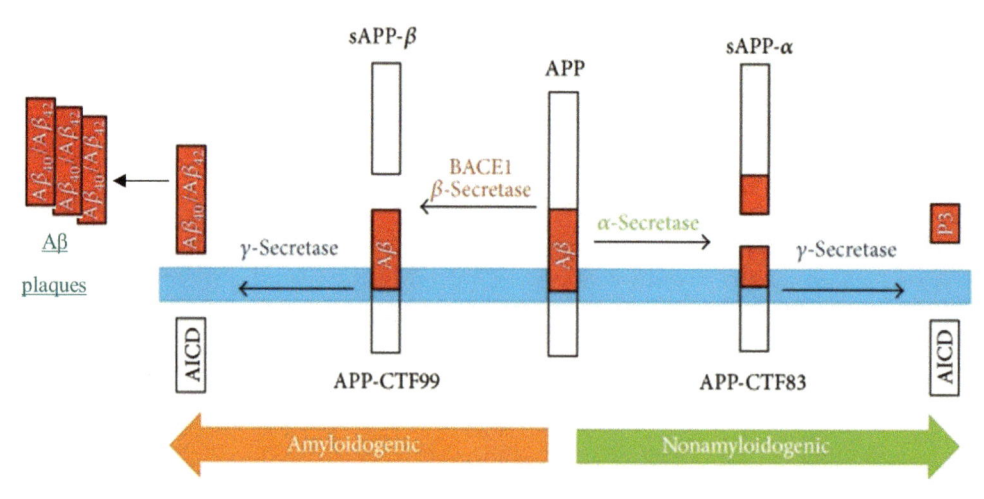

Figure 20.11 APP can be cleaved through the action of secretases to generate pathological and nonpathological fragments. Mutations in APP cause AD due to enhanced pathological processing. (From Wang et al., 2012.)

Aβ peptides, suggesting the AD-causing mutations are pathogenic gain-of-function mutations (Sun, Zhou, et al., 2017). The identification of causative familial AD mutations led to the amyloid cascade hypothesis (Figure 20.12), which has been the most widely accepted theory of AD. First proposed in the early 1990s (Beyreuther and Masters, 1991; Hardy and Allsop, 1991; Hardy and Higgins, 1992; Selkoe, 1991), it suggests that Aβ is the primary cause of AD. As the field has evolved, the hypothesis has been repeatedly updated to accommodate new findings such as sporadic AD risk factors and activation of microglial cells in the AD brain (Dourlen et al., 2019; Selkoe and Hardy, 2016).

20.8.2 In vitro and in vivo modeling with AD-causing mutations inform on AD pathomechanisms

Much of the current understanding of AD pathogenesis and the amyloid cascade hypothesis (in particular, the role of FAD-causing mutations) has come from studies of disease models, particularly transgenic mice. Interestingly, no FAD mutations have fully recapitulated the disease's pathological hallmarks in animal models, although each model has yielded useful insight. Other animal species are being considered as potential AD models (Box 20.6).

Very recently, in silico approaches have added to our ability to model diseases (Box 20.7).

20.8.2.1 APP processing studies in human-relevant cell models

Evidence for a role for APP mutations in Aβ generation comes from in vitro models of disease, including human induced pluripotent stem cells (iPSCs). iPSCs can be derived from AD patients and directed to differentiate into a variety of cell types, including neurons, which can be cultured together or separately. The relative ease of genetic manipulations compared with in vivo models (for example CRISPR correcting mutations) make stem cells an accessible way to model AD. Several groups have differentiated iPSCs with *APP* and *PS1* mutations into neurons, and these show an increased Aβ42:Aβ40 ratio and in some cases elevated phosphorylated tau (Arber et al., 2019; Israel et al., 2012; Ochalek et al., 2017). iPSCs generated from sporadic AD patients have also been differentiated into neurons and astrocytes. Cells from different patients vary

significantly but broadly show increased levels of Aβ (reviewed in Rowland, Hooper, and Kellett, 2018).

A landmark in AD disease modeling with human cells involved the use of a hydrogel matrix as a substrate and iPSCs overexpressing *PS1* and *APP* mutations (Choi et al., 2014; Kim et al., 2015). These cells expressed extremely high levels of Aβ, which became trapped within the matrix and induced the formation of amyloid plaques and hyperphosphorylated, insoluble, silver-positive tau aggregates. These aggregates were confirmed to be tau filaments by electron microscopy, providing further evidence that aberrant APP processing is upstream of tau pathology. Of note, parallel 2D adherent cultures did not develop plaques or tau aggregates. Other groups have since extended this work, adding nonneuronal cells and producing self-organizing cerebral organoids, which generate Aβ plaques and silver-positive tau aggregates (Park et al., 2018). While iPSC organoids are a significant advance, some features of the AD brain have yet to be modeled in 3D cultures, although this has not precluded their use for drug screening (Brownjohn et al., 2017). While a 3D model of hippocampal structures has not yet been created from iPSC cells, hippocampal cells within an organoid have been generated from human embryonic stem cells (Scheff et al., 2006).

20.8.2.2 AD-related pathology studies in mouse models

Much of our understanding of the role of *APP* and *PS1* mutations in amyloid pathology comes from studies using mice and rat models. In the absence of genetic modifications, mice and rats do not develop any AD-like pathology. However, animal models with amyloid pathology have been created by modification of the genes affected by FAD-causing mutations, demonstrating that these genes are involved in the generation of amyloid. Genetically engineered rodent models recapitulate several pathological hallmarks of AD, such as Aβ plaques throughout the hippocampal formation and cortex, astrocytosis and microgliosis closely associated with plaques, synaptic degeneration, and progressive cognitive deficits. Hyperphosphorylated tau accumulates in dystrophic neurites associated with plaques, but overt tau pathology in the form of neuropil threads or somatodendritic tangles is not seen, and importantly neither is neuronal loss. An extensive listing of mouse models of

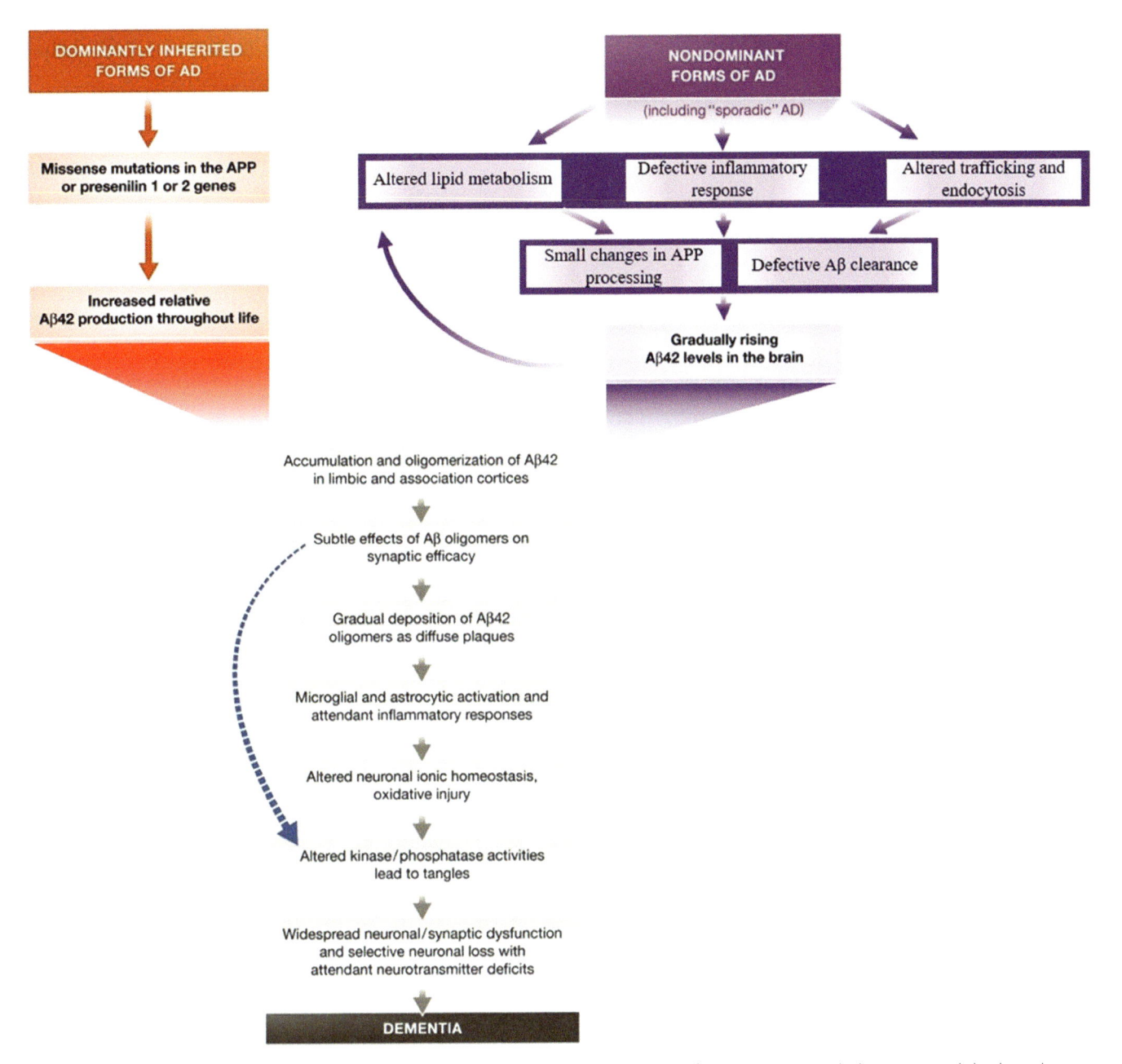

Figure 20.12 The amyloid cascade hypothesis. Aβ generated from proteolytic processing of APP causes tau pathology, neuronal death, and dementia. In the case of familial AD, dominant mutations in APP or PS1 genes cause a relative increase in Aβ42; in other forms of AD, a combination of genetic and environmental risk factors results in an increase in Aβ42 in the brain. Aβ affects several processes including synaptic activity, microglial activation, and the activity of kinases and phosphatases, leading to aberrant tau phosphorylation and tau pathology. It also feeds back to further enhance Aβ42 levels. The cascade eventually leads to neuronal loss and cell death. (Modified from Figure 1 in Selkoe and Hardy, 2016).

AD-related genes is available at https://www.alzforum.org/research-models/alzheimers-disease.

20.8.2.3 Mutations in APP cause hippocampal dysfunction

Despite the limited neurodegeneration seen in most APP animal models, cognitive deficits are consistent with hippocampal dysfunction, as seen in human AD. In vitro studies using hippocampal slices prepared from transgenic mice overexpressing human mutant APP have demonstrated alterations in synaptic transmission and LTP (Larson et al., 1999), while in vivo studies showed impaired induction and maintenance of LTP in CA1 (Giacchino et al., 2000) and impaired presynaptic function. Although the severity

of these deficits increased with age and with the onset of plaque pathology, they were evident in young mice before the development of amyloid plaques, indicating that defects of hippocampal synaptic transmission precede and are independent of overt plaque pathology. This was an important observation as it directed attention away from plaques as being the primary toxic lesion and instigated a search for toxic soluble Aβ species, such as oligomers (Chen et al., 2017; Lesne et al., 2006; Liu, Reed, et al., 2015; Selkoe, 2008; Sengupta, Nilson, and Kayed, 2016; Yang et al., 2017) or APP cleavage fragments (Nhan, Chiang, and Koo, 2015; Jiang et al., 2016). Several studies have demonstrated significant network dysfunction that seems to replicate what has been seen in human

---

Box 20.6 Alternative models

The mouse (*Mus musculus*) is the most frequently used vertebrate species for genetically engineered models of AD. Other model organisms include the rat (*Rattus norvegicus*), sea lamprey (*Petromyzon marinus*), zebrafish (*Danio rerio*), sheep (Handley et al. 2016; Yan et al. 2018), pig (Lee et al. 2017), Fruit fly (*Drosophila melanogaster*), and worm (*Caenorhabditis elegans*)

AD is unique to humans (Platt, Reeves, and Murphy 2013; Toledano et al. 2014). However, amyloid pathology is observed during aging in many species, and both plaques and tau pathology have been seen in aged dolphin (Gunn-Moore et al. 2018). Dogs show age-related cognitive decline and Aβ pathology (Head 2013), and the small rodent *Octodon degus* shows age-dependent amyloid and tau pathology, cognitive decline, and neuroinflammation (Castro-Fuentes and Socas-Perez 2013; Hurley et al. 2018).

Attempts are currently underway to create transgenic nonhuman primate (NHP) models of AD. NHPs such as macaques are genetically and anatomically closer than other species to humans, and they age in a similar fashion (Verdier et al. 2015). Although NHPs develop some cerebral amyloidosis and dementia with aging, tauopathy is minimal (Van Dam and De Deyn 2017) and many dissimilarities with human AD have been noted (Heuer et al. 2012; Oikawa, Kimura, and Yanagisawa 2010). It has proven difficult to correlate the cognitive and behavioral deficits observed in aged NHPs with the neuropathological features seen in the human AD brain (Toledano et al. 2014; Van Dam and De Deyn 2017). Furthermore, there is very little evidence indicating AD-like cognitive decline in NHP models (Jebelli and Piers 2015). With the advent of CRISPR-Cas9 genetic manipulation technologies, transgenic NHPs are being developed that are expected to show enhanced and relevant AD phenotypes. However, many disparities have been pointed out between transgenic and natural animal models (Cavanaugh, Pippin, and Barnard 2014), which might also apply to genetically modified NHPs.

Box 20.7 In silico models

A vast amount of data on AD is being generated from genetic, imaging, and "omic" studies, which has huge potential to be used to create computer simulations of disease processes (Rollo et al. 2016). For example, in silico models that can predict the concentrations of molecules over time in a given network have been used to model amyloid plaque formation (Helal et al. 2014). Other studies have modeled cross-talk between critical AD-related cell types (Puri and Li 2010), which highlighted the role of inflammatory cells in AD.

In silico models of neural circuits (artificial neural networks) and of the hippocampus have been created (Hines and Carnevale 1997). Artificial hippocampal circuits can be adapted for modeling of the hippocampus in AD by removing specific synaptic connections to artificially degrade some of the synapses (Swietlik et al. 2019). In silico models have also been created of the spread of disease from the hippocampus through the rest of the brain. These models are typically composed of "nodes," which represent neurons, with arcs or links to represent the axons/dendrites and synapses. These models can predict the atrophy seen in late-stage AD brains (Raj et al. 2015). In particular, a combination of data from imaging studies identifying disease-associated patterns of brain atrophy with models of neural networks has helped to identify factors causing specific networks to be more vulnerable to AD (Warren et al. 2013; Zhou et al. 2012). Mathematical models have been used to test predictions of mechanisms underlying tauopathy spread in AD (Meisl et al. 2021).

Artificial neural networks can also be used in combination with imaging data in the diagnosis of AD (Page et al. 1996; Swietlik and Bialowas 2019). Other in silico models of AD focus on investigating the aggregation or clearance of the key proteins involved in AD pathologies, Aβ and tau (Proctor et al. 2013).

---

fMRI studies (Sperling et al., 2009). Mutant APP transgenic mice were shown to have spontaneous nonconvulsive seizure activity in cortical and hippocampal networks (Greicius et al., 2004; Palop et al., 2007).

20.8.2.4 Mutations in APP cause hippocampal-dependent cognitive deficits

APP mutant mice have been subjected to a wide range of cognitive and behavioral tests (Lalonde, Fukuchi, and Strazielle, 2012; Webster et al., 2014). The first lines of mice overexpressing mutant APP showed deficits of spatial memory by 9 to 10 months of age, as well as impaired LTP (Ashe, 2001; Chapman et al., 1999; Chen et al., 2000; Cheng et al., 2007; Dodart et al., 1999; Hsiao et al., 1996). Recent studies have shown that memory impairment in transgenic mice expressing Aβ can result from impaired retrieval in hippocampal memory engram cells rather than a deficit in information storage (Roy et al., 2016).

20.8.2.5 Variants in APOE causes hippocampal deficits

Much of our understanding of APOE4 as a genetic risk factor has come from animal model studies. *APOE4* knockin mice have been created that express the human *APOE4* allele under the control of a mouse promotor (Hamanaka et al., 2000; Mann et al., 2004; Sullivan et al., 1997). These mice show hippocampal defects even at a young age; compared with *APOE3* mice, spine density in CA1 is reduced at 3 or 4 months, suggesting that synaptic impairment occurs early in these mice (Rodriguez, Burns, et al., 2013; Sun,

He, et al., 2017). Structural changes in hippocampal circuits correspond with deficits in spatial memory in APOE4 mice, with E4 mice showing impaired performance in the Barnes maze test, the Morris watermaze test, and an object–place recognition task (in which mice usually display a preference for the familiar object that has been relocated) (Grootendorst et al., 2005; Rodriguez, Burns, et al., 2013). However, other studies have shown no alterations in dendritic spines in the hippocampus of 1-year-old APOE4 mice (Dumanis et al., 2009). Electrophysiology studies on hippocampal slices from APOE knockin mice have showed no alteration of baseline synaptic transmission in 5- or 24-month-old APOE4 mice compared with APOE3 mice (Korwek et al., 2009; Yun et al., 2007). However, APOE4 mice show reduced LTP in the performant path (Trommer et al., 2004) and stronger LTP in CA1 when neurons in CA3 are stimulated (Korwek et al., 2009).

20.8.3 Genome-wide association studies highlight potential disease mechanism convergence

More recently, genome-wide association studies (GWAS) and whole-exome/whole-genome sequencing have identified numerous genetic risk factors for sporadic, late-onset AD (Karch and Goate, 2015) (Figure 20.13). Genetic factors are thought to account for 56%–79% of sporadic AD risk, and more than 50 different risk loci have now been identified (Gatz et al., 2006; Sims, Hill, and Williams, 2020; for an up-to-date list see alzgene.org). These genes affect a range of cellular processes, including innate immune function and inflammation, endocytosis and trafficking, and cholesterol and lipid metabolism (Figure 20.13). However, several genes identified in GWAS do not fit easily into these categories, and other pathways are being highlighted; recent analyses have also implicated tau metabolism as an important pathway (Kunkle et al., 2019).

20.8.3.1 Innate immune function and inflammation

Neuroinflammation, as evidenced largely by microglial activation, is thought to be an important process in the course of AD, possibly preceding other pathological events, including amyloid plaque formation (Heneka et al., 2013; Heneka et al., 2015). The explosion of GWAS genes expressed in glia has given new urgency to studying neuron–glia interactions in the etiology of AD (De Strooper and Karran, 2016; Henstridge, Hyman, and Spires-Jones, 2019). Gliosis has been consistently seen in the brains of AD patients since Alzheimer's time but for many years this was assumed to be a consequence rather than cause of disease. Some PET radioligands, including PK-11195, which binds specifically to the peripheral benzodiazepine binding receptor associated with microglial activity, can be used to visualize microglial activation. In subjects with AD, significant microglial activation is seen across the frontal, temporal, parietal and occipital cortices, but is notably absent in the hippocampus, consistent with amyloid PET results (Edison et al., 2008).

The identification of AD risk genes expressed in astrocytes and microglia, and the strong epidemiologic links between vascular risk factors and AD risk, suggest that nonneuronal cell types may be involved in disease initiation. This likely reflects a failure to effectively clear pathological proteins as well as direct interactions with synapses and neurons that may drive neurodegenerative processes. Much of the biology underpinning these processes is being explored in model systems, and more work will be needed to determine its

relevance to human disease. However, there is strong evidence that microglia in particular influence neurodegeneration via multiple mechanisms.

Microglia and astrocytes are the main inflammatory cells of the brain and exist on a spectrum between activated and inactivated states. Activated astrocytes and microglia secrete proinflammatory cytokines, which act to stimulate the clearance of cellular debris or protein aggregates. However, excessive astrocyte activation can lead to neuronal damage and eventual neuronal death (Heneka et al., 2015). In AD, microglia surround Aβ plaques (Bolmont et al., 2008; Itagaki et al., 1989; Stalder et al., 1999) and are activated by Aβ. This could serve to stimulate Aβ clearance and prevent the plaques from seeding throughout the brain (Bard et al., 2000). However, if this results in chronic neuroinflammation, it could lead to neuronal damage and death. There is evidence that both enhancing and suppressing neuroinflammation in AD models can be beneficial: expression of the inflammatory mediator interferon-γ in mouse models enhanced glial activation, resulting in a reduced Aβ plaque burden (Ghosh et al., 2013), whereas knockout of a chemokine receptor, reducing inflammatory signaling, prevented neuronal loss (Fuhrmann et al., 2010). Knockout of the *NLRP3* gene, which is important for the formation of the inflammation-initiating protein complex (the inflammasome), reduced Aβ deposition and prevented spatial memory impairments in APP/PS mice (Tejera et al., 2019). In reality, it is likely that different mechanisms are important at different stages of the disease. This has led to the suggestion that Aβ aggregates can initiate an inflammatory phenotype that serves to clear the aggregates, whereas the continued inflammation is responsible for neuronal degeneration and AD progression. Consistent

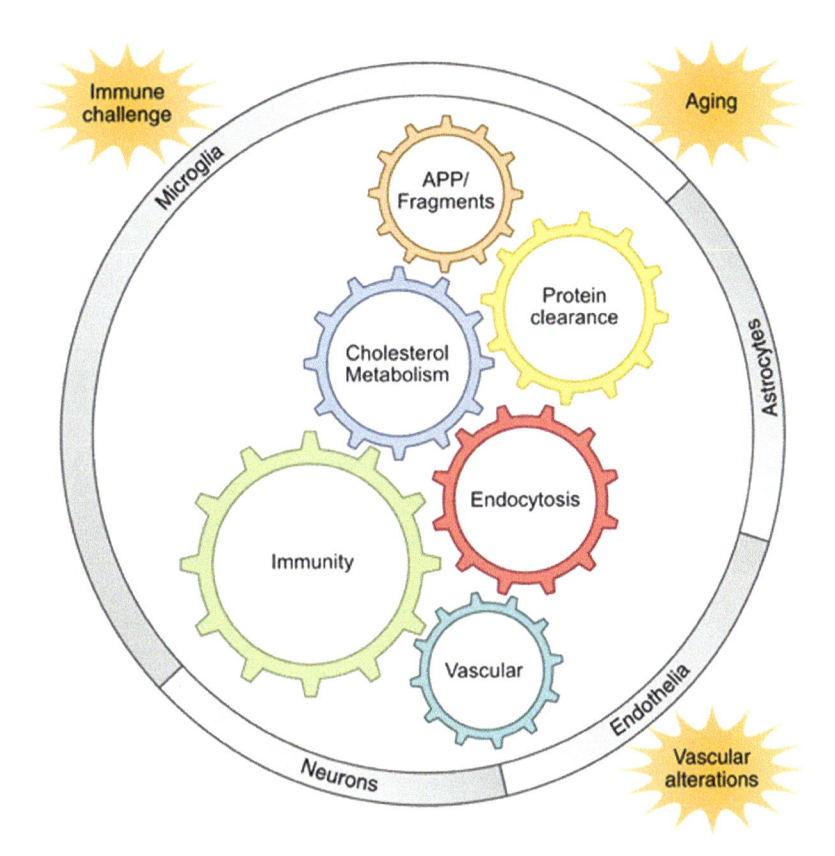

Figure 20.13 Environmental risk factors and genetic risk factors identified from GWAS studies for sporadic AD highlight specific biological mechanisms and pathways that play a role in the development of AD. (Modified from Sims et al., 2020.)

with this idea, high levels of CSF tumor necrosis factor-α (TNFα) in MCI patients is associated with an increased risk of conversion to AD (Tarkowski et al., 2003).

One of the most significant, recently identified risk genes for AD is *TREM2*. *TREM2* encodes an innate immune system receptor that is expressed on microglia and plays a role in activating the inflammatory phenotype of microglia and the initiation of phagocytosis (Gratuze, Leyns, and Holtzman, 2018). Point mutations in *TREM2* are rare but confer a large (2- to 4.5-fold) increased risk of developing AD (Guerreiro et al., 2013; Jonsson et al., 2013). *TREM2* point mutations are associated with reduced hippocampal volume in healthy adults and adults with MCI (Lupton et al., 2016; Rajagopalan, Hibar, and Thompson, 2013). Initial mouse models used CRISPR to introduce AD-linked *TREM2* point mutations directly into mouse *TREM2*, which resulted in altered splicing and reduced expression of TREM2 (Cheng-Hathaway et al., 2018). Later studies showed these changes to be specific to mouse TREM2, and the same point mutation does not affect expression of human TREM2 (Xiang et al., 2018), meaning these mouse models are modeling TREM2 deficiency, rather than the effect of the AD-linked mutation. APP/TREM 2 mutant mice had reduced microglial activation and reduced microglial density surrounding amyloid plaques in the hippocampus. However, there was no change in the total plaque area in the hippocampus (Song et al., 2018). Together, this suggests AD-linked TREM2 mutations have a loss-of-function phenotype and that increased activation of microglia would be beneficial to AD (Song et al., 2018). In vitro studies of TREM2 corroborate this finding, as the *TREM2* R47H mutant shows reduced binding to ligands (Atagi et al., 2015; Bailey, DeVaux, and Farzan, 2015; Kober et al., 2016; Yeh et al., 2016) and leads to reduced uptake of Aβ by microglia (Yeh et al., 2016).

As *TREM2* variants appear to cause loss of function, several studies have investigated the effect of reduction of TREM2 on disease progression. Studies on *TREM2* knockout AD mouse models appear to show that TREM2 has opposite roles at the onset of disease and later in disease progression. In young mice at the onset of disease, decreased TREM2 expression resulted in less Aβ pathology in the hippocampus; in older mice, by contrast, decreased TREM2 expression results in more Aβ pathology (Jay et al., 2017; Jay et al., 2015; Wang et al., 2015).

20.8.3.2 Endocytosis and trafficking

Several GWAS genes implicated in AD, for example *BIN1, CD2AP, PICALM,* and *SORL1,* have roles in intracellular trafficking. Interestingly, enlargement of early endosomes is the first pathology seen in AD brains (Cataldo et al., 2000), which suggests that dysfunctional trafficking occurs very early in the disease process (Figure 20.14). Early endosomes are the hub of several intracellular trafficking pathways. Protein cargoes can be trafficked into early endosomes from the cell surface (via endocytosis) and directly from the secretory pathway, and away from early endosomes either back to the cell surface, to the Golgi, or to late endosomes and lysosomes for degradation (Kimura and Yanagisawa, 2018). Enlarged early endosomes suggest an impairment in the transport of proteins, leading to accumulation in the early endosome; this could have effects on several cellular processes, including protein clearance and synaptic vesicle recycling (Kimura and Yanagisawa, 2018). Proteins derived from genes identified by GWAS studies function at several

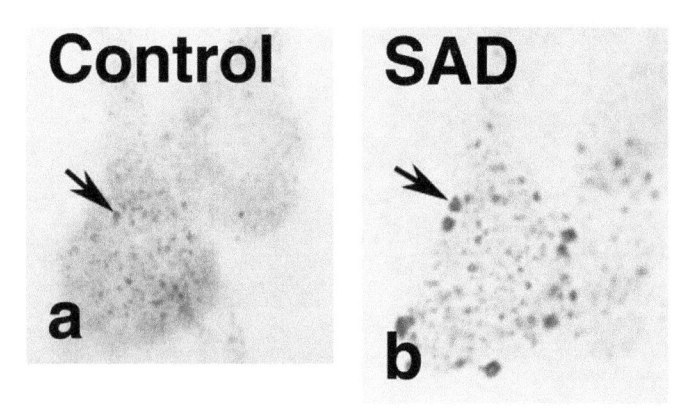

Figure 20.14 Enlarged endosomes (arrow) in neurons from sporadic AD (SAD) cases and controls. (From (Cataldo et al., 2000.)

points in this pathway: SORL1 mediates trafficking between the late Golgi and early endosomes, and both PICALM and BIN1 have been implicated in clathrin-mediated endocytosis (Karch and Goate, 2015). Furthermore, altering the expression of BIN1 or SORLA results in enlargement of early endosomes, as seen in AD (Calafate et al., 2016; Knupp et al., 2020).

Alterations in the endocytic pathway have implications for APP processing and the generation of Aβ. APP normally resides in the trans-Golgi network and is proteolytically processed when it is trafficked to the cell surface or to early endosomes. β-Cleavage of APP, the first step in generation of Aβ, occurs in early endosomes, so an increase in endosomal APP results in increased β-cleavage and Aβ generation (reviewed in Haass et al., 2012). SORLA plays a major role in the retrograde trafficking of APP from endosomes to the trans-Golgi network, and knockdown of SORLA or loss-of-function mutations result in an increase in β-cleavage (Andersen et al., 2005; Fjorback et al., 2012; Herskowitz et al., 2012). BIN1 also affects APP processing, by influencing the trafficking of the β-cleaving enzyme BACE1, reducing lysosomal degradation of BACE1 and increasing endosomal BACE1 levels (Miyagawa et al., 2016). Furthermore, APP proteolysis products, in particular the β-C-terminal fragment resulting from β-cleavage of APP, cause trafficking dysfunctions and enlargement of endosomes (Kwart et al., 2019).

Trafficking dysfunctions have implications beyond amyloid pathology, as recycling of vesicles is also vital for synaptic function and cell signaling. For example, loss of BIN1 in vitro results in a decrease in cell surface AMPA receptors and alterations in synaptic transmission (Schurmann et al., 2019). BIN1 may also play a role in the missorting of tau seen early in AD. BIN1 binds to tau, and this interaction is affected by phosphorylation of both tau and BIN1 (Chapuis et al., 2013; Glennon et al., 2020; Lasorsa et al., 2018; Malki et al., 2017; Sartori et al., 2019). In postmortem AD brains, tau mislocalizes from cytoplasmic to synaptic compartments, and this increase in synaptic tau correlates with the loss of BIN1 from cytoplasmic cellular compartments (Glennon et al., 2020). Furthermore, loss of BIN1 in vitro also results in an increase in phosphorylated tau in synaptic fractions (Glennon et al., 2020), and increased expression of BIN1 in vivo reduced tau mislocalization and rescued spatial memory deficits in a tau-expressing mouse model of AD (Sartori et al., 2019). BIN1 has also been implicated in the spread of tau pathology throughout the brain. BIN1 is present on tau seeding-competent exosomes purified from AD CSF (Crotti et al., 2019), and inhibition of BIN1 expression reduces tau secretion from neurons in vitro (Glennon et al., 2020) and increases tau uptake by neurons (Calafate et al., 2016). In addition, reduction of microglia BIN1 expression in vivo reduced the spread of tau pathology in male mice expressing tau with the pathogenic P301S mutation (Crotti et al., 2019).

20.8.3.3 Cholesterol and lipid metabolism

Several AD risk genes, including *APOE, CLU,* and *ABCA7,* are involved in the metabolism of cholesterol and other lipids. Cholesterol and lipids form the bulk of cell membranes and are therefore vital for membrane-dependent processes such as synaptic function, including synaptic plasticity and LTP. In fact, the brain contains 23% of the total body cholesterol (Loera-Valencia et al., 2019). Levels of several lipids are altered in AD brain in a region-specific way, further implicating their involvement in the disease process (Testa et al., 2016; Winkler et al., 2012), and lipid droplets accumulate in glial cells in AD (Foley, 2010). Hippocampal function and cholesterol are linked: induction of LTP in ex vivo hippocampal slices leads to upregulation of lipid synthesis, while loss of cholesterol from hippocampal slices reduces LTP and synaptic transmission (Frank et al., 2008; Koudinov and Koudinova, 2001). Cholesterol loss causes spatial memory deficits in aged rats, which can be rescued by administration of cholesterol to the brain (Martin et al., 2014).

CNS and somatic cholesterol are independent. In the brain, cholesterol is synthesized by astrocytes, which also synthesize APOE, the largest genetic risk factor for sporadic AD. APOE transports cholesterol from astrocytes to other cells of the brain (Boyles et al., 1985; Pitas et al., 1987). Cholesterol and other lipids can influence APP processing and Aβ pathology. APP and all the secretases that process it are intramembrane proteins (Steiner, Fluhrer, and Haass, 2008), and the Aβ-generating γ-cleavage of APP occurs within the lipid bilayer. Amyloidogenic processing of APP takes place within cholesterol-rich lipid microdomains of the cell membrane (Ehehalt et al., 2003), where both β- and γ-secretase are preferentially located (Riddell et al., 2001; Vetrivel et al., 2004). Furthermore, the thickness of the lipid bilayer (which is partly dependent on its lipid content) affects γ-secretase cleavage of APP (Winkler et al., 2012). Cholesterol levels have also been linked to Aβ pathology in vivo: induction of high cholesterol levels in mutant APP mice leads to an increase in the number of Aβ plaques (Shie et al., 2002) and altered proteolytic processing of APP (Refolo et al., 2000). A link between lipid metabolism and tau is less well documented. However, tau has been found in Aβ-containing lipid rafts along with APOE in mouse models (Kawarabayashi et al., 2004), and inhibitors of cholesterol synthesis also inhibited tau phosphorylation in an in vitro stem cell model of AD (van der Kant et al., 2019). Further evidence for a link between cholesterol pathways and tau pathology has come from APOE mouse models (Shi, Yamada, et al., 2017).

20.8.4 GWAS-implicated pathways are not independent

While AD GWAS genes have been classed into different pathways playing different roles in the development of AD, these pathways are not distinct and converge at several points (Figure 20.15). For example, APOE, which is generally considered part of the set of lipoproteins involved in cholesterol metabolism, also affects endosomal trafficking: the APOE4 allele causes enlarged early endosomes in aged mice, reduces cell-surface expression of the insulin receptor (Zhao et al., 2017), reduces cell-surface levels of LRP1, impairing uptake and degradation of Aβ by astrocytes (Prasad and Rao, 2018), and affects calcium signaling by influencing cell-surface expression of the NMDA receptor, thereby altering LTP in mouse hippocampal slices (Chen et al., 2010). SORL1, which has a major role in APP trafficking, is also a cholesterol receptor, and APOE is also a ligand for SORL1 (Holtzman, Herz, and Bu, 2012). APOE is also a ligand for the inflammatory receptor TREM2, and AD-associated TREM2 mutations have a reduced affinity for APOE. Mice fed a high cholesterol diet develop activated microglia and astrocytes and have increased levels of proinflammatory cytokines, showing

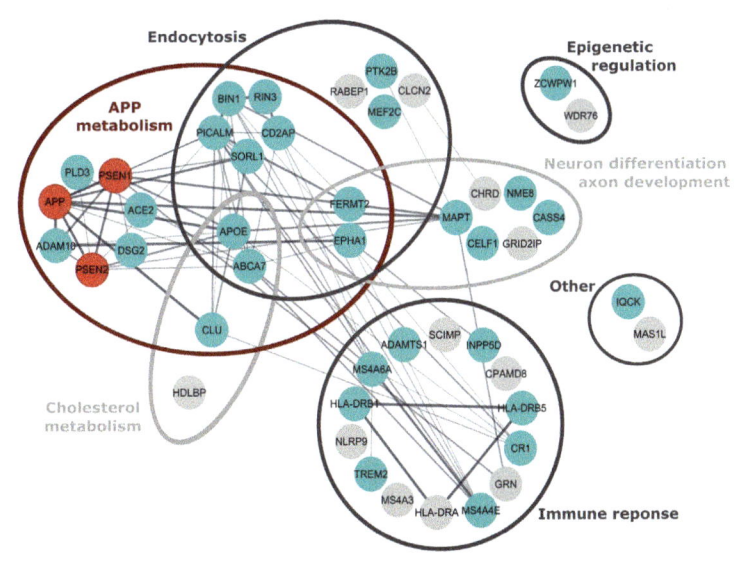

Figure 20.15 AD risk genes have overlapping risk mechanisms. (Figure 2 from Van Acker et al., 2019.)

that high cholesterol levels can influence inflammatory pathways (Thirumangalakudi et al., 2008).

20.9 Therapeutic approaches to treat or prevent AD

20.9.1 Symptom-modifying therapeutics

Most drugs in development for AD focus on pathways leading to neurotoxicity by targeting either Aβ, tau, neurotransmission, or inflammation (Figure 20.16). The first approved drug treatments for AD targeted neurotransmitters and aimed to prevent either cholinergic deficits in the AD brain or glutamate-induced excitotoxicity. Enhancing cholinergic transmission was achieved by inhibiting breakdown of acetylcholine with acetylcholinesterase inhibitors, later

marketed as donepezil, galantamine, and rivastigmine. However, while these can lead to an improvement in AD symptoms in some patients, they are not disease-modifying therapies and do not slow down disease progression. Prevention of Aβ-induced excitotoxicity has been attempted using NMDA receptor antagonists. Currently the only approved NMDA receptor antagonist is memantine, which, like acetylcholinesterase inhibitors, can provide some symptomatic benefits but is beneficial only in late-stage AD (Cummings, Feldman, and Scheltens, 2019; Lao et al., 2019).

20.9.2 Disease-modifying therapeutics

20.9.2.1 Anti-Aβ/amyloid

Drugs currently approved or in clinical trials predominantly target amyloid/Aβ at the early stages of the disease (Cummings et al., 2023). Amyloid-targeting therapies aim to reduce the Aβ burden

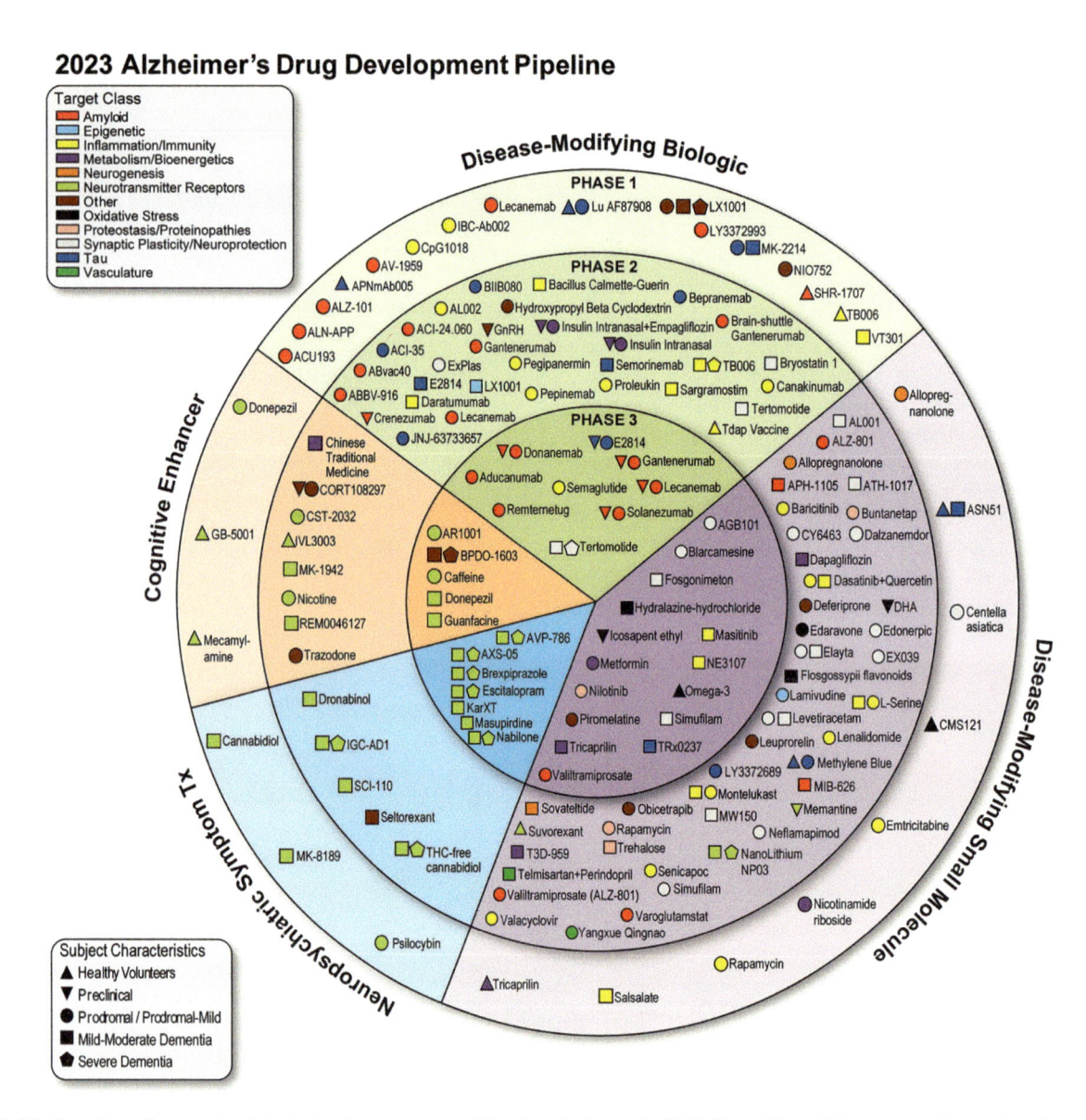

Figure 20.16 Overview of agents in clinical trials for treatment of Alzheimer's disease in 2023 (from ClinicalTrials.gov as of the index date of January 1, 2023). The inner ring shows Phase 3 agents; the middle ring comprises Phase 2 agents; the outer ring presents Phase 1 therapies; agents in green areas are biologics; agents in purple are disease-modifying small molecules; agents in orange areas are symptomatic agents addressing cognitive enhancement or behavioral and neuropsychiatric symptoms; the shape of the icon shows the population of the trial; the icon color shows the CADRO-based class of the agent ("Other" category includes CADRO classes that have three or fewer agents in trials). CADRO, Common Alzheimer's Disease Research Ontology; Tx, treatment. (Figure © J Cummings; M de la Flor, PhD, Illustrator). (Figure and legend from Cummings et al., 2023.)

in the brain, usually by reducing its production (by inhibiting β- or γ- secretase) or by enhancing its degradation or clearance. One of the most promising mechanisms for enhancing Aβ clearance is immunotherapy, where patients are treated with Aβ-directed antibodies that then target Aβ for destruction by the immune system. Several different therapeutics have been developed that target different parts of the Aβ peptide. Earlier generations of these therapeutics, for example bapineuzumab and solanezumab, reached phase III clinical trials, where they were found to successfully reduce both Aβ plaques and phosphorylated tau levels. However, trials were eventually terminated due to a lack of an effect on cognition (Cummings, Feldman, and Scheltens, 2019; Doody et al., 2014; Lao et al., 2019; Liu, Schmidt, et al., 2015). The accelerated approval program allows the approval of drugs that "fill an unmet clinical need based on a surrogate endpoint" (FDA.gov). Aducanumab (Aduhelm) was the first therapy to receive accelerated approval as a treatment for Alzheimer's disease from the US Food and Drug Administration (FDA) in 2021, and its approval was a landmark event for the Alzheimer's field. It was however not approved for use in Europe and the United Kingdom after the EU drug regulator, the European Medicines Agency (EMA), declined to license it. Aduhelm was discontinued by its manufacturer (Biogen) in 2024, to allow the manufacturer to focus on other drug priorities. In 2023 the Aβ targeting antibody Lecanemab (Leqembi) was the first traditionally approved therapy by the FDA, for people in the earliest stages of AD who showed evidence of Aβ elevation. Ongoing trials aim to continue to assess the efficacy of Leqembi on cognitive and functional measures, in extended trials. One issue associated with anti-Aβ therapies is the development of amyloid-related imaging abnormalities with edema (ARIA), or fluid formation on the brain. Although usually asymptomatic, this side effect is not understood and continues to be a concern.

Other Aβ-targeting therapies have attempted to inhibit β- or γ- secretase. The γ-secretase inhibitor semagacestat was found to effectively reduce Aβ (Henley et al., 2009). However, the catalytic component of γ-secretase, PS1, is involved in the cleavage of multiple substrates, and γ-secretase inhibitors were found to have multiple side effects. Furthermore, semagacestat did not have a significant effect on cognition, ultimately leading to phase III trials being terminated (Doody et al., 2013; Lao et al., 2019). Inhibition of the β-secretase BACE1 was initially a less common therapeutic strategy as the large active site of BACE1 made drug design challenging (Lao et al., 2019; Vassar, 2014). These issues have since been overcome and BACE1 inhibitors reached phase II and III clinical trials (Neumann et al., 2018), where they were shown to reduce CSF and plasma Aβ levels. However, BACE1 inhibitors have failed to show cognitive benefit despite demonstrating an Aβ-lowering effect and trials were terminated (Egan et al., 2019).

20.9.2.2 Anti-tau/NFTs

Therapies targeting tau pathology aim to reduce tau aggregation, reduce tau phosphorylation, or enhance tau clearance. Anti-tau aggregation therapies have to date not shown any benefit in phase III clinical trials for moderate to severe AD, although trials are continuing (Cummings et al., 2023; Gauthier et al., 2016). Immunotherapy is also being investigated as a way to target pathological tau species for degradation (Cummings et al., 2023). In mouse models, anti-tau antibodies clear pathological tau and reduce cognitive impairments (Yanamandra et al., 2015; Yanamandra

et al., 2013), and they are safe for use in humans (Novak et al., 2017). Several anti-tau immunotherapies are currently in phase II/III clinical trials (Cummings et al., 2023). As aberrantly phosphorylated tau is a hallmark of AD, the kinases that phosphorylate tau are also potential therapeutic targets. However, the GSK-3β inhibitor tideglusib showed no clinical benefits in phase II trials (Lovestone et al., 2015; Medina, 2018). Phase II trials of inhibitors targeting other tau kinases are currently ongoing (Cummings et al., 2023).

20.9.3 Other targets

Other AD-targeting therapeutics are based on insights from studies that have highlighted key pathways involved in the development of AD, such as the chronic inflammation present in AD brains. Epidemiological studies suggest that chronic use of nonsteroidal anti-inflammatory drugs (NSAIDs) reduces the risk of AD development. However, randomized, controlled clinical trials have failed to identify to demonstrate any benefit of the NSAIDs tested for AD (Jaturapatporn et al., 2012; Meyer et al., 2019). Several other anti-inflammatory drug candidates with a variety of modes of action are in various stages of clinical trials (Cummings et al., 2023; Yiannopoulou and Papageorgiou, 2020).

20.9.4 Overview

The development of AD therapeutics has been challenging, and to date the only disease-modifying approaches that have been approved target Aβ (Aducanumab/Lecanemab), through immunotherapy. As AD is a complex disease involving multiple pathological mechanisms, combinations of therapies are currently under investigation (Cummings et al. 2023). Additionally, as biomarkers evolve and their relationships to the underlying disease become better understood, it is possible to stratify patients by, for example, amyloid or tangle load, before they are accepted to clinical trials. Clinical trials on specific cohorts of patients with known familial AD mutations are also underway and are expected to reveal new insights into AD pathology. Given the current ordering of events demonstrated from biomarker studies, it is likely that the most robust effects of anti-amyloid therapeutics will need to be very early during the disease course, ideally before pathological tau forms have spread from the hippocampal formation to the neocortex. Significantly more work is therefore needed to understand why this region of the brain is so vulnerable to the etiological events that trigger AD, and how we can diagnose the earliest stages, currently considered preclinical, when we have the greatest chance of preventing the catastrophic decline that occurs once disease pathology has taken hold. There is much discussion in the field of how to define "success" in clinical treatment or prevention, with a call for less emphasis on cognitive metrics and more emphasis on increasing the health-span. The goal of delivering effective treatments, or even a cure, for AD will only be achieved by further fostering the partnerships between research funders, academics, clinicians, the pharmaceutical industry, and—most of all—the individual patients and patient charities whose contribution to research is fundamental and necessary for success.

20.9.5 Future perspectives

In the clinical sphere, the anticipated advent of a wide range of disease-modifying drugs will accelerate current efforts to detect AD in its earliest stages, further shifting the diagnosis of AD away from a clinically defined entity and toward a biologically defined disorder requiring in vivo evidence of neurodegeneration in association with amyloid and tau pathology. Earlier detection approaches will see legacy, pen-and-paper tests increasingly replaced by digital tools, not just for testing cognition but also other functions, and behaviors not testable in current clinical practice, such as navigation and sleep. These next-generation approaches will benefit from guidelines aimed at maximizing inclusivity and diversity, to ensure usability across different cultures and demographics, while remote assessment will aid initiatives for accurate disease detection at scale. The hope and expectation is that the application of machine learning and AI to these high throughput, multidimensional, datasets will not only extract additional diagnostic features but also deliver personalized "fingerprints" of disease for detection and management of AD on an individual level.

Beyond early detection, future efforts will be targeted toward primary prevention of disease with focus on those potentially modifiable factors that affect risk, and also progression of disease such as diet and lifestyle. The technological revolution will drive improvements in the care of people with cognitive impairment of dementia. While efforts to maintain or enhance cognitive function in the context of neurodegenerative disease are relatively embryonic at present, there is greater current interest in the use of tech to support everyday activities and maintain autonomy in the context of dementia. Such usages range from passive sensing systems for home monitoring, with alerts for falls or malnutrition, through to more complex active assistive devices such as wearable robotics for mobility.

In conclusion, the diagnosis and management of AD is entering a new phase that promises better outcomes for those affected, driven by neuroscientific and technological advances. The emerging challenge will be to maximize access to these improvements across the global population and avoid the risk that such advances result in a two-tiered inequality of haves and have-nots.

REFERENCES

Acosta, D., F. Powell, Y. Zhao, A. Raj. 2018. Regional vulnerability in Alzheimer's disease: the role of cell-autonomous and transneuronal processes. *Alzheimers Dement*, 14: 797–810.

Ahmed, Z., J. Cooper, T. K. Murray, K. Garn, E. McNaughton, H. Clarke, S. Parhizkar, M. A. Ward, A. Cavallini, S. Jackson, et al. 2014. A novel in vivo model of tau propagation with rapid and progressive neurofibrillary tangle pathology: the pattern of spread is determined by connectivity, not proximity. *Acta Neuropathol*, 127: 667–683.

Albert, M. S., S. T. DeKosky, D. Dickson, B. Dubois, H. H. Feldman, N. C. Fox, A. Gamst, D. M. Holtzman, W. J. Jagust, R. C. Petersen, et al. 2011. The diagnosis of mild cognitive impairment due to Alzheimer's disease: recommendations from the National Institute on Aging-Alzheimer's Association workgroups on diagnostic guidelines for Alzheimer's disease. *Alzheimers Dement*, 7: 270–279.

Allison, S. L., A. M. Fagan, J. C. Morris, D. Head. 2016. Spatial navigation in preclinical Alzheimer's disease. *J Alzheimers Dis*, 52: 77–90.

Ally, B. A., E. P. Hussey, P. C. Ko, R. J. Molitor. 2013. Pattern separation and pattern completion in Alzheimer's disease: evidence of rapid forgetting in amnestic mild cognitive impairment. *Hippocampus*, 23: 1246–1258.

Altomare, D., C. Ferrari, A. Caroli, S. Galluzzi, A. Prestia, W. M. van der Flier, R. Ossenkoppele, B. Van Berckel, F. Barkhof, C. E. Teunissen, et al., Initiative Alzheimer's Disease Neuroimaging.

2019. Prognostic value of Alzheimer's biomarkers in mild cognitive impairment: the effect of age at onset. *J Neurol*, 266: 2535–2545.

American Psychiatric Association. 2013. *Diagnostic and Statistical Manual of Mental Disorders*. Fifth Edition. Washington, DC: American Psychiatric Association.

Andersen, O. M., J. Reiche, V. Schmidt, M. Gotthardt, R. Spoelgen, J. Behlke, C. A. von Arnim, T. Breiderhoff, P. Jansen, X. Wu, et al. 2005. Neuronal sorting protein-related receptor sorLA/LR11 regulates processing of the amyloid precursor protein. *Proc Natl Acad Sci U S A*, 102: 13461–13466.

Arber, C., J. Toombs, C. Lovejoy, N. S. Ryan, R. W. Paterson, N. Willumsen, E. Gkanatsiou, E. Portelius, K. Blennow, A. Heslegrave, et al. 2019. Familial Alzheimer's disease patient-derived neurons reveal distinct mutation-specific effects on amyloid beta. *Mol Psychiatry*, 25: 2919–2931.

Arevalo-Rodriguez, I., N. Smailagic, I. Figuls M. Roque, A. Ciapponi, E. Sanchez-Perez, A. Giannakou, O. L. Pedraza, X. Bonfill Cosp, S. Cullum. 2015. Mini-Mental State Examination (MMSE) for the detection of Alzheimer's disease and other dementias in people with mild cognitive impairment (MCI). *Cochrane Database Syst Rev*, CD010783. doi:10.1002/14651858.CD010783.pub3. PMID: 34313331 F

Ashe, K. H. 2001. Learning and memory in transgenic mice modeling Alzheimer's disease. *Learn Mem*, 8: 301–308.

Ashton, N. J., M. Ide, H. Zetterberg, K. Blennow. 2019. Salivary biomarkers for Alzheimer's disease and related disorders. *Neurol Ther*, 8: 83–94.

Atagi, Y., C. C. Liu, M. M. Painter, X. F. Chen, C. Verbeeck, H. Zheng, X. Li, R. Rademakers, S. S. Kang, H. Xu, et al. 2015. Apolipoprotein E is a ligand for triggering receptor expressed on myeloid cells 2 (TREM2). *J Biol Chem*, 290: 26043–26050.

Bailey, C. C., L. B. DeVaux, M. Farzan. 2015. The triggering receptor expressed on myeloid cells 2 binds apolipoprotein E. *J Biol Chem*, 290: 26033–26042.

Ball, M. J. 1987. Morphometric analyses of neuronal populations and dendritic extent in normal aging and dementia of Alzheimer type: a frank appraisal of the difficulties. *Neurobiol Aging*, 8: 564–565.

Barbeau, E., M. Didic, E. Tramoni, O. Felician, S. Joubert, A. Sontheimer, M. Ceccaldi, M. Poncet. 2004. Evaluation of visual recognition memory in MCI patients. *Neurology*, 62: 1317–1322.

Bard, F., C. Cannon, R. Barbour, R. L. Burke, D. Games, H. Grajeda, T. Guido, K. Hu, J. Huang, K. Johnson-Wood, et al. 2000. Peripherally administered antibodies against amyloid beta-peptide enter the central nervous system and reduce pathology in a mouse model of Alzheimer disease. *Nat Med*, 6: 916–919.

Bateman, R. J., C. Xiong, T. L. Benzinger, A. M. Fagan, A. Goate, N. C. Fox, D. S. Marcus, N. J. Cairns, X. Xie, T. M. Blazey, et al., Network Dominantly Inherited Alzheimer. 2012. Clinical and biomarker changes in dominantly inherited Alzheimer's disease. *N Engl J Med*, 367: 795–804.

Benedet, A. L., N. J. Ashton, T. A. Pascoal, A. Leuzy, S. Mathotaarachchi, M. S. Kang, J. Therriault, M. Savard, M. Chamoun, M. Scholl, et al. 2019. Plasma neurofilament light associates with Alzheimer's disease metabolic decline in amyloid-positive individuals. *Alzheimers Dement (Amst)*, 11: 679–689.

Benilova, I., and B. De Strooper. 2013. Neuroscience. Promiscuous Alzheimer's amyloid: yet another partner. *Science*, 341: 1354–1355.

Bereczki, E., R. M. Branca, P. T. Francis, J. B. Pereira, J. H. Baek, T. Hortobagyi, B. Winblad, C. Ballard, J. Lehtio, D. Aarsland. 2018. Synaptic markers of cognitive decline in neurodegenerative diseases: a proteomic approach. *Brain*, 141: 582–595.

Berron, D., D. van Westen, R. Ossenkoppele, O. Strandberg, O. Hansson. 2020. Medial temporal lobe connectivity and its associations with cognition in early Alzheimer's disease. *Brain*, 143: 1233–1248.

Beyreuther, K., C. L. Masters. 1991. Amyloid precursor protein (APP) and beta A4 amyloid in the etiology of Alzheimer's disease: precursor-product relationships in the derangement of neuronal function. *Brain Pathol*, 1: 241–251.

Bird, C. M., D. Chan, T. Hartley, Y. A. Pijnenburg, M. N. Rossor, N. Burgess. 2010. Topographical short-term memory differentiates Alzheimer's disease from frontotemporal lobar degeneration. *Hippocampus*, 20: 1154–1169.

Bittar, A., U. Sengupta, R. Kayed. 2018. Prospects for strain-specific immunotherapy in Alzheimer's disease and tauopathies. *NPJ Vaccines*, 3: 9.

Blennow, K., M. J. de Leon, H. Zetterberg. 2006. Alzheimer's disease. *Lancet*, 368: 387–403.

Blennow, K., H. Hampel, M. Weiner, H. Zetterberg. 2010. Cerebrospinal fluid and plasma biomarkers in Alzheimer disease. *Nat Rev Neurol*, 6: 131–144.

Bolmont, T., F. Haiss, D. Eicke, R. Radde, C. A. Mathis, W. E. Klunk, S. Kohsaka, M. Jucker, M. E. Calhoun. 2008. Dynamics of the microglial/amyloid interaction indicate a role in plaque maintenance. *J Neurosci*, 28: 4283–4292.

Bordi, M., M. J. Berg, P. S. Mohan, C. M. Peterhoff, M. J. Alldred, S. Che, S. D. Ginsberg, R. A. Nixon. 2016. Autophagy flux in CA1 neurons of Alzheimer hippocampus: increased induction overburdens failing lysosomes to propel neuritic dystrophy. *Autophagy*, 12: 2467–2483.

Botcher, N. A., J. E. Falck, A. M. Thomson, A. Mercer. 2014. Distribution of interneurons in the CA2 region of the rat hippocampus. *Front Neuroanat*, 8: 104.

Boyles, J. K., R. E. Pitas, E. Wilson, R. W. Mahley, J. M. Taylor. 1985. Apolipoprotein E associated with astrocytic glia of the central nervous system and with nonmyelinating glia of the peripheral nervous system. *J Clin Invest*, 76: 1501–1513.

Braak, H., E. Braak. 1991. Neuropathological stageing of Alzheimer-related changes. *Acta Neuropathol*, 82: 239–259.

Braak, H., K. Del Tredici. 2015. The preclinical phase of the pathological process underlying sporadic Alzheimer's disease. *Brain*, 138: 2814–2833.

Braak, H., U. Rub, C. Schultz, K. Del Tredici. 2006. Vulnerability of cortical neurons to Alzheimer's and Parkinson's diseases. *J Alzheimers Dis*, 9: 35–44.

Braak, H., D. R. Thal, E. Ghebremedhin, K. Del Tredici. 2011. Stages of the pathologic process in Alzheimer disease: age categories from 1 to 100 years. *J Neuropathol Exp Neurol*, 70: 960–969.

Brandt, J Benedict RHB. 2001. Hopkins Verbal Learning Test—Revised: professional manual. *Psychological Assessment Resources*.

Breen, K. C., M. Bruce, B. H. Anderton. 1991. Beta amyloid precursor protein mediates neuronal cell-cell and cell-surface adhesion. *J Neurosci Res*, 28: 90–100.

Brinkmalm, A., G. Brinkmalm, W. G. Honer, J. A. Moreno, J. Jakobsson, G. R. Mallucci, H. Zetterberg, K. Blennow, A. Ohrfelt. 2014. Targeting synaptic pathology with a novel affinity mass spectrometry approach. *Mol Cell Proteomics*, 13: 2584–2592.

Brown, J., G. Pengas, K. Dawson, L. A. Brown, P. Clatworthy. 2009. Self administered cognitive screening test (TYM) for detection of Alzheimer's disease: cross sectional study. *BMJ*, 338: b2030.

Brownjohn, P. W., J. Smith, E. Portelius, L. Serneels, H. Kvartsberg, B. De Strooper, K. Blennow, H. Zetterberg, F. J. Livesey. 2017. Phenotypic screening identifies modulators of amyloid precursor protein processing in human stem cell models of Alzheimer's disease. *Stem Cell Reports*, 8: 870–882.

Buckley, R. F., B. Hanseeuw, A. P. Schultz, P. Vannini, S. L. Aghjayan, M. J. Properzi, J. D. Jackson, E. C. Mormino, D. M. Rentz, R. A. Sperling, et al. 2017. Region-Specific association of subjective cognitive decline with tauopathy independent of global beta-amyloid burden. *JAMA Neurol*, 74: 1455–1463.

Buckner, R. L. 2004. Memory and executive function in aging and AD: multiple factors that cause decline and reserve factors that compensate. *Neuron*, 44: 195–208.

Busche, M. A., G. Eichhoff, H. Adelsberger, D. Abramowski, K. H. Wiederhold, C. Haass, M. Staufenbiel, A. Konnerth, O. Garaschuk. 2008. Clusters of hyperactive neurons near amyloid plaques in a mouse model of Alzheimer's disease. *Science*, 321: 1686–1689.

Busche, M. A., S. Wegmann, S. Dujardin, C. Commins, J. Schiantarelli, N. Klickstein, T. V. Kamath, G. A. Carlson, I. Nelken, B. T. Hyman. 2019. Tau impairs neural circuits, dominating amyloid-beta effects, in Alzheimer models in vivo. *Nat Neurosci*, 22: 57–64.

Buschke, H. 1984. Cued recall in amnesia. *J Clin Neuropsychol*, 6: 433–440.

Bush, D., C. Barry, D. Manson, N. Burgess 2015. Using grid cells for navigation. *Neuron*, 87: 507–520.

Cacucci, F., M. Yi, T. J. Wills, P. Chapman, J. O'Keefe. 2008. Place cell firing correlates with memory deficits and amyloid plaque burden in Tg2576 Alzheimer mouse model. *Proc Natl Acad Sci U S A*, 105: 7863–7868.

Calafate, S., W. Flavin, P. Verstreken, D. Moechars. 2016. Loss of Bin1 promotes the propagation of tau pathology. *Cell Rep*, 17: 931–940.

Campion, D., J. M. Flaman, A. Brice, D. Hannequin, B. Dubois, C. Martin, V. Moreau, F. Charbonnier, O. Didierjean, S. Tardieu, et al. 1995. Mutations of the presenilin I gene in families with early-onset Alzheimer's disease. *Hum Mol Genet*, 4: 2373–2377.

Castro-Fuentes, R., R. Socas-Perez. 2013. Octodon degus: a strong attractor for Alzheimer research. *Basic Clin Neurosci*, 4: 91–96.

Cataldo, A. M., C. M. Peterhoff, J. C. Troncoso, T. Gomez-Isla, B. T. Hyman, R. A. Nixon. 2000. Endocytic pathway abnormalities precede amyloid beta deposition in sporadic Alzheimer's disease and Down syndrome: differential effects of APOE genotype and presenilin mutations. *Am J Pathol*, 157: 277–286.

Cavanaugh, S. E., J. J. Pippin, N. D. Barnard. 2014. Animal models of Alzheimer disease: historical pitfalls and a path forward. *Altex*, 31: 279–302.

Cembrowski, M. S., N. Spruston. 2019. Heterogeneity within classical cell types is the rule: lessons from hippocampal pyramidal neurons. *Nat Rev Neurosci*, 20: 193–204.

Cerami, C., B. Dubois, M. Boccardi, A. U. Monsch, J. F. Demonet, S. F. Cappa, Biomarkers Geneva Task Force for the Roadmap of Alzheimer's. 2017. Clinical validity of delayed recall tests as a gateway biomarker for Alzheimer's disease in the context of a structured 5-phase development framework. *Neurobiol Aging*, 52: 153–166.

Chan, D., N. C. Fox, R. I. Scahill, W. R. Crum, J. L. Whitwell, G. Leschziner, A. M. Rossor, J. M. Stevens, L. Cipolotti, M. N. Rossor. 2001. Patterns of temporal lobe atrophy in semantic dementia and Alzheimer's disease. *Ann Neurol*, 49: 433–442.

Chapman, P. F., G. L. White, M. W. Jones, D. Cooper-Blacketer, V. J. Marshall, M. Irizarry, L. Younkin, M. A. Good, T. V. Bliss, B. T. Hyman, et al. 1999. Impaired synaptic plasticity and learning in aged amyloid precursor protein transgenic mice. *Nat Neurosci*, 2: 271–276.

Chapuis, J., F. Hansmannel, M. Gistelinck, A. Mounier, C. Van Cauwenberghe, K. V. Kolen, F. Geller, Y. Sottejeau, D. Harold, P. Dourlen, et al., Gerad consortium. 2013. Increased expression of

BIN1 mediates Alzheimer genetic risk by modulating tau pathology. *Mol Psychiatry*, **18**: 1225–1234.

Chartier-Harlin, M. C., F. Crawford, H. Houlden, A. Warren, D. Hughes, L. Fidani, A. Goate, M. Rossor, P. Roques, J. Hardy, et al. 1991. Early-onset Alzheimer's disease caused by mutations at codon 717 of the beta-amyloid precursor protein gene. *Nature*, **353**: 844–846.

Chen, G., K. S. Chen, J. Knox, J. Inglis, A. Bernard, S. J. Martin, A. Justice, L. McConlogue, D. Games, S. B. Freedman, et al. 2000. A learning deficit related to age and beta-amyloid plaques in a mouse model of Alzheimer's disease. *Nature*, **408**: 975–979.

Chen, G. F., T. H. Xu, Y. Yan, Y. R. Zhou, Y. Jiang, K. Melcher, H. E. Xu. 2017. Amyloid beta: structure, biology and structure-based therapeutic development. *Acta Pharmacol Sin*, **38**: 1205–1235.

Chen, M. K., A. P. Mecca, M. Naganawa, S. J. Finnema, T. Toyonaga, S. F. Lin, S. Najafzadeh, J. Ropchan, Y. Lu, J. W. McDonald, et al. 2018. Assessing synaptic density in Alzheimer disease with synaptic vesicle glycoprotein 2A positron emission tomographic imaging. *JAMA Neurol*, **75**: 1215–1224.

Chen, Y., M. S. Durakoglugil, X. Xian, J. Herz. 2010. ApoE4 reduces glutamate receptor function and synaptic plasticity by selectively impairing APOE receptor recycling. *Proc Natl Acad Sci U S A*, **107**: 12011–12016.

Cheng, I. H., K. Scearce-Levie, J. Legleiter, J. J. Palop, H. Gerstein, N. Bien-Ly, J. Puolivali, S. Lesne, K. H. Ashe, P. J. Muchowski, et al. 2007. Accelerating amyloid-beta fibrillization reduces oligomer levels and functional deficits in Alzheimer disease mouse models. *J Biol Chem*, **282**: 23818–23828.

Cheng-Hathaway, P. J., E. G. Reed-Geaghan, T. R. Jay, B. T. Casali, S. M. Bemiller, S. S. Puntambekar, V. E. von Saucken, R. Y. Williams, J. C. Karlo, M. Moutinho, et al. 2018. The Trem2 R47H variant confers loss-of-function-like phenotypes in Alzheimer's disease. *Mol Neurodegener*, **13**: 29.

Chetelat, G., B. Desgranges, V. de la Sayette, F. Viader, K. Berkouk, B. Landeau, C. Lalevee, F. Le Doze, B. Dupuy, D. Hannequin, et al. 2003. Dissociating atrophy and hypometabolism impact on episodic memory in mild cognitive impairment. *Brain*, **126**: 1955–1967.

Chibnik, L. B., F. J. Wolters, K. Backman, A. Beiser, C. Berr, J. C. Bis, E. Boerwinkle, D. Bos, C. Brayne, J. F. Dartigues, et al. 2017. Trends in the incidence of dementia: design and methods in the Alzheimer Cohorts Consortium. *Eur J Epidemiol*, **32**: 931–938.

Choi, S. H., E. Bylykbashi, Z. K. Chatila, S. W. Lee, B. Pulli, G. D. Clemenson, E. Kim, A. Rompala, M. K. Oram, C. Asselin, et al. 2018. Combined adult neurogenesis and BDNF mimic exercise effects on cognition in an Alzheimer's mouse model. *Science*, 361.

Choi, S. H., Y. H. Kim, M. Hebisch, C. Sliwinski, S. Lee, C. D'Avanzo, H. Chen, B. Hooli, C. Asselin, J. Muffat, et al. 2014. A three-dimensional human neural cell culture model of Alzheimer's disease. *Nature*, **515**: 274–278.

Cleary, J. P., D. M. Walsh, J. J. Hofmeister, G. M. Shankar, M. A. Kuskowski, D. J. Selkoe, K. H. Ashe. 2005. Natural oligomers of the amyloid-beta protein specifically disrupt cognitive function. *Nat Neurosci*, **8**: 79–84.

Colom-Cadena, M., T. Spires-Jones, H. Zetterberg, K. Blennow, A. Caggiano, S. T. DeKosky, H. Fillit, J. E. Harrison, L. S. Schneider, P. Scheltens, et al., Group Synaptic Health Endpoints Working. 2020. The clinical promise of biomarkers of synapse damage or loss in Alzheimer's disease. *Alzheimers Res Ther*, **12**: 21.

Corder, E. H., A. M. Saunders, W. J. Strittmatter, D. E. Schmechel, P. C. Gaskell, G. W. Small, A. D. Roses, J. L. Haines, M. A. Pericak-Vance. 1993. Gene dose of apolipoprotein E type 4 allele and the risk of Alzheimer's disease in late onset families. *Science*, **261**: 921–923.

Crotti, A., H. R. Sait, K. M. McAvoy, K. Estrada, A. Ergun, S. Szak, G. Marsh, L. Jandreski, M. Peterson, T. L. Reynolds, et al. 2019. BIN1 favors the spreading of Tau via extracellular vesicles. *Sci Rep*, **9**: 9477.

Cummings, J., H. H. Feldman, P. Scheltens. 2019. The "rights" of precision drug development for Alzheimer's disease. *Alzheimers Res Ther*, **11**: 76.

Cummings, J., Zhou, Y., Lee, G., Zhong, K., Fonseca, J., and F. Cheng. 2023. Alzheimer's disease drug development pipeline: 2023. *Alzheimers Dement (N Y)*, **9**: e12385.

Davies, D. C., N. Horwood, S. L. Isaacs, D. M. Mann. 1992. The effect of age and Alzheimer's disease on pyramidal neuron density in the individual fields of the hippocampal formation. *Acta Neuropathol*, **83**: 510–517.

de Calignon, A., M. Polydoro, M. Suarez-Calvet, C. William, D. H. Adamowicz, K. J. Kopeikina, R. Pitstick, N. Sahara, K. H. Ashe, G. A. Carlson, et al. 2012. Propagation of tau pathology in a model of early Alzheimer's disease. *Neuron*, **73**: 685–697.

De Strooper, B., W. Annaert. 2000. Proteolytic processing and cell biological functions of the amyloid precursor protein. *J Cell Sci*, 113 (Pt 11): 1857–1870.

De Strooper, B., W. Annaert, P. Cupers, P. Saftig, K. Craessaerts, J. S. Mumm, E. H. Schroeter, V. Schrijvers, M. S. Wolfe, W. J. Ray, et al. 1999. A presenilin-1-dependent gamma-secretase-like protease mediates release of Notch intracellular domain. *Nature*, **398**: 518–522.

De Strooper, B., E. Karran. 2016. The cellular phase of Alzheimer's disease. *Cell*, **164**: 603–615.

De Strooper, B., P. Saftig, K. Craessaerts, H. Vanderstichele, G. Guhde, W. Annaert, K. Von Figura, F. Van Leuven. 1998. Deficiency of presenilin-1 inhibits the normal cleavage of amyloid precursor protein. *Nature*, **391**: 387–390.

Dejanovic, B., M. A. Huntley, A. De Maziere, W. J. Meilandt, T. Wu, K. Srinivasan, Z. Jiang, V. Gandham, B. A. Friedman, H. Ngu, et al. 2018. Changes in the synaptic proteome in tauopathy and rescue of tau-induced synapse loss by C1q antibodies. *Neuron*, **100**: 1322–1336 e7.

DeKosky, S. T., S. W. Scheff. 1990. Synapse loss in frontal cortex biopsies in Alzheimer's disease: correlation with cognitive severity. *Ann Neurol*, **27**: 457–464.

DeKosky, S. T., S. W. Scheff, S. D. Styren. 1996. Structural correlates of cognition in dementia: quantification and assessment of synapse change. *Neurodegeneration*, **5**: 417–421.

Delis, D. C., Kramer, J. H., Kaplan, E., Ober, B. A. 1987. The California Verbal Learning Test: Research Edition, Adult Version. San Antonio, TX: The Psychological Corporation.

Del Tredici, K., H. Braak. 2020. To stage, or not to stage. *Curr Opin Neurobiol*, **61**: 10–22.

Deng, W., C. Xing, R. David, D. Mastroeni, M. Ning, E. H. Lo, P. D. Coleman. 2019. AmpliSeq transcriptome of laser captured neurons from Alzheimer brain: comparison of single cell versus neuron pools. *Aging Dis*, **10**: 1146–1158.

de Wilde, M. C., C. R. Overk, J. W. Sijben, E. Masliah. 2016. Meta-analysis of synaptic pathology in Alzheimer's disease reveals selective molecular vesicular machinery vulnerability. *Alzheimers Dement*, **12**: 633–644.

Dhindsa, K., V. Drobinin, J. King, G. B. Hall, N. Burgess, S. Becker. 2014. Examining the role of the temporo-parietal network in memory, imagery, and viewpoint transformations. *Front Hum Neurosci*, **8**: 709.

Dodart, J. C., H. Meziane, C. Mathis, K. R. Bales, S. M. Paul, A. Ungerer. 1999. Behavioral disturbances in transgenic mice overexpressing the V717F beta-amyloid precursor protein. *Behav Neurosci*, **113**: 982–990.

Doebler, J. A., W. R. Markesbery, A. Anthony, R. E. Rhoads. 1987. Neuronal RNA in relation to neuronal loss and neurofibrillary pathology in the hippocampus in Alzheimer's disease. *J Neuropathol Exp Neurol*, **46**: 28–39.

Donohue, M. C., R. A. Sperling, D. P. Salmon, D. M. Rentz, R. Raman, R. G. Thomas, M. Weiner, P. S. Aisen, Biomarkers Australian Imaging, Ageing Lifestyle Flagship Study of, Initiative Alzheimer's Disease Neuroimaging, and Study Alzheimer's Disease Cooperative. 2014. The preclinical Alzheimer cognitive composite: measuring amyloid-related decline. *JAMA Neurol*, **71**: 961–970.

Doody, R. S., R. Raman, M. Farlow, T. Iwatsubo, B. Vellas, S. Joffe, K. Kieburtz, F. He, X. Sun, R. G. Thomas, et al., Group Semagacestat Study. 2013. A phase 3 trial of semagacestat for treatment of Alzheimer's disease. *N Engl J Med*, **369**: 341–350.

Doody, R. S., R. G. Thomas, M. Farlow, T. Iwatsubo, B. Vellas, S. Joffe, K. Kieburtz, R. Raman, X. Sun, P. S. Aisen, et al., Committee Alzheimer's Disease Cooperative Study Steering, and Group Solanezumab Study. 2014. Phase 3 trials of solanezumab for mild-to-moderate Alzheimer's disease. *N Engl J Med*, **370**: 311–321.

Dourlen, P., D. Kilinc, N. Malmanche, J. Chapuis, J. C. Lambert. 2019. The new genetic landscape of Alzheimer's disease: from amyloid cascade to genetically driven synaptic failure hypothesis?. *Acta Neuropathol*, **138**: 221–236.

Dubois, B., H. H. Feldman, C. Jacova, J. L. Cummings, S. T. Dekosky, P. Barberger-Gateau, A. Delacourte, G. Frisoni, N. C. Fox, D. Galasko, et al. 2010. Revising the definition of Alzheimer's disease: a new lexicon. *Lancet Neurol*, **9**: 1118–1127.

Dubois, B., H. H. Feldman, C. Jacova, H. Hampel, J. L. Molinuevo, K. Blennow, S. T. DeKosky, S. Gauthier, D. Selkoe, R. Bateman, et al. 2014. Advancing research diagnostic criteria for Alzheimer's disease: the IWG-2 criteria. *Lancet Neurol*, **13**: 614–629.

Dumanis, S. B., J. A. Tesoriero, L. W. Babus, M. T. Nguyen, J. H. Trotter, M. J. Ladu, E. J. Weeber, R. S. Turner, B. Xu, G. W. Rebeck, et al. 2009. ApoE4 decreases spine density and dendritic complexity in cortical neurons in vivo. *J Neurosci*, **29**: 15317–15322.

Duvernoy, H. M. 2005. The Human Hippocampus: Functional Anatomy, Vascularization and Serial Sections with MRI. Berlin; Heidelberg: Springer-Verlag.

Edison, P., H. A. Archer, A. Gerhard, R. Hinz, N. Pavese, F. E. Turkheimer, A. Hammers, Y. F. Tai, N. Fox, A. Kennedy et al. 2008. Microglia, amyloid, and cognition in Alzheimer's disease: An [11C](R)PK11195-PET and [11C]PIB-PET study. *Neurobiol Dis*, **32**: 412–419.

Egan, M. F., J. Kost, T. Voss, Y. Mukai, P. S. Aisen, J. L. Cummings, P. N. Tariot, B. Vellas, C. H. van Dyck, M. Boada, et al. 2019. Randomized trial of verubecestat for prodromal Alzheimer's disease. *N Engl J Med*, **380**: 1408–1420.

Ehehalt, R., P. Keller, C. Haass, C. Thiele, K. Simons. 2003. Amyloidogenic processing of the Alzheimer beta-amyloid precursor protein depends on lipid rafts. *J Cell Biol*, **160**: 113–123.

Finnema, S. J., N. B. Nabulsi, T. Eid, K. Detyniecki, S. F. Lin, M. K. Chen, R. Dhaher, D. Matuskey, E. Baum, D. Holden, et al. 2016. Imaging synaptic density in the living human brain. *Sci Transl Med*, **8**: 348ra96.

Fjorback, A. W., M. Seaman, C. Gustafsen, A. Mehmedbasic, S. Gokool, C. Wu, D. Militz, V. Schmidt, P. Madsen, J. R. Nyengaard, et al. 2012. Retromer binds the FANSHY sorting motif in SorLA to regulate amyloid precursor protein sorting and processing. *J Neurosci*, **32**: 1467–1480.

Fleminger, S., D. L. Oliver, S. Lovestone, S. Rabe-Hesketh, A. Giora. 2003. Head injury as a risk factor for Alzheimer's disease: the evidence 10 years on; a partial replication. *J Neurol Neurosurg Psychiatry*, **74**: 857–862.

Foley, P. 2010. Lipids in Alzheimer's disease: a century-old story. *Biochim Biophys Acta*, **1801**: 750–753.

Folstein, M. F., S. E. Folstein, P. R. McHugh. 1975. "Mini-mental state": a practical method for grading the cognitive state of patients for the clinician. *J Psychiatr Res*, **12**: 189–198.

Forgrave, L. M., M. Ma, J. R. Best, M. L. DeMarco. 2019. The diagnostic performance of neurofilament light chain in CSF and blood for Alzheimer's disease, frontotemporal dementia, and amyotrophic lateral sclerosis: a systematic review and meta-analysis. *Alzheimers Dement (Amst)*, **11**: 730–743.

Foster, N. L., J. L. Heidebrink, C. M. Clark, W. J. Jagust, S. E. Arnold, N. R. Barbas, C. S. DeCarli, R. S. Turner, R. A. Koeppe, R. Higdon, et al. 2007. FDG-PET improves accuracy in distinguishing frontotemporal dementia and Alzheimer's disease. *Brain*, **130**: 2616–2635.

Fox, N. C., E. K. Warrington, P. A. Freeborough, P. Hartikainen, A. M. Kennedy, J. M. Stevens, M. N. Rossor. 1996. Presymptomatic hippocampal atrophy in Alzheimer's disease: a longitudinal MRI study. *Brain*, **119**: 2001–2007.

Frank, C., S. Rufini, V. Tancredi, R. Forcina, D. Grossi, G. D'Arcangelo. 2008. Cholesterol depletion inhibits synaptic transmission and synaptic plasticity in rat hippocampus. *Exp Neurol*, **212**: 407–414.

Frisoni, G. B., M. Bocchetta, G. Chetelat, G. D. Rabinovici, M. J. de Leon, J. Kaye, E. M. Reiman, P. Scheltens, F. Barkhof, S. E. Black, et al., I. STAART's NeuroImaging Professional Interest Area. 2013. Imaging markers for Alzheimer disease: which vs how. *Neurology*, **81**: 487–500.

Frisoni, G. B., D. Perani, S. Bastianello, G. Bernardi, C. Porteri, M. Boccardi, S. F. Cappa, M. Trabucchi, A. Padovani. 2017. Biomarkers for the diagnosis of Alzheimer's disease in clinical practice: an Italian intersocietal roadmap. *Neurobiol Aging*, **52**: 119–131.

Fu, H., J. Hardy, K. E. Duff. 2018. Selective vulnerability in neurodegenerative diseases. *Nat Neurosci*, **21**: 1350–1358.

Fu, H., G. A. Rodriguez, M. Herman, S. Emrani, E. Nahmani, G. Barrett, H. Y. Figueroa, E. Goldberg, S. A. Hussaini, K. E. Duff. 2017. Tau pathology induces excitatory neuron loss, grid cell dysfunction, and spatial memory deficits reminiscent of early Alzheimer's disease. *Neuron*, **93**: 533–541 e5.

Fu, H., A. Possenti, R. Freer, Y. Nakano, N. C. Hernandez Villegas, M. Tang, P. V. M. Cauhy, B.A. Lassus, Shuo Chen, S. L. Fowler, H. Y. Figueroa, et al. 2019. A tau homeostasis signature is linked with the cellular and regional vulnerability of excitatory neurons to tau pathology. *Nat Neurosci*, **22**: 47–56.

Fuhrmann, M., T. Bittner, C. K. Jung, S. Burgold, R. M. Page, G. Mitteregger, C. Haass, F. M. LaFerla, H. Kretzschmar, J. Herms. 2010. Microglial Cx3cr1 knockout prevents neuron loss in a mouse model of Alzheimer's disease. *Nat Neurosci*, **13**: 411–413.

Fung, C. W., J. Guo, H. Fu, H. Y. Figueroa, E. E. Konofagou, K. E. Duff. 2020. Atrophy associated with tau pathology precedes overt cell death in a mouse model of progressive tauopathy. *Sci Adv*, 6(42).

Gan, L., M. R. Cookson, L. Petrucelli, and A. R. La Spada. 2018. Converging pathways in neurodegeneration, from genetics to mechanisms. *Nat Neurosci*, **21**: 1300–1309.

Ganguli, M., B. E. Snitz, J. A. Saxton, C. C. Chang, C. W. Lee, J. Vander Bilt, T. F. Hughes, D. A. Loewenstein, F. W. Unverzagt, R. C. Petersen. 2011. Outcomes of mild cognitive impairment by definition: a population study. *Arch Neurol*, **68**: 761–767.

Gatz, M., C. A. Reynolds, L. Fratiglioni, B. Johansson, J. A. Mortimer, S. Berg, A. Fiske, N. L. Pedersen. 2006. Role of genes and environments for explaining Alzheimer disease. *Arch Gen Psychiatry*, **63**: 168–174.

Gauthier, S., H. H. Feldman, L. S. Schneider, G. K. Wilcock, G. B. Frisoni, J. H. Hardlund, H. J. Moebius, P. Bentham, K. A. Kook,

D. J. Wischik, et al. 2016. Efficacy and safety of tau-aggregation inhibitor therapy in patients with mild or moderate Alzheimer's disease: a randomised, controlled, double-blind, parallel-arm, phase 3 trial. *Lancet*, **388**: 2873–2884.

Gerschutz, A., H. Heinsen, E. Grunblatt, A. K. Wagner, J. Bartl, C. Meissner, A. J. Fallgatter, S. Al-Sarraj, C. Troakes, I. Ferrer, et al. 2014. Neuron-specific alterations in signal transduction pathways associated with Alzheimer's disease. *J Alzheimers Dis*, **40**: 135–142.

Ghag, G., N. Bhatt, D. V. Cantu, M. J. Guerrero-Munoz, A. Ellsworth, U. Sengupta, R. Kayed. 2018. Soluble tau aggregates, not large fibrils, are the toxic species that display seeding and cross-seeding behavior. *Protein Sci*, **27**: 1901–1909.

Ghosh, S., M. D. Wu, S. S. Shaftel, S. Kyrkanides, F. M. LaFerla, J. A. Olschowka, and M. K. O'Banion. 2013. Sustained interleukin-1beta overexpression exacerbates tau pathology despite reduced amyloid burden in an Alzheimer's mouse model. *J Neurosci*, **33**: 5053–5064.

Giacchino, J., J. R. Criado, D. Games, S. Henriksen. 2000. In vivo synaptic transmission in young and aged amyloid precursor protein transgenic mice. *Brain Res*, **876**: 185–190.

Ginsberg, S. D., S. Che, S. E. Counts, E. J. Mufson. 2006. Single cell gene expression profiling in Alzheimer's disease. *NeuroRx*, **3**: 302–318.

Ginsberg, S. D., S. E. Hemby, V. M. Lee, J. H. Eberwine, J. Q. Trojanowski. 2000. Expression profile of transcripts in Alzheimer's disease tangle-bearing CA1 neurons. *Ann Neurol*, **48**: 77–87.

Glennon, E. B., D. H. Lau, R. M. C. Gabriele, M. F. Taylor, C. Troakes, S. Opie-Martin, C. Elliott, R. Killick, D. P. Hanger, B. G. Perez-Nievas, et al. 2020. Bridging Integrator-1 protein loss in Alzheimer's disease promotes synaptic tau accumulation and disrupts tau release. *Brain Commun*, 2(1).

Glodzik-Sobanska, L., B. Reisberg, S. De Santi, J. S. Babb, E. Pirraglia, K. E. Rich, M. Brys, M. J. de Leon. 2007. Subjective memory complaints: presence, severity and future outcome in normal older subjects. *Dement Geriatr Cogn Disord*, **24**: 177–184.

Gomez-Isla, T., J. L. Price, D. W. McKeel, Jr, J. C. Morris, J. H. Growdon, B. T. Hyman. 1996. Profound loss of layer II entorhinal cortex neurons occurs in very mild Alzheimer's disease. *J Neurosci*, **16**: 4491–4500.

Gratuze, M., C. E. G. Leyns, D. M. Holtzman. 2018. New insights into the role of TREM2 in Alzheimer's disease. *Mol Neurodegener*, **13**: 66.

Greicius, M. D., G. Srivastava, A. L. Reiss, V. Menon. 2004. Default-mode network activity distinguishes Alzheimer's disease from healthy aging: evidence from functional MRI. *Proc Natl Acad Sci U S A*, **101**: 4637–4642.

Grootendorst, J., A. Bour, E. Vogel, C. Kelche, P. M. Sullivan, J. C. Dodart, K. Bales, C. Mathis. 2005. Human APOE targeted replacement mouse lines: h-apoE4 and h-apoE3 mice differ on spatial memory performance and avoidance behavior. *Behav Brain Res*, **159**: 1–14.

Grundman, M., R. Morgan, J. D. Lickliter, L. S. Schneider, S. DeKosky, N. J. Izzo, R. Guttendorf, M. Higgin, J. Pribyl, K. Mozzoni, et al. 2019. A phase 1 clinical trial of the sigma-2 receptor complex allosteric antagonist CT1812, a novel therapeutic candidate for Alzheimer's disease. *Alzheimers Dement (N Y)*, **5**: 20–26.

Guerreiro, R., A. Wojtas, J. Bras, M. Carrasquillo, E. Rogaeva, E. Majounie, C. Cruchaga, C. Sassi, J. S. Kauwe, S. Younkin, et al., Group Alzheimer Genetic Analysis. 2013. TREM2 variants in Alzheimer's disease. *N Engl J Med*, **368**: 117–127.

Gunn-Moore, D., O. Kaidanovich-Beilin, M. C. Gallego Iradi, F. Gunn-Moore, S. Lovestone. 2018. Alzheimer's disease in humans and other animals: a consequence of postreproductive life span and longevity rather than aging. *Alzheimers Dement*, **14**: 195–204.

Haass, C., C. Kaether, G. Thinakaran, S. Sisodia. 2012. Trafficking and proteolytic processing of APP. *Cold Spring Harb Perspect Med*, 2: a006270.

Haberman, R. P., A. Branch, M. Gallagher. 2017. Targeting neural hyperactivity as a treatment to stem progression of late-onset Alzheimer's disease. *Neurotherapeutics*, **14**: 662–676.

Hamanaka, H., Y. Katoh-Fukui, K. Suzuki, M. Kobayashi, R. Suzuki, Y. Motegi, Y. Nakahara, A. Takeshita, M. Kawai, K. Ishiguro, et al. 2000. Altered cholesterol metabolism in human apolipoprotein E4 knock-in mice. *Hum Mol Genet*, **9**: 353–361.

Handley, R. R., S. J. Reid, S. Patassini, S. R. Rudiger, V. Obolonkin, C. J. McLaughlan, J. C. Jacobsen, J. F. Gusella, M. E. MacDonald, H. J. Waldvogel, et al. 2016. Metabolic disruption identified in the Huntington's disease transgenic sheep model. *Sci Rep*, 6(20681).

Hanseeuw, B. J., R. A. Betensky, H. I. L. Jacobs, A. P. Schultz, J. Sepulcre, J. A. Becker, D. M. O. Cosio, M. Farrell, Y. T. Quiroz, E. C. Mormino, et al. 2019. Association of amyloid and tau with cognition in preclinical Alzheimer disease: a longitudinal study. *JAMA Neurol*, **76**: 915–924.

Hara, M., K. Hirokawa, S. Kamei, T. Uchihara. 2013. Isoform transition from four-repeat to three-repeat tau underlies dendrosomatic and regional progression of neurofibrillary pathology. *Acta Neuropathol*, **125**: 565–579.

Hardy, J. A., G. A. Higgins. 1992. Alzheimer's disease: the amyloid cascade hypothesis. *Science*, **256**: 184–185.

Hardy, J., and D. Allsop. 1991. Amyloid deposition as the central event in the aetiology of Alzheimer's disease. *Trends Pharmacol Sci*, **12**: 383–388.

Harper, L., G. G. Fumagalli, F. Barkhof, P. Scheltens, J. T. O'Brien, F. Bouwman, E. J. Burton, J. D. Rohrer, N. C. Fox, G. R. Ridgway, et al. 2016. MRI visual rating scales in the diagnosis of dementia: evaluation in 184 post-mortem confirmed cases. *Brain*, **139**: 1211–1225.

Harris, J. A., A. Koyama, S. Maeda, K. Ho, N. Devidze, D. B. Dubal, G. Q. Yu, E. Masliah, L. Mucke. 2012. Human P301L-mutant tau expression in mouse entorhinal-hippocampal network causes tau aggregation and presynaptic pathology but no cognitive deficits. *PLoS One*, 7: e45881.

Hartley, T., C. M. Bird, D. Chan, L. Cipolotti, M. Husain, F. Vargha-Khadem, N. Burgess. 2007. The hippocampus is required for short-term topographical memory in humans. *Hippocampus*, **17**: 34–48.

Hawkins, B. E., S. Krishnamurthy, D. L. Castillo-Carranza, U. Sengupta, D. S. Prough, G. R. Jackson, D. S. DeWitt, R. Kayed. 2013. Rapid accumulation of endogenous tau oligomers in a rat model of traumatic brain injury: possible link between traumatic brain injury and sporadic tauopathies. *J Biol Chem*, **288**: 17042–17050.

Head, E. 2013. A canine model of human aging and Alzheimer's disease. *Biochim Biophys Acta*, **1832**: 1384–1389.

Helal, M., E. Hingant, L. Pujo-Menjouet, G. F. Webb. 2014. Alzheimer's disease: analysis of a mathematical model incorporating the role of prions. *J Math Biol*, **69**: 1207–1235.

Heneka, M. T., M. J. Carson, J. El Khoury, G. E. Landreth, F. Brosseron, D. L. Feinstein, A. H. Jacobs, T. Wyss-Coray, J. Vitorica, R. M. Ransohoff, et al. 2015. Neuroinflammation in Alzheimer's disease. *Lancet Neurol*, **14**: 388–405.

Heneka, M. T., M. P. Kummer, A. Stutz, A. Delekate, S. Schwartz, A. Vieira-Saecker, A. Griep, D. Axt, A. Remus, T. C. Tzeng, et al. 2013. NLRP3 is activated in Alzheimer's disease and contributes to pathology in APP/PS1 mice. *Nature*, **493**: 674–678.

Henley, D. B., P. C. May, R. A. Dean, E. R. Siemers. 2009. Development of semagacestat (LY450139), a functional gamma-secretase inhibitor, for the treatment of Alzheimer's disease. *Expert Opin Pharmacother*, **10**: 1657–1664.

Henneman, W. J., J. D. Sluimer, J. Barnes, W. M. van der Flier, I. C. Sluimer, N. C. Fox, P. Scheltens, H. Vrenken, F. Barkhof. 2009. Hippocampal atrophy rates in Alzheimer disease: added value over whole brain volume measures. *Neurology*, 72: 999–1007.

Henstridge, C. M., B. T. Hyman, T. L. Spires-Jones. 2019. Beyond the neuron-cellular interactions early in Alzheimer disease pathogenesis. *Nat Rev Neurosci*, 20: 94–108.

Henstridge, C. M., M. Tzioras, R. C. Paolicelli. 2019. Glial contribution to excitatory and inhibitory synapse loss in neurodegeneration. *Front Cell Neurosci*, 13: 63.

Herskowitz, J. H., K. Offe, A. Deshpande, R. A. Kahn, A. I. Levey, J. J. Lah. 2012. GGA1-mediated endocytic traffic of LR11/SorLA alters APP intracellular distribution and amyloid-beta production. *Mol Biol Cell*, 23: 2645–2657.

Heuer, E., R. F. Rosen, A. Cintron, L. C. Walker. 2012. Nonhuman primate models of Alzheimer-like cerebral proteopathy. *Curr Pharm Des*, 18: 1159–1169.

Hines, M. L., N. T. Carnevale. 1997. The NEURON simulation environment. *Neural Comput*, 9: 1179–209.

Holtzman, D. M., J. Herz, G. Bu. 2012. Apolipoprotein E and apolipoprotein E receptors: normal biology and roles in Alzheimer disease. *Cold Spring Harb Perspect Med*, 2: a006312.

Hong, S., V. F. Beja-Glasser, B. M. Nfonoyim, A. Frouin, S. Li, S. Ramakrishnan, K. M. Merry, Q. Shi, A. Rosenthal, B. A. Barres, et al. 2016. Complement and microglia mediate early synapse loss in Alzheimer mouse models. *Science*, 352: 712–716.

Howett, D., A. Castegnaro, K. Krzywicka, J. Hagman, D. Marchment, R. Henson, M. Rio, J. A. King, N. Burgess, D. Chan. 2019. Differentiation of mild cognitive impairment using an entorhinal cortex-based test of virtual reality navigation. *Brain*, 142: 1751–1766.

Hsiao, K., P. Chapman, S. Nilsen, C. Eckman, Y. Harigaya, S. Younkin, F. Yang, G. Cole. 1996. Correlative memory deficits, Abeta elevation, and amyloid plaques in transgenic mice. *Science*, 274: 99–102.

Hsieh, H., J. Boehm, C. Sato, T. Iwatsubo, T. Tomita, S. Sisodia, R. Malinow. 2006. AMPAR removal underlies Abeta-induced synaptic depression and dendritic spine loss. *Neuron*, 52: 831–843.

Hudry, E., J. Dashkoff, A. D. Roe, S. Takeda, R. M. Koffie, T. Hashimoto, M. Scheel, T. Spires-Jones, M. Arbel-Ornath, R. Betensky, et al. 2013. Gene transfer of human APOE isoforms results in differential modulation of amyloid deposition and neurotoxicity in mouse brain. *Sci Transl Med*, 5: 212ra161.

Hudry, E., J. Klickstein, C. Cannavo, R. Jackson, A. Muzikansky, S. Gandhi, D. Urick, T. Sargent, L. Wrobleski, A. D. Roe, et al. 2019. Opposing roles of apolipoprotein E in aging and neurodegeneration. *Life Sci Alliance*, 2(1).

Hurley, M. J., R. M. J. Deacon, K. Beyer, E. Ioannou, A. Ibanez, J. L. Teeling, P. Cogram. 2018. The long-lived Octodon degus as a rodent drug discovery model for Alzheimer's and other age-related diseases. *Pharmacol Ther*, 188: 36–44.

Hyman, B. T., C. H. Phelps, T. G. Beach, E. H. Bigio, N. J. Cairns, M. C. Carrillo, D. W. Dickson, C. Duyckaerts, M. P. Frosch, E. Masliah, et al. 2012. National Institute on Aging-Alzheimer's Association guidelines for the neuropathologic assessment of Alzheimer's disease. *Alzheimers Dement*, 8: 1–13.

Hyman, B. T., J. Q. Trojanowski. 1997. Consensus recommendations for the postmortem diagnosis of Alzheimer disease from the National Institute on Aging and the Reagan Institute Working Group on diagnostic criteria for the neuropathological assessment of Alzheimer disease. *J Neuropathol Exp Neurol*, 56: 1095–1097.

Hyman, B. T., G. W. Van Hoesen, A. R. Damasio. 1990. Memory-related neural systems in Alzheimer's disease: an anatomic study. *Neurology*, 40: 1721–1730.

Insel, P. S., M. C. Donohue, R. Sperling, O. Hansson, N. Mattsson-Carlgren. 2020. The A4 study: beta-amyloid and cognition in 4432 cognitively unimpaired adults. *Ann Clin Transl Neurol*, 7: 776–785.

Iseki, E., R. Yamamoto, N. Murayama, M. Minegishi, T. Togo, O. Katsuse, K. Kosaka, H. Akiyama, K. Tsuchiya, R. de Silva, L. Andrew, H. Arai. 2006. Immunohistochemical investigation of neurofibrillary tangles and their tau isoforms in brains of limbic neurofibrillary tangle dementia. *Neurosci Lett*, 405: 29–33.

Ismail, Z., E. E. Smith, Y. Geda, D. Sultzer, H. Brodaty, G. Smith, L. Aguera-Ortiz, R. Sweet, D. Miller, C. G. Lyketsos, Istaart Neuropsychiatric Symptoms Professional Interest Area. 2016. Neuropsychiatric symptoms as early manifestations of emergent dementia: provisional diagnostic criteria for mild behavioral impairment. *Alzheimers Dement*, 12: 195–202.

Israel, M. A., S. H. Yuan, C. Bardy, S. M. Reyna, Y. Mu, C. Herrera, M. P. Hefferan, S. Van Gorp, K. L. Nazor, F. S. Boscolo, et al. 2012. Probing sporadic and familial Alzheimer's disease using induced pluripotent stem cells. *Nature*, 482: 216–220.

Itagaki, S., P. L. McGeer, H. Akiyama, S. Zhu, D. Selkoe. 1989. Relationship of microglia and astrocytes to amyloid deposits of Alzheimer disease. *J Neuroimmunol*, 24: 173–182.

Ittner, A., L. M. Ittner. 2018. Dendritic tau in Alzheimer's disease. *Neuron*, 99: 13–27.

Ittner, L. M., Y. D. Ke, F. Delerue, M. Bi, A. Gladbach, J. van Eersel, H. Wolfing, B. C. Chieng, M. J. Christie, I. A. Napier, et al. 2010. Dendritic function of tau mediates amyloid-beta toxicity in Alzheimer's disease mouse models. *Cell*, 142: 387–397.

Izzo, N. J., C. M. Yuede, K. M. LaBarbera, C. S. Limegrover, C. Rehak, R. Yurko, L. Waybright, G. Look, G. Rishton, H. Safferstein, et al. 2021. Preclinical and clinical biomarker studies of CT1812: A novel approach to Alzheimer's disease modification. *Alzheimers Dement*, 17: 1365–1382.

Jack, C. R., Jr, J. Barnes, M. A. Bernstein, B. J. Borowski, J. Brewer, S. Clegg, A. M. Dale, O. Carmichael, C. Ching, C. DeCarli, et al. 2015. Magnetic resonance imaging in Alzheimer's Disease Neuroimaging Initiative 2. *Alzheimers Dement*, 11: 740–756.

Jack, C. R., Jr, D. A. Bennett, K. Blennow, M. C. Carrillo, B. Dunn, S. B. Haeberlein, D. M. Holtzman, W. Jagust, F. Jessen, J. Karlawish, et al. 2018. NIA-AA Research Framework: Toward a biological definition of Alzheimer's disease. *Alzheimers Dement*, 14: 535–562.

Jack, C. R., Jr, M. A. Bernstein, N. C. Fox, P. Thompson, G. Alexander, D. Harvey, B. Borowski, P. J. Britson, L. Whitwell J, C. Ward, et al. 2008. The Alzheimer's Disease Neuroimaging Initiative (ADNI): MRI methods. *J Magn Reson Imaging*, 27: 685–691.

Jacobs, H. I. L., J. C. Augustinack, A. P. Schultz, B. J. Hanseeuw, J. Locascio, R. E. Amariglio, K. V. Papp, D. M. Rentz, R. A. Sperling, K. A. Johnson. 2020. The presubiculum links incipient amyloid and tau pathology to memory function in older persons. *Neurology*, 94: e1916–e28.

Jankowsky, J. L., H. Zheng. 2017. Practical considerations for choosing a mouse model of Alzheimer's disease. *Mol Neurodegener*, 12: 89.

Janus, C., J. Pearson, J. McLaurin, P. M. Mathews, Y. Jiang, S. D. Schmidt, M. A. Chishti, P. Horne, D. Heslin, J. French, et al. 2000. A beta peptide immunization reduces behavioural impairment and plaques in a model of Alzheimer's disease. *Nature*, 408: 979–982.

Jaturapatporn, D., M. G. Isaac, J. McCleery, N. Tabet. 2012. Aspirin, steroidal and non-steroidal anti-inflammatory drugs for the treatment of Alzheimer's disease. *Cochrane Database Syst Rev*, CD006378. doi:10.1002/14651858.CD006378.pub2

Jay, T. R., A. M. Hirsch, M. L. Broihier, C. M. Miller, L. E. Neilson, R. M. Ransohoff, B. T. Lamb, G. E. Landreth. 2017. Disease progression-dependent effects of TREM2 deficiency in a mouse model of Alzheimer's disease. *J Neurosci*, 37: 637–647.

Jay, T. R., C. M. Miller, P. J. Cheng, L. C. Graham, S. Bemiller, M. L. Broihier, G. Xu, D. Margevicius, J. C. Karlo, G. L. Sousa, et al. 2015. TREM2 deficiency eliminates TREM2+ inflammatory macrophages and ameliorates pathology in Alzheimer's disease mouse models. *J Exp Med*, 212: 287–295.

Jebelli, J. D., T. M. Piers. 2015. Amyloid-β oligomers unveil a novel primate model of sporadic Alzheimer's disease. *Front Neurosci*, 9.

Jessen, F., R. E. Amariglio, R. F. Buckley, W. M. van der Flier, Y. Han, J. L. Molinuevo, L. Rabin, D. M. Rentz, O. Rodriguez-Gomez, A. J. Saykin, et al. 2020. The characterisation of subjective cognitive decline. *Lancet Neurol*, 19: 271–278.

Jessen, F., R. E. Amariglio, M. van Boxtel, M. Breteler, M. Ceccaldi, G. Chetelat, B. Dubois, C. Dufouil, K. A. Ellis, W. M. van der Flier, et al., Group Subjective Cognitive Decline Initiative Working. 2014. A conceptual framework for research on subjective cognitive decline in preclinical Alzheimer's disease. *Alzheimers Dement*, 10: 844–852.

Jiang, Y., A. Rigoglioso, C. M. Peterhoff, M. Pawlik, Y. Sato, C. Bleiwas, P. Stavrides, J. F. Smiley, S. D. Ginsberg, P. M. Mathews, et al. 2016. Partial BACE1 reduction in a Down syndrome mouse model blocks Alzheimer-related endosomal anomalies and cholinergic neurodegeneration: role of APP-CTF. *Neurobiol Aging*, 39: 90–98.

Jicha, G. A., J. E. Parisi, D. W. Dickson, K. Johnson, R. Cha, R. J. Ivnik, E. G. Tangalos, B. F. Boeve, D. S. Knopman, H. Braak, et al. 2006. Neuropathologic outcome of mild cognitive impairment following progression to clinical dementia. *Arch Neurol*, 63: 674–681.

Johnson, K. A., A. Schultz, R. A. Betensky, J. A. Becker, J. Sepulcre, D. Rentz, E. Mormino, J. Chhatwal, R. Amariglio, K. Papp, et al. 2016. Tau positron emission tomographic imaging in aging and early Alzheimer disease. *Ann Neurol*, 79: 110–119.

Johnson, K. A., R. A. Sperling, C. M. Gidicsin, J. S. Carmasin, J. E. Maye, R. E. Coleman, E. M. Reiman, M. N. Sabbagh, C. H. Sadowsky, A. S. Fleisher, et al., Av A. study group. 2013. Florbetapir (F18-AV-45) PET to assess amyloid burden in Alzheimer's disease dementia, mild cognitive impairment, and normal aging. *Alzheimers Dement*, 9: S72–S83.

Jonsson, T., J. K. Atwal, S. Steinberg, J. Snaedal, P. V. Jonsson, S. Bjornsson, H. Stefansson, P. Sulem, D. Gudbjartsson, J. Maloney, et al. 2012. A mutation in APP protects against Alzheimer's disease and age-related cognitive decline. *Nature*, 488: 96–99.

Jonsson, T., H. Stefansson, S. Steinberg, I. Jonsdottir, P. V. Jonsson, J. Snaedal, S. Bjornsson, J. Huttenlocher, A. I. Levey, J. J. Lah, et al. 2013. Variant of TREM2 associated with the risk of Alzheimer's disease. *N Engl J Med*, 368: 107–116.

Kanak, D. J., G. M. Rose, H. P. Zaveri, P. R. Patrylo. 2013. Altered network timing in the CA3-CA1 circuit of hippocampal slices from aged mice. *PloS One*, 8: e61364.

Karch, C. M., A. M. Goate. 2015. Alzheimer's disease risk genes and mechanisms of disease pathogenesis. *Biol Psychiatry*, 77: 43–51.

Karikari, T. K., T. A. Pascoal, N. J. Ashton, S. Janelidze, A. L. Benedet, J. L. Rodriguez, M. Chamoun, M. Savard, M. S. Kang, J. Therriault, et al. 2020. Blood phosphorylated tau 181 as a biomarker for Alzheimer's disease: a diagnostic performance and prediction modelling study using data from four prospective cohorts. *Lancet Neurol*, 19: 422–433.

Kawarabayashi, T., M. Shoji, L. H. Younkin, L. Wen-Lang, D. W. Dickson, T. Murakami, E. Matsubara, K. Abe, K. H. Ashe, S. G. Younkin. 2004. Dimeric amyloid beta protein rapidly accumulates in lipid rafts followed by apolipoprotein E and phosphorylated tau accumulation in the Tg2576 mouse model of Alzheimer's disease. *J Neurosci*, 24: 3801–3809.

Keren-Shaul, H., A. Spinrad, A. Weiner, O. Matcovitch-Natan, R. Dvir-Szternfeld, T. K. Ulland, E. David, K. Baruch, D. Lara-Astaiso, B. Toth, et al. 2017. A unique microglia type associated with restricting development of Alzheimer's disease. *Cell*, 169: 1276–1290 e17.

Khan, U. A., L. Liu, F. A. Provenzano, D. E. Berman, C. P. Profaci, R. Sloan, R. Mayeux, K. E. Duff, S. A. Small. 2014. Molecular drivers and cortical spread of lateral entorhinal cortex dysfunction in preclinical Alzheimer's disease. *Nat Neurosci*, 17: 304–311.

Kim, H. G., S. Park, H. Y. Rhee, K. M. Lee, C. W. Ryu, S. J. Rhee, S. Y. Lee, Y. Wang, G. H. Jahng. 2017. Quantitative susceptibility mapping to evaluate the early stage of Alzheimer's disease. *Neuroimage Clin*, 16: 429–438.

Kim, Y. H., S. H. Choi, C. D'Avanzo, M. Hebisch, C. Sliwinski, E. Bylykbashi, K. J. Washicosky, J. B. Klee, O. Brustle, R. E. Tanzi, D. Y. Kim. 2015. A 3D human neural cell culture system for modeling Alzheimer's disease. *Nat Protoc*, 10: 985–1006.

Kimura, N., K. Yanagisawa. 2018. Traffic jam hypothesis: Relationship between endocytic dysfunction and Alzheimer's disease. *Neurochem Int*, 119: 35–41.

Klunk, W. E., H. Engler, A. Nordberg, Y. Wang, G. Blomqvist, D. P. Holt, M. Bergström, I. Savitcheva, G. F. Huang, S. Estrada, et al. 2004. Imaging brain amyloid in Alzheimer's disease with Pittsburgh Compound-B. *Ann Neurol*, 55: 306–319.

Knupp, A., S. Mishra, R. Martinez, J. E. Braggin, M. Szabo, C. Kinoshita, D. W. Hailey, S. A. Small, S. Jayadev, J. E. Young. 2020. Depletion of the AD risk gene SORL1 selectively impairs neuronal endosomal traffic independent of amyloidogenic APP processing. *Cell Rep*, 31: 107719.

Kober, D. L., J. M. Alexander-Brett, C. M. Karch, C. Cruchaga, M. Colonna, M. J. Holtzman, T. J. Brett. 2016. Neurodegenerative disease mutations in TREM2 reveal a functional surface and distinct loss-of-function mechanisms. *Elife*, 5.

Koepsell, T. D., S. E. Monsell. 2012. Reversion from mild cognitive impairment to normal or near-normal cognition: risk factors and prognosis. *Neurology*, 79: 1591–1598.

Koffie, R. M., T. Hashimoto, H. C. Tai, K. R. Kay, A. Serrano-Pozo, D. Joyner, S. Hou, K. J. Kopeikina, M. P. Frosch, V. M. Lee, et al. 2012. Apolipoprotein E4 effects in Alzheimer's disease are mediated by synaptotoxic oligomeric amyloid-beta. *Brain*, 135: 2155–2168.

Koffie, R. M., M. Meyer-Luehmann, T. Hashimoto, K. W. Adams, M. L. Mielke, M. Garcia-Alloza, K. D. Micheva, S. J. Smith, M. L. Kim, V. M. Lee, et al. 2009. Oligomeric amyloid beta associates with postsynaptic densities and correlates with excitatory synapse loss near senile plaques. *Proc Natl Acad Sci U S A*, 106: 4012–4017.

Kohler, S., S. E. Black, M. Sinden, C. Szekely, D. Kidron, J. L. Parker, J. K. Foster, M. Moscovitch, G. Winocour, J. P. Szalai, et al. 1998. Memory impairments associated with hippocampal versus parahippocampal-gyrus atrophy: an MR volumetry study in Alzheimer's disease. *Neuropsychologia*, 36: 901–914.

Kopeikina, K. J., G. A. Carlson, R. Pitstick, A. E. Ludvigson, A. Peters, J. I. Luebke, R. M. Koffie, M. P. Frosch, B. T. Hyman, T. L. Spires-Jones. 2011. Tau accumulation causes mitochondrial distribution deficits in neurons in a mouse model of tauopathy and in human Alzheimer's disease brain. *Am J Pathol*, 179: 2071–2082.

Kopeikina, K. J., M. Polydoro, H. C. Tai, E. Yaeger, G. A. Carlson, R. Pitstick, B. T. Hyman, and T. L. Spires-Jones. 2013. Synaptic alterations in the rTg4510 mouse model of tauopathy. *J Comp Neurol*, 521: 1334–1353.

Korwek, K. M., J. H. Trotter, M. J. Ladu, P. M. Sullivan, E. J. Weeber. 2009. APOE isoform-dependent changes in hippocampal synaptic function. *Mol Neurodegener*, 4: 21.

Koudinov, A. R., N. V. Koudinova. 2001. Essential role for cholesterol in synaptic plasticity and neuronal degeneration. *FASEB J*, 15: 1858–1860.

Kourtis, L. C., O. B. Regele, J. M. Wright, G. B. Jones. 2019. Digital biomarkers for Alzheimer's disease: the mobile/ wearable devices opportunity. *NPJ Digit Med*, 2. doi:10.1038/s41746-019-0084-2. Epub 2019 Feb 21.

Koychev, I., R. N. Gunn, A. Firouzian, J. Lawson, G. Zamboni, B. Ridha, B. J. Sahakian, J. B. Rowe, A. Thomas, L. Rochester, et al. 2017. PET tau and amyloid-beta burden in mild Alzheimer's disease: divergent relationship with age, cognition, and cerebrospinal fluid biomarkers. *J Alzheimers Dis*, 60: 283–293.

Kuchibhotla, K. V., S. T. Goldman, C. R. Lattarulo, H. Y. Wu, B. T. Hyman, B. J. Bacskai. 2008. Abeta plaques lead to aberrant regulation of calcium homeostasis in vivo resulting in structural and functional disruption of neuronal networks. *Neuron*, 59: 214–225.

Kuchibhotla, K. V., S. Wegmann, K. J. Kopeikina, J. Hawkes, N. Rudinskiy, M. L. Andermann, T. L. Spires-Jones, B. J. Bacskai, B. T. Hyman. 2014. Neurofibrillary tangle-bearing neurons are functionally integrated in cortical circuits in vivo. *Proc Natl Acad Sci U S A*, 111: 510–514.

Kunkle, B. W., B. Grenier-Boley, R. Sims, J. C. Bis, V. Damotte, A. C. Naj, A. Boland, M. Vronskaya, S. J. van der Lee, A. Amlie-Wolf, et al., Consortium Alzheimer Disease Genetics, Initiative European Alzheimer's Disease, Heart Cohorts for, Consortium Aging Research in Genomic Epidemiology, Genetic, Polygenic Environmental Risk in Ad/Defining Genetic, and Consortium Environmental Risk for Alzheimer's Disease. 2019. Genetic meta-analysis of diagnosed Alzheimer's disease identifies new risk loci and implicates Abeta, tau, immunity and lipid processing. *Nat Genet*, 51: 414–430.

Kunz, L., T. N. Schröder, H. Lee, C. Montag, B. Lachmann, R. Sariyska, M. Reuter, R. Stirnberg, T. Stöcker, P. C. Messing-Floeter, et al. 2015. Reduced grid-cell-like representations in adults at genetic risk for Alzheimer's disease. *Science*, 350: 430–433.

Kvartsberg, H., F. H. Duits, M. Ingelsson, N. Andreasen, A. Ohrfelt, K. Andersson, G. Brinkmalm, L. Lannfelt, L. Minthon, O. Hansson, et al. 2015. Cerebrospinal fluid levels of the synaptic protein neurogranin correlates with cognitive decline in prodromal Alzheimer's disease. *Alzheimers Dement*, 11: 1180–1190.

Kwart, D., A. Gregg, C. Scheckel, E. A. Murphy, D. Paquet, M. Duffield, J. Fak, O. Olsen, R. B. Darnell, M. Tessier-Lavigne. 2019. A large panel of isogenic APP and PSEN1 mutant human iPSC neurons reveals shared endosomal abnormalities mediated by APP beta-CTFs, not Abeta. *Neuron*, 104: 256–270 e5.

Lacor, P. N., M. C. Buniel, P. W. Furlow, A. S. Clemente, P. T. Velasco, M. Wood, K. L. Viola, W. L. Klein. 2007. Abeta oligomer-induced aberrations in synapse composition, shape, and density provide a molecular basis for loss of connectivity in Alzheimer's disease. *J Neurosci*, 27: 796–807.

Laczo, J., R. Andel, M. Vyhnalek, K. Vlcek, Z. Nedelska, V. Matoska, I. Gazova, I. Mokrisova, K. Sheardova, J. Hort. 2014. APOE and spatial navigation in amnestic MCI: results from a computer-based test. *Neuropsychology*, 28: 676–684.

Lalonde, R., K. Fukuchi, C. Strazielle. 2012. APP transgenic mice for modelling behavioural and psychological symptoms of dementia (BPSD). *Neurosci Biobehav Rev*, 36: 1357–1375.

Lambert, M. P., A. K. Barlow, B. A. Chromy, C. Edwards, R. Freed, M. Liosatos, T. E. Morgan, I. Rozovsky, B. Trommer, K. L. Viola, et al. 1998. Diffusible, nonfibrillar ligands derived from Abeta1-42 are potent central nervous system neurotoxins. *Proc Natl Acad Sci U S A*, 95: 6448–6453.

Lao, K., N. Ji, X. Zhang, W. Qiao, Z. Tang, X. Gou. 2019. Drug development for Alzheimer's disease: review. *J Drug Target*, 27: 164–173.

Larson, J., G. Lynch, D. Games, P. Seubert. 1999. Alterations in synaptic transmission and long-term potentiation in hippocampal slices from young and aged PDAPP mice. *Brain Res*, 840: 23–35.

Lasagna-Reeves, C. A., D. L. Castillo-Carranza, U. Sengupta, A. L. Clos, G. R. Jackson, R. Kayed. 2011. Tau oligomers impair memory and induce synaptic and mitochondrial dysfunction in wild-type mice. *Mol Neurodegener*, 6: 39.

Lasorsa, A., I. Malki, F. X. Cantrelle, H. Merzougui, E. Boll, J. C. Lambert, I. Landrieu. 2018. Structural basis of tau interaction with BIN1 and regulation by tau phosphorylation. *Front Mol Neurosci*, 11: 421.

Lee, S. E., H. Hyun, M. R. Park, Y. Choi, Y. J. Son, Y. G. Park, S. G. Jeong, M. Y. Shin, H. J. Ha, H. S. Hong, et al. 2017. Production of transgenic pig as an Alzheimer's disease model using a multi-cistronic vector system. *PLoS One*, 12.

Lehmann, M., P. M. Ghosh, C. Madison, A. Karydas, G. Coppola, J. P. O'Neil, Y. Huang, B. L. Miller, W. J. Jagust, G. D. Rabinovici. 2014. Greater medial temporal hypometabolism and lower cortical amyloid burden in ApoE4-positive AD patients. *J Neurol Neurosurg Psychiatry*, 85: 266–273.

Lesne, S., M. T. Koh, L. Kotilinek, R. Kayed, C. G. Glabe, A. Yang, M. Gallagher, K. H. Ashe. 2006. A specific amyloid-beta protein assembly in the brain impairs memory. *Nature*, 440: 352–357.

Levine, T. F., S. L. Allison, M. Stojanovic, A. M. Fagan, J. C. Morris, D. Head. 2020. Spatial navigation ability predicts progression of dementia symptomatology. *Alzheimers Dement*, 16: 491–500.

Levy-Lahad, E., W. Wasco, P. Poorkaj, D. M. Romano, J. Oshima, W. H. Pettingell, C. E. Yu, P. D. Jondro, S. D. Schmidt, K. Wang, et al. 1995. Candidate gene for the chromosome 1 familial Alzheimer's disease locus. *Science*, 269: 973–977.

Li, S., S. Hong, N. E. Shepardson, D. M. Walsh, G. M. Shankar, D. Selkoe. 2009. Soluble oligomers of amyloid beta protein facilitate hippocampal long-term depression by disrupting neuronal glutamate uptake. *Neuron*, 62: 788–801.

Liang, Y., Y. Pertzov, J. M. Nicholas, S. M. Henley, S. Crutch, F. Woodward, K. Leung, N. C. Fox, M. Husain. 2016. Visual short-term memory binding deficit in familial Alzheimer's disease. *Cortex*, 78: 150–164.

Lithfous, S., A. Dufour, O. Despres. 2013. Spatial navigation in normal aging and the prodromal stage of Alzheimer's disease: insights from imaging and behavioral studies. *Ageing Res Rev*, 12: 201–213.

Litvinchuk, A., Y. W. Wan, D. B. Swartzlander, F. Chen, A. Cole, N. E. Propson, Q. Wang, B. Zhang, Z. Liu, H. Zheng. 2018. Complement C3aR inactivation attenuates tau pathology and reverses an immune network deregulated in tauopathy models and Alzheimer's disease. *Neuron*, 100: 1337–1353 e5.

Liu, E., M. E. Schmidt, R. Margolin, R. Sperling, R. Koeppe, N. S. Mason, W. E. Klunk, C. A. Mathis, S. Salloway, N. C. Fox, et al., Bapineuzumab, and Investigators Clinical Trial. 2015. Amyloid-beta 11C-PiB-PET imaging results from 2 randomized bapineuzumab phase 3 AD trials. *Neurology*, 85: 692–700.

Liu, L., V. Drouet, J. W. Wu, M. P. Witter, S. A. Small, C. Clelland, K. Duff. 2012. Trans-synaptic spread of tau pathology in vivo. *PLoS One*, 7: e31302.

Liu, P., M. N. Reed, L. A. Kotilinek, M. K. Grant, C. L. Forster, W. Qiang, S. L. Shapiro, J. H. Reichl, A. C. Chiang, J. L. Jankowsky, et al. 2015. Quaternary structure defines a large class of amyloid-beta oligomers neutralized by sequestration. *Cell Rep*, 11: 1760–1771.

Liu, Y., G. Spulber, K. K. Lehtimaki, M. Kononen, I. Hallikainen, H. Grohn, M. Kivipelto, M. Hallikainen, R. Vanninen, H. Soininen. 2011. Diffusion tensor imaging and tract-based spatial statistics in Alzheimer's disease and mild cognitive impairment. *Neurobiol Aging*, 32: 1558–1571.

Liu, Z., C. Lv, W. Zhao, Y. Song, D. Pei, T. Xu. 2012. NR2B-containing NMDA receptors expression and their relationship to apoptosis in hippocampus of Alzheimer's disease-like rats. *Neurochem Res*, 37: 1420–1427.

Livingston, G., A. Sommerlad, V. Orgeta, S. G. Costafreda, J. Huntley, D. Ames, C. Ballard, S. Banerjee, A. Burns, J. Cohen-Mansfield, et al. 2017. Dementia prevention, intervention, and care. *Lancet*, 390: 2673–2734.

Lleo, A., R. Nunez-Llaves, D. Alcolea, C. Chiva, D. Balateu-Panos, M. Colom-Cadena, G. Gomez-Giro, L. Munoz, M. Querol-Vilaseca, J. Pegueroles, et al. 2019. Changes in synaptic proteins precede neurodegeneration markers in preclinical Alzheimer's disease cerebrospinal fluid. *Mol Cell Proteomics*, 18: 546–560.

Loera-Valencia, R., J. Goikolea, C. Parrado-Fernandez, P. Merino-Serrais, S. Maioli. 2019. Alterations in cholesterol metabolism as a risk factor for developing Alzheimer's disease: Potential novel targets for treatment. *J Steroid Biochem Mol Biol*, 190: 104–114.

Lohith, T. G., I. Bennacef, R. Vandenberghe, M. Vandenbulcke, C. A. Salinas, R. Declercq, T. Reynders, N. F. Telan-Choing, K. Riffel, S. Celen, et al. 2019. Brain imaging of Alzheimer dementia patients and elderly controls with (18)F-MK-6240, a PET tracer targeting neurofibrillary tangles. *J Nucl Med*, 60: 107–114.

Lombardi, G., G. Crescioli, E. Cavedo, E. Lucenteforte, G. Casazza, A. G. Bellatorre, C. Lista, G. Costantino, G. Frisoni, G. Virgili, et al. 2020. Structural magnetic resonance imaging for the early diagnosis of dementia due to Alzheimer's disease in people with mild cognitive impairment. *Cochrane Database Syst Rev*, 3: CD009628.

Londono, A. C., F. X. Castellanos, A. Arbelaez, A. Ruiz, D. C. Aguirre-Acevedo, A. M. Richardson, S. Easteal, B. A. Lidbury, M. Arcos-Burgos, F. Lopera. 2014. An 1H-MRS framework predicts the onset of Alzheimer's disease symptoms in PSEN1 mutation carriers. *Alzheimers Dement*, 10: 552–561.

Lovestone, S., M. Boada, B. Dubois, M. Hull, J. O. Rinne, H. J. Huppertz, M. Calero, M. V. Andres, B. Gomez-Carrillo, T. Leon, et al., Argo investigators. 2015. A phase II trial of tideglusib in Alzheimer's disease. *J Alzheimers Dis*, 45: 75–88.

Lupton, M. K., L. Strike, N. K. Hansell, W. Wen, K. A. Mather, N. J. Armstrong, A. Thalamuthu, K. L. McMahon, G. I. de Zubicaray, A. A. Assareh, et al. 2016. The effect of increased genetic risk for Alzheimer's disease on hippocampal and amygdala volume. *Neurobiol Aging*, 40: 68–77.

Lussier, F. Z., T. A. Pascoal, M. Chamoun, J. Therriault, C. Tissot, M. Savard, M. S. Kang, S. Mathotaarachchi, A. L. Benedet, M. Parsons, et al. 2020. Mild behavioral impairment is associated with beta-amyloid but not tau or neurodegeneration in cognitively intact elderly individuals. *Alzheimers Dement*, 16: 192–199.

Ma, Y., S. Zhang, J. Li, D. M. Zheng, Y. Guo, J. Feng, W. D. Ren. 2014. Predictive accuracy of amyloid imaging for progression from mild cognitive impairment to Alzheimer disease with different lengths of follow-up: a meta-analysis. [Corrected]. *Medicine (Baltimore)*, 93: e150.

Machulda, M. M., H. A. Ward, B. Borowski, J. L. Gunter, R. H. Cha, P. C. O'Brien, R. C. Petersen, B. F. Boeve, D. Knopman, D. F. Tang-Wai, et al. 2003. Comparison of memory fMRI response among normal, MCI, and Alzheimer's patients. *Neurology*, 61: 500–506.

Malki, I., F. X. Cantrelle, Y. Sottejeau, G. Lippens, J. C. Lambert, I. Landrieu. 2017. Regulation of the interaction between the neuronal BIN1 isoform 1 and Tau proteins - role of the SH3 domain. *FEBS J*, 284: 3218–3229.

Mann, K. M., F. E. Thorngate, Y. Katoh-Fukui, H. Hamanaka, D. L. Williams, S. Fujita, B. T. Lamb. 2004. Independent effects of APOE on cholesterol metabolism and brain Abeta levels in an Alzheimer disease mouse model. *Hum Mol Genet*, 13: 1959–1968.

Markesbery, W. R., F. A. Schmitt, R. J. Kryscio, D. G. Davis, C. D. Smith, D. R. Wekstein. 2006. Neuropathologic substrate of mild cognitive impairment. *Arch Neurol*, 63: 38–46.

Marschallinger, J., T. Iram, M. Zardeneta, S. E. Lee, B. Lehallier, M. S. Haney, J. V. Pluvinage, V. Mathur, O. Hahn, D. W. Morgens, et al. 2020. Lipid-droplet-accumulating microglia represent a dysfunctional and proinflammatory state in the aging brain. *Nat Neurosci*, 23: 194–208.

Martin, M. G., T. Ahmed, A. Korovaichuk, C. Venero, S. A. Menchon, I. Salas, S. Munck, O. Herreras, D. Balschun, C. G. Dotti. 2014. Constitutive hippocampal cholesterol loss underlies poor cognition in old rodents. *EMBO Mol Med*, 6: 902–917.

Maruta, C., M. Guerreiro, A. de Mendonca, J. Hort, P. Scheltens. 2011. The use of neuropsychological tests across Europe: the need for a consensus in the use of assessment tools for dementia. *Eur J Neurol*, 18: 279–285.

Massa, F., R. Meli, S. Morbelli, F. Nobili, M. Pardini. 2019. Serum neurofilament light chain rate of change in Alzheimer's disease: potentials applications and notes of caution. *Ann Transl Med*, 7: S133.

Matsuda, H. 2001. Cerebral blood flow and metabolic abnormalities in Alzheimer's disease. *Ann Nucl Med*, 15: 85–92.

Matthews, F. E., B. C. Stephan, I. G. McKeith, J. Bond, C. Brayne, Function Medical Research Council Cognitive, and Study Ageing. 2008. Two-year progression from mild cognitive impairment to dementia: to what extent do different definitions agree? *J Am Geriatr Soc*, 56: 1424–1433.

Matthews, F. E., B. C. Stephan, L. Robinson, C. Jagger, L. E. Barnes, A. Arthur, C. Brayne, Function Cognitive, and Collaboration Ageing Studies. 2016. A two decade dementia incidence comparison from the Cognitive Function and Ageing Studies I and II. *Nat Commun*, 7: 11398.

Mattiasson, G., H. Friberg, M. Hansson, E. Elmer, T. Wieloch. 2003. Flow cytometric analysis of mitochondria from CA1 and CA3 regions of rat hippocampus reveals differences in permeability transition pore activation. *J Neurochem*, 87: 532–544.

Mattsson, N., N. C. Cullen, U. Andreasson, H. Zetterberg, K. Blennow. 2019. Association between longitudinal plasma neurofilament light and neurodegeneration in patients with Alzheimer disease. *JAMA Neurol*, 76: 791–799.

Mattsson, N., S. Palmqvist, E. Stomrud, J. Vogel, and O. Hansson. 2019. Staging beta-amyloid pathology with amyloid positron emission tomography. *JAMA Neurol*, 76: 1319–1329.

McDonald, J. M., G. M. Savva, C. Brayne, A. T. Welzel, G. Forster, G. M. Shankar, D. J. Selkoe, P. G. Ince, D. M. Walsh, Function Medical Research Council Cognitive, and Study Ageing. 2010. The presence of sodium dodecyl sulphate-stable Abeta dimers is strongly associated with Alzheimer-type dementia. *Brain*, 133: 1328–1341.

McInnes, J., K. Wierda, A. Snellinx, L. Bounti, Y. C. Wang, I. C. Stancu, N. Apostolo, K. Gevaert, I. Dewachter, T. L. Spires-Jones, et al. 2018. Synaptogyrin-3 mediates presynaptic dysfunction induced by tau. *Neuron*, 97: 823–835 e8.

McKhann, G., D. Drachman, M. Folstein, R. Katzman, D. Price, E. M. Stadlan. 1984. Clinical diagnosis of Alzheimer's disease: report of the NINCDS-ADRDA Work Group under the auspices of Department of Health and Human Services Task Force on Alzheimer's Disease. *Neurology*, 34: 939–944.

McKhann, G. M., D. S. Knopman, H. Chertkow, B. T. Hyman, C. R. Jack, Jr, C. H. Kawas, W. E. Klunk, W. J. Koroshetz, J. J. Manly, R. Mayeux, et al. 2011. The diagnosis of dementia due to Alzheimer's disease: recommendations from the National Institute on Aging-Alzheimer's Association workgroups on diagnostic guidelines for Alzheimer's disease. *Alzheimers Dement*, 7: 263–269.

Medina, M. 2018. An overview on the clinical development of tau-based therapeutics. *Int J Mol Sci*, 19.

Meisl, G., E. Hidari, K. Allinson, T. Rittman, S. L. DeVos, J. S. Sanchez, C. K. Xu, K. E. Duff, K. A. Johnson, J. B. Rowe, et al. 2021. In vivo rate-determining steps of tau seed accumulation in Alzheimer's disease. *Sci Adv*, 7: eabh1448.

Menkes-Caspi, N., H. G. Yamin, V. Kellner, T. L. Spires-Jones, D. Cohen, E. A. Stern. 2015. Pathological tau disrupts ongoing network activity. *Neuron*, 85: 959–966.

Metzler-Baddeley, C. 2007. A review of cognitive impairments in dementia with Lewy bodies relative to Alzheimer's disease and Parkinson's disease with dementia. *Cortex*, 43: 583–600.

Meyer, P. F., J. Tremblay-Mercier, J. Leoutsakos, C. Madjar, M. E. Lafaille-Maignan, M. Savard, P. Rosa-Neto, J. Poirier, P. Etienne, et al., Prevent-Ad Research Group. 2019. INTREPAD: A randomized trial of naproxen to slow progress of presymptomatic Alzheimer disease. *Neurology*, 92: e2070–e80.

Miebach, L., S. Wolfsgruber, A. Polcher, O. Peters, F. Menne, K. Luther, E. Incesoy, J. Priller, E. Spruth, S. Altenstein, et al. 2019. Which features of subjective cognitive decline are related to amyloid pathology? Findings from the DELCODE study. *Alzheimers Res Ther*, 11: 66.

Mielke, M. M., O. C. Okonkwo, K. Oishi, S. Mori, S. Tighe, M. I. Miller, C. Ceritoglu, T. Brown, M. Albert, C. G. Lyketsos. 2012. Fornix integrity and hippocampal volume predict memory decline and progression to Alzheimer's disease. *Alzheimers Dement*, 8: 105–113.

Miller, M. I., J. T. Ratnanather, D. J. Tward, T. Brown, D. S. Lee, M. Ketcha, K. Mori, M. C. Wang, S. Mori, M. S. Albert, et al., Biocard Research Team. 2015. Network neurodegeneration in Alzheimer's disease via MRI based shape diffeomorphometry and high-field atlasing. *Front Bioeng Biotechnol*, 3: 54.

Milward, E. A., R. Papadopoulos, S. J. Fuller, R. D. Moir, D. Small, K. Beyreuther, C. L. Masters. 1992. The amyloid protein precursor of Alzheimer's disease is a mediator of the effects of nerve growth factor on neurite outgrowth. *Neuron*, 9: 129–137.

Minoshima, S., N. L. Foster, A. A. Sima, K. A. Frey, R. L. Albin, D. E. Kuhl. 2001. Alzheimer's disease versus dementia with Lewy bodies: cerebral metabolic distinction with autopsy confirmation. *Ann Neurol*, 50: 358–365.

Mioshi, E., K. Dawson, J. Mitchell, R. Arnold, J. R. Hodges. 2006. The Addenbrooke's Cognitive Examination Revised (ACE-R): a brief cognitive test battery for dementia screening. *Int J Geriatr Psychiatry*, 21: 1078–1085.

Mitchell, A. J., M. Shiri-Feshki. 2009. Rate of progression of mild cognitive impairment to dementia: meta-analysis of 41 robust inception cohort studies. *Acta Psychiatr Scand*, 119: 252–265.

Miyagawa, T., I. Ebinuma, Y. Morohashi, Y. Hori, M. Young Chang, H. Hattori, T. Maehara, S. Yokoshima, T. Fukuyama, S. Tsuji, et al. 2016. BIN1 regulates BACE1 intracellular trafficking and amyloid-beta production. *Hum Mol Genet*, 25: 2948–2958.

Mizuseki, K., S. Royer, K. Diba, and G. Buzsaki. 2012. Activity dynamics and behavioral correlates of CA3 and CA1 hippocampal pyramidal neurons. *Hippocampus*, 22: 1659–1680.

Mohs, R. C., W. G. Rosen, K. L. Davis. 1983. The Alzheimer's disease assessment scale: an instrument for assessing treatment efficacy. *Psychopharmacol Bull*, 19: 448–450.

Mokrisova, I., J. Laczo, R. Andel, I. Gazova, M. Vyhnalek, Z. Nedelska, D. Levcik, J. Cerman, K. Vlcek, J. Hort. 2016. Real-space path integration is impaired in Alzheimer's disease and mild cognitive impairment. *Behav Brain Res*, 307: 150–158.

Montagne, A., S. R. Barnes, M. D. Sweeney, M. R. Halliday, A. P. Sagare, Z. Zhao, A. W. Toga, R. E. Jacobs, C. Y. Liu, L. Amezcua, et al. 2015. Blood-brain barrier breakdown in the aging human hippocampus. *Neuron*, 85: 296–302.

Montagne, A., D. A. Nation, J. Pa, M. D. Sweeney, A. W. Toga, B. V. Zlokovic. 2016. Brain imaging of neurovascular dysfunction in Alzheimer's disease. *Acta Neuropathol*, 131: 687–707.

Moodley, K., L. Minati, V. Contarino, S. Prioni, R. Wood, R. Cooper, L. D'Incerti, F. Tagliavini, D. Chan. 2015. Diagnostic differentiation of mild cognitive impairment due to Alzheimer's disease using a hippocampus-dependent test of spatial memory. *Hippocampus*, 25: 939–951.

Morganti, F., S. Stefanini, G. Riva. 2013. From allo- to egocentric spatial ability in early Alzheimer's disease: a study with virtual reality spatial tasks. *Cogn Neurosci*, 4: 171–180.

Morrison, B. M., P. R. Hof, J. H. Morrison. 1998. Determinants of neuronal vulnerability in neurodegenerative diseases. *Ann Neurol*, 44: S32–S44.

Muddapu, V. R., S. A. P. Dharshini, V. S. Chakravarthy, M. M. Gromiha. 2020. Neurodegenerative diseases: is metabolic deficiency the root cause? *Front Neurosci*, 14: 213.

Muratore, C. R., C. Zhou, M. Liao, M. A. Fernandez, W. M. Taylor, V. N. Lagomarsino, R. V. Pearse, 2nd, H. C. Rice, J. M. Negri, A. He, et al. 2017. Cell-type Dependent Alzheimer's disease phenotypes: probing the biology of selective neuronal vulnerability. *Stem Cell Reports*, 9: 1868–1884.

Nasreddine, Z. S., N. A. Phillips, V. Bedirian, S. Charbonneau, V. Whitehead, I. Collin, J. L. Cummings, H. Chertkow. 2005. The Montreal Cognitive Assessment, MoCA: a brief screening tool for mild cognitive impairment. *J Am Geriatr Soc*, 53: 695–699.

Neumann, U., M. Ufer, L. H. Jacobson, M. L. Rouzade-Dominguez, G. Huledal, C. Kolly, R. M. Lüönd, R. Machauer, S. J. Veenstra, K. Hurth, et al. 2018. The BACE-1 inhibitor CNP520 for prevention trials in Alzheimer's disease. *EMBO Mol Med*, 10.

Newton, C., M. Pope, C. Rua, R. Henson, Z. Ji, N. Burgess, et al. 2024. Entorhinal-based path integration selectively predicts midlife risk of Alzheimer's disease. *Alzheimers Dement*, 20: 2779–2793.

Nhan, H. S., K. Chiang, E. H. Koo. 2015. The multifaceted nature of amyloid precursor protein and its proteolytic fragments: friends and foes. *Acta Neuropathol*, 129: 1–19.

Novak, P., R. Schmidt, E. Kontsekova, N. Zilka, B. Kovacech, R. Skrabana, Z. Vince-Kazmerova, S. Katina, L. Fialova, M. Prcina, et al. 2017. Safety and immunogenicity of the tau vaccine AADvac1 in patients with Alzheimer's disease: a randomised, double-blind, placebo-controlled, phase 1 trial. *Lancet Neurol*, 16: 123–134.

Nurdal, V., A. Wearn, M. Knight, R. Kauppinen, E. Coulthard. 2020. Prospective memory in prodromal Alzheimer's disease: Real world relevance and correlations with cortical thickness and hippocampal subfield volumes. *Neuroimage Clin*, 26: 102226.

O'Brien, J. T., M. J. Firbank, K. Ritchie, K. Wells, G. B. Williams, C. W. Ritchie, L. Su. 2020. Association between midlife dementia risk factors and longitudinal brain atrophy: the PREVENT-Dementia study. *J Neurol Neurosurg Psychiatry*, 91: 158–161.

Ochalek, A., B. Mihalik, H. X. Avci, A. Chandrasekaran, A. Teglasi, I. Bock, M. L. Giudice, Z. Tancos, K. Molnar, L. Laszlo, et al. 2017. Neurons derived from sporadic Alzheimer's disease iPSCs reveal elevated TAU hyperphosphorylation, increased amyloid levels, and GSK3B activation. *Alzheimers Res Ther*, 9: 90.

Oh, M. M., D. Simkin, J. F. Disterhoft. 2016. Intrinsic hippocampal excitability changes of opposite signs and different origins in CA1 and CA3 pyramidal neurons underlie aging-related cognitive deficits. *Front Syst Neurosci*, 10: 52.

Oikawa, N., N. Kimura, K. Yanagisawa. 2010. Alzheimer-type tau pathology in advanced aged nonhuman primate brains harboring substantial amyloid deposition. *Brain Res*, 1315: 137–149.

Olsson, B., R. Lautner, U. Andreasson, A. Ohrfelt, E. Portelius, M. Bjerke, M. Holtta, C. Rosen, C. Olsson, G. Strobel, et al. 2016. CSF and blood biomarkers for the diagnosis of Alzheimer's disease: a systematic review and meta-analysis. *Lancet Neurol*, 15: 673–684.

Ormond, J., J. O'Keefe. 2022. Hippocampal place cells have goal-oriented vector fields during navigation. *Nature*, 607: 741–746.

Osterrieth, P. A. 1944. Le test de copie d'une figure complexe; contribution à l'étude de la perception et de la mémoire [Test of copying a complex figure; contribution to the study of perception and memory]. *Archives de Psychologie*, 30: 206–356.

Page, M. P., R. J. Howard, J. T. O'Brien, M. S. Buxton-Thomas, A. D. Pickering. 1996. Use of neural networks in brain SPECT to diagnose Alzheimer's disease. *J Nucl Med*, 37: 195–200.

Palmqvist, S., S. Janelidze, E. Stomrud, H. Zetterberg, J. Karl, K. Zink, T. Bittner, N. Mattsson, U. Eichenlaub, K. Blennow, O. Hansson. 2019. Performance of fully automated plasma assays as screening tests for Alzheimer disease-related beta-amyloid status. *JAMA Neurol*, 76: 1319–1329.

Palop, J. J., J. Chin, E. D. Roberson, J. Wang, M. T. Thwin, N. Bien-Ly, J. Yoo, K. O. Ho, G. Q. Yu, A. Kreitzer, et al. 2007. Aberrant excitatory neuronal activity and compensatory remodeling of inhibitory hippocampal circuits in mouse models of Alzheimer's disease. *Neuron*, 55: 697–711.

Park, J., I. Wetzel, I. Marriott, D. Dreau, C. D'Avanzo, D. Y. Kim, R. E. Tanzi, H. Cho. 2018. A 3D human triculture system modeling neurodegeneration and neuroinflammation in Alzheimer's disease. *Nat Neurosci*, 21: 941–951.

Parker, T. D., D. M. Cash, C. A. S. Lane, K. Lu, I. B. Malone, J. M. Nicholas, S. N. James, A. Keshavan, H. Murray-Smith, A. Wong, et al. 2019. Hippocampal subfield volumes and pre-clinical Alzheimer's disease in 408 cognitively normal adults born in 1946. *PLoS One*, 14: e0224030.

Parra, M. A., S. Abrahams, K. Fabi, R. Logie, S. Luzzi, S. Della Sala. 2009. Short-term memory binding deficits in Alzheimer's disease. *Brain*, 132: 1057–1066.

Parra, M. A., S. Abrahams, R. H. Logie, L. G. Mendez, F. Lopera, and S. Della Sala. 2010. Visual short-term memory binding deficits in familial Alzheimer's disease. *Brain*, 133: 2702–2713.

Pekeles, H., H. Y. Qureshi, H. K. Paudel, H. M. Schipper, M. Gornistky, H. Chertkow. 2019. Development and validation of a salivary tau biomarker in Alzheimer's disease. *Alzheimers Dement (Amst)*, 11: 53–60.

Pengas, G., K. Patterson, R. J. Arnold, C. M. Bird, N. Burgess, P. J. Nestor. 2010. Lost and found: bespoke memory testing for Alzheimer's disease and semantic dementia. *J Alzheimers Dis*, 21: 1347–1365.

Perez-Nievas, B. G., T. D. Stein, H. C. Tai, O. Dols-Icardo, T. C. Scotton, I. Barroeta-Espar, L. Fernandez-Carballo, E. L. de Munain, J. Perez, M. Marquie, et al. 2013. Dissecting phenotypic traits linked to human resilience to Alzheimer's pathology. *Brain*, 136: 2510–2526.

Pericak-Vance, M. A., J. L. Bebout, P. C. Gaskell, Jr, L. H. Yamaoka, W. Y. Hung, M. J. Alberts, A. P. Walker, R. J. Bartlett, C. A. Haynes, K. A. Welsh, et al. 1991. Linkage studies in familial Alzheimer disease: evidence for chromosome 19 linkage. *Am J Hum Genet*, 48: 1034–1050.

Petersen, R. C. 2004. Mild cognitive impairment as a diagnostic entity. *J Intern Med*, 256: 183–194.

Petersen, R. C., G. E. Smith, S. C. Waring, R. J. Ivnik, E. G. Tangalos, E. Kokmen. 1999. Mild cognitive impairment: clinical characterization and outcome. *Arch Neurol*, 56: 303–308.

Pickett, E. K., A. G. Herrmann, J. McQueen, K. Abt, O. Dando, J. Tulloch, P. Jain, S. Dunnett, S. Sohrabi, M. P. Fjeldstad, et al. 2019. Amyloid beta and tau cooperate to cause reversible behavioral and transcriptional deficits in a model of Alzheimer's disease. *Cell Rep*, 29: 3592–604 e5.

Pickett, E. K., J. Rose, C. McCrory, C. A. McKenzie, D. King, C. Smith, T. H. Gillingwater, C. M. Henstridge, T. L. Spires-Jones. 2018. Region-specific depletion of synaptic mitochondria in the brains of patients with Alzheimer's disease. *Acta Neuropathol*, 136: 747–757.

Pink, A., G. B. Stokin, M. M. Bartley, R. O. Roberts, O. Sochor, M. M. Machulda, J. Krell-Roesch, D. S. Knopman, J. I. Acosta, T. J. Christianson, et al. 2015. Neuropsychiatric symptoms, APOE epsilon4, and the risk of incident dementia: a population-based study. *Neurology*, 84: 935–943.

Pitas, R. E., J. K. Boyles, S. H. Lee, D. Foss, R. W. Mahley. 1987. Astrocytes synthesize apolipoprotein E and metabolize apolipoprotein E-containing lipoproteins. *Biochim Biophys Acta*, 917: 148–161.

Platt, T. L., V. L. Reeves, M. P. Murphy. 2013. Transgenic models of Alzheimer's disease: better utilization of existing models through viral transgenesis. *Biochim Biophys Acta*, 1832: 1437–1448.

Polydoro, M., C. M. Acker, K. Duff, P. E. Castillo, P. Davies. 2009. Age-dependent impairment of cognitive and synaptic function in the htau mouse model of tau pathology. *J Neurosci*, 29: 10741–10749.

Pontecorvo, M. J., M. D. Devous, I. Kennedy, M. Navitsky, M. Lu, N. Galante, S. Salloway, P. M. Doraiswamy, S. Southekal, A. K. Arora, et al. 2019. A multicentre longitudinal study of flortaucipir (18F) in normal ageing, mild cognitive impairment and Alzheimer's disease dementia. *Brain*, 142: 1723–1735.

Pooler, A. M., M. Polydoro, E. A. Maury, S. B. Nicholls, S. M. Reddy, S. Wegmann, C. William, L. Saqran, O. Cagsal-Getkin, R. Pitstick, et al. 2015. Amyloid accelerates tau propagation and toxicity in a model of early Alzheimer's disease. *Acta Neuropathol Commun*, 3: 14.

Portelius, E., B. Olsson, K. Hoglund, N. C. Cullen, H. Kvartsberg, U. Andreasson, H. Zetterberg, A. Sandelius, L. M. Shaw, V. M. Y. Lee, et al. 2018. Cerebrospinal fluid neurogranin concentration in neurodegeneration: relation to clinical phenotypes and neuropathology. *Acta Neuropathol*, 136: 363–376.

Potier, B., P. Krzywkowski, Y. Lamour, P. Dutar. 1994. Loss of calbindin-immunoreactivity in CA1 hippocampal stratum radiatum and stratum lacunosum-moleculare interneurons in the aged rat. *Brain Res*, 661: 181–188.

Prasad, H., R. Rao. 2018. Amyloid clearance defect in ApoE4 astrocytes is reversed by epigenetic correction of endosomal pH. *Proc Natl Acad Sci U S A*, 115: E6640–E49.

Prestia, A., A. Caroli, W. M. van der Flier, R. Ossenkoppele, B. Van Berckel, F. Barkhof, C. E. Teunissen, A. E. Wall, S. F. Carter, M. Scholl, et al. 2013. Prediction of dementia in MCI patients based on core diagnostic markers for Alzheimer disease. *Neurology*, 80: 1048–1056.

Prince, M., R. Bryce, E. Albanese, A. Wimo, W. Ribeiro, C. P. Ferri. 2013. The global prevalence of dementia: a systematic review and metaanalysis. *Alzheimers Dement*, 9: 63–75 e2.

Proctor, C. J., D. Boche, D. A. Gray, J. A. Nicoll. 2013. Investigating interventions in Alzheimer's disease with computer simulation models. *PLoS One*, 8: e73631.

Provenzano, F. A., J. Muraskin, G. Tosto, A. Narkhede, B. T. Wasserman, E. Y. Griffith, V. A. Guzman, I. B. Meier, M. E. Zimmerman, A. M. Brickman, Initiative Alzheimer's Disease Neuroimaging. 2013. White matter hyperintensities and cerebral amyloidosis: necessary and sufficient for clinical expression of Alzheimer disease?. *JAMA Neurol*, 70: 455–461.

Puri, I. K., L. Li. 2010. Mathematical modeling for the pathogenesis of Alzheimer's disease. *PLoS One*, 5: e15176.

Radenovic, L., A. Korenic, G. Maleeva, I. Osadchenko, T. Kovalenko, G. Skibo. 2011. Comparative ultrastructural analysis of mitochondria in the CA1 and CA3 hippocampal pyramidal cells following global ischemia in Mongolian gerbils. *Anat Rec (Hoboken)*, **294**: 1057–1065.

Raichle, M. E., A. M. MacLeod, A. Z. Snyder, W. J. Powers, D. A. Gusnard, G. L. Shulman. 2001. A default mode of brain function. *Proc Natl Acad Sci U S A*, **98**: 676–682.

Raj, A., E. LoCastro, A. Kuceyeski, D. Tosun, N. Relkin, M. Weiner, Initiative Alzheimer's Disease Neuroimaging. 2015. Network diffusion model of progression predicts longitudinal patterns of atrophy and metabolism in Alzheimer's disease. *Cell Rep*, **10**: 359–369.

Rajagopalan, P., D. P. Hibar, P. M. Thompson. 2013. TREM2 and neurodegenerative disease. *N Engl J Med*, **369**: 1565–1567.

Randolph, C., M. C. Tierney, E. Mohr, T. N. Chase. 1998. The Repeatable Battery for the Assessment of Neuropsychological Status (RBANS): preliminary clinical validity. *J Clin Exp Neuropsychol*, **20**: 310–319.

Refolo, L. M., B. Malester, J. LaFrancois, T. Bryant-Thomas, R. Wang, G. S. Tint, K. Sambamurti, K. Duff, M. A. Pappolla. 2000. Hypercholesterolemia accelerates the Alzheimer's amyloid pathology in a transgenic mouse model. *Neurobiol Dis*, **7**: 321–331.

Reisberg, B., M. B. Shulman, C. Torossian, L. Leng, W. Zhu. 2010. Outcome over seven years of healthy adults with and without subjective cognitive impairment. *Alzheimers Dement*, **6**: 11–24.

Reitz, C., C. Brayne, R. Mayeux. 2011. Epidemiology of Alzheimer disease. *Nat Rev Neurol*, **7**: 137–152.

Rey, A. 1941. L'examen psychologique dans les cas d'encéphalopathie traumatique. (Les problems.) [The psychological examination in cases of traumatic encepholopathy. Problems]. *Archives de Psychologie*, **28**: 215–285.

Richards, M., I. J. Deary. 2005. A life course approach to cognitive reserve: a model for cognitive aging and development?. *Ann Neurol*, **58**: 617–622.

Riddell, D. R., G. Christie, I. Hussain, C. Dingwall. 2001. Compartmentalization of beta-secretase (Asp2) into low-buoyant density, noncaveolar lipid rafts. *Curr Biol*, **11**: 1288–1293.

Ritchie, C., N. Smailagic, A. H. Noel-Storr, O. Ukoumunne, E. C. Ladds, S. Martin. 2017. CSF tau and the CSF tau/ABeta ratio for the diagnosis of Alzheimer's disease dementia and other dementias in people with mild cognitive impairment (MCI). *Cochrane Database Syst Rev*, **3**: CD010803.

Ritchie, K., I. Carriere, D. Howett, L. Su, M. Hornberger, J. T. O'Brien, C. W. Ritchie, D. Chan. 2018. Allocentric and egocentric spatial processing in middle-aged adults at high risk of late-onset Alzheimer's Disease: the PREVENT Dementia Study. *J Alzheimers Dis*, **65**: 885–896.

Roberson, E. D., B. Halabisky, J. W. Yoo, J. Yao, J. Chin, F. Yan, T. Wu, P. Hamto, N. Devidze, G. Q. Yu, et al. 2011. Amyloid-beta/Fyn-induced synaptic, network, and cognitive impairments depend on tau levels in multiple mouse models of Alzheimer's disease. *J Neurosci*, **31**: 700–711.

Roberson, E. D., K. Scearce-Levie, J. J. Palop, F. Yan, I. H. Cheng, T. Wu, H. Gerstein, G. Q. Yu, L. Mucke. 2007. Reducing endogenous tau ameliorates amyloid beta-induced deficits in an Alzheimer's disease mouse model. *Science*, **316**: 750–754.

Rocher, A. B., J. L. Crimins, J. M. Amatrudo, M. S. Kinson, M. A. Todd-Brown, J. Lewis, J. I. Luebke. 2010. Structural and functional changes in tau mutant mice neurons are not linked to the presence of NFTs. *Exp Neurol*, **223**: 385–393.

Rodriguez, G. A., M. P. Burns, E. J. Weeber, G. W. Rebeck. 2013. Young APOE4 targeted replacement mice exhibit poor spatial learning and memory, with reduced dendritic spine density in the medial entorhinal cortex. *Learn Mem*, **20**: 256–266.

Rodriguez, J. J., H. N. Noristani, T. Hilditch, M. Olabarria, C. Y. Yeh, J. Witton, A. Verkhratsky. 2013. Increased densities of resting and activated microglia in the dentate gyrus follow senile plaque formation in the CA1 subfield of the hippocampus in the triple transgenic model of Alzheimer's disease. *Neurosci Lett*, **552**: 129–134.

Roehr, S., A. Pabst, T. Luck, S. G. Riedel-Heller. 2018. Is dementia incidence declining in high-income countries? A systematic review and meta-analysis. *Clin Epidemiol*, **10**: 1233–1247.

Rogaev, E. I., R. Sherrington, E. A. Rogaeva, G. Levesque, M. Ikeda, Y. Liang, H. Chi, C. Lin, K. Holman, T. Tsuda, et al. 1995. Familial Alzheimer's disease in kindreds with missense mutations in a gene on chromosome 1 related to the Alzheimer's disease type 3 gene. *Nature*, **376**: 775–778.

Rollo, J. L., N. Banihashemi, F. Vafaee, J. W. Crawford, Z. Kuncic, R. M. Holsinger. 2016. Unraveling the mechanistic complexity of Alzheimer's disease through systems biology. *Alzheimers Dement*, **12**: 708–718.

Rowland, H. A., N. M. Hooper, K. A. B. Kellett. 2018. Modelling sporadic Alzheimer's disease using induced pluripotent stem cells. *Neurochem Res*, **43**: 2179–2198.

Roy, D. S., A. Arons, T. I. Mitchell, M. Pignatelli, T. J. Ryan, S. Tonegawa. 2016. Memory retrieval by activating engram cells in mouse models of early Alzheimer's disease. *Nature*, **531**: 508–512.

Sachdev, P., R. Kalaria, J. O'Brien, I. Skoog, S. Alladi, S. E. Black, D. Blacker, D. G. Blazer, C. Chen, H. Chui, et al., International Society for Vascular Behavioural and Cognitive Disorders. 2014. Diagnostic criteria for vascular cognitive disorders: a VASCOG statement. *Alzheimer Dis Assoc Disord*, **28**: 206–218.

Sachdev, P. S., D. M. Lipnicki, J. Crawford, S. Reppermund, N. A. Kochan, J. N. Trollor, W. Wen, B. Draper, M. J. Slavin, K. Kang, et al., Ageing Study Team Sydney Memory. 2013. Factors predicting reversion from mild cognitive impairment to normal cognitive functioning: a population-based study. *PLoS One*, **8**: e59649.

Santacruz, K., J. Lewis, T. Spires, J. Paulson, L. Kotilinek, M. Ingelsson, A. Guimaraes, M. DeTure, M. Ramsden, E. McGowan, et al. 2005. Tau suppression in a neurodegenerative mouse model improves memory function. *Science*, **309**: 476–481.

Sarazin, M., V. Chauvire, E. Gerardin, O. Colliot, S. Kinkingnehun, L. C. de Souza, L. Hugonot-Diener, L. Garnero, S. Lehericy, M. Chupin, et al. 2010. The amnestic syndrome of hippocampal type in Alzheimer's disease: an MRI study. *J Alzheimers Dis*, **22**: 285–294.

Sartori, M., T. Mendes, S. Desai, A. Lasorsa, A. Herledan, N. Malmanche, P. Makinen, M. Marttinen, I. Malki, J. Chapuis, et al. 2019. BIN1 recovers tauopathy-induced long-term memory deficits in mice and interacts with Tau through Thr(348) phosphorylation. *Acta Neuropathol*, **138**: 631–652.

Saxena, S., P. Caroni. 2011. Selective neuronal vulnerability in neurodegenerative diseases: from stressor thresholds to degeneration. *Neuron*, **71**: 35–48.

Saykin, A. J., H. A. Wishart, L. A. Rabin, R. B. Santulli, L. A. Flashman, J. D. West, T. L. McHugh, A. C. Mamourian. 2006. Older adults with cognitive complaints show brain atrophy similar to that of amnestic MCI. *Neurology*, **67**: 834–842.

Scheff, S. W., S. T. DeKosky, D. A. Price. 1990. Quantitative assessment of cortical synaptic density in Alzheimer's disease. *Neurobiol Aging*, **11**: 29–37.

Scheff, S. W., D. A. Price, F. A. Schmitt, E. J. Mufson. 2006. Hippocampal synaptic loss in early Alzheimer's disease and mild cognitive impairment. *Neurobiol Aging*, **27**: 1372–1384.

with lipid rafts in post-Golgi and endosome membranes. *J Biol Chem*, **279**: 44945–44954.

Visser, P. J., P. Scheltens, F. R. Verhey, B. Schmand, L. J. Launer, J. Jolles, C. Jonker. 1999. Medial temporal lobe atrophy and memory dysfunction as predictors for dementia in subjects with mild cognitive impairment. *J Neurol*, **246**: 477–485.

Visser, P. J., F. Verhey, D. L. Knol, P. Scheltens, L. O. Wahlund, Y. Freund-Levi, M. Tsolaki, L. Minthon, A. K. Wallin, H. Hampel, et al. 2009. Prevalence and prognostic value of CSF markers of Alzheimer's disease pathology in patients with subjective cognitive impairment or mild cognitive impairment in the DESCRIPA study: a prospective cohort study. *Lancet Neurol*, **8**: 619–627.

Vogels, T., A. Leuzy, C. Cicognola, N. J. Ashton, T. Smolek, M. Novak, K. Blennow, H. Zetterberg, T. Hromadka, N. Zilka, et al. 2020. Propagation of tau pathology: integrating insights from postmortem and in vivo studies. *Biol Psychiatry*, **87**: 808–818.

Walsh, D. M., I. Klyubin, J. V. Fadeeva, W. K. Cullen, R. Anwyl, M. S. Wolfe, M. J. Rowan, D. J. Selkoe. 2002. Naturally secreted oligomers of amyloid beta protein potently inhibit hippocampal long-term potentiation in vivo. *Nature*, **416**: 535–539.

Wang, H., A. Megill, K. He, A. Kirkwood, H. K. Lee. 2012. Consequences of inhibiting amyloid precursor protein processing enzymes on synaptic function and plasticity. *Neural Plast*, **2012**: 272374.

Wang, X., R. Pal, X. W. Chen, N. Limpeanchob, K. N. Kumar, E. K. Michaelis. 2005. High intrinsic oxidative stress may underlie selective vulnerability of the hippocampal CA1 region. *Brain Res Mol Brain Res*, **140**: 120–126.

Wang, Y., M. Cella, K. Mallinson, J. D. Ulrich, K. L. Young, M. L. Robinette, S. Gilfillan, G. M. Krishnan, S. Sudhakar, B. H. Zinselmeyer, et al. 2015. TREM2 lipid sensing sustains the microglial response in an Alzheimer's disease model. *Cell*, **160**: 1061–1071.

Wang, Y., M. P. Mattson. 2014. L-type Ca2+ currents at CA1 synapses, but not CA3 or dentate granule neuron synapses, are increased in 3xTgAD mice in an age-dependent manner. *Neurobiol Aging*, **35**: 88–95.

Wang, Z. T., C. Zhang, Y. J. Wang, Q. Dong, L. Tan, J. T. Yu. 2020. Selective neuronal vulnerability in Alzheimer's disease. *Ageing Res Rev*, **62**: 101114.

Warren, J. D., J. D. Rohrer, J. M. Schott, N. C. Fox, J. Hardy, M. N. Rossor. 2013. Molecular nexopathies: a new paradigm of neurodegenerative disease. *Trends Neurosci*, **36**: 561–569.

Webster, S. J., A. D. Bachstetter, P. T. Nelson, F. A. Schmitt, L. J. Van Eldik. 2014. Using mice to model Alzheimer's dementia: an overview of the clinical disease and the preclinical behavioral changes in 10 mouse models. *Front Genet*, **5**: 88.

Weissberger, G. H., J. V. Strong, K. B. Stefanidis, M. J. Summers, M. W. Bondi, N. H. Stricker. 2017. Diagnostic accuracy of memory measures in Alzheimer's dementia and mild cognitive impairment: a systematic review and meta-analysis. *Neuropsychol Rev*, **27**: 354–388.

West, M. J., P. D. Coleman, D. G. Flood, J. C. Troncoso. 1994. Differences in the pattern of hippocampal neuronal loss in normal ageing and Alzheimer's disease. *Lancet*, **344**: 769–772.

Westwood, S., A. L. Baird, S. N. Anand, A. J. Nevado-Holgado, A. Kormilitzin, L. Shi, A. Hye, N. J. Ashton, A. R. Morgan, I. Bos, et al. 2020. Validation of plasma proteomic biomarkers relating to brain amyloid burden in the EMIF-Alzheimer's Disease Multimodal Biomarker Discovery Cohort. *J Alzheimers Dis*, **74**: 213–225.

Wilde, G. J., A. K. Pringle, P. Wright, F. Iannotti. 1997. Differential vulnerability of the CA1 and CA3 subfields of the hippocampus to superoxide and hydroxyl radicals in vitro. *J Neurochem*, **69**: 883–886.

Winkler, E., F. Kamp, J. Scheuring, A. Ebke, A. Fukumori, H. Steiner. 2012. Generation of Alzheimer disease-associated amyloid beta42/43 peptide by gamma-secretase can be inhibited directly by modulation of membrane thickness. *J Biol Chem*, **287**: 21326–21334.

Wisse, L. E., G. J. Biessels, S. M. Heringa, H. J. Kuijf, D. H. Koek, P. R. Luijten, M. I. Geerlings, Group Utrecht Vascular Cognitive Impairment Study. 2014. Hippocampal subfield volumes at 7T in early Alzheimer's disease and normal aging. *Neurobiol Aging*, **35**: 2039–2045.

Wolfe, M. S., W. Xia, B. L. Ostaszewski, T. S. Diehl, W. T. Kimberly, D. J. Selkoe. 1999. Two transmembrane aspartates in presenilin-1 required for presenilin endoproteolysis and gamma-secretase activity. *Nature*, **398**: 513–517.

Wolfsgruber, S., A. Polcher, A. Koppara, L. Kleineidam, L. Frolich, O. Peters, M. Hull, E. Ruther, J. Wiltfang, W. Maier, et al. 2017. Cerebrospinal fluid biomarkers and clinical progression in patients with subjective cognitive decline and mild cognitive impairment. *J Alzheimers Dis*, **58**: 939–950.

Wood, R. A., K. K. Moodley, C. Lever, L. Minati, D. Chan. 2016. Allocentric spatial memory testing predicts conversion from mild cognitive impairment to dementia: an initial proof-of-concept study. *Front Neurol*, **7**: 215.

Wu, L., D. Sun. 2017. Adherence to Mediterranean diet and risk of developing cognitive disorders: an updated systematic review and meta-analysis of prospective cohort studies. *Sci Rep*, **7**: 41317.

Xiang, X., T. M. Piers, B. Wefers, K. Zhu, A. Mallach, B. Brunner, G. Kleinberger, W. Song, M. Colonna, J. Herms, et al. 2018. The Trem2 R47H Alzheimer's risk variant impairs splicing and reduces Trem2 mRNA and protein in mice but not in humans. *Mol Neurodegener*, **13**: 49.

Yamazaki, Y., N. Zhao, T. R. Caulfield, C. C. Liu, G. Bu. 2019. Apolipoprotein E and Alzheimer disease: pathobiology and targeting strategies. *Nat Rev Neurol*, **15**: 501–518.

Yan, S., Z. Tu, Z. Liu, N. Fan, H. Yang, S. Yang, W. Yang, Y. Zhao, Z. Ouyang, C. Lai, et al. 2018. A Huntingtin knockin pig model recapitulates features of selective neurodegeneration in Huntington's disease. *Cell*, **173**: 989–1002.e13.

Yanamandra, K., H. Jiang, T. E. Mahan, S. E. Maloney, D. F. Wozniak, M. I. Diamond, D. M. Holtzman. 2015. Anti-tau antibody reduces insoluble tau and decreases brain atrophy. *Ann Clin Transl Neurol*, **2**: 278–288.

Yanamandra, K., N. Kfoury, H. Jiang, T. E. Mahan, S. Ma, S. E. Maloney, D. F. Wozniak, M. I. Diamond, D. M. Holtzman. 2013. Anti-tau antibodies that block tau aggregate seeding in vitro markedly decrease pathology and improve cognition in vivo. *Neuron*, **80**: 402–414.

Yang, T., S. Li, H. Xu, D. M. Walsh, D. J. Selkoe. 2017. Large soluble oligomers of amyloid beta-protein from Alzheimer brain are far less neuroactive than the smaller oligomers to which they dissociate. *J Neurosci*, **37**: 152–163.

Yeh, F. L., Y. Wang, I. Tom, L. C. Gonzalez, M. Sheng. 2016. TREM2 binds to apolipoproteins, including APOE and CLU/APOJ, and thereby facilitates uptake of amyloid-beta by microglia. *Neuron*, **91**: 328–340.

Yew, B., S. Alladi, M. Shailaja, J. R. Hodges, M. Hornberger. 2013. Lost and forgotten? Orientation versus memory in Alzheimer's disease and frontotemporal dementia. *J Alzheimers Dis*, **33**: 473–481.

Yiannopoulou, K. G., S. G. Papageorgiou. 2020. Current and future treatments in Alzheimer disease: an update. *J Cent Nerv Syst Dis*, **12**: 1179573520907397.

Yoshiyama, Y., M. Higuchi, B. Zhang, S. M. Huang, N. Iwata, T. C. Saido, J. Maeda, T. Suhara, J. Q. Trojanowski, V. M. Lee. 2007. Synapse loss and microglial activation precede tangles in a P301S tauopathy mouse model. *Neuron*, **53**: 337–351.

Yuan, Y., Z. X. Gu, W. S. Wei. 2009. Fluorodeoxyglucose-positron-emission tomography, single-photon emission tomography, and structural MR imaging for prediction of rapid conversion to Alzheimer disease in patients with mild cognitive impairment: a meta-analysis. *AJNR Am J Neuroradiol*, **30**: 404–410.

Yun, S. H., K. A. Park, S. Kwon, C. S. Woolley, P. M. Sullivan, J. F. Pasternak, B. L. Trommer. 2007. Estradiol enhances long term potentiation in hippocampal slices from aged apoE4-TR mice. *Hippocampus*, **17**: 1153–1157.

Zhang, Z., P. Nadeau, W. Song, D. Donoviel, M. Yuan, A. Bernstein, B. A. Yankner. 2000. Presenilins are required for gamma-secretase cleavage of beta-APP and transmembrane cleavage of Notch-1. *Nat Cell Biol*, **2**: 463–465.

Zhao, N., C. C. Liu, A. J. Van Ingelgom, Y. A. Martens, C. Linares, J. A. Knight, M. M. Painter, P. M. Sullivan, G. Bu. 2017. Apolipoprotein E4 impairs neuronal insulin signaling by trapping insulin receptor in the endosomes. *Neuron*, **96**: 115–129 e5.

Zhou, F. C., Y. Y. Wang, W. Zheng, Q. Zhang, G. S. Ungvari, C. H. Ng, J. Zhang, Y. T. Xiang. 2017. Prospective memory deficits in patients with depression: a meta-analysis. *J Affect Disord*, **220**: 79–85.

Zhou, J., E. D. Gennatas, J. H. Kramer, B. L. Miller, W. W. Seeley. 2012. Predicting regional neurodegeneration from the healthy brain functional connectome. *Neuron*, **73**: 1216–1227.

Zhou, L., J. McInnes, K. Wierda, M. Holt, A. G. Herrmann, R. J. Jackson, Y. C. Wang, J. Swerts, J. Beyens, K. Miskiewicz, et al. 2017. Tau association with synaptic vesicles causes presynaptic dysfunction. *Nat Commun*, **8**: 15295.

Zoltowska, K. M., O. Berezovska. 2018. Dynamic nature of presenilin1/gamma-secretase: implication for Alzheimer's disease pathogenesis. *Mol Neurobiol*, **55**: 2275–2284.

Index